Y0-BRQ-528

NURSING CARE OF THE PATIENT WITH MEDICAL-SURGICAL DISORDERS

Edited by HARRIET COSTON MOIDEL, R.N., B.S., M.A.

Associate Professor of Medical-Surgical Nursing
School of Nursing
University of California at Los Angeles

GLADYS E. SORENSEN, B.S., M.S., ED.D.

Dean and Professor of Nursing
College of Nursing
The University of Arizona, Tucson, Arizona

ELIZABETH C. GIBLIN, B.S., M.N., ED.D.

Professor and Director of the Medical-Surgical Nursing Program
School of Nursing, University of Washington
Seattle, Washington

MARGARET A. KAUFMANN, R.N., B.S.N., M.S., ED.D.

Professor of Nursing, School of Nursing
University of Colorado, Denver, Colorado

WITH CONTRIBUTIONS BY
THIRTY-SIX NURSE SPECIALISTS

NURSING CARE OF THE PATIENT WITH MEDICAL- SURGICAL DISORDERS

McGRAW-HILL BOOK COMPANY

A Blakiston Publication

New York · St. Louis · San Francisco · Düsseldorf · Johannesburg · Kuala Lumpur · London
Mexico · Montreal · New Delhi · Panama · Rio de Janeiro · Singapore · Sidney · Toronto

NURSING CARE OF
THE PATIENT WITH MEDICAL-SURGICAL
DISORDERS

1 2 3 4 5 6 7 8 9 0 V H V H 7 9 8 7 6 5 4 3 2 1 0

This book was set in Medallion by
Westcott & Thomson, Inc.,
and printed on permanent paper and
bound by Von Hoffmann Press, Inc.
The designer was Wladislaw Finne;
the drawings were done by John Cordes, J. & R. Technical Services, Inc.
The editors were Joseph J. Brehm and Bernice Heller.
Robert R. Laffler supervised production.

*To three deans who made it possible
for us to work together and
gave us support and encouragement
in the writing of this book:*

PEARL P. COULTER

*Dean Emeritus
College of Nursing
The University of Arizona*

LULU WOLF HASSENPLUG

*Dean Emeritus
School of Nursing
University of California at Los Angeles*

MARY S. TSCHUDIN

*Dean Emeritus
School of Nursing
University of Washington*

PREFACE

This textbook is presented to students of professional nursing as a basis for a cohesive and continuing approach to learning in the nursing care of adults. It is grounded upon the broad concept of nursing as a professional undertaking based upon knowledge that permits and facilitates sound judgment in the assessment, implementation, and evaluation of nursing care.

Three basic and interlocking purposes are inherent in the development of the text. These are:

A. To present the care components of nursing—its nature, its functions, and its process.
B. To present basic concepts of health, illness, and nursing care which are pertinent to and utilizable in all aspects of nursing care of the adult patient in a medical-surgical setting.
C. To present disease conditions and the particular nursing care requirements requirements related thereto.

The text is not intended to be encyclopedic in nature. Rather it should be utilized in conjunction with related references, such as those focused on medicine and medical science, pharmacology, or nutrition wherein extensive detail and specificity may be found.

The relationship the parts bear to each other is one of a flow from the general to the particular. Parts I through IV provide basic and common care information for the chapters in Part V. Part V deals with specifics related to diseases and is not intended to be used without reference to the basic materials in the preceding parts.

The repetition that occurs from one part to the next has been planned to lend added emphasis and clarification and to present the material from the viewpoint of the objectives of each part.

Part I   presents the philosophy and focus of nursing upon which the text is based.
Part II   presents a basic understanding of man in health and illness as an informational foundation, and
Part III presents basic concepts of disease and treatment which further develop a common foundation of knowledge upon which the nurse may draw and against which she may compare, contrast, evaluate, and predict in specific illness situations.
Part IV   presents significant manifestations that occur in a variety of illness situations in terms of the physiological and psychological mechanisms that underlie them and give direction to nursing action. This section provides the nurse with a reservoir of broadly applicable information

that will help her assess care requirements for the individual patient and to plan appropriate nursing intervention based on a comprehension of concepts and relationships rather than upon memorization of specifics and isolates.

Part V   presents particular information related to the disease itself and its nursing management to supplement the common care knowledge of Parts I through IV.

Each part of the text is intended to be used in conjunction with all other parts and therefore will include cross-references between the basic knowledge sections and the specific knowledge sections. Though the intent is for the parts of the book to support each other, it is conceivable that some portions could be utilized separately, depending upon the learning objectives of a particular course. The text could also be used as a reference book for nurse practitioners.

The text utilizes a multiple authorship in order to bring together the thinking of nurses expert in their fields from across the country. This approach naturally results in variations in both style and differential emphasis on various aspects of the content. These variations allow the student to develop the ability to utilize information presented from several vantage points and thereby increase the flexibility of her intellect.

HARRIET COSTON MOIDEL
GLADYS E. SORENSEN
ELIZABETH C. GIBLIN
MARGARET A. KAUFMANN

ACKNOWLEDGMENTS

We acknowledge the unfailing support and encouragement given us by the members of our families throughout the many months spent in the planning and preparation of this book, without which it could not have been written. In particular, we thank Mitchel Moidel for his interested concern, patience, and good humor.

We are greatly appreciative of the splendid contributions made by the invited authors, as well as the cooperative spirit all of them displayed. Since all held full-time positions at the time they wrote their contributions, this book represents a real sacrifice of their time and energy. Their families, too, helped significantly in this endeavor by offering a full measure of support and affection to the author-member.

We express appreciation to our respective secretaries, Mrs. Geraldine F. Schaefer, Mrs. Marian V. Burson, Mrs. Johanna Gaedeke, and Mrs. Esther Gaskill, who carefully typed and retyped manuscripts, proofread manuscripts, and assisted us with voluminous correspondence.

We are grateful to the McGraw-Hill Book Company for the freedom to produce the type of book we desired and for their constant cooperation and assistance.

HARRIET COSTON MOIDEL
GLADYS E. SORENSEN
ELIZABETH C. GIBLIN
MARGARET A. KAUFMANN

CONTRIBUTORS

RUTH E. BARSTOW, R.N., M.S.
Instructor, Nursing Service Education, Veterans Administration Hospital, Livermore, California.

EM OLIVIA BEVIS, R.N., B.S., M.A.
Associate Professor of Nursing, San Jose State College, San Jose, California.

JUANITA A. BOOTH, R.N., P.H.N., B.S., M.A.
Director, Associate Degree Nursing Program, Cuesta College, San Luis Obispo, California.

PAULINE BRUNO, R.N., M.S.N.
Assistant Professor of Nursing, School of Nursing, University of Washington, Seattle, Washington.

WILDA G. CHAMBERS, B.Sc.Ed., S.M.
Associate Professor, The Ohio State University, Columbus, Ohio.

MARY ALICE CHELGREN, B.S., M.Ed.
Predoctoral Lecturer in Nursing, University of Washington, Seattle, Washington.

PATRICIA FELTZ COHEN, R.N., B.S.G.N., M.A., Ed.M.
Formerly Instructor of Nursing, School of Nursing, University of California at Los Angeles.

DORIS COLEMAN, R.N., B.S.N., M.S.N.
Consultant to Continuation Education Department, School of Nursing, University of Colorado, Denver, Colorado.

ROSEMARY PRINCE COOMBS, B.Sc.N., M.N.
Clinical Nurse Specialist in Cardiac Surgery, Ottawa Civic Hospital, Ottawa, Ontario.

MARCIA LYN DALE, B.S.N., M.N.
Associate Professor, University of Wyoming, Laramie, Wyoming.

SISTER M. AGNITA CLAIRE DAY, S.S.M., B.S.N., M.S.N.
Professor of Nursing, School of Nursing and Health Services, Department of Nursing, St. Louis University, St. Louis, Missouri.

HONOR B. DUFOUR, R.N., B.S., M.ED.
Professor of Nursing, San Jose State College, San Jose, California.

VIRGINIA L. EARLES, M.S.
Professor of Medical-Surgical Nursing, University of Massachusetts, Amherst, Massachusetts.

ANNETTE EZELL, M.S.
Assistant Professor of Nursing, Orvis School of Nursing, University of Nevada, Reno, Nevada.

MAGDALENE FULLER, R.N., M.S.
Associate Professor, School of Nursing, Indiana University, Indianapolis, Indiana.

M. ARLENE GARDNER, B.S., M.A.
Formerly Associate Professor of Nursing, Frances Payne Bolton School of Nursing, Case Western Reserve University, Cleveland, Ohio.

BARBARA ANN GRUTTER, B.S., M.S.
Formerly Visiting Assistant Professor, School of Nursing, Seton Hall University, South Orange, New Jersey.

ISOBEL DUNCAN HARTLEY, B.S.N., M.N.
Assistant Professor of Nursing, University Extension Division, Bureau of Continuing Professional Education, Rutgers-The State University, New Brunswick, New Jersey.

DOROTHY OLSON HOSHAW, R.N., B.S., M.S.
Instructor, School of Nursing, University of Washington, Seattle, Washington.

LOIS NUGENT HOUGH, R.N., B.S.N.ED., M.S.
Formerly Assistant Professor, School of Nursing, University of Colorado, Denver, Colorado.

MARY S. KLEINKNECHT, R.N., M.ED.
Associate Chief, Nursing Service for Education, Veterans Administration Hospital, Fresno, California.

LOUISE W. MANSFIELD, R.N., B.S.ED., M.A.
Professor of Medical-Surgical Nursing, School of Nursing, University of Washington, Seattle, Washington.

DOROTHY M. MARTIN, R.N., M.S.
Professor of Nursing, Loma Linda University, Loma Linda, California.

KATHLEEN MIKAN, B.S., M.S.
Assistant Professor, School of Nursing, Michigan State University, East Lansing, Michigan.

PAMELA HOLSCLAW MITCHELL, B.S.N., M.S.
Assistant Professor, University of Washington, Seattle, Washington.

MARTHA CHEW PEAKE, MAJ, AUS (Ret.), R.N., B.S.N.
Public Health Nurse, Anne Arundel County, Maryland Department of Health.

ELIZABETH FORD PITORAK, R.N., B.S.N., M.S.N.
Associate Professor of Nursing, Frances Payne Bolton School of Nursing, Case Western Reserve University, Cleveland, Ohio.

IRENE E. POLLERT, R.N., B.S., M.S.
Associate Professor, School of Nursing, Indiana University, Indianapolis, Indiana.

PHYLLIS E. PORTER, R.N., B.S., M.S.
Assistant Professor, University of Bridgeport, Bridgeport, Connecticut.

ARLENE M. PUTT, R.N., B.S., ED.M., ED.D.
Associate Professor of Nursing, College of Nursing, The University of Arizona, Tucson, Arizona.

BETSY EELLS RAY, B.S.N., M.S.
Assistant Professor, The University of Texas Nursing School, Austin, Texas.

GERALDINE SKINNER, R.N., M.S.
Professor of Nursing, School of Nursing, and Project Director, Continuing Education Services for the School of Nursing, University of Michigan, Ann Arbor, Michigan.

GRACE TOEWS, R.N., B.S.N., M.A.ED.
Associate Professor of Medical-Surgical Nursing, School of Nursing, University of Colorado, Denver, Colorado.

MARGARET A. WILLIAMS, R.N., B.S., M.S.
Berkeley, California.

MARY OPAL WOLANIN, B.A., M.P.A.
Associate Professor, College of Nursing, The University of Arizona, Tucson, Arizona.

LOUISE F. WORSTER, R.N., B.S., M.A.
David O. McKay Hospital, Ogden, Utah.

CONTENTS

Part V   Nursing Care of Patients

NURSING CARE OF THE PATIENT WITH MEDICAL-SURGICAL DISORDERS

PART I
THE NURSE
AND HER
PRACTICE

PURPOSE

To present the editors' general philosophy of nursing upon which this book is based.

To show the place of nursing in total health care.

To orient the reader to the definition, scope, and limitation of the area covered in the book.

To discuss briefly the nurse and the skills and abilities she needs to render care of a professional nature.

To present the various roles the nurse plays from that of an independent practitioner to the assistant of the physician.

To present the scope of functions of the nurse as viewed by the authors. The process of nursing is presented which will be applicable in all nursing situations regardless of patient diagnosis or setting in which the patient is found.

Part I is designed to provide the reader with a feeling tone for what nursing is, who the nurse is, and what she does. The remainder of the book is then based on this philosophy and definition of nursing, the nurse, and the nurse's function. The entire book is based on the idea of nursing as being a patient-centered service with the nurse having independent, collaborative, and assistive roles and utilizing a problem-solving approach to each patient situation.

CHAPTER 1
A CONCEPT
OF NURSING

GLADYS E. SORENSEN

Nursing is one of the health professions that provide a special type of service to society. It renders help to both the sick and the well in times of crisis or stress. More often than not the tendency is to think of nursing as assistance only to persons who are ill or disabled. But this is not always the case. Individuals who are well benefit from nursing also, through various programs of prevention of disease or disability, and the promotion of health.

Since other health care professions also provide a direct service to individuals and their families, the special type of service extended by nursing must be defined in differentiating nursing services from the services provided by the other health professions. The definition of nursing as presented below not only identifies the special type of service extended by nursing but delineates as well the philosophy of nursing basic to this book.

A Definition of Nursing

Nursing is the process of assisting individuals who are ill or disabled to perform those activities of daily living which they normally perform but which they presently cannot because of their current disability. These nursing activities are carried out through direct contact with patients and often are referred to as the *ministrations,* or *care aspect,* of nursing. It is through these nursing ministrations that the nurse conveys to the patient her concern for him as an individual. These ministrations are the one aspect of patient care not shared with other health professionals.

Nursing is more than this, however. It is teaching and counseling the patient and his family toward understanding and coping with disability. It is encouraging, supporting, and listening to the patient and his family in ways that provide emotional support in their time of stress. It is being able to recognize signs of and to attempt to prevent further illness or injury. It is assisting the patient in maintaining the capabilities he possesses and preventing disability from recurring by applying specific nursing measures. It is restoring the patient to his home and community, insofar as it is possible, in a state of improved health. In essence, nursing is assisting, doing for the patient, teaching and counseling, attempting to prevent illness, and promoting health, whenever the need arises. Except for the nursing ministrations, the aspects of patient care, as defined above, are shared to a greater or lesser degree with other members of the health team, depending upon the patient situation. Many of the goals in patient care are common to a number of health team members, though the way each of the health professions contributes to the goals varies.

Underlying the philosophy that nursing is a special type of direct service to patients is the conviction that the patient plays an active part in the overall plan for his care and is to be encouraged to do for himself as much as he is capable of doing within the limits of his condition and his capabilities. In addition, the patient is recognized as a member of a family and a community, with problems inherent in his role in each of these social units.

The Place of Nursing in Total Health Care

In addition to the aspect of nursing just described is that facet of nursing in which the nurse collaborates with others to provide total health care. Implicit in the concept of total health or comprehensive patient care is the team approach. Each member of the health team has a definite role and an understanding of the role of every other member, enabling all members to coordinate their efforts toward accomplishment of comprehensive patient care.

The physician is the recognized leader of the health team. He evaluates the patient, makes a medical diagnosis, and prescribes a plan for therapy. All members of the health team must know the medical goals for the patient if they are to contribute to their fullest, since the responsibilities of each member of the health team are carried out within the context of the patient situation and the physician's plan for therapy.

The nurse is an integral part of the team. As stated earlier in this chapter, certain aspects of patient care fall solely under the jurisdiction of the nurse. The other team members expect the nurse to perform these services as her responsibility. For some of these services to the patient, such as bathing, feeding, making him comfortable, being a good listener, and providing emotional support, the nurse usually does not need special orders from the physician. Before initiating other aspects of patient care, however, the nurse needs to have orders from the physician. These other aspects of care generally relate to administration of medications, preparation for diagnostic tests, and carrying out some areas of patient teaching.

In addition to the nurse and the physician, and depending upon the needs of the patient, other members of the health profession are called on to assist the patient. Some of the team members, e.g., the social worker and the clergy, may be contacted directly by the nurse. Usually, though, team members' services are requested by the physician, and they receive orders from him to carry out a treatment or a diagnostic measure. Others, such as the psychologist or another physician, are usually requested by the physician to see the patient for assistance in evaluating the patient and his needs. The physical therapist, the occupational therapist, the dietitian, the social worker, the clinical psychologist, the vocational counselor, and the clergy all contribute to the welfare of the patient and his family. Besides these persons, others who may come in contact with the patient are the laboratory, oxygen therapy, and x-ray technicians. The nurse needs to understand the aims of each member of the team, know which members are available in her situation, know when to request help from them or when to suggest to the physician the need for their assistance, and be able to complement and supplement their activities as she works with the patient.

The working relationship between the nurse and the other health team members is not the same as the working relationship that pertains between the nurse and the physician. That is to say, there are no prescribed orders moving in either direction between the nurse and the other team members as there are between the nurse and the physician. Therefore, the nurse and the other team members need to build a working relationship among themselves that is beneficial to the patient. After making their initial evaluation of a patient's needs, the team members may move, from time to time, from a primary to a secondary place on the team. With one patient, for example, nursing care may take precedence; with another patient, physical therapy may fill the greatest need. With each patient, however, just as the physician remains in the picture, so does the nurse. In all cases, there is always some nursing assistance which must be identified and provided.

The nursing unit provides the basic unit for the care of the patient, and the nurses carry the responsibility for the welfare of the patient between his visits to or from the other team members. This welfare involves not only providing for the patient's basic needs, but also contributing to control of the environment. The nurse is the one person who is privileged to be with the patient over a long period of time. Thus, she has a special place on the health team. She is frequently the first person, beyond the patient's own physician, to establish a relationship with the patient and his family, whether in the hospital, home, or office setting. She may be the one to explain to, or clarify for, the patient the physician's prescription, including why and what he can expect when the physician advises the use of the services of other members of the team. She may be the one to prepare the patient either physically or emotionally for the contributions these persons will make to his care. She may be the only person who is to continually observe and report on the patient's condition, which means that the patient may or may not require the services of additional team members. For example, because the patient is having respiratory problems, the nurse will request the oxygen therapist to come ahead of schedule; or as a result of the nurse's observation that the patient has a fever, physical therapy will be postponed. The nurse also observes and reports the patient's reactions to the services provided by other team members. For example, the dietitian has provided a diet, but the patient refuses to eat the planned meal and asks for some substitution of foods. Or the patient becomes nauseated and the nurse suspects it may be a side effect of prescribed medication. In all of these instances it is the responsibility of the nurse to communicate with the team member concerned. Nursing thus has a dual responsibility—to the patient for direct, individual care, and to the other members of the team for the successful coordination of all aspects of patient care.

Specialty Fields in Medicine

Knowledge of the terminology used in the medical profession to designate specialty fields is basic to the nursing student's understanding of the scope of medical-surgical nursing. Medicine is the science of treating disease. In a restricted sense it refers to internal medicine, that branch of the healing art which deals with internal diseases and treats them by nonsurgical measures. The specialist in this branch of medicine is called an *internist.* Surgery is the branch of medicine which treats diseases by means of surgical procedures, including manipulation.

Within each of these branches of medicine, there are specialties that pertain to the care of patients with diseases or dysfunctions of specific systems of the body. These specialties and the specialists in the field are usually identified by a term which designates the specific organ system or type of tissue being studied and treated. For example, the specialist who studies and treats diseases of the heart is called a *cardiologist,* and his specialty field is known as *cardiology;* similarly, the specialist in *neurology*—the science and study of diseases and the treatment of the nervous system—is a *neurologist;* the specialist in *gynecology*—the science and study of diseases and treatment of reproductive organs in women—is a *gynecologist;* and the specialist in *orthopedics*—the science and study of diseases and treatment of the locomotive apparatus—is an *orthopedist.*

Certain other specialists are concerned with the diagnosis, the therapeutic research, the treatment, and the study of problems presented by patients. For example, the *anesthesiologist* specializes in the field of *anesthesiology*—the science and study of the administration of local and general anesthetics to produce the various types of anesthesia; the field of the *pathologist* is *pathology*—the study of the nature of disease, its causes, its processes, and its effects, together with the associated alterations of structure and function; and the *radiologist* is concerned with *radiology*—the science dealing with radioactive substances, rays and other ionizing radiations, and with their utilization in the diagnosis and treatment of disease.

MEDICAL-SURGICAL NURSING

Within the field of nursing, medical-surgical nursing is recognized as one broad area of specialization. Although the nurse in medical-surgical nursing does not specialize to the extent that the physician specializes in medicine and surgery, the expanding knowledge in these branches of medicine may eventually require greater specialization on the part of the nurse. Medical-surgical nursing encompasses the nursing care of the patient who is being treated either medically or surgically, or by a combination of these methods. It includes the nursing care of the patient in the operating room, the recovery room, the intensive care unit, and the medical and surgical units of the hospital. The scope and skills of medical-surgical nursing are also utilized in the care of patients in other situations, such as in clinics, in doctors' offices, in homes, and in industry.

Nursing care of patients whom the physician has classified as medical or surgical is presented in combination in this text, because all nursing care, in essence, is based on knowledge from the basic sciences and utilizes many common understandings and many of the same nursing measures, whether the patient is being treated medically or surgically. Frequently, the patient is under medical therapy until the decision is made to treat him surgically; and after surgery, his treatment is again medical. The physical and emotional factors that may cause or contribute to a disease are the same, or similar, in the majority of patients with that specific disease. In some cases medical therapies, such as medications or special diets, relieve or remove the cause; in other cases, surgical removal of the involved area is necessary. The basic nursing care, the diagnostic measures, and the manifestations of disease in the medical and in the surgical patient may be the same. For example, not every patient with a peptic ulcer requires surgery. Neither can every patient with an ulcer be treated conservatively, so that at times surgical intervention is necessary. Yet there are many commonalities in the care of the patient with an ulcer, whether he is being treated medically or surgically. This combined approach also enables the nursing student to view the patient as an individual who is in need of nursing care, regardless of the physician's choice of treatment.

The term *medical-surgical patient* is applied to the patient who is being treated for a disease or condition that is classified as both medical and surgical, according to the universal definition of medicine and surgery. Many of the considerations discussed in this text will apply to both the child and the adult. The focus is on the adult, however, and the special problems involved in the nursing care of children are not presented herein.

The Nursing Practitioner

In the preceding paragraphs nursing has been defined, the place of nursing in total patient care has been described, and the scope of medical-surgical nursing has been delineated. Since nursing cannot exist without a practitioner, it seems appropriate, as part of this introductory chapter, to present an overview of the characteristics of the professional nurse who is responsible for providing nursing care. Because her skills, abilities, understandings, and approaches to the patient influence the patient's progress, the professional nurse must possess certain qualifications. These qualifications include the following:

1. Ability to assess a patient situation, make accurate judgments, and take action, all based on her understanding of scientific knowledge and cause-and-effect relationships.

2. Respect for the individual differences and rights of each patient.

3. Knowledge and understanding of her own background, beliefs, values, culture, and education and their influence on her reactions to patients and nursing.

4. Knowledge that what she says and does, and how she speaks and behaves, influence the patient's reaction.

5. Recognition of her limitations in providing all the care a patient needs, and willingness to seek assistance from persons qualified in other fields.

6. Skill in observing, communicating, and reporting.

7. Ability to evaluate the care she has given, and the desire and ability to improve this care.

8. Motivation to keep up-to-date in nursing and related areas, and applying what she learns to nursing.

9. Understanding and knowledge of health and disease.

10. Understanding the potential effect of both the physical and the interpersonal environments on the patient's well-being.

11. Understanding, knowledge, and skill in nursing measures in general and specific situations.

12. Sensitivity to clues presented by a patient, and the ability to recognize a patient's changing nursing needs, as the nursing care needed by a patient is rarely static.

13. Feeling of responsibility for using her skills, and knowledge to assist the patient who is unable to care for many of his own needs.

14. Ability to work with other team members.

No attempt has been made to present a complete list of the desirable characteristics, including leadership skills and responsibility to the profession. Rather, this list relates only to the characteristics important to a consideration of nursing as a direct service to patients and the nurse's work as that of a clinician. The knowledges and skills related to leadership and management of groups of patients and personnel are outside the scope of a textbook on medical-surgical nursing.

CHAPTER 2
THE NURSE'S VARYING ROLES

GLADYS E. SORENSEN

The independent role
The assistive role
The collaborative role
Moving from role to role
The role in which the patient may place the nurse
Legal aspects related to the nurse's role

As she participates in providing patient care, the nurse is guided and influenced by the obligations and accepted ways of behavior considered appropriate for a person in her position. These obligations and ways of behavior are known as her *role*. In addition, the expectations and interpretations of others also condition her behavior. Certain aspects of the nurse's role are defined by law and by local policies in the institution or agency in which she works. The profession of nursing, through its national organizations—The National League for Nursing and the American Nurses' Association—also influences the nurse's perception of her role through the expression of guidelines such as "What People Can Expect of Modern Nursing Service," "Code for Professional Nursing," and "A Position Paper."

The roles of the nurse may be presented from a number of standpoints. In this textbook they will be considered from the viewpoint of her responsibilities as a member of the health team. In the first chapter, in describing the place of nursing in total health care, the roles of the nurse as a team member were alluded to. In general, there are three chief roles: (1) independent, (2) assistive, and (3) collaborative. Within each of these three main roles there are further roles, such as teacher, counselor, comforter, and leader.

The Independent Role

Certain activities specifically fall within the province of nursing for which the nurse needs no direction. Providing comfort and support through nursing ministrations and through listening and responding properly, and offering skillful assessment, evaluation, and appropriate intervention are all within the realm of the independent role of the nurse. The nursing activities that are part of the independent role are learned by the nurse as a student. Her skill in performing them increases as she gains experience as a nurse. In performing these independent activities the nurse applies what she has learned in the various science and nursing courses she has taken. In the independent role the nurse relies on her own powers of observation and perception and then acts in certain ways as a result of her judgment of the situation, based on her learning and experience. The independent role overlaps the assistive and collaborative roles to the extent that the nurse makes certain independent judgments when working with the physician and other team members and does not follow orders blindly.

The Assistive Role

The assistive role of the nurse requires her to carry out the physician's orders for therapy and to contribute in any other way toward his goal of the patient's recovery or cure. The nurse's chief concern is always for the patient, and everything she does in assisting the physician is directed toward her concern for the patient and his well-being. There are both independent and dependent aspects in this role. For example, the independent aspect requires her to make observations of changes in the patient's condition and report these observations to the physician in order to help him evaluate the patient and continue with the therapy. In the dependent aspect, the nurse helps the physician to accomplish a treatment or procedure. This assistance may range from setting up supplies and equipment for him to giving actual assistance during the procedure. An example of an assistive activity that combines dependent and independent aspects is the administration of medications. The nurse is dependent in that the physician prescribes the medication through a written order. However, she uses judgment in determining whether or not the dosage is within the amount usually prescribed for most patients, and seeks clarification from the physician if she has any questions; or in the case of a p.r.n. medication the physician's order provides the nurse with some leeway in deciding when the patient needs the medicine. Just as any leader places great reliance on his fellow workers, so the physician relies greatly on the nurse to fulfill his orders in a safe manner and to notify him of any inability to carry out his orders or of any unusual circumstances surrounding the patient.

The Collaborative Role

The collaborative role is one in which the nurse works with other members of the health team in meeting the objectives of patient care. In this role the nurse assists others, or they assist her, and neither gives formal direction to the other as occurs in the assistive role. In the collaborative role the nurse seeks help from, and supplements, supports, and plans with, other members of the health team, including the physician. For example, she may ask the physical therapist to help her initiate range of motion exercises with a bedfast patient, or she may reinforce or clarify the teaching of the dietitian. This means that the nurse needs to be aware of what other team members are doing for the patient. As was stated in Chapter 1, these other team members also need direction from the physician for whatever they are to do for the patient. In some instances, as with the social worker, the other team member may not be aware that his services are needed unless the nurse so notifies him. Thus, the collaborative role of the nurse places her in the position of both helping and receiving the help of others for the good of the patient. The collaborative role also calls for the nurse to be the coordinator of patient care, to share responsibility with other health team members, and to plan with them, both within and without the hospital, to provide continuity of care.

Moving from Role to Role

The nurse may find herself occupying a number of roles, some of which may be performed almost simultaneously. How she may move from one role to another in just one morning's time is illustrated as follows: In her *independent* role the nurse receives a report about a patient from another nurse, makes observations of the patient as she talks with him, and plans for his morning care and how it will be accomplished. In her *assistive* role, she sets up and assists the physician with a lumbar puncture. She demonstrates the independent aspect of this activity by giving emotional support to the patient as the procedure progresses. During the morning she also assists another patient with exercises he was taught by the physical therapist, thus assuming the *collaborative* role. She also finds herself in the *teacher* role as she corrects, when necessary, the manner in which the patient performs the exercises. When a nurse aide comes to the nurse for guidance on how to help a patient out of bed, the nurse finds herself in the *leadership* role. As the nurse moves in and out of a number of roles, she may find that the physician expects her to act in one way, the physical therapist in another way, and the aide in still another way. In these situations the nurse may respond either in accordance with expectations or as she feels she should respond on the basis of her past learning and experience.

The Role in Which the Patient May Place the Nurse

Depending on his past experience with nurses or what he has heard and read about them, the patient also has expectations of the nurse and may place her in a variety of roles as he progresses through his illness. Thus, he may expect her to be kind and sympathetic or cold and efficient. He may expect her to give him complete physical care whether or not he wants it. It may be necessary for the nurse to clarify for the patient what her role is and what he can expect from her as a nurse. In addition to this perceived role, the patient may unconsciously view the nurse as someone else and not as a person in her own right. To the patient, the nurse may be a mother figure, a sibling, or a figure outside the family. He is apt to relate to the nurse as he would to the person he has in mind. When this is the case the nurse needs to help the patient become aware of likenesses and differences and to regard her as an individual nurse.

Legal Aspects Related to the Nurse's Role

There are legal aspects related to the various roles in nursing. Certain phases of the nurse's role have been legally defined, and every activity of the nurse in the performance of her nursing services is the subject of potential analysis by the law. Lesnik defines nursing from the legal standpoint as being composed of independent and dependent functions which are determined on the basis of whether or not a physician's legal order is needed before the nurse may perform the function. He lists the following six independent areas of nursing functions: (1) supervision of a patient, (2) observation of symptoms and reactions, (3) recording and reporting, (4) supervision and direction of auxiliary workers, (5) application and execution of nursing procedures and techniques, and (6) health direction and educational and social services, including activities of psychological significance. Lesnik lists the application and execution of legal orders of physicians concerning treatments and medications, including an understanding of cause and effect, as dependent functions under the direction or supervision of a licensed physician.

Negligence. Negligence in nursing practice is defined as conduct which fails to meet a standard recognized by law for the protection of persons against unreasonable risks of harm. This conduct involves either doing something wrong or failing to do something that ought to be done. If harm results from failure to adhere to this standard, the nurse can be accused of malpractice and liability can be imposed. Professional persons, because of their specialized education, are held to a different and higher standard than laymen. A nurse is expected to utilize her professional knowledge in giving care. Both nursing students and graduates may be held legally responsible for their own nursing actions in their assistive and independent roles. The nurse should exercise due care and not attempt to do things for which she does not have preparation. She is obligated to question the physician when she is not certain of his orders or when his order seems to be contrary to usual procedure. The nurse is expected to be aware of the consequences of her carrying out a physician's order. Knowing what she is doing, how to do it, and why it should be done is the nurse's safeguard against suits for malpractice.

Medical Practice versus Nursing Practice. Another area to be considered by the nurse in her independent and assistive roles is that of the pressures for nurses to undertake responsibility for some of the activities that once were considered the prerogative of the physician. To reemphasize, the nurse must know why a given therapy has been prescribed and what its effects should be, both expected and untoward. In some situations, the line of demarcation between medical practice and nursing practice is not easy to delineate. The nurse could be held liable for practicing medicine without a license if she is not aware of which areas are properly in the realm of nursing practice and which are in the realm of medical practice. In some hospitals the nurse is expected to carry out procedures which in other hospitals would be considered the sole responsibility of the physician. Policies differ from one geographic region of the country to another because of legal statutes. The nurse must learn not only regional policies but local hospital policies pertinent to each type of health care situation in order to protect herself from accusations of practicing medicine.

Bibliography

Lesnik, Milton J. and B. Anderson: *Nursing Practice and the Law,* 2d ed. Philadelphia: J. B. Lippincott Company, 1962.

A Position Paper. American Nurses' Association. New York, 1965.

Code for Nurses with Interpretive Statements. American Nurses' Association. New York, 1968.

What People Can Expect of a Modern Nursing Service. National League for Nursing. New York, 1958.

CHAPTER 3
THE NURSE'S FUNCTIONS

MARGARET A. KAUFMANN

Nursing has taken its place as an important health profession. With the assumption of such a position comes an increasing responsibility for the health and welfare of those served by the profession. Nursing practice seeks to fulfill this responsibility, with its inherent obligation, duty, and accountability through its functions. The term *function* itself is a broad and general designation for the characteristic and expected activities of an agent or class of agents. Functions themselves are defined in a range from broad categories of responsibilities embodying the philosophy and purpose of those responsibilities to highly specific descriptions of activities performed in a particular circumstance.

The Nature of Nursing Functions

The components of nursing practice may usefully be classified somewhat as they are in the American Nurses' Association position paper on education for nursing as falling within three areas of responsibility: (1) the provision of care to the patient, (2) the support of cure (or the amelioration of disease) for the patient, and (3) the coordination of the purposes and processes of nursing with those of other health care agents and agencies. These functional areas are interlocking and usually operate simultaneously. At first glance they may appear deceptively clear in their intent, but in actuality their purposes and natures are quite complex.

The functions are complex because the facets within them are fluid and highly dependent upon the utilization of knowledge and judgment in combination with perceptual, organizational, and technological skills. The knowledge base underlying the functions is a diversified one which draws from the basic and applied sciences both natural and behavioral and encompasses not just general but also specific kinds of information. Nursing judgments are made within a constantly changing situation which presents numbers of variables, many of which are only moderately predictable. The illness situations which arise frequently do not follow the textbook pictures presented of them. Further, nursing is carried on within an interpersonal situation which is also multifaceted and complex, involving not only many patients and their families but also the full range of health worker groups. Patients' needs, desires, and goals vary widely. Health workers, although they have the same goals of care and cure of the patient, have different points of emphasis and different methods of operation which do not always meld harmoniously.

The functions of nursing are basic to its practice and therefore applicable to all categories of personnel who engage in nursing activities. There is, however, a marked difference in the numbers and kinds of activities performed by the various personnel groups, both in the amount of knowledge, skill, and judgment required to carry them out and in the nature of the responsibility inherent in them. The nurse aide, for example, carries out limited and specified activities of a noncritical nature under the direct guidance and supervision of the nurse, whose responsibility it is to see that they are carried out correctly and that they are not beyond the scope of the individual performing them. The licensed vocational (practical) nurse is prepared to undertake activities of a somewhat broader scope but of a procedural or technical nature requiring manual skill and basic knowledge of the act, its purposes, and its dangers, but not entailing the use of abstract judgments. The licensed vocational nurse, too, works under the guidance of the professional nurse, who carries the major responsibility for the welfare of the patient, although she does have sufficient training to be accountable for the safety and effectiveness of her actions.

Within the scope of the nursing functions there are interwoven aspects of the technical and professional dimensions of performance and responsibility. The kinds of behaviors which are technical and those which are professional are much discussed, often without either equanimity or consensus. Too often it is implied that something technical in nature is somehow less worthy. In this discussion the technical nurse and the professional nurse are considered equally worthy and equally purposeful, and both are essential to the practice of nursing. In both types of nursing, however, there is some variance in the amount and kind of preparation necessary and in the nature of the responsibilities they entail.

Professional nursing and technical nursing require different degrees of knowledge, involve varying amounts of judgment, and carry different degrees of responsibility. The professional dimensions of nursing require the exercise of independent judgment based on knowledge and an analytical assessment of the total nursing situation. The term *professional* itself implies that the individual possesses a body of specialized knowledge and skill, that he (she) will be able to make rational decisions and take appropriate action within the sphere of his functions, that he will assume responsibility for the consequences of his judgments and actions, and that he will work toward the development of new knowledge.

The professional functions of nursing encompass the physical, the psychological, and the social dimensions of the person, and also the physical and interpersonal environment which surrounds him. They are not limited to one particular aspect or activity of patient care. They take into account relevant elements from the patient's past and project his future in order to give breadth and depth to the planning of nursing care. Pursuits of this nature require knowledge from several fields, especially the natural and behavioral sciences, and the adapting of that knowledge to nursing practice. This broad base of understanding is essential in making sound clinical judgments relative to the kinds and amounts of nursing care needed by many different patients who are subject to a great variety of factors influencing their illness, treatment, and health care in general.

The technical dimensions, which also involve elements of the physical, psychological, and social, relate to the working methods or manner of performance of the art and science of nursing. The facts and principles from the natural and behavioral sciences are applied in a skillful manner in a situation for which the components have been defined or prescribed. The technical activities are employed largely in the implementation of the designated plans of nursing and medical care. They do not require the degree of independent assessment and critical judgment implicit in professional function. Some of the technical aspects of nursing are rather elementary but many more of them require appreciable depth in specialized knowledge and skill for their performance.

In nursing practice the indispensable element is purpose. Without purpose the activities of nursing rapidly become fixed and mechanical, task-centered, and subject to whatever positive or negative pressures the situation may bring to bear upon them. Purpose breathes life into function and makes possible nursing which is patient-centered in fact as well as in name. The needs of each patient are individually and continually analyzed. Overall goals take into account not just the illness status and medical therapeutic program, but also the well areas of the individual which need to be maintained and enhanced. The various aspects of the patient as a person, a family member, and a member of a community are considered and guidance in health care both for recovery and for prevention becomes a part of the nursing program. The purposes set forth, whether their accomplishment be slow or rapid, make each nursing action meaningful, so that nursing becomes in a true sense therapeutic.

Nursing functions, while maintaining their patient-centered and therapeutic orientation, may be either direct or indirect in nature. The nurse may work directly in a one-to-one relationship with the patient, giving him his physical care or interacting with him as a person. Or she may work through others, as is the case when the nursing team leader plans and guides for a group of patients care which is actually implemented by her team members. She may also operate indirectly yet in the patient's behalf through her general clinical unit activities by conferring with the physician, clarifying medical orders, and preparing equipment and supplies for therapeutic procedures. Nursing is a fundamental and integral part of a patient's total health care program. Each of its components contributes to this whole, and should not become an end in itself.

The Scope of Nursing Functions

Nursing in the modern world is in a state of evolution. Many knowledgeable persons are analyzing it—but throughout the analyses nursing must still be practiced. That practice takes place in a milieu characterized by an apparent paradox: On the one hand, patients are rapidly discharged from the hospital, perhaps even in 1 to 3 days following some surgical procedures. This situation presses the nurse to establish and accomplish her care objectives in a short period. On the other hand, nursing practice is confronted by the admission of increasing numbers of persons in the older age groups who have illnesses of a chronic nature and who have a decreased physical capacity to deal with those illnesses. The practice situation is further complicated by the increasing pressure from many physicians to have the nurse take over many of the routine medical functions of the doctor in order to facilitate his ability to manage the increasing demands placed upon medicine. Similarly, the professional nurse is handing on to the practical nurse and even to the aide many of her routine (and sometimes not routine) functional activities. When, where, how, and whether to assume activities through delegation from medicine or from hospital management, and when, where, how, and whether to delegate activities to other health care personnel are matters for continuing consideration in determining the scope of professional nursing functions.

CARE AS A NURSING FUNCTION

Care is the keystone of the nursing functions, and contains elements of both cure and coordination. The care function, multidimensional in its facets and its goals, may be implemented in a variety of ways, but always embodies principles of safety and comfort of the patient and of his environment.

Care which embodies quality is designed for each patient in relation to his specific circumstance. The particularization of nursing care is one of the great skills of nursing because it requires an acuteness of perception and an ability to differentiate small variations, coupled with proficiency in implementation. True individualization of care goes beyond the point of simple variation in approach between patients.

The care function deals with the whole patient as a unit, not with just one aspect of him. It involves understanding and support, supplying to the patient what he needs when he needs it, but not impinging upon him where no need exists. The care therefore embodies selective intervention based on assessment of the biopsychosocial status and requirements of the individual in relation to his health-illness status. The scope of the nurse's knowledge and her ability to see relationships is most clearly reflected in the implementation of the care function because it is here that learnings from psychology and sociology, chemistry, bacteriology, normal and pathological anatomy, and physiology—indeed from all the sciences and the humanities—are blended into a harmonious whole.

Care is predicated upon the actual and the perceived ability of the individual to manage for himself his basic and important human requirements, physical and psychosocial. The person who can successfully handle these requirements in their entirety has no need for care. When he can handle only some of the total range of requirements or only parts of certain of his needs, he then has selective needs for care. The latter is true of almost all patients. An example is found in the hospitalized person who can eat and assimilate his food well, but, because he is in the hospital, has no access to its purchase or preparation. His need is to have food made available to him. It is through assessment that the nurse determines the kind and extent of the care needs of each patient.

Patient perception as well as nurse perception plays a role in need determination. Not infrequently a patient does not recognize a need for help in a particular area; for example, dental hygiene, but the nurse does. The first requirement of the patient then becomes one of interpretation of the situation and its meaning for him so that he will recognize the need and desire assistance. Only when a person's safety or well-being (or that of others as when communicable disease is a factor) is truly in jeopardy should particular aspects of care be forced upon him. The physiological or psychological response to forcing may well be more detrimental than the omission of the desired action. This is one of the considerations which underlie the relaxation of physical restrictions placed upon patients with acute myocardial infarctions. In situations where nurse and patient differ in their recognition of a need for care, the nurse would be well advised to examine both her cultural and value systems and those of the patient to be assured that a genuine health problem exists and not just a divergence in preferred living patterns. Eating patterns, bathing habits, and certain aspects of morality and modesty are frequent areas where cultural and social norms of patient and nurse may conflict.

In a sense all nursing is therapy since its intent is to foster the well-being of the patient. The therapeutic dimensions of care exist even though the purpose may be specified as provision of comfort or maintenance of the patient at a certain point rather than allow deterioration, and support of whatever natural function exists. As a part of its therapeutic undergirding, nursing care has as great a concern with the well areas of the patient as it has with the sick areas. This emphasis is unique to nursing inasmuch as other members of the health professions have the greater part of their attention directed toward diagnosis and remedy of dysfunction.

In an approach to nursing care that follows a wellness-illness and a selective patient need for assistance perspective, it can be very useful to make an assay of all human systems, physical and psychosocial (including the perceptual, motivational, and coping mechanisms). The patient is thereby reviewed essentially from head to foot in relation to his overt functional ability and his psychological status. What is his self-help ability? To what degree is his body maintaining itself? To what extent can the patient accomplish his activities of daily living independently, from the standpoint of both his inherent capacity and his medical program? Many patients can actually *do* a lot for themselves, but are restricted from activity as a part of their medical therapy. When physical incapacity is great the patient may need to be bathed, toileted, even fed. The nurse may have to assume full care for a fairly long period in a functional disability such as a severe cerebrovascular accident, or only briefly as when high fatigue and pain levels occur, e.g., immediately following surgery. Where feasible the nurse encourages the patient to participate in a few nonstressful activities at planned intervals while she skillfully completes the greatest portion of care.

The nurse notes many things as she assesses physical care requirements. What is the respiratory capacity? Is the patient hypoxic? Is the hypoxia a consequence of restrictive positioning; of bronchial secretions which could be relieved by turning, coughing, and deep breathing; of diminished cardiac capacity aggravated by energy demands which extend beyond the body's capacity to supply adequate oxygen to the tissues? What is the state of the patient's elimination: will measures such as increased fluid intake, daily ambulation, guidance in food selection be of benefit? Is an enema necessary or should the doctor be consulted about ordering a laxative? Is the patient able to move about in bed by himself? Does he move his arms and particularly his legs sufficiently to maintain muscle tone and good venous return? If not, why? Is it physical incapacity, the influence of discomfort, or lack of motivation that limits his motion? He may need instruction and encouragement, or he may need to be placed on a schedule for turning and exercise. What is the patient's capacity to protect himself? Is the body able to ward off infection normally or has general debility or a specific condition such as leukemia reduced this ability? Is the patient particularly vulnerable in one area as is, for example, a patient with burns who is readily susceptible to infection? Can the patient guard himself against injury from falls, burns, or abrasions? In any of these situations where actual or potential imbalances exist, the care function of the nurse includes both protecting the patient against untoward occurrences stemming from the imbalance and instituting therapeutic efforts to alleviate the imbalance.

Concurrent with a comprehensive physical assessment, the patient's physical and interpersonal environment deserves consideration. Physiological and psychological comfort and safety as well as the therapeutic potential of nursing care measures are dependent upon this environment. The environmental situation can better be viewed as an aggregation of innumerable small yet distinct areas rather than as one or two global areas. It is often the little things that make a big difference—the tightness of the sheet over the feet, the light shining in the eyes. Because nursing has realistic limitations in the hospital resources available to it and in personnel, time, and energy, the nurse following her assessment of the environment must make some judgments and decisions related to the favorable aspects of the situation which should be retained, the unfavorable aspects which need to be changed, and the noncritical aspects which she can afford not to deal with or can set aside for a time.

Nursing care, as "environmental engineering," is concerned with everything that relates to the patient, physically and perceptually. Is the bed linen clean and dry? Are the pillows and supportive devices placed well for comfort and for anatomical positioning? Is the bed equipped with adequate safety and self-help devices such as side rails, foot board, trapeze; and are these things being used correctly? Is the patient's stand placed so that he can reach the things on it, such as the glass of water? What is the temperature in the room? Are ventilation and lighting adequate? What does the patient see from his bed: heaps of equipment left lying around, half-dead flowers, nothing but a blank and dreary wall? Are his roommates compatible or does the illness, behavior, or therapeutic program of one patient affect the others, diverting their energy from restoring their own wellness to reacting against the environment? Do the people giving care deal with the patients as individuals or as "jobs to be done"? Do they work with the patient during treatment or just with the task? The therapeutic use of self is an important element of care. Personnel who are rough, or careless, or inconsiderate, or unfriendly, or who use the patient to meet their own needs, or who do not like a particular patient are not helpful to the patient, even though they may get the work done. They may need instruction, guidance, or a change of assignment in order to increase their effectiveness and also to increase the personal rewards they get from their care-giving activities.

Also within the purview of the environment is the sensory stimulation the patient receives. Even the very sick individual needs some sensory input to support his feelings of humanness and worth. The dying patient, for example, is one who is often left quite alone except when being given treatments. Patients who are recovering can also benefit from increased amounts of balanced stimulation. Mild sensory deprivation can cause an amorphous, unmotivated state which may go unobserved; severe deprivation has been shown to give rise to inappropriate behavior and even hallucinations.

Another important area of concern inherent in the care function is what might be termed the patient's *human status*. All individuals, whatever their origins or present situations, are deserving of consideration of their rights and dignity as human beings. Too often when a person places himself, or is placed, in the hands of nursing or any other health-care group, he is regarded in whole or in part as having given up his right to modesty, privacy, knowledge of his situation, and participation in decision-making. Patients are at times exposed physically or psychologically, poked, prodded, told what to do but not why, talked about but not to, and otherwise ignored. Therapeutic care will reverse this situation. It strives to give the person, through concern demonstrated by words, by action, and by attitude, the feeling that he has worth no matter what capacities have been stripped from him, for example, his ability to speak or to control his bladder, or regardless of how cantankerous he may become. Maximum effort is made to have the patient and his family understand through explanation and guidance the "what" and the "why" of what is going on around him and happening to him and to involve him in the planning for and progress of his own care. Implementation of this aspect of care involves at least some, and sometimes a great deal of, interaction with the physician and consideration of his methods and goals in order to arrive at an effective manner of working with the patient.

The care function is as much an intellectual undertaking as it is an implementive one because the nurse works with the total human being. She deals with his perceptual schema, his modes of communication, and his coping mechanisms, as a means of determining constructive approaches to his care. Much depends upon a patient's past experience, his formal and informal learning, and his native intelligence. What does a patient actually see in a situation? Is, for example, the nurse who inquires into his family relationships or his personal feelings seen as being inordinately curious or wanting to learn in order to help him in some specific way? Is turning and coughing following chest surgery viewed as a form of modern torture, or is it recognized as being worth the discomfort it can cause? Advance preparation of the patient, with interpretation at his level of understanding and linked to past or anticipated experiences which have value to him, will help a great deal in making a patient an active participant in his own care. He becomes motivated. Getting a patient to "want to" often spells the difference between success and failure in having him do or learn something which will be to his benefit without spending his energy in resisting or setting up a block to eventual cooperation. Time spent in motivating is time saved in the long run.

Just as patients perceive things differently so, too, do they communicate in a variety of ways. Uncooperativeness may not be that at all, but rather, an indication of lack of understanding or of fear. Words cannot always be taken at their face value, nor can behavior. The nurse is faced with the necessity of trying to determine whether the patient's actions actually mean what they seem to mean. A common example is the patient who says a thing is "all right" or a certain nurse is "nice," not because he feels it is true but because he is afraid that if he "complains" his light will not be answered when he needs something.

The importance of making an interpretation of the meaning of patient behavior is recognized, but its hazards must be taken into account as well. Attitudes can be read into an act, a word, or a situation which do not, in fact, exist. A woman does not *have to have* psychological problems regarding her femininity because her uterus was removed. A man is not necessarily depressed because he turns to the wall and will not talk. He may be tired, or he may not be a conversationalist. He has a right to be what he is. Care flounders just as much when attempts are made to force patients into the mold of favored theories, as it does when the valid possibilities for meaning and reaction in people are not taken into account and analyzed in relation to the individual patient. Patients do have different modes of coping with physical and interpersonal situations. Some of these may be both sound and successful; others may be deemed poor by an observer but may be successful from the patient's viewpoint (for example, he may "get his way" by yelling). When coping mechanisms are unsuccessful, the patient is placed in a situation of rising frustration with waste of physical and psychic energy.

A third large area of concern in the care function is life style. Analysis of the patient's life style guides the individualization of nursing care and aids in the establishment of goals or objectives for that care. It takes into consideration the concept the patient has of himself, the cultural and social values he holds, and the milieu in which he normally lives. It considers his religious preference and practices, his educational level, his economic status, and his vocation.

All these factors can make a difference in the nature of the care plan and its implementation. It is, for example, virtually useless to discuss dietary matters with a patient from the viewpoint of foods he dislikes and will not eat, those he cannot afford, or those that conflict with his cultural and family eating patterns. His health care regarding nutrition would better be drived from an exploration of those habits, his illness problem, and his general and specific physiological condition (e.g., is he diabetic or edentulous?), and then designed on the basis of what elements in his diet can be retained and built upon, what should be changed, and what suggestions for change will actually be effective.

The ways in which a patient views himself as regards his perceived and his actual self-help ability influence the focus and components of care. Some individuals see themselves as having a greater capacity than their physical state warrants and will, for example, attempt to resume normal activities too soon after surgery or will overtax a heart in congestive failure. Others may think they know all about their illness and therapy and will ignore medical and nursing advice. Still others will come to believe they can do almost nothing and will lead unnecessarily restricted lives. These problems challenge the nurse's capacity to guide, instruct, and motivate her patients in a constructive fashion.

The care requirements of another type of patient may have a different focus. The patient may see himself as having little worth as a person, as no longer desirable to his spouse, as incapable of caring for himself. Sometimes the family may think these things too. Here the nurse not only has a number of attitudes to work with, but she must seek to establish a program for maintaining existing function and reestablishing as much capacity as possible in the affected areas in order to approach the problem from both dimensions. This can be a long and arduous task in severe disabilities such as cerebrovascular accident and paraplegia. The program requires the efforts of the entire health team. Here, as in all care, the nurse activates principles of timing, of continuity, of motivation, and of realistic expectation so that a patient does not receive a great deal of attention one day and very little the next, so that he is challenged but not beyond the point of achieving at least a little recognizable success; so that he is not led to expect the impossible or pushed to do what he cannot possibly do; so that his program of activities is timed to meet his periods of greatest physical and psychological readiness.

Some patients will indeed require all the knowledge, skill, and resources the nurse can mobilize to contribute to their health care, but there are others for whom illness or injury is merely a brief interlude. They have been well-functioning individuals before they entered the hospital and will continue to be so after they leave. Their physical and psychological care can be good without being extensive. It is important to point out, however, that because a patient does not seem to need much nursing care, he is not to be left unattended. The nurse must maintain an awareness of each patient so that she will know what his needs are. Then, should they change, she can formulate or alter her plan of care and intervention appropriately.

The care-giving function is a complex, challenging, and goal-directed responsibility which is essentially rehabilitative and preventive in nature. Maintenance, support, and restoration embodied in the care-giving and cure-supportive actions of nursing are fused to keep the well areas well and directly or indirectly bring the areas affected by disease back to the greatest possible function. In her care function the nurse uses herself as guide, counselor, comforter, teacher, sounding board, and ministrator through word, touch, empathy, and action. She recognizes when resources beyond those she possesses are needed and works with other members of the health team to provide them. She evaluates care priorities for individuals and for groups, and is conscious of the timing of her actions so that they take place at points of need and readiness for the patient. She utilizes consistency as principle to give care the flow, the balance, and the predictability basic to effectiveness. Through the care function the uniqueness of nursing in the health professions is demonstrated.

CURE AS A NURSING FUNCTION

Cure and care are not mutually exclusive, because so much inherent in care makes a vital contribution to cure. Cure in this chapter will be viewed primarily from the perspective of its role in the support of medical therapy.

The instrumental activities of cure should not hold the primary position in nursing, but they often do. A demonstration by the nurse of efficiency and skill in administering treatments and medications has high value to the physician, of course, since these activities further his goals, but they also carry prestige for many nurses who view them as the core of nursing. Most of the cure-related activities were and still are, under certain circumstances, done by the physician. They would not now really need to be done by nurses at all, but could be taken over by medical technicians unless these activities are fused with *care,* the patient thereby gaining a double benefit.

The foregoing is not intended to depreciate the nursing activities of cure but rather to bring them into a rational perspective in the totality of nursing. The nurse has many important responsibilities within her cure function. She needs much knowledge of considerable depth, observational and judgmental abilities, and technical skill to fulfill them.

To participate in cure effectively, the nurse requires a clear understanding of the physician's overall goals as well as the effect he hopes to achieve through a particular therapy. This knowledge provides her with a basis for two kinds of observation: overall patient progress, and the particular and more immediate response of the patient to the specific therapeutic measure. The pertinence and accuracy of these observations depend upon an understanding of the nature of the pathophysiology involved and the particular way it is manifested in the patient and upon knowledge of the therapy itself, i.e., what effects may be expected from it, what untoward reactions can occur, and what changes in physiological or psychological behavior of the patient might alert the nurse to an incipient problem. Changes in vital signs, skin color, or temperature, dermal eruptions, or wheezing respirations are overt warning signals. Other changes are more subtle. Alterations in interpersonal behavior, such as lethargy in a normally talkative person, might indicate an incipient drug reaction. Often it is the nurse who first notes change in the patient and so must decide whether the development is noncritical and can be handled independently or whether the physician should be notified and medical assessment and intervention sought.

The increased use of experimental drugs has opened an area of additional concern for the nurse. Physicians themselves are not entirely sure just what the effects of such drugs will be. Literature on these drugs is not always available on the clinical unit. It then becomes the nurse's responsibility to obtain from the doctor or the pharmacist enough information to enable her to administer the medication properly and observe the patient adequately in order to ensure his safety.

Allied to the responsibility of the nurse for knowledgeable observation is the responsibility for communication, verbally and in writing. Any questions which arise relative to the nature of a physician's order, its intent, the appropriateness of a dosage as it is written, when to begin or end a particular therapeutic sequence, the timing of treatments with respect to the patient's fatigue level, or any other aspect of his care program must be asked. The nurse is legally responsible for her actions in all areas where she should have knowledge of what is correct and what is safe for the patient. Verification therefore becomes an essential part of nursing action.

Observations by the nurse are limited in value unless they are transmitted. Clear, concise records are necessary, including data on the patient's response to treatment as well as the particulars of the treatment or medication, the amounts, the times, and the frequency. Verbal communication supplements the written record in many ways. It conveys a message instantly in a critical situation; it allows for discussion of problems, clarification of purpose, planning of ways of working with the patient. It helps maintain awareness of the patient's particular situation and is of value not only to the physician but to the members of the nursing team and to other health workers as well.

An important aspect of the nurse's function in cure is her skill: skill not only in performing but also in preparing the patient for a particular intervention and in caring for him afterward. Skill embodies safety—safety of body, of tissue, of function, and of psyche. Equipment must be used correctly so that it achieves the purpose for which it was intended: for example, intermittent positive pressure breathing apparatus is checked for any leaks which will cause it to malfunction, and its gauges are checked for the delivery of proper pressure; sterile dressings do not touch unsterile areas nor are they handled with the fingers. Precautions are taken not to injure tissues during a procedure, such as may occur in probing with a urinary catheter or forcefully injecting irrigating fluid into a ureteral catheter. Tubes are secured in a manner which will provide for optimum drainage yet will not pull on or press against tissue, or otherwise annoy the patient. For example, a nasogastric tube is taped in such a way that it does not rub the tip of the nose or pass before the patient's eye, constantly distracting vision. The patient is guided to understand what a procedure is and what to expect during and following it in efforts to reduce any anxiety it may engender.

One goal in cure is to make its contributory procedures as easy and comfortable for the patient as possible. The patient may be given a rest period between his bath and ambulation, administered a pain medication in advance cf having to cough following chest or abdominal surgery so that he is physically more capable of coughing effectively, or placed in a position fostering relaxation of the muscle site before an intramuscular injection is administered. Explanations of procedures and support to the patient during the procedure should be a routine part of every therapeutic action. The *care* function is actually a part of the *cure* function and operates in harmony with it.

COORDINATION AS A NURSING FUNCTION

Coordination might be viewed as the "glue" which holds the nursing and health care programs together and the "grease" which keeps them moving smoothly. The nursing function has an admirable opportunity to act as facilitator and communicator throughout the scope of patient care inasmuch as it focuses upon the totality of that care and not upon a segment thereof, and its contacts with the patient are more contiguous in nature than are those of other health workers.

Nursing should be a prime activator in the achievement of comprehensive, patient-centered care through its coordinative role. It does, however, encounter some limiting factors with which it must deal to achieve the goal. First, nursing itself is not an automatically integrated whole. It is made up of nurses, and nurses are individual and different persons. Communication and synchronization between nurses does not occur spontaneously. It must be planned for and worked at. Second, the hospital and its departments may assume a preemptive position in the total schema so that its operational procedures and policies can and often do take precedence over patient need, thus causing the health care process to become hospital-centered. The care situation can easily become personnel-centered, as well, when nurses and doctors give priority to their particular preferences and convenience rather than to patient requirements. From a realistic point of view, efficiency, economy, and the priorities of some situations over others make it impossible for a health agency or its personnel to be totally responsive to all the wants and specialized needs of each patient, but where a philosophy of patient-centeredness is truly functional, a constructive balance can be achieved. Nursing is an important factor in establishing this balance.

Many difficulties in health care implementation occur as a result of lack of awareness, poor communication, inadequate planning, and insufficient interpretation. The collaborative role of the nurse embodies an effort to seek out these kinds of problems and their possible causes, to review them with the appropriate person or department, and to use herself as an agent of change, instituting cooperative planning and demonstrating constructive action. The nurse may be the only one who is actually aware that a patient is scheduled to have laboratory work done, have an x-ray examination, and receive physical therapy all in the same morning. A brief interpretive discussion with the doctor, or a phone call to one of the therapeutic departments concerned, could initiate a rescheduling which would save the patient from arriving at his noontime meal too exhausted to eat. In another instance, the nurse might inform a therapeutic department of the condition of a patient who is particularly weak or in considerable discomfort so that he is not called to the department in advance of its readiness for him and does not have to sit in a wheel chair or lie on a stretcher for an extended period.

Utilization of resource agencies and personnel is an element of the coordinative function, which is usually undertaken in consultation with the physician. Such consultation serves not only to secure his approval but also to keep him abreast of patient status from the nursing perspective, and alerts him to any present or potential problems which have come to the attention of the nurse. Through her frequent contacts with the patient and her close involvement in his total care, the nurse may be better able than the doctor to become aware of instances when the assistance of the physical therapist, the dietitian, or the medical social worker, as examples, might be of value.

Of particular importance is the preparation of the patient for discharge and the assessment of his ability to manage his continuing care at home. Referral to the visiting nurse service in the patient's area of residence might permit shortening of hospitalization by a day or two, or make the difference between the establishment of successful and unsuccessful living patterns at home. Guidance in the management and irrigation of a colostomy, follow-up instruction in the self-administration of insulin, and teaching a family the care of a parent with residual impairment from a cerebrovascular accident are examples of the use of a health resource to bridge care from hospital to home. Effective referrals to the visiting nurse service cannot be made at the last minute. A good deal of information about the patient and his medical care program must be communicated. The agency must be able to plan for evaluation of the home situation and equipment and to arrange to have a nurse available for the patient's arrival home, and not at some time after he and his family have gotten themselves into an almost irreparable state of confusion and frustration.

Conferences which encourage sharing of information, identification of problems, and cooperative planning are of considerable importance in health care coordination. Frequent meetings of the health team and regular nursing team conferences, planned in advance and having particular patients or issues selected for discussion, are extremely helpful in individualizing patient care, developing therapeutic care programs, and identifying and resolving problems of policy or procedure which may adversely affect patient care, whether that care be medical or nursing in nature. Conferences also provide an excellent opportunity for health care personnel to get to know each other and each other's values, goals, and perspectives, and for each team member to gain a sense of belonging and productivity in his job. Interpersonal problems and misinterpretations of meaning or intent can do more to dissolve an otherwise cohesive organization than almost anything else.

A not very frequently discussed aspect of coordination of care surrounds the patient's family and his visitors. Often they become the "lost souls" of the hospital when they might well be a valuable therapeutic resource. Visitors, whether family or friends, sometimes exhaust patients by overlong or ill-timed visits, or by expecting them to talk beyond their capacities. Visitors may also upset patients with inappropriate topics of conversation, suggestions contradictory to the physician's plan of therapy, discussions of family problems with which the patient cannot at the moment cope, and the like. With guidance from the nurse, these visits could be pleasant, beneficial, nonfatiguing experiences for the patient giving him, for example, an opportunity to be as self-centered as he needs to be, yet gently guiding him away from dwelling excessively on his problems. Families could, if they wished, become involved in selected aspects of the patient's care, if given proper interpretation and teaching. They could then feel they were being of some help and would also gain support and understanding in their concern for the patient.

Although the nurse works with the health team as a whole, the largest part of her coordinative responsibilities lies within the scope of nursing itself. Through her activities of teaching and supervision, and through the constant evaluation of the nursing practice carried out in her clinical unit, the professional nurse can accomplish a great deal in unifying the activities of all levels of nursing personnel and developing a team which works together to provide safe, therapeutic, comfort-giving nursing to all the patients under its care.

Implementation of Nursing Functions

Many methods can be used in performing nursing functions so long as the goal is clear. Nursing, as has been said, is a purposeful activity having its focus upon the patient. Purpose if it is to be effectively achieved cannot be left to chance. Therefore planning becomes essential. Basic to planning is a determination of the nature and components of the situation with which the planning will be concerned. The value of the plan is reflected in its implementation, and the effectiveness of the total process is determined through evaluation. Evaluation at a professional level is not confined to an analysis of final outcome but is an ongoing and integral process which may lead to revision of goal or method at any time during the nursing process.

The implementation of the nursing functions follows what is essentially the problem-solving method: (1) Delineating the focal or problem area to be considered; (2) gathering evidence relevant to the area of focus in an orderly and inclusive way; (3) identifying both nursing problems and nursing care requirements with their causative and contributory factors; (4) specifying the plan or approach to be utilized in meeting the identified problems and care requirements; (5) implementing the plan; and (6) evaluating its components and outcome. The problem-solving method provides for a systematic and comprehensive approach to nursing care which allows for focus upon the individual patient, or nursing problem, and provides a mechanism by which the relevant may be separated from the irrelevant on the basis of actuality, rather than of conjecture.

THE NURSING CARE PLAN

The formulation of a nursing care plan begins with assessment and arrives at conclusions. Its intent is to bring analysis and logical thinking to bear upon the problems and process of patient care. It is a means of providing for a determination of the patient's needs and the inclusion of the necessary components of nursing care in an organized and effective fashion. A well-developed care plan will conserve the time and energy of both nurse and patient, as well as make constructive use of the available health care resources. The plan serves to coordinate the efforts of all the persons engaged in the care of the patient, to unify their approaches, and to provide for effective progression and revision of care in accordance with the patient's needs and progress.

An important aspect of the planning process is the identification of nursing problems and the development of a nursing diagnosis. A *nursing problem* may be considered a situation or circumstance related to the patient in which he has an actual or potential need for care, which he cannot meet for himself, and which is within the scope of nursing function (Abdellah). A given patient may have many nursing problems simultaneously or sequentially. A *nursing diagnosis* is not to be confused with a medical diagnosis. Though it takes into account the disease, it does not determine what the disease is or differentiate it from other diseases. That is the function of the physician. Because nursing is still in the early stages of development of classifications, or typologies, for nursing entities, there are few words or phrases which summarize a body of information and signs and symptoms such as the physician has in the naming of diseases, for example, *appendicitis, tuberculosis, congestive heart failure.* A nursing diagnosis may therefore have to be a descriptive and interpretive sentence or paragraph which offers a summary and an evaluation of the nature of the patient's condition, classifying and differentiating the identified nursing problems. The nursing diagnosis represents the conclusions arrived at by the nurse as a result of her analysis of the total patient care situation and its particular relationship to nursing functions. A single patient may have several nursing diagnoses just as he may have several medical diagnoses. However, differing from the medical diagnosis which, once determined, remains constant, the nursing diagnosis is subject to change as the patient proceeds through his illness experience.

An approach to the development of a nursing diagnosis and care plan, which embodies an analysis of the patient's care-need situation and leads to the determination of care goals and requirements, is presented in the "Nursing Analysis" which follows.

Nursing Analysis

    I. Person profile
        A. Biographical data: age, sex, marital status, number of children (age, sex), race, religion, military service (branch, length)
        B. Family constellation and status, relevant family and marital history, present members of household

C. Location and nature of residence, living arrangements, length of time at residence, areas of past residence
D. Educational level and history
E. Occupation and occupational history, preferred occupation (if relevant)
F. Economic status
G. Interests, hobbies, recreational preferences
H. Health habits and beliefs: sleep, physical activity, nutrition, elimination, hygiene, health supervision, drugs (e.g., cathartics, alcohol, tranquilizers); smoking, concept of health, concept of illness
I. Physical limitations
J. Estimate of personality characteristics and emotional state
K. Estimate of present and potential reaction to stress
L. Family response to patient's illness

II. Medical profile
A. Overview of patient's health-illness status
B. Diagnosis: primary, secondary
C. Diagnostic tests and results
D. Physician's objectives and therapeutic plan
E. Medical history, signs and symptoms, variations from the classic picture of the disease
F. Therapies: medical, surgical; response to therapy
G. Prognosis and potential health status

III. Nursing objectives
A. Rationale of nursing objectives
   1. Assessment of basic human requirements (needs)
   2. Estimate of self-help ability
   3. Manifestations of nursing problems
B. Nursing diagnosis
C. Objectives for nursing care
   1. Immediate
   2. Intermediate
   3. Long-range
   4. Plans for home care
D. Relationships of nursing objectives to physician objectives

IV. Nursing-care requirements
A. Immediate
   1. To meet basic needs
   2. To support self-help ability
   3. To support medical diagnostic and therapeutic program
   4. Priorities in care requirements
B. Intermediate
   1. To meet basic needs
   2. To support self-help ability
   3. To support medical diagnostic and therapeutic programs

4. Priorities in care requirements
C. Long-range and home care
   1. To meet basic needs
   2. To support self-help ability
   3. To support diagnostic and therapeutic programs
   4. Priorities in care requirements

The first section of the Nursing Analysis, the *person profile,* is in essence a nursing history. It deals with the nature of the whole person, where and how he normally lives, what he likes and does not like, what his reactions to his health and his illness are. This information is utilized by the professional nurse in two important ways: first, to "custom tailor," insofar as possible, the patient's nursing care program to the patient and his preferences; second, to guide her in the all-important guidance-teaching dimension of her function, wherein she must judge how much and what kind of teaching is needed and determine the most feasible means for accomplishing it.

A nursing history is also very valuable in that it brings the patient and/or his family into active partnership in the design of his care. The patient is thereby looked upon as *someone,* not as *something.* A nursing history is very much patient-centered, while the medical history is largely focused upon the determination of the existence and scope of pathology.

The second section of the Nursing Analysis bears on the medical dimensions of the patient's health-illness situation. It represents an essential dimension in the development of a nursing care plan.

It is in the third and fourth sections of the Nursing Analysis that creative nursing care is generated through the processes of analysis, synthesis, and evaluation for the planning and activation of individualized, therapeutic nursing care.

Planning is a continuing process. As the patient care circumstances change, the care plan must be changed. A plan of care known only to the one who conceived it is of minimal value inasmuch as the entire care of the patient is not undertaken by a single individual, even in private duty nursing, because no one nurse stays with a patient 24 hours a day, 7 days a week. Word-of-mouth communication is not adequate because it easily becomes omissive and does not always reach each individual who is concerned with the care of the patient.

Care plans must be written, and herein lie some difficulties. Hospital nursing services, even today, are infrequently structured to provide adequate time for initially developing, and maintaining, the care plans for each patient. Work activities become preemptive, and too many people still believe that a nurse who is sitting and thinking is not working, even though the patient will benefit from her thought processes. Nurses themselves may be frustrated in their efforts to develop a balance between the preparation of a plan of care which attempts to be all-inclusive and so becomes cumbersome and one which is so brief and general that it loses pertinence and fails to serve as a guide to nursing action. Mastery of the care plan lies in developing the skill to abstract from the total assessment data the salient factors and formulate them into concise statements of the desired goal and the actions necessary to achieve it. Care plans are not intended to be complex and esoteric but rather to be simple, straightforward guides which are useful to the nursing staff and beneficial to the patient. They are means by which duplication of data gathering and nursing action can be avoided, while overall completeness and progression of care is more nearly assured.

The nursing care plan is generally written by one person to give it internal consistency, but it is most productively developed on the basis of consultation and discussion with members of the nursing staff, the physician, and other concerned health workers. Its format is usually determined in accordance with the requirements of the particular agency in which it is to be used. A separate, more extensive form can be used in conjunction with the Kardex (or other card system) or the plan may be incorporated into the Kardex. A limitation in the use of the Kardex occurs only when it is employed primarily for noting medications, treatments, and activity limitations, and little that is actually nursing care is included. Figure 3-1 presents a sample Kardex nursing care card which within its space limitations provides for notation of the patient's therapies and diagnostic tests, objectives of nursing care and related care requirements, limited information about the patient himself, and some data related to the medical prescription for the patient and to the patient's self-help abilities in the areas of diet, activity, and self-care.

Planning blends directly into implementation. The care plan for each patient is correlated with the overall organization of care for all patients assigned to the nursing team or unit, and assignments for various segments of the care are made to the nursing personnel. Judgments are made concerning the priorities of care needs among the group of patients as well as for individual patients. An assessment is made of the capabilities of each member of the team so that work assignments can be made to harmonize with the nature of the patient care requirements, the abilities of the personnel, and the amount of responsibility they may rightly assume. A team leader may decide to give a bath to a particular patient so that she may make a detailed assessment of his status or provide him with the benefit of her expert skill in a particular area. She may decide to work with a licensed vocational nurse in order to assume the professional dimensions of the care which should not be delegated.

In nursing, the unanticipated is commonplace. Emergencies arise, new patients are admitted, personnel are absent because of illness, operations are scheduled or canceled at the last minute, new treatments are ordered, doctors are delayed, and well-laid plans for the day must be changed on the spot. The nurse must be able to accommodate these variations and carry out the immediate program of action without losing sight of the nursing goal. This kind of flexibility is an important part of implementation.

The planning and the implementation of nursing care is brought to full circle with its evaluation. Evaluation is done both in retrospect and as an ongoing appraisal of the assessment, planning, and intervention aspects of nursing care. By this means, the nurse judges whether to continue a program of care in accordance with the original plan, or whether other approaches and interventions might be more successful. She reviews her nursing activities after completing

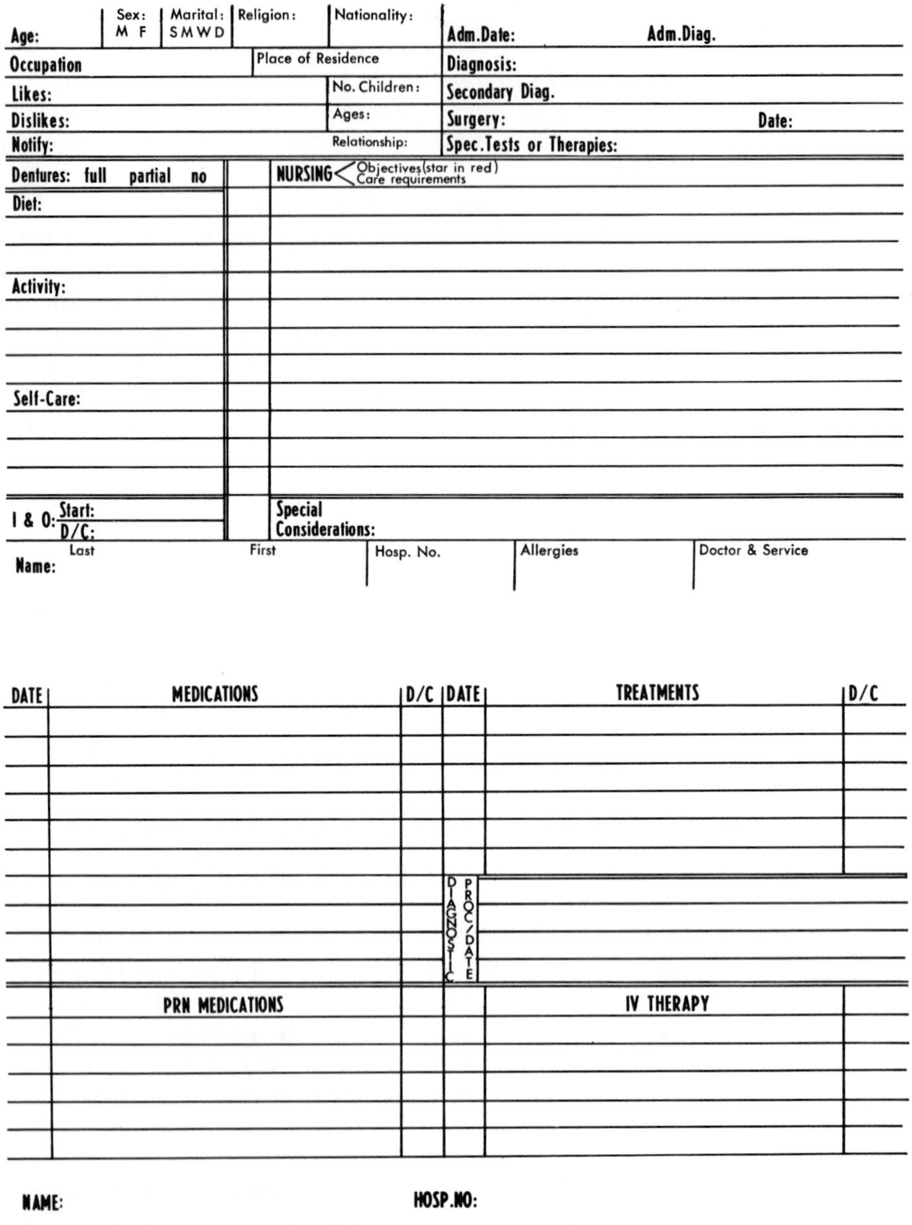

Age:	Sex: M F	Marital: S M W D	Religion:	Nationality:	Adm.Date:		Adm.Diag.
Occupation			Place of Residence		Diagnosis:		
Likes:				No. Children:	Secondary Diag.		
Dislikes:				Ages:	Surgery:		Date:
Notify:				Relationship:	Spec.Tests or Therapies:		

Dentures: full partial no	NURSING ⟨ Objectives(star in red) Care requirements
Diet:	
Activity:	
Self-Care:	
I & O: Start: D/C:	Special Considerations:

Name:	Last	First	Hosp. No.	Allergies	Doctor & Service

DATE	MEDICATIONS	D/C	DATE	TREATMENTS	D/C
			DIAGNOSTIC	PROC/DATE	
	PRN MEDICATIONS			IV THERAPY	

NAME: HOSP.NO:

Figure 3-1
Sample Kardex nursing
care card.

them, and reassesses the patient so that she can improve and refine her practice in the future; and so that she will be aware of which modes of planning and intervention were most successful and whether the nursing care has accomplished its goals. If part of the plan was not effective, she seeks to understand why it was not. Time spent in thoughtful review of past activity and outcome means time saved and enhanced efficiency for the future.

Skills Needed to Implement Nursing Functions

The skills of professional nursing practice are not just technical and procedural, although these are of considerable importance. The rapid development of physiological monitoring devices has markedly increased the complexity of the technical skill area and established a need for specialized training, such as that now provided in intensive cardiac care units.

A large number of the skills required of the professional nurse are intellectual, interpersonal, and judgmental in their nature. The development of these skills begins with the study of liberal arts courses such as English, speech, and philosophy, and the behavioral sciences such as psychology and sociology, and is supported in selected areas by the knowledge acquired through study in the natural sciences. These skills accrue and are enhanced throughout the nursing program and the nursing experience and through continued learning by the graduate nurse in her professional practice.

OBSERVATION SKILLS

Observation involves looking and listening. Both are trained operations based on knowledge and developed through experience. The observation skills of the nurse are inclusive and perceptive. In her visual observations the nurse unobtrusively focuses upon many things, gross and minute. She notes the physical state of the patient from head to toe, his vision, his hearing, his breathing. She is aware of his position, his movements, the expression on his face and in his eyes, the way he acts and responds, the things he has around him. She is concerned as well with any signs and symptoms of disease or malfunction of the body or mind. She looks for changes between one observation and another, from one day to the next.

Skill in observation lies not alone in looking into pertinent areas and seeing many things, but in relating one observation to another, in separating the important and critical factors from the normal and natural. Discrimination can make one observation good; lack of it can make another observation poor. The little changes, the seemingly irrelevant acts, the new and almost unnoticeable symptom that appears in a location distant from the site of the patient's disease are often the most pertinent observations.

Discriminative observation is based not only on an understanding of where to look, but also of what to look for. A knowledge of the norms of physical function in health and at the various age levels, along with a concept of human behavioral patterns and their usual or expected response to stress, sharpens observation and increases the probability of detecting an incipient problem. The same is true for a knowledge of the disease process in general and the patient's disease or disability in particular. Visual observation may go on without auditory observation when the patient is silent. Listening, however, should always be accompanied by visual observation so that nonverbal communication is not overlooked. The expression, the gesture, or the body position may support or belie what is being said.

Listening seems a simple enough act, but it is deceptive. Sometimes people do not listen at all. They are thinking of something else, or what they will say next, or how to "talk someone into something." They never get the message of the words they half hear. Other people hear what they want to hear—not what is actually being said. A nurse may make her own interpretation of the patient's words without ever trying to find out what meaning the patient himself attaches to them. Often a phrase or two, "Will you tell me a little more about that?" "I'm not quite sure what you mean," "You're terribly upset," will lead the patient to express himself more fully and so make clearer his thoughts and feelings. The voice may say, "I'm not worried," while the tonal quality and the fidgeting fingers say, "I'm scared to death." So the nurse listens to what lies behind the words and to the themes of the conversation. She listens to the particular choice of words and notes the facial expressions that go with them. She also evaluates what is being said against the realities of the situation. Imagination may cause one patient to build up a circumstance while another may underplay or brush off a condition because he is embarrassed or does not want to be a nuisance. Through all her observations the nurse blends objective clinical judgment with a kind of perception Frances Reiter calls *seeing it from the patient's side of the eyes.*

COMMUNICATION SKILLS

The nature of communication is a vast subject which can only be touched upon here. The nurse is engaged in communication constantly, both as a giver and as a receiver. Communication is the transmission of ideas, information, feelings, and attitudes. It has three basic elements: (1) the source or sender of the message, (2) the message itself, and (3) the receiver of the communication. The sender formulates the message, which embodies his concept of its meaning. It is then transmitted verbally, in writing, by gesture, or by any other signal which can be interpreted. The receiver acquires the message and interprets it within his own frame of reference. All parties to communication, whether sending or receiving messages, are influenced by two factors which affect the formulation of a message and the interpretation of it. These are the conscious and the subconscious—the things that slip in unintentionally, without awareness, such as feelings, values, and attitudes. The nurse skilled in communication strives to reduce the areas of the subconscious in her own communication and to detect and comprehend what lies behind the acts and messages of the patient. She will not always be successful. She will not always be correct. However, the more knowledge she has of the theory and dynamics of human behavior, the more resources she will have to draw upon in assessing and understanding her own behavior and that of the patient. She will also be better able to recognize when she is going too far and invading the realm of the psychiatrist, when she is making judgments based on too few facts, or when she is making interpretations of the meaning of behavior the source of which she has neither the knowledge nor the skill to determine.

Communication in nursing is achieved by observation, by discussion, conference, and interview, and by recording and reporting. Interviewing skills are used extensively by nurses because the nature of their interaction with patients is purposive. The more formal type of interview is sometimes used in nursing when the nurse actually sits down and talks with the patient face to face. More often the interview is informal in that the nurse is simultaneously engaged in other activities. The conversation may go on while the nurse is physically active, or she may cease her activity for a time and concentrate on the discussion. An interview may be quite direct in nature, as it is when particular facts or information is sought, or when instructions, information, or immediate reassurance is given. It may be of an indirect nature when it involves appraisal, assessment, or counseling; when it deals with the exploration of topics of concern to the patient or nurse; or when it has to do with feelings, attitudes, and ideas.

The preferred methodological approach to an interview is an indirect and open-ended one in which the patient is given the initiative and an effort is made to induce spontaneity. The nurse may give verbal leads or focus upon charged areas, but she keeps her activity to a minimum insofar as possible. The actual amount of verbal activity varies. Maurice Greenhill describes three levels used in interviewing. The first is low verbal activity, wherein the nurse uses sounds for prompting and acknowledgment. She may also give verbal leads by repeating words or phrases of the patient, by using incomplete sentences, and by employing general focusing or direction-giving statements, but these she keeps to a minimum. The second level, moderate verbal activity, is one in which the nurse engages in somewhat greater verbal productivity in the exploration of pertinent topics and in focusing upon feelings. The third or high verbal activity level is concerned with the direct information-getting and -giving activities, direct questions being asked or specific instructions given. The nurse may also engage in persistent focusing statements if the patient is either uncommunicative or appears to be ready to reveal some charged information.

The choice of verbal activity level is dependent upon the information desired and the response of the patient. In general, however, marked verbal activity by the nurse is to be avoided. It holds pitfalls for the unskilled or the unwary. Knowingly or unknowingly, verbal activity may be based on provocation of an emotional response in the patient. It may also result in promotion of the nurse's private purposes or ideas. These are not a part of a professional interaction. The nurse who talks too much may become involved with excessive probing or forcing of the patient; she may be led to give unrestricted advice or offer premature explanations or interpretations, some of which may be based on guesses, hunches, or private theories. She may become involved in pure socialization which though pleasant may well be unproductive. Socialization undertaken for the purpose of diversional therapy is of a different order from that which reflects an interview.

In her interviewing activities, the nurse responds to verbal and nonverbal cues which aid her in directing and focusing the conversation. She may note the repetition of statements or questions, see indications of emotion by expression, tone, or changes in motor activity. She may become aware of irrelevant or bizarre statements, the avoidance of certain topics, or the omission of particular details. Then, based on her judgment of what will benefit the interview and how much the patient can tolerate, she may give him leads to further communication. These may be of low intensity, as in the clarification or restatement of a point, or in the posing of an open-ended question. If she is skillful and feels it is justified, she may use one of the forcing methods such as direct questioning, complete silence, challenging, or blocking of other emotional outlets, as by tapping the fingers or fussing with the bedclothes or other objects. In counseling circles there is considerable disagreement about whether forcing methods should be employed. They are designed to arouse some anxiety and motivate learning, but they can easily destroy a permissive atmosphere and interrupt the development of rapport between nurse and patient. They should be used only by an individual who has achieved sufficient skill in assessment so that she can judge the patient's readiness for and probable reaction to such methods.

In talking with patients, just as in any other of her activities, the nurse should have an objective in mind. The objective may be a broad one when she wishes to assess the general aspects of a patient's interests and feelings. It may be quite specific when she wants to know how much a person understands about his illness, his reaction to approaching surgery, why he is upset after visits from his family, why he resists parts of his medical therapy, or any number of other things. When she has an objective in mind she can bring up the general area of concern and direct the patient's comments toward it.

The nature of the questions and statements the nurse makes to the patient is of considerable importance. If the questions and statements are threatening or challenging, particularly at first, they will inhibit rather than enhance communication. If they are couched in language the patient does not understand, he will not be able to respond or will answer according to what he guesses the meaning to be. Questions which are not carefully phrased may bias the response. They may telegraph to the patient the answer the nurse wants to hear and never disclose the patient's real feelings. "Mrs. Jones, don't you think it would be a good idea to get up and walk a little?" "Yes, nurse." But Mrs. Jones really thinks that walking is a poor idea—her stitches might break. "Mrs. Jones, how do you feel about getting up and walking a little this morning?" "Oh, no, honey, I'm afraid if I move that much, my stitches will come loose." Then the nurse can explain to Mrs. Jones about the strength of her incision and the benefit she can gain through exercise without the fear of harm.

The relationship the nurse gains with the patient makes a great difference in communication. If that relationship is empathic and understanding, the inclination to communicate freely is increased. If the nurse seems uninterested and the patient has developed no trust in her, he may be reluctant to talk at all or may make irrelevant comments which obscure his real concern.

Interviewing skills are used constantly in talking with patients but they are also of importance in the process of communication between nurses themselves and with other members of the health team. Feelings, attitudes, and hidden areas of concern are present in these interactions too. A conference or discussion may never achieve its purpose if these factors are not considered. Talking things over, exchanging information, and reviewing various points of view and planning together are important modes of communication among health team members. Patient care may be fragmented, its quality and continuity jeopardized, when conferences among health workers are fruitless.

Recording and reporting are other avenues of communication used extensively by the nurse. Whether spoken or written, the message should be clear and precise. It should include relevant material and be free of irrelevant and judgmental words. It should also be free of words that have so many meanings that they can be variously interpreted. Concise, objective descriptions convey the clearest meaning. If an opinion is offered, it should be indicated as such. A classic example of poor recording may be found frequently in the nursing notes: "Patient had a good night." Mr. Brown slept several hours and had medication for pain only once and so it may have been a good night for him. The same circumstances for Mr. Grey might indicate it was not a good night at all. "Mrs. Green is anxious." Does anxiousness mean the same thing to the nurse who reads the report as it does to the one who wrote it? "Mrs. Green called the nurse every hour. Her requests were to raise the shade, lower the shade, fluff the pillows, change the water. She licked her lips and twisted her handkerchief almost constantly. She always had one more request, just as the nurse was leaving the room." Such a description of Mrs. Green is longer but it tells much more about her. It also gives a basis for comparing her actions from one day to the next. A verbal or written report which tells nothing is not worth making. One which contains perceptive observations is of great service to the nurse in assessing and planning nursing care.

INTERPERSONAL SKILLS

Understanding oneself is an underlying element in the development of interpersonal skills. The nurse who is able to recognize her own values, attitudes, and beliefs, and who understands that she does react, and something about the reasons why she reacts as she does to different people and situations is much better able to maintain her individuality and still use herself as a positive, therapeutic force in the care of the patient. She can more easily be a constructive participant in the planning and implementation of nursing and health care. The ability to recognize how one is affected by others reduces the amount of spontaneous and uncontrolled reactions and permits more purposive action. A spontaneous reaction may be either "toward" or "away from." Often the negative reactions, withdrawal from a patient or antagonism toward a colleague, are thought of as the ones which need alleviation and well they may. However, the "moving toward" actions also merit analysis. It is quite possible to be oversolicitous, overprotective, too ready to "go along," and so reduce the adequacy of a patient and usurp his rightful and necessary independence.

A second phase of interpersonal skill development lies in becoming aware of how others are affected by one's words and actions. Do the words chosen or the phrasing of a question convey a meaning not intended? Does one's manner or mannerisms give a false impression? Actions which are more or less usual or normal for an individual may be interpreted by another as threatening or condescending, antagonistic or uninterested, and thus cause a person to withdraw or act defensively.

Patients are people under stress as a result of their illness and of their having been removed from their normal environments and living patterns. They frequently have considerable inability to communicate their needs, at least until a favorable relationship has been established with someone. Because the nurse is with the patient a great deal, she is logically that person.

The relationship develops as the patient gains a sense of trust in the nurse, a feeling that she has some concern for him as an individual and as a person of worth. Often, the supplying of physical wants is a first step, but it must be followed by talking with and listening to the patient, drawing out his real feelings and concerns, and approaching him in a nonjudgmental manner. The nurse who rates a patient as "good" or "bad," according to her own values and denies him the right to his own ways and beliefs will have difficulty in establishing more than a superficial and contrived relationship.

Patients do not always understand the purpose of the activities engaged in by the nurse or doctor and so may need some explanation or interpretation. They may also have some needs quite different from the ones seen and acted upon by the medical and nursing staffs. Reacting to the patient as he seems to be on the surface may lead the nurse to conclude that the patient is disagreeable, uncooperative, stupid, "not all there," fussy, and the like. If the nurse, through observation, interview, and interpersonal interaction, can find out what the patient is really concerned about, she may find him to be quite a different sort of person and she will have a realistic basis upon which to begin helping him understand his problems and meet his needs.

Nursing care is in a large measure an interaction because it takes place between one person—the nurse—and another person—the patient. Nursing care is intended to benefit the patient, but whether its full potential is realized or not may be quite dependent on the nurse's ability to utilize the interactive process. Can she show the patient she has confidence in him? Can she permit him the rights of a human being to make some decisions and even to solve his own problems or refuse her help, if he so chooses? Does she help the patient recover his health and his independence as rapidly as possible, or does she slow his progress and make him dependent upon her by treating him like a child, doing for him what he can learn to do for himself, or neglecting to provide him activities or teach him ways in which he could regain strength and function more rapidly? Too often a patient is left in a hospital gown when he could wear his own pajamas, or placed in a chair when he could walk a little, or not shown exercises for arms, legs, or hands which would help him regain their full use provided that they are not contraindicated by his medical therapy. When these things happen, the nurse may well be meeting her own needs instead of the patient's and ultimately both she and the patient suffer loss.

TEACHING SKILLS

Teaching skills are of importance because they are brought into play both in the planning activities of the nursing and health teams and in determining the components and timing of each nursing care plan. Teaching skills are developed through application of principles of learning and selection of a productive method of presenting the material. Formal or informal teaching begins as most efforts in nursing do—with an objective in mind. What is to be taught? What kinds of behaviors are expected of the learner who has learned?

Some kind of organization and structure is also necessary to establish a logical sequence for presenting the material and to develop the relationships between various points of information. The presentation must be developed and phrased in ways which are clear and understandable. Some information is comprehended more easily when it is discussed, other information can be told by one person to another, still other information is most easily learned when it is demonstrated.

The learner's readiness to learn must be determined. Is he interested? Does he need the information? Is his mind on something different? Has his energy been used up in some other way? The person, be he patient or staff member, probably will not learn if he is not ready and if he is not motivated. It will then be necessary to start with a subject that is of interest or concern and to work toward the desired objective by showing that it is worth achieving.

One must also find out what the learner already knows, what he does not know, and the amount of misinformation he may have. This concept is called *starting where the learner is*. It relates to finding out the areas of interest and determining the learner's areas of knowledge and experience. Is a discussion of theory appropriate, or are practical examples better? The kind of language used is important. Medical terminology is confusing to those who are not familiar with it. Colloquial terms may be the only understandable ones to some persons, whereas others may find them uninformative, even offensive.

It is generally a good idea to start with the simpler aspects of the matter under consideration and then get into its more complex aspects. In this the nurse must use some judgment and evaluate the learner's response. What is simple for one individual may not be so for another. In addition, it is helpful to begin with something familiar, for example, a skill or knowledge area the person has already acquired. This skill can then be used as a bridge to new and unfamiliar activities or information.

Repetition is of value in teaching if it is not carried to the point of boredom. It serves to reinforce the important elements of the material presented. Some sort of reward or indication of approval will also enhance the learning process, particularly if it comes soon after the learner has made the kind of response the teaching was intended to bring out. This kind of reinforcement may consist of a word or two of praise or recognition of a correct performance. In situations where the correct response has not been made by the learner, it is useful to find something which can be commended at the time a correction is made. Most people respond more favorably to success than they do to failure, and they do not respond at all well to indications that they lack intelligence.

Nurses whether they recognize it or not are teaching almost constantly. Not infrequently, more is learned by the patient from the nurse's actions and attitude, from the things to which she attaches importance and the things she passes by, than from her conscious and intentional teaching activities. No part of nursing is a casual act.

MANAGEMENT SKILLS

Management skills are inherent in patient-centered professional nursing care. They include organization and coordination, and direction and supervision. Their focus is upon that care, however, and not upon the running of the hospital per se.

These skills are extensively used by the team leader and are more fully described in the literature on that subject than they can be in this small section.

Organization and coordination flow through an individual patient assignment just as they do in the multiperson, multipatient assignment patterns of team nursing. These skills involve the spacing of activities so that all the necessary ones can be accomplished in their most productive order without conflict and overlap. Organization and coordination are dependent upon prediction of needs and preparation for meeting them. They therefore involve the acquisition of appropriate resources in personnel, supplies, and equipment, the establishment of work patterns for personnel, and clarification of the scope and individual components of each person's assignment. They also are dependent upon the synchronization of hospital policies related to personnel and procedures with the proposed nursing care program.

Direction and supervision have a triple focus: upon patient care, upon personnel, and upon the environment. The professional nurse is called upon to make decisions and take action in all three areas. The skills of directing and supervising draw upon the nurse's abilities in observation, teaching, guidance, communication, and interpersonal interaction. The nurse becomes involved in the process of delegation, not just of tasks, but also of authority and responsibility for the accomplishment of nursing actions while still retaining her professional responsibility for being assured that what she delegates is accomplished safely and effectively.

Management in nursing care is in many respects a matter of quality control. It seeks the cooperation of coworkers and looks toward the generation of new ideas, methods, and better techniques to enhance the therapeutic effectiveness of nursing.

Use of the Computer—A Skill for the Future

The age of the computer has arrived. Extensive studies are now being undertaken in the use of computers on clinical units, for example, in processing physician's prescriptions for medication and establishing a record of their administration to patients. The day is approaching when nursing observations and recordings will be handled by computers. Both basic nursing curricula and hospital in-service education programs will be faced with the necessity of including material on the nature and use of computers so that nurses will be able to effectively utilize this efficient and accurate adjunct to patient care.

Bibliography

Aasterud, Margaret: Explanation to the Patient. *Nursing Forum,* 2:4: 36–44, 1963.

Abdellah, Faye G. et al.: *Patient-Centered Approaches to Nursing.* New York: The Macmillan Company, 1960, p. 7.

Allport, Gordon W.: *Becoming.* New Haven: Yale University Press, 1955.

American Nurses Association: First Position on Education for Nursing. *American Journal of Nursing,* 65:12:106–111, December, 1965.

Baziak, Anna: Prospects for Change in

Nursing. *Nursing Forum,* 6:2:135–154, 1967.

Beland, Irene L.: *Clinical Nursing: Pathophysiological and Psychosocial Approaches.* New York: The Macmillan Company, 1965. 1: Introduction, pp. 1–34.

Bird, Brian: *Talking with Patients.* Philadelphia: J. B. Lippincott Co., 1955.

Blum, Richard H.: *The Mangement of the Doctor-Patient Relationship.* New York: McGraw-Hill Book Company, 1960.

Brown, Esther Lucile: *New Dimensions of Patient Care.* New York: Russell Sage Foundation, 1964. Part I: The Use of the Physical and Social Environment of the General Hospital for Therapeutic Purposes; Part II: Improving Staff Motivation and Competence in the General Hospital; Part III: Patients as People.

Dietrich, Betty J. and Doris I. Miller: Nursing Leadership—A Theoretical Framework. *Nursing Outlook,* 14:8:52–55, August, 1966.

Durand, Mary and Rosemary Prince: Nursing Diagnosis: Process and Decision. *Nursing Forum,* 5:4:50–64, 1966.

Elder, Ruth G.: What Is the Patient Saying? *Nursing Forum,* 2:1:25–37, 1963.

Folta, Jeannette R. and Edith S. Deck: *A Sociological Framework for Patient Care.* New York: John Wiley & Sons, Inc., 1966.

Francis, Gloria M.: This Thing Called Problem Solving. *Journal of Nursing Education,* 6:4:27–30, 1967.

Georgopoulos, Basil S.: The Hospital System and Nursing: Some Basic Problems and Issues. *Nursing Forum,* 5:3:8–35, 1966.

Greenhill, Maurice H.: Interviewing with a Purpose. *American Journal of Nursing,* 56:10:1259–1262, October, 1956.

Hadley, Betty Jo: The Dynamic Interactionist Concept of Role. *Journal of Nursing Education,* 6:2:5–10, 24–25, April, 1967.

Hanebuth, Lorna and David Stoppel: The Use and Abuse of Principles. *Nursing Forum,* 7:3:309–313, 1968.

Hassenplug, Lulu W.: A Message to Members. in Memo to Members, Department of Baccalaureate and Higher Degree Programs, National League for Nursing. New York, October, 1966.

Henderson, Virginia: *The Nature of Nursing.* New York: The Macmillan Company, 1966.

International Council of Nurses: *Basic Principles of Nursing Care.* Prepared by Virginia Henderson. London, England: ICN House, 1 Dean Trench Street, Westminster, 1960.

Johnson, Dorothy E.: Competence in Practice: Technical and Professional. *Nursing Outlook,* 14:30–33, October, 1966.

Johnson, Dorothy E.: Powerlessness: A Significant Determinant in Patient Behavior. *Journal of Nursing Education,* 6:2:17, 1967.

Johnson, Dorothy E., Joan A. Wilcox, and Harriet C. Moidel: The Clinical Specialist as a Practitioner. *American Journal of Nursing,* 67:11: 2298–2303, November, 1967.

Johnson, Jean E., Rhetaugh G. Dumas, and Barbara A. Johnson: Interpersonal Relations: The Essence of Nursing Care. *Nursing Forum,* 6:3:325–334, 1967.

Komorita, Nori I.: Nursing Diagnosis. *American Journal of Nursing,* 63:12:82–86, December, 1963.

Kreuter, Frances: What Is Good Nursing Care? *Nursing Outlook,* 5:302, May, 1957.

Kron, Thora: *Nursing Team Leadership,* 2d ed. Philadelphia: W. B. Saunders Company, 1966.

Lambertsen, Eleanor C.: *Nursing Team Organization and Functioning.* New York: Bureau of Publications, Teachers College, Columbia University, 1953.

Lederer, Henry D.: How the Sick View Their World. in E. Gartly Jaco (Ed.): *Patients, Physicians and Illness.* New York: The Free Press of Glencoe, Inc., 1958.

Levine, Myra E.: Four Conservation Principles in Nursing. *Nursing Forum,* 6:1:45–59, 1967.

Little, Dolores: The Nurse Specialist. *American Journal of Nursing,* 67:3:552–556, March, 1967.

Little, Dolores and Doris Carnevali: Nursing Care Plans, Let's Be Practical about Them. *Nursing Forum,* 6:1:61–76, 1967.

McCain, Faye: Nursing by Assessment—Not Intuition. *American Journal of Nursing,* 65:4:82–84, April, 1965.

Melody, Mary and Genevieve Clark: Walking-Planning Rounds. *American Journal of Nursing.* 67:4:771–773, April, 1967.

Pellegrino, Edmund D.: Better Patient Care—Better Physician-Nurse Communication. in *Blueprint for Progress in Hospital Nursing.* Proceedings of the 1962 Regional Conferences Sponsored by the Department of Hospital Nursing, National League for Nursing, and the Regional Councils of State Leagues for Nursing, pp. 69–74.

Peterson, Grace: *Working with Others for Patient Care.* Dubuque, Iowa: William C. Brown, 1968.

Reiter, Frances K.: The Clinical Nursing Approach. *Nursing Forum,* 5:1:39–44, 1966.

Rothberg, June S.: Why Nursing Diagnosis? *American Journal of Nursing,* 67:5:1040–1042, May, 1967.

Shanks, Mary D. and Dorothy A. Kennedy: *The Theory and Practice of Nursing Service Administration.* New York: McGraw-Hill Book Company, 1965.

Skipper, James K.: Barriers to Communication between Patients and Hospital Functionaries. *Nursing Forum,* 3:1:14–21, 1963.

Skipper, James K. and Robert C. Leonard (Eds.): *Social Interaction and Patient Care.* Philadelphia: J. B. Lippincott Company, 1965.

Taylor, Carol D.: The Hospital Patient's Social Dilemma. *American Journal of Nursing,* 65:10:96–99, October, 1965.

Wiedenbach, Ernestine: *Clinical Nursing, A Helping Art.* New York: Springer Publishing Co., Inc., 1964.

PART II
THE PATIENT AND FAMILY IN HEALTH AND ILLNESS

PURPOSE

To present basic concepts of health and factors that influence health or an individual's definition of health.

To present society's view of illness and some general approaches to how society cares for its ill.

Part II defines health and the social forces and cultural aspects that influence one's health beliefs and attitudes toward care.

The normal physiological needs and psychological needs and drives of the adult are discussed, to alert the student to the usual needs of people and to note differences or alterations in typical responses to need caused by illness.

Because of the increasing number of older people in our society, material on aging is given additional emphasis.

The functions of the family, in terms of what might be considered ideal, and the effects of support or lack of support from the family are touched upon.

Part II presents an overview of studies done by psychologists, sociologists, and nurses; the references at the end provide greater detail for understanding this aspect of patients and their care.

CHAPTER 4
BASIC CONCEPTS OF HEALTH; REACTIONS TO ILLNESS

MARY OPAL WOLANIN

The three dimensions of the concept of health embody all facets of the anatomical, physiological, and psychological status of the individual. A definition of health, however, is based as much upon one's philosophy of life as it is on the scientific knowledge accumulated by the various disciplines. The most commonly accepted and understood definition of health is "the absence of disease" and implies that the human organism is in a state of equilibrium, that all its components are functioning according to the norm for that organism. But as the sciences uncover new facets of the human organism, the existing definition of health must be broadened. The social context also provides concepts and attitudes and further shapes the definition of health.

Sources of Definitions of Health

The study of man and his nature is an endless one. It is approached by many disciplines and each adds knowledge at a rapid rate. The nurse, as her own knowledge increases in scope, finds that she too has access to a special kind of information about man, information which is realized through her own observations during the nursing process. As she coordinates her findings with those from the sciences and the humanities, she draws conclusions regarding the health and nature of man. She begins to define the terms *health* and *illness* as they relate to the total human being. The more extensive the nurse's background knowledge and the wider her experience, the broader her understanding of the implications of health and illness as relative terms with multiple meanings.

Definitions rely on the shared meaning of words and the ideas they represent. Because a word has a specific concept for one person, it becomes easy for him to assume that others share the same concept when that word is used. When pertaining to objects this statement is true. A cup has certain qualities understood by all who comprehend the English language. Within the range of cups, however, one person may think of a dainty piece of Haviland china, another may think of folding aluminum cups as used by campers, and still another may envision a gourd dipper. In each case, the individual's experience has colored his understanding of the word. In the areas of subjective feelings the variations may be greater. Can the nurse be sure, for example, that *nausea* describes the feeling the patient is experiencing? The term *health* may have different connotations for the nurse and her patient. The basic concepts of health in the adult, as used in this textbook, will attempt to delineate a shared meaning.

In the preamble to its constitution, the World Health Organization defines health as follows: "Health is a state of complete physical, mental and social well-being, not merely the absence of disease or infirmity."

The term *well-being* in this definition needs elaboration for it is used to characterize the human event, which is the life of man and which occurs in many different circumstances. Halbert Dunn prefers the term *wellness,* which he sees as an integrated or harmonious interaction of body, mind, and spirit and which he further interprets as existing in degrees or levels. This concept considers the genetic limitations with which an individual is born, the environment in which he must function, and the final outcome of the interactions of body, mind, and

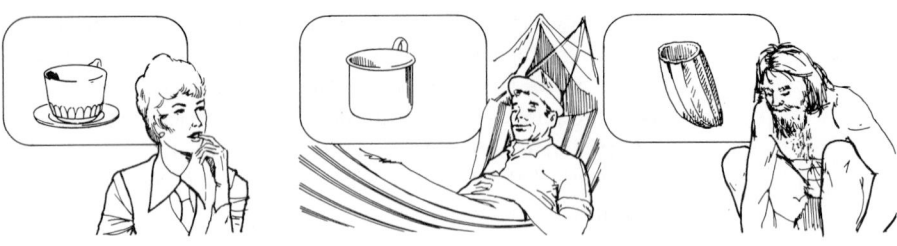

Figure 4–1
Subjective interpreta-
tion of objective fact.
Three possible connota-
tions of the word
"cup."

spirit. Spirit is the force which gives meaning to life. Dunn defines high-level wellness as "an integrated method of functioning which is oriented toward maximizing the potential of which the individual is capable, within the environment where he is functioning."

There may be many interferences with the total functioning of the human being, and these may have physical, economic, or other causes. For example, a child may be genetically destined to suffer mental retardation from the lack of one enzyme. This limitation thwarts his striving for many goals in which intellectual achievement is a factor. A child reared in a slum area may be so culturally deprived that his intelligence is never developed to its potential. A child with hookworm disease may be physically unable to cope with the demands of his environment.

Interrelatedness of Body, Mind, and Spirit

Mind, body, and motivation (spirit) are inseparable. A dysfunction in any one of these elements may result in a dysfunction in the other two. The despair that follows physical incapacity and the fear and anxiety that accompany the unknown in illness are readily apparent to the nurse. The physical component of mental illness is seen in the responses of the autonomic nervous system and the endocrine glands to stressful situations. The physical zest which expresses happiness and health contrasts with the slowed physical processes that spell depression. Prolonged anxiety is reflected in pathologic states.

Each individual must find a purpose in life and determine a meaning for his own life. Purpose gives meaning because it provides an opportunity to express uniqueness and to feel valued. Perhaps this is the key to the dignity of the individual as he interrelates with others on the basis of his own worth. Thus well-being involves a zest for living in which each day is greeted as an opportunity for further learning and understanding.

Health and Adaptation

If one perceives the concept of health as integrated function which maximizes the potential of the individual, variations in the human capacity may be accounted for, not as illnesses, but as limitations of potential. Early in the twentieth century, the diabetic was considered ill, handicapped, and unable to adjust harmoniously to his environment. Later, with insulin replacement therapy and better diet, the diabetic became enabled to attain a purposeful life to nearly the same degree as the normal individual.

Conversely, the individual is ill, although his physiological functioning is adequate, if his social relationships are such that he is unable to find meaning or purpose in life. The lack of harmonious relationships sets him aside from the mainstream of life and he lives in a closed world of distrust and suspicion.

Adaptation may be seen as a measure of one's ability to develop to his potential; inability of tissue or mind or motivation to adapt, as illness; and total inability to adapt, as death. Adaptation may involve the efforts of many significant persons as well as those of the individual: parents, spouse, friends, and those having specialized knowledge and skill in specific fields.

Social Factors Determine Attitudes Toward Health

Attitudes that determine in part whether an individual will interpret a disability as a hindrance or as a challenge for adjusting depend on factors within the culture. If the society views his condition as a form of illness the affected person will do likewise. For example, a patient who has made a satisfactory recovery from a stroke may feel ready to resume the activities of daily living. But if, upon his return home, his wife refuses to allow him the independence that comes from self-care, he will shortly see himself as his wife sees him, that is, as a helpless, hopeless individual who cannot recover.

Business firms that refuse to employ handicapped people have established a societal attitude regarding well-being. The healthy man who is refused employment because he is near retirement age may see his advancing years as constituting an unhealthy state, when in actuality the firm may be attempting to protect its pension fund.

Social norms change. With the constant advances of science, the hopeless condition of yesterday becomes the medically controllable condition of today. In epilepsy, for example, marriage and employment were formerly proscribed, whereas today the epileptic's record of medical control is used as the criterion by which the degree of his participation in normal activity may be measured.

Another source of influence is folk practice. Certain folk customs are unscientific yet may still be practiced among certain cultures which have not advanced beyond that level. Others at one time had or still may have a certain degree of validity, such as the proscription of pork (Jews and Moslems) and proscription of coffee and liquor (Mormons).

Still another factor which determines to some extent the individual's concept of health is the communications media, particularly the advertising and public relations industry. The "medical advice" thereby disseminated is accepted as authentic by numbers of people and helps to shape their concept of health.

Integrating the Patient's Concept of Health into Nursing Practice

Many factors are seen to influence the individual's concept of health. The individual as a patient brings these concepts with him when he enters the hospital environment. The nurse has important responsibilities in this area. Without criticizing the patient, censuring him, or behaving moralistically toward him, the nurse tries to understand his background which gave rise to his concept of health and which may be entirely different from her own. When dealing with controversial health practices or practices which are contrary to accepted medical knowledge the nurse attempts to devise a plan of caring for the patient which will in no way threaten his system of beliefs. This plan will allow ample consideration of the patient's individual health practices and will build upon those areas which are in agreement with good medical practice.

Social Correlates of Basic Human Needs

To appreciate the total effect of illness on the normal adult and his family, it is necessary to know first how the normal adult functions in health and then to mention briefly the role of the family.

All normal adults have a number of basic needs, although there are certain differences in the way they are met which arise from such factors as differences in geographical location, socioeconomic status, local customs or traditions, and ethnic groupings.

NUTRITION

The normal nutritive needs of the adult are supplied by a well-balanced diet consisting of protein, carbohydrate, fat, minerals, vitamins, and water. There are differences in need resulting from sex and age: the active adult engaged in hard physical labor will utilize many calories, whereas the older adult or one who leads a sedentary life will require fewer calories to balance his expenditure of energy. Illness may impose variations in intake to meet special requirements, e.g., renal disease or hyperpyrexia.

Nutrition involves more than making the necessary nutrients available to the cells of the body. Food has social value as well as physiological value. For example, during infancy and childhood the human being is dependent upon others for his food. He comes to associate food with mother, love, and warmth, and at this early stage unpleasant surroundings and implications of rejection affect his appetite. Another example of the social significance of food is seen in the lavish attention to food and food service given to celebrate a marriage.

SLEEP

While the universality of sleep indicates that it is a physiologic process, no firm theory has been promulgated as to its actual cause. The individual need for sleep is affected by such factors as age, temperament, sex, fatigue, habit, presence or absence of stimuli, and by the inherent operation of the circadian cycle (Latin: circa, about; dies, day). Illness may have a profound influence on sleep, causing an increase or a decrease in the length of sleep and altering its depth and quality. The newborn infant may sleep as much as 18 to 20 hours in each 24-hour period; the youth of 18 years may require not more than 7 hours of sleep in each 24-hour period; and during periods of intense mental activity, such as studying for an examination or writing an important paper, he may sleep as little as 3 or 4 hours in a 24-hour period.

OXYGEN AND CARBON DIOXIDE

At birth a mechanism of respiration is set in motion that could continue without interruption for at least 100 years if the organism were otherwise able to survive that span of years. The efficiency of the respiratory system can be seen in the way it allows the human organism to adapt to different environmental conditions. The numbers of erythrocytes and the amount of hemoglobin in the blood are sufficient in the given environmental circumstance to carry oxygen to the tissues. At very high altitudes the number of erythrocytes is increased to meet the increased demands of the organism. The human being has been shown to be capable of adapting to elevations above 24,000 feet with the aid of 100 percent oxygen (for example, in the conquest of Mount Everest, which rises 29,029 feet). At the altitudes reached by today's jet planes, which climb 29,000 to 33,000 feet within a few minutes, there is no time for the human organism to adapt gradually to the decreased oxygen pressure. Formerly, acute altitude sickness occurred: the pilot generally experienced either fatigue, depression, and sleepiness, or outbursts of hilarity, inappropriate pugnacity, or laughter; and in either case the resulting poor judgment could be the cause of a fatal accident. Today the high-altitude jet plane incorporates in its design the pressurized cabin, which ensures maintenance of oxygen pressure similar to the pressure at the earth's surface. Similarly, in the submarine the pressurized cabin maintains the proper oxygen pressure for human existence many feet below sea level.

DIGESTION AND ELIMINATION

Both mechanical and chemical means are utilized in the digestive process. The foods eaten are broken down into particles small enough to be absorbed by the circulating blood and used by the cells. The fecal material—the substances remaining after digestion (undigested foods, bacteria, mucus, and water)—is eliminated.

Habits of elimination are highly individual. In one case a daily bowel movement may be normal; in another, only two or three bowel movements per week. Since bowel function is under cortical control, the stool remains in the rectum until a convenient time and place for evacuation become available. Bowel training patterns vary, but the attitude learned from the mother tends to become fixed as the attitudes of the individual during his entire life. If the mother's attitude toward normal elimination conveyed the idea of shame to the young child, he may grow up with this feeling. Similarly, bladder function is under cortical control, and with time the child learns to await the availability of a convenient time and place before emptying the bladder. Here, too, the mother who in subtle ways conveys the notion that there is something shameful about bladder function implants an idea in her child's mind that may be carried through life.

REST AND ACTIVITY

The present meaning of the word *quick* denotes motion or action. The word also represents living, as in the term *quickening*, which is used to describe the first awareness of fetal movement. All forms of animal life respond to their environment in movement. The organism demands activity; restraint produces restlessness and in many animals rebellion.

The muscular strength and coordination of the adult result in some measure from the training and play he experienced during childhood and adolescence.

All activity is purposeful or goal-directed. Movement not controlled by the conscious will is mediated by the autonomic nervous system and sustains the organism, as during sleep. Purposeful action or activity which the individual views as goal directed is the principal voluntary type of physical activity. This activity involves the coordinated action of many muscles under the conscious direction of the individual will. It is not possible to direct each muscle singly or in sequence. Movement is a harmonious coordination of many parts acting in unison.

Purposeful activity may involve prescribed exercises in addition to the activities of daily living, and in this sense activity is a learned need. The goal in doing a particular exercise is to accomplish a specific purpose, so that motivation is dependent upon the value of that purpose to the individual.

Muscular activity falls into two principal categories: (1) isotonic activity which involves shortening of the muscle body to external force, and (2) isometric activity, which involves the creation of force within the muscle without changing its shape (contraction). In walking there is isotonic contraction of the same muscles that stabilize the joint during isometric contraction for standing.

Psychosocial Factors in Adult Motivation

PROTECTION

Throughout the ages man has sought protection or security from forces over which he has little control. He looked to the stable elements of life to give him a feeling of safety. Man makes positive efforts to maintain safety in a number of ways and in so doing commits himself to a total community effort. He settles in favorable temperature ranges and builds houses suited to the particular terrain and environmental conditions. He undertakes research into the causes of disease and disability and uses the findings of this research in planning prophylaxis and cure. Regulations concerning such matters as sanitation, housing, traffic, water supply, and lighting are the visible expression of man's concern for safety and his commitment to responsibility for the safety of others.

LOVE

Probably no subject has been so thoroughly analyzed in literature as love. Perhaps this attention indicates the proper place of love in the life of man. No reference to the adult and his family in health would be complete without acknowledging the primacy of love in a person's "becoming." The concept of Confucius, in which a person "wishing to establish his own character, also seeks to establish the character of others, and wishing to succeed, also seeks to help others succeed," is one of giving, in which the giver grows through giving. Love is a reciprocal relationship, mutually satisfying, wherein each person gives and accepts love.

The loving relationship, which is so meaningful to a person, involves a *significant other* with whom the person feels accepted and valued as himself. Lindeman hypothesized that even a very small influence exerted by a *significant person* during a crisis may be enough to decide the outcome, toward either mental health or mental illness. Many of us can recall instances in which the support of the *significant other* became the factor which contributed to health. Rejection by the person with whom this loving relationship is held may take with it the motivation for living, for love gives meaning and purpose to life. The individual who sees himself through the eyes of the valued person in his life and beholds a useless unwanted individual may accept this evaluation as his own.

FRUSTRATION, HOSTILITY, AND AGGRESSION

It is the life experience of man to frequently "find the cookie jar out of reach on the top shelf." Drives, which are the basis for goal-directed activity, are suddenly blocked and a state of internal tension develops which is termed *frustration*. In an effort to relieve that tension man usually follows one of several courses: aggression, regression, withdrawal, apathy, or stereotyped behavior. The *frustration-aggression* hypothesis states that aggression is the naturally dominant response to frustration, although the reverse is not true. Aggression may be defined as a class of responses designed to relieve the initial tension produced by a barrier to the goal which is potentially injurious *if* the responses are directed at a vulnerable object. The man who is refused a job because he does not have the proper qualifications may physically attack the personnel director who is perceived as blocking the goal. On the other hand, if he has been punished for such behavior in the past, or if this aggressive response increases rather than decreases the tension which is present, he may be inhibited from overt action directed toward the primary frustrating agent. Instead he may choose a target which will not fight back; for example, prejudice against a minority group may be an acceptable way of expressing his aggressive feelings. This response, termed *object displacement*, may or may not be successful in relieving the original frustration, depending on whether or not the displaced response is socially approved and consistent with the internal values of the individual.

THE UNKNOWN AND UNEXPECTED

Earlier in this chapter, the dynamic interaction between man and his environment was described, as he adapted to those parts of his life which acted as strains. He worked toward an equilibrium in which he felt comfort. In the social world he combined with others to create a community which offered safety and protection. Responses which man makes to fear and loneliness are similar to those which are made to the unknown. Man asks to be understood as he tries to express his uncertainty. He may try to hide his concern behind a shield of aggressiveness or withdrawal, but with each he is expressing his helplessness and inability to control, manipulate, or adapt to the unknown. He is concerned that he may not have the ability to act or react as he should, for he cannot prepare for the unknown. At all times he is interacting with his environment, but to one in which he sees no pattern of the familiar.

The adult in health reacts to anxiety and fear according to the degree in which he sees himself able to cope. Anxiety may be seen as a necessary force to arouse the state of tension by which one makes adaptations to the strains and stresses of life. Concern as a positive force allows discomfort, but only to the degree that mobilization of the individual's own forces can be brought to bear on the strain.

There is no fine line which one can draw between the end of useful states of tension and the beginning of disorganizing ones, but at some point on the continuum, the mobilized forces cease to have purpose in a constructive sense. Instead there are diffuse actions made as the person approaches the panic end of the spectrum. No useful behavior is observed, but the familiar "fight or flight" pattern is intensified into complete withdrawal or aggressive outbursts which appear to be unrelated to the event. When thinking becomes immobilized the person may no longer be able to apply normal rational problem-solving approaches to the situation. Only the person with his particular constellation of experience, beliefs, and viewpoints can understand the threat to his total person, his self-concept. The observer who is familiar with the individual's past patterns of behavior may become aware of inconsistencies or the inappropriateness of the present behavior and thereby identify the presence of overwhelming anxiety with which the individual is no longer able to cope in an effective manner.

A widespread cultural belief is that illness is a result of evil. This was and is stimulated by some religious beliefs, and by the inheritance of modes of rearing children. In order to control the child's behavior the parent may say, "If you climb that tree when I tell you not to, you will fall and get hurt." If the child should slip and injure himself, the injury may be associated in his mind as punishment for wrong-doing. Promiscuous sex activity is frowned upon in our culture. School sex education, parental warnings, and the church teach that venereal disease follows such sexual contact. The connection is obvious: wrong-doing brings disease. Although these are cultural efforts to preserve the integrity of the family, a lifetime attitude is taught which associates illness with wrong-doing. Illness then may cause guilt feelings in the individual which arouse anxiety.

The impact of human interaction may be a strong neutralizing force in anxiety. Reassurance may be impossible, even unrealistic, but empathy and a willingness to share the experience tend to aid the fearful person to face his anxiety and cope with it. Emotional support during a period of anxiety gives a feeling of being valued, of being protected, and of trust that one has resources to use against the feeling of helplessness. It allows mobilization of the individual's energy for action to adapt. Approval is the pattern of acceptance which the individual learns in the parental home as a child. Emotional support which includes acceptance helps the anxious person to regain a feeling of worth and leads to self-understanding, which is impossible when one is caught in the grip of fear.

COMMUNICATION–LONELINESS

Communication is a means of reaching out toward another being, a sharing of some part of the self. The form may be spoken or written words, touch, an inflection, an expression such as a wink, or the many countless ways one uses to share his attitudes and feelings. Tardiness for an appointment speaks eloquently of the individual's value for another's time. A nurse's spotless appearance tells a patient that she values the image of the nurse as an example of a person who practices cleanliness.

To tell is not enough. Communication must have a responsive listener. People who are accustomed to speaking before an audience find speaking on television most difficult because there is no feedback. Ordinarily the listener is watched carefully to see how he reacts to the message; his response tells the speaker whether his message has met with agreement, disagreement, or, even worse, complete indifference. It is important to note that even though words may be carefully chosen the general feeling tone which pervades the voice, expression, and posture serves to convey a nonverbal message which may conflict with or support the verbal message.

Communication is the basis of interaction between individuals and within social groups. Effective communication can result in successful relationships with others, whereas a breakdown in communication can result in psychological isolation and a feeling of loneliness. Probably the loneliest people in the world are not those who live alone on a desert island, but the persons who live among happy, busy groups with whom they are unable to successfully communicate.

Several factors contribute to the inability to communicate meaningfully with others. Physical handicaps, such as impaired hearing or vision, may significantly reduce the person's ability to receive and interpret messages in a correct manner. Patients with aphasia become frustrated when their attempts to communicate are never understood or are greeted with indifference and finally ignored. Thus, physical limitations may force the individual to withdraw from further social interactions leading to a form of social isolation.

Social isolation presents many problems to individuals, especially if they have previously been incorporated within close-knit groups. The older person, whose circle of friends continually diminishes through death and other forms of separation, may have a need for companionship which is expressed through reminiscence of earlier years. The lack of stimulation in his own world makes the past his greatest source of enjoyment, for from his memories he can select happy, dramatic, and pleasurable events. When he attempts to share these memories with others his tales may bring indifference from the listener, and eventual avoidance. His world narrows to a smaller and smaller circle of responding individuals until, in the extreme case, he reaches the epitome of loneliness—complete social isolation. The recluse who leaves her estate for the care of an animal reveals the need for companionship during her later years which no human being supplied. As the motor and sensory abilities diminish with aging, the person becomes less able to develop new relationships to replace earlier ones. This is the tragedy of the lonely aged person in our society.

Mental illness involves in part an inability to relate to others. These people, unable to interact successfully, may have developed their own fantasy world to replace reality which they no longer share with those around them. Individuals with language barriers may be lonely because they cannot communicate verbally with those in their environment. To some people this is no handicap, for they find ways of establishing relationships with others which do not require the verbal interaction.

Loneliness may be the result of a loss of motivation or a sense of estrangement from the environment. The feeling of not belonging, of being an outsider, may have two distinct effects on the individual's behavior. It can either increase his drive toward social contact and perhaps initiate significant changes in his behavior, or it can lead to withdrawal and further isolation. All individuals, at one time or another, have been lonely and apart from those around them. It is important to be aware of the conditions which will reinforce or counteract this feeling, thus enabling the individual to realize complete fulfillment of his need for meaningful relationships.

SEXUALITY

Human sexuality, that is, sexual motivation, is a powerful force that is based on two main factors, the sex hormones and learned behavior. In the male, the testis, and in the female, the ovary, secrete hormones that regulate the development of the secondary sex characteristics of the body. At maturity the body form, hair distribution, voice, and adult sex organs are developed. By the time he has reached young adulthood, the individual understands the prescribed and approved expressions of sexuality as regards dating, courtship, marriage, friendship, and business relations.

Functions of the Family

The family has several functions: biological, economic, protection, and socialization. In its *biological* function, it exercises control of the sexual behavior of its adult members in some way, and provides for the bearing and physical rearing of its children. In the United States, for example, a child is considered legitimate only if it is born into a family, i.e., born to a legally married husband and wife. Sexual relations outside this relationship are frowned upon, although in recent years changes in this attitude have been taking place. In its *economic* function, the family provides the necessities of food, shelter, and clothing for its members until they reach the age of economic independence. In its *protection* function the family ensures the health and welfare of its members either by providing such care itself or by delegating this care to various other individuals or agencies. In its *socialization* function the family serves as a mediator between the child and his culture. The family is the chief influence over the child's early behavior, attitudes, and

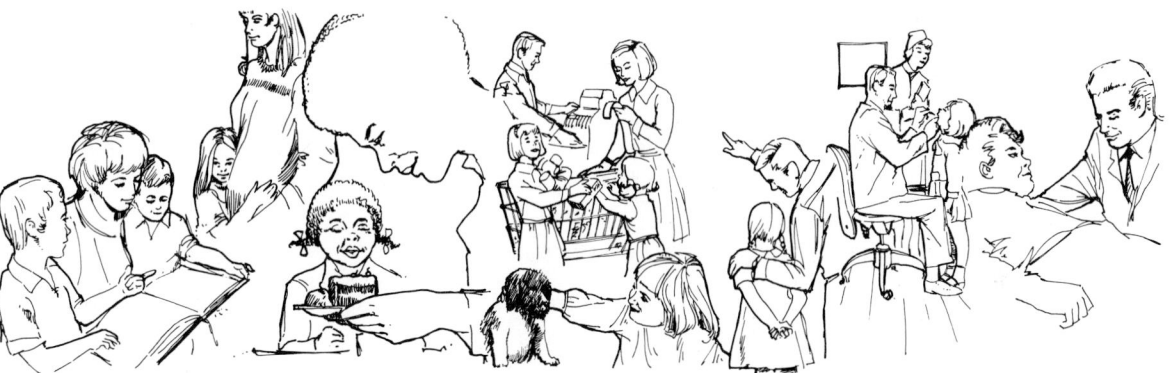

*Figure 4–2
The nuclear family unit
has evolved as the most
satisfactory instrument
for serving the needs of
its members.*

beliefs. Even though as he grows older the child spends a large part of his time with his peers, he continues to spend many hours of each day with the other members of the family; their interaction is the groundwork upon which the child's later attitudes will be built.

The family transmits its moral code to the child, taking responsibility for developing socially approved behavior. In this transitional area, however, the school now takes over a portion of the character-forming function of the family, and attitudes may be formed in proportion to the time spent in school. For example, the student who remains in school for 19 years—the length of time usually necessary to obtain a doctoral degree—has been exposed to attitudes taught by educators and his peers to a greater extent than those of his family.

The affectional function of the family serves both the personal needs of its members and its socialization function. Within the family circle one learns to love and be loved. The individual's feeling of worth and acceptance is dependent upon this basic affectional foundation. His ability to relate to the greater human family rests upon his earlier experience within the nuclear family.

Aging

In western Europe, Canada, and the United States advances in the health sciences have combined with urbanization to make highly visible the number of persons over 65 years of age and the problems—physical, emotional, economic, and social —associated with aging.

The term *aging* is often used to designate the end result of a series of changes that may proceed in a definite pattern through chronological age. Many authorities, however, regard aging as a life process wherein one "dies a little" each day after birth. Another view is that aging is a process beginning with early adulthood and proceeding at various individual and social levels which are relatively independent of chronological age, except as a limiting factor. A different concept and one for which present studies offer much support does not view aging as an unfavorable change correlated with the passage of time and terminating in death. Rather, it acknowledges that different faculties and qualities of the human organism reach their prime at different rates, and as each faculty reaches its zenith, there is another still to reach its zenith. In order to understand the nature of change in later years one must understand the interrelation of different aspects of the aging process as a whole. Perhaps the key characteristic of all aging is the reduction in the reserve capacities of the body to return to normal quickly after a disturbance in equilibrium has occurred.

SOCIAL DEFINITION OF AGING

The time when aging is believed to take place is determined by the pattern of behaviors expected from the aged in his culture. In agricultural societies, loss of vigor in the aging person was met by assigning him tasks requiring less strength while maintaining him as the head of the household and community. In industrialized societies, a man's productivity is a measure of his importance and determines his place in the family and community. With automation the decreased need for certain skills, coupled with the constant need for retraining to remain employable, has encouraged industry generally to adopt a rigid retirement age, which is 65 years for men and 62 to 65 for women. Retirement implies a decision on the part of society regarding lack of fitness of old people to perform a culturally significant role. It may affect the man performing at his peak and the man who has barely been able to complete his career.

THE INDIVIDUAL'S SELF-CONCEPT

Certain investigations have suggested that the human being sees himself in relation to time as in a photograph, in which time is fixed at an earlier point and does not move forward. Contrast this to viewing oneself in a mirror, which instantly reflects, and our apparent disregard of chronological time in relation to aging is clarified. Since the self-concept may be dependent upon peer relationships, retirement may mark the moment when the individual regards himself as old. Whether retirement is voluntary or forced, certain problems arise that produce changes in self-concept and result in an admission of aging: loss of capacity to master the environment and one's physical self, and increasing isolation.

SUCCESSFUL AGING

Simmons described the desires of the aging among 71 preliterate cultures as follows: (1) to prolong life, (2) to conserve energy through release from work and through rest, (3) to remain active participants in social life, (4) to safeguard such prerogatives as property, authority, and prestige, and (5) eventually, to depart life honorably and with a good prospect for a new existence in the hereafter. Successful aging should allow the maintenance of human dignity, which is central to the five universal desires, while attainment of them would result in maximum satisfaction and happiness.

Two theories for successful aging are offered: (1) The activity theory, in which the activities of middle age are maintained as long as possible, and finally other activities are substituted for the work, clubs, and friends that are given up. This

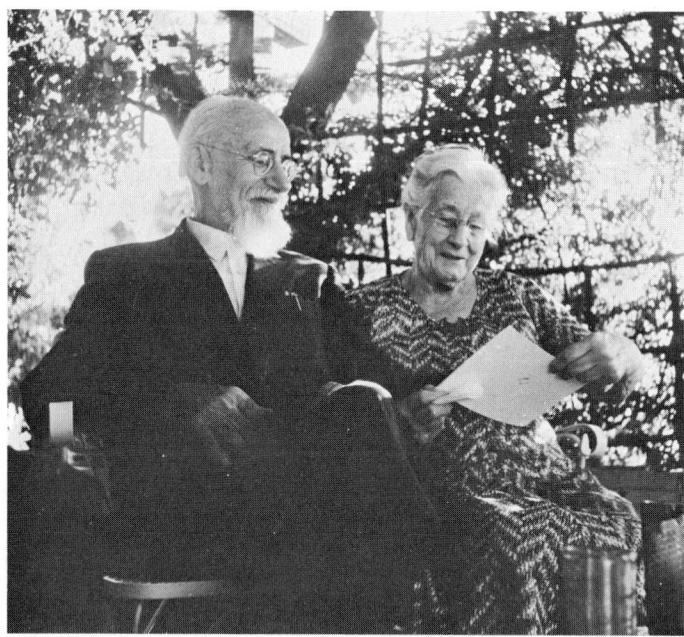

Figure 4-3
Successful aging. This
elderly couple find satis-
faction in shared inter-
ests. Both are in their
eighties, yet retain a zest
for living and learning.
(Courtesy Paul Kuiper.)

theory offers middle age as the model of desirable social and personal development which would inhibit the development of aging and would be desirable in its own right. (2) The disengagement theory. This theory recognizes that as the individual grows older he gradually withdraws from the activities of middle age. There is said to be a concomitant withdrawal on the part of society. When the aging process is complete the state of equilibrium which existed during middle life between society and the individual is replaced by a state of greater distance. The individual transfers much of his energy to thoughts of his own inner life: his memories, his fantasies, and his image of himself as he *was*.

PHYSICAL CORRELATES OF AGING

The aged are represented by many points on the continuum from physically fit to acute illness and disability among which are (1) physically active with no apparent illness, (2) physically active with chronic disease or disability that does not prevent function, (3) physically disabled with chronic disease or disability, and (4) acutely ill. Each of these categories could be subdivided again and again.

Although few carefully done studies of aging are presently available and much research remains to be done, certain generalizations can be made at this time:

Normal health in the older person encompasses satisfactory compensation to altered tissue function and structure.

Caloric requirement is less because muscular activity is decreased and metabolism is reduced. Marked change in diet is unnecessary unless there is systemic disease or local lesions of the gastrointestinal tract. Provision of adequate proteins, vitamins, minerals, and fluids is especially important to meet the needs of aging tissues.

Under resting conditions the oxygen consumption of functioning cells does not change significantly with age, although a reduction in basal oxygen uptake may be attributed to gradual loss of cellular elements.

The mechanism for preventing heat loss is less efficient in the older person, and there may be decreased heat production.

There are wide variations in pulse rates of aging individuals. In general there is a decrease in mean pulse rate with increased age, and the rate may not represent a reaction to a disease process.

Aging is not accompanied by anemia. The presence of anemia indicates a need for treatment because of its aggravating effect upon cardiac disease and cerebral arteriosclerosis. Arteriosclerosis causes an increase in systolic blood pressure and a slight increase in diastolic pressure which is not true hypertension. The blood pressure must be correlated with the physical findings as a whole before its significance can be understood.

Atrophy of the epidermis and a gradual decrease in the sebaceous gland secretions result in a dull dry appearance of the skin. Tissue cells are reduced and replaced by fat or connective tissue so that there is a loss of elasticity. Brown pigmented areas appear over the thinning skin, especially in exposed areas such as the face and hands.

The Digestive Tract. In the absence of gross pathology, the aged individual can enjoy a normal diet, eating the usual foods at the usual times. The stress of a gross departure from usual food intake, either quantitative as in starvation or overeating, or qualitative, as in eating undesirable foods, is responded to in much the same manner as by the younger person. Even the loss of dentition apparently can be compensated for, since many aged individuals chew foods with their gums alone. Provision of adequate fluids seems to be essential for normal digestion and elimination of metabolic wastes.

The Respiratory Tract. A decrease in the elastic tissue of the lungs and tracheobronchial tree leads to fibrosis and a reduction in vital capacity. There is a decreased oxygen uptake resulting from this factor and from the reduced cardiac output. The maximum breathing capacity shows a decline of 40 percent between the ages of 20 and 80 (Shock).

Renal Efficiency. The flow of blood plasma through the kidney declines by about 55 percent with aging, with the filtration rate and secretory capacity declining similarly. The entire process is slower yet remains efficient.

Hormone Function. This factor is difficult to measure. The thyroid continues to manufacture and release thyroxine. Stimulation of the adrenal cortex produces less increase in adrenal activity which may partially account for the reduced ability to respond to stress. There is decreased ability to excrete glucose.

Fluid Intake. Fluid intake must be closely regulated for normal cell function. In the older person any change in, for example, total blood volume, acidity, or osmotic pressure imposes a much longer recovery period than in a younger person.

Coordination between Systems. Coordination of systems is generally reduced. Neural impulse shows little change with age, while cardiac output decreases considerably. Loss of cells results in a decrease in organ weight. Since some cell loss is replaced by connective tissue, the decrease is greater than is indicated by weight loss. Changes in the muscle fiber are indicated by the strength of the hand grip which is markedly decreased after the sixth decade.

SOCIAL AND ECONOMIC CORRELATES OF AGING

Change of Goals

With aging there is a realization that the goals of youth may have been unrealistic and that the only future goal is to meet death in a peaceful manner. Financial ambition and a desire for power and prestige may give way to a desire for personal friendships. The person whose greatest satisfaction in a monotonous and unhappy work experience was gained from picking up his paycheck at the week's end may welcome his pension and the release from the drudgery of his job. Another person who gained great satisfaction from the creative work he performed may find life quite empty after these challenges cease to exist.

Change in Social Abilities

Loneliness in old age may progress to the point that fantasy takes supremacy over reality. The aged and lonely person may retreat to an infant-like self-preoccupation. If social contacts have always been difficult they may now become impossible. If there is no one who loves him and feels involved with him his sense of interpersonal responsibility decreases and with the loss of responsibility judgment may falter, for judgment and responsibility are closely related. Increased dependency fosters suggestibleness—the aging person may respond favorably to anybody who pays attention to him or promises him what he wishes for.

Societal View of Illness

If *health* is considered as *well-being*, which is further defined as ability to adapt to one's environment in a meaningful manner, then *illness* may be seen as a condition at the other end of a continuum ranging from perfect physical, emotional, and social adaptation to death, or the total lack of adaptation. The duration of illness may be extremely short, as a period of syncope, or exceedingly long, as the chronic disease of a lifetime.

The sick individual has resources that can be called upon to assist him in his own maintenance and restoration, and that may offer the most effective means of coping with his illness. One of these is the constant striving toward independence and self-realization which all normal persons possess. The basic assumption that each individual acts according to what seems best at the moment is necessary if one is to accept the individual and his apparent lack of judgment which may have led to illness.

Illness is a psychosocial phenomenon that is usually stressful and disruptive to the normal pattern of living. According to Parsons, the sick person is one who cannot fulfill his usual responsibilities in the social group. He needs help in the form of a therapeutic process. The incapacity is seen not as a function of his conscious decision making, but as something he could not prevent. This status carries certain obligations: the sick person must make an effort to regain wellness, he must cooperate with others who can help him get well, and he must seek technically competent help in the therapeutic process. With advances in medical science and care, greater numbers of people today reach maturity, and illness thus becomes a constant with which society must deal.

Labor has demanded safety regulations to prevent illness in the form of industrial accidents, but insists on medical care in preference to salary increases. Health insurance, which paradoxically means insurance against the costs of illness, is an accepted necessity. The care of the sick and disabled is an important occupation in the United States today. In many cities the health care industry employs more people than any other.

In most twentieth century cultures the family recognizes that an illness has occurred and makes efforts to assume the tasks of the sick member and to ensure that he receives care. Industry recognizes illness by defining the period of sick leave for which wages are paid.

Among the primitive cultures in America, the element of mystery still clings to illness. Religious symbolism is used to exorcize the cause of the illness. The Navajo invites the medicine man to participate in a *sing* at which tribal members gather. The patient and the principal tribal leaders meet with the medicine man in a *hogan* where a sand painting is constructed with symbolic figures. At the end of the day, the sand painting is destroyed. According to the Navajo custom, those who attend must be fed to satisfaction or the spells cast by the medicine man will be ineffective.

The sick role in Oriental culture was studied in an enclave in New York City known as Chinatown. Regarding the attitudes and health practices of these Chinese, the author says:

> The traditional Chinese view of the etiology of disease is something apart from our own in which pathogenic organisms are responsible for many conditions. The Chinese stress harmony and moderation as the means of maintaining good health, and immoderation as the cause of most pathology. The seven emotions, diet, physical activity and behavior in general, contribute to one's state of health, and all of these are more or less subject to human direction. Other factors such as age, economic level and the elements of nature are also important but since they are not subject to human control, give rise to a fatalistic attitude. . . .
>
> Among most Chinese, one is not either ill or well, as in Western Society, because illness and wellbeing are but two parts of the same continuum. One may be less well today than yesterday or twenty years ago, but since most conditions are caused by an imbalance in diet or too strong emotional feeling, bodily functions may be brought back into harmony through the application of self restraint and the use of proper medicines. . . .[1]

A third subculture views God as the prevailing force for destiny, causes, and

---

[1] Stuart H. Cattell: *Health, Welfare and Social Organization in Chinatown*. A report prepared for the Chinatown Public Health Nursing Demonstration of the Department of Public Affairs Community Service Society of New York, 105 East 22nd Street, New York City, August 1962, p. 70. This research demonstrates the problem of viewing various cultures from a white middle-class urban orientation and offers a very rewarding study of attempts by the Chinese to bridge cultural gaps.

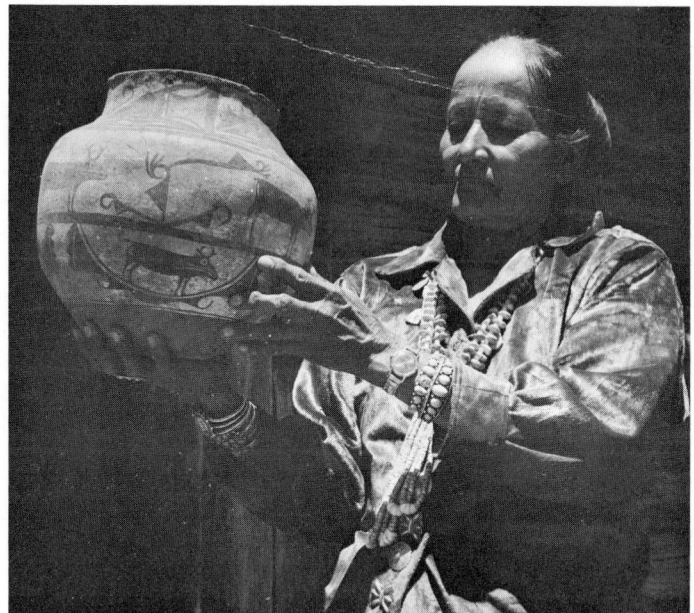

Figure 4-4
The Navajo woman feels
pride, dignity, and self-
worth as she displays a
hand-wrought cooking
vessel. The modern
wristwatch she wears
exemplifies acculturation.
(Courtesy Paul Kuiper.)

cures. The following excerpt is from an interview in which a woman responded to the question whether a person can get well without treatment as follows:

> Answer: any person who turns himself over to the Lord, any person regardless of who it might be. If this person turns himself over to the Lord, and asks Him only, and is confident that He will cure her (sic), He will cure her.
> Question: And if they do this are they sure that they will get well, or not?
> Answer: Yes, if they have truthfully, faithfully, asked Him. "Well, are You going to cure me; You did this; You cure me."
> And He will cure them. He has to.[2]

The United States is rich in a diversity of peoples from many areas of the world, and the interested person has opportunities to learn about many systems of beliefs and values.

The Patient's Attitude and Reaction to Illness

The person faced with inability to meet the demands of daily life because of change in his physical, emotional, or social condition reacts on the basis of his

---

[2] Robert C. Hanson and Lyle Saunders, with the collaboration of Marion Hotopp: *Nurse-Patient Communication, A Manual for Public Health Nurses in Northern New Mexico.* The Bureau of Sociological Research, Institute of Behavioral Science, University of Colorado, Boulder, Colorado, and the New Mexico State Public Health Department, Santa Fe, 1964, p. 60. Study of a group of Spanish-Americans who traveled up the Rio Grande Valley many generations ago and settled in a mountainous area which isolated them from acculturation by the eastern American; they retained their language and the beliefs of the original Spanish settlers. This excellent study illustrates the way in which the nurse may investigate the culture of her patients in efforts to recognize the communication barrier which frequently arises out of totally different concepts of causation of disease.

personality, his present situation, and his future. A simple cold may provide a welcome excuse to stay at home to the child who is unhappy at school. It poses no threat to his future. On the other hand, the aging widow, who has managed to maintain a comfortable existence in her own home, will see a cold as a problem in maintaining independence if she must seek help to meet her daily needs. If complications such as pneumonia follow, her future might take on a totally new aspect as she surrenders control over her existence. Each person can react only as he perceives the illness in light of his life experience.

The individual will draw on the mechanisms that have served in other stressful events and utilize them to meet the new situation. If the culture attaches blame and stigma to illness as being of one's own doing, then the individual may respond with great courage and bravery, since the guilt he cannot face may force denial or a need for punishment. For the person whose strong dependency needs cannot be met within the expectancies of his role in life, illness may gratify the urge to be taken care of. This would be interpreted not as indulgence, but as conformity to the strictly regulated existence that accompanies illness.

THE PATIENT'S REACTION TO THE UNKNOWN

Every individual develops a system of beliefs and behavior which brings his physical and emotional needs into equilibrium with the demands of his environment. When these patterns of adaptation are threatened or disrupted, anxiety is generated and the individual believes himself unable to pursue the usual activities that fulfill his emotional needs. His behavior is then designed to prevent, avoid, or decrease injury—not only to the body and mind but also to his basic adaptive patterns and their social implications.

The person as a patient has graver threats to his self-image when illness—the unknown—strikes and leaves him dependent and helpless. Important activities of the patient's daily life and social existence are interrupted. There is a threat to one's capacity to be loved if illness changes roles and relationships, conflicts over dependency arise, and there may be tensions over handling of hostility as well as feelings of personal inadequacy.

When a breakdown in health is first perceived, one may organize his defenses to adapt to the threat. Most people adhere to a belief of some sort in order to explain what has happened, even if this belief is not expressed directly, in an effort to decrease the anxiety aroused by a threat of the unknown. They seek to understand or control the situation. Self-blame is frequently expressed in such comments as "didn't take care of myself," "thinking evil," or "pent-up emotions." Projective beliefs may establish the cause to be a vengeful god. The patient may resign himself to "God's will."

When the diagnosis has been made and need for therapy established, many of the anticipatory fears acquire a sense of reality. Cut off from the usual source of emotional gratification, the patient may feel trapped and helpless. Signs of panic may occur upon his admission to hospital or the beginning of treatment, ranging from complete submissiveness or withdrawal to hyperactivity. Nightmares occur and appetites falter. Sleep is fitful and restless. The patient is attempting to adjust to an environment which he feels is hostile and injurious.

THE NURSE'S ROLE IN CARING FOR THE ANXIOUS PATIENT

The patient who has had close relationships and warm affections throughout his illness may be less giving, yet is preserved from withdrawing all feelings into himself in service of self-maintenance.

The nurse meets anxiety within her culture's established pattern. If she has learned to recognize and deal with anxiety as expressed by the patient she may not be threatened by inconsistency in behavior. She will be able to understand it in the context of the patient's situation. She will investigate, examine, and define. Through various nursing actions she will explore further until the patient's tension is relieved. If, however, she does not recognize this tension as the patient's expression of anxiety, she may feel threatened by contact with him. Superficial interaction, which will not relieve the patient's tension but may relieve her own, will meet her needs. On the other hand, her own undefined anxiety expressed as dissatisfaction and feelings of failure may make nursing a chore instead of the challenging and helping profession it should be.

STAGES OF ILLNESS

Certain patterns of reaction to illness seem to be common among all patients and families. Illness may strike suddenly, during which there is no prodromal period or preparation. On the other hand, the onset may be insidious, while the patient recognizes a loss or change in his ability to adjust to his environment. He may meet this with appropriate action, or with some form of psychological defense which essentially denies change in condition, prolonging the prodromal period to the onset of unmistakable illness. From our knowledge of the adult in health, we may expect the patient to follow older patterns of behavior to a degree appropriate to the threat posed by the illness. The need to be an independent person may prove insurmountable in the face of incapacitating illness, but acceptance of the fact may never be expressed except in behavior such as acts of aggression or denial as the patient tries to cope with his anxiety.

At some point in the preillness period, the patient "accepts" the existence of his disease enough to seek help; or, in the event of his complete incapacity, the family or the community may seek help for him. What will happen depends upon his culture, the form of help available, and the support of the significant other. The sick world becomes his world, with its restrictions on activity, decision making, and independence. The hospital setting provides an atmosphere resembling the childhood period when activity, decision making, and independence were restricted by parents. The patient may react with behavior used in childhood. He may be so concerned with self that he forgets all former interests. His world is patient-centered and he is the patient.

The illness may end in one or two of three directions: recovery, chronic illness, or death. If recovery, a period of convalescence is required, during which the patient makes graded steps back to his potential activity level. Services of many helpers may be involved as physical restoration is sought; motivation is promoted by counseling, welfare is examined by social workers, and an effort is made to rehabilitate the patient to his highest level. Not only physical ability is required.

Motivation to become a contributing member of society may be the factor which allows the patient to leave the protected and sheltered existence of illness.

If the illness becomes chronic, the family circle may close without the patient. He no longer shares the same world as his family members who are free to come and go. Stereotyped relationships develop. The patient is given a separate room, perhaps with a television set on which he must depend for stimulation and recreation. The family members pursue their own interests, leaving the patient to become more and more self-centered and illness-involved. The two worlds merge at few points; increasing divergence in interests separates the two. An accommodation has been reached which continues until grave illness captures the family's attention and the patient dies.

HELPING THE PATIENT FACE LOSS OR DEATH

Because of the anxiety the patient experiences when he faces the loss of a body part, he may refuse to sleep. His fear of the unknown—death—tells him that sleep requires surrender of control. On the other hand, he may demand drugs to prevent awareness of the situation, as he takes flight from fear by avoiding consciousness.

Perception may become distorted. Anesthesia is a form of sleep which is welcomed to spare the experience of a mutilation to the self. An intrusive procedure such as cystoscopy is a mutilation: a part of the body is exposed to view which is inaccessible under ordinary circumstances, and its integrity is violated. The pain which follows cystoscopy is proof to the patient that his tissue has been insulted. Depending upon the value the patient assigns the procedure, he may welcome the sleep, or in his ambivalence, he may equate this sleep with death. In heart-lung surgery, the anesthetist assumes responsibility for oxygenating tissue, and in any surgical procedure the anesthetist is prepared to maintain oxygenation if the patient's own respiratory system is inadequate. This knowledge may be recognized on an intellectual level by the patient, but never incorporated into his feeling self.

The work of Jeanne Quint has revealed the thinking, feeling person behind the patient's facade. In her research with patients who have undergone mastectomy, she has found bewilderment, fear of asking, and aloneness. Profound depression follows this loss of total body integrity. The doctor may be embarrassed because he too cannot face the problem. The nurse is relieved if the patient is cheerful and denies the facts. The professional members of the health team may abandon the patient by disregarding her stress signals, and insist on maintaining a superficial atmosphere of hope and reassurance which leaves them feeling uninvolved and comfortable.

Few nurses have a philosophy of death, or have faced their own feelings regarding their death or the dying of their patient. Yet both nurse and patient can grow in understanding of life when they share in this, the final experience of life. The patient need not lose his independence and ability to maintain control of his life if he can approach dying with honor. If he knows that he is valued as a person, that he will be assisted until the end, he is no longer alone but shares with another this final step. If avoidance tactics are utilized by nurses they cannot share this final experience. Instead of avoiding, they need to provide the patient and the family an opportunity to discuss their feelings about death, if they so desire.

The studies of Strauss and Quint indicate that it is a part of the nursing culture to deny death and dying. The nurse should understand how her own feelings about death may blind her to the need of assisting her patient as he is dying. The patient has a need to prepare for this final act. He will discuss it with those who will listen, and the nurse who stays with him helps him to face his end. It is not reassurance that he needs but assurance that he will be protected. Words are rarely less useful or deeds more communicative than those actions which tell the dying person that he will not be abandoned. Religious solace is never to be overlooked at this time, but before the minister comes and after he leaves, the nurse remains to sustain the patient's faith in himself as he faces death.

The Family's Reaction to Illness

Many factors enter into family attitudes toward illness:
1. Past experience with illness
2. Role of the patient as a family member
3. Threat to future of the sick member and to the family (disability with loss of ability to function or possible infection of another member, as in tuberculosis)
4. Affectional patterns between the sick member and other members
5. Socioeconomic threat created by the illness
6. Family's orientation toward illness and health (representative of the culture)
7. Conditions under which the illness occurred (car accident caused by careless driving, promiscuous sexual contact)
8. Attitudes and beliefs about death
9. Type of illness (some illnesses are "respectable," others, such as venereal disease and some emotional disorders, bear stigma or fear)
10. Period of disability
11. Cultural pattern of disease causation

Where affectional patterns are strong, even a lengthy illness will not threaten the status of the sick member. But if there is little affection among family members, hostility may be expressed toward the patient for being ill and lead to withdrawal of love as a punishment. The nurse will see family contacts decrease to fewer and shorter visits with eventual rejection when an unloved family member becomes chronically ill and unable to fill his former roles.

For the family and the patient attitudes and reaction to illness are modified as their personal situations change and new aspects enter into the patient-family relationship.

Occasionally the remark, "What did I do to deserve this," indicates the persistence of the old belief that illness is a punishment for sin. The Chinese philosophy of illness and the results of the study in northern New Mexico may show variations of this belief. In many instances, however, the connection between carelessness and illness is quite obvious, as when a patient disregards the implicit directions of a physician or takes risks in an unsafe situation.

ROLE CHANGE, MODIFICATION, OR REVERSAL DURING ILLNESS

Although the sick role allows release from usual responsibilities, it demands an effort by the patient to recover and resume his responsibilities. Illness may alter relationships within the family temporarily, e.g., the father accepts "mothering" from his daughter, or the wife cares for her disabled husband as if he were a child. As the restoration to health continues, it is expected that the patient will resume his previous roles; but his family and associates may not accept him with his residual disabilities, or he may not be able to face previous responsibilities with his limited energy and ability. In a study on role modification of the disabled male, Christopherson pointed out several trends.[3] He asked husband and wife to rate the husband's predisability characteristics and abilities. In most instances the predisability scores were similar. If the wives rated their husbands significantly higher on the postdisability scoring than the husbands rated themselves, the husbands seemed to show humility and loss of self-esteem which could be helped by support from the wives if they recognized the need. These men were retrainable, and 80 percent returned to work. However, if the wives rated their husbands significantly lower than the husbands rated themselves, the men were found to be uniformly bitter, arrogant, and insensitive to their situations. They "sat around the house" all day waiting for their working wives to come home and do the housework.

If affection, common goals, and adequate communication between the members of the family exist, adjustments can be made by which the role of the disabled member allows him to operate within the limitations imposed by his illness. He will still be valued as an important member. Although by common agreement in the household involved, when a couple feel that their own economy is best served by having the wife become the breadwinner, and the husband the homemaker, traditional cultural views of these roles are not met. Such a household will be seen as a nonconforming relationship, rather than a harmonious one.

Hospitalization and Its Meanings

THE HOSPITAL ENVIRONMENT

The hospital is a special subculture with its own roles, customs, attitudes, and beliefs. The expectation of the patient's role has been internalized by the personnel who have defined the rights and privileges of the patient. Usually the responsibility toward the patient is written into a code of policies; however, many policies have never been formalized. Personnel who work with many patients have a clear understanding of these hospital relationships, but the patient and his family usually are made aware of the existence of these policies only by breaching them. The policy of removing all medications brought by a patient has safety implications for the nursing staff and the patient. Unless this policy is ex-

---

[3] Victor A. Christopherson and Daniel Schwartz: *Role Modification of the Disabled Male*. Project 755, Vocational Rehabilitation Administration, U.S. Department of Health, Education, and Welfare, University of Arizona, Tucson, November, 1963.

plained to the patient and his family in a way that they can understand, it may represent an unpardonable insult to their intelligence and integrity or, at the extreme, a form of robbery until the medications are returned at discharge. The patient loses autonomy; he obediently submits to the hypodermic needle or an enema, neither of which he has asked for. Often he does not know their value. The visiting hours may limit the companionship an elderly person has from his working son.

The patient and his family learn of the restrictions and advantages enjoyed in special units. The progressive care unit assures the patient and his family that everything possible is being done to help the patient recover. The intensive care unit, in which the family is limited to brief visits, may be appreciated by the patient who needs constant care, yet deprive him of support from a loved one. Families anxiously watch each person who comes out of the unit for news of their sick member. Patient and family spend anxious moments trying to determine the regulations of each special service and its flexibility for meeting special needs. Acceptance and warmth from personnel enable families to trust nursing service when they leave.

LOSS OF INDEPENDENCE

Some hospitals give the newly admitted patient a booklet explaining some of the general regulations to which he will be subject. Nonetheless, for the individual who enters the hospital for the first time, a new world, without familiar guideposts, must be faced.

One of the principal sources of the patient's feeling of dependence lies in not knowing what is expected of him. Such a state makes him totally dependent upon the hospital personnel for interpretation and explanation. He wants to know what he is to do and what they will do. The illness itself imposes a dependency upon the patient, and he feels he has lost control over his life situation and given up his independence.

SOCIAL ISOLATION

The hospital restricts the social relationships of the patient with several aims in view:
1. To protect the patient from fatigue caused by excessive visiting
2. To protect children from the sights and sounds of the hospital
3. To protect visitors of all ages from possible infection
4. To plan the best possible procedures for patient care

Hospitalization acts as a barrier to social contact. Organizations have formalized their obligations to a sick fellow member into carefully defined "rules" about the "right" thing to do. In the case of infectious diseases, social contact may be restricted to sending the member cards. The family may remain at the bedside continually at the beginning of a long illness, but gradually the pattern becomes one of fewer and shorter visits. Frequently the result is social isolation. Rarely, in illnesses which last longer than a few weeks, do the patients continue to maintain contact with their social groups. An exception is the occasional dramatic illness of a member of the family who has had unsatisfactory social relations. The change in the situation allows the patient to become the center of attention in a new and meaningful relationship. Family and friends, who have not exerted themselves to maintain contact over a long period, seem to feel the necessity to make up for this deficiency while he is in the hospital. Yet when the patient is discharged to his home the former distant relationship is resumed—a situation which the patient anticipates when he reluctantly leaves the hospital to go back to his lonely existence.

THE PATIENT'S VIEW OF HOSPITAL PERSONNEL

The patient, who is helpless and therefore asking for help, places himself at the moment of life-threatening events in the hands of those whom he must trust. Other than the intensely personal relationships within the family, perhaps no relationship is as emotionally charged as that of the patient and the people to whom he surrenders his body and individuality as an independent person. The physician may be looked upon as a father figure who can do no wrong. A nurse may be seen as a mother-surrogate. The ego demands that life-threatening situations, when loss of control over one's being is involved, be placed in the hands of worthy persons. Child-like submission, overt aggression, and rebellion all represent bowing to authority. The patient watches every movement and expression and listens to every word in an effort to test the validity of his expectations. Most patients are desperately afraid of being alone and try to be "good" patients who will not offend the omnipotent figures on whom they must rely.

If his dependency needs are not met, the patient may respond with aggression in an effort to force the support needed. Patients questioned about their expectations of a nurse anticipated personalized care, good personality, and prompt and efficient care. Knowledge was inferred in the responses which the patient felt were appropriate to him (Tagliacozzo). The patient and the family's expectancies have come from many sources: the patient's own need, past experience, and communication through mass media. Reactions depend in part upon the patient's ability to adjust to the degree of anxiety and meaning attached to his illness, and the reality of the situation in relation to his expectancies. If he sees himself as being able to cope, he may dismiss the disappointment of not having his needs met. Self-expression is repressed in an effort to maintain the atmosphere least threatening to the patient's image of his patient-self.

PREVIOUS HOSPITALIZATIONS

The patient who enters a hospital for the second time brings with him the sum total of his earlier hospital experience. It cannot be assumed that previous experience will cause the family to have less anxiety regarding the quality of care to be given for the second or succeeding hospitalizations; indeed, the reverse may be true. The inability of the family to secure information and help during the first experience will color their reaction to the second, while the patient will anticipate the new experience according to his remembrance of an earlier hospitalization. Hospital personnel should know methods of protecting the patient from having to cope with the hospital situation in addition to having to cope with his illness.

MEETING THE COSTS OF HOSPITALIZATION

Hospital care costs have risen rapidly during the past 20 years. Some of the reasons for this increase include the following:

1. Decrease in hours worked, following the pattern of industry, and resulting in a need for more personnel because of shorter working hours
2. Employment of more specialized technical personnel
3. Invention of new equipment which is expensive but must be retained on a standby basis
4. Employment of diagnostic and treatment procedures which require expensive equipment and highly trained personnel, e.g., radioactive isotopes and heart-lung machines
5. Increases in employee salaries
6. Improved quality of care
7. Employment of better techniques and processes for disease prevention within the hospital itself, such as climate control, better sterilization procedures, segregation of infective patients and materials, use of disposable equipment

During this same period the average patient's stay in the hospital has dropped almost as sharply as the costs have risen. At one time a patient remained in bed for 14 days following a simple appendectomy; today the patient leaves the hospital in 3 to 5 days and recovers in his home. Nonetheless, certain long, expensive illnesses require prolonged use of life-saving measures. The average family budget cannot tolerate the expense of preventive medical care plus a few weeks of intensive care in a hospital. Insurance companies refer to prolonged illnesses and disabilities as *catastrophic,* e.g., cancer, poliomyelitis, and tuberculosis. However, to the average family without health insurance, illness that lasts over several weeks and requires specialized medical intervention is catastrophic. In addition to the loss of savings, there may be prolonged loss of income if the sick member is the breadwinner. If the member is the mother of children who still need her care, the father may choose to remain at home rather than allow the disruptive influence of strangers on children who are threatened by the illness of their mother. His income will be sacrificed to maintain family unity.

The lower-income family may have few alternatives. For many families the medical care that characterizes the midtwentieth century is not even a dream, and certainly not a reality. Densely populated areas maintain tax-supported hospitals for patients who cannot afford needed care. Scattered populations may have no resource available. Inhabitants of rural areas in the United States are served if there is the money to pay for care and if good roads eliminate the barriers of distance. The poor in rural areas cannot afford care, whereas the poor in suburban areas have care which ranges from excellent, in the research and medical centers connected with schools of medicine, to none.

The principle that all health care must be paid for is the basis for the following:

(1) Private medical care in which the patient pays the expenses from his own funds. (2) Insurance with coverage provided through either private contracts, paid by the individual, or group coverage in which the individual risk is shared by the entire group. Almost all employers of more than 10 employees provide such coverage as a fringe benefit. (3) Payment for health and illness care may be tax-supported, usually by a governmental unit large enough to face the problem of caring for a number of poor. Cities, counties, and states all have various methods of meeting this responsibility. The federal government provides health care for war veterans, for members of the military services, and for American Indians on reservations. In addition, research carried on by the National Institutes of Health results in constant improvement in health care. (4) Voluntary organizations, foundations, and citizens who make a bequest or endow a memorial all contribute to reducing hospital costs, so the capital costs of the hospital are rarely reflected in the patient's bill. The actual cost of patient care is very high, and construction costs for new hospital facilities must be borne by the community through fund drives and other financial arrangements.

Whether the patient himself bears the expense of illness, or it is carried through support or insurance, prolonged illness costs far more than the hospital bill represents. Loss of income, the additional expense of buying services to replace the sick member's contribution to the family, and the additional needs of the sick member not borne by insurance all have an impact on the family economy. If the sick member cannot return to his old position, vocational retraining may be necessary to enable him to become an independent earning person again. Or he may require services having no productive value except his welfare as he consumes instead of contributing.

Medicare

On July 30, 1965, when President Lyndon Johnson signed House of Representatives Bill 6675, the 89th Congress terminated 20 years of debate over the principle of paying for the medical care of American citizens who are over 65 through the use of Social Security funds. All members of that age group came under the bill's provisions regardless of their own employment record. On July 1, 1966, the bill became law as did a voluntary insurance plan for medical expense at a cost of $6 a month, later increased to $8, half to be paid by the individual and half by the federal government. For the first time one group of United States citizens is eligible for health care regardless of ability to pay.

Assistive Agencies

The kinds of agencies on which a person can depend for help with the cost of illness differ according to where he lives and the resources of his community. Many types of assistance are available through the federal government on a matching basis for funds to be administered by the state, i.e., the Kerr-Mills bill (1962) for medical care for the medically indigent. Not all states have provided the machinery to put this bill into effect. In the typical metropolitan area, government aid through tax support is available, and many voluntary organizations assist in giving services. Groups like the Shriners make orthopedic care available to children. The United States, unlike many European countries, does not provide uniform care to all citizens regardless of their geographical location. The nurse is forced to explore each community to learn of the facilities available for a particular person. The social worker is a resource to which she can turn.

Bibliography

The Adult in Health

Dubos, Rene: *Mirage of Health.* Garden City, New York: Doubleday & Co., Inc., 1961.

Dunn, Halbert L.: *High-Level Wellness.* Arlington, Virginia: R. W. Benter Co., 1961.

Kleitman, N.: *Sleep and Wakefulness,* rev. ed., Chicago: The University of Chicago Press, 1963.

Maslow, Abraham H.: *Motivation and Personality.* New York: Harper & Brothers, 1954.

Murphy, Gardner: *Human Potentialities.* New York: Basic Books, Inc., Publishers, 1958.

Schaefer, Karl E. (Ed.): *Man's Dependence on the Earthly Atmosphere.* New York: The Macmillan Company, 1962.

Strand, Fleur L.: *Modern Physiology, the Clinical and Structural Basis of Function.* New York: The Macmillan Company, 1965.

Taylor, Norman B.: *Basic Physiology and Anatomy.* New York: G. P. Putnam's Sons, 1965.

Toman, Walter: Family Constellation as a Basic Personality Determinant. *Journal of Individual Psychology,* Vol. 15, 1959.

Circadian Cycle

Halberg, Franz: Physiological Rhythms. in James D. Hardy (Ed.): *Physiological Problems in Space Exploration.* Springfield, Ill.: Charles C Thomas, Publisher, 1964.

Stephens, Gwen Jones: The Time Factor. *American Journal of Nursing,* 65:5:177–82, May, 1965.

Communication

Bender, Ruth E.: Communicating with Deaf Adults. *American Journal of Nursing,* 66:4:757–60, April, 1966.

Lewis, Garland K.: Communication: A Factor in Meeting Emotional Crises. *Nursing Outlook,* 13:8:36–39, August, 1965.

Schramm, Wilbur (Ed.): *The Science of Human Communication.* New York: Basic Books, Inc., Publishers, 1963.

Nutrition

Burton, Benjamin T.: *The Heinz Handbook of Nutrition in Health and Disease,* 2d ed. New York: McGraw-Hill Book Company, 1965.

Sex

Winakur, George (Ed.): *Determinants of Human Sexual Behavior.* Springfield, Ill.: Charles C Thomas, Publisher, 1963.

Marriage and Family Living

Duvall, Evelyn Willis: *Family Development,* 2d ed. Philadelphia: J. B. Lippincott Company, 1962.

Sociocultural

Gardner, John W.: *Self-Renewal: The Individual and the Innovative Society.* New York: Harper & Row, Publishers, Incorporated, 1963–64.

Lee, Dorothy: *Freedom and Culture, A Unique View of the Individual in His Society,* Englewood Cliffs, N.J.: Prentice-Hall, Inc., 1959.

Linton, Ralph (Ed.): *The Science of Man in the World Crisis.* New York: Columbia University Press, 1945.

Montagu, M. F. Ashley: *The Direction of Human Development.* New York: Harper & Brothers, 1955.

Paul, Benjamin D. (Ed.): *Health, Culture and Community.* New York: Russell Sage Foundation, 1955.

Aging

Burgess, Ernest W. (Ed.): *Aging in Western Societies.* Chicago: The University of Chicago Press, 1960.

Shock, Nathan W. (Ed.): *Biological Aspects of Aging.* New York: Columbia University Press, 1962.

Tibbitts, Clark (Ed.): *A Handbook of Social Gerontology.* Chicago: The University of Chicago Press, 1960.

The Adult in Illness

Brown, Esther Lucile: *Newer Dimensions of Patient Care.* New York: Russell Sage Foundation. Part 1, 1961; Part 3, 1963.

Jaco, Gartly E. (Ed.): *Patients, Physicians and Illness,* New York: The Free Press of Glencoe, Inc., 1958.

King, Stanley H.: *Perceptions of Illness and Medical Practice.* New York: Russell Sage Foundation, 1962.

Paul, Benjamin D. (Ed.): *Health, Culture and Community.* New York: Russell Sage Foundation, 1955.

Saunders, Lyle: *Cultural Differences and Medical Care: The Case of the Spanish Speaking People of the Southwest.* New York: Russell Sage Foundation, 1954

Tagliacozzo, Daisy: The Nurse from the Patient's Point of View. in James K. Skipper and Robert C. Leonard (Eds.): *Social Interaction and Patient Care.* Philadelphia: J. B. Lippincott Company, 1965.

Adaptation to chronic disease

Leshan, Laurence: The World of the Patient in Severe Pain of Long Duration. *Journal of Chronic Disease,* 17:2:119–125, February, 1964.

Lindeman, Erich: The Meaning of Crisis in Individual and Family Living.

Teachers College Board, 57:2:315, February, 1956.

Menninger, Karl: *The Vital Balance.* New York: The Viking Press, Inc., 1963.

Otto, Herbert A.: The Human Potentialities of Nurses and Patients. *Nursing Outlook,* 13:8:32–35, August, 1965.

Anxiety

Davis, Marcella Zaleski: Patients in Limbo. *American Journal of Nursing,* 66:4:746–748, April, 1966.

Hechman, Maru K.: What If It Were I? *American Journal of Nursing,* 66:4:768–769, April, 1966.

Nehren, Jeanette and Naomi R. Gilliam: Separation Anxiety. *American Journal of Nursing,* 65:1:109–112, January, 1965.

Taylor, Carol D.: The Hospital Patient's Social Dilemma. *American Journal of Nursing,* 65:10:96–99, October, 1965.

Titchner, James L. and Maurice Levine: *Surgery as a Human Experience.* New York: Oxford University Press, 1960.

Death and Dying

Baher, Joan M. and Karen C. Sorenson: A Patient's Concern with Death. *American Journal of Nursing,* 63:7:90–92, July, 1963.

Davidson, Ramona Powell: To Give Care in Terminal Illness. *American Journal of Nursing,* 66:1:70–75, January, 1966.

Engle, G. L.: Grief and Grieving. *American Journal of Nursing,* 64:9:93–98, September, 1964.

Glaser, Barney G. and Anselm Strauss: *Awareness of Dying.* Chicago: Aldine Publishing Company, 1965.

What Can I Say? Film distributed through ANA-NLN Film Service. Tucson: University of Arizona College of Nursing.

PART III
BASIC CONCEPTS OF DISEASE AND ITS MANAGEMENT

PURPOSE

To present a basic concept of disease which can be utilized throughout the remainder of the text.

To present the causative factors of disease.

To present diagnostic and therapeutic regimens related to disease.

To introduce the general concept of rehabilitation.

Part III presents generalities important to the understanding of disease and its management. In addition, it presents classifications of diagnostic measures that the nurse assists with, either by preparing the patient in advance or by providing necessary nursing measures, if any, after the procedures. Emphasis is placed on her knowing what information to seek and its importance, rather than on learning the details of each and every test.

Treatments are presented also according to general classifications and purpose with examples of their application.

Lastly, a general concept of rehabilitation is presented with stress on the fact that all of nursing is directed toward rehabilitation of the patient.

CHAPTER 5
A CONCEPT OF DISEASE

GLADYS E. SORENSEN

What is disease? Do patient and physician always agree as to when disease is present? What is the difference between health and disease? Can a diagnosis of a specific disease be established for each patient?

In Part II, concepts of health and descriptions of the adult in health and illness were presented. This chapter deals with concepts of disease in general and definitions of the terminology and factors relating to an understanding of disease.

The characteristics of normal structure and function of the body are learned through the study of anatomy and physiology. Changes in these anatomical or physiological characteristics signify the presence of disease. Often it is difficult to recognize disease when the changes in structure or function are slight, although it is easy to recognize extremes in change. The line of demarcation between health and disease is not always readily determined.

What the physician may label as disease the patient may not. According to the results of one study, many people believe that as long as they are still able to eat, sleep, and "keep going" they are not ill and will reject the idea that a physical examination is necessary to determine health status (Apple).

A Definition of Disease

Disease has been defined in several ways. The medical dictionaries define disease as the failure of adaptive mechanisms of an organism to adequately counteract the stimuli or stresses to which it is subject, resulting in disturbance in function or structure of any part, organ, or system of the body. Boyd writes that to the patient it means "dis-ease, dis-comfort, dis-harmony with his environment"; to the physician, a variety of signs and symptoms; and to the pathologist, structural changes or lesions which may be gross or microscopic. He states further that disease should be considered as disordered function rather than changed structure, a concept involving in the last analysis the chemistry of cells and tissues. Peery and Miller define disease simply as any disturbance of the structure or function of the body or its constituent parts. In the previous section health is described as a state of balance or a state of dynamic equilibrium in which homeostasis is maintained. In opposition to this state of balance, Hopps believes that the most useful concept of disease is that of imbalance, which produces change in cells, tissues, and organs. He believes that in the future attention will be given to homeostasis of the organism, and thus will facilitate the recognition of disease and make it possible to control disease in its incipient form before the body's autoregulative processes have been pushed to the breaking point.

Lack of adaptation to the environment is another way of describing disease. Harrison states that disease represents a faulty or inadequate adaptation of the organism to its environment. The faulty adaptation may be to physical forces, microorganisms, or disruption of customs and habit or social environment. This concept is in line with May's belief that disease is alteration of living cells or tissues that jeopardizes their survival in their environment, and that disease is synonymous with maladjustment to the environment. Selye talks specifically about "diseases of adaptation" as those not so much the direct result of external agents but the consequences of the body's inability to meet these agents by adequate adaptive reactions.

According to Stambul disease is the result of alterations in the chemical composition of either the tissues or the surrounding medium or of both, and that such alterations are caused by derangements of the agencies controlling the exchanges between the tissue cells and their environment. These agencies are the autonomic nervous system, the endocrine system, and the electrolytes. Disease is the result of loss of the dynamic biochemical equilibrium of the body and must be associated with disturbances of these regulating mechanisms.

In brief, disease may be defined as imbalance of the autoregulative processes in the body resulting in disturbance of any cells, tissue, organ, or system in the body and in lack of adaptation or maladjustment of the individual to the environment. It is manifested by alteration in or loss of function and/or structure of the constituent parts of the body. It is caused by environmental forces—physical, biological, and sociocultural.

The final emphasis of the study of disease must be on the individual as a whole and not just on a small bit of tissue or alteration in function. It should also be kept in mind that all systems and tissues of the body are interdependent, and when one cell or tissue or system in the individual is affected others are apt to be also.

Definitions of Clinical Terms

Sign, Symptom, and Syndrome. Any disease is usually manifested by specific signs and symptoms. A *sign* is any objective evidence or physical manifestation of a disease such as cyanosis or swelling observed in the patient. It may be seen, felt, heard, smelled, or detected by special methods such as taking blood pressure with a sphygmomanometer and auscultating with a stethoscope. A *symptom* is a phenomenon felt by the patient which leads to complaints by the patient such as pain or dizziness. It is of a subjective nature from the standpoint of the patient as contrasted to an objective sign observed by someone else. A *syndrome* is a group of signs and symptoms, which, when considered together, characterize a disease or lesion. An example of this is Stokes-Adams syndrome in which the group of signs and symptoms occurring together are a slowed pulse with syncopal attacks or convulsive seizures. The bradycardia is due to heart block and the cerebral symptoms are a direct result of hypoxia caused by the inadequate circulation to the brain from the slowed heart rate.

Etiology and Pathogenesis. Etiology refers to the causes of the disease, both direct and predisposing, while pathogenesis refers to the production and development of a disease, including sequence of processes or events from inception to development of the characteristic lesion or disease. The changes brought about by the etiologic agents result in pathophysiology, which is manifested by signs and symptoms characteristic of the disease. In some diseases, such as early cancer, there may be lesions with no obvious symptoms.

Dysfunction. Dysfunction may be defined as any abnormality or impairment of function. This may include hyperfunction, hypofunction, or complete lack of function of an organ or part of the body.

Lesion. Lesion may be defined as discontinuity of tissue, loss of function of a part, or structural alteration in tissues which occurs with disease and distinguishes one disease from another.

Diagnosis. Diagnosis comes from the Greek word meaning "deciding." Medical diagnosing is the art or act of determining the nature of a disease. Diagnosis refers to the decision reached.

Prognosis. This is the prediction of the duration, course, and termination of a disease based on all information available in the individual case and knowledge of how the disease behaves generally.

Morbidity. Morbidity means the condition of being diseased. Morbidity statistics refer to the ratio of sick to well persons in a community.

Mortality. Mortality refers to the condition or quality of being subject to death. Mortality statistics refer to the ratio of the total number of deaths to the total population.

Illness and Sickness. These two terms may be used synonymously and mean disease or disorder.

Classification of Disease

Diseases may be classified as to system of the body involved, the pathology of the disease, the etiology, or the dysfunction produced. Under the auspices of the American Medical Association, a system of classifying diseases has been adopted in order to have some logical means of presenting clinical names and terms for diseases used in the field of medicine. This system of classification is published as *Standard Nomenclature of Diseases and Operations.* In this nomenclature the method of classification is based on two elements: the portion or system of the body concerned, such as respiratory or digestive; and the etiology of the disorder, such as diseases due to trauma or diseases secondary to circulatory disturbances. Each classification contains subclassifications and all classifications have a code number which enables record librarians to code patients' records according to a standard method. This makes it possible for anyone to ask for a group of records by diagnosis or etiology for study, review, and research. The student will find the "Nomenclature" a useful reference for comprehending relationships of disease and etiology.

Patterns of Disease

A study of the history of health and disease shows that there are varying patterns of occurrence of disease and death from one period of time to another. The pattern depends upon the advancement of scientific knowledge—vaccination to protect against specific disease, development of new drugs, new surgical techniques, discovery of causes of disease; geographic conditions; economic conditions; wars;

average age of the population; and other factors. For example, in the United States in the late 1800s diphtheria was prevalent, causing a large number of deaths. By the early 1900s, with the introduction of diphtheria antitoxin, the incidence and death rate dropped markedly. Other communicable diseases were also rampant in previous times and were responsible for a great number of persons being ill or permanently disabled as well as for a large number of deaths. Another example of change is the decline in rheumatic fever deaths. According to the National Health Education Committee figures, the number dropped from 3.5 deaths per 100,000 population in 1935 to 0.5 per 100,000 in 1958 with the wide distribution of penicillin. Today the degenerative diseases are more prevalent, with cardiovascular conditions being the leading cause of death. Medical research is working on this problem, and the result may be that in the future some other disease may hold first place in morbidity and mortality figures.

Age plays a role in incidence and presenting picture of disease. Statistics concerning the causes of death by age indicate that immaturity is the leading cause of death in infants; accidents, in children and young adults through age 34; and cardiovascular diseases, after the age of 34.

Sex also plays a role in disease incidence, some diseases being more common in one sex than the other. Rheumatoid arthritis is more often seen in women than in men. Both sexes are susceptible to cancer of the breast, but it occurs more frequently in women than in men. Statistics show that causes of death differ by sex. For example, in 1966, in persons 15 to 19 years of age, the first cause of death, accidents, is the same for both males and females, but almost four times as many males as females died from accidents. The second cause of death, malignant neoplasms, is also the same, but again more males than females in this age bracket died from this cause—about eight males to every five females. The third, fourth, and fifth causes of death for males were homicide, suicide, and cardiovascular-renal diseases; for females, the third, fourth, and fifth causes of death in the same age bracket were cardiovascular-renal diseases, homicide, and congenital malformations (vital statistics of the United States).

Race is believed to be a factor in the occurrence of some diseases, though it is difficult to separate the effects of race from culture, economic factors, and geographic considerations.

Socioeconomic factors and customs enter into the picture of disease. Poverty-stricken families are more apt to have diseases caused by malnutrition and poor hygienic conditions than families with financial security. Families with ready access to physicians and health clinics and who utilize these services have less illness than those with little or no medical care available. In some cultures old customs and beliefs keep the members from profiting from the use of modern medicine.

Geographic location influences the types of disease suffered by people in a given region. In the United States it has been shown that the incidence of rheumatic fever is higher in the New England and some of the Rocky Mountain states than elsewhere and is thought to be due to considerable variations of temperature within short periods of time. Coccidioidomycosis, more commonly known as *valley fever,* is found almost exclusively in the southwestern part of the United

States. The factors of time in history, age, sex, race, socioeconomics, culture and customs, and geographic regions all enter into the picture of disease as we know it today.

Epidemiology

Epidemiology is the study of the occurrence and distribution of disease, with the underlying purpose being control and prevention of disease. Such study was first developed in efforts to understand and control communicable diseases, but its scope has been broadened so that it now entails study of occurrence of disease in any form or degree of prevalence. The American Public Health Association provides a broader definition: epidemiology is the study of populations in relation to their environment and way of living. It is particularly applicable to the study of chronic illnesses and is one of the most hopeful approaches toward learning how to prevent and alleviate the human and social consequences of chronic illness.

Anderson states that epidemiology considers all factors that contribute to the occurrence of disease, including the secondary factors which may be economic, sociological, political, or even religious. It includes the problem of treatment and early care to lessen or reduce the likelihood of permanent changes in the body. Epidemiology attempts to consider all factors that may directly or indirectly cause or contribute to disease in either the individual or the community. The study of the cause and effect of these many factors indicates which factors favor the development and existence of disease. Disease can, in some instances, be controlled before the cause is established. In epidemiology energies are directed toward those etiologic agents or predisposing factors that can be controlled most readily while study goes on to identify those that are more obscure.

The nurse contributes to epidemiology through observations of the patient, including listening to what the patient relates about himself, his family, or his community, and reporting these observations to the physician. Carefully collecting specimens for diagnosis, participating in treatment and rehabilitation, and teaching the patient and his family about prevention and control may all be a part of the nurse's role in epidemiology.

Ecology

Ecology is the science of organisms as affected by factors in their environment. More specifically, as mentioned by May in *The Ecology of Human Diseases*, the ecology of human disease deals with the relationship between disease and the geographical environment in which it occurs. The social as well as the physical environment is taken into account. Disease cannot occur without a combination of three factors converging in time and space. These are stimuli from the environment, response from the host, and the culture of the individual (May in *Studies in Human Ecology*). In this respect ecology is very similar to epidemiology as shown by Schuman, who has stated that the most important principle in epidemiology is that of the host-agent-environment relationship. Ecology contributes a great deal to epidemiology.

May in *Studies in Human Ecology* classified stimuli from the environment considered by ecology as (1) physical factors (heat, humidity, radiation, and static electricity), (2) biological factors (viruses and bacteria) which in turn are dependent upon some of the physical factors just mentioned, and (3) cultural and social patterns that can create emotional stress, can protect a group against certain stimuli, or can expose them or leave them exposed to others. These three groups of stimuli from the environment—physical, biological, and cultural—can singly or in combination produce disease in man.

Ecologists are also interested in the host. In the study of human disease the host, of course, is man. The responses from the host are to a great extent dependent on his genetic makeup. The influence of culture on individuals has been discussed in the preceding section dealing with the adult in health and illness.

Acute Disease

A disease is said to be acute when it has a rapid onset, pronounced symptoms, usually is severe in its immediate effects, and runs a short course. It may or may not have sequelae or become chronic. Some chronic illnesses have an acute phase during a period of exacerbation.

Chronic Disease

Diseases that persist for a long time or for which there is no known cure or hope of recovery, though they may be controlled, are referred to as *chronic diseases*. This type of illness is not confined to old age. It strikes at any age level. However, more chronic illness occurs in older than younger individuals and the incidence of chronic illness is increasing due to the greater number of persons over 65 in the population today. The U.S. Public Health Service publishes statistics periodically on the size of this problem.

In *Chronic Illness in the United States,* the Commission on Chronic Illness has listed a number of impairments or deviations from normal one or more of which characterize chronic disease: (1) are permanent, (2) leave residual disability, (3) are caused by nonreversible pathological alteration, (4) require special training of the patient for rehabilitation, (5) may be expected to require a long period of supervision, observation, or care.

Chronic illness may also be characterized by periods of *remission*, a time when the disease process seems to be quiescent and the patient experiences few difficulties, and periods of *exacerbation*, a time when there is an increase in disease activity.

The problem of chronic disease in the United States is revealed by the mounting death rate from cardiovascular diseases and cancer and disabilities from neuromuscular and pulmonary disease. There is need to concentrate on measures to prevent long-term disabling effects from diseases that as yet have not been controlled or eradicated. One such measure is to encourage people to have periodic examinations in order to discover illness in its early phase. Another is to initiate treatment to restore damaged function and promote independence of the afflicted individual.

Chronic disease and its aftermath—permanent disability and suffering, financial burden, and emotional distress—often overwhelm many individuals and their families. They cannot stand up alone under its impact, and need help. In this country provision is made for such assistance in a variety of ways. In addition to all that medical care, hospitalization, and other patient-care facilities have to offer to individuals and their families in the fight against disease, voluntary health organizations and government-sponsored programs direct their energies toward the problem of chronic illness.

Private voluntary agencies such as the American Heart Association and the American Cancer Society have as their major aims the education of both lay and professional persons, and research into the cure and prevention of disease. They seldom offer services directly to individuals, though they do help sponsor clinics and provide certain types of equipment to hospitals and clinics which aid in patient care.

Government or official agencies such as the U.S. Public Health Service also have education and research as one of their aims in the control and prevention of chronic diseases. The American Public Health Association has a Committee on Chronic Disease and Rehabilitation which was established in 1957. This committee offers guidance to state and local health departments in their programs for control of chronic disease. Chronic diseases cannot be controlled without long-term sustained effort, and both voluntary and official agencies contribute greatly to this effort. As pointed out in *Chronic Illness in the United States,* an effective means for organizing chronic disease activities is one which integrates all phases and stages of attack—prevention, early detection, treatment, rehabilitation, and research—into programs that recognize the commonalities among chronic disabilities. The nurse should be aware of and utilize the services of both the voluntary and official agencies for the benefit of the patient, his family and the community, and keep herself up-to-date on the latest advances in the services they have to offer. Pamphlets suitable for the education of both professional and lay persons are available from the majority of the agencies. The nurse can also contribute by participating in and supporting the activities of these agencies.

Outcome of Disease

Diseases do not affect all persons equally, and the outcome or prognosis can range from complete recovery to death. This outcome depends upon the severity or virulence, the amount of involvement of body tissue, the area or organ of the body involved, the effectiveness of the body's defense mechanisms, the effectiveness of the treatment used to combat the disease, and whether or not there is any known form of therapy. Relating this to epidemiology and ecology it could be said that there is no known cure at this time for some diseases and that the outcome depends upon the characteristics of the agent, the host, and the environment. A number of stages of adjustment between recovery and death may occur, depending upon the particular situation.

Recovery. Recovery from disease implies that the person has no observable or known after effects from his illness. There is an apparent restoration to the pre-illness state. In some individuals recovery takes place spontaneously, as a result of the healing powers within the body. In others rest, medication, diet, and other therapies (which will be discussed in later chapters) contribute to recovery.

Readjustment. With some persons the damage or change in cells, tissues, and organs is such that they cannot return to the predisease level of function. In many cases the body is able to adjust and the person learns to compensate for his disability. This may involve a nonprogressive structural change such as amputation of a limb following an injury. The person learns a new way of life in order to live with his disability. A new balance is established and disease is no longer considered to be present. The illness may be a functional change, such as diabetes mellitus. In this case the person takes medication and is on a special diet to control or maintain his balance. If he maintains his new balance he also may no longer be thought of as having disease in the strictest sense of the word. In one of the illustrations cited, no further therapy is required once the patient has changed his pattern of living to adjust to his loss of limb, but in the other the patient's readjustment involves taking medicine and watching his diet for the rest of his life if he expects to maintain his new state of balance. This is a simplified example for the purpose of illustration. The readjustments in the examples given are far from simple for the patient and involve emotional as well as physiological adjustment.

Progression. Other diseases can be of a progressive nature. In illnesses such as multiple sclerosis and some cancers there are progressive changes. There may be periods of exacerbation which discourage the patient, alternating with periods of remission which make the patient hopeful, but in the long run he gradually becomes worse and may progress to complete disability or death. Even if the disease itself is not the actual cause of death, the patient had become much more susceptible to infections which led to his death and to which he may not have succumbed had the original illness not been present.

A progressive disease is usually much more difficult for the patient to adjust to than a nonprogressive one as there is no point at which he can hope for permanent stabilization and adjustment to the disability. Later chapters will discuss therapies, including rehabilitation and the role of the nurse in care of patients who need help in readjusting to permanent and progressive changes in body function.

Death. Death occurs when the etiologic agent and the disease process are so great that the body defenses are overwhelmed. Death may occur very suddenly due to heart failure as with a massive myocardial infarct, severe trauma to the brain causing damage to vital centers, or severe hemorrhage cutting off blood supply to vital centers and organs, or by obstruction of the airway causing asphyxiation. Death may occur gradually when it is due to a prolonged disease which finally overcomes both the ability of the body to adjust and the medical therapy that has been prescribed.

Somatic death is death of the body as a whole and ensues when respiration and heart action cease. In sudden death these will be the two main manifestations observed in the patient.

With the advent of transplantation of the heart and other vital organs that must be removed from the donor immediately upon his death and transplanted into the recipient to assure viability of the organs, the decision whether or not death of the donor has occurred has raised new questions and issues concerning a definition of somatic death. Groups of physicians in several areas of the world are attempting to establish guidelines.

When death comes at the end of a protracted illness more gradual changes occur which can be recognized as signs of impending death. These signs usually are related to slowing of or difficulty in respiratory and circulatory systems. Manifestations of disease including signs of death are presented in detail in Part IV.

The Nurse, and Care of the Individual with Disease

The general concepts and principles expressed in Part I on nursing and those in Part II on the adult in health and illness are applicable when the nurse cares for the acutely ill patient, the chronically ill, or the dying, and are not repeated at this time. The chapters that follow go into detail on the nursing care of patients with specific imbalances and diseases of the various systems.

Bibliography

American Medical Association: *Standard Nomenclature of Diseases and Operations,* 5th ed. New York: McGraw-Hill Book Company, 1961.

Anderson, Gaylord W., et al.: *Communicable Disease Control,* 4th ed. New York: The Macmillian Company, 1962, pp. 14–15.

Apple, Dorrian (Ed.): *Sociological Studies of Health and Sickness.* New York: McGraw-Hill Book Company, 1960, p. 34.

Boyd, William: *An Introduction to the Study of Disease.* Philadelphia: Lea & Febiger, 1962, pp. 47–48.

Chronic Disease and Rehabilitation. The American Public Health Association. New York, 1960, pp. 8–9.

Chronic Illness in the United States. Vol. I, *Prevention of Chronic Illness.* Cambridge: Harvard University Press, 1957, p. 4; pp. 6–7; pp. 78–79.

Facts on the Major Killing and Crippling Diseases in the United States Today. The National Health Education Committee, Inc. New York, 1961.

Harrison, T. R. (Ed.): *Principles of Internal Medicine,* 5th ed. New York: McGraw-Hill Book Company, 1966, p. 183.

Hopps, Howard C.: *Principles of Pathology,* 2d ed. New York: Appleton Century Crofts, 1964, pp. 3–41.

May, Jacques M.: *The Ecology of Human Disease.* New York: MD Publications, Inc., 1958, p. xxiii; p. 1.

May, Jacques M. (Ed.): *Studies in Disease Ecology.* New York: Hafner Publishing Company, Inc., 1961, p. xvi.

Peery, Thomas and Frank Miller, Jr.: *Pathology, a Dynamic Introduction to Medicine and Surgery.* Boston: Little, Brown and Company, 1961.

Schuman, Leonard M.: Epidemiology—

The Problem Defined and Principles. in Marjorie Corrigan and Lucille Corcoran (Eds.): *Epidemiology in Nursing.* Washington, D.C.: Catholic University of America Press, 1960, p. 11.

Selye, Hans: *The Stress of Life.* New York: McGraw-Hill Book Company, 1956, pp. 66–67.

Stambul, Joseph: *The Mechanisms of Disease.* New York: Froben Press, 1952, p. xviii.

U.S. Department of Health, Education, and Welfare, Public Health Service, National Center for Health Statistics. *Mortality.* Vol. II, Part B. Vital Statistics of the United States, 1963. Washington, D.C.: U.S. Government Printing office, 1968.

CHAPTER 6
CAUSATIVE FACTORS OF DISEASE

PAULINE BRUNO

Precipitating and contributory causes of disease
Characteristics related to damaging effect
Extrinsic agents and effects
Intrinsic agents and effects

Throughout life, human beings constantly adjust to potentially harmful factors in both the external and internal environments. This constant adjustment maintains the individual in a state of relative balance of body structure and function. Consider the changes in chemical composition of body fluids and the demands made on homeostatic mechanisms in the following situation. A 19-year-old student arises an hour earlier than usual after going to bed an hour later than usual; she eats three slices of bacon (high sodium content) and an egg, and drinks two cups of coffee. Her anxiety level is high as she tries to study for an examination, knowing she is unprepared. When brushing her teeth, the student traumatizes the mucous membrane, and some of the pathogens normally, or abnormally, present in the oral cavity are absorbed into the bloodstream. It is a rainy, damp day, requiring increased heat production by the body as the student waits for the bus. There is no time for lunch as she dashes to an appointment at the beauty salon in preparation for a postexamination dance that evening.

What are some of the adjustments the body had to make? The sodium level had to be maintained within normal limits; under the stimulus of anxiety and caffeine, there was stimulation of the nervous system which, in turn, stimulated adrenal activity. Epinephrine production would increase heart action. Bacteria in the bloodstream had to be destroyed; loss of body heat had to be prevented. Blood glucose level had to be maintained even though no food was ingested at the normal lunch time, when the stomach cells expected to receive food and when breakfast food had been used up because of the influence of epinephrine on metabolic rate. Despite all this, the student maintained a balance in body function, and she was not unique. Most people are capable during their life span of usually adjusting to the almost continuous variations in constituents of body fluids resulting from the activities of daily living in a complex society. Eventually, adaptive mechanisms falter and temporary illness, permanent disability, or uncontrollable disease results.

Why is it that some people are ill more often than others during a lifetime, and why do some persons die at an early age while others do not? What are some of the factors that influence whether a person will maintain normal function and structure or if pathological processes will occur? What changes are brought about by these factors? What are some of the responses of cells and tissues to harmful agents?

Precipitating and Contributory Causes of Disease

The presence of an etiologic or causative agent does not mean that a pathological process will eventuate. It is obvious that a cold does not develop in everyone exposed to cold viruses and cancer of the lung does not develop in everyone who smokes. An etiologic agent is one that possesses the potential for producing injury or disease. For disease to occur, the host must be susceptible to the agent, and the environmental conditions must be favorable to the action of the agent or unfavorable to host resistance. These, then, are the three general classifications of factors influencing the development of the disease: the characteristics of the injurious or etiologic agent, the susceptibility of the person, and the prevailing environmental conditions during the time of exposure to the causative agent.

The interrelationships of these three general factors in the development of disease are expressed in the concept of etiology. The concept of etiology embraces the idea of precipitating and contributory causes, that is, a potentially harmful agent acting on a susceptible host. The origin or source of any of the three general factors influencing the development of disease may be from within or from outside the individual. In the above illustrative example of actions of a college student, an inciting or precipitating cause of disease could be the pathogens present in the oral cavity. The presence of cold viruses is essential for this acute catarrhal infection of the respiratory tract to develop. The inciting agent of most infectious diseases is known, but there are many other diseases for which the inciting agent has yet to be identified, if there is one such agent. Many times pathogens are present and disease does not develop. The necessary contributing factors are missing.

Contributory, or predisposing, causes are complex and often operative over a prolonged period of time. They prepare the way or weaken the host, thus making it possible for the inciting agent to exert its harmful effect, or they increase the possibility of host exposure to the inciting agent.

One of the earliest recognitions of the relationship of occupation to the development of a specific disease was made by Sir Percival Potts near the end of the eighteenth century. He recognized the relationship between scrotal cancer and the occupation of chimney sweep. This observation served to direct research toward the carcinogenic action of chemicals. Obviously, the occupation prolonged the contact with the potentially harmful agent, thereby enhancing the action of the agent.

Unsanitary living conditions provide a favorable environment for the growth of pathogenic organisms. Persons living in this type of environment are exposed to a large number of a particular harmful organism and to a variety of organisms. Survival and growth of organisms in the host are favored, since such persons commonly have below optimum internal defense mechanisms because of poor nutrition and perhaps the presence of other diseases.

Economic and sociocultural patterns and values in a family and community determine sanitary practices and also psychological pressures on an individual and family. Psychological pressures to excel or to conform to certain standards can create anxiety and fears that stimulate nervous system and endocrine gland activity. Prolonged overactivity of glandular cells stimulated by the nervous system can cause increased secretory activity and chemical changes in body fluids. Some other cells may be damaged by this change in quantity of normal secretions. For instance, frequent repression of feelings of frustration, anger, resentment, and impatience can increase vagal stimulation, which in turn increases production of hydrochloric acid by glandular cells of the stomach. Prolonged contact with excessive hydrochloric acid produces chemical damage to other cells lining the stomach. In this instance, psychological components could be a contributing factor in the development of disease.

Characteristics Related to Damaging Effect

The damaging effects of factors that contribute to or cause disease are related to particular characteristics. These characteristics are the quality and quantity of the harmful agent, the location and extent of the injury, and the period of time in life when or over which the injury occurs. Quantity refers to the amount of exposure to a harmful agent. For instance, a blood glucose level of 700 mg per 100 ml of blood would be more damaging to central nervous system cells than would a rise of 400 mg per 100 ml, and the presence of many staphylococci in a wound is potentially more dangerous than the presence of a few such organisms. Quality refers to the potency of the injurious agent. A few tetanus bacilli are potentially more harmful than a few pyocyaneous organisms because of the nature of the toxins that are elaborated.

The location and extent of injury influence the ability of the individual to maintain bodily function within normal limits. The vital nature of brain function in maintenance of life makes it obvious that a severe blow to the head may be more life-threatening than a blow of the same force to a lower extremity. Some body sites are more vital to the well-being of the whole than are other sites. The extent of damaged body tissue also influences the ability of the person to maintain physiological balance. For instance, a person with a first degree sunburn of the face may readily adjust to this situation, whereas a third degree burn of an extremity would necessitate medical therapy.

The influence of time on the development of disease can be considered from various aspects. In many prolonged disease processes, such as cancer, reactions to early changes are much less evident than are changes that occur near the terminal stages of the disease. The acute and chronic stages of an infectious process will also show variations in tissue reactions with time. Elderly persons and infants are more susceptible to some harmful agents than are young adults.

The factors that contribute to or cause disease may be viewed as arising from conditions outside the host (extrinsic) or from conditions existing within the individual (intrinsic). Extrinsic factors include biological, physical, and chemical agents and the more nebulous socioeconomic, cultural, and psychologic forces. These factors are interrelated, since low economic status may mean living in substandard housing and may increase one's exposure to biological and physical agents. Examples of extrinsic agents are pathogens, physical force, excesses of heat and cold, ionizing radiation, smoke, gas fumes, acids, and alkalies. Intrinsic factors include personality, genetic influences, nutritional status, metabolic activity, age, sex, and previous illness. It is the interaction of all of these factors that determines if health or illness will prevail. Some of the potentially harmful agents and their effects on cells and tissues will be discussed. This discussion will provide a basis for the consideration of response mechanisms which will follow.

Extrinsic Agents and Effects

Biological or animate agents are the pathogens present in the external environment and as normal flora on the skin and mucous membrane, and in the gastrointestinal tract. An infection requires the presence of a pathogenic organism. The ability of the pathogen to multiply in the host is the major characteristic influencing the extent of tissue damage. Pathogens interfere with the normal metabolic activity of cells. Viruses enter cells and by direct reproduction of themselves, inhibit normal cell activities. Bacteria produce toxins that injure or kill host cells and provide favorable conditions for invasion of further organisms. The toxin may be released by living bacteria (exotoxins) or upon the death of the organism (endotoxin). Some toxins have an affinity for particular tissues; for examples, tetanus toxin affects motor nerve cells. Toxins may destroy parenchymal cells or cells involved with defense mechanisms. The toxicity of the elaborated substance is different for each pathogen and for various strains of a particular pathogen. Some bacteria have or produce potentially antigenic components that are helpful to them by interfering with phagocytosis, destroying defense cells, or promoting spread in the tissues. For instance, leukocidins are toxin components produced by *Staphylococcus aureus* which interfere with phagocytic action of leukocytes and may even destroy leukocytes. Pneumonococcus organisms have a capsule that interferes with phagocytosis. Two enzymes produced by some bacteria are hyaluronidase, which promotes spread by digesting mucopolysaccharide, and collagenase, which dissolves collagen. The injurious characteristics of particular pathogens influence the intensity of the inflammatory response and the effectiveness of defense mechanisms. The characteristics of some organisms make them resistant to body defense mechanisms and medical therapy. Knowing the characteristics of pneumococcal organisms, a nurse would be using good judgment when guarding against placing a surgical patient or any patient particularly susceptible to infection in the same room with a patient with pneumococcal pneumonia.

Bacteria may remain localized or may enter the bloodstream and be disseminated throughout the body. Asymptomatic presence of a small number of bacteria in the bloodstream is known as *bacteremia*. This occurs relatively often from no more than too-vigorous tooth brushing and other slight trauma to mucous membrane and skin.

Pyemia is the result of invasion of the bloodstream by embolic particles of pus-producing bacteria. The most frequent offender is *Staphylococcus aureus*. Usually, the process is that of local infection, with thrombi forming in the vessels at the site of infection and inflammation. Later, emboli may break off from the thrombus and carry infected particles to distant sites. Abscesses may develop in many different locations in the body.

Septicemia is the result of invasion of the bloodstream by multiplying, toxin-producing bacteria. This may lead to death or establishment of multiple foci of proliferating bacteria. The organisms compete with the cells of many vital organs for nutrients and release toxins into the interstitial spaces surrounding these cells. When the organisms gain control, the normal cells, lacking nutrients and being exposed to toxins, undergo degenerative changes or necrosis. Infection may involve any organ, resulting in inhibition of normal function.

Pathogens may spread through lymph channels to local and regional lymph nodes. If the organisms are not phagocytosed by the nonmotile phagocytic cells in the interstices of the regional node, they may move onward to the thoracic duct and empty into the circulation. The efficiency of the phagocytic cells in the lymph node varies inversely with the rate of lymph flow. Rest of an infected part keeps the lymph flow slow and permits more effective action by the reticulo-endothelial cells. Once the organisms are in the bloodstream, the phagocytic cells

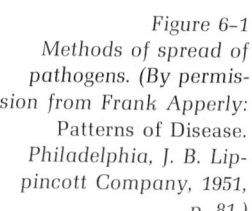

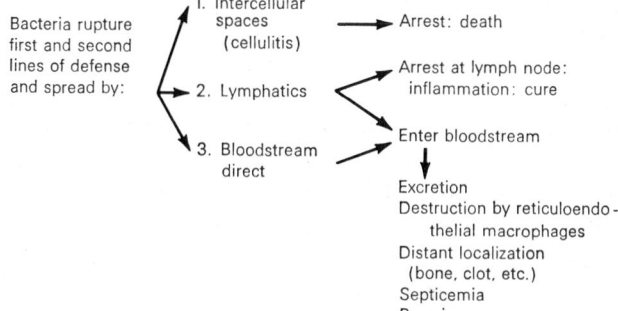

Figure 6–1
Methods of spread of
pathogens. (By permis-
sion from Frank Apperly:
Patterns of Disease.
Philadelphia, J. B. Lip-
pincott Company, 1951,
p. 81.)

in the other organs of the reticuloendothelial system, particularly the liver and spleen, will have an opportunity to inhibit their multiplication and spread. Methods of spread are depicted in Figure 6–1.

Extrinsic agents may also be of a physical or chemical nature (inanimate). The most important characteristic of these agents relative to the severity of damage inflicted is the amount of the force. Mechanical force, such as is sustained in a car accident, disrupts cell membranes, causing cell death, or interferes with the ability of cells to obtain or use necessary nutrients. The blow may contuse or lacerate tissues, including skin, blood vessels, and nerves, and may fracture bones. The break in skin surfaces predisposes to infection, and blood vessel damage may result in severe external or internal hemorrhage. The extent of tissue damage is proportional to the force of the blow. Accidents, especially car accidents, are a leading cause of death and disability in the United States.

Mechanical force is the physical agent that most often causes injury, but other physical agents are a source of danger to man. There is a narrow range of temperature tolerable to human beings. Excessive heat, or burning, may coagulate the protein in cells and may even carbonize tissue. High body temperature (fever) increases the rate of cell metabolic activity and cell needs for oxygen and other nutrients. The increase of metabolic rate (7 percent with each degree of temperature elevation) may be too great for the blood to adequately remove toxic waste products and supply necessary oxygen. Exposure to high environmental temperature for a period of time may overburden the temperature-regulating mechanisms of the body and result in heat stroke. Ultraviolet rays from the sun damage skin tissues, especially skin with little melanin pigmentation. It is common knowledge that persons who have light complexions (little melanin) are more readily traumatized by exposure to sunlight than are persons with darker skins.

Exposure to cold constricts blood vessels and in so doing inhibits blood flow and oxygenation of tissues. A decreased oxygen supply slows the metabolic rate of cells and decreases their functional efficiency, that is, they may become more susceptible to the harmful action of other injurious agents. Decreased functional efficiency of the cells of the respiratory tract during the winter months in a cold climate probably contributes to the increased prevalence of respiratory tract infections. Exposure to extreme degrees of low temperature and for a prolonged period of time injures capillary endothelium and alters its permeability, damaging the interior of cells and causing disruption of cell structure and death of cells. As plasma fluid shifts to interstitial spaces, the red cells clump together and inhibit blood flow which decreases oxygenation of tissues.

In the past 20 years, there has been an increase in the amount of ionizing radiation to which the population is exposed. Various forms of ionizing electromagnetic and particulate radiation are present in the environment as cosmic rays and from manmade sources such as x-rays. Ionizing radiations cause ejection of electrons from some atoms. These electrons attach to other atoms but, in so doing, change or unbalance electrical charges. This action may change the molecular structure of cell compounds, including cell water. Harmful chemicals may be formed in the cell, causing interference with biochemical processes. It is also possible that the ionizing radiation may alter the all-important nucleoprotein molecules of the genes. In this event, there could be permanent modification of the offspring of the affected cell. The final effect of ionizing radiation may be a temporary depression of cell function, a permanent change in cell structure or function manifested in the offspring of damaged cells, or death of cells. Radioactive fallout from nuclear explosions, diagnostic and therapeutic use of x-rays, and radioactive isotopes in medicine and their use in industry magnify the need for knowledge regarding their biologic effects.

The second group of extrinsic inanimate etiologic agents is chemical substances. Chemicals, like ionizing radiation, are being studied intensively in medical research. One reason for increased interest and concern is the awareness of health hazards from air pollution. Contamination of the air by smoke, dust, and exhaust fumes, especially in heavily industrialized areas, has increased the incidence of respiratory diseases. Cigarette smoke is related to the incidence of epidermoid carcinoma of the lung, and some chemicals used in industry are known to be associated with the development of other types of cancer. Chemical poisons are many; this is a subject of specialized knowledge. Chemical poisons include carbon monoxide gas, phenol, lye, fumes from cleaning fluids, insecticides, bacteria toxins, and many drugs used therapeutically but toxic in excessive doses. All these agents are relatively common in the environment, and ultimately all act to interfere with metabolic processes of cells. Some toxic chemicals exert their effect at the site of local contact, such as irritants and corrosives, while other chemicals cause damage only after being absorbed into the tissues. Gases, fumes, and sprays may be inhaled into the respiratory tract or they may be absorbed into the bloodstream through the mucous membrane lining the oral or nasal passages. Chemicals may be swallowed, causing local tissue damage, or the drug may be absorbed from the gastrointestinal tract, causing damage to distant tissues. The ingestion of household lye destroys tissues in the oral cavity, esophagus, and stomach, whereas an overdose of barbiturate drugs acts by depressing the central nervous system.

The period of time required for chemicals to act ranges on a continuum from almost immediately, such as carbon monoxide, to prolonged. Examples of the latter are lead and silica, which accumulate in the body and cause tissue damage sometimes over a period of years. Tissue damage from chemicals in polluted air and which are associated with the development of cancer usually requires long-term exposure in susceptible individuals. Any chemical substance, if in high enough concentration, is potentially capable of causing injury. Even a salt solution in high concentration is toxic to body tissues, which is why untreated sea water is not a source of water supply for human use.

Intrinsic Agents and Effects

Intrinsic conditions may contribute to or cause disease. As mentioned earlier, one of the factors influencing internal conditions is the genetic inheritance of the individual. Genes are nucleoproteins that control the biochemical activities of cells and the potential of the person to adapt to adverse forces. An inherited abnormality is one that depends on the presence of a particular gene or group of genes in the chromosomes of the affected person. The defect can involve an entire chromosome or a portion of a chromosome or a single gene that controls a major body function or characteristic. The defective chromosome or gene may be responsible for initiating the disorder, or the presence of other factors may be required before a defect is manifested. Mongolism is an inherited disorder brought about by the presence of an extra autosomal chromosome. The chromosome defect is the initiating cause of this developmental defect. However, not all developmental defects are genetic in origin. Some developmental malformations may be due to an abnormal intrauterine environment or to as yet unidentified causes. An abnormal intrauterine environment may be caused by the presence of chemical toxins from the mother which interfere with fetal cell growth and development.

Genes not only play a role in the development of the embryo but also control cell activity throughout life. They control protein synthesis and, since enzymes are proteins, they also control enzymatic activity. It is to be expected that genetic inheritance influences the development of metabolic disorders. Genetic factors are known to contribute to the development of diabetes mellitus, a relatively common metabolic disorder.

In some situations, heredity seems to increase either susceptibility or resistance to an inciting agent. For instance, the offspring of parents in both of whom cancer develops seem to have a higher incidence of cancer than the offspring of parents in neither of whom cancer develops. This observation holds for infections also, as some individuals and families seldom have infectious diseases, and others are highly susceptible to pathogenic organisms. The hereditary factors that promote resistance to disease are not known at the present time.

Nutritional status influences adaptation to harmful agents. The adequacy of dietary intake often depends on economic and cultural factors, but the use of absorbed nutrients by cells depends on internal environmental factors, such as blood flow and efficiency of cell metabolism. The latter, as was mentioned above, is influenced by genetic inheritance. Cells need a daily adequate supply of fats, carbohydrates, proteins, vitamins, and minerals to carry out normal metabolic activities. A deficiency of an essential amino acid or vitamin may interfere with cell synthesis of protein or with enzymatically controlled reactions within cells. Dietary deficiencies can also contribute to the development of other diseases, especially infectious diseases. Malnutrition inhibits the synthesis of antibodies that are protein in nature and are essential in overcoming pathogenic organisms. Excesses of particular nutrients are known in some instances to interfere with metabolism of the substances leading to abnormal accumulations of normal substances within cells, such as fat. Changes in cell structure and function result from prolonged deprivation or excess of the nutrients and oxygen needed for normal cell metabolism.

Genetic influences and nutritional deficiencies and excesses have been noted as intrinsic factors that interfere with cell metabolism. Metabolic disturbances may also occur with disturbed function of endocrine glands and with bodily chemical derangements such as electrolyte and pH abnormalities of body fluids. This latter situation may be secondary to another disease process. For instance, respiratory disease that inhibits removal of carbon dioxide by the lungs results in an acidotic state in the blood. Chemical change interferes with functioning of other cells in the body, especially nerve cells.

Age and sex were mentioned earlier as intrinsic factors that influence the development of disease. Aging causes wear and tear on body cells, as injurious forces are met daily and balance is maintained. Over the years subtle changes gradually accumulate and slow down or interfere with defense reactions. Some cellular changes that occur with aging are termed *physiologic* because they seem to be a normal part of the aging process, but they may interfere with defense mechanisms. For instance, the change in activity of stomach cells decreases the formation of hydrochloric acid, which interferes with both digestive processes and the combating of ingested pathogens. Variations in the susceptibility of males and females to particular diseases point to sex as a contributing factor. Obviously, hormonal differences exist between the sexes, and this may be a factor in the differing incidence of some diseases such as cancer of reproductive organs, but it does not explain the difference in incidence of cancer of the lungs and ulcers of the stomach. Perhaps sociocultural and psychological factors are also operating in these situations.

CHAPTER 7

THE MEDICAL DIAGNOSTIC PROCESS

MARGARET A. KAUFMANN

Making a diagnosis is one of the most challenging and exacting responsibilities of the physician. He must combine the art and the science of medicine with his personal resources of perceptiveness, thoroughness, and investigative skill. From signs and symptoms, from distinct or indistinct clues arising from the appearance, behavior, or comments of the patient, from laboratory data and test results he must arrive at a decision relative to the nature of an illness.

Medical diagnosis has two interrelated dimensions implicit within it: the *process* by which the diagnosis is made and the *decision* (commonly called the *diagnosis*) to which the process leads.[1] In making a diagnosis the physician goes through what is essentially a problem solving process. He makes observations and some tentative judgments. These are subjected to further testing, delineation of the clinical picture, and refining of judgments until a decision is reached, a decision that is open to reevaluation in relation to the interaction of the disease and the patient, response to therapy, or to the acquisision of additional data relevant to the problem. Some diagnoses are easily achieved, as when the etiology and clinical picture of the disease are clear and well defined, the signs and symptoms demonstrated by the patient are definite, and the diagnostic tests (e.g., x-ray film of a fractured bone) are revealing. Other diagnoses are made with increasing difficulty and uncertainty depending upon what is known of the etiologic agent, how well the clinical picture and its various components can be defined, what variations can occur between patients and within different environments, and how widespread, masked, obscure, or imitative of other diseases the disease or disease process may be. Depending on the circumstances, the physician may achieve his diagnostic goal rapidly or he may have to search for a long time, exploring many different avenues to complete the diagnosis. At times, even with the scientific aids of modern medicine he may not be able to make as clear and specific a determination of the medical problem as he would like. The patient must then be guided by both physician and nurse to understand why he does not have a precise diagnosis and why the diagnostic process may be a lengthy one.

However small or great the problem, the diagnostic goal of the physician is to determine with maximum accuracy the particular nature and extent of disease or injury affecting the patient. Physicians characteristically seek to achieve this goal in ways that cause the patient the least discomfort and the least expense in both time and money. They will therefore select those diagnostic modalities which are accomplished with the greatest ease and rapidity, which cause the least discomfort, and which are the least costly to the extent that these means are fully adequate in achieving the diagnostic goal.

The medical profession is continually seeking new ways of enhancing the accuracy of diagnosis and in speeding its process. One such investigation, still in its formative period, is in the use of the computer. The computer provides the physician with an extensive memory bank and a means of correlating many pieces of information. It is limited, however, by the nature of the instructions that can be given it to guide its performance. Definitions of disease are still in many respects

---

[1] A valuable discussion of the concepts of process and decision in medical diagnosis may be found in Ralph L. Engle and B. J. Davis: Medical Diagnosis: Past, Present and Future. Part I: Present Concepts of the Meaning and Limitations of Medical Diagnosis. *Archives of Internal Medicine,* 112:512–519, October, 1963.

diffuse and their symptomatology is vague. Medicine has not yet developed means of describing adequately for computer use such subtle clues as pallor, the look in the eyes, or the state of the patient which the physician only senses. The computer can assist with some of the deductive aspects of diagnosis but the inductive portions, the thinking and judgment, have not nor may they ever be reduced to a computer model and program.

A prevailing characteristic of medical diagnosis is orderliness. The diagnosis begins with a search for all facts and information that may be medically relevant. It continues through a variety of investigative procedures initiated by the physical examination, and undergoes a series of analyses and judgments by the physician as it moves toward its goal.

Several diagnostic approaches may be undertaken either singly or in combination. Primary among these is the *differential* diagnosis, the distinguishing between two or more diseases having similar characteristics through a comparison of their symptoms. This concept of differentiation among diseases is a part of all diagnoses. Other types of diagnosis include the following: *physical* diagnosis, accomplished by inspection, palpation, percussion, and auscultation; *clinical* diagnosis, derived from the patient's history and physical examination; *laboratory and microscopic* diagnosis, made through tests and examinations of body tissues, fluids, or excretions; and *anatomic* or *pathologic* diagnosis, based on recognition of anatomic alterations and the study of structural lesions.

The Medical History

The diagnostic process begins with the medical history which embodies the physical, psychological, and social histories to the end that all information that may have a bearing on the medical problem and state of health is obtained. The history is focused primarily upon the patient himself but also includes any information about his family which may have a bearing upon his illness or indicate a hereditary disposition toward a particular condition.

Included in the history are personal data and social history such as age, sex, occupation, and marital status, and personal history such as birthplace, residence, habits (e.g., diet; use of drugs, tobacco, stimulants; amount of physical exercise; idiosyncrasies such as nail biting). The patient's chief complaint is noted and followed by a description of the onset, characteristics, and course of the present illness. A record is also made of previous illnesses, injuries, acute infections (including those of childhood), allergies, and the like.

Most important is the account of the symptoms that brought the patient to the physician. These symptoms are described with varying degrees of objectivity and completeness. Certain symptoms may be omitted or distorted by reason of the patient's fear, tension, or misconception, or he may simply forget them. Others may be reported but may seem unimportant or unrelated to the problem at hand. No symptom should be disregarded as irrelevant, nor should any statement made by the patient be passed by without scrutiny. The seemingly unimportant sometimes supplies the ultimate clue to the diagnostic problem.

Although the medical history is taken by the physician, the nurse may make an important contribution to it. In many instances, and particularly within the hospital, the nurse sees the patient before the physician does. She can make him comfortable and at ease so that he will be somewhat relaxed and better able to describe his condition when the physician arrives. The nurse can also inform the patient that his history will be taken, explain its nature and importance, and help him bring to mind the things he will want to tell the doctor. In the case of community hospitals where there is no intern or resident program the largest portion of the history and physical examination may have been accomplished in the physician's office prior to the patient's admission, but the nurse in the hospital still can help in securing information.

The nurse serves as a resource to the physician through her roles of observer and interviewer. As she cares for the patient she may note physical or behavioral symptoms that were not mentioned to the doctor. The patient may reveal bits of information or bring out problems that he did not mention during the history-taking. The nurse may also pick up verbal and nonverbal clues to the patient's physical or emotional state, to his family relationships, or to his or his family's medical history which may be pertinent. Frequently, in the relaxed atmosphere of nursing care, or because he may feel more comfortable talking with the nurse than with the doctor, the patient will reveal information that might be critical. This level of observation requires that the nurse have a working knowledge of both normal and pathophysiological states of health and of the psychosocial aspects of health and illness.

The history provides an excellent resource for the nurse, as well as for the doctor. It offers her clues to her independent nursing assessment and enables her to save the patient from having to reiterate statements. She can approach the patient not as a stranger but as someone who already knows him slightly. She is better able to determine and meet his nursing care requirements as she combines her knowledge of him with her general knowledge of illness and of man as a social being.

The Physical Examination

A physical examination is done in conjunction with the history-taking. All investigations of the body are considered parts of the physical examination; thus the physician may use the stethoscope, the ophthalmoscope, or the roentgenograph to study body parts and functions, and laboratory specimens of body tissues and fluids.

Several methods of examination are employed. The physician supplements his

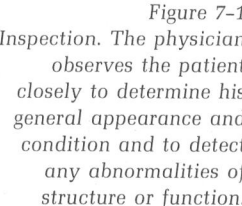

Figure 7–1 Inspection. The physician observes the patient closely to determine his general appearance and condition and to detect any abnormalities of structure or function.

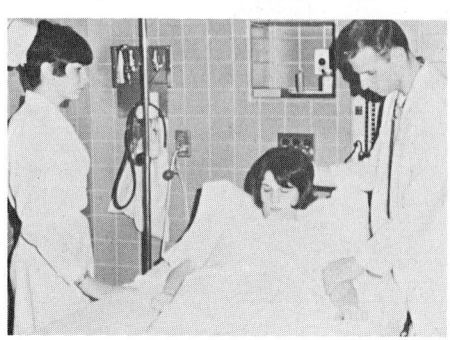

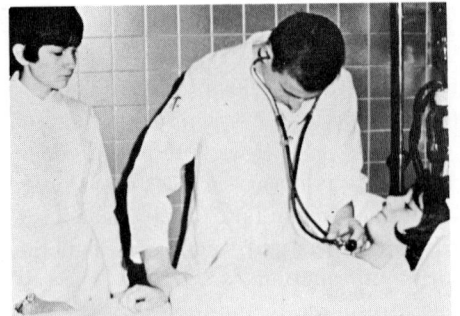

Figure 7-2
Auscultation. The hands
are employed to feel or
examine soft parts of the
body. Palpation is utilized
to determine relative
size and condition of
many glands.

own powers of sight, hearing, touch, and smell with the use of instruments. The four important types of examination utilizing the senses are inspection, palpation, auscultation, and percussion. *Inspection* is observation with the naked eye. Notation is made of any visible deviation from normal such as change in size, shape, color, or position. The presence of scars or rashes and observable evidence of malfunction such as hand tremor is noted. The ophthalmoscope or the otoscope may be used to visualize the internal aspects of the eye or ear. *Palpation* is feeling with the hands. Certain abdominal organs may be felt by exerting pressure on the abdomen; the soft tissues are explored manually; and the pulses are detected by digital pressure. *Percussion* is the production of sound by tapping the body surface with the hand. It is employed primarily in examining the chest and abdomen which, being "hollow," have a characteristic sound when tapped. *Auscultation* means listening to body sounds either with the ear placed against the body or with the aid of a stethoscope.

Figure 7-3
Palpation. The physician
places a finger of his
right hand firmly against
the part being examined.
He taps this finger
smartly with the finger-
tips of his left hand,
producing various
resonant sounds.
These sounds offer clues
to the condition of the
underlying area.

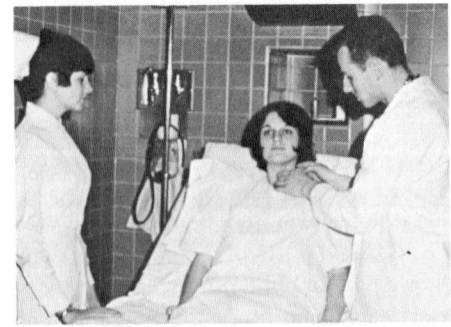

Figure 7-4
Percussion. This method
is used to detect and
study sounds arising
from various organs,
chiefly the lungs and
heart. With the aid of
the stethoscope, the phy-
sician can hear sounds
not easily detected by the
ear alone.

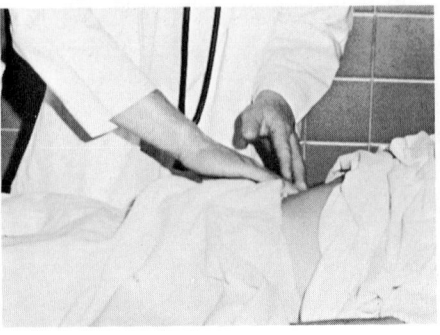

Certain aspects of body function may require more extensive study than can be carried out by the physician at the bedside. In these instances special tests or laboratory procedures are undertaken, usually within several days following the physical examination.

As she has in obtaining the history, the nurse has important functions connected with the physical examination. One of these is interpreting the examination to the patient and perhaps to the family. To some patients a physical examination is a familiar experience, whereas to others it may be new and frightening or embarrassing. If the procedure is new, the patient will benefit from a clear and reasonably full explanation given at a level and in terms he is able to understand. Nonetheless, whether he is familiar or unfamiliar with the physical examination, each patient should, whenever possible, know the approximate time when the doctor may be expected and should be given an opportunity to ask any questions or express whatever concerns he may have prior to the examination. A well-prepared patient is much more at ease and far better able to cooperate with the doctor and help him achieve a complete and accurate examination.

A second function of the nurse is to assist with the examination itself. She may or may not be present during the examination. During certain parts of the examination, particularly of the male genitalia, the doctor will wish to be alone with the patient. On the other hand, the nurse is always present when a female patient is given a pelvic examination. When the nurse is present, she plays two important roles. The first is supporter, guide, and comforter for the patient. The second is assistant to the physician by such means as preparing the examination room, positioning the patient, and procuring needed supplies and equipment. In her assistive function the nurse may carry out parts of the examination, as when she takes and records the temperature, pulse, and respiration, and when she obtains specimens for laboratory testing such as urine and feces.

The physical examination has a number of components. First, general observations are made of both the physical and the emotional states. These include the character and build of the body, bodily movement, facial expression, behavior, and the like. The height, weight, and vital signs are checked. The physician then undertakes a systematic and detailed examination of each readily accessible body part and function. He notes any special diagnostic measures he wishes to undertake at a later date, such as laboratory tests, x-ray examinations, and electrocardiograms. The neurological system is subjected to a routine evaluation, but should there be any untoward findings or should the patient's disorder be a neurological one, a special neurological examination is undertaken. The basic components of the neurological examination are summarized in Table 7-1 (A detailed description of the physical examination can be found in a textbook on physical diagnosis.)

The neurological examination is a fairly long one and may be tedious or tiring to the patient. It may also cause him some apprehension as he carries out unfamiliar tasks and makes unaccustomed responses. The patient will be helped to relax and to respond in his customary manner if he is given an explanation of the examination and permitted a rest period before it is undertaken.

For the most part, the basic physical examination is not painful, although palpation may cause discomfort in the abdominal and pelvic areas. The nurse can help alleviate discomfort by encouraging the patient to relax or by suggesting that

TABLE 7-1
Summary of Basic
Components of
Neurological
Examination*

FUNCTION OR STRUCTURE TESTED	AREA OF OBSERVATION	TYPE OF TEST
CEREBRAL FUNCTION	Behavior, emotional status, intellectual performance and thought content, level of consciousness	Observation of appearance Observation of physical and emotional behavior Response to questions and to mental tasks (e.g., repeating number series)
	Cortical function: sensory interpretation, motor integration	Recognition of objects by sight, sound, feel Carrying out of motor acts
	Language	Communication in and response to spoken and written language
CRANIAL NERVE FUNCTION	I Olfactory nerve	Recognition of familiar odors
	II Optic nerve	Visual acuity Ophthalmoscopic examination of fundus Visual fields
	III Oculomotor nerve IV Trochlear nerve VI Abducens nerve } these three nerves are generally tested together	Observation of pupil size, shape, equality, reaction to light Range and direction of ocular motion
	V Trigeminal nerve	Facial sensation—touch, warmth, cold Equality of sensation on both sides of face Maxillary reflex Corneal reflex
	VII Facial nerve	Facial muscle symmetry: at rest, in motion Ability to taste sweet and salt
	VIII Acoustic nerve: cochlear part : vestibular part (not routinely tested)	Hearing (watch tick) Lateralization of sound (tuning fork) Air and bone conduction
	IX Glossopharyngeal nerve X Vagus nerve } tested together	Pharyngeal gag reflex; palatal reflex Ability to swallow Symmetrical movement of vocal cords Clarity of speech
	XI Accessory nerve	Strength and size of sternocleidomastoid and trapezius muscles
	XII Hypoglossal nerve	Lateral deviation, atrophy, or tremor of tongue
CEREBELLAR FUNCTION	Balance and coordination	Touch finger to nose, to examiner's finger (eyes open and closed) Rapidly alternating movements (e.g., pat knees) Make figure-of-eight movement with foot

TABLE 7-1 *Summary of Basic Components of Neurological Examination* (Continued)

MOTOR FUNCTION	Muscle size, tone, strength		Measurement of muscle size
	Abnormal movements		Inspection for abnormal movements
			Joint flexion and extension : without and against resistance
SENSORY FUNCTION	Tactile sense		Sensitivity to light touch (wisp of cotton)
	Temperature sensitivity		Response to hot and cold objects
	Vibration sensitivity		Ability to feel vibration (tuning fork)
	Superficial pain		Response to pinprick
	Deep pressure pain		Response to squeezing forearm and calf muscles and Achilles tendon
	Position and motion		Identification of position of passively moved fingers and toes (eyes closed)
	Discriminatory sense	: two point	Two-point touch : varying distances apart : different parts of body
		: single point	Single point touch to various parts of body
		: extinction	Recognition of two points of touch on opposite sides of body
		: texture	Recognition of material by feel
		: stereognostic	Recognition of familiar objects by feel
REFLEXES	Superficial reflexes	: upper and lower abdominal	Response to stroking skin in specified area with a moderately sharp object
		: cremasteric	
		: plantar	
		: gluteal	
	Deep reflexes	: biceps	Contraction response to tapping a tendon or bony prominence, sudden muscle stretching
		: brachioradialis	
		: triceps	
		: patellar	
		: Achilles	
	Pathological		
	Babinski : pyramidal tract pathology (Chaddock, Oppenheim, and Gordon reflexes elicit same response)		Stroke lateral aspect of sole of foot: big toe dorsiflexes, toes fan out
	Hoffman : muscular hypertonia		Flick distal phalanx of middle finger: thumb flexes

* For details of the neurological examination, the reader is referred to a neurology textbook or to Francis A. Vazuka: Essentials of the Neurological Examination. Philadelphia: Smith, Kline and French Laboratories, 1962.

he breathe through his mouth which tends to bring about relaxation during the pelvic or rectal examination. She can also alert the physician if she has noted that the patient seems tense, nervous, or particularly sensitive to physical manipulation. A matter-of-fact approach to the examination which nevertheless reflects concern for the patient will help reduce his embarrassment and achieve a complete and accurate examination.

The physical examination is important to the physician because it aids him in making the diagnosis. It is important to the patient because its findings will influence his medical treatment and his subsequent state of health. It is important to the nurse because it will guide her in planning and implementing her nursing care. The physical examination therefore is worth the constructive attention of the nursing staff.

Tools and Techniques That Aid in Diagnosis

The diagnostic tools available today range from the fairly simple to the very complex. This chapter cannot hope to discuss them all in detail but will merely attempt to classify them.

EXAMINATION BY GENERAL SENSE PERCEPTION PROCEDURES

The general sense perception procedures are, in the main, used in the physical examination. The physician inspects the external surface of the body for abnormalities, views the ear canal and tympanic membrane with the aid of an otoscope, and examines the oral cavity and pharynx with the naked eye to detect changes in color or structure such as inflammation of the tonsils or adenoids. The fundus of the eye is examined by means of the ophthalmoscope to determine the presence of disorders of the retina, blood vessels, and optic nerve. The eye offers a number of clues to diagnosis such as the possible occurrence of papilledema in hypertension or brain tumor, the constricted arterioles of hypertension, the tiny aneurysms that may occur in diabetes, and the arteriosclerotic changes that closely parallel similar changes in the brain and elsewhere in the body.

With the aid of a stethoscope the physician assesses function of the heart, the lungs, and the intestinal tract. In listening to the heart the physician notes both its sounds and its rhythm. He may hear a reduction in parts of the sound patterns as occurs in severe ischemic heart attack or the gallop rhythm characteristic of congestive failure. He may hear premature or fibrillatory beats, the murmurs that accompany valvular dysfunction, or the friction rub of pericarditis. In the chest he may hear diminished breath sounds or the abnormal sounds known as rales, which can occur in such diseases as pneumonia, bronchiectasis, and pulmonary tuberculosis. In the abdomen he will listen for decreased bowel sounds indicating inadequate peristalsis such as occurs in ileus, or the increased bowel sounds of obstruction.

EXAMINATION BY VISUALIZATION PROCEDURES

Visualization procedures extend the physician's perceptual capacities. These procedures may be divided into three general categories: (1) the *direct* procedures, in which the physician views the interior of certain body cavities with the aid of special instruments; (2) the *indirect* procedures, in which the physician examines body structures roentgenographically; and (3) the *transformed* procedures, in which electrical activity or sound waves originated by or reflected by the body are portrayed visually on strip charts and/or oscilloscope, and in which radioisotope activity is visualized by scanning and counting devices.

Direct Visualization

The direct visual procedures are accomplished with instruments generally called *scopes* (-scope, a combining form denoting an *instrument for seeing or examining*). All scopes have the same basic structure: an aperture for viewing, and a light source. Some are equipped with magnifying lenses for viewing structures too small or indistinct to be seen otherwise. The ophthalmoscope has a flat head; the otoscope has a short funnel that is inserted into the ear canal; the scopes used in examining deep body cavities are straight or flexible tubes of various diameters. Advances in the field of fiber optics have resulted in the development of flexible scopes that utilize a revolutionary optical system by which visual images are transmitted through a bundle of tiny glass fibers, thus providing a considerably greater range of visibility within a body cavity. Some scopes are equipped with attachments such as biopsy forceps, cautery tips, or grasping forceps. The full name of the scope identifies the area to be viewed, e.g., bronchoscope. Commonly used scopes are described next (Fig. 7–5).

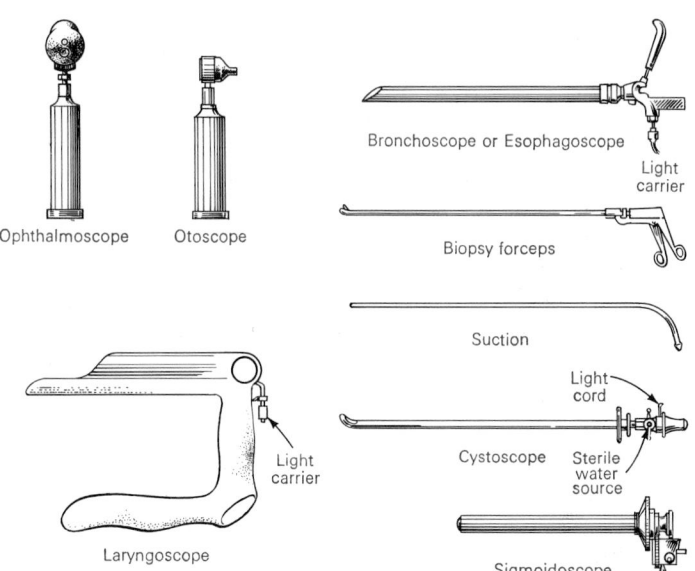

Figure 7–5
Some scopes frequently used in the physical examination.

The laryngoscope visualizes the larynx and vocal cords. It is used in making a biopsy of the larynx and vocal cords, and in the insertion of an endotracheal tube for administering an anesthetic. The bronchoscope is used in inspecting the trachea and bronchial tree. A biopsy forceps can be inserted through the bronchoscope for procuring a tissue specimen. The esophagoscope or endoscope is used in visualizing the length of the esophagus and the interior of the stomach. Biopsy may also be done during this procedure.

The laryngoscope, bronchoscope, and esophagoscope are inserted through the oral cavity. Laryngoscopy and esophagoscopy frequently are sterile procedures, and bronchoscopy almost always is sterile. The throat is anesthetized, unless a general anesthetic is used. The neck is fully hyperextended to provide a straight passage for insertion of the scope. Relaxation of the neck muscles facilitates passage of the scope and tends to diminish the patient's discomfort.

Nursing Care. Nursing care is of considerable importance in these procedures. Although it is the physician's responsibility to explain the procedure to the patient, it is the nurse who provides interpretive support. The patient should have a realistic understanding of what is to occur and should be given an opportunity to express his concerns. These concerns often center around anticipated pain and interference with breathing. Too much or too detailed explanation may, however, induce fright rather than the intended reassurance, so the nurse must exercise perception and judgment in preparing the patient psychologically.

Before the procedure is begun, food and fluids are withheld and a sedative is administered. Following the procedure, if a general anesthetic has been administered, the usual postoperative regimen is followed. If a topical anesthetic has been used in the throat area, the patient will be awake but special precautions regarding fluid intake are necessary, since the anesthetic interferes with normal closure of the glottis and aspiration can occur. For this reason the stomach must be empty before a local anesthetic is administered and the nurse must restrain the patient from drinking until sensation and the swallowing reflex return. These can be determined by offering the patient small sips of water. Immediately following the procedure the patient may require an analgesic; this should be administered parenterally. Special attention to mouth care will help alleviate dryness and discomfort and diminish the desire for fluids.

Postprocedural discomfort may be felt in the area of the head, neck, throat, and possibly the teeth, due to the position of the head during the procedure, throat irritation from passage of the instrument (particularly if the patient had struggled against its insertion), and from the pressure of the tube against the upper teeth during the procedure. The nurse helps the patient by arranging him in a comfortable position with good head and shoulder support, massaging the neck muscles, and administering an analgesic if necessary.

The cystoscope is an instrument of small diameter containing magnifying lenses and a tiny light. It is inserted through the urethra for visualization of the interior of the bladder. The very small ureteral catheter may be inserted through the cystoscope if the physician wishes to explore the ureter. Cystoscopy is always a sterile procedure. The bladder should be emptied in advance of the procedure.

PROCTOSCOPE AND SIGMOIDOSCOPE

These scopes have a wide diameter. They are available in short lengths for viewing the rectum, and longer lengths for viewing the sigmoid. They are inserted through the anus and afford direct vision. Tissue specimens may be obtained in this way. It is essential that the bowel be empty, and the physician may order enemas in preparation for the procedure. These are generally clean procedures, rather than sterile ones.

Nursing Care. Cystoscopy and proctosigmoidoscopy may cause the patient embarrassment because of the anatomical area to be examined. It is helpful to him if the nurse's explanations are matter-of-fact yet sympathetic. The nurse also ensures adequate draping and privacy during the procedures. A surgical preparation of the area is necessary for a cystoscopy.

Indirect Visualization

The indirect visual procedures commonly employed are roentgenography and fluoroscopy. They permit visualization of virtually all important areas of the body. Both methods utilize roentgen rays (commonly called *x-rays*). Roentgen rays pass through body tissues with various degrees of translucency. Fatty tissue is relatively radiotranslucent; muscle, connective tissue, and cartilage are less so. Bone is moderately opaque. Thus, both normal and abnormal structures can be studied through their images, which are captured on x-ray film.

X-rays are used extensively in detecting skeletal fractures, pulmonary lesions such as neoplasms and tuberculous and atelectatic areas, and the presence of fluid. Films can be made at various depths of structure such as the lung; thus serial films (planigrams) demonstrate the depth of, for example, a tuberculous cavity.

The fluoroscope projects the image onto a screen and permits study of the form and motion of internal structures of the body.

When greater visibility than that obtainable on a flat plate x-ray film is desired a contrast medium is introduced to outline a particular structure. The medium may be negative (air, oxygen, or helium) or a positive radiopaque substance (e.g., barium sulfate or iodine salts such as Telepaque and Diodrast). The *dyes*, as these substances are called, are selected on the basis of their metabolization and excretion. The contrast medium is administered orally, intravenously, or directly into a structure through its orifice, as into the lung through the bronchus.

A number of x-ray studies utilizing contrast media are employed to visualize various body structures and systems. Table 7-2 presents common radiological diagnostic procedures.

Transformed Visualization

The transformed procedures are visual in the sense that they present to the physician a graphic representation of a structure and/or its function. The graphs are

TABLE 7-2
Summary of Common Radiological Procedures

SYSTEM	STRUCTURE	PROCEDURE	MEDIUM	NURSING CONSIDERATIONS
NERVOUS Brain	Ventricles	Ventriculogram	Air: injected directly into ventricles	Patient will have had head shaved and burr holes made in skull; headache may follow; patient to lie flat
	Ventricles and meningeal spaces	Pneumoencephalogram	Air: injected into subarachnoid space	Headache may follow; patient to lie flat
	Subarachnoid spaces and ventricles	Encephalogram	Air: introduced by lumbar puncture	Headache may follow; patient to lie flat. Observe for signs of increased intracranial pressure or convulsion
	Cerebral vessels	Cerebral angiogram	Dye: injected into carotid or vertebral arteries	Observe neck for obstruction from swelling. Check movement of extremities and facial mobility
Spine	Spinal subarachnoid space	Myelogram	Air or dye: introduced by lumbar puncture	Observe for signs of meningeal irritation. If air used, position patient flat for several hours. If dye used and not removed, elevate head to prevent flow of dye to brain
GASTROINTESTINAL Upper	Esophagus Stomach Duodenum	Barium swallow	Barium sulfate: taken by mouth	Patient fasted for procedure. Stools may be light in color for following few days. Observe for constipation following procedure
Lower	Colon Rectum	Barium enema	Barium sulfate: given by enema	Before examination: bowel cleared by enemas. After examination: retained barium can cause constipation and impaction; cathartics and/or enemas may be required
	Polypoid masses	Double contrast	Air: injected into colon after expulsion of barium	

TABLE 7-2
Summary of Common
Radiological Procedures
(Continued)

SYSTEM	STRUCTURE	PROCEDURE	MEDIUM	NURSING CONSIDERATIONS
Biliary	Gallbladder	Cholecystogram	Dye: by mouth or intravenously Fatty meal (e.g., cream) following first x-ray series	Before examination: cathartics and enemas to empty gastrointestinal tract for better visualization : fats withheld at evening meal : patient fasted for procedure Dye tablets (given preceding evening) may cause mild diarrhea
	Cystic, hepatic, common ducts	Cholangiogram	Dye: injected directly into biliary tree, or intravenously (less frequent)	Rarely, bile peritonitis may result from leakage into peritoneal cavity via needle tract
RENAL	Kidney Renal pelves Ureters, Bladder	Intravenous pyelogram Retrograde pyelogram	Dye: injected intravenously or by ureteral catheter	Patient fasted Gastrointestinal tract may be cleared by enemas During and after procedure: observe for any signs of reaction to intravenously administered dye (skin flushing, nausea, abdomenal cramps)
CARDIOVASCULAR	Heart and great vessels	Cardioangiogram	Dye: injected into heart by cardiac catheter	Patient will require postoperative cardiac catheterization care
		Angiocardiogram	Dye: injected intravenously	
	Arteries and veins	Venogram Arteriogram Aortogram	Dye: injected into desired area of vascular system	
RESPIRATORY	Lungs	Bronchogram	Dye: instilled into bronchi intratracheally	After procedure: patient placed on postural drainage for removal of oily dye substance

translations of physical energy forms, primarily electricity, but also sound and radiation waves. The more common of these procedures are described below.

The *electrocardiogram* (ECG or EKG) is a graphic record made by the electro-cardiograph of the electrical potential differences due to cardiac action, taken from body surfaces. Alterations of the normal pattern are significant. The ECG is particularly useful in detecting abnormalities of cardiac rhythm and conduction defects such as may occur in hypoxia, electrolyte imbalance, or from drugs such as digitalis. The electrocardiogram also helps demonstrate hypertrophy of one of the cardiac chambers and the development of necrosis in myocardial infarction, since conduction is slowed in hypertrophied tissue and absent in necrotic tissue. Lead wires placed on specific areas of the trunk and extremities transmit electrical activity through a stylus which records the activity on a strip chart or through a cardioscope which protrays the cardiac activity as "blips" of light on the screen.

The *electroencephalogram* (EEG) affords a record of the electrical activity of the brain. The EEG records abnormal patterns such as those of idiopathic epilepsy and can demonstrate the focus of certain neoplastic, hemorrhagic, or traumatic brain lesions. In the EEG lead wires from electrodes are placed on specific areas of the head, and the electrical activity is then recorded on a strip chart. Electrodes may also be surgically implanted in the brain substance to afford a more precise picture of the electrical activity in specific areas, for example, in the temporal lobe when a focal lesion is suspected as the cause of epilepsy.

The *electromyogram* (EMG) is a record of the response of a muscle to an electric stimulation. Electromyography is somewhat limited because of the great variations in muscle tissue. A normal response in one area does not guarantee the absence of pathology in another nearby site.

Sound

The use of *sound* is increasing as a diagnostic modality.

Audiometry is employed in the assessment of sensitivity and discrimination in hearing. It affords information that aids in the differential diagnosis of hearing loss.

In *echoencephalography* ultrasound is projected against the reflecting surfaces of the skull and brain, primarily the bones of the skull and the midline structures of the brain. A graphic record is made of the distance between the reflecting surface and the receiving unit. Thus, information may be gained relative to a shift of the midline structures in respect to their distance from the skull.

Palencephalography through the use of highly sensitive microphones provides a record of the sounds of blood flowing in the head. Normally these sounds are bilaterally equal but in the presence of a neoplasm or hematoma the sounds are altered in the affected area.

Radioisotopes are important diagnostic aids. A radioisotope is a radioactive isotope, generally of a stable element. Certain isotopes of normally stable elements exist naturally in radioactive form, but many are prepared artificially by bombardment in a nuclear reactor or other device.

Tracer doses of the isotope are administered to the patient. The choice of isotope is based on the isotope affinity for the tissue to be studied, e.g., radioiodine (^{131}I) locates in thyroid tissue. A counter, such as the scintiscanner, is used to note the amount of radioactive substance taken up by the target tissue. Abnormalities are detected by evaluation of the amount of radioactive material taken up by the particular tissue.

ANALYSIS OF BODY CONSTITUENTS

Many kinds of tests are performed upon the body constituents in order to determine deviations from normal in components and/or function. Tests are made of the blood, lymph, gastrointestinal secretions, and bronchial secretions; the urine, feces, and perspiration; and the various tissues. From these determinations the physician seeks relationships between the laboratory findings and the existence of disease. Certain disease conditions produce characteristic changes in the body constituents. In other situations the chemical and microscopic analyses may suggest one or several possible disorders. Table 7-3 presents a summary of the major body constituents that are frequently examined, the means by which the specimen is obtained, and the nature of the examination. For a more detailed description of test methodologies, purposes, and norms the student is referred to a laboratory text and diagnostic procedure manual.

The laboratory analyses of body constituents are individual for each type of test performed and for the specific constituent tested. The analytical methods most frequently employed are chemical, physical, and microscopic. The range of normal values varies according to the methods followed by the individual laboratory. The student should familiarize herself with the normal range of the particular laboratory before interpreting the results.

The majority of specimens are obtained by the laboratory technician or by the physician, with the common exception of urine, which is frequently procured by the nurse. It may be necessary to add a preservative or other agent to the collection container, or to employ a special method of handling in order to protect and preserve the specimen components. Such requirements are specified for the individual test and must be observed if the analysis is to be satisfactory. Test results in many cases can be affected by the drugs a patient has taken within the preceding 72 hours; because of the current proliferation of drugs, the physician may not be aware of these effects. The clinical pathologist in charge of the laboratory should be notified of the drugs the patient is receiving.

TESTS OF FUNCTION

Many functional analyses are accomplished by means of constituent analyses. Table 7-4 presents a summary of the common functional tests that are not accomplished through constituent analysis, e.g., many of the tests for liver, kidney, and metabolic functions, and certain cardiac functions.

These kinds of function tests generally are used in combination with other diagnostic modalities, rather than alone.

ANALYSIS USING INTEGUMENTARY COMPONENTS

Analyses of components of the integumentary system are made chiefly to determine the existence and extent of contact between the patient and a particular organism. Serum sensitivity and allergen tests, for example, are accomplished by introducing a minute amount of the test material into the tissues, usually intradermally, and observing for a reaction. Skin tests also aid in diagnosis of communicable diseases

TABLE 7-3 Summary of Body Constituent Analyses

CONSTITUENT	MEANS OF OBTAINING SAMPLE	SUBSTANCE OR MECHANISM OF EXAMINATION
BLOOD	Venepuncture Finger puncture	Cell counts: kinds and number Tests: for chemical and biological constituents, normal and abnormal Tests: for bleeding, clotting, circulation times Tests: for functional test drug levels Blood types Cell behavior (e.g., fragility) Organism cultures
CEREBROSPINAL FLUID	Lumbar puncture Cisternal puncture Ventricular puncture	Cell counts Chemical and biological constituents Pressure (lumbar puncture)
FECES	Stool sample	Blood Biological and chemical constituents, e.g., urobilinogen Parasites (warm specimen) Bulk
FLUIDS AND EXUDATES		
Abscess, cyst, tissue exudate	Aspiration, swab smear	Organisms
Gastric	Aspiration (via stomach tube)	Acid content Neoplastic cells Organisms, e.g., tubercle bacillus
Respiratory: bronchial	Aspiration (via bronchoscope) Sputum collection	Organisms Neoplastic cells
Nasopharyngeal	Swab smear	Organisms
Serous and pyogenic fluids	Pleural: thoracentesis Peritoneal: paracentesis Pericardial: aspiration	Chemical and biological constituents Quantity Organisms
Vaginal and cervical	Swab smears	Organisms Neoplastic cells
TISSUE		
Bone marrow	Needle aspiration biopsy: sternum, iliac crest	Cells; chemical constituents
Liver	Needle biopsy	Nature of tissue
Soft tissue, breast	Surgical biopsy; needle biopsy	Nature of tissue and cells
Other: bits of tissue may be taken from a variety of sites within the body and from its surfaces	Surgical biopsy Balloon studies: gastric scrapings	Nature of tissue and cells
URINE	Single specimens: voided, clean catch, catheterized Fractional collection Time collections	Sugar; acetone; pH; specific gravity Cells

TABLE 7-4
Summary of Common
Functional Tests*

FUNCTION TESTED	TYPE OF TEST	NATURE OF TEST
BLADDER	Cystometry	Recording of intravesicular pressure by measured filling and emptying of bladder, via catheter and pressure-measuring instrument
CARDIAC	Exercise tolerance	Blood pressure apparatus and electrocardiograph are attached to patient. Patient walks up and down a 9- to 10-inch step for 10 minutes. Preceding and following rest the electrocardiogram, blood pressure, and pulse are checked
CIRCULATION	Circulation time	Measurement of rate of blood flow: arm to lung, arm to tongue. A test substance is injected i.v.—patient reports the appearance of taste, warmth, smell, or he coughs according to the effect of the test agent
	Pressures: intracardiac Pressures: intraarterial	Insertion of pressure sensing device into vessel or into heart via cardiac catheter
METABOLIC RATE	Basal metabolism	Patient at complete rest, breathes into a machine which measures oxygen consumption; from this measurement heat production is computed
NEUROLOGICAL	Neurological examination	See Table 7-1
	Caloric: vestibular function	Cold and hot water injected into auditory canal, patient observed for nystagmos
	Sweat test: sympathetic nervous system lesions	Skin in test area painted with iodine and dusted with starch, pilocarpine administered and patient observed for sweating (starch darkens with sweating)

* This table does not include functional tests done by constituent analyses.

such as diphtheria, scarlet fever, pertussis, and tuberculosis, and certain fungal infections such as brucellosis, tularemia, coccidioidomycosis, and histoplasmosis. The presence of mycotic disorders is determined through laboratory examinations of clippings or scrapings from the hair, nails, skin, and mucocutaneous tissues, or of excretions such as sputum or pus.

Uses of Diagnostic Information

The information gained during the diagnostic process is important to the physician in several ways. It guides his initial determination of the nature and extent of disease. The data thereby gathered allow him to proceed confidently yet cautiously to the next step. Developments in modern medicine bring increasing accuracy to test results, yet the physician remains aware of the possibility of inaccuracy through errors in specimen collection or in technique of analysis. He is aware also that many tests are suggestive only and may point to several diseases. He knows too that a single test may be insufficient to confirm a diagnosis. Nonetheless, when test results are considered along with the patient's history and results of the physical examination, and these are viewed in light of the physician's clinical judgment, the speed and accuracy of diagnosis are markedly increased.

The value of laboratory tests is not limited to the diagnostic process. The tests contribute also to the physician's ongoing assessment of the course of the disease. Test results aid the physician in selecting therapy to be prescribed, they assist him in measuring the patient's response to the therapeutic program, and they guide his decisions to maintain, alter, or discontinue a particular form of therapy. By means of laboratory tests, trial and error has been very greatly reduced in the practice of medicine.

The Nurse's Role in the Diagnostic Process

As one observes the rapidity with which laboratory technicians enter and leave a patient's room and the speed and perfunctoriness with which patients are whisked to various diagnostic departments in the hospital, one might well gain the impression that the nurse has only a minor role in the patient's diagnostic process and that this role is chiefly that of physician's assistant. Such, however, is not or should not be the case. All three facets of the nursing function—care, cure, and coordination—come into play with special emphasis upon the *care* dimension. This dimension is the most meaningful to the patient and the one most frequently overlooked by the nurse.

The diagnostic period is stressful for any patient because it approaches the point at which a health problem may definitely be shown to exist. In almost all patients the strain increases proportionately with the degree of physical and/or psychological involvement and the anticipated seriousness of the condition, and with the time, expense, complexity, and indefiniteness involved in the diagnostic process. It is therefore important for the nurse as a part of her care function to use her judgment in determining the need to spend time with the patient; time for talking with him and offering an appropriate explanation of his diagnostic program or particular test, time for listening to him and allowing him to ask questions and express his concerns, even though this may take a little while. The patient will need to know what to expect during a particular procedure, and quite often he will need a clear explanation of how he is to participate in the procedure. The latter is particularly important if he is to maintain a particular position as for a lumbar puncture or a thoracentesis, or if he is to be given the responsibility of collecting any specimens such as urine or sputum himself.

In addition to his psychological and instructional preparation the patient may require a particular type of physical preparation for which the nurse is responsible. He may also need some special care or observation following a particular procedure as in the management of the absent swallowing reflex following bronchoscopy or barium swallow. The nurse must also consider the scheduling of tests in order to ensure that the patient does not become exhausted by them or miss a series of meals as a result. At times the nurse may have to intercede on his behalf.

The care responsibilities of the nurse are equally important during a diagnostic procedure in which she participates. While it is true that the physician needs the nurse's active assistance, too often he becomes the sole focus of her attention when in fact the patient should be her primary concern. The patient may well need assurance by touch or by word, by some action to increase his physical comfort, or through guidance in following the physician's instructions. Above all he needs to know that he is not just an object being worked upon. Determining in advance the nature of the diagnostic procedure, and the preparation of the patient, the environment, and the equipment needed, will do much to help the nurse direct her attention to the patient during the procedure. Each act of care, comfort, and coordination the nurse performs contributes in a positive way to the therapeutic dimension of the diagnostic process by increasing the safety, accuracy, and effectiveness of the particular procedure.

To fulfil her responsibilities in the medical diagnostic process, the nurse should try to seek answers to a number of questions in advance of each procedure. The following list will serve as a guide.

In preparation for the procedure:

What is the nature and purpose of the test or procedure; what method will be utilized?

What equipment will be required and how will it be obtained; is a prepared tray available; is additional equipment or supplies needed; is the procedure a sterile or a clean one?

Will specimens be taken; when and how often; are they to be sterile or clean; what kinds of containers are needed, and are preservatives or special solutions necessary; who will procure the specimen (i.e., physician, nurse, or technician); must the specimen be handled in a particular way (e.g., refrigeration, warmth); should the specimen be taken to the laboratory immediately?

What kinds of test request forms are needed; who is responsible for preparing them; is written consent of the patient necessary, and who is responsible for obtaining it?

Who will perform the procedure (i.e., physician or technician); is the test one of the few performed by the nurse (e.g., testing urine for sugar, acetone, or specific gravity)?

Where will the procedure be done (i.e., patient's room, treatment room, diagnostic department)?

For what time is the procedure scheduled?

In preparation of the patient:

What kinds of explanation and interpretation are necessary; what has been the nature of the physician's discussion with the patient and with his family?

Is any physical preparation necessary (e.g., hexachlorophene scrub, shave of operative area, enema, laxative)?

Is food to be withheld, and if so, when; is a special diet required?

Is fluid to be withheld, and if so, when?

Are any medications to be ordered, either before the procedure or as part of it?

Is the patient receiving any medications that will affect the test results; who should be informed of this; should a medication be discontinued within a particular period before the procedure; should smoking be restricted?

During the procedure:

What assistance from the nurse will be needed by the patient and by the physician?

Are there special measures to be taken in respect to care of the patient or the equipment?

Are untoward reactions to be anticipated; should emergency equipment be available?

Who will be responsible for the disposition of specimens?

After the procedure:

What care will the patient need; what observations should be made?

Are untoward reactions to be anticipated?

Are follow-up procedures to be performed?

When may the patient resume intake of food and fluids?

What are the implications of the diagnostic findings for the patient's health status and for his nursing management?

It is important that the nurse possess all the information necessary to ensure her fulfilling her responsibilities. If a procedure is not correctly done, it may have to be repeated, thus causing delay and additional discomfort and expense to the patient. False results can lead to inaccurate diagnoses or failure to detect a pathological condition. If specimens are not collected on time or in sufficient amount the studies made of them may give erroneous results. If the specimens are not preserved correctly a change in their constituents results. So many diagnostic tests and procedures are currently available that it is virtually impossible for the nurse to remember the details of all of them. Therefore she should familiarize herself with the tests commonly used on her unit and keep at hand a reference manual of all widely used diagnostic procedures.

Diagnostic findings provide useful information for the nurse in her initial and continuing assessment of the patient. They serve as guides to the planning and implementation of care. In interpreting diagnostic findings, the nurse will draw upon her knowledge of normal anatomy and physiology and of pathophysiology. The physician may also be a valuable resource in this regard, by simplifying and interpreting particular findings. Through such communication the physician can come to appreciate the nurse's concern for his patient and her interest in providing knowledgeable, constructive care. Thereby the collaborative effort of nurse-physician, medical therapy-nursing therapy is enhanced.

Bibliography

Conn, Howard F., Robert J. Clohecy, and Rex B. Conn, Jr. (Eds.): *Current Diagnosis.* Philadelphia: W. B. Saunders Company, 1967.

Cooper, Philip: *Ward Procedures and Techniques.* New York: Appleton Century Crofts, 1967.

deGutiérrez-Mahoney, C. G. and Esta Carini: *Neurological and Neurosurgical Nursing,* 4th ed. St. Louis: The C. V. Mosby Company, 1965.

Engle, Ralph L. Jr. and B. J. Davis: Medical Diagnosis: Present, Past, and Future. Part I: Present Concepts of the Meaning and Limitations of Medical Diagnosis; Part II: Philosophical Foundations and Historical Development of Our Concepts of Health, Disease, and Diagnosis; Part III: Diagnosis in the Future, including a Critique on the Use of Electronic Computers as Diagnostic Aids to the Physician. *Archives of Internal Medicine,* 112:512–519; 520–529; 530–546, October, 1963.

French, Ruth: *Nurse's Guide to Diagnostic Procedures,* 2d ed. New York: McGraw-Hill Book Company, 1967.

Harrison, T. R. (Ed.): *Principles of Internal Medicine,* 5th ed. New York: McGraw-Hill Book Company, 1966.

Hochstein, Elliot and Albert L. Rubin: *Physical Diagnosis.* New York: McGraw-Hill Book Company, 1964.

Prior, John A. and Jack S. Silberstein: *Physical Diagnosis, The History and Physical Examination of the Patient.* St. Louis: The C. V. Mosby Company, 1963.

Saunders, William H., William H. Havener, Carol J. Fair, and Josephine T. Hickey: *Nursing Care in Eye, Ear, Nose and Throat Disorders,* 2d ed. St. Louis: The C. V. Mosby Company, 1968.

Selzer, Arthur: *The Heart.* Berkeley and Los Angeles: University of California Press, 1966.

Vazuka, Francis A: *Essentials of the Neurological Examination.* Philadelphia: Smith, Kline and French Laboratories, 1962.

CHAPTER 8
THERAPIES FOR DISEASE

MARGARET A. KAUFMANN

The nature of therapy
Therapeutic modalities
BIOLOGICAL AND CHEMICAL AGENTS
PHYSICAL AGENTS
PSYCHICAL AGENTS

The term *therapy* is a broad one referring to that which has healing, curative, or preventive power. The term is often used interchangeably with *treatment,* the means employed in effecting the management or cure of disease or the repair of injury.

The Nature of Therapy

Therapy, like diagnosis, has two interrelated dimensions: process and decision. The therapeutic process is one of assessment, intervention, and evaluation or, more simply put, deciding what to do, doing it, judging its effectiveness, and deciding whether to continue or to revise the treatment. Normally the initiation of therapy proceeds from the physician's diagnosis. Therapy may, however, begin in advance of the diagnosis when the doctor's initial impression of the problem or the urgency of the presenting signs and symptoms leads him to decide that some intervention should or must be undertaken before a complete diagnostic study can be completed. For example, early shock apparently may be due to internal bleeding, but the source of the bleeding may not be immediately discernible. The physician would administer a blood transfusion or other fluid therapy first, then seek the source of the problem.

The therapeutic process evolves through intervention and evaluation, toward increasing precision and effectiveness. Diagnosis and therapy are closely related. Precise diagnosis permits the physician to utilize precise therapy. His intent is to be as specific as possible, directing his treatment plan toward elimination of the underlying cause of the medical problem. This specificity is possible when the therapeutic modalities known to be effective for particular disease conditions are available. In other circumstances therapy may have to be of a less specific nature and designed to aid the body, or, as in psychotherapy, the mind, to mobilize its own healing forces. Therapy may also be directed toward the relief of symptoms. Many therapies have elements of both the specific and the nonspecific within their scope, depending upon the circumstances for which they are utilized. Nutritional therapy is of this order. It may be prescribed for its general constitutional effect or for a particular purpose, such as the administration of thiamine in beriberi. Rest, too, may be a nonspecific therapy, when used in support of the body's natural restorative powers, or a highly specific one, as in the treatment of myocardial infarction. Whether specific or nonspecific, therapy is always purposeful. It is intended to aid in the accomplishment of some purpose: replacement of a necessary body constituent, repair of an anatomical structure, removal of a neoplasm, relief of a symptom, maintenance of muscle tone, or improvement in the general state of the body tissue and function.

Many approaches are taken to therapy. These can be grouped generally according to their purpose. Table 8-1 presents the main kinds of therapeutic approaches and their purposes. Several of the categories tend to incorporate concepts of a similar nature and thus overlap. This is virtually unavoidable since therapeutic approaches have not been developed to the point where they are clear, distinct, and mutually exclusive.

The therapeutic approaches mentioned are utilized singly and in combination. For example, while a patient is in traction for reduction and repair of a femoral

APPROACH	PURPOSE
Prevention (prophylaxis)	Intervention before the occurrence of a problem, e.g., immunization, water fluoridation, regular health examination, range of motion exercises, vitamin therapy, mental hygiene
Removal (extirpation)	Complete removal or surgical destruction, e.g., surgical excision, some forms of drainage, antimicrobial drugs
Replacement	Restoration of or supplying of an equivalent, e.g., blood transfusion, fluid and electrolyte therapy, administration of hormones, vitamins, minerals
Substitution	Permanent replacement of or provision of an alternate form for a part or substance, e.g., prosthesis (limb, heart valve), surgical revision (ileal bladder), insulin therapy (chemical equivalent)
Repair	Return to original or correct form, e.g., setting a fracture, surgical repair (laceration, cleft lip, fistula, hernia)
Reduction (minimization)	Decreasing amount, e.g., drainage, diuretics, restoration of dislocation, muscle relaxants, antihypertensive drugs, traction
Restoration	Return to a more nearly normal condition or state of health, e.g., certain cardiac drugs, physical therapies, nutritive or hormonal supplements, rest
Inhibition	Checking or restraining an action of an organ, cell, or chemical agent, e.g., cholinergic blocking agents, vagotomy, radiation, antiinfective drugs, vaccines
Support	Directed toward a general constitutional effect, of a nonspecific nature, e.g., maintenance of fluids, nutriments, vitamins, drugs; rest; certain physical, occupational, and psychotherapies
Palliation	Relief or moderation, e.g., drug or surgical relief of pain, partial excision of growths, radiation of malignant tumor, antineoplastic drugs

TABLE 8-1
Therapeutic Approaches and Purposes

neck fracture he may also be receiving supportive therapy such as protein supplementation.

The desired result of therapy is complete cure. Cure is not always possible to achieve, however, and the therapeutic goal must be shifted to that which is the best attainable. It may mean substitution of a pharmacologic agent or a prosthesis for a natural part of substance. It may mean minimization of an untoward reaction or support of the remaining body function without materially affecting its repair. Perhaps the most that can be achieved in some situations is palliation when other therapies are no longer effective.

Because cure is not always attainable, the institution of prevention where possible is the most desirable of all approaches. Prevention avoids problems and maintains the individual in a normal state. Preventive techniques are useful in detecting disorders early when the cure potential is best. Recognition of the importance of prevention is demonstrated by the development of preventive medicine as a specialty in medicine.

Throughout the therapeutic process the physician *prescribes* and *evaluates*. He must know whether and to what extent his intervention is successful. Accordingly, he determines whether to modify, maintain, or discontinue his program of therapy. He employs objective observation, subjective reports of the patient, tests, examinations, information provided him by the nurse, and his own clinical judgment to accomplish this end. In all therapies the physician considers the individual patient and the course of the disease in him. Patients do not always present the classic picture of a particular disease, nor do they always respond to therapy in the anticipated manner. This is true particularly in dealing with pharmacologic agents. The patient may have no response to a certain agent, as occurs in resistance to some antibiotics. A drug may be toxic to the patient, or he may be allergic to a particular drug. A particular therapy may be inadequate in the management of a medical problem and the physician will find it necessary to employ two or more therapeutic approaches. In, for example, congestive heart failure, a digitalis glycoside preparation may aid heart function but diuretics may have to be administered to assist in reducing edema. In the treatment of a malignant neoplasm it may be impossible to surgically remove the original growth and the metastatic ones, and radiation therapy will be required as a further treatment.

In prescribing medical therapy the physician considers the patient, the disease or injury, and the therapeutic agent. He tries to give the patient the most effective treatment with the least possible discomfort, inconvenience, and expense. Because the work of the nurse and the physician is closely interrelated, the physician's efforts to help the patient are greatly affected by the knowledge, ability, and concern which the nurse brings to bear upon the care she gives.

Therapeutic Modalities

There are numerous therapeutic techniques and agents and new ones are developed with great frequency. This chapter will not attempt to enumerate or describe particular therapeutic agents and techniques but rather will present the important categories of therapeutic modalities.

A large number of therapeutic agents act systemically, i.e., they are circulated in the bloodstream, and some have an affinity for a specific organ or area of the body. Other agents are topical, i.e., they are applied to the surface of the body. Other therapeutic agents are psychical, i.e., they deal with the mind and the emotions. Therapeutic agents can be categorized on the basis of their composition into three large groups: the biological and chemical agents, the physical agents, and the psychical agents. Although there is considerable diversity of action within each group, all contribute to the achievement of the physician's therapeutic purpose. Thus they are employed in prevention, removal, replacement, substitution, repair, reduction, restoration, inhibition, support, and palliation.

BIOLOGICAL AND CHEMICAL AGENTS

The biological and chemical agents comprise the largest group, and chief among them are the pharmacologic agents. The pharmacologic agents have both specific and general actions. They cause stimulation, depression, inhibition, destruction. They supplement, replace, and counteract. They cause alterations in growth, function, and sensation. They induce calm or arousal, sleepiness or wakefulness. They replicate the actions of substances normally present in the body. In certain circumstances they can be harmful.

The biological and chemical agents occur as solids, semisolids, fluids, and gases. Some are biological substances, some are inorganic. They can be applied externally, inhaled, ingested, or injected. The nurse needs considerable working knowledge of the forms and actions of drugs so that she can deal with them safely and effectively in patient care. (It is not the intent of this chapter to deal with specific pharmacological content [for this the reader is referred to a text book on the subject] but rather to point up the scope of therapeutic agents.)

The nutritional substances compose one portion of the biological and chemical group. They are utilized both as the basis for particular diets, e.g., diabetic, low-sodium, and as supplements to the diet, e.g., postsurgery diet high in protein and vitamin C.

PHYSICAL AGENTS

The chief physical agents are temperature and energy. Heat, cold, wetness, and dryness are physical agents.

Force, a manifestation of energy, has several uses in therapy. Pressure is utilized to aid respiration; i.e., pressure can be applied through the trachea (Bennett and Bird respirators), or externally to the thorax and abdomen (Drinker and chest respirators). Pressure is employed to produce hemostasis (Sengstaken tube, pressure dressing or tourniquet). Pressure is used to reduce blood flow (dry phlebotomy for massive pulmonary edema). Pressure is also used to stabilize (the truss). Traction, another form of force, is employed, for example, in the reduction of dislocation and fractures, and treatment of spasms. The active exercises, passive movement, and massage which are performed in physical therapy are applications of force.

Radiation is another manifestation of energy. Roentgen rays, ultraviolet rays, and infrared rays are forms of radiation energy. Ultrasound and light amplification (laser) are other forms of radiation energy.

Vibration, a periodic movement in alternately opposite directions from a point of equilibrium, is employed in some types of physical therapy.

Surgery and surgical treatments can be considered physical agents, since both involve the use of force (i.e., cutting) to accomplish a particular purpose in therapy. Whatever its extent, in all its forms surgery involves invasion of the body surface, whether by an incision through several layers of body substance, a slicing of a thin layer of the epidermis, or a puncture (penetration) used in certain drainage procedures and biopsy techniques.

PSYCHICAL AGENTS

The psychical agents are employed in the treatment of medical and surgical disorders as well as in psychiatric illnesses. Psychotherapy, psychoanalysis, and group therapy are the most widely known forms of psychical, or psychiatric, therapy. Electroshock therapy, insulin shock therapy, and pentylenetetrazol (Metrazol) therapy incorporate biological and chemical agents in the management of psychiatric illnesses.

Recreational therapy, occupational-vocational therapy, and music therapy might also be considered as psychical agents, although they do not fall strictly into this category.

Bibliography

Ayres, Stephen M. and Stanley Giannelli, Jr.: *Care of the Critically Ill.* New York: Appleton Century Crofts, 1967.

Brain, Sir Russell: *Clinical Neurology.* London: Oxford University Press, 1960.

Brainerd, Henry, Sheldon Margen, and Milton J. Chatton: *Current Diagnosis and Treatment.* Los Altos, California: Lange Medical Publications, 1969.

Burton, Benjamin T.: *The Heinz Handbook of Nutrition.* New York: McGraw-Hill Book Company, 1965.

Cooper, Philip: *Ward Procedures and Techniques.* New York: Appleton Century Crofts, 1967.

Goodman, Louis S. and Alfred Gilman (Eds.): *The Pharmacological Basis of Therapeutics,* 3d ed. New York: The Macmillan Company, 1965.

Goth, Andres: *Medical Pharmacology,* 4th ed. St. Louis: The C. V. Mosby Company, 1968.

Greenwood, Maud E.: *Medical Physics,* 2d ed. Philadelphia: F. A. Davis Company, 1966.

Harrison, T. R. (Ed.): *Principles of Internal Medicine,* 5th ed. New York: McGraw-Hill Book Company, 1966.

Harkins, Henry N. et al. (Eds.): *Surgery, Principles and Practice,* 2d ed. Philadelphia: J. B. Lippincott Company, 1961.

Whitehouse, Fredrick A.: The Concept of Therapy. *Rehabilitation Literature,* 28:8:238–247, August, 1967.

CHAPTER 9
THE REHABILITATION PROCESS

GERALDINE SKINNER

Rehabilitation for the aged and disabled is a major health movement. Like other specialists concerned about health, the nurse is involved with programs whose aim is to restore disabled persons to the best possible level of function. Although rehabilitation centers have been constructed and many physical therapy services have been established in general hospitals during recent years, the process of rehabilitation is an integral part of most nursing activities, since numerous nursing measures have as their goal the prevention of deformities or the provision of support to the patient during his curative program.

The Scope of Rehabilitation

Rehabilitation is the process of restoration to previous capacities. By contrast, *habilitation* is the process employed initially in the child with, for example, cerebral palsy, who must learn new skills. Every patient requires some physical rehabilitation during and following an acute illness. The goal in *all* patient care is to prevent disability and to help the patient regain the greatest possible degree of independent function in the shortest possible time with the least possible effort on the part of the patient and all those assisting him.

Although efforts at rehabilitation have been made for many centuries, rehabilitation did not gain status as a specialty until after World War II. The many techniques developed during that war gave impetus to rehabilitation efforts. Initially programs were developed for patients with critical physical disabilities, such as paraplegia, quadriplegia, amputations, and rheumatoid arthritis. Still further impetus has been given to this movement with the recent enactment of broad social legislation providing for medical assistance to the aged and indigent. Increased emphasis on the care of the patient following a cerebrovascular accident, which commonly resulted in hemiplegia and aphasia, has greatly expanded the need for rehabilitative care during the acute illness as well as later during the rehabilitation period.

The concept of rehabilitation has significantly changed the general attitude toward health care in the hospital. In the medical approach to the care of the acutely ill patient, deviations from normal are identified through diagnostic procedures. Thus, emphasis is placed upon functions the patient has lost through his illness. Rehabilitation, however, has changed the approach from the question, "What is wrong with the patient?" to the question "What physical, psychological, and intellectual assets does the patient still possess?" As one passes through the door of a rehabilitation unit one is immediately struck by the air of hopefulness. Here the personnel are not as concerned with how the patient acquired his disability as with what he has left to work with. How the patient became disabled is of little significance for his future *provided that the disability is a stable, rather than a progressive, one.* The patient with multiple sclerosis, for example, may be a candidate for rehabilitation during periods of remission, but will not be such a candidate during periods of exacerbation. This is true also of the patient with rheumatoid arthritis.

One authority has stated, "Rehabilitation is a service combining medical, surgical, nursing, occupational therapy, physical therapy, clinical psychology, vocational rehabilitation and other specialties combined into one integrated program of patient care. It is designed to improve a patient's physical and functional status or *to prevent loss of such function.* This cannot be achieved by one of the disciplines alone but *requires the combination of all or most of them.* The total program is directed and supervised by the physician."[1]

The statement describes the rehabilitation process as it takes place in a special center or unit. It is important that the rehabilitation process be begun at the time of the injury or the onset of the illness, if it is to be effective. *The basic concepts of nursing rehabilitation should therefore be applied in all nursing care.* Many of these concepts are discussed throughout the text. This chapter presents general concepts in rehabilitation nursing and outlines nursing responsibilities and rehabilitation techniques.

It is the patient who undergoes the process of rehabilitation—the process is not one in which something is done to him. He must be motivated to perform the activities and must participate in the development of the total treatment and care plan; otherwise it cannot succeed. The patient rehabilitates himself, and the members of the health team assist in motivating him and in carrying out the program that has been agreed upon by everyone concerned.

The rehabilitation team is headed by a physician, who may be a *physiatrist,* one highly trained in physical medicine, or a specialist in another branch of medicine or surgery. An orthopedic surgeon or a neurologist, for example, may head the team. The number of health workers on the team may vary at different stages of the process.

The Nurse's Role in the Rehabilitation Program

Because of her special relationship to the patient, the nurse may play a dual role (see Figure 9–1). First, she applies her skill to the care of all patients. She might be called a *generalist* as she applies both curative and preventive measures under the direction of the patient's physician.

Second, the nurse functions as a rehabilitation nursing specialist when she is participating as a member of a team organized to provide rehabilitation services. Here, too, her role is a multifaceted one in contrast to that held by other members of the team. She serves as *care coordinator* between the patient, the physician, and other members of the care team. The professional nurse and members of her nursing care team (staff nurses, practical nurses, and aides) are in a unique position because of their close proximity to the patient and 24-hour contact with him. Thus the nurse can learn of his hopes, fears, and ambitions, sees the effect of therapy *daily,* and has many opportunities to support him both physically and emotionally. She meets his family and teaches and interprets care to both family and patient. The physician relies upon her to see that the total program is well integrated. She can make the patient's needs known to the physician and to other members of the therapy team.

As she participates in rehabilitation nursing, the nurse finds that she must learn

[1] John Affeldt, in speech presented to nursing staff at Rancho Los Amigos Hospital, Downey, California, June, 1963.

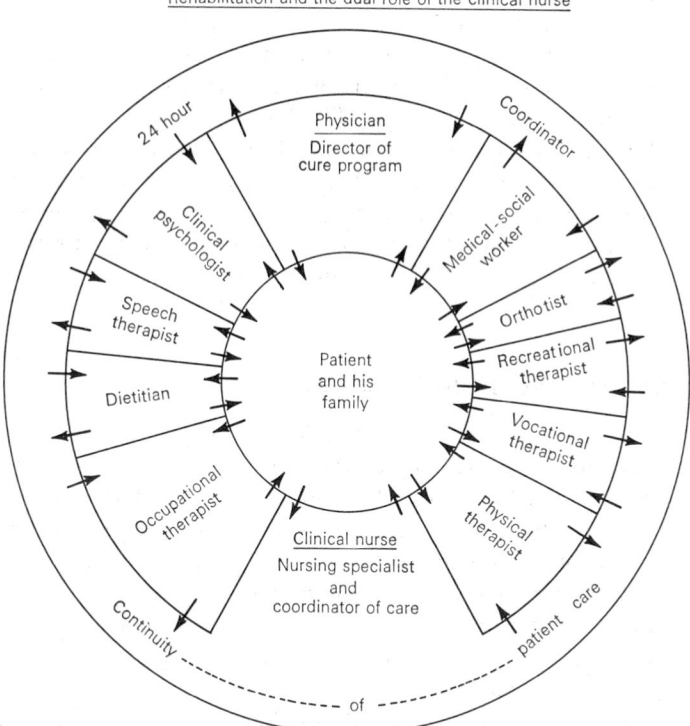

Rehabilitation and the dual role of the clinical nurse

Figure 9–1
Dual role of the clinical
nurse in rehabilitation
therapy.

to communicate her knowledge of the patient, especially during team conferences. She is the one person who sees the effect of the entire program upon the patient. Her value as an effective rehabilitator depends largely upon how she sees her role in relation to the patient and the various members of the team. She is far more than a custodian of physical care during the absence of other specialists.

THE NURSE AS SPECIALIST

Figure 9–1 depicts the nurse's dual role of nursing specialist and coordinator of patient care. As a specialist she has a number of responsibilities. She maintains the integrity of the skin or treats decubitus ulcers. She assists in bowel and bladder training if the patient is incontinent. These responsibilities are discussed more fully later in the chapter.

THE NURSE AS COORDINATOR

In her role of coordinator the nurse supports the staff members in their activities. When the physical therapist is working with an arthritic patient to reduce flexion contractures in his knees and to build up muscle strength in preparation for walking, the nurse helps in this effort by having the patient keep his knees extended at all times of the day and night. To allow him to place pillows under his knees for even one night may undo many hours of physical therapy effort.

Both therapist and nurse strive to motivate the patient toward increasing his independent actions. The nurse and the occupational therapist work with the patient on a program of activities of daily living. For example, the patient may be learning to feed himself with special feeding tools. The occupational therapist has designed the tools and taught the patient how to use them effectively, but the members of the nursing team guide the patient in his eating activities three times a day in the patient unit. The nurse supports and coordinates each new activity and provides psychological support, guiding the patient through periods of discouragement, and informs the staff of his readiness for the next step in rehabilitation. She helps patient and family to accept program goals.

Prevention and Rehabilitation

The most important contribution the nurse can make toward the recovery of patients in her care is the provision of good preventive nursing care. "The expertness with which this role a nursing staff performs during the early stages of a patient's illness can well mean the difference between whether he will remain many weeks or months in the hospital, often depleting his family's financial resources" (Skinner) or will be rehabilitated and back on the job within a matter of weeks. Many patients are being rehabilitated at a tremendous cost to their families and to the state or local government because preventive care techniques were not applied by nursing personnel. The nursing literature of the 1940s is rich in information concerning the prevention of disabilities due to poor posture, poor body mechanics, incorrect positioning in bed, lack of beneficial exercises, and deformities due to use of improper furniture. The rehabilitation movement has made a major contribution to health care by refocusing attention upon the preventive care.

Some disabilities that commonly develop when inadequate attention is given to preventive nursing care are as follows:

Adhesions and stiffness of the shoulder joint following radical breast surgery

External rotation of the "good" hip due to lack of support during traction or bed care for fractured hip

Hip dislocation following prolonged side positioning for decubitus ulcer care, especially likely to occur in thin, elderly individuals

Flexion contractures of the hips, knees, wrists, and elbows in the patient with rheumatoid arthritis or who has had a leg amputated

Drop foot or drop wrist following prolonged illness and inadequate foot and wrist support

Decubitus ulcers in patients with neurological disorders who have not been turned often enough or been given adequate skin care

Many other examples could be given, and the student will be able to add others as she studies the nursing care of patients with medical-surgical conditions. To provide good preventive care, the nurse must make a systematic assessment of the patient, give thoughtful, purposeful action at the bedside, teach members of the nursing team to implement the nursing care plan, and teach the patient to perform the indicated activities.

Some preventive and curative measures that the medical-surgical nurse can carry out are as follows:

Maintain the patient's normal joint action throughout illness by exercising all uninvolved joints through their normal range of motion. This activity is part of basic nursing care. *A doctor's written order should not be required.* When a nurse exercises a joint she does so *only* to the point of pain, even when a doctor's order has been given. The physical therapist carries the joint motion or muscle stretching past the point of pain.

Teaching bed exercises to all patients. These exercises may include the following:

1. Deep breathing exercises. (If the patient cannot carry out deep breathing exercises the physician may prescribe intermittent positive pressure breathing therapy using the Bird or Bennett respirator. If an inhalation therapist is not available the nurse usually assists.)

2. Gluteal tightening.

3. Abdominal tightening.

4. Quadriceps setting.

5. Foot circling, with emphasis on dorsiflexing the ankle.

The last three exercises help prepare the patient for ambulation, which requires stabilization of the trunk, knees, hips, and ankles, and thus help the patient to ambulate. They also help to maintain muscle tone, stimulate the circulation, and prevent joint stiffness and muscle contractures.

Maintain the patient in proper alignment in the supine, prone, and side-lying positions.

Reposition the patient frequently to prevent muscle stiffness and maintain muscle tone.

Prevent decubitus ulcers in all patients, and be particularly watchful with neurological and neurosurgical patients.

Supervise or administer special measures as ordered by the physician. Such measures might include the following:

1. Exercise the affected arm following breast surgery.

2. Early ambulation, if indicated, following cerebral vascular accident.

3. Use of commode by patient with myocardial infarction.

4. Correct use of walkers and wheel chairs.

5. Correct techniques in crutch-walking and use of canes.

Rehabilitation for the Short-Term Patient

A large number of patients with medical or surgical conditions, particularly those in the younger age groups, are hospitalized for only 4 or 5 days. A short hospitalization period allows the nurse all too little time to develop and execute sound nursing care plans. The short-term patient may need a minimum of restorative services before he can return to a normal life, yet his need for them may be acute. Consequently it is essential that the nurse spend what time she has with the patient purposefully. This requires prompt, systematic assessment of the patient and a plan of action. Purposeful, intelligent teaching, tailored to the patient's needs and level of understanding, can do much to reduce the patient's fears, the stress of the situation, and the time spent in the hospital. Such teaching frequently speeds recovery, both in the hospital and at home, and in some instances will avert a further hospitalization for the same disorder.

The nursing care plan is discussed in another chapter. It is helpful in rehabilitation nursing to prepare an outline of the nursing care plan and to place this outline on a clip board at the foot of the patient's bed or on a small blackboard or bulletin board fastened above the head of the bed where it can be readily seen by all personnel. All members of the nursing and health team are thereby apprised of activities that the patient may do for himself. The patient is encouraged to function independently and personnel are discouraged from doing more for the patient than is to his advantage. *Increasing independence of the patient is a key concept of rehabilitation.*

When preparing such a list, both at the bedside and on the Kardex or other device, the nurse should stress positive concepts. Her outline might include, for example, items such as these:

Can read well using right eye

Can perform abdominal tightening, quadriceps setting, and ankle dorsiflexion exercises

Can lie comfortably in prone position if given assistance in turning

Can raise buttocks off the bed by use of trapeze bar

Can ambulate most easily when holding cane in right hand

Can feed self with use of adaptive spoon

Can irrigate colostomy by sitting in straight chair before toilet

Can administer own insulin if given assistance in reading syringe

Can use telephone and intercommunication system

Can use sliding board to move self into wheel chair (leave board withing reach of patient)

Is a partial aphasic but understands what is said to him

Can use alphabet board to communicate

Has learned to write with left hand

Is learning to type on typewriter at bedside

Can move from wheel chair back to bed

Spouse comes in to assist patient in self-feeding of evening meal

All too often nursing personnel learn vital information concerning the patient but do not record it so that it can be used in a meaningful way. The nurse and members of her team should be expert listeners, skilled in grasping the meaning of all that the patient is trying to convey to them. Much information may also be gathered through nonverbal communication. This pertinent information, compiled in a useful form, may save the patient and the staff much time and frustration as it indicates the patient's abilities and provides direction for nursing care.

Psychological Considerations in Rehabilitation

Earlier in this chapter it was mentioned that the nurse has many opportunities to provide emotional support because of her unique relationship with the patient. The sick individual is a person in trouble. He needs much psychological support. Rehabilitation personnel frequently find that the loss of a limb or a breast is not as disabling as is the mental attitude of the patient, his family, and the hospital staff toward that loss. It is essential that the nurse possess adequate knowledge about general reactions to stress and crippling, so that she can deal with the individual patient's personality and his response to his life experiences. It is logical that the nurse serve as a therapeutic listener. Rarely is a clinical psychologist or psychiatrist available to assist the patient in meeting the problems surrounding illness or surgery. The patient needs to express his fears of the present and future, readjust his self-image, and accept his disability. Only then is he able to make any appreciable strides toward independence and health. The nurse must recognize her limitations and not let herself become deeply emotionally involved with the patient's problems, because if she cannot retain objectivity she will lose her therapeutic usefulness to the patient. She can relay much pertinent information to the physician, who may request assistance from the psychologist or the psychiatrist, if he believes such is indicated. When this is done the nurse may deem it important that she too obtain assistance as to how she and other members of her nursing team can best approach and support the patient.

In most instances the nurse can best serve her patient by maintaining a friendly (objective) approach. Empathy and nonjudgmental listening may provide sufficient emotional support and assistance to the patient for resolution of his emotional reactions to a change in body image due to the loss of a body part and the disfigurement or crippling. The nurse should maintain honesty and a consistent attitude toward the patient. Although, in his efforts to solve his personal problems, he may express hostility toward her, the nurse should continue to accept him. Rejection and recrimination must be avoided at all costs. The loss of nursing support at this time could be detrimental to his recovery. Acceptance of the patient for what he is and feels at each stage in his rehabilitation leads to progress and increased motivation toward attainment of independence and health.

Skin Care

Skin breakdown and partial or total loss of bladder and bowel control may be associated with injury and serious illness. These interfere with rehabilitation, and it is chiefly the nurse's responsibility to prevent, control, and treat them.

The condition of the patient's skin depends upon his age, his general physical condition, his nutritional status, his state of ambulation, the presence or absence of neurological disease or injury, his general muscle tone, and other factors. Debilitating diseases such as diabetes mellitus and generalized arteriosclerosis may make him susceptible to circulatory problems and skin breakdown. A careful examination of the patient's integumentary system at the time of the initial nursing assessment will point up the need for special nursing measures to prevent skin breakdown which might make it necessary to discontinue some portions of the therapeutic program.

If the patient is very thin and his bony prominences stand out, this should be noted, and the color and tone of the skin in these areas should be recorded. Redness over a bony prominence should be noted and nursing orders written to turn the patient every 2 hours until redness disappears. His weight should be kept off the reddened area if possible. The area should be massaged and bathed frequently to stimulate the circulation to local tissue.

The elderly patient may have poor skin tone, and this should be noted. It may be necessary to apply an after-bath oil. The skin may be thin because of atrophy. It may be sallow or muddy and may be wrinkled. Decreased circulation and atrophy can give the skin a pale, shiny appearance. Elevation of an extremity may improve the circulation. The nurse should be extremely careful in turning and moving the patient, as denudation readily occurs and gives rise to decubitus ulcers. The nurse should always try to prevent skin breakdown, rather than cure decubitus ulcers.

Many words have been written on the treatment of decubitus ulcers, yet no treatment is entirely successful. Nursing personnel continue to search for a magic formula for curing decubitus ulcers, but *the best therapy is the prevention of skin breakdown.* This requires planning and consistent effort but is far superior to the prolonged therapy needed for the cure of a decubitus ulcer. The nurse must recognize that most decubitus ulcers are a consequence of poor circulation to the skin and subcutaneous tissues of a local area which reduces nutrients to the cells and inhibits removal of waste products. The poor circulation may be due to blockage of blood to an area, generalized atherosclerosis, or a neurological deficiency. In addition, an adequate intake of protein is essential for the maintenance of an intact integumentary system. The following measures can be used to promote circulation and prevent pressure on body parts:

1. Turning the patient according to a regular schedule, and arranging him in proper alignment at all times. This may be done periodically (every 20 minutes to 2 hours) by turning him from the supine position to side-lying to prone to supine. The patient may be in bed, on an orthopedic frame, or in a CircOlectric bed.

2. Employing a mechanical device such as an alternating pressure mattress or a rocking bed. A rocking bed that has been slowed to a barely perceptible movement has been shown to be most effective in helping to maintain circulation to skin areas sufficient to prevent decubitus ulcer formation.

3. Frequent washing and massaging of the skin, with special consideration when reddened areas have appeared in the skin, keeps irritation of the skin from causing breakdown. The skin must be kept clean or bacterial growth increases. The use of mild soap containing hexachlorophene is advantageous.

4. The use of Diaperene lotion and Diaperene in the laundry with the bed linen has helped to reduce skin irritation in the presence of urinary incontinence. This decreases bacterial breakdown of urinary products into irritating ammoniacal substances.

5. The use of sheepskin, especially in elderly and emaciated patients, reduces pressure over bony prominences. The use of air rings and "donuts" should be discouraged, since they form rings of pressure on the skin and this decreases circulation.

Incontinence

Injury to the spinal cord can cause a neurogenic bladder; the reader is referred to appropriate textbooks for detailed information on treatment of the neurogenic bladder. Less has been written about periodic or partial loss of bladder and/or bowel control. Partial loss of control may prevent the patient from being accepted for rehabilitation training. Nurses and nurse aides should understand the nature of the condition. In many instances partial loss of control is regarded as a result of the patient's willful neglect, but it may be that the patient himself does not understand the cause, and he should not be considered at fault.

Management of the patient with spinal cord injury is clear-cut. In medical disorders that predispose to loss of bowel and/or bladder control the management of incontinence may be a more difficult problem. Several medical disorders may produce varying degrees of neurogenic bladder, disturbed bowel tone, or reduced rectal sphincter control. Partial or periodic loss of control is especially likely to develop in older patients with chronic illness. Diabetes mellitus, for example, may be accompanied by a sufficient degree of neurological involvement to produce bladder atonicity and overflow incontinence. There may be a diminution in sensory function which interferes with the normal voiding mechanism. Frequently, in generalized arteriosclerosis, there is neurogenic involvement causing periodic loss of bowel and bladder control. Cerebral arteriosclerosis may affect the micturition center in the brain and produce periodic loss of control of urination. Incontinence is frequently associated with a cerebrovascular accident which may improve as the patient's general condition improves. With hemiplegia urinary incontinence is frequently periodic because the brain damage is unilateral, affecting the micturition center on one side of the brain, while the other side of the brain and the micturition center are not affected. The nurse should bear in mind that some of these patients will regain control through training, but not all of them will. Each patient with incontinence should undergo a thorough neurological examination so that the nursing program can be based on his physiological condition.

It is a rare adult who does not prefer to maintain complete independence, including control of the urinary bladder and the bowel. Very rarely is incontinence based on psychological disturbances; even in the so-called senile patient there usually is an organic or pathological basis for the incontinence. It is never possible to predict that complete control will be regained.

The lower bowel, the rectum, the detrusor muscle of the bladder, the internal and external urinary sphincters, the penis or the vulva, and the inner aspects of the thighs are innervated by the pudendal nerve plexus whose origin is the sacral plexus. These nerves contain both sensory and motor fibers, so injury to them or disease affecting them can result in incontinence.

During the course of an acute illness urinary incontinence may develop and an indwelling catheter may be inserted to avoid skin irritation from urine constituents, to facilitate nursing care, or to obtain an accurate record of urinary output. Intermittent bladder drainage is utilized to maintain bladder muscle tonicity by preventing overdistention of the bladder, thereby protecting the detrusor muscle. This is accomplished by clamping and unclamping the catheter or connecting drainage tube at specified time intervals to permit periodic filling and emptying of the bladder. (Continuous drainage over a period of time may cause the bladder to skrink to a nonfunctional size.) As the patient's condition improves the physician may consider removing the catheter, and the nurse may be responsible for assessing the patient's ability to control urination. One method for testing the patient's neurological status is to prick the inner aspect of the patient's thighs and the vulva or the base of the penis with a pin. If sensation is present the patient's motor ability is probably present, since the pudendal nerve is a mixed nerve, and he may be able to exercise voluntary control of the urinary sphincters. If sensation is lacking the prognosis for sphincter control is poor.

Methods other than an indwelling catheter should be used when possible. A schedule of periodic attempts to void can be instituted. A commode or toilet rather than a bedpan should be used whenever possible, since this permits the patient to assume the normal posture for voiding, use of abdominal muscles is facilitated, and there is a beneficial psychological effect. When a patient has a progressive disease, it may be necessary to utilize an external catheter and leg urinal (for the male patient), or rubberized pants or incontinent pads (for the female patient), or an indwelling catheter may be employed as the last resort. Fluid intake of at least 2,500 ml is necessary to promote urinary drainage and reduce the possibility of urinary tract infection.

Bowel control may be easier to accomplish than bladder control. The patient should be encouraged to drink at least 250 ml of fluid early in the morning on an empty stomach to stimulate reflex action in the lower bowel. It is helpful to give 60 to 100 ml of prune juice with breakfast. Immediately following breakfast the patient should be placed on a toilet or commode. The sitting position will increase intra-abdominal pressure and facilitate evacuation. If the patient is unable to defecate, a glycerine or bisacodyl (Dulcolax) suppository may be administered as prescribed by the physician. Adequate oral fluid intake should be maintained to ensure that the feces will be soft. The nurse should utilize the patient's evacuation habits in establishing a bowel control regimen. Stool softeners and products that provide bulk, such as psyllium hydrophilic mucilloid (Metamucil), may benefit the patient.

The lower colon is atonic in many elderly patients, and in those who are bedridden the large bowel may be filled with feces. Frequently the patient has diarrhea. The rectum may be impacted. It may be necessary to administer a cathartic along with suppositories to rid the bowel of this fecal matter. The treatment may be carried out over a period of several days. The physician or nurse should perform an abdominal examination followed by a rectal examination. Simple palpation of the abdomen may be sufficient to reveal the presence of a mass in the descending colon, and impaction may be found on rectal examination. An oil enema may be administered, but large fluid enemas should not be given, as they cause distention of the colon and aggravate the problem. A well-planned routine for bladder and bowel care may eventuate in regained control. With this control, the patient will also develop an improved sleep pattern and will experience fewer skin problems.

Bibliography

A Handbook of Rehabilitative Nursing Techniques in Hemiplegia. Kenney Rehabilitation Institute. Minneapolis, 1964.

Allgire, Mildred J. and Ruth R. Denny: *Nurses Can Give and Teach Rehabilitation.* New York: Springer Publishing Co., Inc., 1960.

Asher, Richard A. J.: The Dangers of Going to Bed. *California's Health,* 16:8, October 15, 1958.

Hirschberg, Gerald G., Leon Lewis, and Dorothy Thomas: *Rehabilitation.* Philadelphia: J. B. Lippincott Company, 1964.

Hurd, Georgina G.: Teaching the Hemiplegic Self Care. *American Journal of Nursing,* 62:9:64-68, September, 1962.

Kessler, Henry H.: *Rehabilitation of the Physically Handicapped,* rev. ed. New York: Columbia University Press, 1953.

Larson, Carroll B. and Marjorie Gould: *Calderwood's Orthopedic Nursing,* 6th ed. St. Louis: The C. V. Mosby Company, 1965.

Lowman, Edward W.: *Self Help Devices for the Arthritic.* New York: The Institute of Physical Medicine and Rehabilitation—New York University, 1954.

Madden, Barbara Williams and John E. Affeldt: To Prevent Helplessness and Deformities. *American Journal of Nursing,* 62:12:59-61, December, 1962.

Morrissey, Alice B.: *Rehabilitation Nursing.* New York: G. P. Putnam's Sons, 1951.

Morrissey, Alice B. and Muriel E. Zimmerman: Helps for the Handicapped. *American Journal of Nursing,* 53:3:316-318, March, 1953; 53:4:454-456, April, 1953.

Newton, Kathleen: *Geriatric Nursing,* 4th ed. St. Louis: The C. V. Mosby Company, 1966.

Plaisted, Lena M.: The Clinical Specialist in Rehabilitation. *American Journal of Nursing,* 69:3:562-564, March, 1969.

Skinner, Geraldine: The Nurse—Key Figure in Preventive and Restorative Care. *Hospitals,* 35:52-56, January, 1961.

U.S. Department of Health, Education, and Welfare, Public Health Service: *Strike Back at Stroke.* Washington, D.C.: U. S. Government Printing Office, 1960.

U.S. Department of Health, Education, and Welfare, Public Health Service: *Strike Back at Arthritis.* Washington, D.C.: U. S. Government Printing Office.

Wagner, Berniece: The Nursing Care Plan. *Nursing Outlook,* 9:172, March, 1961.

PART IV
SIGNIFICANT MANIFESTATIONS OF DISEASE REQUIRING NURSING ACTION

PURPOSE

Part IV focuses on the physiological response to disease-producing factors and the various manifestations of imbalance, commonly classified as physical signs and symptoms or unusual behavior. The mechanism of the manifestation is described accompanied by the related medical therapy and nursing care functions.

The intent is to provide the rationale and practical guide for general nursing action to alleviate the manifestations. The content is classified according to a systematic approach that the nurse can use to observe, evaluate, report, and record the patient's manifestations of dysfunction and to use as a basis for arriving at a nursing diagnosis and plan of care.

It is the nurse's responsibility to understand the normal range of well-being and recognize individual differences, as presented in Parts II and III, so that she can recognize deviations from normal or the usual behavior of the patient which are discussed in this section.

The manifestations of imbalance herein discussed can occur when there is pathophysiology in various body systems and may be present in a variety of medical diagnoses. The reader is referred to Part V for specific manifestations of a particular disease and the related specific nursing care.

CHAPTER 10
HOW THE NURSE LEARNS WHICH IMBALANCE IS PRESENT

LOUISE W. MANSFIELD

Observation and Communication

It is highly important that the nurse be able to recognize manifestations of imbalance in the patient's condition. The patient expects the nurse to see and know how he is getting along and whether or not his progress is satisfactory, and to take action as necessary for his protection. The physician also depends on the nurse to know the condition of the patient, to be aware of the signs that indicate a change, to recognize the signs as those associated with improvement or deterioration in the patient's condition, and to take appropriate action to safeguard the patient's welfare. The action may consist of accurately and promptly reporting to the physician any change or the performance of a nursing activity aimed at correcting the imbalance. It might consist of employing a drug or treatment previously prescribed by the physician to be administered by the nurse when, in her opinion, the patient's condition warrants its use.

There are a variety of sources that the nurse should utilize in making her overall assessment of the patient in order to learn about existing imbalances.

THE PATIENT

First and foremost as a source of information is the patient himself. What he says, how he says it, and how he reacts or behaves in the situation are all important clues to be observed and incorporated in making decisions about his plan of care. As well as listening to the patient and observing his behavior, the nurse selectively attends to those stimuli or factors in the situation which are likely to have special significance in relation to the patient's health, while at the same time remaining aware of other events in the situation. By recalling and applying previously acquired knowledge, the nurse decides which factors should be scrutinized and evaluated in a scientific manner. She uses the sense of touch in recognizing temperature, moisture, and palpable characteristics of the patient's body and of situational objects. She depends upon the sense of smell in detecting and discriminating characteristic odors of food, medication, smoke, drainage, and metabolic waste products. Abnormal variations of sound are heard and recognized as physiological clues, moist or labored respirations, the cry of a newborn infant with cerebral birth injury, or a change in the cardiac rhythm recorded on a monitor. By visual perception the nurse observes color, size, and shape of body parts, as well as position of objects in the clinical setting and interprets these in relation to the total situation. She learns to recognize characteristic facial expressions, posture, and body positions that are commonly associated with pain or fatigue or other physical states, and to be alert to the atypical patient or situation in which the ordinary signs are not manifested.

THE FAMILY

The patient's family can also be a valuable source of reference, particularly if the patient is too ill to respond or to provide information. They can add to knowledge concerning the patient's illness, as well as provide information as to his likes and dislikes. The nurse can also use her contact with the family to validate information regarding the patient.

THE PATIENT'S CHART

The patient's chart or record is a written source that can provide several aids to discovering imbalances.

Diagnostic Studies. Reports of laboratory work, x-ray studies, and other studies can sometimes provide the nurse with clues to imbalances. For example, the nurse may observe that the patient's urine appears concentrated, note the laboratory report of increased specific gravity, and take steps to correct this through increasing his oral fluid intake if there are no contraindications by reason of the patient's condition or medical plan for care.

Results of laboratory work may also direct the nurse to notify the physician about medications, such as reports of prothrombin time and need for an anticoagulant.

In addition to guiding her to take direct action, such reports will also add to the nurse's understanding of the patient, as, for instance, an electrocardiographic report stating that there is evidence of digitalis intoxication present.

Physician's History and Physical and Progress Notes. The report of the history and physical examination can provide the nurse with an understanding of the patient and the degree of his illness, as well as the physician's plan of therapy. This should not preclude the nurse's talking with the physician for further exploration and planning, but will give details and background to facilitate the planning with the physician for care of the patient.

Reports of Other Team Members. In addition to the physician's reports in the chart, there may be reports of other persons, such as the social worker, whose notes will aid the nurse in her total understanding of the patient, the situation he comes from, and the environment to which he will return, any or all of which may have contributed to the present imbalance.

Likewise, the report in the chart of the physical therapist's evaluation can provide the nurse with knowledge of physical limitations that need to be considered in the nursing plan of care.

Conversations with Health Team Members. Along with reports of health team members, a verbal exchange can also be a valuable source of information about the patient. Whoever is concerned with the patient and contributing to his care can be helpful to the nurse in her search for knowledge of the patient.

The Use of Problem-Solving in Nursing

The existence or development of physiological or psychological imbalance may or may not represent a nursing problem and require nursing action. The nurse must be able to recognize manifestations of abnormal function and to determine which imbalance is present. She must also then be able to decide whether or not nursing action is required and if so, which nursing actions are most appropriate for the particular patient and situation. Such differentiation requires sequential steps in thinking which are described as *problem-solving*. A detailed discussion of nursing actions appropriate to specific nursing problems arising in medical and surgical disease conditions is found in Part V of this textbook. The steps in problem-solving are presented here since the thought process is the same for our present concern of determining which imbalance is present and for determining appropriate nursing action.

A nursing problem is a need, arising from a condition faced by the patient and/or family, which the nurse can help him or them to meet through the performance of her professional functions. This definition is based on the concept of nursing and the unique function of the nurse as developed by Henderson and others.

The practice of nursing is concerned with problems that affect the health of the patient and family and require direct nursing action, e.g., assisting the patient and family, for their solution. But it must also be recognized that not all problems in a given situation are *nursing* problems. In working with patients and families, the nurse becomes aware of patients' problems that may not be of concern to her as she assists them in meeting their health needs. Some situations involve problems of working relationships between members of the health team, or problems of medical therapy which are related to and may affect the nursing problem but need to be recognized and differentiated from the nursing problem because their solution involves actions other than nursing actions.

STEPS IN PROBLEM-SOLVING

Problem-solving is discussed here as a process of critical thinking which is used in nursing in recognizing imbalances that may be present and deciding *when* nursing action should be taken and *what* nursing action is most appropriate. With continued experience in patient care, the nursing student develops the habit of identifying the problems presented in any situation and thinking through to action based on scientific facts and principles.

The following outline of steps in problem-solving is similar to that described by other writers in education, engineering, and human relations.

1. Recognize, limit, and define the problem or problems presented by the given situation.
2. Collect relevant facts and principles.
3. Formulate alternate courses of action or possible solutions to the problem.
4. Select the best course of action or solution.
5. Follow through on the selected course of action.
6. Evaluate the outcome.

1. Recognize and Define the Problem. It has been said that a problem well defined is half solved. Though the statement may not be quantitatively exact, it emphasizes the importance of the first step in the process. In order to think clearly and think through to a solution one must have the problem clearly defined. This accomplishment is preceded by an awareness or recognition of the existence of the problem, whether an imbalance or a need. A further step may be to limit the scope of the problem or subdivide it into two or more problems in order to provide a clearer statement of the problem and to facilitate critical thinking about it.

Since nursing problems are derived from needs of patients which require nursing action, a useful approach to recognizing and defining the nursing problem in a given situation is to ask, "What are the specific needs of this patient which require nursing action to meet them?" or "What physiological or emotional imbalances are manifested by the patient?" In a complex patient-care situation it is necessary to identify the nursing problem in relation to each need or condition of the patient which requires nursing action. For the beginning student in nursing these problems are best stated in "how to" form which directly calls for nursing action as the solution to each problem.

Examples of problems defined in this manner:

1. How to allay Mrs. A's anxiety regarding the cardiac catheterization procedure?

2. How to assist Mr. B. with bowel elimination with a minimum of physical exertion and emotional stress?

A nursing problem may be defined in different forms according to the thinking of the individual. Problem No. 2 could be stated in an alternate form: How can physical and emotional stress be minimized for Mr. B. in relation to bowel elimination?

Problem recognition requires a total awareness of the situation, the patient, the family, the nurse herself, other personnel, and all factors that are influencing the patient. It requires the use of observation and communication skills for a broad survey of the situation. The number of nursing problems for any patient is determined by the extent of his needs and the complexity of his situation.

2. Collect Relevant Facts and Principles. Much of the essential information used in solving a nursing problem will have been previously learned in formal education and by experience in caring for patients. Thus, some recall of previously acquired scientific knowledge pertinent to the situation occurs almost simultaneously with recognition of the problem and is used in arriving at a clear definition of the problem. This is followed by conscious recall of additional relevant information and a determination of the need for further information from other sources.

In some situations the nursing problem requires immediate decision and nursing action. In this case, decision and action are based entirely on present knowledge of the situation with recall and application of previously learned facts and principles. A science principle has been defined as generally accepted fact or a fundamental truth that can be used as a guide to action (Nordmark and Rohweder) and as "a delineation of a relationship between two facts that explains phenomena, guides actions and predicts outcomes of actions" (Wandelt). It is the professional nurse's available knowledge of the scientific facts and principles which prepares her for the responsibility and the task of making on-the-spot decisions in solving nursing problems. She also uses observation and communication skills in collecting pertinent information from the patient and family.

When the solution of a nursing problem does not call for immediate decision and action or when the problem is likely to present itself repeatedly, the nurse obtains additional information from other sources in order to plan the best course of action. She uses literature of nursing, medicine, and the biological and behavioral sciences, and the sources described earlier in this chapter.

3. Formulate Alternate Courses of Action or Possible Solutions to the Problem. At this stage in the solution of a nursing problem, the nurse considers available information relevant to the problem and looks for principles that point or guide her to a specific course of action. One or more pertinent facts from the patient situation may guide her to a course of action, or these facts along with relevant principles from basic sciences may point to an appropriate solution for the problem at hand.

The definitions of science principles stated earlier imply that a nurse should be able to consider facts and principles relevant to a given situation and, by the process of deductive thinking, recognize a course of action based on scientific principles.

The identification of alternate solutions to a nursing problem before the final determination of a course of action is a most important step toward ensuring better care for the individual patient. This step in problem-solving also provides for the improvement of patient care in general by developing better methods, better equipment, and better ways for nursing personnel to work together. Improvement in patient care goes hand-in-hand with problem-solving based on scientific principles. For example, in a given situation the problem, "How is a moist, sterile compress applied," is better answered by a scientifically developed procedure for the specific setting than by the statement, "This is how we do it here." The procedure will provide for the use of selected and tested equipment and a procedural method based on scientific principles. Such scientific development of method ensures the effectiveness of the procedure as well as the safety and comfort of the patient.

When the nursing problem requires immediate decision and action the consideration of alternate solutions becomes an on-the-spot mental process of recalling scientific facts and principles that are relevant to the situation and recognizing the possible courses of action. With these possible courses of action in mind, one is ready to take the next step—selecting the best or most reasonable course of action for helping the patient in the situation. *Situation* is used here to include the physical setting, the patient with his personality, physical condition, and health problem, the family, the staff, and all factors which affect the solution to the problem.

4. Select the Best Course of Action or Solution. The selection of the best or most appropriate nursing actions to meet the needs recognized in the defined nursing problem requires critical thinking and decision-making. The decision will take into consideration all situational factors and may require the nurse to make some value judgments relative to the patient's welfare and rehabilitation potential. The selection of one best course of action from two or more alternatives usually requires further application of scientific principles and additional factual information from the patient. It may even require a restatement of the problem and another survey of the situation. At this state of problem-solving one needs and appreciates the science principle or nursing principle that clearly states a relationship between two things and predicts outcomes. The nurse must be able to predict the outcome of her actions before she can decide and follow through. At the present stage in the development of nursing science there are too few nursing literature sources that make needed scientific knowledge available in the form of principles readily usable in problem solving. And those which are available as principles—statements which may guide to action—rarely predict the outcome. The nursing student often finds that she must formulate available scientific knowledge into her own statement of a principle that guides to action. Whether by available principles or through her own organization of scientific knowledge in order to show relationships and predict outcomes, the nurse must now compare and contrast the possible solutions, weigh the probabilities, and make an important decision. As a professional nurse she also assumes the responsibility for her decision. She is then ready to follow through with the selected course of action.

5. *Follow Through with the Selected Course of Action.* As the nurse performs those nursing actions which were selected as the best solution to the problem, she continues to observe the patient and the situation. Through this contact with the patient she may note essential information that was not available before. The patient's condition may change or other important factors of the situation may change within a few minutes' time. These changes may necessitate a reconsideration of the selected plan of action. They might indicate that one of the alternatives is now the plan of choice, or they may require restatement of the nursing problem itself. These changing aspects of the nursing situation demand that the nurse be an astute and continual observer as she works with the patient.

This observation of the patient and the situation also provides the means of evaluating the outcome of the selected plan of action, which is the last step in the process of problem solving.

6. *Evaluate the Outcome.* The final step in problem-solving seeks to answer the question: "How effective were these nursing actions in helping the patient with the need out of which the problem arose?" Did the cooperative action of nurse and patient resolve the need or tend to restore balance in a system that had been in a state of imbalance? If the problem was concerned with patient comfort, how comfortable was he after the selected nursing action? If the problem related to fluid balance, what was the patient's state of hydration following the selected plan of action? Suppose the nursing problem with a helpless patient was that of preventing decubitus ulcers. How successful was the plan? What criteria may be used in a day-to-day evaluation of the effectiveness of the plan?

Scientific evaluation of the effectiveness of nursing care has developed as a product of recognition of the independent functions of nursing. The opportunity for improvement in nursing care, whether for the individual patient or as a general goal of nursing, is lost if the solution to the nursing problem is not evaluated and these results are not used.

After defining a nursing problem, thinking it through, and taking appropriate action based on scientific principles, the nurse will find that evaluating the outcome is not as easy as checking the answer to an algebra problem in the back of the book. However, in either case a failure to do so results in repetition of errors.

It should be noted that the thought processes used in problem-solving do not always proceed in a straight line from definition of the problem to the selection of the most appropriate plan and action on it. There is often a circular process of returning to previous steps for redefinition of the problem and seeking further information and further use of scientific principles as guides to action and selection of the best course of action. The following situation illustrates this process of continued observation, Step 2, and redefinition of the nursing problem, Step 1, while the nurse is selecting a solution or acting upon a selected solution.

PROBLEM-SOLVING SITUATION

At the scene of an accident a nursing student found no one assisting an unconscious young man whose pulse was perceptible but who was cyanotic and apneic. These observed facts indicated his need for respiratory assistance. The student's recall of scientific knowledge regarding brain cell damage with pro- longed hypoxia and the relative efficiency of various methods of artificial res- piration guided her to the appropriate action of instituting mouth-to-mouth ventilation without delay. In checking the mouth for a clear airway, she dis- covered that blood was present in the oropharynx, but the patient then clenched his teeth so firmly she could not open them again to remove this blood. The nursing problem, which had been, "How can I assist the patient's respiratory efforts?" had now to be defined in relation to the two alternatives and their associated risks. Should the student attempt to ventilate the patient's lungs despite the risk of complications that might result from aspiration, or should she position him with his head lower than his chest to favor drainage before proceeding with mouth-to-mouth resuscitation? In making this decision, she recalled that the cells of the cerebral cortex may be damaged after as little as 30 seconds' oxygen deprivation and may be irreparably damaged after 5 minutes' oxygen deprivation. The fact of obvious cyanosis, due to a reduction in the hemoglobin content of the blood, indicated that the patient had been apneic for a few minutes. Ventilation must be provided by some means with all possible haste. The student weighed the possible consequences of brain damage against those of pulmonary complications and decided that the latter posed a lesser threat to the patient's welfare. She could not delay to position the patient; she elevated his chin and proceeded with mouth-to-mouth ventilation. She was able to force air into his lungs and after a few breaths he began to breathe spontaneously.

The student used observed situational information and her recall of scientific facts and principles as guides to alternative actions. She then made further ob- servations and used the additional information gained thereby and other scientific principles in selecting the best course of action, i.e., immediate mouth-to-mouth ventilation. When she attempted to follow through on the selected plan of action the complication of foreign material being present in the airway was recognized. This new situation required reconsideration of the original problem in relation to possible complications, and a decision regarding loss of time to position the patient. Immediate evaluation of the outcome indicated that she was successful in assisting his respiratory efforts, thereby reducing the danger of further brain damage from hypoxia. Nonetheless, the student recognized that injury to the cerebral cortex could result, since the length of the period of apnea was not known and the patient was cyanotic when found.

Bibliography

Abdellah, Faye G., Almeda Martin, Irene L. Beland, and Ruth V. Matheney: *Patient-Centered Approaches to Nursing.* New York: The Macmillan Company, 1960.

Harmer, Bertha and Virginia Henderson: *Textbook of the Principles and Practice of Nursing,* 5th ed. New York: The Macmillan Company, 1955.

Henderson, Virginia: The Nature of Nursing. *American Journal of Nursing,* 64:8:62–68, August, 1964.

Nordmark, Madelyn Titus and Anne W. Rohweder: *Science Principles Applied to Nursing,* 2d ed. Philadelphia: J. B. Lippincott Company, 1967.

Wandelt, Mabel: Quest for the Elusive Principle. *Nursing Outlook,* 12:5; 48, May, 1964.

CHAPTER 11

PHYSIOLOGICAL RESPONSES TO DISEASE-PRODUCING AGENTS

PAULINE BRUNO*

* Dr. George Martin, Associate Professor, Department of Pathology, University of Washington, reviewed this chapter and made valuable suggestions. Dolly Ito, Assistant Professor, School of Nursing, Seattle University, and Janet Erickson, formerly Assistant Professor, University of California School of Nursing, served as consultants.

The physiological response to harmful agents is a complex series of dynamic changes set into motion by an initiating agent in conjunction with contributing factors and may terminate in restoration of structure and function, in adjustment to permanent structural and/or functional changes, or in death. By means of adaptive mechanisms, the body attempts to overcome or adjust to the damaging effects of harmful agents and restore structural and functional balance. Responses of the body to injury are related to the concept of cellular and humoral basis of disease. Injurious agents disrupt normal cell metabolic processes, and the products of metabolic disturbances are spread throughout the body through the medium of interstitial and vascular fluid. This concept helps to explain why diverse injurious agents may stimulate a common type of response.

Reaction to injury may have a rapid onset, as occurs with physical trauma and some infections, or the process may progress slowly over a period of years, as happens in some blood vessel disorders. When the process is slow and the body compensates for the defect, the individual is often unaware that the disorder is present. The reaction to injury may be of a permanent nature, that is, once damage has been inflicted, that process cannot be reversed. If the response is temporary, it may be reversible or reparable. Structural changes in the cells of the wall of blood vessels are permanent, whereas a break in the continuity of bone is reparable. Response may also be considered in relation to the local reaction (reaction at the site of injury), and the systemic reaction (the total body reactions throughout the nervous system and humoral responses).

Responses may be either specific to or characteristic of a causative agent or a common, nonspecific reaction to injury. Characteristic tissue responses occur in tuberculous lesions and the rash of scarlet fever, but these and most responses include certain basic common denominators. The inflammatory response is an example of a common denominator.

The response mechanisms selected for discussion in this chapter are those encountered most frequently in nursing and are the neuroendocrine responses, inflammatory response, responses to alterations in blood volume, and cellular responses (hypertrophy, atrophy, neoplasia). The remainder of the chapter will focus on these basic pathologic processes, the various agents that may initiate a particular process, and the aims of medical and nursing therapy.

Neuroendocrine Responses

The terms *injury*, *trauma*, and *stress* are used interchangeably to refer to any condition or situation that is a threat to the well-being of the individual, whether physical or psychological, and either an actuality or perceived as such by the individual.

CAUSATIVE AGENTS

Factors that may initiate neuroendocrine responses of varying degree and duration are injuries of a physical, chemical, biological, or psychological nature. Examples of these injuries are intense heat or cold, forceful blows, surgery, loss of blood volume, internal or external chemical poisons, infections, and psychological stresses such as speaking before a group of people and as a nursing student being assigned to care for a critically ill patient.

The person who is sick often perceives the illness as a threat to his well-being and becomes fearful. The fear as well as the disease process may stimulate neuroendocrine responses. Factors that seem to intensify the degree of neuroendocrine response are fear, apprehension, pain, extent and type of trauma (e.g., bone injury and burns), presence of high fever, youth, and a preinjury state of good nutrition. Young, well-nourished males respond more intensely than do women, elderly persons, and poorly nourished individuals. A nurse can expect that patients will differ in the manifestations of neuroendocrine response because of the presence or absence of some of these influencing factors. Patients need individualized nursing care to support and keep the response within desired limits.

Some situations commonly encountered in nursing in which the patient may manifest signs and symptoms of neuroendocrine responses are on admission to the hospital, throughout a surgical experience, during diagnostic tests, and when seriously ill. The operative procedure is usually a relatively controlled stressful experience, as contrasted with the stress of accidental injury, overwhelming bacterial invasions, or sudden psychological trauma.

RESPONSE MECHANISMS

In 1914, Dr. W. B. Cannon demonstrated that the adrenal medulla responded to threatening situations of fear, hunger, pain, and rage with a release of epinephrine (adrenalin) and, as later determined, norepinephrine (noradrenalin). Epinephrine and norepinephrine produce effects similar to those obtained by stimulation of the sympathetic nervous system. This mobilization of body reserves was labeled the *fight or flight* reaction, since it provides the energy and blood flow needed to fight an aggressor or flee from the danger. For instance, one may retreat quickly from the path of an oncoming car (flight) and in the event of bodily invasion by pathogenic organisms fight by producing antibodies. Since Cannon's initial work, research has enlarged the scope of knowledge regarding neuroendocrine responses.

Dr. Hans Selye did much of the research on the stress syndrome or, as he labeled it, *the general adaptation syndrome*. This response is thought to be brought into play with the occurrence of either external or internal exaggerated change, that is, a change not within the realm of normal for the individual. The injurious agents have a common feature, that of acting as stress on the body as a whole. The general adaptation syndrome is thought to evolve in three stages: (1) the alarm reaction, during which the defensive forces are mobilized, (2) the stage of resistance, which reflects full adaptation to the stressor (the individual adapts and reestablishes balance), and (3) the stage of exhaustion, which inexorably follows if the stressor is severe enough and applied for a sufficient length of time, since the adaptation energy or adaptability of a living being is always finite.

Sympathoadrenal Medullary Response

The sympathoadrenal medullary response is an almost immediate protective reaction to injury. The functional changes are brought about by the action of epinephrine and norepinephrine. It is thought that the harmful agent stimulates receptor nerve endings, causing transmission of nerve impulses to the cerebral cortex where they are interpreted. Impulses are then sent to the hypothalamus and, via the autonomic nervous system, to arterioles and to the adrenal medulla. Norepinephrine is released at postganglionic sympathetic nerve endings in effector organs. The adrenal medulla responds with an increased secretion of epinephrine and norepinephrine into the bloodstream, augmenting that produced by the sympathetic nervous system. These hormones have a sympathomimetic effect of stimulating contraction of muscles in the walls of arterioles in the skin and mucous membrane and of dilating coronary and skeletal muscle and lung arterioles. Dilatation of these arterioles increases blood flow to meet cell needs resulting from an increased metabolic rate. Constriction of skin and mucous membrane arterioles increases peripheral resistance and narrows the pulse pressure, thereby helping to maintain blood pressure and to shunt blood to other parts of the body.

Epinephrine stimulates heart muscle to contract more forcefully and rapidly, increasing cardiac output and contributing to maintenance of blood pressure and to meeting the demands of tissues for oxygen. Carbon dioxide-oxygen exchange in the lungs is increased because epinephrine relaxes smooth muscle of lung bronchioles, the bronchioles dilate, and alveolar ventilation increases. There is need for increased gas exchange because of the increased metabolic rate of most cells of the body. Glucose is made available to muscle for the performance of work by an action of epinephrine which promotes conversion of liver glycogen to glucose (glycogenolysis) and causes a rise in blood level. The radial muscles of the iris are stimulated by epinephrine, resulting in dilatation of the pupil and increased visual acuity. Increased perspiration may occur since sweat glands are innervated by the sympathetic nervous system. By contrast with these accelerated body activities, there is depression of muscle activity along the gastrointestinal tract, resulting in a slowing down of digestive processes and intestinal peristalsis. These effects of sympathoadrenal medullary response to trauma are manifested in signs and symptoms that give the doctor and nurse evidence of what is happening and on which therapy is based. It is evident that some of these manifestations are an increase in pulse rate and force; increased blood pressure; restlessness; dilated pupils; cold, pale, moist skin; decreased appetite; and perhaps abdominal distention. (See Figure 11–1.) The sympathoadrenal medullary response is usually a relatively short-term response that protects the body in emergency situations. There is individual variation in the frequency of stimulation of this phase of neuroendocrine response and in the degree of intensity of the response. In relatively severe injuries the cortical portion of the adrenal gland plays a vital role.

Adrenocortical Response

Increased production of certain cortical hormones is an essential response to injury for the maintenance of life and repair of damaged tissues. The hormones are the

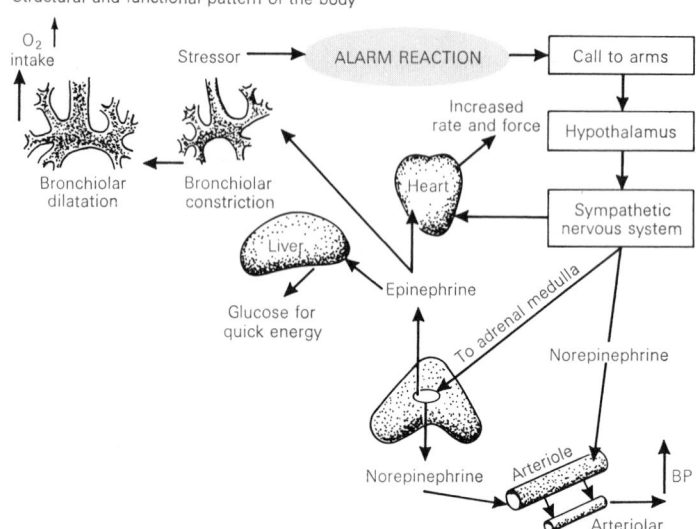

Structural and functional pattern of the body

Figure 11–1
The sympathetic-adrenal
medullary responses to
stressors. (By permission
of Katherine J. Bordicks:
Patterns of Shock. New
York: The Macmillan
Company, 1965, p. 29.)

glucocorticoids, such as cortisone and hydrocortisone, and the mineralocorticoids, such as deoxycorticosterone acetate (DOCA) and aldosterone. Secretion of the hormones by the adrenal cortex is thought to be regulated by other hormones released in particular areas of the brain. Stimulation of the adenohypophysis (anterior pituitary) by the blood level of corticotropin-releasing factor in the hypophyseal portal system results in the release of adrenocorticotropic hormone (ACTH). The adrenal cortex responds to ACTH with an increased secretion of glucocorticoids and, in particular, cortisol (hydrocortisone).

Metabolic responses to the increased production of glucocorticoids are (1) gluconeogenesis, (2) an increased rate of protein catabolism, and (3) increased rate of fat catabolism. The mechanisms by which these effects are obtained are unknown at this time. Increased catabolism of protein in body cells may provide injured tissues with necessary amino acids for synthesis of other compounds necessary for cell life. It is known that liver cells can use the mobilized amino acids to form new proteins and glucose. The increased formation of glucose is sometimes evidenced in hyperglycemia and glycosuria. A drop in eosinophil count below the normal 2 to 4 percent of total white cells parallels the increased secretion of glucocorticoids. The reason for this is not known at this time. Increased protein catabolism leads to a negative nitrogen balance; the extent of nitrogen loss seems to be directly related to the severity of the injury. Urinary nitrogen excretion may range from 12 to 25 g per day (normal 10 to 12 g). A less intense response occurs in elderly, malnourished individuals than in young, healthy ones. The state of negative nitrogen balance reverses itself as the person progresses toward recovery from injury. The purpose of these metabolic responses is thought to be to provide cells with a ready supply of compounds needed for energy and for synthesis of substances vital to various tissues of the body.

Regulation of secretion of the mineralocorticoids is thought to be by glomerulotropin, a hormone released from neuronal centers in either the diencephalon or mesencephalon. The neuronal centers respond to one or more of three conditions: (1) an above-normal extracellular concentration of potassium, (2) a below-normal extracellular concentration of sodium, and (3) a below-normal extracellular fluid volume. Any or all three of these conditions may be present in a variety of traumatic situations. For instance, hemorrhage or severe blood loss with surgery may so decrease the extracellular fluid volume and the sodium concentration that these changes stimulate the mechanisms that promote secretion of mineralocorticoids, particularly aldosterone.

The major effects of aldosterone in the early post-trauma period are increased reabsorption of sodium and chloride by the kidney tubules and decreased potassium reabsorption. Sodium reabsorption stimulates the thirst drive and the affected person drinks fluids, if this is possible. This action replenishes the decrease in circulating volume and prevents excess concentration of sodium. Reabsorption of water usually accompanies sodium reabsorption. Excessive sodium and chloride reabsorption and potassium excretion may precipitate acid-base imbalance unless other regulatory mechanisms are functioning adequately. The goal of mineralocorticoid activity is maintenance of fluid and electrolyte balance. This is also a purpose of the antidiuretic hormone secreted by the neurohypophysis.

Neurohypophyseal Hormone

Antidiuretic hormone (ADH) is thought to be formed in certain portions of the hypothalamus and transported along nerve fibers to cells of the neurohypophysis (posterior pituitary) where it is stored. When extracellular fluid becomes more concentrated than normal, specialized nerve cells in the hypothalamus become excited and transmit impulses to the neurohypophysis. This gland responds by releasing antidiuretic hormone into the bloodstream. ADH acts on cells of the distal and collecting renal tubules to increase their premeability to water. This action conserves water and dilutes the extracellular fluid. For instance, surgical trauma may cause a loss of extracellular fluid without a corresponding loss of electrolytes or plasma proteins. In response to this condition, nerve impulses are transmitted to the neurohypophysis and ADH is released. Conversely, when extracellular fluid concentration drops below normal, the response is a depression of nerve impulses and of the secretion of ADH. The effect of this response is increased water loss through the kidneys. ADH acts in conjunction with other hormones to maintain fluid and electrolyte balance. (See Figure 11-2.)

AIMS OF THERAPY

The broad aims of medical and nursing therapy are prevention of an imbalanced neuroendocrine response to injury and support of the normal defense reactions. This therapy is based on knowledge of situations that might precipitate the response, knowledge of factors that intensify the reaction, and understanding of the response mechanisms. For instance, the alarm reaction may be stimulated when the surgeon informs the patient that surgery is indicated and may be manifested as a transitory increase in heart rate, blood pressure, and perspiration. The degree and duration of response would be influenced by the patient's personality and past experiences,

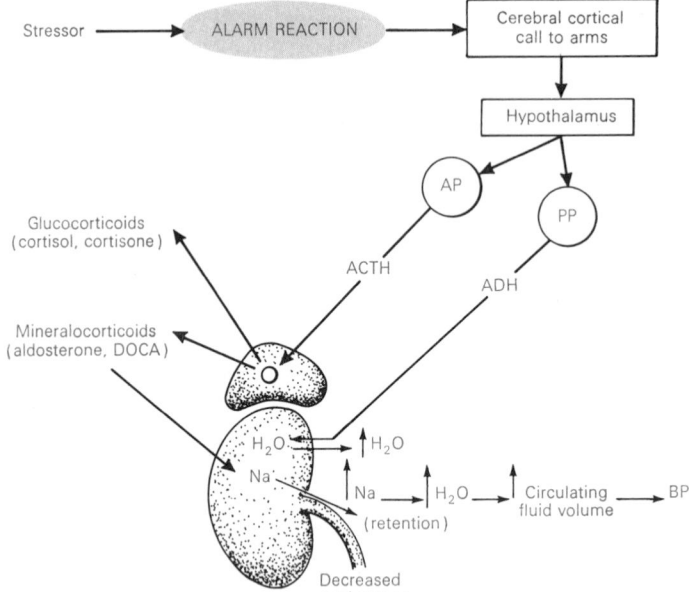

Stressor ⟶ ALARM REACTION ⟶ Cerebral cortical call to arms

Hypothalamus

AP

PP

Glucocorticoids (cortisol, cortisone)

Mineralocorticoids (aldosterone, DOCA)

ACTH

ADH

H_2O

H_2O

Na^+

$Na \longrightarrow H_2O \longrightarrow$ Circulating fluid volume $\longrightarrow$ BP
(retention)

Decreased renal output

*Figure 11–2
The adrenocortical and
ADH responses to stres-
sors. (By permission of
Katherine J. Bordicks:
Patterns of Shock. New
York: The Macmillan
Company, 1965, p. 34.)*

by the physical problem necessitating surgery, and by the explanation given by the surgeon and office nurse of the surgical and hospital procedures. Encouraging the patient to verbalize his reaction to the physical problem and the forthcoming operative experience will help to decrease fear and anxiety. Apprehension is known to intensify the neuroendocrine response. Drugs are used in some situations to reduce anxiety and depress the adrenal medullary response. Sedatives, preoperative analgesics, and cerebral depressants decrease cerebral sensitivity to stimuli which in turn may decrease the degree of neuroendocrine and metabolic responses.

Postsurgical evidence of neuroendocrine and metabolic reaction of the body to trauma may last from 4 to 20 days or longer, depending upon the extensiveness of the operative procedure and individual variations in perception of and reaction to surgery. The effect of adrenocorticoid activity is catabolism of protein tissue and a negative nitrogen balance, increased potassium loss in the urine, retention of sodium and water, and oliguria. Concurrent with these changes, the sympathetic response depresses cellular function along the gastrointestinal tract and there is a decrease or lack of peristalsis; the patient is listless, has no interest in his surroundings, and has little or no appetite. When the patient is able to eat, nutrition becomes an aspect of therapy. The protein that has been broken down by the action of glucocorticoids must be replaced by body cells.

The surgeon evaluates what the patient is attempting to do for himself and plans for supportive therapy, such as administration of intravenous fluids with the addition of potassium chloride, the use of nasogastric suction to prevent distention due to lack of peristalsis, and the use of analgesics for the relief of the stress of pain. The nurse assists the doctor in evaluating what the patient is attempting to do for himself by observing and reporting signs and symptoms of the effectiveness of the neuroendocrine response, such as intake and output, vital signs, and self-activity.

Neuroendocrine responses are general body reactions to nonspecific injurious agents. The purposes of the response are assumed to be maintenance of fluid and electrolyte balance, and provision of body cells with nutrients for energy and for repair of damaged tissues. While these responses involve the total organism, the body also has a local response to nonspecific injurious agents, namely, inflammation.

Inflammatory Response

Inflammation is a dynamic process involving cellular and vascular responses to tissue injury by diverse injurious agents. The well-known manifestations of inflammation (heat, redness, and swelling) are caused by the vascular component of the inflammatory response. These signs are observable when the injury is to external body tissues. Although not directly observable, the same responses and signs occur with internal tissue injury. Inflammation of a part is designated by the suffix -*itis*. For instance, the word *hepatitis* means inflammation of the liver.

The purposes of the inflammatory response are to neutralize or destroy the inciting agent and to promote repair of damaged tissues. Coordinated cellular and vascular changes usually make it possible to accomplish these goals. The response

Figure 11-3 Outline of inflammatory response. (By permission of Howard C. Hopps: Principles of Pathology. New York: Appleton Century Crofts, 1964, p. 186.)

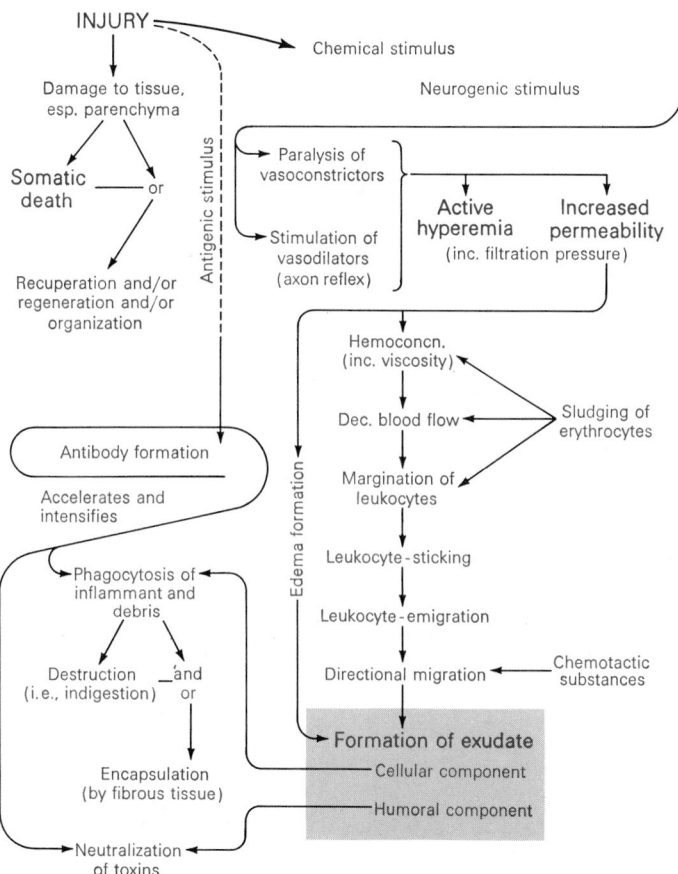

is a commonly occurring defense mechanism that is essential for the maintenance of life. Without this mechanism the human organism would be defenseless against the many potentially harmful agents in the environment. The inflammatory response is outlined in Figure 11-3.

CAUSATIVE AGENTS AND EFFECTS

The stimuli for the inflammatory process are chemical substances released by injured tissues. Any tissue injury causes some inflammatory response. The known sources of tissue injury include extrinsic agents of a physical, biological, and chemical nature, intrinsic agents, and a combination of extrinsic and intrinsic agents. Examples of extrinsic etiologic agents are excesses of heat and cold, ionizing radiation, physical force, smoke, gas fumes, acids and alkalies, and toxins from pathogenic organisms. Some intrinsic agents are excesses of digestive enzymes and breakdown products from dead tissue. The well-known inflammation that occurs with an allergy is of both extrinsic and intrinsic origin. The allergen or antigen is of extrinsic origin, but the antibody is intrinsic. All these agents cause cell damage. Antigen-antibody reactions and pathogens will be emphasized in the following discussion because of some special characteristics of inflammation caused by these agents.

Principal *extrinsic* instigators of the inflammatory response are pathogens. The specific characteristics of pathogens which are different from characteristics of most other extrinsic causative agents are (1) proliferation in human tissues, thereby providing a constant source of toxins and a prolonged duration of injurious action; (2) liberation of substances that interfere with the action of phagocytic cells, and (3) ability to travel and reproduce, permitting spread throughout the body.

Intrinsic factors that may incite an inflammatory response are (1) cell deprivation of oxygen and nutrients, (2) inadequate removal from interstitial spaces of products of cell metabolism, (3) presence of abnormal substances in blood and interstitial fluids, and (4) presence of insufficient or excessive amounts of normal substances in body fluids. These situations may result from insufficient blood flow to or from a body part and from altered function of particular tissues.

The effects of inadequate blood flow are interference with nutrient and oxygen supply to tissues, depression of metabolism and functional activity of cells, and inadequate removal of metabolic waste products, including carbon dioxide, from interstitial spaces. Hypoxia and accumulation of toxic waste products provide the chemical stimulus for inflammation. Interference with blood flow can occur in many disorders. An example of this is obstruction within a vessel, such as a thrombus (intravascular clot). Myocardial infarction (death of an area of heart muscle) is frequently caused by thrombus occlusion of a coronary vessel. The accumulation of products of cell death initiates an inflammatory response. Inflammation of intrinsic source occurs when tissues occasionally produce toxic metabolic products for no known reason.

The combined actions of *extrinsic* and *intrinsic* substances that result in tissue injury are the antigen-antibody complexes. The basis for the action is the ability of an antigen to incite antibody production by particular cells. Once antibody has been produced it reacts with its homologous antigen in a highly specific manner. The basis for immunity from some infectious diseases is the ability of specific antibody to combine with its bacterial antigen and neutralize or prevent bacterial action. This type of antigen-antibody reaction, as will be recalled from the study of microbiology and physiology, is known as *immunity*. The effects of antigen-antibody reaction are (1) to alter the biological activity of the antigen, such as neutralizing bacterial toxins, (2) to form clusters of antigen-antibody complexes which act as foreign bodies and attract phagocytic leukocytes or interfere with tissue nutrition, and (3) to stimulate enzyme systems within cells resulting in the release of histamine and other chemical compounds. The last effect heightens the inflammatory process and is particularly important in the hypersensitive type of antigen-antibody reactions, whereas the first two effects occur most often in immunity. The first two effects may occur so quickly following invasion by pathogenic organisms that the inflammatory reaction to these potentially harmful agents is very mild or almost nonexistent, since the pathogens are not allowed to exert their harmful effects on tissues.

The beneficial nature of immunity is in contrast to the apparently detrimental nature of hypersensitivity, though both are antigen-antibody reactions. In some hypersensitive reactions the antibodies are thought to represent an abnormal hereditary reaction to normal environmental antigen. Hay fever and bronchial asthma are the best known of these disorders. This tendency to become sensitive to a particular pollen, dust, food, or other allergen is a lifetime characteristic. If the allergen is continuously present in the environment, it becomes a constant source of stimuli for the inflammatory response. The site of greatest antigen-antibody concentration is termed the *shock organ* and is usually the site of antigen penetration, such as the nasal mucosa in hay fever. The resulting tissue injury causes the characteristic inflammatory response of hay fever (swollen nasal mucous membrane and increased mucous secretions).

Other hypersensitive reactions are apparently the result of normal response to unusual stimuli. These antigen-antibody reactions occur within a short period of time following a second or subsequent inoculation with the sensitizing antigen. Antigenic substances do not incite antibody formation in all human beings; immunologically competent cells of an individual do not respond to every antigen with the production of antibody. For example, some, but not all, persons develop antibodies to penicillin and will have an antigen-antibody reaction of varying intensity to a second or subsequent administration of the drug. The stimulus for the reaction is thought to be tissue injury from the antigen-antibody complex. The intensity of the inflammatory response varies directly with the intensity of the tissue injury.

In antigen-antibody reactions the inciting antigen is usually a substance foreign to the individual, but in some disorders it appears that the antigen is a factor within the body which becomes antigenic. These disorders are known as *autosensitive diseases*. One theory of causation is that there may be an alteration in tissue protein as a result of chemical changes in the body, and the changed protein is then capable of stimulating antibody production. This antigen material contained within a person's own tissues becomes a chronic source of stimulus for inflammation. One rather common disorder that may be of this nature is rheumatoid arthritis. There are currently many unknown factors in regard to the causation and mechanisms of development of autosensitive reactions.

RESPONSE MECHANISMS

The three components of the inflammatory response are vascular changes, formation of exudate, and cellular activity. These changes are the basis for the manifestations of inflammation, and underlie supportive and restorative medical and nursing therapy.

Vascular changes start immediately after injury. The first response is an immediate, transient vasoconstriction that decreases blood flow at the local area of injury. This response is apparent only under experimental conditions and is rapidly reversed to vasodilatation. Chemical agents that stimulate vascular responses include histamine, which is released by granules in basophilic or mast cells, and bradykinin, an enzyme present in plasma and other substances. Histamine is thought to excite a local axon reflex that stimulates arteriole and capillary dilatation in the injured area. The action of histamine seems to be most pronounced immediately after injury. Opening up of closed capillaries and dilatation of the central capillary bed increases the blood flow in the area and increases hydrostatic pressure in the vessels. Increased hydrostatic pressure forces more than the usual amount of fluid into interstitial spaces. Usually about an hour after the initiation of the inflammatory process the flow of blood slows down even below the normal rate, but the dilatation of vessels continues. Venule constriction is thought to occur, elevating hydrostatic pressure at the venule end of the capillary and inhibiting movement of interstitial fluid back into vessels. As fluid is lost to interstitial spaces, cellular concentrations in the blood increase, the blood becomes more viscous, and rapidity of flow decreases. The blood cells become closely packed, especially in the capillaries, and stasis of blood may occur. An increase in the amount of blood in vessels is termed *hyperemia* or *congestion*.

The second component of the inflammatory response is *formation of exudate*. The term *exudate* refers to extravascular formation of plasma fluid, cellular elements, and proteins. The formation of exudate begins almost immediately and continues for a few days, depending upon the extent and severity of trauma. It results from the increased hydrostatic pressure, capillary permeability, and osmotic pressure of interstitial tissues. Normally, the movement of water and solutes such as salt, glucose, amino acids, albumin, and other small molecules across the capillary wall is balanced by the return flow into the blood and lymph vessels. There is a constant movement of interstitial fluid, but no excess accumulation in this space. Increased capillary permeability permits the large protein molecules, fibrinogen and globulin, to move into the interstitial spaces. This increases the osmotic pressure of tissue fluid, which acts in conjunction with the increased hydrostatic pressure to promote movement of plasma fluid into interstitial spaces. Loss of protein from the circulating blood decreases capillary osmotic pressure which normally acts at the venule end of the capillary to draw interstitial fluid back into the vascular bed. The effectiveness of plasma osmotic pressure is lessened when plasma protein moves into interstitial spaces. The imbalance in forces controlling the movement of plasma results in edema, an excess of fluid in interstitial spaces. Such edema may be manifested as a localized swelling. The height of inflammation may occur many hours and even days after initial injury. The exudate serves to dilute the toxic cell metabolites elaborated by injured tissues and bacteria (if they are present). Inflammatory exudate examined in the laboratory is found to have a high protein count, a high specific gravity, perhaps a few red blood cells, and many white blood cells. Some of the proteins present in the exudate may be from the breakdown of injured cells and loss of cytoplasmic protein, but most are plasma proteins due to increased capillary permeability.

Vasodilatation, increased blood supply, and increased capillary permeability explain some of the manifestations of inflammation, namely, rubor (redness), calor (heat), tumor (swelling), and pain. A throbbing type of pain may be present if the congestion is severe and the pulsating wave from heart contraction is the propulsive force. The chemical mediators of vasodilatation and increased vessel permeability are thought to stimulate sensory nerve endings in the area, resulting in pain. One method of preventing excessive congestion and swelling may be obtained by applications of cold in the early postinjury period. Cold stimulates vasoconstriction, and to varying extent offsets the normal vasodilatation response and inhibits edema formation.

The swelling that is apparent at the site of inflammation is caused by distention of interstitial tissue with inflammatory exudate as well as by hyperemia. Accumulation of inflammatory exudate may have two detrimental effects on cells in the area. (1) The rate of transfer of oxygen and nutrients to cells and of waste products from cells to the blood is slowed down. The increased quantity of interstitial fluid increases the distance substances must travel to reach cells, and nutrition may be impaired. (2) Excess interstitial fluid may cause compression of tissues and interference with their function. In inflammation of the lung, for example, compression of blood vessels, which impairs blood flow, can result in interference with the oxygen-carbon dioxide exchange across the alveolar membrane. The distention of interstitial tissues with fluid may also irritate nerve endings, resulting in sensations of pain in the inflamed area.

Inflammation may be classified according to the character of the inflammatory exudate. The exudate is classified as *serous* if it is a watery secretion, such as occurs with a skin blister or burn. This exudate is present early in the course of inflammation and contains relatively few inflammatory cells but does contain protein. In appearance it may be a pinkish yellow—pinkish because a few red cells may be present. This type of exudate is secreted by the cells lining the peritoneal and pleural cavities and is the type of discharge present on a clean surgical wound dressing. Drainage that has a definite reddish color contains a large number of erythrocytes and is termed *sanguineous* or *serosanguineous*.

A fibrinous exudate is one characterized by the loss of a considerable amount of fibrinogen into interstitial spaces at the site of inflammation. This is usually associated with more severe, prolonged reactions. The endothelial lining of blood vessels is injured, and fibrinogen is readily lost into interstitial spaces, where it is precipitated as fibrin. It forms a dull gray, sticky, stringy membrane over the serous surfaces. Fibrinous exudate is common in chronic inflammation and may be present in open wounds when skin edges cannot be approximated with sutures.

Catarrhal inflammation is a copious outpouring of mucinous exudate such as occurs with a common cold and some allergic reactions. The exudate is whitish, thick, and ropy. Inflammation of tissues in which mucous cells are present will produce a catarrhal exudate; therefore, this type of exudate would be expected in inflammatory processes occurring in the respiratory and gastrointestinal tracts.

Suppurative or purulent exudate contains pus or purulent drainage. Purulent exudate consists of dead and dying bacteria, phagocytic cells, and necrotic tissue cells that have been liquefied by the action of autolytic enzymes. Pus is a thick, foul-smelling secretion of different colors, depending on the type of organism present. When the exudate has a yellow color, it usually indicates a staphylococcus organism; grayish white, a streptococcus; and a greenish color indicates the presence of a pyocyaneous organism. The various types of exudates may be present at different periods of the inflammatory process, or they may coexist at a particular period. For example, the initial exudate following a burn may be serous, but eventually it may become seropurulent or serofibrinous. The nurse assists the doctor in his evaluation of therapy by reporting the amount and character of exudate from wounds or body cavities and by obtaining specimens of wound drainage for laboratory study.

The third component of the inflammatory response is *cellular* activity. Normally, the blood cells flow along in the center of the plasma. With loss of plasma to interstitial spaces and increased concentration of cells, the red blood cells adhere to each other and become densely packed in the center of the stream, pushing the white cells to the periphery. As plasma seeps out of the dilated, permeable vessels, there is less and less fluid available in the peripheral flow, and the white cells come in contact with the vessel wall. It is thought that a thin layer of fibrin is deposited on the endothelial wall and perhaps on the endothelial cell membrane. The fibrin is sticky, causing the white cells to adhere to the vessel (margination). This is the first stage in the movement of white cells through the endothelial wall. The polymorphonuclear leukocytes are the first cells to send out pseudopods between the endothelial cells and eventually by ameboid movement to travel into the interstitial spaces. These cells are small and motile in comparison to the lymphocytes and monocytes. They start this movement about 2 to 4 hours after the onset of the inflammatory reaction. Not only do the cells emigrate through the capillary endothelium, but they also move toward the site of injury. The mechanism that directs the leukocytes is termed *chemotaxis*. Chemotaxis is a positive physical attraction exhibited by most inflammatory chemical substances. Leukotoxin is a protein fraction released from injured tissues and present in the inflammatory exudate which has been shown to attract white blood cells. The effect of chemotropic attraction is the accumulation of polymorphonuclear leukocytes at the foci of injury in the early phases of inflammation.

Monocytes also immigrate into the inflammatory area but at a much slower pace. Usually monocytes begin to accumulate at about the second or third day after injury. Monocytes and histiocytes gradually move into the area of plasma fluid, dead tissue cells, and perhaps bacteria. Some red blood cells may be forced through the permeable capillary wall by the elevated hydrostatic pressure, a process known as *diapedesis*. Extravasation of red blood cells is usually slight, except when there has been extensive vascular damage.

The role of the polymorphonuclear leukocytes and monocytes in the acute inflammatory process is to phagocytose foreign substances at the site of tissue trauma.

*Figure 11–4
Successive stages in
phagocytosis. (By per-
mission of Howard C.
Hopps: Principles of
Pathology. New York:
Appleton Century Crofts,
1964, p. 193.)*

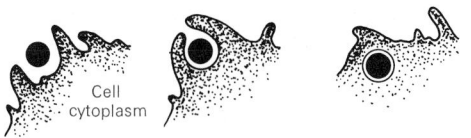

(See Figure 11-4.) The histiocyte, a motile connective tissue cell, assists with the phagocytic function. The polymorphonuclear leukocyte contains hydrolytic enzymes that work in an acid medium to digest the foreign substances which the cell phagocytoses. When the neutrophil dies, it liberates proteolytic enzymes to dissolve itself and foreign substances. The inflammatory process stimulates a release of mature polymorphonuclear leukocytes from stores in the body and also promotes an increase in the speed of formation of cells in the bone marrow. This action accounts for the increased white blood cell count during an inflammatory response.

The monocytes and histiocytes (macrophages) are a second line of defense. They have a greater power of phagocytosis than the neutrophils and contain cell enzymes that function in both acid and alkaline media. Macrophages have the ability to produce more enzymes, an ability not shared by the neutrophil. The monocytes remove waste materials before the actual repair process starts. The cellular activity increases the swelling of interstitial tissues and influences the character of the exudate and the duration of time when swelling is present. The injured area feels warm to the touch, if the injury is on the external body surface. Increased chemical activity with release of energy in the form of heat contributes to the elevated tissue temperature that occurs with inflammation. The four cardinal signs and symptoms of inflammation are heat, redness, swelling, and pain, but a fifth indicator, loss of function, is usually present. This loss results from cellular injury and from depression of normal cellular function. Sensations of pain with movement cause the person to protect against these sensations by such means as splinting the affected part. Thus, the tissues are not subjected to further injury and the beneficial effects of the inflammatory process are promoted.

Systemic manifestations are usually present during an inflammatory response. One sign is temperature elevation. Theories to explain the cause of fever are that (1) it is an indication of dehydration caused by movement of fluid into the interstitial spaces and a resulting depletion of extracellular volume, and (2) polymorphonuclear leukocytes release a substance called *pyrogen*, which acts on the temperature-regulating center, raising the level at which the body cooling processes are activated. The elevated temperature increases the metabolic rate of cells and their need for oxygen and nutrients; therefore rapid heart and respiratory rates may be present. Perspiration is increased to permit some loss of body heat and to keep the fever from becoming extremely high, but this means increased fluid loss. Replacement of fluid loss and provision of adequate caloric intake are indicated. The laboratory studies would reveal an elevation of white cells and an increased sedimentation rate. The change in sedimentation rate possibly occurs because the increased concentration of protein antibodies promotes adherence to red blood cells and hastens their rate of settling out.

The toxic metabolites from injured tissues, bacteria, and possibly polymorphonuclear leukocytes enter the circulation and lymph drainage and are thought to account for general feelings of lassitude, weakness, apathy, and malaise. The severity of the systemic manifestations of inflammation varies with the extent and severity of trauma and with the causative agent. The systemic manifestations following surgical trauma may be slight, but when the causative agent is a pathogen, the manifestations may be intense.

CHRONIC RESPONSE MECHANISMS

Inflammatory responses are either *acute* or *chronic*. These terms are used with two frames of reference. In one respect they refer to temporal sequence, that is, an acute infection is one that occurs here and now. The process lasts for a short time (from days to a few weeks) by contrast with a chronic infection which may be present for weeks, months, and even years. The second frame of reference is in regard to the type of cell response at the site of inflammation. An acute inflammatory process is characterized by the presence of polymorphonuclear leukocytes and some macrophages. The predominant cells at the site of a chronic inflammatory process are lymphocytes, plasma cells, macrophages, and fibroblasts. In chronic inflammation there is a continuous interaction between phagocytic cells and the injurious agent. Around the periphery of the inflamed tissue are fibroblasts and fibrocytes with interlacing strands of reticulum and collagen, abundant ground substance, and newly formed blood vessels. This is an attempt to confine the area of inflammation and to repair tissue damage. Pathogens may cause chronic inflammation when either the biologic agent is very persistent or the defenses of the host are ineffective. The tubercle bacillus is one such hardy organism.

Figure 11–5 Outcomes of injury. (By permission of Howard C. Hopps: Principles of Pathology. New York: Appleton Century Crofts, 1964, p. 296.)

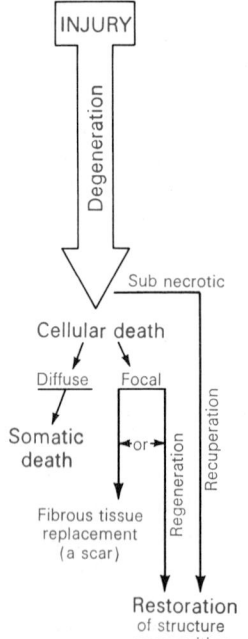

REPARATIVE MECHANISMS

The inflammatory response is usually a reversible, defensive reaction that gradually subsides as tissues recover from injury. The intensity and duration of the reversible components of the process, vascular dilatation and increased permeability, formation of fluid exudate, and cellular activity vary with the severity of the injury. Abatement of these components of the inflammatory response involves specific changes. The neutrophils and macrophages phagocytose and digest the products of cellular injury, capillary dilatation gradually subsides, the fluid exudate is reabsorbed into the blood or removed through lymph drainage, and damaged cells recover and once again carry on their normal functions. These damaged cells may be supporting, stromal cells, or if the injury was to a vital organ, the degenerative changes in the parenchymal cells are reversed. When the injury causes the death of some cells, regeneration is a necessary part of recovery, as contrasted with recuperation of cells and tissues when injury causes reversible cell degeneration but no cell destruction. (See Figure 11-5.)

Repair consists of replacement of an area of tissue destruction with new healthy cells. The new cells are derived from parenchymal cells and/or connective tissue stroma of the injured tissue. For example, when tubular cells of the kidney are destroyed, the remaining healthy tubular lining epithelial cells may proliferate and replace the destroyed cells, or the fibrous stroma supporting the tubules may be the source of tissue to fill in the defect. If proliferation of the lining epithelial cells (parenchymal elements) predominates, then almost perfect reconstruction takes place with normal function being maintained. If proliferation of connective tissue is dominant, then repair is by fibrous scar tissue and there is loss of tubular function in the affected area. The extent to which parenchymal elements and connective tissue stroma replace themselves in the normal pattern during the reparative process determines whether the outcome is reconstitution with maintenance of function, scarring with loss of function, or something intermediate between these two extremes. The damaged area seldom returns to its original state, as some excess of fibrous tissue formation is invariably present.

Factors determining whether the predominant type of reconstruction will be regeneration or fibrous tissue substitution are (1) the type of cell affected, (2) the extent of tissue damage, (3) the architectural pattern of tissue, and (4) the duration of injury. Different types of cells vary in their regenerative capacity. Fibrous tissue has a great regenerative capacity and is a very tough, resistant tissue, whereas parenchymal cells are more fragile and regeneration is more easily delayed by suboptimal environmental conditions, such as marginal blood supply. Based on regenerative capacity, parenchymal cells may be classified as labile, stable, or permanent. Labile cells are cells that constantly regenerate and replace themselves throughout life. This is a normal physiological process readily adapted for use when there is tissue damage. Labile cells in the body are the cells of the epidermis, of the mucous membranes lining the gastrointestinal, respiratory, and genitourinary tracts, of the serous membranes overlying body organs and lining body cavities (pleura, peritoneal), and of bone marrow and lymph nodes. Stable cells retain their capacity for mitotic division, but at adolescence they ordinarily either cease multiplying or proceed at a much slower pace. In this category are parenchymal cells of liver, pancreas, thyroid, kidney, and adrenal organs. These cells are capable of regeneration following tissue damage. Permanent cells are incapable of regeneration once formation of the organ or tissue structure has been completed. Neurons in the central nervous system and muscle cells are believed to be permanent. Function that is lost because of nerve cell damage cannot be regained; if the damage is to a peripheral fiber and the neuron itself is not damaged, then regeneration of the fiber may occur. The type of cell that is damaged influences the regenerative process, as cells incapable of mitotic division cannot replace themselves.

A second factor influencing the outcome of regeneration is the extent of tissue damage. For example, extensive destruction of tubular epithelial cells of a kidney may mean that too few viable cells remain to undergo mitosis and repair the damage. In this instance, replacement by fibrous tissue substitution would dominate. This type of repair would also predominate in the healing of extensive external wounds such as burns. Minimal tissue trauma as occurs with a surgical incision heals rapidly and with little scar formation.

The architecture of the damaged organ influences regeneration, for not only must the primary functional cells replace themselves with like cells, but they must arrange themselves so that they are in the necessary relationship to ducts and to blood vessels. Regeneration in the liver requires bile ducts and blood vessels to so arrange themselves that bile can be excreted as well as formed. Regeneration must follow the normal organizational pattern of the organ; to do this, the rate of regeneration of the various types of cells must be synchronized. This may be a deterrent to adequate reconstruction, as each type of cell has a different rate of mitosis. Extensive tissue damage necessitates more complex organizational regeneration of cells than does slight damage. Understanding regenerative powers and processes of various body tissues is basic to understanding problems related to healing of specific organs. For example, one cannot aim to restore the function of damaged cerebral cells and the skeletal muscles these neurons control, since nerve cells do not regenerate. In a patient with cirrhosis of the liver, the complex structure of the liver and limitations for adequate regeneration permit understanding of the permanent damage that may occur.

The fourth factor affecting reparative processes is the duration of trauma. When the agent causing tissue damage persists for a prolonged period of time, a chronic inflammatory response takes place. Repair in chronic inflammation differs from the healing process following self-limiting trauma and acute inflammation. One difference is that the injurious agent, the inflammatory cells, and the reparative cells may be present concurrently at the site of a chronic inflammatory process. The injurious agent may be viable, such as tuberculosis organisms, or nonviable, such as silicon dust, which is a chronic respiratory tract irritant. The inflammatory cells are usually in the center of the damaged tissue and there is active proliferation and migration of fibroblasts and endothelial cells from the outer margins of the damaged area. These cells move into the damaged site, and under a microscope are seen to be present along with mononuclear inflammatory cells. A second difference of repair in chronic inflammation is that healing is by fibrous substitution, since the environment is usually unfavorable to parenchymal cell regeneration. The formation of fibrous scar tissue around the periphery often results in structural deformity because of the inelastic quality of fibrous tissue. When chronic inflammation is present in body cavities, fibrin may adhere to the outer membrane of organs and may attach to more than one organ, causing adhesions. Healing by fibrous tissue substitution occurs with chronic inflammation as well as when the architectural pattern of the organ is not maintained during repair.

In a surgical incision, there is minimal blood vessel and cell destruction, and following the surgical procedure the edges of the tissues are reapproximated with sutures. This is apparent externally, but a similar process occurs internally when tissue edges are approximated with sutures, such as in resection of a segment of bowel and anastomosis of remaining bowel. Healing in this favorable environment takes place by what is known as *primary union* or *union by first intention*. The inflammatory process, including blood and serum exudate, accumulation of polymorphonuclear leukocytes, and formation of fibrin clot, takes place along the suture line in the first 24 to 48 hours after surgery. The fibrin clot serves to seal off the wound and protect it from bacterial invasion. It also prevents further loss of fluid and provides a pathway for fibroblasts to follow as they move into the wound area at a later period. Shrinkage of the wound size is brought about by migration of epithelial cells from the wound edges out over the wound surface during the first 24 hours. The process of proliferation of epithelial cells and then of migration of the fibroblasts present in the outer fringe of damaged connective tissue commences about the second or third day after injury. These cells move into the incision area along the course of the fibrin strands and tracts made by the preceding leukocytes.

About the same time that fibroblast activity starts, proliferation of endothelial cells lining capillaries close to the wound edges also starts. Solid endothelial buds begin to protrude from the ends of these capillaries, but soon the buds become canalized and anastomose with other buds. Vascularization continues inward, toward the center of the damaged area. Lymphatic capillaries are reestablished by a process similar to vascular development. As the reparative process proceeds, the fibroblasts and endothelial buds of blood and lymph capillaries replace the neutrophils and macrophages. The autolytic action of the enzymes released by neutrophils and tissue cells breaks down the protein that was present in these cells into amino acids and polypeptides; these substances then provide nourishment for the incoming fibroblasts and endothelial cells.

The strength of the tissue undergoing repair depends on the development of intercellular fibers. Fibroblasts are essential for the production of fine fibers, which are chains of globular protein molecules. Glucocorticoids are thought to depress the production of fine fibers by fibroblasts and thus to minimize the formation of fibrous scar tissue. At first, these fine fiber strands have no precise arrangement, but as the reparative process continues, they tend to become arranged along the lines of stress at the wound site. Collagen fibers are thought to form from the coming together of fine fibers in a parallel arrangement. In this way, they give strength to the eventual scar. The formation of collagen fibers is slowed down when there is a deficiency of vitamin C. About 8 days after surgery most surgical wounds have considerable collagen support and proliferation of surface epithelial cells is completed.

The reparative process continues over a period of months with the rate of activity at the site slowly decreasing. Alterations in cell population occur: the fibers become coarser and stronger, the number of fibroblasts decreases, and tissues contract to squeeze capillaries and cause them to collapse and again become blind-ended sprouts. The outward appearance of the wound changes from a bright pink to a pale, contracted scar. (See Figure 11-6.)

Healing by *secondary union* or *secondary intention* means that wound edges are not approximated. It may occur internally or externally. Some examples of situations where healing is by second intention are death of a portion of heart muscle, peptic ulcers, infected wounds, second and third degree burns, and

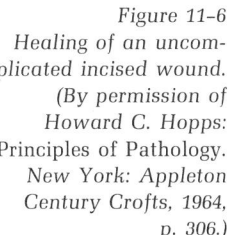

Figure 11–6 Healing of an uncomplicated incised wound. (By permission of Howard C. Hopps: Principles of Pathology. New York: Appleton Century Crofts, 1964, p. 306.)

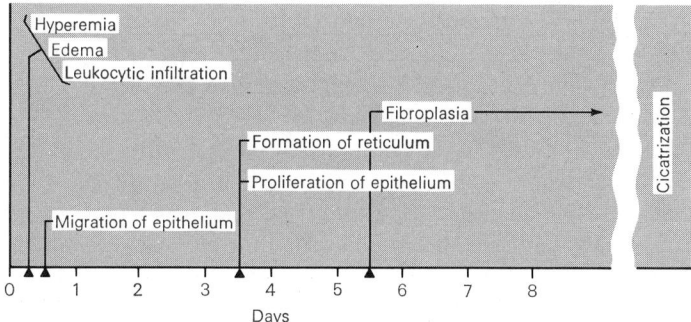

decubitus ulcers. This type of repair occurs when there has been extensive destruction of epithelial and underlying tissues and skin edges cannot be approximated, or when the tissue damage is internal.

An open wound heals in an upward direction from its depths. Granulation tissue proliferates from the less traumatized tissue at the bottom of the wound. Granulation tissue is the name given to the reparative fibrous connective tissue, including blood vessels and lymphatics. It is the same tissue that is present in wounds that heal by first intention. In that case, however, the granulation tissue is not visible; it is of lesser extent and the healing process is more rapid. In healing of surface wounds by second intention, the moist, friable, red, granular surface is visible during the prolonged healing process. The growth of capillaries is great if infection is present, since an extensive blood supply is needed to supply the phagocytic cells necessary for the defensive inflammatory part of the process. A layer of pus containing many leukocytes and macrophages may overlie the granulation tissue. Fibroblasts and many endothelial buds grow upward, and epithelial cells grow inward from the periphery to eventually cover the granulation tissue. Granulation can advance only as rapidly as the debris is cleared, and complete healing cannot occur as long as infection and necrotic tissue are present. If the tissue defect penetrated through the full dermal thickness, no sweat glands or hair follicles will be present in the healed surface epithelial tissue. When the defect is large, the reparative process may take months. The end result of healing by secondary union is a large irregular, indurated, contracted, pale area as contrasted with the fine linear scar that remains after healing by primary union. Observation of healed areas of burned tissue or decubitus ulcers provides visual reinforcement of the characteristics of a wound healed by secondary intention. Frequent dressing changes are often needed when an external wound heals by secondary union. Responsibility for changing the dressing and for observing and reporting the appearance of the healing tissue is usually delegated to nurses; therefore the nurse must be able to recognize the appearance of both normal and abnormal wounds.

Thus, repair by secondary union differs from repair by primary union in the following ways: (1) a larger tissue defect is present, (2) a prolonged inflammatory response may be necessary to remove tissue debris, and (3) healing requires a longer period of time and is characterized by more extensive formation of granulation tissue and scar formation. Connective tissue regeneration is not the total picture in injury to internal organs. When the injury has been to both parenchymal cells and supporting stroma, reconstruction may include both regeneration and fibrous tissue substitution.

Harmful effects occur when *parenchymal cell regeneration* is inadequate and *fibrous tissue substitution* fills in the defect. The loss of parenchymal cells decreases the amount of tissue available for the performance of necessary functions. For example, fibrous tissue healing of a portion of the liver decreases the number of cells available for the production of bile and storage of glycogen. Fibrous tissue substitution in repair of stomach ulcers may result in stenosis of the pyloric sphincter and even obstruction of flow of gastric contents into the duodenum. Replacement of traumatized muscle, tendon, and loose areolar connective tissue with fibrous substitution eventuates in joint contractures. For instance, healing of second and third degree burns (partial and full thickness of skin) may result

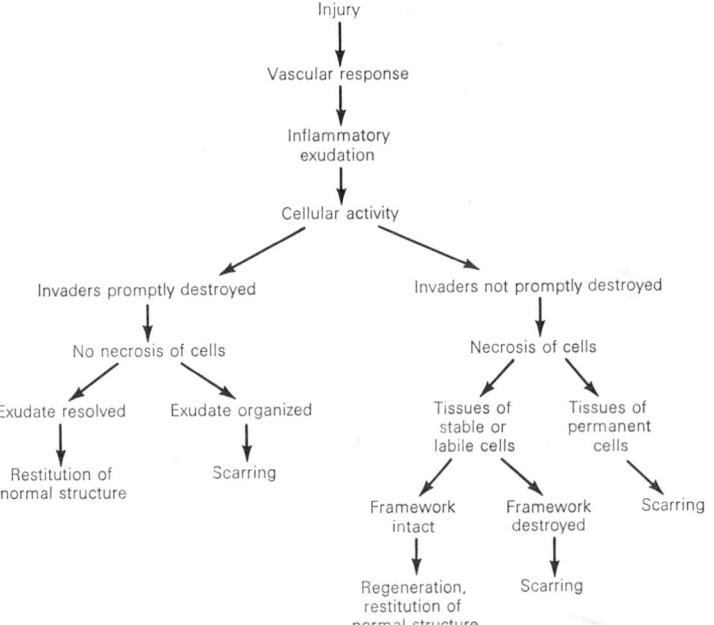

Figure 11-7 Reconstitution of damaged cells. (By permission of Stanley Robbins and Sir Roy Cameron: Textbook of Pathology. Philadelphia, W. B. Saunders Company, 1967, p. 71.)

in contractures that interfere with normal function of the extremities, unless skin grafting during the healing process is successful in preventing extensive healing by granulation and eventual scar contraction.

There are beneficial effects of healing by fibrous tissue substitution. The interweaving of fibrin strands forms a barrier to the movement of bacteria and/or toxic metabolic products out of the area of tissue damage, thereby preventing dissemination of harmful substances throughout the body. In fractures of bone, fibrous tissue provides support to damaged structures, and this tissue is necessary in filling in defects and restoring continuity of tissues or organs.

The reconstitution of damaged tissue is depicted in Figure 11-7.

Variations in Response Mechanisms Due to Pathogenic Action

The inflammatory response that occurs when the causative agent is a pathogen may have specific characteristics. One such characteristic is the ability of cells to react to viral invasion with the production of *interferon*. Interferon is a protein which cells invaded by a virus are capable of producing and releasing to other cells. The presence of interferon in other cells enables them to produce a protein that inhibits the entrance of viruses released on the death of invaded cells. This appears to be a cell defense mechanism against viral invasion. The inflammatory reaction with viral infection is less marked than with bacterial infections, perhaps because it is not initiated until the virus causes cell death and releases toxic metabolites. The tissue damage from cell death by viral activity may be greater than the tissue damage from bacterial infections despite the more intense inflammatory reaction that accompanies bacterial infections. Some pathogenic organisms result in *abscess formation*. In this situation the toxic metabolites produced by the living, proliferating bacteria destroy normal tissue cells and the bacteria may have control for a period of time. Leukocytes do carry on phagocytic activity but it may not be effective until antibodies are produced in sufficient quantity to neutralize bacterial toxins. Leukocytes die and release proteolytic enzymes that promote digestion of the products of bacterial and cellular debris. The products of autolytic digestion of bacteria and leukocytes become liquefied and form a core or center of partially digested and dying bacteria, leukocytic cells, and stromal and parenchymal cells. Bacterial action and core formation differentiate inflammatory response accompanied by abscess formation from the other inflammatory responses. Purulent exudate, discussed earlier, is present in abscess formation. Around the edge of the core or abscess are the larger phagocytic cells, the macrophages. Fibrinogen exuded from the serum coagulates, forming fibrin strands interwoven in the interstitial spaces. This layered arrangement helps to confine the process and to prevent its spread, though some of the soluble products of the reaction do move through the fibrin strands and enter the lymphatics and the bloodstream. The staphylococcus organism is one which commonly causes abscess formation. The process of removal of inflammatory debris by absorption into lymphatic drainage and reabsorption into the blood proceeds slowly.

Cellulitis is a spreading, diffuse type of inflammation that is most likely to occur in loose connective tissue that has few barriers to dissemination of exudate. The injurious agent is often the beta streptococcus organism, which produces large amounts of hyaluronidase and fibrinolysins. Hyaluronidase is an enzyme that promotes hydrolysis of the mucopolysaccharides of the ground substance, thus permitting diffusion of exudate throughout a wide area of subcutaneous tissue. Fibrinolysins dissolve the fibrinous exudate and permit spread of toxins and bacteria throughout a wide area of tissue. Cellulitis appears as a diffuse, swollen, reddened area. It frequently affects the soft tissues of the face and neck and may result in interference with respiration and ability to chew and swallow.

Spread of pathogens is possible if phagocytic cells are ineffective in their action. Motile phagocytic cells may ingest the foreign pathogen but be unable to digest it in the absence of antibodies. The motile phagocytic cell would move along to lymph nodes where the cell dies and liberates the still-living bacillus, which then sets up new foci of infection. The process of controlling the infection with specific antibodies plus host native defenses may take days or even weeks. During the time it takes for the host to gain control, the individual manifests both local and systemic signs and symptoms of an infectious process. The tubercle bacillus spreads in this manner. Four specific characteristics that may be present if the agent causing an inflammatory response is a pathogen are production of interferon, abscess formation, cellulitis, and pathogen spread.

Variations in Response Mechanisms Due to Antigen-Antibody Reaction

The response mechanisms that occur when a causative factor is an antigen-antibody reaction may have specific characteristics. Antigen that pierces the skin or mucous membrane barrier either makes its way in solution to a regional lymph node or is brought there by a cell. Before an antigen-antibody reaction can occur, antibody must be produced by particular cells. The process of antibody formation is associated with increased activity in lymph nodes. In particular, antibody production seems to be an activity of lymphocytes and plasma cells. The lymph node cells may release the antibody (a protein compound) into the blood or the antibody may remain within the cell. Antibody released into the blood may stay in solution or may become fixed to specific blood cells. The antibodies that mediate the majority of antigen-antibody reactions are the various types of serum immune globulins.

Immunity is the beneficial antigen-antibody response that is man's second line of defense against pathogens. The antibodies to most bacteria and viruses circulate in the bloodstream, but the antibodies to tuberculosis and some other pathogens are contained within cells. Acquired immunity is specific host resistance obtained by previous contact with a particular antigen. The previous contact may be either by an immunizing injection of dead or attenuated pathogens or may occur in the course of a particular disease.

The pathogen as an antigen incites the production of specific antibodies, but the process requires time; therefore, the phagocytic cells and nonspecific antibodies in serum that are part of the inflammatory exudate are the major defense mechanisms until specific antibodies are produced. The specific antibodies of acquired resistance have a very potent action as compared to the slight degree of potency of the general antibodies that are part of the defense mechanisms of the inflammatory response. While the potency of action of the two types of antibodies differs, there is a similarity of action in that both specific and general antibodies have the same type of resistive mechanisms. Specific opsonins permit rapid phagocytosis, bactericidal substances kill bacteria quickly, and antitoxins rapidly neutralize toxins. This is the same type of action as the general antibodies exhibit, but the process is generally accelerated and more potent. The ability to produce specific antibody may be retained by the progeny of the lymphatic and plasma cells and may protect the person against further infection with the particular pathogen. A second contact with the pathogen results in rapid production of antibody by the lymph node cells. Some infectious diseases are followed by permanent immunity, but others evoke little antibody reaction and reinfection is possible. Long-lasting immunity is obtained following an attack of German measles (rubella), but little immunity is present following a cold. It is not currently known why there is considerable variation in the duration of immunity stimulated by contact with the various pathogens.

Much of the control of infectious diseases is due to the development of vaccines that stimulate antibody reaction and provide actively acquired immunity. Obtaining immunizing injections at recommended intervals is part of preventive health practice. This practice makes possible the presence of specific antibodies prior to contact with the particular pathogen.

Resistance to pathogens may also be acquired passively. This process is used to combat some infectious agents once they have become established. The infected person is given passive immunity by injections of the serum of an actively immunized animal. The serum is known as an *antitoxin*. The serum is partially purified as part of the preparation for injecting it into human beings; however, some foreign (horse) proteins usually remain. The inflammatory response initiated by an immune type of antigen-antibody reaction is relatively slight. The reaction prevents pathogens from causing tissue damage; therefore, there is little stimulus for the inflammatory process.

Hypersensitivity reactions of a humoral type are referred to as *immediate re-*

actions, to distinguish them from the delayed reaction of cellular response. The *humoral* type of hypersensitivity disorders that are primarily related to known hereditary influences is designated *atopic disease*. When a person with atopic disease is skin-tested to determine the offending antigen or antigens, an immediate urticarial wheal is produced at the site of injection. This is thought to be due to the action of histamine. Histamine and heparin are present in the granules of mast cells and are released from the cells as a result of mechanical and chemical stimuli such as antigen-antibody reaction. Histamine is one of the chemical mediators of the inflammatory response.

A second type of humoral hypersensitivity reaction is the normal response to an unusual stimulus. The most commonly encountered reactions of this type are serum sickness and anaphylactic shock. Serum sickness is a syndrome resulting from the combination in the body of antigens of an injected foreign serum and the respective specific antibody formed by the recipient. For example, a person receives a first dose of tetanus antitoxin produced by horses, and the antigen in the horse serum becomes attached to tissue cells and also enters reticuloendothelial cells where antibodies are produced. Approximately 7 to 10 days later, the antibodies are released into the blood and come in contact with the antigens that are still present in the joints, skin, and other tissues. The inflammatory response occurs in these tissues. The disorder is manifested by joint pains, malaise, fever, lymph node swelling, and other signs of inflammation. On exposure to a second dose of antitoxin, symptoms of serum sickness would occur in a few hours to a few days, since the latent period for formation of antibodies is shorter with a second inoculation.

Anaphylaxis is a term meaning *the opposite of protection*. Anaphylactic shock is a diffuse, life-threatening, rapidly occurring antigen-antibody reaction to a second or later contact with an antigen. The reaction occurs throughout the body almost immediately after the antigen enters the circulatory system and encounters antibody. The reaction stimulates a generalized response of the vascular component of inflammation. A union between antigen and antibody can exert this injurious effect only if one or the other of them has previously become incorporated into the membrane or cytoplasm of certain exposed cells (Wright). The nature of the anaphylactic disturbance is still uncertain. It is known that certain pharmacologically active substances are liberated into the surrounding fluid by the antigen-antibody combination. Histamine and heparin are two potent agents that have been identified in the analysis of shocked organs. The release of potent pharmacologic agents in anaphylaxis results in a simulation of cholinergic response. Manifestations of the response are tearing, sneezing, itching, urticaria, contraction of smooth muscles, especially the smooth muscles of the bronchi and bronchioles (bronchospasm), generalized vasodilatation, and increased capillary permeability. Systemic vasodilatation and increased capillary permeability cause a sharp fall in cardiac output and arterial pressure resulting in a drop in blood pressure and edema, particularly laryngeal edema. Unless treated promptly with epinephrine (vasoconstrictor effect) and antihistamines, the person dies of asphyxia and vascular collapse. The body does have the ability to detoxify the potent agents that are released; however, the effectiveness of this ability is dependent on the amount of the noxious agent released within a given period of time. The effect of a hypersensitivity reaction is dependent upon the amount and rate of histamine release. A quantity of foreign serum given to a sensitive person may be harmless if given slowly over a period of time, but might cause anaphylactic shock if given intravenously. For instance, a person who has a positive sensitive reaction to an intradermal test dose of tetanus antitoxin may be given small doses of the antitoxin over a period of time in order to provide the desired immunity.

Cellular antigen-antibody responses are also known as *delayed sensitivity reactions*. Less is known about this type of response than is known of the humoral type. The reaction is characterized by a time span of 12 to 72 hours between the time of antigen contact and the signs of inflammatory reaction. The delayed reaction to an intradermal antigen injection is characterized by the appearance of local blanching with a surrounding area of redness. The area immediately over the site of injection is often tender to finger tap. The delay in the reaction appears to be the result of a need for participation in the reaction by lymphocytes and perhaps monocytes. Time is required for these wandering cells to accumulate at the test site and for their direct interaction with the test material. The exact mechanism of reaction at the site of antigen injection is unknown at present. An example of the delayed sensitivity reaction is the tuberculin skin test which, when positive, gives evidence of previous contact with the tubercle bacillus. Other delayed sensitivity reactions are contact dermatitis and drug sensitivities. In these two situations it is thought that a chemical substance combines with a host protein, and the host protein becomes antigenic, stimulating the production of antibodies which then react with antigen. Continued contact with the chemical increases the severity of the inflammatory response. The inflammatory response to tissue injury from hypersensitive antigen-antibody reactions is usually intense and may be generalized.

AIMS OF THERAPY

Medicine and nursing are concerned with the prevention of tissue injury as well as the care of persons who have sustained an injury. Both aspects of medical and nursing therapy are dependent on knowledge of harmful agents and their effects. Preventive measures may be carried out in community agencies or within the hospital environment. The nurse is carrying out preventive functions in the community when counseling a family regarding environmental accident hazards, immunizations, methods of preventing spread of infectious diseases, and when assisting in administration of immunization programs.

In the hospital, prevention of trauma is obtained by the use of safety measures, judicious application of principles of asepsis and barrier techniques, and by control of environmental factors such as ventilation and cleanliness. Protection of the patient from infection and tissue trauma is one purpose in providing hygienic care. This care helps to maintain an intact skin and mucous membrane and a decreased bacterial flora of these tissues. Measures to promote adequate circulation and respiration protect against trauma. The nurse assists in minimizing the possibility of the hypersensitivity type of antigen-antibody reaction by determining if the patient has had reactions to known sensitizing agents such as penicillin and diagnostic dyes and by sensitivity testing prior to administering these agents.

Treatment of a patient with an inflammatory condition is aimed at (1) eliminating the stimulus for inflammation, (2) supporting the normal defense mechanism, and (3) promoting recovery. The doctor may accomplish removal of the source of stimuli by surgical excision. Surgical excision would be the treatment of an inflamed organ (e.g., an inflamed appendix) that could be removed without threatening the life of the individual. Surgical debridement of a traumatic wound removes dead tissue that would otherwise be a source of toxic metabolites. Drug and diet therapy may be prescribed when disturbances in cell function seem to be the source of tissue injury. For instance, excessive secretion of hydrochloric acid in the stomach may be treated with drugs to depress secretion and by diet to avoid cell irritation. When the source of tissue injury is accumulated toxic metabolites in interstitial tissues because of disturbances in blood flow, therapy is aimed at improving vascular dynamics.

Therapy to eliminate pathogenic agents includes identification of the offending organism and prescription of specific organism-sensitive chemotherapeutic agents. Impregnating bacterial cultures with various antibiotics will demonstrate the relative sensitivity or resistance of the bacteria to the particular agents, and therapy can be based on this specific information. The nurse assists the doctor in this restorative therapy by administering the antibiotic prescribed. Antibiotics must be given on time; the intervals between administrations are usually equal over a 24-hour period in order to maintain effective blood levels.

Not all infectious agents are susceptible to the action of antibiotics. Identification of the offending agent, such as a virus, may be possible by determining antibody titers or levels in the blood, or by observing a cytopathogenic effect in tissue culture. Elevation of the antibody level may indicate infection with the particular organism. Assistance in combating this organism may be provided by administration of antitoxins. In some instances this assistance may be provided for prophylactic reasons without waiting for an elevated titer following exposure to the virus. A pregnant woman may receive prophylactic gamma globulin immediately after exposure to the German measles virus. (Infection of the fetus with this virus during the first trimester of pregnancy frequently results in serious malformations.)

Elimination of harmful effects of some antigen-antibody reactions may be accomplished by a series of injections of minute amounts of sensitizing antigen. The body has the ability to detoxify substances released as a result of a sensitive antigen-antibody reaction provided that only small amounts of the substances are released at one time.

Support of normal defense mechanisms may be provided by various measures. Intermittent applications of cold in the period immediately following injury is advantageous in some situations, since cold promotes vasoconstriction. Vasoconstriction of blood vessels is in opposition to the normal events in the inflammatory response. Vasoconstriction delays and inhibits the formation of fluid exudate. In some situations this is desirable since it prevents excessive swelling. For instance, this technique is prescribed by some doctors following delivery to minimize perineal swelling. Depression of exudate formation decreases tissue distention and stimulus of pain fibers.

Physical and psychological rest and relaxation obtain a state of basal metabolism which permits body defenses to concentrate activity at the site of trauma. Nurses assist in minimizing functional demands on body tissues when a relaxing physical environment is established, and when listening to the patient and permitting verbalizations of emotional reactions to illness. Rest of the affected part minimizes stimuli to sensory nerve endings, thereby both decreasing pain and preventing further tissue trauma. Elevation of the part, if possible, tends to lower the arteriole hydrostatic pressure and decrease the extent of edema formation. Pain is less intense if tissues are not greatly distended with fluid. This position promotes by gravity venous and lymphatic drainage of metabolic toxins from the injured area. Pillows and slings aid in immobilizing a part, and bed cradles keep the weight of clothing off injured tissues. The judicious use of analgesics ordered on a "whenever necessary" basis provides for patient comfort.

Support of the inflammatory process may be obtained in some situations by intermittent applications of heat to the site of injury. Heat stimulates vasodilatation, and the resulting increase in blood flow brings fluids, antitoxins, and inflammatory cells to the area, dilutes toxins present at the site of injury, and aids in removing the products of cellular debris. Heat increases tissue temperature, which increases the rate of metabolic activity of cells and may promote repair of tissue damage. This therapy is usually prescribed at the site of infection.

Supportive measures include maintenance of high fluid intake to replace what is lost through perspiration and adequate nutritional intake to meet increased metabolic needs. Fluid replacement by intravenous therapy is sometimes indicated because of the severity of the trauma. Extensive loss of exudate, as with burns, is one example of a situation calling for this type of replacement. Intravenous fluids replenish fluids lost from the circulating blood, thereby preventing dehydration. Fluids also dilute toxins present at the site of injury or in the bloodstream.

Therapy aimed at promoting recovery includes minimizing the danger of further injury or infection. If an open wound is present, a dressing may be applied to inhibit the entrance of organisms and the nurse may be expected to cleanse the wound daily, using aseptic technique, and to make pertinent observations. These data enable the nurse to decide if the doctor should examine the wound and if any changes in treatment are indicated. The patient with an open wound should be in a private room and protective isolation should be maintained.

The accelerated cell activity that is part of the inflammatory process necessitates an increase in the cell supply of nutrients. This is obtained from nutritional intake. If infection is present, antibodies may have to be synthesized, requiring amino acids and other substances derived from food. Dead cells must be replaced by proliferation of healthy cells on the periphery of the injured area. The nurse promotes restoration of damaged tissue when she assists the patient in selecting foods with a high protein and adequate vitamin content and when she promotes adequate intake of fluids between meals.

Self-care activities are mentally and physically beneficial to the patient, but nursing judgment is needed to determine the extent of these activities. Data for evaluating the severity of the inflammatory process and the desirability of fostering self-care are provided by laboratory reports, vital signs, appearance of the patient, patient interests outside of self, the location of the inflammatory process, and the effect of increased functional demands with activity, e.g., involving the heart.

Restorative nursing measures include having the necessary emergency drugs readily available when known sensitizing agents are being administered. Prompt recognition of adverse signs and symptoms and administration of vasoconstrictor and antihistaminic drugs are essential in restoring equilibrium.

Medical and nursing goals must be within the realm of what is physiologically possible to attain. For example, the patient who has had damage to certain brain cells cannot be expected to regain the function previously performed by the particular tissue, though it may be possible to train other nondamaged tissues to take over the function of the disturbed tissue. The nursing goals are aimed at helping the patient to live as independently as the tissue damage and training permit.

Healing by fibrous substitution disrupts the normal function of the damaged tissue; therefore the doctor may try to minimize this type of healing, for instance, by grafting skin on burned patients. Nursing assistance in minimizing the disturbance in normal function is accomplished by positioning to prevent contractures and assisting with preventive exercises after the grafts have healed.

The medical and nursing goals and actions described are based on an understanding of the inflammatory response and are aimed at assisting in eliminating the stimulus for inflammation, supporting defense mechanisms, and promoting recovery.

Responses to Changes in Blood Volume

Injurious agents interfere with vascular stability by damaging the structure or function of the heart, vessels, or blood constituents. Tissue trauma can result in abnormal circulating volume and/or changes in rate of blood flow. The volume may be in excess (overfilling of vessels) or deficient in amount (blood loss, or shift in fluid to interstitial spaces). The rate of flow may increase as with muscle activity or may slow as in the later phases of the inflammatory response. Local congestion occurs in the inflammatory process and in situations where the injurious agent interferes with venous outflow from an area. Local congestion was discussed in the preceding section. The focus in this section is on systemic and local decrease in circulating volume and systemic congestion.

CAUSATIVE AGENTS AND THEIR EFFECTS

Injurious agents may bring about a decrease in systemic blood volume in three ways: (1) by disrupting vessel continuity, (2) by promoting vasodilatation and/or marked increase in permeability of capillaries and the movement of blood or fluid through vessel walls, and (3) by disturbing normal clotting mechanisms.

Physical trauma is a common extrinsic cause of severance of blood vessels. Lacerations, penetrating wounds and fractures resulting from forceful blows, gunshot wounds, or knife injuries may disrupt the continuity of vessel walls. Intrinsic causes include chemical erosions (ulcerations) of vascular tissues along the gastrointestinal tract; infectious agents, such as tubercle bacilli, which damage vessel walls; congenital or acquired areas of tissue weakness (varicosities or aneurysms), which may rupture with increased pressure; and a slipped ligature following surgery or with opening of vessels that were apparently closed during surgery because of low blood pressure and therefore not tied off. One reason for taking vital signs frequently of patients in the immediate postoperative period is the need for early detection of hemorrhage.

A break in the continuity of the wall of a blood vessel results in loss of blood into serous cavities or surrounding tissues or onto the external surface if there is also a break in the continuity of the skin or mucous membrane. The blood loss may be from a ruptured capillary, vein, or artery. If from a capillary, it will be a steady oozing, as contrasted with the steady flow of dark red blood from a vein and the pulsating bright red flow from the arterial end of the system. The amount of bleeding into tissues is variable. *Petechiae* are minute capillary hemorrhages appearing as red dots about the size of a pinpoint. *Ecchymosis* results from greater blood loss as occurs with a bruise, and is characterized by a dark red to yellow color as red blood cells break down. *Purpura* is characterized by large purplish areas of skin or mucous membrane, resulting from an oozing of blood into tissues. Arterial bleeding may rapidly decrease the amount of circulating volume and threaten survival of the individual. Blood loss with venous or capillary bleeding may also be life-threatening, but usually depletes blood volume over a longer period of time than arterial bleeding. Injurious agents may cause vasodilatation and/or increased capillary permeability, thereby effecting a decrease in circulating volume. An excessive shift of plasma fluid to body cavities or interstitial spaces, as may occur with inflammatory or congestive disorders, can cause a decrease in circulating volume. Examples are the shift of fluid to the abdominal cavity in peritonitis and ascites, to the pulmonary alveoli in pulmonary edema, and to the interstitial spaces following massive burns.

Marked increase in capillary permeability to blood cells may be caused by deficiency of vitamin C, by some bacterial toxins, and by increased intracapillary pressure. Erythrocytes may escape from between the endothelial cells, probably due to a change in the intercellular cement which is thought to bind the endothelial cells.

Disorders in the normal clotting mechanisms may disrupt the normal defense mechanisms set into action when vessel trauma occurs, namely, clumping of platelets and sealing off of minor breaks in capillaries. Hemophilia is caused by a genetic defect that is manifested in a deficiency of one of the plasma factors essential to the clotting process. Deficiency in clotting processes also occurs when intestinal bacteria are unable to produce vitamin K or when there is an absence of bile salts that are necessary for absorption of vitamin K from the intestine. Vitamin K is required by the liver for the formation of prothrombin.

Three factors influence the effects of a decrease in circulating blood volume. These factors are time, quantity of loss, and site of bleeding. The time factor refers to the rapidity of blood loss; sudden loss of more than 500 ml can precipitate manifestations of volume inadequacy, whereas loss of more than this amount over a period of days or weeks may not be readily apparent. Compensatory mechanisms may permit adequate adjustment for some time to chronic loss.

As indicated, a sudden loss of blood volume is a threat to life. If such loss is 35 percent of the total blood volume, it may be fatal unless immediate replacement is available. Loss of erythrocytes with hemorrhage decreases the oxygen-carrying component of the blood. This may lead to fainting, since the central nervous system is particularly sensitive to hypoxia.

The site of blood loss is an important factor. If this loss occurs within a closed space, a small loss may be serious because of the pressure exerted on vital structures in the area and not because the quantity of loss is a threat to the body as a whole. The brain may be irreversibly damaged with loss of a relatively small amount of blood into this tissue, especially if it occurs near the brain stem. Hemorrhage into the pleural or pericardial cavity may cause collapse of the lungs or inhibition of dilatation of the heart, and thereby precipitate death.

RESPONSE MECHANISMS

The two major defense mechanisms that control bleeding and maintain essential body functions when there is disruption of vessel continuity are *coagulation of blood* and *vasomotor compensations.* Control of bleeding starts with contraction and retraction of severed blood vessels. This elastic recoil capacity of vessels causes a decrease in the size of the lumen from which blood flows and causes the end of the vessel to be buried in damaged tissue. Damaged tissues and platelets secrete the enzyme *thrombokinase,* which is necessary for the conversion of prothrombin to thrombin in the clotting process. The elastic recoil of a vessel is a homeostatic response, but may be a detriment during surgery when it may be difficult to locate retracted severed vessels.

The process of clot formation depends on the ability of normally functioning platelets to clump together at the site of breaks in the wall of capillaries and seal the hole. The platelets (thrombocytes) release epinephrine and other compounds that promote vasoconstriction, as well as enzymes that promote the sequence of chemical changes which results in conversion of serum fibrinogen to fibrin. The fibrin is initially deposited as a loose network of strands that incorporate platelets. The platelets participate both in initiating the clotting mechanisms and in forming the fibrin-retracted clot. The plasma factors that are essential in the clotting process include two produced by the liver: prothrombin, which is made only when adequate vitamin K is present, and fibrinogen. Normally, the formation of thrombin from prothrombin requires about 10 seconds. The whole process of coagulation of venous blood requires between 5 and 10 minutes. The clot is a mechanical block to the flow of blood from a vessel. The primary or temporary clot, if undisturbed, becomes an inherent part of the vessel by the process of fibrous consolidation. This prevents dislodgment of the clot and rehemorrhage. (The reader may wish to review the clotting process in a physiology textbook.)

The clot itself will retract, but it is a space-occupying mass and will cause pressure on surrounding tissue. It also provides pressure at the end of the severed vessel or vessels and in this way helps to stop further bleeding. Clot pressure can compress cells and other blood vessels and interfere with normal metabolic processes. Cell function may be depressed, and death of some cells probably will ensue. The speed of reabsorption of fluid that escaped into tissues varies with the site of loss. The clot is handled similarly to that of a foreign body in tissues. The phagocytic cells migrate into the area and digest the erythrocytes, releasing within the phagocytic cell an insoluble iron-containing pigment (hemosiderin). This pigment within macrophages gives the yellowish color to bruised areas during healing. The pigment changes to a brown color and may remain in the fibrocytes or in the interstitial spaces of the scar tissue that forms in the healing process. The fluid portion is readily absorbed through lymph and capillaries.

Compensatory vasomotor mechanisms serve to maintain essential body functions when there is disruption of vessel continuity. The loss of blood and drop in blood pressure from hemorrhage decrease the stimulation of the pressoreceptor organs of the afferent vagus nerve in the aorta and the carotid sinuses. This decreases the nerve impulses being sent to the cardiac (inhibitory) and vasomotor (vasoconstrictor) centers in the medulla. Peripheral arteriole vasoconstriction is promoted by the decrease in the stimulation of the pressoreceptor. The adrenal medulla responds to blood loss with an increase in the production of epinephrine. This compound also promotes vasoconstriction. These mechanisms serve to shunt blood flow away from the skin and less vital organs and to maintain flow to the brain and heart. They decrease the size of the vascular space and by so doing maintain adequate filling of essential vessels and of the heart.

The manifestations of decreased circulating volume reflect the action of adaptive mechanisms. The above-mentioned inhibition of vagal stimulation to the heart results in an increase in heart rate, and a decrease in volume of output is indicated in the weak or faint pulsation. Peripheral arteriolar vasoconstriction is evidenced in a pale, cold skin and slow response to the blanching test—capillary filling following pressure on the nailbeds or skin. This compensatory mechanism may maintain blood pressure despite a rather severe blood loss, though there is usually a slight drop in systolic pressure. The fall in systolic pressure reflects the decrease in circulating volume. Diastolic pressure is usually maintained at the same level because of arteriolar constriction, therefore a narrowing of pulse pressure is often observed.

The decrease in parasympathetic activity and the increase in sympathetic that are part of the neuroendocrine response to trauma function during blood loss to inhibit gastrointestinal activity. There is vasoconstriction of vessels along the alimentary canal, causing decreased cell activity and retarding ability to absorb oral fluids. Thirst may be present because of loss of circulating volume. Constriction of renal arterioles assists in maintaining systemic blood volume, but the decrease in renal flow is reflected in decreased formation of glomerular filtrate. This mechanism is manifested as oliguria. Kidney hypoxia is thought to induce the formation of vasoexcitor material (VEM), which promotes peripheral vasoconstriction. Vasoconstriction also reduces the capillary blood flow and capillary hydrostatic pressure, thereby permitting the capillary osmotic pressure to exert a pull on interstitial fluid. The movement of fluid from interstitial spaces helps to restore blood volume, though hemodilution occurs. This mechanism requires several hours to occur; therefore, in the first few hours after initiation of bleeding the hemoglobin level, red blood cell count, and hematocrit will be about normal. These will decrease as hemodilution occurs.

Increased epinephrine output and glycolysis can, as noted in the discussion of the neuroendocrine response, increase mental alertness and cause restlessness. The seriousness of the situation is recognized by the patient, and feelings of anxiety and fear may be apparent.

If protective mechanisms and medical therapy are sufficient to maintain or restore blood pressure to functional levels, the person is said to be in a state of *compensated shock.* In the event of acute blood loss, the aim of therapy is to prevent shock, but this is not always possible.

Shock may be defined as *a state of disproportion between circulating blood volume and the available vascular space.* Failure of protective mechanisms or of medical therapy to control the precipitating factors in the event of hemorrhage may result in shock. Various injurious agents, other than those that disrupt vascular continuity, may precipitate a shock state. Normally, in health, the capillary bed is not completely open. At any particular moment some of the capillaries in the organ are open and some are collapsed. If all the capillaries and venules were dilated with blood at the same time, there would be an insufficient amount to fill the heart and to stimulate heart contractions. Shock can occur when there is tremendous dilatation of the capillary bed, permitting stagnation of blood in these vessels, or when there is a vast decrease in the amount of circulating volume. In both situations there is a disparity between circulating volume and the vascular space. Shock may be categorized as hypovolemic (loss of fluid volume) or normovolemic (dilatation of capillary bed).

Two relatively common situations that the nurse encounters and in which she needs to be alert to signs and symptoms indicating possible hypovolemic shock are in caring for patients postoperatively and in caring for patients with bleeding gastric or intestinal ulcers. In both situations there is danger of hemorrhage and resulting shock. Hypovolemic shock may also be precipitated by situations in which there is an extensive loss of body fluids, such as severe vomiting and diarrhea.

Normovolemic shock occurs when there is a disproportionate increase in the vascular space because of inability to maintain vessel tone. Loss of vessel tone leads to failure of venous blood return to the heart and a resulting decrease in cardiac output and filling of arteries. This type of shock may be a complication of intense toxic bacterial infections, inadequate function of the adrenal cortex, and anaphylaxis. Shock intervenes when homeostatic mechanisms and supportive medical therapy fail to compensate for changes in vascular dynamics.

The essential feature of shock is increasing tissue hypoxia because of decreased circulation. Tissue hypoxia leads to altered chemical activity of cells, decreased aerobic metabolism, and accumulation of cellular catabolites, including lactic acid in tissue spaces.[1] The toxic catabolites, as in the inflammatory process, stimulate reflex vasodilatation and increased permeability of capillaries. (See Figure 11-8.) This event opposes protective responses since it leads to an increase in blood flow and a loss of fluid to interstitial spaces. The increasing severity of the situation is manifested by a falling blood pressure. A drop below 80 systolic is considered life-threatening. At this level renal blood flow is severely decreased,

Figure 11-8
Effects of decreased circulation. (By permission of Howard C. Hopps:
Principles of Pathology.
New York: Appleton Century Crofts, 1964,
p. 27.)

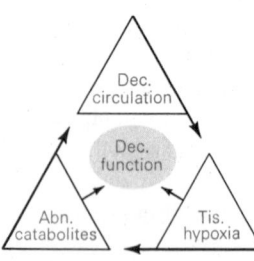

[1] Lactic acid is normally reconverted to pyruvic acid, some of which is degraded to carbon dioxide and water in the citric acid cycle to supply energy for reconversion of other pyruvic acid molecules and to glycogen.

which may precipitate injury to renal tubules with resulting oliguria or anuria, the skin becomes an ashen color, and there may be cyanosis of nailbeds and lips due to hypoxia. Depressed metabolic rate and heat production are noted in a falling temperature. As the venous return diminishes and the blood pressure falls, the myocardium is no longer receiving the necessary amount of blood, and depression of myocardial cell activity results. The low stroke output is manifested in a change from a weak, rapid pulse to a slow, thready pulse accompanied by a feeling of great weakness. The accumulation of carbon dioxide in the blood increases the respiratory rate, which helps to compensate for hypoxia, but in progressive shock cerebral hypoxia results in depressed function of nerve cells, decreased ability to comprehend what is spoken, mental apathy, and eventually coma. Death may ensue.

AIMS OF THERAPY

The aims of medical therapy in hemorrhage are to control the bleeding, provide an adequate blood volume, support homeostatic mechanisms, and prevent shock.

Bleeding may be controlled by direct pressure, elevating the injured part, applying cold, and when possible by suturing the vessel. These measures promote clotting by decreasing the forcefulness of blood escape from the injured vessel. This permits platelets, red blood cells, and fibrinogen to adhere to the vessel wall. The protective mechanisms will be supported by immobilization of the involved area and by inactivity of the body as a whole.

An adequate circulating volume is obtained through replacement with whole blood, plasma, dextran, normal saline, or other intravenous fluids. The amount and quality of replacement must be balanced in accordance with quantity loss and effectiveness of homeostatic mechanisms. Laboratory tests and nursing observations aid the doctor in calculating the patient's requirements for fluid replacement. Frequent observations and recording of signs and symptoms, accurate records of intake and output, maintenance of intravenous infusions at the desired rate of flow, and prevention of infiltration are nursing responsibilities.

Prevention or reversal of the shock process is obtained by therapies that support stabilizing mechanisms. These include use of vasopressor drugs for limited periods of time to stimulate peripheral vasoconstriction, thereby helping to maintain blood pressure at adequate levels; however, vasodilator drugs supplemented with fluid therapy may be used to ensure adequate perfusion of all tissues; oxygen therapy to promote gas exchange with minimal exertion of respiratory muscles by making available a higher than normal concentration of oxygen to circulating red cells; judicious use of analgesics to depress response to pain stimuli; and positioning to promote blood flow to vital centers without inhibiting the effectiveness of respiratory excursion. Nursing functions include administration of prescribed therapies and observations to evaluate their effectiveness. To detect evidence that shock is developing or increasing in intensity, it is necessary to observe for specific signs and symptoms. The care of patients with loss of blood volume is discussed in detail elsewhere.

Nursing measures, medical therapy, and the patient's protective mechanisms working together should control blood loss or compensate for a shift of body fluid.

The patient's return to a previous level of health includes a convalescent period during which recuperation from the secondary effects of hemorrhage occurs. The liver synthesizes plasma proteins to replace those lost with hemorrhage and restore blood osmotic pressure. The decrease in circulating red blood cells stimulates the bone marrow to increase production of erythrocytes. Anemia will be present for a period of time following hemorrhage, since the iron present in the hemoglobin of red cells is also in need of replacement.

Independent nursing functions during the recuperative phase are related to patient activity and nutrition. Explanations regarding desired activity and assistance with planning daily routines may be indicated. Activity must be adjusted to the body's ability to perform without undue fatigue. Any increase in activity increases the metabolic rate and oxygen needs of cells and puts added strain on the heart to circulate the blood faster; since the number of red blood cells is decreased, the rate of blood flow must be increased to keep up with tissue demand for oxygen and for carbon dioxide removal. The cardiac muscle is likewise attempting to work harder without an increase in supply of oxygen. The patient should be helped to realize that a regimen of decreased activity and daily rest periods is to be expected for weeks or even a month or two, depending on the severity of the hemorrhage and the precipitating cause.

Temporary replacement of erythrocytes and plasma proteins is accomplished by whole blood transfusion, but permanent replacement is accomplished by activity of body cells. These cells require proteins, vitamins, and iron to carry out their functions. A discussion with the patient regarding dietary habits and nutrients needed and the foods that contain these nutrients is usually indicated.

Response to Local Decrease in Blood Supply

Another action of injurious agents on the vascular system is to precipitate changes in the amount of blood present in a local area. Blood flow is either promoted or depressed. Local hyperemia or congestion is part of the inflammatory response which was discussed in the preceding section.

Insufficient blood flow to a local area may be brought about by a decrease in size of vessel lumen and by obstruction to flow. Injurious agents that cause a decrease in size of vessel lumen are excessive cold, which injures capillary endothelium and stimulates arteriolar vasoconstriction; metabolic disturbances, which result in a thickening of the intima of vessel; and compression of capillaries from external sources such as tumors or prolonged immobility. It is a nursing responsibility to prevent formation of decubitus ulcers over bony prominences by frequently changing the patient's position in order to prevent prolonged compression of the capillaries. Hypothermia therapy is relatively common and necessitates special nursing measures to prevent death of tissues from inadequate blood flow.

Obstruction to flow is often caused by a thrombus. Clot formation may be caused by any agent—physical, chemical, biological, or metabolic—that interferes with the normal protective mechanisms of a continuous flow of blood over a smooth endothelial lining of heart and vessels. Physical blows, vessel ligation during surgery, extreme cold, burns, and bacterial toxins are all agents that roughen the lining of the vessel and permit adherence of platelets. Metabolic disturbances such as abnormal deposition of lipids in the arterial intima interfere with the smoothness of the vessel lining. Calcified deposits on the valves of the heart as an aftermath of an inflammatory process may initiate platelet rupture and thrombus formation. Any increase in blood viscosity predisposes to clot formation. The nurse is responsible for assisting in the prevention of blood stasis and its sequela, clot formation. Fostering patient self-activity and early ambulation are two measures that promote blood flow.

A local deficiency or occlusion of blood supply to tissues due to gradual or sudden interference with blood flow is termed *ischemia*. Since tissues have a high oxidative metabolism and no means for storing oxygen, they are dependent upon a continuous circulation for survival. The effects of ischemia are dependent upon the sensitivity of the particular tissue to oxygen lack, the pattern of blood supply to the part, and the length of time for the development of partial or complete occlusion of blood flow. The many types of cells in the body are not equally susceptible to a decrease in oxygen supply. The parenchymatous tissue is usually more susceptible than is connective tissue. Brain tissue is especially sensitive to oxygen deprivation, being incapable of surviving more than 4 or 5 minutes without sufficient oxygen. Kidney, myocardium, and liver are also especially sensitive to oxygen lack. By contrast, bone tissue may survive oxygen deprivation for hours.

Tissues with more than one source of blood supply, such as the liver (hepatic artery and portal vein) are seldom severely affected by a decrease in blood supply from one source. Other tissues, such as the stomach, have sufficient collateral circulation to maintain blood flow, even when there is an obstruction within a particular vessel. Tissues with only one source of blood supply, such as the kidney, are particularly susceptible to ischemia, since a main artery branches to supply a relatively large peripheral area of tissue.

The effects of gradual diminution of blood supply and deprivation of oxygen to tissues supplied are of two kinds: first, there is a depression of normal cell function and of resistance to injury from other sources. For instance, physical trauma to a toe of an individual with thickening and narrowing of lower extremity arterial blood vessels may result in infection and death of damaged tissues because the narrowed vessels are unable to supply the increased amount of oxygenated blood necessary to repair tissue injury to ward off infection.

A second effect of chronic ischemia is stimulation of collateral circulation which may occur when there is gradual occlusion of a coronary artery from thrombus formation or progression of an atherosclerotic plaque. This is a homeostatic mechanism that functions to preserve tissue viability.

Sudden and complete occlusion of a main artery usually causes infarction. An *infarct* is an area of dead tissue resulting from a sudden occlusion of blood supply. An infarct may occur in the liver or lungs, organs that have a double vascular supply, and in organs with a single vascular supply. There may be relatively little effect from sudden obstruction of a major vein because of extensive collateral circulation, although occlusion of the vena cava, the mesenteric vein, or the portal vein will lead to death of tissues because of the extensive area experiencing a decrease in circulation. If capillary damage is extensive, as occurs with burning or freezing of a body area, the circulation to the area ceases and cell death ensues.

The development of an area of infarction is as follows: A sudden occlusion of blood supply causes progressive hypoxia of tissue as the available blood supply is used up. Metabolic waste products accumulate in interstitial spaces and stimulate dilatation of collateral vessels. This is followed by increased blood flow in the collateral vessels and from these vessels to the dilated, atonic capillaries that have been deprived of blood flow as a result of the occlusion; the capillaries become engorged with static blood. This collateral flow is sufficient to engorge the affected area with blood but inadequate to meet the needs of tissues in the area for a more continuous supply of oxygen and removal of waste products; ischemia results. The ischemic condition affects the engorged capillaries, the connective tissue stroma, and the parenchymal cells. Engorgement of capillaries gives the area a red color, but as oxygen is used up the area becomes deep bluish red. The capillary wall may rupture, spilling blood into the area, especially if the area is one with considerable interstitial space. If the affected tissue has little interstitial space, this space may be filled with edema fluid, which exerts pressure on the capillaries and inhibits rupture or diapedesis of erythrocytes. If the blocked vessel is an artery, the infarcted area would be white, as contrasted to the reddened area when interstitial spaces are more numerous or when a vein is obstructed.

Death of cells follows engorgement of the ischemic area. Hypoxia and the chemical toxins released on cell death stimulate the inflammatory process. Inflammatory changes, namely, vasodilatation and increased capillary permeability, formation of exudate, cellular activity, and repair, take place over a period of time. The effects from infarction are destruction of tissue and disturbance of fluid and electrolyte balance, and there may be secondary infection since destruction of tissues containing pathogens permits general dissemination of toxic products throughout the body. Infarction may occur in any tissue or organ of the body. It is discussed in the appropriate sections of Part V.

AIMS OF THERAPY

Therapeutic aims for patients with inadequate blood supply to a local area are to increase the blood supply, prevent extension of the causative process, remove devitalized tissue, support adaptive mechanisms, and promote reparative processes. The particular therapy depends on the causative agent. In some situations it may be possible to increase blood supply to the part by surgical removal of obstructive lesions such as thrombi or tumors causing external pressure. Development of collateral circulation may be promoted by vessel grafts around sites of obstruction and by surgical sympathectomy to inhibit vasoconstriction. Heat may be applied when vessels are capable of responding with vasodilatation.

Extension of the injurious process may be prevented by anticoagulant therapy when thrombus is the precipitating agent. Teaching a patient safety and hygienic measures may bring about inhibition of extension of tissue trauma when narrowed, thickened vessels cause depression or blood flow to a part. Sometimes the source of trauma may be eliminated surgically, as when a twisted or kinked loop is causing infarction of a section of bowel.

Support of protective mechanisms and repair processes is obtained by specific regimens of rest and activity, relief of ischemic pain, maintenance of fluid and electrolyte balance, promotion of adequate nutritional intake, and prevention of superimposed infection. Rest decreases tissue needs for blood supply, specific exercise programs stimulate collateral circulation and prevent venous stasis, and relief of pain decreases the intensity of neuroendocrine response to trauma. Pain stimulates the neuroendocrine response, which in turn promotes vasoconstriction and may further inhibit blood flow to a part.

Responses Leading to Increase in Systemic Blood Volume

An increase in systemic blood volume (systemic congestion) occurs when injurious agents have caused a disturbance of function of an organ through which all blood must pass, namely, the heart and lungs. Interference with circulation through the heart and/or lungs leads to congestion of vessels behind the obstructive process. Some causes of interference with blood flow are the following: (1) Degenerative changes in coronary arteries. Injurious agents may cause narrowing of vessels which decreases blood flow to the myocardium. Hypoxia of heart muscle prevents adequate contraction and emptying of the ventricles. (2) Inflammation of heart valves as may occur with rheumatic fever. Scarring and stenosis that are part of the repair process may cause impairment of heart valve function. These tissue changes may interfere with blood flow by inhibiting the amount of flow through the valve and/or by permitting backward regurgitation of blood through the damaged valve. (3) Congenital anomalies. Structural defects of the heart or great vessels may interfere with the normal path of blood flow and with the rate of flow through the heart and lungs. (4) Thickening of the intima and loss of elasticity of vessel wall place an increased demand on the heart to pump blood out against an elevated arterial pressure. The heart cannot compensate indefinitely, and eventually the force of heart contraction is insufficient to empty the ventricle and blood flow is slowed.

The process of development of systemic passive congestion is usually explained on the basis of whether the flow is inhibited on the right or the left side of the heart. The following theories have not been proven. If the defect is on the right side and there is not adequate flow of blood out of the right ventricle, the amount and pressure of blood in the right ventricle and auricle increase. The increased hydrostatic pressure is transferred along the vena cava and to the veins draining into the vena cava. This leads to slowing of venous return to the heart. When the vessel hydrostatic pressure is elevated sufficiently, there is edema formation, since reabsorption of interstitial fluid into the venule end of the capillary is inhibited. The liver and abdominal organs become edematous. The signs of systemic passive congestion include engorgement of all veins, with this being particularly evident in dilated, full neck veins, abdominal discomfort from congestion of the liver and spleen, and indigestion from congestion of the intestine. Edema of the sacral area, feet, and ankles is evidenced by a swollen, tense, taut, and shiny appearance.

When the obstructive lesion is on the left side of the heart, the venous congestion is thought to occur first in the pulmonary circulation. Chronic pulmonary congestion leads to degenerative changes (increase of connective tissue and fibrosis) and to slight hemorrhages per diapedesis in the alveoli. The changes in the alveolar septa inhibit oxygen-carbon dioxide exchange, as does the increased fluid (edema) in the pulmonary interstitial spaces, and even alveoli. These changes cause the the respiration to be moist, rapid, and shallow. Dilatation of pulmonary veins stimulates a neurogenic mechanism that results in labored respirations. The engorged bronchi and increased mucus secretions produce a chronic cough. Eventually, the increased pressure in the pulmonary circulation is reflected backward to the right side of the heart and to the systemic circulation.

Hypoxia of the kidneys results when there is inadequate outflow of blood from the left ventricle. The hypoxic kidneys elaborate a humoral agent that stimulates the production of aldosterone by the adrenal cortex. Aldosterone, it will be recalled, acts on the renal tubules to promote reabsorption of sodium, thereby increasing the osmotic pressure of the blood. In turn, the rise in osmotic pressure activates the regulating mechanism in the hypothalamus to stimulate the posterior pituitary to secrete ADH. The elevated ADH level in the blood results in water reabsorption by the renal tubules and an increase in blood volume. This increase elevates the capillary hydrostatic pressure, and more fluid is pushed into interstitial spaces. The increased blood volume slows the flow of blood, and further tissue hypoxia ensues.

Passive hyperemia is apt to be a chronic, long-standing response to changes in structure and/or function of the heart or lungs. Prolonged general congestion results in characteristic structural and functional changes in the affected tissues. Engorgement of veins and capillaries inhibits reabsorption of interstitial fluid and results in edema of the affected tissues, causing increase in weight and size of the organ and of the body.

Blood flow through the tissues is slowed as is the exchange of oxygen, nutrients, and metabolic waste products between the blood and the cells. Absorption of medication given into edematous tissues is delayed. An increase in fibrous connective tissue leads to thickening and loss of distensibility of the organ and to impairment of normal function of the edematous tissues.

Some relationships between cause and effect in tissue reaction to chronic passive congestion are depicted in Figure 11-9.

AIMS OF THERAPY

When systemic congestion is present therapeutic aims are to support heart and lung action; to prevent further tissue and organ damage from engorgement of vessels; to maintain fluid and electrolyte balance; and to repair damaged tissues, if possible. Further tissue damage from hypoxia may be prevented by prescribing

Figure 11–9 Cause-and-effect relationships in tissue reaction to passive congestion. (By permission of Howard C. Hopps: Principles of Pathology. New York: Appleton Century Crofts, 1964, p. 41.)

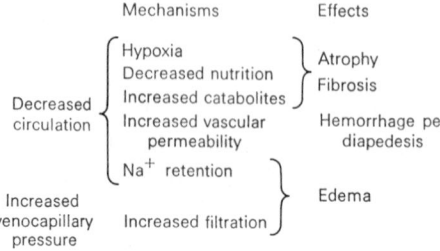

medications to strengthen heart action or to decrease arterial resistance to the outflow of blood from the heart. Rest and decreased activity lower the tissue needs for nutrients and oxygen and thereby decrease the energy demands on the heart and lungs. Promotion of adequate oxygenation of blood with minimal effort is obtained through oxygen therapy and intermittent positive pressure breathing. Diuretics and low-sodium diet are used to promote excretion of fluid and prevent its further accumulation. It may be possible to repair or correct incompetent heart valves or congenital heart defects by surgical techniques. Specific therapies are discussed in appropriate chapters of Part V.

Cellular Responses to Injury

The cell is the basic unit of the human body, but no cell can function without assistance from the vascular, hormonal, nervous, and gastrointestinal systems. Food must be ingested, digested, absorbed, and carried to the cells by the blood; hormones produced by cells comprising specific organs stimulate other cells to activity; nerve impulses aid in regulation of cell activity; and the waste products of this activity must be removed. The well-being of the individual is dependent upon the interrelated functions of the body parts. This statement applies to the body as a whole and to the cell as a unit. Although various organelles within the cell are sensitive to particular injurious substances, the integrity of the cell as a unit depends upon the interrelated functioning of its various constituents. The cell functions of synthesis and energy production are carried on over a 24-hour-period, day after day. Despite daily internal and external environment variations, the cells are maintained in a stable fluid and electrolyte medium and with the necessary nutrients to perform their functions.

CAUSATIVE AGENTS AND EFFECTS

The health of cells depends on the nutrient and oxygen supply, a stable fluid and electrolyte medium, humoral and/or nerve stimulation, and removal of waste products from the surrounding interstitial fluid. It is possible for injurious agents to disrupt normal cell function by disturbing any of these four required conditions. Interference with adequate nutrients reaching the cell may be brought about by inadequate dietary intake, defective digestion or absorption, interference with blood flow, or interference with oxygenation of blood. The presence of chemical or bacterial toxins causing disruption of enzyme formation, and interference with electron transport mechanism, are intracellular conditions that may interfere with the utilization nutrients by the cell. A change in nerve or hormonal stimuli, of either an excess or deficiency nature, may result in a change in cell metabolism. When vascular changes result in inadequate removal of waste products of cell metabolism, these products act as toxins to the cell. Depression of cell function and change in structure eventuate. Physical trauma to the cell such as electrical currents, ionizing radiations, temperature excesses, and forceful blows may cause rupture of the cell membrane. If the cell's reserve capacities are not too badly damaged, the autoregulative mechanisms will repair and replace the damaged cell area, but, if the injury is severe, structural and chemical disorganization of the cell will occur. Cell responses to injury are an increase or decrease in size or number of cells and alterations in function and structure.

RESPONSE MECHANISMS

Hypertrophy, hyperplasia, and metaplasia are adaptive cell responses to humoral or functional demands for an increase or change in function. Both hypertrophy and hyperplasia are increases in the size of an organ or tissue. The difference in these two states is the means of obtaining the increase in size. *Hypertrophy* is an increase in individual cell size, whereas *hyperplasia* is an increase in the number of cells. *Metaplasia* refers to a transformation of cell type.

Hypertrophy and hyperplasia occur separately or concurrently in a particular tissue. Hypertrophy can occur in most tissues or organs, but hyperplasia can occur only in those tissues or organs in which cellular proliferation is possible. Therefore, hypertrophy usually occurs without significant hyperplasia in cardiac and skeletal muscles. Hyperplasia is a controlled, purposeful increase in the number of cells and usually occurs in tissues whose cell population normally replaces itself, such as bone marrow and lymphoid tissue.

The major causes of hypertrophy and hyperplasia are an increased work load and increased hormonal stimulation. When, for example, the heart needs to contract forcefully for a prolonged period of time against an elevated blood pressure, the heart muscle responds by an increase in size. Hypertrophy of upper arm muscles results from prolonged use of crutches. Hyperplasia is a response to a particular stimulus, and removal of the stimulus is followed by a return to the normal rate of proliferation.

Since proliferation of cells which occurs in hyperplasia is associated with cellular differentiation, there is a concurrent increase in organ function. That is, hyperplastic changes in endocrine glands means that there is an increase in glandular secretion. Likewise, hyperplastic changes in mucous membrane result in an increase in mucous secretion, and bone marrow hyperplasia brings about an increased production of blood cells.

The effects of hypertrophy and hyperplasia are beneficial if the need for increased function is met. However, there are limits to the extent of hypertrophy that is possible, since the vascular supply to hypertrophied tissue does not necessarily increase proportionately. As a result, the hypertrophied muscle cells may cease to function effectively. Hyperplasia is also limited, since it is a controlled response confined to a range of normal.

Metaplasia usually occurs in response to chronic injury, the new type of tissue being more resistant to the injurious agent. Metaplasia may occur in epithelial and in mesenchymal tissues. The change is possible, because some primitive germinative cells are retained in the specialized tissues and have the potential of differentiating into other types of cells. For example, the chronic irritation of the bronchus that occurs when work is performed in a smoky environment may stimulate a gradual change in the respiratory epithelial tissue from columnar to squamous cells. The squamous cells are more resistant to trauma, but this change has a detrimental aspect, in that the mucous cells of columnar epithelium are replaced; therefore, less mucus secretion is available to entrap dust particles and move them out of the respiratory tract. The effects, then, of metaplasia will depend on the function of the displaced cells and the protective properties of the new type of cell. These three responses—hypertrophy, hyperplasia, and metaplasia—are cell reactions to demands for an increase or change in function of particular tissues or organs. By contrast, a cellular change of an opposing nature is often initiated by injurious agents.

Atrophy is a decrease in organ or tissue size due to a decrease in number and/or size of component cells. The failure to maintain normal size may be caused by (1) nutrutional or oxygen inadequacies, (2) a decrease in demand for cell function, or (3) a decrease in hormonal stimulation. Atrophy is a slow process. When cells do not have the materials needed for anabolic processes, a general debilitation of the body results. *Disuse atrophy* refers to cell changes caused by a decrease in stimulation for function. Lack of innervation and prolonged immobilization may precipitate atrophic changes. Prolonged bed rest or immobilization in traction results in muscle atrophy, as does an injury to the brain or spinal cord which destroys nerve cells and thereby prevents innervation of muscles. There is decreased stimulus for cell function, since muscles are not contracting and blood flow is at a minimum. The result is a decrease in muscle mass. Continued use is essential for maintaining the function of cells.

Usually the atrophic process is reversible if the underlying cause is corrected, as by improving nutritional intake and blood flow to the part, or by a gradual return to physical activity. The process is also to some extent preventable. Nursing actions to prevent muscle atrophy include scheduled exercise periods to stimulate circulation and promote muscle function to whatever extent is possible.

The ultimate in irreversible cell changes is death of cells in an area of the body. The structure of the cell undergoes a sequence of changes, resulting in a rupture of nuclear membrane and finally a disappearance of cell membrane. During this time the disrupted cell enzyme systems are promoting self-digestion of cell constituents, and the cell is unable to carry out its normal activities.

Cell death may occur over a period of time, or it may be instantaneous. When it is instantaneous the structural pattern of the cell is maintained. Rapid fixation of tissue specimens obtained during surgical procedures precipitates cellular proteins and stops enzymatic functions, so the appearance of the cell is preserved. The pathologist can then study the cells and make inferences regarding the disease process. Causative agents may directly disrupt cell function, or they may damage cells indirectly by interfering with blood supply to the part. *Gangrene* is massive ischemic necrosis of tissues with or without the presence of saprophytic microorganisms. It is a process of decomposition of dead tissues which may result from gradual or sudden occlusion of blood supply to the part. When ischemia is present over a period of time, the tissues atrophy prior to becoming gangrenous. In this situation the gangrene is dry, that is, there is little liquefaction of tissue, the tissues are dehydrated, and no organisms have been able to survive in the hypoxic tissues. The affected part is black and atrophied, and a line of demarcation of viable tissue is present. Dry gangrene is a complication of arteriosclerosis and is often seen in diabetics, who are prone to manifest severe arteriosclerosis. When gangrene results from rapid occlusion of a vessel or when an infection is present, moist gangrene occurs. The necrotic area is partly liquefied as a result of bacterial action and the presence of fluid in the tissues. In moist (wet) gangrene, there is usually no definite line of demarcation. The tissue is reddish black, and there may be a moist purulent discharge.

Any injurious agent that acts over a prolonged period of time or with sufficient intensity may cause cell death, but the extent and distribution of cell necrosis produced by a particular agent is variable. In general, all agents act by disruption of normal cell activities.

It is obvious that there are two effects of necrosis, namely, a loss of function of the affected tissue and a predisposition to infection in the tissue. The factors affecting the course of events in a necrotic area are the extent or amount of dead tissue, the nature or kind of dead tissue, the blood supply to the area, and the causative agent. For example, in a diabetic patient with complicating vascular disease who bruises a toe, an infection may develop in the area and the necrosis may spread, because the blood supply to the part was inadequate. By contrast, in a healthy person who slams a door on a finger, the injured necrotic area would readily heal. The person who has an infarction of a small area of the myocardium has a better chance of recovering than does the person who has massive destruction of heart muscle. Evidence of the extent of tissue necrosis may be obtained by determining the enzyme level in the serum. Since cellular enzymes such as glutamic oxaloacetic transaminase (SGOT) and lactic dehydrogenase (LDH) are released into the bloodstream upon destruction of the cell, the blood level of these particular enzymes will rise when necrosis occurs. Laboratory studies of SGOT and LDH are often ordered when the doctor suspects death of tissues of the liver, pancreas, or myocardium.

The result of tissue necrosis is usually autolysis or self-digestion of the cells and digestion of cell debris by other enzymes, such as the proteolytic enzymes liberated by dying leukocytes followed by encapsulation of the unabsorbed debris by fibrous tissue and then regeneration and repair of tissue.

AIMS OF THERAPY

The aims of therapy for patients with cell responses of increased function are dependent on the underlying cause. No therapy is indicated when the stimulus is within normal limits, such as the response to increased muscle activity with the use of crutches. Compensatory change in response to stimuli from pathological conditions as in the previous example of hypertrophied heart muscle is supported by therapy. The therapy is directed toward correcting or controlling the pathological condition stimulating the increased function, thereby maintaining the demands within the compensatory limits of the target organ. For instance, drugs may be use to lower blood pressure which then decreases the stimulus for cardiac muscle hypertrophy.

Aims of therapy in situations where the response is inhibition of cell function depend on the underlying cause of the disability. In general these aims are (1) to remove the cause when possible, (2) to provide for replacement of cell function, (3) to prevent extension of the retrogressive process, (4) to prevent superimposed infection, and (5) to promote repair of damaged tissues. Elimination of the initiating cause is usually possible when cell degeneration and/or necrosis is brought about by physical trauma or biologic agents. If atrophic or degenerative processes are precipitated by inadequacies of nutritional intake and/or physical inactivity, there may be a favorable response to diet therapy and increased activity.

In many situations it is not possible to remove the cause, as for example in diabetes mellitus. The genetic defect that contributes to the development of this degenerative condition of islet cells of the pancreas cannot be removed. In this condition secretory cells are not able to function normally. Replacement or supplement therapy may be effective in maintaining an adequate supply of hormone.

Degenerative changes may proceed over a period of time with some permanent tissue changes before therapy is sought. Therapy is aimed at preventing extension of the process. For instance, in degeneration of the liver associated with the inadequate nutrition that may accompany chronic alcoholism, some liver damage is permanent. Treatment with adequate diet may help to prevent further extension of the process. In certain irreversible degenerative kidney conditions, therapy is focused on accomplishment of organ function by means of mechanical devices such as the artificial kidney.

In other situations, extension of degenerative or necrotic processes may be inhibited by therapy that increases circulation to the part. Surgical procedures to remove obstructing thrombi or to perform bypass vessel grafts may be indicated. Exercises, applications of heat, and position may also promote circulation. Anticoagulants may be prescribed to prevent intravascular clotting processes that interfere with circulation to a part.

Barrier techniques are used in the hospital to prevent infection of devitalized tissues such as occurs in burns. Patients with deficient circulation to a part are taught self-care measures to protect against infection and to promote blood flow to the part. Repair of damaged tissue is fostered by decreasing functional demands on the affected part. Rest, both physical and psychological, is essential.

Neoplastic Response

Neoplasia is a cellular response to injurious agents. For emphasis, it is considered apart from the cellular responses discussed in the preceding section. Neoplasia is the second leading cause of death in the United States, and it is essential that the nurse have a basic understanding of its nature.

The meaning of the word *neoplasia* is *new formation*, but in medical science this word usually carries with it the connotation of a nonbeneficial new growth. This new growth is individualistic in the respect that is proliferates without regard for the well-being of the organism as a whole and apparently has no useful function in the body. There is a range of differences in the various characteristics of neoplastic cells, and it is on the basis of these differences that neoplasms are classified into two major types, benign and malignant.

The benign neoplasm is one which usually grows slowly and remains localized. It is separated from the tissue of origin by a fibrous capsule, and the neoplastic cells are similar in structure to the cell of origin. This is the neoplasm which the lay person considers to be harmless. However, complications may result from the

*Figure 11–10
Variations in cell size
and shape, and varia-
tions in the size of nu-
cleus and nucleolus,
between normal cells
and malignant cells. (By
permission of Howard C.
Hopps: Principles of
Pathology. New York:
Appleton Century Crofts,
1964, pp. 326–327.)*

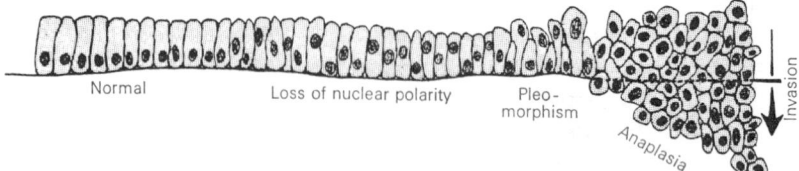

*Figure 11–11
Characteristics of malig-
nant cells. (By permission
of Howard C. Hopps:
Principles of Pathology.
New York: Appleton
Century Crofts, 1964, pp.
326–327.)*

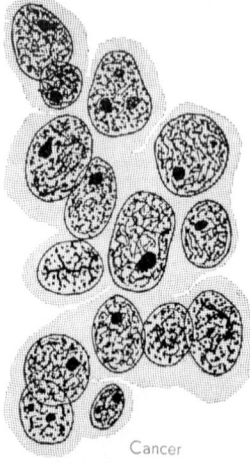

presence of benign neoplasms because of mechanical pressure on surrounding structures or from excessive production of secretions, if this is the nature of the cells of origin. Benign neoplasms expand and push other tissues aside, causing compression of these tissues and of their vascular supply. The location of the benign neoplasm influences whether the growth will be detrimental to the well-being of the person. For example, a benign neoplasm of supporting glial tissue in the brain may cause destruction of vital tissue and may not be removable surgically because this would necessitate destruction of vital tissue in the approach to the neoplasm. The cells of a benign neoplasm arising in an endocrine gland may secrete hormones as do the normal cells. An excess of hormone such as insulin from a benign pancreatic tumor would cause hypoglycemia and its attendant symptoms.

Malignant neoplasms, by contrast to benign ones, are always a threat to the existence of the person because they invade throughout the tissue of origin and spread to other parts of the body. Malignant cells apparently do not respond to growth control factors that tell a cell not to divide. The process of spread to distant sites is termed *metastasis.* Microscopically, malignant cells show varying degrees of change from normal structure. The cells of malignant tissue have an abnormal arrangement and are of varying sizes and shapes (pleomorphism). The rate of growth of malignant cells is usually more rapid than that of benign cells. Benign cells may eventually cease to grow. Unfortunately for the host, malignant cells reproduce cells like themselves and seldom cease growing. There is a spectrum of neoplasms from most benign to most malignant. The microscopic structural differences from one cancer cell to another are variations in degree, not in kind. All malignant neoplasms show a lack of organization, differences in cell size and shape, and variations in the size of nucleus and nucleolus, though each malignant neoplasm shows variations within each of these characteristics. (See Figures 11-10 and 11-11.)

Some of the terminology commonly used by both lay and medical personnel when discussing neoplasms is rather confusing. The word *tumor,* which means *swelling,* is used frequently by lay persons when referring to a malignant neoplasm, perhaps because this term seems less frightening than the term *malignancy* or *cancer.* Cancer is a term commonly used by both lay and medical personnel, as synonymous with any malignant neoplasm.

The ability to understand medical and nursing literature on the subject of neoplasms presupposes a knowledge of how neoplasms are named. Benign tumors are named by adding the suffix "-oma" to the name of the cell of origin. Malignant tumors are termed *carcinomas* if they arise from epithelial cells and *sarcomas* if they arise from cells of connective tissue origin. This term may be followed by the name of the involved organ. The nomenclature applicable to the more com-

TISSUE OF ORIGIN	BENIGN	MALIGNANT	COMMON SITES
TUMORS OF MESENCHYMAL ORIGIN *Connective Tissue*			
Fibrous	Fibroma	Fibrosarcoma	
Cartilage	Chondroma	Chondrosarcoma	
Bone	Osteoma	Osteosarcoma	
Adipose	Lipoma	Liposarcoma	
Muscle			
Smooth	Leiomyoma	Leiomyosarcoma	Uterus, stomach
Striated	Rhabdomyoma	Rhabdomyosarcoma	
Hematopoietic		Leukemia Lymphosarcoma	
Lymphoid and reticuloendothelial tissue		Lymphosarcoma Hodgkin's disease	
Nerve Tissue Neuroglia		*Glioma †Glioblastoma	Brain
Nerve sheaths	Neurofibroma	Neurofibrosarcoma	
Nerve cells	Ganglioneuroma	Neuroblastoma Retinoblastoma	
TUMORS OF EPITHELIAL ORIGIN *Pavement Epithelium*	Papilloma	Squamous cell carcinoma	Skin, cervix, buccal mucosa, esophagus, larynx
		Basal cell carcinoma	Skin
		Transitional cell carcinoma	Urinary bladder, ureter, renal pelvis
Mucous Membrane	Polyp	Adenocarcinoma	Bronchus, colon, stomach
Glandular Epithelium	Adenoma	Adenocarcinoma	Breast, thyroid, adrenal, kidney, pancreas

TABLE 11-1
Nomenclature in common benign and malignant neoplasms

* Generally considered malignant because of their local invasiveness and lethality.
† An "undifferentiated" highly malignant glioma.

mon benign and malignant neoplasms, including the type of cell origin and common sites of occurrence, is summarized in Table 11-1.

CAUSATIVE AGENTS AND THEIR EFFECTS

Carcinogens are agents that act on normal cells to initiate a malignant neoplastic change or permit the selective proliferation of malignant cells by means of differential toxicity, in the case of certain chemical carcinogens (Prelin). Many variables seem to play a role in determining if a particular carcinogen will exert an initiating action on an individual.

Experimental research on carcinogenic agents is, of course, performed on animals. The results of animal research cannot be assumed to be applicable to human beings but they provide clues for study of cancer in man. Experimental studies have indicated that cancer may be produced by chemical, physical, and biological agents that are present in the environment to varying extents. The environment in an industrial city, a mining area, and a radiologic laboratory will contain differing amounts of these agents. Chemical agents that have been identified as carcinogens include hydrocarbons, arsenic, chromates, and aromatic amines produced in the dye industry. The number of coal tar and other carcinogenic products in our present industrial and atmospheric environments is constantly increasing. It seems that the external environment of modern society is becoming a health hazard.

The source of chemical carcinogens may be within the body. For instance, custom dictates that Jewish males be circumcised shortly after birth, and cancer of the penis is virtually absent in this group. This fact is attributed to the lack of accumulation of secretions under the prepuce. These normal secretions are apparently slightly carcinogenic and the custom of circumcision prevents the secretions from accumulating and becoming a source of constant irritation.

Physical agents capable of initiating cell changes that result in cancer are ultraviolet rays and ionizing radiation. Prolonged exposure to ultraviolet rays or sunlight produces cancer of the exposed skin in some individuals. The incidence of skin cancer is greater among persons living in sunny southern states such as Texas and California than it is in persons residing in northern industrial cities that have fewer brilliant sunny days. The incidence of skin cancer is also higher in farmers than in city dwellers. It seems that the intensity of sunlight and the duration of exposure are factors that influence the carcinogenic action of ultraviolet rays. Another variable influencing the ability of sunlight to produce cancer is skin coloring, a hereditary factor. The incidence of cancer among Nordic populations is much greater than among Negro populations. Apparently, melanin pigment in the skin is a protective barrier against the carcinogenic action of sunlight.

Ionizing radiation exerts a carcinogenic effect on skin and other body tissues. The skin cancer effect was observed in persons instrumental in the discovery and early therapeutic use of radium. Precautions have been devised to decrease this hazard in industry and medical therapy but perhaps these precautions are not sufficient, since the incidence of leukemia (a neoplastic change in leukocytes) is higher among radiologists (doctors who specialize in radiation therapy) than among members of the medical profession as a whole.

Research findings indicate that some viruses are probably initiating agents in the development of cancer in man. Viruses are known to produce malignant neoplasms in mice, chickens, and rabbits. In man, the benign papilloma commonly known as a *wart* is caused by a virus and this virus does have biologic similarities to the papilloma virus of rabbits, but this fact leads to further research rather than to general conclusions. Research related to viral implications in the occurrence of clusters of cases of leukemia in human beings living in certain geographic areas has not definitely proved a virus to be a causative agent, but the implication is strong. Investigators of the viral etiology of cancer point out the similarity between normal intracellular structures and the structure of viruses. It is postulated that viruses invade the cell and shift or block metabolic pathways and in this way initiate the development of cancer or they may introduce some new genetic material. Proponents of the viral theory propose that other carcinogens act by inciting to activity a latent virus already present in cells. It is true that viruses are composed of nucleoproteins as are the genetic components of cells. To date, there is only suggestive evidence of the role of viruses in the production of human cancer. In animal experiments with viral agents both species specificity and tissue specificity have been demonstrated. Injection of cell-free filtrates of cancerous tumors of cottontail rabbits produces cancer in other cottontail rabbits but not in domestic rabbits. Tissue specificity has been domonstrated in this animal and in others through intravenous injection of cell-free filtrates from tumors into the same species of animals, with the result that cancer develops only in the same type of tissue from which the filtrate was obtained. It may be that there is a critical point in the relationship of host resistance and virus virulence that must be reached for the production of cancer. The answer to the etiologic role of viral agents in the development of cancer will be forthcoming.

Individual susceptibility to carcinogens is a broad term that encompasses many intrinsic variables. Animal experiments and studies of human beings indicate that some cancers are genetically transmitted. Mammary cancer occurs almost inevitably in some strains of mice. In human beings retinoblastomas and multiple neurofibromas have been shown to follow Mendelian principles of heredity. Studies of the chromosomal characteristics of some leukemic patients now reveal that some of these disorders of white blood cells may be genetically transmitted. The genetic defect is found on the same chromosome that is implicated in the transmission of mongolism. This may explain the high incidence of chronic myelocytic leukemia in persons with mongolism. More often the hereditary influences seem to be "disposition toward" instead of a relatively well-defined genetic defect. For instance, the incidence of cancer among the offspring of parents who died of cancer is greater than the incidence in offspring of parents who died of other causes. Clinical histories of persons with a diagnosis of cancer often reveal that other family members have also had cancer.

It has been said that everyone will have cancer if he lives long enough. The incidence of cancer does increase with increasing age, but with increasing age one also has been exposed for a longer period of time to agents that produce cancerous change. The wear and tear of life may influence resistance to harmful agents. It is of interest that the peak incidence of cancer of a particular type occurs at different ages. The peak incidence of prostatic cancer is over age 70, that of bone cancer is between 15 and 25 years, and cancer of the female sex organs occurs most often in the 50 to 55 age bracket. Currently there is no scientific explanation of these data.

Sometimes hormone production offers a possible explanation of the differing incidences between males and females of cancer in a particular organ. Hormones do influence the development of cancers in sex organs. Estrogen excess has been implicated in the development of breast cancer in premenopausal women. Disturbances in hormonal balance have also been implicated in the development of cancer of the uterus and the prostate, but hormones do not explain why cancer of the lung and the stomach develops more often in men than in women.

It is evident from the foregoing discussion that our present level of knowledge permits the conclusion that carcinogenesis is influenced by a number of factors. A way of considering the relationship between intrinsic and extrinsic causative factors is presented in the schema at the end of this paragraph.[2] If the extrinsic or environmental factors are overwhelming, cancer may develop even though the person's inherent disposition is slight. The reverse is also true; a strong inherent disposition and the presence of a weak environmental stimulus may also result in cancer.

$$E \times i = C \qquad \text{Key: E, e} = \text{extrinsic}$$
$$e \times I = C \qquad \text{Key: I, i} = \text{intrinsic}$$
$$E \times I = C \qquad \text{Key: c} = \text{no cancer}$$
$$e \times i = c \qquad \text{Key: C} = \text{cancer}$$

Despite the dissimilarities of injurious agents, the changes they incite seem to be of a similar nature. Horsfall believes current research to indicate that inciting agents produce their effect by causing a disturbance in the genetic mechanisms, perhaps the nucleic acids, and that this is responsible for the formation of other abnormal cell materials and the permanent transfer of the same changes to daughter cells. The process of producing an abnormality in the genetic material may require a period of time. The prolonged duration of exposure to an inciting agent such as ionizing radiation seems to support this possibility. It may be that once a change has occurred in the genetic material, this material is quiescent until it receives a stimulus from other promoting factors. It is apparent that not everyone who is exposed to inciting agents will have cancer; it may be that a promoting factor (or factors) is present in some individuals and not in others.

It seems that some carcinogens require prolonged exposure to bring about a progression of changes from normalcy to malignancy. A number of factors operate in the development of cancer and it may be that some factors act during the latent period to permit proliferation of malignant cells. An analogous situation is the presence of the herpes simplex virus. At some period in life most persons come in contact with this virus, an initiating agent. If the body defenses are lowered at this time this serves as a favorable variable to the virus, permitting it to become established in cells of the skin and mucous membrane around the lips and nostrils. At a later period of time, exposure to cold or to strong sunlight (two of many nonspecific factors) permits activation of the virus to cause cell damage and produce the well-known symptoms of the cold sore. Here the analogy ends, for this virus can be brought under control, but the cancer cell continues to produce cancer cells.

The reasons for the process of continuous, unrestrained growth that is a characteristic of malignant tumors are still unknown. This reflects the fact that the reason normal cells cease to proliferate when they have replaced damaged tis-

---

[2] From Hopps.

sue is also unknown. Normal cells are apparently restrained from further multi-plication when they are no longer free to move in one plane; they do not pile up on top of each other. This restriction is known as *contact inhibition.* Cancer cells are obviously less influenced by the control devices that inhibit proliferation; they do grow on top of one another. It is thought that the outside surfaces of cells may influence the organization of cells in multicellular organisms.

The origin of both malignant and benign neoplasms may be any of the stromal or parenchymal cell types. It is relatively rare that neoplastic cells are of neuronal origin. This may be related to the fact that nerve cells have a highly specialized function and little regenerative capacity.

The person is often unaware of what is happening in the early stages of malignant growth. Exceptions to this would be neoplasms of the skin, and even though these should be apparent, they may be overlooked. As a malignant growth invades adjacent tissues it may, like the benign growth, disturb normal functions because of location and/or mechanical pressure. A neoplasm growing into the lumen of the bowel may interfere with the passage of intestinal contents and be evidenced by changes in bowel habits. The body does react to the disturbance, for in a sense the neoplasm is a foreign body. The inflammatory reaction is usually mild but persistent and results in the production of fibrous tissue. In benign tumors this fibrous tissue encircles the slowly proliferating cells and provides a capsule for the tumor. In malignant tumors the cells propagate rapidly and irregular extensions into tissues occur, therefore no capsule can form but rather the fibrous tissue is interwoven with the neoplastic cells.

There are seven relatively early signs of the presence of a malignant neoplasm. The American Cancer Society has as one of its functions the education of the public in regard to these. The signals reflect (1) proliferation, (2) mechanical obstruction of a lumen, and (3) ulceration of the malignant tissue. The center of malignant tissue may become necrotic, and may ulcerate and bleed because the growth of capillaries into tumor tissue has not been adequate to meet the nutritive requirements of the cells. Neoplastic cells like normal cells will die from inadequate nutrition. The dead tissue sloughs, leaving an area of capillary oozing or frank bleeding if larger vessels are involved. The danger signals are as follows: (1) any unusual bleeding or discharge, (2) any sore that does not heal, (3) a change in normal bowel habits, (4) persistent indigestion or difficulty in swallowing, (5) any change in a wart or mole, (6) a lump or thickening in the breast or elsewhere, and (7) persistent hoarseness. Prompt investigation by a physician of any of these symptoms is essential if treatment is to be effective. The metastatic character of malignant neoplasms is the reason for avoiding delay in seeking medical attention.

The prognosis in a patient with cancer is related to the degree of dedifferentia-tion of cells. This characteristic is the basis for the designations of grade given to malignant lesions. The grade designations range from I to IV, with grade I in-dicating that the cell closely resembles the normal cell of the tissue of origin and grade IV meaning that the cell has a bizarre shape and size, that it is very atypical. A grade IV lesion is more apt to grow rapidly and metastasize sooner than a grade I, therefore the prognosis would be guarded.

The metastatic process may occur by direct invasion, by lymphatic or vascular invasion, or by seeding in serous cavities. Because malignant growths are not encapsulated, the reproducing cells are capable of invading adjacent tissues by following lines of tissue planes. The proliferating cells at the site of origin will push aside normal cells and be disseminated through the various tissue layers. For example, a cancer of the epithelial lining of the stomach may invade the cells of the basement membrane, the muscle layer, and the serosal surface. The malignant cells may gain access to the perineural lymphatics and grow along them for a considerable distance. The growing cells compress the nerve bundles and cause degeneration of distal nerve fibers. Compression of the nerve bundle stimulates nerve impulses that are interpreted as pain in the cerebral cortex. The malignant cells are motile and are able to invade the wall of lymphatics and proliferate along the lumen, and may break off and be carried to the regional lymph nodes where they continue to proliferate. Other malignant cells may invade veins and from the wall of the vein be carried as emboli to other organs. For example, malignant cells from the stomach or intestine would be carried by the portal circulation to the liver where the cells would reproduce and establish a metastatic focus. Cellular emboli that invade systemic veins may metastasize to the lungs.

Malignant neoplasms occurring in serous cavities spread by seeding cells that drop from the surface of the afflicted organ. For example, malignant cells that invade the stomach wall may slough off the surface and drop to the pelvic cavity. These cell emboli may be sufficient in number to establish a metastatic focus on an ovary, the sigmoid colon, or the mesentery. Malignant cells lack cohesiveness, and the outer cells are readily loosened from the main mass of cells. The muscular action of the wall of the stomach may dislodge some cells.

Tumors of epithelial origin tend to be disseminated by invasion of lymphatic and lymph nodes. This is the reason that axillary lymph node dissection is part of the surgical treatment of cancer of the breast. Tumors of mesenchymal origin spread by blood vessel invasion and emboli rather than by invasion of lymphatics. This method of spread may result in distant metastases that are difficult to treat surgically.

A metastatic focus may arise in tissues whose function is more readily disturbed than that of the primary site and the initial symptoms of disease may be referable to the secondary site. This sometimes happens with metastasis of prostatic cancer to vertebrae. Bone is an inelastic tissue, and pain from a space-occupying lesion such as a metastatic focus may be severe.

The person who is afflicted with a malignant growth is often unable to rapidly mobilize body defenses against other injurious agents. Pathogenic organisms easily become established when the host's resistance is low and he is unable to produce antibodies and phagocytes. It is not uncommon for infections to become established in the lungs or other tissues of the body including the neoplasm. When infections occur, the causative organism destroys neoplastic cells just as it does normal cells.

Malignant neoplasms have a great need for amino acids to carry on cell proliferation. These cells are capable of obtaining the amino acids they need for reproduction to the detriment of normal cells. It is not understood why neoplasms have first priority on the nutrients that are available for cell growth. The neoplasm continues to proliferate while other body cells decrease in size and function for lack of adequate amino acids. The person loses an extreme amount of weight and becomes weak and emaciated; his skin has a gray, waxen appearance. Anemia is evident in a low red blood cell count. The anemia is partially explained by the slow persistent seepage of blood from ulcerated tissue at the site of neoplastic growth but it is usually greater than can be attributed to this reason only. These signs and symptoms comprise what is known as the *cachexia of malignancy.*

Malignant neoplasms may affect the body in various ways. Hopps lists these effects as (1) disfigurement, (2) mechanical interference with normal function, (3) interference with normal tissue function by tissue replacement, (4) discontinuity of structure, (5) nutritional competition, (6) function of the neoplastic cell itself, and (7) psychic disturbances. The preceding discussion of the malignant process has mentioned effects that fit each of these categories with the exception of psychic disturbances, but much has been written on the subject of emotional reactions to cancer.

The diagnosis of cancer carries with it a connotation of prolonged, debilitating, painful death that evokes fear in most persons, both lay persons and those with medical knowledge. This outlook is understandable since medical science has yet to pinpoint a causative agent, and in fact it appears that there is no one agent responsible for the development of a malignant neoplasm—therefore there are no specific means of preventing or curing cancer. Knowledge that metastasis may have occurred before warning symptoms were noticed sometimes deters people from seeking medical attention because the situation is perceived to be hopeless. Most people in an educated country like the United States realize that once extensive metastasis has occurred curative treatment is not possible.

Uncertainty about the course of illness is another factor affecting emotional reactions to a malignant disease. A surgeon cannot definitely state that all of a tumor was removed because metastasis may have occurred and yet not be apparent at the time of treatment. The effectiveness of surgery, radiation therapy, or chemotherapy cannot be accurately predicted; even the same type of malignant tumor may respond differently to these methods of destroying cancer cells.

In general, four outcomes are possible in malignant neoplasia. (1) The disease may spread rapidly, may be resistant to treatment, and may quickly terminate in death. (2) All diseased tissue may be removed, and the patient apparently cured. (3) The primary growth may be removed, but metastatic lesions may produce slowly debilitating effects and death. (4) The neoplasm may be held in check for a number of years, and the affected person may succumb to the effects of some other disease. Lay persons are often aware of the variance in the course of malignant diseases and derive hope from the fact that some people have apparently been cured. One cannot expect patients to have a set pattern of emotional reactions to the diagnosis, treatment, and course of a malignant illness. In general, emotional reactions to the diagnosis of malignant neoplasms are influenced by the current status of knowledge regarding them. These reactions are discussed in detail in other chapters.

AIMS OF THERAPY

The goals of medical care are early diagnosis and complete removal of the malignant lesion. If these are not possible then the goal becomes one of inhibiting the rate of growth and spread of the lesion and promoting patient comfort. The methods of treatment are surgical excision, destruction of malignant cells with radiation therapy, and palliation with the use of radiation, hormone therapy, and anticancer drugs. These therapies are discussed elsewhere.

The goals of nursing care are to promote among lay persons positive attitudes and actions regarding preventive measures and examinations for early diagnosis and accurate knowledge about cancer; to teach self-care following particular types of surgical treatment; to provide physical and emotional care for the patient receiving curative and palliative treatment and the patient for whom treatment is not possible; and to provide support to the family of the afflicted individual. This care includes maintenance and support of body functions and emotional well-being, and when therapy permits, restoration and rehabilitation to maximum potential for assumption of his previous role in the family and society. Specific nursing measures relative to the site of the lesion and the particular medical therapy are discussed in the appropriate chapters in Part V.

Summary

This chapter has focused on factors that contribute to or cause disease or dysfunction and bodily responses to these injurious agents. The content is summarized in the following principles:

1. Disease or dysfunctions result when there is an imbalance between the harmful effects of injurious agents and the defense mechanisms of the host. It is a dynamic, ever-changing process.

2. By means of adaptive mechanisms, the body attempts to overcome or adjust to the damaging effects of harmful agents and restore structural and functional balance.

3. Injurious agents are present in both the extrinsic and intrinsic environments. They are of a physical, biological, chemical, sociocultural, psychological, or hereditary nature.

4. In essence, all disease is a result of metabolic defects within cells. Metabolic disturbances result in alterations of cell function and structure.

5. Characteristics influencing the effect of factors that contribute to or cause disease are the quality and quantity of the agent, the location and extent of injury, and the period of time of the injury.

6. Neuroendocrine responses are vital, systemic reactions to nonspecific injurious agents.

7. The magnitude of the neuroendocrine response is usually proportional to the magnitude of the trauma.

8. The purposes of neuroendocrine responses are to maintain circulatory stability and to provide nutrients for energy and repair of damaged tissues.

9. Neuroendocrine responses involve (a) sympathoadrenal medullary activity and the release of norepinephrine and epinephrine. These hormones prepare the body for fight or flight. (b) Adrenocortical activity is mediated through the hypothalamus and adenohypophysis. Glucocorticoids secreted by the adrenal cortex

increase catabolism of protein, carbohydrate, and fat. (c) Mineralocorticoids are secreted in response to adrenocortical stimulation from neuronal cells in either the diencephalon or mesencephalon. The mineralocorticoids promote reabsorption of sodium and excretion of potassium by renal tubules. (d) Antidiuretic hormone is released by the neurohypophysis in response to stimuli from neuronal cells in the hypothalamus. This hormone acts on cells of the distal and collecting renal tubules to increase their permeability to water.

10. Inflammation is a protective local response to diverse injurious agents. It occurs at the site of most bodily injuries.

11. The inflammatory process consists of vascular, cellular, and exudative changes that tend to localize the injury, destroy the harmful agent, and digest the products of cellular debris.

12. The manifestations of inflammation (heat, swelling, redness, pain) reflect the vascular changes of increased dilatation and permeability of capillaries. (a) The ability to replace injured tissues with like cells in the same organization is dependent on the extent of injury, the regenerative capacity of the affected cells, and the complexity of the organizational pattern of the tissues. (b) Healing by fibrous tissue substitution results in contraction and scarring. (c) Adequate nutrition, especially amino acids and vitamin C, is essential for regeneration of connective tissue and parenchymal cells. (d) The healing process progresses from the inflammatory process; there is no sharp line of demarcation between these two.

13. Human beings have certain natural barriers that inhibit pathogenic invasion.

14. Pathogens cause cell damage by the production of toxins or intracellular enzymes that disturb normal metabolic activity.

15. Factors essential to production of infectious disease are the presence of a causative agent, a reservoir for the agent, a mode of escape from the reservoir, and a means of transmission and entry into a susceptible host.

16. Host defenses against pathogens include nonspecific and specific antibodies, as well as phagocytic action of cells that participate in the inflammatory response.

17. Pathogenic toxins stimulate a systemic as well as a local response.

18. Immune responses involve the reaction of an antigen with its particular antibody.

19. Immunity to some pathogens may be acquired by either artificial or natural contact with the particular antigenic organism which results in production of specific antibodies.

20. Humoral or immediate antigen-antibody reactions take place when the antibody is present in circulating body fluids. Cellular or delayed responses are thought to occur when the antibody is present within lymphoid cells and must be transported to the site of antigen presence.

21. The hypersensitive humoral or cellular antigen-antibody reaction stimulates an intense inflammatory response. The hypersensitive reaction depends on previous contact with a sensitizing antigen to which the individual produces specific antibodies.

22. Individual susceptibility to the stimulus of antigenic substances varies from none to marked response to many substances. There is no means of predicting individual response to antigens.

23. Skin testing with minute amounts of sensitizing antigen permits prediction of possible hypersensitive reaction, but this method is not feasible for use with all possible antigenic substances.

24. An intact circulatory system is essential for the well-being of the human being. It provides for an exchange of materials between the external and internal environments and between the organs of the internal environment.

25. Disruption of the continuity of vessels initiates protective local and systemic responses that control blood loss and maintain blood flow to vital organs. These responses are concerned with clotting of blood and contraction of the vascular bed.

26. Secondary protective mechanisms following blood loss are aimed at restoration of blood osmotic pressure and replacement of erythrocytes. These mechanisms function over a period of time.

27. Decreased circulation of blood to a part causes inadequate oxygenation and nutrient supply of the receptive tissues and a depression of tissue function and/or altered structure.

28. Any interference with blood flow through the heart or lungs is reflected in the vascular system throughout the body. Slowing of blood flow and elevation of venous pressure result in systemic passive congestion. Congestion of tissues interferes with nutrient exchange and causes depression of cell function.

29. Hypertrophy and hyperplasia are adaptive mechanisms by which cells respond to stimuli for increased function.

30. Atrophy is a cellular response to decreased stimuli for function or to prolonged decreased blood flow below maintenance requirements.

31. The excess accumulation within cells of normal metabolic products or of metabolic products not normal to the cell disrupts cell function.

32. The process is often reversible but may go on to necrosis.

33. Necrosis of cells occurs when injurious agents disrupt the cell membrane, interfere with normal intracellular metabolism, or interfere with the cell supply of necessary nutrients and oxygen. Any of these agents in sufficient quantity may cause cell death. The systemic effect from cell necrosis is dependent upon the extent of damaged tissue, the location of injury, and the regenerative capacity of damaged cells.

34. The development of neoplastic changes within cells is influenced by the presence of an inciting agent, an intrinsic predisposition, and favorable environmental conditions.

35. Malignant neoplasms may arise in any tissue of the body.

36. Cancer spreads by direct invasion and by metastasis.

37. There is a spectrum of neoplasms from most benign to most malignant.

38. All malignant neoplasms have a lack of organization, differences in cell size and shape, and variations in the size of nucleus and nucleolus, though each neoplasm shows variations within each of these characteristics.

39. It appears that a carcinogen acting in the presence of a favorable variable may initiate or potentiate a chemical change in a group of cells and at a later period in time a nonspecific agent (a promoter) may activate the potential of the cell for the cancer process.

40. As a malignant growth invades tissues it may disrupt normal functions because

of its location and/or mechanical pressure, or because of erosion of the wall of the blood vessels.

41. The person with a malignant neoplasm often is unable to mobilize body defenses against other injurious agents.

42. Many, but not all, types of cancer can be treated successfully if detected early in the course of the disease.

Bibliography

Books

Anderson, W. A. D. (Ed.): *Pathology,* 5th ed. Vol. I. St. Louis: The C. V. Mosby Company, 1966.

Apperly, Frank L.: *Patterns of Disease,* Philadelphia: J. B. Lippincott Company, 1951.

Bajusz, E. and Jasmin, G. (Eds.): *Major Problems in Neuroendocrinology.* New York: S. Karger, 1964.

Beland, Irene: *Clinical Nursing: Pathophysiological and Psychosocial Approaches,* New York: The Macmillan Company, 1965.

Best, Charles and Taylor, Norman: *The Physiological Basis of Medical Practice,* 8th ed. Baltimore: The Williams & Wilkins Company, 1966.

Black, Maurice and Bernard Wagner: *Dynamic Pathology.* St. Louis: The C. V. Mosby Company, 1964.

Bordicks, Katherine: *Patterns of Shock.* New York: The Macmillan Company, 1965.

Boyd, William: *An Introduction to the Study of Disease.* Philadelphia: Lea & Febiger, 1962.

Cannon, Walter: *The Wisdom of the Body.* London: K. Paul Company, 1932.

Florey, Sir Howard: *General Pathology,* 3d ed. Philadelphia: W. B. Saunders Company, 1962.

Guyton, Arthur: *Textbook of Medical Physiology,* 3d ed. Philadelphia: W. B. Saunders Company, 1966.

Hardy, James D: *Pathophysiology in Surgery.* Baltimore: The Williams & Wilkins Company, 1958.

Hopps, Howard C.: *Principles of Pathol-* ogy, 2d ed. New York: Appleton Century Crofts, 1964.

Horsfall, Frank Jr. and Tamm, Igor: *Viral and Rickettsial Infections of Man.* Philadelphia: J. B. Lippincott Company, 1965.

Landells, John: *Essential Principles of Pathology,* Philadelphia: J. B. Lippincott Company, 1959.

Montgomery, George: *Textbook of Pathology,* Vol. I. Edinburgh: E & S Livingstone Ltd., 1965.

Morehead, Robert: *Human Pathology.* New York: McGraw-Hill Book Company, 1965.

Moyer, Carl, et al.: *Surgery: Principles and Practice,* 3d ed. Philadelphia: J. B. Lippincott Company, 1965.

Perry, Thomas M. and Frank N. Miller: *Pathology.* Boston: Little, Brown and Company, 1961.

Robbins, Stanley: *Textbook of Pathology,* 3d ed. Philadelphia: W. B. Saunders Company, 1967.

Selye, Hans: *The Stress of Life.* New York: McGraw-Hill Book Company, 1956.

Shafer, Kathleen, et al.: *Medical-Surgical Nursing,* 4th ed. St. Louis: The C. V. Mosby Company, 1967.

Smith, Edward, et al.: *Principles of Human Pathology.* New York: Oxford University Press, 1959.

Sodeman, William: *Pathologic Physiology,* 2d ed. Philadelphia: W. B. Saunders Company, 1956.

Tuttle, W. W. and Byron Schottelius: *Textbook of Physiology,* 16th ed. St. Louis: The C. V. Mosby Company, 1969.

Watson, J. D.: *Molecular Biology of the*

Gene. New York: W. A. Benjamin, Inc., 1965, Chap. 16.

Winson, Travis and Chester Hyman: *A Primer of Peripheral Vascular Disease.* Philadelphia: Lea & Febiger, 1965.

Wright, G. Paling: *An Introduction to Pathology,* 3d ed. London: Longmans, Green & Co., Ltd., 1958.

Zimmerman, Bernard: Surgical Metabolism and Electrolyte Balance. in Davis, Loyal (Ed.): *Christopher's Textbook of Surgery,* 9th ed. Philadelphia: W. B. Saunders Company, 1968.

Articles

Basic and Clinical Immunology. *Medical Clinics of North America,* November, 1965.

Bennett, Herman: Burns, First Aid and Emergency Care. *American Journal of Nursing,* 62:10;96–100, October, 1962.

Cohn, Howard: Hemostasis and Blood Coagulation. *American Journal of Nursing,* 65:2:116–119, February, 1965.

Cuthbertson, D. T.: Metabolic Effects of Injury and Their Nutritional Implications. *Nursing Times,* 146–147, January 29, 1965; pp. 179–180, February 5, 1965.

Davis, Marcella: Patients in Limbo. *American Journal of Nursing,* 66:4:746–749, April, 1966.

Frohman, I. Phillips: The Adrenocorticosteroids. *American Journal of Nursing,* 64:11:120–123, 1964.

Hildreth, Eugene: Some Common Allergic Emergencies. *Medical Clinics*

of North America, 1313–1323, September, 1966.

Horsfall, Frank: Unifying Concept of the Origin of Cancer. *Medical Clinics of North America,* 869–874, May, 1966.

Kottke, Frederick and Russel Blanchard: Bedrest Begets Bedrest. *Nursing Forum,* 3:3:56–72, 1964.

Miller, Daniel G. and Leonard Korngold: Monoclonal Immunoglobulins in Cancer. *Medical Clinics of North America,* 667–674, May, 1966.

Moore, George: Cancer: 100 Different Diseases. *American Journal of Nursing,* 66:4:749–753, April, 1966.

Newton, William: The Biologic Basis of Tissue Transplantation. *Surgical Clinics of North America,* 45:2:393–406, April, 1965.

Prehn, Richmond: Cancer Antigens in Tumors Induced by Chemicals. *Federation Proceedings,* 24:5:1018, September-October, 1965.

Prehn, Richmond: Role of Immunity in the Biology of Cancer. *Proceedings National Cancer Conference,* 97–104, 1965.

Schneewind, John H.: Surgical Physiology of Trauma. *Surgical Clinics of North America,* 42:1:79–90, February, 1962.

Selye, Hans: The Stress Syndrome. *American Journal of Nursing,* 65: 3:97–99, March, 1965.

Simeone, F.A: Shock: Its Nature and Treatment. *American Journal of Nursing,* 66:6:1286, June, 1966.

Snively, W. D.: Toward a Better Understanding of Body Fluid Disturbances. *Nursing Forum,* 3:1:61–77, 1964.

Stephens, Gwen: The Time Factor. *American Journal of Nursing,* 65: 5:77–82, May, 1965.

CHAPTER 12
ALTERATIONS IN VITAL SIGNS AND ASSOCIATED RESPIRATORY MANIFESTATIONS

LOUISE W. MANSFIELD

This chapter includes a discussion of vital signs as a group because it is often convenient to make observations of temperature, pulse, and respiration at the same time and also because they are so interrelated that a variation in one sign is usually considered in relation to the others. Following the discussion of alteration in body temperature, pulse rate and blood pressure are considered together. Respiration is discussed in this chapter along with common disturbances in respiratory functions.

Observation of vital signs is an independent nursing function, a part of the continued nursing assessment. It is the responsibility of every nurse to develop the ability to observe, accurately measure, and report those symptoms which are included in the group known as *vital signs*. Some points regarding observation of temperature, blood pressure, pulse, and respiration will be included here but techniques for observation of these signs are more fully presented in introductory nursing textbooks. The nursing care for surgical patients with respiratory problems is presented more fully elsewhere.

Alterations in Body Temperature

Fever has been recognized as a cardinal sign of disease since the time of Hippocrates. Early physicians recognized and evaluated fever by touch. In the first part of the seventeenth century, a crude clinical thermometer was invented by an Italian professor, Sanctorius; Gabriel Fahrenheit produced a mercurial instrument for measuring temperature in 1714. The medical possibilities of clinical thermometry were not realized until late in the nineteenth century; today body temperature is probably the most frequently observed index of physical function.

Body temperature is a measure of the heat content of the body expressed in degrees on a centigrade or Fahrenheit scale. It is indeed a vital sign because of the relatively small range within which physiological processes can operate, and any departure from the normal range, 36.5° to 37.5° C, is a cardinal sign of disease. The rate of chemical reactions *in vivo* and *in vitro* is increased by approximately 10 percent for each degree centigrade temperature increase. Body heat must be regulated within a narrow range because enzyme systems are temperature-sensitive to the extent that a rise or fall of a few degrees may completely inhibit their activity, interrupt metabolism, and result in death. Tissue proteins are heat-sensitive and become irreversibly inactivated at the upper limits of the physiological temperature range. Central nervous system function is impaired by a variation of 4° C (9° F) above or below the normal range; and with the exception of artificial regulation and medical care, survival is limited to a range of approximately 8° C above and 10° C below normal (DuBois). Convulsions are common at temperatures above 41° C (105.8° F).

Body temperature is an indefinite term, since the temperature of tissues varies considerably according to the site and state of activity of the tissue at the time of measurement. However, for clinical purposes, the term is commonly used to refer to temperature measured in the mouth, rectum, axilla, or esophagus. The normal range of oral temperature in resting man is said to be 36.5° to 37.5° C (97.7° to 99.5° F), with the average at 37° C (98.6° F). Rectal temperature is usually about 1 Fahrenheit degree (.55° C) higher and axillary temperature 1 Fahrenheit degree lower. Body temperature varies 0.5° to 2.0° F during each 24-hour period, following a diurnal pattern with the highest temperature in the late afternoon and the lowest during sleep and early morning hours. The commonly accepted low normal of 36.5° C (97.7° F) for oral temperature is questionable. Early morning readings lower than this are often observed and should be measured and reported accurately. For clinical purposes 99.5° F (37.5° C) is generally accepted as the normal upper limit for oral temperatures. Bennett says that in the case of a person who has been lying in bed it is safe to regard an oral temperature above 98.6° F as an indication of disease. For a person who has been engaged in moderate activity a temperature above 99.0° F has the same significance.

Because of its convenience the oral method is most commonly used for clinical temperature measurement. The measured rectal temperature is generally higher; it has been thought that the rectum is better isolated from external temperature changes. However, recent research has demonstrated that oral temperature reflects changes in the temperature of the arterial blood better than rectal temperature (Cranston). It has been suggested that rectal temperature may be affected by the temperature of blood in the pelvic veins close to the rectal wall. When the lower extremities are cold, cooled blood in these vessels may lower the temperature of the area (DuBois; Mead). In a recent nursing study it was found that rectal temperatures measured with the temperature-probe angled toward the anterior rectal wall were higher than those taken with the probe angled posteriorly (Tate). It is thought that this may explain the common experience of nurses in finding a difference between rectal temperature readings obtained with a glass clinical thermometer in comparison to those from an indwelling electrical probe. This finding has implications for temperature determination with hypothermic or other acutely ill patients in intensive care units where temperature is monitored continuously. A better indication of central body temperature can be obtained at a depth of at least 3 inches with the thermometer or probe angled anteriorly.

Fever, or pyrexia, is characterized by temperatures above the usual range of normal. Fever levels may result from strenuous muscular exercise, hot baths, or exposure to an extremely hot environment; however, the term *fever* is generally reserved for elevations in body temperature due to disease. An elevated body temperature is a cardinal sign of disease because all disease conditions in which fever occurs seem to have one feature in common, namely, tissue injury.

NURSING RESPONSIBILITIES IN RELATION TO ABNORMAL BODY TEMPERATURE

The nurse is responsible for accurate determination, reporting, and recording of all vital signs, whether she performs these determinations herself or delegates them to other members of the nursing staff. In the hospital situation these are usually performed at scheduled times; however, abnormal elevation of body temperature is such a sensitive and reliable indicator of disease that it warrants continued alertness on the part of the nurse, and the temperature should be determined at unscheduled times whenever the nurse observes any indication of fever. An unexpected level or sudden rise in temperature is promptly reported to the physician in order that early treatment may be instituted to counteract the fever and also that the disease condition may be diagnosed and definitive treatment begun. The graphic temperature record is useful in diagnosing the type and severity of disease and in assessing the patient's response to therapy.

For moderate variation in body temperature the nurse will perform independent nursing actions aimed at increasing the comfort of the patient and assisting in maintenance of physiological homeostasis. The patient with serious alteration in body temperature may need to be protected by the use of special therapies prescribed by the physician. To be able to give effective nursing care in either of those situations, the professional nurse must have a good understanding of the physiological processes that regulate body temperature and the pathophysiology associated with fever. The reader is referred to the textbooks and references listed at the end of this chapter for review of the physiology of temperature control.

PATHOPHYSIOLOGY OF FEVER

The thermoregulatory mechanism functions quite well over a range of 6 or 7 degrees C in health, in disease, and during strenuous physical exercise; this is illustrated in Figure 12-1. In febrile disease and during and immediately after strenuous physical exercise the internal body temperature may be elevated 1 or 2 degrees C while the temperature adjusting mechanisms are functioning to return the temperature to normal, or in the case of febrile disease to maintain it at a new "set point" which is somewhere above normal and which varies according to the type and severity of the disease. Above and below this normal range of temperature regulation thermoregulatory control continues to function, although with impaired efficiency. The body much more vigorously defends against overheating than against cooling; the protective significance of this is apparent when

Figure 12–1
Extremes of body temperature and zones of temperature regulation. (By permission of Eugene F. DuBois: Fever and the Regulation of Body Temperature. Springfield, Ill., Charles C Thomas Publisher, 1948.)

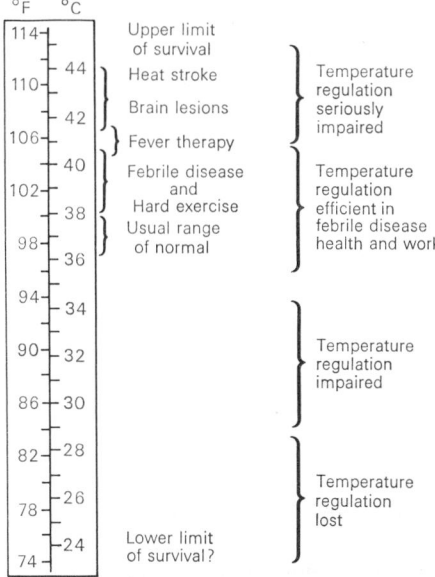

the upper and lower limits of survival of thermal extremes are compared (see Figure 12-1). Irreversible changes occur and thermal death results when internal body temperatures exceed 44° or 45° C, but hypothermia with internal temperatures below 24° C can be tolerated provided that intensive medical support is available. Temperature regulation is almost completely lost at 30° C; the subject becomes poikilothermic, and rewarming will not occur unless heat is supplied from external sources (Brengelmann). However, at high temperatures, above 41° C (106° F), the rate of cell metabolism is so greatly increased because of the temperature itself that no amount of physiological regulation can overcome the very rapid rate of heat production. The resulting vicious circle of heat production is a medical emergency and death will occur within a few hours unless pharmacological and physical means are used to supplement the patient's own cooling mechanisms.

With fever the rise in body temperature is not due to a breakdown of the temperature regulation system. The physiological mechanisms that control heat gain and heat loss function normally except that the physiological thermostat seems to be set to maintain the temperature at a higher level than normal. When the set point of the thermostat is adjusted upward the individual then responds as if he were cold. Surface heat loss is minimized by vasoconstriction and heat production may be increased by shivering. The individual feels cold and may put on more clothing or bedding or turn up the room heat. As a result the body gains heat until the new set point is reached and then regulates heat gain and heat loss around that level until the thermostat is reset.

Fever, or pyrexia, is an elevation of body temperature due to disease. The terms *hyperpyrexia* and *hyperthermia* usually refer to temperature elevations of 41° C (106° F) and above. Body temperature may be elevated to fever level by strenuous physical exercise or hot baths. Children are especially susceptible to temperature elevation due to physical exercise or emotional excitement. It is important to remember that children have a normal temperature slightly higher than that of adults and higher fever levels during illness than are usully seen in adult patients. Elderly persons, on the other hand, tend to have a lower normal temperature and their fever response in illness is somewhat less than that which would be seen in a healthy young adult with a comparable disease process.

Fevers may be classified according to their pattern of rise and fall as intermittent, remittent, and continuous. A fever characterized by wide fluctuations with the temperature rising each day but falling to normal or below at some time during the day is known as *intermittent fever* and is also referred to as *septic fever*. This pattern is seen with abscesses and malaria.

A remittent fever has a pattern of a rise in temperature each day followed by a decrease but remaining above normal. This type of fever is common during an infectious process, particularly if the infection is not responding to therapeutic measures. When the temperature remains elevated for several days with only slight fluctuations similar to those seen in normal temperature this is sometimes termed a *continuous fever*. A relapsing fever has a pattern of alternating periods of fever and normal temperature, each period lasting 1 or more days. The Pel-Ebstein fever seen in some patients with Hodgkin's disease is an example (Atkins).

Tissue injury is a factor common to nearly all febrile diseases. For this reason fever may be considered a physiological response to tissue injury. It is thought that fever results when the set point of the hypothalamic thermostat is adjusted upward by the effect of one or more products of tissue injury. Experimental evidence indicates that the temperature-regulating centers in the hypothalamic area may be affected directly by bacterial toxins and also indirectly by products of tissue injury such as endogenous pyrogen of polymorphonuclear leukocytes.

For a better appreciation of the fact that fever is a physiological response to tissue injury, it may be well to enumerate some types of tissue injury that cause fever. Any infectious disease process may cause fever regardless of the causative organism. Extensive surgical procedures, crushing injuries, and radiation are associated with elevated temperature as a result of mechanical injury to tissues. Vascular accidents occurring at any location in the body are usually associated with some fever. Tissue injury in the area where the blood supply has been impaired probably accounts for the elevated temperatures seen in patients following myocardial infarction, cerebral hemorrhage or thrombosis, and occlusion of a peripheral vessel. Many types of neoplasms can cause fever, and disorders of the hematopoietic system are marked by intermittent bouts of fever. In addition to these a number of inflammatory diseases and acute metabolic disorders are capable of producing fever (Bennett).

In spite of the frequent occurrence of fever and its wide clinical use as an index of the course of the disease and the patient's response to treatment, the physiological significance of fever is still not well understood. Much work has been done in an attempt to answer the question as to whether or not fever in disease is beneficial. In 1948 in a well-known monograph on fever, DuBois wrote, "There is always the possibility, not yet proved, that the defenses of the body are increased at high temperatures. There is still much to be learned about fever." In 1952 Selle stated that there was increasing evidence to indicate that fever is protective and beneficial and hastens recovery from infection. It has long been known that artificially induced fever is of value in the treatment of certain infectious diseases. Fever therapy was commonly used in the treatment of gonorrhea and syphilis before antibiotics were available. The lack of fever in elderly or debilitated patients with infectious diseases is considered an unfavorable prognostic sign. It is possible that the increased metabolic rate associated with fever increases the production of immune bodies and phagocytosis; however, it has not been conclusively demonstrated that fever increases these or other defense mechanisms of the body or serves any useful purpose. Fever is generally considered to be disadvantageous to the patient because of the accompanying pathophysiological changes. For example, the fever response with malignant disease accelerates weight loss and causes malaise. Following a myocardial infarction fever increases the metabolic rate, thereby placing an extra load on the damaged myocardium (Atkins).

For temperature elevations of moderate degree, the planning of patient care that will provide physical comfort and maintenance of homeostasis is usually an independent nursing responsibility. Higher temperature elevations represent problems that require specific medical therapies and nursing measures prescribed by the physician. These include the use of hypothermia mattresses, cooling baths, and antipyretic drugs. In the presence of fever, antipyretic drugs have the effect of resetting the hypothalamic thermostat at a lower level, thus activating the physiological mechanisms for decreasing body temperature. Aspirin, 300 to 600 mg, is the drug most frequently employed for antipyretic effect. It may be administered either orally or by rectal suppository. The effect of aspirin seems to be proportional to the degree of fever, the higher the temperature the more it will be decreased, and temperatures within the normal range are unaffected by the administration of aspirin.

TEMPERATURE RISE WITH CHILL

A chill often marks the onset of fever associated with infectious processes. The involuntary muscular activity produces heat and increases body temperature, although a sudden rise in body temperature may also occur without a noticeable shaking chill. In either case the resulting fever is due to accumulation of body heat after the thermostat has been reset at a higher level. When chilling does occur it is usually of shorter duration than the period of increased heat production and conservation by which the body temperature is raised to the higher level. During a chill the patient is extremely uncomfortable because he feels cold; he tends to seek extra clothing and bedding. A chilled patient often prefers a curled-up side-lying position in bed. This position favors isometric contraction of large flexor muscles and also conserves heat by reducing the amount of heat lost by radiation and convection. Similarly, animals exposed to cold assume a spheroid form, which markedly reduces the area of exposed skin. During the period of increased heat production and conservation the skin is usually cool, pale, and covered with "goose-flesh," the vestigial form of piloerection. With peripheral vasoconstriction and decreased blood flow in the capillaries there is more complete removal of oxygen from the blood, resulting in the cyanosis sometimes seen. The shaking phase of a chill usually lasts 10 to 40 minutes and there is a rapid rise of body temperature of 1° to 4° C (2° to 7° F).

Nursing care of the patient during a chill consists of careful observation and nursing measures aimed at increasing the patient's comfort. Since the chief source of discomfort is the patient's sensation of coldness, extra blankets should be applied immediately. Prewarmed blankets are especially comforting. A hot water bottle applied to the feet and another at the back, high up between the shoulders, will do much to increase the patient's comfort. These measures will not increase the eventual height of the patient's fever because the physiological mechanisms for heat gain will be reversed as soon as the central temperature reaches the new set level. Vigorous shivering is an efficient though exhausting means of heat production. The suggested nursing measures, while adding to the patient's comfort, will also conserve his expenditure of energy by shortening the time required to bring the body temperature to the new level.

The onset of a chill should be promptly reported to the patient's physician because diagnostic blood cultures may be indicated. Atkins states that the ideal time for blood cultures would be 1 hour before the onset of the chill since there is a time lag during which thermoregulatory centers are affected by the pyrogens. Obviously this is not possible; however, it is not advisable to wait until the height of the chill or the height of the fever which usually follows the end of the chill by ½ to 1 hour. The nurse should observe and report the severity and duration of the chill and the color and general condition of the patient, and take rectal temperatures at 15-minute intervals during the chill. Oral temperatures are less reliable and unsafe due to mouth breathing and chattering of the teeth with shivering. With the increase in metabolism and oxygen consumption there is increased ventilation and heart rate. It is difficult and sometimes impossible to determine rate of pulse and respiration during active chilling.

Following the chill the temperature should be taken at intervals of 15 to 30 minutes until a peak elevation has been reached, and somewhat less often during the next few hours, depending on the trend of the patient's temperature. If the patient's temperature is rising rapidly and approaching a level that may require the use of special protective therapies, it should be evaluated and reported to the physician at more frequent intervals. Following a chill, or sudden rise in temperature without a chill, the temperature may remain elevated or subside to a lower fever level and be regulated around that point varying according to the activity of the patient, the time of day, and the disease process.

NURSING CARE OF THE FEBRILE PATIENT

Nursing care of the febrile patient requires a number of independent nursing actions to assist the patient in maintaining or regaining homeostasis and to provide for his comfort. Following a sudden increase in body temperature or with any febrile condition considerable quantities of heat must be dissipated. This is accomplished primarily by evaporative and convective heat loss through increased sweating and peripheral vasodilatation. Thus, the process of transfer of excess heat from the interior to the surface of the body requires increased cardiac output for the work of temperature regulation. In the absence of fever a similar work load is imposed upon the cardiovascular system when environmental temperature is high and increased sweating is required for the elimination of normal body heat. When air conditioning is not available cardiac patients are sometimes placed in a cooled oxygen tent to reduce the physiological cost of temperature control.

Activities of the febrile patient should be planned to minimize exertion and allow for rest. Interaction with visitors and other patients should also be taken into consideration since emotional excitement tends to increase body temperature. The necessity for establishing a medical diagnosis and therapy often requires the acutely ill febrile patient to undergo a number of stressful procedures that represent large energy expenditures. The nurse, more than any other member of the health team, is responsible for planning the patient's total activities to minimize stress and fatigue.

The fact that the rate of tissue metabolism increases cumulatively by approximately 10 percent for each centigrade degree of fever indicates that the febrile patient has specific nutritional needs. Feedings should be small, nutritious, and easily digested. High-caloric liquids meet these requirements, providing both food and fluid. Since mild acidosis is common with fever, the use of citrus juices and carbonated beverages is favored. Their weak organic acids have an alkaline effect in the body.

Fluid lost by evaporation in the process of heat elimination must be replaced to prevent dehydration, electrolyte imbalance, and decreased urinary output. The patient should be frequently encouraged to take fluids by mouth unless this is contraindicated by the medical diagnosis. Parenteral administration of fluids may also be necessary to supplement oral intake and correct electrolyte imbalances. The recording of fluid intake and output is an important responsibility in the care of febrile patients. It is expected that the increased loss of fluids through sensible and insensible perspiration will be taken into consideration by physicians and nurses in using the record as a guide for fluid administration. All members of the nursing staff involved with caring for the patient should be aware of the significance of highly concentrated urine. In some hospitals a hydrometer is kept in the patient's bathroom or the utility room, and specific gravity may be easily determined when the urine appears to be concentrated.

Constipation may become a problem with the patient who has a continued fever. An enema is usually physically and emotionally stressful and for this reason a mild laxative may be ordered. Also, less energy will be expended if the patient can be assisted in using a bedside commode rather than a bedpan (Benton).

Headache, photophobia, and a feeling of general malaise are symptoms commonly experienced by the patient with an elevated temperature. Perception of fever varies widely from one individual to another; some persons may be aware of fevers of low grade, whereas others may have high fever with delirium without being aware that they have fever. Delirium seldom occurs with temperatures less than 40° C (104° F); however, protective bed rails are advised for adults with fever above 39° C (102.2° F). High fevers are associated with convulsions, particularly in children at the onset of acute infectious diseases.

Because of increased evaporation from skin and mucous membranes, the febrile patient requires special mouth and skin care. Frequent cleansing of the teeth, gums, and tongue with a soft brush is necessary to prevent accumulation of sordes. A clean mouth will contribute much to the comfort of the patient and facilitate adequate fluid and food intake.

Herpetic lesions in and around the mouth and nose may be a source of discomfort to the febrile patient. "Fever blisters" are produced by the herpes simplex virus and are not directly related to any other infection the patient may have. The latent herpes virus seems to become active and produce lesions when there is a rise in body temperature or a general lowering of resistance. These lesions are characteristically quite painful during the first day or two after their appearance. They are small, watery blisters occurring singly or in clusters on the lips, around the mouth, and inside the nose. They may also occur inside the mouth on the buccal mucosa. After 2 or 3 days the lesions become dry and crusted; they are then more noticeable but less painful. Local application of compound tincture of benzoin or proprietary preparations is useful in alleviating the discomfort from these lesions during the first 2 or 3 days.

The febrile patient who perspires freely will be more comfortable if the moisture and solid products of sweating are removed by frequent bathing and change of clothing and linens. Both comfort and heat dissipation are improved in a well-ventilated room, but the patient should not be in a direct draft of rapidly moving air.

HYPERTHERMIA: PATHOPHYSIOLOGY AND PATIENT CARE

Body temperatures of 41° C (106° F) and upward are usually classified as hyperthermia or hyperpyrexia. It will be noted in Figure 12-1 that temperature regulation is impaired in this range. Fevers of this degree occur with heat stroke, also known as sun stroke, and with neurogenic hyperthermia.

Heat stroke results from prolonged exposure to high environmental temperature such as hot boiler rooms or continued exposure to sunlight on a very hot day. The temperature-regulating center may be functioning but the body is still gaining heat from the outside faster than it is losing heat. As tissue temperature rises by heat gain from the environment the metabolism of all cells increases according to the van't Hoff principle, which states that the velocity of chemical reactions is proportional to the temperature at which they occur. These two sources of heat gain outweigh the effect of the physiological mechanisms for heat loss with the result that body temperature rises. At around 42° C (107.6° F), the rate of cell metabolism is approximately 50 percent higher than that of tissues at normal temperature (Hopps). At temperatures above 41° C (106° F) there appears to be a failure of the thermoregulatory center resulting in a sudden onset of symptoms characterized by collapse, high fever, and absence of sweating. The heat-regulating mechanisms are no longer able to dissipate the excessive heat being produced, and the body temperature continues to rise in a vicious circle. Death will result within a few hours unless the temperature rise is checked by artificial means and the temperature brought back within the range of normal regulation.

Elderly persons and patients with arteriosclerosis and impaired cardiac reserve are more susceptible to heat stroke. Heat stroke should not be confused with heat prostration or exhaustion, or with heat cramps. These conditions are also the result of the failure to adjust adequately to a hot environment; however, they are not associated with marked elevation of body temperature.

Neurogenic hyperthermia refers to conditions in which the rise of body temperature to the range of hyperthermia is due primarily to malfunction of the thermoregulatory center and occurs in the absence of environmental heat stress. Hyperthermias of this type may occur following head injury, surgical procedures near the hypothalamus, following a cerebral vascular accident, and from other brain lesions and tumors. Temperature control can be affected by brain tumors located at some distance from the hypothalamus, possibly by compression or interruption of neurogenic tracts. It has been suggested that the failure to regulate temperature may be an effect of hypoxic injury to the hypothalamus, with the result that its thermostatic function fails. This results in loss of control of the normal mechanisms for heat transfer and evaporative cooling.

Measurements of oxygen consumption with fever have indicated an increase in oxygen requirement of approximately 13 percent for each centigrade degree rise in body temperature or 7 percent for 1 degree Fahrenheit. This would mean that the hyperthermic patient with a temperature of 41° C would have an oxygen requirement approximately 50 percent greater than his tissues normally need. At least three other factors may contribute to hypoxia in the acute hyperthermic patient. The oxygen-combining capacity of hemoglobin is diminished, and there is also an increased rate of blood flow which reduces the available time for oxygen transfer. In addition to this, the patient is often hyperventilating and a respiratory alkalosis develops. Alkalosis is associated with increased affinity of hemoglobin for oxygen, thus interfering with the release of oxygen to the tissues (Hopps).

Since brain tissue is highly susceptible to hypoxia, it is obvious that immediate and sometimes extreme artificial measures must be employed to control and lower the body temperature. The physician may prescribe the use of antipyretic drugs with the possibility of some response from the thermoregulatory center. Cooling sponge or tub baths and a hypothermia blanket are often used. Since antipyretic drugs seem to obtain their effect through action on the hypothalamic centers and by means of the normal physiological processes, they are of little value in hyperthermias resulting from loss of temperature control due to hypoxia or injury of the hypothalamic centers. They are most useful when the fever is due to the effect of pyrogens acting upon the temperature-regulating center and are not effective in patients suffering from heat stroke or neurogenic hyperthermia.

The temperature-lowering effect of a cold sponge bath or tub bath is the result of heat loss by conduction and evaporation; body heat is transferred from the skin surface to the bathing solution and some is lost as the heat of vaporization. In an emergency, a patient may be immersed in a tub of ice water to arrest a rapid rise in body temperature. Ataractic drugs may be used to prevent shivering, which produces heat and counteracts the desired effect of body cooling. The cold bath should be continued for the length of time prescribed by the physician or until the temperature reaches a prescribed level. It is difficult to evaluate the effectiveness of this procedure, especially when it is used in conjunction with antipyretic drugs. If the skin is cold during a temperature elevation, sponge friction massage may improve cutaneous vasodilatation thus bringing more warm blood to the surface to be cooled. A cooling sponge of too-brief duration and poorly administered may only stimulate shivering and result in more heat production than heat loss.

A *tepid* sponge is often administered to accomplish heat loss by evaporative cooling. This procedure is more easily tolerated than a cold bath and may be more effective, since it is less likely to evoke shivering. The bathing solution may be water, alcohol, or a mixture of these. Since effective cooling depends upon continued evaporation of moisture into the air, a well-ventilated room is essential and the effectiveness of the procedure may be increased by the use of an electric fan to keep air in motion in the room. The patient's temperature, pulse, and respiratory rate should be checked frequently. In the event of irregularity of cardiac rhythm or a marked change in rate, the procedure should be discontinued and the physician informed regarding the temperature response and other changes in vital signs.

A hypothermia blanket is often used to maintain body temperature within a prescribed range. Temperature reduction is accomplished by conduction and convection, heat being transferred from the body surface to the cooling unit. Room air should be comfortably cool and the patient's clothing and bedding adjusted to prevent shivering. This equipment is commonly used to control temperature in patients who have undergone cardiovascular surgery or neurosurgery. Nursing responsibilities in connection with its use are further discussed in Part V.

Alterations in Pulse and Blood Pressure

The pulse is a force wave resulting from systolic ejection of blood from the ventricle. This wave conducted through the blood in the arteries, arterioles, and to a limited extent in the capillaries is responsible for pulsatile flow in the arterial side of the circulatory system. The rate, strength, and rhythm characteristics of these pulsations can be evaluated by palpation of larger arteries lying close to the body surface or of smaller arteries that can be partially compressed against bone. The fact that the characteristics of the pulse can be easily determined at several points on the body surface and without the use of specialized equipment accounts for its frequent use as an indicator of cardiovascular function, as well as a means of evaluating peripheral circulation. The professional nurse should be able to palpate the pulse at the carotid, temporal, brachial, and radial arteries, at the femoral artery in the groin, the popliteal, dorsalis pedis, and posterior tibial arteries.

Pulse and blood pressure evaluation are a part of the assessment of patient welfare which the nurse does on her first contact with the patient and repeats often as a measure of progress and an index of response to therapy, to activity, and to stressful procedures. "Pulse taking" at scheduled times with the evaluation of temperature and respiration or with blood pressure usually consists of counting the pulse rate for 15 or 30 seconds and multiplying to obtain a minute rate based on the period counted. The fact that regularly scheduled pulse determinations are routinely assigned to technical and auxiliary nursing personnel does not decrease the importance of accurate observation of the characteristics of the pulse. Pulse taking is sometimes used as an "opener" in nurse-patient communications or as a "cover" for other observations of the patient's welfare and response to therapy. For the acutely ill patient this simple and often-repeated procedure provides physical contact and the attention of a professional nurse which may, of itself, be reassuring or, if injudiciously used, may arouse anxiety in some patients.

It has been suggested that heart rate may change as a result of the patient's awareness that his pulse is being counted. This question and also the accuracy of counting for a longer or shorter counting interval are now being investigated.

The pulse may vary abnormally as to strength, rate, and rhythm. The strength characteristic is better evaluated by determination of the blood pressure, and changes in rate and rhythm are more precisely studied by a cardiotachometer or electrocardiographic monitor. However, the most frequent evaluation of pulse characteristics is by palpation of the radial artery.

PULSE RATE

The rate and strength characteristics of the pulse wave are reflections of the frequency and force of systolic ejection from the left ventricle. The pulse is normally regular in rhythm with no detectable difference in intervals between pulsations. Included in the range of normal are slight variations in rhythm arising from the sinoatrial node. These may be seen on the electrocardiogram but are not usually noticeable in pulse counting. Because circulatory demand is directly related to the rate of metabolism, there are normal physiological variations in the heart rate related to age, sex, physical activity, and the body temperature. The normal resting heart rate usually falls between 60 and 80 beats per minute, occasionally 50 and 60; rates less than 50 per minute are rarely seen in healthy persons with the exception of athletes. Resting rates of 80 to 100 per minute are sometimes seen in healthy persons.

Cardiac output in milliliters of blood pumped per minute is the product of stroke volume and heart rate: $CO_{ml/min} = SV_{ml} \times HR/min$. Since any increase in metabolism results in an increased demand for cardiac output, it is also associated with an increase in heart rate. Faster heart rates are seen in children, who have a higher basic metabolic rate than adults. Rapid heart rates occur in adults during periods of increased metabolism such as strenuous physical exercise, fever, or hyperthyroid condition. Slow heart rates are seen with hypothermia, hypothyroidism, and any condition of general metabolic depression.

When the radial pulse rate is less than 60 per minute an apical rate should be taken to determine whether this represents a true bradycardia or a pulse deficit, which occurs when some beats audible at the apex of the heart are not palpable at a peripheral artery. When an apical rate less than 60 beats per minute is observed in a new patient or if it represents a change for a patient, the nurse will consult the physician for instructions before further administration of digitalis, ouabain, or other medications that affect heart rate.

The occurrence of rapid pulse rates without fever or other evidence of increased metabolic rate is an indication of serious physiological imbalance and suggests the possibility of inefficient cardiac function due to disease of the heart itself, a decrease in circulating blood volume, response to neuroendocrine stimulation, or an unrecognized disease process. Pulse rates in excess of 100 beats per minute in the absence of heart disease or other recognized disease processes call for diagnostic consideration by both nurse and physician. For possible explanation of the increased heart rate and also as a guide to therapy the nurse should assess the patient's state of hydration and note the record of fluid intake and output.

The increase in heart rate occurring with hemorrhage, shock, or severe dehydration is a physiological response of the cardiovascular system which tends to compensate for the decrease in stroke volume. With the decrease in circulating blood volume characteristic of shock and hemorrhage, there is a decrease in venous return and a decrease in diastolic filling of the ventricle; the resulting decrease in force and volume of systolic ejection results in a weaker pulse, thus accounting for the rapid weak pulse seen in shock and hemorrhage.

Rapid pulse rates may also reflect the cardiac response to physically or emotionally stressful stimuli such as pain, fear, worry, and anxiety. For example, the severe discomfort experienced by a patient with an overly distended bladder, or concern for an acutely ill patient in the same room, may be manifested by rapid heart rates until the cause of the stress is relieved. Cardiovascular responses to these stimuli are mediated by neuroendocrine pathways, i.e., stimulation of the sympathetic nervous system and increase in circulating catecholamines.

PULSE RHYTHM AND STRENGTH

As a means of evaluating cardiac function, the rhythm and force of the pulse waves may be more important than the rate. Rapid ventricular ejection into an arterial system where the diastolic pressure is low produces a full and bounding pulse. This water-hammer pulse occurs with severe aortic regurgitation and with some congenital defects. Irregular rhythm of the palpated pulse may reflect either a true arrhythmia from abnormal electrical activity of the heart, or changes in stroke volume. An irregular pulse is noted when some ventricular contractions are so weak, or the systolic ejection volume is so small, that the conducted pulse wave is not palpable at the peripheral artery. This pulse may be irregular in both rhythm and force, and is usually associated with a pulse deficit. A pulse is described as irregular in strength when the force of the pulse wave varies from one beat to another and irregular in rhythm when the interval between pulse waves varies in length. When a pulse is irregular in rhythm, the variation in strength or fullness of the pulse wave is the result of differences in time for diastolic filling of the left ventricle and therefore differences in the volume of systolic ejection.

Bigeminal rhythm, characterized by two pulsations close together followed by a longer pause, is caused by premature contractions in response to an ectopic pacemaker usually in the ventricle. Other irregularities in pulse force and rhythm occur with ectopic beats, atrial fibrillation, and other defects of electrical conduction in the heart. The physician should be informed regarding irregularities in rhythm; this is of special importance for the myocardial infarction patient in whom arrhythmias may precipitate ventricular fibrillation or cardiac arrest. Electrocardiographic monitoring and antiarrhythmia therapy may be indicated to restore normal rhythm and prevent further deterioration of cardiac function or cardiac arrest. (Abnormalities in heart disease are further discussed in Chapter 23.)

In caring for patients with peripheral vascular disease and after vascular surgery, evaluation of the pulse in the involved extremity is an important nursing procedure. Information regarding the patency of an artery or an arterial graft is obtained by evaluating the strength of the pulse at a given site in comparison with the other extremity or at a more proximal site. Evaluation of local skin color and temperature is done at the same time as a further measure of adequate circulation for the area involved.

ALTERATION IN BLOOD PRESSURE

The pressure of the blood in the arterial system is maintained within narrow limits over a wide range of activity and physical surroundings. With maintenance of normal pressure the blood is circulated through the pulmonary and systemic systems transporting oxygen and nutrients to tissues and removing carbon dioxide and metabolic wastes. The pressure increases with physical activity and falls if there is a large loss of blood; however, these factors are adjusted by physiological systems to provide the homeostatic environment necessary for cell metabolism.

Systemic arterial blood pressure represents a force which is the result of cardiac output and the resistance of the peripheral vascular system. The term *blood pressure* usually refers to pressures within the systemic arterial system. Pressures within the pulmonary system, heart, or veins are identified as pulmonary artery pressure, ventricular pressure, or venous pressure.

Blood pressure, measured and expressed in millimeters of mercury, is the force exerted by the blood on the walls of the vessels. Thus a pressure of 120 mm mercury means that the force of the blood at this measurement site would support a column of mercury 120 mm in height.

Normal blood pressure averages from 120/80 in young adults to 150/90 in old age. The *systolic pressure* of 120 mm mercury represents the peak pressure of the blood against the wall of the vessel as the result of left ventricular contraction.

The *diastolic pressure* of 80 mm mercury is the lowest pressure exerted on the vessel wall at this site during the cardiac cycle; it is the force of the blood itself against the arterial wall with the aortic valve closed and the heart in diastole. *Pulse pressure*, the difference between these two readings, represents the range of pressure in the arteries during the events of the cardiac cycle.

The *mean arterial pressure*, which is the effective blood pressure, is slightly lower than the arithmetical mean of the systolic and diastolic pressures. It can be determined by the use of an intra-arterial catheter and mercury manometer or by electronic equipment. It is sometimes estimated as two-thirds of the diastolic pressure plus one-third of the systolic pressure, thus allowing for the longer period of diastole in the cardiac cycle. This is illustrated by the formula:

$$\text{Mean arterial pressure} = \frac{\text{Systolic pressure} + 2\,(\text{diastolic pressure})}{3}$$

With a blood pressure of 120/80, the mean arterial pressure is approximately 93 mm Hg $\dfrac{120 + 2(80)}{3} = 93.3$

In considering the consequence of hypotension, it is well to remember that mean arterial pressure is lower than systolic pressure and serious tissue damage can result if the effective perfusing pressure remains low for more than a few minutes. For example, kidney function requires a mean arterial pressure of about 70 mm mercury. Oliguria or anuria may result when the mean arterial pressure is lower, followed by renal tubular necrosis if the period of low pressure is prolonged.

BLOOD PRESSURE DETERMINATION

Information gained from blood pressure determination is important to patient welfare in that it serves as a diagnostic aid and guide to therapy for both physician and nurse. For the hospitalized patient it is sometimes repeated so often as to become an annoyance and a source of physical and emotional stress. If used injudiciously it may disturb the patient's rest to the extent that recovery is jeopardized or delayed. Recognizing the value of blood pressure information and also the stress imposed upon the patient, the nurse will consult with the physician regarding frequency of measurement during periods of rest and sleep.

Blood pressure is useful only to the extent that it is accurate. Research has shown considerable variation in observer accuracy in blood pressure determination (Wilcox). For review of technique of accurate blood pressure determination the reader is referred to sources listed at the end of this chapter.

Particular attention is directed to the report entitled "Recommendations for Human Blood Pressure Determination by Sphygmomanometers." This official report of a committee of the American Heart Association discusses equipment, lists common errors and how to avoid them, and recommends certain standards for accuracy of measurement and recording. A major change is indicated in that the point of *muffling* rather than *disappearance* of sound is recommended as the best index of diastolic pressure. The report states that if there is a difference in mercury level for those two sounds both readings should be recorded, e.g., 136/80/72. If muffling and disappearance of sound occur at the same level, the pressure should be recorded as 140/78/78.

Numerous studies comparing direct (intra-arterial) and indirect measurement of blood pressure have shown that the muffling sound is heard at 7 to 10 mm mercury above the intra-arterial diastolic pressure. However, the point of disappearance of sound may fall near or far below the intra-arterial diastolic pressure. The latter sound is subject to variations related to the position of the stethoscope over the artery, the sound frequency characteristics of the stethoscope, and the auditory acuity of the observer.

A number of physical and emotional factors may affect blood pressure. Since resting level blood pressure is usually desired, these factors should be avoided or controlled as much as possible. Anxiety and excitement, emotionally disturbing sights and sounds, or unpleasant interpersonal relationships tend to raise the blood pressure. Physical stresses such as a cold environment, an overly distended bladder, or pain can cause variations in blood pressure. The nurse should relieve these discomforts and allow a period of stabilization before blood pressure is determined. It is suggested in the Recommendations that resting level blood pressure be determined 5 minutes after postural change and 30 minutes after eating or smoking.

NURSING RESPONSIBILITIES IN RELATION TO ALTERATIONS IN BLOOD PRESSURE

When blood pressure is significantly altered the nurse makes further observations for assessment of patient welfare. In doing so it should be remembered that the pressure of the blood within the arterial system may be considered as the result of three factors: (1) Volume of the circulating blood. (2) Output of the heart. (3) Resistance to flow which results from (a) the integrity of the "closed" circulatory system—no rapid blood loss; (b) the characteristics of the system at the time— dilated or constricted; (c) elasticity of the vessels; (d) viscosity of the blood.

Figure 12-2 illustrates these three factors with contributory aspects and general nursing activities. Blood volume changes are normally brought about slowly, over a period of hours, regulated by the kidneys and endocrine system. The use of intravenous infusion of fluids, blood, plasma, solutions, and other blood volume expanders allows adjustment of the circulating blood volume within a few minutes.

Cardiac output is dependent upon the volume of blood returning to the right atrium and the efficiency of the pump in moving this venous return. Cardiac output affects the pressure of the blood, especially the systolic pressure, with each cardiac cycle. Thus systolic changes occur within a few seconds, in fact from one systolic ejection to another.

The resistance factor accounts for change in blood pressure within a matter of minutes by vasoconstriction and vasodilatation. These changes in the lumen of the vessels are under neuroendocrine control. Blood pressure is also directly related to viscosity in that more viscous blood, as with hemoconcentration, offers more resistance to flow than does blood with less viscosity. The viscosity factor is of lesser, though still significant, importance in the control of blood pressure. In

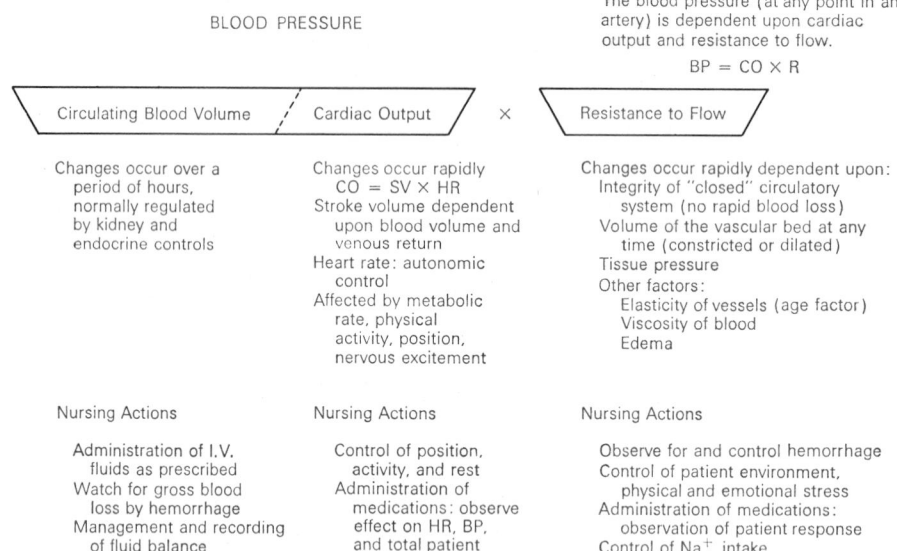

The blood pressure (at any point in an artery) is dependent upon cardiac output and resistance to flow.

$$BP = CO \times R$$

Circulating Blood Volume / Cardiac Output		×	Resistance to Flow
Changes occur over a period of hours, normally regulated by kidney and endocrine controls	Changes occur rapidly CO = SV × HR Stroke volume dependent upon blood volume and venous return Heart rate: autonomic control Affected by metabolic rate, physical activity, position, nervous excitement		Changes occur rapidly dependent upon: Integrity of "closed" circulatory system (no rapid blood loss) Volume of the vascular bed at any time (constricted or dilated) Tissue pressure Other factors: Elasticity of vessels (age factor) Viscosity of blood Edema
Nursing Actions	Nursing Actions		Nursing Actions
Administration of I.V. fluids as prescribed Watch for gross blood loss by hemorrhage Management and recording of fluid balance Control of Na⁺ intake	Control of position, activity, and rest Administration of medications: observe effect on HR, BP, and total patient response		Observe for and control hemorrhage Control of patient environment, physical and emotional stress Administration of medications: observation of patient response Control of Na⁺ intake

Figure 12–2 Nursing actions in relation to factors of blood pressure maintenance and control.

older persons the normal, slowly developing loss of elasticity contributes to higher arterial pressure.

An important principle of circulatory dynamics is that blood pressure is the product of cardiac output and the total resistance to flow within the system. It can be expressed by the equation:

Blood pressure = Cardiac output × total peripheral resistance

Remembering that cardiac output is dependent upon circulating blood volume, one can see that an increase in either cardiac output or vascular resistance will bring about an increase in blood pressure. A decrease in either of these will tend to lower blood pressure.

In working with a patient whose blood pressure is abnormally high or low, the nurse should keep in mind the above factors and also be aware of the general disease conditions with which each of these alterations is associated. This knowledge is a guide in making purposeful observations for other manifestations of illness. More importantly, knowing the factors involved in blood pressure regulation she is able to assist both patient and physician in the overall plan for therapy, or in case of emergency, take independent action to bring the blood pressure back toward the normal range.

Acute hypertension occurs with head injury or circulatory overload and is a medical emergency requiring specific treatment prescribed by the physician. Chronic hypertension occurs as a primary manifestation of essential hypertension and secondary to cardiovascular and kidney disease. Care of the hypertensive patient includes administration of specific medications or other prescribed therapy. Nursing care is planned to control physical activity and environmental stress, thus limiting the demand for increased cardiac output and neuroendocrine response to stress. Specific treatment and nursing care are discussed at length in Part V.

Acute hypotension of short duration occurs with syncope. Abnormally low arterial pressures are associated with shock, hemorrhage, acute heart attack, and cerebrovascular accidents. General nursing measures include placing the patient in a recumbent position and keeping him comfortably warm until specific treatment such as blood volume replacement and medications can be administered.

Orthostatic hypotension may occur in patients who have been confined to bed rest for a period of 2 weeks or longer. For this reason sudden changes in position are to be avoided in working with chronically ill patients and patients convalescing from acute illness. Slower movements with brief rest periods allow for adjustment of blood flow to the central nervous system.

Chronic hypotension is seen in patients with thyroid hypofunction, malignant neoplasms, or other debilitating disease.

Alterations in Respiration and Associated Respiratory Disturbances

The assessment of respiratory function includes much more than counting the patient's respiration as a ritualistic part of the "TPR" routine. If the patient's illness warrants hospitalization for treatment of illness or for diagnostic studies, this vital function should be carefully observed. In the actuely ill or postoperative patient observation of respiratory function is one of the most important nursing responsibilities. Abnormal breathing or a change in respiratory pattern is, indeed, a vital sign and emergency measures may be required to restore and maintain adequate gaseous exchange.

Respiration involves the processes of ventilation, diffusion, pulmonary perfusion, transport, and gaseous exchange at metabolizing tissue sites. Nursing requires a clear understanding of these processes. The focus of this discussion is on ventilation, since the observation and facilitation of this aspect of respiration is a primary nursing responsibility. Nursing activities in relation to cough and other protective mechanisms are introduced here. References listed at the end of this chapter are suggested for further reading regarding common respiratory disturbances. Nursing responsibilities in relation to respiratory function in surgical patients and specific nursing care of patients with respiratory diseases are discussed elsewhere.

ABNORMAL CHARACTERISTICS OF RESPIRATION

Normal breathing, *eupnea,* is characterized by quiet, regular respirations of moderate excursion at a rate of 12 to 20 per minute interrupted at frequent intervals by a sigh. *Sighing* consists of taking a deep breath of two to three times the average tidal volume for that individual at rest. In adults sighing occurs normally about six to 10 times per hour. This irregularity in the pattern of breathing is important for the maintenance of normal lung function. It appears that shallow, constant tidal volume breathing leads to progressive collapse of the alveoli, and the maintenance of normal ventilation depends upon periodic deep breaths for reinflation of collapsed air spaces (Bendixen, 1964). The sighing component of breathing provides the physiological basis for the frequently performed nursing action of "deep breathing" or hyperinflation in which the nurse assists—coaches, encourages—the patient with this important activity. When spontaneous sighing is absent and deep-breathing exercises are not effective, mechanical equipment must be used to provide periodic hyperinflation, thus providing immediate increase in ventilation and also preventing further alveolar collapse and atelectasis. It is suggested that infants and children should have more frequent hyperinflation than adults (Bendixen, 1964). A normal yawn or sigh is characterized by a momentary "hold" at the end of inspiration and this technique is used in assisting patients with deep breathing without mechanical aids. It has been shown that a "single breath, hold" is more effective in raising arterial oxygen tension than either a single deep breath or repeated deep breaths without the inspiratory hold (Ward).

Morphine appears to have a profound depressant effect upon the frequency of sighing. The side effect of morphine in depressing the depth and rate of breathing has long been known. More recently it was shown that postoperative patients after intravenous administration of morphine, in doses that did not depress the frequency or depth of breathing, did not sigh for approximately 1 hour, and the frequency of sighing was markedly reduced for at least 3 hours (Egbert). At this time it is not known to what extent this is true with other medications; however, the nurse is advised to assume that spontaneous sighing will be absent or severely depressed and to encourage frequent deep breathing for all postoperative patients receiving analgesic medications.

Position may be an important factor in preventing hypoxemia. Maintenance of normal oxygen tension at approximately 100 mm mercury in the arterial blood is dependent upon perfusion as well as ventilation. In general, dependent areas of the lung are better perfused than uppermost areas for any position. Total lung perfusion is greater in supine position than in sitting or standing position. On the other hand, tidal volume is somewhat greater in an upright rather than a lying position. Ventilation-perfusion ratios vary throughout the lung according to the state of alveolar ventilation and local perfusion of the alveolar capillaries.

A recent study has shown that in the supine position normal volunteers, as well as chronic lung and thoracotomy patients, had suboptimal ventilation-perfusion relationships. In every instance turning the subject to a lateral position resulted in increase in oxygen tension, the increase being greater for patients breathing oxygen. This research has important implications for nursing in relation to positioning and turning acutely ill patients. If there is any possibility of impaired respiratory function, the patient should be positioned on his side and turned frequently from one side to the other, not from side to back (Clauss; Medical News in *American Journal of Nursing* [p. 2596]).

Minute ventilation, or minute respiratory volume, is the quantity of air moved in and out of the respiratory tract per minute. This is not to be confused with alveolar ventilation, which is always much less because of the anatomic dead space. Minute ventilation equals the tidal volume times the respiratory rate. *Hyperventilation* and *hypoventilation* are correctly used to describe increase and decrease in the minute respiratory volume. Hyperventilation usually involves an increase in both rate and depth of breathing. It should be noted that a patient with rapid shallow respirations is more correctly described as tachypneic rather than hyperventilating. By reason of the anatomic dead space, rapid shallow respiratory cycles may fail to accomplish the essential function of breathing, ventilation of the alveoli. The result of alveolar hypoventilation is hypoxemia and tissue hypoxia, which are manifested by anxiety, restlessness, confusion, and cyanosis. A second result of alveolar hypoventilation is carbon dioxide retention, hypercapnia, and respiratory acidosis. The hypoxic and hypercapnic effects of hypoventilation are increased by inadequate capillary perfusion or any interference with the diffusion of oxygen and carbon dioxide through the alveolar membrane. Thus patients with either chronic respiratory or cardiovascular disease are more likely to become hypoxic than those with normal cardiac and respiratory function.

The nurse plays a major role in the prevention of respiratory insufficiency due to inadequate alveolar ventilation. It is not enough to be alert for restlessness, cyanosis, and other signs of hypoxia after it has developed. Hypoventilation is to be avoided in any patient, but it can produce serious consequences in geriatric patients and in patients with recognized cardiovascular or chronic respiratory disease. Some of the common causes of hypoventilation are as follows: (1) loss of sighing and decrease in tidal volume by depressant action of anesthesia, narcotics, or sedatives; (2) shallow, guarded breathing due to painful chest or upper abdominal incision; (3) bed position that inhibits chest expansion and movement of the diaphragm thereby reducing ventilation; (4) partial or complete airway obstruction by loose dentures, tongue or other soft tissues, from laryngeal edema, occlusion or displacement of a tracheostomy cannula, or pressure from dressings; (5) failure or improper functioning of mechanical ventilating equipment. These factors should be kept in mind while observing the depth and rate of breathing, uniformity of chest expansion, color of skin, lips, and nailbeds, and watching for signs of central nervous system hypoxia. Comroe states that respiratory rate itself is not very valuable as an index of useful ventilation because either rapid or slow rates may be associated with hyperventilation or hypoventilation, depending upon other factors.

Pallor may be a sign of respiratory insufficiency, although variation in skin shade is more directly related to the state of vasoconstriction or dilatation of the capillary bed. *Cyanosis* is a dark blue or purplish discoloration of the skin usually due to excessive amounts of unsaturated hemoglobin in the capillaries. It may be seen with either decreased oxygenation of hemoglobin or decreased rate of flow. Cyanosis is discussed in Chapter 13.

Cyanosis is often observed in the nailbeds before it is noticeable in the skin. In black or other dark-complexioned persons cyanosis cannot be detected in the skin but can be observed in the mucous membranes of the mouth and may show in the lips and nailbeds.

Tachypnea and *bradypnea,* to use the common prefixes for rapid and slow, respectively, are the correct terms for increased and decreased rates of breathing. *Polypnea* also refers to a rapid rate of respiration. *Hyperpnea* and *hypopnea* are used to describe increase and decrease in depth of respiration.

Short periods of *apnea,* cessation of breathing, occur with periodic breathing, an abnormal respiratory pattern seen in patients with certain disease conditions.

Periodic breathing is characterized by a short period of deep breathing followed by a period of apnea or very shallow respirations with the cycle repeating itself. In *Cheyne-Stokes respiration,* the most common form of periodic breathing, each succeeding breath becomes more shallow until a period of apnea occurs. After a few seconds, usually less than a minute, shallow respiratory movements begin again increasing in depth with each breath until full, deep respirations are reached and the declining phase of the cycle begins again. This abnormal respiratory pattern is common in moribund patients but may also occur during sleep in geriatric patients and patients suffering from cardiovascular disease.

Dyspnea is a subjective sensation of respiratory distress, sometimes described as air hunger or shortness of breath. It is defined as "the awareness of respiratory distress or of unusual breathlessness" (Wright). Thus the unconscious patient whose breathing is noisy and appears to be labored or difficult is not, in the strictest sense of the word, dyspneic, though the term is often used to describe such breathing. When the lungs and chest wall, normally compliant and easily distensible, lose some of their compliance, the work of breathing is increased. Dyspnea may be associated with any condition that increases the work of breathing—atelectasis, tracheal or bronchial obstruction, or limited movement of the chest or diaphragm. It may also occur on an emotional basis. Some persons are abnormally afraid of not being able to get enough fresh air; they may feel dyspneic in a crowded room or elevator even though it is well ventilated.

The dyspneic patient first attempts to take one or more deep breaths; if the unpleasant sensation is not relieved he may continue to hyperventilate, developing respiratory alkalosis as he blows off carbon dioxide. In observing the dyspneic patient it is necessary to determine whether he is actually using his inspiratory reserve or whether his respirations are rapid and shallow, i.e., tachypneic. Actual hyperventilation will help to relieve the sensation, depending upon the cause of the dyspnea; shallow breathing moves air in and out of the anatomic dead space without ventilating the alveoli.

The comfort and ventilatory efficiency of the dyspneic patient are often improved in a sitting position, which lowers the diaphragm and allows some increase in both tidal volume and vital capacity. It has been shown that both these measures are greater in the sitting than in the supine position. McCarthy and others have found that resting subjects had greater vital capacity at back rest positions than in supine or other recumbent positions (Comroe; McCarthy).

Many cardiac patients become dyspneic after a few minutes without supporting pillows or when their back rest is lowered. The flat position allows increased return of pooled blood from the lower extremities and trunk to the heart and pulmonary circulation. Pulmonary congestion results if the diseased heart is unable to pump the increased quantity of blood; this type of dyspnea is known as *orthopnea.*

Other common signs observed in patients with respiratory disorders include *rales, wheezing, stridor,* and *stertor. Rales* are abnormal sounds produced by air passing through accumulations of fluid in air passages. They are sometimes audible without the aid of a stethoscope or may be felt by placing the hand against the chest wall. They are usually heard by stethoscope, and nurses caring for acutely ill cardiac patients or other patients in intensive care units are expected to use this means of evaluating change in the patient's condition. Rales are fairly common in patients with chronic respiratory or cardiac disease, but a change in the sound or extension of the area involved should be called to the attention of the physician. The development of rales in cardiac patients or elderly patients during intravenous administration of fluids is a sign of acute pulmonary edema. Since the resulting interference with gaseous exchange at the alveolar membrane may produce hypoxemia, the infusion should immediately be discontinued or reduced to a very slow rate, to keep open, and the patient's physician notified.

Wheezes, whistling or sighing sounds associated with breathing, indicate partial obstruction of air passages due to spasm, edema, foreign body, tumor, or external pressure. Expiratory wheezing is often heard in asthmatic patients. Audible rales and wheezes are often a sign that the patient needs to cough or be suctioned to remove secretions.

Stridor is the harsh crowing sound associated with laryngeal spasm or laryngeal edema. It may also occur with tracheobronchitis, accompanied by a "croupy" cough. The patient should be watched closely for other signs of respiratory embarrassment, such as substernal retraction with inspiration, anxious appearance, pallor, and cyanosis. An emergency tracheostomy tray should be kept in the patient's room or readily available on the nursing unit.

Stertor, or stertorous respiration, is the term used to describe the raspy rattling sound produced by breathing through the mouth, or mouth and nose at the same time, causing vibration of the soft palate. Commonly known as *snoring,* this occurs in many healthy people, and is more common in the supine position. Sometimes the patient himself is awakened frequently by this increase in airway resistance, or the sonorous sounds may be disturbing to other patients. The nurse may be able to assist this patient and others nearby by repositioning him in a side-lying position with the head well back. This hyperextends the airway, allowing more room for air flow through the relaxed walls and muscles of the pharynx.

A hoarse voice is associated with edema, pressure, or inflammation of the vocal cords. Other voice changes may occur when resonance of the chest and nasal sinuses is affected by colds or other respiratory diseases.

PROTECTIVE RESPIRATORY MECHANISMS

Sneezing, coughing, and throat clearing are protective reflexes that serve to remove foreign matter, noxious substances, and excessive secretions from respiratory passageways. The sighing mechanism, discussed above with patterns of respiration, prevents gradual collapse of the alveoli by periodic hyperinflation to two or three times the tidal volume. It is important to remember that most anesthetic and analgesic agents and sedatives have a depressant effect on coughing, sighing, and depth and rate of breathing.

Sneezing is stimulated by irritation of nasal mucosa; a quick inspiration is followed by expiratory block by the uvula and soft palate rather than at the larynx as in coughing. A sudden explosive release of air through the nose and mouth helps to remove the irritant substance. During the act of sneezing or coughing the mouth and nose should be loosely covered with disposable tissue to prevent droplet spread to other persons and into the surrounding air. It is important, however, that the mouth be kept open and no pressure be applied to the nose. Stifling a sneeze or cough at the pharyngeal level or at the nose and lips predisposes to middle ear and sinus infections as a result of forcing air and secretions into the nasal sinuses and the eustachian tubes. The common cold and resulting secondary infections constitute a major health problem in the United States. Nurses and other health workers should take every opportunity to teach patients how to protect themselves and others during coughing and sneezing.

Sneezing is important as a prodromal sign of upper respiratory infection. Its occurrence in a hospitalized preoperative patient suggests further observation of signs and symptoms and prompt notification of the patient's physician if other signs of a cold are found. In this event elective surgery is usually rescheduled for a later date. The patient is usually emotionally ready for his surgery at the scheduled date, and this change of plans because of a "little sneeze" may be hard for patient and family to accept. The nurse can help to lessen their psychological and physiological letdown. She can help the patient to feel that his worth and his safety are of such importance that the decision was right and was made for his welfare.

Repeated sneezing accompanied by nasal discharge and lacrimation is a common manifestation of allergic reactions to pollens or other foreign proteins. The symptomatic and specific treatment of allergies and infection of the upper respiratory tract are discussed in Chapter 22.

Throat clearing and *coughing* are adjuncts of the normal respiratory toilet. Excessive secretions from cells lining the tracheobronchial tree along with foreign particles and tissue debris engulfed in the mucous blanket are moved toward the pharynx by constant beating action of the cilia. This normal cleansing process is drastically interfered with by smoking, which stimulates increased secretion of mucus and also slows the ciliary action that should work to remove it (Turner; Hopps). Drying also greatly reduces the mobility of the mucous secretions, thereby increasing the chance of upper respiratory tract infection. For this reason it is important that room air in homes and hospitals be humidified. Dry, heated air is considered a major factor in the increased incidence of upper respiratory infections during winter months.

Tracheobronchial secretions enter the pharynx by action of the cilia, assisted by coughing or clearing the throat, and are swallowed or expectorated. Cough and throat clearing become abnormally frequent when secretions are increased in amount or hard to raise, or when irritants other than normal secretions are stimulating these reflexes.

Cough is described according to sound, as harsh, brassy, or croupy; but more important is a description according to its productiveness. When no secretions are loosened or raised the cough is dry, tight, or unproductive; it is loose or productive when sputum is raised even though it may not be expectorated.

Cough is a symptom usually associated with inflammation, infection, or chemical irritation, and its treatment depends upon the specific cause. When further observation and diagnostic studies are needed to determine the cause of illness, these may take priority over relieving the symptom. A dry, unproductive cough may disturb the patient's rest and serve no useful purpose. For the postoperative patient coughing is painful and, if prolonged, may interfere with normal healing of the surgical wound. Coughing may be suppressed or controlled by medication, but a productive cough usually should not be suppressed unless it is excessive and exhausting because of thick, tenacious sputum. In this case expectorant medications are used to loosen and reduce the viscosity of the secretions, and nursing care is aimed at encouraging and assisting the patient with coughing. In some instances the patient has little reserve strength for coughing but the cough is productive of secretions that must be removed. The nurse and physician can plan a schedule that allows intervals for facilitation of cough, perhaps assisted by expectorant medication and postural drainage, alternating with intervals for rest. Codeine has long been the most commonly used cough depressant. Several newer non-narcotic medications are said to suppress cough by depression of the cough center without depressing respiration and without any sedative action or habit-forming potential.

Turning, coughing, and deep-breathing exercises are important nursing care functions aimed at the prevention of respiratory complications in postoperative patients. These procedures are discussed in Chapter 21. Specific nursing care for patients with cough and other respiratory disturbances must be based on the cause and the plan for medical care of the disease. These are discussed with respiratory diseases in Chapter 22.

Bibliography

Temperature

Atkins, Elisha: Fever. in Cyril Mitchell MacBryde: *Signs and Symptoms* 4th ed. Philadelphia: J. B. Lippincott Company, 1964, pp. 442–468.

Bennett, Ivan L., Jr.: Alterations in Body Temperature. in T. R. Harrison (Ed.): *Principles of Internal Medicine,* 5th ed. New York: McGraw-Hill Book Company, 1966, pp. 50–59.

Benton, Joseph G., Henry Brown, and Howard A. Rusk: Energy Expended by Patients on the Bedpan and Bedside Commode. *Journal of American Medical Association,* 144:1443–1447, December 23, 1950.

Brengelmann, George and Arthur C. Brown: Temperature Regulation, pp. 1050–1069. in T. Ruch and H. Patton: *Physiology and Biophysics.* Philadelphia: W. B. Saunders Company, 1965.

Cranston, W. I.: Temperature Regulation. *British Medical Journal,* 5505:69–75, July 9, 1966.

DuBois, Eugene F.: *Fever and the Regulation of Body Temperature.* Springfield, Ill. Charles C Thomas, Publisher, 1948.

Guyton, Arthur C.: *Textbook of Medical Physiology,* 3d ed. Philadelphia: W. B. Saunders Company, 1966.

Hopps, Howard C.: *Principles of Pathology,* 2d ed. New York: Appleton Century Crofts, 1964.

Mead, Jere and C. Lawrence Bonmarito: Reliability of Rectal Temperatures as an Index of Internal Body Temperature. *Journal of Applied Physiology,* 2:97–109, August, 1949.

Selle, W. A.: *Body Temperature, Its Changes with Environment, Disease, and Therapy.* Springfield, Ill.: Charles C Thomas Publisher, 1952.

Tate, Gayle V.: *Effects of Variation of Angle and Depth of Thermometer Insertion on Rectal Temperature Readings.* Unpublished Master's Thesis. Seattle: University of Washington, 1968.

Pulse and Blood Pressure

Burch, George E. and Nicholas P. De Pasquale: *Primer of Clinical Measurement of Blood Pressure.* St. Louis: The C. V. Mosby Company, 1962.

Kirkendall, Walter M., Alan C. Burton, Federick H. Epstein, and Edward O. Freis; Recommendations for Human

Blood Pressure Determination by Sphygmomanometers. *Circulation,* 36:980–988, December, 1967.

Programmed Instruction: Correcting Common Errors in Blood Pressure Measurement. *American Journal of Nursing,* 65:10:133–164, October, 1965.

Recommendations for Human Blood Pressure Determination by Sphygmomanometers. American Heart Association, New York: 1967.

Sphygmomanometers, Principles and Precepts. Copiague, New York: W. A. Baum Company, Inc.

Wilcox, Jane: Observer Factors in the Measurement of Blood Pressure. *Nursing Research,* 10:4–17, Winter, 1961.

Respiration

Ayres, Stephan M. and Stanley Giannelli: Respiration, pp. 3–41. in *Care of the Critically Ill.* New York: Appleton Century Crofts, 1967.

Bendixen, H. H., et al.: Pattern of Ventilation in Young Adults. *Journal of Applied Physiology,* 19:195–198, 1964.

Bendixen, H. H., et al.: *Respiratory Care,* St. Louis: The C. V. Mosby Company, 1965.

Betson, Carol: Blood Gases. *American Journal of Nursing,* 68:5:1010–1012, May, 1968.

Cherniak, R. M. and L. Cherniak: *Respiration in Health and Disease.* Philadelphia: W. B. Saunders Company, 1961.

Clauss, Roy H., et al.: Effects of Changing Body Position upon Ventilation-Perfusion Relationships. *Circulation,* Supplement II to Vols. 37 and 38: 214; 217, April, 1968.

Comroe, Julius H., et al.: *The Lung:* *Clinical Physiology and Pulmonary Function Tests,* 2d ed. Chicago: Year Book Medical Publishers, Inc., 1962.

Egbert, L. D. and H. H. Bendixen: Effect of Morphine on Breathing Pattern. *Journal of American Medical Association,* 188:485–488, May, 1964.

Guyton, Arthur C.: *Textbook of Medical Physiology,* 3d ed. Philadelphia: W. B. Saunders Company, 1966.

Hopps, Howard C.: *Principles of Pathology,* 2d ed. New York: Appleton Century Crofts, 1964.

Kurihara, Marie: Assessment and Maintenance of Adequate Respiration. *Nursing Clinics of North America,* 3:1:65–76, March, 1968.

Larson, Elaine; The Patient with Acute Pulmonary Edema. *American Journal of Nursing,* 68:5:1019–1021, May, 1968.

McCarthy, Rosemary: The Metabolic Cost of Maintaining Five Fixed Body Positions. *Nursing Research,* 17: 6:539–544, November–December, 1968.

Modell, Walter: *Relief of Symptoms,* 2d ed. St. Louis: The C. V. Mosby Company, 1961.

Turn Side to Side, Not Side to Back. *American Journal of Nursing,* 67:12:2596, December, 1967.

Turner, Howard G.: The Anatomy and Physiology of Normal Respiration. *Nursing Clinics of North America,* 3:3:383–401, September, 1968.

Ward, Richard J., et al.: An Evaluation of Postoperative Respiratory Maneuvers. *Surgery, Gynecology, and Obstetrics,* 123:51–54, July, 1966.

Wright, George W.: Dyspnea, pp. 63–69. in T. R. Harrison (Ed.): *Principles of Internal Medicine,* 5th ed. New York: McGraw-Hill Book Company, 1966.

CHAPTER 13
ALTERATIONS IN PHYSICAL APPEARANCE

BARBARA ANN GRUTTER

Certain deviations from physiologic balance are manifested by alterations in the appearance of the human form. Changes in color, texture, and contour of the body surface are relatively easily observable. Many of these manifestations are symptomatic of problems about which there is a considerable amount of knowledge. The solutions to the problems and the intervention measures employed are reasonably well standardized, as are the nursing techniques and approaches utilized in alleviating the manifestations. The observation and interpretation of visual clues are part of the systematic assessment of the patient. This chapter discusses some of the more common alterations in physical appearance. These include alterations in color, local temperature, texture, and size or shape.

Alterations in Color

Abnormal color of the individual's skin and/or mucous membranes may be observed as a generalized state or may be confined to a localized area, depending upon the factors that are causing the abnormality and amount of melanin in the skin. For dark-skinned individuals, significant color changes may be observable only in the mucous membranes and the sclera.

PALLOR

The color of the skin is an important sign of changes in the peripheral circulation, since to some extent the color is attributable to the cutaneous vessels down to and including the subpapillary plexus. The vessels of the plexus are located parallel to the surface of the skin and thus significantly influence skin color. Pallor or a light pink color of the skin is evident when the blood vessels are partially constricted or of moderate tone and the blood flow through them is normal or rapid. When little blood is present in the subpapillary venous plexus, the skin becomes transparent and takes on the color of the subcutaneous connective tissue. This tissue is composed chiefly of collagen fibers with a whitish hue. The skin then has an ashen white pallor. Such skin color may occur in times of circulatory stress such as during strenuous exercise, following severe hemorrhage, and in some anxiety states. Vasoconstriction of cutaneous vessels diverts blood from the skin to meet the circulatory demands of other parts of the body.

The anemic patient often presents a pale appearance. This is particularly evident in the fingernail beds, the mucous membranes, and the conjunctiva. The deficiency in hemoglobin allows the whiteness of the subcutaneous tissues to manifest itself through the skin. Also, cutaneous vasoconstriction frequently occurs in anemia, which further decreases the amount of hemoglobin in the superficial tissues.

Acute arterial occlusion of an extremity will produce symptoms including pallor, cyanosis, and mottling of the affected part. These symptoms are transitory since, if circulation is not readily restored, tissue death rapidly occurs. The affected extremity will be cold. The absence of a pulse in the extremity is one of the earliest signs of an acute arterial occlusion.

Medical therapy is directed toward elimination of the cause of the pallor while supporting body maintenance during the crisis period. Definitive medical and nursing measures are discussed in other chapters dealing with shock, anemia, and disorders of peripheral circulation.

FLUSHING OR REDNESS

Excessive blood flow through skin vessels causes the skin to turn red. Rapid flow decreases normal deoxygenation which usually occurs in the skin, thus giving the skin a redder than normal color. Dilatation of the blood vessels brings greater amounts of the oxygenated blood into the surface area. Vasodilatation occurs through release of sympathetic vasoconstrictor tone as well as through sympathetic vasodilator fibers supplying arterioles of most areas of the skin.

Vasodilatation of skin vessels is effected by these various mechanisms in order to cool the body. Body heat is brought to the skin with the surface diversion of blood. The excess heat is then lost to the environment.

Increased metabolism in the skin activates another regulatory mechanism, the local autoregulatory mechanism, which causes local dilatation of skin vessels. This mechanism, also termed *reactive hyperemia,* is inherent in the tissues and responds to local blood flow and metabolism. Occlusion or decrease in the arterial blood supply of a body part results in stimulation of the reactive hyperemic mechanism. Increased blood flow occurs in the muscle and skin, thereby producing an obvious local hyperemia.

Prolonged or unrelieved pressure may decrease and finally occlude the arterial blood supply. A reactive hyperemia over weight-bearing surfaces, particularly bony prominences, is a premonitory sign of the development of a decubitus ulcer (pressure sore). Swelling under an encircling bandage or cast on an extremity may cause pressure on the underlying blood vessels.

Injury involving skin area which evokes an inflammatory response causes a local hyperemia. During the early phase of the inflammatory reaction, blood vessels dilate and blood flows rapidly through the tissues. Thus an intense localized redness of the skin may indicate beginning inflammation.

Cutaneous vasodilatation producing a red or flushed appearance may also result from alcoholic intake, a febrile reaction to systemic infection, and certain emotional states. The head and neck appear particularly flushed, since arterial blood flow and capillary perfusion in these areas are comparatively great.

Nurse's Action. The nurse should support the body's temperature-regulating activity through such measures as preventing drafts while allowing exposure of the skin to the environment. Heat loss would thus be effected mainly through radiation and conduction. Understanding of this temperature-regulating function of the skin is basic to the intelligent use of tepid water or alcohol sponge baths in febrile states. Specific aspects of the nursing care of the febrile patient were discussed in the preceding chapter.

Hyperemia from prolonged or unrelieved pressure is preventable. The skin over bony prominences in inactive patients should be carefully inspected several times a day. Frequent changes of position will help prevent development of decubitus ulcers. The frequency of position changes should be guided by the appearance of the skin.

CYANOSIS

Cyanosis is a bluish color of the skin and mucous membranes. The color derives from the presence of excessive amounts of reduced or deoxygenated hemoglobin in the blood of the superficial vessels. Hemoglobin not combined with oxygen is a very dark blue color. Cyanosis usually is indicative of a localized or generalized hypoxia.

The most important determinant of the degree of cyanosis is the absolute concentration of deoxygenated hemoglobin in the arterial blood. Normally there is 2.5 g of reduced hemoglobin in 100 ml of capillary blood. It has been suggested that cyanosis does not become perceptible until the mean concentration of reduced hemoglobin in the capillaries is almost double the normal value. Because of the deficiency of hemoglobin in anemia, hypoxia may be present without any evidence of cyanosis.

The clinical manifestation of cyanosis is also dependent upon the number and size of the surface capillaries. Cyanosis is readily detected when the skin vessels are dilated and blood is circulating through them.

The rate of blood flow through the skin further influences the degree of cyanosis. Normally, the metabolism of the skin is minimal and little deoxygenation occurs as the blood traverses the skin capillaries. When blood flow in the skin is abnormally slow, however, greater quantities of hemoglobin are reduced, causing cyanosis to develop or become intensified.

Pigmentation and skin thickness can modify or hide cyanosis. Thus the bluish color can best be appreciated where the skin is thin, unpigmented, and vascular. Such areas include the ear lobes, cutaneous surfaces of the lips, and fingernail beds. In individuals with dark skin, cyanosis can be observed in the mucous membranes of the mouth and the palpebral conjunctiva.

The significance of cyanosis depends upon the underlying pathology. Failure of the respiratory, circulatory, or nervous system may contribute to its development. Localized cyanosis may result from the excessive removal of oxygen from the blood which occurs with venous stasis. Abnormal reduction of oxygenated hemoglobin in cutaneous vessels is also observed when the skin is exposed to cold. The resulting constriction of skin vessels causes a retardation of blood flow and oxygen is removed more completely before the blood leaves the capillaries. The capillaries then contain large amounts of dark, deoxygenated blood giving the skin a bluish hue. Extreme cold, on the other hand, retards the use of oxygen by the tissues and an intensely red skin may be observed.

Physician's Action. Medical therapy is directed toward correction of the underlying disorder. This is covered in greater detail in subsequent chapters, in which diseases of the respiratory, circulatory, and nervous systems are discussed.

Generally, though, the detection of cyanosis may be interpreted as an indicator of hypoxia. Oxygen therapy is indicated when the cyanosis is due to the unsaturation of hemoglobin after passage through the pulmonary capillary bed. Conditions of this nature include (1) atmospheric anoxia, (2) disturbances in oxygen diffusion between the alveoli and the blood, and (3) anoxia of hypoventilation. It should be noted that the use of oxygen in chronic hypoventilation anoxia can be extremely dangerous. Oxygen lack becomes the primary stimulus to respiration and the administration of oxygen may eliminate this stimulus, resulting in respiratory failure. This is discussed in greater detail in relation to the patient with chronic obstructive lung disease.

Nurse's Action. The patient needs to be protected from the effects of oxygen deficiency of either a local or general nature. The nurse must be able to recognize the signs that indicate an oxygen lack and to take appropriate action to correct the situation.

When cyanosis is indicative of a generalized hypoxic state, certain nursing activities are suggested. The patency of the airway must be maintained and the possibility of obstruction by the tongue or by secretions should be considered and prevented. An unconscious patient should be positioned in a side-lying or prone position, with the head turned to one side to prevent the relaxed tongue from obstructing the airway. Obstructing secretions may be removed by having the patient cough, or by suctioning. The patient's position should be observed and adjusted to ensure adequate ventilation. Provision for physical rest is important to decrease the metabolic demands of the body for oxygen. Efforts are made to decrease cardiac demands, since the heart is already attempting to compensate for the hypoxia by an increase in rate. Safety needs of the patient must be considered, since the nervous system reacts to the hypoxia with symptoms which may include headache, fatigue, lassitude, apathy, depression, excitement, euphoria, irritability, insomnia, defective judgment, memory loss, poor muscle coordination, and stupor. The many technical responsibilities of care of the patient receiving oxygen therapy also are included in the nursing plan.

Localized cyanosis indicates impaired nutrition to the area or part. Poorly nourished tissue is very vulnerable to trauma and must be protected from environmental hazards that may injure it. When the cyanosis results from stasis of blood, nursing activity includes efforts to prevent thrombosis. Periodic leg exercises, frequent position change, avoidance of pressure in the popliteal space, and assurance of an adequate fluid intake are vital aspects of the care of the patient with lower extremity stasis.

Observation of the skin for cyanosis or a mottled appearance and of sensory changes is an important nursing responsibility in the therapeutic application of cold. The appearance of any or all of these symptoms should be reported and the treatment terminated. Tissue damage and destruction must be avoided through the proper application of cold. This includes a schedule of alternate applications of cold which must be followed.

JAUNDICE

Most of the bilirubin produced in the body is the result of the breakdown by the reticuloendothelial system of hemoglobin from mature erythrocytes. Normally the bilirubin is processed by the liver and excreted in the bile. Accumulation of bilirubin in the body usually results from impaired excretion of bilirubin by the liver, overproduction of this pigment in hemolytic states, or biliary tract obstruction. *Hyperbilirubinemia* is the accumulation of bilirubin in the blood. Bilirubin is capable of passing through capillary walls and penetrating cell membranes, thus producing a discoloration of body tissues. The visible yellow discoloration of the skin, sclerae, and mucous membranes is *jaundice*.

Medical and surgical intervention is aimed toward correction of the cause of the jaundice. This is discussed in subsequent chapters concerned with blood, liver, and gallbladder diseases.

Nurse's Action. Jaundice in itself presents certain implications for nursing care. The patient and his family will undoubtedly be concerned about this distortion in his appearance. An explanation of the jaundice as a symptom of the illness is indicated. The nurse also needs to be sensitive to the patient's feelings about his altered appearance and to offer him support in coping with his feelings.

Pruritus may or may not accompany the jaundice. In the patient with obstruction of intra- or extrahepatic biliary channels, whole bile is regurgitated into the blood. The pigment fraction of the bile causes the jaundice, and other biliary constituents in the blood and tissues probably cause the itching. The physician will probably prescribe measures to relieve the itching. A cool environment, tepid water sponge baths, gentle rubbing of the area, application of powder, and diversional activities may also be indicated. Care of the nails to reduce the mechanical trauma and danger of infection due to scratching should be included.

Certain significant observations of the jaundiced patient should routinely be made by the nurse. These observations may offer clues to the diagnosis and to progression of the disease. The depth of jaundice should be carefully noted. The color, odor, and character of the feces and the color of the urine should be reported and recorded. Certain derivatives of bilirubin are responsible for the brown color of feces. Failure of adequate amounts of bile to reach the intestine affects fat digestion and absorption, producing fatty, bulky, and foul-smelling stools. In some jaundiced patients bilirubin or its derivatives may be excreted in larger than normal amounts by the kidney, resulting in an amber to brown urine.

A bleeding tendency may be noted in certain jaundiced patients. The nurse should check the prothrombin time. Absence of bile in the gastrointestinal tract may cause a deficit of vitamin K, necessary for prothrombin synthesis. Further, liver damage may be so extensive that the cells are unable to produce prothrombin and related compounds. Thus the nurse observes for evidences of bleeding and takes special care to effect hemostasis at any bleeding sites.

ECCHYMOSIS

An *ecchymosis* or *bruise* is formed when bleeding occurs beneath the skin and the blood diffuses throughout an area of the subcutaneous tissue. An initial purplish-blue or blue discoloration is noted. This accounts for the commonly used descriptive term, "black and blue mark". As the blood pigments break down, bilirubin and biliverdin are formed. The bilirubin in the tissue produces an area of yellow discoloration, and the combination of bilirubin and biliverdin causes a yellowish-green hue.

The cause of subcutaneous bleeding may be of an extrinsic or intrinsic nature. External physical force may result in disruption of blood vessels with bleeding into surrounding tissue. Such damage to soft tissue and blood vessels is a *contusion*. Ecchymoses may also occur spontaneously and are symptomatic of some disorder of the blood vascular system occurring in various conditions. The term *purpura* is used to describe such spontaneous bleeding.

The free blood in the tissue acts as a foreign substance and stimulates an inflammatory response.

Physician's Action. Subcutaneous hemorrhage of spontaneous origin is treated through treatment of the underlying disease state. Ecchymosis due to external trauma may be treated with heat applications and administration of proteolytic enzymes. The objective of therapy is to improve local circulation, which will hasten the absorption of blood and lymph from the subcutaneous tissue. This serves to promote healing and to reduce local pain. There is some controversy as to the efficacy of proteolytic enzyme preparations in accomplishing these ends.

Nurse's Action. Observation of ecchymotic areas should include attention to location, size, and coloring. The coloring gives some indication of the recency of occurrence. The patient should be questioned about the cause of the bruise. Prevention of infection in the ecchymotic area is important, especially in debilitated patients and when the skin is broken. The extravasated blood serves as an excellent medium for bacterial growth. Additional nursing care activities that might be indicated are discussed later in this chapter in the section dealing with inflammatory edema.

Alterations in Size and Shape

EDEMA

A change in the normal contour and size of an area of the body surface may be a manifestation of an excessive accumulation of fluid in the interstitial spaces—edema.

This abnormal fluid accumulation is due to some disturbance in the mechanisms that control the inward and outward flow of fluid through the capillary wall. Absorption is exceeded by filtration and the increased volume of interstitial fluid distends the interstitial spaces, causing a visible increase in the bulk of the involved tissues.

A number of physiological disturbances may cause or contribute to the development of edema. These include an elevation in the capillary hydrostatic pressure, a deficiency in plasma proteins, and an increase in proteins in the interstitial spaces. Increased hydrostatic pressure in the capillaries may be due to an obstruction in the venous return, as from swelling under a cast or other restrictive dressing. Venous valvular insufficiency or a failure of the heart to pump blood forward will lead to an increase in the hydrostatic pressure in the venules. Such edema is characteristically prominent in dependent areas and will pit from pressure on the swollen tissue.

A deficiency in serum proteins may be caused by an abnormal loss of albumin through the kidneys or from exudates. A dietary deficiency of proteins or a deficiency in the formation of albumin in liver will also cause or contribute to a decrease in serum proteins. The protein content of the interstitial fluids will be increased by an obstruction to lymphatic drainage or by an increase in the permeability of the capillary wall which may occur with any inflammatory process.

Another type of edema which visibly alters the physical appearance is *ascites*. This is the abnormal collection of fluid in the peritoneal cavity which may or may not be a part of generalized edema. This can be recognized by the appearance of pale, shiny skin over a distended abdomen, and the shifting of the fluid with a change in position.

Nurse's Action. Certain activities of the nurse are indicated regardless of the cause of the extracellular edema. The excess fluid in the tissues compromises the blood supply thereby causing direct pressure on the capillaries. The increased interstitial fluid interferes with the diffusion of oxygen delivered to the tissues. The transport of cellular wastes to the blood is also disturbed. Thus cellular nutrition may be severely limited, making the tissue vulnerable to injury and lessening its capacity to adapt to increased demands.

Generally edema appears first in the skin and subcutaneous tissues, which are poorly protected against the effects of hydrostatic pressure. The decreased vitality of the skin is immediately evident by its taut and shining appearance. Nursing efforts must be exerted to preserve the integrity of the intact skin. Prevention of breakdown and subsequent infection is paramount. Once the bacteria enter the tissue, the edema fluid provides a good culture medium for their growth. The body's natural defenses against bacteria are deficient, since the edema fluid dilutes certain bactericidal substances derived from blood and lymph. The skin of the edematous areas must be kept clean, well lubricated, and free of external pressure. In generalized edema the swelling frequently appears first in dependent parts of the body as a result of gravity. Areas requiring special attention would therefore be the feet and ankles of the ambulatory patient and the sacrum, buttocks, and genitalia of the bedridden individual.

Edema in the area of a joint creates a splint-like effect, thereby limiting mobility. The patient may require assistance with certain activities because of this limitation. The ambulatory patient with lower extremity edema must be protected from injury. The feet tend to be heavy and clumsy and frequently the shoes fit poorly. The muscles of edematous legs are often very painful during exercise. Normal anatomical position of the edematous part should be maintained and periodic range of motion exercises carried out if not contraindicated by the underlying disease.

Some general therapeutic approaches are used to relieve the swelling and edema associated with an inflammatory process. The nurse assists the patient in achieving immobility of the area. The limitations imposed will dictate the patient's needs for nursing. Until the area of injury is well walled-off and localized, it should be protected from trauma. The development of inflammation should proceed undisturbed. The nurse teaches the patient that boils, furuncles, and similar inflamed areas should not be squeezed or manipulated.

Certain nursing care activities are directed toward the maintenance of circulation in the area of inflammation. Edema of inflamed tissues causes pressure on veins, restricting venous return. The affected part should be elevated, if possible, in order to allow gravity to facilitate venous return. Swelling of an extremity beneath a cast or constricting bandage is particularly hazardous. With minimal space for tissue expansion, pressure is referred inward, causing compression of veins and arteries. Elevation of the extremity and frequent observation of the distal portion for evidence of circulatory failure are important nursing activities. Indications of circulatory complications include cyanosis or pallor, coldness, swelling, pain, altered sensation, and disturbed motor function. The physician should be notified, as it may be necessary to cut the cast or to loosen the bandage. Another nursing function to enhance circulation in inflammation is the safe application of heat.

Evidence of extension of inflammation due to invasion of microorganisms must be noted. Involvement of adjacent tissue results in a cellulitis. Swelling of nearby lymph nodes indicates that organisms have entered the lymph channels. Observation of systemic responses, i.e., fever, malaise, muscle weakness, lassitude, and tachycardia, is an important indication of escape into the lymphatics and bloodstream of products of inflammatory reaction, substances secreted by bacteria, or bacteria themselves. The entrance of bacteria into the general circulation may cause a very serious extension of the disease.

ATROPHY

Atrophy is an acquired decrease in the size of a normally developed tissue or organ. The change occurs through a reduction in cell size, a decrease in the total number of cells, or a combination of the two. The normal shape and form of the atrophied part persists. When skeletal muscle is involved, decreased size is usually associated with decreased functional capacity.

Atrophy occurs as a result of disuse, malnutrition, or ischemia. Diminution in muscle mass due to inactivity can be observed in an extremity that has been immobilized in a plaster cast for a period of time. Atrophy of denervated skeletal muscle also results from inactivity or diminished function. Atrophy of skin and deeper structures can result from chronic circulatory insufficiency.

Physician's Action. Therapy is directed toward alleviation of the cause. This might include improvement of nutrition or circulation to a part, electrotherapy to denervated muscle, or a program of physiotherapy.

Nurse's Action. Assistance with a program of exercise is probably the single most important responsibility of the nurse in preventing or treating atrophy. Exercises prescribed by the physician are carried out by the physical therapist, the nurse, and the patient. The role of the nurse is to carry out passive exercise, to teach the patient and his family specific exercises, to encourage the patient, and to see that the program is followed. Attention to safety needs is important, since the atrophied muscle is a weakened muscle. Further, atrophied tissue resulting from malnutrition and ischemia would be especially vulnerable to injury and would have a limited capacity to adapt to increased demands.

HYPERTROPHY

Hypertrophy is an increase in the volume of a tissue or organ produced entirely by the enlargement of the existing cells. A visible alteration in the size of the part is caused by hypertrophy of skeletal muscle due to marked physical activity. This can be seen when weakness of muscles of one lower extremity increases the work load and causes hypertrophy of the muscles of the unaffected extremity. The increase in skeletal muscle mass increases the functional capacity of the part.

Local Temperature Changes of Inflammation

Reference has already been made to the localized increase in blood flow occurring as part of the inflammatory response to tissue injury. The blood moves rapidly through dilated vessels, bringing body heat to the surface. Some increased heat may also be caused by the increased metabolic activity of the area. These factors, then, cause an elevation in the temperature of the affected part.

Therapeutic approaches and nursing activities have already been discussed in relation to inflammatory edema. Edema and local heat are two of the cardinal signs of inflammation, the body's defensive reaction against injury.

Alterations in Skin Texture

DEHYDRATION

In *dehydration* the volume of body fluids, and particularly the volume of extra-cellular fluid, is decreased. In a very general way, such a state results from an insufficient intake, excessive losses from normal or abnormal routes, or a combination of the two. Electrolyte imbalance occurs concomitantly with the fluid reduction.

Observation of the dehydrated individual reveals a loss of skin turgor and elasticity. The skin appears dry, wrinkled, and loose. When it is picked up between the fingers, it tends to stick together and to retain the pinched shape or to return slowly to the original position. This is a result of the loss of subcutaneous fat and water from the deeper layers of the skin. The mucous membranes of the mouth are dry and parched and the tongue is shrunken and wrinkled. Other findings include weight loss, weakness, lassitude, thirst, anorexia, nausea and vomiting, scant and concentrated urinary output, faintness, fever, weak pulse, and hypo-tension. The condition may further deteriorate to shock and coma. Renal failure is a dreaded development.

Physician's Action. Dehydration without circulatory impairment may often be treated by increasing the oral intake of fluid and sodium chloride. If oral alimenta-tion is not possible or the dehydration is of a more serious nature, parenteral administration of fluids and electrolytes is instituted. Possible disturbances in the acid-base balance are corrected. Expansion of the circulating blood volume is indicated when shock is present or impending. Therapy is further directed toward the correction of the disorder responsible for precipitating the dehydration. Specific consideration of the management of dehydration and disturbed fluid balance is discussed in conjunction with the diseases in which these problems are of major importance.

Nurse's Action. Nursing attention to fluid intake is particularly important in the prevention of dehydration. To encourage or to force fluids is to establish and follow a schedule of fluid intake. Such a schedule is based upon the optimum intake desired, the type of fluid permitted and available, the likes and dislikes of the individual, and the waking hours of the particular patient. Salty foods and fluids would probably be indicated when sodium loss is high. The condition of the patient dictates the amount of nursing assistance he requires to follow such a schedule.

Certain patients are especially susceptible to dehydration. Careful observation is important in the care of patients with presenting problems of diaphoresis, fever, coma, confusion, lethargy, diarrhea, and rapid mouth breathing.

Other nursing activities include the following: (1) assisting with parenteral replacement therapy; (2) accurately recording intake, output, and weight; (3) periodically monitoring urinary output; (4) preventing skin breakdown; and (5) giving attention to oral hygiene.

DIAPHORESIS

Diaphoresis is profuse or drenching sweating. Large quantities of sweat are secreted onto the skin surface by the sweat glands. Stimulation of the anterior hypothalamus excites sweating. Impulses to the skin are transmitted by the sympathetic nerves of the autonomic nervous system.

Diaphoresis occurs during overheating of the body, during a febrile disease, and in certain emotional states. It is frequently associated with cutaneous vasodilation. Water secreted by the sweat glands in the form of perspiration evaporates from the body surface, causing cooling.

Profuse localized sweating of the forehead, palms of the hands, and soles of the feet may be noted in conjunction with certain nervous or fearful states. Such sweating due to psychic influences may be accompanied by constriction of skin blood vessels. Diaphoresis and peripheral vasoconstriction may also occur in profound shock states.

Nurse's Action. Discussion of nursing intervention is limited to the manifestation of diaphoresis as a temperature-reducing mechanism. Intelligent nursing care of a diaphoretic patient is based on an understanding of the following facts: (1) When the temperature of the external environment equals or exceeds the body temperature, the only means by which the body can rid itself of heat is evaporation. (2) The rate of evaporation, and thus the evaporative loss of body heat, is controlled by the moisture content or humidity of the surrounding air. (3) The use of clothing or body covering pervious to moisture allows almost normal loss of heat from the body by evaporation.

Nursing, then, is concerned with the temperature, humidity, and movement of air in the immediate environment of the patient. Alteration of environmental conditions within the nurse's control might include thermostatic regulation of temperature, maintenance of optimal ventilation, and possibly the use of fans. Heat loss is facilitated by maximum exposure of skin to the environment. Therefore, the body should be lightly and sparsely covered. The use of plastic or waterproof fabrics next to the body is contraindicated, since such materials block the loss of heat by evaporation. The evaporative loss of heat must be promoted in a safe and comfortable manner for the patient. Periodic sponge baths and linen change are welcome comfort measures.

Diaphoresis over a period of time may cause a significant loss of water, sodium, and chloride from the body. The nurse needs to observe for dehydration, dizziness, headache, fainting, postural hypotension, lethargy, diarrhea, abdominal cramps, and muscle weakness and cramping. The nurse assists in the oral and parenteral replacement of losses.

Elevation of body temperature was discussed in some detail in the preceding chapter.

SCAR FORMATION

New scar tissue is bright pink to purple because of the presence of abundant blood vessels. An "old" scar is hard and white.

Scar tissue is inelastic. It tends to contract when subjected to moderate stress. This shortening of the scar can cause deformity and partial loss of function.

Physician's Action. Plastic surgery is the therapy of choice for scars that are unsightly or cause limitation of function.

Nurse's Action. Newly formed scar tissue must be protected from external trauma. When scarring is extensive, as might occur in the healing of burns, nursing efforts must be directed toward the prevention of contractures of the affected part. The patient should be taught to avoid irritation of mature scars. Any change in the character of the scar should be reported to the physician, since this may be a manifestation of beginning cancer.

Bibliography

Books

Beland, Irene: *Clinical Nursing: Pathophysiological and Psychosocial Approaches.* New York: The Macmillan Company, 1965.

Best, Charles H. and Norman B. Taylor: *The Physiological Basis of Medical Practice,* 8th ed. Baltimore: The Williams & Wilkins Company, 1966.

Brooks, Stuart: *Basic Facts of Body Water and Ions,* 3d ed. New York: Springer Publishing Co., Inc., 1968.

Cecil, Russell L. and Robert F. Loeb (Eds.): *A Textbook of Medicine,* 12th ed. Philadelphia: W. B. Saunders Company, 1967.

Guyton, Arthur C: *Textbook of Medical Physiology,* 3d ed. Philadelphia: W. B. Saunders Company, 1966.

Harmer, Bertha and Virginia Henderson: *Textbook of the Principles and Practice of Nursing,* 5th ed. New York: The Macmillan Company, 1955.

Hopps, Howard C: *Principles of Pathology,* 2d ed. New York: Appleton Century Crofts, 1964.

Perez-Tamayo, Ruy: *Mechanisms of Disease.* Philadelphia: W. B. Saunders Company, 1961.

Smith, Dorothy W. and Claudia S. Gips: *Care of the Adult Patient,* 2d ed. Philadelphia: J. B. Lippincott Company, 1966.

Articles

Hayter, Jean: Impaired Liver Function and Related Nursing Care. *American Journal of Nursing,* 68:11:2374–2379, November, 1968.

Page, Robert G: Differential Diagnosis of Peripheral Edema. *Hospital Medicine,* 2:55–68, December, 1966.

Turner, Howard C: The Anatomy and Physiology of Normal Respiration. *Nursing Clinics of North America,* 3:383–401, September, 1968.

Zimmerman, Hyman J: The Differential Diagnosis of Jaundice. *Medical Clinics of North America,* 52:1417–1443, November, 1968.

CHAPTER 14
BODY POSITION, MUSCLE TONE, AND MOVEMENT

PHYLLIS E. PORTER

The elements of body position, muscle tone, and movement and the interrelatedness are in large measure determinants of the ability or inability, effectiveness or in-effectiveness, ease or dis-ease with which a person functions. In itself, each element plays an important role in maintaining equilibrium; together, they act to ensure the internal and external equilibrium of man in his environment. Because of the interrelatedness of these elements, factors that interrupt the function and upset the equilibrium of one of these elements result in interruption and imbalance of one or both of the other elements—in addition to altering the effectiveness of the three elements in functioning together to produce harmony, efficiency, and economy of action. Yet in an increasingly complex era of medical technology and treatment with its concomitant influence on nursing practice, the importance of equilibrium within and between body position, muscle tone, and movement is often disregarded.

Alteration in body position, muscle tone, and movement may result from such direct causes as injury or disease with resultant loss of or change in function. Equally significant and frequent, however, is loss of or change in function resulting from disuse or misuse that occurs while medical and nursing attention is focused upon the cure of disease or injury to another part of the body. In such an instance, the patient may find that he has recovered from an acute life-threatening episode only to face a new problem such as disruption of normal body position, loss of muscle tone, or limitation in normal movement—entirely because of inadequate planning for maintenance of normal function in these three areas. It cannot be denied that in some specific instances, the treatment of the acute or life-threatening problem may necessitate the disuse or misuse of a part or parts. When such a measure is necessary, then frequent assessment and reevaluation must be made to ensure that the measure is not continued longer than is therapeutically necessary. The determination of such needs should be made by the members of the therapy team, who must fully realize the potentially harmful consequences of the treatment to body position, muscle tone, and movement.

Body Position in Health

Body position may be defined simply as the placement or arrangement of body parts. Placement or arrangement is commonly seen in relation to two major areas: the arrangement or placement of the parts individually to each other, and the arrangement or placement of all the parts in relation to the immediate physical environment. In the former sense, the position of a part is described, for example, as abducted, adducted, flexed, or extended, and in the latter sense, as standing, sitting, or lying.

The term *body alignment* is similar to *body position,* and the terms often are used synonymously. In nursing, however, the former term is frequently used to describe the position of the parts in relation to each other, particularly as regards the patient who is in bed. *Posture* is a third term that can be used synonymously with body position or body alignment. Posture is said to be dynamic or static. If the person is standing, walking, or moving, then he is said to be in dynamic posture. On the other hand, if the person is lying in bed, then his posture is described as static posture.

That the person is always in some state of position, alignment, or posture is evident, but these become further imbued with quality or value. Thus the person is described as having good posture or conversely as being in a state of poor body alignment. In the standing position, good posture or alignment is often described in relation to physiological functioning. Fuerst and Wolff convey this concept when they describe good body alignment as alignment of body parts which enhances musculoskeletal balance, operation, and physiologic functioning. These criteria of good posture can then be applied to any of the positions of standing, sitting, or lying.

ELEMENTS OF GOOD ALIGNMENT

Before the nurse can logically appreciate the effects of disease and/or injury upon posture, she must be aware of the elements contributing to good body alignment. Since the body is made up of segments, good alignment in the standing position occurs when the segments are centered over each other; thus the center of gravity of each body segment is centered over its supporting base. In this position, the body is best able to maintain stability and balance. When good alignment is not maintained, then muscles and bones are placed in positions of functional disadvantage, resulting in added strain upon these structures in their efforts to maintain stability and support.

In addition to greater stability, better balance, and ease of motion, good posture offers other advantages to the body as a whole. As described by Broer, good segmental alignment of the body in the standing position has these results: the feet are straight ahead and a few inches apart; the knees are slightly flexed, with the patellae pointing forward; the pelvis is balanced in a neutral position between flexion and extension; the shoulders are level; and the head is balanced on the shoulders with the chin level.

In the sitting position, the principles of segmental alignment remain the same for the trunk, but because sitting enlarges the base of support and lowers the center of gravity, there is generally less strain than in the standing position. The hips should be well back in the chair so that the back is supported, the knees should be at right angles, and the feet should be supported or flat on the floor. Modifications of the sitting position occur depending upon whether the person is at work while sitting or is relaxing in an easy chair.

GENERAL EFFECTS OF GOOD ALIGNMENT

Much has been written about good posture and its effects on the total health of the individual. The ultimate therapeutic aim would be for all persons to be able to achieve a state of "normal" posture. The difficulty then becomes to define and recognize normal posture. Cooper and Glassow introduce the physiological concept of normal as being that condition which permits the organs and systems of the body to function efficiently. In this respect, body posture then affects physiological functions. However, among people who have extensively studied the relationship of good posture to normal health, there is no clear-cut agreement about the specific effects and the degree to which good posture affects normal body functions. One of the difficulties in determining the effects of good posture on health has been that many of the studies in this area have concerned themselves primarily with posture in the standing position. In his discussion of the effects of posture on health, Karpovich reiterates the disadvantages commonly attributed to poor posture as including such problems as a decrease in lung capacity, poor circulation, kinks in the intestine, and even albuminuria. Conversely, then, good posture should result in an increased lung capacity, a more efficient circulation, and better functioning of internal organs. This, however, has yet to be proven.

Nonetheless, certain facts are known about posture and its relation to the physiological whole. It has been substantiated that the energy requirements of lying, sitting, and standing differ. According to Cooper and Glassow, the rigid military posture requires about 20 percent more energy than does a relaxed standing position, and a relaxed standing position requires about 10 percent more energy than an extremely relaxed standing position. Moreover, the energy requirement of a completely relaxed standing position is approximately equal to that of sitting or lying. Cooper and Glassow add that assumption of the erect rigid posture is followed by an increase in blood pressure, which suggests a change in circulatory efficiency. The change in respiratory efficiency is more difficult to assess but is believed not to be great. Thus it may be concluded that the rigid erect posture is not normal, since the efficiency of the respiratory and circulatory systems is reduced— yet when individuals consciously try to achieve "good posture," it is often this rigid erect posture which they are trying to emulate.

Pathological disruption of normal posture and body alignment must be considered, including extremes of curvature and malalignment. It is not known to what degree such deviations are possible without impairing health or interfering with the efficiency of vital organs, but it is probable that minor deviations have little effect on health and the efficient functioning of vital organs.

With knowledge of the foregoing factors, the nurse should have a better understanding of good posture so that she can apply this knowledge to the care of her patients.

FACTORS THAT INFLUENCE ALIGNMENT

According to Cooper and Glassow, normal posture is that which is best suited to the individual in relation to his specific condition and the circumstances of his environment.

Using the foregoing definition, one can easily recognize several factors that influence an individual's posture at a given time. In a situation that demands alertness or readiness for action, the normal posture is likely to be erect but not rigid. Appropriately, fatigue may give rise to a slouched posture. Distress due to difficult emotional situations may also be expressed in a drooping posture. Thus, normal posture reflects the individual's state of readiness, his physical state, or his mental state. Every individual will display different postures at different times, and each posture will be a normal one for the specific situation. Recognition of these individual differences is as essential to the assessment of the individual's postural state as is an arbitrary standard against which to compare his posture.

Body Position in Illness

All health problems have either a direct or an indirect effect upon body position. In her dealing with patients the nurse utilizes her knowledge of body position to prevent poor body position, maintain normal body alignment, and in some instances to help restore normal body position.

Since every patient is always in some state of body alignment, the nurse should comprehend the great importance of maintaining normal body position in her patients. She should see herself as aiding therapy by assessing positioning needs, planning for normal body position, and implementing therapeutic positioning. In most instances, positioning of the patient is an independent therapeutic nursing measure; therefore, except when circumstances dictate otherwise, the nurse positions the patient without the physician's order.[1] Positioning is an important area of independent nursing practice, and carries significant nursing responsibilities.

ASSESSING POSITIONING NEEDS

The first responsibility is to assess the patient's position and his positioning needs. During the assessment process the nurse can ask herself such critical questions as these: What is the patient's position? Why is he in this position? What is the relationship of his medical or surgical problem to his positioning needs? What problems can I predict will occur if proper positioning techniques are not employed? What actions must I take to prevent these problems? To make such an assessment the nurse will have to have a sound knowledge of the scientific and theoretical framework of nursing as well as a knowledge of the individual patient. She will consider such factors as the sex, age, diagnosis, and general condition of the patient as well as any contraindications to specific positions.

For example, in answering her first question, she will find out whether the patient is standing (and therefore probably ambulatory), sitting, or lying. How did he get where he is? Was he able to accomplish this himself? Did he need help and, if so, how much? Is he in good alignment? Suppose that she finds the patient curled up in bed. Why? If she pursues her second question she may find out that the patient is in pain, or is cold, or has spastic paralysis. What are the implications for positioning needs of such medical-surgical problems as a mastectomy, congestive heart failure, or a spinal cord injury? The knowledgeable nurse will predict that a hip flexion, abduction, external rotation contracture will develop in the patient with a midthigh amputation unless she positions his stump in an extended, neutral or slightly internally rotated, adducted position. Or she can predict that in the patient with a cerebrovascular accident flexion contractures of the upper and lower extremities will develop unless she positions him therapeutically. Hence a critical assessment of the patient's positioning is the first step in ensuring that the patient's body position will be as near normal as his specific problems will allow.

---

[1] In circumstances of direct pathological consequences and treatment, as in certain fractures and surgical procedures, the nurse should consult the physician for specific positioning directions to the affected part or parts.

PLANNING FOR POSITIONING NEEDS

The second responsibility is for planning the positioning needs of the patient. How much of the patient's positioning needs is he able to assume himself? The patient who is ambulatory and who has little interference in normal neuromusculo-skeletal function may be able to meet his positioning needs with little assistance from the nursing staff. He may require supervision and teaching rather than direct nursing intervention. Some patients are less able to meet their total needs for positioning, but with some help can meet some of their needs. Perhaps they need to be reminded to change position or encouraged to assume positions that are not as comfortable as other positions. Perhaps they need physical assistance in changing position, or in getting in and out of bed, or in transferring to a wheel chair. Do their positioning needs require the use of added or special equipment such as a pillow, a foot board, a trochanter roll, or a Stryker frame? The extent and type of such assistance and equipment must be planned for in providing nursing care for these patients.

Patients assume many positions accidentally or spontaneously, and these positions have little or no purpose. Positioning becomes purposeful when the patient's positioning needs have been assessed and a plan has been made for meeting these needs. In addition to providing the means for positioning and assuring that positioning will be purposeful, planning will ensure the degree and frequency with which positioning is carried out. If the patient is ambulatory, a rigid schedule for positioning may not be needed. If the patient is in a wheel chair, perhaps he will need verbal supervision at specified intervals to make certain that he is changing his position frequently enough to reduce pressure on the ischial tuberosities and the sacrum. The paraplegic patient may have to raise himself from the seat of his wheel chair as frequently as every 30 minutes for a full minute to prevent the formation of pressure sores. If the patient is comatose, a more rigid schedule will be required which specifies both the time and the position of the patient. He will have to be repositioned at least every 2 hours, and turned on all four sides (anterior, posterior, and two sides) in rotation to obtain the maximum benefits.

PLANNING FOR THERAPEUTIC POSITIONING

The third area of responsibility is providing that positioning be therapeutic. Therapeutic positioning may be defined as positioning that enhances healing. Positioning as a nursing measure thus gains a positive dimension. Therapeutic positioning is based upon the individual needs of the patient. This view reinforces the nurse's responsibility to assess and plan for the positioning needs of the patient. Positioning can be nontherapeutic, as well as therapeutic; moreover, in the majority of situations where the positioning is not therapeutic it probably will be detrimental. While there may be some disagreement concerning the value of good posture to health, there can be no disagreement that the effects of non-therapeutic positioning are detrimental to the health of the patient.

Some patients assume therapeutic positions without guidance. Hence therapeutic positioning may be spontaneous or accidental as described in relation to purposeful positioning. The dyspneic patient who assumes the orthopneic position illustrates this point. Unfortunately, however, patients with equal frequency choose positions that are not therapeutic. The patient who wants his stump elevated on a pillow for comfort illustrates how a patient given a free choice might choose a non-therapeutic position. Since the patient will always be in some state of body position, it is a nursing responsibility to ensure that the patient's position is chosen specifically for its therapeutic aims—it will be purposeful therapeutic positioning.

The aims or goals of therapeutic positioning will differ according to each patient situation. By viewing goals and aims in relation to specific objectives, the nurse can classify these objectives as prevention, maintenance, and restoration of function. Accordingly, therapeutic positioning may be a preventive, a maintenance, or a restorative measure depending upon the positioning needs of the patient.

Ideally, all patients coming under the care of the nurse would need positioning that is primarily oriented toward preventing deformities. This assumes that such patients have no preexisting deformities, nor would their current condition proscribe the institution of preventive positioning measures. The goal then would be to prevent deformity—to ensure that the patient recovers from his acute illness with normal posture or body position as has previously been described. Although all patients may suffer some degree of incapacity if proper positioning techniques are not instituted, those who may be harmed most are those who are confined to bed. The dangers of bed rest and the resultant disuse phenomena are well known. With proper positioning, many of the problems of disuse can be eliminated or minimized to a degree that deformity is not permanent. Disuse complications, either temporary or permanent, develop because purposeful therapeutic positioning measures have not been instituted. These complications include postural malalignment and deformities of the trunk such as scoliosis, kyphosis, or lordosis; circulatory problems such as stasis or dependent edema; hypostatic pneumonia; muscle contractures, and ankylosis of joints; and finally decubitus ulcers or pressure sores.

The maintenance of proper body position as the second objective of therapeutic positioning is complementary or corollary to the aim of prevention. Indeed it is often difficult to differentiate the two. By carrying out preventive positioning the nurse surely is maintaining the patient's normal body posture. If, however, the patient has already experienced some degree of deformity, then the objective is to maintain him in as near normal a state as possible, as in caring for patients with long-term problems, chronic illnesses, or permanent disabilities particularly of a progressive nature. By maintaining the patient at his present level of capability, further deterioration is halted and in some instances restorative measures can then be undertaken. In progressively deteriorating diseases such as multiple sclerosis, it is not always possible to prevent deformity, nor is it always possible to institute restorative measures; under such circumstances the most logical objective is to maintain as much function as possible.

With patients who have experienced deformity of one type or another, its alleviation may become the prime goal of care. Here the aim of therapeutic positioning is to restore function. At times the nurse can act independently to implement restorative positioning, but more frequently she will act as one member of the therapy team concerned with therapeutic positioning. Other team members include the physician, the physical therapist, and the occupational therapist. The nurse then cooperates with the other team members. In this situation, she may also be responsible for ensuring that the entire nursing team works cooperatively with the therapy team.

The following tables illustrate therapeutic positioning for the patient confined to bed and for the patient in a wheel chair. They are intended to serve as a guide in assessing common positioning needs, in showing common deviations from therapeutic positions, and in determining nursing intervention to prevent deformity. Such charts of course cannot be comprehensive. Modifications must be made in relation to the individual patient and his positioning needs and problems. It must be stressed that no position maintained without change is therapeutic. Change of position is as essential as the position itself. Change should be made in the position of the individual body parts that comprise each complete body position as well as from one postion to another.

TABLE 14-1

*Positioning the Patient
in the Supine Position*

PART OF BODY	THERAPEUTIC POSITION	COMMON DEVIATIONS OR PROBLEMS	NURSING INTERVENTION TO PREVENT DEFORMITY
HEAD	Neutral or extended	Flexion; hyperextension	Avoid excessive use of pillows; place pillows so that both shoulders and head are supported in a continuous line
UPPER ARM Shoulder joint	Slight abduction; neutral rotation	Adduction; internal rotation	Position with pillow or bath blanket so that the arm is slightly abducted and slightly externally rotated
FOREARM Elbow; radio-ulnar joint	Extension; slight supination or slight flexion	Too much flexion	Maintain in extension or slight flexion; provide for alteration in supination and pronation
WRISTS	Extension or slight hyperextension	Flexion and adduction (ulnar deviation)	Support wrists in "cockup" (extended to hyperextended) position
FINGERS AND THUMBS	Functional position: slight finger flexion and thumb opposition	Extension or extreme flexion	Provide for grasp position—fingers slightly flexed and in opposition to thumb; hand roll may be used
TRUNK	Maintenance of normal curvature	Flexion and hyperextension; exaggeration of normal curves (kyphosis and lordosis)	Firm mattress or bed board; use of pillows or other devices (such as small pad under lumbar area) to maintain normal curvature
HIPS	Extension; neutral rotation; neither abducted nor adducted	Flexion; external rotation; abduction or adduction	Use of trochanter roll to prevent external rotation, maintain neutral rotation without abduction or adduction
KNEES	Extension or slight flexion	Hyperextension; too much flexion	Avoid large pillows or rolls under knees; small flat roll or pad to prevent hyperextension
FEET	Neutral or slight dorsiflexion	Plantar flexion (foot drop); pressure on heels	Use of foot board or other supportive device to maintain functional position; heels off end of mattress or slightly elevated by thin pad supporting entire calf

TABLE 14-2
*Positioning the Patient
in the Side-Lying
Position*

PART OF BODY	THERAPEUTIC POSITION	COMMON DEVIATIONS OR PROBLEMS	NURSING INTERVENTION TO PREVENT DEFORMITY
HEAD	Neutral or extended	Hyperextension; forward and lateral flexion	Avoid excessive use of pillows; place pillows so that head is supported level and in neutral position
UPPER ARM	*Superior arm*—slight hyperextension or forward flexion in varying degrees	*Superior*—extension, lack of opportunity for hyperextension or flexion horizontal adduction	*Superior*—support with pillow in flexion or hyperextension and level or in slight abduction
	Inferior arm—flexed and in front of patient	*Inferior*—caught under patient because of lack of flexion	*Inferior*—check for comfort and unnatural pressure or strain
FOREARM Elbow; radio-ulnar joint	*Superior*—extended or flexion of not more than 90°; pronated	*Superior*—lack of support with resulting strain	*Superior*—provide adequate support in therapeutic position
	Inferior—flexed and supinated	*Inferior*—caught under patient	*Inferior*—be sure it is not caught under patient
WRISTS	*Superior*—extension or slight hyperextension	*Superior*—flexion	*Superior*—support wrist in "cock-up" (extended to hyperextended) position
	Inferior—extension	*Inferior*—flexion	Make sure wrist is in extension
FINGERS AND THUMBS	Functional position—fingers slightly flexed and thumbs in opposition	Extension; too much flexion	Provide for grasp position with fingers slightly flexed and thumb in opposition; *inferior*—use of hand roll; *superior*—hand roll or fingers curved over supporting pillow
TRUNK	Maintenance of normal curvature	Flexion; hyperextension; scoliosis; rotation	Firm mattress or bed board; use pillows or other devices to maintain normal curvature and rotation; adjust hips and shoulders far enough under patient so that line of gravity falls anteriorly thus eliminating necessity of using supporting pillows along back
HIPS	*Superior*—flexed at 90° and level with body; anterior to inferior leg	*Superior*—too much flexion; adducted because of lack of support; resting on inferior leg	*Superior*—prevent extreme flexion; support with pillows anterior to inferior leg and level with body
	Inferior—slightly flexed or extended; posterior to superior leg, and well under patient	Too much flexion; not far enough under patient; underneath superior leg	Prevent extreme flexion; place well under patient and posterior to superior leg
KNEES	*Superior leg*—at right angle to hip level with body; anterior to inferior leg	*Superior*—flexion more than 90°; resting on anterior leg; not level with body	*Superior*—support on pillow level with body and anterior to inferior leg; flexed at about 90°
	Inferior—extended or slightly flexed and posterior to superior leg	*Inferior*—flexion of more than 45°; under superior leg	*Inferior*—place posterior to superior leg and in extended or slightly flexed position
FEET	Functional (neutral position); foot of extended leg may be against foot board	Plantar flexion; lack of adequate support for superior foot	Maintain functional position; support foot of superior leg adequately.

TABLE 14-3
*Positioning the Patient
in the Prone Position*

PART OF BODY	THERAPEUTIC POSITION	COMMON DEVIATIONS OR PROBLEMS	NURSING INTERVENTION TO PREVENT DEFORMITY
HEAD	Extended; lateral rotation	None usual; potential hyperextension	Caution: if patient cannot control head movement be sure that his face is not in the mattress and that he can breathe
UPPER ARMS Shoulder joint	Over the head in varying degrees of flexion, abduction, and external rotation	Extended at sides; extreme internal rotation	Small pillows or pads under the shoulders for support; encourage therapeutic position, sometimes a difficult position to maintain without encouragement
LOWER ARM Elbow; radio-ulnar joint	Varying degrees of flexion; pronation with slight degree of supination possible for variation		Maintain therapeutic position
WRISTS	Extension or slight hyperextension	Flexion	Support wrist in "cockup" (extended to hyperextended) position
FINGERS AND THUMBS	Extension or slight flexion	Flexion	Provide for extension or provide for grasp position, fingers flexed and in opposition to thumb; may use hand roll
TRUNK	Extension	None usual; potential lordosis	Small pillow or pad under the abdomen
HIPS	Extension; neutral rotation; neither abducted nor adducted	External rotation	Use of a trochanter roll to prevent external rotation
KNEES	Extended or slightly flexed	Too much flexion	Flex knee by placing small pillow under lower leg
FEET	Neutral	Plantar flexion	Position patient so that feet hang over the mattress or place pillow under lower leg so that knees are flexed (about 45°), allowing feet to be in neutral position

Muscle Tone

Preservation of muscle tone is an important nursing function whenever such preservation is physiologically possible. There are three types of muscle tissue: striated, smooth, and cardiac. We shall be concerned only with striated muscle, which is also commonly called voluntary or skeletal muscle.

Muscle tone or *tonus* refers to the condition or state of the muscle, and is a term often used to describe its firmness or tautness. The physiological basis of muscle tone is attributed to a variety of factors. Early definitions of muscle tone described it as a continuous state of partial contraction. Each muscle and muscle group is composed of individual muscle fibers. Both the individual muscle fibers and the muscle groups, as well as the individual muscles, have the properties of tone and contractility. It was felt that numbers of muscle fibers within the muscle groups alternated in their contractions resulting in constant firmness of tone of the muscle.

TABLE 14-4
Positioning the Patient
in the Sitting Position
(Chair or Wheel Chair)

PART OF BODY	THERAPEUTIC POSITION	COMMON DEVIATIONS OR PROBLEMS	NURSING INTERVENTION TO PREVENT DEFORMITY
HEAD	Neutral or extended and balanced on shoulders	Forward and lateral flexion; hyperextension	Support head in therapeutic position if the patient is unable to maintain support without aid
SHOULDERS	Maintained upright and level	Slouched forward; not level—elevation or depression of one	Provide for support in therapeutic position if patient is unable to maintain this himself; be sure that support does not result in elevation of one or both shoulders
LOWER ARM	Supported on arms of chair if patient is unable to control it	Lack of support with resulting strain on shoulder joint with possible subluxation	Position on arms of chair or with support; consider possibility of using sling if movement of arms cannot be controlled
WRISTS	Extension or slight hyperextension	Flexion	Maintain in extension by supporting on arm of chair, or in a sling if one is being used
FINGERS AND THUMBS	Flexed over end of chair arm in functional position	Extension; too much flexion	Provide for therapeutic position
TRUNK	Normal posture and good alignment; back supported against back of chair	Forward and lateral flexion	Provide for proper trunk support if patient is unable to accomplish this
HIPS	Flexed at 90° and placed against back of chair	Not far enough back in chair, patient slides forward	Maintain hips at 90° flexion and place patient well back in chair; strap patient in this position if he is unable to maintain it without aid
KNEES	Flexed at 90° unless there is specific need for them to be placed otherwise	Become extended when hips are not back in chair and patient slides forward	Maintain in the therapeutic position; place small pillow or roll between the knees if hip adduction is a problem
FEET	Neutral	Plantar flexion	Support feet flat on floor or foot rest of wheel chair; have patient wear shoes

In this manner the muscle maintained its tone, but the muscle and muscle groups did not become fatigued.

Later evidence suggested that this explanation of muscle tone was too simple and did not explain sufficiently the physiology inherent in muscle tone. Guyton attributes muscle tone entirely to the action potential of the muscle fiber, since skeletal muscle is not known to contract without stimulation. This potential accounts for the tautness of muscle. Other bases for muscle tone have been attributed to the physical property of elasticity in the muscle, to the normal condition or turgor of the muscle, and to continuous low-frequency electrical discharges emanating from the muscle. An abnormally high concentration of carbon dioxide affects muscle tone, as does a variation in hydrogen ion concentration. In addition to the direct physiological basis for muscle tone in the muscle tissue, tonus appears to be an integrated function of centers in the spinal cord and brain. It is also known that the general condition or health of the individual affects normal muscle tone.

Normal muscle tone is of functional importance to health. The highest degree of muscle tone consistently found in the human being is in the antigravity skeletal muscles, including the muscles of the back and the muscles supporting the head in an erect and upright position. In addition to its characteristic firmness, muscle tone in skeletal muscles maintains a slight but steady pull on the attachment of muscles and also serves to maintain firmness of the abdominal wall, thereby exerting pressure on the abdominal viscera. Muscle tone directly influences the ease, speed, and rhythm of movement.

Although there may be some controversy about the basis of muscle tone, it is agreed that normal skeletal muscle does have a condition of tautness or firmness. The nurse is concerned with the maintenance of this normal tone. Muscle tone is related to the ability of the muscle to work. The primary work of skeletal muscles is to accomplish motion. The ability of muscles to perform work depends upon an intact neuromusculoskeletal system, adequate nutrition, circulation, and ventilation. Although the remaining discussion in this section will be limited to the muscles themselves, it must be remembered that an interruption of any of the foregoing factors can affect the ability of the muscle to work.

CHANGES IN MUSCLE TONE

Muscle tissue responds to a stimulus to work. If the muscle is continually called upon to perform more work than usual, its response will take the form of *hypertrophy*. Hypertrophy results in an increased capacity to perform work. The weight lifter is an example of this phenomenon. Conversely, when the muscle is unable or not called upon to work, it shrinks and loses its capacity to perform work. Initially, muscle weakness ensues. If this process is not interrupted, the muscle will continue to shrink. This is called *muscle atrophy,* or, commonly, *disuse atrophy.* Common causes of disuse atrophy include nerve denervation, enforced bed rest or chair rest, restriction of activity because of external or environmental causes, mental illness such as catatonia, and immobilization resulting from the use of such devices as casts and braces.

Pathophysiological Disorders That Cause Changes in Muscle Tone

A number of pathophysiological disorders can also give rise to changes in normal muscle tone. Early reduction in the efficiency of muscle tissue is first manifested as muscle weakness. This may be of minor significance or may be an early indication of progressively severe disorders. Temporary muscle weakness of minor importance can occur following fatigue from overexertion, minor acute infections such as the common cold, or surgery. In these instances the weakness is temporary, and normal muscle tone and strength returns usually without specific treatment.

Muscle weakness may be the first symptom of a pathologic process, in which case the weakness may remain relatively stable or may progress depending upon the underlying disease. In either instance treatment and nursing actions correspond to the nursing measures indicated for the specific disorders. Hence muscle weakness may accompany systemic disturbances (e.g., acute inflammatory and infective processes, potassium depletion), disease of the cardiovascular system (e.g., rheumatic fever and acute bacterial endocarditis), blood disturbances (e.g., anemia and leukemia), and practically all diseases of the neuromusculoskeletal system (e.g., arthritis, fractures, myasthenia gravis, muscular dystrophy, multiple sclerosis, poliomyelitis, and other paralytic disorders). The exact mechanism of muscle weakness following denervation is not known, but it is most likely related to the inability of the muscle to maintain tension.

Paralytic disturbances result in alteration of normal muscle tone even though the muscle tissue itself is not the direct site of pathology. The two major types of change in muscle tone following paralysis are described in relation to the type of paralysis. The patient is described as having either flaccid or spastic paralysis, or both combined. The muscles themselves are said to be flaccid or spastic.

Flaccid paralysis occurs as a result of lower motor neuron damage or destruction. The lower motor neuron is composed of the ventral horn cell of the spinal cord and its projection or nerve to the effector unit—the muscle. In other words, there is damage to the final common nerve pathway. Lesions here produce a decrease or loss of muscle tone, decrease or absence of the tendon reflexes, and muscle atrophy. The nurse can easily recognize flaccid paralysis because of the characteristic appearance of the muscle. A flaccid muscle loses its resilience and its ability to maintain its normal shape. It is limp and flabby, hanging loosely because of its own weight. Flaccid paralysis is seen in patients with poliomyelitis and in some patients with spinal cord injuries.

Spastic paralysis is seen in patients with upper motor neuron damage or destruction. The term *upper motor neuron* refers to nerve cells of the pyramidal tract and the cerebral cortex which terminate in the ventral horn of the spinal cord. This is sometimes also called the *corticospinal tract*. Lesions in this area result in excessive preservation of reflexes, impairing voluntary motion. There is an exaggeration of the stretch reflex because of impairment of the central inhibitory influences that normally reduce the stretch reflex. This results in involuntary contraction of muscle and spasm. Very slight stimulation will initiate contraction in the stretched muscle. A persistent spasm is *tonic spasm*. Alternate contraction and relaxation of the muscle is *clonic spasm*. Spastic paralysis is also easily recognized by the nurse. Loss of voluntary movement accompanied by increase in muscle tone and spasticity is characteristic of spastic paralysis. The muscle offers resistance to stretch or motion and the limbs are stiff. Spastic paralysis is seen in patients with damage to the cerebral cortex and in patients with incomplete spinal cord lesions.

Because of the complex nature of the nervous system, some patients with injury or disease of the nervous system exhibit both spastic and flaccid paralysis. However, the characteristics of flaccid and spastic paralysis are quite readily recognized in spite of the complexity of the disorder of which they are a part.

Mass involvement and disruption of normal muscle tone occurs during convulsions and more specifically those convulsions designated as *grand mal seizures*. Convulsions of this type can be produced by any number of factors that result in a diffuse assault on the brain causing disorder of the cerebral metabolism. Seizures, although dramatic in themselves, are usually considered symptomatic of an underlying problem. Such factors as a disturbance in the nutritional status of the cerebral cortex, decreased cerebral blood flow, disturbance of cardiac rhythm, neuronal discharge from irritative or anoxic ischemic processes, electric current, and drugs may all produce convulsions. During a convulsion, the muscle tone is greatly increased to the point of extreme spasticity and rigidity. The patient is literally convulsed by the tonic and clonic muscle spasms. Fortunately, in most instances seizures are of a short duration and occur episodically. Treatment and nursing care depend upon the cause of the convulsion whenever specific causes can be determined. For specific nursing care measures of the patient having a convulsion the reader is referred to Part V.

EVALUATING MUSCLE TONE

One of the objectives of therapeutic nursing care is to maintain normal muscle tone whenever this is possible. Most patients with whom the nurse comes in contact will have experienced a change in their everyday routine, and their exercise patterns will be affected by this change. This change will affect normal muscle tone and thereby the ability of the patient's skeletal muscles to perform work. The patient's specific health problem may interfere with or alter the ability of the muscle to work as a direct result of injury or disease to the neuromusculoskeletal system or indirectly as the result of rigid enforcement of bed rest, which ultimately affects normal muscle tone, as previously explained. Normal muscle tone and strength are best maintained with proper exercise. Provision should be made for exercise within the limitations of the patient's capabilities and the restrictions imposed by his specific pathophysiological problem.

The first step in providing for the patient to receive appropriate exercise is to assess his muscle tone and strength. In some instances the nurse may work independently in making this assessment, but more frequently she will work collaboratively with and under the direction of such team members as the physician, the physical therapist, and the occupational therapist.

One common method of evaluating muscle tone and strength is to grade the muscle from *0* to *normal* depending upon its ability to accomplish motion as follows: *0,* no contraction is seen or felt; *trace,* the muscle can be felt to tighten but cannot produce movement; *poor,* the muscle can produce motion if the force of gravity is eliminated, but cannot move against gravity; *fair,* the muscle can move against gravity; *good,* the motion can be accomplished against gravity and/or some outside resistance; and *normal,* the muscle can move against greater resistance (Rusk). Although this is a subjective method of testing muscle strength, it does provide a basis upon which the patient's progress can be measured. The nurse can assess muscle weakness and grossly evaluate the muscle. She is also able to grossly determine the patient's state of muscle tone as being firm and taut, or soft and flabby, and whether paralysis is flaccid or spastic. More detailed evaluation and muscle testing must be made by therapists trained in making such evaluations. The type, extent, and degree of the exercise program will be determined by the total health problems of the patient. Assessment and reevaluation by the team must be made as the patient's health needs change.

The most common types of exercise with which the nurse should be familiar and with which she will most commonly be concerned include passive exercise, active exercise, active-assistive exercise, resistive exercise, static or setting exercise, and range of motion exercise.

EXERCISES

Passive Exercise

Passive exercise is the exercise accomplished by power other than the contraction of the muscles of the part being exercised. It may be accomplished by another person (such as the nurse), by the use of equipment, or by the patient himself when he exercises a paralyzed arm with his unaffected extremity. Passive exercise is necessary to maintain the full range of motion in each joint. Passive exercise prevents adaptive shortening of muscles, prevents joint contractures, and aids in circulation. Passive exercise preserves the essential function of mobility in the joints. Nonetheless, it is important for the nurse to remember that passive exercise will not prevent muscle atrophy nor will it preserve muscle tone or strengthen muscles. In performing passive motion there are a few basic techniques of which the nurse should be aware: (1) Avoid handling the muscle at the muscle belly; rather, support the joints above and below the joint being moved by either cupping or cradling the extremity. (2) Move the uninvolved extremity (as in the hemiplegic patient) before moving the involved extremity. This technique will give some indication of the patient's normal range of motion. (3) Motion should never go beyond the point of pain, unless there is specific direction for this. (4) In moving the extremities of the patient with flaccid paralysis, care should be taken to avoid stretching the flaccid muscle and damaging the muscle and disrupting the joint. (5) In moving the extremities of the patient with spastic paralysis, care should be taken not to move the extremity too quickly and thereby prevent the initiation of a clonus reaction. If the muscle becomes spastic and rigid, returning to the starting point or waiting until the spasm subsides will result in a greater degree of movement.

Active Exercise

Active exercise is exercise or motion accomplished by contraction of the muscle. The patient accomplishes the motion without the assistance of the nurse, or other personal or mechanical means. Active exercise preserves normal muscle function and strength and normal joint function. It contributes greatly to the prevention of disuse atrophy and should be encouraged to the fullest possible extent.

Active-Assistive Exercise

Active-assistive exercises are exercises in which the patient carries out motions to his fullest capabilities and then is assisted to complete them. Again, assistance may be in the form of personal or mechanical assistance. They allow the patient to perform up to the limits of his capabilities and at the same time ensure that full range of motion will be accomplished. They encourage maintenance and restoration of normal function. The nurse must remember to assist the patient only when he is no longer capable of moving or exercising without assistance.

Resistive Exercise

In *resistive exercises*, the patient accomplishes active motion against resistance. The resistance may be manual as in exerting pressure against the motion, or it may be mechanical as by adding weight. Resistive exercises increase muscle strength. They are not usually considered independent therapeutic nursing measures, but may be done under the direction of the physician or the therapist. They are indicated when there is a need to increase the strength and function of specific muscles or groups of muscles.

Static or Setting Exercise

In *setting exercises*, the muscle is contracted but no motion takes place. The muscles are tightened, held for a short period, and then relaxed. The procedure is repeated several times. Setting exercises help to prevent muscle atrophy and maintain muscle strength when movement is not possible. For example, the patient with a long leg cast may practice quadriceps setting exercises under his cast. Gluteal and abdominal setting exercises are frequently done, as are triceps and biceps setting exercises. Unless contraindicated (as discussed under range of motion exercises), the establishment of setting exercises can usually be considered an independent nursing measure. The concept of setting exercises is sometimes difficult for the patient to comprehend. Having him think about the muscles involved sometimes helps him to perform the exercises. Suggestions such as "tighten your muscle" or "pinch your muscle under my hand" while the nurse touches the specific muscle, and "push against my hand" and "hold your muscle tight" may help the patient to understand what is expected.

Range of Motion Exercise

Range of motion exercises are instituted to provide full range of motion to each joint in the body. Their purpose is to preserve full range of motion of each joint. They prevent contractural deformities of the joints and adaptive shortening of the muscles, maintain muscle tone, and enhance venous and lymphatic flow.

Range of motion to unaffected parts and parts not directly involved with the site of pathology can be considered as an independent nursing measure. However, range of joint motion to parts directly affected by pathology would not be considered an independent nursing function, but should be instituted only under the guidance of the physician. In the patient with a cerebrovascular accident, the nurse should institute range of motion to both his nonaffected side and his affected side. Although paralysis certainly is the result of pathology, the site of pathology is the brain, therefore the nurse can institute range of joint motion to the patient's affected side as an independent therapeutic nursing measure. The nurse usually should not decide independently to perform range of motion for a patient with a fractured

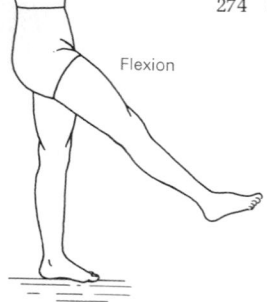

Figure 14-1

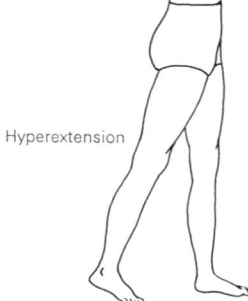

Figure 14-2

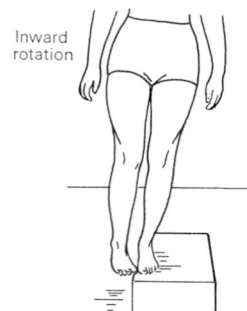

Figure 14-3

Figure 14-4

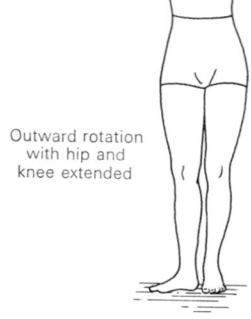

hip, or one with a radical mastectomy, until she has received permission from the physician, because these are sites of direct pathology and/or surgical intervention. Common instances when it is best for the nurse to collaborate with the physician before instituting range of motion include the presence of swelling, inflammation, pain, new tissue formation as in surgery or burns, and complicating disturbances such as respiratory and cardiac involvement. When the nurse believes the patient is ready for range of motion exercises, she has a responsibility to discuss with the physician the advisability of instituting such measures as soon as feasible. Criteria she may use in determining the patient's readiness for exercises include (1) reduction in complicating circumstances of a respiratory or cardiac nature; (2) reduction in swelling, inflammation, and pain; and/or (3) healing that has progressed to the point where exercise will no longer disrupt surgical incisions, callus formation, and healing of burns.

Before instituting range of motion exercises the nurse must consider the normal movements of each joint and the attached muscles. Joint movements are defined as follows:

flexion	Movement to decrease the angle of a joint
extension	Movement to increase the angle of a joint
hyperextension	Extension beyond the ordinary range
rotation	Movement of a part around its axis
inward rotation	Turning inward toward the center
outward rotation	Turning outward away from the center
circumduction	The distal part of a limb moving in a circle, the proximal end fixed
abduction	Movement away from the midline of the body
adduction	Movement toward the midline of the body
pronation	Turning downward
supination	Turning upward

Movements of the hip, most of which are accompanied by movements of the pelvis, are flexion, extension, hyperextension, inward rotation, outward rotation, circumduction, abduction, and adduction. See Figures 14-1 to 14-5.

Movements of the shoulder are flexion toward and above the shoulder level, extension and hyperextension, abduction to and above shoulder level, adduction, inward and outward rotation, and circumduction. See Figures 14-6 to 14-13.

Movements of the knee and elbow are flexion and extension. See Figures 14-14 and 14-15.

Movements of the forearm are supination and pronation. See Figure 14-16.

Movements of the ankle are dorsal flexion and plantar flexion. See Figure 14-17.

Movements of the foot are eversion (pronation) and inversion (supination). See Figure 14-18.

Movements of the toes are adduction and abduction, flexion, and extension. See Figures 14-19 and 14-20.

Movements of the wrist are flexion, extension and hyperextension, and radial flexion (abduction) and ulnar flexion (adduction). See Figures 14-21 and 14-22.

Figures 14-1 through 14-31 were suggested by illustrations from Margaret Winters: *Protective Body Mechanics in Daily Life and in Nursing*, and are used by permission of W. B. Saunders Company, Philadelphia.

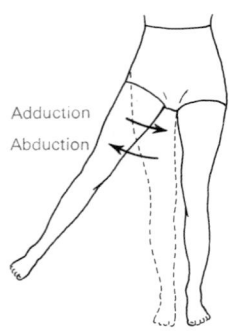

Figure 14–5

Movements of the fingers are flexion, extension, abduction, and adduction. See Figures 14-23 and 14-24. Movements of the thumb are abduction, adduction, opposition of thumb to fifth finger, flexion, and extension. See Figures 14-25 and 14-26.

Movements of the cervical spine are flexion, extension, hyperextension, lateral flexion, and rotation. See Fgures 14-27 to 14-30.

Movements of the trunk are flexion, extension, hyperextension, lateral flexion, and rotation. See Figures 14-31 to 14-34.

Range of motion exercises may be accomplished passively, actively, or by means of active-assistive exercise. If the patient remains in bed for a week or longer, activities and exercises for joint movement should be instituted. The patient should perform the exercises himself to the degree that he is able. Exercise of some of the joints can be accomplished through daily activities such as brushing the teeth, combing the hair, feeding oneself, bathing oneself, getting on and off the bedpan while in back-lying position (by flexing the knees, placing the feet on the mattress, and lifting the hips while pushing the feet on the mattress). In such cases it may be necessary only to provide the opportunity to perform the activities, and specific exercises may not be required. When specific exercises are carried out, each should be done three to five times for two or three times a day.

When passive exercise is given, the body part is held at the joint with firm easy pressure, and slow smooth movements are made to move the joint through

Figure 14–6

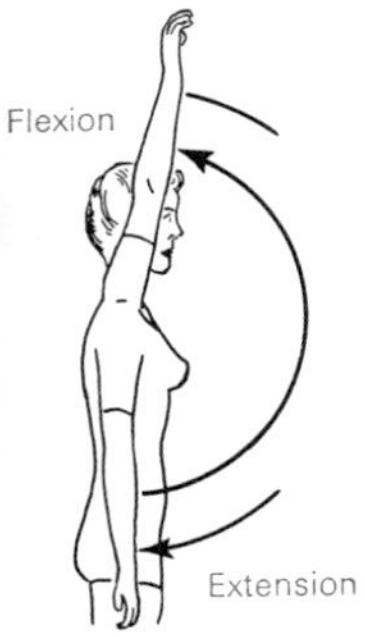

Figure 14–7

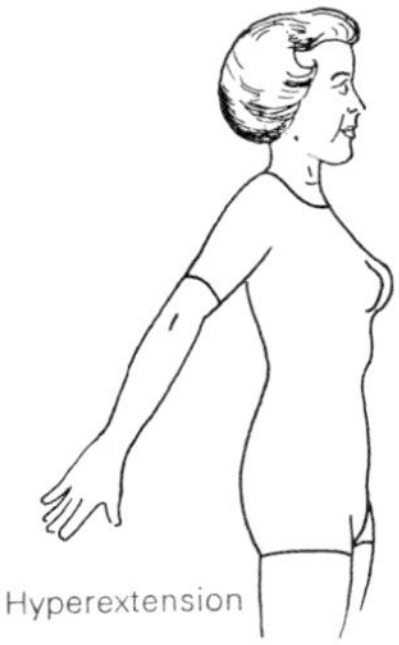

Figure 14–8

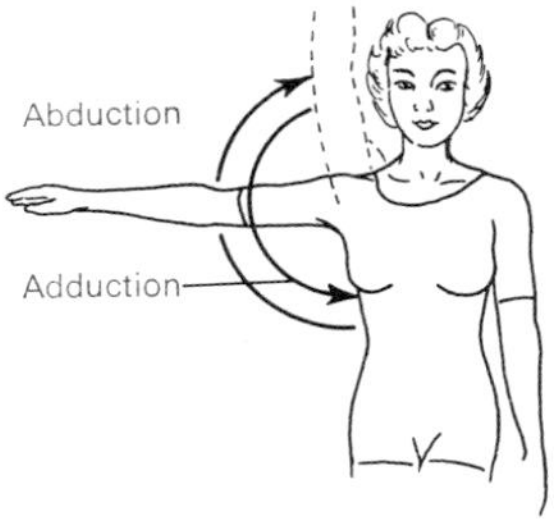

Figure 14–9

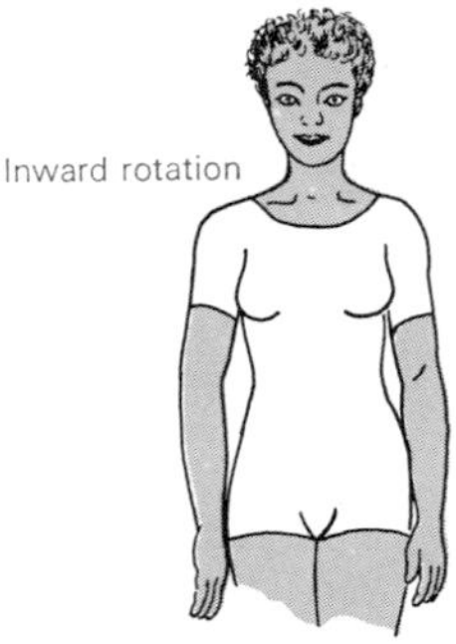

Figure 14–10

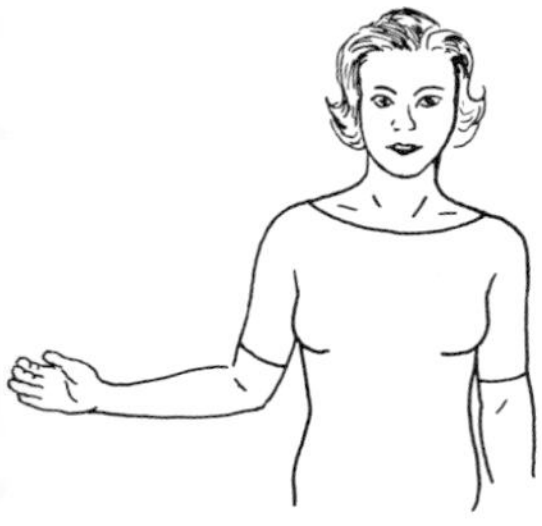

Outward rotation of shoulder joint with shoulder adducted and elbow flexed

Figure 14–11

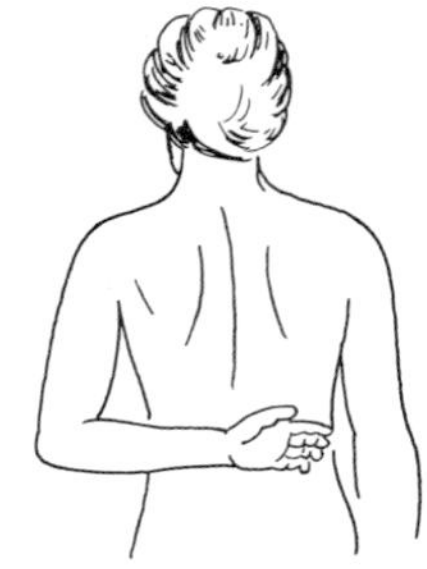

Inward rotation (left) with humerus in slight abduction and hyperextension, elbow flexed

Figure 14–12

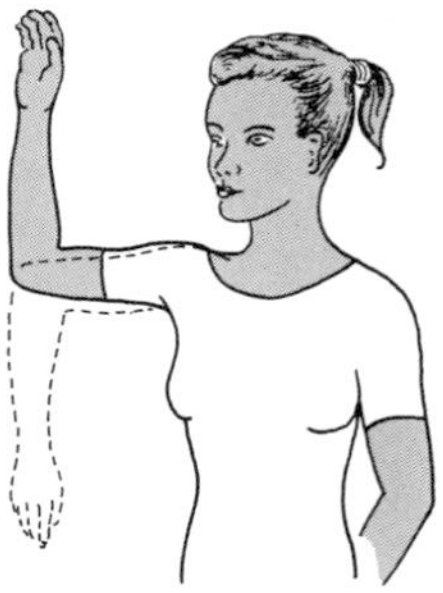

Outward rotation of shoulder joint with arm abducted to shoulder level, elbow flexed

Figure 14–13

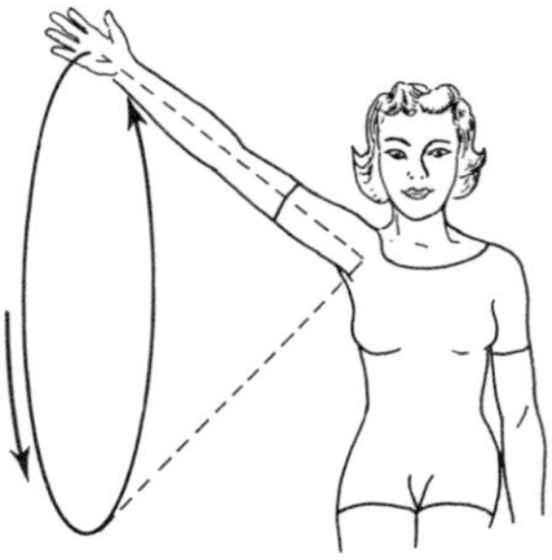

Circumduction

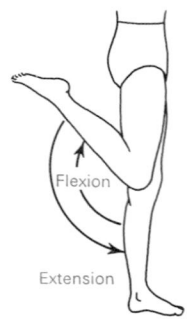

Figure 14–14

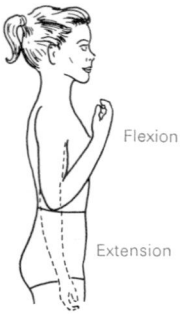

Figure 14–15

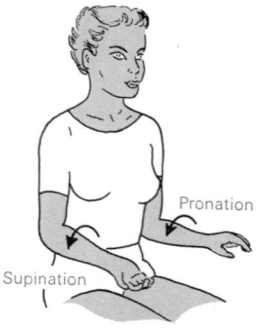

Figure 14–16

Figure 14–17

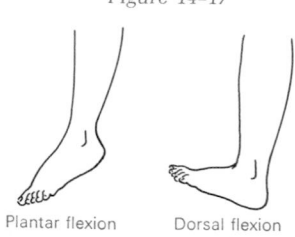

the *patient's* full range of motion, which is the *pain-free* range of movement. When pain occurs the movement of the joint is beyond the patient's range of motion and the exercise becomes a stretching exercise which is therapeutic in nature and requires a prescription from the physician. While passive exercise is given, the patient can be taught each exercise and its purpose so that he can perform the exercises himself as early as possible.

Suggested exercises for each body part follow.

SHOULDER

Shoulder exercises should be carried out without use of a pillow under the head.

1. Raise one arm (or both) upward over the head (elbow straight) as far as possible.

2. Move one arm (or both) sideways, with elbow straight, as far as possible, then move the arm slowly toward the head, moving the elbow as close to the head as possible.

3. Hang the arm over the side of the bed and move it in a circular motion.

4. Move arm sideways and then move arm slowly across the chest, and with elbow slightly flexed move hand and arm to or beyond the opposite shoulder.

FOREARM AND ELBOW

1. Starting with arm flat on the bed, flex the elbow and touch the shoulder with the fingers. Supinate the forearm by turning the palm of the hand toward the face as the hand comes toward the shoulder; pronate the forearm by turning the palm of the hand toward the feet as the elbow is extended in returning to the starting position.

WRIST

1. Bend wrist down and return to neutral position.
2. Bend wrist up and return to neutral position.
3. Move wrist toward ulnar side.
4. Move wrist toward radial side.

FINGERS

1. Make a fist, with thumb out, then straighten hand.
2. Extend the fingers and thumb so that a "fan" is formed, then bring the fingers and thumb together.
3. With fingers straight, bend the thumb into the palm of the hand, move the thumb back so that it points away from the hand, and move the thumb in a circle.
4. Touch the tip of each finger with the thumb.

HIP AND KNEE

1. Start with leg extended, bend (flex) knee and move knee toward the chest, pointing toes upward; when the knee is as close to the chest as possible straighten (extend) the knee and return to starting position.

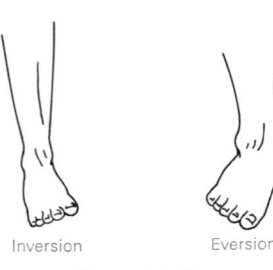

Inversion   Eversion

Figure 14–18

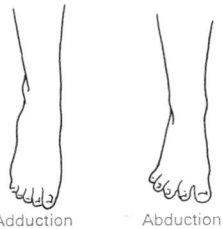

Adduction   Abduction

Figure 14–19

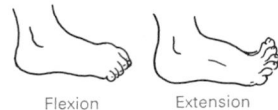

Flexion   Extension

Figure 14–20

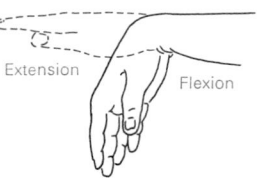

Extension   Flexion

Figure 14–21

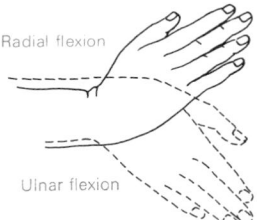

Radial flexion

Ulnar flexion

Figure 14–22

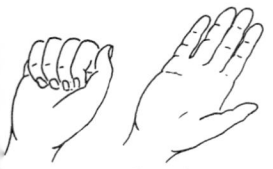

Flexion   Extension

Figure 14–23

Figure 14–24

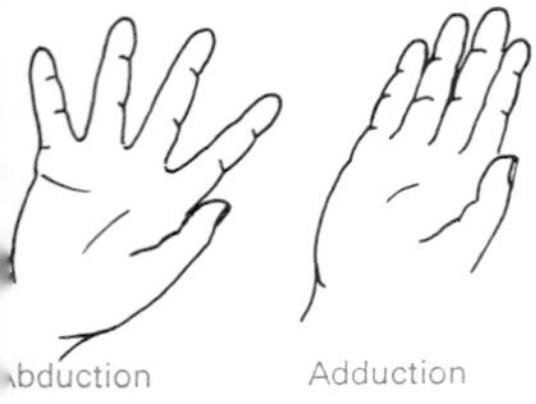

Abduction   Adduction

2. With knee and ankle straight, roll leg in and roll leg out, or turn both legs inward until toes touch and turn both legs outward until heels touch.

3. With knee and ankle straight and toes pointed up, move leg outward toward the side of the bed (foot toward the corner of the bed) and then move the leg toward the other side of the bed, over the other leg.

ANKLE

1. Move foot in a circular motion, clockwise and counterclockwise, starting with foot pointed downward, circle to the side, circle to point foot upward, and circle to the side.

TOES

1. Bend the toes up and down.

EXERCISE AS PART OF NURSING CARE

When the nurse performs passive or active-assistive exercises, they can be combined with other nursing care such as during the bath, with evening care, or while changing the patient's position. Several exercises can be accomplished during the bath. While washing the patient's face, ears, and neck, turning the head from side to side provides rotation, and moving the head back and forth (chin to chest) provides flexion, extension, and hyperextension of the neck. When bathing the axilla, outward (external) rotation and abduction of the shoulder and elbow flexion can be accomplished, and while bathing the undersurface of the arm, shoulder flexion and elbow extension can be performed. If the patient's forearm is brought across his abdomen, inward (internal) rotation of the shoulder takes place, and while bathing the forearm, pronation and supination can be accomplished. In bathing the hand (or when the patient holds and uses the washcloth) wrist flexion and extension, finger flexion, extension, abduction, and adduction and all the movements of the thumb can be performed. Moving the leg out from the body, as while draping the patient, provides abduction of the hip. Turning the leg inward while washing and drying provides inward rotation of the hip, and the hip can be placed in outward rotation for washing and drying the inner surface of the leg. When placing the foot in the bath basin, knee and hip flexion and extension are accomplished. In bathing the foot, dorsal flexion and plantar flexion of the ankle and flexion, extension, adduction, and abduction of the toes can be performed.

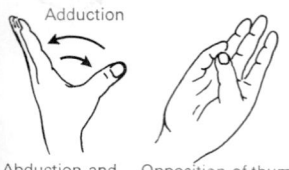

Adduction

Abduction and adduction   Opposition of thumb to little finger

Figure 14–25

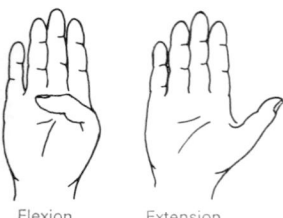

Flexion   Extension

Figure 14–26

Movement

Movement is essential to full participation in daily activities. The importance of normal body position and normal muscle strength has been discussed. Their normal function is prerequisite to normal movement. Further, the ability to move depends in large measure on the intact functioning of the neuromusculoskeletal system. Efficiency in movement will be reduced when there is interference in any of the structures necessary for motion. Motion in the human body is largely accomplished by the integrated functions of the nerves, muscles, bones, and joints. These act together to perform both single and multiple motions, which are accomplished largely through a system of levers. By recognizing the importance of the leverage system in motion, the nurse and the patient can achieve the maximum potential for movement even when there may be some disruption in the normal mechanisms and structures of movement.

Postural deformities reduce the efficiency of the leverage system, thus making it more difficult for even normal muscles to work. Hence the maintenance of normal posture assumes importance if normal ability to move is to be maintained. Likewise, loss of muscle tone and strength will result in diminished effectiveness for movement. Hence the maintenance of normal muscle strength also assumes importance if normal ability to move is to be maintained.

If the above requisites are met, most patients who have experienced no direct pathology to the neuromusculoskeletal system will recover with little or no impairment in their ability to move. However, other patients will experience limitation of motion for a number of reasons. Movement is usually associated with the ability to ambulate, yet many patients who may be unable to walk will be able to accomplish some degree of independent movement, and this should be encouraged within the limits of their capabilities. In order to encourage this, the nurse will have to expand her concept of mobility.

Seriously impaired patients may be able to achieve independence only in moving and turning in bed. Such activity should be encouraged because it helps to prevent disuse problems and contributes to the patient's self-esteem.

Less seriously impaired persons may not be able to move normally, yet are able to get from one place to another. Some patients are able to move independently from bed to wheel chair. The essential value of ambulation is the ability to get

Figure 14–27

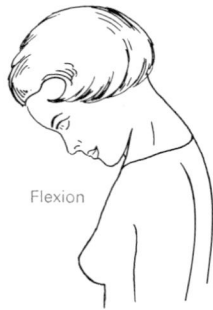

Flexion

Figure 14–28

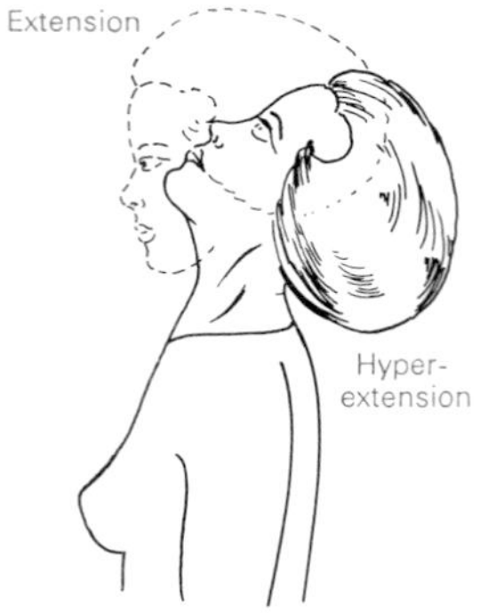

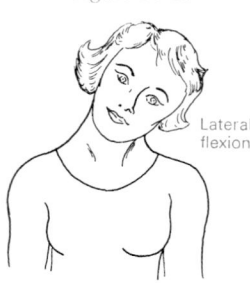

Extension

Hyper-extension

Figure 14–29

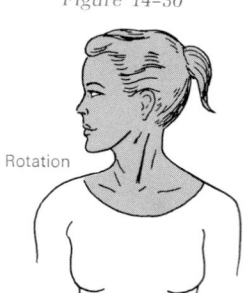

Lateral flexion

Figure 14–30

Rotation

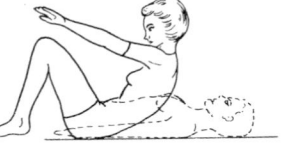

Flexion of the spine*

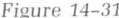

* The hips are flexed to rule out the action of the hip flexor muscles

Figure 14–31

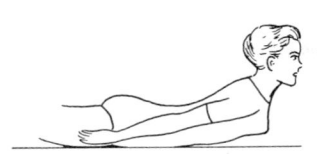

Hyperextension of the spine

Figure 14–32

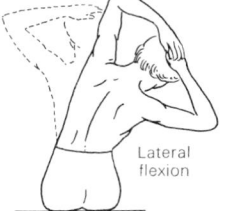

Lateral flexion

Figure 14–33

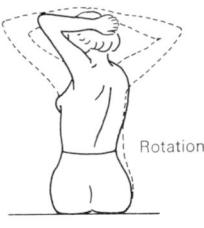

Rotation

Figure 14–34

from one place to another. If the patient can do this through another means of locomotion, then the essential value of mobility is maintained. The use of wheel chairs, walkers, crutches, and canes, although inconvenient and at times limiting, does allow the patient independence in locomotion.

Patients who have experienced paralysis, spasticity, weakness, excessive movement (such as the cerebral palsied), and gait disturbance comprise a significant segment of the population whose normal means of locomotion has changed. The nurse who can help the patient adjust to a new level or means of mobility will greatly increase his ability to participate more fully in normal activities.

Bibliography

Beland, Irene L: *Clinical Nursing: Pathophysiological and Psychosocial Approaches.* New York: The Macmillan Company, 1965.

Broer, Marion R: *Efficiency of Human Movement.* Philadelphia: W. B. Saunders Company, 1966.

Brunner, Lillian Sholtis, et al.: *Textbook of Medical-Surgical Nursing.* Philadelphia: J. B. Lippincott Company, 1964.

Buchwald, Edith: *Physical Rehabilitation for Daily Living.* New York: McGraw-Hill Book Company, 1952.

Cooper, John M. and Ruth B. Glassow: *Kinesiology.* St. Louis: The C. V. Mosby Company, 1963.

deGutierrez-Mahoney, C. G. and Esta Carini: *Neurological and Neurosurgical Nursing.* St. Louis: The C. V. Mosby Company, 1960.

Fash, Bernice: *Body Mechanics in Nursing Arts.* New York: McGraw-Hill Book Company, 1946.

Forster, Francis M: *Synopsis of Neurology.* St. Louis: The C. V. Mosby Company, 1966.

Fuerst, Elinor V. and LuVerne Wolff: *Fundamentals of Nursing.* Philadelphia: J. B. Lippincott Company, 1964.

Greisheimer, Esther M: *Physiology and Anatomy.* Philadelphia: J. B. Lippincott Company, 1955.

Guyton, Arthur C: *Textbook of Medical Physiology,* 2d ed. Philadelphia: W. B. Saunders Company, 1961.

Hirschberg, Gerald G., Leon Lewis, and Dorothy Thomas: *Rehabilitation.* Philadelphia: J. B. Lippincott Company, 1964.

Kimber, Diana Clifford, et al.: *Anatomy and Physiology.* New York: The Macmillan Company, 1966.

Karpavich, Peter V.: *Physiology of Muscular Activity.* Philadelphia: W. B. Saunders Company, 1965.

Myers, Julian S: *An Orientation to*

Chronic Disease and Disability. New York: The Macmillan Company, 1965.

Newton, Kathleen and Helen C. Anderson: *Geriatric Nursing.* St. Louis: C. V. Mosby Company, 1966.

Rehabilitative Aspects of Nursing. National League for Nursing. New York, 1966.

Rusk, Howard A: *Rehabilitation Medicine.* St. Louis: The C.V. Mosby Company, 1958.

Shafer, Kathleen Newton, et al.: *Medical-Surgical Nursing.* St. Louis: The C. V. Mosby Company, 1961.

Sodeman, William A.: *Pathologic Physiology.* Philadelphia: W. B. Saunders Company, 1961.

Winters, Margaret Campbell: *Protective Body Mechanics in Daily Life and in Nursing.* Philadelphia: W. B. Saunders Company, 1952.

Wyburn, G. M: *The Nervous System.* New York: Academic Press, 1960.

CHAPTER 15
ABNORMAL SENSATIONS

SISTER M. AGNITA CLAIRE DAY

Man receives information concerning objects in the external world by means of sensory receptors that transmit impulses to the sensory cortex via the thalamus and give rise to a number of primary sensations, such as light, sound, touch, pressure, pain, temperature, and kinesthetic sensations. From the primary sensations the higher parts of the nervous system organize sensations into perceptions of recognizable objects. These are more complex integrations. There is considerable evidence that even so-called simple sensations are not conscious appreciation of a single sensory excitation, but are modified by the central nervous system control of sensory inputs. If pathological conditions affect the receptors, the afferent nerves, the pathways in the spinal cord, the brain stem, the thalamus, or the sensory cortex, sensory impulses are either blocked or so modified that normal perception is altered, giving rise to unpleasant or unusual sensations.

Because unusual sensations are largely subjective in nature and, in general, are identified because of the patient's awareness of his own state, it may be somewhat difficult for the nurse to evaluate their true significance. Such sensations may have a profound meaning for the patient and a marked effect on his behavior, even though there may be very little other objective evidence of their presence. On the other hand, symptoms such as severe pain may produce observable physiological signs—at times so acute that they should be considered potential danger signals. For these the nurse must be constantly on the alert. No matter how bizarre the symptoms may seem, it is well to remember that in the majority of instances there is an organic explanation for them, very often related to the integrity of the nervous system. Even if the case should be a psychogenic one, as occasionally happens, the patient still *has* the symptoms and may need even more support to cope with them than the person who has a known organic lesion. A certain relief is experienced in just knowing that there is a physical cause for the symptoms.

Considerable information about the patient's problems and behavior can be obtained from his family and friends by the use of a few judicious questions. The content of these observations may be invaluable in giving support to a plan of nursing care or in altering it to meet specific needs. Other important sources of data include the physician's history and physical examination (from which at least a tentative medical diagnosis can be obtained) and his initial and subsequent orders for treatment, reports of laboratory tests, roentgenograms, and other special procedures. Perhaps most important of all in making reliable judgments about the patient's condition is the nurse's own ability to be an empathic listener and an accurate observer, so that she may sift and analyze the information thus obtained to fit it into a unified pattern. From this pattern, the plan of nursing care can be derived, tailored to fit the individual patient.

Pain

One of the more common yet one of the most difficult symptoms with which the nurse must deal is that of pain. The majority of persons face pain with fear and dread and are affected in many ways by its occurrence. The more thorough understanding the nurse has of its nature, its significance to the patient, and her own psychological reactions to the specific situation in which it occurs, the greater the support and assurance she is able to give the patient and the better does she appreciate her own role in the management of pain.

DEFINITION OF PAIN

Pain might be defined as a disagreeable sensation produced by the action of stimuli of a harmful nature. The pain perception may be (and usually is) accompanied by a feeling or emotional state as well as by reactions of a physical nature.

DUAL ASPECTS OF PAIN
(PAIN PERCEPTION VS. PAIN REACTION)

In considering pain, it is most necessary to distinguish between pain sensation or perception and pain reaction. These are actually two different entities. The ultimate perception of pain depends more upon its interpretation in the cerebral cortex than upon the characteristics of the original stimulus. The pain reaction, on the other hand, may be more severe than the actual perception would seem to warrant, because of the many associations and meanings the pain experience may have for the patient.

Such information as the location and intensity of pain, its quality, the time of its occurrence, and other significant concomitant findings help differentiate its possible causes. Accurate evaluation of its character and significance is essential to proper treatment and nursing care. While most types of pain are physical in origin, two types of psychogenic pain may occur: (1) the conversion pain of hysteria, and (2) functional pain resulting from emotional disorders.

THE ANATOMY AND PHYSIOLOGY OF PAIN

End-Organs

The receptor endings are said to be fine, branching nerve endings belonging to the delta group of A fibers and the small C fibers, which form plexuses within the skin. There is a rich distribution of these plexuses over the body surface, but relatively fewer pain fibers exist in the deep somatic structures and viscera; there are none in the parenchyma of the central nervous system or lungs, which are insensitive to pain.

Sensory Units

The sensory units consist of many fine branching endings, all ramifications of a single sensory fiber connected with a cell body in the dorsal root ganglion. The distribution of each cutaneous unit covers an area of approximately 1 sq cm, but there is considerable overlapping of units in any given area.

Nerves Conducting Pain Impulses

Impulses travel along peripheral nerves to nerve plexuses, to dorsal root ganglia, to posterior roots of the spinal nerves, and to the lateral filaments of the spinal cord. Impulses for touch and pressure travel over similar routes, except that they travel in the medial filaments of the spinal cord. Pain may be superficial or deep. Some of the deep pain impulses are carried by pain fibers attached to the blood vessels, which then join an adjacent autonomic nerve to enter the dorsal root.

Central Pathways

The afferent fibers that mediate temperature, pain, and probably itching enter Lissauer's tract (the dorsolateral fasciculus), which lies between the tip of the dorsal column and the surface of the cord, and split immediately to form ascending and descending branches that run for one or at most two or three segments before terminating on sensory posterior horn cells or forming reflex connections in the gray matter of the cord. The descending branches seem to be primarily for reflex connections. The ascending fibers also send collaterals to cells in the spinal gray matter to make reflex connections. Over these reflex arcs the input on the pain fibers may cause reflex muscle spasm and vasoconstriction in the area from which the pain sensation has originated. The secondary sensory neurons arise in the posterior horn, cross by way of the anterior commissure, and ascend in the *lateral spinothalamic tract* to the posterolateral ventral nucleus of the thalamus.

The afferent fibers that mediate coarse touch and pressure are somewhat larger than those for pain and temperature. They enter the cord in the medial part of the root and bifurcate in the dorsal funiculus. The descending branches make reflex connections. The ascending branches may extend several segments from their level of entry before ending on cells in the nucleus proprius of the dorsal horn. Secondary neurons pass to the opposite side of the cord to the *ventral spinothalamic tract.* These two pathways come together in the medulla and ascend together in the spinal lemniscus to the thalamus.

From the thalamus tertiary neurons run to the cortex. Their chief terminal is the sensory cortex, although some fibers go to the precentral gyrus and other widely scattered gyri. Pain and crude touch can be experienced in the thalamus, even though the cortical centers are damaged, but the cortex is necessary for fine discrimination, accurate localization, and interpretation of stimuli.

Collaterals are also given off from the spinothalamic pathways to the reticular

*Figure 15–1
A, Diagram of dorsal root fibers for pain and temperature conduction and reflex connections. B, Diagram of ipsilateral pain conduction. DSC, dorsal spinocerebellar tract; FC, fasciculus cuneatus; FG, fasciculus gracilis; LST, lateral spinothalamic tract; SMF, somatic motor fiber; VMF, visceral motor fiber; VSC, ventral spinocerebellar tract; VST, ventral spinothalamic tract. (Redrawn from T. L. Peele: The Neuroanatomic Basis for Clinical Neurology. New York: McGraw-Hill Book Company, 1962.)*

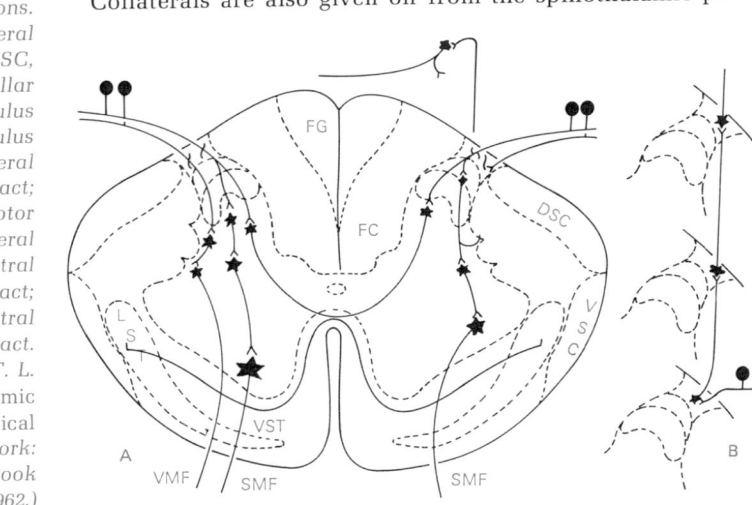

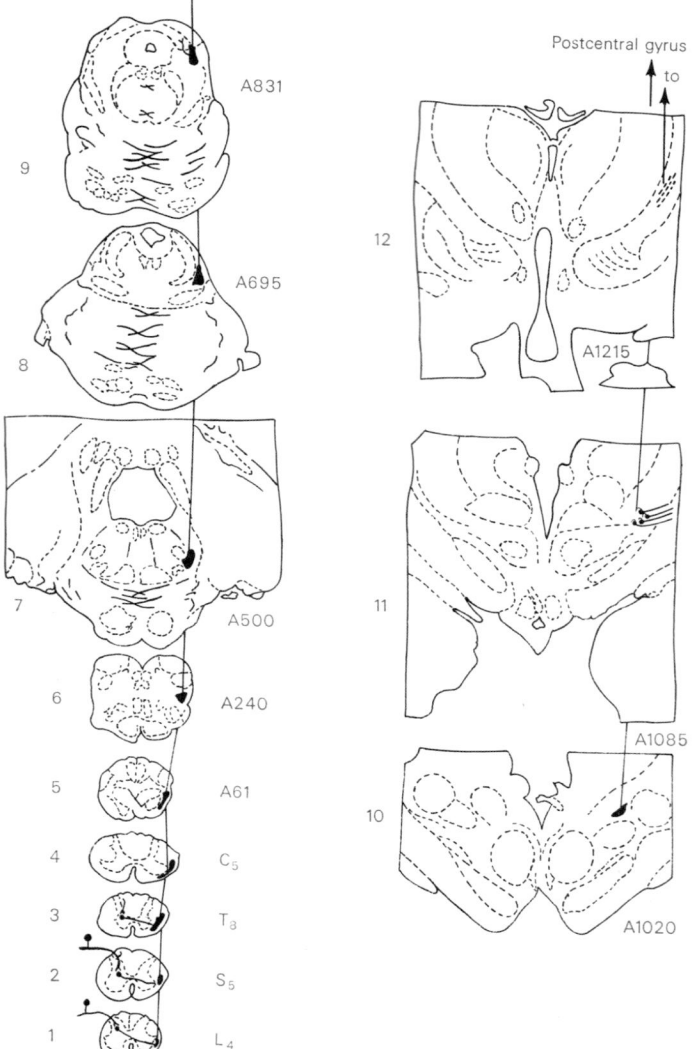

Figure 15–2 Diagram of the spinothalamic and spinotectal tracts. Impulses traversing these paths traverse one to three or more spinal segments on the side of entry before crossing. This is illustrated in the small figures 1, 2, and 3. The serial numbers, such as A1020, refer to the sections of a human brain stem series. (Redrawn from T. L. Peele: The Neuroanatomic Basis for Clinical Neurology. New York: McGraw-Hill Book Company, 1962.)

formation throughout the brain stem and possibly in the spinal cord which are transmitted to primitive nuclei in the thalamus and thence via the corona radiata to the cortex of the parietal and frontal lobes. It is thought that this system serves to alert the mind to the general situation rather than to contribute sensory data.

Effective Stimuli

Effective stimuli can be mechanical, thermal, electrical, or chemical in character. Evidence available at present indicates that tissue tension or chemical irritants, or both, comprise an adequate stimulus to initiate nerve impulses of pain. Pain is a warning that tissue damage is in progress and is an indication of the rate of tissue damage rather than an indication of potential or existing injury to the tissues or the seriousness of the damage.

Injury to the tissues may release or cause to be formed several pain-producing agents. If present in high enough concentrations, these substances may cause pain by direct stimulation of nerve endings. If present in lower concentrations they may sensitize nerve endings to produce *primary hyperalgesia*, that is, increased sensitiveness to pain. Present evidence suggests that histamine, serotonin, and certain plasma pain-producing substances may act singly or in combination to produce this effect chemically. The intensity of the stimulus and the intensity of the pain are correlated.

Pain Threshold

The threshold of pain is not far from the intensity causing tissue damage, and some authors and researchers believe that they are one and the same thing, that the appearance of pain indicates the beginning of damage to the fiber endings. The stimulus of radiant heat applied to the skin is a convenient and easily controlled method of experimentally measuring pain thresholds. In many such studies the threshold of pain perception has been demonstrated to be remarkably constant in large numbers of people. If, however, the subjects of these tests were unable to focus their attention on the test because of fatigue, lethargy, defects in ability to concentrate, suggestibility, or prejudice, the pain threshold varied widely and unpredictably. The threshold was not only not constant from man to man, but was not constant in the same person at different periods of time, probably because the experience and value judgment of the individual entered unavoidably into the experimental situation.

Pain Perception

The thalamus is important in the integration of pain. Although there is an awareness of pain at the thalamic level, the sensory cortex is essential for distinction of the point of origin of the stimulus and the quality, degree, and extension of the pain. Increasing the intensity of the stimulus results in perception of increasing degrees of pain, but the spreading of noxious stimuli over a larger area apparently does not increase the intensity of the resulting pain. Both the extension and the duration of the pain stimuli are important, however, in determining the overall reaction to pain.

Descriptive words that express the quality, intensity, and duration of pain include the following:

1. Quality: burning, pricking, aching, or various combinations of these qualities.
2. Intensity: expressed in dols; ranges from 0 to 10½ for pricking pain or aching pain. The scale for burning pain has not been defined.
3. Extension: localization on the body, that is, the "size and shape" of the pain. Deep pain seems to be three-dimensional or space-occupying, superficial pain to seem more like a point along a line.
4. Duration: includes all temporal aspects of pain such as cramping, lightning, throbbing, and pulsating, plus the time of onset and duration.

Factors That Tend to Influence Pain Perception

No matter what the site of origin, certain factors tend to influence a person's psychological response to pain and thus to influence his perception of it.

Integrity of the nervous system is essential, for end-organs, conductive pathways, and perceptive centers must be intact for pain to be experienced. One's *state of consciousness* is also a determining factor, and the numerous stages of consciousness range from deep coma on the one hand to intense alertness on the other. The meaning or interpretation of any sensory stimulus, such as pain, depends to a great extent upon the person's position in the spectrum of consciousness at the time the stimulus occurs. The *total pain load* is also significant, for the pain experience is intensified when the messages reach the perceptive centers over many pathways. More profound reactions can be expected with greater intensity of pain.

The person's *past and present experiences* have a symbolic significance that may modify the pain experience, either enhancing it or negating it as something important to him. *Training* in meeting pain can be very influential in the patient's total reaction. Persons who because of ethnic group, education, or previous environment have been taught that pain is to be accepted without a show of emotion are less apt to exhibit weeping, crying out, or "fight or flight" reactions; those not so trained may show violent reactions. This point is extremely important for the nurse to remember in dealing with patients in pain. The person who shows the least external evidence may actually be experiencing the most intense pain, and the nurse must learn to judge by his physiological reactions the actual extent of the pain stimulus.

Conditioning through previous experience with pain may either increase or decrease a person's reaction to pain. Intense fear of a pain-producing situation and anticipation of its repetition can cause profound emotional reactions accompanied by vomiting, syncope, and similar symptoms. On the other hand, repeated experience with pain may develop fortitude or resignation with progressive decrease in the patient's psychological and emotional response. Knowledge and understanding of the *origin* and *significance* of pain can do much to alleviate the severity of a psychological reaction. Uncertainty or fear merely exaggerates responses. This, too, is a point that the nurse should remember in her reassurance of the patient. One can face a known situation, even an extremely difficult one, much more readily than one can face the unknown.

Attention and *distraction* exert a profound influence in modifying reactions to pain. One's awareness of pain is greatly decreased by distraction and greatly increased by focusing one's attention on it. All persons have frequent experiences attesting to the significance of this phenomenon. *Fatigue* can change the reaction to pain in various ways. Weariness and exhaustion may be so great that attention wanders from an injury. On the other hand, fatigue may sometimes so vitiate a person's powers of resistance and self-control that even minor discomfort precipitates profound psychological reactions, such as crying out, weeping, and attempting flight or withdrawal.

Anxiety, tension, and *fear* increase the suffering experienced by the person who has pain. Likewise, measures to relieve anxiety can dissociate pain from the response to it. In other words, pain is still perceived, but the suffering induced by it is reduced or even abolished.

Pain associated with pleasureable emotion may cease to be recognized as pain. "Natural childbirth" is partially based on this principle. *Religious or hysterical mental states* may cause considerable dissociation of pain perception from the reaction to pain. *Suggestion,* however, has not been demonstrated to alter reactions to pain in experimental studies on both normal and psychoneurotic patients as had been expected. *Hypnosis* is sometimes effective, but must be used with caution.

One of the most important factors influencing the pain reaction is the *significance of pain to the affected person.* Transitory pain is usually soon forgotten, but chronic or long-continued pain may affect the personality of the person who experiences it. MacBryde stresses the following patterns of reaction. The affected person may become (1) resigned, patient, with a brave "carry on" attitude; (2) resigned, but depressed, with resultant withdrawal, a "give-up" attitude and even suicidal tendencies; (3) stoic, indifferent to his own pain and consequently often indifferent to that of others; (4) vindictive, revengeful, wanting to strike back. Cruelty to self and to others may become manifestations of this reaction.

TYPES OF PAIN
Superficial Pain

Two types of cutaneous pain have been described by a number of investigators: (1) pain with abrupt onset and a sharp, pricking quality, and (2) pain with a slower onset and a burning quality. It has been postulated that the first type is carried by the large myelinated fibers conducting at rates between 10 and 90 M per second, while the second is caused by stimulation of the small C fibers with conducting rates of 0.5 to 2 M per second. These two types of pain can be dissociated to some extent and can occur separately. It has been demonstrated experimentally that the C fibers are the last to be blocked by asphyxia, but the first to be blocked by cocaine, that is, cocaine applied topically blocks the slow pain component first. Morphine is more effective against continuous dull pain than sharp intermittent pain, although its effect is central in its action.

Superficial pain, sometimes called *direct pain,* can be localized accurately to the point of disturbance. It may be associated with hyperalgesia, paresthesia, analgesia, tickling or itching, and possibly with temperature changes in the skin. All these modalities actually assist in localization of the pain because one learns to interpret the location of common cutaneous sensations.

Deep Pain

Deep pain differs from superficial pain in *quality,* in that it feels deeper and has a duller, aching nature. In *duration* it tends to persist for longer periods of time than superficial pain. *Localization* is more diffuse, usually seeming to originate in a wider area, and the site of origin is less accurately perceived. It is sometimes spoken of as three-dimensional in nature, that is, it seems to occupy space. Those structures more commonly stimulated by contacts that give rise to sensory impulses (muscles, periosteum of bones lying near the surface) can be located with reasonable accuracy.

Three kinds of deep pain are recognized: (1) true visceral or somatic pain, (2) referred pain, and (3) pain from secondary muscle contractions.

Previously it was believed that the viscera have little or no innervation with pain fibers. More recent research, however, has demonstrated sensory end-organs in the viscera which resemble those in the somatic structures but are less varied in type. Naked branching terminals are in great preponderance and are probably nociceptive in nature. When strongly or abnormally stimulated, these are thought to mediate conscious sensations of *visceral pain* and possibly of temperature. Some structures resembling the Pacinian corpuscles of the integument have been noted in certain organs and apparently respond to pressure. Sensory endings occurring in the walls of blood vessels seem to be important in the reflex control of blood flow to an organ and in mediating conscious sensations of pain from the organ. Visceral pain is peculiar in its mode of origin in that it is caused by spastic contraction of smooth muscle and not by ordinary traumatic stimuli such as cutting. Elliott states that fibers from the naked nerve endings of the viscera are small and unmyelinated and that the majority eventually join the spinal nerves via the white rami. Pain messages from regions where the segmental nerves have no white rami (that is, the esophagus above the sternal notch and the lowest pelvic viscera) travel in the vagus and pelvic nerve respectively. The visceral afferent fibers have cell bodies in the dorsal root or cranial nerve sensory ganglia like the somatic afferents. Some fibers end on somatic motor neurons to contribute to reflexes such as coughing or vomiting; others end on visceral motor neurons to mediate visceral reflex control; still others synapse with dorsal horn neurons that give off secondary axons to ascending sensory paths. These latter fibers mediate such conscious visceral sensations as occur. The secondary fibers seem to run chiefly in the lateral spinothalamic tract as both crossed and uncrossed components. In the brain stem many fibers apparently pass into the reticular formation. Terminals on the thalamus are similar to the somatic terminals and follow the same projections to the sensory cortex.

Pain of segmental distribution associated with segmental tenderness of the skin is due to *somatic* rather than visceral disease in a large number of cases, and may be from muscles, tendons, joints, and similar structures.

Referred pain from a visceral lesion may give the impression of pain in a somatic area, usually the skin, and sometimes far distant from the actual lesion. This is explained by what has been called the *dermatome rule,* that is, the two areas embryologically have arisen from the same segmental level. For example, the pain from angina pectoris is referred to the inner side of the left arm. Referred pain may also come from deep lesions in the joints, tendons, and muscles, as well as from the viscera, and follows the same segmental distribution. In addition to the anatomically related type of referred pain, there is also a "learned" type, in which pain may be referred to the site of some recent injury, such as a scar or a new filling in a tooth. In all these forms referred pain is clinically important and offers a clue to proper diagnosis and treatment. At least three theories concerning the mechanism of referred pain have been proposed. The so-called convergence theories seem to be the most widely accepted at present.

Figure 15–3 Mechanism of referred pain and referred hyperalgesia. (Redrawn from A. C. Guyton: Textbook of Medical Physiology, 3d ed. Philadelphia: W. B. Saunders Company, 1966.)

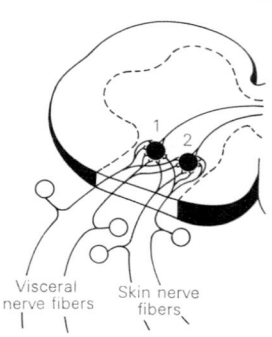

Visceral nerve fibers   Skin nerve fibers

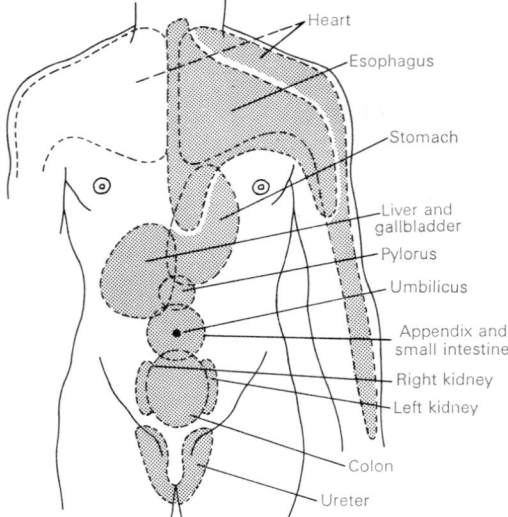

Figure 15–4
Surface areas of referred
pain from different
visceral organs. (Redrawn
from A. C. Guyton:
Textbook of Medical
Physiology, 3d ed.
Philadelphia: W. B.
Saunders Company,
1966.)

Elliott states that according to the convergence theories, alarm messages from the viscera radiate in the central nervous system not only to visceral-sensory fields (and thence to visceral reflex arcs and ascending paths) but also to nearby somato-sensory fields. What happens to the somatosensory fields has been variously interpreted: (1) According to the "convergence-facilitation" theory, the visceral messages merely lower the threshold of the somatosensory neurons; the somatosensory messages due to trivial stimuli then can easily fire these neurons. (2) According to the "convergence-projection" theory, impulses can themselves fire the somatosensory neurons without somatic reinforcement. In either case, deceptive messages pass up somatosensory ascending paths (lemnisci), to the thalamus and sensory cortex. Anatomical data support the convergence theory.

Pain from *secondary muscle contraction* is the end result of transmission of impulses over reflex arcs at the spinal level which cause muscle spasm, and therefore pain. Impulses traveling over autonomic reflex pathways may cause vasoconstriction and diaphoresis. Vasoconstriction and muscle spasm also result in ischemia of the muscle and ischemia, in turn, is probably responsible for most of the pain. These reactions may be of considerable assistance in identifying the source of the pain, but may also need specific treatment to eliminate the additional discomfort created by them.

Central Pain

Central pain is perceived by the subject when no peripheral cause exists. It may be due to organic lesions in the sensory gray matter and/or sensory tracts of the nervous system, but most frequently is due to persistence of perception after a peripheral stimulus has ceased. It frequently occurs in injury to nerve trunks as in "phantom limb" following amputation. Lesions of the thalamus or spinothalamic tracts may cause constant or frequently recurring pain that is poorly localized and may even affect one entire side of the body or an entire limb.

CLINICAL MANIFESTATIONS OF PAIN

Since pain and discomfort are subjective phenomena, the patient's reaction to them should be carefully studied in order to provide diagnostic clues and to expedite institution of proper therapy. Under certain conditions pain may be either facilitated or inhibited. Such reactions may be important as an aid to determining the severity of the pain.

Facilitated Pain

After continued or repeated stimulation, the sense-perceptive centers in the brain become hypersensitive and the habitual pain pathways respond to even slight changes in barometric pressure and possibly temperature. The cortical threshold as a whole also may be lowered as well as locally. This lowered threshold is responsible for the generalized hyperalgesia frequently found in illnesses such as malaria and influenza.

Inhibited Pain

Certain individuals seem very much less sensitive to pain than others. This can be caused by a number of factors, such as age, training, and learned emotional reactive components. The infant seldom feels pain to the same degree as the adult, who has developed greater sensitivity through learned emotional attitudes. On the other hand, habituation and exposure to a rigorous environment usually diminish pain perception. Education and protection may cause increased sensitivity. Control by will power is often effective in inhibiting pain reactions. Persons of certain ethnic groups seem to be less sensitive to pain than others. For example, Anglo-Saxon and Nordic types seem less sensitive to pain than Semites and Latins. Again, these reactions may be due to cultural and social patterns rather than to actual changes in pain thresholds. All these factors must be taken into consideration, however, in developing an understanding of a particular patient's reaction.

Severity of Pain

An estimate of the severity of the patient's pain must be based on a number of factors, including one's *general impressions* of the patient's general sensitivity (estimated on the basis of age, ethnicity, training, emotional state, and cultural patterns as mentioned above). The face can present a typical picture of pain, with pallor, furrowed forehead, drawn lips and clenched teeth, fixed eyes and dilated pupils. Pallor is probably due to reflex vasoconstriction. The furrowed forehead, drawn lips, and clenched teeth may be due to reflex muscle spasm or to an effort (which may be either conscious or unconscious) to diminish the pain by projecting other inhibiting stimuli. The *body position* may give a clue to the location of the pain, as the person usually assumes the position that affords the greatest comfort. Such positions as knees drawn up (in severe, colicky abdominal pain) and a limb held in a protected rigid position are examples. *Muscular rigidity* or involuntary muscle spasm frequently occurs with fractures and represents a response over reflex arcs mediated at the spinal level, as discussed above. General *body activity* usually ceases in very severe pain, although some patients may respond with extreme restlessness, rolling about in bed, and similar manifestations. *Blood pressure* and *pulse rate* are usually increased by reflex effects on the autonomic nervous system. In severe pain, however, peripheral vasoconstriction may be so severe that the blood pressure falls and shock may occur. Severe pain is often accompanied by other associated signs such as vomiting, fever, and sweating, which are also the result of reflex connections at the spinal level.

Emotional reactions, such as fear, excitement, anger, depression, weeping, and other comparable states reflect the significance of the pain to the subject; the greater the significance, the stronger the reaction. Anxiety increases the intensity of the pain and the emotional response to it, sometimes setting up a vicious circle in which the anxiety increases the pain and the pain increases the anxiety until the patient is completely exhausted. Such positive feedback mechanisms must be broken into by therapeutic relief of the pain. One must also remember that the patient's description of the pain is not so reliable as the objective signs noted, for he may consciously or unconsciously minimize or exaggerate his pain.

Quality of Pain

A number of characteristic or descriptive words used to describe pain may be associated with specific locations or conditions. MacBryde lists the following:

In aneurysmal erosion: boring, pounding.

In bones: deep, aching, boring.

In muscles: sore aching.

In colic: twisting, griping, cramping; recurs in waves.

In angina: compression, constriction, comes with exertion, feeling of great weight, agonizing, fear of impending death, and similar terms.

In pleuritis: stabbing, knife-like; occurs with each breath.

In peptic ulcer: burning, sharp, associated with hunger, relieved by food or alkali; frequently occurs at night.

In tabes: lightning-like, shooting, stabbing, girdle pains.

In neuralgia: sharp, cutting, paroxysmal, intermittent.

In neuritis: burning, stabbing.

In causalgia: burning, peculiar stinging.

In burns, blisters, and superficial skin lesions: burning, smarting, stinging.

Time of Occurrence

The time of occurrence of the pain may be quite significant in diagnosing its cause. Terms used to describe qualities usually involve a time dimension. Terms signifying momentary pain include sticking, pricking, flashing, shooting, stabbing; those indicating a longer duration include burning, throbbing, boring, cramping, crushing. Pain from organic disease is seldom constant; it frequently is periodic or even seasonal. Peptic ulcer seems to recur in the spring or fall, or to recur at intervals of weeks to months and then occur daily for several weeks. Gallbladder pain tends to occur in severe attacks with a tendency toward relative freedom from symptoms for weeks or months.

The time of day at which a pain consistently occurs may be important in diagnosing its cause. For example, certain pains are made worse by activity and therefore tend to occur during the day. Examples include neurasthenic pain, locomotor pain (as in rheumatism, sciatica, and flatfoot), eye pain, gastrointestinal pain, and morning sinus pain due to lack of adequate drainage during the night. *Night* pain is usually indicative of organic disease, especially if it is severe enough to awaken the person from sleep or to keep him from sleeping.

Adverse Physical Effects of Pain

Because of its widespread physiological effects on the nervous system and circulation, pain may produce profound disturbances in the function of vital organs. Shock from severe pain may be drastic enough to cause death. Because of its reflex effect on the blood vessels, pain may cause a significant decrease in the blood supply to the kidneys with a failure of kidney function and a fall in urinary output. Physiological responses to pain via the autonomic nervous system may adversely affect heart function. Peripheral nerve damage may cause tissue changes in the area of distribution of the nerve, such as muscular atrophy.

Adverse Psychological Effects of Pain

The adverse psychological effects of pain include mobilization for resistance or flight, with anger and/or fear as the dominant emotions. This is a protective mechanism. On the other hand, pain may result in immobilization or withdrawal, with feelings of weakness, sickness, and near-panic. If pain is repeated or prolonged, fear, depression, insomnia, anorexia, irritability, and nervous tension may appear. Interruption of pain or abolishment of it may have a profound beneficial effect on the patient's morale and emotional balance.

Function of Pain

Normally, pain operates as an alerting device or alarm signal that warns of the imminence of danger, the presence of peripheral damage, or of central distress. The perception of pain is a part of a protective mechanism that sets in operation defensive or withdrawal actions valuable in preserving the integrity of the organism. Very occasionally, pain sensations are congenitally absent, and a child so afflicted is in constant danger of severe trauma because he is completely unaware of the danger of many situations that normally cause pain.

RATIONALE FOR THE TREATMENT OF PAIN

Pain perception can be abolished or at least greatly minimized by preventing sensory impulses from reaching the sensory cortex or by depressing the cortex itself. This can usually be accomplished by the judicious use of drugs. In intractable pain that refuses to respond to drugs, surgical intervention may be advisable.

Drugs may act anywhere along the sensory pathways to block pain impulses. The more potent analgesics, such as morphine and its derivatives, and some of the synthetic drugs, such as meperidine and methadone, increase the threshold for pain by depressing sensory cortical areas, but without loss of consciousness. Morphine is the drug of choice for relieving severe visceral pain. Besides elevating the pain threshold, morphine elevates the mood and alters the reaction to pain. Anxiety, fear, and worry are usually abolished and are frequently replaced by relaxation and a feeling of comfort and tranquility. For this reason, the drug readily can become habit-forming. It also has a selective effect on the medullary centers, depressing the respiratory and cough centers while stimulating the vomiting and vagus centers. When morphine is administered, therefore, the nurse must be on the alert for possible respiratory depression; it should never be given in conditions in which the respiratory center is already depressed, as in brain tumors. The reflex centers of the spinal cord are stimulated by morphine, but the depressant action of the drug on the brain antagonizes this reaction in man. It causes marked constriction of the pupils of the eyes; impulses that travel by way of the oculomotor nerve produce spasms of the sphincter muscles of the iris. Morphine also increases the tone of the smooth muscle of the gastrointestinal tract, the billary tract, and the urinary tract. It decreases metabolism and lowers body temperature (Musser and Shubkagel).

Some of the less potent analgesics such as the salicylates and the synthetic drugs acetanilid, phenacetin, and aminopyrine are also antipyretic. It is believed that their antipyretic effect is mediated by way of the hypothalamus to speed up heat elimination through increased radiation of heat from the skin and increased sweating. Analgesia seems to result from the action of these drugs in the region of the thalamus, blocking or interfering with the pain impulses carried over the spinothalamic tracts, thus interfering with the relay of pain impulses from the thalamus to the cerebral cortex (Musser and Shubkagel).

Local anesthetics, which block pain impulses from local areas to which they have been applied, have a selective action on nerve fibers and interfere with nerve conductivity. Drugs such as cocaine and its synthetic derivatives act specifically on the sensory nerves or nerve endings; other drugs such as ethyl chloride produce their effect by chilling or freezing the area to which they are applied, thus lowering the ability of the local nerve fibers to transmit pain impulses (Musser and Shubkagel).

If intractable pain cannot be controlled by drugs, surgical intervention may be advisable. One of the more common procedures is chordotomy or more accurately, spinothalamic tractotomy. Since the lateral spinothalmic tract travels near the surface of the cord, it is not too difficult a procedure to sever the fibers of the tract, thus preventing the passage of pain impulses to the higher centers. Section of the tract in the medulla and midbrain has also been carried out to ensure relief of the upper parts of the body. Pain sensations from the viscera seem to have rather extensive representation in both ipsilateral and contralateral tracts. It may be necessary in these cases to carry out a bilateral incision to relieve the pain, and it may be necessary to carry the incision deeply enough to penetrate the gray matter of the cord before relief is obtained. Frontal lobotomy, in which the fibers to the frontal lobe are severed, has also been used at times. While this operation probably does not abolish the pain, the patient ignores the pain and seems to be little affected by it.

THE NURSE'S ROLE IN THE MANAGEMENT OF PAIN

When the nurse as a person perceives a patient she does so in the light of her own experience and the meaning she attaches to such perceptions; that is, she is not a completely objective interpreter of the patient's behavior. If she has experienced no pain in her own life, she can have little personal understanding of how it affects the patient. Her perception may not agree with the patient's point of view; therefore, on the basis of her scientific background and professional experience, she must acquire skill in identifying the *real* problem in order to meet the patient's needs. He often manifests anxiety and fear by repeated requests for small services rather than by saying directly, "I need to talk to someone about my problems," or, "I need something to relieve my pain." Or he may be completely stoic in his responses and deny that he has any needs, even when the objective signs tell the skilled observer that the very opposite is true.

The three basic steps to be followed in the solution of any problem include assessment of the situation, active intervention, and evaluation.

ASSESSMENT OF THE SITUATION

The nurse's original reaction must be explored with the patient in order to determine its validity. She must not only strive to interpret the clinical meaning of a particular pain, but must assess its meaning to the patient and his total personality. Since pain is a subjective manifestation, the accuracy of the nurse's information will depend to a great extent on her skill in framing questions and in eliciting answers to them. Her powers of observation must be developed to the point where she is aware of and able to identify and evaluate the pertinent external signs described in the earlier part of this chapter. All this information must be synthesized into a judgment that forms the basis for devising a plan of nursing care. She must also become aware of the secondary factors that increase pain, such as pressure on tender areas, uncomfortable positions, localized hypoxia, and excessive light and noise in the room or close surroundings.

ACTIVE INTERVENTION

Active intervention embodies those actions which tend to alleviate or diminish pain. It may be involved with the psychological and sociocultural components of pain as well as the physiological. In other words, the patient's reaction as well as his perception of pain must be considered in deciding upon a course of action. Perhaps only listening to the person, reassuring him, and making him physically comfortable will be all that is needed. Very severe pain, however, may require immediate administration of a p.r.n. narcotic such as morphine to interrupt a severe, even dangerous reaction. The decision and choice of the appropriate intervention requires expert nursing judgment.

EVALUATION

Evaluation must follow intervention; that is, it is a deliberate process used by the nurse to determine the effect of her care upon the patient. If her intervention was successful, why was it successful? Is the patient relaxed, apparently comfortable, even sleeping? Morphine does not have a sedative effect as such, but the relief of pain it provides enables the patient to sleep. Could the intervention have been more successful if another choice had been made? For example, did the patient really need a sedative rather than a narcotic? Or should they have been given in combination to produce the best effect? If the intervention was unsuccessful, with the patient still complaining of severe pain, restlessness, and anxiety, wherein did the failure lie and what further exploration of the problem is necessary in order to achieve success?

It is true that one cannot hope to relieve all pain, at all times, for all people. When pain is severe, recurrent, or chronic, interpretation of the pain experience with all its aspects is quite complex, and the nurse must learn to use herself as a therapeutic agent in those cases in which drugs are no longer effective. To do this, she must face and come to terms with her own anxiety and frustration because she cannot banish pain entirely, and must communicate her support generously and courageously to aid the patient to develop a philosophy of pain with which he can face an uncertain future.

Itching (Pruritus)

DEFINITION OF ITCHING

Itching is an unpleasant cutaneous sensation that produces the desire to scratch and signals damage to the epidermis.

MECHANISM OF ITCHING

The sensation of itching arises in free nerve endings (probably fine plexuses of the small C fibers) in the epidermis or corresponding layer of the transitional mucous membrane. Impulses are thought to be mediated by the same pathways as those subserving pain, although itching is a sensation distinct from pain, and sometimes is much more difficult to tolerate. It is not a universal sensation, however, but seems to be limited to the skin and mucous membranes. There is increased responsiveness to itching at the mucocutaneous junctions of the anus, the external auditory canal, and the nostrils, although the entire skin is able to receive impulses that lead to the perception of the itching.

The nerve endings can be stimulated by chemical, mechanical, thermic, and electric stimuli arising from the outside as well as from within the tissues. If the stimulus also irritates the walls of the capillaries or epidermal cells, an inflammatory lesion develops with a state of increased excitability of nerve endings in that area. Inadequate stimuli such as light touch, light stroking, light pressure, and similar mechanisms elicit an intense itching sensation, and the more the area is scratched, the more itching excitability is increased, and a vicious circle is established. Itching is especially aggravated if a proliferative response of the epidermis occurs.

Itching is aggravated by vasodilatation, therefore by heat, mechanical friction or irritation, and similar stimuli. It is also aggravated by venous stasis, tissue anoxia, and local sweating. It is lessened by cold applications, corticotropin (ACTH), adrenocorticoids, local anesthetics, and at times by ultraviolet or x-ray irradiation.

The perception of itching has an integrating center in the hypothalamus whose excitability can be influenced by drugs and at times by central stimuli that are psychogenic in nature. Production of histamine and histamine liberators in the tissues causes itching that can be relieved by the administration of antihistaminic drugs. Certain other cellular enzymes, especially proteinases, may also be chemical stimuli for itching.

ANALYSIS OF ITCHING AS A SYNDROME

Important diagnostic criteria can be elicited by questioning the patient: "Are you disturbed in your sleep by itching, and do you awaken to find yourself scratching?" "Can you forget about your itching in the daytime when your attention is distracted?" "Can you stop scratching easily when you make up your mind to do so?" "Does itching arise only in certain situations?"

MacBryde classifies cutaneous disorders as (1) obligate itching disorders, which are recognized as such only if they definitely disturb the patient at night and interfere with his sleep. These conditions include pediculosis, scabies, contact dermatitis, and similar conditions. (2) Facultative itching disorders include dry skin, psoriasis, and pruritus due to diabetes and similar conditions. (3) Nonitching disorders, such as developmental anomalies and neoplasms, also occur.

The nurse must be on the alert for scratch marks or other lesions on patients who suffer from pruritus, for these may have definite diagnostic value. Scratch marks are not found in a number of skin lesions; scratching techniques seem to vary according to the condition involved. Elevated, itching papules are torn off with the fingernails as soon as they are formed; in scabies the entire lesion is torn off. In neurotic excoriations, normal skin is irritated by digging and picking. Linear scratch marks may occur when scratching with the fingernails is uninhibited. These marks may be secondarily infected with pyogenic organisms. All such marks should be carefully described by the nurse and recorded on the patient's chart, since they may be important diagnostic criteria and/or prognostic signs.

CLINICAL MANIFESTATIONS OF ITCHING

Generalized Pruritus

Generalized pruritus may be due to a number of conditions. *Tissue anoxia* is often responsible for "senile pruritus" and is usually due to venous stasis. Tissue anoxia may cause pruritus in younger persons as well. *Asteatosis,* a decrease in sebaceous gland activity with drying of the skin, is most prominent in winter and causes a mild itching, especially when the skin is exposed to abrupt changes of temperature. It usually can be remedied by curtailing soap and water and massaging with a lubricant such as an ointment base containing cholesterol or its derivatives. Lanolin is a useful application.

Allergic manifestations may be eczematous in nature, with the reaction taking place in the epidermal cells and promoting vesicle formation, or urticarial with wheal lesions.

Pruritus is rather commonly of *psychogenic origin*. It may occur as *parasitophobia*, in which one's attention is centered on crawling parasites, although very little real itching accompanies this condition. *Neurotic excoriations* are formed because of a compulsion to pick at the skin until actual lesions are formed, and to keep them active by further picking and scratching. Such excoriations may also become secondarily infected. In neurodermatitis an increased itching sensibility occurs, although this condition is more commonly localized than general in nature. A type of emotional urticaria sometimes known as the *cholinergic* type is caused by an allergy to acetylcholine, which is released in the skin in response to emotional stimuli or to heat.

Pruritus during pregnancy is characterized by an abrupt onset with early generalization and intense itching both day and night. Fortunately, it disappears within the first few days following delivery and there are no accompanying skin changes. This condition apparently is caused by fetal metabolic products that are toxic to the mother. Administration of suberythematous doses of generalized ultraviolet irradiation is thought to be one of the most useful methods of treatment. Other types of pruritus occasionally occur during pregnancy.

Diabetic pruritus may be the first symptom of the disease noticed by the patient. It is usually caused by increased drying of the skin, although the mechanism by which this is produced is not well understood. Monilial infections involving the skin folds are sometimes present causing additional damage to the skin.

Pruritus is present in about 20 to 25 percent of *jaundiced* patients because of disturbances in liver function. There seems to be no correlation between the mechanism by which the jaundice arose and the degree of pruritus. It occurs also in *liver disease without jaundice* and can be caused by an increase in bile acids in the blood. Symptomatic relief can often be obtained with suberythematous doses of ultraviolet or small doses of soft x-ray. Biliary drainage may end the itching. Generalized pruritus may occur in lymphoblastoma and malignant tumors, myeloid and lymphatic leukemias, mycosis fungoides, and Hodgkin's disease. Pruritus may also occur in renal insufficiency because of retention of nitrogenous materials in the blood.

Localized Pruritus

Localized prutitus occurs most commonly at the mucocutaneous junctions of the anus, vulva, ear canals, and nostrils. *Pruritus ani* is associated with neurodermatitis in about 50 percent of the cases, but there is also an idiopathic type. It may also occur with hemorrhoids or with venous stasis in the anal region. It can usually be controlled by mild sedatives and local measures. *Pruritus vulvae* is commonly a functional condition, but it may be caused by local inflammation and irritation. It causes a great deal of anguish to its victims. Pruritus of the *ear canals* is usually caused by neurodermatitis or by fungus infections, but can be caused by excess wax accumulation in the ear canal. Pruritus of the *nostrils* may be caused by intestinal parasites in children, it may be allergic in origin, or it may be of central origin when intracranial pressure is increased.

RATIONALE FOR THE TREATMENT OF ITCHING

The cause of the pruritus must be determined and treated promptly. Because scratching of the skin may cause excoriations and secondary infections, local remedies such as wet dressings, lotions, ointments, and similar medications are also indicated. Hot wet dressings may be used when infection is present. Because heat frequently intensifies the itching, however, cold wet dressings may be more soothing. Sometimes cool water alone is sufficient to relieve itching. Other solutions commonly used include Burow's solution (aluminum acetate solution), which is diluted with 10 to 40 parts of water before application. It is of value in acute inflammatory conditions, edema, and vesicular dermatoses. Boric acid solution 2 percent is frequently used in contact and atopic dermatitis, but should not be used on denuded skin areas because of the danger of absorption. Potassium permanganate solution 1:5,000 or 1:10,000 is used in weeping, blistered, and denuded areas as an antiseptic, astringent, and keratolytic. Other solutions include normal saline, milk, starch, and oatmeal (used in oatmeal baths). Local anesthetics may be used, but one must be aware of the danger of sensitization to these preparations and the necessity for close observation whenever they are in use. Topical steroids are useful in reducing the inflammatory component, and topical antibiotics may be helpful if infection is present. Calamine lotion and lotions containing camphor, menthol, or phenol frequently are soothing to an itching area. Antihistamines can be used to good advantage if the condition is allergic in nature. Systemic drugs that may be of some value in treating pruritus include the tranquilizers or mild sedation to lessen the severity of the reaction (which might be compared with the pain reaction, since it is of a similar nature in many ways). Systemic anti-inflammatory steroids may also be useful and are frequently used.

THE NURSE'S ROLE IN THE MANAGEMENT OF ITCHING

The same problem-solving method of assessment, intervention, and evaluation suggested for the management of pain should be used in the care of the patient with pruritus. Since the patient is often completely exhausted both mentally and physically by severe itching, psychological and emotional support plays a very important part in the nurse's approach. The greatest favor she can do for the patient, however, is to promptly apply the drugs or treatments ordered by the physician, as outlined above, to allay the symptoms as soon as possible.

The patient must be taught the importance of avoiding further trauma to the sensitive skin, and as a preventive measure his fingernails should be cut sufficiently short that it is impossible for him to use them to scratch. He should be urged to use other measures as substitutes for scratching, such as applying firm pressure to the area. If possible, some diversion should be provided to distract his attention from the desire to scratch. If he is an outpatient, he should be warned about the irritating effect of too-frequent use of soap and water on dry or irritated skin and should be instructed not to use strong friction over the irritated area. If he is hospitalized, the same information can be given during actual care so that the nurse also teaches by example. All stimuli that may increase itching, such as heat, perspiration, and light stroking over the irritated area, must be scrupulously avoided.

Light loose clothing should be worn. If the patient must be in bed, old smooth linens should be used on the bed in preference to new and rougher material. Room temperature and humidity also should be controlled; a cool temperature (68° to 70° F) plus a fairly low humidity (30 to 40 percent) seem to be the most conducive to rest.

All irritated skin should be closely observed for the effect of local applications or of drugs given systemically. Not all persons' skin responds in the same way and a preparation that is successful for one may be irritating rather than soothing to another. A description of any changes should be made a part of the patient's record and the doctor should be kept informed of his progress. If the cause of the condition is unknown, the nurse may be able to make a contribution to the final diagnosis by exploring with the patient any known contacts (or possible contacts) with allergens which might have caused the reaction.

The treatment and care of specific skin diseases are discussed in Chapter 28.

Hyperesthesia, Numbness and Tingling, Anesthesia

Since hyperesthesia, numbness and tingling, and anesthesia are abnormal manifestations of the same modality (touch), they can be considered together as making up a continuum between two extremes, with normal sensory responses approximately midway between hyperesthesia and anesthesia on such a scale. The sensations of numbness and tingling are more closely related to anesthesia, but do not represent complete loss of sensation. The terms *hyperalgesia* and *analgesia* bear the same relationship to the sensation of pain and may be closely related to hyperesthesia and anesthesia. They do not necessarily occur together, however.

DEFINITIONS

Hyperesthesia is defined as the unusual or pathological sensitivity of the skin to ordinary touch stimuli. *Numbness and tingling* represent a partial loss of touch sensation accompanied by a spontaneous sticking and pricking sensation in the same area. *Anesthesia* is complete loss of the sensation of touch. If sensation is merely diminished and not completely absent, it is termed *hypesthesia*.

ANATOMICAL AND PHYSIOLOGICAL CONSIDERATIONS: DERMAL SEGMENTATION

The segmentation of the spinal cord and the peripheral distribution of the nerves to the skin form a map upon which the level of sensory disturbances can be fairly well localized. The *dermatome distribution* is somewhat different from that of the individual "named" nerves, however, since these nerves may contain fibers from several dermatomes. For example, the nerves supplying the hand and arm are derived from the brachial plexus and supply specific portions of the hand and arm, while a dermatome segment that runs the entire length of the hand and arm and includes a portion of the shoulders represents the innervation from a single spinal segment.

In describing a dermatome, the cord is divided into arbitrary segments, one for each spinal nerve with its dorsal and ventral roots. There are eight cervical segments (C1 to C8), 12 thoracic (T1 to T12), five lumbar (L1 to L5), five sacral (S1 to S5), and one (very occasionally two) coccygeal (Co). Since the spinal cord is shorter than the vertebral canal, these segments are not at the level of the corresponding vertebrae, with the exception of a few cervical segments, but are from one to three vertebral levels higher as one goes from thoracic to sacral segments. There is also considerable overlapping of the areas supplied by single spinal nerves, so that damage to a single spinal nerve probably produces hypesthesia rather than complete anesthesia along the dermatome it supplies.

Some general knowledge of dermatome distribution is useful to the nurse in assessing symptoms reported by a patient with sensory defects. The following general areas of sensory innervation are fairly simple to remember:

1. The cervical segments C1 to C4 supply the back of the head, the entire neck, and the shoulders. (The face is supplied by the three branches of the fifth cranial nerve, the trigeminal.) The cervical segments C5 to C7 supply the lateral aspects of the arm; the inner aspect is supplied by C8 and T1.

2. The throacic segments T1 to T12 supply the trunk. Two valuable landmarks occur at the levels of T4 and T10. The segment T4 encircles the trunk at the nipple line anteriorly and slightly higher posteriorly. The segment T10 encircles the trunk at the level of the umbilicus.

3. The lumbar segments L1 to L4 supply the inner and anterior surfaces of the hips and thighs from above downward; L5, S1, and S2 supply the outer and posterior surfaces of the thighs.

4. The sacral segments S2 to S5 supply the perineum; the coccygeal segment (Co) supplies the base of the spine.

CLINICAL MANIFESTATIONS

Pathology at one or more segmental dermatome levels will be reflected by sensory disturbances below the level of the lesion if the posterior root, the spinothalamic tracts, or the dorsal columns of the cord are involved. Some motor disturbances are also present if the sensory input of a reflex arc at the spinal level is severely damaged. Because of the overlapping of segments, involvement of a single dermatome is rarely noticed by a person unless pain along the distribution also occurs.

Since the pathways for pain and temperature (lateral spinothalamic) and coarse touch (ventral spinothalamic) cross in the same segment they enter, or within a few segments above or below this level, injuries to these pathways on one side of the body give rise to symptoms on the opposite side of the body below the level of the lesion.

The pathways for fine touch discrimination and proprioception travel up the dorsal columns of the cord and do not cross until the secondary neurons leave the nucleus gracilis and nucleus cuneatus in the lower medulla. They decussate in the medulla as the internal arcuate fibers and ascend by way of the medial lemniscus to the posterolateral ventral nucleus of the thalamus. Tertiary fibers run from the thalamus to the sensory cortex and other scattered areas of the cortex. Lesions of these path-

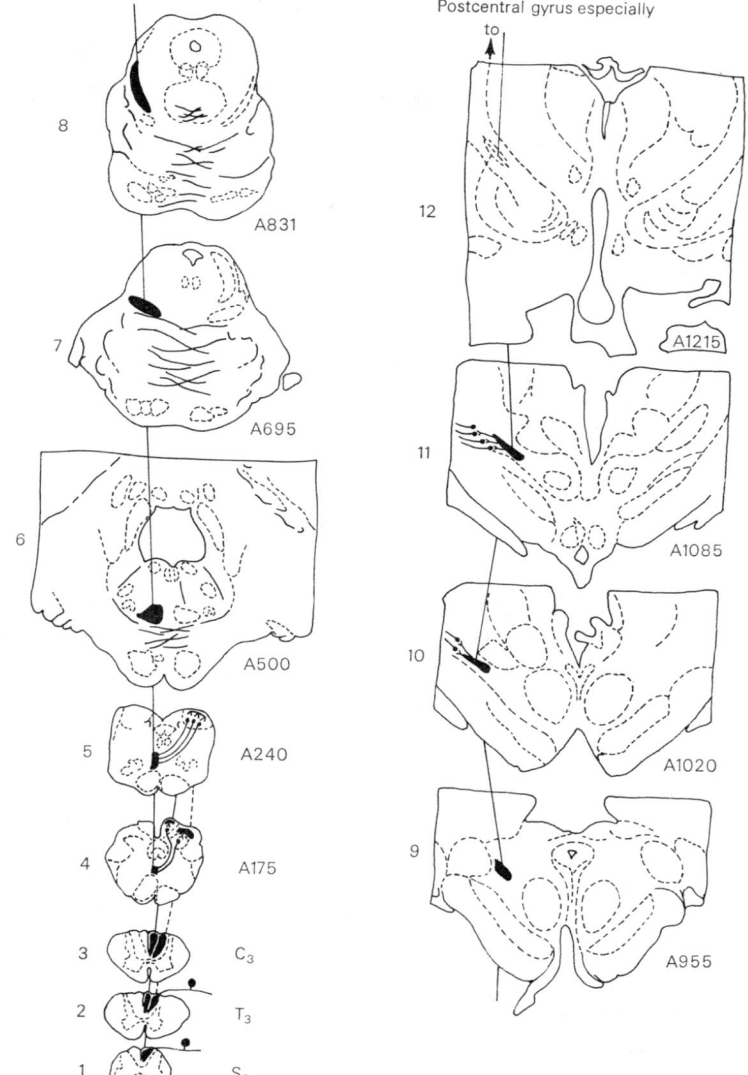

*Figure 15–5
Diagram of the medial
lemniscus. The serial
numbers, such as A1215,
refer to the sections of a
human brain stem series.
(Redrawn from T. L.
Peele: The Neuroanatomic
Basis for Clinical
Neurology. New York:
McGraw-Hill Book
Company, 1962.)*

ways below the medulla are reflected by a deficit on the same side of the body below the lesion. Lesions of the medulla or of the medial lemniscus above the decussation of the arcuate fibers would give rise to deficits on the opposite side of the body. Involvement of the dorsal columns also gives rise to a loss of position sense and vibration; there is not a complete loss of touch because of the fibers that run via the ventral spinothalamic pathway.

Hysterical anesthesia or malingering may be suspected if the area of reported involvement does not follow the pattern of the dermatomes or of the individual "named" nerves. It most frequently takes the form of a "stocking or glove" anesthesia or a complete hemianesthesia (including the face on the same side). The boundary line of anesthesia is sharply demarcated from the normal zone. This is particularly apparent in the stocking or glove type. In addition to the nonanatomic distribution of anesthesia there is often almost a minute-by-minute change in the line of demarcation from normal sensation. This is particularly evident at the time of neurological examination when response to pinprick and light touch is tested. A shifting line of demarcation is always suggestive of hysteria or malingering.

If the patient should be a malingerer—and this is becoming more frequent in cases in which accident compensation is involved—the nurse may notice reactions that do not parallel the deficits claimed. Such a patient is not always completely on guard or may actually forget some of the details of his story. The average person knows nothing about dermatome or nerve distribution and is completely unaware that his fabricated symptoms do not follow the anatomical pattern. All discrepancies noted should be charted and called to the attention of the physician, as discrepancies may be important medicolegal evidence. In most true cases of sensory loss there is also a reflection in motor deficits and reflex responses because of the damage to afferent components of reflex arcs.

COMMON SENSORY SYNDROMES

A number of common sensory syndromes can be recognized by the nurse who is alert to the significance of the symptoms described by the patient. These syndromes are characteristic of peripheral nerve involvement, spinal cord involvement, or involvement of higher centers.

Peripheral Nerve Involvement

Peripheral nerve involvement may be due to injury of a single peripheral nerve, to involvement of multiple peripheral nerves (polyneuropathy), or to nerve root involvement. All these present fairly characteristic syndromes, which the nurse will be able to recognize after some experience with this type of injury. In a *single peripheral nerve injury,* symptoms will vary according to the type of nerve involved, that is, whether the fibers are predominantly muscular, cutaneous, or mixed. Proprioception and cutaneous sensitivity may be affected separately because of a difference in the distribution of the fibers within various nerves. Because of the overlapping of adjacent nerve endings, the area of sensory loss is less than the actual cutaneous distribution of the damaged nerve. This may be manifested by a central area of complete loss of sensation, which becomes less marked toward the periphery of the involved area. This, of course, becomes apparent at the time of neurological examination.

Polyneuropathy, or multiple peripheral nerve involvement, usually includes the loss or impairment of all sensory modalities in the area of distribution. Some modalities may be impaired more than others; for example, the sensation of touch may be impaired more than that of pain. The extremities are most frequently affected, especially the feet and legs. The hands sometimes are affected, but the abdomen, thorax, and face are rarely involved. The phrase "stocking and glove anesthesia" is also used to describe the symptoms of this type of lesion, but it differs from the type found in hysteria by the tendency of the sensory loss to shade off gradually over a considerable vertical line of limb, while that in hysteria shows a sharp line of demarcation between normal and abnormal responses to stimulation.

Injury to a *single dorsal root* does not cause complete loss of sensation, but various degrees of impairment. When two or more roots are involved, the zone of sensory loss will follow the segmental distribution, in which there is almost complete loss of pain and touch surrounded by a zone of hyperesthesia and hyperalgesia. If the ventral roots are involved, muscle paralysis and motor loss will occur. The latter is also true if the dorsal roots are completely severed, because of the complete interruption of the afferent arm of the reflex arc.

Spinal Cord Involvement

Symptoms resulting from spinal cord involvement may differ vastly, depending upon the level and the extent of the involvement. With *complete transection of the cord,* which seems to be occurring more frequently today as a result of serious automobile accidents, all forms of sensation are abolished below a level that roughly corresponds to the segmental level of the lesion. There usually is a narrow margin of hyperesthesia and hyperalgesia at the upper margin of the area of sensory loss, corresponding to the collateral distribution of the primary neurons. In a peripheral cord lesion in which the area of damage evolves from the periphery of the cord toward the center, the lower extremities are usually involved first, followed by ascending levels of sensory loss. When a lesion progresses from the center of the cord toward the periphery, changes usually occur in the reverse order because of the lamination of the pathways, with fibers that carry impulses from the lower extremities lying at the outer border of the cord. Since motor pathways are also destroyed, there will also be paralysis below the level of the lesion.

Hemisection of the cord (Brown-Séquard syndrome) shows a different distribution of involvement from complete transection. If the lesion is above the level of complete decussation of pain and temperature fibers (at about T10), there is a loss of pain and temperature on the side opposite the lesion beginning one or two segments below, that is, below the level of normal collaterals. Proprioception, vibratory sense, and touch sensations are lost on the same side as the lesion. There will be ipsilateral motor paralysis also, since this level is below the pyramidal decussation in the medulla. Because touch fibers from one side of the body are distributed via tracts on both sides of the spinal cord, the sensation of touch will be least affected and deficits in touch will not be so noticeable unless the involvement is very extensive.

Lesions of the *central gray matter* of the cord, such as syringomyelia, produce symptoms that vary according to the location of the lesion within the cord. The lesion may cause a loss of pain and temperature over a segmental pattern of distribution without the loss of touch. If the lesion is more extensive, loss of touch and areflexia may also occur.

In *posterior column lesions* there is usually a loss of vibratory and position sense on the same side, below the level of the lesion, without loss of pain, temperature, or touch sensations. Loss of position sense due to interruption of proprioceptive fibers may also affect two-point discrimination and judgment of the size, shape, and weight of objects. Paresthesias are a common symptom. Even though motor pathways are not involved, posterior column lesions are accompanied by ataxia and loss of equilibrium because of the loss of the sensory component.

Anterior and *lateral column lesions* may cause loss of pain and temperature sensations without loss of position sense or other proprioceptive modalities. Paralysis of motor function usually accompanies this syndrome, since the corticospinal pathways are also located in this region.

Involvement of Higher Centers

Symptoms of involvement of the higher centers vary according to the location of the lesion, that is, whether it be brain stem, thalamus, or cerebral cortex. In lesions of the *medulla* and *lower pons,* there is usually a disturbance of pain and temperature on one side of the face and on the opposite side of the body, because of the location of the major nuclei in the brain stem. If high in the *pons* or *midbrain,* a lesion may cause loss of all superficial sensation over the entire contralateral side of the body. Disturbances of cranial nerve function will also be manifested at this level.

Lesions of the thalamus give rise to more profound symptoms, because of its nature as an integrating center. Involvement of the posterolateral ventral nucleus causes diminution or loss of *all* forms of sensation on the opposite side of the body. Position sense is most profoundly affected and deep sensory loss may be more pronounced than superficial loss. Such a lesion may also cause spontaneous pain or discomfort (thalamic pain) on the same side of the face but on the opposite side of the body. Usually there is an elevated threshold for sensory stimuli, but once such sensations are evoked, they are more lingering and unpleasant than ordinary sensations.

Lesions of the *sensory cortex* do not cause a complete loss of pain or other sensations, but rather impair one's ability to localize pain and to make fine discriminations. Lesions of the *parietal cortex* are accompanied by symptoms of asteriognosis, loss of position sense, changes in the threshold of two-point discrimination, and a general inattentiveness to sensory stimuli on the opposite side of the body. Involvement of the other sensory modalities may fluctuate, at one time being very apparent, at others inconsistent and irregular.

Sensory manifestations in *hysteria* are also of central origin. Complete hemianesthesia (including the face on the same side) is a common finding in hysteria and is usually accompanied by hemianalgesia as well, but is not necessarily associated with hemiplegia. As in the peripheral type of anesthesia, hemianesthesia can usually be differentiated from a true organic deficit by the discrepancies between the type of loss described and the anatomical sensory distribution. Organic hemianesthesia may occur with a complete transection high in the brain stem, but this is accompanied by motor deficits as well.

RATIONALE FOR TREATMENT

At this point it might be well to reemphasize the fact that while we have considered sensory symptoms almost exclusively in the preceding discussion, pure organic sensory deficits rarely occur without motor involvement as well, so that in the actual diagnosis of the condition present motor deficits must be considered as well as sensory.

Since sensory deficits exist in many conditions, there is no single method or rationale of treatment. Collins emphasizes the point that in making a neurological diagnosis it is important to rule out first (or to recognize) those diseases that can be treated.

THE NURSE'S ROLE IN THE MANAGEMENT OF SENSORY SYNDROMES

Certain problems are involved in the care of any patient with a sensory deficit regardless of the formal diagnosis. These might be reviewed at this time.

Physical Care

Meticulous care of the skin is an important part of the personal hygiene of the patient suffering from a sensory syndrome. Because of poor circulation with resulting ischemia of body tissues, the area that has lost cutaneous sensitivity may break down more readily than normal tissue. The impairment of circulation increases the likelihood of decubitus ulcers if the patient remains in one position for any length of time, for the weight of his body still further curtails the circulation. If he is confined to bed or wheel chair, his position should be changed at intervals of 1 or 2 hours. Light massage to the skin should be give each time the patient is turned, with special attention given to any reddened areas and bony prominences. An alternating pressure mattress, foam rubber mattress, or sheepskin under the bony prominences aids in relieving pressure. If the patient is ambulatory, anesthetic skin areas should be checked regularly for possible unnoticed trauma, and he should be taught to carry out this procedure at home. The patient with sensory deficits needs continuous protection from mechanical trauma or burns of the involved area, since severe tissue damage can occur without his being aware of the danger. Fractures have gone unnoticed after falls, and simple fractures have been compounded by weight-bearing on an injured extremity.

Maintenance of good body mechanics is essential to prevent deformities. This is particularly true of the bed patient with a related paralysis or severe motor deficit. A board should be used at the foot of the bed against which the feet can be positioned to prevent foot drop. All pressure of bedclothing should be kept off the involved area; a bed cradle may be useful, if involvement is extensive. If general sensation and position sense have been lost in the lower extremities, the patient is usually unaware of the position of the legs and feet unless he observes them visually, and he may be unable to control their position even though he is aware of it. Under these circumstances the nurse must be particularly alert to his needs. Patients who have suffered a fracture of the spine with resulting spinal cord damage may be positioned on a Stryker frame.

Whenever possible, the patient should be encouraged to carry out independently as many of his activities of daily living as fall within his capabilities. Passive range of motion of the extremities should be carried out whenever necessary (or possible) to prevent contractures and to improve circulation. Physical therapy may be of value.

Specific nursing care activities will depend to a great extend upon the neurological diagnosis and the particular circumstances created by each organic deficit, whether the treatment of choice is medical or surgical, and whether the condition is one that can be treated. If the condition is progressive without hope of recovery, even greater nursing skill is necessary to make the patient as comfortable as possible and to maintain his morale.

Psychological and Emotional Factors

One of the important factors that the nurse must constantly keep in mind is the effect of sensory deprivation on the patient. The person who experiences even minor local areas of sensory deficit needs a great deal of psychological support and reassurance. As with the patient who experiences pain, the total reaction to sensory deficits is much more important than the perception of the physical symptoms. The effect of major sensory deficits on some persons is at times almost overwhelming. The reaction is compounded if the person is also aware that his condition is incurable and may be progressive. Whenever it is possible to instruct the patient about the causes of his peculiar symptoms, it should be done. It is far easier to face a *known* "enemy" than to face the unknown. As with pain, the patient must be aided to formulate a philosophy of suffering which will enable him to face the future with courage. If his condition is hopeless, he should not be given false hopes for a cure. On the other hand, he may be encouraged by the research that is going on in many areas, for perhaps a cure *will* be found within his lifetime.

To understand some of the patient's reactions, it would be well for the nurse to review a few of the many studies on sensory deprivation which have been made during the past few years. Studies made on normal persons deprived of sensory contacts have demonstrated that absence of these normal stimuli evoked some rather profound reactions, such as a seeming loss of sensation in the arms and legs, a feeling of disembodiment, sensations of the bed moving, visual and auditory hallucinations, and difficulty in thinking. Suggestions made to the subjects about reactions to be expected seemed to enhance the abnormal effects experienced (Pollard). Effects on body image have been reported in both normal and schizophrenic subjects in which normal persons experienced disorganization of body boundary awareness and stress, whereas the schizophrenic subjects experienced more realistic body boundaries than usual (Reitman and Cleveland).

Almost all nurses have experienced the demoralizing effects of immobility on a previously normal patient, such as the elderly patient with a fractured hip who is confined in a body cast or in traction, the patient with cataracts who has both eyes covered and who suddenly panics, the patient with poliomyelitis who is confined in a respirator and is dependent upon it for every respiration. Jackson suggests that increased contact with the nursing personnel, with other patients, and with the family, plus initiation of occupational therapy as soon as the patient is capable, can do much to offset the effects of isolation, immobilization, sedation, and sensory attenuation. Teaching the patient to compensate for various types of sensory deprivation should be a primary nursing therapeutic function.

The hysterical patient with loss of sensation should receive adequate psychiatric treatment. It may be possible for the nurse to effect some change in his reaction to his sensory disturbance by the use of positive suggestion, just as negative suggestions may cause enhancement of the symptoms by centering the patient's thoughts on them. The nurse needs to exercise the greatest prudence when dealing with the hysterical patient. For details of care, an appropriate textbook on psychiatry or psychiatric nursing should be consulted.

In evaluating the success of her care of the patient with sensory deficits, the nurse may judge by his degree of physical and mental comfort, the condition of his skin, the absence of contractures and other deformities, his willingness to cooperate in his care and treatment, his efforts to carry out his activities of daily living, and his general attitude toward his illness. This type of patient may tax all the skill and ingenuity the nurse possesses in order to meet his needs adequately.

Dizziness and Vertigo

Dizziness and vertigo might be considered as the sensory component of certain disorders of equilibrium and gait. The motor components and disturbances of gait frequently associated with vertigo are discussed elsewhere.

DEFINITIONS

Dizziness is a term usually used to describe a sensation of giddiness, unsteadiness on the feet, swimming sensations, lightheadedness, a sensation of movement, and similar symptoms. One needs to get a detailed description of this complaint to determine whether or not true vertigo exists. A feeling of lightheadedness can be brought about by hyperventilation or may be associated with anemia. This is not true vertigo.

True *vertigo* consists of hallucinations of movement, either of the subject himself or of his surroundings. This includes sensations such as spinning of the body, falling or being pushed suddenly and forcefully, or the surroundings revolving about the person in a specific direction. In severe attacks, as occur with acute labyrinthitis, the person may fall to the ground, completely unable to maintain his equilibrium; at times he may even be in a state of mild shock because of the intensity of the reflex effects.

If vertigo is pronounced, equilibrium is always affected and attempts to sit, stand, or walk only aggravate the symptoms. There is, therefore, a tendency for the victim to remain in the recumbent position and to move as little as possible. Coordination of individual movements of the limb is not impaired, however, even though the person's gait may be ataxic. True vertigo is usually accompanied by a number of associated symptoms such as nausea, vomiting, sweating, headache, and pallor because of reflex effects on the autonomic nervous system. Actual loss of consciousness may occur, but is very rare. Symptoms are made worse by movements of any kind, but especially by assuming an upright position from the horizontal more rapidly than usual.

MECHANISMS OF VERTIGO

Vestibular function is related to the maintenance of equilibrium and includes both a sense of "gravity" and one of "acceleration." Any change in the angle of the head from a vertical position is detected by the gravity receptors; any increase or decrease in linear motion or angular acceleration is detected by the receptors for the sense of acceleration. The chief function of the vestibular mechanism seems to be to "set" the body in a standard upright position and to return it to this position when it has been displaced. In carrying out this function the vestibular mechanism does so through an elaborate set of reflex arcs.

The receptors for the vestibular system lie within the utricle, saccule, and semicircular canals of the inner ear. Ciliated receptor cells in the utricular maculae are probably those that detect gravitational changes. The saccular maculae may respond to changes in gravity, but more recent research suggests that they also detect low-frequency vibrations. The semicircular canals respond to angular acceleration.

The ciliated cells of the utricular maculae extend into a gelatinous substance in which small calcareous particles, the otoliths, are embedded. As the head changes position, so does the gravitational pull on the otoliths. This pull, in turn, stimulates the receptor cells in such a way that the change in position is noted. Unless such a change is carried out voluntarily, the stimulus sets in motion the reflex that returns the head to its upright position. When the subject is upside down the maximum pull of the otoliths on the cilia is exerted; when the head is upright stimulation is minimal.

The three semicircular canals of each vestibule lie in three planes and at approximate right angles to each other. The lateral or horizontal canal actually slopes downward and backward at an angle of 20° to 30°. The anterior and posterior canals are vertical, perpendicular to the plane of the lateral canal, and are at right angles to each other. They are joined medially somewhat like the covers of an open book. The posterior canal slopes backward and laterally; the anterior canal slopes forward and laterally in oblique planes. At the end of each semicircular canal where it joins the utricle is an enlargement called the *ampulla*. Each ampulla contains a patch of specialized epithelial cells covering a transverse ridge, the crista, which forms a partial barrier across the cavity. The cilia projecting from the epithelial cells of the crista form a long brush-like tuft embedded in a gelatinous mass, the cupola, which moves back and forth with currents set up in the endolymph by movement. Thus any movement of the head in any direction or acceleration or deceleration of the head in a straight line sets up currents in the endolymph which sway the cupola in a specific direction and thus fire characteristic patterns of neurons which are recognized centrally.

Nerve fibers from the cristae and maculae have their cell bodies in the vestibular ganglion. The vestibular nerve forms a part of the eighth cranial nerve and travels through the internal auditory meatus, as the medial portion of this nerve, to the cerebellopontine angle, then separates from the cochlear portion of the nerve on entering the brain stem. Apart from a few fibers that pass directly to the cerebellum, the greater number of fibers terminate in the four cellular masses that comprise the vestibular nuclei. These extend from the pons to the upper part of the medulla and are located in the floor and lateral walls of the fourth ventricle. From the vestibular nuclei secondary tracts are given off to the cerebellum, the ocular nuclei, the spinal cord, and the cerebral cortex. The so-called flocculonodular lobe of the cerebellar cortex receives large numbers of these fibers, and in turn sends fibers to the vestibular nuclei; it is entirely vestibular in function and is primarily concerned with the unconscious maintenance of equilibrium. Fibers from the vestibular nuclei also pass to the cerebral cortex for conscious sensations of balance and posture. Although the course of these fibers is not yet definitely established, vestibular stimulation by rotation or galvanic current gives rise to action potentials that have been recorded from the superior temporal gyrus just rostral to the primary auditory cortex.

Vertigo can result from stimulation of the labyrinth or irritation of any part of the vestibular system. It can be produced by spinning the subject around in a revolving chair, then stopping the chair abruptly, or by irrigating the ear canal with hot or cold water to set up convection currents in the endolymph. The latter procedure is used in the standard caloric tests. Failure of these stimuli to produce vertigo and nystagmus usually indicates a block in the vestibular system. Irritation occurring with lesions involving the labyrinths may be accompanied by incoordination of gross movements, including falling, past pointing, and nystagmus (involuntary movements of the eyes). Nystagmus has two components, a fast movement and a slow movement. The direction of the slow component in labyrinthine nystagmus is toward the more active labyrinth and is most pronounced when the eyes are turned away from the involved labyrinth. This is an important diagnostic criterion, for it differs from the nystagmus that occurs with brain stem lesions. Blocking of vestibular function usually causes a loss of muscle tone on the ipsilateral side of the body, with a tendency to lose balance toward that side.

CLINICAL SIGNIFICANCE OF VERTIGO AND DIZZINESS

Vertigo and dizziness accompany many pathological conditions, most of which, however, involve irritation or blocking of the vestibular pathways. *Aural vertigo* is an involvement of the labyrinths which tends to occur in paroxysmal attacks and can be either inflammatory or noninflammatory in nature. The *inflammatory type,* an acute labyrinthitis, may give rise to very severe symptoms. The sensation of vertigo is usually aggravated by movement of the head. Nausea, vomiting, and nystagmus may be present during the acute stage. Recovery is gradual over a period of a few days to weeks. In chronic cases vertigo sometimes is extended over a period of several years. Involvement of the vestibular nerve, thought to be caused by a virus infection, is termed *vestibular neuronitis.* Vertigo can also occur with other acute, toxic inflammatory conditions. Of the *noninflammatory types* of aural vertigo, Ménière's disease is the most common. The symptoms are caused by a fluid imbalance within the labyrinth causing increased endolymphatic pressure. The attacks of vertigo are usually accompanied by tinnitus and deafness. The cause is unknown.

Vertigo with *lesions of the eighth cranial nerve* is a late and inconstant symptom of lesions of the eighth nerve. It may be caused by an acoustic neuroma or vascular anomalies pressing against the nerve. These produce more severe symptoms than a lesion of the nerve itself. Vertigo may also be accompanied by tinnitus and deafness because of the proximity of the cochlear components of the nerve.

Vertigo with *lesions of the brain stem* is frequently more severe in nature than the aural type. Lesions involving the vestibular nuclei usually produce very severe vertigo. Such lesions are most frequently the result of vascular accidents with occlusion of either the anterior inferior or posterior inferior cerebellar arteries. It may also occur with multiple sclerosis, tumors of the brain stem, or other brain stem lesions. This type of vertigo lasts much longer than aural vertigo and may affect equilibrium over long periods of time.

Vertigo or dizziness with *lesions of the cerebellum* is not so common and there is no substantial evidence that cerebellar lesions per se give rise to true vertigo, even though they may be accompanied by disturbances of equilibrium which are very severe. When it does accompany a cerebellar lesion, there is usually evidence that structures of the brain stem are also involved, as with a cerebellopontine angle tumor.

True vertigo is uncommon with supratentorial lesions, such as lesions of the forebrain, but may occur when the intracranial pressure is elevated. It is an occasional rare accompaniment of epilepsy or migraine. It may occur with certain temporal lobe lesions.

Next to headache, *post-traumatic dizziness* is the most common complaint following head injury, occurring with a frequency of 39 to 60 percent. True vertigo is uncommon. The sensations usually are less specific and are described as disturbances of equilibrium, unsteadiness, faintness, or dizziness. The symptom usually occurs in attacks without nausea or vomiting and may be precipitated by changes in posture, stooping, straining, or similar exertion and not by movements of the head alone.

True vertigo is rare in *cardiovascular* or *cerebrovascular disease,* but sensations usually described as dizziness related to changes in posture occur more frequently, and are probably due to cerebral ischemia.

A number of *drugs* may cause vertigo. A toxic disturbance of the vestibular mechanisms may be caused by quinine, salicylates, alcohol, streptomycin, and a number of other drugs that produce deafness, tinnitus, and vertigo.

A *psychogenic* form of dizziness may occur as a continuous sensation that may last for weeks or months. It is unaccompanied by loss of balance, staggering, or other evidence of disequilibrium. In such cases it may be a symbolic reflection of the person's sense of insecurity. One should guard against interpreting dizziness as psychogenic, however, until all other possibilities have been ruled out.

Ocular dizziness and motion sickness frequently occur. *Ocular disorders* are not a common cause of true vertigo, but may give rise to sensations of unsteadiness, staggering, and even nausea. *Motion sickness* is apparently a direct result of stimulation of the labyrinths by excessive motion and produces characteristic vertigo, nausea, and vomiting.

RATIONALE FOR THE TREATMENT OF VERTIGO

The treatment of vertigo is dependent upon the cause. If an acute inflammatory condition is present, especially if accompanied by an infection of the middle ear, antibiotics may be helpful. Bed rest and sedation are generally helpful. Drugs such as phenobarbital and chlorpromazine hydrochloride (Thorazine) assist in controlling symptoms.

A number of measures are used in the treatment of Ménière's syndrome. No specific treatment is available, but general measures include a salt-free diet and administration of ammonium chloride to alter fluid balance; nicotinic acid has been found useful. Antihistiminic drugs such as dimenhydrinate (Dramamine) and diphenhydramine (Benadryl) are of benefit to some patients. In severe cases that do not respond to medication, section of the vestibular portion of the eighth nerve may be carried out. Drugs used in the treatment of motion sickness include the belladonna alkaloids, cyclizine hydrochloride, meclazine hydrochloride, and similar drugs.

Vertigo due to lesions of the brain stem or other central nervous system lesions can be treated only symptomatically, unless caused by an operable tumor pressing against the vestibular nerve or brain stem. Under these circumstances removal of the tumor may relieve the symptoms.

If the vertigo is due to circulatory deficiency of the inner ear, vasodilator drugs may be of some benefit. Drugs such as nicotinic acid and nylidrin hydrochloride seem to be the most effective.

THE NURSE'S ROLE IN THE MANAGEMENT OF VERTIGO

Nursing care is largely symptomatic and depends upon the degree to which the patient is incapacitated. If complete bed rest is necessary, the nurse should make every effort to provide as much rest as possible for the patient and to avoid movements that may aggravate the symptoms. The patient is frequently able to find a position of the head which will decrease the severity of the vertigo. Drugs should be administered as ordered, and should be given on time, since the patient may be dependent upon these for minimizing his symptoms.

The nurse's powers of observation are important, since a changing picture of symptoms may show progression of a lesion or give information previously unnoted. Any new symptoms should be recorded and reported.

From the psychological point of view, a sympathetic understanding of the patient's problems is essential. Such symptoms, especially if prolonged, can be very demoralizing, and support and reassurance are absolutely essential. A cold and unsympathetic nurse has no place in the care of this type of patient.

The nurse must realize that overreaching, awkwardness in handling objects, dropping objects frequently, and slowness of movement are a part of the total syndrome. The degree and frequency of these symptoms gives some evidence as to the severity of the lesion. Some compensation for disequilibrium and imbalance can be achieved by deliberate use of the neck reflexes, placing the head in such a postion as will counteract the abnormal manifestations, and the patient can be taught to use these reflexes deliberately to achieve such compensation. This is especially important if he must learn to live with an inoperable lesion. The nurse's knowledge and understanding of such conditions will enable her to use her best judgment in meeting any problems presented by such patients.

Faintness

DEFINITION OF FAINTNESS

Faintness is to be distinguished from fainting or syncope (a transient loss of consciousness caused by reversible disturbances of cerebral function). Faintness might be considered an incomplete faint and is characterized by a sensation of weakness and dizziness and of impending loss of consciousness.

POSSIBLE CAUSES OF FAINTNESS
WITHOUT LOSS OF CONSCIOUSNESS

Anxiety Accompanied by Hyperventilation

One of the most common causes of recurrent faintness without loss of consciousness is anxiety accompanied by hyperventilation. This sensation is not relieved by recumbency, as is syncope, but it can be alleviated by voluntary control of respiration to reduce hyperventilation. It frequently can be reproduced by having the patient deliberately hyperventilate for 2 or 3 minutes. The symptoms apparently are due to the loss of carbon dioxide as a result of hyperventilation and release of epinephrine initiated by the emotional disturbance.

Postural Faintness

A sensation of giddiness and weakness frequently accompanies a sudden change in position from the recumbent to the upright. This type of postural faintness is especially likely to occur when patients have been on bed rest and are being ambulated for the first time. It is usually caused by a transient instability of the blood pressure caused by sluggish vasomotor reflexes.

Hypoglycemia

A mild hypoglycemia may cause sensations of weakness and faintness. It is usually associated with excessive insulin secretion in response to an elevated blood glucose following eating or excitement. It occurs most commonly in connection with anxiety and increased nervous tension. It may occur when concentrated carbohydrates are ingested, thus stimulating rapid insulin production. In functional hypoglycemia, morning fasting blood sugars are usually within the normal limits in contradistinction to the low fasting blood sugars that may occur with pancreatic tumor.

Acute Internal Hemorrhage

Faintness and weakness may be a symptom of acute internal hemorrhage if the blood loss is not very sudden and very severe. If pain is absent, faintness may be one of the earliest symptoms of internal hemorrhage. Hemorrhage should not be overlooked as a possible cause of faintness in persons with known peptic ulcers or following accidents in which there has been trauma to the abdomen.

Cerebral Ischemia

Arteriosclerotic narrowing of the cerebral vessels or localized vasospasm may cause cerebral ischemia with accompanying numbness and weakness of one side of the body, faintness and weakness, thickness of speech, and similar symptoms. Such transient ischemic attacks are usually indicative of cerebral thrombosis and are considered prodromata of an impending thrombotic stroke.

RATIONALE FOR THE TREATMENT OF FAINTNESS

The type of treatment given depends upon the causative factor, and the physician makes every attempt to arrive at an accurate differential diagnosis. This may be made more difficult because the physician frequently is not present when such episodes occur and must rely on observations made and information given by others, plus the condition of the patient at the time he is examined. The physician's knowledge of the patient's history and present diagnosis frequently gives the necessary clues to recognition of the cause.

Usually no specific treatment is necessary with the hyperventilation syndrome, although the underlying anxiety may require psychiatric treatment. On the other hand, simple reassurance of the patient that there is no serious organic condition present may be sufficient to satisfy his fears. Sometimes the patient can be convinced of his own part in causing the symptoms by having him hyperventilate under observation for 2 or 3 minutes, or until the syndrome is reproduced. Once he has determined to his own satisfaction that it is within his power to create such symptoms at will, he will no longer be afraid of them and will know how to handle them.

With postural faintness, the physician may wish to rule out serious cardiac conditions, chronic vasomotor instability, and similar conditions. If the condition is more than transitory, or if it occurs frequently, other causes will be investigated.

For mild hypoglycemic attacks, the best treatment is food to absorb the effects of excess insulin. Orange juice with sugar is a good emergency treatment, although one may run the risk of precipitating another attack if too much carbohydrate is given. As a precaution, one might use the sweetened orange juice as emergency treatment and follow this with some food that is high in fat and protein.

If further examination of the patient points to acute internal hemorrhage or to cerebral ischemia, immediate surgical intervention may be indicated. In carotid artery thrombosis, removal of the clot surgically can be a life-saving measure.

THE NURSE'S ROLE IN THE MANAGEMENT OF FAINTNESS

The role of the nurse as well as that of the physician depends upon the causative factor. She is more frequently present when such episodes occur than is the physician; therefore accurate observation and reporting is essential at all times.

The hyperventilation syndrome is frequently observed in persons who are emotionally upset, especially if they have been crying or sobbing uncontrollably. They become frightened by the symptoms of hyperventilation and frequently set up a vicious circle of forced breathing followed by still more pronounced symptoms. This syndrome may be encountered more frequently outside the hospital than among hospitalized patients. An alert nurse who is aware of the hyperventilation syndrome, which is fairly easily recognized, is in an excellent position to calm and reassure the person by explaining the probable cause of the symptoms and to work with him to reestablish normal breathing. Holding the breath as long as possible or breathing into a paper bag may be helpful in overcoming the carbon dioxide deficit more rapidly. Once the person is aware of what factors produce the syndrome, he usually can control the symptoms voluntarily.

The nurse should guard against postural faintness at any time, especially when ambulating a patient for the first time after an extended period of bed rest. Raising him slowly to the sitting position and allowing him to sit on the side of the bed for a few minutes with the feet dangling before permitting further exertion is a good preventive measure. If the patient experiences faintness in the sitting position, his head should be lowered between his knees. If he seems likely to lose consciousness, it is fairly simple to swing him back around on the bed to a recumbent position and to loosen any tight clothing until the faintness has passed. This precautionary measure may save the patient a severe fall. If he does not recover rapidly, some other cause of the faintness may be present and the physician should be called at once. In the meantime, the patient's pulse and blood pressure should be checked frequently and he should be observed carefully for signs of respiratory failure, cardiac arrest, or other unusual symptoms.

If at any time the nurse observes symptoms that correspond to those usually present with hypoglycemia, possible internal hemorrhage, or cerebral ischemia the physician should be notified at once. Hypoglycemia should be suspected when the faintness occurs after the ingestion of carbohydrates. Faintness from internal hemorrhage usually will be accompanied by a rising and weakening pulse rate, increased respiration, and a fall in blood pressure. Cerebral ischemia causes other characteristic symptoms in addition to faintness. The patient may experience unilateral weakness, numbness and tingling of the extremities, and loss of motor power in addition to the sensory changes. Symptoms usually depend upon which cerebral vessel is involved. Thrombosis of the internal carotid artery may cause symptoms typical of a stroke. Since it is often possible to remove a clot surgically from this artery, promptness in reporting such symptoms is important. The sooner such surgery can be performed, the less permanent brain damage will occur.

Palpitation

DEFINITION OF PALPITATION

Palpitation is an unpleasant sensation of the heart's action. It may occur whether the heartbeat is slow or fast, regular or irregular, although it occurs more frequently when the heart action is irregular.

CAUSES OF PALPITATION; CLINICAL SIGNIFICANCE

The sensation is thought to be brought about by any unusually forceful closure of the atrioventricular valves; therefore, it can occur in any clinical condition in which there is an increased stroke volume. Some of the more important conditions in which palpitation occurs include extrasystoles, ectopic tachycardias (with the exception of ventricular tachycardia), and other organic heart conditions affecting stroke volume and rate. Thyrotoxicosis, anemia, fever, hypoglycemia, and the ingestion of certain drugs may also be causative factors. The most common cause of palpitation, however, is as a manifestation of the anxiety state. In this condition it is usually transitory in nature, but it may become chronic as in neurocirculatory asthenia.

RATIONALE FOR THE TREATMENT OF PALPITATION

Treatment depends upon the underlying cause. Palpitation of itself is not a diagnostic symptom since it occurs in many conditions, and is usually explained only after a thorough physical examination. If the physician has determined that there is a functional cause for the symptoms, his explanation may be sufficient to reassure the patient of its harmlessness. The true neurasthenic usually is not satisfied with such an explanation, however, and may go from doctor to doctor, convinced that he has a serious heart condition. If palpitation should accompany an organic heart condition, treatment will depend upon the condition present.

THE NURSE'S ROLE IN THE MANAGEMENT OF PALPITATION

Even though palpitation is often functional in nature, a complaint of this symptom should not be overlooked by the nurse and should be reported to the physician along with any other accompanying signs and symptoms. If the physician has determined that the condition is not serious and has explained the probable cause to the patient, further reinforcement will be advisable, for the patient usually feels the need of further discussion with someone who can give him reassurance. Even though there is no serious organic difficulty, such patients are usually very apprehensive.

If the palpitation is due to an anxiety reaction, the person frequently can be taught to control this symptom by breathing very slowly and deeply, and prolonging expiration. This not only focuses his attention on something besides his unpleasant sensation, but actually will slow heart action reflexly and make it nore regular.

The care of patients with heart conditions, including the irregularities of rhythm, is covered in Chapter 23.

Fatigue, Lethargy

DEFINITION OF FATIGUE AND LETHARGY

The terms *fatigue* and *lethargy* usually refer to a feeling of weakness or tiredness. They include a wide variety of conditions that involve a decrement in potential or actual capacity for work. There is usually a loss of interest and ambition and a disinclination to work or even to play; there is difficulty in initiating activity and also in sustaining it.

TYPES OF FATIGUE

Fatigue falls into three distinct categories: (1) Pathological fatigue stems from organic illness. (2) Physiological fatigue results from chemical reactions in the blood, such as an accumulation of the byproducts of muscular activity, depletion of glycogen, and other metabolic changes. (3) Psychological fatigue is the most common kind of fatigue, and accounted for as many as 80 percent of the subjects complaining of fatigue who were studied in several experimental projects. It seems to result from such psychological states as anxiety, boredom, inner conflicts, and similar emotional states.

PATHOPHYSIOLOGY OF FATIGUE

Susceptibility to fatigue depends upon the degree of stability and integration of the whole person. Some authorities believe that one's fatigue pattern is inherited and that there are definite differences in the energy potential of different individuals, probably created by metabolic reserve deficiencies. Symptoms of fatigue may occur with deficiencies of oxygen or glucose in the blood. Disturbances of carbo-hydrate metabolism may be responsible for the glucose deficit. Anoxia may be due to defects of the heart and circulation. Disturbances of regulation of hydrogen ion concentration and the amount and nature of serum calcium, sodium, and potassium are also important factors in fatigue.

"Normal" fatigue appears only after strenuous work (either physical or mental) giving rise to such effects as (1) a series of physiological changes in the body probably produced by chemical changes in the blood, (2) reduced output of work, and (3) subjective feelings of tiredness and weariness and possibly dissatisfaction. With normal fatigue, rest usually restores the person's sense of well-being; with pathological fatigue, one frequently is more tired on rising in the morning than when he went to bed. The psychopathology of fatigue and lethargy is similar to that of nervousness, and they frequently occur together. By far the greatest number of chronic cases of fatigue accompany some type of psychiatric disorder such as manic-depressive psychosis, schizophrenia, and the psychoneuroses (anxiety states, hysteria, obsessive-compulsive states, hypochondriasis, and anorexia nervosa).

Of the organic conditions with which fatigue is associated, neurological and endocrine conditions are the most common. The neurological disorders include (1) cerebrovascular disorders, (2) sequelae to head injury, (3) postencephalitic disorders, (4) multiple sclerosis, and (5) many others in which loss of muscle tone and blocking of sensory pathways may occur.

Among the endocrine disorders that may be responsible for fatigue are the following: (1) Hyper- or hypothyroidism, usually more pronounced in the latter. In marked hypothyroidism lethargy is a prevailing symptom and there is a slowing down of body movements as well. A tendency toward soreness of the muscles also may be noted at times. (2) Pituitary disorders such as hypopituitarism and acromegaly give rise to marked fatigue as does (3) ovarian dysfunction with lack of estrogen production. (4) Testicular dysfunction with lessened production of testosterone has a similar effect. (5) Pancreatic disorders such as hypoglycemia, diabetes mellitus, and carcinoma of the pancreas may be the chief offenders, or the fatigue may be due to (6) adrenocortical deficiency.

Other possible causes include (1) circulatory conditions with cerebral circulatory insufficiency, (2) anemia, (3) nutritional deficiencies, either from lack of proper food intake or from metabolic defects, (4) drug addiction (alcohol, morphine, cocaine, bromides, barbiturates), and (5) aging, with general constitutional changes.

RATIONALE FOR THE TREATMENT OF FATIGUE

With so many possible causes, it is important that the true cause of fatigue be determined. If the cause is physiological as a result of physical or mental over-exertion, additional rest should be advocated in order to prevent possible complications. In times of particular stress, persons may resort to one of the amphetamines, caffeine, or one of the preparations sold at drugstores for the purpose of offsetting drowsiness and lethargy. Such drugs may be useful if the patient is depressed, but should be taken only under medical supervision, for they so mask the symptoms of fatigue that a person may become completely exhausted before realizing that fatigue has occurred.

If fatigue is due to an organic condition, all those conditions already mentioned must be ruled out in order to make an accurate diagnosis. There is very little that can be done to relieve this symptom in the neurological conditions mentioned. Endocrine disorders should be treated by replacement therapy. Nutritional deficiencies are treated by adequate diet and vitamin supplements as indicated. Psychiatric conditions should have adequate treatment.

THE NURSE'S ROLE IN THE MANAGEMENT OF FATIGUE

The exact role of the nurse depends somewhat upon the cause of fatigue. The person suffering fatigue and lethargy needs reassurance, kindness, and sympathetic understanding, with an opportunity to discuss his problems with a perceptive listener. He also needs plenty of additional rest and should be provided with periods of quiet during which he can sleep. If the cause is organic, supportive or replacement therapy usually will be carried out. When the patient is receiving hormones he should be observed for possible symptoms of overdosage.

The nurse may be in a position to be of more assistance to the person suffering from psychological fatigue. If this symptom is not due to an overt psychiatric condition, the patient frequently can be taught to handle his own problems. He should be encouraged to face his situation squarely and to analyze those situations in which fatigue most frequently occurs. He should ask himself, "What are the main stress situations in my life which cause fatigue? When do I possess the most energy during the day? How well do I adapt to trying circumstances?" The answers to these questions may give the proper approach to treatment. It has been suggested that one's daily tasks be so spaced that the most demanding ones coincide with those times when one's energy is at its peak. If this approach is impossible because one has no control over his working conditions, he must try to build up his psychological resistance by positive rather than negative attitudes toward his problems. Mild mental depression frequently can be dissipated by physical exercise. Relaxation can often be attained by taking a walk, listening to quiet music, or engaging in pleasant conversation. The nurse can apply these general principles to her own daily life and has an excellent opportunity to instruct others in their use.

Common Sensations Associated with Fluid and Nutritional Balances

A group of sensations, namely, thirst, hunger, anorexia, nausea, and vomiting, which are associated with the fluid and nutritional balances of the body are described in detail in Chapters 18 and 19.

Conclusion

The unusual sensations discussed in this chapter are the ones which will be most frequently encountered by the nurse. Accurate information about the causes and effects of certain neurological as well as other conditions which cause peculiar sensory symptoms will enable the nurse to collaborate with the physician on a much more intelligent basis, make her own nursing diagnosis more meaningful, and devise more effective plans for nursing care. The ability to correlate such knowledge with the symptoms demonstrated by the patient and with the effects of treatments administered is one of the marks of the professional nurse. Her sympathy, support, and understanding of the patient may be the one factor that stands between the patient and panic or despair at the unknown. Her assistance and instruction can be one of the most important factors in the rehabilitation of such patients, or, if the condition is progressive, in assisting them to meet the future with courage and resignation. If one can help a patient to help himself a little longer, or to develop compensatory mechanisms for deficits that may otherwise be almost completely disabling, including a sound personal philosophy of suffering, it can be a source of tremendous satisfaction to the nurse. Then all expenditure of effort seems well worth while.

Bibliography

General

Boncia, John J.: *The Management of Pain.* Philadelphia: Lea & Febiger, 1954.

Collins, R. Douglas: *Illustrated Manual of Neurological Diagnosis.* Philadelphia: J. B. Lippincott Company, 1962.

Dupratal, Margaret: *A Key to Happiness —The Art of Suffering.* Milwaukee: Bruce Publishing Company, 1943.

Elliott, H. Chandler: *Textbook of Neuroanatomy.* Philadelphia: J. B. Lippincott Company, 1964.

Grollman, Arthur (Ed.): *The Functional*

Pathology of Disease: The Physiologic Basis of Clinical Medicine, 2d ed. New York: McGraw-Hill Book Company, 1963.

Guyton, Arthur C.: *Textbook of Medical Physiology,* 2d ed. Philadelphia: W. B. Saunders Company, 1961.

Guyton, Arthur C.: *Function of the Human Body,* 3d ed. Philadelphia. W. B. Saunders Company, 1969.

Harrison, T. R. (Ed.): *Principles of Internal Medicine,* 5th ed. New York: McGraw-Hill Book Company, 1966.

Lief, H. I., F. V. Lief, and N. R. Lief: *The Psychological Basis of Medical Practice,* New York: Paul B. Hoeber, Inc., 1963.

MacBryde, Cyril M. (Ed.): *Signs and Symptoms: Applied Pathologic Physiology and Clinical Interpretation,* 2d ed. Philadelphia: J. B. Lippincott Company, 1964.

Mayo Clinic and Mayo Foundation: *Clinical Examinations in Neurology,* 2d ed. Philadelphia: W. B. Saunders Company, 1963.

Musser, Ruth D. and Betty Lou Shubkagel: *Pharmacology and Therapeutics,* 3d ed. New York: The Macmillan Company, 1965.

Nodine, J. H. and J. H. Moyer: *Psychosomatic Medicine.* Philadelphia: Lea & Febiger, 1962.

Ochs, Sidney: *Elements of Neurophysiology.* New York: John Wiley & Sons, Inc., 1965.

Peele, Talmage L.: *The Neuroanatomic Basis for Clinical Neurology,* 2d ed. New York: McGraw-Hill Book Company, 1962.

Ruch, T., H. Patton, J. W. Woodbury, and A. L. Towe: *Neurophysiology.* Philadelphia: W. B. Saunders Company, 1961.

Sauerbach, Fred and Hans Wenke: *Pain, Its Meaning and Significance,* 2d ed. London: George Allen & Unwin, Ltd., 1963.

Steegman, A. T.: *Examination of the Nervous System: A Student's Guide,* 2d ed. Chicago: Year Book Medical Publishers, Inc., 1962.

Pain

Agbert, L. D., et al.: Reduction of Postoperative Pain by Encouragement and Instruction of Patients. *New England Journal of Medicine,* 252: 285–327, April 16, 1964.

Alstead, Stanley: Pain and Analgesia: The Philosophic Background. *Practitioner,* 184:5–9, January, 1960.

Bain, Barbara: The Therapeutic Role of the Staff Nurse. *Nursing Forum,* 2:2:10–11, 1963.

Berber, Th. X.: The Effects of Hypnosis on Pain. A Critical Review of Experimental and Clinical Findings. *British Journal of Medical Hypnotism.* 15:4:30–37, 1964.

Dunlap, Marjorie: Pain and Its Alleviation. UCLA School of Nursing Monograph, 1962.

Friedman, Arnold P.: Headache and Allergy. *American Journal of Nursing,* 64:4:117, 1964.

Friedman, Arnold P.: Reflections on the Problems of Headache. *Journal of the American Medical Association,* 190:1:445–447, 1964.

Friedman, Arnold P.: Newer Drugs in the Treatment of Headaches. *Medical Clinics of North America,* 48:2:445–447, March, 1964.

Gillis, Leon: The Management of the Painful Amputation Stump and a New Theory for Phantom Phenomena. *British Journal of Surgery,* 51:88, February, 1964.

Gillis, Leon: Amputation Stump and Phantom Pain. *Modern Medicine,* 37, July, 1964.

Hyman, Robert J.: Commonly Overlooked Causes of Abdominal Pain. *Consultant,* 2:10:37–40, 1962.

Kaufmann, Margaret A. and Dorothy E. Brown: Pain Has Many Faces. *American Journal of Nursing,* 61: 1:48–51, January, 1961.

Master, Arthur M.: the Spectrum of

Anginal and Myocardial Chest Pain. *Journal of the American Medical Association,* 187:12, 1964.

Negrin, J.: Interference with Frontal Lobe Function for the Relief of Intractable Pain. *Journal of the International College of Surgeons,* 42: 516–519, November, 1964.

Petrie, A., W. Collins, and P. Solomon: The Tolerance for Pain and Sensory Deprivation. *American Journal of Psychology,* 73:80–90, March, 1960.

Pope John XXIII: The Meaning of Suffering: A Gift. *The Pope Speaks,* 5:331–334, June, 1959.

Shaw, R. S.: Pathological Malingering: The Painful Disabled Extremity. *New England Journal of Medicine,* 21:1, July 2, 1964.

Sloan, A. B.: Psychological Aspects of Headache. *Canadian Medical Association Journal,* 91:17:905, October, 1964.

Wang, Richard I.: Control of Pain. *American Journal of Medical Science,* 246:590–609, November, 1963.

Zbrowski, Mark: Cultural Components in Response to Pain. *Journal of Social Issues,* 8:16–30, 1952.

Itching (Pruritus)

Carey, J. B. and G. Williams: Therapy for Pruritus of Jaundice. *Journal of the American Medical Association,* 176:432–435, 1961.

Epecki, O. L. and A. N. Okore: A Pattern of Pruritus Due to Chloroquine. *Archives of Dermatology,* 89:631–632, April, 1964.

Epstein, E. and J. Pinski: A Blind Study. *Archives of Dermatology,* 89:631–632, April, 1964.

Scott, O.: The Problem of Pruritus. *Practitioner,* 192:1151:645–651, 1964.

Shelly, W. B. and R. P. Arthur: Neurohistology and Neurophysiology of Itch Sensation in Man. *Archives of Dermatology,* 76:296–323, 1957.

Wilkinson, R. T., et al.: Psychological and Physiological Responses to Raised Body Temperature. *Journal of Applied Psychology,* 19:2:287–291, March, 1964.

Hyperesthesia, Analgesia, and Sensory Deprivation

Bennett, D. R., et al.: Sleep Deprivation: Neurological and Encephalographic Effects. *Areospace Medicine,* 35:9: 888–890, September, 1964.

Benzinger, Theodore H.: Origins of Conscious Sensations of Warm or Cold in Man. *Areospace Medicine,* 34:3:248–249, March, 1963.

Jackson, C. W., J. C. Pollard, and E. W. Kansky: The Application of Findings from Experimental Sensory Deprivation to Cases of Clinical Sensory Deprivation. *American Journal of Medical Science,* 243:558–564, May, 1962.

Kenna, J. C.: Sensory Deprivation Phenomena: Critical Review and Explanatory Models. *Proceedings of the Royal Society of Medicine,* 55:1005–1010, 1962.

Krosnick, Arthur: Diabetic Neuropathy. *American Journal of Nursing,* 64:7: 106, July, 1964.

Leskind, Eugene: A Second Look at Sensory Deprivation. *Digest of Neurology and Psychiatry,* 1964:268, June-July.

Marshall, J.: The Natural History of Transient Ischemic Cerebrovascular Attacks. *Quarterly Journal of Medicine,* 33:131, July, 1964.

Melzak, R. G., G. Rose, and D. McGinty: Skin Sensitivity to Thermal Stimuli. *Areospace Medicine,* 34:3:275, March, 1963.

Pollard, John C., et al.: Studies on Sensory Deprivation. *Archives of General Psychiatry,* 8:435–454, May, 1963.

Pollock, I. W., F. M. Ochberg, and E. Meyer: Effect of Deprivation of Sight on Subjective Time Sense. *Psychosomatic Medicine,* 27:1:71–79, January-February, 1965.

Poser, C. M.: Psychiatric Manifestations

of Cerebrovascular Insufficiency. *Diseases of the Nervous System,* 25:10:611–617, October, 1964.

Reitman, E. E. and S. Cleveland: Changes in Body Image following Sensory Deprivation in Schizophrenia and Control Groups. *Journal of Abnormal and Social Psychology,* 68:2:168–176, 1964.

Zubek, J. P.: Effects of Prolonged Sensory and Perceptual Deprivation. *British Medical Bulletin,* 20:1:38–42, January, 1964.

Zukerman, M., et al.: Stress Response in Total and Partial Perceptual Isolation. *Psychosomatic Medicine,* 26:3:250–256, May-June, 1964.

Vertigo and Dizziness

Barber, H. O.: Positional Nystagmus: Testing and Interpretation. *Transactions of the American Otological Society,* 52:248–268, 1964.

Brown, J. L.: Orientation to the Vertical during Water Immersion. *Areospace Medicine,* 32:209–217, February, 1961.

Cohen, L. A.: Human Spatial Orientation and Its Critical Role in Space Travel. *Areospace Medicine,* 35:11:1054–1057, November, 1964.

Cramer, R. L., P. J. Dowd, and D. B. Helms: Vestibular Responses to Oscillation about the Yaw Axis. *Areospace Medicine,* 34:1031–1034, November, 1963.

Lushman, A. W.: Epidemic Vertigo with Oculomotor Complications. *Lancet,* 1:228, 1955.

Schuhneck, H. F.: The Pathology of Several Disorders of the Inner Ear Which Cause Vertigo. *Southern Medical Journal,* 57:10:1161–1167, October, 1964.

Shuster, Benjamin H.: Dizziness—Your Body's Warning Light. *Today's Health,* 41:2:50, February, 1963.

Faintness and Palpitation

Elrick, H., et al.: Plasma Insulin Response to Oral and Intravenous Glucose Administration. *Journal of Clinical Endocrinology and Metabolism,* 24:2:1076, 1964.

George, W. K., et al.: Hyperventilation and Serum Calcium. *New England Journal of Medicine,* 272:4:214, January 28, 1965.

Leeman, C. P.: Neurocirculatory Asthenia. *New England Journal of Medicine,* 272:16:862 April 22, 1965.

Miller, Perry B., et al.: Modifications of the Effects of Two Weeks Bed Rest Upon Circulatory Functions in Man. *Areospace Medicine,* 35:10:931–938, 1964.

Strano, L. J., et al.: Adrenal Response to Hypoglycemia. *Endocrinology,* 74: 656–657, 1965.

Wachenberg, B., et al.: On the Mechanism of Insulin Hypersensitivity in Adrenocortical Insufficiency. *Diabetes,* 13:2:169–176, March-April, 1964.

Fatigue and Lethargy

Gambill, E. E.: Doctor, Why am I So Tired? *Postgraduate Medicine,* September, 1964.

Hausberger, D. and I. Rodbard: Relation between Pain and Fatigue in Contracting Ischemic Muscle. *American Journal of Cardiology,* 8:481–484, 1961.

Neylon, Margaret P.: Anxiety. *American Journal of Nursing,* 62:5:110–111, May, 1962.

Pierson, W. R. and A. Lockhard: Fatigue, Work Decrement and Endurance of Women in a Simple Repetitive Task. *Areospace Medicine,* 35:8:724–795, 1964.

Roberts, Hyman: Fatigue as an Elusive Organic Problem. *Consultant,* 64:5: 30–33, 1964.

CHAPTER 16
VARIATIONS FROM EXPECTED STATE OF ALERTNESS

WILDA G. CHAMBERS*

* William Hunt, M.D., Chairman of the Department of Neurosurgery, The Ohio State University, acted as consultant in the preparation of this chapter.

Man is distinguished from other animals by his marked ability to adapt to changing circumstances. His intelligence enables him to know what is going on and his part in it. He is watchful and ready to act. The biologist calls this state of man *awareness;* the psychologist, *alertness.* Both may refer to it as *consciousness.* Variations from this state may be minimal or maximal and may last minutes, months, or even years. Coma, stupor, delirium, and confusion have been identified by some authors as variations from alertness. The limits of these variations are not discrete, and use of these terms in describing patient behavior is discouraged for that reason.

The content of this chapter is primarily concerned with nursing the patient who is unconscious. If the nurse can give effective care to the unconscious patient, she can make appropriate modifications for the person whose symptoms indicate partial consciousness.

Consciousness and Unconsciousness

Consciousness is associated with brain function, and is concerned with awareness and responsiveness. It involves many kinds of nervous activity. In normal circumstances we are, actually or potentially, conscious of sights, sounds, touch, smell, anger, fear, interest, excitement, memories, ideas, thoughts, images, sleepiness. In abnormal circumstances consciousness may include disordered sensations like pain and giddiness; disordered perceptions such as illusions and hallucinations; and disordered memories and ideational states (Brain, 1958). Consciousness is maintained in amnesia, dreams, hypnotic reveries, and daydreams (Abramson, 1951). Sleep is cited as an example of both consciousness and unconsciousness, or as intermittent unconsciousness (Lennox). Normally, sleep is characterized by a loss of critical reaction to stimuli of the environment (Brock and Krieger). Kleitman believes that consciousness occurs in sleep as well as in wakefulness (Abramson, 1954). These concepts of consciousness have been highlighted in this introduction in the hope that the reader will be motivated to study them further.

Consciousness is maintained through a neural network believed to originate in the thalamus and the cerebral cortex. It is thought that the thalamus sorts out and interprets the afferent impulses from receptors for heat, cold, pain, touch, and muscle sense and the cerebral cortex is concerned with interpretation of refined impulses (Carlson et al.). Brain in 1958 stated that consciousness occurs as a result of the integrative neural process of the cerebral cortex which in turn is dependent upon the integrity of diencephalic and brain stem activity. Walter believes that at least six interacting systems are concerned with sensation and consciousness: (1) specific afferent pathways, (2) devious paralemniscal byways passing through the brain stem reticular formations, (3) pyramidal motor thoroughfare, (4) parapyramidal detours, (5) reticular traffic and route controls with ascending and descending patrols, (6) central censorship channels whereby the central mechanisms block or promote access to themselves in varying circumstances.

Allen concluded that full consciousness and higher cerebral activities were dependent upon integration and communication between the cerebral cortex, the higher brain stem, and the hypothalamus and other structures near it.

Unconsciousness results from impairment of the neural system that maintains consciousness. Something has altered the functioning of the alerting system. A number of conditions may impair consciousness, and these will be described in Part V. For quick reference, Sears suggests the following list of representative causes:

A   alcohol, apoplexy, anesthesia, angina
E   epilepsy, eclampsia, encephalitis, electricity
I   injury, insulin, infection
O   opium and other poisons
U   uremia
D   diabetes, drowning

What causes an individual to lose consciousness? The causative factors are ischemia, toxemia, and compression of the brain stem. The brain is a very active organ and requires a continuous and abundant supply of oxygen and nutrients to function and to survive. If the brain is denied oxygen for even a few minutes, mental and physical impairment follows. Some authorities say that the maximum time the brain cells can survive without oxygen is 2 minutes; others, 3 to 4 minutes. Toxemia is caused by invading microorganisms (as in encephalitis) or disturbances of acid-base balance (as in uremia, diabetes). Compression of the brain stem is brought about by the pressure of edema, a blood clot, or by an abnormal growth.

In summary, consciousness means awareness of or responsiveness to the environment. It is dependent upon an intact neural system. When the intactness of the neural system is interrupted and severely damaged, unconsciousness occurs. There are degrees of consciousness and unconsciousness, but these degrees are not always exactly measurable. Therefore, the nurse's written and verbal observations should provide a complete and vivid description of the patient's status at a given time.

Nursing Care of the Unconscious Patient

The nurse has unlimited opportunity to test her skills in three chief areas of nursing practice in the care of unconscious patients. These areas are *observation, ministration,* and *communication.* The nurse needs to know what to look for and how to observe. Her observations provide her with certain information she needs in order to plan her nursing care and to evaluate the effectiveness of what she has done. In addition, the information she collects helps the physician in establishing a diagnosis or in determining the prognosis. The specific observations that the nurse is expected to make, report, and record are elaborated upon in the next several paragraphs.

EVALUATION OF THE NEUROLOGICAL STATUS
OF THE PATIENT

The nurse's evaluation of the neurological status of a patient involves testing certain sensory and motor functions of the nervous system and observing and/or

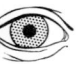
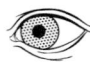

Figure 16–1
Right eye does not devi-
ate centrally. Cranial
nerve VI involved.

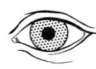

Figure 16–2
Note miosis of right pupil
and mild ptosis of eye-
lid. Sympathetic paraly-
sis.

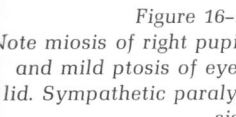
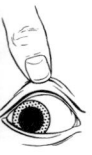
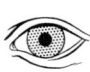

Figure 16–3
Right pupil dilated and
may be fixed. Eye is di-
rected downward and
outward. There may be
partial or complete
ptosis of eyelid. Cranial
nerve III involved.

measuring others (Table 16-1). The material pertains to adults, although it is applicable to children who are 6 years of age and older.

These tests are considered specific for determining the patient's status on the continuum of consciousness to unconsciousness. Additional data are needed, however, to complete the picture. These data include measurements of temperature, pulse, respiration, and blood pressure, and observations of certain body functions. This series of measurements and observations is listed in Table 16-2 along with the possible findings. As they are read, the student should think about the physiology of the central and autonomic nervous systems and try to predict the measurements in a given pathologic condition. She might ask herself, for example, what the measurements of temperature, pulse, respiration, and blood pressure might be in insulin shock. What would the condition of the skin be in insulin shock? Why does the patient who has had a complete stroke have a slightly elevated temperature, slurred speech, and incontinence of urine and stool?

Convulsions may occur because of oxygen and glucose deficits, acid-base imbalance, and edema. Laboratory reports may give clues about the possibility of convulsions, particularly the reports pertaining to the electroencephalogram, blood sugar, and urinalysis. In addition, the nurse watches for convulsions whenever the patient has a progressive elevation of blood pressure, nausea and vomiting, somnolence, mental confusion, and muscular twitchings. Details about observation of the patient while he is in a convulsive state are given in Chapter 29.

A partial or complete neurological evaluation is done at intervals. The frequency with which it is to be done is usually prescribed by the physician. If he does not prescribe the frequency, evaluation is made every hour as long as there is a fluctuation in any of the signs or symptoms. When significant changes occur, the nurse assumes responsibility for repeating the evaluation as often as necessary to collect enough information to show what is happening. In all cases, the complete evaluation should be made at the beginning and end of each 8-hour shift or of each tour of duty to determine whether the patient's condition has improved, worsened, or stabilized.

The nurse is not expected to interpret the meaning of all the information procured from her evaluation, but she is expected to recognize significant findings and bring them to the physician's attention. Fluctuations or rapid changes in any of the factors are of significance. Headache, dizziness, vomiting, convulsions, and memory loss are also indicative of significant change in the patient's status. According to Thompson, memory is the chief criterion for determining whether a person is fully conscious or in automatism (possessed of all faculties except recall), and Allen supports this judgment.

Communication about the patient's state is apt to be clearer when specific descriptive information is reported or recorded. For example, the notation, "At 12:30 A.M. patient tried to get out of bed; wants to get his breakfast," is more descriptive than "Patient seems confused, restless, thirsty."

In his book, *Episode*, Eric Hodgins describes quite vividly the medical neurological examinations he underwent while being treated for a cerebrovascular accident. He tells how he came to hate the words *Wednesday* and *electricity* as he was asked to say them so frequently. Other patients probably have similar feelings. Explanation of why one is testing helps to alleviate such feelings.

TABLE 16-1
*Tests to Determine
Neurological Status*

TEST	METHOD	OBSERVATION AND RECORDING	STRUCTURES TESTED
Eye response (See Figures 16-1 to 16-3)	If eyes are closed, try to open by lifting upper lid with thumb	Note speed of closure; whether there is a blink, flicker, or tremor of eyelids in response to light, sudden movement, or sudden noise	Cranial nerves III (oculomotor), IV (trochlear), VI (abducens)
Pupillary response	Have patient look at distant object and cover one eye; flash light from flashlight in other eye; repeat for opposite eye	Normally, pupils are central, equal in size, and constrict in response to light; abnormally, pupils may be constricted and respond to light or may be dilated and not respond to light	Cranial nerve III (parasympathetic fibers)
Motor ability	Observe for movements in absence of stimulus	Movements may be aimless or be automatic, e.g., rubbing the chin constantly; there may be tremors, twitching, spasms; patient may be immobile; musculature may be flaccid or normal.	Motor area of cerebral cortex, pyramidal and extrapyramidal tracts
	Have patient hold arms straight out in front with palms up	Note whether both arms can be kept in this position or whether there is pronator drift (forearm turns so that palm of hand faces downward)	
	Have patient flex knees and keep them slightly apart; request patient to wink, stick out tongue, wrinkle his nose and forehead, and smile	Note whether lower extremities can be maintained in this position or whether they drift to the side; note ability to comply with these requests and whether there is similar response on both sides of the face	Cranial nerves V (trigeminal), VII (facial), IX (glossopharyngeal), X (vagus), XI (hypoglossal)
Response to painful stimuli	Prick with pin or apply pressure over root of fingernail or grasp small bit of skin on inner aspect of arm and twist	Normally, the person will flinch or try to withdraw from the stimulus	Somatic sensory area of cerebral cortex
Response to questions relating to orientation	Call name in normal tones; progress to a shout and at the same time shake patient;	May respond, may only open eyes, may make no response	Frontal and temporal areas of cerebral cortex
	Ask him to state his name, where he is, the date, the time of day	Note which of these he can do	

FACTOR	POSSIBLE FINDINGS
Pulse	Rapid to slow; bounding to feeble
Respirations	Slow, deep, irregular, stertorous; thoracic or abdominal in origin or alternation from one to the other
Temperature	Subnormal to elevated
Blood pressure	Shock level to elevated
Skin	Moist to dry; warm to cold
Sphincter control	Loss or partial loss of control of urinary bladder or anal sphincters
Verbalization	Groans, mutters, unable to form words; slurred speech
Emotional response	Tendency to stubbornness; quick to anger; inappropriate laughter
Intellectual response	Memory impaired or lost; judgment faulty; responses vague or absent; retells stories as if they were personal experiences

TABLE 16-2
*Measurement of
Neurological Status*

MINISTRATIONS

The unconscious patient is completely dependent on others for maintenance of his physiological status. Function of all body systems must be maintained and he must be fed. He must be protected from harm. At the same time every effort must be made to help him become oriented and move toward the conscious state.

Positioning and Turning

The pulmonary tree must be kept free of drainage so that oxygen and carbon dioxide exchange can occur. This can be accomplished through positioning the patient so the tongue falls forward, turning him from side to side, and aspirating secretions or encouraging him to cough. Except in the case of certain head injuries or a specific decision by the physician, the patient is kept on one side with his head raised 15 to 20 degrees. The head should be lowered periodically to permit clearance of the bronchi. Care should be taken to ensure free excursion of the thorax. The patient should be turned every hour and at the same time helped to cough. Slapping him on the back stimulates coughing. Aspiration may be necessary to clear the bronchi of mucus or to stimulate coughing. If a tracheostomy has been done, aseptic technique is to be observed during aspiration (Plum and Dunning). If both nasal and tracheal catheters are used, they should be maintained separately. Therefore, set-ups for both the nasal catheter and the tracheal catheter are essential. If airways are used, these must be removed, cleansed, and replaced at least once a day and more often if necessary.

Care of the Skin

Constant vigilance is necessary to keep the skin intact and in a healthy state. The skin is likely to break down for several reasons. There is pressure against it because the patient is confined to bed. Lack of muscle tone causes the body to become a dead weight. Flaccid muscles do not maintain the usual muscle mass between bones and skin and, in time, muscles tend to atrophy with disuse. Circulation is decreased because the patient is not active. There may be insufficient protein intake and incontinence of urine and stool; these increase the likelihood of skin breakdown. The occurrence of decubitus ulcers is often attributed to poor nursing care. This is not always the case, as these ulcers may occur in spite of meticulous nursing. In a study of 35 patients, Mulholland found that protein metabolism plays an important role in the occurrence of decubitus ulcers. Avoidance of pressure is the key to effective skin care. Husain found that pressure distributed evenly over a large area of the body is much less damaging to the tissues than localized or point pressure, and that low pressure maintained for long periods of time produces more tissue damage than high pressure for short periods. The time factor is more important than pressure intensity. The shearing force[1] that occurs when the head of the bed is raised and the weight shifts to the sacrum has been pointed out as an example of pressure intensity. Pressure against the ischial tuberosities is increased when the head of the bed is elevated, and the pressure is even greater when the patient is sitting upright in a chair (Reichel).

The pressure-relieving measures necessary in a given case can be easily assessed by sliding one's hand between the patient's body and the bed. Wherever there is space for the hand, the space should be filled with soft padding of some kind.[2] This padding distributes the pressure over a larger area and obviates point pressure. Synthetic or natural sheepskins, silicone gel pads, alternating pressure mattresses and chair pads, and foam rubber pads are useful for relieving pressure. Because wrinkles and crumbs also create pressure, the bed linen should be taut and free of extraneous particles.

The frequency for turning a patient to alleviate pressure is determined by the nurse, the guideline for this being the length of time required for pressure signs to appear and disappear. It may be necessary to turn the patient as often as every 15 minutes in order to prevent pressure signs. He should remain in a given position no more than 2 hours, even though his skin shows no redness. Some evidence suggests that skin breakdown tends to occur when there is constant pressure for 2 hours. Since the side position is the recommended one for the unconscious bedridden patient, the use of half-lateral and full-lateral positions permits four changes.

The skin is washed as necessary to keep it clean. Nondrying soaps, bath oils, and body lotions are useful to maintain normal state and prevent dryness. When the skin is dry, breaks may occur in the epidermis and permit microorganisms to enter.

Whenever the patient is turned, the nurse should make certain that his position assures good body alignment. Precautions against contractures must be taken and the hips and feet supported in order to prevent external hip rotation and foot drop. The upper extremities should be kept slightly abducted to prevent the development of a frozen shoulder, and the fingers should be supported with a hand roll to prevent contracture of the fingers.

---

[1] The sacral skin remains relatively fixed because of friction of the skin and bed. Tissue between the skin and superficial fascia is interlocked and unyielding. The deeper portion of the superficial fascia is rather loose and mobile in the sacral region and it slides easily in relation to the deep fascia, which is well anchored. The shearing force is concentrated in the deeper portion of the superficial fascia; this stretches the blood vessels and may lead to angulation.

[2] Suggestion made by William Hunt, M.D., Professor and Chairman of the Department of Neurosurgery, The Ohio State University.

Bladder and Bowel Function

There is apt to be urinary incontinence with motor loss and bladder distention with sensory loss. In either case an indwelling catheter is usually ordered. When this is so, maintenance of the drainage system is to be carried out in a manner to prevent infection. Assurance of dependent drainage, constant bladder rinse, and avoidance of long use of a catheter are considered preventive measures. Of course none of these measures will be effective if a faulty technique is used in inserting the catheter. The amount of fluid intake and the urinary output should be checked to see if they are approximately equal. The urine should be examined for deviation from the normal straw color and clear appearance.

It is the nurse's responsibility to observe for adequate bowel elimination. Incontinence follows motor loss, and oozing or impaction may follow sensory loss. Impaction can be avoided by procuring orders for and administering medication when necessary. Wetting agents such as dioctyl sodium sulfosuccinate (Colase), oil-based rectal suppositories, or low pressure enemas have all been found to be effective for bowel elimination. Knowledge of the usual frequency and time of bowel elimination is helpful in making plans for the use of aids to elimination.

If drug intoxication is the cause of unconsciousness, urine and vomitus should be saved for analysis of the drug level.

Prevention of Muscle Atrophy

Nonuse of muscles leads to loss of tone and stiffness of joints. Putting the extremities through full range of motion exercises twice a day is sufficient to prevent these occurrences. Passive exercise promotes circulation and helps to prevent thrombus formation. Chair sitting may be prescribed, particularly if the unconscious state is prolonged, to relieve pressure areas caused by bed rest and to serve as a stimulus in orientation toward wellness. The patient should be positioned so that there is no pressure on the popliteal area. A chair that has a back high enough to support the head is preferable, but such support can be improvised if one is not available. In these situations, special attention must be given to keeping the patient upright and to preventing falls from the chair. A bath blanket or a narrow cotton strap can be used to provide this security. If the strap is used, it should be centered at the back of the neck; each end should be brought forward and under an arm, and tied at the back of the chair. An alternating pressure pad or a 2-inch foam rubber pad on the seat permits a longer period in the chair. Kosiak measured the magnitude and distribution of pressure at the skin surface over the entire sitting area of subjects on various types of chairs and found that the pressure was over 300 mm mercury in the area of the tuberosities on unpadded flat and contour surfaces. The pressure under the tuberosities decreased to 160 mm mercury when a 2-inch foam rubber pad was used on a flat surface. The 2-inch foam rubber was effective in distributing pressure to all sitting surfaces. Pressure in the average range of capillary pressure[3] is provided by using a contour chair

---

[3] The average blood pressure in an arteriolar limb is 23 mm mercury; at the end of the loop, 20 mm; and at the venous end, 12 mm (Landis, 1930).

equipped with an alternating pressure pad cycled to permit intermittent circulation to the area (Kosiak). The skin should be examined for redness and marks that denote pressure during and at the end of the sitting period. Support for the arms can be provided by a table or overchair board. Sandbags or blocks under the front legs of a chair tilt it backward and thus help to keep the patient in better alignment.

Care of Eyes, Nose, and Throat

The eyes should be examined for dryness and signs of inflammation. If these are present, the physician should be notified. He will probably prescribe an ointment, a lubricant, and/or irrigations. The cornea should be protected from dirt and other particles as long as the eye is insensitive. A shield made from x-ray film can be used for this purpose. The physician may suture the eyelids together, or the lids may be approximated with a butterfly tape (deGutierrez-Mahoney and Carini).

The nostrils must be kept free of crusts and lubricated as necessary. If a nasogastric tube is in the nose, the opening of the nostril should be frequently lubricated. A water-soluble lubricant is used in case a droplet should get into the tracheobronchial tree. Oil droplets are not absorbed readily by lung tissue.

Mouth care must be given often enough to keep the mucous membranes moist and free of debris. Oral hygiene is more effective when the teeth, gums, and tongue are brushed rather than swabbed.[4] It is necessary to use a water-soluble lubricant for all the mucous membranes of the mouth and the lips. If a patient wears dentures, these should be removed if there is motor loss of the facial muscles, since there is danger that the dentures will become dislodged and occlude the airway.

Nutritional State

Usually the unconscious patient is fed intravenously at first and by a nasogastric tube later. Tube feedings include any mixture of foods liquid enough to pass through a nasogastric tube. Generally, they include puréed meat, fruit, and vegetables, milk and milk products, cream, eggs, and vitamins. Foods from regular diets are being used increasingly for tube feedings since electric blenders have become available. When food is liquefied in a blender, the fiber content is preserved and normal bowel function is aided (Arkansas Diet Manual). In some institutions the nurse is responsible for inserting the nasogastric tube. If so, she must verify that the tube is actually in the stomach. Even when the nurse does not have to pass the tube initially, it is essential that she verify that the tube is in the stomach before each feeding. Verification may be made by withdrawing some gastric fluid and testing it on litmus paper (Ansell). The contents of the stomach are normally acid, and the litmus paper should turn red. It is also recommended that the nurse listen for epigastric gurgle with a stethoscope (Meyers). About 30 ml of water is given prior to the feeding, and 60 to 100 ml of water after the feeding. Water should be given before the feeding to test the patency of the tube, and after the

---

[4] Brushing is not done if the patient has a blood dyscrasia or a gum disorder.

feeding to rinse the tube and prevent accumulation of food particles that would attract pathogens. The physician prescribes the total number of calories and amount to be fed for the 24-hour period. He also specifies the amount and frequency of single feedings. Ordinarily, the feedings are ordered to be given at 3-to-4-hour intervals and in amounts of 300 to 350 ml. If the feedings for the 24-hour period are stored in one container, the container is shaken well before a single feeding is poured. After the single feeding is poured, the remainder is returned to the re-frigerator immediately. Putting single feedings in separate containers at the time of preparation is helpful. Single feedings should be warmed to body temperature before they are given to the patient; they are said to be tolerated better when warm rather than cold. A patient's tolerance to tube feedings can be established by giving him one-third of the total feeding on the first day; one-half on the second day; and the total amount on the third day. Giving the total feeding more rapidly than this, or giving single feedings too rapidly or in too large amounts, may cause diarrhea and/or distention. Special care must be taken against aspiration when the patient is hyperactive. Special care also must be given to the intake of water when the patient is receiving high-protein feedings. If sufficient water is not given, azotemia may develop (Pareira). Comfortable anchorage of the nasogastric tube is accomplished by securing the tube to the nose with a Y-shaped piece of adhesive or Micropore tape and then carrying the tube across the cheek, under the ear lobe, and up behind the ear to the forehead. After the tube has been bent back on itself and secured with a rubber band, it is anchored to the forehead with trans-parent or Micropore tape (deGutierrez-Mahoney and Carini). Disposable naso-gastric tubes are recommended, since the inner surface of any tubing is difficult to clean and the cost of these tubes is about the same as for rubber tubing. A question is often asked about the length of time a nasogastric tube should remain in place. Erb has recommended that the tube be removed only when necessary for the patient's comfort and safety. According to Pereira, polyvinyl nasogastric tubes can be left in place for 4 months without clogging or causing irritation. However, rubber connections, glass drips, and containers must be cleansed and replaced every 24 hours.

Control of the Environment

The patient's room must be kept free of drafts and warm enough for comfort. If he is elderly, it may be necessary to maintain a higher room temperature than is usual.

If the patient has a marked temperature elevation or is given hypothermia therapy, the top bed covers are removed. A bikini is used to cover the genitalia, and a towel to cover the breasts in women.

The patient's restlessness or hyperactivity may be controlled by providing a quiet environment and offering reassuring verbalization. Restraint ordinarily increases rather than decreases restlessness. Soft restraints may be used in situa-tions where a gentle reminder is insufficient for achieving quietness and protection from self-harm. Side rails are used to provide security; they should be padded in case the patient comes in contact with them. if the patient is noisy, he should be placed in a soundproof room for the benefit of other patients. If such accommodations are not available, he may be placed in a section of the nursing unit where the fewest patients are located.

Every procedure requires attention to the safety of the unconscious patient. Bed rails are kept up to prevent falls from the bed. When the patient is sitting in a chair, falling is prevented by anchoring the chair and tying the patient in. Precautions are taken to prevent aspiration into the tracheobronchial tree, to avoid pressure to prominent body points, and to guard against infection and trauma. For patients who regain consciousness but are depressed, sharp objects or other items that could be used in suicidal attempts are removed from the room or locked in a safe place in the room. If convulsions are likely to occur, a padded mouth gag should be taped to the head of the bed or some other place where it is clearly visible. The gag is taped loosely so that it can be grasped quickly. A transparent container can be attached to the head of the bed and used as a holder for the gag.

COMMUNICATION

It can never be assumed that the unconscious patient is unable to hear. All verbal communication in his presence should be made as though every word might be heard. Hearing is one of the last senses to be lost with unconsciousness, if not the last one. Variance in the sequence and duration of consciousness and unconsciousness has been found (Allen). We cannot be sure where the patient is on the continuum between consciousness and unconsciousness at any given time. Thus, the nurse explains in simple terms what she is about to do for and to the patient. As he becomes more alert the nurse expands her explanations and constantly tests his ability to comprehend. If there is aphasia, particular attention must be given to ways of teaching the patient how to redevelop his speaking skill. In some situations the nurse may have the main responsibility for this teaching, but in most situations the help of a speech therapist can be obtained. The needs of the patient will be met insofar as the plan of nursing care is agreed to and communicated to all who are involved in implementing the plan. Likewise, nursing observations are useful to others insofar as they are reported and recorded.

Bibliography

Abramson, Harold A. (Ed.): *Problems of Consciousness.* Transactions of the Second Conference March 19–20, 1951. New York: Josiah Macy, Jr. Foundation, 1951.

Abramson, Harold A. (Ed.): *Problems of Consciousness.* Transactions of the Fifth Conference March 22, 23, and 24, 1954. New York: Josiah Macy, Jr. Foundation, 1954.

Allen, I. M.: Dissociation of the Conscious State and Its Content with Special Reference to Cortical and Total Brain Function. *New Zealand Medical Journal,* 59:102–110, February, 1960.

Ansell, Susan E. A.: Feeding the Unconscious Patient. *Nursing Times,* 60:311–312, March, 1964.

Arkansas Diet Manual, 3d ed. Little Rock, Arkansas: Nutrition Service Arkansas State Board of Health, 1962.

Baker, A. B. (Ed.): *Clinical Neurology,*

2d ed. Vol. I. New York: Harper & Brothers, 1962.

Brain, Russell: The Physiological Basis of Consciousness. *Brain,* 81:426–455, 1958.

Brain, W. R.: *Clinical Neurology,* 2d ed. New York: Oxford University Press, 1964.

Brock, Samuel and Howard P. Krieger: *The Basis of Clinical Neurology,* 4th ed. Baltimore: The Williams and Wilkins Company, 1963.

Butts, Clarence L. and Vesta E. Carney: The Unresponsive Patient. *American Journal of Nursing,* 67:1886–1887, September, 1967.

Carlson, Anton J., Victor Johnson, and H. Mead Cavert: *The Machinery of the Body,* 5th ed. Chicago: University of Chicago Press, 1961.

Cipriano, Mary Elizabeth: A Study of Ten Nurses' Performance and Understanding of the Craniotomy Check Procedure while Caring for Selected Neurological and Neurosurgical Patients. Unpublished Master's Thesis. Columbus, Ohio: Department of Nursing, The Ohio State University, 1963.

deGutierrez-Mahoney, C. G. and Esta Carini: *Neurological and Neurosurgical Nursing,* 4th ed. St. Louis: The C. V. Mosby Company, 1965.

Erb, Alma, et al.: Nasal Gavage. *American Journal of Nursing,* 51:39–40, January, 1951.

Fason, M. Fitzpatrick: Controlling Bacterial Growth in Tube Feedings. *American Journal of Nursing,* 67: 1246–1247, June, 1967.

Ganong, William F.: *Review of Medical Physiology,* 3d ed. Los Altos, Calif.: Lange Medical Publications, 1967.

Goldie, L. and J. M. Green: Changes in Mode of Respiration as an Indication of Level of Consciousness. *Nature,* 189:581–582, February 18, 1961.

Hodgins, Eric: *Episode.* New York: Atheneum Publishers, 1964.

Husain, Tafuzzul: An Experiental Study of Some Pressure Effects on Tissues with Reference to Bedsore Problem. *Journal of Pathology and Bacteriology,* 66:347–358, October, 1953.

Kosiak, Michael, et al.: Evaluation of Pressure as a Factor in the Prediction of Ischial Ulcers. *Archives of Physical Medicine and Rehabilitation,* 39:623–629, October, 1958.

Lendis, Eugene: Micro-Injection Studies of Capillary Blood Pressure in Human Skin. *Heart,* 15:209–228, 1930.

Martin, Christopher M. and Edward N. Bookrajian: Bacteriuria Prevention after Indwelling Urinary Catheterization. *Archives of Internal Medicine,* 110:703–711, November, 1962.

Meyers, Mary Emma: Nursing the Comatose Patient. *American Journal of Nursing,* 54:716–718, June, 1954.

Mulholland, J. H., et al.: Protein Metabolism and Bed Sores. *Annals of Surgery,* 118:1015–1023, December, 1943.

O'Leary, James L. and William M. Landau: Coma and Convulsion. in Cyril Mitchell MacBryde (Ed.): *Signs and Symptoms: Applied Pathologic Physiology and Clinical Interpretation,* 4th ed. Philadelphia: J. B. Lippincott Company, 1964.

Pareira, Morton D., et al.: Therapeutic Nutrition with Tube Feeding. *Journal of the American Medical Association,* 156:810–816, October 30, 1954.

Plum, F. and M. F. Dunning: Technics for Minimizing Trauma to the Tracheobronchial Tree after Tracheostomy. *New England Journal of Medicine,* 254:193–200, February 2, 1956.

Poynter, F. N. L.: *The History and Philosophy of Knowledge of the Brain and Its Functions.* Springfield, Ill.: Charles C Thomas, Publisher, 1957.

Reichel, Samuel M.: Shearing Force as a Factor in Decubital Ulcers in Paraplegics. *Journal of the American Medical Association,* 166:762–763, February 15, 1958.

Schiffmann, Wanda: Neurological Evaluation of the Child. *Canadian Nurse,*

57:329–334; 462–466, April and May, 1961.

Sears, Gordon: The Management of the Unconscious Patient. *Practitioner,* 187:41–45, July, 1961.

Stevenson, Joanne C.: *Tracheostomy Suctioning—An Experimental Study.* Columbus, Ohio: Research Founda-

tion, The Ohio State University, 1967.

Thompson, Raymond K.: Head Injuries. *Maryland State Medical Journal,* 12:101–103, March, 1963.

Walter, W. Gray: The Control of Consciousness. *Anaesthesia,* 15:105–122, April, 1960.

CHAPTER 17
ABNORMAL BEHAVIORAL RESPONSES

VIRGINIA L. EARLES

The behavior of patients doubtless presents the greatest potential for an infinite variety of any category of data with which the nurse deals. At the same time, the behavioral responses during illness or hospitalization are the responses regarding which the nurse has the greatest responsibility for appropriate reaction and the greatest opportunity for assisting the patient. The vast potential for the seemingly endless variety of human behavior and the nurse's responsibility for acting in response to behavior demand a framework for use in classifying the observed behavior and making some reasonable diagnosis as to its source and meaning.

Fortunately there is sufficient repetition of common elements as well as a limitation to man's ability to express himself behaviorally which make it possible to develop a framework for viewing behavioral responses. An experienced clinician is aware of this. The repeated patterns of behavior and what has been learned about them add much to one's diagnostic ability in a new situation. This chapter proposes a way of thinking about behavior of patients which will assist the nurse to consider all possible facets and to respond effectively.

Sources of Patient Behavior

Human behavior is described and explained in many frameworks. The particular frame of reference for the psychologist, the neurologist, or the sociologist facilitates theoretical development and research in the field. The professional person working with the patient must appreciate that his overt behavior is influenced by forces included in the theories of all these fields of study. The emotional feeling of the patient, which is influenced by his psychological development, must be expressed through his neurophysiological system. Expression of emotion in behavior therefore can be altered or blocked by altered function of the neurophysiological system. Similarly, neurological malfunction may cause behavior that mimics behavior usually thought of as psychological in origin.

The six major areas to be considered as sources of overt human behavior among patients are (1) neurological status, (2) metabolic status, (3) degree of physical comfort, (4) intellectual capacity, (5) psychological state, and (6) culture or learned behavior. None of these factors controls behavior exclusively; each, however, is extremely important in explaining the observed behavior.

NEUROLOGICAL DISTURBANCES

Behavior that seems abnormal may be due to organic lesions of the central nervous system, particularly the brain. Often this potential source of behavior change is overlooked unless one works with a patient population in which this type of problem occurs frequently. One of the areas in which change occurs most frequently is intellectual activity. This kind of change is associated with cerebral damage or dysfunction. The intellectual changes are difficult to detect since they usually are slowly progressive. The patient attempts to compensate for his losses in an effort to deny them to himself and to prevent others from learning about them. The most frequent and earliest intellectual deficit due to organic cerebral injury is loss of memory. This loss is retrogressive in nature. Memory for the most recent events and most recently acquired information is the poorest. Memory for events or learned facts from previous years is much better. This is true of patients with localized damage to the brain, such as a tumor, or of older persons whose cerebral functioning is poor as a result of circulatory or degenerative changes. This type of memory loss can be determined by the patient's ability to remember the most recent events, such as what he ate at a recent meal, names of persons around him, what he did the night before. The patient may attempt to compensate for this loss by getting others to "fill in the gaps." He may ask questions or respond to questions in such a way that someone else will provide the information. The patient might say, "The nurse who brought my breakfast was very nice!" The respondent says, "Oh, you mean Miss B." The patient now knows the name for the moment and can call Miss B. by name.

The second major area of deficit in intellectual functioning is conceptualization and abstract thinking. The patient can understand and react to concrete objects, directions, or actions, but cannot relate these to their larger context. For example, he may be able to recognize an object as an apple or a peach but not to move from that to a higher level of abstraction, and understand that they are fruits. Or, the patient may recognize that his meal contains no sugar or dessert but cannot connect this with the concept of sugar consumption being related to a disease process. This kind of deficit is usually associated with other evidence of severe neurological deficit and is particularly evident in some forms of aphasia, since language and high levels of concept formation are so fully integrated in the nervous system.

Another early manifestation of difficulty with intellectual activities is loss of simple mathematical ability. This function is studied whenever a complete neurological examination is done. It can be detected by the patient's ability to subtract when he cannot rely on his memory of addition or multiplication tables, as determined by the direction: "Subtract 7 from 100," or by evidence of difficulty with monetary change or the number of pills remaining.

The second major area of behavioral change related to organic brain disease is affect, or mood manifestations. Most common is the tendency toward emotional lability: quick shifts from sadness to elation, sudden anger or rage, outbursts of laughter and gaiety. Also characteristic is an inappropriate response, such as laughing in a serious situation and crying when happy events occur. This kind of lability and inappropriate response occur also in certain psychotic states. The neurological source for this kind of emotional response is the hypothalamus. The damage may be to the hypothalamus directly, or there may be disturbed interaction between the cerebrum and the hypothalamus. If the damage is hypothalamic, there may be other evidence for this source, such as alterations in appetite, sexual aggressiveness, and sleep patterns. Since most manifestations of this behavior seem unrestrained and unrelated to reality, the behavior can be threatening to persons working with the patients unless those persons understand the source of the behavior.

The third general area of behavioral change related to organic brain disease is the capacity for handling sensory intake. The most frequent manifestation of alteration in this area is evidenced by disorientation and misinterpretation of sensory stimuli. Alterations usually arise from circulatory disturbance, degenerative change due to aging, toxic states, or extreme emotional states such as severe anxiety or panic, and may arise from marked reduction in sensory stimulation such as isolation or immobilization.

The most common clinical situation in which the inability to cope with sensory stimuli is evident is seen in the patient with vascular changes sufficient to reduce the blood supply to the brain or with degenerative changes due to aging. Frequently these two states occur concomitantly. These individuals may function quite well in their ordinary life situations in which all stimuli are well known and activities have a regular pattern. However, when hospitalized, they are in a situation in which practically all sensory stimuli are unfamiliar, and their pattern of regular activities is disrupted. The result is disorientation. They do not know where they are, the time of day or the day of the week; nor can they clearly determine what is going on in the environment. Such a situation can be greatly aggravated if sedatives or other central nervous system depressants are administered. It is also made worse if the environment is arranged in such a way that the meaning of sensory intake is made obscure, as by poor lighting, absence of a clock or a calendar, change in activities that reduces perception of night and day, sameness of rooms, indiscriminate use of auditory equipment, and the human voice so pitched that the sound is heard but not understood.

Aphasia bears mention, since it is a fairly frequent outcome of cerebral damage. Complete or nearly complete expressive aphasia is quite apparent. Frequent outbursts of crying, anger, and laughter are quite characteristic. These may be disturbing to the nurse unless they are understood. This form of emotional expression may be due to a combination of factors, such as inability to express oneself verbally, frustration because of blocked communication, and the organic lesion that has caused the aphasia.

Receptive aphasia, in which the patient does not comprehend the spoken word, may cause alterations in behavior. The patient may not respond to verbal commands or may respond inappropriately to verbal communication. Receptive aphasia may be overlooked unless one is alert to the possibility. Usually it occurs in conjunction with expressive aphasia. If a patient with any form of aphasia does not respond to attempts at verbal communication or seems to resist direction and help, it may be that he does not comprehend anything said to him. Other forms of communication, such as touch, or the use of symbols, drawings, or writing, should be tried. Failure of the patient to respond to directions may be perceived to be part of the emotional reaction when actually the primary problem is one of communication.

The functioning of the brain as well as the brain tissue is greatly affected by altered metabolic states. Alterations in behavior can therefore be anticipated with metabolic imbalance. Only a few of the most frequent causes of behavioral changes due to metabolic problems will be mentioned here.

INFECTIONS

Most serious infectious processes are early associated with lassitude and diminished activity. If the infection is not controlled by antibiotic therapy and it is allowed to run its full course, the disease may be characterized by confusion and delirium. The degree of delirium can be correlated with the degree of fever. Both of these manifestations reflect a hypermetabolic state during the period of infection. Since the advent of antibiotics the nurse sees fewer patients with delirium due to infection. It still occurs, however. The patient becomes restless, has difficulty in sleeping, and moves from mild disorientation to severe confusion. The confusion adds to the restlessness, and the patient pulls at the bedclothes, pulls down the oxygen equipment, and attempts to get out of bed. He shows remarkable strength at this point, seemingly beyond that which his severe illness should allow. Needless to say, such energy expenditure is not helpful. It takes great skill on the part of the nurse to handle the patient. Nursing measures in such a situation are discussed later.

HYPOXIA

Another physiological cause of altered behavior is hypoxia. If the hypoxia is mild and chronic, the patient will compensate by reduction in the amount and rate of activity. If the hypoxia is due to poor respiratory ventilation, he may be reluctant to talk, since talking inhibits his maximum effort for ventilation. Forcing conversation can be very trying to the patient. If the hypoxia develops acutely, the patient will show signs of fear and panic. He will become extremely restless and active as he attempts to surmount the difficulty. Since this hyperactivity denotes severe hypoxia, it usually does not last long without resolution one way or another. For a short period, however, the nurse must deal with the paradox of a patient severely deprived of oxygen yet extremely restless and overactive, for example, the patient with acute pulmonary edema who has acute oxygen deprivation and is so restless that it is difficult to institute treatment.

ELECTROLYTE IMBALANCE

Electrolyte imbalance may be a factor in determining behavioral changes. Loss of essential electrolytes generally is characterized by weakness, fatigue, drowsiness, and difficulty in mentation. Marked loss of water or sodium may result in extreme confusion and delirium. Potassium deficiency causes decreased motor activity because of muscle weakness. An excess of calcium may cause mental confusion and slurred speech. Such problems should be anticipated in most seriously ill patients, and particularly patients who have had surgery, those whose oral intake of food and fluids is restricted and who are being fed intravenously, those with severe burns, those with cardiovascular or renal disease, and those with adrenal insufficiency. Acidosis and alkalosis lead to altered states of consciousness.

HYPOGLYCEMIA

Hypoglycemia can give rise to abrupt changes in behavior, as when excessive insulin has been administered. The patient feels shaky, he perspires, he is weak, and he may exhibit marked changes in behavior. He may become irritable and belligerent. Occasionally he will seem intoxicated as with alcohol. If he appears intoxicated he may be treated accordingly, whether he is hospitalized or not, since very serious consequences may result without treatment. Administration of glucose by vein or by mouth should remedy the situation forthwith; if it does not, in all probability another basis for the hypoglycemia must be sought.

DISTURBANCES DUE TO DRUGS

Drugs that act on the central nervous system are an ever-present source of behavioral change. Marked alterations may be due to overdosage, idiosyncrasy, or withdrawal effects. These drugs either stimulate or depress the central nervous system, and in either case the effect is excessive. For example, using phenobarbital in therapeutic dosage will sedate the patient and relieve his anxiety, whereas overdosage will make him comatose. Sudden withdrawal of phenobarbital after a period of continued use will cause central nervous hyperactivity.

With patients who have received few drugs, administration of relatively small amounts may cause considerable effect. It is not unusual to see a patient who is receiving small amounts of phenobarbital become slowed, drowsy, and somnolent. The nurse must constantly observe for such effects, which may be highly undesirable in relation to the basic illness.

Barbiturates deserve special attention because they are used so commonly outside the hospital and barbiturate overdosage is a common cause of hospitalization. Mild intoxication causes impairment and slowing of all mental function. Judgment is poor. There may be ataxia and dysarthria. The person is drowsy or sleeping but can be aroused. Severe poisoning with barbiturates leads to coma and death, usually from respiratory failure. Individuals who use barbiturates habitually may have difficulty with mentation, and may be confused and show increased emotional instability. Withdrawal from barbiturates following habituation may lead to severe illness. The potential for barbiturate withdrawal symptoms is high in the newly hospitalized patient, since barbiturates are widely used by the "normal" population. In addition, the hospitalized patient is denied his usual sources of drugs, and often hospital personnel fail to inquire whether or not the patient has been taking them. Even if there is a record of previous use, the drug may not be ordered. Within 24 hours of withdrawal the patient becomes restless and anxious. Tremors and weakness in the limbs develop. After 24 hours there may be uncontrollable shaking and muscular twitching, without loss of consciousness. This may be followed in the next 24 hours by insomnia and grand mal seizures. If this series of events is not interrupted, between the third and seventh day a state simulating a psychosis may follow with vivid hallucinations and strong delusions.

Other widely used central nervous system depressants that require careful observation are narcotics, tranquilizers, and alcohol. The stimulants of greatest importance are the psychic energizers (amphetamines). Tranquilizers and psychic energizers are also being used increasingly by the general population. Withdrawal from these drugs may cause reactive symptomatology.

ALCOHOLISM

Alcohol deserves particular attention since alcoholism and withdrawal causes much abnormal behavior among hospitalized patients. Alcoholics who are hospitalized for illness or surgery need special care to avert severe withdrawal symptoms. In the past hospitalization in general medical settings was often denied because of the difficulty in handling the withdrawal symptoms. This need not be true, since with careful use of sedation, vitamins, and fluids, the withdrawal phase can be controlled.

In general, delirium tremens gives rise to typical withdrawal symptoms from central nervous system depressants. Some specific characteristics are not fully explained but are probably related to the metabolic problems of electrolyte imbalance and vitamin depletion. The first signs of impending delirium tremens are insomnia and restlessness, which are often quite in contrast to the patient's previous behavior. This restlessness is relentless and progressive. Tremor also develops. The combination of tremor overactivity causes numerous small accidents. The water glass is knocked over. The bedpan is dropped. Pills are lost among the bedclothes. Clothing is burned by cigarettes. The restlessness proceeds rapidly to disorientation and then delirium. Characteristically, the patient attempts to leave the hospital. He may get out of bed and be found on the elevator or stairs, or wandering about in the hallway looking for a bus.

The delirium is severe and is characterized by frightening hallucinations, most often of snakes, bugs, or animals. These are so horrifying to the patient that he panics and attempts to get away. He may take any avenue of escape at this point—including a window. Restraint during this period may be unendurable. The aggressive, occasionally assaultive behavior exhibited by a badly frightened patient at this point is most often caused by efforts to restrain and immobilize him. Hence it is essential that impending delirium tremens be recognized so that appropriate sedation may be given. Uncontrolled delirium tremens in itself is a threatening development, but in the sick person and the one recovering from surgery, it is life-threatening.

VITAMIN DEFICIENCY

Vitamin deficiency, although rare in the United States, does occur. If severe, it may result in marked behavioral changes. Thiamine deficiency may result in severe anxiety manifestations and confusion. Niacin depletion may cause tremor, confusion, and delirium. Scurvy may be associated with negativism and severe depression. Despite its infrequency in the United States, it should not be overlooked as a possibility in alcoholics or patients with diseases of malabsorption.

STATE OF PHYSICAL COMFORT

A source of behavior often overlooked is the state of the patient's physical comfort. Pain has considerable influence upon overt behavior. Excruciating pain may cause overactivity, pacing the floor, rolling in bed, even beating the head on the wall. Certain kinds of severe pain may cause immobility, e.g., severe anginal pain or acute abdominal pain with spasm of smooth muscle causing temporary immobilization. The patient in severe pain tends to concentrate on enduring it. He does not respond to other stimuli, he may not understand what is said to him or who is present with him, and he tends to become uncommunicative and to have little concern for what is going on about him.

Chronic pain tends to cause irritability with episodes of aggressive behavior, since the tolerance for frustration is reduced.

Since aggressive physical behavior is usually controlled, such aggression most often is channeled through verbal action. The patient may make excessive demands on the nurse, be overtly critical, deride one person in front of another, be sarcastic, or use other forms of verbal aggressive behavior. If he is blocked in this attempt, he may resort to physical means such as throwing things or dropping articles on the floor. He might pull out his intravenous therapy equipment, disrupt his traction, make a suicidal gesture, or take other drastic action that may harm him. The extreme action would be to commit physical harm on others. This is rare unless precipitated by drugs or delirium. It can occur, however, if all the other modes of behavior described have been unsuccessful in eliminating the anger. If the aggressive behavior is prolonged as a result of the chronicity of the condition, it is easy to see why the patient, through his verbal behavior, may tend to alienate others. Such alienation will provoke even further behavioral changes by the patient.

Other sources of discomfort such as immobilization, casts, poor positioning, and intubation may cause similar behavior. The patient becomes preoccupied and irritable. His usual concern for the well-being of others or his own well-being is gradually lessened as discomfort is prolonged. He may attempt to defy treatment measures by removing the source of his discomfort despite the potential outcome, or if this is not possible, he may seek to retaliate by striking out verbally at whoever is nearby.

INTELLECTUAL CAPACITY

The present discussion of intellectual capacity does not deal with persons whose intellectual deficits are due to their disease. Intellectual development plays an important role in patient behavior. Nursing personnel frequently cause the patient to feel frustrated by assuming that he has greater (or less) intellectual capacity than is the case. This frustration leads to aggressive behavior toward the perpetrator or someone else. For example, if the nurse attempts to teach a patient with below-normal intelligence to prepare and administer his own insulin, she may insist that he meet a level of comprehension which he cannot do. He may become angry at this insistence that he perform at a level beyond his ability. On the other hand, if he cannot express anger directly, he may be forced to behave as though the action is of no real importance. He might indicate that he probably will not do it, both verbally and by failing to perform it while in the hospital or clinic. If the nurse attempts to teach the same procedure to an individual with normal or above-normal intelligence and fails to respond to his curiosity about the basis for the action, a similar reaction of anger and frustration may occur. Again, the patient may have above normal intelligence but little formal schooling. He may have the same amount of curiosity as another better educated patient, yet the supposition might be made that he lacks the understanding needed to be told all the facts.

THE CULTURE

The last main source of patient behavior is his culture. The effects of socialization and growth and development in a specific culture have been discussed in Part II. The patient's acculturation in regard to his sex role, family role, the meaning of illness, and appropriate ways of handling pain and illness is thus superimposed on the other factors previously discussed.

Effects of Stress upon Patient Behavior

All the factors previously discussed are extremely important, but it is their inter-action with the personality of the individual which finally determines his behavior. The patient as an individual and a family member has been discussed in Part II. Certain defense mechanisms and sources of personality development are mentioned in that section.

When an individual becomes ill and is hospitalized, he is subjected to considerable additional stress regardless of his personality and success in adjustments. The effect of this additional stress must be considered in interpreting the patient's behavior. The sources of this stress are many: There is the stress of the illness itself and the therapy employed in treating it. There is the possibility, whether remote or imminent, that he will die. Pain and discomfort are very likely to occur and usually are anticipated by the patient. He cannot control what is being done. He loses his identity. The hospital personnel do not react as his family and close associates do. He is separated from persons with whom he enjoys the most meaning-ful relationships. He is in an unfamiliar social structure and does not know "the rules of the game." Nor does he have a clear understanding of his role. Finally, he must face the outcome of his illness and the necessity of returning to his former position in life.

What are the potential outcomes when these added stresses are exerted on the individual? (1) He may be able to endure the stress without experiencing special problems. He will be aware of the need for added energy expenditure in with-standing the situation, and be able to manage without great difficulty. (2) The stress will be sufficient to cause a breakdown in the usual defense mechanisms with resultant severe anxiety. For example, he might deny that he has a malignant neoplasm. As the day of the scheduled surgery approaches, the reality of events may now override his efforts at denial, and the full impact of the situation may cause great anxiety. (3) The absence of his customary environment and the presence of the rather restrictive environment of the hospital may make it impossible for him to call upon his usual defenses, and thus give rise to increased anxiety. For example, the patient may always have overreacted to his strong need for dependency by showing extreme independence. He does not permit anyone to help him. His inability to function in an extremely independent fashion creates great anxiety.

The added stress of the hospital situation plus the potential activation of un-conscious anxiety may bring into focus new defense mechanisms or may cause reactivation of earlier defense mechanisms. Thus, the two chief reactions to the added stress are (1) intensification of anxiety and (2) intensification or adoption of defense mechanisms.

FEAR AND ANXIETY

Fear is an important determinant of behavior. It produces behavior very much like that of anxiety. Fear combined with anxiety may have even greater effects on behavior.

The observable symptoms of anxiety are restlessness, jumpiness, and overtalkativeness. The patient often does not seem to hear what is said to him, but keeps talking as though no one else had spoken. Preoccupation with one theme is common. If one listens carefully, one may find that he tries to avoid certain topics. His attention on matters outside his own concerns is short. He seems to be unaware of many things going on about him, and at the same time may be overly concerned with something in the environment which he perceives as threatening him. In moderate anxiety the patient's pulse is rapid and he perspires freely. Palpitation and dizziness may then develop. In extreme anxiety bordering on panic, the patient may be overactive; he misinterprets sensory stimuli, talks incoherently, and responds inappropriately to external stimuli. Finally he becomes completely disorganized and may move about purposelessly or become immobile. He may attempt to flee or may become psychotic. He may try to jump out a window, yet have no desire to commit suicide.

DENIAL

Denial, as mentioned, is a common defense mechanism during illness. In fact, its use can be helpful in certain situations, such as imminent death or loss of body parts. Euphoria, an exaggerated sense of well-being, may be regarded as an extension of denial in that the patient is unconcerned about any aspect of his life situation. Euphoria is rarely seen in the nonpsychiatric setting; when it does occur in relation to physical illness, it may represent a transient reaction or sense of extreme well-being resulting from the resolution of a problem or relief from anxiety through the use of some adaptive defense mechanism. For instance, a patient who is depressed and contemplating suicide may temporarily experience marked well-being once he has reached the decision to commit suicide. Or he may experience great relief simulating euphoria when his severe anxiety has been relieved by successful denial or rationalization.

FRUSTRATION

Frustration may give rise to aggressive and hostile behavior. Although frustration is occasionally felt by all normal individuals, it may be greatly increased during illness and hospitalization. The reasons for this are many, but perhaps the chief one is that the patient is cut off from his usual sources of gratification of needs. (Occasionally, of course, the reverse may be true, and hospitalization may reduce frustrations that were considerable in the patient's usual life setting.) The added stress of hospitalization, already discussed, will lower the patient's tolerance to frustration, and the resultant aggressive behavior will most often be expressed verbally. Verbal aggressiveness may not be directed at a particular person, but may be generalized. In some cases the patient may direct his aggressiveness toward the nurse in place of the doctor. The patient may sense that verbal aggressiveness toward medical or nursing personnel may result in their withholding of services, and try to suppress it. In most cases the nurse can assume that verbal aggression toward her signifies either extreme frustration at her behavior or displacement from some other source. However, if the nurse has acted purposefully in order to make the patient feel he can express himself without risking loss of care, his aggressiveness may be considerably reduced. By contrast, physical aggression is generally associated with altered metabolic and neurologic states.

Response of Nurse to Observed Behavior

In order to respond to patient behavior in a way that will alleviate discomfort and be therapeutic, the nurse must have an orderly way of viewing this behavior. First she observes the patient's actions. After analyzing them she makes decisions as to possible responses. If the meaning of the behavior is obscure, the nurse must try to clarify it by interacting with the patient. If the meaning seems clear, the nurse may take initial action immediately. She might, for example, decide that the patient is disoriented because of oversedation, and act to relieve this as a first step. A particular expression of behavior may be attributable to several causative factors, thus a decision as to the most pertinent one requires additional information. This would include all that is known about the patient's physiological state obtained from the patient's chart, from the doctor, and from direct observation as described elsewhere. In addition, it would be necessary to gain as much knowledge as possible from the family and the patient about his customary behavioral responses. For instance, it is very helpful to know the patient's pattern of sleep. Perhaps he always is up prowling around part of each night at home and his similar behavior in the hospital is quite normal.

It is also important to determine what the patient and family are experiencing concerning fears, apprehensions, and resentment. One might discover, for instance, that the patient's family is pressing him to have surgery in their strong desire for him to be well. He, on the other hand, may be quite dubious about the wisdom of his having it done and is acquiescing only to please them. Knowing this from the patient and his family can be very helpful in understanding the patient's restless, purposeless activity or his angry outbursts toward personnel.

The importance of change in behavior over a period of time cannot be overemphasized, i.e., what has preceded, at what point changes have occurred, and the rate at which change is occurring. This is one of the reasons why data should be gathered and recorded in descriptive terms. If one finds only the diagnostic impression in the nurse's recordings from the previous day, it is very difficult to evaluate subsequent behavior. For example, the nurse should note that the patient was disoriented yesterday and that he has improved (or worsened) in this behavior today. Or she may note a sudden change from the patient's customary behavior.

When the several inferences about the cause of the behavior have been made, the nurse must decide which is the most probable, what action is to be taken, the subsequent course of action, if necessary, and what additional data she will need for future action.

A clinical illustration will demonstrate the process. A 69-year-old man, newly admitted to the hospital, is disoriented at night. He does not know where he is and keeps getting up to look for the bathroom. He is in a room by himself. The nurse thinks through the possibilities. Is his restlessness caused by illness? He has an inguinal hernia, which makes this unlikely. However, because of his age there may be some cerebrovascular insufficiency that could account for his behavior. Has he had any sedation? According to the chart he has not. The nurse makes a mental note to be sure that he does not receive any sedatives until his disorientation is explained. Has he ever been in the hospital before? The chart indicates he has not. Perhaps the new environment and his reduced mentation caused by the vascular disease have resulted in difficulties in orienting himself. If the light in his room was turned on, he might reorient himself. Another possibility is that he has too little sensory stimulation being alone in his room, or that he is frightened or anxious about something. If efforts at reorientation and keeping the light on are not helpful, the next step would be either to move him to an area where there is more sensory stimulation or to spend some time talking with him in efforts to learn the cause of the problem. If these actions prove inappropriate, the nurse continues to reevaluate the situation and take further actions.

General Principles of Nursing Action

There are general actions the nurse can take which are therapeutic in all situations, and these can relieve the problem temporarily while she seeks more definitive measures. She can help the patient to reorient himself in several ways. All sensory stimuli must be clearly comprehensible. Adequate lighting is very helpful, as is a reduction in mixed auditory stimuli. Excessive auditory stimulation may add to the patient's disorientation, e.g., if one person talks quietly with him the effect may be calming, but the stimulation produced by the sound of personnel talking at a distance, paging systems, radios, and the noises of running hospital equipment will add to the patient's confusion. Repeated efforts should be made to inform him where he is, the time of day, and who is in his presence. A large clock should be clearly visible. These measures are helpful even when the patient is severely disoriented. If he is delirious, such reminders, repeated every few minutes, serve to reassure him.

If the patient is hyperactive, he should be allowed as much space and freedom of movement as possible. Attempts to restrain him at this time only add to his difficulties, and often result in further activity, assaultive behavior, or attempts to flee. Furthermore, he will become physically exhausted. If he cannot be moved to a safe place, the nurse can move about his room with him. If he is not frightened by efforts to restrain him, he usually can be distracted from taking any action that will endanger him. If the cause of the extreme overactivity is known and sedation is not contraindicated, then it should be used to its maximum therapeutic effect; this applies also to mild overactivity. The patient who is well oriented may be provided opportunities for purposeful physical activity which will expend his energy in something other than pacing the floor.

Generally, the patient who is hypoactive because of depression or some other cause receives much less attention than the hyperactive one. He is not as troublesome to the personnel, and they do not fear for his safety. Usually it is not possible to force, cajole, or encourage such a patient to increase his activity. However, it is extremely important to make a continuous effort to reach the patient through verbal interaction, by including him in group activities and by generally acting as though one anticipated his returning interest in his surroundings.

The depressed patient is often quite aware of what is going on, and being left unstimulated, he may think that his feelings of unworthiness are thus confirmed. If his withdrawal and inactivity have an organic basis, a reduction in stimuli resulting from his being left alone will tend to aggravate the situation.

With a patient whose intellectual capacity is deficient, perhaps the most important principle underlying nursing action is that the action should serve to reduce his sense of frustration. Inability to perform intellectually leads to other failures of performance.

Bibliography

Arieti, Silvano: *American Handbook of Psychiatry.* New York: Basic Books, Inc., Publishers, 1966.

Gellhorn, Ernst and G. N. Loofbourrow: *Emotions and Emotional Disorders.* New York: Paul B. Hoeber, Inc., 1963.

Goldberger, Emanual: *A Primer of Water, Electrolyte and Acid-Base Syn-dromes,* 2d ed. Philadelphia: Lea & Febiger, 1962.

Goodman, Louis and Alfred Gilman: *The Pharmacological Basis of Therapeutics,* 3d ed. New York: The Macmillan Company, 1965.

Merritt, Hiram H.: *A Textbook of Neurology,* 4th ed. Philadelphia: Lea & Febiger, 1967.

CHAPTER 18
ABNORMALITIES IN GASTROINTESTINAL AND URINARY OUTPUT

ELIZABETH C. GIBLIN

This discussion of abnormal or unusual excretions and discharges is limited to those that may occur with pathophysiology of more than one system of the body. The problems of vomiting, diarrhea, constipation, flatulence, polyuria, oliguria, and anuria are included. The basic factors that may cause or contribute to the pathophysiology are discussed, and the medical treatment and nursing care plan are presented in relation to these factors. Significant observations that may be made to judge the nature and the severity of the problem and to evaluate the outcomes of the medical and nursing therapy have been included. Primary emphasis has been placed on therapies that may be used to minimize and alleviate the factors that may cause or contribute to the disturbance. Detailed explanation for the occurrence of these symptoms in specific diseases has been purposely left for Part Five.

Vomiting

Vomiting is a symptom seen in patients with a variety of medical and surgical conditions. It is a protective mechanism designed to remove potentially harmful ingested substances. Severe or prolonged vomiting may, however, result in the loss of fluid and electrolytes with consequent dehydration and electrolyte depletion.

Studies have shown that the highest incidence of vomiting occurs in children and adolescents. Thereafter it tends to decrease with age. The incidence is higher in women than men. An increased incidence is found in postoperative patients with a history of motion sickness or of previous postoperative vomiting, and in female patients who have surgery during the third or fourth week of their menstrual cycle.

Vomiting is usually preceded by nausea. The individual may feel weak, dizzy, and/or faint. Increased salivation, frequent swallowing, tachycardia, diaphoresis, and pallor may be observed. Irregular rapid respirations and retching may occur prior to the onset of vomiting.

The act of vomiting consists of simple or forceful regurgitation of the stomach contents, either with or without retching. It is accomplished by the relaxation of the stomach and of the cardiac and esophageal sphincters followed by contraction of the abdominal muscles and the diaphragm. Normally, the glottis closes to prevent aspiration of the emesis into the trachea and lower respiratory passages. Unfortunately, the glottis may fail to close in patients with impaired reflexes such as those who are unconscious or who have had a cerebrovascular occlusion.

The act of vomiting raises the intraocular, intracranial, and intra-abdominal pressures, thus increasing the danger of bleeding following intraocular surgery, head injuries, or intracranial surgery. Following abdominal surgery, the danger of wound separation or dehiscence is increased by vomiting.

FACTORS CAUSING VOMITING

Vomiting is a reflex response. The integrative vomiting center in the medulla may be excited by impulses from any one or a combination of three general sources. These include stimulation of afferent nerves from the stomach, intestines, or other viscera; stimulation of the higher centers of the brain; and stimulation of the chemoreceptor trigger zone.

Afferent impulses may be initiated by irritation of the gastrointestinal mucosa;

by distention of the pylorus, intestines, colon, biliary ducts, or gallbladder; by inflammation or congestion of the abdominal viscera; by occlusion of coronary vessels; and by sufficiently painful stimuli from any portion of the body. Mechanical stimulation of the posterior pharynx or stimulation of the vestibular nerves from sudden change in position may also initiate vomiting.

Impulses from the higher centers of the brain are initiated by disagreeable sights, sounds, odors, and tastes, and by feelings of discouragement, hopelessness, fear, and depression.

The chemoreceptor trigger zone is stimulated by chemicals circulating in the blood. These include exogenous toxins from contaminated foods; ingested poisons and drugs such as apomorphine, morphine, meperidine, digitalis; and some general anesthetic agents. Sensitivity to these drugs varies with both the individual and the dose. Circulating endogenous toxins from infections, uremia, ketosis, and therapeutic radiation may also stimulate the chemoreceptor zone.

Finally, vomiting may be caused by hypoxia of the vomiting center, which occurs with a fall in blood pressure, increased intracranial pressure, or high-altitude sickness.

A number of these factors may act concurrently to contribute to the severity of the vomiting episode. Thus, certain anesthetic agents may initiate vomiting as a result of stimulation of the chemoreceptor zone. The severity may be increased by the presence of unrelieved pain and the patient's feelings of discouragement or other adverse feelings.

MEDICAL TREATMENT

The physician considers the potential cause of vomiting and its possible ill effects in his plan of care. Antiemetic drugs may be prescribed to depress the sensitivity of the vomiting center or of the chemoreceptor trigger zone. They are used to prevent vomiting as well as to relieve it. Drugs used may include sedatives, anticholinergics, antihistamines, and phenothiazines.

Antihistamines are particularly effective for suppressing vestibular irritability. Phenothiazines, on the other hand, appear to suppress the chemoreceptor trigger zone. Therapeutic doses of anticholinergics depress gastrointestinal motility and result in delayed emptying time. Sedatives initiate general relaxation and allay apprehension.

Nasogastric intubation with intermittent or continuous suction may be prescribed to prevent distention as well as for its relief. If distention is due to obstruction, surgery may be necessary. Treatment for other causes of vomiting will depend on the specific findings and recommendations of the physician. The treatment for ingested poisons is discussed in Chapter 33.

Since considerable fluid and electrolytes may be lost in the vomitus, the physician will prescribe parenteral therapy to provide the necessary replacements when the patient is unable to take oral fluids or food.

NURSING CARE

The nursing care plan for patients with the problem of vomiting is designed to complement and supplement the medical management. The aims are to prevent or minimize factors that may cause or contribute to vomiting and to prevent or minimize the possible ill effects that may result from vomiting.

The characteristics of the emesis, the associated signs and symptoms, and the circumstances under which vomiting occurs provide clues to factors that may cause or contribute to the severity of the vomiting. Information should be obtained on the frequency, duration, type, amount, and character of the emesis. Important characteristics of the vomitus include the color; the odor; and the presence of bright red blood or blood clots, coffee-ground-like material, food particles, or bile or fecal material. Fecal materials are often found in the emesis with obstructions in the intestinal tract. The presence or absence of nausea, retching, projectile vomiting, abdominal cramps, or diarrhea should be noted.

Specific prodromal signs or symptoms usually occur with vomiting. These may include increased salivation or frequent swallowing, tachycardia, diaphoresis, pallor, irregular rapid respirations, and complaints of dizziness, faintness, nausea, or weakness.

The relation of vomiting to the medications taken prior to its onset, to pain, to change in position, and to the feeling state of the patient should be elicited. When food poisoning is suspected, the specific foods, including the amount and time when eaten in relation to the onset of vomiting, should be obtained.

Changes in the characteristics of the emesis, and the frequency and amount of the emesis, and the associated signs and symptoms provide one basis for evaluating the effectiveness of the medical and nursing care.

Aspiration of vomitus is a hazard for patients with defective reflexes, especially those who are unconscious or even semiconscious. Unless it is contraindicated, such patients are positioned on either side with the head flexed and supported during the vomiting episode to prevent aspiration, and the head of the bed may be lowered to promote flow of the emesis by gravity. The emesis may need to be suctioned from the mouth and nose. Suction equipment should be available at the bedside for such patients. Artificial dentures are often removed to prevent obstruction of the airway during retching.

A number of nursing actions may be used to reduce the severity of vomiting. The conscious patient can be encouraged to pant to help suppress the vomiting reflex. Placing the patient in the prone position may arrest postanesthetic vomiting. Antiemetic drugs should be administered at the precise time intervals specified in the doctor's order to maintain an effective blood level. Prescribed medications should be used judiciously to control pain. The patient's position should be changed slowly to minimize vestibular stimulation. To minimize the psychogenic factors, as well as for esthetic comfort, the emesis basin should be emptied and cleaned immediately following each vomiting episode. The patient should be provided with mouthwash to rinse his mouth, and assisted as necessary. Soiled linen should be removed and the room ventilated well. The patient should be protected from other disagreeable odors, sights, and sounds. The nurse should not smoke or wear strong perfumes when caring for these patients. Room deodorants may be used to minimize disagreeable odors from draining wounds or burns; the room deodorant itself should not produce a disagreeable odor.

The patency of indwelling gastric tubes is maintained by irrigation as often as necessary in order to ensure relief of the distention. Normal saline is used for irrigation to minimize the electrolyte loss. Patients with indwelling nasogastric tubes are provided with isotonic ice chips to keep their mouth and throat moist. Ice made from plain water should be avoided.

A careful fluid balance record is to be maintained on all patients who vomit repeatedly or whose therapy includes use of indwelling nasogastric tubes.

When intravenous therapy is prescribed, the rate of flow will be governed by the amount of emesis and frequency of vomiting as well as by the fluid loss from other sources. Signs and symptoms of dehydration or electrolyte disturbances should be reported and recorded in order to help evaluate the adequacy of fluid replacement.

Unless contraindicated, fluid loss from vomiting is replaced by oral intake of fluid as soon as the patient can tolerate it. Cold or hot fluids are usually better tolerated than tepid ones. Tea and carbonated beverages have been found to be easily tolerated and helpful in alleviating the nausea. Broth may be used to replace some of the electrolyte loss. When the patient is able to take food, small amounts are give at first to minimize the distention of the stomach.

When morphine or meperidine is prescribed, its effect is evaluated in relation to the relief of pain and occurrence of vomiting. If vomiting continues, the physician may reduce the dosage, discontinue the drug, or substitute another.

Vomiting may be beneficial for the individual who has ingested potentially harmful and irritating substances. However, it is contraindicated following ingestion of certain substances. The treatment of ingestion of potentially harmful substances is discussed in detail in Chapter 33. Vomiting may be induced by mechanically stimulating the posterior pharynx or by distending the stomach with large quantities of liquids designed to neutralize or dilute the ingested substance.

GENERAL PRINCIPLES UNDERLYING THE NURSING CARE PLAN

Vomiting occurs with many systemic conditions. Early recognition and treatment of the underlying disease may forestall the occurrence of vomiting. Providing a pleasant physical environment, free from disagreeable odors, sights, and sounds, will help to prevent its occurence. Early recognition of the patient's concerns and provision of support perceived by the patient as emotionally supportive can also be expected to help prevent vomiting. The administration of the prescribed medication at the appropriate time cannot be emphasized too strongly.

An effective nursing care plan for the patient who has the problem of vomiting is based on careful observation of the patient and his environment. Careful and accurate reporting and recording of the observations made, procedures used, and effects on the patient are of value not only to the doctor, but also to the nursing staff who will subsequently be giving nursing care to the patient.

Abnormal Stools

Although vomiting usually occurs with acute illness, abnormalities in the frequency and consistency of the stools may occur as an acute or a chronic condition. The consistency and amount of stools is related to food and fluid intake and the rate of transport of the food residue through the intestinal tract. Rapid propulsion results in a liquid or semiliquid stool; very slow propulsion results in a stool containing little water. There is a wide variation in the pattern of defecation among normal, healthy individuals. A range of from three bowel movements a day to only three a week was found in a study of over 1,000 healthy factory workers (Connell et al.). Changes in an individual's normal pattern of frequency and/or content of meals may be expected to result in changes in his defecation pattern.

Diarrhea

Diarrhea is a term indicating the frequent passage of unformed stools. It reflects an increase in peristaltic motility of either the small or the large intestine, and it may reflect an impairment in digestion and absorption and an increase in intestinal secrections. With severe diarrhea, the large loss of fluid and electrolytes, i.e., potassium, sodium, and bicarbonate, can lead to circulatory failure from the resulting hypovolemia and electrolyte disturbances.

FACTORS CAUSING DIARRHEA

Diarrhea may be caused by a number of factors. Essentially, these may either increase the peristaltic activity or decrease the tone of the intestine. Rapid peristaltic activity in the small intestine may result in incomplete digestion, particularly of proteins and fats, and impaired absorption of both fluids and nutrients. The consistency of the stool will depend upon whether the pathology occurs in the small intestine or the colon and is directly related to the rate of transport of the contents. The stools tend to be large with involvement of the small bowel and small with pathology of the colon.

The duration of diarrhea will vary depending upon the cause and the effectiveness of the therapy. In acute conditions the diarrhea may last for only 1 to 3 days. In other conditions it may be prolonged or may become chronic.

Inflammation or congestion of any portion of the intestines may increase the irritability of the intrinsic nerve plexuses and increase peristalsis. Inflammation may be caused by infectious organisms, including bacteria, parasites, and viruses; by ingestion of foods contaminated with bacterial toxins; and by the presence of abnormal products of digestion, such as fatty acids and partially digested proteins, which may be found with malabsorption syndromes. Congestion or edema of the intestines may occur with circulatory failure or food allergies.

Emotional tension may either cause or contribute to the severity of diarrhea. Feelings of anger, resentment, hostility, anxiety, fear, and worry have been found to be associated with episodes of diarrhea and with increases in congestion and hypermotility of the intestines. These feelings may not be expressed verbally.

Some chemicals may cause diarrhea. These include irritant cathartics and ingested poisons. A deficiency of ionized calcium which may be found with renal failure or with parathyroid deficiency increases the neuromuscular excitability, causing diarrhea.

Other factors have been found to contribute to the severity of diarrhea. These include a diet containing foods high in roughage, such as whole grain cereals and raw fruits and vegetables, highly seasoned foods, fried foods, and foods that cause the formation of gas, such as cabbage, cauliflower, and baked beans. These foods may serve as irritants to sensitive mucosa. The presence of polyps or neoplasms may cause alternating diarrhea and constipation.

Diagnosis of the possible causes and evaluation of the severity of diarrhea is based on the history of the onset, the frequency, and the characteristics of the stools, as well as the accompanying signs, symptoms, and laboratory findings. Proctoscopic and x-ray studies may also be necessary. The latter may include a barium enema or an upper gastrointestinal study. A warm stool specimen is necessary to detect the presence of bacteria or parasites.

MEDICAL TREATMENT

Medical therapy is designed to eliminate the cause of the diarrhea, to reduce the peristaltic hyperactivity, and to restore fluid and electrolyte balance as necessary. Medications frequently ordered include antibiotics or chemotherapeutic agents to eliminate infections; demulcents to absorb toxins and coat the mucosa and thus reduce its irritability; anticholinergics to reduce the parasympathetic tone; sedatives or tranquilizers to relieve emotional tension; and enzymes to replace deficiencies in malabsorption syndromes. Special diets may be ordered to eliminate food allergies and foods that may be irritating. During an acute infection all food and fluids may be withheld for a period of time in order to reduce peristaltic activity. Parenteral therapy may be employed during acute episodes of diarrhea to provide necessary replacements of fluids and specific electrolytes.

NURSING CARE

The nursing care plan for patients with a problem of diarrhea is dependent upon the severity of diarrhea and the factors that may be causing or contributing to it. Observations of the characteristics of the stools, accompanying signs and symptoms, the patient's emotional state, and the laboratory findings provide a basis for defining the severity of the problem and for evaluating the results of the medical and nursing therapies.

Significant characteristics of the stool include the amount, color, and consistency; the presence of partially digested foods, mucus, exudate, and blood; any characteristic odor; and accompanying flatus. With acute infections the onset is usually sudden; the stools are watery, and may contain mucus and blood. Mucus, blood, and exudates may also appear in the stool in chronic inflammatory conditions. Stools associated with incomplete digestion of proteins and fats are typically large, frothy, greasy appearing, malodorous, and frequently accompanied by flatus. The physician may wish to examine an abnormal stool specimen. Before discarding a specimen, the nurse should find out whether it is to be saved.

Accompanying signs and symptoms may include anorexia, nausea and vomiting, abdominal tenderness, cramping pain, distention, urgency, and tenesmus. Tenesmus is a sharp cramp in the left lower quadrant associated with straining at stool which is partially relieved by defecation. The precise location of the abdominal tenderness may indicate the site of the inflammation. Other signs and symptoms may include fever, leukocytosis, malaise, weakness, and weight loss. The volume and specific gravity of the urine provide a basis for evaluating the adequacy of fluid replacement. Urinary output of less than 1,500 ml in 24 hours should be reported to the physician.

Nursing care is designed to help decrease the severity of diarrhea, to help prevent fluid and electrolyte deficiencies, to minimize the discomfort associated with diarrhea, and to prevent the spread of infectious diarrhea. Prevention of the development of diarrhea associated with specific diseases is discussed in Part Five.

In order to help decrease the severity of diarrhea, both physiological and psychological factors should be considered. Careful timing of the administration of prescribed drugs may be expected to reduce the number and quantity of loose stools. The aim of nursing therapies is to minimize stimulation of peristalsis. During an acute attack of diarrhea, all food and fluid may be withheld for a least 24 hours. When the patient is able to take oral fluids and food, peristaltic activity may be decreased by avoiding the administration of either hot or iced fluids and by giving only small amounts of fluids and food at a time. Consideration should be given to selecting fluids to help replace the electrolytes as well as the water loss. Warm weak tea, broth, and orange and tomato juices have been recommended. The broth and juices will help replace the lost sodium and potassium. Buttermilk and yogurt may change the bacterial flora in the intestinal tract and reduce the irritation to the mucosa. Bland foods are encouraged following an acute attack. The frequency of oral intake as well as the quantity to be encouraged will be governed by the frequency and consistency of the stools. Guides for the dietary management of specific diseases causing diarrhea may be found in a nutrition textbook.

Encouraging the patient to lie flat in bed and to relax his abdominal muscles may help to slow peristaltic activity following meals.

Psychological factors that may contribute to the severity of both acute and chronic diarrhea must also be considered. These may include a feeling of discomfort associated with the diarrhea itself and feelings about the medical care situation. Provision of a readily available clean bedpan, privacy, and a well-ventilated room, and the use of deodorizers as necessary will help allay feelings of discomfort associated with diarrhea. Lack of information or misconceptions regarding expected care and diagnostic tests may be another source of stress. Changes in daily routines which are necessitated by the medical plan should be clarified. Providing emotional support as indicated may be therapeutic.

Frequent passage of loose stools may cause perianal irritation and discomfort. Such discomfort may be reduced by the use of soft toilet tissues or facial tissues and by gently washing the area following each stool. Careful hand washing by the patient and the personnel and isolation of the bedpan and contaminated linen must be carried out whenever diarrhea is caused by an infectious organism. The stools may have to be disinfected if the sewage disposal system is inadequate.

GENERAL PRINCIPLES UNDERLYING THE NURSING CARE PLAN

The nursing care of patients with problems of diarrhea will vary depending upon the medical diagnosis and the specific factors that may be causing or contributing to the problem. The history of the onset; careful observation of the frequency and characteristics of the stools; associated signs and symptoms; and the emotional state of the patient provide the basis for identifying the severity of the problem and planning for the nursing care. The nursing care is designed to minimize peristaltic activity through attention to both physiological and psychological factors that may be involved. The care plan will also consider the fluid and electrolyte and nutritional needs of the patient, and prevention of perianal discomfort and spread of infectious organisms to others.

Constipation

Constipation may be defined as undue delay in the passage of feces. It usually results in the passage of dry stools. A delay in the passage of stools may be expected whenever there is a prolonged interval between meals or when less than the usual amount of roughage is included in an individual's diet. Changes in the particular individual's pattern of defecation must be considered in identifying a problem of constipation.

Constipation occurs from prolonged retention of food residue in the colon or rectum, with resulting increased absorption of water and passage of dry, hard stools. Some individuals consider themselves constipated if they fail to have a daily bowel movement. Others define constipation as a smaller than normal stool or the feeling of incomplete emptying of the rectum. Self-treatment with cathartics or enemas may be used by such individuals.

It should be recalled that the defecation reflex is stimulated by the pressure of feces entering the rectum from peristaltic activity in the colon. This reflex can be voluntarily suppressed. Evacuation of the stool is aided by contraction of the diaphragm, abdominal, and perineal muscles.

FACTORS CAUSING CONSTIPATION

Constipation may be associated with a variety of systemic diseases, with emotional stress, and with pathology of the colon and rectum as well as with irregularity of meal patterns. Constipation may be caused by any one or a combination of factors. These include a lack of regularity, a lack of sufficient bulk to stimulate the defecation reflex, impaired propulsion of feces, weak abdominal muscles, and an impaired defecation reflex.

The lack of regularity may be due to failure to establish or maintain a habitual time for defecation. The lack of sufficient bulk may be due to insufficient bulk in the diet or to habitual use of cathartics or enemata. A slow propulsion of feces occurs with a decrease in motility of the bowel or with hypertonicity. A delayed propulsion of the intestinal contents has been found with emotional tension and feelings of anger, depression, and fear, and with pain. It has also been found to result from the administration of some drugs, including opiates, anticholinergics, and ganglionic blocking agents, and from inflammation of the intestines or of other abdominal viscera. Mechanical obstruction from lesions within the bowel lumen or from external pressure by abdominal tumors or a gravid uterus may also retard the propulsion of feces.

Prolonged inactivity, as with bed rest and general debility, results in weakness of the abdominal and perineal muscles which impairs the evacuation of feces.

The defecation reflex may be suppressed by painful rectal or anal lesions. Finally, constipation may result from neurological pathology that impairs the defecation reflex. This may occur with pathology of the peripheral nerves, the spinal cord, or the central nervous system.

Considerable muscular exertion is required to provide sufficient intra-abdominal pressure to evacuate hard, dry stools. Chronic constipation may result in fecal impactions, particularly in older patients or those with neurological impairments. Such impactions are characterized by frequent stimulations for defecation and by the passage of small amounts of loose stool which may be mistaken for diarrhea. A digital examination will detect the mass filling of the rectum.

Constipation may be associated with a coated tongue and a foul breath, with abdominal discomfort, anorexia, nausea, flatulence, headache, malaise, weakness, and restlessness. These manifestations have been attributed to prolonged distention of the rectum and to anxiety aroused by constipation. These symptoms were found to disappear within an hour following defecation (Davenport).

MEDICAL TREATMENT

The medical management of a problem of constipation is dependent upon the causative factors and the associated pathology, if any. Proctoscopic examinations, barium studies, and a search for occult blood in the stool are used to rule out pathology in the bowel. Cancer will be suspected. With chronic constipation the diagnosis is aided by analysis of the patient's dietary and defecation patterns, his use of laxatives or enemas, mode of living, and emotional problems.

When constipation is associated with systemic diseases, cathartics may be ordered to help restore the normal defecation pattern. Cathartics may include those that stimulate the intrinsic nerves directly or indirectly to improve peristalsis, or those that aid defecation by softening and lubricating the feces. A saline enema may be ordered for every second or third day. Sedatives or tranquilizers may be ordered to allay emotional tension. Antispasmodics may be ordered for patients with hypertonic or spastic colons.

Dietary modifications will depend upon the factors causing the constipation. Bulk-producing foods may be encouraged to increase peristalsis; however, low-residue diets may be ordered for patients with hypertonic or spastic colons. Regularity of meals and defecation time and moderate exercise may be encouraged.

Information on the frequency, size, and consistency of the stool provides a guide for the medical and nursing care. A stool with a small caliber is characteristic of spastic constipation, which is associated with an increased tone of the colon. Mucus may be present in the stool in this condition. Cancer of the colon is characterized by the presence of occult blood in the stool and alternating constipation and diarrhea. The presence of blood in the stool is an indication of a lesion in the bowel. The patient's emotional reaction and expressed concern about any change in his bowel pattern may also be valuable guides for medical and nursing care.

NURSING CARE

The aim of nursing care is to help identify factors that may be causing or contributing to the constipation and to support or help restore a normal pattern of defecation.

Supportive nursing therapy includes instruction, encouragement, emotional support, and adjustment of routines to support a normal elimination pattern when possible. Information on the normal pattern of defecation and on what the individual does to maintain regularity will provide a basis for planning supportive care. The time of elimination and frequency, content and approximate amount of diet, and amount of activity are all important. Some individuals have their routine bowel movement after drinking a cup of hot coffee or hot lemon juice in water and eating breakfast.

Any alteration in the patient's dietary pattern, activity pattern, or defecation routine provides clues to the possible development of the problem of constipation. In our bowel-conscious society, failure to have the usual bowel movement may be a source of concern to the patient. The patient's understanding of the influence of irregularity of dietary and activity patterns on defecation and of the frequency of bowel movements considered desirable provides a basis for clarifying any misunderstandings and giving needed instructions.

Dietary instruction should include discussion of the value of well-balanced meals including whole grain breads and cereals and both raw and cooked fruits and vegetables, which provide bulk and stimulate peristalsis, thus helping to maintain or reestablish regularity. Patients on limited activity who are selecting their own diets may need encouragement and guidance in diet selection and adequate fluid intake.

Patients with signs or symptoms of spastic constipation may do better on a diet that contains refined breads and cereals and only cooked fruits and vegetables. Their diet should be well balanced, but should exclude foods high in roughage.

Some regular exercise will aid normal defecation. Encourage this in moderation unless it is contraindicated. Bed patients may be permitted to do some exercise. This may be limited to muscle setting of the abdominal and perineal muscles to help maintain their tone. This is particularly important for elderly people. When possible, the patient should have the opportunity to use the toilet or a bedside commode rather than a bedpan. A squatting position requires the least effort for defecation. The use of a footstool may help the patient assume this position. Sufficient uninterrupted time and privacy should be provided to enable the patient to maintain his normal elimination pattern when possible, and he should be encouraged to try to have a movement at his usual time of day within his usual pattern. It should be made clear to the patient that daily bowel movements are unnecessary.

Fluids should be encouraged for patients who are being treated with bulk-producing or saline cathartics. This will help to prevent dehydration and increase the effectiveness of the cathartics.

Patients with chronic constipation may need to reestablish a habitual time for defecation. The specific time for this may be adjusted to suit their responsibilities. The physiologically opportune time for this is after a meal, as peristaltic activity in the colon may be expected to be more active at that time. The patient should be encouraged to allow sufficient time and to avoid the use of laxatives or enemas unless they are specifically ordered by a physician.

Patients with flaccid paralysis and elderly bed patients should be observed for fecal impactions. This should be done very gently. An oil retention enema may be ordered to soften the feces, and may be followed by a saline enema. Repeated tap water enemas should be avoided because they may result in loss of sodium and potassium and thus cause weakness.

GENERAL PRINCIPLES UNDERLYING THE NURSING CARE PLAN

Nursing care is concerned with helping to identify factors that may be causing or contributing to the problem of constipation and with providing support or assistance to help restore normal elimination. Nursing therapy includes clarification of the patient's understanding of factors that influence normal defecation, instruction as needed on the value of regularity of dietary pattern, activity, and a habitual time for defecation, and provision of uninterrupted time and privacy to permit support of normal defecation routines.

Flatulence

Either the failure to pass flatus or the passage of unusual amounts of flatus may indicate a potential problem. The failure to pass flatus, both postoperatively and following a spinal cord injury, may lead to abdominal distention and possibly to an intestinal obstruction. The passage of unusual amounts of foul-smelling flatus is embarrassing to the patient and may be a sign of impaired digestion and absorption.

Gas is a normal constituent of the intestinal tract. It is found both in the stomach and in the colon. About 50 cc is normally present in the stomach and about 100 cc in the colon. Estimates of the amount that is passed as flatus per day vary from 400 cc to 1600 cc.

FACTORS CAUSING FLATULENCE

Intestinal gas is derived from three possible sources. The principal source is air swallowed along with food, fluid, or frothy saliva. The other sources are gas formed during digestion and gas formed by the action of bacteria on partially digested foods. The amount that is formed from bacterial action depends on the diet and on the rate of peristalsis.

Flatus is normally odorless; however, the action of bacteria on certain ingested foods gives it a characteristic odor. Foods that have been found to increase the amount of flatus include broccoli, brussels sprouts, cabbage, cauliflower, cucumber, kohlrabi, lima beans, navy beans, onions, radishes, turnips, and melons. Excess intake of either raw fruits or raw vegetables may cause distressing flatus.

Some individuals find that the intake of milk, especially malted milk, may cause increased flatulence. This has been attributed to a deficiency of the enzyme lactase.

The accumulation of gas from swallowed air has been found to be influenced by posture, eating habits, and amount of salivation. More air is swallowed when the individual is in a supine position than in an upright one, and when eating rapidly, bolting foods, gulping liquids, drinking through a straw, or drinking carbonated beverages in a supine position. Chewing gum and smoking excessively increase salivation and the amount of air swallowed. The most common cause of aerophagia is said to be emotional tension associated with feelings of nervousness, apprehension, anxiety, resentment, or grief.

The accumulation of gas in the intestinal tract may cause considerable discomfort. It is normally relieved by belching or by passing flatus. Abdominal distention can reduce respiratory ventilation as a result of pressure on the diaphragm.

The movement of gas through the intestine provides an indication of its peristaltic activity. This may be detected by hearing soft crepitations, slow rumbles, or explosive sounds, and by the passage of flatus. Loss of motility of any segment of the intestine may result in the rapid accumulation of gas, causing cramping, abdominal pain, and abdominal distention. Unfortunately, the pressure of the gas may cause a spasm of the adjacent distal segment, which may further block peristaltic activity and can result in intestinal obstruction.

A number of factors may cause or contribute to loss of effective motility and peristalsis and hence predispose to gaseous distention. These include administration of some anesthetic agents or opiates; a low serum potassium; hypoxia of a segment of the intestine or a generalized hypoxemia; and spinal cord trauma.

MEDICAL TREATMENT

Patients in whom gaseous distention is expected to develop may be treated prophylactically with gastric intubation to remove swallowed air. Food and fluids may be withheld until flatus is passed. Patients in whom distention develops and who fail to pass flatus may be treated by intestinal intubation to relieve the distention or may be given a medication such as physostigmine or vasopressin (Pitressen) to stimulate peristalsis. A rectal tube or a low enema may be ordered to help remove the flatus from the colon.

NURSING CARE

Nursing care is designed to help detect the problem of gaseous distention, to help the patient minimize the amount of air swallowed, and to stimulate peristalsis.

Observation on postoperative or other patients on complete bed rest should include the presence or absence of the passage of flatus, abdominal distention, or any cramping pain.

When possible, the patient should sit up to drink fluids from a glass, rather than drink through a straw. Keeping the patient's mouth moist by frequent rinsing will help decrease the amount of air swallowed. Chewing gum and smoking should be avoided.

Less air enters the stomach when the individual is in the prone position than in the supine position, and the air that has been swallowed can be better eructated in the prone position.

Frequent change of position, turning, and walking help stimulate peristalsis and thus help prevent or relieve discomfort from gaseous distention.

The discomfort from distention may also be relieved by helping the patient relax his abdominal muscles. This is said to result in a reflex relaxation of spasm of the intestine. A side-lying position with the knees flexed promotes abdominal relaxation. The patient can be taught to consciously relax his abdominal wall. This should be done prior to surgery. Unless contraindicated, external heat may be used to help relieve spasm of the intestine. The patient should be expected to pass flatus when the spasm subsides.

In some individuals emotional tension may slow peristalsis and thus contribute to the problem of gaseous distention. Nursing therapy that may be useful includes listening to the patient's concerns, clarifying his misconceptions, and providing information about what he can do for himself and what will be done for him.

Individuals who have chronic problems of excessive or foul-smelling flatus should have a dietary history taken. Information regarding foods that may be contributing to this problem should be provided.

Early return of bowel sounds, absence of abdominal distention or of abdominal cramps, and passage of normal amounts of flatus provide evidence of successful prevention or alleviation of the problem of abdominal distention.

GENERAL PRINCIPLES UNDERLYING THE NURSING CARE PLAN

The failure to pass flatus may indicate the absence of effective paristaltic activity of the intestines. This may result in gaseous distention. The principal source of the gas is swallowed air. The amount of air swallowed may be increased by frequent swallowing of saliva, drinking through a straw, drinking in a supine position, and by emotional tension.

Nursing care is designed to help minimize the amount of air swallowed and to increase peristalsis. The use of the prone position will aid eructation of swallowed air, and frequent change of position or encouraging the patient to walk, when permitted, will help to stimulate peristalsis.

Chronic problems with gaseous distention and the passage of increased amounts of flatus may be related to the action of bacteria on certain foods. Information regarding foods that may contribute to this problem should be provided.

Abnormal Urinary Output

Among the most important of the abnormal discharges are marked alterations in the volume and characteristics of the urinary output. The volume of urine may be expected to vary depending upon the amount of fluid lost from the skin, lungs, and gastrointestinal tract—which are obligatory losses—and the amount of food and fluid intake. It should be recalled that two of the important functions of the kidneys are to maintain a constant volume and composition of body water and electrolytes and to excrete the waste products of protein catabolism. A daily minimum urinary output of 400 to 500 ml is essential to excrete the metabolic wastes from protein in the diet and from endogenous protein metabolism.

The volume of urinary output depends upon the concentrating power of the kidneys as well as the solute load of waste products to be excreted. The normal daily urinary output is about 1200 to 1500 ml. The daily intake and output may be expected to vary from individual to individual and from day to day under

WATER INTAKE		WATER EXCRETION	
In fluids	1500 ml approx.	Urine	1500 ml
In solid food	800 ml	Insensible perspiration	600 ml
In a mixed 2,500-calorie diet (from oxidation of hydrogen)	300 ml approx.	Vaporization from lungs	400 ml
		In feces	100 ml
Total	2600 ml approx.	Total	2600 ml

TABLE 18-1
Daily Water Balance   (Adapted by permission from Emanuel Goldberger: *A Primer of Water, Electrolyte and Acid-Base Syndromes,* 3d ed. Philadelphia: Lea & Febiger, 1965.)

different circumstances in the same individual, depending on the obligatory losses, the body temperature, and the specific food and fluid intake. Table 18-1 presents some *average* figures for the normal intake and output balance.

In disease states the volume of urine may vary from 0 to 10 liters or more a day. Both extremes are potentially life-threatening. Such alterations in urinary output may occur as acute or chronic conditions.

A comparison of the volume, specific gravity or osmolarity, pH, and sugar content of the first specimen of urine voided in the morning, with other specimens taken at specified intervals during the day, may assist in the diagnosis. A fresh urine specimen should be used to measure the pH because of the chemical changes that may occur over time.

Both deficiencies and excesses of urinary output may be accompanied by changes in the electrolyte composition of the intracellular and extracellular body fluids. These changes may occur as a result of abnormal losses of fluid from the gastro-intestinal tract, the skin, and/or the kidneys. Marked changes will be ultimately reflected in the electrolyte content of the plasma. Table 18-2 summarizes the range of water and electrolytes that may be lost from the gastrointestinal tract or the skin and the normal electrolytes in the blood plasma.

Changes in the concentration of sodium in the extracellular fluids will affect the volume of fluid in both the intracellular and extracellular spaces. This can usually be detected by changes in the serum proteins and hematocrit as well as signs and symptoms of circulatory insufficiency or overload.

Deviations in the normal electrolyte composition of body fluids have been found to be associated with signs and symptoms of altered physiological function of a number of other body systems. The presence of specific signs and symptoms serves as a clue to the possible fluid and electrolyte disturbance and provides a guide for the medical therapy.

Polyuria

Polyuria is the passage of excessive quantities of urine. This can lead to dehydra-tion, electrolyte deficiency, and circulatory deficiency. Polyuria may develop as

FLUID	AVERAGE VOLUME (ml/24 hr)	ELECTROLYTE CONCENTRATIONS (meq/liter)			
		Na+	K+	CL	HCO3–
Blood plasma		136–145	3.5–5.5	98–106	23–28
Gastric juice*	2500				
achlorhydric		8–120	1–30	100	20
containing HCl		10–110	1–32	8–55	0
Bile	700–1000	134–156	3.9–6.3	83–110	38
Pancreatic juice	>1000	113–153	2.6–7.4	54–95	110
Small bowel (Miller-Abbott suction)	3000	72–120	3.5–6.8	69–127	30
Ileostomy					
(a) recent	100–4000	112–142	4.5–14	93–122	30
(b) adapted	100–500	50	3	20	15–30
Cecostomy	100–3000	48–116	11.1–28.3	35–70	15
Feces	100	<10	<10	<15	<15
Sweat	500–4000	30–70	0–5	30–70	0

TABLE 18-2
Water and Electrolyte Losses in Gastrointestinal Secretions and in Sweat

* Electrolyte concentrations in gastric juice vary greatly. The concentration of sodium may be almost equal to that of chloride in patients with hypoacidity. This is a frequent finding in elderly patients. (Adapted by permission from Emanuel Goldberger: *A Primer of Water, Electrolyte and Acid-Base Syndromes*, 3d ed. Philadelphia: Lea & Febiger, 1965.)

a result of an inadequate reabsorption of water by the kidney tubules or from an increase in solute load. It may occur as a transient state or as a chronic condition.

FACTORS CAUSING POLYURIA

A number of factors may cause or contribute to polyuria. A transient polyuria may occur with the rapid administration of fluid, either parenterally or orally, with a high protein diet from the consequent increase in urea, or with the administration of diuretics. Polyuria may also occur with the ingestion of water and alcohol, both of which suppress the secretion of antidiuretic hormone.

A deficient reabsorption of water by the kidneys may occur from a lack of secretion of the antidiuretic hormone, as is seen in diabetes insipidus. Such a deficiency may also occur from the lack of response of the kidney tubules to the antidiuretic hormone, which may occur with chronic renal disease, hypokalemia, and hypercalcemia and as a congenital condition. The daily urinary output may be 3.5 to 10 liters or more. Such patients have polydipsia and will become rapidly dehydrated if fluids are withheld.

A number of factors can cause or contribute to an increased solute load and thus cause polyuria. These include an elevated blood sugar and ketone bodies in diabetes mellitus; elevated urea and other waste products as a result of the protein catabolism occurring from infections; an accumulation of water, urea, and other waste products and electrolytes during severe oliguria; and conditions leading to excess sodium, potassium, or calcium loss in the urine. Psychogenic water drinking is a final factor that may cause polyuria.

Polyuria can lead to dehydration, electrolyte deficiencies, and circulatory deficiency. Signs and symptoms of dehydration which may be seen in patients with polyuria include thirst, absence of saliva, dry mouth, a furrowed tongue, difficulty in phonation, lack of tissue turgor, a dry skin, and weight loss. Symptoms related to electrolyte deficits include weakness, muscle cramps and muscle twitching, personality changes, somnolence, confusion, hallucinations, and delirium. Convulsions and coma may occur with severe electrolyte deficits. Circulatory deficiency may be manifested by an elevation in serum proteins and hematocrit and by a weak, rapid pulse, a decrease in filling of neck veins, and hypotension.

MEDICAL MANAGEMENT

The medical management is designed to correct or control the primary disorder causing the polyuria and to prevent dehydration and electrolyte deficiencies. The specific fluid replacement will be guided by the amount of output, weight changes, and by laboratory findings including hematocrit, serum proteins, serum electrolytes, blood urea nitrogen, and possibly by the specific gravity, pH, sodium, potassium, or chloride content of the urine.

NURSING CARE

One of the major aims of nursing care for patients with polyuria is to help prevent fluid and electrolyte deficiencies. In order to accomplish this, a careful assessment of the patient's problem must be made and an adequate intake of oral or parenteral fluids ensured.

The seriousness of the problem of polyuria may be judged by changes in the volume and characteristics of the urine in comparison with the intake of fluids, weight changes, circulatory status, and the presence of any manifestations of fluid and electrolyte abnormalities. These should be assessed periodically and the findings recorded for future comparisons. The frequency of such assessments will depend upon the seriousness of the patient's fluid and electrolyte deficits.

The relation between a high urinary output, a high rate of fluid intake, and the administration of diuretics should be investigated, reported, and recorded.

The amount and rate of parenteral fluid intake should be checked with the physician's order. If the urine becomes pale and has a low specific gravity, the rate of the intravenous flow should be questioned. It may be reduced and then reevaluated by testing another urine specimen.

For patients with chronic polyuria, the selection of oral fluids will be based on a consideration of the electrolytes that are being lost and the patient's preferences. The patient's understanding of his fluid replacement needs should be assessed. His selection of fluids and his dietary intake should be observed to make sure that he is getting the replacements needed.

The adequacy of his fluid replacement may be judged by daily weights, an accurate intake and output record, and the presence or absence of signs and symptoms of fluid and electrolyte deficiencies.

The discussion of nursing care requirements for patients with dehydration will be included in the problem of oliguria.

Oliguria and Anuria

Oliguria denotes a diminished excretion of urine. For an adult it signifies a urinary output of less than 400 ml a day or not more than 15 to 20 ml per hour. Strictly speaking, *anuria* means the complete absence of urinary output, but this term is also used to denote an output of less than 100 ml a day. Oliguria may occur in a variety of systemic conditions as well as in primary renal disease.

Considered from a physiological standpoint, oliguria may occur as a result of either a decreased glomerular filtration rate or an increased reabsorption of water and sodium in the renal tubules. Both mechanisms may be involved. The glomerular filtration rate may be decreased in patients who have a low cardiac output, a diminished circulating volume, and/or a decreased blood pressure, and in patients who have an acute renal insufficiency. Anuria may reflect a severe oliguric state or the retention of urine in the bladder. A urinary tract obstruction will cause anuria.

Oliguria may occur as an acute or a chronic state. Prolonged oliguria is a potential threat to life due to the accumulation of the catabolic waste products from protein metabolism with the resulting elevation in serum potassium and metabolic acidosis. An excess intake of fluid in relation to the total output will cause an overhydration and a hyponatremia. Death may occur from fatal cardiac arrhythmias and pulmonary edema.

FACTORS CAUSING OLIGURIA

A number of factors may cause or contribute to oliguria in patients with normal kidney function. These include a loss of blood, as from hemorrhage; a loss of blood plasma, as from burns; or an abnormal loss of water and electrolytes from the gastrointestinal tract, the skin, or the lungs. Unless adequate replacements are given, such losses cause a reduction in circulating blood volume and blood pressure, a reduced glomerular filtration rate, and an increased reabsorption of water and sodium due to stimulation of secretion of antidiuretic hormone and aldosterone. The urine will be concentrated and have a specific gravity above 1.020. Prolonged hypotension can cause renal failure.

Sources of abnormal losses from the gastrointestinal tract include vomiting, diarrhea, intubation, or an ileus. Several liters of fluids may be sequestered in the intestines as a result of a paralytic ileus or an intestinal obstruction. With such losses not only may oliguria develop but also electrolyte disturbances. These will vary depending on the specific electrolytes lost.

Abnormal losses from the lungs or the skin may contribute to oliguria. They may also cause dehydration. Increased losses of water from the lungs may be expected in patients with a fever or with hyperventilation. The insensible loss may be doubled with such conditions. Fever, sweating, or a high environmental temperature will increase the water loss from the skin.

An inadequate intake of fluids may also contribute to the development of oliguria. This can be a hazard for patients who are on tube feedings or patients who are unable to respond to thirst.

A number of other factors have been found to contribute to a diminished urine formation in patients with normal kidney function. These include unrelieved pain, trauma, the administration of general anesthetics and some drugs including morphine, meperidine, and barbiturates, and positive-pressure breathing. The patient's feeling state has been found to influence the reabsorption of water and sodium, and hence the amount of urine formed. Feelings of anxiety, apprehension, fear, and of emotional tension associated with situations perceived as threatening by the patient have been associated with a diminished urinary output.

Oliguria is a common manifestation of all types of acute renal disease. These are discussed in detail in Chapter 24. A prolonged period of renal ischemia or nephrotoxicity may cause acute renal insufficiency and the resulting oliguria or anuria. The urine is characterized by a low or fixed specific gravity.

And finally, any obstruction to the flow of urine in the ureters, bladder, or urethra may cause an oliguria. If the obstruction is acute it will cause a total anuria. Among the more common factors causing obstructions are renal calculi, blood clots, enlarged prostate, and sphincter spasms. These conditions are discussed in greater detail in Chapter 24.

Hyperkalemia and metabolic acidosis may develop in patients with severe or prolonged oliguria as a result of the accumulation of potassium and acid products of protein catabolism. A hyponatremia associated with an accumulation of excess body water may also develop. These complications have been found to be associated with a number of symptoms of circulatory, central nervous system, gastrointestinal, muscular, and respiratory disturbances. The specific symptoms exhibited depend upon the severity of the electrolyte disturbances.

Manifestations of circulatory disturbances that may develop include specific electrocardiographic changes, arrhythmias, a decreased pulse rate, and engorged neck veins. A number of symptoms referable to the central nervous system may be observed. Such patients may complain of headache and they may be irritable, agitated, confused, disoriented, depressed, lethargic, drowsy, or stuporous and finally may become comatose.

Such gastrointestinal symptoms as anorexia, nausea, vomiting, diarrhea, and abdominal cramps may develop. The patient may complain of weakness and muscle cramps. Muscular weakness and muscle twitching may be observed. Flaccid paralysis, beginning in the extremities, is occasionally seen. Weakness of the respiratory muscles and difficulty with phonation may also be seen. The respirations may be slow and deep—the so-called Kussmaul respirations. An acetone odor may be detected on the breath.

Diagnosis of the possible causes and severity of oliguria is based on the history of the onset; the characteristics of the urine, particularly its color, appearance, specific gravity or osmolarity, and pH; laboratory findings including the hematocrit, serum proteins, blood urea nitrogen, and electrolytes; and accompanying signs and symptoms. Catheterization may be necessary to rule out a urinary obstruction.

MEDICAL MANAGEMENT

The medical therapy used in relation to the oliguria is designed to support the patient's circulation and to prevent further complications. For patients with a circulatory insufficiency the fluid replacement is guided by the amount and sources of the fluid loss. The rate of replacement is guided by the hourly urinary output, serial venous pressure changes, the hematocrit, and weight changes.

For patients with acute renal insufficiency, the aim of the medical therapy is to minimize the catabolic waste products that have to be excreted by the kidneys, to remove toxic waste products, and to prevent overhydration and circulatory failure. Supportive therapy usually includes a protein-sparing diet containing a minimum of 100 g of carbohydrate and no potassium or protein. Medications should be potassium-free. The patient may be given 50 percent glucose flavored with orange, lemon, or lime that has been either iced or frozen. When the serum potassium is elevated, the physician may order 10 percent glucose with insulin to be given intravenously to promote the movement of potassium into cells. Sodium lactate may be used to correct metabolic acidosis. Dialysis may be employed to remove toxic waste products. Antibiotics may be given to prevent infections. Fluids are restricted to prevent a circulatory overload. The amount of fluid intake is governed by the rate of output and an estimate of insensible loss.

NURSING CARE

One of the most important nursing responsibilities in caring for patients with acute oliguria is the periodic accurate assessment of fluid losses and the volume and rate of fluid intake. The aim of nursing care is to help minimize factors that may cause or contribute to oliguria as well as to help prevent complications.

In order to help assess the severity of the oliguria and the fluid and electrolyte deficiencies or excesses, the volume, specific gravity, and pH of the urine must be measured and recorded at specified intervals. This may be done hourly for the acutely ill patient. The output from vomiting, diarrhea, or tubal drainage must also be measured and recorded. Fluids used for enemas or for irrigating indwelling tubes or catheters must be measured. The amount of fluid that fails to return should be added to the daily intake record.

Loss of blood as a cause or contributing factor to oliguria may be assessed by observing the color of drainage from wounds, suction, vomitus, urine, and feces. Dressings may be weighed to estimate the plasma and blood loss through this route.

The possibility of a retention of urine should be considered. The patient's complaints of discomfort in the lower abdomen provide a valuable clue. A distention of the bladder may be detected by careful palpation and observation of the abdomen. An indwelling catheter may be irrigated with small amounts of normal saline, or a prescribed fluid, to check for an obstruction from blood clots or calculi. Results should be charted.

Further decreases in the volume or an increase in the specific gravity of the urine following the administration of morphine, barbiturates, or analgesics should be evaluated and recorded. If this occurs, the physician should be consulted before another dose is given. The rate of parenteral fluid intake must be carefully monitored. Pulmonary edema may develop in patients with severe oliguria and metabolic acidosis. The development of vascular overload leading to pulmonary edema may be recognized by an increased pulse rate, engorged neck veins, or an increase in the central venous pressure to 15 to 20 cm of water. Symptoms of pulmonary edema include rales, wheezing, frothy sputum, and dyspnea.

When a 10 percent infusion of glucose is ordered it should be given to minimize the irritation of the vein. In order to prevent insulin overshoot, the rate of flow should be gradually decreased before the infusion is discontinued.

The effectiveness of sodium lactate may be evaluated by changes in the respiratory rate and depth. These should both decrease when the metabolic acidosis has been neutralized.

For patients on a prescribed restricted oral fluid intake, the careful spacing of fluids throughout the day may help to minimize the discomfort of thirst. Consideration must be given to the amount of fluids which may be taken with oral medications in planning for the distribution of fluids during the day. It has been found that less fluid is taken per tablet or capsule when medications are taken with meals and when they are given less frequently. A dry mouth and the absence of saliva increase the amount of fluid taken with medications. Patients on a restricted daily intake of water tend to take a higher volume of water with their medications than others (Holmes).

When the patient is able to take his own fluids he must understand the amount of restriction. His preferences for specific permissible fluids should be elicited. Any restrictions on electrolyte and protein intake must be considered in selecting fluids to be given.

A number of nursing actions may be carried out to help minimize factors that contribute to the severity of oliguria. For patients on gastrointestinal suction, the loss from intestinal secretions will be minimized by using isotonic solutions, preferably normal saline, for irrigating the tubes, by using isotonic substances to make ice chips for moistening the patient's mouth, and by preventing the smell of food from entering the patient's room. Unless it is contraindicated, the patient's bed should be kept in a flat position in order to decrease the stimulus for antidiuretic hormone and to minimize postural hypotension. Keeping the patient who is bleeding quiet and avoiding sudden changes in his blood pressure will help minimize dislodgment of clots that help arrest bleeding.

Preventing infections, providing rest, and allaying anxiety will help to minimize protein catabolism and hence help to reduce the magnitude of hyperkalemia and metabolic acidosis in patients with acute renal failure. Allaying anxiety and pain may also help to reduce the amount of antidiuretic hormone secretion and hence the amount of water reabsorbed.

Preventing infection will also help to minimize the fluid loss from the lungs and the skin. Patients with severe or prolonged oliguria and hyperkalemia are likely candidates for a pulmonary infection because of their decreased ability to cough. These patients should be protected from exposure to personnel or other patients with infections. Careful medical asepsis must be used in caring for such patients. Aseptic precautions must be carried out in catheterization or irrigation of the catheter.

Patients with oliguria may also be dehydrated. This condition may be recognized by a shrunken tongue with longitudinal folds or furrows and a loss of elasticity or tissue turgor as measured by pinching the skin over the sternum, clavicle, or tibia. The mucous membranes of the mouth may be dry and saliva may be absent. The skin tends to be dry also. Parotitis may develop in these patients. Frequent mouth care with half-strength hydrogen peroxide has been found effective for improving the condition of the mouth. Keeping the mouth moist will help allay thirst. Oil emulsion in the bath water is useful for the dry skin.

GENERAL PRINCIPLES UNDERLYING THE NURSING CARE PLAN

The importance of accurate measurement and recording of intake and of specific fluid losses cannot be overemphasized. Such information, along with the signs and symptoms of fluid and electrolyte disturbance, provides a guide to the medical therapy and the nursing care. Periodic measurements of the volume and specific gravity of the urinary output, together with an assessment of the blood pressure, pulse, venous pressure, or neck vein collapse or engorgement, provide a guide to the adequacy of fluid intake. The signs and symptoms of fluid and electrolyte disturbances should be expected to subside with successful therapy.

The aim of nursing care is to help minimize factors that may contribute to the polyuria or oliguria and to minimize the discomfort from thirst, dry mouth, and dry skin. Prevention of infection is particularly important for patients with oliguria. The patient's preference and his understanding of permissible oral fluids should be considered in planning for the spacing of fluids during the day.

Bibliography

Books of General Interest

Beeson, Paul B. and Walsh McDermott (Eds.): *Cecil-Loeb Textbook of Medicine,* 12th ed. Philadelphia: W. B. Saunders Company, 1967.

Davenport, Horace W.: *Physiology of the Digestive Tract,* 2d ed. Chicago: Year Book Medical Publishers, Inc., 1966.

Goldberger, Emanuel: *A Primer of Water Electrolyte and Acid-Base Syndromes,* 3d ed. Philadelphia: Lea & Febiger, 1965.

Goodman, Louis Sanford and Alfred Gilman: *The Pharmacological Basis of Therapeutics,* 3d ed. New York: The Macmillan Company, 1965.

Hamburger, Jean, et al.: *Nephrology,* Vol. 1. Philadelphia: W. B. Saunders Company, 1968.

Harrison, T. R. (Ed.): *Principles of Internal Medicine,* 5th ed. New York: McGraw-Hill Book Company, 1966.

MacBryde, Cyril M. (Ed.): *Signs and Symptoms,* 4th ed. Philadelphia: J. B. Lippincott Company, 1964.

Maxwell, Morton H. and Charles R. Kleeman: *Clinical Disorders of Fluid and Electrolyte Metabolism.* New York: McGraw-Hill Book Company, 1962.

Metheny, Norma Milligan and William D. Snively: *Nurses' Handbook of Fluid Balance.* Philadelphia: J. B. Lippincott Company, 1967.

Shafer, Kathleen Newton, Janet R. Sawyer, Audrey M. McCluskey, and Edna Lifgren Beck: *Medical-Surgical Nursing,* 4th ed. Saint Louis: The C. V. Mosby Company, 1967.

Smith, Dorothy W. and Claudia D. Gips: *Care of the Adult Patient,* 2d ed. Philadelphia: J. B. Lippincott Company, 1966.

Vomiting

Borison, Herbert L. and S. C. Wang: Physiology and Pharmacology of Vomiting. *Pharmacological Review,* 5:193–230, June, 1953.

Cummins, Alvin I.: The Physiology of Symptoms; III. Nausea and Vomiting. *American Journal of Digestive Diseases,* New Series, 3:10:709–721, October, 1958.

Downs, Howard S.: The Control of Vomiting. *American Journal of Nursing,* 66:76–82, January, 1966.

McCarthy, Rosemary T.: Vomiting. *Nursing Forum,* 3:1:49–59, 1964.

Purkis, Ian E.: Factors That Influence Postoperative Vomiting. *Canadian Anaesthetists' Society Journal,* 11:335–353, July, 1964.

Wilbur, Dwight L.: Functional Disturbances of the Gastrointestinal Tract. in Gordon McHardy (Ed.): *Current Gastroenterology.* New York: Paul B. Hoeber, Inc., 1962, pp. 221–232.

Abnormal Stools

Connell, A. M., Claire Hilton, G. Irvine, J. E. Lennard-Jones, and J. J. Misiewicz: Variations of Bowel Habit in Two Population Samples. *British Medical Journal,* 2:1095–1099, November 6, 1965.

Cooke, W. T. and C. T. G. Flear: Treatment of Electrolyte Disturbance Associated with Malabsorption. *Modern Treatment,* 2:400–406, March, 1965.

Grace, William J., Stewart Wolf, and Harold G. Wolff: Life Situations, Emotions, and Colonic Function. *Gastroenterology,* 14:1:93–107, January, 1950.

Kirshen, Martin M.: Constipation, *American Journal of Proctology,* 13:5:291–296, October, 1962.

Sherbanuik, Richard W.: The Physiology of Diarrhea. *Canadian Medical Association Journal,* 91:1–6, July, 1964.

Thomas, J. Earl: The Autonomic Nervous System in Gastrointestinal Disease. *Journal of the American Medical Association,* 157:3:209–212, January 15, 1955.

Turner, A. C.: Traveller's Diarrhoea: A Survey of Symptoms, Occurrence, and Possible Prophylaxis. *British Medical Journal,* 4:653–654, December 16, 1967.

Wangell, Anders G. and Donald J. Deller: Intestinal Motility in Man; III. Mechanisms of Constipation and Diarrhea with Particular Reference to the Irritable Colon Syndrome. *Gastroenterology,* 48:1:69–84, January, 1965.

Weijers, H. A. and J. H. van de Kamer: Causes of Diarrhoea in Disturbed Digestion. *Bibliotheca Nutritio et Dieta,* 7:233–242, March, 1965.

Flatulence

Gall, L. S.: The Role of the Intestinal Flora on Gas Production. *Annals of New York Academy of Science,* 150:27–30, February 26, 1968.

Hood, J. H.: Clinical Considerations of Intestinal Gas. *Annals of Surgery,* 163:3:359–366, March, 1966.

Roth, James L.: The Symptom Patterns of Gaseousness. *Annals of New York Academy of Science,* 150:109–126, February 26, 1968.

Abnormal Urinary Output

Barnes, Robert and William W. Schottstaedt: The Relation of Emotional State to Renal Excretion of Water and Electrolytes in Patients with Congestive Heart Failure. *American Journal of Medicine,* 29:2:217–227, August, 1960.

Brun, Claus, E. O. E. Knudsen, and Fleming Raaschou: The Influence of Posture on the Kidney Function; 1. The Fall of Diuresis in the Erect Posture. *Acta Medica Scandinavica,* 122:315–331, 1945.

Gault, Henry, Michael Dixson, Michael Doyle, and Walter Cohen: Hypernatremia, Azotemia, and Dehydration Due to High-Protein Tube Feeding. *Annals of Internal Medicine,* 68:4: 778–791, April, 1968.

Holmes, Joseph H., Visith Sitprya, Pamela Walker, and James Simpson: Fluid Intake with Medication. *Archives of Internal Medicine,* 116:813–818, December, 1965.

Lapides, Jack, Richard B. Bourne, and Lloyd R. MacLean: Clinical Signs of Dehydration and Extracellular Fluid Loss. *Journal of the American Medical Association,* 191:5:141–143, February 1, 1965.

Mandell, Arnold: Psychogenic Retention of Water. *American Heart Journal,* 65:4:572–573, April, 1963.

Moralejo, Richard V.: Fluid Balance. *Canadian Nurse,* 58:1075–1078, December, 1962.

Moran, Walter H., et al.: The Relationship of Antidiuretic Hormone Secretion to Surgical Stress. *Surgery,* 56:99–108, 1964.

Passos, Joyce Y. and Lucy M. Brand: Effects of Agents Used for Oral Hygiene. *Nursing Research,* 15:3: 196–202, Summer, 1966.

Pearson, J. B.: Water and Electrolyte Balance. *Nursing Times,* 63:415–418, March 31, 1967.

Schottstaedt, William, William Grace, and Harold G. Wolff: Life Situations, Behavioral Patterns and Renal Excretion of Fluid and Electrolytes. *Journal of the American Medical Association,* 157:1485–1488, April 23, 1955.

Snively, W. D. and B. Becker: Body Fluids and Neuro-Psychologic Disturbances. *Psychosomatics,* 9:6:295–305, November-December, 1968.

Thomas, S.: Some Effects of Change of Posture on H_2O and Electrolyte Excretion by Human Kidney. *Journal of Physiology,* 139:3:337–352, December, 1957.

CHAPTER 19
DISTURBANCES OF INTAKE OF FOOD AND FLUID

DOROTHY OLSON HOSHAW

Manifestations of disturbances of food and fluid intake
HYPERPHAGIA AND ANOREXIA
POLYDIPSIA
DYSPHAGIA

A complex of possible causative factors and sequential body response mechanisms comes into play in patients who demonstrate disturbances of food and fluid intake. The key to the interrelatedness of these mechanisms is thought to be the physiological functioning of the hunger and thirst centers that have been demonstrated in the hypothalamus. Physical and psychological stimuli act on these centers and stimulate or depress their function, causing the sensations of thirst, appetite and hunger, and satiety. Excessive stimulation or inhibition of these centers results in symptoms of hyperphagia, anorexia, or polydipsia, and indicates the presence of a pathophysiological process.

Normally, eating is a voluntary act mediated by sensations of appetite, hunger, and satiety. Specifically defined, appetite is a person's psychological need for food, whether there is a physiological need for food intake or not. It is tempered by one's food likes and dislikes, one's mood of the moment, one's environment, and many other emotional factors. Hunger is the body's organic, physiological need for food —the basic, life-sustaining drive that motivates food intake. It can be present with or without appetite, just as appetite can be present with or without hunger.

Satiety, on the other hand, is the cessation of one's desire for food as a result of adequate intake. It is inherent in that warm, pleasant feeling of satisfaction and the complete lack of interest in food that one experiences after having eaten a hearty meal.

Much research has been done in efforts to define the specific nature of the homeostatic mechanisms involved in hunger, appetite, and satiety; and though few specifics have been demonstrated clearly, feeding and satiety centers have been demonstrated in the hypothalamus. It is thought that these centers are the site of homeostatic regulation of food intake. Various stimuli are relayed to the controlling centers, and these stimuli trigger reflexive feedback. For instance, about 3 to 5 hours after one has eaten, the nerve endings in the walls of the stomach are stimulated by the emptiness of the stomach, and these receptors send impulses to the feeding center in the hypothalamus which indicate a need for food. The feeding center reflexively causes the stomach to begin to contract—contractions interpreted as "hunger pangs"—and simultaneously stimulates thoughts of food—appetite. After food intake, the stretch receptors in the wall of the stomach are stimulated by the distention of the stomach and send stimuli to the feeding and satiety center inhibiting thoughts of more food intake and stimulating sensations of satiety. In this way, the feeding and satiety centers are sensitive to stimuli from various local sources which cause either stimulation or inhibition of the desire for food.

Along with the local sources of stimuli, various metabolic mechanisms have been demonstrated such as the glucostatic mechanism. In this case it is hypothesized that there are glucoreceptors in the hypothalamic feeding center which are sensitive to blood glucose levels. The decrease in available blood glucose that occurs between meals is picked up by the glucose-sensitive cells, and they initiate impulses that stimulate sensations of hunger.

Another metabolic mechanism that has been hypothesized is the thermostatic mechanism. There is a slight increase in body temperature upon eating, due to the specific dynamic action of foods, which is too small to record clinically but which seems to be a factor in limiting food intake. It is felt that the feeding and satiety centers are sensitive to this temperature change related to eating and thus work to regulate the balance of food intake with energy output—inherent factors in the total metabolism of the body.

In addition to the physiological mechanisms that act on the feeding and satiety centers, there is also the strong influence of the psychological mechanisms. Appetite is psychogenically oriented and, though usually related to hunger, can be completely disassociated from it. Emotional stress, such as anxiety, guilt, or depression, can completely depress the feeding center even to the point of starvation.

The eating environment is important, and the influence of previous experiences a person has had with food or situations related to eating tempers his appetite. Food likes and dislikes are more often than not the key to appetite, and determine to a large extent what one eats and does not eat. Culture and religion are also decisive mediators of food habits. Mexicans, for instance, traditionally eat hot, chili-spiced foods and find much of the lightly seasoned foods in the United States tasteless and unpalatable. Most of us in the United States, on the other hand, find it almost "incompatible with life" to eat some of the favorite Mexican condiments, because they are simply too hot. Thus eating is mediated by many physiological and psychological factors.

Manifestations of Disturbances of Food and Fluid Intake

HYPERPHAGIA AND ANOREXIA

Common manifestations of disturbances of food intake are *hyperphagia*, a symptom denoting excessive food intake, and *anorexia*, a symptom involving a loss of appetite which causes an absence of food intake. Both these symptoms pose challenging patient problems that must be dealt with by nursing approaches that are based on an understanding of the underlying pathophysiology and complement the physician's therapeutic plan.

It has been experimentally shown in animals that a destructive lesion of nuclei in the ventromedial aspect of the hypothalamus (the satiety center) causes food intake far beyond that needed, and subsequent gross obesity. Likewise, a destructive lesion of the lateral hypothalamic nuclei (the hunger center) can inhibit food intake to the point of emaciation and starvation. Destructive hypothalamic lesions are rarely seen in human beings, however, and the underlying causes of hyperphagia and anorexia in patients are more commonly related to local gastrointestinal stimuli or metabolic derangements, or are the results of influences from the higher psychic centers, any one of which can cause an inhibition or stimulation of the feeding center.

An example of a metabolic disorder causing hyperphagia is the hyperphagia of untreated diabetes. In this disease, the symptom is due to an insufficient production of insulin which interferes with the ability of cells to utilize the available blood glucose, despite adequate carbohydrate intake. This inability to utilize the available blood glucose is seemingly true for the glucoreceptor cells in the hypothalamus as well, rendering them insensitive to the hyperglycemia and causing them to continue to stimulate food intake. The hyperphagia, then, is a manifestation of the pathophysiological changes that accompany diabetes. The physician's rationale for therapy is to control the underlying metabolic deficit by administering insulin or one of the hypoglycemic agents and by prescribing a controlled diabetic diet. The nurse, in turn, supplements the physician's therapeutic plan by such observations as those related to assessing the insulin therapy or watching for signs and symptoms of insulin shock or diabetic coma. This, then, is an example of treating hyperphagia by treating the underlying disease process.

Another example of a metabolic cause of hyperphagia is seen in the patient with hyperthyroidism. In this case there is an overproduction of thyroid hormone which greatly increases the body's metabolic rate and, in turn, increases the body's demand for food to support the increase in metabolism. Here again, the treatment of choice is to treat the underlying metabolic deficit by decreasing the amount of thyroid being produced, through the use of drugs, or through the surgical removal of part or all of the thyroid gland. In this case, the nursing approach would be to see that the patient ingested enough high-carbohydrate, high-protein, vitamin-enriched foods to support the increased metabolism and prevent excessive weight loss; whereas with the diabetic, excessive intake of high-carbohydrate and high-caloric foods must be prevented, because of the resultant hyperglycemia.

The psychological factors related to disturbances of food intake are receiving greater recognition through clinical and laboratory research. In the case of obesity, most authorities agree that the cause is predominantly related to an excessive appetite and not to a fundamental metabolic defect. It is a problem of an excessive desire for food and is unrelated to physiological need.

Therapeutically, the physician tends to approach obesity in four basic ways: by recommending and prescribing a reduced food intake, increasing exercise, prescribing appetite depressants, and providing psychotherapy or emotional support. Because of the common problem of a chronic intake of calories beyond the body's metabolic need and a resultant excessive storage of fat in body tissue, a reduction diet is basic. By means of a diet, the caloric intake can be controlled to provide enough intake of essential nutrients to maintain optimum health and, at the same time, facilitate the gradual use of the fat stores by the body. In conjunction with the diet, appetite suppressants are sometimes prescribed to be taken at specific intervals during the day. These can help to decrease the desire for more food and promote a feeling of satisfaction with the amount of food allocated for each meal by the diet, but they are not very often an effective replacement for will power. Planned exercise is also an important part of a reduction regimen, because a decrease in exercise is often a contributing cause of obesity. The "middle-age bulge," for instance, is more often than not the result of decreased activity without a decrease in the amount of food intake to match the reduced metabolic need.

There is also the difficult problem of dealing therapeutically with the often very complex emotional causes of excessive food intake. Sometimes close supervision and general emotional support on the part of the doctor are adequate, but in many cases there are severe, deep-seated psychological problems that require long-term psychotherapy preceding, or in conjunction with, a reduction regimen.

Effectively supporting the doctor's therapeutic approach to obesity is the nurse's responsibility. Instruction in diet is frequently an initial and on-going responsibility of the nurse. Also, there is the need for the nurse to provide continual encouragement for the patient as he tries to readjust his eating habits and work through his frustrations and problems related to dieting. A familiarity with some of the everyday problems such as those described by Little and Gray in relation to what they faced and experienced during their dieting regimens can help the nurse become aware of what to anticipate in patients. It also enables her to warn the patients of what to anticipate in themselves.

Facilitating group therapy for obese patients can also be a nursing approach when done under the direction of a psychiatrist. The group situation provides an opportunity for obese patients to give each other group support and comradeship by sharing their feelings about their obesity and the problems and frustrations they are having with their dieting regimens.

Anorexia, as a symptom, results in a loss of body weight. It may be due either to some underlying pathology such as leukemia or hepatitis or to the side effects of a therapeutic treatment being used, such as cobalt therapy, or it may be of unknown etiology. It may be either a short-term problem or a chronic problem which leads to excessive weight loss and emaciation. Whatever the predisposing cause, anorexia is usually the result of a depression of the appetite center in the hypothalamus associated with a reflexive hypofunction of the stomach. This is manifested by a relaxation of the muscles of the stomach, causing hypomotility, pallor of the mucosa of the stomach, and hypoacidity. The depression of the feeding center in the hypothalamus can be from central nervous system origin, such as the psychic centers or the sensory centers, both of which have a definite influence on a person's appetite.

Such psychogenic factors as disgusting or obnoxious sights, smells, or tastes, mental depression, emotional stress, fear, and pain are known to cause anorexia and, reflexively, to cause the hypoactivity and hypotonicity of the stomach. There can be direct inhibition of the center from substances in the blood, such as toxins from acute and chronic infections, the accumulation of abnormal metabolites, or direct ischemia of the center, as in the case of increased intracranial pressure and anemia. Local visceral pathology, such as conditions that cause a dilatation of the stomach, congestion or edema of the walls of the stomach, or congestion of other closely associated organs, may stimulate nerve endings with resultant depression of feeding centers. But, whatever the cause, anorexia can lead to a vicious circle with increasing malnutrition and debilitation, if the patient fails to eat.

As with hyperphagia, the rationale for treatment of anorexia by the physician is related to the underlying pathophysiology. Most often this involves specifically treating the organic disease entity either therapeutically or palliatively, such as using medication to decrease pain, treating the cause of infection, or drilling burr holes to relieve the cause of increased intracranial pressure. Certain appetite stimulants can be administered, but anorexia, as an isolated symptom, is a difficult problem to treat directly.

In the case of the symptom complex, anorexia nervosa (a psychogenic malnutrition), or in the case of acute mental depression, psychotherapy is usually necessary to deal with the deep-seated emotional problems associated with eating which are causing the anorexia.

The rationale for the nurse's approach to the problem of anorexia should be basically related to the immediate cause of the anorexia. However, even if the cause of the anorexia is unknown, there are measures that a nurse can take to

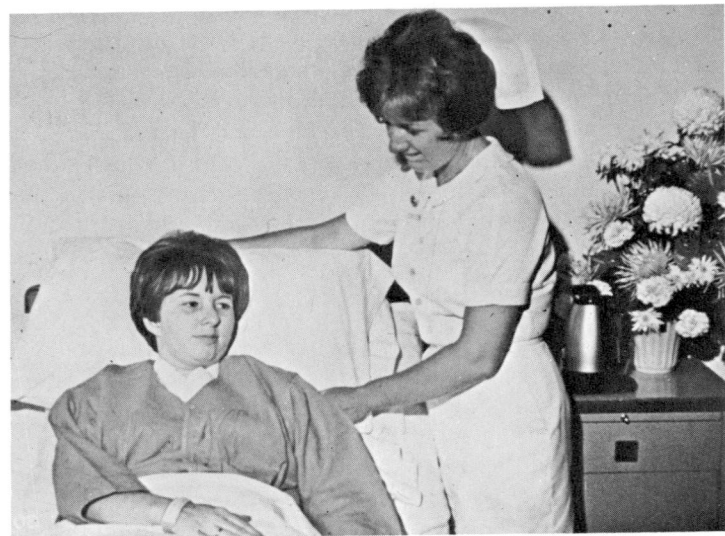

*Figure 19–1
The nurse can take sev-
eral simple measures to
encourage the anorectic
patient to eat, such as
straightening the bed
linens and elevating the
back rest.*

increase the appeal of food for an anorectic patient and make the environment for eating as pleasant and conducive to eating as possible (Figs. 19-1 and 19-2).

It is important to ascertain the food likes and dislikes of the patient and see that he gets what seems desirable to him, if possible. Also, an attractive tray with the food prepared and served in an appealing manner can stimulate the patient's desire to eat. Placing the patient in a room or a ward away from unpleasant smells, sounds, or sights might help. Avoid changing dressings just before meals or carrying out malodorous treatments that might produce sensory stimuli that would depress appetite. Providing for oral hygiene before meals and scheduling medications that might depress the appetite so that their effects interfere as little as possible with mealtimes are other beneficial nursing actions. Frequent small feedings of solids or liquids increase oral intake. Also, when a patient has to be fed, this assistance should be carried out in a pleasant and unhurried manner.

*Figure 19–2
An attractive tray will
help to stimulate the pa-
tient's appetite. All necessary items are properly
arranged on the tray.*

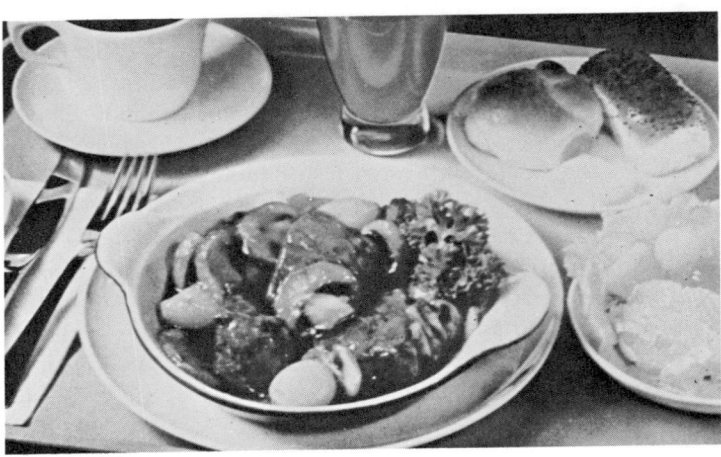

A nursing practice based on physiological principles is to start an anorectic patient's meal with an appetizer in the form of a small serving of food or liquid. If a short time span is permitted before the next course, the appetizer may cause the stomach to begin to contract and may combat the hypomotility and hypoacidity typical of anorexia. Dietary teaching may be necessary for the patient and, not infrequently, for the family as well. In cases in which stresses such as fear, severe depression, or psychoses are causing the anorexia, a therapeutic approach of emotional support and encouragement on the part of the nurse is important.

POLYDIPSIA

As with food intake, fluid intake is a voluntary act requiring specific sensations that indicate the need for fluid or that enough fluid has been taken in. Normally, homeostatic mechanisms such as sensations of thirst and selective reabsorption of fluid and electrolytes in the kidney tubules control the amount of fluid taken in and the amount excreted. The total fluid intake should approximate the total fluid output over a 24-hour period of time. This maintains the extracellular fluid volume in a consistent concentration and volume and, in turn, maintains the homeostasis of the intracellular fluid.

Thirst is a generalized sensation indicating the need for fluid intake. It can be caused by dryness of the oropharyngeal mucous membranes and a decrease in saliva production, by a decrease in extracellular fluid volume, or by cellular dehydration. A thirst center has been demonstrated in the hypothalamus which, as with the eating center, can trigger reflex actions that motivate or inhibit fluid intake. It is hypothesized that the cells in this hypothalamic center are osmoreceptors that are sensitive to solute concentration of circulating body fluids and to variations in fluid content of tissue cells themselves. It seems that the source of the antidiuretic hormone and the osmoreceptors of the thirst center are closely approximated in location and in physiological function, and that the thirst-neurohypophyseal-renal axis is the primary mechanism maintaining the solute concentration of the body's extracellular fluid in a constant state.

Basically, thirst indicates an underlying need for water, but it does not always indicate a deficit in the water content of the body. For instance, a patient who has had fluid withheld because of surgery but whose fluid intake has been maintained by adequate administration of intravenous fluids might experience extreme thirst. This thirst can be caused by dryness of the mouth from the effect of a drug such as atropine, and the lack of oral fluids to moisten the membranes. An effective means of alleviating the thirst is to keep the oropharyngeal membranes moist by frequently rinsing the mouth with water or a dilute mouthwash solution, and by keeping the lips and tongue moist with a damp, cold sponge or small amounts of ice chips. These techniques are also effective with patients who have had severe fluid and electrolyte disturbances from renal or hepatic disorders and an accompanying dryness of the oral mucous membranes. These patients tend to retain large amounts of water in various tissues such as the soft tissues of their extremities or in their peritoneal cavity, and yet experience severe thirst. The thirst is due to cellular dehydration from the abnormal osmolarity of the extracellular solutes, and if the patients drink excessive amounts of water, this further compounds the fluid imbalance.

Polydipsia, as a symptom, is indicative of various pathophysiological disorders. Diabetes mellitus is one in which the excretion of high quantities of glucose by the kidneys osmotically causes the excretion of high quantities of water. Thus, the untreated diabetic finds that he is constantly thirsty and drinking water, a homeostatic response to prevent severe dehydration that would otherwise occur as he lost more and more water in his urine. In diabetes insipidus, there is a failure of production of the antidiuretic hormone (vasopressin) by the anterior hypophysis, which controls the permeability of the collecting tubules of the kidney. This results in an uncontrolled loss of water through the kidneys and a secondary polydipsia due to the tendency toward dehydration. In these cases, the physician's treatment of choice is to treat the underlying disease by administering insulin for the diabetes mellitus and vasopressin for the diabetes insipidus. In fact, any condition causing a diminished extracellular fluid volume, such as hemorrhage, severe diaphoresis, renal or intestinal fluid loss, or a change in body fluid distribution, as in severe burns, causes thirst and the desire for increased fluid intake. Medical treatment focuses on correcting the underlying condition causing the thirst, as well as correcting the fluid and electrolyte imbalance.

The nursing approach to thirst and polydipsia relates to the underlying cause of the symptom and the physician's therapeutic plan. It is basically aimed at restoring or maintaining body fluid balance. As previously mentioned, in cases of extreme thirst in which the administration of oral fluids would be detrimental —for instance, postoperatively—the nursing measures are geared toward decreasing the local sensations of thirst in the mouth and pharynx, in the hope of allaying the patient's discomfort. When large amounts of fluid are being excreted and must be replaced, as with the patient with diabetes insipidus, the nurse's responsibility is to administer an adequate amount of fluid as indicated necessary by the patient's output. This might necessitate conscientiously encouraging the patient to drink, if the sensation of thirst is absent, and seeing that a certain amount is taken (forcing fluids), or by regulating the infusion of the intravenous fluid therapy as ordered by the doctor. Basic to any problem of fluid imbalance or potential imbalance is the nurse's responsibility for keeping an accurate record of the patient's intake and output, including all the means by which the patient is receiving and losing fluids, and in utilizing the information in initiating and planning nursing care.

In addition to the physiological causes of polydipsia, there are cases of psychogenic polydipsia that can lead to water intoxication, a hysterical condition in which the patient drinks excessive quantities of water for no apparent reason. It is manifested by irritability, confusion, convulsions, and then coma, symptoms caused by a decrease in the osmolarity of the extracellular fluid causing cellular hydration. To alleviate this problem, the patient has to be prevented from drinking the massive quantities of water that he is inclined to drink, and the underlying emotional problems have to be explored and dealt with psychiatrically. Actually, most of the acute cases of water intoxication per se occur in patients in the immediate postoperative period who have been given excessive quantities of fluids intravenously. This is preventable by the careful regulation of fluids by both the doctor in ordering fluids and the nurse in regulating the intravenous infusions.

DYSPHAGIA

Swallowing is a process initiated by voluntary action under central nervous system control and carried through by reflex action. The tongue pushes the bolus of food to be swallowed to the back of the mouth toward the pharyngoesophageal sphincter. This stimulates the sphincter to relax. The soft palate moves up to close the nasopharynx to keep food from entering the nares, the vocal cords close together, and the epiglottis moves back to cover the aperture of the larynx and prevent food from entering the trachea. Then the pharyngeal contraction moves the bolus of food through the cricopharyngeal sphincter into the upper part of the esophagus. There an esophageal peristaltic contraction is stimulated and the bolus of food moves down the esophagus, through the gastroesophageal sphincter, and into the stomach.

Any difficulty in the swallowing process is denoted as *dysphagia,* a symptom characterized by the inability to pass food or fluid from the mouth to the stomach or by pain associated with some aspect of swallowing. It can be due to mechanical obstruction of the esophagus, a disturbance in the neuromuscular mechanisms involved in swallowing, some problem in the mouth, larynx, or pharynx which causes pain or prevents the movement of food into the esophagus, or a psychological problem that prevents normal swallowing from taking place.

If possible, a surgical approach is used to treat esophageal obstructions or strictures and, depending on the underlying cause, this is frequently the treatment of choice as well for lesions of the mouth, larynx, or pharynx which cause pain upon swallowing. In dysphagia caused by disturbances of the neuromuscular mechanisms such as is seen in amyotrophic lateral sclerosis, Guillain-Barré syndrome, and multiple sclerosis, and also in disturbances of the smooth muscle and fibers of the esophagus as is seen in scleroderma, no known definitive medical treatment is readily available. In these cases, the dysphagia is treated palliatively, as by inserting a feeding tube. In globus hystericus, muscle spasm causes the patient to feel a lump in his throat which interferes with swallowing. The treatment of choice is to deal with the underlying psychological problem, which is usually related to emotional stress and fatigue.

Dysphagia can actually be manifested in various ways. The difficulty may be specific to foods of a certain consistency; for instance, a patient may have no trouble swallowing thick, viscous liquids or semisolids, whereas he might have great difficulty in swallowing thin liquids. Another patient might find liquids in general easier to swallow than solids, or he might find that only periodically does he have difficulty and between times he experiences no dysphagia at all. In any case, it is important that the nurse observe and inquire into the nature of the dysphagia. She must also note the existence and timing of any regurgitation that occurs after food or fluid intake, what the regurgitated material looks like, any complaints by the patient of feelings of food sticking in the throat or the esophagus and, if pain is present, where it is localized and to what aspect of swallowing it is related.

In addition to making pertinent observations, the nurse must also be concerned with maintaining the dysphagic patient's intake, whether by providing foods of the consistency the patient can swallow, by positioning him in a manner that facilitates his swallowing, or by arranging matters so that the patient is not rushed during his meals and has adequate privacy if he is embarrassed by his inability to eat neatly without drooling or losing food from his mouth. The nurse must also be alert to any indications of choking or coughing, especially in patients with neuromuscular disturbances, since there is always the serious danger of food or fluid being aspirated into the trachea if the swallowing reflex fails. Any escape of food or fluid through the nares should be immediately noted, as this may be an indication that there is a paralysis of the soft palate, and all oral intake should be discontinued until the doctor has seen the patient. In a case in which swallowing is completely inhibited, the patient must usually be fed through a nasogastric feeding tube; or, if tube feeding is to be a permanent means of food intake, a surgically placed gastrostomy tube is used.

Bibliography

Books

Beland, Irene: *Clinical Nursing: Pathophysiological and Psychosocial Approaches.* New York: The Macmillan Company, 1965.

Best, C. H. and N. Taylor: *The Physiological Basis of Medical Practice,* 8th ed. Baltimore: The Williams & Wilkins Company, 1966.

Guyton, A. C.: *Textbook of Medical Physiology,* 3d ed. Philadelphia: W. B. Saunders Company, 1966.

Harrison, T. R. (Ed.): *Principles of Internal Medicine,* 5th ed. New York: McGraw-Hill Book Company, 1966.

MacBryde, Cyril: *Signs and Symptoms: Applied Pathologic Physiology and Clinical Interpretation,* 4th ed. Philadelphia: J. B. Lippincott Company, 1964.

Ruch, T. C. and H. D. Patton: *Physiology and Biophysics,* 19th ed. Philadelphia: W. B. Saunders Company, 1965.

Shafer, Kathleen, Janet Sawyer, Audrey McCluskey, and Edna Beck: *Medical-Surgical Nursing,* 4th ed. St. Louis: The C. V. Mosby Company, 1967.

Thompson, R. F.: *Foundations of Physiological Psychology.* New York: Harper & Row, Publishers, Incorporated, 1967.

Articles

Bewley, T. H.: Acute Water Intoxication from Compulsive Water Drinking. *British Medical Journal,* II:864, October 2, 1964.

Brobeck, J. K.: Neural Basis of Hunger, Appetite and Satiety. *Journal of Gastroenterology,* 32:169–174, 1957.

Brosin, H. W.: Psychiatric Aspects of Obesity. *Journal of American Medical Association,* 155:1238–1239, 1954.

Bruch, Hilda: Psychological Aspects of Overeating and Obesity. *Psychosomatics,* 15:5:269–274, September-October, 1964.

Fischer, R. A., G. W. Ellison, W. R. Thayer, H. M. Spiro, and G. H. Glaser: Esophological Motility in Neuromuscular Disorders. *Annals of Internal Medicine,* 63:2:229–248, August, 1965.

Kelly, M. L.: Esophageal Motor Function Physiology as Reflected by Intraluminal Manometric Studies. *Ameri-*

can *Journal of Digestive Diseases,* New Series 9:8:553–565, August, 1964.

Little, Dolores and Florence Gray: It's Not a Matter of Will Power. *American Journal of Nursing,* 61:11:101–103, November, 1961.

Loeb, L.: The Clinical Cause of Anorexia Nervosa. *Psychosomatics,* 6:345–347, November-December, 1964.

Mayer, Jean: Some Aspects of the Problem of Regulation of Food Intake and Obesity. *New England Journal of Medicine,* 274:11:610–616, March 17, 1966.

Miller, C. H.: Current Understanding of Eating and Dieting. *Psychosomatics,* 2:119–126, March-April, 1964.

Stevenson, J. A. F.: The Hypothalamus in the Regulation of Energy and Water Balance. *Physiologist,* 7:4:305–318, November, 1964.

Texter, E. C.: Motility in the Gastrointestinal Tract. *Journal of the American Medical Association,* 184:640–647, May, 1963.

PART V

NURSING CARE OF PATIENTS

PURPOSE

The purpose of Part V is to provide knowledge of specific diseases and the nursing care of patients with these diseases.

The nurse needs information about disease, not only to provide quality patient care but to talk intelligently with the physician and to understand his plan of treatment.

For the most part, this section does not reiterate material from the first four parts but repeats where it seems important for added emphasis. Some repetition was included so that Part V could stand alone for the nurse who already has an understanding of materials presented in the first four parts. An attempt has been made to avoid too much repetition, but a certain amount is thought to increase learning. There may still need to be reference to the first four parts to recall some of the generalities that may apply to the specifics in Part V. The discussion of the disease is limited to those aspects which, in the opinion of the authors, the nurse needs to know about in order to have a rationale for planning and providing nursing care. Further details about disease should be sought in other textbooks.

ORGANIZATION OF MATERIAL

The material is organized, for the most part, under three broad headings: the disease description, which includes definition, incidence, etiology, pathology, manifestation, diagnosis, and course and prognosis; medical treatment; and nursing care specific for the patient with the particular disease. The material is presented by major systems in which the pathology originates even though the disease may eventually affect other systems of the body.

The diseases are not presented in any order of importance, and the reader may start with any of the chapters as desired. It is recognized that many patients have multiple diagnoses, but for clarity and ease in discussion, diseases and nursing care are discussed as distinct entities.

RELATIONSHIP TO FIRST FOUR PARTS

The reader will also want to relate Part V to the preceding four parts. Some of this she will need to find for herself; some she will be guided to through reference to another part or chapter.

For example, Part I, Chapter 3, discusses the nurse's functions. These functions should be kept in mind as the approach to nursing in any consideration of patient care in any of the chapters in Part V.

In Part II, Chapter 4, the psychological defense mechanisms are discussed. One or more of these may be observed in any of the patients described in Part V regardless of the patient's specific disease.

In Part III, Chapters 7 and 8 give general diagnostic and treatment measures, some of which are used in a number of the diseases described in Part V.

Part IV sets forth the common manifestations of illness, a number of which occur in several of the diseases discussed in Part V; e.g., edema (Part IV, Chapter 15) is one of the clinical manifestations seen in some of the diseases covered in Part V, Chapter 23 (cardiovascular) and Chapter 24 (renal). Therefore the general knowledge of edema is not repeated in Chapters 23 and 24, but the reader is referred to Part IV, and only the specifics of edema as they relate to patients with diseases of the cardiovascular and renal systems are found in those chapters. It is hoped that the reader will distinguish from the first four parts the commonalties in patient problems and nursing approach and then identify the specifics related to patients with particular diseases from Part V.

As an example, the following table presents one patient problem and illustrates one common or general nursing approach and why it is helpful, as well as specific nursing approaches and medical treatment based on knowledge of the actual disease process in the patient.

DYSPNEA AS A PROBLEM OF A PATIENT
PART I

GENERAL PROBLEM	GENERAL NURSING ACTION AND BASIS
(Some possible causes)	
Hypersensitivity of Hering-Breuer reflex →↓ tidal volume	Observe depth and rate of respirations, equality of chest movement, and presence of rales (or inspiratory or expiratory wheezes) in order to help identify the extent of the pathophysiology and the patient's response to therapy
Increased work in breathing with fatigue of respiratory muscle	
Alveolar hypoventilation with hypoxemia and hypercapnia	Position patient to provide optimal ventilation and perfusion
	Provide rest to decrease oxygen withdrawal and thus decrease hypoxemia
	Administer oxygen as ordered to alleviate hypoxemia
Obstructed airway	Encourage patient to take a series of slow deep breaths to ventilate the alveoli and move secretions into the bronchi
	Encourage patient to cough after breathing deeply to remove any obstructing secretions
	When patient is unable to cough up secretions, suction airway as necessary
	Encourage fluid intake to help liquefy secretions
	Administer liquefying agents as ordered
	Administer bronchodilators as ordered
Anxiety or apprehension	Observe for presence of pain or anxiety which may cause or contribute to dyspnea
	Allay emotional stress to reduce stimulus respiratory drive and to help reduce metabolic rate, thus reducing hypoxemia and hypercapnia

PART II

MEDICAL DIAGNOSIS AND PATHOPHYSIOLOGY	SPECIFIC NURSING ACTION AND MEDICAL TREATMENT AND THEIR BASES
Emphysema Dyspnea due primarily to:	Encourage patient to exhale using his diaphragm and abdominal muscles and keeping lips pursed to increase ventilation and minimize collapse of bronchioles
1. Alveolar hypoventilation from:	
a. Increased residual volume	
b. Increased airway resistance from partial collapse of bronchioles during expiration	

MEDICAL DIAGNOSIS AND PATHOPHYSIOLOGY	SPECIFIC NURSING ACTION AND MEDICAL TREATMENT AND THEIR BASES
2. Possible obstructing secretions	To help prevent or remove obstructing secretions: 1. Administer liquefying agents as ordered 2. Encourage fluid intake to help liquefy secretions 3. Use postural drainage 4. Endotracheal suction may be used when patient is unable to cough up secretions
3. Increased work of breathing	Use a respirator as ordered to decrease work of breathing
Congestive Heart Failure Dyspnea due to acute generalized pulmonary edema associated with acute left-sided heart failure from increased filling load and/or loss of strength causing:	
1. Hypersensitivity of Hering-Breuer reflex from pulmonary edema	1. A. To reduce venous return: 1) Use sitting position with feet lowered 2) Apply alternating tourniquet to extremities as ordered 3) Administer diuretics as ordered 4) Encourage patient to avoid coughing or straining to prevent sudden increase in venous return 5) Decrease response to respiratory drive from Hering-Breuer reflex and anxiety by administration of morphine as ordered B. To strengthen myocardium: 1) Administer digitalis as ordered 2) Administer oxygen as ordered
2. Possible obstructed airway from edema in the bronchi and bronchioles and possible bronchial spasm	2. Administer bronchodilators as ordered to relieve bronchospasm
Asthma Dyspnea due to obstructed airway from:	
1. Bronchial spasm	1. A. Administer bronchodilators, i.e., epinephrine, aminophylline, as ordered to reduce bronchospasm B. Try to allay anxiety in order to help reduce bronchial spasm C. Administer sedatives and tranquilizers as ordered to control anxiety which may contribute to bronchospasm
2. Bronchial secretions	2. A. Encourage patient to expire slowly to help ↑ tidal volume and remove secretions B. Eliminate cigarette smoke from environment to reduce irritation to the mucosa and amount of secretions produced
3. Edema of bronchial mucosa	3. A. Eliminate possible allergens from the environment B. Support patient in a sitting position to increase vital capacity

CHAPTER 20
THE MEDICAL PATIENT

DOROTHY M. MARTIN

This chapter is concerned with the medical patient and general aspects of his nursing care. A medical patient is any person who is receiving diagnostic, therapeutic, or supportive care that is not surgical or psychiatric therapy or care directly related to the maternity cycle. For the purposes of this textbook he would also be an adult, but as far as the scope of the general definition is concerned, there are children as well as adults who are medical patients. The medical patient then is not necessarily hospitalized. He may be at home, attending a clinic, in a nursing home, or in a rehabilitation center. However, most of the discussion in this chapter will focus upon the hospitalized patient. Many of the things to be discussed here do have applications for the surgical, maternity, psychiatric, and pediatric patient, which is an interesting commentary on the general applicability of core nursing knowledge. The purpose of this chapter is to emphasize and bring into focus the nursing problems of a general nature which are frequently encountered in the care of medical patients. Most of them have been dealt with in detail in previous chapters and will only be mentioned here. Others have not yet been discussed so will be rather thoroughly explored.

General Considerations

People do not "plan" to have a medical illness develop. Some surgical experiences are elective, and many others are considered and planned for long before the nurse sees the patient in the hospital. Thus, when the nurse first sees a medical patient, the patient has seldom had time to work through his feelings about his illness. His behavior may signify denial, frustration, fear, depression, hostility, or other manifestations.

Almost every medical patient's encounter with his illness is an overwhelmingly stressful event. Whether his hospitalization is a growth experience or a psychic and physical disaster will depend predominantly upon the resources he himself brings to the situation. However, among the medical "helping" persons available to the patient, the nurse will frequently play a major role in supporting coping patterns that will help the patient regain or maintain his integrity as an individual.

The nurse will be responsible for assessing the patient's needs and developing a plan of nursing care. This care will probably include giving medications, carrying out the physician's orders, and preparing the patient for diagnostic tests that may be unpleasant, uninteresting, and even painful. There will also be nursing interventions that she initiates in order to avoid undesirable complications, and they may be uncomfortable at the time. Her skill in developing a relationship of trust will be instrumental in assisting the patient through the difficult experience of illness.

Diagnostic Procedures

A great variety of diagnostic procedures may be ordered for medical patients, and the nurse should always stop to check the bed-tag alert system before giving food or fluids or moving a patient. The nurse's awareness that a patient may often need to have a forthcoming test explained more than once will alert her to covert cues that he may display. No doubt someone told him about the test the night before, but because of anxiety he may not have heard; maybe he has simply forgotten; or perhaps he was never given an explanation or a chance to ask questions or express his feelings about it.

As the results of diagnostic tests are reported, they will be of benefit to the nurse in her evaluation and reassessment of the plan for nursing care.

Medications

A major mode of therapy for the medical patient is the use of drugs; in fact it is not uncommon for the patient to receive several different drugs both by mouth and by injection daily. The administration of medications prescribed by the physician is a nursing responsibility that requires knowledge of the drug, the patient, and the altered physiology of the patient.

The nurse should have knowledge of the mode of action, the average dose, the anticipated effects, the untoward effects, the contraindications for use, and the methods of administration of each drug she administers. The timing and specific methods of drug administration must take into consideration the action and pur- pose of the drug and the special considerations of the patient. Some drugs must be given at specific time intervals in order to maintain a therapeutic blood level (e.g., penicillin) or to obtain effectiveness at calculated time intervals (e.g., insulin preparations, diuretics). Some drugs must be given before or after meals for maximum effectiveness; some drugs should be given with milk or other specific fluids to protect the gastric mucosa. Some drugs are given for specific symptoms if they occur, such as analgesics or narcotics for pain or sedatives for sleepless- ness. Many drugs do not necessitate precise timing, e.g., 1-hour delay in admin- istration will not seriously hamper the ultimate effectiveness nor will administra- tion with food or fluids or other drugs.

Concern for the patient and his comfort should be considered in planning the timing and mode of administration of drugs. If the patient is receiving several in- jections daily for several days, the site of the injection should be altered each time and/or the nurse should judge whether or not two drugs can be mixed in order to give one rather than two injections; the judgment would be based on whether or not the two drugs are compatible when mixed, whether or not both drugs will be effective if given together, and the total volume of the solution to be injected. Some patients cannot swallow a single pill, several pills, or large pills or capsules with ease, in which case alternatives should be considered. Perhaps the drug can be prepared by the pharmacy in liquid form; perhaps the pill can be crushed and the resulting powder mixed in a small amount of fruit juice or some food product that will not affect the drug but will counteract the bitter taste; per- haps the pill or capsule can be given in a spoonful or more of applesauce, Jell-O or custard, if such foods are not contraindicated. If a patient must take several pills several times a day he may prefer to take all of them at one time every 3 or 4 hours or have the timing spaced so that he can take one pill at a time over a period of 2 to 4 hours. On the other hand, the nurse may decide to administer one pill each hour as a vehicle for observing and communicating with the patient, e.g., the patient who is anxious, apprehensive, seriously ill, or lonely such as a patient who is terminally ill or in isolation. At times the administration of medications must be altered in relation to other events in the patient's therapeutic program such as treatments, diagnostic procedures, and physical therapy, and to allow time for meals, rest, exercise, and sleep. If the patient is nauseated and/or vomiting oral medication may be withheld for a period, a dose may be omitted, or perhaps the drug may be given by injection. In this situation, as in other situations when the patient cannot or should not receive a drug (e.g., an allergic reaction), the nurse must report the circumstances to the physician and request written directions, since this entails a basic change in his original prescription.

The nurse has the responsibility and the right to talk with the physician to clarify his prescription of a drug and/or the dosage when the written order is not legible, or when she has knowledge about the patient's physical condition which may suggest that the use of the prescribed drug or dosage would be contraindicated. The nurse has the right to refuse to administer a drug or a dose of a drug if, on the basis of her knowledge and after discussing the situation and prescription with the physician, she believes the drug will be injurious to the patient. The practice of professional nursing requires the use of nursing judgment based on knowledge of cause and effect of the nurse's actions; this is implied or explicit in the nurse licensing act of each state. If the nurse does not understand the possible effects of her act it could be held that she is not exercising nursing judgment. If injury of the patient results from her act she could be held liable for negligence (professional malpractice). An individual is always responsible for his own actions and this responsibility cannot be transferred to or accepted by another individual; therefore, the nurse could not be excused from negligence on the basis that the physician prescribed the drug or the dose when she knowingly administered a medication that could cause injury. In such a situation both the physician and the nurse may be liable. If the nurse makes an error in drug administration such as misunderstanding a verbal order, misreading the written order, giving the incorrect dose, or giving the medication to the wrong patient, or omits giving a prescribed drug, she may be held liable if her act or her failure to act injures the patient.

Diet, Intake and Output

It is the unusual medical patient who has a good appetite, although some long-term chronically ill patients may even have problems of excessive weight gain. It can be an important and creative task to find ways to spark lagging appetites. The idea has been proposed that a loss of appetite is a sign of the body's inability to deal effectively with food. Therefore, food should not be forced, or urged unduly, upon an anorectic patient. Special therapeutic diets are frequently ordered and these ought to be eaten completely; the nurse should record the amount of each food the patient ate or did not eat if the patient is on a calculated diet. Even for regular diets the nurse should observe and record a fair estimate of the amount of food the patient has eaten at each meal. The nurse should be informed of dietary limitations and food likes and dislikes of each patient so that she may select or have the patient select appropriate foods and fluids for between-meal nourishment, for administering oral medications, or for encouraging fluid intake. If the consistency or type of food is inappropriate for the patient, the dietitian should be notified.

For some patients fluid intake and output should be observed and a balance sheet kept as indicated. If the patient is perspiring a qualitative estimate of the amount and frequency should also be recorded. The patient's dysfunction may create a fluid or electrolyte imbalance, even though intake and output *amounts* are normal. Therefore, alert observation for symptoms of abnormalities is indicated.

Patient Teaching

The principles of patient teaching have been discussed in Part I in relation to the function of the nurse. The opportunities for both incidental and planned teaching should be utilized, especially for those patients whose stay in the hospital is several weeks or months in length and who need assistance in adjusting to new patterns of living.

As part of the nursing care plan for each patient, consideration should be given to those things he needs to learn in order to facilitate his full rehabilitation after he returns home. The following brief checklist will provide a reminder of those general areas about which a patient may need further knowledge if he is to experience the desired changes in behavior after his return home:

1. Modifications in diet

   Conferences can be arranged with the dietitian and whoever will be preparing the meals at home as well as with the patient himself.

2. Medications and treatments to be continued at home

   a. The patient's understanding of the medication and treatment regimen to be continued at home should be carefully evaluated.

   b. Symptoms of toxic effects of medications should be described, if it is important for the patient to recognize and report early signs of toxicity.

   c. Opportunity should be provided in the hospital for the patient or an appropriate family member to actually do the dressing, treatment, irrigation, or other task that he will be expected to continue at home.

3. Follow-up appointments

   If the patient needs to have laboratory tests performed, the time should be written on his home care plan. The nurse can assist the patient in making plans so that he has assurance of a means of transportation to obtain such a laboratory test or to keep a doctor's appointment.

4. Prevention of illness and promotion of health

   This topic covers an immensely broad area and in a general way was discussed in a previous chapter. The nurse can discuss with the physician those areas in which the patient should be instructed to carry out special precautions because of the insult to his health which his illness has caused.

5. Modifications in daily living

   The patient's limitations and prognosis will provide a baseline for planning instruction in this regard, and a multidiscipline case conference will result in the optimum planning for the patient's benefit.

The teaching plan for each patient will be an individualized integrated part of the total plan of nursing care that arises out of her assessment and continual reevaluation of his needs.

The Bed Patient

EFFECTS OF BED REST AND IMMOBILIZATION

For most people, the daily retirement to bed is a pleasantly anticipated event and getting out of it again an often difficult task! Yet it has been suggested by numerous writers that bed rest holds many hazards. Is it the recumbent or horizontal position per se that is hazardous; the time involved; the degree of absolute immobility of a limb or the entire body; associated factors of isolation, deprivation, and change of social role? Does bed rest hold the same dangers for a young healthy person as for the elderly, or for someone who has undergone major surgery or a traumatic injury?

In 1960, the U.S. Public Health Service reported that disability from immobilization was one of 10 *preventable* health problems and with *then* existing knowledge, such disability could be reduced by 50 to 75 percent.[1] Is this reduction largely a nursing responsibility?

In this chapter we will attempt to answer each of these questions, and will begin by examining the physiological and psychological effects of bed rest and immobilization.

The normal physiological position for man is the *active erect*. However, most physiological measurements have been made with the subject lying supine. Numerous papers describe the effects of changing from the supine to the erect position. Can the results simply be reversed to find the effects of changing from the erect to the supine? Many studies report on physiological functions with the subject in the *passive erect* position, i.e., supported on a tilt table, so the normal contraction of the antigravity muscles is not occurring (contraction of muscles has a massaging effect on veins, and increases central blood volume). With the subject on a tilt table, not all the proprioceptive reflexes are called into action that would be were the subject required to stand erect alone. What are the effects immediately, after 1 hour, or after 3 weeks or longer of remaining inactive in a horizontal position? Obviously one must look carefully at the experimental conditions under which data have been obtained and make interpretations and generalizations cautiously.

The topics discussed in this chapter have been chosen for their relation to the student's background study and their relevance to nursing practice.

Metabolic and Hormonal Functions

It seems appropriate to discuss metabolic and hormonal effects of bed rest first, since any change in metabolic function will intensify or counteract the direction of change occurring in any body system. For example, if positional change alone causes a decrease in cardiac output, then if metabolic needs are reduced, this will

---

[1] Public Health Service Hearings before the House Committee on Appropriations, 86th Congress, Second Session 1960, pp. 1205–1212.

result in a further reduction in cardiac output, because cardiac output varies directly with metabolic rate.

Some functional changes associated with prolonged immobility of several weeks' duration include reduced metabolic demands, muscle atrophy with resulting protein catabolism, bone demineralization, and slight changes in fluid and electrolyte patterns (Deitrick et al.).

When erect, one is normally moving about and reacting to his environment, both emotionally and physically. When one goes to bed, many changes are really the result of a reduction in the amount of exercise and opportunity to interact with people and with variations in the surroundings. A change in posture is therefore a change in level of activity as well as in body position.

Two interesting experimental studies have been carried out with normal healthy individuals subjected to several weeks of bed rest. Deitrick and others in 1948 studied in great detail the physiological and biochemical changes occurring in four healthy young men who were immobilized in bilateral hip spica casts for 6 weeks. Birkhead and his group in 1963 studied certain effects produced by 42 days of continuous supine complete bed rest on four healthy young men. Much of our knowledge of the effects of bed rest and immobilization on healthy subjects comes from the results of these two studies.

Deitrick's subjects showed a 6.9 percent decline in *basal* metabolic rate, which is certainly only a very slight fall. However, the difference between the *total* metabolic demand during average ambulatory activity and during immobilization is considerable. Estimates of the caloric expenditure during minimal activity of an ambulatory adult are usually given as about 125 Cal per hour compared to about 80 Cal per hour for the person who is lying still in bed. Light exercise will increase the caloric expenditure to 175 Cal per hour and extreme exertion will increase it to 600 Cal per hour (White et al.).

When man is normally active and receiving adequate nutrition, he is in positive nitrogen balance. That is, he is taking in more nitrogen than he is excreting. Nitrogen metabolism gives some indication of the state of protein metabolism. Dietrick's subjects showed a significant increase in urinary nitrogen but Birkhead's group did not. The explanation probably lies in the actual immobilization in casts in the one

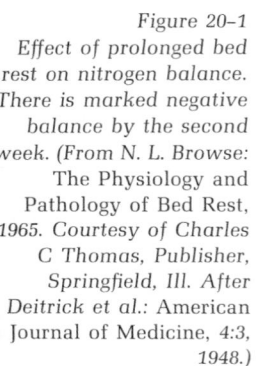

Figure 20-1
Effect of prolonged bed rest on nitrogen balance. There is marked negative balance by the second week. (From N. L. Browse: The Physiology and Pathology of Bed Rest, 1965. Courtesy of Charles C Thomas, Publisher, Springfield, Ill. After Deitrick et al.: American Journal of Medicine, 4:3, 1948.)

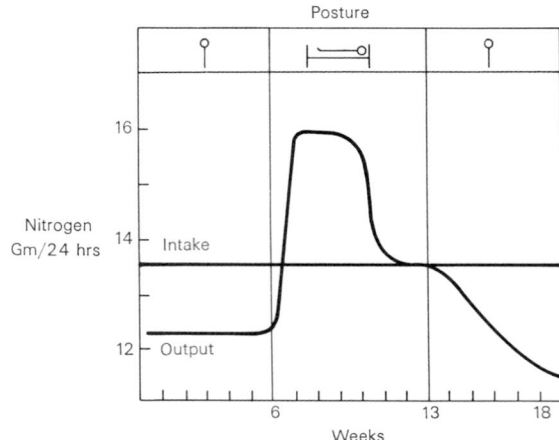

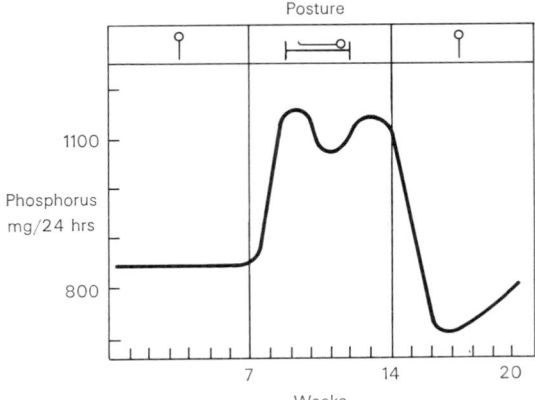

Figure 20-2
Effect of prolonged bed
rest on urinary excretion
of phosphorus. There are
two peaks, the first
corresponding to the
peak of negative nitrogen
balance, the second to
the peak of negative
calcium balance. (From
N. L. Browse: The
Physiology and Pathology
of Bed Rest, 1965.
Courtesy of Charles C
Thomas, Publisher,
Springfield, Ill. After
Deitrick et al.: American
Journal of Medicine, 4:3,
1948.)

group and the allowance of freedom of movement in bed by the other group. Therefore, it could be expected that the latter group would have less muscle atrophy, and consequently less loss of nitrogen, phosphorus, and sulfur (see Figures 20-1 and 20-2).

Deitrick's group was maintained on a 2,500 calorie diet, which is greater than the basal caloric requirement for a man resting in bed. The ratio of protein to carbohydrate in the diet was increased also. Steady weight was maintained for the group in spite of loss of appetite. The provision of a diet of caloric value greater than basal requirement probably accounted for the maintenance of body weight in the presence of the loss of muscle mass, as indicated by negative nitrogen balance. If caloric intake were reduced below body requirements anorexia could well produce a decrease in weight because of loss of body fat stores and perhaps even greater loss of protein.

During prolonged bed rest there is progressive increase in calcium excretion within the first 6 days and it reaches a maximum in about 3 to 4 weeks. The negative calcium balance continues during the period of immobilization (see Figure 20-3). Most investigators interpret this calcium loss to be due to a disuse osteoporosis.

Figure 20-3
Effect of prolonged bed
rest on calcium balance.
The peak of negative
balance is not reached
until the sixth week of
bed rest. (From N. L.
Browse: The Physiology
and Pathology of Bed
Rest, 1965. Courtesy
Charles C Thomas,
Publisher, Springfield, Ill.
After Deitrick et al.:
American Journal of
Medicine, 4:3, 1948.)

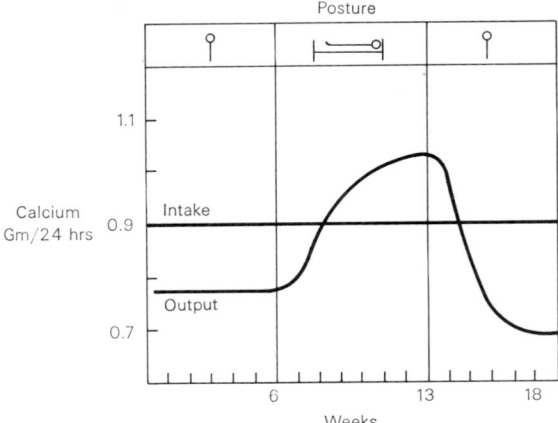

Further discussion of the mechanism involved is given later with the discussion of the changes affecting the musculoskeletal system.

The internal temperature of the body is maintained at a very constant level ($\pm$ about 0.5° C) mainly by controlling heat loss at the external surface. The heat loss through the expired air, feces, and urine is obligatory. Heat loss occurs by conduction, convection, radiation, and surface evaporation. The relative importance of each depends on (1) the environmental temperature, humidity, and air movement and (2) the rate of internal production of heat (Selkurt).

Since total metabolism is brought nearer basal levels when a person is in bed, the total heat production falls. When the environmental temperature is low, in order to maintain body temperature in comfort, relatively more bedclothes will be required than ordinary clothes for an ambulant person, for at least two reasons: (1) because of the decreased heat production of the recumbent patient; (2) because the bedclothes are more loose-fitting than ordinary clothes and, since the layer of air next to the skin is not as tightly trapped, more heat can be lost to the surrounding air.

On the other hand, when the environmental temperature is higher than usual comfort levels for the ambulant person, there will be a lessened gradient of temperature between the heat source (the patient) and the surrounding environment. If the bedclothes are not loose about the patient, air between him and the bed-clothes becomes warmed very readily. Since the horizontal position also causes a relative dilatation of skin blood vessels, the patient will increase his perspiration rate. The trapped air becomes both warmed and more humid. Since humid air is more of a barrier to radiated heat loss than dry air, one means of heat loss is diminished and he perspires even more.

Sweating when one is ambulant and normally clothed is most marked in those parts of the body unable to radiate, e.g., the axillae and groin, the places where skin surfaces touch. In bed, the entire inner surfaces of the arms and legs may be in apposition to other skin surfaces. Accumulation of perspiration may also be increased under the breasts, in the folds of the neck, where the body rests upon the bed, and in any areas where circulation of air is prevented.

As well as increased loss of electrolytes, particularly sodium, potassium, and chloride, the excessive sweating may cause psychological discomfort and increased danger of skin irritation. Perspiration of weight-bearing skin surfaces will also increase the friction and shearing forces on the skin when one is moving in bed.

The adrenal mineralocorticoid aldosterone (particularly concerned with electrolyte balance and control of sodium and potassium levels) shows a diurnal rhythm. Wolfe has shown this variation from day to night to be due to changes in posture. An increase in blood volume, which occurs on assuming the horizontal position, probably depresses ADH (antidiuretic hormone) secretion and aldosterone secretion via a low pressure volume receptor-pituitary reflex, osmoreceptors, and the renin mechanism of the juxtaglomerular apparatus in the kidney. These reflex and hormonal mechanisms are therefore important in maintaining homeostatic levels of body fluids and electrolytes whether the individual is erect or supine. Although normally these diurnal variations are marked, when a person is confined to bed for long periods a new dynamic equilibrium of blood volume is reached and there is a near-constant production of aldosterone varying with metabolic needs.

The adrenal glucocorticoids and epinephrine and norepenephrine also show diurnal variations, but no consistent pattern during prolonged bed rest has been documented.

Stress reactions are commonly associated with immobilization and illness. Therefore, changes in the above hormones as well as antidiuretic hormone may occur in the immobilized patient, and their psychological and physiological effects as well as other manifestations of stress may be anticipated.

The Function of the Heart and Circulation

Cardiovascular homeostasis is maintained in health by compensating adjustments in great part mediated by reflexes that maintain the heart and circulatory functions physiologically effective under widely varying conditions and demands, e.g., anything that causes an increase in blood pressure will activate the baroreceptor reflexes (of the carotid sinus and aortic arch) which will quickly cause changes that bring the pressure back to the "set" level. On the other hand, the cardiac output may increase five times and the muscle blood flow 30 times in response to vigorous exercise.

In the accompanying graphs (see Figure 20–4) the major compensations for gravitational effects are illustrated. In general we can assume the graphical interpretation to be correct, if not in exact percentages at least in direction of change, if we read from right to left, i.e., a change from upright to the supine position.

*Figure 20–4
Effect on the cardio-
vascular system of rising
from the supine position
to the upright position.
The figures are average
changes. Changes in
abdominal resistance and
limb resistance and in
blood pressure are
variable from individual
to individual. (Courtesy
of Donald E. Gregg, in
Charles H. Taylor and
Norman B. Best: The
Physiological Basis of
Medical Practice, 8th ed.
Baltimore, The Williams
& Wilkins Company,
1966.)*

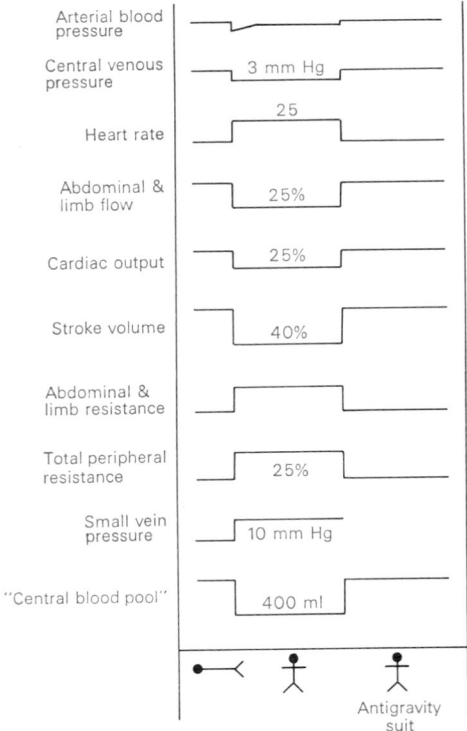

These changes illustrated are immediate changes that occur when one assumes the alternate position.

If there were *no* compensatory cardiovascular changes, the reduction in cardiac output due to pooling of the blood in the venous capacitance vessels of the lower extremities on standing would lead to reduction of cerebral blood flow to the extent that consciousness would be lost.

The major compensations that occur on assumption of the upright position are triggered by the drop in blood pressure in the carotid sinus and aortic arch. Reflexly, sympathetic stimulation causes an increase in heart rate and the strength of contraction is increased, both helping to maintain cardiac output. Sympathetic impulses cause arteriolar constriction, helping to maintain blood pressure. With prolonged increases in venous pressure there is venoconstriction, particularly of the lower extremity, which decreases the capacity of the veins and thus diminishes venous pooling. This latter response is weak and cannot be consistently demonstrated experimentally (Gauer and Thron).

The changes illustrated in Figure 20-4 are those occurring during tilt table or passive standing and they are immediate changes. When a person stands actively erect, using his muscles to maintain erect posture, the muscle activity squeezes blood from those veins running in proximity to the muscles. The valves allow blood to flow only toward the heart, but not retrogradely. Thus with exercise, superficial veins are emptied into deep veins, the pressure gradient encouraging flow.

In the cerebral circulation there are additional compensatory changes that produce a decrease in cerebral vascular resistance and an increase in oxygen extraction, so cerebral blood flow decreases only slightly with change to the standing position and oxygen consumption remains about the same. Thus by a number of reflexes the vital function of the brain is ensured because the oxygen delivered to the brain remains approximately constant.

When one lies down, the heart rate falls immediately; however, the cardiac output rises. Cardiac output is the product of heart rate and stroke volume. Therefore, the stroke volume increases (percentage-wise) even more than cardiac output. It is generally thought that the increase in stroke volume when one is recumbent is due to an increase in the central volume, resulting from orthostatic shifts in the distribution of blood. That is, blood that has been pooled in the capacitance vessels of the lower extremities is now shifted centrally. Sjostrand reports that the blood volume of the heart and lungs increases by 25 percent when one is lying down. Therefore, the heart is filled more during diastole and expels a greater amount with each beat (stroke volume).

A function of the heart is to supply blood, with its oxygen, to the tissues. The metabolic rate is a measure of tissue oxygen requirements, and the cardiac output has been shown to vary directly with the basal metabolic rate. As discussed in the previous section, total metabolic requirements are certainly less when one is at bed rest than when ambulant; therefore with prolonged rest the reduction in activity will cause a new dynamic equilibrium to be reached with the cardiac output at a lower level.

To summarize the arguments of the last few paragraphs, then, we can say that the change in position from standing to lying will cause an increase in cardiac output, but the decrease in muscular activity with lying down will tend to result in a decrease in cardiac output. Sitting up quietly produces very similar hydrostatic and reflex changes to those occurring with standing. At the same time, it is possible to reduce activity to a minimum. Therefore, the net reduction in cardiac output and cardiac work could be expected to be greatest in a supported resting sitting position.

Coe has studied the cardiac work (approximately stroke volume times arterial pressure) and he reports that the work done by the heart with the subject in the supine or recumbent position is 30 percent greater than that done when sitting up in a chair, supported and relaxed.

When the Valsalva maneuver is performed (expiratory effort against a closed glottis), the intrathoracic pressure is raised, which reduces the venous return and filling pressure of the heart. There is intense vaso- and venoconstriction from reflex discharge. During the straining period the cardiac output and coronary blood flow fall, but when the maneuver lasts only a few seconds this ordinarily produces no overt effect in a person with a normal heart. When the glottis is opened and there is a sudden increase of venous return, cardiac output and blood pressure may increase tremendously for several seconds (Burton). The dangers involved are, then, those of an excessive load upon a weakened heart, or cerebral hemorrhage in persons with cerebrovascular disease when the blood pressure is suddenly tremendously increased. When confined to bed, one frequently uses the arms to aid movements of the trunk. Such movements are more effective if the glottis is closed and the chest fixed, thus producing an involuntary Valsalva maneuver. Another situation that produces the same effect is getting on and off the bedpan and particularly straining at stool.

Dietrick found that normal subjects who had experienced prolonged bed rest had no significant change in arterial blood pressure. It is widely documented that persons with essential hypertension will usually have a significant lowering of their arterial blood pressure after being horizontal for some time.

The peripheral resistance falls upon one's lying down. The main vessels involved are those of the muscles and splanchnic bed (mesentery and intestinal wall). The mechanism is probably mainly mediated through the baroreceptor reflexes.

Changes in vascular resistance and hydrostatic pressure associated with lying down alter the distribution of blood within the body. The largest amount of blood that leaves the legs (approximately 11 percent of total blood volume) enters the thorax, increasing the blood volume in the lungs and heart. Thus the effect of this sudden inflow of blood to the central areas of the circulation is similar to that of a sudden blood transfusion. Elevating the legs above the horizontal intensifies such effect (Sjostrand). This obviously involves hazards for a patient with cardiac or respiratory disease.

Healthy volunteers confined to bed rest but allowed to move about freely showed no significant change during the period of inactivity in venous velocity in the legs. Wright et al. studied two groups of postoperative ambulant patients. The group who ambulated showed no significant decrease in venous velocity, whereas the other group who were confined to bed did. Wright also studied 42 medical patients (ages 22 to 87) who had noncardiac and nontraumatic injuries but were on bed rest for at least 3 weeks. Their venous velocity remained approximately constant and showed no significant difference from normal. However, a group of 22 medical patients (ages 39 to 80) with hemiplegia had a slight decrease in venous velocity in the unaffected leg and an average decrease of 65 percent in the affected leg. Wright's explanation was that postsurgical patients confined to bed have fear and pain, and tend to be very still. Wright believed that the first group of medical patients moved about in bed freely enough to maintain a normal circulation in the legs, but the group with hemiplegia moved less and the greater decrease in velocity seen in the affected limb was due to lack of the massaging effect of active muscular contraction.

Many workers report that there is an overall increase in hemostatic efficiency following trauma, hemorrhage, or increased adrenal activity (stress would be one condition that would produce increased adrenal activity). Wessler says that clotting time is shortened, fibrinogen values are elevated, and platelet "stickiness" is increased. The precise mechanisms are unknown, but teleologically they would be aimed at reducing the risk of hemorrhage in traumatic states or when trauma would be threatened.

Several theories have been proposed to explain the mechanism for the development of intravascular clotting. One theory propounds that endothelial damage and the agglutination of platelets are the major precipitating factors. Another presumes that a condition of hypercoagulability exists and in the presence of a retarded blood flow thrombosis may be initiated which can slowly or rapidly progress to massive thrombosis in the large vessels. Seegers hypothesizes that homeostasis may be maintained by a continuous clotting process that is counterbalanced by fibrinolysis and neutralization of coagulation products. Such a dynamic process requires continuous flow and thus the clotting of blood would depend upon the velocity gradient (Seegers).

McLachlin et al. demonstrated roentgenographically (by dye studies) that venous stasis occurs in valve pockets for as long as 60 minutes in elderly supine subjects. Sevitt and Gallagher in a study conducted over a period of a number of years reported on autopsies on 125 patients who died following hip fractures but showed no clinical or autopsy evidence of pulmonary embolism. (All patients showing pulmonary embolism can be presumed to have had thrombosis.) Sixty-five percent of this group had thrombosis of the veins of the lower extremities. Of these 81 patients, thrombosis of calf veins was most common, then ileofemoral, and then popliteal. Sevitt's findings also support the contention that venous stasis plays a major etiological role in venous thrombosis. In fact, it would seem that extreme *local stasis* may occur in dilated veins or valve pockets, even though measured venous velocity may approach normal values.

All nurses are familiar with the dizziness, shakiness, and weakness that patients experience when ambulating after lying in bed for even a few days. The patient is always attended his first time out of bed after bed rest to provide emotional and physical support and because of the danger of syncope. These sensations, and possibly fainting, are caused by postural hypotension and the bodily changes associated with the change to the standing position. As the period of bed rest gets longer the ability of the blood vessels to constrict via reflex sympathetic stimulation diminishes and dizziness and fainting are due to pooling of blood in the abdominal viscera and veins of the legs. Dietrick's subjects showed progressive deterioration in their response to tilt table tests during their immobilization, and after a week began to faint sooner. Birkhead also found decreased tolerance to head-up tilt but a satisfactory cardiovascular response to exercise in the supine position following prolonged bed rest.

The Function of the Lungs

The chest wall and diaphragm are moving structures, and their resting positions vary with posture and are influenced by effects of gravity upon them and upon associated organs. The resting position of the diaphragm is highest when one is supine and lowest when one is sitting, although there will be some variation in degree of difference depending upon body build, obesity, and other factors. According to McMichael and McGibbon, the vital capacity is reduced by about 350 cc upon lying down. This is because of two reasons: (1) the actual chest shape and position of the diaphragm and (2) the increased volume of blood that is shifted to the thorax when one is supine.

When one lies down the bronchiolar diameter is reduced slightly. The bronchioles are held open wider by outward traction from a negative intrapleural pressure. When one assumes the supine position, the diaphragm rises and the blood volume within the thorax increases, thus causing the intrapleural pressure to approach closer to atmospheric, and the diameter of the bronchioles is reduced. The effective inner luminal diameter is reduced even further because the layer of mucus lining the bronchiole becomes disproportionately thicker (see Figure 20-5).

The compliance of the lung refers to the ease with which it distends with increases in filling pressure. Therefore, a decrease in compliance will reduce the total surface area available for blood-air exchange by retarding the expansion rate and/or increasing the work of breathing. Sharp reported that there was no change in compliance with changes in posture in eight normal subjects, but in seven patients with congestive heart failure his measurements for compliance fell an average of 21.9 percent when the body position was changed from sitting to lying. Some respiratory physiologists would say that this was actually an indication of increased resistance due to the method Sharp used to measure compliance. In any case, the *work* of respiration would be increased whether from a decreased compliance or increased resistance. After the congestive heart failure was successfully treated, the decrease in compliance was no longer present with assumption of the horizontal position.

Figure 20–5
Effect of a change in diameter on the lumen of a bronchus. The thickness of the layer of mucus increases as the bronchus constricts and the lumen becomes disproportionately reduced. When the subject lies down there is a slight reduction of bronchiolar diameter; the effect of this upon the lumen will depend upon the amount of mucus present. (From N. L. Browse: The Physiology and Pathology of Bed Rest, 1965. Courtesy of Charles C Thomas, Publisher, Springfield, Ill.)

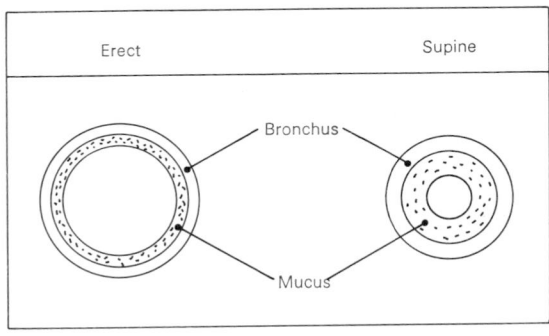

Erect   Supine

Bronchus

Mucus

The minute volume (ventilation rate x tidal volume) usually falls when one lies down, and this probably reflects the decrease in total oxygen consumption as a result of decrease in activity.

The development of muscle weakness generally which occurs during bed rest also affects the muscles involved with the mechanics of respiration, i.e., if they are not exercised maximally occasionally, then some loss of reserve power will occur, and maximum ventilatory capacity would be expected to decline.

The respiratory tract is lined with a high columnar, ciliated epithelium as far as the small bronchioles. These cilia beat in a cephalad direction, continuously sweeping along the mucus, so a net movement occurs in the direction of the trachea and larynx. When the person is upright, although gravity impedes the movement of the mucus somewhat, it does cause the mucus to spread out evenly all around the tube. With the subject in the supine position, gravity tends to draw the mucus downward, distorting the even film into a puddle on the lower side and a thin film on the upper side (see Figure 20-6). Both these conditions impair the function of the cilia: those on the upper side become dry and completely non-functioning; those in the puddle become overwhelmed, causing more mucus to collect. Both areas are more vulnerable to infection, and the increase of mucus in the lumen increases resistance to breathing. If enough mucus collects to obstruct passage of air, local atelectatic areas will occur distal to the obstructed site.

The airways (trachea, bronchi, bronchioles, and alveolar ducts) are dilated reflexly during deep inspiration. Therefore a maximal inspiration *decreases* resistance of the air passages. Exudates in the lumen may act as foreign particles and cause reflex bronchoconstriction, and/or reflexly stimulate coughing. An effective method of moving foreign materials or mucus from the airways up to the throat is by coughing. Coughing begins with a forced expiratory effort against a closed glottis (Valsalva maneuver) which raises the intrathoracic pressure. When the glottis opens abruptly there is a large pressure gradient between alveoli and the upper trachea, resulting in a rapid flow rate. At the same time the high intrathoracic pressure inverts the noncartilaginous portion of the upper trachea, result-

Figure 20-6
Effect of gravity on the distribution of mucus within a bronchus. Excess mucus pools on the dependent side of a horizontal tube; the upper surface may dry out, which predisposes to infection and obstruction. (From N. L. Browse: The Physiology and Pathology of Bed Rest, 1965. Courtesy of Charles C Thomas, Publisher, Springfield, Ill.)

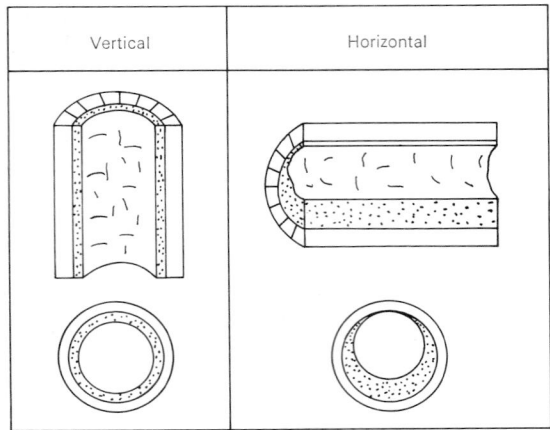

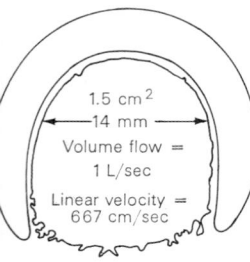

Trachea during normal breathing

1.5 cm^2
←14 mm→
Volume flow =
1 L/sec
Linear velocity =
667 cm/sec

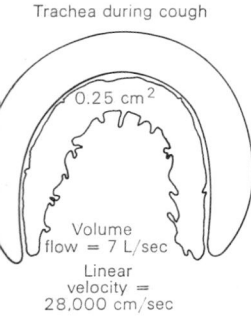

Trachea during cough

0.25 cm^2

Volume
flow = 7 L/sec
Linear
velocity =
28,000 cm/sec

*Figure 20–7
Tracheal air velocity
during cough. The
positive intrathoracic
pressure inverts the
noncartilaginous part of
the intrathoracic trachea
and decreases its cross-
sectional area to one-
sixth of normal. This,
added to a sevenfold
increase in flow rate,
increases the linear
velocity 42-fold, or
approximately 500 miles
per hour! (From
Physiology of Respiration,
by Julius H. Comroe.
Copyright © 1965, Year
Book Medical Publishers,
Inc. Used by permission
of Year Book Medical
Publishers, Inc.)*

ing in a narrowed trachea with a linear velocity of air rushing through it of approximately 500 miles per hour (Comroe)! Because the vital capacity is greater in the erect or sitting posture, coughing is also more effective when one is upright than when lying down, because a larger pressure gradient can be developed between alveoli and upper trachea.

The cilia of the respiratory tract *constantly* and *gently* move the mucus sheet and entrapped particles up to the pharynx where they can be swallowed or expectorated. By contrast, the explosive, tiring cough mechanism removes foreign particles and excessive amounts of mucus that would overwhelm the minute and gentle cilia.

During sleep there is an increase in blood pCO_2 which is greatest during deepest sleep. It is not completely clear why this occurs. Normally, any rise in pCO_2 stimulates receptors that reflexly through the respiratory center cause an increase in respiration which returns the blood pCO_2 to normal levels by the blowing off of more carbon dioxide from the lungs. Browse proposes that one explanation could be that sleep causes an inhibition of the normal activity of the respiratory center.

The Function of the Kidneys and Body Fluid

Claude Bernard's *milieu intérieur* is the body fluid. The organ primarily concerned with maintaining its constancy is the kidney. The meaning of Cannon's concept of homeostasis, although applying to all bodily functions, is particularly well illustrated by many mechanisms that maintain volume and osmotic constancy of body fluids.

In a change from the passive erect to the horizontal position, the renal blood flow increases. The main factors producing this rise are the increased blood volume and cardiac output via reflex activity when one changes to a horizontal position. Movement of the legs while one is standing, by preventing pooling of blood in the legs, causes the standing and supine values to approximate each other more closely, and Ganong points out that a lower extremity positive pressure suit abolishes the difference. Another reason for the increase in renal blood flow with assumption of the horizontal position has been proposed to be reduction in renal resistance, which apparently occurs as a result of reduction in vasoconstrictor tone.

The amount of glomerular filtrate also increases with a change to the horizontal position, but not as much as the renal plasma flow; therefore the filtration fraction decreases, which suggests a reduction in efferent arteriolar tone that could occur with a decrease in sympathetic vasoconstrictor tone as a result of reflexes accompanying the change in posture.

As mentioned in a previous section, aldosterone secretion decreases after assumption of the horizontal position. Wolfe and others have shown that changes in renin (an enzyme released from the juxtaglomerular cells in the kidney) secretion rate also follow postural changes and precede the aldosterone changes. Since it is known that renin releases angiotensin, which in turn stimulates the release of aldosterone from the adrenal cortex, it appears that this is an extremely sensitive and complex mechanism that responds to changes in glomerular filtration rate and sodium load, and plays a major role in sodium and volume control of body fluids (Vander).

The blood is slowly diluted by increased reabsorption of fluid from the tissues which occurs when one lies down, primarily because of a greater reabsorption of tissue fluid as a result of hydrostatic changes associated with assumption of the supine position. Therefore, blood volume increases about 10 percent and the concentration of all the contents is slightly reduced (Sjostrand).

Because of changes in renal blood flow and changes in the blood volume, osmotic pressure, and contents of electrolytes and protein in the blood, the renal functions are also altered directly. These hemodynamic effects on kidney function are extremely complex and not fully understood, but are being studied intensively. The net effect is that after assumption of the horizontal position more glomerular filtrate is formed, and more urine is formed with an increase in sodium excretion which also reflects the effect of the decrease in aldosterone secretion. Aldosterone causes increased reabsorption of sodium in the distal tubules of the kidney, thus conserving body sodium, and the sodium obligates a certain amount of water, thus helping to maintain a constancy of extracellular volume and osmolarity.

The slight decrease in blood osmolarity and increase in blood volume associated with lying down causes reduction in ADH via osmoreceptors in the supraoptic nucleus and left atrial volume receptors. This reduction in ADH then will result in an increase in urine production, and a decrease in its specific gravity.

All the previous changes discussed in renal function and body fluids have been in relation to an immediate change from a passive erect position to a horizontal position. Although there is an initial increase of 10 to 15 percent in blood volume, it is followed by a gradual decrease during the first 3 weeks of bed rest, as the body seeks a new dynamic equilibrium. Browse states that the average urine output tends to remain slightly higher and the specific gravity slightly lower than control values during the period of bed rest. However, this can certainly be altered or reversed if the patient is not supported optimally by nutritional, electrolyte, and fluid intake.

There is a diurnal variation in urine flow associated with sleep. There is a decrease in urine flow during sleep. Filtration rate does fall slightly during sleep as a result of the decreased blood pressure, but this change is not enough to explain the oliguria. Therefore Browse and others postulate mechanisms probably of central origin. Patients in congestive heart failure who are ambulatory sometimes show a reversal of this diurnal variation in urine flow. Apparently the mechanisms producing the oliguria of sleep cannot overcome the stimulus to increased urine flow produced by the change to a horizontal position, in this case on someone who obviously would have the potential of producing an even greater increase in blood volume than normal when lying down because of the retained edema fluid in the lower extremities.

During prolonged bed rest there is little change in urine flow but a large increase in calcium excretion. The chance of calcium being precipitated is therefore much greater and explains the high incidence of renal calculi after prolonged rest in bed. It also points up the importance of adequate fluid intake.

When one is horizontal, gravity impedes the emptying of the calyces into the pelvis of the kidney. Any sediment or solid material is moved with greater difficulty. Therefore very small particles may remain in the kidneys and form the nuclei of stones.

The Function of the Gastrointestinal Tract

There are a few clear-cut studies reporting changes in gastrointestinal function which occur with changes of posture. We know that the immediate effect of one's lying down on blood flow to the intestines is to produce a slight increase.

Deitrick's subjects reported decrease in appetite during immobilization, yet they were able to eat and maintain weight and normal excretory function.

Many patients confined to bed experience problems of constipation. The basis for this dysfunction and nursing measures to prevent and treat it are thoroughly discussed in other chapters.

The Function of the Musculoskeletal System and the Skin

Normal standing is not a passive state, and some muscles must work to maintain the body upright. The principal antigravity muscles are the calf muscles, the quadriceps femori, the glutei, and the erector spinae. In the supine position the muscles that must work against gravity are an entirely different group. When one is in bed, neck flexion is produced by weak anterior neck muscles, which tire quickly. Therefore how welcome it is to the bed patient to have his head supported in a comfortable position!

The normal angle of the foot with the leg is at 90 degrees, but in bed the foot tends to be plantar flexed, and dorsiflexors must contract to counteract this gravity effect. Heavy bedclothes used without a cradle or foot board increase the work of the dorsiflexors or make normal foot position impossible.

The normal healthy individual will shift his position frequently when lying in bed in order to relieve tired muscles. Such activity may be limited or absent in a patient in bed. Muscle atrophy as a result of disuse was discussed briefly in the section on metabolism.

Joint stiffness after a period of immobility is mostly due to muscle atrophy and contraction. For example, knee flexion between 30 degrees and 160 degrees may be easy, but movement from 30 to 20 degrees and 160 to 180 degrees may be painful and difficult. Stillwell points out that if a joint is immobilized for a long time, full range of motion may never be recovered, even after extensive rehabilitation exercises.

New skin areas must adapt to weight-bearing when bed rest is prolonged. The response of the epidermis to rubbing and weight-bearing is thickening of the stratum corneum and increased cohesion between cells; thus the outer layers thicken and the cells in the stratum germinativum increase their division rate. A callus develops. A few weeks of bed rest is usually not long enough to produce callus formation. In fact, often other factors, e.g., moisture, shearing forces, and local reduction of blood flow, cause a decrease in the regenerative capacity of the tissues, so breakdown occurs rather than callus formation. The supine weight-bearing areas are the back of the head, spines of the scapulae, iliac crests, sacrum, femoral trochanters, heels, and elbows. The skin and underlying subcutaneous tissue of most of these areas is not suited for weight-bearing, being soft with loose areolar tissue; the weight cannot be efficiently transmitted to the bones without the intervening tissue being compressed and the blood supply obstructed. Further physiological effects of pressure on vulnerable skin areas are discussed in the section under *nursing care to minimize hazards.*

Normal bone metabolism involves a continual reshaping, with an equilibrium between osteoblastic and osteoclastic activity.

Osteoporosis, a loss of mineral and bone matrix, always occurs during periods of prolonged bed rest. For many years, the explanation for disuse osteoporosis was that weight-bearing and muscle action stimulate osteoblastic activity, so bone formation stops (or is retarded) when muscles are not used and weight-bearing is not occurring. Recent studies seem to indicate that there may be a relation between bone blood flow and osteoporosis, with evidence supporting the idea that inactivity is stimulating to bone destruction, or that activity, by increasing blood flow, inhibits osteoclastic activity.

Regardless of the mechanism, we know that bed rest does produce a negative calcium balance and evidence of osteoporosis when bed rest is prolonged or when immobilization occurs.

Cognitive and Emotional Functions

Does being at bed rest produce a change in psychological function? This may depend on the reason for going to bed, and the degree of incapacity. However, changes that occur in the person's mental and emotional state will depend largely upon how he views the experience of being confined to bed.

It should be useful to look at possible causes of disruption of one's psychological equilibrium which may occur upon being confined to bed. In considering the *physiological* effects of bed rest, we found many specific alterations of function arising largely out of the actual changes from the erect to the horizontal position. In examining the *psychological* effects of bed rest we will do well to look not primarily at the effect of position as such, but at what being confined to bed may *mean* to a patient and the effects that associated conditions may have upon him.

A person's individual psychological structure and ego strength develop throughout his lifetime. Erikson describes personality as developed through a series of "decisive encounters" . . . "conflicts," inner and outer, which the healthy personality weathers, emerging and reemerging with an increased sense of inner unity. Thus the patient comes to the hospital with a concept of himself based upon past experiences. Part of his self-concept is body image—his mental image of his body and its parts. Certain areas of one's body or ideas about it may be charged with emotional interest and energy (Fisher and Cleveland). The American way of life accords high value to virility, youth, beauty, energy, and independence. These values affect most Americans' ideas and perceptions about themselves and their body image. It is difficult for most persons to equate the situation of bed rest with these generally held values of vitality and activity, thus making it particularly difficult in our culture to accept a dependent, helpless role.

In the normal stages of development one moves from dependency ————→ independency ————→ interdependency. Consider a middle-aged man, hospitalized because of an acute myocardial infarction and needing a maximum degree of rest, who behaves like a teenager, insisting that he can do everything for himself. Or there may be the teenager who is on bed rest because of rheumatic fever but is permitted to move freely in bed. Nonetheless he asks to be fed, wants a light left on at night, and generally displays a level of behavior indicating a much earlier period in his psychosocial development. For both these patients, the order confining them to bed threatens their self-image, causes feelings of frustration. Their behavior demonstrates *regression,* which is an attempt to establish psychological equilibrium by returning to an earlier more comfortable level of adaptation.

Frequently the first reaction of a patient to an order for bed rest is *denial.* He uses the mechanism of denial of his illness and need for bed rest because he cannot integrate into his self-image the dependent role he must assume as a helpless, critically ill bed patient, who therefore is no longer the strong capable provider for his family. Because a person on complete bed rest has his personal needs cared for and things done *for* and *to* him as do children, he may feel that he is both treated and perceived to have child-like status. This perception of his change of self-image from healthy, virile provider of his family to that of "child" may result then in immediate and sometimes continued denial of his illness, or to depression over what he perceives as the reality of the situation.

An order for bed rest frequently means to a patient that he must be seriously or critically ill, or he would not be confined to bed. This may be true, but such a perception of the meaning of bed rest can generate a considerable amount of fear and anxiety or intensify feelings of depression. Depression is one of the commonest symptoms associated with immobility or confinement to bed and is present to some extent regardless of the dysfunction or disease that necessitates the bed rest. Solomon reported that even normal subjects in experiments in partial immobilization exhibited degrees of depression. Decrease in sensory stimuli intensify depressive reactions. When the patient's interpretation of his confinement to bed is of a serious or terminal outcome to his illness, then his depression often reaches pathological proportions and thoughts of and efforts at suicide may occur.

Confinement to bed may increase anxiety because of embarrassment over real or imagined lack of privacy to carry out personal grooming and excretory functions. Anxiety may also be increased by fear that some essential to life will not be obtainable while one is in this relatively helpless situation. For instance, just having water available and within reach, or even what we might consider relatively unimportant needs such as to look out the window, may assume great importance to the patient who knows that these things are no longer within his prerogative to obtain independently.

Since denial is frequently the predominant response to an order for bed rest, it is not unusual to have a patient repeatedly found going to the bathroom, up in a chair, or out in the hall, even after repeated explanations as to the importance of and reasons for his remaining in bed. The nurse's efforts to develop a relationship with the patient so that he feels unconditionally accepted will achieve positive results sooner than repeated efforts to "explain to," and "educate" him.

Feelings of separation and loneliness common to illness and hospitalization may be intensified by confinement to bed. The patient must passively wait for those *important to him* to come. There is loss of contact with meaningful and familiar day-to-day activities.

Consider the patient confined to bed in a "typical" hospital room. The *variety* of color, form, light, and sound is distinctly diminished. His opportunities for varied tactile stimuli and interpersonal contact are either severely limited or soon fall into some repetitive hospital routine. This limitation of sensory input may lead to boredom, and even hallucinations and disorientation when extreme (Carlson). Recent studies on sensory deprivation indicate that normal functions of the brain depend on a continuing arousal reaction generated in the reticular formation, which in turn depends upon constant bombardment with sensory stimuli (Heron). In every test on how humans react in a situation where nothing at all is happening, the subject's performance including thought processes was impaired.

Normal subjects in experiments of sensory deprivation and Jackson's study of hospitalized patients showed intense desire for stimuli and bodily motion, increased suggestibility, impairment of organized thinking, oppression and depression, and in extreme cases, hallucination, delusions, and disorientation. Reducing the patterning and meaningful organization of sensory stimuli is called *perceptual deprivation* and has similar effects. Apart from their specific functions, sensory stimuli have the general function of maintaining the arousal level in the midbrain, but Heron points out that they rapidly lose their power to do so if they are restricted to monotonously repeated stimulation from an unchanging environment. Deprivation of social stimuli frequently has the most devastating effect on patients confined to bed. The tragedy is that the patients most in need of an increased amount of interpersonal contact are often avoided by hospital personnel, because of the symptoms they manifest, i.e., depression, hostility, and "obnoxious" and "un-cooperative" behavior. The decrease in sensory stimulation for an immobilized patient or one confined to bed has multiple effects, and when continued for any length of time beyond hours, frequently leads to the serious manifestations described.

As a result of sensory deprivation, the attention of a patient confined to bed is often turned inward, i.e., to his own feelings, and to an overconcern with his own body and its functions. As a result he may exhibit an unusually low pain threshold and tolerance. Psychosomatic manifestations are superimposed on existing illness because of his hypochondriasis. The patient in an intensive care unit may be particularly susceptible to such problems because of the monotonous sounds of monitoring equipment and the multitude of paraphernalia attached to his body, and the personnel's focus on the equipment and his body rather than on him as a person. He may suffer severe deprivation in interpersonal interaction, particularly if he is conscious, reasonably aware of his surroundings, but too weak or frightened to initiate any interaction himself.

A patient who is confined to bed for a very prolonged or indefinite period of time may indulge in self-pity and grieving—a response to the loss of his former way of life or self-concept. The next phase should be a new ego identification, built with self-esteem and within objective limitations of his function and hope of recovery.

PATHOLOGICAL CONDITIONS THAT PRODUCE VARIATIONS IN THE EFFECTS OF BED REST AND IMMOBILIZATION

The first section on *effects* of bed rest and immobilization dealt primarily with physiological and psychological changes that occur as a result of the changes in body position, activity, and opportunity for interaction with people and environment resulting from immobilization or bed rest. The psychological reactions generally associated with any illness or dysfunction treated by bed rest were also considered. The pathological conditions present will obviously also have pronounced effects, but an extensive coverage of these detail differences is not within the scope of this chapter. The following conditions cause definite accentuation of certain hazards associated with bed rest.

The reader is referred to sections of this textbook which discuss the following conditions in further detail in order to provide a basis for thorough understanding. *Unconsciousness* in general causes all the functional effects of changes described in the preceding pages to be maximized because what is occurring is immobilization, except for those things that are *done for the patient.*

When lying on his back, the unconscious patient is in danger of having his airway obstructed by the jaw and tongue falling backward, just because of the pull of gravity, thus closing the oropharynx. This does not occur in the lateral or prone position. Also, aspiration of vomitus by an unconscious patient is almost certain if he is in the supine position.

Paralysis such as quadriplegia and paraplegia increases the predisposition to skin breakdown because no sensation of pain occurs when an area becomes ischemic. A nonparalyzed person frequently makes small shifts in position and weight-bearing as he becomes aware of discomfort on a pressure area. This protective mechanism is not available to the paralyzed individual. Psychological factors related to feelings of helplessness and hopelessness and problems of body image play a major role in assessment of nursing care indicated. Long-term rehabilitation programs involving a multidiscipline approach will influence development of the nursing care plan.

In *hemiplegia* the occurrence of contractions is likely because of the spasticity present. It is important to remember that sensation may still be present on the affected side and the patient particularly uncomfortable because of pressure or poor positioning. Aphasia presents an additional barrier to communication which is a challenge to overcome.

The patient in *congestive heart failure* is one in whom changes in circulatory phenomena are exaggerated when assuming a horizontal position. The position of sitting up in a chair may be particularly helpful to him.

All patients with *cardiac* conditions and the elderly are particularly susceptible to dangers associated with volume overload of the heart and the circulatory changes induced by the Valsalva maneuver. Unnecessary immobility may be instituted by the patient himself because of fear or misunderstanding of his condition.

The *aged and debilitated* may become virtually immobile when put to bed even though it is not necessary that their activity be so restricted. Careful assessment of the reason for an aged person's withdrawn and immobile state will give clues to the appropriate nursing intervention. Just the opposite effect is frequently seen;

that is, an older person who has been calm, quiet, and able to care for his own needs at home begins to hallucinate and be belligerent or hostile when put in a hospital bed. It is not known for sure why the reaction is seen as often as it is in older persons. It may be the result of sensory deprivation, and some controlled studies have shown rapid reversal of psychotic-like symptoms just by increasing sensory input (Jackson and Linton). However, such symptoms often occur very soon after an admission and confinement to bed (within hours) and an alternative explanation may be that the organic brain damage resulting from atherosclerosis and processes associated with aging is minimal enough that in familiar surroundings he can remain in contact and function at a relatively normal level because familiar objects and persons continually help him to reorient himself in spite of a failing memory and some hallucinations. A strange bed; unfamiliar clothes, surroundings, and people—his slim grip on reality is lost, and frank disorientation occurs.

The *incontinent* patient presents many challenges to nursing care, the greatest of which is to prevent the incontinence. Skin frequently moist with urine and/or feces is more likely to develop pressure sores because the moisture increases friction with the bedclothes thus increasing irritation and shearing forces. It also predisposes to rapid development of infection, should any break in the skin occur. An elderly or debilitated person confined to bed for a few days may become incontinent because of acute illness or lack of opportunity to urinate or defecate in privacy or in a normal position. Then he may be *kept in bed because of* his incontinence, or at least not encouraged and assisted to get to the bathroom.

When a *fracture* occurs, a different pattern of calcium and phosphorus metabolism is seen from that with bed rest, and if the patient is in a cast, muscle atrophy is greater than when movement is permitted; therefore an even greater increase in nitrogen loss is seen. *Traumatic injuries* and *surgery* cause bodily reactions that accentuate certain hazards previously discussed.

THE BENEFITS OF BED REST

To Relax the Musculoskeletal System. Rest in bed allows the system that supports the body in the upright position to relax, and is used in numerous orthopedic conditions to relieve strain on muscles and joints and to facilitate immobilization of fractures.

To Alter the Effects of Gravity. Bed rest is useful in treatment of severe varicose veins and venous ulceration. Edema of the legs and ankles is reduced by assumption of the horizontal position, because hydrostatic changes cause an increase in tissue fluid reabsorption.

To Increase Venous Return and Cardiac Output. Probably the most valuable effect of the supine position is in the treatment of shock. Because of reflexes activated by the low blood pressure and/or reduced blood volume, the muscle, splanchnic, and skin vasodilatation that normally is seen when one lies down does not occur and instead, intense vasoconstriction continues as long as the blood pressure is low.

To Decrease Certain Functions. A decrease in general activity results in a decrease in metabolism and concomitant physiological functions, e.g., oxygen consumption, cardiac output, and work of the heart. However, postural change to the horizontal position may cancel this effect on cardiac output, in fact, usually negates it. The same objective can be achieved by support in the sitting position, in which case the reduction in cardiac output and work of the heart is even greater.

To Immobilize a Wound. Bed rest is certainly an invaluable method of treatment for patients after eye operations and for fractures that cannot be immobilized without fixing the entire patient.

To Support. When a patient is very weak or debilitated, rest in bed is the most comfortable way to avoid the additional exertion of fighting against the pull of gravity.

To Relieve Pain. Severe pain alone is seldom an indication for *prolonged* bed rest, although it may be a very useful measure to relax certain muscles and thus relieve pain for limited periods of time. Some types of pain are increased by moving, and the easiest way not to move is to lie quietly in bed.

There are many other conditions and diseases that are frequently treated by bed rest, but any evidence from controlled trials as to the value of treatment with and without bed rest is lacking. We really do not know the value of bed rest in many conditions. We do know that it has many dangers, and this is the subject of the next section.

THE HAZARDS OF BED REST

The hazards of bed rest can be largely deduced from the previous discussion. The following listing will serve as a summary of the most frequently encountered problems.

Psychological Aspects. "Look at a patient lying in bed. What a pathetic picture he makes. The blood clotting in his veins, the lime draining from his bones, the scybola stacking up in his colon, the flesh rotting from his seat, the urine leaking from his distended bladder, and the spirit evaporating from his soul" (Asher).

This is not an exaggerated picture, even though a startling description perhaps. What is the most serious of all these most unpleasant phenomena? I think it is the "spirit evaporating from his soul"—the loss of meaningful purpose and identity. The *results* of forces disrupting psychological equilibrium have already been discussed in a previous section, for it seemed impossible to separate the "physiology" and the "pathology" in describing the mental and emotional changes often associated with bed rest.

Thrombosis and Pulmonary Embolism. At least as early as Virchow, in 1847, it has been suspected that bed rest may cause a sluggishness in venous blood flow, which may predispose to intravascular clotting, this in turn permitting the release of large emboli that enter the circulation and lodge in the pulmonary arteries causing pulmonary embolism. However, not until the last few decades has clear-cut pathological evidence confirmed the described events. It is still uncertain what the mechanism is which initiates the intravascular clot. An overview of relevant findings regarding development of thrombophlebitis has been discussed previously.

If massive emboli are released (usually from deep veins) the main pulmonary artery may be completely occluded with the resultant dramatic symptoms of pulmonary embolism and sudden death. However, more frequently only branches of the pulmonary arteries are occluded and symptoms like those of pulmonary edema occur and later pneumonia may develop, depending upon the size of the emboli and location where they lodge.

Muscular Atrophy, Weakness, and Contractions. Disuse atrophy, especially of the antigravity muscles, occurs. The amount of atrophy is inversely related to the amount of exercise each muscle has received during the period of restricted activity. Muscle size and strength can only be restored again gradually by exercise. Joint stiffness is due primarily to muscular contraction and it may be irreversible.

Disuse Osteoporosis. Even short periods of bed rest cause a negative calcium and phosphorus balance, but prolonged bed rest, and particularly complete immobilization, produces great loss of mineral elements from the bones, so they are brittle and may fracture more readily.

Urinary Tract Calculi. The drain of calcium from the bones predisposes to the development of kidney and bladder stones because most of the calcium lost is excreted by the kidneys and as the concentration increases, small amounts of calcium salts precipitate and form the nuclei for calculus formation.

Urinary Retention and Incontinence. The unnatural position, coupled with attempting micturition in an uncomfortable unnatural way, often causes retention. It is certainly more frequent in older men with prostatic hypertrophy. In elderly patients, we often see retention with overflow or simple incontinence. Problems of incontinence add to the deterioration of morale.

Urinary Tract Infection. Cystitis and ascending pyelonephritis often are complications of retention with overflow. A chronically overstretched bladder may cause trauma to the mucosa and predisposes to infection. If an indwelling catheter is used, it is another potential factor that can produce irritation and predispose to infection.

Loss of Appetite. Anorexia may be expected because of decreased metabolic demand and decreased activity, but probably an even more important factor is the boredom and psychic deterioration mentioned previously.

Constipation and Fecal Impaction. These disturbances are not infrequent complications of bed rest, and are more frequent in the more debilitated, helpless patient. The explanation of mechanisms involved was discussed in an earlier chapter.

Decubitus Ulcers. This is perhaps the one hazard of bed rest which has always been recognized, because it occurs so easily, its presence cannot be overlooked, and treatment is difficult.

Atelectasis and Pneumonia. Pneumonia is the *immediate* cause of death in the majority of elderly patients, those confined to bed for serious and long-term illnesses, and following extensive surgery. Many of the effects of bed rest and immobilization predispose to this complication. Hypostatic pneumonia is descriptive of the etiology in which position favors the pathologic process. The supine position allows collection of bronchial secretions in dependent portions of the lung. The interference with the normal action of cilia in mucus removal and protection of mucous membrane surfaces has been discussed. Expulsive force of coughing is reduced. Inadequate fluid intake or other conditions leading to dehydration as well as neural influences may cause secretions to be thick and tenacious. These conditions lead to bacterial growth, plugging of small and terminal bronchioles with mucus causing local atelectatic areas. Normally, yawning and occasional deep breathing reexpand small atelectatic areas of the lung. The heavily sedated or severely debilitated patient may not breathe deeply and the stimulus to sigh or yawn may be depressed.

Aspiration pneumonia is another hazard caused by improper positioning of unconscious and semiconscious patients and by careless feeding of patients with partial paralysis of the muscles of deglutition. The changes in circulation are also of great importance in development of pulmonary complications especially in patients who already have cardiac or pulmonary disease; e.g., increased blood volume in the lungs may lead to some degree of pulmonary edema and decrease in oxygen—carbon dioxide exchange across the alveolar-capillary membrane. Small pulmonary emboli resulting from venous thrombosis cause pulmonary edema, atelectasis, and/or tissue necrosis locally, thus predisposing to development of pneumonia.

All the above are examples of recumbency in the ill or debilitated patient causing a complication (pneumonia) that would probably never, or seldom, occur in a healthy person subjected to complete immobilization, because the etiological factors are multiple; but in such an ill person, many of these factors are simultaneously present. But bed rest versus activity or even sitting upright may be the deciding factor as to whether his body can cope with the physiological insults.

Postural Hypotension. Vasomotor instability seen *after* a period of bed rest may cause postural hypotension, dizziness, and even syncope because of failure of adequate peripheral vasoconstriction to occur on assumption of the erect position.

Dr. Kenneth Cooper, a U.S. Air Force Major, wrote a book titled *Aerobics*, in which he described his conditioning program and the physiological basis for it. To increase general conditioning, and particularly to improve the function and reserve capacity of the heart and lungs, a regular program of exercise (*entire* body exercise) is necessary. It might be said that bed rest provides a *deconditioning*, in which the reserve capacity of the body is diminished even further. This reflects the capacity of the body to adjust to the demands upon it, to seek a new state of dynamic equilibrium. The adaptability ensures that the body will operate at near maximal levels of efficiency, depending upon the work demand. It provides a means by which a valuable method of treatment may be used, i.e., to reduce total body metabolism over a certain period of time. But along with this valuable possibility for treatment lurk all the hazards that have been described, and many more that did not seem essential information in order to plan intelligent and effective nursing care. No doubt there are other effects of bed rest which produce hazards that have great import for nursing intervention, and further study and research will reveal these.

NURSING CARE TO MINIMIZE HAZARDS

This section is brief, not because it is unimportant, but because the implications for nursing care have been made abundantly clear in the preceding sections. Many of the topics are discussed at length elsewhere in this textbook in relation to other conditions.

Prevention of the multiple undesirable complications that may beset the patient confined to bed rest is largely the responsibility of the nurse. It is true that the easiest solution would appear to be to eliminate the inactivity and the horizontal position. When this is possible this is certainly the nursing measure *par excellence!* However, since for any number of very good reasons this may not be possible, the nurse must then be innovative in maintaining the desirable aspect of the rest prescribed while introducing nursing measures that will counteract, as far as possible, the undesirable effects.

A patient must not be inadvertently permitted to assume bed rest completely and for prolonged periods when it is not necessary. Perhaps this occurs most frequently in the case of chronically ill and elderly patients, or in depressed patients. Just the simple matter of seeing that appropriate clothing is available for ambulation may increase tremendously the amount of time a patient stays out of bed. If a patient does not have his own robe and slippers, these should be as readily available from the hospital linen supply as are hospital gowns.

Psychosocial Needs. Many hospitals are archaic and unrealistic in the lack of provision of areas for patient socialization, eating elsewhere than in bed, and provision for individual and small group activities. The facilities need to be on the patient units so that even the patient who is able to be up only a very limited length of time will have an interesting and pleasant location to go to which is nearby—in fact, not just to "go to" but that will "beckon him" by its desirable appearance, activities, and opportunity for interpersonal contacts. The nurse can be alert to the need to refer patients for occupational therapy or physical therapy who will benefit by the special services offered.

Many undesirable psychological manifestations can be averted by seeing that bed rest does not rob the person of his identity as an individual.

The above provisions of environment and activity will help, but suppose the patient *must* remain in bed *all the time*? Intervention to prevent the undesirable manifestations, whether the patient is allowed some activity or is at complete bed rest, is an interpersonal one—the use of the nurse-patient relationship. This has been interwoven throughout the entire text.

Therapeutic nursing interventions that are very specifically related to the psychosocial needs of the patient confined to bed involve measures that should be instrumental in making his hospitalization a growth experience, increasing his feelings of personal worth and self-respect so that he can modify or reconstruct his self-image (or ego identification and body image) in keeping with his ideals and realistic goals. The nurse needs to be aware of covert behavior and have the ability to interpret covert and not just overt cues.

Since the bedfast or immobile patient cannot move himself so as to experience variations in environment or sensory perception, the innovative nurse will bring the variety and stimulation to him. She can encourage visitation by family members and their participation in the plan of care where appropriate. A clock, calendar, radio, and television would seem to be "musts" unless specifically contraindicated. Planning and participation in his own care will promote movement toward independence. Usually his environment can be extended by a trip to the lounge or porch in wheel chair or bed, and such a daily or more frequent excursion should be high on the priority scale of nursing care, thus increasing his opportunity for increased sensory stimuli and physical mobility.

Experimental studies have demonstrated the facilitating effects of exercise during isolation in counteracting the impairments produced by sensory restriction. The performance of exercises may provide sufficient variability of kinesthetic and proprioceptive stimulation to counteract most of the effects of unvarying stimulation from the visual and auditory sense modalities. It has been shown that somatic (muscle) sensory excitation produces a powerful excitatory influence upon the reticular formation. Certainly the patient should be encouraged to perform as much exercise, and perform it as frequently, as his condition will permit, since it is a powerful deterrent to both physical and psychological complications of bed rest.

The originality and innovative ability of the nurse will be taxed to find meaningful things and ideas to bring to her patients (be they barber, housewife, electrician, teacher, student) that will stimulate them toward independence and will provide intellectual stimulation. Her interest in each of them is the best beginning, and her awareness of their individual needs and resources provides the basis for a careful assessment and plan of action with ongoing evaluation.

Diet and Fluids. Adequate fluid intake should be provided, to assist in maintaining normal fluid and electrolyte patterns and to help prevent renal calculi. If the patient is not taking in enough orally, the physician should be notified so that parenteral fluid and electrolyte replacement can be instituted.

A well-balanced high-protein diet is indicated, even though it should be recognized that excessive protein intake alone cannot correct the negative nitrogen balance. Special therapeutic diets may be ordered as indicated.

GENERAL MEASURES

For the person who must be confined to complete bed rest, the following measures are vital to diminish circulatory, muscular, skin, and respiratory effects of immobility and thus decrease the hazards of thrombosis, decubitus ulcer formation, pneumonia, atelectasis, and muscle wasting and contractions.

Individual Determination of the Need for Turning and Positioning. A schedule of turning every 2 hours has been suggested but is woefully inadequate for some patients. For a person in good general condition, alert and able to move or shift his position even slightly, a longer interval between assisted changes in postion may be satisfactory. To prevent dangers inherent in the Valsalva maneuver, the patient should be instructed to exhale rather than hold his breath when moving in bed. The use of an overbed frame and trapeze will make it easier for the patient to assist in changing his position.

Range of Motion Exercises Several Times Daily. Many patients can be taught to carry these out for themselves. However, a reminder and emotional support are usually needed each day or oftener. During an acute phase of critical illness, the patient's condition may not warrant even the exertion associated with passive range of motion exercises. However, the *time interval* over which this essential activity is omitted should be carefully evaluated by both physician and nurse and the advantages of omission carefully evaluated against the hazards involved.

Deep Breathing and Coughing. These can be much more effectively performed in the sitting or standing position than in the supine position; therefore, if permitted, such positions should be assumed during these exercises.

It is a good idea to include these activities whenever the patient is moved. If the patient is turning himself, then a reminder by the nurse several times a day should suffice *if* the patient understands the purpose and value of these activities, which may be disturbing and even painful to him. Because coughing as usually performed includes the Valsalva maneuver, it may have to be omitted for the cardiac patient, regardless of its inherent value. To avoid dangers inherent in the Valsalva maneuver, the patient should not prolong holding his breath before coughing. Coughing can be performed without preliminary closure of the glottis but it is relatively ineffective in raising tracheobronchial secretions.

There are days when time may be at a premium and a nurse cannot get everything done that needs to be done. If an emergency absorbs 50 percent of her time then there is half as much time remaining for all the usual activities. Her judgment about priorities then becomes of prime importance, for obviously something must be left out. Of the above three very important preventive measures, an occasional time may occur when something must be done faster or be eliminated. Range of motion exercises may be streamlined. Actually they are no longer *complete* range of motion exercises, but we can selectively include those with greatest benefit and need for frequent performance. If the antigravity muscles of the lower extremities are exercised this will also provide an excellent stimulation of venous circulation, e.g., dorsiflexion and plantar flexion of the foot. Many patients who cannot do any of the other range of motion exercises actively may be able to carry these out actively and therefore more frequently, with great benefit. The dorsiflexion position is also used for quadriceps setting or isometric exercise. Frequently a person will hold his breath and strain while doing an isometric exercise, thus producing a Valsalva maneuver. The cardiac patient can be warned against this.

Skin Care. This is an important area for nursing care for the bedfast patient particularly for the following reasons:

1. A clean body, free of odors, gives positive value to self-concept for most Americans, by enhancing self-esteem and body image, through being acceptable to others.

2. Keeping the skin in good condition will promote comfort and avoid pain of irritation and itching. Shaving lotions, cosmetics, deodorants, and talcum powder are more important for the moods of the helpless patient than for any physical benefit they may bestow. Regular shaves, shampoos, and haircuts for men, and shampoos and sets for women, should be arranged. Such provision for the ordinary grooming expectations in our culture are frequently of even greater value to the patient's family than to the patient himself.

Careful nursing assessment will determine if the patient's condition warrants these grooming aids, which are necessities on a long-term basis, but during critical periods may have to be postponed.

3. Decubitus ulcers are an ever-present threat. The undesirable results after the formation of a decubitus ulcer give abundant reasons for *prevention.* The ulcer is painful to the patient and exposes him to all the dangers of infection associated with an open wound. The treatment is time-consuming and thus is ultimately very expensive, because of the time of nursing personnel, the equipment and medications used, and the often necessary extension of a patient's hospital stay. Although decubitus ulcers are discussed in other chapters, it may be helpful to the student to have certain points emphasized, because of the great prevalence of this problem.

A decubitus ulcer is a localized area of cutaneous tissue destruction with or without involvement of underlying structures which has been caused by pressure. The terms *bedsore, pressure sore,* and *decubitus ulcer* are generally used synonymously and interchangeably.

The mechanism of development is simply a matter of external pressure exceeding a level such that internal circulation can no longer supply the nutritional needs of cells in the local tissue. Changes take place in the tissue leading to cellular death with subsequent necrosis and sloughing of tissue. Early signs of damage (which with prompt treatment can heal rapidly without a frank breakdown of the protective intact skin) are redness, itching, and pain. A dark mottled appearance usually signals damage to deeper tissues which may lead to later necrosis and sloughing even though there is no break in the skin when symptoms are first noted.

Any patient in a debilitated, toxic, uremic, or poor nutritional state will be more susceptible to the development of decubitus ulcers. If the blood supply is diminished for any reason, the formation of a pressure area is more likely. Local impairment of circulation through poor positioning, infrequent changes of position, or some pathologic disturbance of circulation are possible predisposing factors. A patient with a generally sluggish peripheral circulation (i.e., shock, congestive heart failure) will also be likely to experience pressure sores.

Persons with neurological disturbances are especially apt to have serious problems in prevention of decubitus ulcers. Paralysis or unconsciousness will prevent the normal shifts of position which one makes when any degree of discomfort is detected. Loss of sensation will prevent the individual from even being alerted to the discomfort. Therefore, even an impairment of circulation sufficiently prolonged to cause cellular death will not provide the usual alerting symptoms of pain and itching.

Fever and any other condition that raises the metabolic requirement will make cellular destruction more likely, given the same blood supply and external pressure factors.

Other internal factors that contribute to ulcer formation include anemia, edema, insufficient supply of protein and essential amino acids, and the absence of the normal muscle and fat over bony prominences.

External factors that may hasten the formation of an ulcer are primarily (1) pressure, (2) shearing forces (produced by abrupt changes in body position while the skin is still in contact with sheet, bed, or chair), and (3) material in contact with the skin, e.g., moisture, bacteria, feces, urine.

The mean capillary pressure is 20 to 30 mm mercury at heart level. These small thin-walled vessels have virtually no means other than this internal pressure to counteract the effects of external applied forces, in maintaining an adequate circulation at the cellular level. The substance of skin, fat, muscle, and subcutaneous tissue offers some cushioning and distribution of externally applied pressure. Kosiak has conducted experiments in animals which demonstrate that ulcer formation can occur after only 45 minutes of constant pressure maintained at 600 mm mercury. If the pressure was held at 150 mm mercury then ulcers did not form unless it was maintained for 12 hours. He recorded the pressure at various points on thighs, ischia, and coccyx in patients with spinal cord injuries who were sitting up. The pressures recorded were in the following ranges: on a wooden office seat, 45 to 400 mm mercury, and on a 2-inch foam rubber pad, 50 to 125 mm, with highest pressure recorded over the ischia and coccyx. Even the minimum pressures were above capillary levels. The highest pressure points would indicate that the conditions for decubitus ulcer formation are present within a relatively short time interval. This points up the fact that the term *bedsore* is really imprecise and misleading, since the pressure sore may occur as readily when one is sitting as in bed, and may also occur under ill-fitting prostheses or casts.

Perhaps a list of nursing measures to prevent the formation of decubitus ulcers will best illustrate the application of information given in the preceding paragraphs.

1. Proper positioning and frequent turning should be carried out with any patient confined to bed.

2. Frequent skin care is necessary, particularly of bodily parts exposed to weight-bearing, e.g., washing and massage with mild, bacteriostatic lotions.

3. Avoid any contact of skin (particularly weight-bearing areas) with irritating secretions, urine, or feces.

4. Keep the skin dry, e.g., avoid overheating and excessive diaphoresis or, if it occurs, change linen and bedding immediately. The moisture not only predisposes to bacterial growth, but also increases friction and shearing forces when movement is attempted.

5. In particularly susceptible individuals an alternating air pressure mattress, sponge rubber, sheepskin, or a silicone gel pad should be used under bony prominences.

6. In susceptible individuals exceptional vigilance must be maintained in positioning and turning, and observation of susceptible skin areas, so that any early signs of skin irritation can be vigorously countered with protective measures.

Decubitus ulcers may occur through negligence, or in spite of what may seem to be heroic measures to prevent them in the susceptible individual. When the skin is broken or when obvious signs of deeper tissue damage appear, the physician should be informed.

The physician's diagnosis of the degree of local extension of a decubitus ulcer, as well as the patient's prognosis, and his evaluation of the general state of health will determine his plan of treatment.

An open sore is invariably considered infected, and bacteriological study will determine the identification of organisms and their antibiotic sensitivity. Radiographic studies will assist in determining the presence and extent of osteitis. The depth and direction of a pressure sore can usually be found by inspection and probing.

Hematological and biochemical studies may be done to assess more accurately the patient's general condition and adequacy of plasma protein levels. A patient with a pressure ulcer suffers protein depletion for several reasons. The anorexia frequently accompanying illness and confinement to bed may result in inadequate dietary intake, particularly of protein. Elderly persons may have had a low protein intake for financial reasons for a prolonged period of time before illness. Pyrexia and sepsis destroy body protein at an accelerated rate. If large amounts of protein-containing pus or exudate drain from the decubitus ulcer, emaciation can occur with alarming speed.

A high-protein, high-calorie diet will make adequate protein available to the body for tissue repair and wound healing. The amino acid methionine has been shown to be essential to proper maturation of collagen in wound healing. Administration of vitamin supplements is usually indicated, particularly vitamin C. Transfusion of whole blood may be indicated when a patient shows a low hemoglobin. Intravenous administration of amino acids is usually neither desirable nor necessary. Additional fluids and protein can be given by nasogastric tube even during sleeping hours, if the patient has difficulty in consuming the amount of food prescribed.

The local treatment of a decubitus ulcer involves, first of all, the complete relief of pressure from the ulcerated area. If positioning and turning of the patient cannot accomplish this, then special devices may be of aid. The production of weightlessness through flotation therapy is described by Pfaudler. A Stryker frame, sawdust bed, or CircOlectric bed may be helpful.

An enzyme, such as Elase, Varidase, Parenzyme, Tryptar, Panafil, or Biozyme, may be prescribed for topical application as a debriding agent to remove clotted blood or fibrinous or purulent material that has accumulated and thereby facilitate normal tissue repair. The first three products are available in powder form, which can be mixed with solution for use as wet dressings. All products are available as ointment except Varidase powder, which is mixed with jelly for local application. Biozyme contains the enzyme trypsin and the antibiotic neomycin. Directions for use are supplied with each drug. Generally, the ointment is applied to the wound once or twice a day and covered with a dry fine mesh gauze square, and the wound is irrigated with a mild cleansing agent to remove the liquefied material before the ointment is reapplied. The "old-fashioned" treatment with the use of granulated sugar, instead of an enzyme ointment, is reported by practicing nurses to be very effective. The wound is lightly packed by sprinkling the sugar into the cavity until it is filled. It is then covered with fine mesh gauze and an ABD pad is secured with nonallergic adhesive tape. After weeping has occurred, the wound is irrigated with a solution of one part hydrogen peroxide 3 percent and three parts normal saline, followed by gentle drying with gauze and air drying, and light packing with gauze fluffs covered by an ABD pad. This treatment is given as often as necessary but at least once every 8 hours. If the wound does not have purulent exudate, treatment with irrigation and packing as described, omitting the application of sugar, is effective. Surgical debridement of necrotic tissue may be necessary. With any treatment the skin and bed linen should be kept dry.

Local application of antibiotics in the form of jelly, ointment, or irrigations may be used after all microscopic dead tissue has been removed and cellular debridement is going forward.

The question of the local application of *any drug* actually accelerating epithelialization and granulation should be put in proper perspective. The only effect shown to be possible by drugs is that of bringing local and systemic factors to a normal level, thus allowing healing to occur at a normal rate. In fact excessive application of foreign materials can only have a depressing effect on healing (Bailey).

The use of externally applied dry heat is often recommended for the purpose of increasing blood supply to the area. The heat will increase the metabolism locally and thus promote tissue repair and healing. However, it will also necessitate an increase of circulation to maintain adequate tissue nutrition and removal of catabolic products. Inflammatory exudation and edema when infection is present may increase tissue tension to a point where blood vessels are occluded. There is frequently a deposit of calcium in the muscles surrounding a pressure ulcer which imparts rigidity to the walls and diminishes the chances of healing.

Dry heat can be provided by an ordinary light bulb in a floor lamp, placed 2 to 3 feet from and directed to the injured area for 15 to 20 minutes two or three times a day. In elderly or debilitated patients or those with a neurological deficit, there may be sensory and/or motor loss at the ulcerated area. Because of the preceding three circumstances, application of external heat should be carried out with extreme caution, with full recognition of the danger that may be involved. If the local heating raises tissue metabolism beyond the ability for local increase of blood supply, further cellular damage will occur. A patient with a neurological deficit may not be able to sense pain, if the heat is causing burning, or to move, even though he may feel an uncomfortable increase in temperature.

To accomplish rehabilitation and promotion of a state of good health and positive nitrogen balance, decubitus ulcers should be healed as quickly as possible. To allow closure by spontaneous healing of a medium to large ulcer requires months of watchful waiting. Large ulcers are a constant source of nitrogen loss and an infection hazard. Therefore the physician will frequently elect to close the ulcer surgically. The ulcer is usually prepared for surgical closure by debridement and clearing of any infection present. The patient's general condition is important; this has been discussed previously. Simple approximation of the wound edges and suturing may be possible. However, methods of closure will frequently involve rotation flaps, skin grafts, and methods of plastic surgical repair.

Constipation and Incontinence. The prevention and solution of problems associated with constipation and urinary retention and incontinence have been discussed elsewhere. Inadequate preventive measures frequently cause elimination needs to become a major problem and the focus of a proportionately great deal of attention by the nursing staff. This compounds the patient's problems related to body image. The sensible goal should be to achieve the same proportion of attention to these functions for the immobilized patient that one devotes to them in the course of ordinary living. If at all possible, assistance to the bathroom or use of a bedside commode should be arranged; otherwise the patient should be placed as near to the normal functional position as possible, e.g., by raising the head of the bed to provide a sitting position on the bedpan. To avoid the danger associated with the Valsalva maneuver, the patient should avoid straining at stool, avoid holding his breath, and breathe through his mouth.

Vasomotor Status. When the time comes to begin ambulation again (especially after prolonged bed rest) the hazards of vasomotor instability should be recalled. The possibilities of weakness and fainting are very real. The patient may fear that he cannot manage out of bed or that his condition will worsen. Elastic bandages on the lower legs have been shown to help stabilize the peripheral circulation. Gradually increasing periods of ambulation, with assistance provided at first, will ensure a positive outcome.

Observation of Patient's Overall Progress. At every contact with a patient, the nurse should maximize her opportunities for reassessment of the patient's condition and for evaluation of how the plan of care is achieving intended goals in meeting present and future needs, and use appropriate nursing interventions. Aware of hazards that may plague the immobilized patient, she will be alert to observe respiration, position, skin condition, fluid intake, evidence of comfort, mood, and environment; she will visit him frequently, listen and interact therapeutically; she will encourage all avenues of sensory stimulation that are acceptable to him and that his condition will permit; and she will work with the patient and help him plan for his optimal rehabilitation. For the patient confined to bed with a terminal illness, she can use the principles to achieve for him the greatest degree of comfort and freedom from pain which is possible, as well as assist him to approach death with peace and serenity.

Controlling the Spread of Communicable Disease

From a nurse's point of view and her particular role in health care, there are two questions that are especially pertinent in relation to the control of the spread of communicable disease. How does she afford the greatest possible protection for other persons from pathogenic organisms originating from a patient with a recognized or unrecognized communicable disease? How does she give the best possible care to a patient who requires isolation? The danger of spread of communicable disease from unrecognized sources is frequently overlooked on a hospital ward, or is given only token attention. On the other hand, when a communicable disease is recognized, in an effort to protect personnel and other patients, the nursing personnel's preoccupation with unfamiliar and cumbersome isolation procedures may compromise the quality of nursing care that the isolated patient receives. Numerous studies have shown that patients in isolation on a general hospital ward frequently feel neglected and depersonalized.

The purpose of this section is to attempt to answer the two questions posed. Specific details of disinfection, sterilization, gowning, and the like are not discussed. Such material is thoroughly covered in other textbooks. The particular physical set-up for an isolation unit as well as detail procedures for concurrent and terminal disinfection are more appropriately treated in the procedure manual for the institution involved. Therefore this textbook presents guiding principles for the care of patients with communicable disease which the perceptive nurse can use to determine details of procedure in a particular situation. The scope of this discussion does *not* include a comprehensive treatment of epidemiological approaches and public health measures that are within the nurse's realm of responsibility in the total community setting.

The control and management of communicable disease is one of the great triumphs of modern medicine. Diphtheria, smallpox, scarlet fever, and more recently poliomyelitis have been virtually eliminated as threats to life and health. Several reasons explain the marked reduction of these diseases, the foremost of which is the discovery and widespread use of immunizing agents. Chemotherapeutic agents have been effective in the control of many communicable diseases for which effective immunization is still unavailable or impractical. In spite of these marked advances, diseases such as tuberculosis, malaria, infectious hepatitis, and the dysenteries still pose serious threats.

Staphylococcal infections also present a serious problem, especially in hospitals. The repeated use of antibiotics has led to the production of increased populations of antibiotic-resistant strains of certain organisms, and one such organism, *Staphylococcus aureus*, has come to constitute a world-wide problem for hospitals and communities. These micrococci are apparently able to survive for months and even years in dust and bedding. Studies have shown that hospital personnel and patients may harbor such organisms in the nasal passages without necessarily manifesting any clinical signs of illness. Other studies have shown hospital floors to be a reservoir of infection. It takes no imagination to realize that nurses' hands may spread such dangerous pathogenic organisms. Thus, it is apparent that the staphylococcus may be uniquely equipped to produce hospital cross-infections. Also, precautions are necessary in the hospital which will not be necessary in the patient's own home, or even in *group* living situations where the population is generally strong and healthy. The most vulnerable persons are the debilitated, the newborn, and those with breaks in the skin.

MEDICAL ASEPSIS

Medical asepsis refers to measures that are used to prevent the transfer of *pathogenic organisms* from one person to another. It does not mean that all equipment that comes in contact with the patient is *sterile;* it does mean that the equipment has been disinfected to destroy all pathogenic microorganisms. We can find countless examples of the practice of medical asepsis in daily living. Individually wrapped straws and toothpicks; sterilization of pillows and mattresses before sale, and labeling that they are sterilized; public health department regulations for beauty salons, barber shops, and restaurants; maternal concern for teaching children to wash their hands after using the toilet; and the homemaker's care to wash her hands before she begins food preparation. Most persons have an understanding of the need to protect themselves and the means by which it can be accomplished, whether or not they have a knowledge of the mode of transmission of pathogenic organisms. They are accustomed to looking critically at sanitation and aseptic practices in a restaurant, motel, or other public place. They will certainly expect no less from the hospital and from medical and nursing personnel when they are patients. For the patient who is not alert to the necessity for such protection for himself and others, the nurse has opportunity to set a good example and do health teaching. Many practices connected with efforts to provide medical asepsis are traditional or ritualistic; effective procedures for medical asepsis must be guided by an understanding of the principles on which they are based. Such basic principles from the study of microbiology and other sciences are not reviewed here.

Although portals of entry and portals of exit for the causative organism vary from disease to disease, some portals are the same for so many diseases that a degree of generalization is possible in developing principles for medical asepsis, and thus for protecting all individuals from the unrecognized case of communicable disease. Any excretion or secretion from the body is likely to be a portal of exit. Therefore such substances and any materials soiled by them are considered contaminated. Any normal opening in the body, even though covered with mucous membrane, is more susceptible to the entrance of many pathogenic organisms into the body than intact skin. Any break in the skin or mucous membrane is a potential portal of entry. Thus the designation of clean and contaminated areas is important in the hospital in *any* area where body excretions or secretions or materials that have been in immediate contact with them are handled, for example, food trays, drinking glasses, soiled linen, soiled utensils, and instruments.

Any material that will contact a mucous membrane or body orifice must be guaranteed to be free of pathogenic organisms. The way in which this is accomplished is not by keeping all equipment and nourishments sterile until they reach the patient, but by measures that assure destruction of pathogenic organisms (sterilization or disinfection) and then preventing contamination by such organisms during storage or transport to the patient (keeping them clean). Covered food trays, covered linen carts, and sterile packaging for many personal items such as straws and washcloths are examples. Many disposable items now available make this objective easier to accomplish.

Individual equipment for each patient is desirable and decreases the chance of cross-contamination because of a break in medical asepsis in sterilization, storage, or handling.

The discerning reader will see a significant area of possible cross-contamination still lurking as a danger to personnel and patients—hands! Patients' hands will always be contaminated to some degree by the organisms they harbor, therefore anything they touch is contaminated. Nurses' hands will of necessity handle many contaminated substances each day, and yet they must also handle clean materials and move from patient to patient.

The hands have been shown to normally have two types of bacterial flora—*transient* and *resident*. Price in 1938 published a report of an extensive study of skin bacteriology. *Transient bacteria* are picked up by the hands during whatever activities the person is engaged in and are loosely attached to the skin and under the fingernails. They can be removed with relative ease by thorough and frequent hand washing. *Resident bacteria* are found on the surface and in the fine creases and are relatively stable in type and number. They are not removed readily by washing with soap and water or use of disinfectants. If enough friction is used with a brush the bacterial count plotted against time can be reduced according to a logarithmic curve. Prolonged friction or excessive and careless use of a brush may damage the skin. Transient bacteria that remain on the skin over a long period of time tend to become part of the resident flora. If such flora contain pathogenic organisms, the nurse's hands may become carriers of these pathogens. Frequent and thorough hand washing will decrease the possibility of transient pathogenic bacteria becoming resident.

Hexachlorophene is a widely used skin disinfectant that is bacteriostatic to most organisms including gram-positive staphylococci and gram-negative microorganisms. It does appear to penetrate crevices and remain on the skin, thus allowing the bacteriostatic action to persist. It is available in cake and liquid soaps and in detergents. It is an ingredient of many popular soaps advertised for their deodorizing property. Its bacteriostatic action interferes with bacterial activity which is largely responsible for decomposition of skin secretions with resultant odors. The regular use of hexachlorophene-containing preparations markedly reduces the number of residual bacteria on the skin, and it is possible to get good results from hand washing in less than half the time formerly recommended.

Most recommended hand washing techniques for medical asepsis suggest a routine for using hand-applied friction on all skin surfaces. When this is done thoroughly, a minimum amount of time will have elapsed. If a brush is used, dry autoclaved brushes should be available; a poor compromise is a brush kept in a disinfectant solution. A brush used repeatedly without sterilization may harbor bacteria, and if used too vigorously may also cause a break in the skin. A nail file or orangewood stick should be available for cleaning under nails.

Careful and frequent hand washing is without doubt the *one best precaution* that the nurse can carry out in preventing cross-contamination between patients. However, it is the precaution that is probably most frequently neglected. In 1932 Pfefferkorn reported that in pediatric, maternity, and contagion units of a hospital nurses washed their hands as many as 69 times daily, while on the medical and surgical services many nurses washed only three times in 10 hours. That year is a long time ago, and perhaps a similar survey today would show a very different situation. We hope so!

All patients should be accorded the protection of recognized medical aseptic procedures. It is desirable then that workers know, and help patients to recognize, clean and contaminated areas, and that nurses (and all attendants) wash their hands after touching any patient or his belongings. A ½- to 1-minute scrub has been recommended when no obvious organic material is on the hands. When there is contamination with secretions, blood, mucus, and so forth, a more thorough procedure of 2 to 3 minutes, preferably done with a brush, should be carried out. Equipment used by many patients should be properly disinfected after each use. Whenever possible the patient can be supplied with individual equipment that can be discarded or thoroughly disinfected when he leaves the hospital.

FACTORS MODIFYING METHODS OF CONTROL

General principles of medical asepsis have been discussed briefly. When a patient is known to have a communicable disease he may be put in isolation. That is, the precautions for any transfer of pathogenic organisms from him to others are made especially secure. There are some diseases in which it is always considered necessary to isolate the patient. For other conditions some variation is seen. Furthermore, besides general isolation, special precautions may be necessary in the handling of excreta, drainage, and the like. In this section, we will attempt to identify the reasons why such variation is practiced and if it is justifiable.

Susceptibility of Population at Risk

We recognize that certain precautions are necessary to protect infants from disease which are unnecessary for adults, i.e., masks and gowns are worn in the nursery to prevent skin infection, and formula and all items that might reach the infant's mouth are sterilized in order to prevent diarrhea. The medical patient may be particularly susceptible to disease invasion because of malnutrition, poor circulation, free-floating anxiety, or his own imposed poor health practices such as smoking or prolonged excessive intake of alcohol. A patient with a break in the skin or an irritated skin area may be particularly susceptible to a staphyloccocal infection.

Whether a patient with pneumonia is put in isolation may well depend upon the susceptibility of other patients on the same ward. If their susceptibility is calculated to be low, then the usual precautions of medical asepsis and the effect of antibiotics and/or chemotherapeutic agents in rapidly producing bacteriostatic effects will be depended upon to reduce to practically nothing the transfer of pathogenic organisms.

Seriousness of the Disease

When a disease is a serious threat to life (i.e., meningitis), or is extremely difficult to cure (i.e., Hansen's disease), even though it is *not* highly communicable, drastic efforts are made to isolate the person having the disease. The common cold, on the other hand, is extremely communicable, but to a healthy child or adult it does not present a serious risk, therefore we seldom find a patient in full isolation because of the common cold. It is well to keep in mind that the common cold may be a very serious risk to a person with lung disease, blood dyscrasia, and a number of other conditions. A nurse with a common cold will therefore do well to isolate herself at home and not endanger any of her patients or coworkers.

Whether it is wise to make decisions on the basis of the factors indicated above is open to question. However, putting a patient in isolation, in itself, presents numerous problems and hazards that will be discussed later.

Mode of Transmission of the Causative Organism

When the nurse knows the routes by which the pathogenic organisms leave the body of the affected person and enter that of the well, then she can intelligently plan measures for prevention and control. The common routes are respiratory tract, alimentary canal, genital tract, conjunctiva, and broken skin (trauma, skin diseases, and surgical wounds).

One precaution is prominently common in all conditions: attendants must carry out proper hand washing after handling anything contaminated with infectious material from the patient, which for the sake of safety must include the patient himself and *all* materials in his immediate area.

Susceptibility of Organism to Disinfecting Agents

Bacteria and viruses respond differently to destructive agents. Anything that inhibits growth or destroys protoplasm will inhibit the growth of microorganisms. But the bacterial strain, stage of development, and other factors will determine the relative destructive effects of chemicals, temperature extremes, light rays, and drying processes. Sterilization with high temperatures and moist heat under pressure is necessary to ensure destruction of spores. By contrast, the gonococcus organism is destroyed at a temperature of 40° C. Its inability to survive outside the body explains its classification as a cause of venereal disease. It is virtually impossible to contract the disease without immediate transfer of the organism from host to recipient. Although infrequently seen since the advent of antibiotics, an acute gonorrheal conjunctivitis is extremely contagious through direct contact.

Since the causative organisms of most common diseases other than wound infections, botulism, and tuberculosis are considered to have vegetative forms only, medical asepsis is attained more readily than surgical asepsis. Mechanical cleansing with soap and water or a disinfectant and exposure to air and/or sunlight is an accepted method for ridding large equipment and walls of pathogenic organisms. Ultraviolet irradiation is effective if it is sufficiently strong or of sufficient length. Since the rays are injurious to skin and particularly to the conjunctiva and eyes, it is difficult to administer enough irradiation in a patient area to produce bactericidal effects.

ISOLATION TECHNIQUES

In the foregoing pages, an attempt has been made to emphasize the importance of and reasons for carrying out sound practices of medical asepsis in the care of *all* patients. When a patient is diagnosed as having a communicable disease, it is usually ordered that he be placed in isolation. This means that the infected person is separated from the uninfected by specific procedures aimed at ensuring that all items that contact him or any of his excretions, secretions, or other wastes will be destroyed, or rendered free of contamination before being considered safe for reuse. The isolation is usually physical as well as procedural, since when a patient is in a private room with bathroom the isolation technique can be carried out more readily. Unfortunately, the isolation is also frequently social as well, and the patient may suffer psychologically. On a general hospital ward the necessity of placing a patient in isolation is ordinarily infrequent, so the associated isolation procedures are cumbersome and unfamiliar to the personnel. The physical layout of the patient unit is usually ill suited to the institution of isolation as well. As a result, the emphasis may be on the procedures of maintaining the isolation technique, rather than upon the patient and his needs.

The symptoms of sensory deprivation, as discussed in this chapter in the section on hazards of bed rest, may well appear in the patient who is isolated. A discerning, sensitive nurse will find time to visit the patient when an isolation procedure is required, and means by which to enrich his sensory intake.

Kline has reported on how one medical center solved this problem by establishing a 17-bed ward with single rooms for individual isolation. The nursing staff on this particular ward was so expert in isolation technique that they were free to concentrate their concern and effort on better patient care.

Each institution will have specific isolation procedures suited to its particular situation. Since a smaller hospital may not be able to provide a ward just for patients with communicable disease, careful planning is necessary to ensure a routine that is simple enough to be readily carried out even though needed infrequently. Use of disposable supplies will help to simplify such procedures.

Foster reports from one hospital's experience that specific inclusion of instruction in their procedure book regarding the following aspects of isolation technique proved helpful: articles necessary in order to set up the isolation unit, when to wear mask and gown, how to enter and leave the unit, proper hand washing, procedures for cleaning up, and instructions to give the patient and his visitors. This *written* information was made operational by required in-service education classes on isolation technique for all personnel, including nursing, attendants, housekeeping, and maintenance.

Many studies have demonstrated that it is impractical to attempt to isolate a patient with a communicable disease other than in a private room with private bathroom. It is ideal to have hand-washing facilities in the hallway, but most general hospitals are not so constructed. Everything in the patient's unit (room and bathroom) should be considered contaminated. Therefore a small table or shelf for supplies (e.g., clean gown, masks) should be outside the room. Paper towels can be used by clean hands to turn off contaminated faucets or open contaminated doors.

The nurse has a responsibility to protect others from a communicable disease, and an equal obligation to explore the patient's understanding of his disease and the feelings that the isolation and precautionary measures may create.

GOWNS

A long-sleeved gown is worn whenever the nurse gives care that would bring her uniform into contact with the patient or *anything* within his unit. Particularly in a situation where the isolation set-up is only occasionally used, single-use technique for gowning is highly desirable, i.e., a gown is used once and then discarded for laundering. It is questionable whether it is possible to reuse a gown without at least some slight contamination of that gown occurring, even with the most careful technique. Therefore, only a few wearings should be permitted before it is discarded, even with the reuse technique.

MASKS

The purpose of using a mask is to filter the air of microorganisms. Microphotographs show that coughing or sneezing discharges thousands of moist particles many feet into the air each of which contains a load of microorganisms. Even talking and breathing normally release a smaller number of these dangerously communicable microparticles. The mask may be worn by the patient, but in most cases it is more practical for the nurse or visitor to be masked.

Many types of plastic, fabric, and gauze masks have been tested. They are described in detail in textbooks of fundamental nursing techniques. The most effective mask yet devised appears to be a close-fitting gauze square of six layers. No mask is effective if it is not used properly. An adequate supply of masks should be kept in the clean area. The mask is always applied with clean hands, removed by the strings with clean hands, and immediately discarded into a special laundry bag, or sack if the mask is disposable. A mask should never be allowed to hang about the neck, or be pocketed and then reused. If a period of prolonged contact is necessary with a patient who has a disease primarily transmitted through the respiratory tract, then a fresh mask can be used at intervals.

DISPOSAL OF BODY DISCHARGES AND EXCRETA

Most modern city sewage systems are equipped to render the sewage free of pathogens after the usual treatment; therefore, special pretreatment of body discharges is usually unnecessary. The local procedures and public health regulations should be consulted, particularly in the case of diseases whose mode of transmission is primarily through the alimentary canal. Werrin and Kronick, in a study of Salmonella control in hospitals, found that the objects most frequently implicated as spreading the disease organism were the hands of patients and personnel, contaminated nasal catheters, face masks, ice in patients' drinks, and spray created by flushing a toilet.

CLEANING AND DISINFECTING DISHES

A frequent complaint of patients in isolation is that the soiled tray, dishes, and leftover food from one meal are left in their room until the time that trays are served at the next meal. A way must be found to avoid such breakdown of good patient care, even though it may be time consuming. It may be difficult to properly handle dishes from one isolated patient in a general hospital, but it need not be the hurdle it frequently is allowed to be. The dishes can be scraped and rinsed immediately, and leftover food flushed down the toilet (if this is permissible by local regulation). The tray and dishes are then carried *directly* to the sterilizer on the ward, or to the kitchen washing and sterilizing equipment. Most hospitals now have set-ups that permit complete sterilization of the tray and dishes without handling by personnel. The important thing to avoid is any interim contamination of clean surfaces or handling by food service personnel.

A simpler solution for the occasional case of isolation is to provide disposable food service containers that can be incinerated after each meal.

LAUNDRY

A small laundry bag can be kept in the patient's unit. It can then be put into a clean larger bag for transit to the laundry. Special marking may or may not be necessary, depending on how soiled laundry is handled en route and at the laundry facility.

Reverse Isolation

For a patient with extremely low resistance to infection, the objective is frequently to provide an environment free of pathogenic organisms in the immediate patient area. Such a technique is referred to as *reverse isolation,* and it is literally just that. The patients for whom such precautions are carried out may be, for example, those who have had organ transplants and are receiving large doses of immunosuppressive drugs, or cancer patients receiving extensive chemotherapy, or patients with severe burns. "Life island," a bed completely enveloped by an air-inflated plastic barrier to environmental microorganisms, is an example of a specialized way in which to carry out reverse isolation. It is also referred to as RES-Care—Regulated Environment for Safety Care (Nichols). The discussion of nursing care during reverse isolation is included with the surgical and disease conditions in which it is used.

Radiation

X-rays, radioisotopes, and radium are being used extensively in medicine as tools for diagnosis and therapy. The nurse, as the health team member often having greatest contact with the patient, must understand the nature of radiation, the purpose in using the radiation source, and how she can give good nursing care to patients undergoing radiation therapy and still protect herself and others from radiation hazards.

Radioactive substances do have potential dangers, but when they are handled properly, their potential benefits far outweigh the risk involved. There is hardly a diagnostic or therapeutic tool known that does not involve some degree of risk to the patient. Radiation is unique in that it also involves a degree of risk for personnel administering the radiation and with certain types of sources for persons associated with the patient as well.

THE NATURE OF RADIATION

Radium-226, a naturally occurring radioactive isotope, was extracted from uranium ore by Marie Curie and has been used in medicine since the turn of the century. Defense and industrial uses, as well as medical use, have spurred research. There are now numerous manmade radioisotopes in use in basic biological research and in clinical medicine.

The atom consists of a dense positively charged core, or nucleus, surrounded by negatively charged electrons that travel at high speed in orbits about the nucleus. The major components of this nucleus are protons and neutrons. A given chemical element may exist in several forms called *isotopes*. The isotopes of an element vary in the number of neutrons in the nucleus. Therefore, for any given element, the atomic number is the same, but the *mass numbers* vary. The mass number is the total number of neutrons plus protons in the nucleus. For example, phosphorus-32, which may be written ^{32}P, has a total of 32 protons and neutrons in its nucleus.

Each element has an optimum proportion of protons and neutrons for maximum stability. Radioactive isotopes have ratios outside this range of stability. The emission of radiation by such an isotope can be divided into three types that have medical significance: alpha (α), negative beta (β), and gamma (γ). Alpha radiation consists of positive particles that are identical with the nucleus of a helium atom (two protons and two neutrons). Negative beta rays are identical with electrons. Gamma rays have no electrical charge and no detectable mass. They are like x-rays and may be considered to be a very energetic form of the sources of radiation which include visible light, ultraviolet and infrared, and radio waves. Most isotopes emit alpha or beta particles and give off gamma radiation.

The *rate* of emission of radiation will determine the *half-life*. Each isotope has a specific and unvarying half-life. Half-life is the time required for one-half of the atoms in a sample of material to *decay* (produce their radioactive emission). There is tremendous variation in the half-lives of various isotopes. Most medically useful radioisotopes to be used in open, unsealed form have relatively short half-lives, that is, of the order of days or weeks.

An x-ray machine produces x-rays by bombardment of a target (metal of high atomic number) with high-speed electrons. The higher the voltage that accelerates the electrons the higher will be the average energy of the x-rays produced. Gamma rays produced as a result of nuclear radiation have energies specific and characteristic for each isotope. This energy is expressed as electron volts: Ke V (thousand electron volts) or Me V (million electron volts). For example, cobalt-60 emits a beta particle of 0.312 Me V and two gamma rays, one of 1.17 Me V and the other of 1.33 Me V. The gamma rays from cobalt-60 will travel farther in a given material than will those of cesium-137 which have an energy of 0.66 Me V (Barnett).

Many of the radioisotopes used in diagnostic studies have a much lower energy spectrum than cobalt and cesium. As x-rays and the radiation given off by radioisotopes pass through matter, the original energy is dissipated by a series of collisions with atoms of the materials through which the radiation is traveling. This absorption of radiation energy by the material through which the radiation passes is called *ionization*. The radiation energy is transferred to the electrons of the material, causing the "excitation" of these electrons, and by collisions actually knocking the electrons out of orbit. The resulting atom is ionized. Radiation that produces such an effect is said to be *ionizing radiation*. This phenomenon is responsible for the damage to biological tissues, or in the case of cancer cells, for their destruction.

Chronic low-level radiation in nonlethal doses is thought to have late effects that include (1) acceleration of the aging process, (2) production of neoplastic disease, and (3) genetic effects (Blahd).

PRINCIPLES OF RADIATION SAFETY

Whether originating from radioisotopes or as x-rays, ionizing radiation is harmful to living tissues. Special units are used to measure and express *amounts of radioactivity* in a sample of radioactive substance, and to measure *radiation dose*, which is the energy absorption in interaction with matter.

Curie (c) is the basic unit for measuring amount of radioactivity. Most amounts of radioisotopes used for *diagnostic* purposes are in the microcurie (μc) range. A *therapeutic* capsule of iodine-131 may be 5 to 10 millicuries (mc). The amount of cobalt-60 in a teletherapy machine used to deliver external radiation treatment may be as high as several thousand curies. The unit to express *exposure* is the *roentgen* (R). The estimated *absorbed dose* is given in *rads* or in *rem* (Barnett).

Even though repair of tissue takes place following radiation injury, it is believed that a certain amount of irreparable injury occurs. Since a certain component of radiation damage is permanent, additive effects may be cumulative over a lifetime.

A number of factors determine the degree of damage from a dose of radiation during one's lifetime. The same dose over a longer time is less damaging than the same dose given all at once. The larger the area of the body exposed to a particular dose, the greater the effect.

Three basic methods can reduce radiation exposure from external sources. They are *distance, time,* and *shielding* (Boeker).

Distance is an effective method of rapidly reducing the danger of exposure. X-ray and gamma radiation intensities from point sources are reduced according

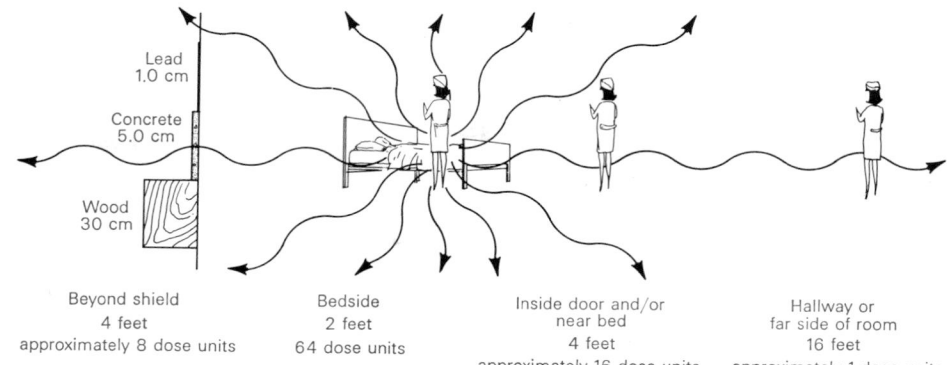

Figure 20–8
Protection offered by
distance and shielding
from radiation hazard
while nurse is caring for
patient with pelvic
radium implant. If
exposure at 2 feet is 64
dose units, then approxi-
mate dose units at
various distances are as
shown, calculated
according to the inverse
square law. Illustrated
are shielding materials
that will reduce radiation
exposure by about one-
half. (Adapted and
redrawn with permission
from E. R. Boeker: The
Nurse in Radiation
Protection. Nursing
Clinics of North America,
N. B. Saunders Company,
Philadelphia, March,
1967.)

Lead
1.0 cm

Concrete
5.0 cm

Wood
30 cm

Beyond shield
4 feet
approximately 8 dose units

Bedside
2 feet
64 dose units

Inside door and/or
near bed
4 feet
approximately 16 dose units

Hallway or
far side of room
16 feet
approximately 1 dose units

to the inverse square law. To a close approximation, then, the inverse square law will apply to calculating the exposure at varying distances from a patient who has a radium implant. Radium is a strong emitter of gamma rays. At 4 feet the intensity is only one-fourth what it was at 2 feet. At 8 feet it is only one-sixteenth and at 16 feet it is only one-sixty-fourth what it was at 2 feet.

Reducing the *time* of exposure is simply a matter of being aware of sources of radiation, and planning ahead so that no more time is spent close to the source than is absolutely necessary.

Shielding is the method employed when time and distance cannot be used to reduce the radiation exposure to safe levels. Gamma and x-rays lose energy when interacting with matter; therefore the denser the matter, the more rays will be absorbed per unit thickness, i.e., 1 cm of lead will attenuate radiation to a much greater degree than will 1 cm of wood.

The danger of radiation from a strong gamma emitter can be likened to the danger of being burned by a very hot fire. If one touches it he will almost certainly be burned, but the farther away one is, the less heat he feels. Also, one can stay near the fire at a "safe" distance for a relatively long time without danger, but at a few inches he will be burned very quickly. A shield of asbestos will protect a person from the heat radiation from a fire; a shielding of lead or other dense material will protect a person from radiation of a gamma emitter.

It is principally gamma rays and x-rays that present a hazard of radiation from external sources, because they can penetrate long distances and relatively dense materials. Most beta rays can penetrate only a few millimeters into the body. The penetration will be in proportion to the energy of the beta rays. However, beta emitters produce a penetrating electromagnetic radiation, called *bremsstrahlung*, which is created as the result of the interaction of beta particles with matter. The amount of bremsstrahlung is in proportion to the energy of the beta rays and the density of the absorbing material. Therefore, materials such as glass, lucite, and aluminum are good beta shields. For practical purposes, alpha particles can be presumed not to penetrate the body at all.

In the x-ray department, the radiologist wears a heavy leaded apron and gloves when performing fluoroscopy. The nurse may wonder why such shielding would not be appropriate and helpful when she is caring for a patient who has had a radium implant or has in his body some other radioactive substance that emits gamma rays of high energy. Such protection is equivalent to only about 0.25 mm sheet lead and is therefore practical only to protect from radiation of relatively low energy such as is encountered in fluoroscopy. Such gloves and aprons would reduce the radiation exposure from radium or cobalt-60 only slightly, allowing 85 to 90 percent to be transmitted (Blatz). The inconvenience of the bulky garment would probably cause the exposure time to be lengthened, thus *increasing* the actual radiation exposure.

Danger of *internal exposure* to radiation arises from entry of radioactive material into the body. It remains in the body until it is excreted, or until, by its decay rate, its radioactivity is exhausted. Therefore, control is a matter of avoiding contamination by radioactive material of anything that would be inhaled, ingested, or absorbed through the skin.

The concept of contamination control is a simple one. To prevent unsealed radioactive materials from entering the body, the same kinds of precautions are used that are instituted to prevent contamination from the causative organism in communicable diseases. The area can be monitored with an appropriate device to determine if it is free from radioactive contamination. (Unfortunately, there is no machine to monitor for bacteria!)

In any institution where radiation therapy is employed, a radiation safety officer will oversee and coordinate efforts to enforce radiation protective measures. In case of an accident, where radioactive material causes contamination of an area or person(s), the officer should be called immediately.

RADIOISOTOPE TRACERS

Tracers are materials used to label specific atoms, molecules, or organs, or some other entity of a "population" so that the labeled species can be followed in its physical movement or in the kinetics of its conversions. Examples of tracers are dyes, radioactive isotopes, and chemical substituent groups.

A radioactive tracer must have certain characteristics to be useful for diagnostic procedures. The quantity of tracer required should be minimal to avoid untoward biological or radiation effects. It should provide the desired information with minimum radiation exposure to the patient. Therefore, most radioisotopes used for diagnosis usually have a relatively short half-life. The quantity of tracer given is of the order of one to several hundred microcuries (μc). Since most detectors detect gamma radiation, a lower energy gamma emitter, with minimal or no alpha and beta emission, is desirable. Many sources list radioisotopes used in diagnosis with the usual dosage range (Blahd).

Because most radioisotopes chosen for use in diagnosis are relatively low energy emitters, and doses are in the microcurie range, patients who have received them do not usually present radiation exposure hazards to other persons. The nurse should determine the route of elimination of the isotope from the patient's body and, if indicated, take precautions in the disposal of urine and other waste matter.

The nurse's most important function in respect to radiation hazards involved is to see that preparation of the patient and scheduling is correct. Errors in these items may necessitate repeat x-ray procedures, which expose the patient and personnel to unnecessary added amounts of radiation as well as additional expense.

Principles concerning radiation safety important to keep in mind in relation to diagnostic x-ray procedures are as follows: (1) Nursing and x-ray personnel should not be in the room with the patient while the x-ray film is taken. Observation areas protected by shielding and leaded glass windows are provided. (2) If it is absolutely necessary for an attendant to be with a patient (such as a child and during fluoroscopy), the attendant should be someone who is not ordinarily exposed to the ionizing radiation in his work activities, and preferably someone past childbearing age, because of the generative organs' particular sensitivity to damage from radiation. In addition, he should be protected by a leaded apron and leaded gloves. (3) A pregnant woman should not be exposed to ionizing radiation for diagnostic or therapeutic purposes unless her physician feels that such examination or treatment is more important for her health or preservation of life than the risk involved.

RADIATION THERAPY

There is much misinformation and lack of information regarding radiation hazards. This situation extends to health workers, including nurses, as well as the general public. The professional nurse is responsible for effective communication with every patient directly or indirectly under her care. She needs to be informed about radiation so that she can provide supportive and appropriately interventive nursing care for patients receiving radiation and their families and assist ancillary workers in developing skills and understanding related to care of patients with radiation.

Therapeutic radiation is administered most frequently to retard abnormal growth of tissue, such as cancer. Ordinarily it is administered in much higher doses than x-ray and radioisotopes used for diagnostic purposes.

This section on radiation is summarized in an outline of the principles of protection during radiation therapy procedures and a broad outline of the principles of nursing care for patients receiving radiation therapy.

Most sealed sources (e.g., radium applicators, radon seeds) are impossible or extremely unlikely to be ingested inadvertently, therefore they present only *external* hazards. The precautions of time, distance, and shielding provide a triple front of defense for personnel.

Unsealed sources (e.g., iodine-131 for thyroid tumors and gold-198 for intracavitary tumors) pose both *external* and *internal* hazards. The key to internal protection is to prevent radioactive material from entering the body through control of contamination.

X-ray and teletherapy with cobalt-60 or radium in the x-ray department present no radiation hazard to personnel who care for the patient *after* the treatment.

No damage will occur to the nurse if she is informed and follows precautionary measures.

For protection of herself and others and to reduce unnecessary fear, the nurse should observe the following principles of radiation safety:

1. Know the type of hazard involved (i.e., high or low energy, type of emitter, how emitted, how excreted) and the applicable protection measures. The radiation safety officer can be consulted when questions arise.

2. Be informed about the radiation safety protocols as set up in the institution where she is working.

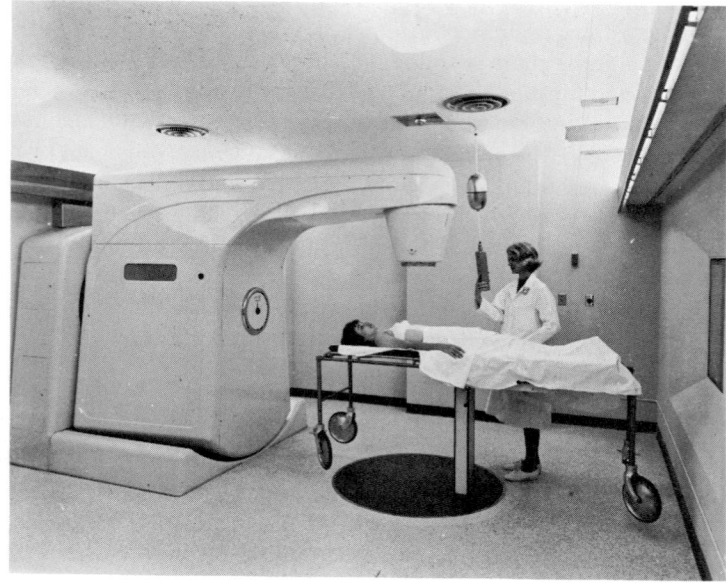

Figure 20–9
Patient in position to
receive therapy from 6
megavoltage linear
accelerator. (Courtesy of
Justin J. Stein, M.D.,
School of Medicine,
U.C.L.A. Center for
Health Sciences.)

3. Observe the precautions of time, distance, and shielding.

4. When a patient needs a considerable amount of direct nursing care, the personnel should be rotated to minimize exposure for any one individual. Necessary nursing care should never be omitted.

5. The patient who will be hospitalized for radiation therapy and his family members should be instructed regarding radiation safety procedures. Understanding nursing care and having frequent contacts with the patient before therapy will help him to accept and realize the necessity for minimal nursing care during his period of isolation.

Figure 20–10
Radiation survey
instruments: Geiger
survey meter and
ionization chamber
survey meter ("cutie
pie"). Both are frequently
used in area monitoring.

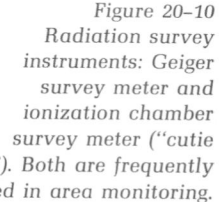

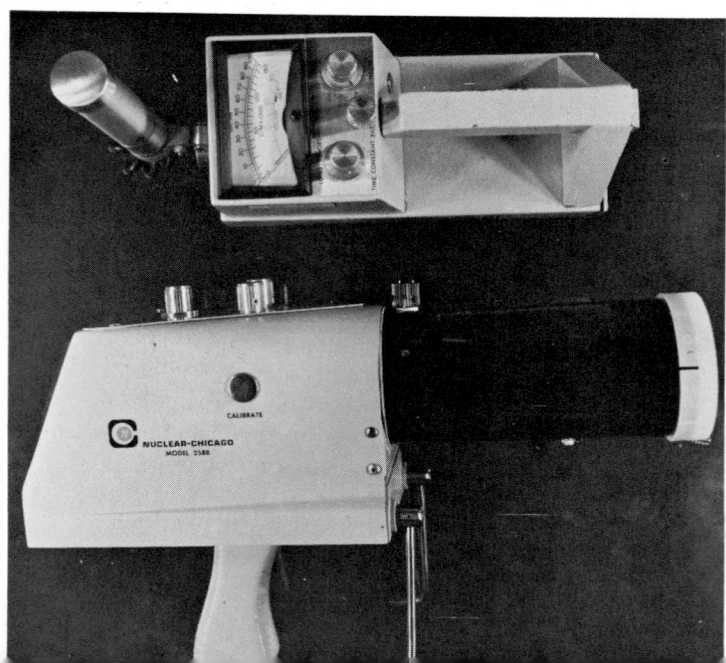

6. If any spillage of radioactive materials or contaminated body fluids occurs, the recommended emergency decontamination procedures should be instituted.

7. Never touch or pick up radioactive sources with the hands—use forceps and transport in a leaded container.

8. Keep the patient and visitors informed about radioactivity and protective barriers necessary. They must understand and cooperate or many persons will be endangered.

9. If a nurse is regularly exposed to radiation sources, she should wear an exposure meter (film badge, dosimeter, pocket chamber) and not exceed the limits of the *maximum permissible dose* (MPD) as recommended by the National Committee for Radiation Protection (NCRP). (See Figure 20-11.)

10. Area monitoring devices should be used if there is a question of contamination having occurred, after cleanup following a spillage, and after a patient is dismissed before the unit is considered safe for occupancy. (See Figure 20-12.)

Radiation therapy is a frightening thing to many people. This may be largely because they do not understand it and do not know what to expect. Also, it may settle a question in a patient's mind as to his fears about the nature of his illness, for he probably sees radiation therapy as a treatment for a malignant tumor, yet radiation therapy is used in treatment of other diseases and the patient's connection of radiation with cancer is not always true. Sensitive, understanding support from the nurse will be important.

The side effects of radiotherapy vary a great deal according to the individual's reaction, and also as to dose and location. For example, radiation to the upper abdomen more frequently results in severe nausea than does radiation to other locations of the body. There is a varying sensitivity of tissues of the body to ionizing radiation. Rapidly dividing cells and those in the process of mitosis are particularly susceptible. This explains the well-known effect of radiation on gonadal tissue. Cancer cells are also rapidly growing and are thus more susceptible to radiation than are normal cells; however, many normal cells are injured and/or destroyed in the process of destroying nearby cancer cells.

Figure 20–11
Personnel monitoring devices: film badge worn on pocket or lapel; dosimeter; film badge worn on wrist.

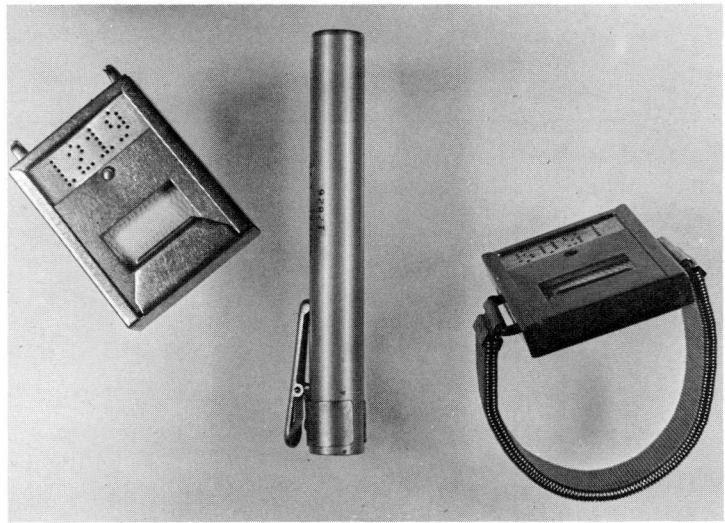

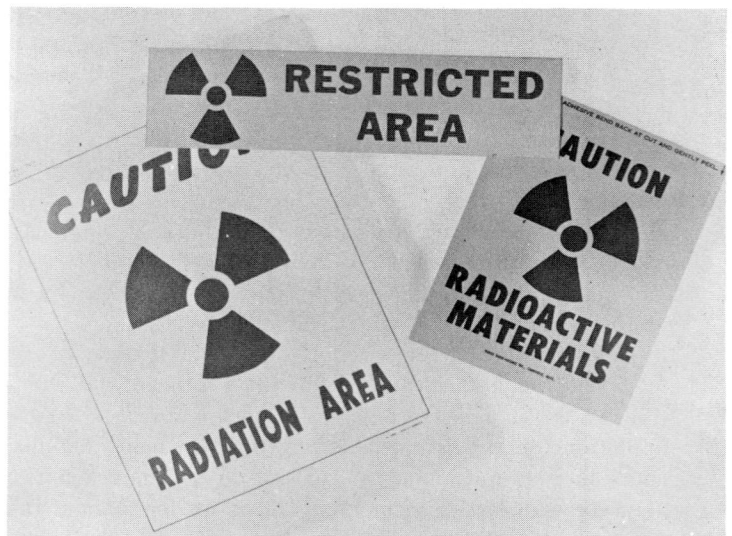

Figure 20–12
Radiation caution signs,
illustrating typical
symbol.

Some effects of radiation are seen within a very short time (i.e., hours, days) and some are seen only after weeks, months, or years. Nausea, malaise, and anorexia are early symptoms. Skin changes, alopecia, scarring, and fibrosis appear later. Supportive nursing care and symptomatic treatment are indicated, for there is nothing that provides a direct antidote to the effects of radiation.

The patient should be instructed to wash a radiated skin area carefully, and not to remove any pencil markings until the series of treatments has been completed. Bland and anesthetic ointments may be prescribed for application to the skin but should not be used without prescription.

Fundamentals regarding the nature of radiation, principles of radiation safety, and nursing care for patients undergoing a difficult and trying method of therapy should be understood by every nurse. She also needs to continue to inform herself about new uses of radioisotopes in medical treatment and diagnosis and her responsibilities in preparation and care of the patient and his family.

Bibliography

Works of General Interest

Asher, Richard A. J.: Dangers of Going to Bed. *British Medical Journal,* 2:967, December 13, 1947.

Bailey, B. N.: *Bedsores.* London: Edward Arnold (Publishers) Ltd., 1967.
Best, Charles H. and Norman Taylor:

The Physiological Basis of Medical Practice. Baltimore: The Williams & Wilkins Company, 1966.

Birkhead, N. C., et al.: Circulatory and Metabolic Effects of Prolonged Bedrest in Healthy Subjects. *Federation Proceedings,* 22:520, March-April, 1963. Abstract.

Browse, N. L.: *Physiology and Pathology of Bedrest.* Springfield, Ill.: Charles C Thomas, Publisher, 1965.

Burton, Alan C.: *Physiology and Biophysics of the Circulation.* Chicago: Year Book Medical Publishers, Inc., 1965.

Carlson, Sylvia: Selected Sensory Input and Life Satisfactions of Immobilized Geriatric Female Patients. American Nurses Association Clinical Sessions. New York: Appleton Century Crofts, 1968.

Coe, S. W.: Cardiac Work and the Chair Treatment of Acute Coronary Thrombosis. *Annals of Internal Medicine,* 40:42, January, 1954.

Comroe, Julius H., Jr.: *Physiology of Respiration.* Chicago: Year Book Medical Publishers, Inc., 1965.

Cooper, Kenneth H.: *Aerobics.* Philadelphia: M. Evans and Company, 1968.

Deitrick, J. E., et al.: Effects of Immobilization upon Various Metabolic and Physiologic Functions of Normal Men. *American Journal of Medicine,* 4:3, January, 1948.

De Meyer, J. A.: The Environment of the Intensive Care Unit. *Nursing Forum,* 6:262, Summer, 1967.

Erikson, Erik: *Identity and the Life Cycle.* New York: International Universities Press, 1959.

Fisher, S. and S. E. Cleveland: *Body Image and Personality.* Princeton, N.J.: D. Van Nostrand Company, Inc., 1958.

Ganong, William F.: *Medical Physiology,* 3d ed. Los Altos, California: Lange Medical Publications, 1967.

Gauer, Otto H. and Hans L. Thron: Postural Changes in the Circulation. in *Handbook of Physiology: Section 2, Circulation, Vol. III.* Washington, D.C.: American Physiological Society, 1965.

Heron, Woodburn: Pathology of Boredom. *Scientific American,* 196:52, 1957.

Holmgren, A. and C. O. Ovenfors: The Heart Volume at Rest and during Muscular Exercise in the Supine and Sitting Position. *Acta Medica Scandinavica,* 167:267, 1960.

Jackson, C. W., J. C. Pollard, and E. W. Kansky: The Application of Findings from Experimental Sensory Deprivation to Cases of Clinical Sensory Deprivation. *American Journal of Medical Science,* 243:558, May, 1962.

Kelly, Mary M.: Exercises for Bedfast Patients. *American Journal of Nursing,* 66:2209, October, 1966.

Kosiak, Michael: Etiology and Pathology of Ischemic Ulcers. *Archives of Physical Medicine,* 40:62, February, 1959.

Kosiak, Michael, et al.: Evaluation of Pressure as a Factor in Production of Ischial Ulcers. *Archives of Physical Medicine,* 39:623, October, 1958.

Levine, Myra E: The Pursuit of Wholeness. *American Journal of Nursing,* 69:93, January, 1969.

Lewis, Edith P.: Four Nurses Who Wanted to Make a Difference. *American Journal of Nursing,* 69:777, April, 1969.

Lewis, Lucile: This I Believe about the Nursing Process. *Nursing Outlook,* 16:26, May, 1968.

Linton, P. H.: Sensory Deprivation in Hospitalized Patients. *Alabama Journal of Medical Science,* 2:256, July, 1965.

Marshall, R. J., J. T. Shepherd, and Y. Wang: The Effect of Changes in Posture and of Graded Exercise on Stroke Volume in Man. *Journal of Clinical Investigation,* 39:1051, 1960.

McLachlin, J. A., et al.: Venous Stasis in the Lower Extremities. *Annals of Surgery,* 152:678, 1960.

McMichael, J., and J. P. McGibbon: Postural Changes in Lung Volume. *Clinical Science,* 4:175, 1939.

Olson, Edith V. (Ed.): The Hazards of Immobility. *American Journal of Nursing,* 67:781, April, 1967.

Pfaudler, Marjorie: Flotation, Displacement, and Decubitus Ulcers. *American Journal of Nursing,* 68:2351, November, 1968.

Pitts, Robert F.: *Physiology of the Kidney and Body Fluids.* Chicago: Year Book Medical Publishers, Inc., 1968.

Pohl, Margaret L.: *Teaching Function of the Nursing Practitioner.* Dubuque, Iowa: Wm. C. Brown, 1968.

Rushmer, R.: Postural Effects on the Baselines of Ventricular Performance. *Circulation,* 20:897, 1959.

Schultz, Duane P.: *Sensory Restriction.* New York: Academic Press, Inc., 1965.

Seegers, Walter H.: Blood Clotting Mechanisms: Three Basic Reactions. *Annual Review of Physiology,* 31:280, 1969.

Selkurt, Ewald E. (Ed.): *Physiology,* 2d ed. Boston: Little, Brown and Company, 1966.

Sevitt, Simon and N. Gallagher: Venous Thrombosis and Pulmonary Embolism. *British Journal of Surgery,* 48:475, March, 1961.

Sharp, J. T.: Effect of Posture on Lung Compliance in Normal Subjects and Patients with Congestive Heart Failure. *Journal of Clinical Investigation,* 38:659, 1959.

Sjostrand, T.: The Volume and Distribution of the Blood. *Physiological Reviews,* 33:202, 1953.

Smith, Dorothy M.: A Clinical Nursing Tool. *American Journal of Nursing,* 68:2384, November, 1968.

Solomon, R., et al.: Sensory Deprivation: A Review. *American Journal of Psychiatry,* 114:357, October, 1957.

Spence, Wayman R., R. D. Burk, and J. W. Roe: Gel Support for Prevention of Decubitus Ulcers. *Archives of Physical Medicine,* 48:283, June, 1967.

Stillwell, D. M., et al.: Atrophy of Quadriceps Muscle Due to Immobilization of Lower Extremity. *Archives of Physical Medicine,* 48:289, June, 1967.

Streeten, D. H. P. and P. J. Speller: The Role of Aldosterone and Vasopressin in the Postural Changes and Renal Excretion in Normal Subjects and Patients with Idiopathic Edema. *Metabolism,* 15:53, 1966.

Taylor, H. L., et al.: Effects of Bedrest on Cardiovascular Function and Work Performance. *Journal of Applied Physiology,* 2:223, November, 1949.

Ullman, M.: Disorders of Body Image after Stroke. *American Journal of Nursing,* 64:89, October, 1964.

Vander, Arthur J.: Control of Renin Release. *Physiological Reviews,* 47:359, 1967.

Wessler, S.: Thrombosis in the Presence of Vascular Stasis. *American Journal of Medicine,* 33:648, 1962.

White, A., P. Handler, and E. L. Smith: *Principles of Biochemistry,* 4th ed. New York: McGraw-Hill Book Company, 1968.

Wolfe, L. K., R. D. Gordon, D. P. Island, and G. W. Liddle: An Analysis of Factors Determining the Circadian Pattern of Aldosterone Excretion. *Journal of Clinical Endocrinology,* 26:1261, 1966.

Wright, H. B., S. B. Osborn, and M. Hayden: Venous Velocity in Bedridden Medical Patients. *Lancet,* 2:699, 1952b.

Care of the Patient in Isolation

Anderson, G. W. and Margaret G. Arnstein: *Communicable Disease Control,* 3d ed. New York: The Macmillan Company, 1953.

Benson, Margaret E.: Handwashing— An Important Part of Medical

Asepsis. *American Journal of Nursing,* 57:1136, September, 1957.

Blank, Irwin H.: Measurement of pH of the Skin Surface. *Journal of Investigative Dermatology,* 2:67, April, 1939.

Bullough, Bonnie: Where Should Isolation Stop? *American Journal of Nursing,* 62:86, October, 1962.

Caswell, H. Taylor: Staphylococcal Infections among Hospital Personnel. *American Journal of Nursing,* 58:822, June, 1958.

Foster, Marion: A Positive Approach to Medical Asepsis. *American Journal of Nursing,* 62:76, April, 1962.

Fuerst, Elinor V. and Lu Verne Wolff: *Fundamentals of Nursing,* 3d ed. Philadelphia: J. B. Lippincott Company, 1964.

Ginsberg, Miriam K. and Maria L. La Conte: Reverse Isolation. *American Journal of Nursing,* 64:88–90, September, 1964.

Harmer, Bertha and Virginia Henderson: *Textbook of Principles and Practice of Nursing,* 5th ed. New York, The Macmillan Company, 1955.

Kline, Patricia A.: Isolating Patients with Staphylococcal Infections. *American Journal of Nursing,* 65:102, January, 1965.

Lester, Mary R.: Every Nurse an Epidemiologist. *American Journal of Nursing,* 57:1434, November, 1957.

Nichols, G. A.: Isolation in a Regulated Environment for Safety. American Nurses Association Clinical Sessions. San Francisco, 1966.

Pfefferkorn, Blanche: Pray, Let Us Wash Our Hands. *American Journal of Nursing,* 32:851, August, 1932.

Price, Philip B.: Bacteriology of Normal Skin; New Quantitative Test Applied to Study the Bacterial Flora and Disinfectant Action of Mechanical Cleansing. *Journal of Infectious Diseases,* 63:301, November–December, 1938.

Rebell, Gerbert, et al.: Factors Affecting the Rapid Disappearance of Bacteria Placed on the Normal Skin. *Journal of Investigative Dermatology,* 14:247, April, 1950.

Roth, J. A.: Ritual and Magic in the Control of Contagion. Dorrian Apple (Ed.): *Sociological Studies of Health and Sickness.* New York: McGraw-Hill Book Company, 1960.

Seidler, Florence M.: Adapting Nursing Procedures for Reverse Isolation. *American Journal of Nursing,* 65:108, June, 1965.

Smendik, Patricia and Cathryn H. Kurtagh: Isolation in the Home. *American Journal of Nursing,* 56:575, May, 1956.

South, Jean: *Tuberculosis Handbook for Public Health Nurses,* rev. ed. New York: National Tuberculosis Association, 1955.

Werrin, M. and D. Kronick: Salmonella Control in Hospitals. *American Journal of Nursing,* 66:528, March, 1966.

Care of the Patient with Radiation Therapy

Barnett, Mark: The Nature of Radiation and Its Effect on Man. *Nursing Clinics of North America,* 2:11, March, 1967.

Blahd, William H.: *Nuclear Medicine.* New York: McGraw-Hill Book Company, 1965.

Blatz, Hanson: *Introduction to Radiological Health.* New York: McGraw-Hill Book Company, 1964.

Boeker, Elisabeth H.: The Nurse in Radiation Protection. *Nursing Clinics of North America,* 2:23, March, 1967.

National Bureau of Standards: *Handbook No. 42, Safe Handling of Radioactive Isotopes.* Washington, D.C.: U.S. Government Printing Office.

Nowak, Patricia Ann: Inservice Education in Radiation Health. *Nursing Clinics of North America,* 2:107, March, 1967.

Smith, Dorothy W. and Claudia D. Gips: *Care of the Adult Patient,* 2d ed. Philadelphia: J. B. Lippincott Company, 1966.

Walker, Elizabeth: Responsibilities of the Hospital Nurse in the Clinical Use of Radiation. *Nursing Clinics of North America,* 2:35, March, 1967.

CHAPTER 21
THE SURGICAL PATIENT

MARCIA LYN DALE AND HARRIET COSTON MOIDEL

This chapter presents a general discussion of the care of the patient undergoing surgical therapy. Care specific to particular surgical procedures is taken up in subsequent chapters of Part V.

Advances in the control of infection, new types of anesthetic agents, and advanced operative techniques have increased the frequency of surgical intervention and the complexity of care of the surgical patient. In order that the surgical patient may be assured the most comfortable route of recovery from the moment he is told surgery is needed until he returns to his accustomed life, a team of professional personnel is engaged in involving him in the surgical experience he will encounter. The nurse, as a member of the team, will play a leading role in his care, since she is the team member who spends the most time with him in the preoperative and postoperative periods and has the opportunity to make acute observations and pertinent suggestions.

Types of Surgery

Surgery is performed for four reasons: cure, diagnosis, palliation, and reconstruction. Each of these reasons will have special implications for the patient and will influence his reaction to the surgical experience. The disease condition for which the surgery is performed, the part of the body which will be operated upon, the length of time between discovery of the need for surgery and the surgical procedure, and the patient's preconceived ideas about the experience will influence his response before and after surgery and the care given by all members of the team.

Most surgical procedures are elective, i.e., the patient can decide, on the basis of medical opinion, whether or not to undergo the surgery. He must make a psychological adaptation to the proposed surgery. Many factors enter into his decision, including financial strain, effect on his business, deferment of his responsibilities, and personal ability to withstand the strain. He may deny the illness or refuse the proposed treatment before adjusting to the reality of the situation. With elective surgery there is some time available for the patient to prepare for the experience and time for the medical evaluation of his health status.

Emergency surgery is performed as a life-saving treatment and on short notice, so the patient has little time to adapt to its necessity. Emergency surgery increases the risk to the patient, since his physical state may not have been thoroughly evaluated and the emergency itself has created physiological responses that have drawn on the body's reserve. The stomach must be completely empty whenever a general anesthetic is to be administered to prevent vomiting and aspiration of gastric contents which are irritating to the bronchial tree and can cause respiratory complications. In an emergency it may not be possible to empty the patient's stomach. The patient should be questioned regarding the time of his last meal and the foods he ate. He may have eaten a meal shortly before, and pain, trauma, or the emotional response may cause slowing or cessation of gastric emptying. On the basis of this information, the physician can decide whether or not gastric suction or lavage may be necessary.

The patient should be questioned concerning allergies to foods or drugs, drugs he is currently taking, and existing disease conditions, so that adequate plans can be made for continuing essential therapy or prescribing different therapy, and preventing complications.

Few emergency situations are so urgent that time cannot be taken to evaluate the patient's condition through routine urine and blood laboratory tests, chest x-ray examination, examination of cardiac and respiratory function, and estimation of fluid and electrolyte loss. At the same time any bleeding should be controlled, and intravenous solution, blood plasma, or whole blood can be administered to restore electrolyte balance or circulating blood volume.

The Preoperative Period

The patient's physical condition is evaluated so that dysfunctions can be corrected or controlled, and the necessary procedures are undertaken to ensure that the surgery will be carried out under the best possible conditions and recovery will be normal.

NUTRITION

The patient's nutritional state is of vital importance to normal recovery and repair of damaged tissues. Adequate nutrition means that all the protein, vitamins, calories, water, and electrolytes needed for homeostasis are provided. If the patient is adequately nourished and has not had much weight loss, surgery can be performed and for the first few postoperative days his body reserves will be utilized to supplement his limited intake. Nutritional therapy will be concerned with replacement of losses due to the trauma of surgery, the effect of the surgery, and the prevention of nutritional deficits. If the patient is malnourished, preoperative nutritional therapy will be required to replace deficits.

Protein Deficiency

Malnutrition usually is due to protein deficiency. It is a serious deficiency in the surgical patient and is the most difficult one to treat. Clinical evidence demonstrates an increase in mortality and morbidity in malnourished patients who have surgery. The unfavorable recovery and prolonged convalescence after surgery is so impressive that surgery is avoided if at all possible until the patient's protein nutrition has been improved.

A brief simplified review of the complex process of protein metabolism provides the basis for understanding the protein requirements of surgical (and medical) patients; for details, physiology and biochemistry texts should be consulted.

NATURE OF PROTEINS

Proteins are intrinsic in all body tissue and physiological processes depend upon protein metabolism. Tissue growth and repair cannot proceed without protein. Plasma proteins affect water balance, the molecules creating colloid osmotic (oncotic) pressure, which at the capillary membrane regulates drawing water from the interstitial space into the vascular space. Cellular regeneration is continuous and requires new amino acids for synthesis of protein.

The protein molecule consists of amino acids linked together, and various proteins contain various amounts and numbers of these amino acids. There are 21 known amino acids. Eight are classified as *essential amino acids*, since they must be supplied by the diet either as free amino acids or as constituents of dietary proteins because they cannot be synthesized by the body. These essential amino acids are methionine, valine, leucine, isoleucine, threonine, phenylalanine, tryptophan, and lysine. Arginine (needed for growth) and histidine (needed for hemoglobin formation) are sometimes listed as essential amino acids, since only small amounts can be synthesized by the body and when large amounts are required they must be supplied by food. The remaining amino acids can be synthesized by the body and are classified as *nonessential amino acids.*

Ingested proteins are broken down by hydrolysis in the gastrointestinal tract by specific enzymes secreted in the gastric juice (e.g., pepsin) and in the pancreatic juice (trypsin and chymotrypsin) and by enzymes of the mucosa of the small intestine to form free amino acids. The free amino acids are absorbed chiefly in the small intestine (vitamin B_6 influences intestinal transport of amino acids) and enter the circulation mainly via the portal blood. They are quickly absorbed by the cells of all tissues and organs to be utilized in synthesis of body proteins.

ROLE OF THE LIVER IN PROTEIN METABOLISM

Synthesis and degradation of protein goes on continuously in all cells, although the liver plays a major role in amino acid metabolism and has a great capacity to take up the circulating amino acids. The liver forms new amino acids and synthesizes proteins and nucleoproteins. The liver is the sole source of some of the plasma proteins (albumins, fibrogen, prothrombin) and the major source of all other plasma proteins with the exception of the gamma globulins (antibody or immune globulins), which are formed in tissues by cells of the reticuloendothelial system. The liver, like other organs and tissues, utilizes the amino acids in regeneration of liver cells. The liver stores proteins that can be broken down to amino acids for protein resynthesis elsewhere in the body.

Amino acids are not stored in the body. The excess—those not used in protein synthesis—are deaminized by the liver, and the amino group (NH_2) is split off, forming ammonia (NH_3), which is converted to urea and excreted in the urine. (The liver converts ammonia from other substances into urea.) The remaining carbon chain (keto acid) is oxidized for caloric value or converted eventually to glucose or to ketone bodies.

This important function of the liver in amino acid (protein) metabolism explains the frequent statement that protein restriction occurs at the expense of the liver and that prolonged liver dysfunction leads to protein deficiency.

CONSEQUENCES OF PROTEIN DEFICIENCY

Various body proteins differ in their composition of amino acids. Protein can be synthesized only when all the necessary component amino acids are available at the same time and in the proper proportions. When an amino acid necessary for a particular protein is not available, the protein is not synthesized and the other amino acids are deaminated like other excess amino acids. The free amino acids from tissue and plasma protein and from ingested protein form the *amino acid pool,* which provides the amino acids to form body protein products. Adequate protein intake is necessary and must supply sufficient essential amino acids daily. In the normal diet 12.5 percent of the total caloric requirement should be supplied from protein and the remainder from carbohydrate and fat to be used for energy thus sparing the protein from supplying energy, and protein foods with essential amino acids should be eaten at each meal. When there is an acute need for body protein products, catabolic processes begin and protein is released from many cells of the body to supply the amino acids.

The patient with protein deficiency has utilized his body protein and does not have a sufficient protein reserve for normal recovery from surgery. Severe protein deficiency can cause physiological derangements of serious nature for surgical patients: contracted blood volume (hypovolemia) and hypoproteinemia (abnormally low concentration of blood protein), which can cause instability of blood pressure and even shock; impaired wound healing, probably due to slowed development of fibroblasts and collagen (wound disruption is more common than in well-nourished patients); hepatic dysfunction, causing interference with production of fibrinogen and prothrombin which are necessary for blood clotting (see Chapter 11); and disturbed antibody formation resulting in reduced resistance to infection (see Chapter 11).

Protein deficiency can result from inadequate intake of food due to anorexia as seen in acute illness, long chronic debilitating illness, or old age, or to severe pain or repeated vomiting, as seen in pyloric obstruction. Inadequate protein intake can also result from inability to purchase sufficient protein foods with a limited income or poor selection of foods because of faulty knowledge of nutrition, but these causes are not as common as the others among surgical patients. Protein deficiency can be due to inability to digest protein as with a lack of pepsin in the stomach, destruction of pancreatic tissue or obstruction of pancreatic ducts limiting the quantity of pancreatic juice reaching the duodenum, or interference with absorption of amino acids in the small intestine (e.g., ulcerative colitis). Excessive loss of protein through urine or drainage from wounds (draining chronic abscess, decubitus ulcer, severe burns) and utilization of ingested or endogenous protein for energy when calories from other sources are not available can create protein deficiency. Chronic blood loss leading to anemia, as with cancer of the gastrointestinal tract, leads to protein depletion.

Several signs of protein deficiency occur before the classic edema of starvation. Loss of weight, muscle wasting, weakness, normocytic or macrocytic anemia, and sometimes hypoalbuminemia are early symptoms. If protein deficiency continues for a long time, dependent edema and eventually generalized edema occur. This is thought to be due to such a severe reduction in circulating blood proteins that colloid osmotic pressure is reduced sufficiently to allow water to collect in the tissues.

Protein deficiency is evaluated on the basis of body weight and laboratory tests for blood plasma concentration and blood volume. Weight loss may be rapid, within a few days, or slowly progressive, within a few months, depending upon the cause of protein depletion. If a person weighs 35 to 50 percent of his normal body weight, protein malnutrition is usually assumed, unless he has been on a therapeutic regimen that could explain the weight loss. The concentration of plasma proteins may be a poor guide to evaluating the protein status of cells, because changes in plasma protein do not occur until after there is considerable change in tissue protein (which may require a period of time) and often there is a compensatory decrease in circulating blood volume with protein deficiency, so the concentration of plasma proteins is normal even though the total plasma and volume are considerably reduced. When the patient has had a rapid loss of protein, plasma concentrations may be low. There is a decrease in albumin, and possibly fibrinogen, due to a decrease in amino acids available to the liver and poor liver function; the globulins are often normal, if total globulins are examined, since the gamma globulins are synthesized in tissue and transported by plasma. Both the blood count and the hematocrit (concentration of red blood cells), which are used to evaluate blood volume, may be normal with hypovolemia that develops slowly or abnormal if protein loss has been rapid.

CORRECTION OF PROTEIN DEFICIENCY

The patient with protein malnutrition is treated preoperatively by diet therapy—a slow process requiring many days or weeks. Varco estimates that 2 weeks of diet therapy is necessary when there has been a weight loss of 25 percent or more of the weight of the previous 3 to 6 months.

If the patient can ingest and utilize food, a high-protein, high-carbohydrate, high-calorie, low-fat diet is given. (Carbohydrates are a more efficient source of calories than are fats.) The foods high in essential amino acids are meat, eggs, milk, and cheese; fish, other dairy products, and cereals are also good sources of protein. Liquid feedings may be used to supplement food intake, especially milk with or without the addition of skim milk powder, which is about 38 percent protein.

Liquid feeding is the best alternative if the patient cannot take food. This consists of a formula that usually combines skim milk (less fat content than whole milk), skim milk powder, eggs (both whole and egg whites), and sugar; it may be flavored. The formula provides 5,000 calories in 3 liters of fluid to be given daily. It may be given orally or by nasogastric tube drip feeding; administration should be slow enough to avoid overfilling of the stomach and regurgitation. Liquid feedings can also be administered via a gastrostomy or jejunostomy.

When one of these methods cannot be utilized, parenteral therapy is employed but this is considerably less effective than ingestion of food products. It is difficult to provide enough calories without creating volume overload and to provide adequate protein substitutes. According to Varco, 200 to 250 g of carbohydrate is given daily in the form of 5 to 20 percent glucose solutions (fructose solutions are also used) to provide calories, thus reducing metabolism of body protein or infused nitrogenous compounds for fuel.

Intravenous fat emulsions such as Lipomul may be given to provide some of the calories. Most such emulsions are composed of soybean oil and contain 10 to 20 percent fat in various concentrations of glucose. According to Wilkinson, the fat emulsions can be given in high concentrations without drawing water from the tissues because they do not have an osmotic effect, as does glucose. These emulsions are administered in 500 ml units and are given at an initial rate of 10 drops per minute; the rate is slowly increased to 100 drops per minute by the end of the first hour. The emulsion should not be mixed with other solutions to be given by infusion. It may be given simultaneously with amino acid mixtures and carbohydrate solutions through a Y tube. The tubing of the bottle of fat emulsion is attached to one branch of the Y tube and the tubing from the other bottle of solution, to the other branch. Portions of one solution can be given while the tubing to the other bottle is clamped. Not more than two units are given daily and not more than 10 to 12 separate infusions. Toxic systemic reactions are indicated by nausea, vomiting, chills, fever, or headache; the infusion should be discontinued if any of these symptoms occur.

Nitrogen-containing compounds such as pure amino acid mixtures, protein hydrolysates, albumin, plasma, and whole blood are available for parenteral administration to control nitrogen balance.

Amino acid solutions are readily available and can be infused or can be taken orally. They have an unpleasant odor and taste that frequently causes nausea and subsequent vomiting even when given parenterally. They must be administered slowly.

Protein hydrolysate mixtures may be administered by infusion or taken orally as a diet supplement. They are commercially prepared by acid or enzymatic hydrolysis of protein, most generally milk or meat. The mixture is given as 5 percent solution with 5 percent (or less) glucose. Usually 1 to 2 liters is administered intravenously slowly at 400 ml per hour during waking hours.

Nitrogen intake may be augmented by repeated daily transfusions of plasma or whole blood, 500 to 1,000 ml, or as much as 2,500 ml in the severely malnourished patient. Transfusions restore blood volume as evaluated by hemoglobin and hematocrit values, and provide plasma proteins. When blood volume has been replenished small daily transfusions of plasma or whole blood (packed red cells for the anemic patient) may be continued along with nitrogen-enriched glucose mixtures. There is no risk of transferring infectious hepatitis with human plasma stored for 6 months at room temperature. Albumin may be infused to increase plasma protein but it is costly.

When parenteral therapy is to be continued for several days small-bore polyethylene tubing may be placed in the vein by a cutdown, thus avoiding frequent insertion and removal of a needle in the veins. When the daily infusion is completed the tubing is flushed with a few milliliters of isotonic saline containing heparin to avoid clotting in the tube, and covered with a sterile dressing. Parenteral feeding should be accomplished within 7 to 10 days if possible.

Correction of protein deficiency can be a slow (1 to 2 weeks), tiresome, and disagreeable process for the patient, who is weak, does not feel well, and is anticipating surgery. He needs understanding, support, and encouragement from the nurse and a little praise for his accomplishment of eating most of his meal or retaining the feeding given by nasogastric tube. Every means of overcoming anorexia should be considered including attractive food service, small servings, and a calm, pleasant environment. Liquid formula is given frequently in small amounts.

It can be made more palatable by the addition of flavoring of the patient's choice. The patient will retain liquid formula given orally or by nasogastric tube more readily if he is in a sitting position; that given by gastrostomy or jejunostomy is easier to administer when he is in a reclining position. Long hours of parenteral administration of fluids, day after day, are not easy to tolerate especially if continuous gastric suction is in operation—the patient may wonder if all the fluids flowing in are not also being removed, without benefit to him. Unless it is contraindicated because of the nature of his illness or his physical ability, the patient can sit in a chair without interfering with the parenteral therapy.

Exact recording of the amount and kind of the food and fluids ingested and a record of output are maintained by the nurse. Weight is checked daily at about the same time each day and on the same scales. A bed scale can be used if the patient does not have the strength to stand. The physician considers this evidence and laboratory reports and patient statements in evaluating the patient's progress, the effectiveness of the therapy, and the plan for the day of surgery.

Hypovitaminosis

Patients who are chronically malnourished may also have hypovitaminosis.

Thiamine (vitamin B_1) is essential for the oxidation of carbohydrates and in maintaining normal gastrointestinal activity. Preoperative deficiency is seen in chronic gastrointestinal and liver diseases. When the patient receives a high-carbohydrate diet or large amounts of intravenous glucose, the body's store of thiamine is utilized and becomes depleted. Vitamins of the B complex (water-soluble vitamins) are used and stored by the body as needed and the excess is excreted in the urine; therefore an excess intake does not have ill effects. With carbodydrate therapy, large amounts of thiamine, 10 to 12 mg daily, or of vitamin B complex are usually given. Oral administration of thiamine is preferred but it can be added to glucose solutions given intravenously.

Vitamin C (ascorbic acid) is essential for wound healing and collagen formation. A deficiency may result from inadequate or poor absorption in the intestinal tract and excess loss from injured tissues. Body storage of vitamin C (a water-soluble vitamin) is limited and the excess is excreted in the urine. Large amounts, 500 mg daily, may be given to saturate the body. It is given orally when possible and may be given parenterally.

Vitamin K is necessary for blood clotting and the production of prothrombin. It is synthesized by intestinal bacteria, and transported to the liver. It is a fat-soluble vitamin and any disorder that diminishes the intestinal absorption of fats or any mechanism that prevents its formation may result in a deficiency. Vitamin K is given by mouth or parenterally.

Loss of Body Fluids

Malnutrition due to excessive loss of body fluids as with repeated vomiting or persistent diarrhea may result in severe loss of electrolytes which will require appropriate replacement therapy.

Obesity

Obesity presents an added surgical risk. Fat deposits have a very limited blood supply so wound healing is slow and infections are more apt to occur. There is an increased incidence of cardiovascular and pulmonary difficulties among obese patients who undergo surgery. Weight reduction is usually recommended in preparation for major surgery.

PSYCHOLOGICAL PREPARATION OF THE PATIENT

Psychological preparation of the patient should begin as soon as he is told that an operation is necessary. Each patient will react to the situation in his own way. In general, the reaction is based on his perception of the degree of immediate threat from the surgery, i.e., the physical, psychological, social, and financial sacrifices and discomforts involved; his perception of the outcome of the surgery, i.e., the degree to which the surgery will ultimately improve his condition or disable him in some way; and on his usual behavior in response to a threat, i.e., withdrawal, denial, bravado, decisive action. Both the physician and the nurse have the responsibility of assisting the patient throughout the entire surgical experience by alleviating fears, reducing or avoiding stressful events, and providing expert care.

The surgeon will explain to the patient the reason for and purpose of the operation, the expected results, and the hazards involved; he will give the patient information about his physical condition and the details of the surgical procedure according to his judgment. The nurse may help the patient understand the situation by giving further explanations and clarifications and by explaining the activities she is performing for him.

In Janis' behavioral studies of surgical patients, data were provided by case studies of 30 hospitalized surgical patients who were interviewed and observed before and after a major operation and questionnaire responses of 150 male college students who had previously experienced major or minor surgery.

An important theoretical assumption concerning the dynamics of stress, derived from numerous studies and analyses of reaction to danger, is that "a person's capacity to assimilate a stressful event without developing residual emotional disturbances depends upon the degree to which he has mentally rehearsed the danger situation in advance and has worked out reassuring concepts which can function effectively to counteract feelings of helplessness (Janis)." If this assumption is applied to surgical patients, preoperative preparation for the frightening events of the surgical experience will allow them to work through psychological defenses in advance (Janis calls this the "work of worrying") with less severe feelings of helplessness and stress reactions.

Janis' interpretive conclusions and hypotheses, based on the above assumption, are numerous and include evidence that lack of information, incomplete or misleading information, and low anticipatory fear are related to feelings of distrust and resentment toward those from whom protective support was expected (doctors and nurses), often due to unexpected and disturbing situations, and to other symptoms of stress reaction such as irritability and sleep disturbances. A person's ability to use anticipatory fear to build defenses and the emotional reactions to the stressful events are also related to his psychological make-up.

Among the 77 questionnaire respondents who had had major surgery, in answer to a question with five possible answers, 55 percent indicated they would prefer being told before surgery "the specific details about all of the unpleasant experiences" to be encountered, 12 percent would prefer being told the specific details about some, but not all, of the unpleasant experiences, 18.5 percent preferred to be given a general idea about unpleasant experiences but not specific details, and 10.5 percent would not want to be told about unpleasant experiences (Janis). The case material also indicated that surgical patients were "hungry" for information and if this was not given by medical authorities the information was sought from other sources such as other patients and friends.

Preparatory Explanations

Preparation includes explanation of certain events that will probably occur, explanation of reasons for certain activities, and provision of explanations sought by the patient. Explanation should not be imposed upon a patient who does not desire it, as indicated directly by a verbal statement or indirectly by ignoring comments, showing lack of interest or inability to deal with the fear, or increased signs of nervousness or worry.

The purpose of preparatory communication is to prevent misconceptions and disappointments or to correct mistaken notions. This requires a skilled, understanding, knowledgeable person to whom the patient can express concerns, fears, and negative feelings and who can help the patient with the "work of worrying." When informing the patient of forthcoming events the nurse should focus on the events *he* will perceive, e.g., preparation of the skin by cleansing, and not on the events he will not perceive, e.g., how surgical drapes are placed, or situations unlikely to occur, e.g., cardiac arrest.

Descriptions of events that may arouse fear should be given gradually over a period of time so that the patient can assimilate and deal with the potential dangers without being overwhelmed.

The nurse must have a general knowledge of the disease being treated, the normal function and current dysfunction of the organs and tissues involved, the anticipated site of the incision, what is to be accomplished by the surgical procedure, and the intended results of the surgery as well as specific information about the patient's physical condition and personality in order to clarify the patient's understanding of actual and anticipated events. The patient's family members, those he considers to be significant and able to assist him, also need information about the patient's condition, the purpose of surgery, and the events of the surgical experience.

The nurse in the surgeon's office or in the surgical clinic should assume responsibility for preparing the patient for anticipated surgery and the hospital experience. Any information she has about the patient's habits, his reaction to stressful situations, and the apparent significance of family members to him should be communicated to the appropriate hospital nurse. She can help by explaining what personal belongings he will need, the hour and specific place of admission, and admission procedures. She may also be responsible for providing instructions regarding prehospitalization preparations (such as diet).

Admission to Hospital

The patient should be admitted to the hospital 1 to 2 days before the scheduled surgery if possible. This applies particularly to aged patients who have not been hospitalized previously. This allows sufficient time for him to become oriented to the strange environment and the hospital personnel and for the personnel to provide unhurried physical and psychological preparation for surgery. Since today it is not always possible or practical to admit a patient more than 12 to 24 hours before surgery, the nurse must make the most of even short contact with the patient.

Information about the patient's habits will permit the hospital team to incorporate it into the patient's care program. The nurse should observe and talk with the patient in order to determine the nature and degree of his stress reaction and assist him in dealing with his anxiety. Common causes of stress in the surgical patient are fear of death, outcome of diagnosis, pain, helplessness, change in body image, finances, and the unknown. The nurse should alert other appropriate professional persons to the patient's concerns as necessary.

The subject of body image is dealt with elsewhere and will not be discussed here, except to say that the nurse should be sensitive to the many implications involved. (See Chapter 4.)

Explanations of preoperative procedures, physical examination, blood drawn for laboratory tests, chest x-ray studies, skin preparation, and enemas are given soon after admission so that the patient will not be surprised as each member of the team arrives and performs various procedures.

Before an anesthetic is given, the patient should be told what will happen. Participation of the anesthesiologist, surgeon, and the nurse in the explanation will contribute to the patient's feeling that he is being given full consideration.

Explanation of postoperative events is given preoperatively because the patient is usually alert, without pain, eager to minimize risks involved, and consequently a motivated learner. An understanding of postsurgical activities will make it easier for him to overcome discomfort and unwillingness to participate during the postoperative period of drowsiness, pain, and fear. Demonstrations and practice periods are helpful.

Usually the patient is transferred to the recovery room after surgery; in some hospitals, to an intensive care unit for several hours before being returned to his room. The patient and family should be told of this practice and given the location of these rooms. A tour of these units and introduction to the personnel who will care for him may be helpful for some patients but fear-producing to others.

Explanations should be given about the procedures routinely performed in the recovery room, such as blood pressure readings and oxygen administration.

Deep breathing, coughing, and turning from side to side are initiated when the patient is in the recovery room, as soon as he is conscious; yet he is drowsy, does not feel well, possibly is in pain, and is afraid to move and therefore is uninterested in performing these activities. Every person knows how to breathe and cough but most do not know how to effectively perform deep breathing and coughing as is required postoperatively. Instruction and practice are given preoperatively. For example: "Breathe deeply and expel the air slowly. Breathe deeply and expel the air slowly again. Take a deep breath and force the air out through your mouth. then take a quick breath and cough from deep in the lungs. While you are doing this, I will stand beside you and put my hands over your incision. That will put a little pressure on the incision and reduce the pain." If possible, have the patient in a sitting position; the erect position allows more room for lung expansion because the abdominal viscera are not pushed against the diaphragm. This position is usually not possible in the immediate postoperative period, so practice in the recumbent position should be tried after the patient has experienced deep coughing. Breathing deeply before coughing stimulates the cough reflex and increases the activity of the tracheal cilia. The patient will be required to do this frequently postoperatively and effective removal of mucus from the lungs is dependent on successful and frequent deep breathing and coughing.

Active body movement and turning is begun even before the patient is conscious to improve circulation and prevent venous stasis; turning also contributes to improved respiratory function. Instruction is given preoperatively when the patient is alert, strong, and free of pain. The exercises include alternate extension and flexion of knee and hip joints, similar to the movements while riding a bicycle (while lying on the side); rotation, flexion, and extension of the feet; and flexion and extension of elbow and shoulder.

PHYSICAL CONDITION OF THE PATIENT

The patient's physical condition is evaluated by the physician with a complete history and physical examination and selected laboratory tests in order to estimate the patient's physiological and psychological capacities for the surgical procedure and recovery and to identify any physiological alterations that must be corrected before surgery or taken into account during the operation and recovery period. The patient may have a disease condition other than the one for which the surgery is performed and which may require treatment or will alter the postoperative therapy. The anesthesiologist also needs this information in order to select the appropriate anesthesia.

The patient must be evaluated and prepared for the anesthetic. One who is considered a poor risk can tolerate a well-administered anesthetic if he has been properly prepared. After the evaluation has been completed, he will be placed in a class or grade according to the amount of risk involved in administering an anesthetic.

Temperature, pulse and respirations, blood pressure, and weight are obtained to provide baseline values and identify any abnormalities. An elevated temperature may indicate an infection, which would increase the risk of surgery. This and any other signs of infection, such as an upper respiratory infection, should be reported to the surgeon.

The routine laboratory tests are urinalysis for specific gravity, albumin, sugar, acetone, and microscopic sediment, and blood tests for red cell differential count, hemoglobin, hematocrit, prothrombin time, and white cell count. A chest roentgenogram is done routinely. These examinations identify any alterations in physiological function.

MEDICATIONS

Any drugs and medications which the patient has been taking should be noted. The patient should be questioned in a systematic manner to help him recall this information. Many surgical patients will be regulated by drugs that must be continued, e.g., insulin, tolbutamide, cortisone, digitalis, thyroid.

Cortisone has been in general use since 1948. It is presently available in so many forms that the patient may not be aware or remember that a medication he is taking contains cortisone. He should be thoroughly questioned about the possibility of cortisone therapy. In cortisone therapy the secretion of ACTH decreases and the adrenal cortex atrophies and does not secrete cortisol (hydrocortisone) in any significant amount. This atrophy is reversible with gradual reduction of cortisone therapy, but abrupt cessation of therapy causes adrenal insufficiency. Continued cortisone therapy is essential for the surgical patient who had been taking it previously, since the atrophied adrenal cortex is not able to respond to the stress of surgery by secreting cortisone. The first 20 hours after surgery is the period of greatest risk of adrenal insufficiency. Symptoms include severe weakness and lethargy, hypotension, dehydration, often an increased temperature, and ultimately coma and vascular collapse. Anorexia, nausea, vomiting, and abdominal pain may occur, but surgical patients frequently have these symptoms postoperatively from other causes. Adrenal insufficiency requires immediate therapy.

Ordinarily, routine medications are withhheld on the day of surgery and all orders are automatically canceled until postoperative orders are written. A review of medications appearing on the patient's chart should indicate whether orders should be obtained for continuing a particular drug.

PREPARATION OF THE SKIN

The skin is thoroughly cleansed in order to minimize the possibility of wound infection from surface bacteria, especially staphylococcal infection. Usually this is accomplished by repeated lathering of the patient's entire body with a soap solution combined with the detergent hexachlorophene (e.g., Septisol), plus shaving of the area and application of an antiseptic in the operating room.

The action of the surface-acting germicide hexachlorophene requires time; two or three applications of the cleansing solution, with a bath or shower when possible, are required. The patient may be given the solution and instructions to cleanse the skin at home once or twice at specific intervals before coming to the hospital, and further cleansing is done the night before surgery or the entire cleansing process may be done at specified intervals after admission. The area to be cleansed should be lathered well with the solution by gentle rubbing, not scrubbing or scratching which would traumatize or irritate the skin, and the lather washed away preferably by shower. Some surgeons prefer to have the entire body cleansed, including scalp, face, axillae, groin, and genital areas, to reduce the bacteria on all surfaces.

Shaving of the skin of the area of incision and a wide surrounding area is usually done to remove all hair, which is an excellent source of bacteria and difficult to cleanse. The shaving is done in two directions in order to pick up the tiny hairs that may flatten to the skin when shaving is done in one direction. Great care should be taken to avoid scratches or abrasions, which can be a source of infection. The hospital procedure book provides instruction for the area to be shaved for each type of operation. The shaving is usually done the afternoon or evening before the operation and, in large hospitals, by a trained technician. It may be followed by soapsuds cleansing of the skin.

The final preparation of the skin is performed in the operating room, and may include another cleansing with soap-hexachlorophene solution before the application of the skin antiseptic. An adhering plastic sheet on the skin of the operative field is commonly used. It is pressed onto the skin surface and is cut as the incision is made, the edges of the sheet adhering to the wound edges. The moist packs applied to wound edges during surgery to prevent the soft tissues from drying do not accumulate bacteria from the skin surrounding the wound covered by the plastic sheet.

OPERATIVE PERMIT

The patient must sign a permit authorizing the physician to perform the operation. The permit protects the patient against unauthorized surgery and the physician and the hospital against claims the patient may make. The physician should explain to the patient the type and extent of the surgery.

The patient has a right to reject, as well as accept, treatment. To make this decision, the patient should be told by the physician the expected results and hazards of the particular surgical procedure. The patient should have a clear understanding of the procedure before signing the permit. If the nurse becomes aware that the patient does not fully comprehend the nature, extent, and risk, she should bring this to the attention of the physician immediately so that the patient can be given appropriate explanation before signing the consent form.

The patient should be asked to sign the permit before being sedated. A witness is needed to the signing of a legal consent in order to testify that the signature is that of the patient, that the patient was aware of his action, and that he signed willingly. Although the nurse at times serves as a witness, it is better policy to utilize another person such as a family member, friend, or the ward clerk to avoid any possible question of bias resulting from her position as a member of the health team and as a hospital employee.

All surgical procedures that involve entering a body cavity require a surgical permit. This includes such procedures as paracentesis and cystoscopy. The physician must perform the operation contemplated and any modification of it must be related to the planned operation without additional risk to the patient. If an extension of the surgery is indicated, it must be in the area of the original incision.

A minor who is married, lives away from home, is self-supporting, and is considered mature may sign a surgical permit in some but not all states. However, if the parents are available it is wise to have them sign. If parents refuse to sign the permit for a child, a court can rule child neglect and order a guardian to take control and custody. A mentally incompetent person cannot give legal consent to surgery. Consent of the nearest relative must be obtained. Both husband and wife are usually required to sign a consent for surgery that will affect the marriage relationship, or produce sterility, except in emergency situations; this may be customary or a legal requirement in some states.

In an emergency situation, a physician can operate without written permission after all efforts have been made to contact the family. The fact that an emergency does exist constitutes consent. Telegrams, telephone conversations, or letters are an acceptable method of securing permission.

IMMEDIATE PREOPERATIVE CARE

Food is usually withheld after the evening meal if surgery is scheduled for the next morning. Fluids are usually withheld after midnight. The purpose is to avoid gastric contents that could be vomited and aspirated during induction of anesthesia, during surgery, or during postoperative return to consciousness. The glottis is relaxed by general anesthesia and the trachea is open, providing opportunity for aspiration of vomitus. Gastric contents entering the respiratory tract are irritating to the mucosa and can plug the alveoli.

Enemas may be given the evening before abdominal surgery. This prevents fecal impaction after surgery, since gastrointestinal motility is considerably reduced during the stress response period following surgery. A full bowel is in greater danger of being punctured during surgery than an empty one. The anesthesia relaxes the sphincters and if the bowel is not empty fecal contents may contaminate the operating table when sphincter control is lost.

The morning of the day of surgery the patient should be given sufficient time to bathe, brush his teeth, comb his hair, and change into a clean gown. The anesthesiologist may prefer that dentures and partial plates be removed because they may fall out of place when the patient is anesthetized and block the airway, or may be broken during intubation. The dentures should be placed in an appropriate container marked with the patient's name, and stored in a safe location. Some anesthesiologists prefer to have the patient's dentures remain in place simply because the patient is embarrassed about his edentulous appearance and because dentures provide some mouth support. The nurse will need to know the anesthesiologist's preference.

Nail polish should be removed from at least one finger on each hand so that the nail beds can be observed for color changes that indicate oxygenation of blood. Lipstick should also be removed for this reason.

Temperature, pulse, and respiration are taken and recorded as discussed earlier. Anxiety may cause an elevation in blood pressure by sympathetic stimulation that constricts the arteries, causing increased peripheral resistance and venous tone, increased blood flow to the heart, and increased cardiac force. A state of relaxation should be achieved, if possible, before the blood pressure is measured. The blood pressure should be taken before the preanesthetic medication is given because it may fall after a large dose of a narcotic has been given.

All jewelry and religious medals should be removed or taped to the patient. If removed, they should be marked with the patient's name and locked in a safe place. The wedding ring can be left on but must be taped to the finger. The patient should be advised that most valuables should not be left in the hospital and that the family take home any large amount of money that is brought to the hospital. The patient will have no need for it and it might be misplaced.

The patient is asked to void just before going to surgery, so that his bladder will be empty. In some instances, depending upon the particular surgical procedure, a retention catheter may be inserted just prior to surgery, or inserted when the patient is brought to the operating room. This will keep the bladder empty and out of the way; an empty bladder is less likely to be punctured during surgery.

The patient may express fears during these final preparations and the nurse should give him the needed time and attention.

Preanesthesia medications usually are given to the patient before he is taken to the operating room. They reduce anxiety during the immediate preoperative period, diminish secretions, reduce autonomic reflex activity, and produce amnesia. Most combine a narcotic (morphine or meperidine), a sedative or phenothiazine (barbiturate, promazine, promethazine hydrochloride), and an agent to lessen secretions (atropine or scopolamine). The drugs should be given at the time and by the route ordered by the physician so that they are effective at the time intended. Drugs may be ordered to be given at a specific time or may be ordered to be given "on call" from the operating room. If there is a change in the operating schedule the patient unit nurse should be informed of any changes in the time for administration of the medications. Generally the medications are given intramuscularly because they quickly reach an area rich in blood supply and their action begins about 20 minutes after injection; if administered subcutaneously absorption is slow and action begins 45 minutes to 1 hour after injection. Some medications can be mixed in the syringe to avoid having to administer two injections. The mixture of drugs must be observed carefully for any signs of precipitation; if precipitation has occurred the mixture must not be given. Not more than 2.5 ml should be given in one intramuscular injection since more than this can cause a reduced rate of absorption and tissue injury. Oral administration is unreliable because the patient's stomach emptying time may be affected by his anxiety and it is desirable to keep the stomach empty.

Anesthesia

The purposes of anesthesia are to block nerve impulses, suppress reflexes, and achieve muscular relaxation, and possibly achieve unconsciousness (general anesthesia). The choice of anesthetic depends on its safety for the patient (physical condition), convenience for the surgeon (area to be incised), and comfort of the patient (length of surgery). Patients generally prefer a rapid, short induction, although some patients have a fear of losing consciousness and want a slow induction.

Usually they want a nonirritating drug that is odorless and provides for a recovery period relatively free from discomfort. The physician is more concerned about muscular relaxation and the amount of bleeding, which are influenced by the drug used. The anesthesiologist is concerned about the safety of the drug, its excretion time, the pathological change it creates, the rate of diffusion, and its side effects.

GENERAL ANESTHESIA

A general anesthetic can be administered intravenously, rectally, or by inhalation. Drugs given intravenously are thiopental sodium (Pentothal Sodium), procaine hydrochloride, alcohol, ether, paraldehyde, and curare. Agents used in rectal administration include ether, barbiturates, paraldehyde, trichlorethanol, and tribromethanol. Inhalation preparations include nitrous oxide, ethylene, ether, cyclopropane, helium, and halothane.

The anesthetic agent is carried by the bloodstream to the brain, where it acts on the neuron membrane to inhibit impulse conduction across the synapses. The physiological changes produced by the anesthetic are described in *stages. Stage I* denotes the change in consciousness. This stage lasts until loss of consciousness. During this stage, the patient is aware of his surroundings and can hear what is being said, so care should be taken as to what is said and done in his presence. Sensory functions become dulled and paralyzed, but reflexes are not impaired. The skin will appear pink or flushed. The pupils react to light and are normal in size. Because of the excitement of induction, the blood pressure may rise slightly. Respirations may be irregular, since the agent is irritating and rapid-acting.

Stage II is the state of delirium or excitement. This stage may be absent in intravenous induction. Consciousness is lost but muscular relaxation is not present. Skeletal muscle tone increases during this period and involuntary motor activity may take place. The skin color varies according to the agent used. Respirations are irregular and exaggerated. At the end of this stage, respirations become regular and deep. Stage II extends to the period of automatic respiration.

Stage III is the state of surgical anesthesia and is divided into four substages called planes. Respirations are entirely automatic because the voluntary pathways are paralyzed. It is during this stage that intubation is done to maintain an airway. A balloon on an endotracheal tube prevents secretions or vomitus from entering the trachea. The intercostal muscles are the first to be paralyzed by the anesthetic agent, followed by the diaphragm. Respiratory obstruction can be due to loss of muscle tone or the irritation of the drug. The reflexes of the respiratory tract are diminished in anatomical order as the anesthesia deepens. The cough reflex and the gag reflex disappear as stage III is reached. Tracheal and bronchial reflexes disappear during stage III. Sensory reflexes are affected in the order of cutaneous, corneal, peritoneal, pharyngeal, and laryngeal. The peripheral nervous system is not affected by a systemic anesthetic. Voluntary movements are absent. Muscle tone progressively diminishes and in plane 4 there is complete relaxation of large muscles. Stage III ends with cessation of spontaneous respiration because of the level of toxins in the central nervous system.

Stage IV is the stage of medullary paralysis and includes respiratory arrest and vasomotor collapse. Artificial respiration must be given to prevent death by asphyxiation.

The recovery period varies according to the type of anesthetic agent used and not on the length of anesthesia. The reflexes return in opposite order to their disappearance, those reflexes affected in stage IV of the induction period being the first to recover. This has implications for nursing care, e.g., in stage I the patient may appear to be unconscious but is able to hear and can hear the nurse's voice.

LOCAL ANESTHESIA

Local anesthetics are used to prevent conduction of nerve impulses. These agents influence the permeability of the cell membrane, preventing sodium ions from moving into the cell and potassium ions from moving outward. Normally the change of ions creates the electrical current necessary for impulse transmission. The effect of the drug lasts until it is eliminated from the body. Two groups of drugs generally are used: alcohols and nitrogenous substances such as procaine and cocaine. The concentration of the drug necessary to prevent impulse transmission is much higher than the amounts used in a general anesthetic, therefore the area in which the drug is used must be limited. The drug is carried by the bloodstream and if the circulating quantity becomes too large, death can ensue. Local anesthesia is referred to as *conduction* or *regional anesthesia*. This classification is further categorized according to the areas of drug administration. In *spinal anesthesia,* for example, the drug is injected into the subarachnoid space, thereby inhibiting impulse conduction in the autonomic, sensory, and motor systems. The effect on the autonomic system may cause a drop in blood pressure. If the drug is injected into the dural sac, the procedure is called *saddle block.* A particular nerve may be blocked after it passes from the vertebral column, and the procedure is named for the nerve involved. If groups of nerves as they branch from the main trunk are blocked the procedure is a *field block.*

Injection of the drug into tissue at the site of surgery is called *infiltration,* or a *local.* If the drug is applied to the mucous membrane it is a *topical anesthetic.* The nerves beneath the area injected are anesthetized.

The duration of a local anesthetic depends on the drug used and the length of time it is in contact with nervous tissue. Vasoconstrictors are often given with the local anesthetic because they prolong and intensify the drug action by decreasing the rate of absorption and permit less drug to be used. This reduces the possibility of a systemic reaction because less of the agent is carried by the bloodstream. The most frequently used vasoconstrictor is epinephrine.

HYPOTHERMIA

Hypothermia may be employed in conjunction with general anesthesia during surgery to decrease the metabolism which in turn reduces the requirement for oxygen. Hypothermia would have a bearing on the amount of anesthetic needed and the rapidity of elimination.

The Postoperative Period

PHYSIOLOGICAL CHANGES IN THE PATIENT

The trauma of surgery elicits neuroendocrine responses as described in Chapter 11. These responses are protective adaptations for survival but also modify the patient's tolerance to administration of fluids and solutes and create the potential for electrolyte imbalance.

With the inception of surgery the anterior pituitary rapidly secretes increased amounts of adrenocorticotropic hormone (ACTH), which is responsible for the secretion of cortisol (hydrocortisone) and partly responsible for the production of aldosterone by the adrenal cortex. The pituitary response is probably initiated by the peripheral nerves transmitting impulses of injury to the central nervous system, and the afferents may also transmit pressure stimuli from blood vessels. The increased cortisol causes changes in organic metabolism resulting in catabolism of tissue protein with increased nitrogen excretion, which can be measured in the urine as urea, an inability to utilize exogenous amino acids for synthesis of body proteins, changes in carbohydrate balance with elevated blood sugar and decreased glucose tolerance, depression of lymphocytes and eosinophils in the blood, and regression of lymphoid tissues.

In the immediate postoperative period, aldosterone can be measured in the urine of surgical patients and returns to basal levels in 2 to 3 days. This hormone plays a part in mineral metabolism, causing sodium and chloride retention, which in turn causes some water retention thus preserving the circulating volume, and potassium excretion, which clears the circulation of potentially toxic concentrations of potassium that can be liberated by destruction of cells.

Surgery is accompanied by the release of large amounts of antidiuretic hormone (ADH) from the posterior pituitary. Elevated blood levels of ADH appear postoperatively and may persist for as long as 3 to 4 days. The blood levels seem to relate to the consequences of the procedure such as the amount of blood loss and the amount of dissection and manipulation which stimulates the visceral afferent autonomic nerves. Release of ADH can be a response to stimuli transmitted from the sensory nerves and results in reduced output of urine, even to the degree of oliguria without shock, during the early postoperative period.

The metabolic changes associated with surgery have been divided into several phases of convalescence by Francis Moore. The first or *injury* phase is characterized by the secretion of adrenal steroids, vasopressin, and vasoactive amines which results in protein catabolism; loss of potassium; and conservation of extracellular fluid, as described above. The patient does not desire to move, usually he has pain, he has no appetite, there is reduced gastrointestinal peristalsis; though thirsty he has an intolerance for water for about 48 hours or more, usually vomiting if water is ingested. The pulse and temperature are slightly elevated probably related to the inflammatory response. This state lasts for 2 to 4 days after major surgery and about 7 days with severe injury. In the second or *turning point* phase there is a return to normal endocrine activity with diuresis of water and sodium and reduced urinary excretion of nitrogen; peristalsis returns to normal, usually with accumulation of flatus; and the pulse and temperature return to normal. The patient's appetite returns and he becomes interested in his surroundings and in other people. The third or *anabolic* phase lasts for 3 to 10 or 12 weeks. The patient has an increasing appetite and eats well and, with the anabolism of protein, muscle substance and strength are restored and slight weight gain begins. He increases his activities and exercise as his strength returns. The end of this phase is indicated by reduction in anabolism with a near normal nitrogen balance (zero) and redeposition of fat. The fourth or *fat gain* phase lasts a few weeks to many months and is dependent on a caloric intake in excess of caloric expenditure. There is resumption of storage of body fat with definite weight gain, then a return to normal weight, and the patient resumes his usual activities and exercise.

WOUND HEALING

The closure of wounds involves two processes. First, is the initial (provisional) closure accomplished by the formation of blood clots sealing the wound, followed by final (definitive) closure accomplished by regeneration of tissue and fibrous substitution.

A clean sharp incised wound destroys a small amount of tissue, severing fibers of collagen and elastica and the blood vessels, which contract and retract into the tissue thus contributing to homeostasis. The larger blood vessels are clamped and tied to stop the bleeding; the smaller capillaries stop bleeding as clots begin to form. In clotting, fibrin strands attach to the damaged blood vessels forming a matrix that entraps the red blood cells, white blood cells, and platelets to form a clot and provides a framework for the fibroblasts. (See Chapter 11.)

The critical period for wound healing is the first 8 to 9 days, during which collagen fibers, blood and lymphatic vessels (granulation tissue), and epithelium are regenerating. Most wound disruptions occur within this time period, because of delayed wound healing, which can be caused by several mechanisms.

Wound healing is classified into three types. In *primary union* (intention) a clean incised wound has been anatomically closed by sutures (or a small, clean superficial wound closed by adhesive bandage) without a gap between the wound margins. The expected result is a hairline scar. In *secondary union* there is a gap between the wound edges which fills in from the bottom and sides with granulation tissue. The scar is not hairline but is much smaller than the original defect, as in traumatic wounds with extensive loss of tissue or with wound infection. In *tertiary healing* an open, granulating wound is repaired by approximation of the edges to assist healing.

Several local factors influence wound healing. A wound requires local arterial and venous blood supply to provide nutrients necessary for manufacturing and maintaining tissue cells and to remove the waste products of inflammation (bacteria, local toxins, dead cells). Local elevated venous pressure interferes with blood flow and may decrease oxygen exchange between the blood and cells and alter the fluid and electrolyte exchange thereby increasing local edema. Adequate venous drainage must be maintained and pressure on and around the wound area should be avoided; injured extremities can be elevated to enhance venous return by use of gravity. In the early stages of wound healing, excessive movement and strain can disrupt clot and tissue formation, so the wounded part is temporarily immobilized and abdominal or thoracic incisions are splinted with light pressure upon them when the patient coughs. Local wound infection will interfere with tissue regeneration by direct action of bacterial toxins and indirectly by systemic response. Precautions preoperatively and postoperatively are taken to avoid infection, e.g., preoperative cleansing of the patient's skin, aseptic technique during surgery and during postoperative care of the wound.

In the absence of food intake during the first few postoperative days body protein, mainly skeletal muscle, is catabolized, providing the amino acids to synthesize the proteins for wound repair. Surgery can be performed upon a patient with depletion of vitamin C because this can be administered parenterally during and following surgery. Postoperative dietary intake of protein is begun as early as possible to provide the essential amino acids necessary for the synthesis of new tissue proteins.

Local wound infection has systemic effects that can delay wound healing. In general, surgery is not performed on patients with active superficial or deep-seated infection because of the possibility of interference with wound healing and the possibility of bacteria from the original infection moving to the wound.

TRANSFUSION

Whole blood is most often given to increase blood volume following hemorrhage, trauma, or burns in order to prevent shock. For surgical patients, whole blood transfusion is administered postoperatively and sometimes during surgery, to replace the estimated blood loss during surgery. The surgeon considers the plasma and blood loss that occurs in the imflammatory response when tissues are injured, i.e., changes in capillary membrane permeability in injured tissue allow plasma proteins, especially albumin, to move from blood to damaged tissue, thus reducing intravascular colloid osmotic pressure and increasing tissue osmotic pressure, which promotes movement of plasma fluid into interstitial spaces. (See Chapter 11.)

Whole blood may be used to treat certain types of anemia, to supply clotting factors, platelets and leukocytes, and as a nutrient to supply plasma proteins and restore colloid osmotic pressure as in hypoproteinemia.

The term *transfusion* generally refers to the administration of whole blood or blood components directly into the bloodstream. The introduction is usually made through the intravenous route although other routes including subcutaneous, intramuscular, intraperitoneal, and intraosseous can be used. At present four methods of transfusion are employed: (1) indirect transfusion in which donor blood stored in a flask is given to the recipient; (2) direct transfusion in which the blood is administered by direct connection (via tubing and needles) between the artery of the donor and the vein of the recipient; (3) exchange transfusion in which the blood of the recipient is replaced by donor blood; (4) reciprocal (or immune) transfusion in which specific immune antibodies in blood of convalescent donor are given to susceptible contacts of an infectious disease (measles, mumps, yellow fever) to provide passive immunity. Indirect transfusion is used most commonly and will be the only method described in this chapter.

Indirect Transfusion

Donor blood to be used in indirect transfusion is withdrawn from the donor vein into a flask and mixed with a mixture of citrate salts (sodium, potassium, and ammonium citrate) to remove the calcium ions from the blood and prevent coagulation. When the blood is received by the recipient the citrate is destroyed by the liver and the blood becomes capable of coagulating. Blood plasma and packed red cells can be prepared from whole blood by a separation process.

Before a blood transfusion is given typing and cross-matching of donor blood and the blood of the recipient are required to assure that the two bloods are compatible. Every individual has antibodies (agglutinins) in his plasma which can cause agglutination (clumping together) and hemolysis (rupture) of injected red cells that contain agglutinogens (antigens) different than those in his own cells. Blood is classified on the basis of the agglutinogens present in the red blood cells which normally cause an immune reaction, called the *ABO blood system,* as follows:

BLOOD TYPE	AGGLUTINOGENS (ANTIGENS)	AGGLUTININS (ANTIBODIES)
O	—	α, β
A	A	β
B	B	α
AB	A,B	None

Type O is considered the universal donor blood because it does not possess agglutinogens and anti-O antibodies rarely develop; therefore, type O cells cannot be agglutinated with any of the agglutinins. Group AB is considered the universal recipient blood because the plasma contains no agglutinins and will not agglutinate any type of donor blood.

As an extra precaution before a blood transfusion is administered, the recipient blood and the donor blood of the same blood type or type O blood are cross-matched for compatibility. Cross-matching is a laboratory test in which cells from the donor blood are mixed with plasma from recipient blood, and vice versa, and if the cells do not agglutinate the two bloods match each other.

Another blood protein that must be considered is the *Rh factor,* which is believed present in about 85 percent of individuals. Blood containing the factor is classified as Rh-positive; blood lacking the factor, as Rh-negative. Isoagglutinins do not develop until an individual with Rh-negative blood receives a transfusion of Rh-positive blood. After Rh-positive blood has been given to a person with Rh-negative blood, the recipient forms Rh antibodies. When a second injection of Rh-positive blood is given, the Rh antibodies cause agglutination and a transfusion reaction.

Hazards are present each time blood is transfused, particularly in patients who have had repeated transfusions because a sensitivity or antibodies may have developed. Despite precautions taken to avoid administration of incompatible blood, errors do occur. Blood from the donor and the recipient is handled repeatedly by personnel of many departments, and errors in collecting samples, use of improperly sterilized equipment, improper transportation of blood samples, errors in laboratory tests, improper storage of blood, and improper administration may occur. In an emergency haste increases the chance of error, cross-matching may not be ordered to save time or because type O blood will be used, or cross-matching tests may be done hurriedly. If several patients in a ward unit are receiving blood, precautions in administration may be carried out hurriedly or ignored.

The nurse has two vital responsibilities: checking the donor blood before administration to see that it is the blood intended for the patient, and observing the patient during the infusion.

When the unit of blood is received from the laboratory department and just before it is administered, two persons (two nurses or a doctor and a nurse) should read and check the cross-match report against the information supplied on the bottle. The type of blood, number on the bottle, and patient's hospital number should agree. Refrigerated blood should be warmed to near room temperature by letting it stand in the room or placing it in a special warmer according to instructions. Blood that has been brought to room temperature, rechilled, and warmed again should not be used, since changes may occur in this blood and when it is administered the risk of a febrile reaction is increased.

The patient's arm should be supported and attached to an arm board to prevent movement that might dislodge the needle from the vein. The first 50 ml of blood is given slowly and with constant observation for a reaction during the first 15 minutes. If large amounts of blood have been lost, the blood can be administered rapidly by drip method, in fact, even pumped into the vein by hand pumping equipment, provided a nurse or doctor is constantly present.

REACTIONS TO TRANSFUSION

Febrile (pyrogenic) reactions are the most common ones. They are usually mild, and may occur during or shortly after the transfusion. These reactions may be caused by small thrombi in the infused blood, insufficient sterilizing of solutions that may contain bacterial pyrogens, improperly cleaned tubing or needles, dead or viable bacteria that have accidentally entered the blood, lysed red cells even though compatible (blood stored improperly or longer than 3 weeks at 4° C), improperly prepared anticoagulant in the blood or reaction to it, or leukoagglutinins of the recipient which may develop after repeated transfusions. The patient has an increased temperature, 100 to 104° F, which may persist for several hours. This may be preceded by a chill and accompanied by headache, nausea and vomiting, weakness, and lumbar pain. The patient is treated symptomatically.

Allergic (urticarial) reactions are reactions to specific allergens in the donor blood. The reaction may be mild with symptoms of itching, skin rash, and uticaria; or it may progress to edema of the face and lips, then to edema of the uvula and laryngeal area, producing respiratory obstruction with symptoms of dyspnea and cyanosis. The transfusion should be stopped immediately and the physician notified. Diphenhydramine hydrochloride (Benadryl), tripelennamine (Pyribenzamine), or epinephrine hydrochloride 1:1,000 may be ordered to alleviate the symptoms and oxygen may be given for dyspnea and cyanosis.

A hemolytic reaction from mismatched blood is a serious event. Wintrobe reports the mortality rate from such reactions as approximately 50 percent; fatal reactions have occurred only when more than 300 ml of blood has been infused. Administration of as little as 10 ml of incompatible blood can cause a hemolytic reaction.

Restlessness, anxiety, sensation of tightness in the chest, and tingling sensations in the back and thighs are warning symptoms. Chills, severe pain in the back, and signs of shock (rapid pulse and decreasing blood pressure) follow. The symptoms vary depending on the amount of blood destroyed. The patient may have profound shock with renal failure.

According to Guyton, the greatest damage is from the free hemoglobin in the plasma which eventually causes plugging of the renal tubules. The first effect is agglutination of red blood cells; the clumps of cells flow through the vessels, plugging the smaller ones. Antibodies of the cell membranes cause disintegration of the red cells which unplugs the vessels and releases large quantities of hemoglobin into the plasma. The hemoglobin molecule is small and can pass through capillary pores, which it does in the glomerular capillaries and enters the kidney tubules. The hemoglobin in the tubules becomes increasingly concentrated as the tubules reabsorb water and electrolytes; finally it precipitates and plugs the tubules, stopping nephron function. The severity of renal failure depends on the number of tubules which have become plugged. In about 2 weeks, if death does not occur, there is automatic disintegration of the hemoglobin plugs and the tubules become functional.

The blood transfusion should be discontinued immediately when symptoms occur, and the physician notified. Whenever a transfusion reaction of any kind occurs the remaining donor blood in the bottle and the tubing should be saved for laboratory examination. Guyton suggests immediate treatment to reduce the development of hemoglobin plugs: administer large quantities of fluids to create water diuresis; administer alkaline substances to create alkaline tubular fluid, which can hold more hemoglobin in solution than acid fluid; administer diuretics to increase the flow of tubular fluid. In severe renal failure treatment with an artificial kidney may be necessary.

BLOOD AND SUBSTITUTES

Transfusions can be given of whole blood or its components. Whole blood is given as a replacement for erythrocytes and plasma. It is considered the best treatment for loss of blood volume due to hemorrhage.

Packed red blood cells are erythrocytes separated from whole blood. This preparation must be typed and cross-matched according to blood type and Rh factor. It is used to replace erythrocytes and raise the hemoglobin, as in the treatment of anemias, or when transfusion of whole blood might cause a circulatory overload.

Platelets can be given by direct transfusion to improve clotting, e.g., in thrombocytopenic purpura.

Blood substitutes can be used in emergencies. Blood plasma is the substitute most frequently employed for restoring blood volume. The protein content of plasma creates colloid osmotic pressure (oncotic pressure) at the capillary membrane thus retaining plasma fluid. It is available in liquid, frozen, and dried forms. Dried plasma has the advantage that it does not necessitate typing or cross-matching and it can be stored and transported easily. Serum is human plasma with the fibrinogen removed. It is used as plasma, but has a lower protein content. Serum albumin is physiologically similar to plasma but the protein content is 96 percent albumin. It is expensive to prepare so is not widely used unless serum protein must be replenished as a means of reducing edema in renal or liver disease.

Plasma Expanders. Plasma expanders are macromolecular solutions having colloidal and osmotic properties similar to plasma. The substances in these solutions are not metabolized by the body so do not replace red blood cells, plasma, or serum proteins. They do restore circulatory volume. Dextran (Expandex, Gentran, Plavolex) is the only substance available for general use in the United States. It is a biosynthetic polysaccharide composed of glucose molecules of varying molecular weights (molecular size).

All preparations of dextran contain molecules of many sizes but each has a different proportion of the molecules and all are identified by the average molecular weight. Dextran 75 (regular dextran) has an average molecular weight of 75,000 with molecules ranging in weight from 25,000 to 200,000. Low molecular weight dextran has an average molecular weight of 45,000 with molecules ranging in weight from 10,000 to 100,000. The large molecular weight molecules are retained in the bloodstream, creating colloid osmotic pressure, whereas the smaller molecules pass through the capillary membrane and are excreted chiefly in the urine; some is excreted through the lungs and feces.

Dextran is given intravenously as a 6 percent or 10 percent solution in isotonic sodium chloride in amounts of 500 to 1,000 ml at a rate of 20 to 40 ml per minute; thus 600 ml is given in 15 to 30 minutes.

Regular dextran has the advantage of remaining in the blood for a relatively long time; 10 to 40 percent is excreted in the urine within 24 hours; 50 to 70 percent is excreted in 3 to 4 days; and the remainder is metabolized. The effect on the blood volume of a single injection of 500 to 1,000 ml continues for about 12 hours. The disadvantages are that more than 1,500 ml may prolong bleeding time, mainly because of overloading the circulation, and the large molecules cause some aggregation of the red blood corpuscles and may subsequently interfere with blood typing and cross-matching. There may be some advantage in the use of low molecular weight dextran because its rapid excretion in the urine increases diuresis and it causes some reduction of aggregation of red cells (after injury red cells tend to aggregate and accumulate in the capillaries) thus freeing red cells in the capillary circulation. The disadvantages are an increased bleeding tendency and shorter duration of increased blood volume because it is rapidly lost in the urine; up to 60 percent may be excreted within 12 hours.

Dextran is a temporary substitute for blood and should not be used repeatedly. It has certain advantages over plasma in that it does not cause allergic reactions, does not require citrate anticoagulant, is quickly available when reconstituted, can be stored for several years, can be prepared commercially, and is relatively cheap.

FLUID AND ELECTROLYTE REPLACEMENT

In restoring body fluids following surgery the first objective is to replace the blood volume lost during surgery, which is accomplished by giving transfusions. The second objective is to restore and maintain fluid and electrolyte balance.

Since food and fluid were withheld beginning 12 hours before surgery and will be withheld for 24 to 48 hours after surgery, the effects of starvation plus the physiological response to injury are taken into account. When food is not ingested the small carbohydrate reserve of the body is utilized for calories followed by oxidation of body protein and fat to produce energy, amino acids, and endogenous water. The physiological response to surgery has been discussed previously.

Parenteral therapy is calculated by considering the patient's baseline requirements of water, calories, electrolytes, vitamins, abnormal losses, and deficits or excesses of these elements.

Calculating Baseline Replacement

WATER

In calculating baseline water replacement, water loss and endogenous water supply are considered. (See Chapter 18.) Insensible loss from skin and lungs ranges from 600 to 1,000 ml when a person is in a comfortable environment and afebrile, but the loss can be much greater with increased metabolic requirements as in fever, response to injury, or a warm environment. It is desirable for a sick person to have a urine output of 1,000 to 1,500 ml daily, since usually his renal function is not optimal and there is an increase in waste products to be excreted by the kidney. To provide for insensible loss and urinary output the normal adult, in bed or on limited activity and deprived of food, will need 1,600 to 2,500 ml of water per day.

Endogenous water (sodium-free and potassium-rich) from the oxidation of body protein and fat will supply some of this water. It is estimated that the patient in bed receiving 400 to 500 calories provided by glucose administration will produce about 150 to 200 ml endogenous water. Conditions that increase metabolism, e.g., fever, trauma, infection, cause an increase in endogenous water production and as much as 1,000 ml can be produced when there is extensive trauma or infection. By subtracting the estimated endogenous water from the total water needed per day and considering the body weight, age, and sex of the patient, the baseline water requirement to be given parenterally will be seen to range from 1,000 to 2,500 ml per day.

On the day of surgery insensible loss is approximately 1,500 to 2,000 ml, urine output will be 500 to 700 ml, and approximately 350 ml of endogenous water is produced. Parenteral replacement of water would be 1,650 to 2,350 ml, the amount varying depending on body size, age, sex, state of preoperative nourishment, extent and type of surgery, amount of bleeding, and amount of blood replacement. Thus, the amount of water given parenterally may be 1,000 to 2,000 ml on the day of surgery.

CALORIES

The baseline requirement of calories is supplied by glucose. If the body does not have carbohydrate for energy production, protein is hydrolyzed to provide energy and to provide the carbon residues to metabolize fat for additional energy. Carbohydrate is given to spare body protein and promote metabolism of fat. One hundred grams of glucose daily will reduce tissue catabolism and prevent starvation acidosis. This can be supplied parenterally by 2 liters of 5 percent glucose or 1 liter of 10 percent glucose in distilled water, the choice depending on the amount of water to be replaced.

It is common practice to provide fluid and calorie requirements parenterally with 2 liters of 5 percent glucose in distilled water on the day of surgery and the first postoperative day. These fluids are given slowly (about 2 ml per minute) to prevent fluid overload and spilling of glucose and to provide a steady source of calories. Often the total amount is given in two infusions spaced about 12 hours apart.

Administration of glucose and protein intravenously during the injury phase after surgery will not prevent protein catabolism and negative nitrogen balance.

SODIUM

Baseline sodium requirements are provided by a *maximum* of 76 mEq of sodium, as provided in 500 ml of 0.9 percent sodium chloride solution. In the injury phase following surgery there is retention of sodium and water and it is not necessary to give sodium parenterally at this time under normal circumstances.

POTASSIUM

Baseline requirement of potassium is 40 mEq, which can be provided by 3 g of potassium chloride dissolved in 1,000 ml of isotonic fluid. In the injury phase the loss of potassium cannot be halted and administration of potassium with oliguria is dangerous; therefore, it is not administered until after renal function has been established and usually only when there is external loss of body fluid as with gastric aspiration.

VITAMINS

Vitamin C and vitamin B complex are both required for wound healing. The well-nourished patient probably has enough of these vitamins stored in the body to meet requirements during the period of injury. Vitamin C is less readily stored in the body; it can be given easily parenterally, it is inexpensive, and the amount the body does not need is immediately excreted. When there is doubt, 100 to 200 mg per day may be added to the infusion solution.

Mechanism of Fluid Loss

Abnormal loss of body fluids is also considered in calculating parenteral therapy.

Deficits may require replacement, and excesses may occur, due to physiological mechanisms or extensive therapy, which require treatment.

Loss of fluid may be through external loss of gastrointestinal secretions, loss of blood as in hemorrhage, loss of interstitial fluid and plasma from extensive wounds, or extensive sweating and internal loss via temporary functional shift of body fluids into areas of traumatized or infected tissue.

Loss of gastrointestinal secretions is a common cause of imbalance of body fluids. Usually the fluid lost is a mixture of secretions from more than one region of the alimentary tract. Loss of secretions from any level of the gastrointestinal tract is loss of water and sodium. All alimentary fluids also contain potassium in amounts as high as or higher than that of plasma. As extracellular fluid and sodium are depleted, intracellular water and potassium move into the extracellular fluid; thus, loss of secretions over a period of time will create serious potassium depletion. Loss of chloride and hydrogen ions or loss of bicarbonate disrupts acid-base equilibrium. (See also Chapter 18.)

Replacement of abnormal losses includes volume-for-volume replacement of water. The source of the secretions must be known for replacement of electrolytes to attain and maintain electrolyte balance and acid-base equilibrium. Serum levels of sodium, potassium, chloride, and bicarbonate (carbon dioxide combining power) indicate alterations of extracellular fluid and indirectly intracellular alterations. Volume loss is measured, and secretions may be saved for laboratory analysis of sodium, potassium, and chloride so that more precise replacement can be instituted.

Normal gastric juice has more chloride than plasma, very little sodium, and relatively high potassium. In repeated excessive vomiting or continuous gastric suction there is loss of chloride and hydrogen ions which is followed by a compensatory rise in the bicarbonate concentration in the extracellular fluid leading to metabolic alkalosis.

Fluid, chloride, potassium, and sodium must be replaced. This may be accomplished by intravenous administration of isotonic saline solution or 5 percent glucose in saline or by adding sodium chloride to glucose solution. Potassium chloride is added to the fluids as soon as renal function has been established after surgery.

Bile, pancreatic juice, and fluid in the small intestines are high in sodium and bicarbonate. These fluids may be lost by small bowel suction, persistent diarrhea, or discharge from fistulas with consequent loss of sodium and bicarbonate which leads to metabolic acidosis. With depletion of sodium in the extracellular fluid, potassium moves out from the intracellular fluid and ultimately there is potassium loss. Fluid, sodium, and bicarbonate must be replaced, usually with sodium solutions with metabolizable anions such as sodium lactate or sodium bicarbonate. If potassium loss is high, it can be replaced by administration of potassium citrate.

During hemorrhage there is a depletion of interstitial fluid, more than can be accounted for by the blood loss alone. In this circumstance blood transfusions are administered to replace blood volume and constituents, and a sodium-containing solution, e.g., lactated Ringer's solution, isotonic saline solution, or 5 percent glucose in saline, given to replace the extracellular fluid and electrolyte deficit.

With surgical dissection and tissue trauma there is an accumulation of interstitial fluid and plasma with the normal extracellular fluid (exudate) in the area of the damaged tissue. The amount of fluid sequestered in the tissues (edema) depends on the type of tissue and the extent of the injury and can be considerable with extensive tissue damage. This process will reach a peak in 36 to 48 hours. This fluid is not available to maintain circulation and hydration and, for the purpose of planning parenteral therapy, is considered as fluid loss in need of replacement. Since extracellular water and electrolytes must be replaced, lactated Ringer's solution or isotonic saline solution is administered, or sodium chloride may be added to glucose solution. In some situations plasma may be given. Replacement is given during the first 24 to 48 hours after surgery. The amount administered depends on the surgical procedure and the patient's size, and is given in addition to the baseline requirements and replacement for external losses.

Postoperative parenteral therapy may include small amounts of sodium containing solutions to compensate for abnormal external loss and for internal loss.

One of the common alterations of fluid and electrolyte balance in surgical patients is an exaggerated water and sodium retention in the extracellular fluid in the traumatized tissue, with a decreased concentration of sodium in the plasma (hyponatremia), termed *dilutional hyponatremia*. This is often accompanied by a decrease in normal intracellular water and potassium with a resulting excess of potassium in the blood (hyperkalemia). This is treated with restriction of water intake. The excess water will be excreted when diuresis begins. Since there has been a loss of intracellular potassium, potassium is given after diuresis begins.

Water loading (also termed *water intoxication* and *hypotonicity*) is due to excessive water intake in a patient unable to excrete water during antidiuresis, usually because of excessive parenteral therapy with glucose and water. Usually it occurs on the first or second postoperative day. There is an abrupt weight gain and fall in urine volume. Drowsiness and weakness are the early symptoms, followed by paralysis, twitchings, convulsions, and coma caused by edema of the brain. Peripheral and pulmonary edema may occur. There is a low concentration of plasma sodium and increase of sodium in the urine, indicating an inappropriate release of sodium from the excess extracellular fluid. The treatment is to stop the intake of water; this is followed by a period of time without fluid intake, or very small volumes of hypertonic glucose solution may be administered slowly. In the absence of pulmonary edema or increased venous pressure, a small volume of hypertonic salt, 300 ml of 3 percent sodium chloride, may be administered to promote renal excretion of water. With increased urine output and insensible loss of water, the patient's status will gradually return to normal.

Measurement of the State of Hydration

Measurement of fluid intake and output and body weight for estimating the volume of body fluids is a nursing responsibility. Urine output is measured, as is loss by vomiting, gastrointestinal suction, and drainage from tubes; sweating is estimated. Postoperatively the urine output should be 25 to 50 ml per hour. The amount is recorded at the time of output and totaled at the end of each 8-hour period. The type and amount of parenteral fluid intake are recorded when a bottle of solution has been administered or at specified time intervals; fluid by mouth including ice chips is recorded when given; and amount of solutions used in irrigating tubes, if not subtracted from the output from the tube, is recorded. The intake is totaled at the end of each 8-hour period.

Change in body weight is the best measure of the state of hydration. Insensible loss and endogenous water are highly variable and unpredictable. The amount of sequestered extracellular fluid varies according to the extent of tissue trauma and is increased in infection; patients with chronic illness before surgery such as cancer, liver disease, or cardiac decompensation may have an expanded extracellular fluid volume before surgery and are likely to have it after surgery. The nurse should observe the patient closely for signs of edema.

The surgical patient may be weighed daily, on the same scales, at the same time of day, and with the same amount of clothing each time. Bed scales can be used if he cannot get out of bed or stand unsupported.

After surgery there is an initial weight gain because of the increased extracellular fluid in the damaged tissue and the necessary replacement therapy. One liter of water gain (or loss) is equal to 1 kg of weight gain (or loss) which equals 2.2 pounds of weight gain (or loss). Patients on parenteral fluids are expected to lose 150 to 300 g per day from oxidation of cellular tissue; the amount varies depending on the patient's initial weight, the extent of injury, and the presence of fever. On the third or fourth postoperative day diuresis begins and the sequestered extracellular fluid is lost in addition to the expected daily weight loss; the weight loss may be as much as 500 g per day. Rapid weight loss greater than this is usually due to excess loss of water and sodium; it may be a favorable sign or one indicating a need requiring for immediate replacement. Continued weight gain or a stable weight for several days postoperatively usually is due to overhydration or an increase in sequestered extracellular fluid because of infection or tissue necrosis.

Early in the anabolic phase, weight loss may continue due to diuresis and early tissue synthesis. With steady tissue anabolism a weight gain of 100 to 300 g per day is expected.

NURSING CARE DURING RECOVERY FROM ANESTHESIA

The purpose of all postoperative care is to establish and maintain the patient's physiological and psychological equilibrium. Consideration must be given to the physiology of the involved tissue or organ and the alterations induced by surgery; the effects of anesthesia; the risks consequent to the surgery; and the patient's perception of his illness and surgical therapy.

The most critical postoperative period is during recovery from anesthesia. During this time special attention is given to the patient's respiratory function, circulatory status, and cardiac function. The stress of surgery is borne by the cardiovascular system, and shock is always a hazard. Blood transfusion and intravenous fluids are administered to replace circulating volume and avoid shock; nonetheless constant observations for signs and symptoms are required. The other important immediate hazard is anoxemia (inadequate oxygen in the blood) due to deficient lung function or inadequate oxygen supply, and several measures are instituted to prevent it.

Most hospitals now have a recovery room adjacent to or near the operating room for specialized care during recovery from anesthesia. Supervision of patient care is usually provided by the anesthesiologist, who accompanies the patient to the recovery room. The room contains equipment generally used during recovery, e.g., oxygen therapy equipment, transfusion apparatus, suction machines, intravenous solutions, and drugs, as well as equipment for emergency use, e.g., tracheostomy trays, resuscitative equipment, and a monitoring device for use with the electrocardiograph. The patient remains in this room until his blood pressure is stabilized, respiratory function is adequate, and he is fully conscious. Depending on the hospital facilities and practices, the patient may remain in the recovery room until ambulatory, he may be transferred to a specially equipped intensive care unit until ambulatory, or he may be returned to his hospital room.

The nurse who receives the patient from the operating room needs to know what surgical procedure was performed, what problems arose that might have a bearing on postoperative care, what fluids and drugs were given, whether or not tubing or drains were inserted and whether they must be attached to drainage apparatus, and what anesthetic agent was used. She needs to be informed of the patient's present condition, the vital signs, the state of consciousness, any complications that might develop, and particular symptoms to watch for. She should be provided with written immediate postoperative orders.

Care must be taken in moving an anesthetized patient from the operating room table to the recovery room bed or cart. Muscles that normally contract with movement are without tone, so there is a possibliity of nerve injury resulting in paralysis. Removal of the patient from the operating table is done slowly, since extreme changes in position, e.g., from the lithotomy position to the horizontal position, may give rise to circulatory collapse.

The patient is placed in the supine or side-lying position depending on the type of surgery, the surgeon's preference, and the needs of postoperative care; the side-lying position is preferred. General anesthesia relaxes the muscles of the pharynx, and when the patient is supine the tongue may fall backward partially closing the air passage. With the patient in the side-lying position, in which his head is turned to the side and no pillow is used, the tongue falls toward the lower cheek, providing a better airway and allowing secretions to drain from the mouth. The patient's hip and knee of one leg are flexed, the other leg is barely flexed to provide stability, and the back is supported by a pillow.

The patient is dressed in a clean gown and covered with lightweight blankets, which are tucked under the mattress at the sides and bottom while he is being transported from the operating room to the recovery room. If a stretcher is used, straps are placed around the patient above the knees and across the chest for safety in transportation. Side rails are raised to prevent him from falling from the bed or cart and they are to remain raised while he is in the recovery room.

The nurse in the recovery room should provide close observation and should never leave the patient alone.

If the patient is unconscious on arrival in the recovery room, the foot of the bed may be elevated slightly to promote evacuation of the tracheobronchial secretions, to reduce venous stagnation in the lower extremities, and to promote stabilization of the blood pressure. The bed remains flat unless the physician has ordered otherwise.

The patient who has had a spinal anesthetic or nerve block is conscious, can maintain an airway, and may be able to change his position; nonetheless it is recommended that he be in a supine position with head and heart at the same level. With a spinal anesthetic he will for a while have no feeling in his lower extremities and will be unable to move them. Spinal anesthesia tends to produce arterial hypotension and headache. With spinal anesthesia the sympathetic afferent fibers to a region of the body have been blocked, therefore constrictor impulses to the veins of the region are blocked. This results in decreased venous tone, pooling of blood, and diminished venous return to the heart which contribute to a decrease in systolic pressure. The decreased venous return may be prevented (or treated) by wrapping the legs in elastic bandages, before the spinal anesthetic is administered, to prevent pooling of blood in the legs, and by elevating the legs after surgery. The so-called spinal headache is thought to be caused by the decreased cerebrospinal fluid pressure.

Airway Maintenance

Maintaining a clear airway is of primary importance; this includes prevention of regurgitation and aspiration of saliva or gastrointestinal contents into the tracheobronchial tree which can cause atelectasis. An artificial hard rubber or plastic airway may be in place in the mouth when the patient arrives in the recovery room. It is a short curved tube that fits between the lips and passes over the base of the tongue into the pharynx, creating an airway from the lips to the pharynx. This tube should be kept in position until the patient begins to push it out as reflexes return.

Respirations are evaluated immediately as to depth and rate. The amount of effort exerted by the patient may indicate the patency of the airway. The nurse may place her hand over the patient's nose and mouth to feel the expired air, but air exchange can be more closely evaluated by placing the ear close to the patient's mouth and listening. Poor volume may be due to an obstruction or insufficient effort. An absence of chest movement would suggest a depression of the respiratory center or paralysis of the chest muscles. An exaggeration in chest movement would indicate an obstruction that is interfering with air passage. Choking and noisy or irregular respirations are also signs of airway obstruction. Obstructions can be due to foreign materials (blood, sputum, or vomitus), soft tissues (tongue, palate, pharynx), or a disorder of the respiratory tract (asthma or emphysema). Nasopharyngeal suction, in which the catheter is passed through the nose into the upper portion of the trachea, is employed to remove excess mucus secretions and stimulate coughing. If the patient is in a supine position his head should be turned to the side to allow secretions to drain from the side of the mouth; his head should be turned sharply and quickly to the side when he vomits. The jaw is pushed forward to prevent the tongue from falling back. This is done by placing the fingers behind the mandibular joint on each side of the jaw and pushing forward on the angle of the jaw, as if to push the lower teeth in front of the upper teeth. This may be done even though the artificial airway is in place. It may be necessary to pull the tongue forward if it has fallen backward by grasping it between pieces of gauze with the fingers.

Respiratory difficulties should be discovered before the late sign of cyanosis.

Oxygen may be administered for cyanosis, but a decrease in cyanosis with oxygen therapy is not an adequate measurement of respiratory function, since the cause of the hypoventilation is not being removed.

In summary, rate and depth of respiration, amount of chest movement, noisy respirations, and cyanosis are to be observed for indications of obstruction and insufficient lung expansion. Increased pulse and restlessness may also point to lack of oxygen.

Cardiovascular Function

Arterial blood pressure and pulse readings are taken and recorded on the patient's arrival in the recovery room and as frequently as every 15 minutes during the first 2 hours for evaluation of cardiovascular function and observation of signs of shock. These measurements should be compared to the preoperative and operative blood pressure and pulse for evaluation of the patient's condition and his return to a normal state. The rate, rhythm, and quality of the pulse should be noted. Not only the blood pressure measurement but also the change from previous measurements should be noted. A systolic pressure of below 90 or persistently fluctuating blood pressure with wide variations should be reported to the physician, unless other instructions have been given to the nurse.

Shock is always a possible complication, usually due to a decreased circulating blood volume. The signs are pallor, rapid and thready pulse, lowered blood pressure, diaphoresis, cold and clammy skin, and oliguria. The decreased blood volume leads to a decreased venous return and a reduction in cardiac output. The blood pressure falls as a result and the peripheral vessels constrict. This causes reduced oxygenation of tissues. Tissue hypoxia stimulates other mechanisms that result in vasodilatation and increase in capillary permeability. This leads to increased blood flow and movement of fluid to interstitial spaces; the blood volume is further reduced. (See Chapter 11.)

Eiseman and Carnes recommend elevation of the patient's legs about 20 degrees with flexion at the hips to promote venous return and while this can be accomplished by elevating the bottom of a gatch bed or by using pillows, elevation of the head and thorax about 5 degrees to promote lowering of the diaphragm can be accomplished by placing a small hard pillow under the head. The patient may be placed in the Trendelenburg position, but this position is not recommended for long periods of time because the diaphragm is elevated by the abdominal viscera, reducing the space for lung expansion and affecting the ventilation capacity. A patient in either of these positions must be observed closely for an obstructed airway and placed in a lateral position to promote removal of secretions. Extremes of position should be avoided. A blanket may be removed to cool the patient, since body heat increases the need for oxygen by increasing the metabolism and excess sweating increases the loss of body fluids. Whole blood is given to replace blood volume; in some circumstances plasma or intravenous fluids may be administered. Oxygen may be administered for maximum oxygenation of the blood. Pain may be alleviated by an analgesic; large doses should not be given since they may decrease respirations.

Hypotension in the absence of other signs may be due to the anesthetic agent.

Elevation of the blood pressure may occur with pain, distended bladder, or restless activity. All these should be evaluated and corrected as necessary.

Nursing Measures after Patient's Status Is Stabilized

After initial observations and assurance that the blood pressure and pulse are satisfactory and the patient has an adequate airway, stat orders, usually for oxygen therapy or drugs, are carried out. Drains or tubes are connected to appropriate drainage bottles, e.g., the catheter is attached to a collecting bottle. Dressings are inspected for drainage in order to provide a basis for comparison with later observations. The nurse may, depending upon the location of the surgery, feel the bedclothes under the patient for bleeding or drainage that may be seeping out under him rather than out the dressing. The intravenous infusion is checked to see if the flow is continuous and at the correct rate. Urine output is noted if a catheter has been inserted; the output should be 25 to 50 ml per hour. If the patient has had lengthy abdominal surgery requiring a great deal of visceral manipulation or if a large quantity of blood has been lost, the urine output may be low in the early postoperative period. An intake and output record is started. The color, warmth, and moistness of the patient's skin are observed and recorded. The patient's temperature is taken as ordered.

All these observations and measurements for evaluating the patient's physiological function during recovery are made repeatedly, and symptoms indicating a steady deterioration or a seemingly slight symptom that recurs repeatedly should be reported to the physician.

The patient recovering from general anesthesia is restless and should be protected from injuring himself but not restrained. Movement of the arm that has been splinted to allow for intravenous infusions will not dislodge the needle; however, the patient may try to pull the needle out. He may roll or turn close to the edge of the bed or try to get out of bed, so the side rails should be raised at all times.

As he returns to consciousness he may begin to talk. The nurse may test his level of consciousness by asking short simple questions; appropriate answers signify comprehension. The patient may make statements (or be asked) about how he feels. These comments should not be ignored by the nurse but should be evaluated along with other observations so that judgments can be made about the care to be given. The patient may be told that his surgery has been completed and that he is now in the recovery room.

PAIN

The patient begins to experience pain as soon as he regains consciousness. The pain may be caused by stimuli from the site of trauma or the operative field. The peripheral stimulus excites the sensory pain nerve endings, which activate the afferent fibers, and when the stimulus reaches the brain, perception of pain follows. Reactions to pain are highly individual. (See Chapter 15.) The skin and subcutaneous structures are rich in end-receptors for pain and pain may arise because skin sutures become increasingly tighter with swelling and inflammation. A tight dressing can interfere with circulation and cause pain. Dissection of muscles during surgery causes more pain than direct cutting of a muscle layer. If heavy

retractors had been used, the patient might experience greater pain. Urinary retention will produce intra-abdominal pain.

Postoperative pain should be relieved by administration of narcotics. Usually
morphine or meperidine (Demerol) is ordered to be given p.r.n. When a choice
of dosage and/or time interval is given in the order for administration, the nurse
must use her judgment as to time and amount. The drug should not be given until
the patient is conscious and his respiratory function is adequate. Pain should be
relieved as quickly as possible, for pain begets pain—the longer the pain is felt
the more severe it becomes, hence greater amounts of drug are required to control
it. Since the patient is drowsy and not alert, a small dose may bring relief if
given soon after pain begins. The drug is administered by hypodermic injection
but may be given intravenously by the physician if quick relief is needed. Children,
geriatric patients, and patients with preexisting respiratory dysfunction or postoperative respiratory difficulties are usually given less than the average dose of
narcotics, because large doses may produce peripheral vasodilation and decreased
respirations. The nurse should carefully observe the effect of the drug upon pain,
restlessness, and respirations.

DEEP BREATHING, COUGHING, AND TURNING

As soon as the patient is conscious, deep breathing, coughing, and turning are
begun to promote pulmonary ventilation, prevent atelectasis caused by obstruction of the bronchial tree by a mucus plug, and prevent postoperative (hypostatic)
pneumonia. Turning of the patient may be started before he is conscious.

Normally, mucus forms an unbroken, moist, sticky surface on the lumen of the
bronchi, bronchioles, and alveolar ducts; ciliary action moves the mucus upward.
This action is impeded by the supine position, slow shallow respirations, and inability to cough. In the supine position puddles of mucus collect on the lower side
of the lumen, while the upper side is dry. The puddles block the bronchioles, so
both areas are susceptible to bacterial infection. (See Chapter 20 for a discussion
of lung function during bed rest.) Atropine given preoperatively to reduce secretions tends to increase mucus viscosity thereby reducing ciliary action. Anesthesia
causes loss of the cough reflex and may directly depress ciliary action, hence
mucus secretions are retained in the bronchial tree. Inhaled anesthetic agents and
intubation may irritate the mucous lining, causing increased secretions. Narcotics
depress the cough reflex and ciliary activity and large amounts reduce respiratory
ventilation. The patient may have shallow breathing because of pain in the operative site with deep respirations.

The patient is requested to take six to 10 deep breaths every 5 to 10 minutes
and to take deep breaths and cough about every 15 minutes. Deep breathing increases the diameter of the airways during inspiration and expiration thus aiding
the upward movement of the mucus, opening small atelectatic areas, and preventing further atelectasis. Coughing causes redistribution of the pooled mucus, keeping the bronchioles moist, and forces the secretions upward. Changing the patient's position every 15 minutes changes the position of the lungs thus aiding in
the redistribution of the mucus. The patient is drowsy, uncomfortable, and concerned about experiencing pain, and probably uninterested and unwilling to per-

form these activities. The nurse must be persistently encouraging in helping him and reducing pain at the incision site by gently holding him during coughing and turning. If the patient has been instructed in these activities before surgery he will perform them more easily in the postoperative period. After repeating these exercises he may expectorate a tenacious mass of mucus. If the mucus is not removed satisfactorily by these methods, intermittent positive pressure breathing or carbon dioxide inhalations may be ordered by the physician. In this early phase the patient will do nothing of his own will; he is dependent upon the nurse to tell him to turn, cough, deep breathe, and so forth.

EXERCISE AND COMFORT MEASURES

As soon as the patient is conscious, exercise of the legs, feet, and arms, through rhythmic up-and-down movements, may be started and repeated every 15 to 30 minutes. The nurse may give passive exercise initially to assist him until he is able to do them himself. The exercises diminish peripheral stasis by aiding venous return and improve cardiac function; this exertion produces deep breathing. Changing the patient's position by turning from side to side also contributes to venous return.

When the patient has completely recovered from the anesthesia and when pulse, respirations, and blood pressure are within normal limits, the blankets applied in the operating room may be removed, and cool sheets placed which usually provide comfort.

EMOTIONAL SUPPORT

Most surgical patients need emotional support during the recovery period. The nurse should answer the patient's questions with reassuring comments—this is not the time for discussion of details. Giving precise attention to the details of his care; telling him of his actual signs of progress; and providing comfort measures such as face washing, a cool washcloth placed on the forehead, comfortable positioning, and relief of pain will help him through this uncomfortable period. The psychological study of Winkelstein demonstrated that affective reactions of patients are reduced during the first hours of awakening from general anesthesia and they are not concerned with the others about them who are sick. Normal emotions and anxiety become apparent after the first 24 hours. However, patients who have had spinal anesthesia or light general anesthesia are awake and alert and are concerned about the condition of the other patients and the procedures observed. The patient should be protected from frightening sights and sounds as much as possible. He may not remember anything that the physician has mentioned about the surgery or the fact that his family has been with him. The nurse may need to offer these explanations a second or third time.

LATER POSTOPERATIVE NURSING CARE

After the patient is fully conscious and the blood pressure is stable, he is transferred to his room or to an intensive care unit by order of the physician. The room should be equipped to meet his needs. The top bedcovers should be fan-folded to one side to facilitate transfer from the cart. An emesis basin should be within easy reach, but not where the patient must look at it; the sight of the emesis basin can suggest nausea and vomiting. Side rails should be raised.

During the first 24 to 48 hours the same observations and care activities as described previously are continued but not as frequently, e.g., measurement of vital signs, regulation of intravenous fluids, relief of pain, deep breathing, coughing and turning, exercises, examination of wound dressing, measurement of intake and output.

Vomiting

Vomiting may follow surgery, but in the absence of complications it should not continue for more than a few hours. Vomiting serves the purpose of emptying the gastrointestinal tract. It may result from the anesthetic agent, irritation to the alimentary tract, or abdominal distention usually secondary to manipulation of the abdominal organs. For the patient who has had abdominal or chest surgery, the nurse should support the wound during retching. The emesis basin is emptied immediately after the patient vomits and he is given mouth care. The bed should be kept clean. The amount of vomitus is recorded as output and the characteristics are described in the nursing notes. If vomiting does not cease in a few hours it should be reported, since it may be an indication of complications.

Micturition

The first urine output may not occur until about 12 hours after surgery; the total 24-hour output is expected to be 500 to 700 ml during the first 24 to 48 hours (the injury phase). The length of time the patient will be allowed to go without voiding depends on the type of surgery performed and the amount of bladder distention; it may be 8, 10, 12, or 16 hours. Overdistention of the bladder should be avoided. Palpation of the abdominal wall over the bladder, the patient's feeling of bladder fullness, and noting the time and amount of previous urine output, if any, will help in determining if the bladder is distended. Every effort is made to avoid catheterization and help the patient exercise control over micturition. Pain should be alleviated, privacy provided, and, if possible, the patient should be placed in the normal position for voiding. The male patient may be allowed to sit up at the edge of the bed or to stand beside the bed. The female patient may be allowed to sit at the edge of the bed with the feet supported on a chair or to use a commode at the bedside. In both situations someone should be in attendance to support the patient and prevent falling or fainting. A warmed bedpan, the sound of running water, or warm packs to the suprapubic area may suggest voiding and help relax the bladder sphincter. Catheterization may be necessary if all other measures fail. Occasionally a patient will void small amounts frequently. If this is the case, the bladder should be observed for distention to be sure that the patient does not have retention with overflow. If the bladder is distended, he will have to be catheterized to relieve the distention, even though he is voiding small amounts of urine. As a rule, the physician will have left an order for this, but if he has not he will have to be called.

About the third or fourth postoperative day diuresis will begin; the urine output is expected to be 1,000 to 1,500 ml or more accompanied by a definite weight loss.

Thirst

Early in the postoperative period the patient is likely to be thirsty. This is because of dryness of the mouth and pharynx resulting from reduction of mucus secretions following the administration of atropine, thick mucus lacking in moisture, dehydration before fluid replacement is completed, lack of fluid intake to moisten the mouth, and mouth breathing. During the first 24 to 48 hours the patient often has an intolerance for water, and water intake causes nausea and vomiting. Cleansing the patient's mouth with mouthwash while being sure that none is swallowed may relieve the dryness. If his thirst is troublesome, the nurse may ask the physician for an order for ice chips, which are given a few at a time and at intervals so that a minimum amount of fluid enters the gastrointestinal tract. When nausea and vomiting have ceased the physician may permit sips of water or hot tea with lemon juice at lengthy intervals or chewing gum or hard candy that may be sucked.

Bed Rest

Browse gives the following reasons for prescribing bed rest for surgical patients: (1) Pain relief: the less movement a patient performs, the less pain he experiences. (2) Support: weakness follows surgery. (3) Wound immobilization. This is rarely required for wound healing but is necessary for healing of fractures and certain types of eye surgery. (4) Overcoming the local effect of gravity.

The patient's position should be changed at least every 2 hours while he is on bed rest. This provides a form of exercise which contributes to increased venous return, aids respiratory ventilation, and relieves pressure on body parts, preventing skin irritation and breakdown. Bed rest gives rise to a number of alterations of function which complicate the patient's physiological state. (See Chapter 20.) The patient begins ambulation as early as possible.

Ambulation

Almost all surgical patients, except those who have an infection, begin ambulation within 24 to 48 hours after operation; some will begin as early as the evening of the operative day. There are several advantages of early ambulation: pain from the operative site disappears more quickly or at least becomes less severe; abdominal distention and voiding difficulties occur less frequently; respiratory exchange is increased; both general and peripheral circulation and gastrointestinal function are improved. The patient's morale is better, once he overcomes the fear of the first attempts, for this is a sign of progress. The hospitalization period is shortened and home convalescence is hastened, thus reducing the cost to the patient.

The patient may have a fear of being out of bed and walking a few steps so quickly after operation. The nurse can support him by reassuring him that ambulation is desirable, that he will be assisted and whatever support is needed will be given, that the sutures will not break, and that ambulation will not hinder healing of the wound. The first step is to have the patient sit at the edge of the bed with his feet on a chair (dangling) for a few minutes. His pulse is taken before and after he sits up to determine how well he tolerates the change in position. A more rapid pulse is expected because of increased cardiac output with exercise and increased return blood flow. The patient may feel faint, and if this happens he should be returned to a horizontal position in the bed immediately and after a short rest period make another attempt to gradually sit up. Fainting is probably due to a reflex dilatation of the arterial tree causing a fall in blood pressure and diminished blood flow to the brain, a temporary reaction to postural change. When the patient can sit up, the next step is to have him stand, with the nurse providing physical support, and then take a few steps away from and back to the bed and return to bed for a rest. The purpose of this activity is to exercise—to walk—not to move to a resting position in a chair. Sitting in a chair has no advantage; venous stasis can occur while the patient is seated in a chair as well as when he is in bed. Each time he is up he should walk a little farther.

The presence of drainage tubes should not limit ambulation. Some tubes can be clamped off and disconnected from the collecting bottle, or the collecting bottle can be carried by the person assisting the patient. If an intravenous infusion is being administered the bottle of fluid can be hung on a portable intravenous standard and pushed along the floor as the patient walks.

The patient is inclined to assume a posture that will protect the incision. For example, a patient with an abdominal incision tends to bend forward slightly and one who has had a thoracotomy drops one shoulder. He should be encouraged to stand straight while walking. An abdominal binder will provide support in cases of abdominal operation, and exercises to strengthen the weakened area may be ordered by the physician.

Diet

Food and fluids may be withheld from 24 to 48 hours until peristalsis has been reestablished as identified by normal bowel sounds, and after the removal of the gastrointestinal tube, if one is present, though there may be a trial period of administering 30 ml of water every hour before the tube is removed. Oral intake is prescribed by the physician; the diet, the amount, and the time it is to be given depend on the type of surgery and the response of the patient.

The first diet may be clear liquid (water, hot tea, clear broth) or full liquid (milk, creamed soups, gelatin, custard) and may include dry toast. The patient then progresses to a soft diet and then to a regular diet. At first he may be hesitant about eating "so soon" after an operation, so eating should be encouraged but not forced. His appetite will return by the third to the fifth day postoperatively and at about the fifth day the regular diet is usually ordered. As soon as food and fluids can be taken orally intravenous infusions can be discontinued. Eating helps to prevent or relieve "gas pains," since gastrointestinal contents stimulate peristalsis. The diet should be adequate in calories to provide energy for reducing tissue catabolism and in protein to supply amino acids for restoring muscle substance and aiding wound healing.

Defecation

Defecation will not begin until gastrointestinal motility is restored and oral intake produces some waste products, though there may be some accumulation of secretions and gaseous material in the intestinal tract during the period of intravenous feeding. Defecation would not be expected until the third or fourth postoperative day; if it does not take place normally the physician may order a small enema. Thereafter the patient should defecate every other day and return to his customary pattern as normal food and fluid intake and activity increase.

Gastrointestinal Distention

Postoperative distention may develop in either of two forms: acute gastric dilatation or inhibitory or mechanical paralysis of the large or small bowel.

Acute gastric dilatation may develop a few days after any type of operation. Fluid continues to accumulate in the stomach. The patient does not vomit large amounts but repeatedly regurgitates small amounts of dark-colored fluid. Suddenly he is dyspneic, slightly cyanotic, and has a rapid and thready pulse and cold clammy skin. When the upper abdomen is percussed tympanic sounds are heard. These symptoms, often mistaken for hemorrhage, should alert the nurse to notify the physician immediately. When the physician inserts a gastric tube there is a gush of air, and a large volume of fluid with coffee-ground material is removed. Suction is used to decompress the stomach, which may contain several liters of fluid. Intravenous fluids to replace water, sodium, and chloride are administered and a blood transfusion may be given. Continuous gastric suction is often employed to prevent this complication following a major operation and until normal intestinal activity returns or ambulation begins.

Manipulation of the abdominal contents during operation produces inhibition of peristalsis for 24 to 48 hours. This may cause postoperative abdominal distention, also termed *inhibitory paralysis* or *ileus* of the large or small bowel, in which there is a temporary loss of the ability of the bowel to contract and empty. This apparently is due to the stimulation of the sympathetic nervous system which prevents movement along the entire gastrointestinal tract by inhibiting the gut wall and exciting the ileocecal sphincter and the internal anal sphincter. Reflex action from irritation to the peritonium will stop intestinal activity. When action of the gastrointestinal tract is inhibited gaseous material (mostly swallowed air), unabsorbed residue from oral intake, saliva, gastric secretions, and bacteria and their end-products accumulate causing distention. This distention excites the pain endings by stretching the tissues. A further cause of pain from distention is possibly due to ischemia resulting from collapse of vessels in the stretched area. The patient may complain of abdominal pain or fullness or inability to pass gas by rectum.

Measures to prevent this complication are the insertion of a gastrointestinal tube before surgery and continuous suction until intestinal activity is restored

(2 to 4 days), withholding food and fluids until peristalsis returns, frequent turning, and exercise in the early postoperative period.

Frequently the gaseous material collects in the colon and insertion of a rectal tube or administration of a small enema may give relief. Tea and dry toast sometimes provide relief, since oral intake may stimulate movement of the intestinal contents. These measures require a physician's order. The condition usually is relieved by ambulation. The distention is seldom severe enough to require the insertion of a gastrointestinal tube for intestinal suction. (See Chapter 18.)

Mechanical obstruction (intestinal obstruction) of the intestinal tract may also occur following abdominal surgery, usually due to a kink in a loop of the intestine. The patient has abdominal pain at shorter and shorter intervals. He may vomit as the intestinal contents are pushed toward the stomach. He does not defecate, and enemas return nearly clear fluid. The physician's examination reveals an abdominal mass and rebound tenderness; the leukocyte count becomes elevated. This complication may be treated by insertion of a Miller-Abbott or similar tube, and application of continuous suction drainage. This may decompress the intestinal tract sufficiently to reduce the inflammatory reaction of the bowel and relieve the obstruction. It may be necessary to treat the obstruction surgically. In either case intravenous fluids to provide water, sodium, and possibly bicarbonate and potassium are administered.

Thrombophlebitis

Phlebitis (inflammation of the vein) may occur as a consequence of intravenous therapy, especially that continued over a long period of time. The symptoms are hyperemia, tenderness, pyrexia, and swelling at the site of the needle or cutdown, possibly with linear extension to the adjacent area, according to the distribution of the vein. Phlebitis can be partially prevented by proper selection of the vein for the intravenous infusion. The largest vein available is chosen because the fluids will be diluted with blood as soon as they enter the vein. With a small vein, the needle is apt to occlude it to the point that blood cannot pass, allowing the fluid to remain undiluted in the vein until it reaches a branch in the vessel. A hypertonic solution is more apt to cause a phlebitis than an isotonic solution, but regardless of the solution used, the needle or indwelling catheter acts like a foreign body connected to the contaminated skin area, abolishing the body's first line of defense—an intact skin surface. The facility with which the needle or catheter was placed in the vein has a bearing on the development of phlebitis.

The injection site should be kept clean. If the indwelling catheter is not in use but remains in the vein it is covered with a sterile gauze pad. It is common practice to remove an indwelling catheter in 72 hours and select a new site for continued infusions. The doctor should be notified of any symptoms of phlebitis so that the site of the needle or catheter can be changed. Local application of hot packs provides relief until the body's normal processes correct the phlebitis.

Venous thrombosis may be manifested as idiopathic phlebothrombosis (intravascular clotting without marked inflammation of the vein) or thrombophlebitis (inflammatory change and thrombus formation in the vein). Elman lists three possible reasons for postoperative development of a thrombus: (1) From an injury to venous endothelium during the surgical procedure. The injury might be caused by restraints or pressure on the calf while the patient was on the operating table. The injury causes release of thrombokinase, a precursor of clot formation. (2) A surgical patient is on bed rest of necessity; this results in a slow venous flow and a statis of blood which precipitates clot formation. (3) Trauma causes an increase in blood coagulability.

The first symptom of venous thrombosis is usually pain or a cramp in the calf, or pain appearing when the foot is dorsiflexed with the knee bent. There is pain at the site with pressure. Later painful swelling and redness of the entire leg occurs and the patient may have a fever. There may be prominent antetibial veins or the inflamed vein may be palpable.

Venous thrombosis is a potentially serious complication because the clot may be dislodged and produce an embolus. It is commonly believed that postoperative pulmonary embolism usually arises in this manner.

Efforts are made to avoid this complication by administering intravenous fluids to prevent concentration of the blood, carrying out leg exercises postoperatively, wrapping the legs with elastic bandage from foot to midthigh previous to or immediately after surgery with removal and rewrapping twice a day, and early ambulation.

Anticoagulant therapy is usually prescribed. Heparin is given intravenously, first in a loading dose followed by an intravenous infusion of 5 percent glucose containing 100 to 200 mg of heparin per liter for 24 to 48 hours. Lee-White clotting time is measured every 4 hours to evaluate and control heparin therapy. Heparin is then given by injection for several days. Bishydroxycoumarin (Dicumarol) or warfarin (Coumadin) may be given by mouth; this treatment is begun before heparin is discontinued because the oral medications are not effective until 24 hours after administration. The physician probably will order the legs wrapped with elastic bandages from toes to groin or elastic stockings to be worn. Venous thrombosis in the ileofemoral area is often treated by thrombectomy.

Wound Care

Prevention of wound infection begins with the preoperative preparation of the skin. The skin cannot be sterilized completely, but the bacterial count can be reduced considerably by cleansing, removal of hair, and application of antiseptics.

As a rule infection of the wound is due to an unrecognized gross contamination, usually from air-borne bacteria, thought to occur in the operating room during the operation. Air-borne bacteria are present in other areas of the hospital but the closed and dressed wound is less susceptible to bacterial invasion. Strict aseptic technique must be observed by all operating room personnel. In the operating room area several measures are taken to reduce the air-borne bacteria. Filtered, treated air is now commonly used. Ultraviolet lamps situated so as to irradiate all areas of the room destroy bacteria if sufficient intensity is maintained. The disadvantage is that the rays can be harmful to personnel working under the ultraviolet light; protective clothing must be worn and exposed areas of the patient protected. Personnel may be required to have shoes to be worn only in the operating room area. Freshly laundered canvas boots with nonporous soles may be worn over the shoes. Only necessary talking in the operating room is the usual practice. Specific rules regarding wearing apparel in operating room suites should be followed. During the operation special techniques are used to protect the wound from bacteria and to prevent drying of the wound edges. Surgery on a patient with an infection or a contaminated wound is performed according to a specific schedule and follows special precautions.

Personnel caring for the patient postoperatively should also take precautions to avoid exposing him to infection. Careful hand washing before and after patient care is necessary. Personnel with colds and other infections should not be permitted in the patient's room. The abdominal dressing should be changed with meticulous attention to details and unnecessary talking should be avoided in order to reduce air-borne bacterial contamination.

The dressing applied to the wound in the operating room varies according to location and type of wound. Sometimes no dressing is applied to a clean incised wound, or a plastic spray dressing is used, which usually is not removed until the metal clips or stitches are removed; a second dressing may or may not be applied. Metal clips are usually removed by the physician between the second and fourth postoperative days and skin sutures are usually removed in 5 to 7 days. It is now common practice to use individually wrapped and sterilized suture and dressing sets for dressing changes. If the initial dressing becomes wet with drainage in the early postoperative days it may be reinforced by placing a sterile dressing over it. The physician should be notified. If dressings are to be changed the physician will write an order. Draining wounds are usually dressed daily by the nurse, using sterile technique, and are held in place with cellulose tape, Montgomery straps, or some other type of tape or binder to prevent irritation caused by daily removal of tape.

Trauma induces inflammation with hyperemia, leukocytosis, and pyrexia. These symptoms do not necessarily indicate a wound infection. The local inflammatory response will continue for 4 to 5 days. If a wound becomes infected the patient usually has a fever and the wound suppurates. He is treated with appropriate antibiotics and placed on bed rest; he may be removed to a separate room and may be placed on isolation. The wound is dressed daily.

A hematoma may develop, creating a large bulge. Should this occur the physician should be notified. The wound is opened over the bulge and the clot evacuated.

Wound disruption (dehiscence) or rupture of an abdominal wound is a serious complication. In disruption the skin remains intact and loops of bowel protrude and can be palpated under the skin. In rupture the skin breaks open and the abdominal viscera are extruded (evisceration).

This complication usually occurs about the seventh postoperative day. The patient will express a feeling that "something gave way." A sudden staining of the dressings with profuse, pink serous drainage occurs. Either condition quickly leads to shock, and the physician should be notified immediately. The patient should be placed in bed immediately and the blood pressure, pulse, and respiration taken. The protruding viscera should be covered with a moist saline sterile dressing.

The patient is given a blood transfusion. A nasogastric tube is inserted and suction begun to evacuate the stomach. If the patient's condition is satisfactory he is taken to the operating room and anesthetized, and surgical repair is performed. If his condition will not tolerate general anesthesia this treatment may be done in the patient's room or the operating room. With sterile technique the viscera are cleansed with sterile warm isotonic saline and returned to the peritoneal cavity. Drains are placed in the wound and the wound is taped with wide adhesive from gluteal fold to the axilla. The nurse provides emotional support to the patient and assists the physician as necessary.

Preparation for Discharge

Patients differ in the degree of concern and anxiety they have or express in the postoperative period. The nurse can be most helpful if she gives immediate attention to the patient's complaints and requests, informs him about activities that are to take place, and provides simple explanations at all times.

The patient may be discharged from the hospital in about 5 to 7 days if complications have not developed; usually this is as soon as he can walk a short distance without assistance and can eat a regular diet. He may be discharged before the skin sutures are removed and, if so, he needs instruction concerning the care of the wound. He should be informed as to when and where the sutures will be removed.

The patient may still be losing weight. He can be told that weight gain is slight at first and may not occur until the second week or later, and return to normal weight may not occur for several weeks (when fat begins to be deposited). Muscle restoration is a relatively slow process so it may be several weeks before the patient regains his usual strength and energy.

Bibliography

Adriani, John: Local Anesthetics. *American Journal of Nursing,* 59:86–88, January, 1959.

Adriani, John: *Techniques and Procedures of Anesthesia,* 3d ed. Springfield, Ill.: Charles C Thomas, Publisher, 1964.

Albert, Somomon, Sumer Chand Jain, Jo Shibuya, and Chalom A. Albert: *The Hematocrit in Clinical Practice.* Springfield, Ill.: Charles C Thomas, Publisher, 1965.

Barbata, Jean C., Deborah M. Jensen, and William G. Patterson: *A Textbook of Medical-Surgical Nursing.* New York: G. P. Putnam's Sons, 1964.

Beal, John M. (Ed.): *Manual of Recovery Room Care,* 2d ed. New York: The Macmillan Company, 1962.

Beland, Irene L.: *Clinical Nursing: Pathophysiological and Psychosocial Approaches.* New York: The Macmillan Company, 1965.

Belinkoff, Stanton: *Manual for the Recovery Room.* Boston: Little, Brown and Company, 1967.

Bird, Brian: Psychological Aspects of Pre-operative and Post-operative Care. *American Journal of Nursing,* 55:685–687, June, 1955.

Breckenridge, Flora J. and Pauline Bruno: Nursing Care of the Anesthetized Patient. *American Journal of Nursing,* 62:74–78, July, 1962.

Brownsberger, Carl N.: Emotional Stress Connected with Surgery. *Nursing Forum,* 4:46–55, 1965.

Browse, Norman L.: *The Physiology and Pathology of Bed Rest.* Springfield,

Ill.: Charles C Thomas, Publisher, 1965.

Carnevali, Doris: Listen to the Patient: To Identify Preoperative Anxiety Requires Skill. *Washington State Journal of Nursing,* 35:2, September, 1963.

Cassady, June R. and John Altrocchi: Patients' Concerns about Surgery. *Nursing Review,* 9:219–221, Fall, 1960.

Council on Pharmacy and Chemistry of the American Medical Association: *Fundamentals of Anesthesia,* 3d ed. Philadelphia: W. B. Saunders Company, 1954.

Cuthbertson, D. P.: Metabolic Effects of Injuries and their Nutritional Implications. Part I, *Nursing Times,* 61:146–147, January 29, 1965; Part II, *Nursing Times,* 61:179–180, February 5, 1965.

Davis, Loyal: *Christopher's Textbook of Surgery,* 9th ed. Philadelphia: W. B. Saunders Company, 1968.

Dumas, Anderson: Psychological Preparation Beneficial—if Based on Individual's Needs. *Hospital Topics,* 42:79, May, 1964.

Dumas, Rhetaugh Graves: Psychological Preparation for Surgery. *American Journal of Nursing,* 63:52–55, August, 1963.

Dumas, Rhetaugh G. and Robert G. Leonard: The Effect of Nursing on the Incidence of Postoperative Vomiting. *Nursing Review,* 12:12–15, Winter, 1963.

Eiseman, B. and M. Carnes: Hemorrhagic and Traumatic Shock. In Henry T. Randall, James D. Hardy, and Francis D. Moore (Eds.): *Manual of Preoperative and Postoperative Care.* Philadelphia: W. B. Saunders Company, 1967.

Elman, Robert: *Surgical Care: A Practical Physiologic Guide.* New York: Appleton Century Crofts, 1951.

Enquist, Irving F.: The Principles of Wound Healing. in Loyal Davis (Ed.): *Christopher's Textbook of Surgery,* 9th ed. Philadelphia: W. B. Saunders Company, 1968.

Fernandez-Herlihy, Luis: Surgery in Patients Taking Corticosteroids. *Hospital Medicine,* 1:6–8, March, 1965.

Friedman, Julius J.: Functional Properties of Blood. in Ewald E. Selkurt (Ed.): *Physiology,* 2d ed. Boston: Little, Brown and Company, 1966.

Gallocher, Josephine: Teaching Your Postoperative Patient to Cough Deeply. *RN,* 25:71, March, 1962.

Ganong, William F.: *Review of Medical Physiology.* Los Altos, California, Lange Medical Publications, 1967, Chap. 27.

Goodman, Louis S. and Alfred Gilman: *The Pharmacological Basis of Therapeutics,* 2d ed. New York: The Macmillan Company, 1956.

Guyton, Arthur C.: *Textbook of Medical Physiology,* 2d ed. Philadelphia: W. B. Saunders Company, 1964.

Hadley, Florence and Katherine J. Bordicks: Respiratory Difficulty: Causes and Care. *American Journal of Nursing,* 62:64–67, October, 1962.

Harrison, T. R. (Ed.): *Principles of Internal Medicine,* 5th ed. New York: McGraw-Hill Book Company, 1962.

Hershey, Nathan: The Patient's Consent. *American Journal of Nursing,* 62:99–101, September, 1962.

Hershey, Nathan: Whose Consent Is Necessary? *American Journal of Nursing,* 62:94–95, October, 1962.

Hershey, Nathan: Informed Consent. *American Journal of Nursing,* 65:101–102, July, 1965.

Hopps, Howard C.: *Principles of Pathology,* 2d ed. New York: Appleton Century Crofts, 1964.

Horgan, Patricia D.: Ultraviolet Helps Keep This O.R. Staph-safe. *RN,* 23:59–64, June, 1960.

Jamieson, R. Ainslie and Andrew W. Kay: *A Textbook of Surgical Physiology,* 2d ed. Baltimore: The Williams & Wilkins Company, 1965.

Janis, Irving Lester: *Psychological Stress;*

Psychoanalytic and Behavioral Studies of Surgical Patients. New York: John Wiley & Sons, Inc., 1958.

Johnson, Barbara: At the Bedside: Supportive Therapy for the Surgical Patient. *Tomorrow's Nurse,* 4:28, August-September, 1963.

Johnson, Brian D.: The Nurse and the Anaesthetic, before Anaesthetic. *Nursing Times,* 57:552–554, May 5, 1961.

Johnson, Brian D.: The Nurse and the Anaesthetic, after Operation: Preserving an Airway. *Nursing Times,* 57:631–633, May 19, 1961.

Kornfield, D. S., S. Zimberg, and J. R. Malm: Psychiatric Complications of Open-Heart Surgery. *New England Journal of Medicine,* 273:287, 1965.

LeMaitre, George and Janet A. Finnegan. *The Patient in Surgery: A Guide for Nurses,* Philadelphia: W. B. Saunders Company, 1965.

Luessenhop, Alfred: Care of the Unconscious Patient. *Nursing Forum,* Vol. IV, No. 3, pp. 6–11, 1965.

Moore, Francis D.: *Metabolic Care of the Surgical Patient.* Philadelphia: W. B. Saunders Company, 1959.

Moore, Francis D.: Metabolic Response to Injury. in Henry T. Randall, James D. Hardy, and Francis D. Moore (Eds.): *Manual of Preoperative and Postoperative Care.* Philadelphia: W. B. Saunders Company, 1967.

Moore, Francis D.: Surgical Nutrition: Parenteral and Oral. in Henry T. Randall, James D. Hardy, and Francis D. Moore (Eds.): *Manual of Preoperative and Postoperative Care.* Philadelphia: W. B. Saunders Company, 1967.

Moore, Ward W.: Endocrine Functions of the Pancreas. in Ewald E. Selkurt (Ed.): *Physiology,* 2d ed. Boston: Little, Brown and Company, 1966.

Moran, John M., Roger P. Atwood, and Marc I. Rowe: A Clinical and Bacteriological Study of Infections Associated with Venous Cut-down.

New England Journal of Medicine, 272:554–560, March 18, 1965.

Nourse, Myron H.: Postoperative Wound Infection. *Lancet,* 1:639–640, March 20, 1965.

Prout, Harry C.: The Modern Concept of Surgical Shock. *American Journal of Nursing,* 58:78–79, January, 1958.

Randall, Henry T.: Fluid and Electrolyte Therapy. in Henry T. Randall, James D. Hardy, and Francis D. Moore (Eds.): *Manual of Preoperative and Postoperative Care.* Philadelphia: W. B. Saunders Company, 1967.

Regan, William A.: The Consent Form and the Borderline Minor. *RN,* 25:58–61, June, 1962.

Regan, William A.: Legal Guideposts in Getting Permission. *RN,* 29:78–86, May, 1966.

Sandiford, H. B. C.: The Management of the Airway of the Unconscious Patient. *Nursing Mirror,* 114:xi–xiii, April 20, 1962.

Sheffer, M. B. and F. E. Greifenstein: Emotional Responses of Patients to Surgery and Anesthesia. *Anesthesiology,* 21:502, 1960.

Sodeman, William A.: Nutritional Factors: Protein and Fat Metabolism. in William A. Sodeman and William A. Sodeman, Jr. (Eds.): *Pathologic Physiology,* 4th ed. Philadelphia: W. B. Saunders Company, 1967.

Sorensen, Gladys: Dependency—A Factor in Patient Care. *American Journal of Nursing,* 66:1761–1763, August, 1966.

Titchener, James L., et al.: Problems of Delay in Seeking Surgical Care. *Journal of American Medical Association,* 160:1187–1193, April 7, 1956.

Titchener, James L. and Maurice Levine: *Surgery As a Human Experience.* New York: Oxford University Press, 1960.

Trail, Ira Davis and J. Victor Monke: Psyche Sequelae of Surgical Change in Body Structure. *Nursing Forum,* 2:3:14–23, 1963.

Use of Blood. Abbott Laboratories, North Chicago, Ill., 1961.

Varco, Richard L.: Principles of Preoperative and Postoperative Care. in Loyal Davis (Ed.): *Christopher's Textbook of Surgery,* 9th ed. Philadelphia: W. B. Saunders Company, 1967.

White, Abraham, Philip Handler, and Emil L. Smith: *Principles of Biochemistry,* 3d ed. New York: McGraw-Hill Book Company, 1964.

Wilkinson, A. W.: *Body Fluids in Surgery,* 3d ed. London: E. & S. Livingstone, Ltd., 1969.

Winkelstein, C., R. S. Blacher, and B. C. Meyer: Psychiatric Observations on Surgical Patients in Recovery Room. *New York State Journal of Medicine,* 65:865, 1965.

Wintrobe, M. M.: Blood Transfusion and Transfusion Reactions. in T. R. Harrison (Ed.): *Principles of Internal Medicine,* 5th ed. New York: McGraw-Hill Book Company, 1966.

Wohl, Michael G. and Robert S. Goodhart (Eds.): *Modern Nutrition in Health and Disease.* Philadelphia: Lea & Febiger, 1955.

Ziffren, Sidney E.: *Management of the Aged Surgical Patient.* Chicago: Year Book Medical Publishers, Inc., 1960.

Zimmermann, Bernard: Surgical Metabolism and Electrolyte Balance. in Loyal Davis (Ed.): *Christopher's Textbook of Surgery,* 9th ed. Philadelphia: W. B. Saunders Company, 1968.

CHAPTER 22
THE PATIENT WITH RESPIRATORY DISEASE

JUANITA A. BOOTH

The respiratory system supplies a basic need of the body for the performance of the normal physiological processes necessary for the maintenance of life. Oxygen is necessary for the metabolic process of oxidation in each cell of the body. The waste materials produced by this process must be eliminated or the individual cells will be inhibited or die, depending upon the extent of the decrease in the oxygen supply and the removal of waste. The components of the respiratory system are the nose, sinuses, pharynx, larynx, trachea, bronchi, bronchioles, alveoli, lungs, pleurae, mediastinum, chest muscles, diaphragm, and the auxiliary structures.

The transport of oxygen is accomplished as follows: Inspired oxygen is carried through the nose, paranasal sinuses, pharynx, larynx, trachea, bronchi, bronchioles, and finally the alveoli where the oxygen is diffused from the alveolar air through the permeable membranes of the alveoli and the capillaries surrounding the alveoli into the blood. The oxygen combines with the hemoglobin in the blood and is carried to the tissue fluid or lymph. The tissue fluid carries the oxygen to the tissue cells where it combines chemically with foods to release energy. This process of combining causes carbon dioxide to be formed. The carbon dioxide is carried by the tissue fluids to the blood and by the blood to the lungs. The carbon dioxide diffuses from the blood into the lung air and is breathed out into the atmosphere. The interchange of oxygen and carbon dioxide within the alveoli is termed *external respiration,* and the interchange of carbon dioxide and oxygen within the tissue cells is termed *internal respiration.* The blood exchanges only a small amount of oxyhemoglobin and carbon dioxide during respiration. Thus the function of respiration is to (1) increase the amount of oxygen in the arterial blood, (2) decrease the amount of carbon dioxide in the venous blood, (3) help regulate acid-base balance through eliminating carbon dioxide and other gases, and (4) help maintain body temperature.

The mechanism of respiration is the process of breathing and is dependent upon (1) the patency of the airway from outside the body to the alveoli of the lungs, (2) the capacity of the thoracic cavity and chest walls to move freely, (3) the size of the thoracic cavity, (4) the elasticity of the lung tissue, (5) the intrapulmonary pressure (760 mm mercury at sea level) and the intrapleural (intrathoracic) pressure (761 to 754 mm mercury at sea level) of the lungs, and (6) the ability of the thoracic muscles to expand and contract. Inspiration results from the contraction of the thoracic muscles pulling the lung tissue outward with the chest wall and downward with the diaphragm, thus allowing atmospheric pressure to push air into the lung, since the intrapulmonary pressure and atmospheric pressure are approximately the same if the intrapleural pressure is normal. If the intrapleural pressure becomes greater than the intrapulmonary pressure the elasticity of the lung is lost and the lung will collapse. Expiration results from the relaxation of the chest muscles and the recoil of the elastic lung tissue. Therefore, as the thoracic muscles contract and relax, air is forced in and out of the lungs. This explanation is oversimplified, but should suffice for the nurse to be able to anticipate and solve the nursing care problems of the patient with a respiratory disorder.

Epidemiology of Respiratory Disorders

The true epidemiology of respiratory illnesses is unknown because (1) most respiratory illnesses are not reportable diseases, (2) the patient may not seek medical assistance, and (3) facilities are not available for collecting all the pertinent data from the many agencies which maintain such data. It has been estimated that approximately 192 million cases of acute respiratory illnesses occur yearly in the United States and that over 12 million individuals have chronic respiratory problems.

Acute respiratory illnesses are endemic, sometimes become epidemic, and occasionally become pandemic. It is estimated that every person in the civilized world has at least one common cold in his lifetime and that most persons have several colds as well as other respiratory problems.

Acute respiratory problems are the most common diseases in the United States. They are estimated to cause the loss of over 220 million work days, 196 million school days, and 10 percent of all deaths. According to the National Tuberculosis and Respiratory Disease Association, of the 10 leading causes of death in 1964, pneumonia and influenza together were the fourth, and tuberculosis was the ninth, for all age groups.

To understand the magnitude of this problem as it affects the economy, education, and family life of our country and the world, one must obtain current data from local, state, national, and international sources. Figures for any specific year will not be quoted because they become obsolete so quickly. The reader should procure current data from the appropriate agencies.

Prevention of Respiratory Disorders

Most respiratory problems are preventable through control of the factors that produce or contribute to disease, imbalance, or dysfunction. Specific factors that contribute to respiratory problems are the following: trauma, obstructions, specific microorganisms, inadequate nutrition and fluid balance, psychological stress and emotional tension, neoplasms, congenital malformations, hypersensitivity, and physical stress. Trauma to the nose, face, throat, or chest can induce a local reaction to the injury which is in direct relationship to the degree of injury. Prevention of accidents can assist in eliminating these injuries. Obstruction of the nose and throat can be eliminated by preventing the inhalation of irritating dust, gases, and foreign bodies, keeping foreign objects out of the nose and mouth, and completely masticating food before trying to swallow it. Problems resulting from infections can be prevented by controlling the etiologic agent, controlling proper nutritional and fluid intake, and having adequate rest. One should avoid excesses of food and fluid, physical stress and fatigue, overexposure to cold or chilling, irritating dust, gases, and pollens, psychological stress and emotional tensions, and exposure to known infectious microorganisms following an illness. Any one or a combination of these factors can give rise to a respiratory problem.

Etiology of Respiratory Disorders

Respiratory problems are created by interruption of the normal anatomical structure, invasion of the nose, throat, and lungs by microorganisms that cause disease, allergy, trauma, or obstruction. The invading microorganism may be communicable or noncommunicable, and it may or may not be positively identified. The etiological agent in some respiratory diseases may be a mixture of several microorganisms. In some cases inflammation may be caused by inhalation of a pollen, gas, or dust. The etiology of trauma and obstruction of the respiratory system is similar to that of other areas of the body.

Pathology of Respiratory Disorders

Pathological reactions involve the mucosa and submucosa and may include the muscle tissue at the site. As in any imbalance or dysfunction, the immediate acute reaction is localized at the site of the injury. The body responses concentrate on immediate recovery; if the infection spreads to adjacent structures the body responses are increased. (See Chapters 11 and 12.)

Clinical Manifestations of Respiratory Disorders

Nasal disturbances in most cases are evidenced immediately. The onset may be abrupt or may occur within 48 hours of the introduction of the etiological factors. Trauma to the nose produces immediate pain at the site of injury, hemorrhage into the surrounding tissue, epistaxis, mouth breathing, swelling, and edema internally and externally. Internal edema or a fracture may cause obstruction of the nasal passages. With obstruction of the nasal canal there is mouth breathing, edema, and at times pain at the site of obstruction. If the obstruction is not removed inflammation occurs, and the individual may become irritable due to the discomfort.

The body responses to nasal and paranasal sinus infections are manifested by a chilling sensation, scratching or burning of the throat, sneezing, watery eyes, watery to purulent rhinorrhea, cough, varying degrees of malaise, pyrexia of 100 to 103° F (37.7 to 39.4° C), anosmia, ageusia, mild to severe headache, aching of back and extremities, sniffling and blowing of the nose, increased rhinorrhea, mouth breathing, excoriation of the external nares, dryness and parching of the lips and tongue, halitosis, irritability, and depression due to body responses and discomfort.

Clinical manifestations of problems of the pharynx, larynx, and trachea also are evidenced immediately except in malignant neoplasms, which have an insidious onset with the development of headache and pain. The onset is abrupt or may occur within 48 hours of the initiation of the etiological factors. Obstruction of the pharynx, larynx, and trachea poses an immediate threat of death, depending upon whether the obstruction is partial or complete and the speed with which therapy is provided. The manifestations of partial obstruction are dyspnea particularly with inspiration, pallor, restlessness, apprehension, fatigue, and (in the absence of therapy) cyanosis and asphyxia. Manifestations of complete sudden obstruction are gasping, flushing followed by pallor, apprehensive expression, clutching and clawing at the throat, and (in the absence of therapy) rapid cyanosis and asphyxia. The body responses to pharyngeal, laryngeal, and tracheal infections are manifested by scratchiness, burning or dryness of the throat, chills, pyrexia of 100 to 105° F (37.7 to 40.5° C), pulse of 100 to 120, headache, malaise, aching of back and extremities, cough, dysphagia, anorexia, halitosis, watery to thick purulent pharyngorrhea, laryngorrhea, or tracheoblennorrhea, unilateral or bilateral cervical lymphadenopathy, irritability, depression, and at times apprehension.

Clinical manifestations of respiratory disorders of the chest may be immediate or long-term. Trauma to the chest is manifested by pain, hemorrhage into the surrounding tissue, pleura or alveoli, pneumothorax or hydrothorax, dyspnea or hemoptysis. If hemoptysis develops and therapy is not initiated immediately asphyxia, shock, and death may result. Complete obstruction or partial obstruction of the bronchi produces coughing and dyspnea, and may cause air entrapment behind the obstruction which in turn causes ballooning of the alveoli and bronchioles.

The body responses to lung infections other than tuberculosis and pneumoconiosis are manifested by tickling in the throat, nonproductive cough or cough producing thin to thick tenacious foul-smelling sputum, pyrexia of 100 to 105° F (37.7 to 40.5° C), progressive dyspnea, fatigue, sore throat, chills, alternate flushing and pallor, halitosis, and possibly pain or pleurisy. The clinical manifestations of tuberculosis and pneumoconiosis will be found in the discussion of these conditions. Both benign and malignant neoplasms have an insidious onset, often masking their presence by manifestations of other respiratory problems.

Diagnosis of Respiratory Disorders

The diagnosis of respiratory problems is made on the facts obtained from the clinical manifestations, physical examination, various diagnostic examinations and tests, laboratory tests, and differential laboratory tests. Several diseases may produce the same early clinical and pathological manifestations and these diseases must be ruled out before a positive diagnosis can be made. This is true of several communicable diseases such as diphtheria, measles, whooping cough, and meningitis. Besides the general physical examination, diagnostic and laboratory examinations include direct visual examination, transillumination of sinuses, laryngoscopy, bronchoscophy, bronchography, fluoroscopy, roentgenography, sectional radiography (planigram, laminagram, tomogram), nasal and throat smear and culture, sputum or gastric study by direct smear, concentration–flotation study, culture or guinea pig inoculation, sedimentation rate, biopsy, skin tests, cold agglutinin, smear cultures in infections of the pharynx and larynx, culture of pleural fluid, and pulmonary function tests. Some of these have been discussed in Chapter 7; a discussion of others follows.

Transillumination of Sinuses

Transillumination of the sinuses enables the physician to see whether a sinus is blocked or contains fluid.

The individual is placed in a darkened room, a beam of light is directed upward through the roof of the mouth while he keeps his lips closed, the light illuminates the structures of the paranasal sinuses. If the individual wears dentures they should be removed. The frontal sinuses are illuminated by directing a beam of light upward through the upper roof of the eye orbit. If there is purulent fluid or a tumor within a cavity the sinus will not be illuminated because of blocking of the light; if fluid is contained within the sinus a dull illumination may outline the fluid level. Blocking of the illumination does not demonstrate the specific nature of the block, but does indicate that such exists and proper drainage is inhibited. The nurse should explain the procedure to the patient and assure him that it is painless.

Bronchoscopy

Bronchoscopy enables the physician to visualize the bronchi. The individual must have nothing by mouth for 8 to 12 hours prior to the examination, and all dental prostheses must be removed prior to the examination. The pharynx, larynx, and trachea are usually anesthetized with a topical anesthetic. A bronchoscope is passed through the mouth, pharynx, larynx, and trachea into the bronchi. The room is darkened. The physician inspects the bronchi directly. He can remove a foreign body or mucus plugs, take a sample of secretions, and take a biopsy specimen of an area within the bronchi.

The patient will find this to be an uncomfortable procedure. The role of the nurse in assisting the patient before, during, and after the procedure is most important. The procedure should be explained to him. The nurse should assure him that he will be able to breathe although his throat will feel full, and that an anesthetic will be used to prevent pain or undue discomfort. The patient must relax the muscles of his throat and swallow as directed or the procedure will be painful and there may be injury to the tissue which can result in painful edema.

The nurse must emphasize the role of the patient. She should instruct him as follows: He is to practice breathing through the nose while keeping the mouth open. He should practice relaxing the muscles of the arms, neck, and chest because tensing the muscles in the throat places muscle pressure against the metal tube of the bronchoscope. This pressure can bruise the throat muscles and delay their return to normal following the procedure. The desire to cough must be suppressed because this also will cause the muscles of the throat to be bruised against the bronchoscope.

The room will be darkened during the procedure so that the physician can see clearly, and the nurse will not leave the patient. He will not have anything by mouth after midnight prior to the day of the procedure in order to prevent aspiration of fluid or food particles either during or following the procedure when his throat is anesthetized. Following the procedure he will not have any fluids or food until his gag reflex has returned; the nurse will test this reflex periodically by inserting an applicator into the back of his throat. Until the gag reflex has returned he must expectorate all saliva rather than swallow it, to prevent aspiration. He will not be able to talk because his vocal cords have been anesthetized and trying to talk will strain these muscles. He will be able to communicate by writing during the short time the anesthesia is in effect.

Prior to the bronchoscopy the nurse should make certain that the patient has good mouth care, that dental prostheses have been removed, and that the prescribed premedications are administered. During the procedure the nurse should assist the patient to relax and to follow the directions of the physician in swallowing. She should remind him to breathe through his nose and allay his fear of asphyxiation. She must not become impatient with him if he has difficulty in following directions, but should remember that he is experiencing much discomfort and is apprehensive about smothering and having pain. He needs support, understanding, and reassurance. Following the procedure the nurse will administer the usual nursing care following any procedure as discussed in Chapter 7, place him in the proper position as indicated by the physician, provide an emesis basin and disposable tissue for his saliva and sputum, provide paper and pencil so he can communicate, and reassure him that he will soon be able to swallow, have fluid and food, and talk. She will test his gag reflex as described. She should be sure his call bell is within reach. The nurse should observe for any indication of difficulty in breathing due to laryngeal edema. If a biopsy was done any excessive bleeding should be reported immediately to the doctor, since a hemorrhage occasionally can result from this procedure.

Bronchography

Bronchography enables the physician to visualize the bronchial tree through x-ray examination. Preparation of the patient prior to this procedure is similar to the preparation for bronchoscopy, i.e., nothing by mouth for 8 to 12 hours prior to the procedure, good mouth care, removal of dental prostheses, patient to breathe deeply and cough to eliminate bronchial secretions, premedications as prescribed, and possibly postural drainage if the patient has thick bronchial secretions.

The pharynx, larynx, and trachea are anesthetized with a topical anesthetic and a laryngoscope is passed through the mouth, pharynx, and larynx into the trachea. A catheter is inserted through the nose into the laryngoscope and bronchi, and radiopaque oil is inserted into the bronchi. The patient is moved and tilted to promote drainage of oil into the bronchioles. X-ray films from various angles are taken. Following this procedure the oil is usually removed by postural drainage.

The function of the nurse in assisting the patient is as described for bronchoscopy:

POSTURAL DRAINAGE

The purpose of postural drainage is to assist the patient in removing bronchial secretions by gravity. The patient lies across the bed on his abdomen with the head and thorax extended downward toward the floor. To prevent the patient from slipping off the bed a chair or stool should be placed between him and the floor so that he may rest his hands and arms upon it to support himself. A sputum receptacle is placed within his reach for collection of secretions drained from the bronchi. If the patient is unable to support himself safely in this position he may be positioned over the knee bend of a Gatch bed with a board placed across the foot of the bedsprings for hand and arm support. If he cannot physically tolerate either of these methods he is positioned on his abdomen with the side of the face extending over the edge of the bed and the foot of the bed raised

12 to 30 inches off the floor. Regardless of which method is used the patient must be protected from falling off or out of the bed. The arms and hands should be protected by padding the leaning board. The bed, leaning board, and floor should be protected from sputum. The nurse must stay with the patient to protect him from falling as he may become dizzy in this position. If dizziness persists the physician should be notified.

After having performed this procedure several times many patients are able to do it unassisted several times daily. The procedure usually is limited to 10 minutes for the first three or four times and the time gradually is increased to 20 minutes. The patient should be encouraged to take several deep breaths and cough to assist in removing secretions. This procedure may be modified by placing the patient on his side.

The procedure should not be done immediately before or after a meal, since the sputum drainage may be foul-tasting and foul-smelling, thus causing loss of appetite before a meal or nausea after a meal.

To assist a patient in removing secretions from a specific area of the lungs other postural positions may be employed. The secretion must be guided into the bronchioles and bronchi. Thus the nurse should be cognizant of the specific area of the lung involved so that she can assist the patient in assuming the proper position. To assist with drainage from the apical segments of the lung the patient is seated in an upright position in bed and a large bolster or pillow is placed so that the patient's chest is at approximately a 60 degree angle from the bed. When the upper lobe is involved the head of the bed is raised to approximately 45 degrees and the patient leans back against the bed. Drainage of the middle lobe of the lung can be improved by placing the patient on the unaffected side without a pillow and elevating the foot of the bed approximately 20 degrees (approximately 16 inches) off the floor. For the lower lobe the same procedure is employed but the foot of the bed is elevated to approximately a 30 degree angle or approximately 20 to 25 inches off the floor. In all postural positions the patient must be encouraged to cough to assist in moving the exudate into the bronchi, trachea, and throat (Fig. 22-1).

Gastric Aspiration

Gastric aspiration enables the physician to obtain laboratory tests of the bronchial secretions when the individual is unable to cough and raise sputum. During sleep the individual swallows all secretions from the mouth, nose, throat, and lungs; therefore an examination of the morning gastric contents may demonstrate the organism causing a lung infection. The patient is given nothing by mouth for 8 to 12 hours prior to the procedure, which is done before breakfast in the morning. A gastric tube is inserted. When the tube is in the stomach a large syringe is attached to the tube and the gastric contents are withdrawn into the syringe. Sometimes sterile water is instilled prior to withdrawal of the stomach contents. From the syringe the contents are transferred to a covered sterile laboratory container. The gastric tube is then removed. The gastric content studies are done by direct smear, concentrate-flotation, culture, and guinea pig inoculation.

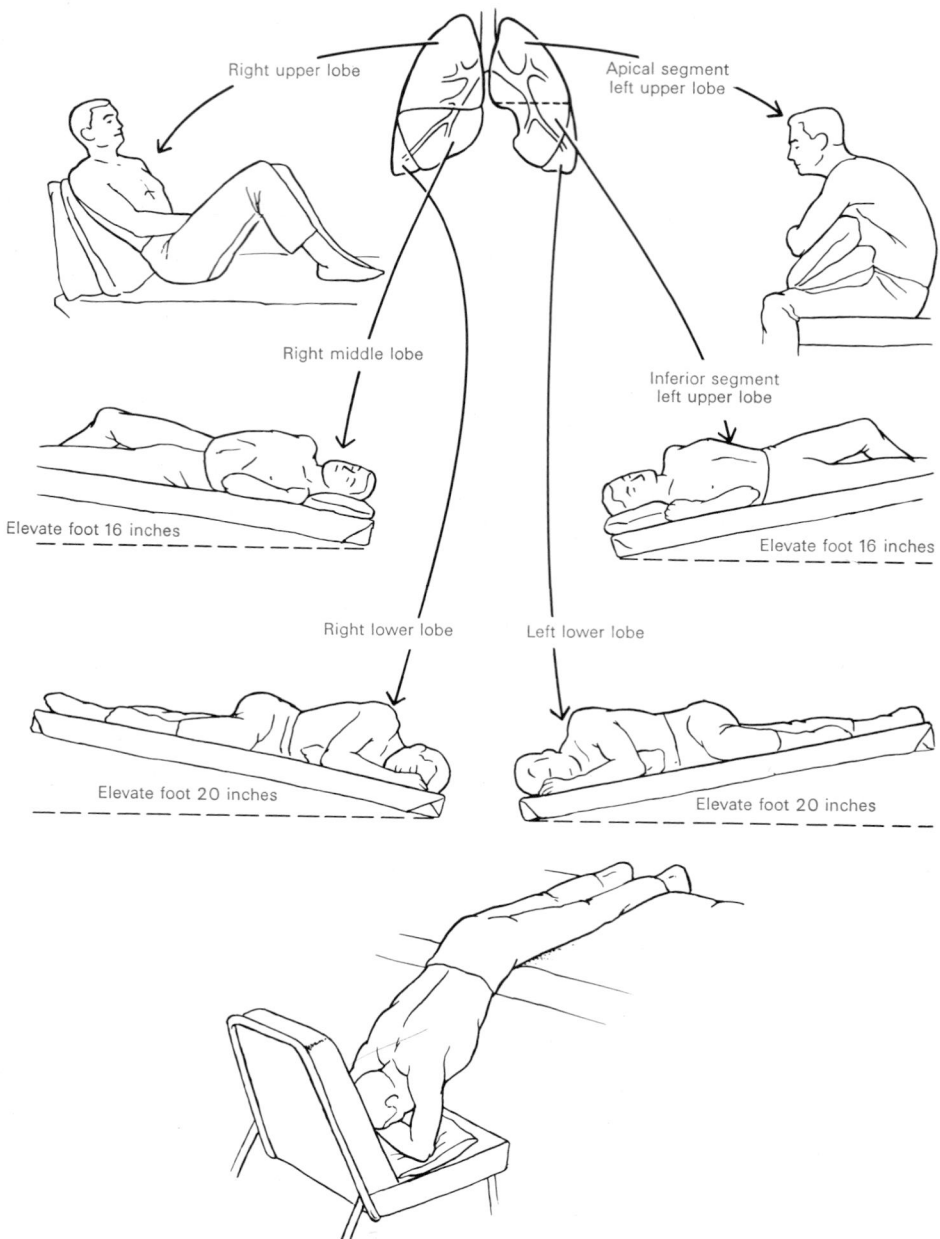

Right upper lobe

Apical segment
left upper lobe

Right middle lobe

Inferior segment
left upper lobe

Elevate foot 16 inches

Elevate foot 16 inches

Right lower lobe   Left lower lobe

Elevate foot 20 inches

Elevate foot 20 inches

*Figure 22–1
The patient coughs and
thus helps move exudate
into the bronchi, trachea,
and throat. (Adapted with
permission from Kathleen
Newton Shafer, Janet R.
Sawyer, Audrey M.
McCluskey, and Edna
Lifgren Beck: Medical-
Surgical Nursing, 4th ed.
St. Louis: The C. V.
Mosby Company, 1964.)*

Predisposing Factors in Respiratory Disorders

Exposure to the etiologic agent, lowered physical resistance to infection due to recent or repeated illnesses, poor nutrition, excessive alcohol ingestion or chronic alcoholism, overexposure to cold, excessive and prolonged emotional disturbances, and certain specific occupations are the predisposing factors. Frequent pregnancies lower resistance.

Treatment of Respiratory Disorders

Respiratory problems are treated both medically and surgically. The treatment depends upon the etiological agent, body response to the problem, extent of physiological and clinical imbalance, extent of anatomical involvement, efficiency of pharmaceutical therapies, recurrences of infection, and immediate threat to life. The overall aim of therapy is to return the individual to as near a healthy status as possible, to lessen his immediate discomfort, to protect him from exposure to communicable diseases, to prevent the spread of infection to other areas of the body, to assist his natural body responses, and to prevent the development of other infections.

TRAUMA

In trauma to the nose, throat, and chest the treatment is similar to that of trauma elsewhere in the body. If there is swelling and edema the application of cold will temporarily contract the capillaries in the area and lessen bleeding into the adjacent tissue. A mild analgesic such as acetylsalicylic acid 0.3 g to 0.6 g (5 to 10 grains) is usually prescribed. If the trauma produces a fracture the treatment will depend upon the location of the fracture.

OBSTRUCTION

Complete obstruction of the pharynx, larynx, or trachea demands emergency procedures. The obstruction must be removed within minutes or the patient will be asphyxiated as a result of anoxia. A sharp slap on the back may cause him to expectorate the obstructing object. It may be possible to reach the obstacle with a long forceps. If the obstacle cannot be removed a tracheostomy should be performed, under aseptic conditions if possible, but if asepsis is not possible it may be performed under any conditions in order to maintain the respiration. The neck is hyperextended backward, a midline incision is made quickly through the skin, the superficial fascia, the pretracheal muscles, the tracheotomic triangle, above the sternal notch and below the thyroid cartilage, and through the third and fourth tracheal rings. The edges of the incision are covered with sterile gauze and the outer cannula of a tracheostomy tube is inserted through the incision into the trachea, guided by the obturator, and held in place by tapes tied around the neck. The obturator is removed and the inner cannula is inserted into the outer cannula. A partial obstruction is treated by attempts to remove the obstruction: if a foreign body it is removed; if the cause is edema, the usual methods of reducing edema are used. However, if the edema is not reduced or continues to increase or the foreign body cannot be removed, a tracheostomy should be done under aseptic conditions.

INFECTION OR INFLAMMATORY REACTION

Therapies employed in treating respiratory problems resulting from infections or inflammatory reactions are supportive, symptomatic, palliative, and specific. Basic therapies are as follows:

Rest or bed rest to assist the body responses in combating the problem, to prevent fatigue, and to lessen the metabolic activity of the cells in all parts of the body and reduce the need for oxygen.

Increased fluid intake to assist in diluting the tissue fluid, especially at the site of the infection, thus reducing the concentration of toxins produced by the inflammatory response; to prevent spread of the infection to the urinary system;[1] to assist in decreasing the pyrexia by increasing moisture available for exhalation; and to dilute sputum to facilitate expectoration.

Balanced diet high in protein, minerals, and vitamins to assist in body repair and to prevent lowering the natural body resistance to infection. Diet may be liquid, semiliquid, soft, or general depending upon the respiratory difficulty and the patient's ability to swallow and breathe. Gaseous foods should be avoided, to prevent distention that will interfere with diaphragmatic motion.

Placing the patient in the most comfortable position for breathing to assist in maintaining an adequate supply of oxygen to the lungs and removing carbon dioxide from the lungs.

Use of mild analgesics, usually a salicylate such as acetylsalicylic acid 0.3 to 0.6 g (5 to 10 grains), for relief of general discomfort and aching.

Use of non-narcotic sedatives and hypnotics for rest and sleep to assist in relieving malaise and fatigue, to assist the body responses in the inflammation reaction, and to assist in decreasing the metabolic activity of the cells.

Good mouth care to lessen the discomfort resulting from mouth breathing and to wash away the topical waste or secretions of the throat and lungs which accumulate in the mouth and prevent reswallowing of microorganisms that may inhibit recovery.

Use of antipyretics to assist in lowering the temperature to normal.

Use of antihistamines to promote dilatation of the bronchial tubes and to depress histamine action in the area.

Nasal and throat irrigations to assist in removing waste materials from the mucous membranes and to stimulate circulation of blood in the area.

Use of antitussives and demulcents of non-narcotic derivatives to lessen nonproductive cough and assist in preventing local and general fatigue.

Use of expectorants and demulcents to assist in liquefying bronchial secretions and aid in eliminating these waste products.

Use of inhalants to assist in liquefying mucous membrane secretions, to assist in eliminating these waste products, and to stimulate increased circulation of blood to the area.

Use of specific antimicrobial therapy to act on specific organisms and assist the body responses to inflammation.

Administration of oxygen to assist the respiration when the patient is unable to inhale an adequate supply.

Use of parenteral therapy to assist in maintaining nutrition and electrolyte and fluid balance.

---

[1] Necrosis produced as the result of an infection may be carried via the blood to the genitourinary tract.

Use of external hot or cold applications to assist in decreasing the edema in the area and to assist in relieving local discomfort.

Cessation of smoking to assist in decreasing irritation of the respiratory tract and inhibition of normal body responses.

Use of suction to remove mucus secretions that are interfering with respirations.

Isolation of the patient if the etiologic agent is communicable.

SURGICAL TREATMENT

Therapy by means of surgical treatment may involve tracheostomy, incision and drainage of abscesses, thoracentesis, or decompression of pneumothorax. *Incision and drainage* of abscesses is accomplished by a surgical incision made into the abscessed area, which is spread open to allow the residual exudate to be removed. Therapeutic doses of sulfonamides or antibiotic drugs may be instilled into the drained area. Drainage may be established by inserting a drain into the area and entirely or partially closing the wound around the drain to allow continued drainage. If a drain is not inserted the incision may be left open or may be partially closed to allow drainage of exudate that may be produced during the reparative process. *Thoracentesis* or chest aspiration is the withdrawal of fluid or exudate from the pleural cavity. Usually it is performed by the physician. The patient sits up in bed and leans over a padded overbed table or the back of a chair padded with a pillow. If the patient is seated on the side of the bed, his feet should be supported by a stool or chair of appropriate height, and not left dangling. If he is debilitated or unable to assume this upright position, he should be placed on his side so that the affected hemithorax is uppermost. Some physicians prefer to have a bolster or pillow placed under the thorax to facilitate separation of the ribs on the upper hemithorax. The side on which thoracentesis is done depends upon the site of the fluid within the pleural cavity. The most frequent site is the seventh interspace below the angle of the scapula in the posterior axillary line. The skin is cleansed with an appropriate antiseptic, and a sterile drape is placed. Using sterile equipment, the physician anesthetizes the site of entry and inserts an aspiration needle through the skin and chest wall into the pleura. Aspiration of the fluid or exudate is performed by maintaining negative pressure in the syringe. *Decompression* of a pneumothorax is discussed in the section on trauma to the chest.

Surgical removal of neoplasms may be performed in all areas of the respiratory tract. Resection is discussed in the section on tuberculosis.

COMPLICATION OF HEMORRHAGE

Hemorrhage can arise as a complication of respiratory disorders any time. After the site of the hemorrhage has been ascertained, the patient should be kept quiet. with the aid of a narcotic or sedative if necessary. He should not cough or clear his throat. If the site of hemorrhage is the pharynx, larynx, or trachea, an ice compress or an ice collar may be applied externally. Nothing is given by mouth until the hemorrhage ceases. If the site is the nose, pressure packing is inserted. Parenteral fluids may be given.

The nurse must remain calm and must reassure the patient that he will not bleed to death. She should stay with him or have someone else stay with him to provide emotional support. The patient's head should be turned to the side so the blood can drain from the mouth. The patient should be kept warm and observed for signs of shock. He should not be disturbed for changing of bed linen; rather, clean linen is added as needed until the hemorrhage has stopped and the patient can safely be moved with assistance. He should not be permitted to sit up or turn over by himself. The mouth is carefully cleaned of dried blood. Later the patient may be given chipped ice to hold in his mouth. Encouraging him to rest and sleep will aid in slowing the circulation of blood to the site of the hemorrhage. He should be discouraged from coughing as this stimulates circulation, increases fatigue, and irritates the site of the hemorrhage, and may cause additional bleeding by dislodging the clot.

Nursing Care of the Patient with a Respiratory Disorder

The goal of nursing care is to help the patient return to as healthy a status as possible, as soon as possible.

The following discussion of nursing care is especially applicable to various respiratory disorders. Thus, only the additional nursing care measures that are specific to or of particular importance in the care of the patient with a respiratory disorder will be discussed. The reader is also referred to the appropriate chapters in Part IV.

SPECIFIC NURSING CARE

The nurse has a number of specific responsibilities in caring for the patient with a respiratory disorder.

Alleviate apprehension and fears relative to the degree of hypoxia. The nursing responsibility is to reassure the patient and family that he will not suffocate, that oxygen will be administered if necessary to assist him in breathing, and that the nurse understands and appreciates his reaction to anoxia. Individuals who are experiencing difficulty in breathing are often fearful of being alone, so the presence of the nurse is reassuring. He may be afraid that no one will know he is unable to breathe or that he will not be able to call anyone in time if his hypoxia increases. Oxygen is a primary need for life and the patient is frightened when threatened by not being able to breathe, because any degree of hypoxia brings the threat of impending death closer. The patient's spiritual adviser often can assist him and lessen his apprehension.

Assist the patient in obtaining a maximum supply of oxygen by inhalation, and in excreting a maximum amount of carbon dioxide by exhalation. The nursing function is to assist the patient in maintaining a patent airway from the atmosphere into the alveoli. If the airway is partially obstructed by sputum the patient should be taught to take several deep breaths and to cough, using the abdominal muscles and the diaphragm so as to use the least amount of energy for the maximum result. This method of coughing utilizes pressure to push the base of the lungs upward and assist in more powerfully exhaling the alveolar air, thereby exerting more pressure and force against the mucus in the bronchioles and bronchi. The cilia then propel the mucus upward into the throat and mouth so that the patient can expectorate it. Deep breathing helps the patient pull more air into the alveoli and stimulates coughing when he has bronchial secretions. If the patient is unable to breathe deeply, intermittent positive pressure breathing or ventilation is prescribed to provide more oxygen, dilate the bronchi, or stimulate coughing for removal of the bronchial secretions. If the patient is unable to cough and raise sputum, postural drainage may be ordered; this procedure is performed by the nurse, as previously described. When the sputum is thick and tenacious and blocking the throat, suction may be used to clear the pharynx, larynx, and trachea. Inhalants, stimulatory expectorants, or bronchodilator drugs may be administered as prescribed by the physician to assist in liquefying the bronchial secretion and lessen the amount of secretion, and to dilate the bronchioles by relaxing the smooth muscle fibers encircling the bronchioles and thereby enlarging the lumen of the passageway.

The patient is positioned to allow for freer expansion of the chest and greater amount of space for the swing of the diaphragm. All parts of the body are supported to prevent fatigue of any group of muscles. The patient may be more comfortable in a semireclining position or an upright position. In either of these positions the pillow is fastened to the top of the bed to prevent it from slipping down and putting pressure on the back of the neck and shoulders and to prevent the head from being forced forward and causing malposition of the larynx and trachea. This development would defeat the purpose of the positioning. The patient is protected from sliding sidewise in the bed, which could cause him to fall out of bed or could cause compression of the lower chest muscles and diaphragm on that side. This again defeats the purpose of positioning. A patient with marked dyspnea may be more comfortable if he sits upright in bed and leans forward. To help him maintain this position without fatigue, a bedside table is placed across the bed and padded with a small pillow; the patient leans forward and supports himself on his arms. If oxygen is prescribed it is administered as discussed elsewhere in this chapter. Adequate ventilation in the patient unit aids him in breathing more easily. Cool fresh air should be constantly circulating to ensure the maximum in oxygen content and maximum removal of carbon dioxide and microorganisms from the environment. Warm air tends to increase the effort needed to breathe.

Minimize the patient's activities thereby minimizing his metabolic activities. Any degree of anoxia causes the patient to be restless and apprehensive; thus he tends to want to move about the room or the bed with quick motions. Both these activities increase the circulation of blood and the metabolic activity of the tissue cells of the involved muscles. Quick contraction of muscle tissue increases the metabolism faster than slow motion because more energy is needed for a sudden contraction. The nurse explains to the patient why rest, especially bed rest, is beneficial to him, and how to relax and rest in order that he may assist in his care and receive maximum benefit from his therapy. She explains that temporarily others will assist him with his activities and that by cooperating with them he is actively participating in his therapy. Rest and bed rest lessen the metabolic processes throughout the body, thereby reducing the oxygen requirements of the body, preventing fatigue, and aiding the body responses to the inflammatory re-action created by the respiratory problem.

Provide an environment that allows the patient the opportunity to profit from the therapy. The nursing goal is to reduce the amount of traffic in the patient area. Both traffic and noise are irritating factors that disturb the patient, prevent him from resting or sleeping, increase his restlessness, produce fatigue, and in-crease his need for oxygen. The nurse limits the number of visitors and the length of time they may visit. If the patient feels that he is the host to the visitor, he will expend more oxygen through the exertion created by his talking to the visitor and his efforts to look alert and to think of subjects to discuss. He must be pro-tected from these interruptions of his therapy which inhibit his recovery.

The patient is protected from chilling or cold, to which he may be more sus-ceptible because of pyrexia and lowered body defenses. These external factors in-crease metabolic activities through the normal protective reactions of the body.

Protect the patient from exposure to other communicable infections. The nursing goal is to prevent further inflammatory processes from developing within the pa-tient that will impede his receiving the maximum benefit from his therapy. Com-municable microorganisms are transmitted into an uninfected individual by in-halation, ingestion, or inoculation. Infection by inoculation is rare and usually occurs as the result of a laboratory or medical accident. Infection by inhalation is the breathing in of contaminated material such as dust or droplets of secretions expelled by the infected individual when he talks, laughs, coughs, sneezes, or sighs. Infection by ingestion is the entrance through the mouth to the gastrointestinal tract of contaminated material such as fluids, food, or objects put into the mouth. Infectious respiratory problems are usually transmitted by inhalation.

Protecting the patient entails reducing traffic and visitors in the patient's en-vironment. Traffic can transport the communicable microorganisms from another environment into the patient's environment or can stir up contaminated dust in the area. Visitors may harbor communicable infectious microorganisms and dis-perse them into the immediate patient environment. They should be requested to stand or sit 3 or more feet from the foot of the patient's bed or, if the patient is sitting in a chair, to stay at least 6 feet from him. Any individual, whether hos-pital employee or visitor, who has signs or symptoms of a communicable infec-tion should be restricted from the patient area, especially if the individual has a respiratory problem. Any interference with respiration interrupts the normal body defenses and its ability to resist infection. Any additional infections increase the body's need for oxygen and thus increase respirations. It is the responsibility of the nurse to protect the patient because he cannot protect himself.

Assist the patient in receiving the required nutrition and fluids. The nursing goal is to stimulate the patient's desire to ingest food and fluids. Patients with respiratory problems usually have loss of appetite, breathing difficulty while mas-ticating food or drinking fluids, and loss of the sense of taste, so food has little or no flavor, or the flavor is altered or may be affected by the odor or taste of sputum. The sense of smell may be lost, so the odor of food or fluid cannot stimu-late a desire for it. Odors within the room may mask the pleasant aroma of the food or fluid. If the patient has lost these senses, much of the stimulation to par-take of food and fluid is lacking. He should have frequent mouth care, especially prior to eating a meal or drinking fluids. The food and fluid should be served in small quantities and attractively prepared. It may be necessary to offer food frequently rather than try to maintain a three-meal-a-day schedule. The nurse should ascertain what foods and fluids the patient enjoys and how he likes them prepared, and should understand any cultural and religious factors that may influence his eating patterns. Food should be easy to masticate and swallow so that the patient who must breathe through his mouth can ingest it. Cool or cold fluids often are pleasant for the patient with an irritated throat. Hot fluids appear sometimes to stimulate sputum-producing cough. The nurse must discuss with the patient the need for nutrition and fluids as part of his therapy and show him how he can cooperate in his therapy.

Keep herself, other nursing personnel, and the physician informed regarding the patient's immediate status. The nursing goal is to make accurate observations, recognize and interpret observations, anticipate untoward reactions, and inform the physician of untoward reactions or clinical manifestations that may indicate an extension of the problem or the development of other problems. The nurse observes the patient and notes whether he is restless, listless, quiet or depressed, in pain, having increased or decreased difficulty in breathing. She notes changes in respiration, whether he is pale or flushed, too cool or too warm, having diaphoresis. She checks the vital signs, and watches for reactions to pharmacologic agents. Any deviation or change in condition that appears to be significant must be reported to the physician immediately. A progress report on the patient's status is given to the physician when he visits the patient.

Prevent the disuse syndrome. The nursing goal is to prevent loss of the ability to use any part of the body due to improper position, lack of motion, or abnormal pressures. The aim of therapy and nursing care is to assist the patient in returning to as near a normal status as possible and not to create any additional problem that will prevent him from carrying on normal activities when his current disease, imbalance, or dysfunction is cured. If a patient must have bed rest as a part of his therapy, then a part of nursing care is to maintain proper positioning, fluid balance, and circulation and to provide passive exercises to maintain muscle tone. The patient must be encouraged to change his position frequently to prevent constant pressure on any group of muscles and nerves, and to do passive exercise to maintain muscle tone and prevent muscle atrophy.

Assist in educating the patient and family regarding his current respiratory problem and their respective roles in therapy and prophylaxis. The nursing goal is to ascertain what the patient and family know about the respiratory problem and whether they understand what they know, to establish communication with them, to communicate at their level of understanding, and to ascertain whether they understand and accept what the physician and nurse are communicating. The nurse is frequently asked to interpret the doctor's statements to the patient and family. Words and phrases of medical terminology frequently are not clear to those outside the medical disciplines. They do not have the background of knowledge or terminology necessary to make the correct interpretations or conclusions from the information presented. The nurse must have the ability to explain it in a meaningful way to the patient and family. She must utilize her knowledge of their culture, education, religion, psychological and emotional reactions, and individual family roles if she is to help them to understand and utilize this information correctly. Her explanations may be given to the patient and family in the hospital or in the home. Some patients with respiratory problems are not hospitalized or may be hospitalized for a short period of time. The acute respiratory problems are usually of short duration and the educational contact with the patient and family is very short, therefore the information exchanged must be clear, concise, and correct to ensure its current application and, it is hoped, its future application in prevention. In long-term respiratory problems the process can take place at a slower pace and in greater depth and breadth.

Administer the specific therapies as prescribed for the patient. The nursing goal is to possess a complete understanding of the principles and procedures of the specific therapies.

SPECIFIC THERAPIES THAT THE NURSE MUST UNDERSTAND

The principles of nursing care are the same in specific therapy as in basic therapy, but application may be different. The application of these principles must encompass new data that have been made available and that may differ from the original or basic premise. Utilization, application, and implementation of these principles change to meet the patient's individual needs. The principles of respiration are the same in patients with respiratory problems as in normal persons—only the application is different. This is true also in administration of drugs.

Oxygen Administration

Oxygen is administered when hypoxia or hyposemia indicates that oxygenation of the blood is insufficient. Oxygen is very drying to the body tissues and usually is administered through a humidifier, via nasal catheter, mask, or tent.

NASAL CATHETER

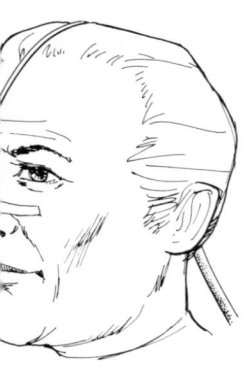

Figure 22–2
Oxygen administration
through nasal catheter.

The nasal catheter is used most frequently (Fig. 22-2). The catheter may be made of metal, rubber, or plastic, rubber or plastic being most often used. The distance from the tip of the patient's nose to the tip of the ear is measured and the catheter is marked at that point. The catheter is lubricated with water and connected to the oxygen supply. The oxygen is set at the proper flow level and allowed to flow through the catheter as the latter is gently inserted through the nostril and passed through the nasal passage until the indicated length has been reached. To ensure that the catheter is in proper position the nurse should have the patient open his mouth and depress his tongue. The tip of the catheter should be visible immediately behind the uvula. If the tip of either a rubber or a plastic catheter is inserted too far it will cause the patient to gag and should be withdrawn until it is in the proper position. The catheter is taped to the side of the face. The oropharyngeal catheter should be changed every 8 hours or whenever it becomes obstructed. The other nostril should be used when the catheter is changed. The same procedure is followed with the metal catheter. Care must be taken not to force the catheter through the nasal passage, to ensure that the delicate mem-

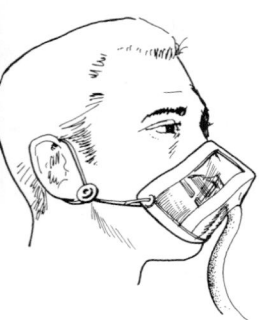

*Figure 22-3
Oxygen administration
through face mask.*

*Figure 22-4
Oxygen regulator.
(Adapted with permission
of the publisher from
Marie M. Seedor: Therapy
with Oxygen and Other
Gases. [New York:
Teachers College Press],
© 1966, Teachers College,
Columbia University.)*

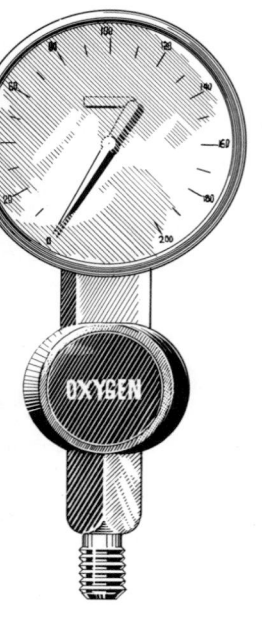

branes of the nasal passage are not damaged. The metal catheter is taped to the forehead. The rate of oxygen flow is ordered by the physician to provide the concentration desired for the individual patient; the usual flow is 4 to 8 liters per minute. The patient should be instructed to breathe through his nose for maximum benefit.

FACE MASK

A face mask may be used if the patient cannot tolerate a nasal catheter or if the nasal passage is obstructed and a catheter cannot be inserted (Fig. 22-3). Various designs of face masks have been devised, the most widely used being the nasal and oronasal types. The nasal mask fits over the nose and the oronasal mask covers both the nose and the mouth. The efficiency of the nasal face mask depends upon the patient's ability to keep his mouth closed. It is used by patients who need to cough or expectorate frequently, those who must be fed orally, and those who have bouts of vomiting. The oronasal mask is used by patients who must breathe through the mouth. The mask is not tolerated well by the apprehensive patient.

Care must be taken to ensure that the mask fits snugly to the facial area and does not leak oxygen around the edges, and that it does not irritate the skin in contact with it. The rate of flow of oxygen is ordered by the physician to provide the desired concentration for the individual patient. The usual flow is 4 to 6 liters per minute.

TENT

An oxygen tent is used when the other methods are not tolerated, or when the patient is critically ill, restless, or uncooperative. The tent is employed in the patient with hyperpyrexia and in the small child. It is fitted over the upper part of the bed and tucked in tightly around the edge of the bed; the fold across the bed is closed by a cotton sheet or blanket. Refrigerated humidified oxygen is forced into the tent, usually with a flush valve to fill the tent rapidly. All openings into the tent must be securely closed at all times and the nurse must administer all nursing care by using the openings provided for this purpose. The temperature inside the tent should be checked frequently to ensure that the patient does not become chilled; proper bedding should be placed over him to keep him warm. The usual temperature is between 65 and 72° F. The physician orders the rate of flow of oxygen. The usual flow is 8 to 12 liters per minute after the tent has been flooded for 2 minutes with a flow of 12 to 15 liters per minute. An oxygen regulator is shown in Figure 22-4. The open-top tents for oxygen administration to children are operated in a similar manner.

CARING FOR THE PATIENT RECEIVING OXYGEN THERAPY

The general nursing care of patients receiving oxygen therapy is as for general nursing care of all patients. The precautions specific to the administration of oxygen therapy are as follows:

Oxygen supports combustion, therefore sparks and open flames must not be allowed in the area.

Electrical appliances in which a "short" may occur and produce sparks are not used in the area. Woolen blankets must not be used, as they may produce sparks.

NO SMOKING signs are posted on the door of the room and in the patient unit and all visitors are prohibited from smoking in the area.

The oxygen source is tested before therapy is begun and frequently thereafter.

If tank oxygen is used the tank must be full when therapy is begun and replacement made before the tank becomes empty.

When a new tank of oxygen is to be started, the cap is removed from the cylinder valve and the valve is loosened slightly until oxygen is expelled in order to protect the oxygen regulator valve and to clear the outlet of any dust before the gauge is attached.

Oil or grease should not be used near the valves or on the nurse's hands as she adjusts the mechanism.

The flow of oxygen is checked frequently to ensure that the correct concentration is maintained.

When a closed oxygen tent is utilized the oxygen must be *turned on* or the patient may be asphyxiated.

If an oxygen tank is used it must be secured to the wall or bed to prevent it from tipping over or falling to the floor.

The danger in a tank falling over is that the valve may break off at the top of the tank. The escaping oxygen then rushes out with great force from a narrow opening and can actually convert the tank into an unguided missile. Then, too, it is obvious that it could cause injury by falling on someone.

Intermittent Positive Pressure Breathing

Intermittent positive pressure breathing therapy (IPPB) is prescribed by the physician and administered by the registered nurse or members of the inhalation therapy department. Before the treatment is begun, the IPPB unit (respirator) is attached to a source of oxygen (tank or wall outlet), the pressure control gauge is set according to the physician's order, the dilution control is set for the prescribed oxygen-air mixture, and, if drugs are to be administered, the medication is placed in the nebulizer of the unit. The special mouthpiece is inserted into the mouth, or an oronasal mask is used; in either case leakage must be prevented. The inspiratory pressure is maintained by the unit and alternates with the patient's expiration of air. The patient commonly is apprehensive about having the mask fitted tightly to his face, since he is already having difficulty in breathing.

The unit has several functions: It increases tidal volume and total minute ventilation, and improves the distribution of the inhaled gas. It increases the arterial oxygen saturation. The unit facilitates the elimination of carbon dioxide and aids in the regulation of the respiratory acid base. It delivers humidified water, detergents, mucolytic agents, bronchodilators, and antibiotics to the terminals of the bronchial tree. It places a volume of gas distal to obstructing secretions and improves the efficiency of coughing. It increases arterial and tissue oxygen tension.

Situations in which IPPB therapy is used include airway obstruction caused by alveolar exudate, secretions, mucosal edema, bronchospasm, unequal and inadequate alveolar ventilation; respiratory arrest; respiratory acidosis; labored breathing.

Usually the physician prescribes the inspiratory pressure in the range of 12 to 20 cm water. The higher pressure is used most frequently. When this therapy is initiated, the pressure range may be 12 to 15 cm water and gradually increased by 1 to 2 cm until the maximum of 20 cm water is reached. In some clinical conditions such as pulmonary edema, hemorrhage, shock, or cardiac failure, a lower inspiratory pressure of 10 to 15 cm is used.

IPPB therapy is usually administered three or four times during each 24-hour interval for 20 minutes each time. The nurse should check the unit frequently to ascertain that the pressure is maintained and there is no leakage in the system. Until the patient has been taught how to use this equipment, the nurse should stay with him to give assurance and emotional support.

The gas mixtures include 100 percent oxygen, oxygen diluted with air, and 40 percent oxygen–60 percent helium. Oxygen diluted with air is the most widely used type. If 100 percent oxygen is used the patient must be observed frequently for symptoms of atelectasis.

Inhalant Therapy

An inhalant may be in the form of drugs or moisture administered to the nose, throat, or lungs by means of steam, an atomizer, or a nebulizer.

Steam generates moisture, which is inhaled. This prevents drying of the mucous membranes, assists in relieving inflammation of the mucous membranes in the nose, sinuses, and larynx, and softens thick tenacious mucus. The moisture also relieves cough. Plain water can be used, or the physician may order that an appropriate agent be added to the water. A steam inhalator will produce moist steam in close proximity to the patient, but the equipment must not be so close to him that the steam might burn him. A tent may be devised from a bath blanket over the head of the bed to concentrate the moisture. All doors and windows should be closed. The inhalator must be kept filled with water or it will boil dry.

An atomizer is used for direct spraying to the nose, throat, or lungs. The patient inhales the fine mist.

Nebulization is achieved by connecting the oxygen tube from the nasal catheter or face mask to the nebulizer. Oxygen flowing through the nebulizer carries the medicated mist to the lungs. In some instances the mouthpiece of the nebulizer is placed in the patient's mouth and with inhalation the medicated mist is pulled into the throat and lungs. The physician prescribes the medication to be used.

Tracheostomy

If tracheal suctioning and bronchoscopy are not sufficient to remove secretions in the severely ill patient, a tracheostomy may be required to allow for suctioning of secretions. Tracheostomy is the surgical creation of an artificial opening from the exterior of the neck through the tracheotomic triangle into the trachea which provides an airway from the exterior of the body into the trachea. The tracheostomy is maintained by the use of a double tube, an outer tube or cannula and an inner tube or cannula. The outer tube is fitted into the passageway with an obturator at the time of the operation to keep the lumen of the incision open and remains in place until the physician changes it. It may be removed and another outer cannula inserted if it becomes clogged with dried secretions that block insertion of the inner tube or interfere with respirations. The inner tube is inserted into the outer tube. These tubes must be clear of mucus secretions to ensure that the patient has a patent airway. The inner tube is removed by the nurse and cleaned as often as necessary to keep it free of secretions.

The inner tube is cleaned by placing it in a container of solution as prescribed by the physician, to soak and loosen the adhering secretions, then placing it in a basin and scrubbing it with a brush until it is clean. It may then be sterilized. If the inner tube is reinserted immediately after cleaning and not sterilized, all excess moisture should be removed to prevent inhalation of fluid into the bronchi. Each tracheostomy set has a minimum of two inner tubes. While one is being cleaned, the other is inserted into the outer tube. A second complete sterile tracheostomy set is kept at the bedside, to be used if the outer cannula must be changed. Each metal set of outer and inner tubes and obturator is matched and the parts should be kept together or they will not fit properly.

If the patient is producing large amounts of mucus or if the mucus is thick and tenacious, the inner tube is removed and the outer tube is suctioned to clear it of all secretions and to assist him in expelling sputum. To suction the tracheostomy passage the inner tube is removed, a catheter that will fit into the outer tube is connected via a Y tube to a suction machine, and the catheter is quickly and gently inserted into the tube as far as the distal end of the tube. The suction machine is started and suction is initiated by placing the thumb over the open branch of the Y tube. The catheter is withdrawn quickly and gently with a rotating motion. If the passageway is not clear the procedure is repeated. If the secretions are thick and tenacious, it may be necessary to repeat the procedure several times and to draw sterile water through the catheter between repetitions to keep the catheter open and the suctioning effective. The suction equipment is kept at the bedside for quick and easy use. It is cleaned following the conclusion of the procedure.

Oxygen is administered to the patient with a tracheostomy as already discussed, except that a special adapter is connected directly to the tracheostomy tube. The end of the adapter fits tightly around the end of the tracheostomy tube and prevents escape of oxygen from around the tube. The nurse must be sure that the adapter is properly attached in order for the patient to receive the maximum benefit.

INCISION AND DRAINAGE

Nursing care for the patient with an incision and drainage is the same as for any surgical patient. The wound should be considered a dirty wound and aseptic technique should be used in cleansing the area, changing the dressing, and disposing of the dressings. The type of drainage should be watched and reported to the physician. If drainage stops the physician should be notified immediately. Antibiotics are administered as prescribed by the physician.

Thoracentesis

The nurse procures the thoracentesis equipment and places the patient in the proper position as described earlier in this chapter. Before the procedure is begun the nurse should explain it to the patient and warn him not to cough during the procedure. During the procedure the nurse should watch the patient for change of skin color and changes in pulse and/or respiratory rate, and report these to the doctor. She may assist in supporting the patient during the thoracentesis. Following the procedure the patient should be closely observed for change in respiratory rate or coughing or expectoration of blood or blood-tinged sputum, and report any of these changes to the physician immediately. A change in the respiratory rate may be indicative of hemorrhage or pneumothorax and the physician will have to administer the proper measures. The dressing at the site of the thoracentesis should be watched for any bleeding and reported to the physician.

DISORDERS OF THE NOSE AND THROAT

Acute Allergic Rhinitis

This condition is also known as *hay fever, vasomotor rhinitis,* and *perennial allergy.*

Acute allergic rhinitis is a hypersensitive reaction of the mucosa of the nasal and paranasal sinuses to an air-borne antigen. In most cases the antigen is a dust or plant pollen. It is estimated that 19 million individuals in the United States have allergies and of these 12½ million have acute allergic rhinitis or asthma. The reaction may be seasonal or perennial. The reaction and treatment are basically similar in both types, except that perennial allergic rhinitis continues throughout the year. Prevention is based on ascertaining the etiological agent and avoiding it.

The agent may be dust from many sources such as feathers, rugs, or curtains; animals; and pollens from plants such as grasses, weeds, trees, or flowers.

The reaction is different from the inflammatory process in that there is dilatation of the blood vessels and swelling of the mucosa and submucosa of the nose and paranasal sinuses and infiltration of eosinophilic and sometimes neutrophilic cells into the submucosa. Histamine is released into the nasal and paranasal sinus mucosa.

The prognosis is good, but repeated attacks may lead to chronic sinusitis, nasal polyps, or asthma. It is estimated that asthma will develop in one-third of these individuals.

There is a sudden onset of persistent sneezing, itching of the nose and sometimes the eyes, watery secretions from the nose and eyes, and obstruction of the nasal passage.

The nasal mucosa appears pale to red, is spongy, and at times is edematous. The usual physical examination is performed. A history of previous allergic reactions may be obtained. Laboratory examination of nasal secretions demonstrates eosinophilic cells. Skin tests may be employed to determine the etiologic agent.

Therapy involves removing the allergen or antigen from the patient's environment; an air purifier is used if the allergen cannot be removed. Symptomatic relief of discomfort may be obtained through use of antihistaminic drugs. If the reaction is severe and continuous, injections of extracts of the allergen may produce hyposensitivity to it. These extracts contain only the antigens or allergens specific to the individual and are administered initially in a dose below the dilution that will cause a reaction to the skin test. Gradually the concentration of the allergen is increased at intervals of 5 to 7 days until the individual can tolerate the maximum concentration. This desensitization period varies with individuals and desensitization must be repeated as necessary.

These patients are rarely hospitalized, therefore the nursing care is mainly one of educating the patient and the public in regard to allergic reaction, administration and reactions to the medication prescribed, and removal of the allergen from the environment. The individual must be reminded to buy or rent a true air purifier rather than an air conditioner.

Infections

ACUTE RHINITIS

Acute rhinitis is also known as *common cold, acute coryza,* or *common upper respiratory infection.*

Acute rhinitis is an infectious disease that is endemic throughout the world. There are no reliable statistics on the incidence of this disease, as it is not reportable and the majority of infected individuals seek medical assistance only when the problem appears to overwhelm them.

Prevention is dependent upon the self-isolation of the infected individual; covering the nose and mouth when sneezing, coughing, laughing, and talking; and the proper disposal or sterilization of all articles contaminated with the discharges of the nose, mouth, and throat. The education of all individuals to these preventive measures and their use by all individuals at the first sign or symptom of the infection is the chief method of controlling this disease. An episode of this infection does not appear to produce any lasting immunity. Various measures including vaccines have been attempted and recommended for preventing acute rhinitis but thus far none have proven to be completely efficacious. These have included polybacterial vaccines, massive doses of vitamin C taken routinely, large doses of multivitamin preparations, or vitamins A and D taken routinely to help prevent the development of acute rhinitis. At this writing there is no prophylaxis that has been proven to be beneficial to the majority of individuals. This infection develops in all age groups. Predisposing factors include lowered resistance to infections as a result of fatigue, overexposure to cold, another recent infection, a coexisting infection, allergic reactions, and the inhalation of irritating dust or gases.

The etiological agent is one of several filterable viruses. The source of infection is the secretions discharged from the nose and throat of an infected individual.

The nasopharyngeal mucosa becomes inflamed followed by edema and engorgement. A clear watery exudate is discharged from the mucosa and excreted through the nose. The exudate may become purulent if the infection continues since there is opportunity for pathogens normally present in the flora of the nose and throat to initiate minor inflammatory reactions. Engorgement of the nasal mucosa may cause temporary unilateral or bilateral nasal obstruction.

Resolution of the infection normally occurs in 4 to 10 days if no extension of the infection or complications from other microorganisms develop. Complications that may develop are acute sinusitis, acute adenoiditis, acute tonsillitis, acute eustachitis, acute laryngitis, acute pharyngitis, acute tracheitis, and acute bronchitis.

The onset is abrupt to 48 hours. It is characterized by a chilling sensation, scratchy throat, sneezing, watering of the eyes, watery rhinorrhea, nonproductive cough, and varying degrees of general malaise. There may be a mild pyrexia, moderate headache, and aching of the back and lower extremities. As the infection progresses there is a temporary loss of the senses of smell and taste; secretions of the nasal mucosa increase in amount and density causing frequent coughing due to local irritation of the pharynx, and frequent blowing and almost constant sniffling of the nose. The external nares become excoriated. Partial or complete obstruction of the nasal passages produces mouth breathing, and the lips and tongue become dry and parched.

Diagnosis is not easily made. Direct visual examination of the nasal mucosa reveals it to be hyperemic, swollen, and covered with a serous exudate. These factors correlated with the clinical manifestations may lead to the diagnosis. However, these factors may be the manifestations of other diseases such as diphtheria, measles, whooping cough, meningitis, streptococcal pharyngitis, influenza, and allergic rhinitis. Laboratory tests are of little value in identifying the etiological agent except that leukocytosis indicates the presence of an infection other than acute rhinitis. A complete physical examination, history, and laboratory tests are performed as in all illnesses.

The aim of therapy is to control the infection, prevent its extension to other anatomical structures, protect the individual from exposure to other communicable diseases, and prevent the exposure and spread of the infection to uninfected individuals. Bed rest for the patient with pyrexia is necessary until the temperature is normal in order to protect him from fatigue, exposure to chilling, and exposure to other infection, and to assist the body responses in combating the infection. A high fluid intake and a balanced light diet are usually prescribed and in most cases acetylsalicylic acid 0.3 to 0.6 g (5 to 10 grains) is prescribed to assist in alleviating the pyrexia and discomfort of the headache, backache, and aching of lower extremities. In the early stages antipyretics and analgesics may be prescribed. Those containing codeine assist in controlling the cough and those that decrease the secretions of the nasal mucosa are useful in decreasing discharges from the nose. When the nasal secretions become thick and purulent, nose drops or a nasal inhaler may be prescribed to facilitate local shrinking and drying of the nasal mucosa but should not be used oftener than every 3 or 4 hours. If a croupy cough or thick tenacious sputum develops, steam inhalations may be prescribed. Expectorants may be ordered to improve the liquefaction of bronchial secretions. The early use of antihistamines has not proven to be successful in aborting the common cold. Antibiotics presently available are not effective against the etiologic agents of acute rhinitis and usually are not prescribed except when bacterial extension or complications are suspected or present.

The infected individual usually is not seen in the hospital. The role of the nurse is to educate the infected individual in how to administer the prescribed therapy, protect other people, and to educate the public to avoid the infection.

CHRONIC HYPERPLASTIC RHINITIS

Chronic hypertrophic rhinitis, chronic coryza, and *polypoid rhinitis* are synonyms.

Chronic hyperplastic rhinitis is a chronic inflammation of the mucosa of the nose and is characterized by thickening and hyperplasia of the nasal mucosa leading to nasal obstruction. Epidemiological figures are not available concerning this respiratory problem.

Preventive measures include avoiding conditions that can result in chronic or recurring nasal irritations, allergic rhinitis, and infections.

The etiologic agent is unknown. Suggested agents include repeated irritation from dusts and chemical fumes, constant cold or excessive dry heat and air, continual infections in the nose or paranasal sinuses, and endocrine imbalance. The role of these factors separately or in combination has not been established. Predisposing factors are repeated upper respiratory infections, chronic sinusitis, nasal obstruction due to septal deviation, bony spurs on the turbinates, and polyps, debility, and poor nasal hygiene.

The changes in the nasal passages are the same as seen in any area of inflammation and hypertrophy. The walls of the blood vessels thicken and dilate, interstitial fibrosis develops, and the mucous glands become enlarged.

The prognosis is fair to good depending on the etiological agent. If the cause is septal deviation or polyps, surgical correction may relieve the condition. Chronic rhinitis is not fatal, but it may predispose to other respiratory problems.

The clinical manifestations are those of nasal obstruction. The individual is unable to breathe through the nose and has a thin watery mucus secretion from the nose and paranasal areas. Usually there is a moderate headache, and the patient is easily fatigued.

A complete physical examination is done. Direct visual examination of the nasal passages reveals red, swollen turbinates. The mucosa often is purplish and coated with a thin sticky secretion. The posterior tips of the turbinates may be swollen and pale. There are no specific laboratory tests.

The goal of therapy is to restore a nasal airway by eliminating infections of the sinuses, pharynx, and larynx with use of the appropriate therapy. If allergy is a factor, desensitization may be carried out. If a septal deviation, a polyp, or hypertrophied turbinates are present they can be removed surgically.

Deviated Septum. Correction of a deviated septum is usually performed under local anesthesia. A bent or deviated septum may be congenital or the result of trauma, a fracture, or recurrent rhinitis. The bony and cartilaginous septa are incised through the nares and the protruding or enlarged section of the bone and cartilage is resected to allow for straightening of the septum. This operation is termed a *submucous resection.* After the incision is sutured, the nasal passage is packed with gauze and held in place with a nasal bandage secured with adhesive tape across the exterior of the nares. If a tampon is used in place of gauze packing, the attached string must be securely taped to the side of the upper lip or lower cheek with adhesive tape to prevent it from slipping through the nasal passage into the pharyngeal area and causing obstruction.

Nasal Polyps. A polyp is a pedunculated nodule composed of neoplastic tissue or other structures and is found especially on mucous membranes. Most nasal polyps are composed of mucous membrane and loose connective tissue. Removal through the nasal passage is accomplished by snipping the connecting fiber where attached to the nasal mucosa. This surgical procedure is a *polypectomy* and may be performed in the physician's office. There is little bleeding and the patient is instructed not to blow the nose for 24 to 48 hours.

Hypertrophied Turbinated Bones. This procedure is similar to a submucous resection except that the hypertrophied turbinates are removed. It is termed a *turbinectomy.*

The nursing care for chronic hyperplastic rhinitis is similar to the nursing care for acute rhinitis except in the patient who has had nasal surgery. The basic nursing care encompasses the nursing care for nasal surgery. This includes the following: nothing by mouth for at least 6 hours preoperatively to prevent nausea and vomiting; preoperative medication with a sedative and an anticholinergic drug such as atropine; enemas preoperatively to empty the lower intestinal tract in order to ensure that postoperatively there will be more rapid evacuation of blood that was swallowed during the surgical procedure.

Postoperatively the nurse has many responsibilities. She checks to be sure that the nasal packing is securely in place; if it slips backward into the pharynx it can cause obstruction. If the packing is slipping or protruding and obstructing the patient's breathing the doctor should be notified immediately.

She observes for hemorrhage or excessive bleeding. This is evidenced by bright red blood on the external dressing or expectoration or vomiting of bright red blood, repeated swallowing, and rapid pulse. Oozing of blood onto the external dressing is normal but soaking of the dressing is a sign of hemorrhage. The nurse should notify the surgeon immediately and bring the emergency dressing tray to the bedside. If the external dressing becomes soiled it may be changed. A soiled dressing is uncomfortable, is disgusting in appearance, and may give off an offensive odor. Thus for the comfort and esthetics of the patient the nurse may remove the adhesive tape and the exterior gauze and replace it. She administers sedatives as prescribed because of the discomfort resulting from the surgery and the pressure packing. She reassures the patient that the packing will be removed in 24 to 48 hours if bleeding has stopped. She encourages the expectoration of any blood oozing into the pharynx, as blood is irritating to the gastrointestinal tract and can produce nausea and vomiting. A cool or ice compress may be applied to the nose. In other respects care is the same as for any surgical patient.

ACUTE SINUSITIS

Acute sinusitis is an inflammation of the accessory nasal sinuses or an infection of one or more of the paranasal sinuses. The epidemiology of this problem is not currently available because the condition is not reportable.

Acute sinusitis is averted by preventing other upper respiratory problems, maintaining a patent nasal airway when the nasal passage is infected, and practicing good dental hygiene.

Acute sinusitis may be initiated by one of several microorganisms. The usual microorganisms infecting the paranasal orifices are filterable viruses of acute rhinitis, staphylococci, streptococci, and pneumococci. The infecting microorganism may invade the sinuses from an infection in the respiratory tract or dental abscess.

The paranasal sinuses respond to the invasion of a microorganism in the same way as any tissue reacts to invasion or injury. The infection and inflammation usually start in one sinus, frequently the maxillary sinus, and spread rapidly to the other paranasal sinuses.

The prognosis is excellent.

The onset of signs and symptoms may be sudden or gradual and concurrent with another infection of the respiratory tract. Characteristic signs and symptoms are moderate to severe headache in the area of one or more of the sinuses, nasal and postnasal discharge of either water or purulent secretions, and general malaise. These manifestations may be quickly followed by pyrexia, vertigo, anorexia, photophobia, anosmia, toothache, impaired hearing, general aching, and periorbital edema. There may be tenderness to pressure in the area of the infected sinuses. Pyrexia varies with the severity of the infection, ranging from 100 to 103° F (37.7 to 39.4° C). If the temperature rises higher than 103° F (39.4 C) it suggests the development of a complicating infection in the respiratory tract.

The diagnosis is made by complete physical examination, direct visual examination of the nasal passage and turbinates, and x-ray study and transillumination of the paranasal sinus.

The aim of therapy is to produce an unobstructed air passage into the nasal and paranasal sinuses thereby providing an adequate drainage tract from the paranasal sinus to the exterior of the body. Febrile patients are placed on bed rest, and fluids are forced. Nose drops, vasoconstrictors, anodynes, antibiotics, and steam inhalations may be prescribed. If the paranasal sinuses are blocked and do not respond to therapy, the physician may suction the nasal passages. When thick tenacious mucus or a purulent discharge is present in the maxillary sinus the physician may irrigate the area by puncturing the antrum. Under local anesthesia a trocar is advanced through the walls of the sinus between the inferior meatus, or a cannula is passed through the ostium of the middle meatus. Usually sterile normal saline is used to irrigate the area and drain back through the cannula and connecting tubing in the nose into a receptacle. The nurse assists with this procedure by supporting the back of the patient's head and holding the head in the proper position as prescribed by the physician. The procedure is usually painless; the nurse can reassure the patient that what he will feel will probably be the pressure exerted in puncturing the antrum or from the cannula.

Malignant Tumors of the Larynx

The most common tumor of the larynx is squamous cell carcinoma, although it is not a leading cause of cancer deaths. For unknown reasons the carcinoma occurs 10 times as often in males as in females and usually after the age of 40.

Means of preventing squamous carcinoma are unknown. Predisposing factors seem to be chronic irritation, chronic laryngitis, continuous straining of the vocal cords, and smoking. Prevention would entail avoiding these predisposing factors. There appears to be evidence that smoking cigarettes and inhaling the smoke is the cause of the disease in some individuals.

The stratified squamous epithelium is thickened, and hyperkeratotic and inflammatory changes at the site are present. The carcinoma usually develops on the anterior third of one vocal cord and continues to spread to other cords. It follows the same growth pattern as other squamous carcinomas. At first there is a lesion at the site; later, there is wrinkling and thickening of the epithelium and gray plaque-like lesions are produced which ulcerate. The carcinoma may involve surrounding areas, the epiglottis, aryepiglottic folds, and the piniform sinuses. A carcinoma arising within the larynx is classified as intrinsic. It may destroy one or all of the vocal cords.

If the diagnosis is made early cure is possible but usually diagnosis is made late; survival studies show that only approximately 25 to 30 percent of patients survive for 5 years.

There may be no early manifestations, or the patient may be aware of a slight scratchiness or lump in the throat when swallowing. He may feel he must clear his throat frequently. Later, progressive hoarseness develops. He may have pain, difficulty in swallowing, and hemoptysis.

Diagnosis is established by direct visualization of the area by mirror or laryngoscopy with biopsy specimen or scrapings from the involved area. The cells are typical cancer cells.

These tumors are treated by x-ray, radiation, and radical surgery to the site.

The nursing care is the same as for any patient with carcinoma. The nurse must be aware of the fears the diagnosis of cancer produce in any patient and give him the psychological and emotional support needed at this time. She should reassure him that the therapy will assist him. The patient will have difficulty in talking and a pad and pencil should be provided at the bedside at all times to prevent him from straining his vocal cords when trying to speak, or after surgery when he will be unable to speak. If a laryngectomy is to be performed, the patient should know he will not be able to speak thereafter. Following surgery, he should be taught to speak through esophageal speech or an artificial larynx. When possible, a member of the local laryngectomee club should work with the patient to demonstrate and teach him how to talk. A speech therapist will work with the patient and the nurse should assist in this therapy when the therapist is not present. Usual tracheostomy care is administered when a tracheostomy has been performed. The patient's resistance is low at this time and the nurse should take necessary precautions against infections. She should assist the patient and teach him how to feed himself with the nasal esophageal catheter. Correct oral hygiene must be carried out before and after all procedures. After surgery the nurse should observe for hemoptysis and report its development immediately to the physician. Antibiotics are administered as prescribed by the physician.

DISORDERS OF THE CHEST

Bronchial Asthma

Asthma, allergic asthma, acute allergic asthma are synonyms.

Asthma is paroxysmal dyspnea. Bronchial asthma is usually defined as recurrent paroxysms of dyspnea with a characteristic wheezing. It is estimated that approximately 12½ million individuals in the United States have acute allergic rhinitis or asthma and that approximately one-third of those having acute allergic rhinitis will later have bronchial asthma.

Prevention is dependent upon avoiding the offending antigen or allergen. When it is impossible to avoid the antigen, hyposensitization or desensitization to the specific allergen should be accomplished as described for acute allergic rhinitis. Predisposing factors are changes in environmental temperature and humidity, exposure to fumes from chemicals, paint, and wax, fatigue and emotional tension, and psychological stress.

The primary etiological factor in bronchial asthma is atopy (an inherited allergic tendency). The etiologic agent is usually described as extrinsic or intrinsic and the reaction is called *extrinsic asthma* or *intrinsic asthma,* i.e., arising from some environmental factor or from within the body. Extrinsic asthma results from the inhalation of allergens such as pollen, animal dander, household dust, feather dust, lint, or insecticides or the ingestion of specific foods, protein, or drugs. Intrinsic asthma is a reaction to an etiological agent that induces respiratory infections such as hemolytic influenza, and pneumococcal and streptococcal infections. Emotional tension may be a predisposing factor to an asthma-like reaction.

Histamine is released into the bronchial mucosa. The bronchi and bronchioles contract in spasms thus narrowing the lumen of the bronchi and bronchioles. There is swelling and edema of the mucosa and the secretion of thick tenacious mucus, with an increase in the size and number of goblet cells in the bronchial epithelium. The muscles of the bronchial walls become hypertrophied and are infiltrated with mononuclear and eosinophilic cells. The submucosa is swollen. There is impaired movement of air through the narrowed bronchial passage, especially outward movement, and air may be trapped causing ballooning of the alveoli.

The prognosis is good since the reaction itself is rarely fatal. However, unless exposure to the allergen is controlled the reaction will recur with each contact. After many such episodes pulmonary emphysema often develops.

Manifestations may develop gradually in intrinsic asthma. In extrinsic asthma, however, the onset is abrupt with dyspnea, a sense of tightness in the chest, a feeling of impending suffocation, wheezing without increased respiration, and a slight dry cough. The patient must sit up to breathe, he has an anxious expression, and he perspires freely. If the reaction does not subside the individual will continue to experience manifestations; the cough will increase and become productive of clear mucus followed by thick tenacious mucus. The patient may expectorate mucus plugs. Usually the reaction subsides within an hour but may continue for several hours. If it is not controlled status asthmaticus may develop. In this stage the patient has severe dyspnea, he must sit up to breathe, he is haggard and anxious, and his chest is distended. He may be cyanotic. All the accessory muscles of respiration are working and diaphoresis is present.

A routine physical examination is done. The patient usually gives a history of previous reactions but if this is the initial attack other respiratory problems must be ruled out, such as a foreign body or a tumor in the bronchi. Sputum studies may demonstrate the presence of eosinophils and Curschmann's spirals. Blood tests may demonstrate the presence of eosinophils. A chest x-ray film may rule out other etiological agents, but is not especially helpful because bronchial asthma has no characteristic roentgenographic manifestations. Occasionally bronchoscopy is performed to rule out the presence of a foreign body or a tumor, but this procedure usually is not carried out during an abrupt fulminating reaction. Skin testing may be helpful in diagnosing an extrinsic cause but not an intrinsic one. Sputum studies may reveal the intrinsic etiological factor but are not specific because micro-organisms are normally present in the throat.

The goal of therapy is to provide immediate symptomatic relief, eliminate the allergen, and prevent future reactions. Medication is prescribed to relax the bronchial spasms immediately. Usually epinephrine is given subcutaneously or intramuscularly; aminophylline may be administered intravenously in status asthmaticus. Bed rest is prescribed as discussed earlier. Fluids are forced to counteract dehydration. Oxygen may be administered in severe prolonged episodes. Intratracheal suction may be performed by the physician to clear the bronchial airway of thick tenacious sputum. If the reaction has an extrinsic basis desensitizing injections may be started when the reaction has subsided. If the reaction has an intrinsic basis the infection is treated with antimicrobials. Antihistamines are usually not prescribed as they appear to be relatively ineffective.

During an acute reaction the nurse should assist the patient in obtaining oxygen as easily as possible. She should place him in a sitting position, place a padded overbed table in front of him for him to lean on, and pull up the bed rail to protect him from falling. His back and sides should be supported with pillows to lessen the strain of maintaining the upright position in bed. She should administer the prescribed medication quickly, and stay with the patient, reassuring him that he will not suffocate and giving him emotional support. His face should be bathed with a cool washcloth to help refresh him and remove perspiration. The area must be kept free of drafts because the patient's skin is damp and the chilling effect may encourage other respiratory problems. Decubitus ulcers should be prevented. When the acute reaction has subsided she should encourage the patient to rest. She should continually observe for possible precipitating causes of the reaction. Traffic in the patient's area and visitors to him should be minimized to decrease exposure of the patient to dust and other possible causative agents. If he is receiving desensitizing or hyposensitizing therapy the nurse must be alert to local or systemic allergic reaction and report it to the physician immediately.

Infections

PNEUMONIA

Pneumonitis is a synonym.

Pneumonia is an inflammation of the lungs. It is endemic throughout the world, especially during inclement weather. It is the fourth leading cause of death in the United States.

Prevention is dependent upon isolating the infected individual when the etiological agent is a bacterium. If the etiological agent is nonbacterial it must be controlled by appropriate measures, such as preventing inhalation of the agent and frequently changing the position of the bedridden patient to prevent hypostatic pneumonia.

Predisposing factors to pneumonia are lowered resistance to infection due to current or recent upper respiratory infection, a debilitating disease, overexposure to chilling, fatigue, alcoholism, trauma to the chest, inhalation of irritating chemical fumes or gases, aspiration of foreign bodies, and inhalation of microorganisms. Pneumonia affects all age groups but is more frequent in the very young and the elderly.

Pneumonia may be caused by a nonbacterial agent, such as inhalation of irritating chemical fumes or gases, or aspiration of any fluid, oily substance, or foreign body, or by a bacterial agent. The microorganism may be a bacillus, coccus, virus, fungus, rickettsia, protozoon, parasite, or an unidentified agent. Bacteria cause the greatest number of cases of pneumonia.

The inflammatory response ensues (see Chapter 11). Briefly, the capillaries are engorged, and the alveoli are partially or completely filled with serous fluid containing red blood cells, polymorphonuclear leukocytes, and bacteria. There is an increase in leukocytes and a decrease in bacteria; the red cells disintegrate and are removed. Gray hepatization occurs, i.e., the lung is gray and of solid consistency, the alveoli are filled with leukocytes, and mononuclear phagocytes appear. Resolution of the inflammatory response occurs with gradual change in the gray color and solid consistency. Dissolved fibrin and liquefied exudate are removed, and air can enter the involved areas. Tissue regeneration takes place.

The prognosis generally is good.

Usually there is an abrupt onset of pyrexia of 102 to 105° F (38.5 to 40.5° C), malaise, chills, diaphoresis, flushed face, headache, chest pain, nonproductive cough followed by production of sputum that may be rust colored. The pulse is 100 to 130 per minute, there is shallow and labored dyspnea with a characteristic grunt on exhalation. Delirium, cyanosis, and anorexia develop. The patient may be nauseated and vomit and tympanites on the affected side may develop.

Physical examination reveals characteristic manifestations; x-ray examination demonstrates opaque areas; laboratory tests of sputum demonstrate the microorganism.

The aim of therapy is to control and cure the infection, prevent the development of complicating problems in other body structures, protect the individual from exposure to other communicable diseases, and prevent exposure and spread of the infection to uninfected individuals. Bed rest during periods of pyrexia is necessary to assist the body responses in combating the infection, and to protect other body structures from overexertion. Fluids are forced and intravenous fluids are given to assist in preventing dehydration. Analgesics for pain may be narcotic or nonnarcotic; morphine sulfate is used sparingly because of its effect on the central respiratory center. Expectorants are employed to raise the sputum, but if no sputum is present, demulcents may be used to control cough. Sedatives or hypnotics may be ordered to encourage sleep. Oxygen therapy by nasal catheter, mask, or tent is usually administered. The specific antibiotic to be employed is determined on the basis of the etiological agent and the organism's sensitivity.

The nursing care is similar to that for any seriously ill patient. The patient must have bed rest. His position is changed frequently in order to maintain good general circulation and prevent pooling of fluids, prevent the development of pressure areas, and ensure comfort. The nurse should bathe the patient during this period. Good mouth care is essential because the patient is breathing through the mouth and raising sputum. The environment should be quiet with a minimum of traffic in order to ensure rest, prevent exposure to other possible causative agents, and prevent exposure of uninfected individuals. The patient should cover his mouth when coughing and should use disposable tissues. If coughing causes pain the nurse may assist in splinting the chest with her hands. When diaphoresis is present, the patient should be kept dry and comfortable by frequent change of bed linen and clothing, and should be protected from exposure to drafts and chilling. Signs and symptoms of sensitivity to the antibiotic must be watched for. Isolation technique should be employed throughout this period (see Chapter 20).

INFLUENZA

Influenza is also known as *flu, la grippe, grippe,* and *catarrhal fever.*

Influenza is an inflammation of the mucous membrane of the respiratory tract. It is sporadic or epidemic throughout the world and has been pandemic. To some degree epidemics can be predicted on the basis of knowledge about the etiological agent. Each year a few cases are reported sporadically throughout the world. The incidence is higher in infants and elderly individuals than in younger age groups.

Four types of filterable viruses have been identified, designated A, B, C, and D. Type A, B, or C is generally the causative organism during epidemics. A limited immunity appears to be produced by each virus which is specific and does not protect against the other strains. The virus is air-borne via secretions from the nose, throat, and mouth. Contaminated articles may contribute also. The incubation period usually is 18 to 36 hours. Predisposing factors are the same as for any communicable disease.

There is an inflammation of the mucous membranes of the respiratory tract which usually is limited to the epithelium. There may be thickening or sloughing of the epithelium.

The prognosis is usually good.

The onset is sudden, with chills or a chilling sensation, pyrexia of 101 to 104° F (38.3 to 40° C). There is generalized aching of the muscles especially of the back and legs, headache, general malaise, and anorexia. The face is flushed, the throat is moderately sore, there is an unproductive cough and moderate coryza, and there may be slight sternal pain. The duration usually is 2 to 5 days.

Diagnosis is based upon the physical examination, direct visual examination of the throat, pharyngeal swabbing, biopsy specimen, and laboratory cultures of secretions.

The treatment is as for any acute respiratory infection as discussed earlier. No specific therapy is available at present.

The patient should be isolated and communicable disease aseptic technique carried out to protect the patient from exposure to other infections and to protect uninfected persons. (See Chapter 20.)

LUNG ABSCESS

Pulmonary abscess is another term often used.

A lung abscess is a localized collection of pus in the lung tissues. It must be differentiated from other disorders of lung tissues. Lung abscess is not a common respiratory problem.

Several organisms may cause this condition, including *Staphylococcus aureus* and *Entamoeba histolytica*. Occlusion due to a neoplasm, intrabronchial foreign body, intrabronchial mucus plug, bronchial obstruction due to embolus, trauma to the chest, and nonspecific infection are other causes. Predisposing factors are infection of the respiratory tract, infection elsewhere in the body, inhalation of a foreign body, and neoplasm in the lung.

Lung abscess usually occurs singly and usually is unilateral. The inflammatory process is characteristic. The abscess ruptures into the bronchus, the material is expectorated, and a cavity remains. If drainage is adequate the walls of the cavity collapse, contract, and heal together. If drainage is inadequate the abscess becomes fibrotic and rigid and healing is delayed. Predisposing factors are malnutrition, alcoholism, or debilitation from a recent or chronic illness.

The prognosis usually is good.

The onset usually is sudden, with malaise, diaphoresis, chills, headache, generalized aching, anorexia, chest pain, and pyrexia. The manifestations are very similar to those of pneumonia. Generally the cough is nonproductive until the abscess ruptures. Hemoptysis may immediately precede rupture.

Physical examination reveals dullness in the area and suppressed fine to medium moist breath sounds. X-ray examination demonstrates a fluid level in the area. Differential diagnosis to rule out other respiratory problems is based on the findings of sputum culture, tonography, bronchoscopy, and bronchography.

Lung abscess is treated like any respiratory infection, as described under therapy in this chapter. The most important aspect of therapy is administration of antibiotics. After the abscess ruptures postural drainage may be prescribed. If the drainage from the abscess is inadequate a surgical resection may be performed.

Nursing care is as for any respiratory problem. Nursing care in surgical resection is discussed under tuberculosis.

COCCIDIOIDOMYCOSIS

Coccidioidal granuloma, valley fever, San Joaquin Valley fever, desert rheumatism, Posadas-Wernicke disease, the bumps are synonyms. Coccidioidomycosis is a highly infectious fungus disease that occurs in a primary and a progressive form. It is endemic in the southern areas of California, Arizona, New Mexico, and western Texas. It appears to affect both sexes in about equal numbers and of all ages. An individual who has had this infection or was exposed to it and inhaled the fungus without having clinical manifestations of the disease appears to have immunity. Negroes, Mexicans, and Filipinos appear to have less resistance than Caucasians.

The causative organism is *Coccidioides immitis*. The spores of the fungus become mixed with the dust of the soil and are inhaled when the dust is blown about. The incubation period is 7 days to 3 weeks. Coccidioidomycosis may be contracted by travelers passing through the area during a period when the air contains dust, especially during a wind storm or on a windy day.

A granulomatous process results from the inhalation of the fungus spores and nodules form on the walls of the bronchi. If these nodules rupture the spores may be disseminated by phagocytes via the blood and lymph and an infectious process may develop at the site where they lodge. In the lungs the process of infection is the same as any other infectious process and with healing there is scar tissue, caseation, and calcification of cavitation.

The prognosis usually is good except when the infection is disseminated throughout the body.

Manifestations are similar to those of other respiratory infections in the early stages. There is pyrexia up to 104° F (40° C), general malaise, general aching of muscles and joints, possibly chest pain on inspiration, and an unproductive cough. Nodules may appear on the forearms and shins which develop rather rapidly, or the infectious process may continue with a resulting breakdown of the tissue and the formation of an ulcer that heals gradually. There may be signs and symptoms of pneumonia or acute bronchitis.

X-ray examination, a positive intradermal coccidioidin test, and demonstration of *C. immitis* in smears from sputum or gastric washings are diagnostic.

Isolation and bed rest until pyrexia subsides are ordered. At present only amphotericin B administered intravenously is useful, but months of treatment may be required. If cavitation does not respond to drug therapy a resection may be performed.

The nurse should maintain communicable disease isolation technique. The fungus forms spores and may be transmitted by dust, so the environment should be kept free of all dust through control of traffic to the area. General nursing care measures should be carried out.

ACUTE BRONCHITIS

Tracheobronchial bronchitis is another term for acute bronchitis.

An acute inflammation of the trachea and bronchi, acute bronchitis occurs frequently in the winter, and it is seen sporadically throughout the world. Predisposing factors are as for other acute respiratory infections; it may develop during the course of another acute respiratory infection.

The etiological agent is usually the same one that caused the preceding respiratory infection, or it may be caused by the inhalation of irritating chemical fumes or irritating dusts.

There is hyperemia of the mucous membranes, desquamation, edema, leukocytic infiltration of the submucosa, and tenacious mucopurulent exudate in the trachea and bronchial tree. The prognosis is usually good. The disease tends to be self-limiting.

The onset is gradual, with coryza, sore throat, malaise, chilliness, and general aching of back and muscles. Symptoms increase with development of a dry unproductive cough, which gradually changes to a productive cough. There is pyrexia of 99 to 102° F (37.2 to 38.8° C). Symptoms subside within 3 to 5 days, with cough persisting for 2 to 3 weeks.

Physical examination and direct examination of the trachea are performed. Laboratory and diagnostic examinations differentiate this disorder from pulmonary tuberculosis, pneumonia, influenza, sinusitis, left heart failure, aortic aneurysm, pericarditis, pleurisy, or other respiratory infections.

Bed rest and forced fluids are prescribed for pyrexia, and a bland diet, sedatives, expectorants, demulcents, or steam inhalation may be prescribed. Analgesics may be prescribed for pain or sore throat, backache, and muscle aching, as well as antibiotics.

The individual is usually kept at home. The nurse's main function is to educate the patient and his family in the administration of drugs and protection of uninfected individuals and the isolation of the patient at home. General nursing care measures are carried out.

Chronic bronchitis or, simply, bronchitis is a long-standing or chronic disease of the tracheobronchial tree. It appears to occur more frequently in England and Wales and less frequently in the United States than in other geographical areas. Men of middle age or older are usually affected. Predisposing factors are recurrent respiratory infections, long exposure to irritating dusts or air pollution, and heavy smoking, especially of cigarettes.

There is no specific agent; any organism causing a respiratory problem except a fungus may be isolated in secretions from the tracheobronchial tree. The cause appears to be prolonged irritation of the mucous membranes of the bronchial tree with damage to the lining of the air passages.

The bronchial wall becomes thick and inelastic and the mucus-secreting glands become enlarged. The wall surface becomes dark red and may be trabeculated, with possible loss of cilia; the epithelium is deformed, being hypertrophied in some places and atrophied in others.

Chronic bronchitis has a poor prognosis. It is a slowly progressive disease which frequently is accompanied by other serious respiratory problems such as pulmonary fibrosis, obstructive emphysema, bronchiectasis, bronchial obstruction, chronic asthma, or chronic sinusitis.

The onset is insidious over a long period of time. The earliest sign usually is a persistent cough with a slight amount of sputum, often mistaken for a cigarette cough. The cough increases if another respiratory problem develops. There is an increase in sputum at night and during inclement weather, and the sputum may be moderate to thin and watery to purulent. The individual is afebrile and there is usually no change in white blood cell count or the erythrocyte sedimentation rate. Gradually the vital capacity diminishes with shortness of breath developing in the late stages of the disease.

Physical examination, laboratory tests, and x-ray examination are unrevealing. The bronchogram demonstrates cylindrical dilatation and irregularity of the bronchial tree. Pulmonary tuberculosis, emphysema, pulmonary fibrosis, bronchiectasis, pulmonary carcinoma, lung abscess, foreign body, silicosis, and fungus diseases must be excluded.

Helpful measures include maintenance of good nutrition, abstention from cigarette smoking, removal of the patient from the area of irritating inhalants, and avoidance of fatigue. During exacerbations expectorants, aerosols, bronchodilators, and antibiotics may be prescribed. A mild cough sedative may be prescribed to control paroxysms of coughing, and postural drainage employed especially if there is a coexisting respiratory infection.

PULMONARY TUBERCULOSIS

Pulmonary tuberculosis is also known as *phthisis, consumption, miner's complaint, tuberculosis,* and *Koch's disease.* Pulmonary tuberculosis is an infectious disease of the parenchyma of the lung, bronchi, bronchioles, alveoli, pleurae, and bronchopulmonary lymph nodes, and is characterized by the formation of tubercles. This disease is endemic throughout the world, and is found more often in urban areas than in rural areas. In the United States, the morbidity and mortality rates have been reduced dramatically in the past several years; currently the mortality rate is 4.1 per 100,000 population.[2] In other areas of the world pulmonary tuberculosis is still a leading cause of death although the use of BCG (bacille Calmette Guérin) vaccine is reducing the incidence. Predisposing factors are poor or overcrowded housing, poor nutrition, overwork, poor ventilation of home or working environment, emotional and psychological stress, lack of sleep, repeated respiratory infections, and in women repeated pregnancies.

Tuberculosis may occur in any part of the body but most often it is a pulmonary infection; this discussion is limited to the pulmonary form.

Primary infection usually occurs in children but can occur in any age group. Second infection or reinfection pulmonary tuberculosis can occur at any age and affects more men than women. In the United States it most commonly infects males 40 years of age or over.

Pulmonary tuberculosis is caused by *Mycobacterium tuberculosis,* which formerly was known as *Koch's bacillus.* This microorganism is spread by inhalation and is disseminated into the air by droplets of excretions from the nose, mouth, throat, and lungs of infected individuals. These droplets are disseminated by coughing, sneezing, talking, laughing, or the expulsion of air from the lungs. *M. tuberculosis* is nonmotile but is transported via air currents to any surface and can remain alive in a favorable environment outside the body for years, although it does not multiply outside the body. Infection by *M. tuberculosis* involves two phases of the disease, namely, a primary infection and a reinfection or second infection. In the primary infection the microorganism is inhaled into the lungs and implanted in the bronchial tree. The usual inflammatory process takes place with healing by resolution, fibrosis, and calcification. These calcified nodules remain permanently in the lungs and may retain live microorganisms within them. As a result the individual manifests an allergic reaction to the protein of *M. tuberculosis.* This allergic reaction will continue as long as live microorganisms remain within the body. Thus a tuberculin test will give a positive reaction.

Second infection or reinfection tuberculosis is usually referred to as *tuberculosis* or *pulmonary tuberculosis.* It results from endogenous or exogenous infection. If endogenous it may be from the primary infection or from tuberculosis in another area of the body; if exogenous it is from inhalation of *M. tuberculosis* after a primary infection has healed.

The remainder of this discussion deals only with second infection or reinfection pulmonary tuberculosis.

[2] National Tuberculosis Association, Tuberculosis Cases and Deaths by State, 1965, September 28, 1967, C-904.

The immediate inflammatory process is as described earlier in this chapter and in Chapter 11, but resolution and healing frequently follow a different course at the stage of suppuration. At this point there is caseation, necrosis, liquefaction, and cavitation and there may be bronchogenic spread to other areas of the lung or to the other lung. Healing may be by resolution. fibrosis, and calcification but when cavitation has developed healing is slow. The cavities are filled with the tubercle bacilli which are expelled via expired air and sputum. Areas of lung tissue may be destroyed and permanently scarred thereby decreasing the area of usable lung tissue for the exchange of gases within the lungs.

The prognosis is good if diagnosis is followed by maximum therapy.

The onset is insidious and clinical manifestations may not develop until after the inflammatory process has caused cavitation. Gradually the individual has a dry or productive cough and expectoration may be scant, thin, and watery to profuse and mucopurulent. Fatigue is noted especially upon arising, and there is general malaise, night sweats, anorexia, irritability, lack of endurance or strength, loss of weight, dyspnea, chest pain, hemoptysis, and in women menstrual disturbances or cessation. Other physical signs are pyrexia of 99 to 104° F (37.2 to 40° C), usually in the afternoon, low blood pressure, and pallor. The fingernails are brittle and there is curving on the long axis over the end of fingers with longitudinal ridges. Occasionally there is clubbing of the ends of the fingers, enlarged cervical lymph nodes, and muscle spasms in neck and shoulders.

Diagnosis is based on findings from the physical examination, history of clinical manifestations, and laboratory demonstration of the presence of M. *tuberculosis* through appropriate cultures. X-ray examination demonstrates the characteristic shadow, and the tuberculin test is positive. Specimens of the secretion may also be obtained by bronchoscopy. Differential diagnosis is necessary to rule out atypical tuberculosis, a disease resembling pulmonary tuberculosis but not responding to the same therapy

The individual is isolated until excretion of M. *tuberculosis* stops completely. The patient is kept on bed rest until the temperature becomes normal and stable. Streptomycin, para-aminosalicylic acid, and isoniazid are usually prescribed. If these cannot be administered because of allergy or other reasons several secondary drugs may be prescribed. If chemotherapy is not effective surgical procedures may be performed including segmental resection, lobectomy, pneumonectomy, thoracoplasty, and pneumoperitoneum. A pneumonectomy is the removal of an entire lung. A thoracoplasty is the removal of several ribs to allow the chest wall to collapse inwardly and collapse permanently a part of the lung. A pneumoperitoneum is the injection of a measured amount of air into the peritoneal cavity just below the diaphragm, pushing the diaphragm and lungs upward on the side where the air is injected, thereby relieving the tension of the lung and preventing full expansion of the lung.

General nursing measures are carried out. To give effective and efficient nursing care the nurse must not be afraid that she will become infected. When strict communicable disease or isolation technique is carried out by the nurse, she is in a safe environment and will not become infected by contact with the microorganism.

Effective nursing care involves assisting the patient in understanding and accepting his diagnosis in order that he may participate in his therapy. Without his assistance and cooperation, the therapy will be ineffective. He must understand the need to protect himself from self-spread or spread to others, and the need to follow the prescribed chemotherapy without interruption. He must understand that interruption to therapy will mean a relapse.

The patient needs strong emotional and psychological support in accepting this interference in his normal living pattern. He must understand that uninterrupted therapy must be maintained when he returns home. The treatment is long-term and may require months of hospitalization or home care with loss of income and changing social relationships.

Nursing Responsibilities in Surgical Resection. Nursing care in surgical resections covers the measures outlined elsewhere. Preoperatively the nurse helps the patient to understand the kind of surgery and the postoperative therapy he will receive in order that he may assist in his therapy. The patient should learn and practice the arm exercises he will have to do postoperatively. He must understand that he will have to cough frequently even though this will hurt. The nurse should teach him the proper way to cough and assist him in coughing with the least amount of pain possible. He must understand that he will have to use the arm on the operative side to prevent the dysfunction syndrome. He must understand that it is normal to have chest tubes and chest drainage following surgery and that he will be receiving medications parenterally and oxygen therapy. The nurse must allow him to express his fears of the surgery and assist him in overcoming his fears.

Postoperatively the nurse helps the patient cough at least every 2 hours by having him sit up and take several deep breaths; she supports and splints his chest over the incision while he coughs. She must be sure that the chest tubes are attached and draining properly; if the tubes are not draining properly she may milk them to clear any obstruction and reestablish drainage.

The surgery has collapsed the lung and interrupted the negative pleural pressure. Drainage of secretions and air from the area and reexpansion of the lung is accomplished through the use of chest tube drainage into a closed drainage system. A water-sealed drainage system is frequently used. The nurse must be sure that there are no leaks in the tubing and that the end of the glass tubing is below the water level of the bottle to prevent air from being sucked into the pleural space. The drainage system must be below the level of the chest so that drainage by gravity can be maintained and fluid and air are not forced back into the pleural space. The system should never be disconnected unless the tubing is clamped off between the chest and the area of disconnection.

The nurse must be sure that the drainage system is clear and allows drainage to flow into the drainage container. The fluid in the water-sealed system will fluctuate if the system is working. This should be checked frequently. If the fluctuation in the drainage container stops, the nurse must immediately check the tubing to see if it is blocked by exudate or obstructed by a kink, or if the patient is lying on it. When exudate is the cause of the blockage, milking the tube often helps to clear it. If the nurse is unable to clear the tube she should request assistance from her supervisor or the physician as quickly as possible. The patient should be encouraged to cough frequently and to breathe deeply in order to facilitate reexpansion of the lung by raising the intrapleural pressure. When the lung

Figure 22-5 A, Water-sealed drainage system. B, Three-bottle drainage system. See text for explanation. (Adapted with permission from Walter Bugden: Pulmonary Resection. American Journal of Nursing, 52:1:39, January, 1952, pp. 38–39.)

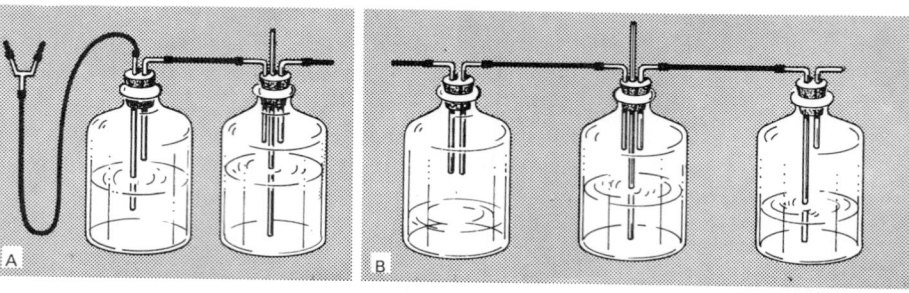

has reexpanded, the fluctuation of the fluid in the drainage bottle will stop, but the nurse must keep in mind that this usually occurs several days after surgery.

In Figure 22-5A, the Y tube is attached to the catheter or catheters that were inserted in the patient's pleural cavity during surgery, and connected with the water-sealed metal tube in the sterile drainage bottle. The bottle contains enough sterile water to cover the end of the metal tube at all times. A right-angle glass tube leads from the drainage bottle to the suction-regulating bottle, which is unsterile and contains tap water. The amount of suction depends on the depth— usually 10 cm—of the water in this bottle; the deeper the water the greater the suction force on the lung. An open glass tube extends from the outside to a point just above the bottom of the suction-regulating bottle. This prevents the development of excessive negative pressure within the system, thus acting as a safety valve. A right-angle glass tube leads from this bottle to the suction machine.

In Figure 22-5B, the first tube at the left is attached to the drainage catheter in the patient's pleural cavity. The drainage bottle is sterile and contains no water. An angulated glass tube leads from the drainage bottle to the suction-regulating bottle, which is unsterile and contains water to a depth of 5 cm. An open glass tube extends from the outside to just above the bottom of the bottle to permit room air to enter the system if negativity greater than 5 cm develops. An angulated glass tube leads from the suction-regulating bottle to an angulated tube, which reaches to about 1 cm from the bottom of a third bottle, which is unsterile and contains water to a depth of 2 cm. The extent of submersion determines the amount of positive pressure. When the tube is submersed more than +1 cm, air is displaced and bubbled off into the room.

The nurse should assist the patient in exercising his arm and in ambulating as prescribed. Non-narcotic sedatives are prescribed for pain and rest. The patient is observed for postsurgical complications.

Bronchogenic Carcinoma

Bronchogenic carcinoma is a malignant tumor occurring in the bronchi. It accounts for approximately 90 percent of carcinoma of the lungs, and in the western world for 10 percent of all male deaths at autopsy (Robbins). There has been a constant increase in the number of diagnosed cases in the past 35 years. The carcinoma is most common in men between the ages of 40 and 70.

The cause of bronchogenic carcinoma is unknown; however, there is evidence that it is associated with exposure to atmospheric fumes or air pollution, air-borne radiation among uranium miners, asbestos inhalation among asbestos workers, metastasis, and cigarette smoking with inhalation of the smoke. There is still much controversy as to whether cigarette smoking is responsible for the steady increase in this disease. The nurse should continue to be informed until proof of the cause is found. Prevention is aided by avoidance of the factors mentioned. Prevention of metastasis is aided by early diagnosis of cancer by means of a yearly complete physical examination.

Primary bronchogenic carcinoma generally arises in and around the hilus of the lung; the majority of lesions originate in the lower trachea, and the rest in the lower bronchi. There is a thickening of the bronchial mucosa which gradually increases until tumor formation and erosion of the area occur.

The prognosis is guarded. Average survival following diagnosis with radiation therapy is approximately 9 months to 2 years. With surgical removal of the primary tumor the patient may survive for 5 to 10 years; a few survive longer.

A chronic cough is usually the first symptom with scant mucoid sputum. Dyspnea arises at some time in the majority of patients. About half the patients complain of chest pain, hemoptysis, loss of weight, pyrexia, wheezing respiration, and cyanosis; clubbing of fingers and toes may occur as the disease progresses. Diagnosis is made by x-ray study, which demonstrates the discrete shadow that is typical, bronchoscopy with either direct visualization, and/or biopsy or microscopic examination of the bronchial secretions obtained during bronchoscopy.

Surgical removal of the tumor is usually the therapy of choice when metastasis to other areas has not occurred. Radiation therapy may be utilized if surgical therapy must be postponed, and may be employed following surgery. With the inoperable or recurrent bronchogenic carcinoma progressively increasing amounts of sedatives and/or narcotics are required to keep the patient comfortable.

The nursing care is the same as for any patient with carcinoma, and following surgical removal of the tumor the nursing care is as for other types of chest surgery. Many patients feel a sense of hopelessness upon learning the diagnosis. They need psychological and emotional support from the nurse. All medications should be given exactly as prescribed.

Other Disorders of the Chest
ATELECTASIS

Atelectasis is a collapsed or airless state of a portion of the lungs caused by occlusion of a bronchus. It occurs when a bronchus is obstructed for any reason.

Obstruction may be caused by a foreign body, mucus plug, bronchial tumor, or enlarged lymph node or extrinsic tumor compressing the bronchi. Limitation of movement of the respiratory muscles, elevation of the diaphragm, accumulations of viscid bronchial secretions, or suppression of the cough reflex may be a cause particularly during or following operations in the upper abdomen.

When the bronchus is occluded the air behind the obstruction is gradually absorbed through the alveoli, and as the air passages retract because of the airless state, the affected area of the lung collapses. If microorganisms are present in the alveoli an inflammatory reaction may develop. The alveolar spaces fill with secretions and cells and the lung may not completely collapse. The lung tissue adjacent to the collapsed or semicollapsed area becomes distended, the mediastinum and heart may be pushed out of alignment from the increased pressure surrounding the involved area, the diaphragm is elevated, and the chest wall flattens. If the obstruction is not relieved and an inflammatory reaction has developed, fibrosis may appear.

Prognosis usually is good. The onset may be sudden or gradual depending upon the cause of the obstruction. In sudden or rapid obstruction of the bronchi or bronchioles such as from a mucus plug or foreign body, there is pain on the affected side, sudden dyspnea and cyanosis, a drop in blood pressure, tachycardia, elevation of temperature, and shock. The patient tends to lie on the affected side. In gradual occlusion such as from a tumor or enlarged lymph node occluding the bronchus, there are no early symptoms; later in the course there is increased dyspnea and weakness.

Examination of the chest reveals dullness to flatness of sound in the involved area, and breath sounds are diminished or absent in that area. The heart is displaced toward the affected side and the trachea is deviated toward the affected side. The roentgenogram demonstrates a solid airless shadow, diminished size of the lung, retraction of the ribs, elevation of the diaphragm, and deviation of the mediastinum. Bronchoscopy may reveal the obstruction if it is in a main bronchus or large bronchi but not if it is in a small bronchus. The condition must be differentiated from spontaneous pneumothorax or massive effusion.

In sudden or acute occlusion the treatment is the immediate removal of the cause if possible. A foreign body or mucus plug if not expelled by coughing or suctioning may be removed with the bronchoscope. The individual is positioned on the uninvolved side to assist in draining the affected area and is encouraged to cough correctly. Antibiotics may be prescribed to combat localized infection. In chronic or gradual obstruction segmental resection or lobectomy may be performed. Broad-spectrum antibiotics are usually prescribed because an infection generally occurs regardless of the cause of the occlusion. Bronchodilators and expectorants may be prescribed.

BRONCHIECTASIS

Bronchiectasis is a dilatation of the bronchi. It is seen in many areas, especially Great Britain, Asia, Africa, India, and the United States. It affects mainly young persons of both sexes. The use of antibiotics for other respiratory disorders appears to have brought about a decrease in the incidence of bronchiectasis in many areas.

There is no specific etiological agent. It may be the result of alveolar agenesis or earlier respiratory infections or obstruction of a bronchus during childhood.

Bronchiectasis may be unilateral or bilateral. The bronchial mucosa becomes infected and ulceration causes dilatation. With healing, scar tissue replaces the original mucosa.

The prognosis is fair to poor according to the individual circumstances.

The onset is insidious, with a dry or slightly productive cough. As the condition progresses the cough and sputum increase to the point where changes in body position, laughing, or talking bring on paroxysms of coughing, and the individual must sit upright for comfort. There are paroxysms of coughing when he arises from sleep. The sputum is purulent and profuse and may have a foul odor. If left standing in a container the sputum will separate into three layers, of which the top is frothy, the middle is turbid and greenish, and the bottom is purulent. Frequently there is hemoptysis and dyspnea on exertion. The patient tires easily and there may be or not be clubbing of the fingers or cyanosis.

Diagnosis is made mainly by bronchography. Pulmonary tuberculosis, chronic bronchitis, and fungus infection must be excluded.

The original respiratory problem must be alleviated by such measures as removing the foreign body or controlling the original infection. Broad-spectrum antibiotics are prescribed to assist in healing any existing respiratory infection and to prevent the occurrence of a new one. Bronchodilator aerosols or detergent aerosols are often prescribed to assist in the expectoration of the bronchial secretions. These are administered by nebulizer or atomizer. Expectorants and mild sedatives to control cough may be prescribed. Postural drainage may be used.

PULMONARY EMPHYSEMA

Diffuse obstructive emphysema is a synonym. The normal air spaces in the lungs are increased. The incidence and mortality have been increasing in recent years, and men above the age of 50 years are most likely to be affected. The specific etiological agent is not known. The condition has been correlated with a history of retention of sputum, bronchial spasms, or repeated infections such as bronchitis, asthma, and bronchopneumonia, which may have caused trapping of air in the distal ends of the bronchioles and alveoli.

The lungs remain distended due to loss of recoil. The walls of the small bronchioles and alveoli are inelastic, thin, and stretched. The alveolar atria are ruptured and the alveoli misshapen. There is an increase in the accumulation of residual air in the alveoli which interferes with gas exchange within the alveoli, and the vital capacity is decreased. The loss of recoil by the lung tissue means that greater pressure must be exerted by the chest muscles and diaphragm in an effort to deflate them. There is a decrease in the arterial oxygen saturation and an increase in arterial carbon dioxide resulting in hypoxia and hypercapnia. This may lead to arterial hypertension, right ventricular hypertrophy, and congestive heart failure.

The progressive nature of the disease and the susceptibility to other respiratory problems which it promotes give rise to a poor prognosis.

The onset is insidious. The individual has a history of wheezing and chronic productive cough. He has dyspnea, which may be mild to severe on exertion, or orthopnea with cyanosis at rest, depending upon the stage of the disease. There may be cyanosis of the lips, nailbeds, and ear lobes and later of the skin. On inspiration the entire chest cage is raised. As the disease progresses these manifestations increase in intensity to the point that each inspiration and expiration requires a maximum of effort and the use of the accessory respiratory muscles. The cough increases and causes fatigability. The patient must sit up in order to breathe.

The clinical manifestations are the key to diagnosis. Pulmonary function tests reveal characteristic changes in vital capacity and gas exchange within the lungs. These tests measure the respiratory cycle by use of a spirometer. A tube or mouthpiece is inserted into the mouth, the nose is closed by a special clamp, and as the patient breathes a kymogram is recorded. The nurse may assist with the procedure. The procedure should be explained to the patient in order that accurate measurements may be obtained.

Tomograms may reveal damage to the alveoli. Tomography is roentgenography of a selected plane; in studies of the chest tomograms are usually taken at 1 or 2 cm through the entire lung area.

A bronchogram reveals marked characteristic changes in the bronchial tree.

Treatment is symptomatic and palliative. The first consideration is to control any existing respiratory infection and to remove any obstructions. The destructive changes within the lungs are irreversible. Expectorants and demulcents are prescribed to thin secretions and assist in raising them. Antibiotics are prescribed to control existing infections or prevent their development. Bronchodilator aerosols may be used to prevent bronchospasm and assist in raising secretions. Intermittent positive pressure breathing or oxygen therapy may be prescribed for relief of anoxia.

Nursing care is as described earlier. The patient requires exceptionally good mouth care because he is breathing through his mouth and expectorating bronchial secretions. The nurse must allow sufficient time in the morning for the patient to clear the bronchial secretions and rest before she serves his breakfast. She should help him and his family plan so that he may live within the limitations of his ability to breathe and move about. They must plan a daily medication schedule, learn how to administer the medications and therapy prescribed, and keep oxygen equipment available. A large supply of disposable tissues should be kept available together with a container for used tissues, and a supply of disposable sputum containers. Instructions should be given for disposing of these articles. The nurse must explain to the family the amount of energy the patient is expending in breathing, talking, and walking in order that they may understand why he is easily fatigued and irritable. She should help them in planning bed rest procedures that will permit him to sit up in bed without expending his energy and will provide easy access to the bathroom. She should prepare them for the long-term problem and how they may help the patient until his condition becomes terminal.

PLEURISY

Pleurisy is also referred to as *fibrinous pleurisy* and *dry pleurisy*. It is an inflammation of the pleura. Pleurisy may appear as a complication of other respiratory infections or trauma to the chest.

There are several causes, the most common being pulmonary tuberculosis. Pleurisy can occur as an extension of any infectious condition of the lung, especially pneumonia, lung abscess, or malignant tumor. It may be due to severe trauma to the chest wall or fracture of a rib or to an infection elsewhere such as rheumatic fever or uremia. Occasionally the cause is unknown.

A small area or the entire pleura may be involved. The inner pleural surfaces between the parietal pleurae become red, sticky, lusterless, and covered with a thin film of fibrin. This produces friction between the two surfaces with each inspiration.

Pleurisy clears with treatment of the cause.

The onset is usually sudden with pain the major symptom. This may vary in intensity from a rather uncomfortable dull aching one to an intense sharp one. It is experienced on inspiration. The patient tries to relieve the pain by taking rapid shallow breaths and limiting the motion of the affected side by clamping his arm against the chest wall in an effort to splint the area. Occasionally there is pyrexia of 101 to 103° F (38.3 to 39.4° C) lasting from 1 to several days; however, the pyrexia may be due to a coexisting infection.

The physical examination reveals pleural friction, which can be heard on listening to the chest sounds. The friction rub and chracteristic pleural pain are diagnostic.

Efforts are made to determine the nature of the existing infection so that therapy can be given to control it. Bed rest is prescribed until the temperature is normal for 1 to several days. Analgesics and mild sedatives are prescribed for pain. The chest wall may be strapped with tape to reduce motion. Dry or moist heat may be prescribed for relief of pain.

General nursing care measures should be given. If heat is applied the nurse must take precautions not to burn the patient; if moist heat is applied the tape strapped on the chest must be kept dry. She must remember that heat may build up under the tape and burn the patient. She helps the patient to cough by assisting him to immobilize the affected side while she splints the chest with her hands.

PULMONARY EMBOLISM AND INFARCTION

A pulmonary embolism is an obstruction of a pulmonary artery, usually caused by a blood clot. Pulmonary infarction is consolidation of the lung parenchyma due to interruption of the blood supply to the area. The infarct may progress to necrosis. The incidence of pulmonary embolism and infarction appears to be increasing; however, the apparent increase may be due in part to improved diagnostic technique. It usually develops after the age of 45 years and more frequently in women than men. It is seen in postoperative patients and in those with heart disease; it can follow pregnancy, hemiplegia, trauma, infection, cancer, and varicose veins.

An embolism from another area of the body, frequently a lower extremity, is carried by the bloodstream to the pulmonary artery. This embolus lodges in the main pulmonary artery or a branch of the pulmonary artery, depending upon the size of the embolus, thereby obstructing blood flow beyond that point. Blockage of the main pulmonary artery causes sudden death. Blockage of a branch of the pulmonary artery causes infarction.

Interruption to the flow of blood in the main pulmonary artery results in pulmonary hypertension, which causes overloading and dilatation of the right side of the heart, poor filling of the left ventricle, and decreased output of blood. With right heart congestion the peripheral circulation collapses; death may ensue. If the embolus is located in a small branch of the pulmonary artery, the area of lung beyond the point of obstruction becomes ischemic, the collapsed artery hemorrhages into the tissue, capillary permeability increases, and there is extravasation of fluid and blood cells into the alveoli. The alveoli are thereby distended. The area involved is usually wedge-shaped, dark red, firm, and airless. Necrosis may develop or the infarction may heal if the area is relatively small.

The prognosis is guarded and is dependent upon the area involved and the amount of lung tissue involved.

The onset may be very sudden. The individual may suddenly lose consciousness and die immediately if the main pulmonary artery is blocked. In other instances the onset is sudden with a sharp pleural pain over the affected area, subsidence of pain followed by cough with bloody sputum, and dyspnea. There is mild pyrexia, general weakness, diaphoresis, rapid pulse, lowering of blood pressure, and an increase in respirations. The symptoms often are similar to those of pneumonia.

Pulmonary embolism and infarction must be differentiated from other respiratory problems. An x-ray study immediately after the incident may not demonstrate any abnormality; later a dense area may be demonstrated similar to that seen in pneumonia. The electrocardiogram may or may not show evidence of congestive heart failure depending on the size of the lung area involved. There may be mild leukocytosis.

Treatment may be medical or surgical. At present, if the area involved is relatively large or more than one area of the lung is involved, immediate open-heart surgery is performed in efforts to remove any other emboli from the heart and in rare cases from the pulmonary artery. (This procedure is still in the developmental stage.) Ligation of the femoral vein or the inferior vena cava may be carried out to prevent migration of emboli to the heart and pulmonary artery.

Medical measures include administration of oxygen, adrenergic drugs to relieve anoxia, and anticoagulants to prevent formation of further emboli. Thrombolytic agents are administered to dissolve emboli present in other areas of the body. Analgesics and sedatives are prescribed for relief of pain and antibiotics are usually prescribed to control infections.

The development of pulmonary embolism and infarction is a life-threatening event. The nurse is responsible for immediately reporting the symptoms to the physician. She should remain with the patient and assist him in achieving a comfortable position, semireclining or upright, with a minimum of body movement, until his condition is evaluated by the physician and specific prescriptions for therapy are given. (See Chapter 23 for nursing care of the patient with congestive heart failure and with cardiac or vascular surgery.)

SILICOSIS

Silicosis is also called *chalicosis, lithosis, schistosis, miner's asthma, grinder's asthma, grinder's rot, potter's asthma, potter's rot,* and *potter's consumption.* This diffuse fibrosis of the lungs is caused by inhalation of crystalline free silica dust. It is a form of pneumoconiosis which is seen in miners, foundry workers, and others employed in work involving exposure to a high concentration of silica dust over a long period. Protective measures in many industries have brought about a decrease in incidence. Some individuals appear to be more susceptible to silicosis than others, but the reason for this has not been determined.

The development of silicosis appears to be dependent upon (1) the size of the dust particles, (2) the percentage and concentration of free silica in the dust, (3) the length of time spent in the environment, and (4) individual susceptibility.

Free crystalline silica is irritating to the walls of the alveoli and stimulates local fibrobastic proliferation and collagen formation in the bronchial tree. Collagen formation leads to the development of small nodules that tend to contract and pull the surrounding tissue together. The untreated condition progresses to massive fibrosis of the lung with deterioration of pulmonary function. There is a decrease in vital capacity, arterial hypoxia, hyperpneic dyspnea, and finally cor pulmonale. Emphysema may be a complicating factor.

The prognosis is dependent upon diagnosis. If the condition is discovered early its progress can be halted. The prognosis then is good, although existing damage is irreversible. If diagnosis is not made until massive fibrosis has developed the prognosis is guarded but the individual may live for several years.

The onset is insidious over a long period of time. There are no symptoms early in the course. Gradually there is shortness of breath on exertion followed by a dry or slightly productive cough. In advanced stages there may be anorexia, malaise, chest pain, disturbed sleep, dyspnea, productive cough, hoarsness, hemoptysis, and cyanosis.

A complete physical examination should include x-ray study of the chest which demonstrates a characteristic pattern when a history of exposure to free silica dust is given. Pulmonary tuberculosis, miliary tuberculosis, siderosis, fungus infection, Hodgkin's disease, berylliosis, and certain pneumonias must be excluded.

In the early stage no treatment is necessary except to remove the individual from the offending environment or institute protective measures. The individual thus may remain on the job.

In the advanced stage of the disease use of bronchodilators and intermittent positive pressure ventilators may be prescribed. It is important that exposure to other respiratory infections be prevented. The individual should not smoke. Symptomatic therapy is prescribed as necessary for cough, malaise, anorexia, and insomnia.

Bibliography

Bates, David and Ronald Christie: *Respiratory Function in Disease.* Philadelphia: W. B. Saunders Company, 1964.

Berlin, Charles I.: Hearing Loss, Palatal Function and Other Factors in Postlaryngectomy Rehabilitation. *Journal of Chronic Diseases,* 17:8:677–684, August, 1964.

Cole, Milton B.: Studies in Emphysema; Long-term Results of Training in Diaphragmatic Breathing on the Course of Obstructive Emphysema. *Archives of Physical Medicine and Rehabilitation,* 43:11:561–564, November, 1962.

Diagnostic Standards and Classification of Tuberculosis. National Tuberculosis Association. New York, 1961.

Fein, Bernard T., Eugenia P. Cox, and Harry E. Malley: Respiration and Physical Exercise in the Treatment of Bronchial Asthma. *Archives of Physical Medicine and Rehabilitation,* 44:5:273–274, May, 1963.

Hass, Albert: Rehabilitation for Emphysema Patients. *Bulletin of National Tuberculosis Association,* 50:4:6–9, April, 1964.

Havener, William H., et al.: *Nursing Care in Eye, Ear, Nose and Throat Disorders,* 2d ed. St. Louis: The C. V. Mosby Company, 1968.

Henry, William M., Jr.: Pulmonary Emphysema. *American Journal of Nursing,* 63:9:88–91, September, 1963.

Introduction to Respiratory Diseases. National Tuberculosis Association, New York, 1964.

Itkin, Irving H.: Exercise for the Asthmatic Patient: Physiologic Changes in the Respiratory System and Effects of Conditioning Exercise Program. *Physical Therapy,* 44:9:815–820, September, 1964.

Jackson, Chevalier and Chevalier L. Jackson: *Diseases of the Nose, Throat and Ear,* 2d ed. Philadelphia: W. B. Saunders Company, 1959.

Johnson, Julian and Charles Kirby: *Surgery of the Chest,* 3d ed. Chicago: Year Book Medical Publishers, Inc., 1964.

Lyght, Charles (Ed.): *The Merck Manual of Diagnosis and Therapy,* 10th ed. Rahway, N. J.: Merck Sharp and Dohme Research Laboratories, 1961.

Robbins, Stanley L.: *Pathology,* 3d ed.

Philadelphia: W. B. Saunders Company, 1967.

Rubin, Eli H., et al.: *Thoracic Diseases.* Philadelphia: W. B. Saunders Company, 1961.

Saunders, William H.: The Larynx. *Ciba Clinical Symposia,* 16:3:67–99, July–September, 1964.

Shames, George H., John Font, and Jack Matthews: Factors Related to Speech Proficiency of the Laryngectomized. *Journal of Speech and Hearing Disorders,* 28:3:273–287, August, 1963.

Ting, Er Ti and M. Henry Williams, Jr.: Mechanics of Breathing is Sarcoidosis of the Lung. *Journal of the American Medical Association,* 192:7:619–624, May 17, 1965.

CHAPTER 23
THE PATIENT WITH CARDIOVASCULAR DISEASE

SECTION 1   DISEASES OF THE HEART

SECTION 1
DISEASES
OF THE
HEART
HARRIET COSTON MOIDEL

Diseases of the heart, hypertension, vascular disorders, and lymphatic disorders affect persons of all ages; they are caused by a variety of agents and only a few are preventable. This is because of a lack of scientific evidence about the complex nature of the causative factors. The length and degree of illness vary considerably. These diseases may be treated by medical and/or surgical therapy. In some instances the treatment can bring the patient to a state of better physiological functioning than previously, as with certain types of valvular heart surgery. In others the treatment may result in sufficient control of the impairment to restore the patient to an earlier level of wellness or to allow him to function at least minimally.

The nursing care of the patient is based on his age, aspects of his general health which contribute to the potential for recovery, areas of his usual pattern of living which can be maintained and those which are altered by the illness, his ability to adjust his pattern of living to the degree imposed by his physical ability or disability, and the effects of the disease and the therapeutic regimen.

Infections

ACUTE RHEUMATIC FEVER
(RHEUMATIC VALVULAR HEART DISEASE)

Definition and Epidemiology

Rheumatic fever is an acute or chronic inflammatory process disseminated in the connective tissue of many organs, especially the heart, joints, and brain.

There are no reliable figures on the incidence of the disease because it is not reportable. It is estimated that 2 to 3 percent of persons who have had group A streptococcal infections of the upper respiratory tract will subsequently manifest rheumatic fever. Since most individuals experience a streptococcal infection in the early years of their life, it is assumed that the incidence is high.

The disease occurs with equal frequency in both sexes, developing primarily between the ages of 2 and 30, and with the highest number of initial attacks between the ages of 7 and 14 years. Once a person has had rheumatic fever, he is especially susceptible to subsequent attacks following streptococcal infections.

Etiology and Prevention

There is considerable evidence that rheumatic fever is precipitated by, if not directly related to, infection with beta-hemolytic, group A streptococcus, especially

547

of the upper respiratory tract. The acute toxic phase of streptococcal infections lasts from 3 to 7 days, and the patient seemingly recovers completely. After a latent period, possibly of 1 to 5 weeks, the patient may present symptoms and signs of illness, but manifestations arise in previously uninvolved areas of the body, such as the joints.

The initial attack of rheumatic fever may be prevented by early and vigorous treatment of the initial group A streptococcal infection with penicillin.

Pathology

One or all three layers of the heart—endocardium, myocardium, and pericardium —may be involved with rheumatic fever. Endocardial involvement is usually manifested in swelling of the valve leaflets, secondary erosion, and deposits of bead-like vegetation, usually along the line of closure. The mitral valve is most commonly affected but, in descending frequency, the aortic and tricuspid valves may be. The pulmonary valve is rarely affected.

The characteristic change in the myocardium is the development of minute nodules called *Aschoff bodies*. According to Rammelkamp, these develop as a result of swelling and fusion of collagenous ground substances of the connective tissues; as the lesions age, fibrosis occurs causing damage to the media of the arteries. The lesions of the pericardium are nonspecific.

The joints become red, swollen, and tender. The tissues are edematous and there is an increase in synovial fluid. The tendons become involved. Subcutaneous nodules may develop and are found usually adherent to tendon sheaths.

Clinical Manifestations and Diagnosis

Rheumatic fever may be insidious or rapid in onset. It is common for the patient to have a streptococcal respiratory infection followed by a latent period of days to weeks, but the symptoms may develop without a latent period. Usually there is malaise followed by fever, perspiration, prostration, and swollen, painful joints (polyarthritis). Some or all of the following signs and symptoms may be present: fever, polyarthritis, carditis, subcutaneous nodules, chorea, erythema marginatum. The presence of two or more of these manifestations is the basis for a positive diagnosis. Dramatic improvement of fever and painful joints with administration of salicylates is also useful as evidence for the diagnosis.

Characteristically the fever is of the relapsing type with a temperature of 100.4° F (38° C) or higher.

Joint pain develops rapidly; the joints are very tender and painful on slight movement. The pain persists for several hours to several days after the swelling subsides. Several joints may become involved simultaneously or may be affected in rapid succession. The ankles, knees, hips, shoulders, elbows, and wrists are most likely to be involved.

The subcutaneous nodules are small, loosely connected to tendon sheaths, and painless; they disappear in a few days to a few weeks. These are most often seen in children.

The rash is migratory; the lesions are flat with irregular margins and typically appear on the warm areas of the body.

Chorea is a common manifestation of rheumatic fever in children. It usually develops slowly and appears late in the illness, and the manifestations are mild.

Carditis is an important feature of the disease, occurring in about half the clinical cases, and usually appears during the first or second week of the illness. Inflammation of the myocardium, the pericardium, and the valves may occur.

There are no laboratory tests that establish rheumatic fever. Laboratory findings associated with infection may be present during the acute phase such as various degrees of anemia, an elevated leukocyte count of 15,000 to 30,000, an elevated sedimentation rate, and elevated C-reactive protein content of the blood. Another nonspecific, yet useful, test is the blood test for elevated titer of an antibody to one or more streptococcal antigens. The antistreptococcal test is repeated at intervals to identify changes in the titer. An elevated titer indicates that the person has recently come in contact with the streptococcus organism but does not distinguish between streptococcal sore throat and rheumatic fever. Similarly, an elevated C-reactive protein will occur with any upper respiratory infection, including a streptococcal infection.

Course and Prognosis

The course of the disease is variable, as is the prognosis. The majority of clinical and laboratory signs of the disease disappear within 4 to 6 weeks. There may be recurrence of rheumatic activity, and rebound is common when steroid therapy has been used and withdrawn.

It is impossible to predict the development of valvular disease following the acute attack of rheumatic fever. Apparently there is no relationship between ultimate damage to the heart and the severity or mildness of the acute attack or of the manifestations of carditis. Disappearance of the murmur on recovery from the acute phase does not indicate that the patient will not have carditis during the next attack or that the valves will not become severely damaged. It is known that those patients who later experience valvular heart disease have had heart murmurs during the acute phase.

A later consequence of the valvular involvement is the gradual progressive narrowing of affected valve(s) over a period of years, often 20 to 30 years. This leads to mitral or aortic stenosis or insufficiency.

Medical Treatment and Nursing Care

The goals of medical treatment are to control the infection, relieve pain in the joints and other symptoms, and protect and minimize damage to the heart. Similarly, the goals of nursing care are to protect the heart by minimizing its work through provision of bed rest, to provide adequate nutrients and fluids to protect the body during fever, to relieve joint pain through medication and protective handling of the joints, and to contribute to the control of the infection.

The purpose of bed rest is not only to minimize the work of the heart but also to reduce the metabolism during infection and fever.

Bed rest must be adhered to for several weeks even though the patient feels well. This is especially difficult when he has signs of carditis which he cannot see or feel. The nurse can help him understand the purpose of the bed rest so that his cooperation is achieved. Certain minimal activities such as turning himself in bed, combing his hair, and possibly brushing his teeth and feeding himself may be allowed according to the doctor's preference. Articles for these activities should be within easy reach. Activities performed by the patient and those done for him by the nurse must be accomplished without his becoming fatigued. Judging fatigue by increased pulse rate may not be applicable when fever is present, since there is an increase in pulse rate with an increase in temperature. Also, salicylates cause a reduction in the pulse rate. The patient should be moved slowly and smoothly, and the painful swollen joints should not be handled except when necessary and with great care. Jarring of the bed should be avoided.

The nurse can provide diversions appropriate to the age and interest of the patient and which do not require a great output of energy, such as reading (provided that the book or magazine can be propped on a overbed table rather than held), radio, television, painting. At this time there is need for visits from family and friends so that social relationships are maintained. The patient must not be near anyone who has an upper respiratory infection.

During fever there is a loss of fluids through perspiration and a high rate of protein metabolism. A large fluid intake must be provided. The diet should be high in protein to replace loss, and high in carbohydrates because of their protein-sparing effect. These factors should be kept in mind when selecting foods for the patient. Consideration should also be given the patient's age and food preferences. Foods that are easily consumed and digested should be offered, such as eggnog, milk, custard, and chopped or ground meat. The fever and pain cause lassitude, which may be demonstrated as a lack of interest in eating; anorexia is often present. Food consumption may be increased through provision of interest, attention, and companionship during mealtimes. The patient will need assistance in eating, and may even have to be fed, in order to reduce his activity and protect the heart, especially if carditis is present. Foods high in sodium content may be contraindicated if cardiac damage is severe and/or if signs of congestive failure are present. (See Chapter 12 for details of care of the febrile patient.)

A course of penicillin therapy is given in adequate amounts to eliminate the streptococcus. The usual amount is 1,200,000 units of benzathine penicillin or 600,000 units of procaine penicillin twice daily by injection for 2 weeks (Rammelkamp). It is necessary to administer the penicillin at the prescribed intervals to attain and maintain an effective blood level.

Salicylates (sodium salicylate or acetylsalicylic acid) or corticosteroids are given to relieve the arthritis and the constitutional symptoms such as anorexia, and to contribute to comfort. They will not, however, alter the duration of the rheumatic attack. Salicylates are given in small doses at frequent intervals. Since the total dose of salicylates may have to be large to ensure maximum effectiveness, the nurse must be constantly observant for symptoms of salicylism. Enteric-coated pills are often ordered so that gastric irritation is reduced.

Long-term Prognosis and Care

Some patients recover completely from rheumatic fever without suffering cardiac damage; in many, chronic valvular heart disease subsequently develops. A prognosis is often withheld until the patient has been observed for many months and periodically examined to evaluate heart function.

It is common for a person who has had rheumatic fever to have a recurrence with subsequent streptococcal infection. This likelihood is increased if he previously had carditis. Repeated attacks usually cause serious cardiac injury. It is most important that all patients who have had the disease attempt to prevent recurrence through prophylaxis and specific health practices. Prophylaxis is begun after the first 2 weeks of intensive penicillin therapy and continued throughout the year and then for an indefinite period, usually years. The most common method is intramuscular injections of benzathine penicillin once a month or sulfadiazine daily. Persons who have had rheumatic valvular disease should also have additional prophylactic penicillin before and after surgical procedures, particularly tooth extractions, to prevent subacute bacterial endocarditis.

All patients should avoid upper respiratory infections, practice good dental care including immediate treatment for cavities and abnormal conditions of the gums, and give immediate attention to any illness.

The nurse provides the initial health teaching or reinforces the physician's teaching so that the patient and his family will gain an understanding of the disease and its treatment. This provides a basis for acceptance of the need for periodic examinations as requested by the physician, for maintaining prophylactic treatment, and for following specific health practices.

Patients who have cardiac damage may be slightly to severely handicapped for varying lengths of time, possibly for the remainder of their lives. The long-term prospect varies according to age, degree and type of heart damage, and degree to which the heart condition can be controlled and further deterioration prevented through a program of therapy planned by the physician.

Corrective surgery for rheumatic valvular disease is possible in some cases. Operations for mitral stenosis are generally quite successful, whereas surgery of the aortic and tricuspid valves is generally less successful. It is reasonable to expect that there will be improvements and new developments in surgery of the heart valves which will extend this type of therapy to more people.

Because of restrictions to physical activity, the patient must adjust his pattern of living not only during the acute phase but also during convalescence, which can extend to a few months. The amount and duration of restriction depend on the degree of heart damage. Even relatively short-term restriction may create adjustment problems of great concern to the patient and family or of serious consequence for the patient. For example, an adolescent may have restrictions in school and play activities which may necessitate a change in educational and occupational goals and hamper his social development. Some school systems provide a home-teacher for such children, and planned quiet social contact with other children of his age may provide some of the needed social interaction. A young adult may have to make a temporary or permanent change in occupation which may pose economic difficulties and changes in family relationships. The nurse can assist the patient and family to make adjustments and find solutions for these situations. For this, information is needed regarding the physical condition of the patient, his interests, capabilities, attitudes, and energy, and the family relationships, resources, and pattern of living. The Crippled Children's Division of the

Federal Children's Bureau, which operates through state and local departments of health, may have resources to assist children, and the local branch of the American Heart Association may be contacted for information on services to adults and children.

Whether the restriction of activity is temporary or permanent, the aim of health personnel, the patient, and family is to have the patient continue his normal life as far as is possible in light of his physical capacity and to prevent unnecessary invalidism. This adjustment is made easier if all those involved place attention and emphasis on what the patient is able to do rather than on what he cannot do.

BACTERIAL ENDOCARDITIS

Definition

Endocarditis is inflammation of the endocardium, the membrane lining the interior of the heart, and of the heart valves, which are specialized endocardial structures. Causative factors of endocarditis may be nonbacterial or bacterial. The most common entity is bacterial endocarditis. Bacterial endocarditis is commonly classified as acute or subacute. The diagnosis of *acute bacterial endocarditis* signifies an infection that has a fulminating onset and a rapid progression, frequently attacks normal valves, and is caused by highly pathogenic microorganisms such as *Staphylococcus aureus*, the pneumococcus, the group A streptococcus, or the gonococcus. The diagnosis of *subacute bacterial endocarditis* commonly refers to the disease that is insidious in onset with a prolonged course, and caused by microorganisms that are of low pathogenicity and indigenous to the body, e.g., *Streptococcus viridans*, a normal inhabitant of the upper respiratory tract, and *Streptococcus faecalis* (enterococcus), a normal inhabitant of the fecal and perineal flora.

Epidemiology, Etiology, and Prevention

Bacterial endocarditis is not a reportable disease, therefore the incidence cannot be estimated with accuracy. Much information about it was accumulated in the preantibiotic era from postmortem studies. According to Dorney, the mortality rate of 98 percent has been reduced to 30 percent since the widespread use of antibiotics; therefore postmortem studies no longer provide data truly representative of the clinical incidence of the disease and the causative organisms.

Subacute bacterial endocarditis usually occurs in persons with a preexisting injury of the heart valves, usually due to rheumatic valvular disease but also due to congenital or syphilitic heart disease and atheromatous changes of the valve. Bacteria circulating in the bloodstream lodge on the surface of a valvular lesion where they multiply, become enmeshed in fibrinous material, and produce vegetations. *Streptococcus viridans* is the most common causative organism. The bacteremia is often secondary to dental extraction, cleaning or filling of teeth, tooth abscess, tonsillectomy, and even the chewing of food by persons with gingival disease or dental infection. This type of endocarditis is decreasing because of the lower incidence of rheumatic fever, use of prophylactic penicillin therapy before dental and genitourinary procedures in patients with valvular disease, and cardiovascular surgery to correct congenital or mechanical defects of the endocardium.

Bacterial endocarditis due to *Streptococcus* faecalis (enterococcus) has increased and, according to Dorney, is the third most common type. It develops most commonly among older men 45 to 60 years old. This disease entity is frequently associated with prostatitis and other genitourinary conditions. This type of bacterial endocarditis is often classified as subacute because *Streptococcus faecalis* is of low virulence, though resistant to antibiotics, and the fever usually low-grade if present. Some writers classify the disease as acute because the bacteria frequently attack normal valves and the valvular damage is rapid.

The second most frequent causative organism of bacterial endocarditis is the staphylococcus, which usually causes acute endocarditis but may also cause the subacute form of the disease. The disease is frequently described in narcotic addicts; also gonococcal and monilial endocarditis occur in this group. Staphylococcal endocarditis may be a serious complication of open heart surgery due to infection from prostheses, grafts, or sutures. Monilial endocarditis is also reported as a complication of open heart surgery. Staphylococcal endocarditis may result from bacteremia due to septic thrombophlebitis or staphylococcal abscesses.

In general, there has been an overall decrease in the incidence of bacterial endocarditis since the advent of antibiotics and a change in the prevalence of the various causative organisms. *Streptococcus viridans* infection, though still the most common, has been reduced. There has been an increase in the incidence of infections due to antibiotic-resistant and unusual organisms such as enterococci, staphylococci, fungi, and Proteus and Pseudomonas organisms which, according to Kerr, appears to be influenced by indiscriminate and/or inadequate antibiotic therapy, steroid therapy, increase in the number of debilitated older hospitalized patients, presence of indwelling venous catheters, and performance of open heart surgery.

Prevention should be vigorously pursued among persons with chronic rheumatic, congenital, arteriosclerotic, and syphilitic valvular heart disease. Upper respiratory infection should be avoided and treated immediately if it occurs. Antibiotics should be given before and after dental manipulation, tonsillectomy, and genitourinary procedures.

Pathology

The basic lesion of bacterial endocarditis is a friable vegetation composed of fibrin, bacteria, platelets, and necrotic substance. The vegetation becomes implanted on the surface of heart valves, the lining of a heart chamber, or the endothelium of a blood vessel. The infection is usually located in areas that have been altered by previous heart disease but can occur on apparently normal surfaces. The left side of the heart is most usually affected, with the mitral valve most frequently involved, followed by the aortic, tricuspid, and pulmonic valves in order of frequency.

The severity of damage depends upon the virulence of the causative organisms and the location, duration, and degree of involvement of the vegetative process. Perforation of the leaflets may occur. There may be secondary spread of the infection to the chordae tendineae which can lead to rupture and serious valvular insufficiency. There may be extension into the valve ring with abscess formation. The healing process is slow with gradual fibrosis, calcification, and endothelialization.

The lesions develop in areas of constant, rapid, forceful circulation. When the left side of the heart is involved, portions of the vegetation may separate from the site of infection; the emboli are then propelled into the systemic circulation and migrate to the brain, spleen, kidney, gastrointestinal tract, or an extremity.

Large renal emboli may occlude a major branch of the renal artery causing a gross infarction; small emboli produce a glomerulitis or a diffuse glomerulonephritis. When the infection involves the right side of the heart, the emboli enter the pulmonary circulation and pulmonary embolic episodes may result.

Clinical Manifestations and Diagnosis

The onset of subacute bacterial endocarditis is gradual and indefinite. Lassitude and low-grade fever are usually the first symptoms that come to the attention of the patient, and may be associated with a failure to completely recover from a sore throat, an upper respiratory infection, a dental extraction, a tonsillectomy, or urethral instrumentation. Because the first symptoms are relatively minor in the eyes of the patient, the infection and vegetative growth processes continue until more severe symptoms cause him to seek medical care.

The classic symptoms of subacute bacterial endocarditis are fever, anemia, heart murmur, petechiae, enlarged spleen, and peripheral embolic manifestations, although not all of them may be present in every case.

Typically the fever is remittent with periods of normal temperature lasting days to weeks. The peak of fever occurs daily at the same time in each 24-hour period, usually in the afternoon or evening. The patient may have chills with the fever, but this is not common.

Because of the prolonged bacteremia, the patient appears to be chronically ill, with associated symptoms of weight loss, anorexia, weakness, and ashen pallor—the "cafe au lait" appearance.

Petechiae may appear on the mucous membranes of the mouth, pharynx, and conjunctiva and anywhere on the skin, especially around the neck, on the hands and wrists, and on the feet and ankles.

Osler's nodes are painful red or purplish subcutaneous papules usually appearing in the pads of the fingers and toes. They are due to endothelial swelling and last from several hours to a few days. These are rarely seen and are not specific to this disease.

An enlarged, nontender spleen is a common manifestation. Arthralgia is relatively common and arthritis similar to that associated with rheumatic fever can occur. When the patient has been ill for some time, there may be clubbing of the fingers.

Symptoms of an embolic episode may occur suddenly, related to the organ affected and the type of involvement. The spleen is the most common site of embolic infarction; there are symptoms of pain in the upper abdomen, sometimes with radiation to the left shoulder, and the spleen is palpable and tender. The next most common organ involved with emboli is the kidney. Pain in the flank, or in the abdomen radiating to the flank, and hematuria signify kidney infarction. Hemiplegia is the most common symptom of an embolic lesion in the brain, though other neurological disturbances may occur. Small peripheral emboli may lodge in the terminal arterioles and suddenly produce gangrenous infarction of the extremities such as fingers, toes, or tip of the nose, whereas larger emboli may cause a peripheral vascular occlusion. When the right side of the heart is affected, cough, pleuritic pain, and hemoptysis are signs of pulmonary emboli.

In acute bacterial endocarditis the symptoms begin abruptly, in response to highly pathogenic organisms, and often the normal heart is involved. The cardiac symptoms progress more rapidly. The fever is often greater, may be intermittent, and often is accompanied by chills. Embolic phenomena are common. Petechiae may be more numerous. Osler's nodes and nodules of the palms and soles are uncommon. Because of the abrupt onset, the symptoms of weight loss and anemia are not present at first but develop rapidly.

Diagnosis often is difficult because the clinical manifestations and laboratory findings are similar to those of other diseases and definitive signs and symptoms often are lacking in the early stages. Blood cultures are done to identify the causative organism before antibiotic therapy is begun. During a 36- to 48-hour period, three to five blood samples of 10 ml are taken at specified intervals for these tests.

Subacute bacterial endocarditis often is difficult to distinguish from acute rheumatic fever with carditis. Bacterial endocarditis following open heart surgery is difficult to diagnose because many of the customary clinical features are absent. The heart murmur is not altered, peripheral emboli, petechiae, and splenic enlargement seldom occur, and anemia is difficult to evaluate during the postsurgical period. A high unexplained fever that persists from 5 to 7 days postoperatively or recurs 4 to 6 weeks after hospitalization is the alerting sign, and blood cultures aid the diagnosis.

Prognosis

The disease is fatal unless treated. The prognosis depends upon how early the diagnosis is made, how quickly therapy is begun, the virulence of the causative organism, and the amount and kind of cardiac damage that occurs.

In many cases the disease has progressed too far before the patient seeks medical care or before a diagnosis can be made because of lack of evidence; the patient does not survive long enough for the antimicrobial therapy to take effect. In patients who have responded well to antibacterial therapy, residual valvular damage, particularly valve perforation or increased insufficiency, leads to congestive failure, which is the most common cause of death. Death also may be due to embolic lesions in vital organs or renal insufficiency.

Medical Treatment

The aims of medical therapy are to immediately and completely eliminate the infecting organism, thus preventing growth of the vegetation and fostering healing, and to protect the heart. Several principles of treatment are generally followed, though differing drug dosages are recommended.

The antibiotic and the length of therapy are selected according to the sensitivity of the causative organism. *Streptococcus viridans* is sensitive to aqueous crystalline penicillin G, and 10 to 12 million units are given daily plus 1 to 2 g streptomycin daily for 2 to 3 weeks (Kerr). The daily dose of aqueous penicillin may be given in divided doses by intramuscular injections every 2, 3, or 4 hours, or intravenously. When the intravenous route is used, 5 percent dextrose and water solution (heparin may be added to prevent local phlebitis) is administered by slow 24-hour continuous intravenous drip via a small needle inserted into a small vein of the hand or arm. The prescribed dose of penicillin may be added to each bottle of intravenous solution or, at specified time intervals, the drug is placed in a burette (drip chamber) which is attached to the infusion tubing and bottle of solution, diluted with a specified amount of intravenous solution, and given by infusion over a period of about 20 minutes.

Streptomycin with penicillin has a synergistic effect upon S. *viridans* and S. *faecalis*. It is given in doses of 0.5 to 1 g every 12 hours by intramuscular injection.

Drug therapy for the more resistant organisms (enterococci and staphylococci) is a combination of a larger number of units of aqueous penicillin G daily plus streptomycin daily for 4 to 6 weeks. Other antibiotics or one of the penicillinase-resistant penicillins may be used for penicillin resistant staphylococcal infections. Gram negative organisms and fungi are treated with the appropriate antibiotic; often near-toxic doses are required to control the infection.

The patient's clinical response, i.e., a feeling of well-being, is the dominant factor in determining which drugs are to be given, the dosage, and the length of therapy. The antibiotic and the duration of therapy are selected according to the sensitivity of the causative organism.

Bacterial endocarditis following open heart surgery is currently treated with the antibiotic appropriate for the suspected organism for 4 to 6 weeks. If recovery does not follow, a second operation is performed to remove the infecting agent, i.e., suture, graft, or prosthesis.

If the patient is allergic to penicillin, penicillin therapy may be combined with a corticosteroid. Emergency equipment, including epinephrine, Solu-Cortef, and a tracheostomy tray, should be available at the bedside when treatment is begun, and careful observations for untoward reactions made. Prednisone may be given orally if itching and rash continue. If the patient has a history of anaphylactic reactions to penicillin, another antibiotic is selected.

Embolic episodes during treatment usually are due to shrinkage and fragmentation of the valvular vegetation as during healing. Generally antibiotic therapy is not discontinued or changed unless there are other signs of uncontrolled infection. Anticoagulant therapy may or may not be instituted by the physician.

Bed rest is indicated when the patient has a fever or when there are cardiac symptoms, such as signs of heart failure or myocarditis. Otherwise physical activity is not limited.

Nursing Care

The aims of nursing care are to carry out the prescribed therapy, provide comfort and care during the fever, provide assistance appropriate to the prescribed physical limitations, observe for characteristic signs and symptoms, and help the patient understand his condition and therapy.

The infecting organism can be eradicated only by maintenance of a high level of antibiotic in the blood, so it is imperative that the medications be administered at the exact time intervals prescribed by the physician. The site of intramuscular injections must be alternated routinely, since the patient will receive a minimum of two injections per day for at least 2 weeks.

The course, height, and accompanying symptoms of the fever response should be observed and recorded. During the acute period, especially in subacute endocarditis, this pattern of fever will probably recur daily. The nurse can anticipate the time of day when the fever will peak and be prepared in advance to give the patient the needed care as follows: promote cooling and give a tepid sponge bath if the peak is high; a blanket and possibly a hot water bottle if chills occur; administer aspirin if ordered; delay the meal when the fever occurs at the meal service hour; provide fluids.

During the acute stage, when the patient is febrile, weak, and anorectic, bed rest is not difficult for him to accept; when, however, the patient feels well, but it is necessary because of cardiac symptoms, the nurse must use ingenuity to gain his acceptance of limitations in physical activity. It may be helpful if she anticipates and schedules activity so as to reduce the number of requests he must make, and explains the reason for imposing bed rest, e.g., a reduction in exercise will reduce the work load of the heart and assist the healing process.

A variety of positions are available to the bed patient who is receiving a continuous intravenous infusion. The tubing must be long enough to allow him to move and turn, the needle must be secured in the vein, and the hand or arm in which the needle is inserted must be immobilized. A hand or arm splint (arm board) is usually applied, with the fingers free so that the patient can exercise them carefully at periodic intervals to prevent the disuse syndrome.

The patient may find it difficult to sleep while the infusion is running, especially for the first few nights. It may help if he assumes his normal sleep position and the arm receiving the infusion is correctly positioned. The nurse should check the needle and the position of the arm at bed time and assure the patient that his position and the infusion will be observed periodically during the night.

The patient will be able to ambulate comfortably with a continuous intravenous infusion utilizing a movable intravenous stand once he has learned how to take the necessary few precautions. He will feel weak and insecure at first and will require the nurse's assistance. The bottle of solution is hung on the hook of a movable standard. The site of insertion must be protected by limiting motion of the arm or hand. When the needle is placed in a small vein of the hand, the patient may be able to keep the hand immobilized by lightly grasping a thickly rolled small towel, or an arm splint can be used. The hand and arm should be held in a position above the waist. The arm, with elbow bent, can be supported in a cloth sling to prevent tiring. The patient uses his free hand to push the stand, keeping it in front of him and to the side of the free arm. For short walks the patient learns to carry the bottle in his free hand, keeping the bottle at the proper height. The patient who feels well, is gaining strength, and feels secure will become adept at getting into and out of bed, sitting in a chair and getting up from it, and going through door-ways without disrupting the infusion.

An embolic episode can occur at any time in the course of the disease and the nurse should observe for the appearance of new signs and symptoms, as stated earlier. The patient should be instructed and encouraged to report any new symptoms immediately, especially pain, which should be identified as to location, type, and duration before the physician is notified.

The lengthy treatment period and hospitalization (2 to 6 weeks) are often difficult for the patient to accept. He becomes weary and annoyed by the need for numerous intramuscular injections and continuous intravenous infusions and does not understand why the drugs must be continued when he feels so well. The nurse can help the patient by explaining the need for the extended period of therapy.

Coronary Artery Disease

CORONARY ATHEROSCLEROSIS

Atherosclerosis, "hardening of the arteries," is a degenerative disease of the arteries in which atheromas (plaques) develop in the arterial wall and lead to increased firmness, narrowing of the lumen, and/or occlusion of the vessel. According to Hopps, the primary arteries affected are those with predominantly elastic media: the aorta and its major branches, the coronary arteries, and the larger arteries of the brain. Since this process is the cause of coronary artery disease, it is appropriately discussed in this section.

The process begins during childhood as fatty streaks in the subintima aligned with the long axis of the vessel. At this stage the process appears to be reversible. The next stage is the development of the atheromas. These are described as *fatty plaques* or *pearly plaques* (fibrous plaques) depending upon whether fat (lipid) or fibrous tissue is predominant. Apparently the fibrous tissue develops in response to a progressive inflammation–healing process. As the plaques accumulate, the lumen of the vessel is progressively reduced in size and its elasticity gradually diminishes. Necrosis, calcification, and vascularization of the plaque, with or without hemorrhage into the plaque or progressive thrombin deposits on the surface of the plaque, are later possibilities. These conditions may lead to thrombosis and total occlusion of the vessel.

Etiology and Epidemiology

Numerous hypotheses have been proposed to explain the cause of atherosclerosis. It seems evident that there are multiple causes and multiple factors. Some of the important factors will be discussed briefly.

A *familial tendency* to atherosclerosis has been demonstrated; in familial hypercholesterolemia and familial hyperlipemia the incidence of coronary atherosclerosis is increased.

Aging is an important factor; atherosclerosis is more prevalent among the aged than the young. The aging process brings metabolic changes and changes in the fibrous tissues which decrease arterial flexibility. These changes appear to increase the rate of atheroma formation.

Certain *hormones* play a part. Coronary atherosclerosis is rare in premenopausal women but after menopause the incidence is approximately equal in men and women. It appears that estrogen decreases the ratio of plasma beta-lipoprotein to alpha-lipoprotein and increases the resistance of the coronary arteries. The incidence of atherosclerosis is higher among persons with diabetes mellitus, probably due to altered lipid metabolism, and among persons with hypothyroidism, in which there is an increase of both alpha- and beta-lipoproteins in the plasma.

The *catecholamines,* epinephrine and norepinephrine, induce the release of nonesterified fatty acids from adipose tissue. According to Olson, this effect, if brisk or prolonged, is sufficient to increase the output of beta-lipoproteins by the liver and to increase the plasma concentration of beta-lipoproteins.

Since emotional stress stimulates the production of catecholamines by the adrenal medulla, this process may help to explain "coronary proneness." There is general agreement that stress is a major factor in the acute occlusive events in arteriosclerotic heart disease and, by implication, plays a role in atherogenesis.

Local *hemodynamic* factors influence the development of the lesions. Hypertensive disease causes increased mechanical stress in the arterial system. The Framingham Study demonstrated that among adults with an arterial pressure of above 160/95 there was a threefold increase in the incidence of coronary artery disease in comparison with normal adults. Plaques commonly develop at points of turbulent arterial flow such as branch points and bifurcation of major vessels.

The *environmental* factors believed to contribute to the atherosclerotic process and which are currently under study are diet, drugs, exercise, occupation, culture and cigarette smoking. Among these, *diet* has been investigated most rigorously and the results of epidemiological studies have shown that population groups with high average plasma-beta-lipoprotein concentration (cholesterol), and who eat diets rich in animal protein, fat, and calories, generally have high rates of coronary artery disease. Of course, the increased risk of coronary heart disease associated with increased serum cholesterol concentration applies to groups and not necessarily to individuals. The upper limit of normal for plasma cholesterol concentration has not been defined; Fredrickson suggests that below the age of 25 a concentration greater than 250 mg per 100 ml is abnormal and beyond age 25 a concentration above 250 to 350 mg per 100 ml is abnormal.

The serum cholesterol level can be raised or lowered significantly by changing the total percentage of fat in the total caloric intake or by changing the ratio of unsaturated to saturated fat in the total fat and caloric intake. Although there is no proof or convincing evidence that coronary artery disease may be prevented or altered by modifying the diet, indirect evidence suggests that this may be beneficial.

Data of life insurance companies and observations of pathologists link increased death rates from cardiovascular disease with *obesity.* The relationship of obesity to coronary atherosclerosis is not clear because both hypertension and hypercholesterolemia are somewhat more prevalent in obese than in nonobese persons and it is difficult to determine the contribution of excess weight to the development of atherosclerosis.

The environmental factors of *drugs, exercise, occupation,* and *culture* continue to be investigated. In general, it appears that physically active persons tend to have fewer and less severe myocardial infarctions than sedentary individuals.

The effect of *cigarette smoking* on atherogenesis is not known but there is conclusive evidence that cigarette smoking is a major risk factor in the occurrence of coronary heart disease. Large-scale prospective studies have demonstrated that men who smoke cigarettes daily have a considerably higher death rate from coronary heart disease than nonsmokers, and the death rate increases progressively with the number of cigarettes smoked. Angina pectoris is equally common in cigarette smokers and nonsmokers (Doyle), though for some individuals smoking can precipitate or aggravate angina.

ISCHEMIC HEART DISEASE

The most common and most easily recognized manifestations of coronary atherosclerosis are angina pectoris and myocardial infarction. Others can occur, such as cardiac standstill and ventricular fibrillation, both of which can cause sudden death, arrhythmias, and conduction defects. Chronic congestive heart failure usually develops in association with some other sign of coronary atherosclerosis. Apparently the manifestation depends upon whether the obstruction is gradual—over a period of years which provides the opportunity for intercoronary collateral circulation to develop—or sudden; the degree of obstruction; and the location of the obstruction.

The basic mechanism is inadequate delivery of oxygen to the myocardial cells via the coronary circulation. Though this is most usually due to narrowing of the coronary arteries by atherosclerosis, other anatomical disorders may have the same effect, such as aortic valve disease (especially stenosis), congenital anomalies, syphilitic aortitis, dissecting aneurysm, arteritis, and embolism (Resnik and Harrison). There are precipitating physiological factors that create an increased need for oxygen in the myocardium or reduce the coronary artery blood flow.

Physical exertion increases cardiac work and is the most common precipitating cause of attacks. There seems to be sufficient evidence that mild exercise, less than the amount that produces pain, is beneficial rather than harmful and presumably assists in developing coronary collateral circulation. Walking on level ground, so that the individual can set his own pace and control the amount of exercise, is often recommended. The type and amount of exercise are increased or adjusted according to the response to activity. Attacks in persons with coronary artery disease are often induced by emotional stress, smoking, eating, cold, or hypoglycemia. Conditions that can increase myocardial oxygen need are myocardial cellular hypertrophy, fever, thyrotoxicosis, anemia, and hypertension.

The clinical syndrome of angina pectoris appears when the oxygen deficiency to the myocardium is temporary and there is no evidence of destruction of muscle fibers. Myocardial infarction occurs when the oxygen deficiency is permanent, complete, and accompanied by necrosis of muscle fibers. However, a person who has angina pectoris can have a myocardial infarction; many of these patients do not have angina upon recovery, probably because the previously ischemic tissue becomes infarcted with loss of pain fibers.

ANGINA PECTORIS

Clinical Manifestations and Diagnosis

The classic symptom of angina is temporary mild to severe steady chest pain on exertion which is relieved by rest. Exertion may be physical and/or emotional inducing chemical responses; rest encompasses physiological rest and cessation of the precipitating event.

The pain of angina is due to a temporary oxygen deficiency in the myocardium. This situation apparently occurs when the narrowed coronary arteries and the collateral circulation are unable to deliver oxygen to the myocardium in circumstances of increased demand for cardiac output or for oxygen.

The pain may be described by patients in a variety of terms; they may consider the sensation discomfort rather than pain. Hence the physician will obtain a detailed history of the kind, location, and duration of the pain and the events associated with its occurrence.

Resnik and Harrison describe the pain as steady, unwavering in quality, and not influenced by breathing, swallowing, or twisting or turning of the body or arms. In many cases the pain is mild rather than severe; often the patient's feeling is one of impending doom. Most commonly the pain is described as a sense of constriction; the patient shows a clenched fist over his sternum—the hallmark of angina described by Dr. Samuel Levine. Other descriptive terms are tightness, aching, squeezing, pressing, heaviness, expanding sensation, choking in the throat, indigestion, and burning. The pain may be confined to the chest or may radiate down one (usually the left) or both arms. Its duration generally is 3 to 5 minutes if the precipitating cause is removed.

Most often the attacks occur during rather than after physical exertion, as in increased exercise. Usually the pain is sufficient warning for the person to stop and rest, and the pain subsides. This type of angina is called "effort" angina, in which a predictable mechanical load will precipitate pain or there is an unpredictable pain response to a given degree of effort (Elliott and Gorlin). In some patients, the pain occurs only in the morning, for example, after a short walk to the garage following breakfast, while more strenuous exercise at any other time does not cause an attack. In some patients the pain occurs immediately following exercise. With "second-wind" angina the pain occurs with initiation of exertion and disappears if the activity is continued.

Often the attack occurs after a meal; the patient assumes it is due to indigestion and delays seeing the physician or does not describe the events accurately. In most cases the pain is precipitated by exercise taken after the meal, but some patients have angina after a meal even though they rest then.

The attack can occur while the patient is at rest and no stimulus is evident, although it is assumed that often there is evidence of sympathetic overactivity manifested by a rise in heart rate and blood pressure (Elliott and Gorlin). It is well known that emotional reactions such as excitement, fear, anxiety, worry, anger, hurry, disturbing thoughts, and stressful life situations can precipitate an anginal attack in many persons probably as a result of the autonomic discharge associated with the emotion. Many patients have attacks during sleep or in the recumbent position, usually called "nocturnal" angina.

The diagnosis of angina is mainly clinical, dependent upon the patient's detailed history and the physician's interpretation of the patient's description of chest pain and the circumstances associated with it. In recent years the development of cine coronary arteriography has greatly advanced the understanding and diagnosis of myocardial ischemia. Transient or serial electrocardiograms may indicate myocardial ischemia. Rapid relief of pain or increased tolerance to exercise is often a means of confirming the diagnosis.

The course and prognosis of angina are uncertain. They appear to depend on the balance between the rate and adequacy of the development of coronary collateral circulation and the progression of obstructive lesions in the coronary arteries. A person may have angina for a period of time after which the symptoms may disappear completely; another may keep the pain under control for many years with treatment; still another may experience a progression in frequency and severity of attacks even with treatment. For all patients, sudden death is always a possibility.

Medical Treatment

The aims of medical treatment are to relieve discomfort, promote collateral circulation, prevent further obstruction by atheromatous deposit, and prevent complications. Again, any associated aggravating condition, particularly obesity, must be detected and treated. Control of physical activity, emotional stress, diet, and drugs is instituted in a regimen tailored to the individual needs.

With the initial attack the patient may have modified bed rest for 2 or 3 weeks while the collateral circulation is developing. Physical activity that induces the pain should be avoided, and if this is not possible, the patient should perform activity slowly and/or take nitroglycerin beforehand. A period of reduced activity or rest should follow an exertion known to precipitate an attack.

Events that create emotional stress should be avoided. If this cannot be achieved, the patient may be able to learn to reduce emotional response to the stimulus, or it may be desirable that he take a tranquilizing drug. Mild physical exertion during a favorite recreational activity, such as golf or swimming, may relieve emotional stress. If the patient knows from experience that a particular event such as a business conference is likely to precipitate an attack, he can take nitroglycerin beforehand.

Many physicians are of the opinion that a low-cholesterol diet is not harmful and may be beneficial; they advise adherence to a fat-restricted or fat-modified diet. The diet may have to be modified if the patient becomes dissatisfied and emotionally upset by such restrictions. There is near unanimity of opinion regarding the importance of weight reduction in the obese person, since it is well accepted that the obesity increases the work load of the heart.

Nitroglycerin, sublingually, is the most important agent in management of angina pectoris. It relieves anginal pain, prevents the pain, and promotes collateral circulation, especially when taken in conjunction with mild exercise. Nitroglycerin has the following effects: it reduces blood pressure, heart size, and mechanical work of the heart; it increases collateral blood flow and improves distribution of coronary flow; it increases the caliber of large blood vessels and reverses spasms; and it reduces coronary arteriolar vasoconstriction (Elliott and Gorlin).

The patient and family should understand that nitroglycerin is not habit-forming and does not lose effectiveness with repeated use; thus it should be taken as often as necessary. Enough nytroglycerin tablets should be taken for each attack of pain to produce the "nitrite effect"—a temporary fullness and throbbing in the head.

There are differences of opinion about the use of tobacco. If smoking induces pain, premature beats, or other cardiovascular symptoms, then smoking should be prohibited. Some authorities believe that all patients with angina should cease cigarette smoking, even though cigarette smoking has not been identified as an angina-precipitating factor; others recommend reduction or withdrawal depending upon the individual reaction.

Nursing Care

The aims of nursing care of the patient with angina pectoris are similar to those of medical therapy. Supporting the medical program with explanations or interpretations of the mechanism that produces the symptoms and the purpose of the various aspects of treatment, as indicated, can help the patient understand and accept his condition and the treatment.

Initially the patient is realistically afraid of the consequences for life or death. Sudden chest pain causes him to immediately think of the possibility of sudden death. Each episode of chest pain creates fear. The nurse may alleviate this fear by staying with him until the pain subsides and administering the nitroglycerin, giving assurance that if the first dose does not bring relief, the next doses will. The patient should be informed that fullness and throbbing of the head will occur but will subside rapidly. With greater experience in taking nitroglycerin the patient gains confidence in its effect and learns to take it every 5 minutes until the nitrite effect occurs and the pain is relieved. Usually in the hospital the patient is given a supply of nitroglycerin which he can self-administer as soon as pain begins. Obviously, he should carry a supply of nitroglycerin tablets with him at all times, and he and his family should be thoroughly instructed in their use.

A modified bed rest regimen usually means that the patient is permitted mild activity such as bathing and feeding himself, periodic chair and bed rest, and a moderate amount of walking, i.e., slowly, for a short distance, on a level surface. The amount of walking is increased as he progresses. The general rule that the patient should follow is to stop exercising if chest pain develops, take nitroglycerin, and rest until the pain and the nitrite effect subside.

The nurse can assist, through observation and talking with the patient and family members, in identifying the characteristics of the pain and the events associated with it. She can help the patient find ways to reduce both the physical exertions and the emotional reactions that trigger the pain. This requires time, patience, and personal interaction. When the patient is hospitalized, the nurse can to some degree control environmental factors and her own behavior to avert events that precipitate an attack. When the patient is at home and going about his usual daily activities he must learn to make adjustments in his pattern of living in order to avoid attacks; when an aggravating stimulus or the reaction to it cannot be averted, he can take nitroglycerin to prevent chest pain.

MYOCARDIAL INFARCTION

The terms *coronary occlusion, coronary thrombosis,* and *myocardial infarction* are often used interchangeably, but there is growing agreement that *myocardial infarction* is most appropriate, since it designates the basic injury to the myocardium which has taken place.

Myocardial infarction is the result of gross inadequacy of oxygen supply to the myocardial cells via the coronary circulation in relation to the needs of the myocardium, developing so rapidly that compensatory flow through collateral channels is inadequate. The oxygen deficiency is permanent and complete. The infarct and anemic necrosis of the heart muscle is usually caused by obstruction (occlusion) of the circulation to an area of the myocardium, usually the result of progressive atherosclerotic narrowing of a coronary artery with or without thrombosis or hemorrhage at the site of a sclerotic plaque. The area of myocardium which was supplied by the occluded vessel undergoes acute degeneration, and infiltration of polymorphonuclear leukocytes takes place. As fibrous replacement occurs, the myocardium becomes thinner. The softening of the infarct is greatest from the fourth to the seventh day, and during this time there is danger of an aneurysm or rupture.

It is 3 to 4 weeks before the scar begins to grow firm through granulation, and 2 to 3 months before a maximum scar is formed. In about 8 to 10 days newly formed capillaries develop from a nonoccluded branch of the injured artery, another main coronary artery, or extracardiac vessels, but it is 2 or 3 weeks before there is a functionally significant collateral circulation.

Clinical Manifestations and Diagnosis

During the first week after the onset of infarction, the most common signs, symptoms, and laboratory findings are the following: pain in the left chest often radiating down the left arm; a drop in blood pressure; profuse perspiration; cool, moist skin; dyspnea; elevation of rectal temperature to 100° F (37.5° C) or more; elevation of pulse rate to 90 or more beats per minute; elevation of sedimentation rate above normal limits; elevation of leukocyte count to 9,500 or more; elevation of certain enzymes.

Chest pain is the most common symptom. It is severe, intense, pressing, prolonged. The patient may describe it as heaviness, tightness, choking, constriction, pressure, or aching. The pain tends to radiate widely down the left arm and to the anterior chest, back, neck, or jaw. It tends to reach a peak rapidly and remains steady. Its duration is variable, lasting from 1 hour to several days; generally it subsides in 12 to 24 hours. The pain is due to anoxia of the viable tissue surrounding the necrosed area which results from the inadequate supply of blood to the myocardium. As the blood supply and accompanying oxygen to the ischemic area of the myocardium become adequate, the pain is relieved. At the onset of pain or shortly thereafter, the patient perspires profusely; the skin becomes pallid, cold, and moist, or ashen. Dyspnea, weakness, faintness, nausea, and vomiting may develop. These symptoms usually subside during the first or second day unless complications such as shock occur. The blood pressure may be normal but commonly it falls within the first hours after the onset of pain and may be preceded by a rise in the systolic pressure for a short period of time.

Usually the heart rate is increased to 100 to 110 beats per minute, especially during the first 48 hours and through the fourth day during the febrile stage; there may be a slow rate of 60 to 70; or the rate may be normal. The pulse rate may be rapid in the presence of shock or heart failure, even when the temperature is normal.

Usually, the patient has a low-grade fever of 100° to 102° F (37.5° to 39° C) rectally which appears on the second or third day; the temperature becomes normal by the seventh or eighth day. Elevated temperature, elevated sedimentation rate, and elevated leukocyte count are evidence of absorption of necrotic material in the myocardium.

The physical examination frequently demonstrates a ventricular diastolic gallop rhythm or atrial gallop and fine and medium moist rales at the bases of the lungs. The systolic pressure may decline to 80 to 90 mm mercury, especially during the first to the fourth day after infarction, but also during the first 2 weeks. This transient hypotension is a common sign and not necessarily a sign of shock, though shock can occur. It may be a week or more before the blood pressure returns to that which is normal for the patient, or it may remain at a lower level than the previous normal.

Cardiac muscle, like other tissues of the body, contains intracellular enzymes; when the tissue is damaged the enzymes are liberated into the serum. Laboratory tests to identify elevated values of certain serum enzymes are used for the diagnosis of myocardial infarction. Tests for serum glutamic oxaloacetic transaminase (SGOT), creatine phosphokinase (CPK), serum lactic dehydrogenase (LDH), and serum alpha-hydroxy-butyrate dehydrogenase (SHBD) are commonly used at present.

Characteristic electrocardiographic alterations in infarction are displacement of ST segments from the baseline, inversion of T waves, and appearance of Q waves. According to Resnick and Harrison, these abnormalities are present in about 80 percent of patients on the first day or two and appear within 7 to 10 days in most of the remaining 20 percent. Myocardial infarction may demonstrate only minor and nonspecific electrocardiographic changes, or none.

After the first day or two the pain has usually disappeared as have other subjective symptoms, and by the fourth day the patient feels much better. It may be difficult to persuade him of the seriousness of his condition and the necessity for several weeks of therapy.

Several severe complications can occur at any time, with the consequence of prolonged recovery, more severe permanent damage to the heart, or death, and more than one such complication is possible. Arrhythmias may occur, some of which are benign and some a potential threat to life. Most develop during the first 3 days of the attack, although they may arise at any time, especially within the first 2 weeks. If shock ensues this is usually at the onset of the attack or during the first week, but it may develop in the second week or later. Shock is described as follows: a systolic blood pressure below 80 to 90 mm mercury in a normotensive person or a decrease in systolic pressure of 30 mm or more below earlier systolic pressure in a previously hypertensive person; low levels of blood pressure persisting for 2 hours or more; and low blood pressure associated with the clinical picture of shock (cold clammy skin, cyanosis or pallor, rapid weak pulse, possibly oliguria or anuria). Congestive heart failure and arrhythmias are frequently associated with shock. The occurrence of shock is a poor prognostic sign; the longer the shock persists the graver the prognosis.

Medical Treatment

The aim of medical therapy is first to relieve the pain and prevent further myocardial damage, then to promote recovery of myocardial function and the emotional and physical rehabilitation of the patient.

RELIEF OF PAIN

Immediate relief of pain is essential. Pain gives rise to further pain reflexively and stimulates the respiratory center, thereby forcing the heart to work harder to maintain cardiac output. The pain is best relieved by opiates. Morphine sulfate, repeated in 4 hours if depression of respirations is not present, is generally used. Morphine antagonists such as N-allylnormorphine hydrochloride (Nalline Hydrochloride) should be available if morphine overdosage with respiratory depression ensues.

Usually an intravenous infusion is started, the solution administered slowly, in order to have an intravenous route for administration of drugs immediately available. During the first 48 hours all drugs are administered intravenously, subcutaneously, or by mouth, avoiding intramuscular injections and the consequent tissue damage that causes liberation of enzymes and interferes with the diagnostic laboratory tests for serum enzymes.

OXYGEN

Oxygen is administered during the first hours after the attack to ensure an adequate supply of oxygen to the myocardium. There is a difference of opinion about the value of oxygen for the relief of pain because it is doubtful that enough oxygen can be administered to sufficiently alter the amount of oxygen to the affected tissue, since the basic difficulty is lack of blood to the tissue. Oxygen is given for respiratory depression, dyspnea, increased respiratory rate, wheezing or cough, and for shock. It is best administered by nasal catheter, with care being taken to prevent air swallowing and gastric dilatation, but it may be given by mask.

BED REST

Initially, complete rest, physical and emotional, is required, to decrease general and cardiac exercise and consumption of oxygen and thereby decrease the work of the damaged heart. The patient should be allowed to assume a position of comfort, and motion in bed need not be restricted. After the pain has been controlled and morphine is no longer needed, diazepam (Valium) may be prescribed to reduce anxiety and tension.

When pain has been relieved, the pulse rate and rhythm are in normal range,

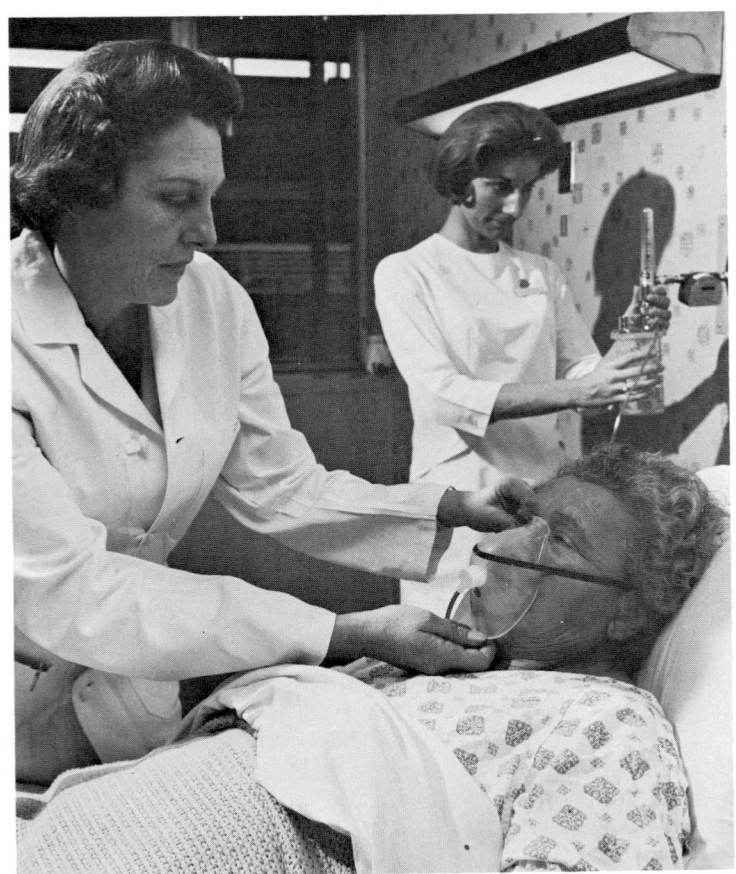

*Figure 23–1
Administration of oxygen
by mask. Note wall oxy-
gen outlet with gauge and
bottle of water to hu-
midify the oxygen.*

and the blood pressure is within a normal range and stable (fluctuating not more than 20 mm mercury), modifications of bed rest may be allowed. The patient may use the bedside commode (if male he may be allowed to void while standing by the bed), and chair rest may be instituted. By *chair rest* is meant that the patient is *assisted* to a comfortable chair by the side of the bed and rests for ½ hour or longer three or four times a day.

During the bed rest period full range of motion exercises of the shoulder joints should be encouraged to prevent the shoulder-hand syndrome. Periodic exercise of the feet, knees, and hips is encouraged to prevent phlebothrombosis; elastic bandages or stockings may be prescribed for the same purpose. The recurrence of pain, rapid or slow pulse rate, irregular heart rhythm, elevation of temperature, abnormal respiratory rate or rhythm, or low or unstable blood pressure may delay chair rest or necessitate a return to bed rest. By trial and error, physical exercise is gradually increased so that by the second or third week following the onset of the attack, moderate ambulation is in progress.

DIET

The diet during the first 24 to 48 hours is usually liquid—including fruit juices—or soft, served in small quantities. The purpose is to provide nourishment that can be easily digested and limits the need for blood supply for the digestive process, thus avoiding cardiac work. Very hot foods and very cold foods should be avoided because they can cause irregularity of the heart beat by stimulating the vagus nerve. Cold causes vasoconstriction and cold liquids increase distention.

After the first few days when the pain and nausea have disappeared, the diet is usually of regular consistency and may be low in salt, saturated fatty acids, and calories.

OTHER MEASURES

Having a bowel movement and particularly straining requires a sudden increase in blood flow and thereby an additional work load for a damaged heart. It is preferable to avoid this exertion during the first 3 days and to facilitate formation of soft feces. For this reason, the diet during the first few days is one that will not provide bulk. Dioctyl sodium sulfosuccinate (DOSS [Colace, Dioxinate]) is generally given to promote formation of a soft stool.

Anticoagulants prevent intravascular coagulation of the blood and venous or mural thrombus formation. Heparin (Liquaemin) may be used initially or for longer-term therapy to prolong the clotting time of blood. The dosage is determined on the basis of blood coagulation time. After the acute period it is usual to change to an oral anticoagulant, i.e., bishydroxycoumarin (Dicumarol) or warfarin sodium (Coumadin), for long-term therapy. These drugs decrease the capacity of the blood to clot by reduction of prothrombin content of the blood. The drug is given in amounts that will maintain the desired elevated blood prothrombin time. The daily dose varies and is calculated and prescribed after the daily prothrombin time has been reported. Vitamin K (Mephyton) should be available for administration to counteract bleeding if it occurs, or if the prothrombin time becomes elevated to dangerous levels. Anticoagulant therapy is usually continued for 3 to 4 weeks and may be continued for months or years.

Shock is treated with oxygen, digitalis, and pressor amines. The patient should be placed in a recumbent position unless there is dyspnea accompanying pulmonary edema, in which case the head of the bed may be elevated to relieve respiratory difficulty. Metaraminol (Aramine) or l-norepinephrine (Levophed) may be given by intravenous infusion, diluted in intravenous solution, and a physician or a nurse should constantly observe the patient, taking the blood pressure, measuring urine volume, and adjusting the rate of infusion as necessary. Digitalis increases heart function and may be given intravenously for rapid digitalization. Inadvertent rapid administration of these drugs can produce hypertension, pulmonary edema, arrhythmias, and further infarction, and symptoms of any of these call for a reduction in rate or discontinuance of the infusion.

Shock can precipitate cardiac arrhythmias and arrhythmias can precipitate shock. Elevation of blood pressure by pressor amines may prevent certain arrhythmias (e.g., atrial tachycardia) but not others (e.g., ventricular tachycardia, ventricular fibrillation) and different therapy may be required.

Each arrhythmia is treated with a specific drug. Because of an unexpectedly high number of episodes of arrhythmia shown by constant electrocardiographic monitoring, many physicians routinely administer quinidine sulfate, 0.2 g, four times a day orally, as a prophylactic measure, especially with frequent atrial or ventricular premature beats per minute. (See Section 1A.)

In the absence of complications, the patient is hospitalized for 3 to 4 weeks as a rule. Caution is exercised during this period while the collateral circulation is developing and the infarct is healing. Constant observations for symptoms of complications are made while the patient gradually resumes moderate activity and exercise. He follows a normal diet except for a reduction in saturated fats and calories to maintain normal weight. Moderate use of alcohol, coffee, and tea is usually allowed. The patient is encouraged to stop smoking.

A period of convalescence at home follows with gradual increase in exercise and several weeks later a return to customary activities and work. The majority of patients are able to resume such activities, perhaps with minor adjustments in diet, an increase in walking (especially if a sedentary life had been the rule), and an increase in rest periods. The outcome depends on the amount of heart damage, the occurrence of complications, and cardiac compensation in relation to metabolic needs.

Nursing Care

The aims of nursing care are to reduce emotional and physical stress, contribute to identification of symptoms, participate in medical therapy, and help the patient to understand the physiological changes that are occurring and their relationship to treatment so that he can accept the therapeutic program.

CONTROL OF ENVIRONMENTAL FACTORS

Emotional stimulation affects the cardiovascular system through autonomic nervous control. Sympathetic (adrenergic) activity increases the heart rate, strengthens the heart beat, and increases the blood pressure; parasympathetic (cholinergic) activity has the opposite effect. The usual reaction to emotion-provoking stimuli is an increase in heart rate, cardiac output, blood pressure, and oxygen consumption.

At the onset of the attack and during the first few days the patient is realistically afraid of the life-threatening physiological changes that have been taking place. He is worried about his survival. He may react to fear through restlessness and active movements, in efforts to "fight for life." Both fear and activity increase the cardiac output and must be minimized. The nurse may help to diminish the patient's fear by her presence, by her attentive, unworried manner, by skillful techniques, by offering explanations of events taking place, by encouraging him to express his concerns, and by giving assurance when this can realistically be done.

The patient may be concerned about whether or not the "right" treatment is being administered in the "right" manner. The nurse can be influential in fostering the patient's trust in the care being given by demonstrating honest concern for him, attending promptly to his symptoms and concerns, and carrying out each procedure with accuracy and confidence. The physical environment should be controlled as far as possible by reducing sights, sounds, and odors that act as emotion-provoking stimuli. The emotional environment can be controlled by avoiding anger, loss of patience, lack of interest, and annoyance as conveyed by tone of voice, lack of attention, etc.

Bed rest during the first weeks is essential and it is the nurse's responsibility to help the patient rest. She can help the patient rest by providing for his physical comfort, as by arranging a comfortable position for him and doing things for him that he cannot do for himself, and by easing his fear, worry, and distress due to his dependency.

Since the patient is placed in a situation of almost complete dependency, there must be a clear understanding among patient, physician, and nurse as to the specific activities the patient is allowed to perform and those the nurse will perform for him. For example, it must be decided whether or not the patient can comb his hair, reach for a glass of water, change his pajamas, brush his teeth, wash his face and hands, and feed himself. Conflicting instructions from different people involved in his care can confuse and disturb him and weaken his trust in his caretakers.

During the first few days, when the patient's attention is on survival and sedation reduces his ability to think, concentrate, and comprehend, the nurse should not expect him to remember explanations or instructions nor should she rely on his self-control. She should expect that it will be necessary to carefully repeat instructions over and over again.

EARLY ACTIVITY

As the acute symptoms subside and the patient feels better, he may be allowed to move, turn, reach, sit in bed, and walk a few steps to the chair to rest or to the bedside commode to have a bowel movement. He must learn to make all physical movements slowly. Exercise is limited, for rest is still essential while the scar is forming and the collateral circulation developing. Within the boundaries of the physician's orders, the nurse initiates and maintains rest patterns for the patient, decides on the extent of his activity at a given moment, and helps him understand the reason for such limitations, thereby helping him to exert self-control, or at least to know why he is being "policed." She is also responsible for teaching him shoulder and leg exercises and for applying elastic bandages when ordered.

As the nurse learns more about the patient, she can judge whether denial of an activity is so upsetting to him that the strong feelings aroused would increase the heart's work. She learns to recognize his signs of fatigue and stops the activity before overexertion occurs. Watching his behavior, she anticipates his wants, thereby saving his energy. Her knowledge and understanding of his personality and behavior can be utilized to help him learn to limit exercise for the present and also gain confidence when exercise is increased.

In carrying out the physician's p.r.n. orders for morphine, the nurse must exercise critical judgment in evaluating the amount of pain the patient is experiencing, i.e., whether it is severe enough to warrant morphine, and how often the morphine should be given. She does not want him to suffer pain, whether severe or mild, because pain increases cardiac output. She must recognize that each patient has an individual tolerance to pain and reacts to pain individually.

VITAL SIGNS

The blood pressure must be measured accurately and at regular intervals. Though the physician prescribes these intervals, the nurse should not hesitate to measure the blood pressure at other times or at greater frequency in the event of a sudden drop of 20 mm mercury, a drop below 100 mm mercury, fluctuation, or the presence of other signs of shock. Lowered blood pressure or shock may give rise to oliguria or anuria, hence the nurse should observe the patient's urinary output.

Pulse rate and rhythm must be conscientiously checked, especially during the first 2 weeks and when the electrocardiographic monitoring system is not in use. Routinely taking an apical rate rather than a radial rate is advisable since the apical rate more accurately measures the heartbeat and thereby the detection of an arrhythmia. It also averts patient alarm caused by the nurse making a change from taking the radial rate to taking the apical rate when the latter method is called for.

ABNORMALITIES OF CARDIAC RATE AND RHYTHM

Abnormalities of heart rate and rhythm are specifically diagnosed by the electrocardiograph but some can be identified through the apical rate. (1) *Premature contractions* are characterized by a single contraction before the regular beat is antic-

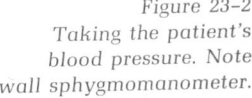

Figure 23–2
Taking the patient's
blood pressure. Note
wall sphygmomanometer.

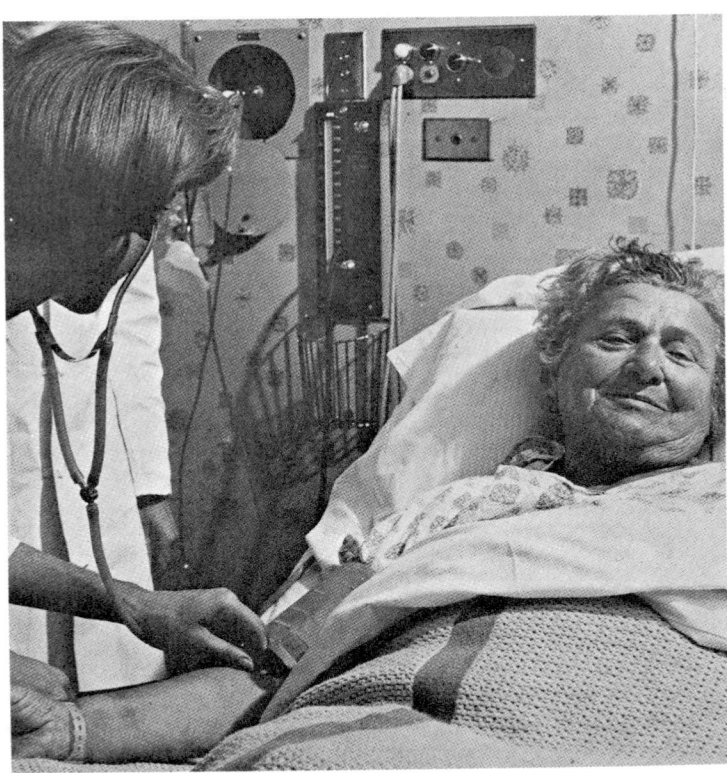

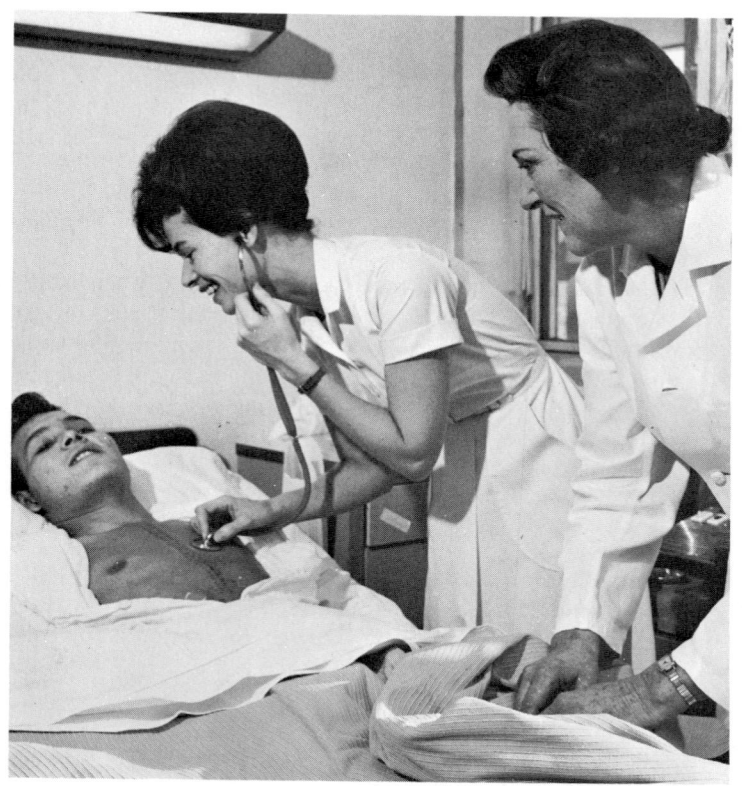

Figure 23–3
Measuring the apical-
dial rate for evaluation
of pulse deficit. Note
incision (healing) made
during prior heart
surgery.

ipated and a slow rate, and are identified by radial or apical pulse and the EKG. (2) *Atrial fibrillation* is characterized by a rapid and irregular pulse with an increased pulse deficit and is identified by apical rate or apical–radial rate and the EKG. (3) *Complete heart block* in which the auricles and ventricles beat independently, is characterized by a slow ventricular rate of 50 (and syncope) and is identified by apical rate and EKG. (4) *Ventricular tachycardia*—a pulse rate of 100 to 200 (usually 140 to 175)—is more easily identified by apical rate than radial rate.

A marked change, to a slow, rapid, or irregular rate, signals a need for the nurse to take the apical rate and report the patient's condition to the physician. Many cardiologists expect the nurse to use initiative in ordering an immediate electrocardiogram when these signs are observed, so that accurate information will be immediately available.

TEMPERATURE

The height and the course of the fever are important prognostic signs. The temperature is taken at regular intervals until the fever has subsided. Rectal measurement of temperature may be preferred for accuracy, but because insertion of the thermometer may induce vagal stimulation the physician may decide upon oral measurement. The patient may have a fever even though he is in shock and his skin feels cold.

OTHER MEASURES

During the first few days the patient may be nauseated and vomit, and may lose his appetite, so food should not be forced upon him. He may be concerned that he is not receiving enough food to help him survive or to recover. The lack of bowel movements can be worrisome, also. This concern not only is based on the cultural concept that one should "keep clean" by having a daily bowel movement but develops also because one of the few personal functions remaining within his power has been denied him. The nurse can help the patient by giving an explanation for the limited diet and temporary avoidance of a bowel movement and help him to avoid straining and the Valsalva maneuver by instructing him to breathe through his mouth while having a bowel movement.

Anticoagulant dosage is determined *after* the laboratory report of coagulation time or prothrombin time is available. If the patient is concerned that daily withdrawal of blood has a serious connotation or will weaken him, the nurse may explain the reason for performing the test and assure him that the small amount of blood removed will quickly be replaced by his body and the loss will not delay his recovery. There is potential danger of hemorrhage when anticoagulants are administered in therapeutic doses, and the nurse must observe for evidence of bleeding such as hematoma, epistaxis, hematuria, tarry stools, petechiae, bleeding gums. The action of an oral anticoagulant persists for 3 to 8 days after it has been discontinued, so continued observation is necessary. If the patient is to continue to take an anticoagulant after discharge from the hospital he should be warned to avoid injuring himself, and to contact his physician immediately if bleeding of any kind occurs. Instructions for taking the drug should be given, including the necessity for having blood tests taken on the specified dates and a reminder to avoid taking aspirin during the period of time he is taking the anticoagulant.

The nurse must continually observe for symptoms of complications such as shock, arrhythmia, embolism, and heart failure which usually develop during the first 2 weeks but may develop at any time. When the patient begins to ambulate she watches for pallor or cyanosis, diaphoresis, cold skin, dyspnea, chest pain, fatigue, increased or slow pulse rate or change in rhythm, and changes in blood pressure. The occurrence of any of these symptoms indicates that the patient should rest. With each increase in activity the nurse observes for symptoms of excessive cardiac work load and complications, while she helps the patient gain confidence in his ability to exercise within his capacity so that he will be able to regulate his activity while convalescing at home.

Clinical Syndromes of Heart Failure

Definitions

General circulatory disturbances may arise in peripheral areas or in the heart. The peripheral disorders are characterized by defective or decreased venous return to the heart (peripheral circulatory failure and low-output syndrome) or by increased venous return (circulatory overload and high-output syndrome). When

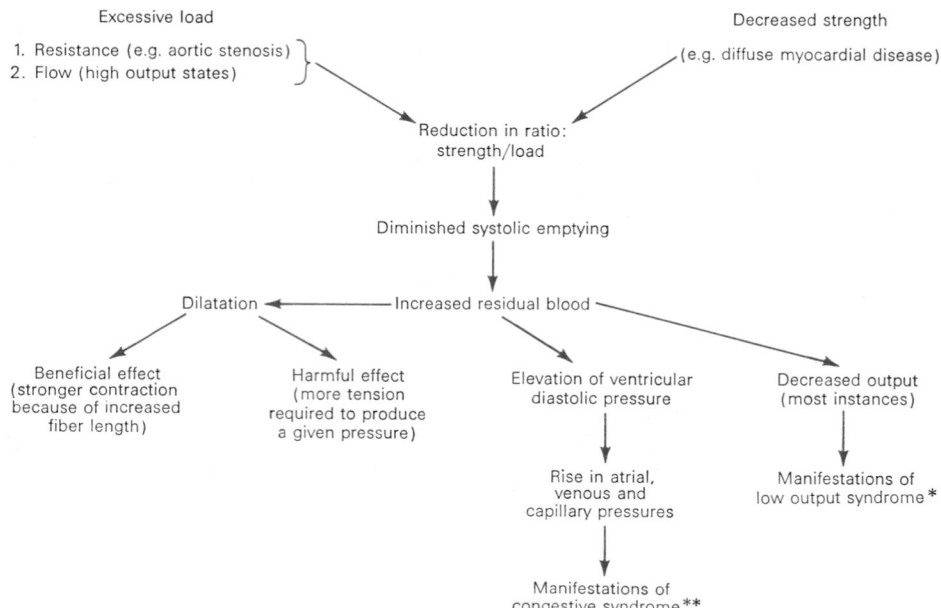

SEQUENCE OF EVENTS IN HEART FAILURE

Excessive load

1. Resistance (e.g. aortic stenosis)
2. Flow (high output states)

Decreased strength
(e.g. diffuse myocardial disease)

Reduction in ratio: strength/load

Diminished systolic emptying

Dilatation ← Increased residual blood

Beneficial effect (stronger contraction because of increased fiber length)

Harmful effect (more tension required to produce a given pressure)

Elevation of ventricular diastolic pressure

Decreased output (most instances)

Rise in atrial, venous and capillary pressures

Manifestations of low output syndrome *

Manifestations of congestive syndrome **

* Not specific for heart failure: These also occur with peripheral circulatory failure.
** Specific for heart failure.

Figure 23–4 Sequence of events in heart failure. (By permission of T. R. Harrison (Ed.): Principles of Internal Medicine, 5th ed. New York: McGraw-Hill Book Company, 1966.)

these disorders are severe or of long duration they may lead to secondary heart failure.

Heart failure or cardiac failure is usually due to a primary disorder of the heart in which the heart is unable to pump an adequate amount of blood to the body in relation to metabolic needs and venous return. This situation may result from an increase in the work load of the heart, a decrease in the strength of the heartbeat, or their combination. Any of these can produce the *low-output syndrome* (forward failure) with symptoms resulting from a marked decrease in cardiac output, e.g., lassitude, fatigue, and decline in blood pressure, or the *congestive syndromes* (backward failure) with symptoms resulting from the elevation of venous pressure behind the failing ventricle, e.g., dyspnea, cardiac dilatation, and venous distention.

Most patients with heart failure have signs and symptoms of both syndromes though either can occur alone. The low-output syndrome may arise from a peripheral circulatory disorder or from the failing heart and does not necessarily indicate heart failure. The manifestations of the congestive syndromes are specific for heart failure.

The term *congestive heart failure* usually refers to a chronic heart failure in which there is abnormal circulatory congestion (backward failure). When this condition has been present for some time there is usually transudation of fluid from the capillaries into the interstitial spaces, i.e., edema. When the manifestations indicate that the pumping ability of the left side of the heart is primarily impaired (dyspnea, pulmonary congestion) the term *left-sided heart failure* is used. Conversely, *right-sided heart failure* indicates primary impairment of the pumping ability of the right side of the heart with manifestations of systemic venous congestion. Left-sided and right-sided failure can occur as separate entities but usually the course of events is the development of left-sided failure causing right-sided failure since, when the pumping ability of one side of the heart is impaired, the output of the other side is secondarily decreased; or both ventricles may fail nearly simultaneously. Usually congestive failure is a chronic condition, developing slowly, with retention of sodium and water by the kidneys, but it may develop acutely.

Latent heart failure refers to heart failure in which the symptoms, chiefly dyspnea, are not apparent at rest but occur under other circumstances when there is an increase in metabolic demands on the work load of the heart, such as exercise, emotional stress, or fever.

Heart failure is said to be *compensated* when the lack of pumping ability of the heart has been counterbalanced by normal compensatory mechanisms, e.g., the cardiovascular reserves (venous blood oxygen reserve, heart rate reserve, systolic volume reserve, and diastolic volume reserve), or by improvement of function through administration of digitalis glycosides.

Etiology

Ventricular failure, atrial failure, or both can cause heart failure. The pumping ability of the heart is mainly the function of the ventricles, and usually the heart failure is initially the result of ventricular failure. The atria make a very minor contribution to the pumping ability of the heart except during times of increased demand on the heart, as in exercise, when their contribution is critical, especially when the usual cardiac reserve and compensatory mechanisms are limited. When the atrium fails to provide adequate filling and distention of the ventricle in relation to the venous return the condition is referred to as *atrial failure*. Atrial failure may be due to a variety of causes but most commonly it occurs secondary to ventricular failure, with mechanical abnormalities in the heart, or in the presence of an arrhythmia.

Heart failure can result from a variety of cardiac or extracardiac disorders or physiological mechanisms that affect cardiac function and ultimately cause a decline in cardiac pumping. A patient may have heart failure from more than one cause and the causes may change during the course of the disease.

Pathophysiology

A number of physiological mechanisms are involved in heart failure; several may be present at one time and all the mechanisms involved are not completely clear. This discussion attempts to summarize the complex physiological changes that occur.

In left ventricular myocardial failure the ventricle fails to contract with sufficient force to eject the appropriate volume of blood per beat (stroke volume) to provide for the filling load upon the ventricle from the atrium. There is diminished systolic emptying of the ventricle with an increase in the volume of residual blood at the end of the contraction—the heart is unable to empty itself. The diminished systolic emptying is usually associated with a reduction in cardiac output which, if severe enough, will cause manifestations of the low-output syndrome (forward failure).

With the diminished systolic emptying there is an abnormal elevation of pressure and an abnormal volume of blood in the ventricle during diastole. The increased end-diastolic pressure and volume in the ventricle secondarily causes an elevation of pressure in the left atrium. Eventually the increased pressure is reflected backward causing, in turn, elevated pressures in the left atrium, pulmonary artery, right ventricle (right ventricular failure may occur), right atrium, veins, and capillaries. These elevated pressures lead to congestion in the pulmonary circuit, with manifestations of left-sided congestive heart failure and/or congestion in the systemic circuit, with manifestations of right-sided congestive heart failure.

The venous and capillary pressures are usually elevated in congestive heart failure. The elevated atrial pressure which is reflected backward causing a rise in venous pressure is probably the initial mechanism.

Various adjustments of the body occur in response to heart failure. Initially the adjustments are similar to homeostatic mechanisms arising in response to circulatory failure from any cause. There is a reflex increase in autonomic sympathetic excitation to most of the arteries and veins of the body and to the heart. The sympathetic (adrenergic) stimulation of the peripheral arteries causes vasomotor regulation so that blood flow to the heart and brain—the essential organs—is maintained at the expense of blood flow to other areas such as skin, kidneys, spleen, and skeletal muscles. The sympathetic stimulation to the veins causes venoconstriction, which increases the venous tone. This increases the venous pressure, which helps to maintain venous return to the heart.

The increased sympathetic stimulation to the heart is associated with an inhibition of parasympathetic activity to the heart. Usually the heart responds with an increase in rate and an increase in the force of myocardial contraction. There is an associated increase in the rate of ventricular relaxation following contraction which contributes to increased ventricular filling.

A later adjustment is retention of salt and water by the kidneys. This may be due to increased reabsorption of sodium and water by the proximal tubules of the kidney associated with decreased renal blood flow and decreased glomerular filtration, and other physiological mechanisms. (See Chapter 11.)

There is an increase in blood volume in congestive heart failure. In addition to retention of water and electrolytes by the kidney there is a slow manufacture of increased amounts of serum proteins by the reticuloendothelial system and a slower increase in red cell production by the bone marrow. The plasma volume increases more rapidly than the red cell mass, because of the comparative length of time for their production; thus the hematocrit tends to fall as heart failure develops. The increase in blood volume contributes to increased venous pressure.

In general, the pressure in the vascular system is elevated by an increase in blood volume and an increase in vasomotor tone. The generalized increase in venous pressure tends to increase transudation of fluid from the capillaries into the interstitial spaces producing edema.

In addition to decreased cardiac output and elevation of ventricular diastolic pressure, with eventual consequences of the congestive syndromes, inability of the heart to empty itself leads to dilatation of the ventricles. Apparently with slight dilatation the beneficial effects predominate and with marked dilatation the harmful effects predominate. Hypertrophy of the ventricular myocardium is a later (chronic) adjustment to heart failure, which may be compensatory.

LOW-OUTPUT SYNDROME (FORWARD FAILURE)

The symptoms of forward failure are due to a pronounced reduction in the cardiac output (the actual amount of blood pumped by the heart per minute). When the cardiac output is decreased there are changes in blood flow to various areas of the body.

The clinical picture depends on the rapidity of physiological changes and the cause of reduced cardiac output. The basic mechanism may be peripheral circulatory failure (a decline in venous return to the heart) and the manifestation may be syncope or shock.

When the basic mechanism is a disorder of the heart with onset of a few seconds to a few minutes the consequence is Adams-Stokes seizure: sudden loss of consciousness, slow heart rate, and transient or permanent atrioventricular block. When the onset is more gradual the result is cardiogenic shock: a drop in systolic blood pressure below 80 to 90 mm mercury, which may last for several hours.

When the onset is slow, perhaps over a period of weeks or months, the chronic low-output syndrome results with symptoms of lassitude, fatigue, loss of muscle strength, and decline in pulse pressure. This syndrome may be due to a cardiac disorder or a peripheral disorder, or may result from treatment for a cardiac disorder. It may occur with congestive heart failure.

CHRONIC CONGESTIVE HEART FAILURE (BACKWARD FAILURE)

Clinical Manifestations and Diagnosis

Backward failure is characterized by long-standing engorgement in the pulmonary and/or systemic vascular beds due to disease of the heart. It rarely involves only the left side of the heart because the sustained elevation of pulmonary vascular pressures, due to impairment of the left side, eventually leads to failure of the right side. It is convenient to separate left-sided heart failure from right-sided failure in discussing the physiological mechanisms and the signs and symptoms that occur.

The manifestations of left-sided heart failure are related to pulmonary congestion. When the left ventricle fails to pump the appropriate volume of blood per minute, the output fails and the residual diastolic volume and pressure rise and ultimately the pulmonary venous pressure increases. If the right ventricle pumps normally there is a redistribution of blood with more entering the pulmonary circulation and less entering the systemic circulation. As the pulmonary capillary pressure (normally 7 to 12 mm mercury at rest) rises and exceeds the plasma oncotic pressure, which is dependent on the concentration of serum proteins and normally is 25 to 30 mm mercury, transudation of fluid out of the pulmonary capillaries to the lung tissue and alveoli occurs. When the rate of lymphatic drainage cannot keep pace with the rate of capillary transudation pulmonary edema develops. Engorgement of the lungs with accumulation of edema fluid and blood increases the work of breathing and impairs the mechanism of ventilation, leading to the common subjective symptom of dyspnea (shortness of breath, breathlessness).

The early symptom is dyspnea on effort, due to inability of the heart to increase its output in response to exercise. Dyspnea on effort is not specific for congestive failure but may occur with other disorders, notably chronic lung disease.

Cardiac asthma is a common complaint. This wheezing is due to edema of the bronchial walls or to bronchospasm, and examination of the lungs reveals basilar rales. Often the patient may not be aware of the wheezing but complains rather of restlessness and cough. Cardiac asthma usually occurs on effort or paroxysmally during the night.

The patient may continue for months or years with symptoms only on effort; then symptoms begin to appear at rest. Dyspnea with exercise is intensified. Orthopnea—difficult breathing in the recumbent position—begins to be felt. Cheyne-Stokes respirations, usually at the onset of sleep, may occur, causing restlessness and insomnia. They are characterized by a phase of rapid, deep breathing followed by a period of apnea.

Paroxysmal nocturnal dyspnea is a common symptom of acute left ventricular failure. It is considered specific if the following pattern occurs: The patient may have had shortness of breath on effort but no symptoms at rest. He retires for sleep and after an hour or more he is suddenly awakened and senses a feeling of suffocation. He sits up on the side of the bed; he may lean forward, get up for a drink of water, or go to the window to get fresh air. At the same time he coughs and pants in the upright position. There may be excessive pallor of the skin, and profuse sweating. The attack may last 10 to 20 minutes. The symptoms subside and the patient returns to bed. No further attacks may take place during the remainder of the night.

Similar episodes may occur in advanced pulmonary emphysema and chronic bronchitis because of increased wheezing or accumulation of bronchial fluids while the patient is lying on his back. Pulmonary emboli and anxiety states may give rise to similar attacks but these usually are not paroxysmal, i.e., occurring for several nights in succession or more than once during the night.

Signs related to pulmonary congestion are basilar rales, pulmonary vascular shadows on x-ray study, reduction in vital capacity, and prolonged circulation time. Diastolic gallop and cardiac enlargement are usually present.

Sustained pulmonary congestion and pulmonary artery hypertension consequent to left heart failure may lead to impairment of right ventricular function. The clinical manifestations of right-sided heart failure are the result of the elevation of systemic venous pressure. Elevated venous pressure is evident in distention of the jugular veins in both the recumbent and the erect position. Another consequence is engorgement of the liver, which becomes tender and painful in response to pressure. Ultimately continuous venous congestion and reduced flow may lead to cirrhosis. The spleen may become enlarged and tender.

Peripheral venous congestion in the skin creates observable cyanosis, due partly to dilatation of venules and partly to impaired oxygenation of the arterial blood.

The accumulation of fluid in the interstitial spaces leads to edema. This may be evidenced first by an increase in weight of 10 to 20 pounds before obvious peripheral edema appears. The ankles and dependent parts of the body begin to swell; in the bedridden patient sacral edema may be prominent. Signs of advanced failure are pitting edema, in which firm finger pressure applied to the edematous region leaves a depression that slowly fills; hydrothorax, a large accumulation of edema in the lung bed; and ascites, accumulation of fluid in the abdomen.

Nausea is a common symptom and may be due to abdominal congestion or to the drugs used in therapy. A fever of one or two degrees is common, probably related to diminished heat loss due to cutaneous vasoconstriction.

The venous pressure is usually elevated when measured, but it may not be because the patient may have begun to improve, or the extracellular fluid volume has been depleted, or there is concurrent peripheral circulatory failure. The urine reflects the renal changes and will contain albumin and/or blood cells and cellular casts.

Prognosis

The outcome of congestive failure is difficult to predict as is the possibility of occurrence of complications. Improvement after a few days of treatment is an important prognostic measurement. The type of underlying heart disease is a factor influencing the outcome; generally failure resulting from mechanical lesions has a more favorable prognosis than failure resulting from coronary artery disease. The circumstances under which the failure develops influence the prognosis. When it has occurred as a result of some situation that can be treated, such as excessive ingestion of salt or increased exercise, the prognosis is generally more favorable than failure that develops without additional stress.

Medical Treatment

The clinical state of the patient with chronic congestive heart failure tends to improve or remain stationary for long periods and then suddenly to worsen due to complications. Attempts are made to prevent curcumstances that could cause increased heart rate or increased cardiac output for the already damaged heart, such as tachycardia, respiratory infections, physical exertion, fever, emotional states, anemia, and excessive ingestion of sodium chloride.

The aims of medical management are to reduce the work load of the heart by reducing metabolic demands through appropriate rest, position, and exercise; to increase the force of the contraction of the heart through administration of digitalis; to reduce congestion through restriction of sodium chloride intake and the use of diuretics; and to remove or treat the precipitating factors including the underlying heart disease.

Both physical rest and emotional rest are needed to reduce the work load of the heart to an appropriate level. The physician and nurse must pay as much attention to situations that cause concern, worry, and emotional stress as to physical exertion.

A combination of bed rest, chair rest, and minimal exercise is employed, depending on the patient's condition. The semirecumbent position in bed (the head of the bed raised as high as is comfortable) reduces dyspnea, probably because of decreased hydrostatic pressure in the lungs and increased vital capacity, reduces metabolic demands of labored breathing, decreases venous return, and promotes transudation of fluid in the dependent parts of the body thus diminishing pulmonary edema. Prolonged bed rest results in poor muscle tone, poor cardiovascular reactivity, venous stasis with predisposition to thromboembolism which can cause pulmonary infarction, and depression and anxiety on resumption of activity. To avoid the disadvantages of bed rest, rest in a comfortable chair near the bed for a specified number of minutes or hours and for a specified number of times a day is frequently prescribed by the physician. Minimal exercise in bed and slow walking to a chair are usually allowed. The general rule is to allow physical exercise that does not produce dyspnea. As the patient improves he gradually assumes more activity and eventually returns to customary or modified daily activities.

USE OF DIGITALIS

Digitalis increases the force of the heart contraction. This creates an increase in cardiac output leading to increased emptying of the heart and increased ventricular filling, and these result in a decrease in atrial, venous, and pulmonary arterial pressures. The renal blood flow and the glomerular filtration rate increase. These changes lead to sodium diuresis. The diuresis causes a decrease in the abnormally elevated circulating blood volume and this contributes to elimination of edema. Digitalis also decreases the ventricular rate when the patient has atrial fibrillation.

The initial dosage of digitalis often is referred to as the *digitalizing dose.* The total dose is based on the severity of symptoms (whether rapid or slow digitalization is needed), tolerance to the drug, and the preparation used. Between doses the patient is observed carefully for untoward effects of the drug; an electrocardiographic "rhythm strip" may be ordered to ascertain the digitalis effect and detect signs of toxicity. If the patient has been receiving digitalis within the preceding 2 weeks (the time required for its complete elimination), a careful survey is made for evidence of digitalis toxicity, potassium depletion, and renal failure before the digitalizing dosage is determined.

After digitalization has been accomplished, the physician prescribes a daily maintenance dose of a digitalis preparation according to the patient's response. Again, the patient is observed for symptoms of digitalis toxicity and potassium depletion while the proper maintenance dose is being established.

Patients who have had digitalis will require permanent digitalis therapy, except for those who have had surgical correction of underlying lesions and those who had temporary heart failure as a complication of a myocardial infarction.

All digitalis preparations have the same action on the heart and all have the same toxic effects. Each preparation has a distinctive time interval for beginning effect, maximum effect, and duration of action.

Digitalis Intoxication. The important symptoms of digitalis intoxication are anorexia, nausea, and vomiting, in that order. (These symptoms can be due to other causes such as local irritation of the gastrointestinal tract, abdominal congestion, potassium salts, ammonium chloride, and opiates.) Other less common symptoms are diarrhea and xanthopsia (yellow vision).

Digitalis intoxication can cause numerous disturbances in cardiac rhythm: premature beats, bigeminy, atrial flutter, severe bradycardia, atrial tachycardia with block, nodal rhythms with tachycardia, ventricular tachycardia, ventricular fibrillation. Arrhythmias are especially likely to occur with potassium depletion. Some changes in cardiac rate and rhythm can be identified by physical findings (pulse rate, apical rate, and heart sounds) but all changes necessitate electrocardiography for identification of the specific disorder. Changes in rate and rhythm, such as slow rate below 60, increased rate either regular or irregular, slight increase in rate rather than slowing with therapy, and changes from rapid rate to regular rate, suggest an arrhythmia, and an electrocardiogram should be made.

With mild symptoms of toxicity (anorexia, nausea, vomiting, diarrhea, infrequent ventricular ectopic beats), withdrawal of digitalis for a few days is the accepted treatment; should an arrhythmia develop, potassium salts are administered unless the patient has renal insufficiency. A protein-rich, carbohydrate-poor diet is recommended, since glucose ingestion causes a fall in plasma potassium. Impaired excretion of digitalis due to increasing cardiac or renal failure is one cause of digitalis intoxication but the most common cause is potassium depletion, which sensitizes the myocardium to the effects of digitalis. Potassium loss generally is due to use of diuretics, but may be due to vomiting, diarrhea, gastric suction, and glucose administered without a potassium supplement.

DIET AND DIURETIC THERAPY

Retention of sodium and water is corrected by restriction of sodium chloride and administration of a diuretic. If the patient is anorectic he may be given sodium-free milk and fruit juices. When he is able to eat, a balanced diet in which sodium is restricted is prescribed. The severity of congestion, the patient's response to treatment, and the choice of diuretic determine the degree of sodium restriction which will be necessary.

Usually the initial diet is restricted to 200 mg or 400 mg of sodium (equivalent to 0.5 g to 1 g of sodium); as congestion is relieved the diet is changed to an 800-mg sodium diet (2 g sodium) and possibly to a "salt-poor" diet (3 g to 5 g sodium). An alternative is to restrict sodium in the diet only slightly at first, and give large doses of diuretics; should heart failure remain uncontrolled the sodium restriction may be increased. The 200-mg and 400-mg sodium diets are tasteless and boring. Commercial sodium-free salt substitutes, vinegar, lemon juice, onion, or onion juice may be used to improve the flavor of foods. Sodium-poor food products such as milk, cereal, bread, and other bakery goods may be used for these diets. Water for drinking should be sodium-poor. A preparation containing vitamin B complex is prescribed if the patient is not eating well. The obese patient must lose weight, since overweight increases the work load of the heart.

The patient is weighed daily so that fluid accumulation and need for diuretic therapy can be measured. A gain of 3 to 4 pounds in a few days indicates a need for diuretic therapy, and a loss of weight acts as a yardstick for judging effectiveness of the therapy.

The type of diuretic and the dose and frequency of administration are determined by the changes in the signs and symptoms of congestion (edema, dyspnea), daily weight, and the dietary intake of sodium. There are several types of diuretics, each having certain advantages and disadvantages related to the time of effectiveness, duration of action, and mechanism of action on the kidneys causing excretion of sodium, chloride, water, and potassium in the urine. Ethacrynic acid (Edecrin) and furosemide (Lasix) are potent and rapid-acting diuretics which are commonly used. Diuresis begins in about 1 hour when the drug is given by mouth and within 5 to 10 minutes when given intravenously. The mercurial diuretics, including meralluride sodium (Mercuhydrin), mercumatilin sodium (Cumertilin), and mercaptomerine sodium (Thiomerin), or thiazide diuretics such as chlorothiazide (Diurel) and its derivatives, may be prescribed.

Potassium and chloride depletion is a common and dangerous result of diuretic therapy and is prevented or treated by giving a potassium supplement, usually potassium chloride in liquid or tablet form, with most diuretics.

Nursing Care

The nurse is responsible for maintaining the prescribed program of bed rest, chair rest, exercise, and walking.

POSITIONING

While in bed, the patient in a semirecumbent position requires support of all body parts. If pillows are to be used they should be placed so that his head, neck, and shoulders are in erect position rather than slumped forward. His arms may be supported on pillows piled high enough to prevent his shoulders from slumping and his chest from sinking. The purpose of this positioning is to provide for optimum chest expansion, thus minimizing dyspnea. A foot board will prevent foot drop and help prevent his sliding down. His position should be changed about every 2 hours, alternating right and left side-lying positions, a comfortable

*Figure 23–5
Resting position for
patient with orthopnea.
Note use of overbed table
and pillows for
positioning.*

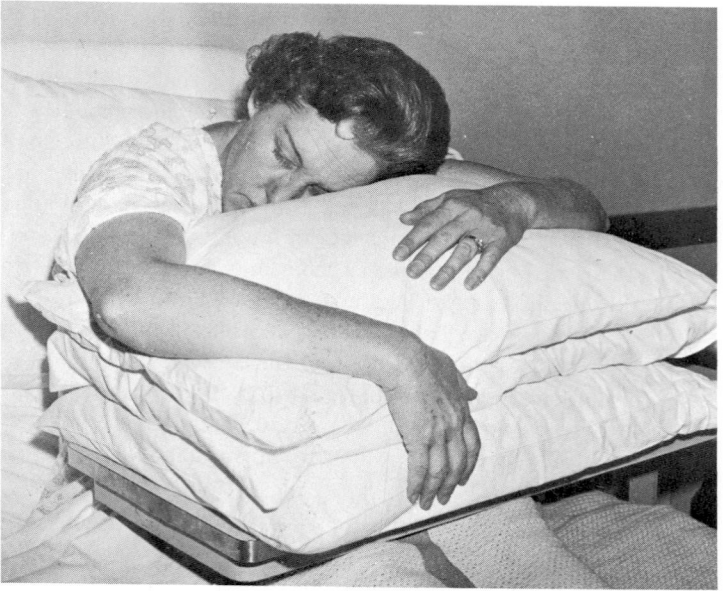

position if the head of the bed is raised and the head and arms are supported by pillows.

The orthopneic patient is helped if positioned in the erect sitting position in bed or with the upper part of the body leaning forward from the hips. The latter position is tiring unless the body is well supported. An overbed table on which a pillow is placed should be arranged across the patient's bed at shoulder height, so that he is supported when leaning forward as described.

His chair should have arms for support while he is sitting and when getting in and out of it. If he is weak and unsteady he should be assisted in getting in and out of bed, in and out of the chair, and in walking.

LIMITATIONS IN ACTIVITY

The very sick patient must be bathed, groomed, and fed; as his condition improves he may do these things himself. Should dyspnea develop during any physical activity the nurse stops the activity immediately. Her close experience with the patient gives the nurse the opportunity to gather the information she needs to help her decide what limitations in activity are necessary. She helps him identify the source of his worries and concerns and by so doing she becomes able to assist in alleviating these problems. She provides honest reassurance, explains events, stays with the patient when he is afraid, and controls the flow of visitors. If it is appropriate she refers the situation to another member of the health team. Oxygen may be required for relief of dyspnea and it should be readily available. The patient can be taught self-administration.

ELASTIC BANDAGES

The skin should be clean and dry before elastic bandages are applied to the leg. The leg should be arranged in a functional position with the knee flexed. Bandaging is begun at the instep, leaving toes exposed for assessment of circulation, and applied toward the trunk in spiral turns and figure-of-eight turns over joints (heel and knee). The bandage is anchored by two circular turns. Each turn of the bandage is applied with even pressure and should overlap the preceding turn for one-half to two-thirds the width of the bandage. The bandage should cover the heel and extend to the knee, or cover the knee, according to the physician's prescription. The physician may prefer elastic stockings to bandages. The bandages or stockings should be removed once every 8 hours and reapplied in 15 to 20 minutes or as ordered by the physician.

OBSERVATIONS OF ACTION OF DIGITALIS

The nurse should be familiar with the action of the digitalis preparation she is administering. She takes an apical pulse rate before administering digitalis; if the rate is below 60 per minute the drug is not given. She must constantly observe for symptoms of digitalis toxicity (anorexia, nausea, vomiting, changes in heart rate and rhythm) and of potassium depletion (anorexia, nausea, muscular weakness especially in the legs, fatigue, irregular pulse). Should these symptoms occur the doctor should be notified, and medications withheld until he has evaluated the situation and given further instructions. A delay of an hour or so in giving digitalis or a diuretic will not be harmful, whereas giving further doses in the presence of these symptoms may be.

Many physicians expect the nurse to take the initiative in obtaining an electrocardiogram rhythm strip when changes in cardiac rate and rhythm occur so that evidence of digitalis toxicity, potassium depletion, and arrhythmia is immediately available. Blood tests also are useful for measuring the serum potassium level.

OTHER MEASURES

Accurate daily recording of weight and intake and output forms the basis for measuring diuresis and adjusting the therapy. The weight should be taken at the same time each day and on the same scale. A bed scale can be used if the patient cannot get out of bed and stand for a few minutes. The intake record should include liquid foods (e.g., soup) as well as fluids, and the output record should include an estimate of the amount of sweating.

The diuretic is given in the morning or according to its mode of action to ensure diuresis during the day rather than at night. The output record provides the necessary information to accomplish this.

A diet severely restricted in sodium is unpleasant. The nurse can help the patient accept it by discussing the significance of the diet in his overall therapy and pointing out that adjustments can be made as he progresses. The diet may be planned to include some or most of the foods that he normally eats. The goal of the program is attainment of a balance of exercise, diet, and medications, and the patient who understands this finds it easier to accept the temporary restrictions placed upon him.

Severe edema of the legs which cannot be controlled by other measures may be relieved by the use of Southey tubes. Usually two tubes are inserted in each leg. The tube consists of a needle with a stylet. It is inserted into the leg after injection of procaine. The stylet is removed and the needle is attached to a sterile infusion set and collects the fluid by gravity flow. The needles are left in place as long as necessary, but seldom longer than 24 hours. Care must be taken to position and move the patient so the needles promote drainage and do not injure him. When the needles are removed the insertion site should be covered with a sterile bandage and any other measures necessary to prevent infection should be carried out. With hydrothorax, thoracentesis may be necessary; with ascites, paracentesis may be.

When the patient goes home he should possess an understanding of his program and what symptoms to observe for. If the doctor has given the instructions, the nurse should be able to clarify them when necessary.

ACUTE PULMONARY EDEMA

Clinical Manifestations and Diagnosis

In acute pulmonary edema the pulmonary congestion has advanced from interstitial pulmonary edema to alveolar pulmonary edema (generalized pulmonary edema). Transudation from the pulmonary capillaries to the lung tissue is so rapid that lymph flow cannot keep pace with transudation and severe pulmonary edema rapidly develops. This situation is due not only to the increased blood volume and sudden increase in blood flow to the heart but probably also to an abrupt decrease in the strength of the heartbeat.

Typically, the dyspnea rapidly becomes progressively worse, the cough becomes more severe, and there may be prolonged expiratory wheezing and a rattling sound from the trachea. Finally there is expectoration of copious, watery, frothy, or blood-tinged sputum. The patient is drowning in his own secretions. He is terrified, filled with dread of impending death. He may sit or stand in the upright position in efforts to breathe. He may feel faint or dizzy. He may be pale and drenched with sweat. His skin may be cold and clammy and cyanotic. Respirations are rapid and deep or shallow. The pulse is rapid. The systolic and diastolic blood pressures may be highly elevated or drop to shock levels. The venous pressure is elevated and the neck veins are distended due to systemic venous constriction. Wheezing, bubbling rales, and rhonchi are heard throughout the lungs on auscultation and obscure the sounds that could identify the underlying heart disease. A chest roentgenogram shows the typical pattern of alveolar pulmonary edema. The symptoms may subside within 15 minutes to several hours.

Many circumstances may initiate the episode: diagnosed or undiagnosed heart disease as in a person whose heart disease has not been previously recognized; following an acute myocardial infarction; malignant hypertension; disorders of rhythm; chronic heart failure. Pulmonary edema can occur in the absence of primary heart disease. Acute pulmonary edema can resemble acute bronchial asthma and distinction may be difficult when the patient's history is not known and the lung sounds mask the heart sounds; however, frothy pink-tinged sputum is not characteristic of acute bronchial asthma.

Medical Treatment

The treatment must be given promptly, with doctor and nurse working calmly and efficiently together so that several measures can be carried out simultaneously.

Most patients are more comfortable in an upright position, preferably in bed (with the head of the bed raised fully) so that other measures can be accomplished more easily; treatment can, however, be initiated with the patient sitting on the edge of the bed or in a chair.

Initially morphine sulfate or a related drug is given to depress respiration and break the cycle of dyspnea → congestion → dyspnea. Usually 10 to 15 mg is given slowly by vein while close observation is made for severe respiratory depression. Morphine antagonists such as nalorphine hydrochloride (Nalline) should be immediately available. (Morphine is contraindicated in pulmonary edema associated with increased intracranial pressure or pulmonary disease.)

Oxygen is administered in high concentration by mask or nasal catheter because severe hypoxia may develop.

Reduction of venous return to the heart can be accomplished in part through application of tourniquets to three extremities. The tourniquets are applied above the knees and above the elbows, sufficiently tight to occlude venous return. Every 15 minutes the tourniquets are rotated by placing a tourniquet on the fourth extremity and releasing one of the others. This is done according to a pattern; e.g., applied to both legs and right arm; removed from left leg and applied to left arm;

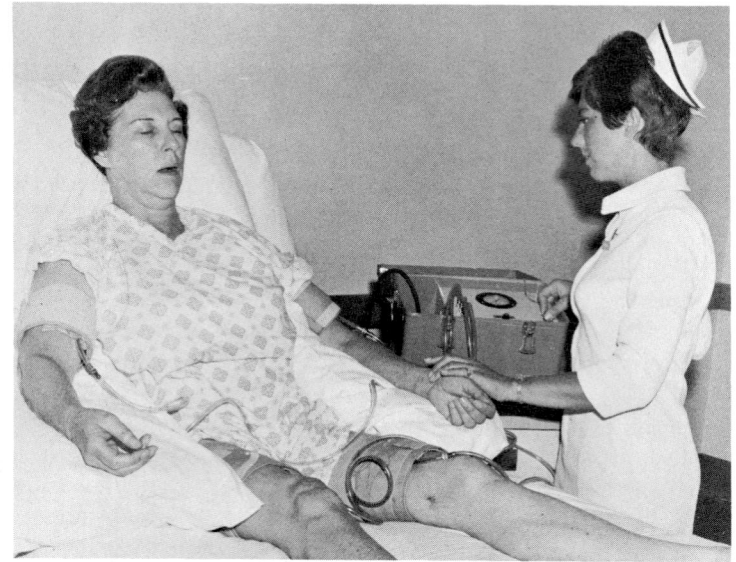

removed from right leg and applied to left leg; removed from right arm and applied to right leg; and so on. Thus, each extremity has a tourniquet applied for a total of 45 minutes out of each hour and 15 minutes of blood flow. Such rotation minimizes the possibility of thrombosis. The tourniquets may consist of rubber tubing, as in a stethoscope or an intravenous set, flat rubber tubing as in a Penrose tube, or blood pressure cuffs. The pattern for releasing tourniquets should be recorded and known to all personnel participating in the patient's care so that there is no confusion or danger of leaving a tourniquet on an extremity for more than 45 minutes of each hour.

Electric automatic rotating tourniquet machines are now available. The amount of pressure in the cuffs is controlled. One cuff is completely deflated automatically and the other cuffs are inflated every 11¼ minutes; complete rotation occurs every 45 minutes. The advantages of the machine over the manual tourniquets are that the pressure is more precise, the pressure can be gradually alternated from one extremity to another, and personnel are freed to perform other care activities.

When the symptoms are severe phlebotomy may be necessary to reduce the circulating blood volume. The amount withdrawn is 200 to 500 ml.

Aminophylline (theophylline ethylenediamine) may be given intravenously in a dose of 0.24 g if the patient does not respond promptly to other measures. This drug increases myocardial contractility and cardiac output for a period of 20 to 30 minutes when given intravenously. It has a vasodilating effect on arteries and veins and a diuretic effect due to increased renal blood flow and glomerular filtration rate. It dilates the bronchioles and relieves bronchospasm.

If the patient had not received digitalis previously, a rapid-acting digitalis preparation is administered intravenously in divided doses at intervals of 1 to 2 hours, depending on his response. If the patient had been receiving digitalis a rapid-acting digitalis preparation may or may not be given. Obviously, observations must be made for signs of digitalis intoxication and potassium depletion.

Edecrin or Lasix may be given intravenously to promote rapid diuresis.

Nursing Care

The nurse's responsibility is to stay with the patient if she is the first person to arrive at his bedside. She should have someone notify the doctor and see that emergency drugs and equipment are immediately available. She should place the patient in a comfortable upright and supported position, administer oxygen, and assist him in expectorating the frothy sputum. The patient is afraid and needs calm, competent help and the comfort of having someone stay with him.

It is usually the nurse's responsibility to manage rotation of tourniquets if they have been prescribed. She is responsible for assisting the doctor with administration of drugs, measuring and recording vital signs, and observing for appearance and disappearance of signs and symptoms.

As soon as the emergency is past, an attempt is made to identify the cause and the precipitating factors. Physical and emotional factors may be contributing factors. The author has observed an attack to occur after the visit of a particular person to a patient, after a patient who lived in a single room in a rooming house was told he was to be discharged "home," and after a patient has had unusual physical exertion. The physician and nurse can try to recall the events of the hour or so preceding the attack, seeking clues to stimuli; the patient probably will not be in a condition to do this until some time later. When the precipitating factors have been identified, efforts should be made to avoid them, or to deal with them appropriately.

Bibliography

Inflammatory Diseases of the Heart

Cluff, Leighton E. and F. Robert Fekety: Bacterial Endocarditis. in T. R. Harrison (Ed.): *Principles of Internal Medicine,* 5th ed. New York: Mc-Graw-Hill Book Company, 1966, pp. 1499–1504.

Cobbs, B. Woodfin: Clinical Recognition and Medical Management of Rheumatic Fever and Valvular Heart Disease. in J. Willis Hurst and R. Bruce Logue (Eds.): *The Heart.* New York: McGraw-Hill Book Company, 1966, pp. 519–609.

Dorney, Edward R.: Endocarditis. in J. Willis Hurst and R. Bruce Logue (Eds.): *The Heart.* New York: Mc-Graw-Hill Book Company, 1966, pp. 875–887.

Eliot, Robert S. and Jesse E. Edwards: Pathology of Rheumatic Heart Disease. in J. Willis Hurst and R. Bruce Logue: *The Heart.* New York:

McGraw-Hill Book Company, 1966, pp. 495–502.

Kerr, Andrew, Jr.: Bacterial Endocarditis Revisited. *Modern Concepts of Cardiovascular Disease,* XXXIII:1:831–836, January, 1964.

Rammelkamp, Charles H.: Hemolytic Streptococcal Infections (including Rheumatic Fever). in T. R. Harrison (Ed.): *Principles of Internal Medicine.* New York: McGraw-Hill Book Company, 1966, pp. 1517–1532.

Sellers, Thomas F., Jr.: Etiology of Rheumatic Heart Disease. in J. Willis Hurst and R. Bruce Logue (Eds.): *The Heart.* New York, McGraw-Hill Book Company, 1966, pp. 491–495.

Selzer, Arthur: *The Heart: Its Function in Health and Disease.* Los Angeles: University of California Press, 1966, pp. 132–144.

Strollerman, G. H.: Current Evaluation of

the Diagnosis, Treatment and Prevention of Rheumatic Fever. *Bulletin on Rheumatic Diseases,* 13:293, 1962.

Coronary Atherosclerosis

Baker, B. M., et al.: The National Diet-Heart Study. *Journal of American Medical Association,* 185:105–106, 1963.

Dawber, T. R., F. E. More, and G. V. Mann: Measuring the Risk of Coronary Heart Disease in Adult Population Groups. The Framingham Study. *American Journal of Public Health,* 47:4, 1957.

Doll, R., and A. B. Hill: Lung Cancer and Other Causes of Death in Relation to Smoking: Second Report on Mortality of British Doctors. *British Medical Journal,* 2:5001:1071–1081, 1956.

Dorn, H. F.: Tobacco Consumption and Mortality from Cancer and Other Diseases. *Public Health Reports,* 74:581, 1959.

Doyle, J. T., et al.: Prospective Study of Degenerative Cardiovascular Disease in Albany: Report of Three Years' Experience—I. Ischemic Heart Disease. *American Journal of Public Health,* 47:(Suppl. April, 1957): 25, 1957.

Doyle, J. T., et al.: The Relationship of Cigarette Smoking to Coronary Heart Disease: The Second Report of the Combined Experience of Albany, N.Y., and Framingham, Mass. Studies. *Journal of American Medical Association,* 190:886, 1964.

Doyle, J. T.: Etiology of Coronary Disease: Risk Factors Influencing Coronary Disease. *Modern Concepts of Cardiovascular Disease,* 35:4:81–86, April, 1966.

Doyle, J. T.: The Effects of Tobacco on the Cardiovascular System. in J. W. Hurst and R. B. Logue (Eds.): *The Heart.* New York: McGraw-Hill Book Company, 1966, pp. 1120–1123.

Fredrickson, Donald S.: Lipidosis and Xanthomatosis. in T. R. Harrison

(Ed.): *Principles of Internal Medicine,* 5th ed. New York: McGraw-Hill Book Company, 1966, pp. 578, 579.

Hammond, E. C.: The Effects of Smoking. *Scientific American,* 207:1:39–51, July, 1962.

Hopps, Howard C.: *Principles of Pathology,* 2d ed. New York: Appleton Century Crofts, 1964, p. 131.

Olson, Robert E.: Etiology of Coronary Atherosclerosis. in J. W. Hurst and R. B. Logue (Eds.): *The Heart.* New York: McGraw-Hill Book Company, 1966, pp. 622–627.

Olson, R. E., et al.: The Effect of Low-protein Diets upon Serum Cholesterol in Man. *American Journal of Clinical Nutrition,* 6:310, 1958.

Rosenman, R. H., et al.: A Predictive Study of Coronary Heart Disease. *Journal of American Medical Association,* 189:15–22, July, 1964.

Rosenman, R. H., et al.: Coronary Heart Disease in the Western Collaborative Group Study. *Journal of American Medical Association,* 195:86–92, January, 1966.

Saltzer, Arthur: *The Heart: Its Function in Health and Disease.* Los Angeles: University of California Press, 1966, pp. 157–159.

U.S. Department of Health, Education, and Welfare, Public Health Service, National Center for Health Statistics: *Mortality.* Vol. II, Part B. Statistics of the United States, 1964. Washington, D.C.: U.S. Government Printing Office, 1966, pp. 7–116; 7–120–7–122.

Yudkin, M.: Dietary Carbohydrate and Ischemic Heart Disease. *American Heart Journal* 66:835, 1963.

Ischemic Heart Disease

Elliott, W. C., and R. Gorlin: The Coronary Circulation, Myocardial Ischemia, and Angina Pectoris (Part II). *Modern Concepts of Cardiovascular Disease,* 35:11:117–122, November, 1966.

Resnik, W. H., and T. R. Harrison:

Ischemic Heart Disease. in T. R. Harrison (Eds): *Principles of Internal Medicine*, 5th ed. New York: McGraw-Hill Book Company, 1966, pp. 828–829.

Angina Pectoris

Bailey, C. P., A. May, and W. M. Lemmon: Survival after Coronary Endarterectomy in Man. *Journal of American Medical Association*, 164:641, 1957.

Cine Coronary Arteriography. Committee on Professional Education, American Heart Association. New York, 1962.

Dilley, R. B., et al.: Treatment of Coronary Occlusive Disease by Endarterectomy. *Journal of Thoracic Cardiovascular Surgery*, 50:511, 1965.

Effler, D. B., et al.: Coronary Endarterotomy with Patch-Graft Reconstruction: Clinical Experience with 34 Cases. *Annals of Surgery*, 162:590, 1965.

Effler, D. B., et al.: Myocardial Revascularization by Vineberg's Internal Mammary Artery Implant: Evaluation of Post-operative Results. *Journal of Thoracic Cardiovascular Surgery*, 50:527, 1965.

Elliott, W. C., and R. Gorlin: The Coronary Circulation, Myocardial Ischemia and Angina Pectoris (Part I). *Modern Concepts of Cardiovascular Disease*, 35:10:111–116, October, 1966.

Elliott, W. C., and R. Gorlin: The Coronary Circulation, Myocardial Ischemia, and Angina Pectoris (Part II). *Modern Concepts of Cardiovascular Disease*, 35:11:117–122, November, 1966.

Logue, R. B., and J. W. Hurst: Clinical Recognition of Coronary Atherosclerosis and Its Complications. in J. W. Hurst and R. B. Logue (Eds.): *The Heart*. New York: McGraw-Hill Book Company, 1966, pp. 669–678.

Nowlin, J. B., et al.: Association of Nocturnal Angina Pectoris with Dreaming. *Annals of Internal Medicine*, 63:1040, 1965.

Resnik, W. H., and T. R. Harrison: Ischemic Heart Disease. in T. R. Harrison (Ed.): *Principles of Internal Medicine*, 5th ed. New York: McGraw-Hill Book Company, 1966, pp. 829–833.

Sabiston, David C., Jr.: Role of Surgery in the Management of Myocardial Ischemia. *Modern Concepts of Cardiovascular Disease*, 35:12:123–127, December, 1966.

Sabiston, D. C., Jr., et al.: Proximal Endarterectomy, Arterial Reconstruction for Coronary Occlusion at Aortic Origin. *Archives of Surgery*, 91:758, 1965.

Sewell, W. H.: Results of 122 Mammary Pedicle Implantations for Angina Pectoris. *Annals of Thoracic Surgery*, 2:17, 1966.

Sones, F. Mason, Jr.: Cine Coronary Arteriography. in J. W. Hurst and R. B. Logue (Eds.): *The Heart*. New York: McGraw-Hill Book Company, 1966, pp. 701–709.

Vineberg, A. M.: Experimental Background of Myocardial Revascularization by Internal Mammary Artery Implantation and Supplementary Technics with Its Clinical Application in 125 Patients: A Review and Critical Appraisal. *Annals of Surgery*, 159:185, 1964.

Wood, P. W., et al.: The Effort Test in Angina Pectoris. *British Heart Journal*, 12:363, 1950.

Myocardial Infarction

Cross, Joseph C.: Back to Work after Myocardial Infarction. *American Journal of Nursing*, 62:2:58, February, 1962.

Day, Hughes W.: Acute Coronary Care—A Five Year Report. *American Journal of Cardiology*, 21:2:252–257, February, 1968.

Hall, Lydia and Genrose Alfano: Myocardial Infarction: Incapacitation or Rehabilitation? *American Journal of*

Nursing, 64:11:C20–C25, November, 1964.

Hazeltine, Louise S.: Myocardial Infarction: The Weeks of Healing. *American Journal of Nursing,* 64:11:C14–C20, November, 1964.

Killip, Thomas, III, and John T. Kimball: Treatment of Myocardial Infarction in a Coronary Care Unit: A Two Year Experience with 250 Patients. *American Journal of Cardiology,* 20:4:457–465, October, 1967.

Kinlein, M. Lucille: Myocardial Infarction: The Critical Hours. *American Journal of Nursing,* 64:11:C10–C13, November, 1964.

Levine, Samuel A: *Clinical Heart Disease,* 5th ed. Philadelphia: W. B. Saunders Company, 1958, pp. 131–163.

Logue, R. Bruce and J. Willis Hurst: Clinical Recognition of Coronary Atherosclerosis and Its Complications. in J. W. Hurst and R. B. Logue (Eds.): *The Heart.* New York: McGraw-Hill Book Company, 1966, pp. 679–696.

Logue, R. Bruce and J. Willis Hurst: Management of Coronary Atherosclerosis and Its Complications. in J. W. Hurst and R. B. Logue (Eds.): *The Heart.* New York: McGraw-Hill Book Company, 1966, pp. 717–725.

MacMillan, Robert L., et al.: Changing Perspectives in Coronary Care: A Five Year Study. *American Journal of Cardiology,* 20:4:451–457, October, 1967.

Modell, Walter, et al.: *Handbook of Cardiology for Nurses,* 5th ed. New York: Springer Publishing Co., Inc., 1966, pp. 76–102; 300–301.

Resnik, William H., and T. R. Harrison: Ischemic Heart Disease. in T. R. Harrison (Ed.): *Principles of Internal Medicine,* 5th ed. New York: McGraw-Hill Book Company, 1966, pp. 837–841.

Ruskin, Arthur: *Physiological Cardiology.* Springfield, Ill.: Charles C

Thomas, Publisher, 1953, pp. 128–134.

Wolff, Ilse S.: Myocardial Infarction: The Experience. *American Journal of Nursing,* 64:11:C3–C9, November, 1964.

Wright, Irving S.: *Myocardial Infarction.* New York: Grune & Stratton, Inc., 1954, pp. 60–198.

Clinical Syndromes of Heart Failure

Goldberg, Leon I.: Pharmacology of Cardiovascular Drugs. in J. W. Hurst and R. B. Logue (Eds.): *The Heart.* New York: McGraw-Hill Book Company, 1966, pp. 1136–1150.

Harrison, T. R., and William H. Resnik: The Congestive Syndromes: Acute Pulmonary Edema. in T. R. Harrison (Ed.): *Principles of Internal Medicine,* 5th ed. New York: McGraw-Hill Book Company, 1966, pp. 792–793.

Harrison, T. R., T. J. Reeven, and L. L. Hefner: The Congestive Syndromes: Chronic Heart Failure. in T. R. Harrison (Ed.): *Principles of Internal Medicine,* 5th ed. New York: McGraw-Hill Book Company, 1966, pp. 793–803.

Logue, R. Bruce and J. Willis Hurst: Etiology and Clinical Recognition of Heart Failure. in J. W. Hurst and R. B. Logue (Eds.): *The Heart.* New York: McGraw-Hill Book Company, 1966, pp. 248–269.

Logue, R. Bruce and J. Willis Hurst: Treatment of Heart Failure. in J. W. Hurst and R. B. Logue (Eds.): *The Heart.* New York: McGraw-Hill Book Company, 1966, pp. 269–282.

McIntyre, Hattie Mildred: Clinical Nursing and the Congestive Heart Failure Patient. *Cardio-Vascular Nursing,* 3:5:19–24, September-October, 1967.

Reeves, T. J., L. L. Hefner, and T. R. Harrison: Heart Failure: Pathophysiology and Classification. in T. R. Harrison (Ed.): *Principles of Internal Medicine,*

5th ed. New York: McGraw-Hill Book Company, 1966, pp. 778–786.

Resnik, William H., and T. R. Harrison: The High-Output and Low-Output Syndromes. in T. R. Harrison (Ed.): *Principles of Internal Medicine,* 5th ed. New York: McGraw-Hill Book Company, 1966, pp. 787–791.

Schlant, Robert C.: Altered Physiology of Cardiovascular System in Heart Failure. in J. W. Hurst and R. B. Logue (Eds.): *The Heart.* New York: McGraw-Hill Book Company, 1966, pp. 224–234.

Selkurt, Ewald E.: Pathological Physiology of the Cardiovascular System: Congestive Failure. in Ewald E. Selkurt (Ed.): *Physiology,* 2d ed. Boston: Little, Brown and Company, 1966, pp. 407–415.

Tuttle, Elbert P., Jr.: Hormonal Factors in the Edema of Heart Failure. in J. W. Hurst and R. B. Logue (Eds.): *The Heart.* New York: McGraw-Hill Book Company, 1966, pp. 239–244.

Waters, William C., III: Disturbance of Inorganic Metabolism in Heart Failure. in J. W. Hurst and R. B. Logue (Eds.): *The Heart.* New York: McGraw-Hill Book Company, 1966, pp. 244–248.

SECTION 1A DISEASES OF THE HEART

R U T H   E .   B A R S T O W *

* The author acknowledges the contribution of Barbara Minckley, who prepared the illustrations for this section.

Disorders of Rhythm

Important physiological attributes of the heart are automatism and rhythmicity. The muscle automatically contracts, rests, and contracts again with a definite rhythm. This activity goes on without extrinsic stimuli. During an average life span, the heart may contract more than 2.6 billion times.

Normally, the heartbeat is initiated in the sinoatrial (SA) node, which lies in the right atrium near the superior vena cava entrance. The node is composed of a specialized bundle of muscle fibers and might be thought of as a generator that sends out electrical impulses on a regularly recurring basis. It is called the *pacemaker*, since it controls the rate of initiation of the heartbeat. A normal conduction pathway exists, yet each muscle cell or portion of the pathway is capable of initiating the electrical impulse to which the rest of the heart responds.

The pacemaker impulse spreads radially over the atria, and the excitable muscle contracts. When the impulse nears the coronary sinus and the atrioventricular opening, another specialized group of cells, the atrioventricular (AV) node, is energized. This node transmits the impulse over the bundle of His, its right and left branches, and their division into plexuses around the Purkinje cells, and ultimately to the fine fibrils that stimulate the individual cells of the ventricles to contract. The normal cardiac cycle—one heartbeat—consists of three phases taking place in 0.8 second, according to Gray. The duration of the atrial contraction is 0.1 second; of the ventricular systole, 0.3 second; of complete diastole, 0.4 second. During diastole, the heart is in a refractory period and cannot respond to stimulation. Each phase of the cycle has a unique electrical pattern, which can be recorded on the electrocardiogram. (See Figure 23-7.)

While the heartbeat is not initiated by extrinsic stimulation, its rate and force vary with impulses from the sympathetic trunk and vagal branches that form the cardiac plexus of the autonomic nervous system.

Cardiac arrhythmias occur in both health and disease. They may be persistent or transitory, regular or irregular, malignant or benign. Only a few significant arrhythmias will be considered here since space does not permit full discussion of all of them. (See Figure 23-8.)

CHANGES IN SINUS RATE

The heart responds to changes in bodily needs by adjusting its rate. With increased demand (as in physical exercise), the vagi are depressed or the sympathetic chain is stimulated, and the heart rate increases. *Sinus tachycardia* exists when the rate is between 100 and 160 beats per minute. It occurs commonly with exercise, excitement, and eating; it may be associated with anemia, infection, myocardial infarction, and hyperthyroidism. Usually, sinus tachycardia is treated by having the individual rest; however, sedation may be required. Any underlying disease should be treated.

With decreased demand for oxygen, the heart rate slows. A decrease below 60 is termed *sinus bradycardia*. As a rule, it occurs with the subject at rest, but it may be associated with malnutrition, jaundice, digitalis intoxication, increased intracranial pressure, and carotid sinus pressure. Individuals who experience

*Figure 23–7
Schematic drawing of
cardiac cycle and
corresponding electro-
cardiographic pattern.
P wave, atrial contrac-
tion; Q, R, S complex,
ventricular contraction;
T wave, retreat of
excitation wave; S-A
node, sinoatrial node;
A-V node, atrioventricular
node; A-V bundle,
atrioventricular bundle.*

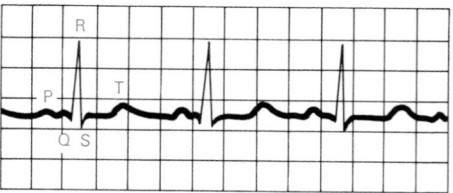

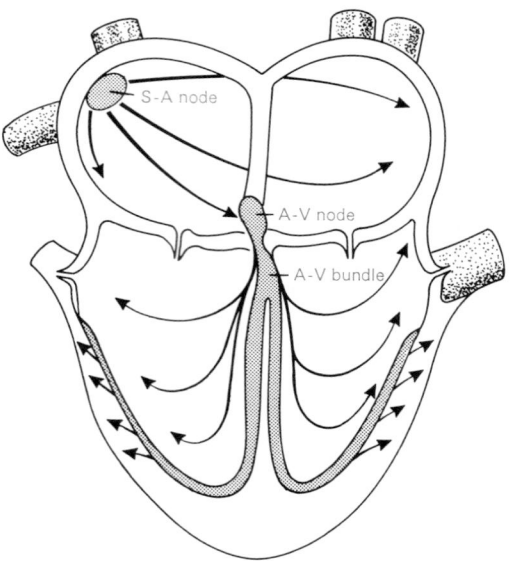

episodes of bradycardia should be cautioned not to stand still for long periods or wear tight-fitting clothes, especially collars. They should lie down if they feel faint. In a few cases it may be necessary to administer atropine regularly, but in most cases no treatment is necessary.

PREMATURE CONTRACTIONS

Irritability of any chamber of the heart, due to local ischemia, pressure from calcified plaques, dilatation or hypertrophy of a chamber, electrolyte imbalance, or drug toxicity, causes release of impulse before the normal sinus discharge—a premature beat. The wave may be transmitted throughout the heart or to portions of it. Whether or not the impulse is strong enough to be felt at the radial pulse depends upon its time of occurrence in the cardiac cycle. The premature contraction may be full and strong, or weak; frequently it follows the normal beat so closely that the beats appear to be joined—"coupled." The compensatory pause that follows further emphasizes the event. Atrial premature contractions occur most often in young adults, ventricular ones in older persons. Premature contractions may be insignificant and may be related to ingestion of coffee or alcohol, excessive smoking, lack of sleep, or stress; or they may point to an underlying

Figure 23-8
Electrocardiographic
patterns of common
arrhythmias.

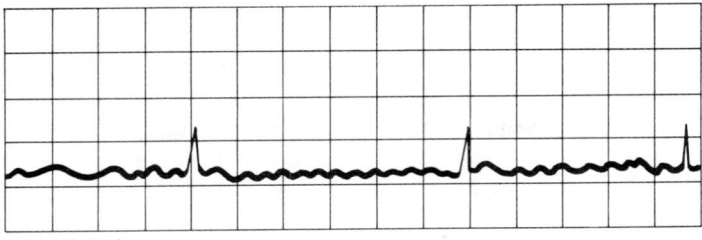

Atrial fibrillation

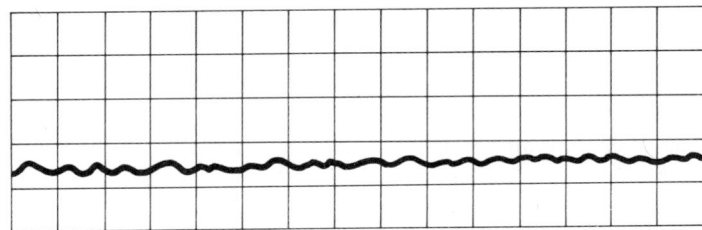

Ventricular fibrillation

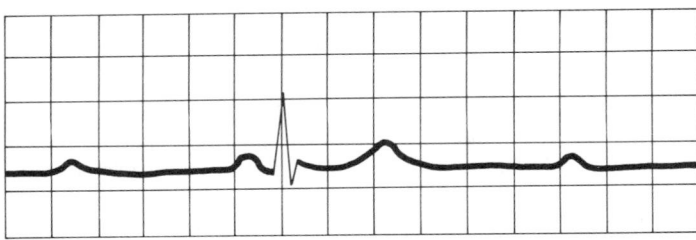

Heart block

heart disease or an infection. Usually there is no circulatory deficit. The individual becomes aware of the action of his heart; it "turns over" or "flutters" in his chest. Palpitations, a "catch" in the throat, and cough frequently are associated manifestations. No treatment is necessary unless the premature contractions occur so often that they cause anxiety. If removal of stimulants or stress is not corrective, a sedative is given. Frequently occurring premature ventricular contractions (PVC), especially when associated with ischemic heart disease, warn of impending ventricular tachycardia or fibrillation and should receive more definitive treatment, as described in the section on ventricular tachycardia.

PAROXYSMAL TACHYCARDIA

In paroxysmal tachycardia the heart rate is increased to 160 to 220 beats per minute. The tachycardia may be of atrial, AV nodal, or ventricular origin. Characteristically, the onset is sudden and the disappearance abrupt, though it may persist for days.

Atrial Tachycardia

Atrial paroxysms occur most often in young adults, whereas ventricular paroxysms occur in older persons. Again, stimulants, stress, and infectious processes are implicated, but in many cases heart disease is present.

The patient is aware that something is wrong. The heart rate is so rapid that cardiac output and vital capacity are decreased. With a rapid rate, the length of each phase of the cycle is shortened; diastole is too brief to permit complete filling of the ventricles, so the amount of blood pumped forward during each systole is lessened. A decrease in the amount of oxygenated blood reaching the peripheral structures causes weakness and syncope. Dyspnea results from the pulmonary congestion. The patient is apprehensive and may become nauseated and vomit; he may lose consciousness.

No treatment is necessary if the incident is transitory. Simple measures to stimulate the vagus nerve may be employed, e.g., leaning over, breathing or holding the breath against the closed glottis, or exerting pressure against the eyes or the carotid sinus. (The last one of these is not taught to patients because carotid pressure may cause an asystole that requires immediate treatment with atropine or epinephrine.) The patient with recurrent attacks of atrial (supraventricular) tachycardia is taught these and other measures that are related to alterations in hemodynamics which may cause a significant change in blood flow. Circulation slows and gravity acts to cause pooling of large quantities of blood in the abdomen and lower extremities. A sudden movement or a change from sitting to standing posture may initiate the aberrant rhythm. Frequent mild exercise and avoidance of prolonged periods of sitting are helpful measures. If severe attacks occur often in spite of precautionary measures, the patient is placed on bed rest and digitalized. It may be necessary to administer quinidine or procaine amide hydrochloride to decrease muscle irritability and conduction time. Synchronized d-c countershock after digitalization may be employed if other methods are not successful.

Ventricular Tachycardia

In ventricular paroxysmal tachycardia, the patient appears and often is more ill. The condition rarely develops in the normal heart. The majority of patients have a history of old or recent myocardial infarction; many of them are in congestive heart failure; some are reacting to toxic doses of digitalis, quinidine, procaine amide, or chloroquine.

The attacks typically begin with sporadic premature ventricular contractions increasing to six or more in brief "runs," i.e., six or more premature contractions appear between longer periods of normal contractions. The paroxysms may last a few seconds and return or may persist for minutes, hours, or days. The death rate in ventricular paroxysmal tachycardia is relatively high because it may lead abruptly to ventricular fibrillation or arrest; therefore treatment should be initiated as soon as the diagnosis is made.

The symptoms are similar to those described under atrial paroxysms but the patient is more obviously ill. Frequently he is already hospitalized for the underlying heart condition.

Cardiac monitoring should be started and the patient should have constant professional attendance. The arrhythmia is identified by the ECG. The ventricular complexes look much like PVCs and the rate is usually between 140 to 175, although it may go as high as 250. The nurse who notes the arrhythmia should notify the physician immediately. Vital signs should be taken frequently, since congestive heart failure or shock may occur. The physician will usually give a drug to decrease myocardial excitability, probably procaine amide 300 to 500 mg intravenously, or lidocaine 70 mg intravenously followed by an intravenous infusion of lidocaine in 5 percent dextrose and water, at a rate that provides 2 to 4 mg of drug per minute. Countershock may be employed if these measures are not effective.

FIBRILLATION

Fibrillation is spontaneous uncoordinated contraction of individual muscle fibers of the heart.

Atrial Fibrillation

Atrial fibrillation is the most common arrhythmia for which treatment is required. The SA node no longer controls pacing; multiple excitation waves, emanating from irritable foci, course around the atria causing rapid, chaotic twitching. The AV node does not transmit all the impulses and the ventricles cannot respond to all those which are transmitted, so the ventricular rate is erratic. This situation is directly related to the refractory periods of these tissues. If an atrial wave reaches the AV node during its refractory period, the impulse will not be transmitted. Since the refractory periods of the tissues vary, an impulse that crosses the AV node may not be sufficient to stimulate the resting ventricle. The rate is too fast to permit the heart chambers to fill, with the result that not enough blood is propelled forward to create a radial pulse with each systolic contraction, and a *pulse deficit* occurs. The pulse deficit is the difference between the apical and radial pulses. Heart action is wasted and the cardiac output decreases.

Atrial fibrillation is frequently associated with mitral stenosis, ischemic heart disease, or other cardiac conditions; thyrotoxicosis; digitalis toxicity; electrolyte imbalance; excessive ingestion of alcohol, coffee, or food; excessive smoking or stress; it may follow myocardial infarction. It may be chronic, paroxysmal, or an isolated attack.

The individual may have no symptoms. In fact atrial fibrillation may exist for years without heart failure if the ventricular rate is slow enough. The patient may be aware of the irregular beat and also of heart movement in his chest or fullness and fluttering in the neck. He will manifest signs and symptoms of decreased cardiac output as described previously.

Treatment is directed toward increasing circulatory efficiency. Patients with symptoms are placed on bed rest and digitalized to slow the ventricular rate.

Quinidine sulfate or procaine amide hydrochloride (Pronestyl) can be administered if fibrillation does not cease with the administration of digitalis. Both produce similar effects although through different mechanisms. Quinidine acts directly on the myocardium; the refractory period of the muscle fibers is prolonged, so contraction cannot occur with the multiple excitation waves. Pronestyl decreases myocardial excitability and conduction time and prolongs atrial refractory periods. Both drugs are potentially dangerous, since overdoses cause ventricular fibrillation. Conversion to normal sinus rhythm may cause dislodgment of mural (wall) thrombi formed by the slowly eddying currents of blood in the atria during fibrillation. Cardiac standstill may result if there is complete depression of the AV node. Warning symptoms of toxicity are nausea, vomiting, respiratory distress, headache, vertigo, and tinnitus. Side effects occur less frequently with Pronestyl, but agranulocytosis may be produced which may be fatal.

CARDIOVERSION

The physician may choose to bring about reversion of atrial fibrillation by administering electric countershock from a defibrillator, a technique known as *cardioversion*. The machine delivers direct current through electrodes placed on the chest wall with sufficient intensity to induce defibrillation of the muscle. The synchronizer is so adjusted that the shock is delivered in exact relation to the patient's cardiac cycle. Cardiac activity is monitored continuously. The defibrillator causes all the heart cells to be stimulated simultaneously by a strong electric impulse and therefore to be depolarized simultaneously. All cardiac activity is stopped and the pacemaker thus can resume its normal function.

In preparation for cardioversion, the patient is given a sedative and light anesthesia is induced. Quinidine sulfate is administered before and after the procedure.

Atrial Flutter

Atrial flutter denotes an atrial rate of 200 to 360 beats per minute. The beat is regular. Again, because of their refractory periods, neither the AV node nor the ventricle can respond to all impulses. Usually a constant ratio between atrial and ventricular rates occurs, commonly 2:1. After digitalization, the block deepens to 3:1 or 4:1; the decreased rate of ventricular contraction provides adequate circulation. Atrial flutter is usually found in older persons with heart disease. Treatment is similar to that of fibrillation.

When other methods are ineffective and congestive heart failure has supervened, it is sometimes necessary to bring about reversion to normal sinus rhythm (NSR) with a defibrillator.

Ventricular Fibrillation

Ventricular fibrillation is the most dangerous arrhythmia, since the ineffectual rapid twitching of the ventricle cannot support circulation and is incompatible with life unless of momentary duration. Ventricular fibrillation is a cause of sudden death, especially in the heart severely damaged by coronary artery disease. Overdosages of Pronestyl, quinidine, or a quinidine-digitalis combination can also cause ventricular fibrillation. The fibrillation can occur following other arrhythmias and is seen in the dying patient.

The patient is pulseless, blood pressure is undetectable, and coma supervenes rapidly. *Prompt action is necessary to maintain life.* An airway is established with an S tube (an oropharyngeal airway with an extension to permit mouth-to-mouth resuscitation without contact between the mouths of the operator and patient) or endotracheal tube. Respiration is assisted by mouth-to-mouth resuscitation, a mechanical ventilator, such as the Bird or Bennett intermittent positive pressure breathing respirators, or pulmonator bag. The pulmonator bag is a rubber bag that can be squeezed to force air into the patient's lungs. An oxygen source can be attached to the air inlet. The outlet fitting permits attachment to either an oronasal mask or an endotracheal tube. External cardiac massage is performed to maintain circulation. The defibrillator is employed as follows: electrodes are placed on the anterior chest wall and a high-intensity shock is given to produce sudden depolarization of the heart.

With frequent episodes it may be necessary to utilize an external pacemaker. Digitalis, quinidine, and Pronestyl are useful in preventing ventricular fibrillation.

With the availability of coronary care units, the patient can be observed by cardiac monitor and an arrhythmia that could lead to ventricular fibrillation is terminated before the fibrillation occurs. Premature ventricular contractions and ventricular tachycardia may be treated as described previously. The best treatment for ventricular fibrillation is prevention.

NURSING CARE OF PATIENTS WITH ARRHYTHMIAS

The nurse has two chief concerns: to create an atmosphere that is conducive to reducing stress and self-concern in the patient and to make nursing observations that will assist the physician in his diagnosis and treatment.

The nurse should understand and begin to recognize the common aberrations of rhythm. To do this, she counts the pulse carefully for 1 minute and notes alterations in regularity, volume, rate, and character. She listens to the apical pulse through the stethoscope and palpates the radial pulse at the same time. If the pulses appear to have different rhythms, she requests another person to count simultaneously and calculate the pulse deficit. If an arrhythmia has occurred or circumstances suggest that it is imminent, a cardiac monitor should be employed. The nurse should learn to distinguish between a transitory relatively harmless aberration and a life-threatening arrhythmia. It should be remembered that a keenly observant nurse who knows her patient is more valuable than a monitor.

Arrhythmias can cause impairment of circulation, especially if chronic, long-standing, and the result of a cardiac disease. The reason for this is that the amount of circulating blood is reduced. Moderate increases in heart rate will affect the output of blood per beat (stroke volume) but not the total output of blood per minute (minute volume). An extremely rapid rhythm, particularly an irregular one, causes diminution of both stroke and minute volumes. There may be little or no impairment, increasing impairment, or virtual standstill as in ventricular fibrillation. According to Loeb, impairment of circulation to the brain causing ischemia will result in confused or inattentive behavior, vertigo, syncope, restlessness, convulsions, coma, and finally death. Peripheral circulatory failure will cause pallor or cyanosis, diaphoresis, and hypotension. These symptoms of shock are usually late and generally found with myocardial failure.

Cardiac action is directly influenced by the electrolyte levels. With an increase above normal in potassium (hyperkalemia) the heart muscle becomes toxic. The refractory period is prolonged, conduction is impaired, and the end result may be cardiac arrest in diastole. With a decrease below normal in potassium (hypokalemia), arrhythmias, especially ventricular or atrial premature contractions, may develop. One of the effects of digitalis, especially when used with diuretics, is to decrease the serum potassium. Besides having irregularities in heart rhythm, the patient becomes hallucinatory and overtalkative, and has weak, limp extremities.

The presence of acidosis or alkalosis and alterations of electrolyte balance can produce fatal arrhythmias.

An episode of arrhythmia should be reported immediately and carefully documented. The time of onset and the signs and symptoms elicited are important diagnostic aids for the physician. Some arrhythmias are so similar that the electrocardiograph provides the only definitive method of diagnosis. The doctor may leave orders for a "stat EKG" for the occasion when an episode is observed in his absence. If the patient is being monitored, "rhythm strips" are easily obtained as most monitors provide a method of attachment to an electrocardiograph. Some systems are equipped to produce an EKG printout every 15 to 30 minutes so that a permanent record is available. Others include a "memory loop" that will reproduce a record of the last minute of monitoring prior to an arrhythmia that sets off the alarm system. Monitors with alarm systems have a heart rate meter that is set at the upper and lower limits of acceptable heart rate, e.g., 30 as the low limit and 150 as the high limit. When the heart rate drops below or increases above these limits, a buzzer will sound.

If a patient is being monitored and there is an alarm system that is audible at the bedside, he should be given special instructions so that he will not be unduly disturbed if the alarm does sound. He should be told that he is the best judge of the way he feels. Even if the alarm goes off, he is probably all right if he feels no different subjectively. Rolling over or moving about vigorously will produce false alarms. If the electrodes become loosened or disconnected or if the paste under them becomes dry, an alarm will sound. The patient should be reassured that someone will attend him immediately. Some patients have found that taking an electrode off is an effective way of getting immediate assistance! This should be discouraged, of course; the best method is to answer his call bell promptly.

Drugs used in the treatment of one arrhythmia may cause another more dangerous arrhythmia. The nurse must observe the patient closely for signs of toxicity. If cardiac arrest occurs, the nurse should establish and maintain an airway, give mouth-to-mouth resuscitation, and administer oxygen. If hospital policy allows it, the nurse trained in these techniques may perform external cardiac massage and use the defibrillator. After the physician arrives she supplies him with necessary drugs, equipment, and assistance.

The patient's psychological problem induced by the stress of the situation may be more difficult to deal with than the physical ones. In his narrowed world, he is constantly reminded of his heart. If he lies quietly, he can feel pulsation in his large arteries. This preoccupation may cause enough anxiety to generate premature contractions, and the patient becomes aware of the flutter in his chest. He goes to sleep with the beat of his heart in his ear. His behavior may become neurotic.

The therapeutic team and the patient's family can cooperate to enlarge his world. After he has passed through the stages of denial, realization, and despair, he can be helped to reorganize his self-concept so as to acknowledge the damaged heart. His adjustment depends on both his inner resources and the attitudes of those around him. Frequent visits by calm, assured, and reassuring personnel will help. He should be allowed the maximum activity within his limitations; he can be helped to learn what he may do. At first, short-term goals such as getting out of bed for the first time can be emphasized; later, the focus is on long-term goals. The patient should be encouraged to plan ahead and to believe that death is far away. Allowing him to "talk through" his anxiety will enable him to draw on inner resources for problem-solving. Visiting nurses can assist in caring for the patient following his discharge from the hospital.

Heart Block

Heart block is an obstruction to the passage of the electrical impulse from the atria to the ventricles. Block can occur in one of the bundle branches but usually occurs at the AV node or in the main bundle. The block can range from simple delay to complete block. (See Figure 23–8.)

Heart block can occur in almost any disease affecting the heart, such as rheumatic fever, arteriosclerosis, myocardial infarction, diphtheria, syphilis, hypertension, and congenital heart diseases. It is caused by structural damage, vagal effects that may be functional, drug toxicity, and nutritional changes.

The degree of the block is described by a ratio in which the first number indicates the atrial beats and the second number the ventricular beats. A first degree block, 1:1, indicates a pause or delay. A second-degree, partial or incomplete, block means that some atrial impulses are blocked so one beat in four, five, six, seven, or eight is skipped. The ratio might be 5:4. In a high-degree block, every second or third impulse is not responded to by the ventricles and a 2:1 or 3:1 block exists. In complete block (third degree), there is no atrioventricular association and the ventricles beat in an inherent rhythm which is approximately half the normal sinus rhythm. A bundle branch block is a delay along one of the branches causing asynchronous ventricular depolarization.

DEGREES OF BLOCK

First-degree block is asymptomatic. Second-degree block may cause palpitations of subjective awareness of the pause. A high-degree block may cause dyspnea, but rarely heart failure. If the underlying condition is treatable the block will disappear.

Complete heart block may have other causes but is most commonly found in arteriosclerotic heart disease. Since arteriosclerosis is a manifestation of aging, complete heart block is a serious disorder. The block may become chronic and present no symptoms if the person learns to live within the limits of his circulatory capability; if imprudent, he has exertional dyspnea. Another patient may become completely incapacitated or suffer from Stokes-Adams syndrome. When the pacemaker shifts from the atria to the ventricles there is a pause before idioventricular pacing begins. During this interval the symptoms ascribed to Stokes-Adams syndrome appear. The patient may experience dizziness or faintness and become pale, hesitant in speech, and unsteady in gait. If the ventricular asystole persists longer than 15 seconds, loss of consciousness, cyanosis, and convulsions occur. The attacks are precipitated by excessive exertion, excitement, or electrolyte imbalance, according to Abrams and Hudson. Between attacks, the pulse rate characteristically is 30 to 40 beats per minute.

If the attacks are infrequent, they may be prevented by administration of isoproterenol hydrochloride (Isuprel), 15 mg sublingually several times daily, or ephedrine sulfate, 20 to 30 mg orally three times daily. During an acute attack, ephedrine in oil or molar sodium lactate may be given for prolonged effect. Uncontrolled attacks ultimately lead to death.

Pacemakers

With the development of the implantable artificial pacemaker, the prognosis in heart block has improved. The artificial pacemaker is a reliable substitute for the ventricular pacemaker. The atria continue to contract automatically and their impulses usually have no effect upon the ventricles. The ventricles beat independently because of the presence of the block, and the electrical pacemaker ensures that the beat will be continuous, strong, and regular.

In the artificial pacemaker, an electrical impulse is discharged from the battery through a stimulating electrode (anode, or positive charge) into or through the myocardium to an indifferent electrode (cathode, or negative charge). This electrode returns the impulse to the energy source. Thus, an electrical circuit is established which stimulates the ventricles to contract. Placement of the pacemaker

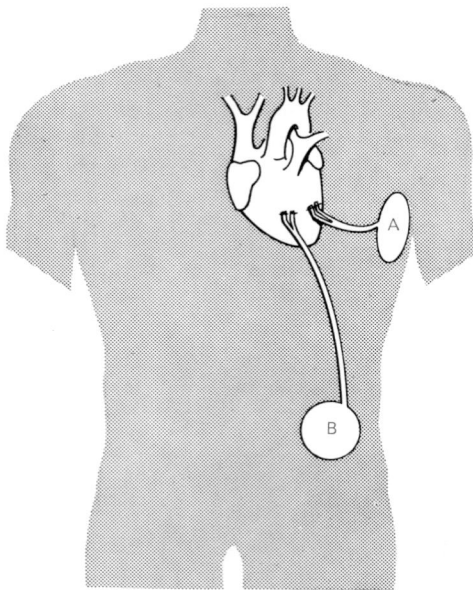

Figure 23–9
Relative positioning of two types of pacemaker implants: A, axillary; B, abdominal.

unit and the electrodes varies with the type used and the circumstances of each case. (See Figure 23–9.)

An external pacemaker can be used preoperatively or during an emergency. It may be set to operate continuously or attached to a special monitor that will sound an alarm when the pulse rate drops and activate the pacemaker so that it functions until reset by the doctor. A band is placed around the chest and two electrodes with a ground are fixed to it. Electrical impulses from the unit stimulate the heart to beat at a set rate. The resultant twitching of chest muscles may be quite uncomfortable. The skin is marked and the electrodes are repositioned as necessary. Small ulcers may appear on the skin under the electrodes. A doctor's order is needed for preventive care, which includes removal of the electrodes, simple soap and water cleansing of the skin, application of alcohol and, after the skin is thoroughly dry, of electrode paste, and replacement of the electrodes. If the transvenous catheter electrode described below is used these ulcerations will not develop, and only the site of the percutaneous puncture will require meticulous attention. The painful stimulation of chest muscles does not occur with this type of pacing. Transvenous electrodes are used more frequently than chest electrodes.

The patient should be encouraged to express his fears and preconceived ideas about the pacemaker. He may have experienced relief of symptoms if the external pacemaker has been used. The nurse can assist him by answering his questions and can call upon her knowledge of the behavioral sciences to help him overcome his fears.

Several types of internal pacemakers are available. The one described by Zoll is a transistorized mercury-cell battery unit that is placed in a molded epoxy resin case enclosed in a Teflon mesh envelope. The wires are coated with Teflon and enclosed in silicone rubber up to the bipolar platinum needle electrodes. Each bipolar electrode is capable of assuming the total work of stimulating the heart so that in effect a "spare" is installed. This is reassuring to the patient.

In the transthoracic approach, the electrodes are imbedded in the myocardium after the wires have been brought into position through a tunnel created under the muscles to the site of pacemaker implantation. Zoll suggests imbedding the electrodes in the axilla behind the border of the pectoralis muscle. Another procedure is to implant them in the abdominal wall over the external oblique muscle. The rate of electrical impulse is set between 70 and 90 per minute. This normal rate is thought preferable to slower rates, which cause compensatory hypertrophy of the heart. The unit measures 6.5 x 6.9 x 1.7 cm and weighs 170 g. The pacemaker should last for 2 to 5 years.

The pacemaker just described is being worn by many patients. During the past few years, a transvenous type has been used increasingly for temporary or permanent installation. One of its chief advantages is that the entire procedure can be done with the patient under local anesthesia; a thoracotomy is unnecessary, so many patients who are poor surgical risks can be treated effectively. A catheter bearing the electrodes is inserted into the external jugular or subclavian vein and manipulated into place under fluoroscopic guidance into the apical wall of the right ventricle. The pacemaker unit usually is imbedded over the pectoralis.

The pacemaker can be one of three types: an asynchronous fixed rate unit described by Zoll; a synchronous type used to replace the AV nodal conduction system when atrial activity is adequate; the stand-by or demand pacemaker, which functions only when asystole occurs and ceases when spontaneous activity resumes.

The asynchronous unit was the first one designed; its drawback is that its rate does not vary regardless of the patient's physical activity or the activity of the intrinsic electrical system of the heart. Occasionally there is competition between the two electrical systems and it is possible for an electrical discharge from the artificial pacemaker to occur at the wrong phase of the cardiac cycle and result in ventricular fibrillation. More frequently a tachycardia can occur as a result of the double beat of intrinsic and pacemaker stimulation. The pacemaker can be turned off manually with a special needle.

The synchronous type responds to atrial activity, bypasses the AV node, and stimulates the ventricles. Its rate varies with changing physiological needs of the body. It works best in the younger, more active patient who still has a relatively intact myocardium; the older patient is not as likely to benefit.

The demand pacemaker probably will be the one most often used. At least 25 percent of patients who use pacemakers are in normal sinus rhythm part of the time. A reliable mechanical pacemaker that is activated only when there is too long an interval between beats is the best means of coping with this intermittent activity.

Postoperatively, nursing care includes the usual measures that promote surgical recovery. If the transthoracic approach has been utilized, underwater seal drainage bottles will be used. Care of these is similar to that for thoracotomy cases. Total drainage is approximately 200 to 500 ml during the first 12 to 15 hours. Usually the tubes are removed on the first or second postoperative day. Special attention is given to observation of the electrocardiogram monitor and recognition of the pacemaker pattern. The ventricles may beat intermittently of their own accord; if this becomes troublesome, the impulses may be suppressed by quinidine. If the demand pacemaker is used this is not a problem. Its action must be observed and annotated, however. The pulse rate should continue to be checked after the monitor is turned off. If the battery fails, the pulse rate slows down; if the timing mechanism fails, the pulse rate increases. The patient's temperature should be measured, because an elevation may mean that the tissues are rejecting the unit.

The patient should be taught to measure his pulse during convalescence and to consult his physician if the rate changes. He should be reassured that the battery can be replaced quickly and simply. The rate and amplitude can be adjusted in some units by simple percutaneous puncture with a special needle if the need arises, e.g., during an infection when metabolism is increased. The goals of the therapeutic team have been met when the patient goes home with a feeling of confidence about his future.

Congenital Anomalies

Congenital anomalies, or structural deviations, of the heart are a result of faulty embryonic development. The heart develops from a premature heart tube that folds upon itself, grows, fuses in some places, and divides in others; it becomes fully developed in structure and function only after birth.

The pathophysiology of congenital anomalies is easier to understand if one remembers that the circulatory system is a closed one and that strictures or abnormal openings anywhere within the system will affect the other parts. Normally the right heart collects and propels venous blood to the lungs at a pressure of approximately 25 mm mercury; the left heart collects and propels oxygenated blood to the body at a pressure of approximately 130 mm mercury.

ATRIAL SEPTAL DEFECTS

The most common anomaly found in young adults is an atrial septal flaw. All or part of the tissue separating the atria may fail to develop. The foramen ovale, important during fetal life for diverting oxygenated blood away from the inactive lungs to the greater circulation, may not close at birth. Oxygenated blood will flow from the left atrium to the right atrium. If the defect is small symptoms may not develop and treatment is unnecessary. If it is large excessive blood will be loaded in the right heart and pulmonary circuit. Pulmonary congestion develops, lower respiratory infections become common, growth and development may be retarded, exertional dyspnea appears, and in time right heart failure intervenes. The treatment consists of prophylactic administration of antibiotics during infections. Individuals who require surgery for relief of symptoms are usually operated on between the ages of 5 and 15 years. The defect is sutured or closed with a patch graft. The operation is accomplished under direct vision, which has been made possible by the development of extracorporeal circulation. Another name for extracorporeal circulation is *cardiopulmonary bypass.* During surgery the heart and lungs are allowed to rest and the blood is oxygenated and circulated through the body by a special machine (Fig. 23–10).

VENTRICULAR SEPTAL DEFECTS

Ventricular septal defects are the most common congenital cardiac lesions. The ventricular septum grows from the apex upward; the opening may be low or high. Blood is shunted from left to right and symptoms are like those of atrial septal defects. If the increase in pulmonary circulation leads to pulmonary hypertension, or if there is a pulmonic stenosis, the shunt may become balanced with equal flow in both directions. This balance is easily upset by exercise or increased pulmonary hypertension. The blood is then shunted from right to left and cyanosis develops. When pulmonary resistance (hypertension) has reached this point surgical repair is not possible. Closure of the defect would quickly lead to right-sided heart failure; the condition is treated medically by supportive measures. Surgical repair is accomplished under direct vision (Fig. 23–10).

PATENT DUCTUS ARTERIOSUS

During fetal life the ductus arteriosus channels blood from the pulmonary artery to the aorta. After birth the ductus arteriosus usually constricts. Occasionally it remains open. Then, after birth, aortic pressure suddenly becomes five times greater than pulmonary artery pressure, so blood is forced through the open ductus and into the pulmonary artery and thence into the lungs. The extra blood causes pulmonary congestion. The end-result is increased pulmonary resistance to blood flow from the heart, and finally pulmonary hypertension. Both ventricles manifest strain. Exertional dyspnea, palpitations, and increased susceptibility to colds are characteristic symptoms, and a machinery murmur is pathognomonic. If the condition is untreated, death usually occurs in the second decade from heart failure. Treatment is by simple closure and should be performed when the child is 3 to 4 years old. After the third decade, arteriosclerosis of the aorta may make the operation hazardous (Fig. 23–10).

COARCTATION OF THE AORTA

Coarctation of the aorta is a congenital narrowing of the aortic arch which is usually found near the ductus arteriosus. It is believed to be caused by overgrowth of tissue when the ductus closes. Coarctation gives rise to hypertension in the upper extremities, since the arteries supplying them branch proximally to the defect. There is hypotension and absence of the femoral pulsation in the lower extremities.

The incidence of coarctation is 1 in 1,000 births. Heart failure occurs in the infant early if the lumen is critically narrowed. The adult may be asymptomatic if the lesion is not severe and if adequate collateral circulation has developed. There may be syncope, chest pain, and weakness and fatigue of the legs. Coarctation may be the cause of an aortic aneurysm, a cerebrovascular accident, or heart failure and may predispose the patient to subacute bacterial endocarditis. It is treated by excising the narrowed area and accomplishing an end-to-end anastomosis of the remaining segments of the aorta. If the excised area is too large to allow approximation without tension, the defect is bridged with a prosthetic graft (Fig. 23–10).

TETRALOGY OF FALLOT

Tetralogy of Fallot consists of a high ventricular septal opening, an aorta that arises from both of the ventricles, pulmonic valve stenosis, and right ventricular hypertrophy. If the pulmonic stenosis is severe, a collateral circulation must develop to carry blood to the lungs. The right ventricle enlarges in efforts to force blood through the stenotic opening. The aorta receives both oxygenated and unoxygenated blood. The patient has clubbed fingers and toes and is cyanotic from birth due to the decrease in oxygen in the peripheral blood. A compensatory increase in red blood cells, polycythemia, occurs. The hematocrit may be high and thrombi may be formed.

The child's activity is limited due to dyspnea. He squats frequently while at play, thereby decreasing venous return to the heart and relieving the dyspnea. The goal of medical treatment is to decrease venous return to the heart and hyperventilation through bed rest and administration of oxygen and morphine. The patient is hydrated to relieve hemoconcentration. Surgical treatment is directed toward providing better oxygenation and improving circulation. In 1944 Drs. Blalock and Taussig created an artificial patent ductus by dividing the subclavian

*Figure 23-10
Common congenital
anomalies: A, atrial
septal defect; B, ven-
tricular septal defect; C,
overriding aorta; D,
ventricular septal defect;
E, pulmonary stenosis;
F, right ventricular
hypertrophy.*

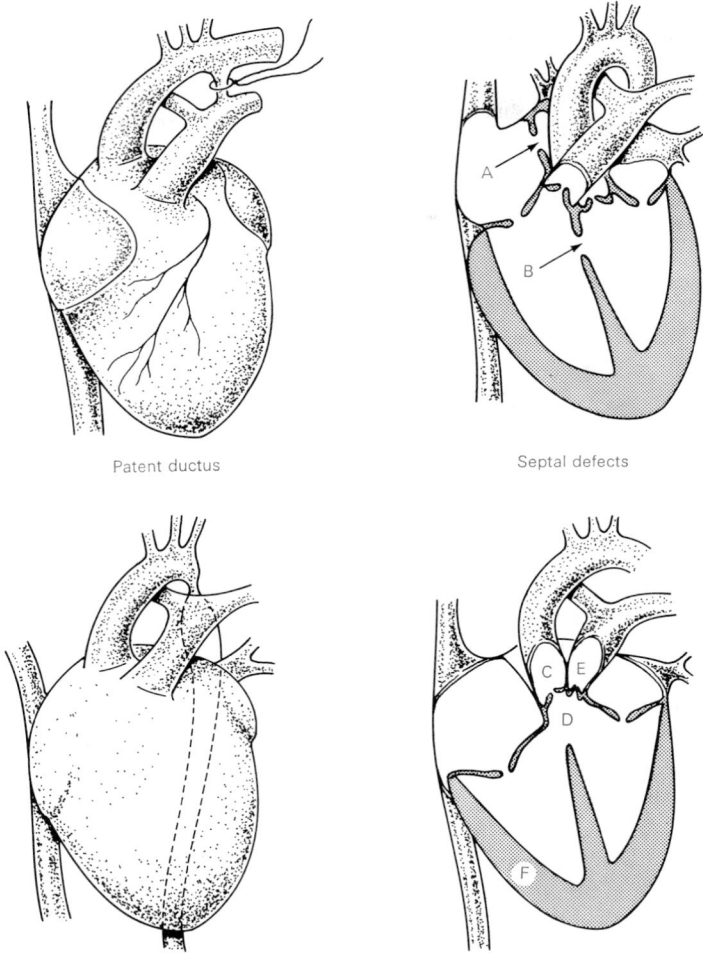

Patent ductus

Septal defects

Coarctation of aorta

Tetralogy of fallot

artery and anastomosing it to the pulmonary artery. Today correction of the defects is being accomplished under direct vision (Fig. 23-10).

Numerous other congenital anomalies exist some of which are treated with varying degrees of success by surgical methods and some of which are incompatible
with life. The interested reader is referred to cardiology textbooks for appropriate
discussions of these defects.

Valvular Defects

The valves of the heart lie between the upper and lower chambers of the heart
and in the blood vessels as they leave the ventricles. Their function is to keep
blood flowing in the proper direction. If a valve is stenotic or narrowed, the work

of the chamber behind it is increased. If it is insufficient or widened, the work of both chambers is increased.

Rheumatic fever is the single most frequent cause of valvular defects. Syphilis, congenital heart disease, healed subacute bacterial endocarditis, arteriosclerosis, and trauma are other etiologic factors.

MITRAL VALVULAR DISEASE

Mitral valvular disease comprises more than one-half of all cases of valvular disease. The mitral valve occurs between the left atrium and ventricle. The free borders of its two leaflets are attached to the ventricle by the chordae tendineae, which are controlled by the papillary muscles. During systole, these structures hold the leaflets closed, but allow them to float freely apart as soon as diastole begins. It is not known why rheumatic fever causing a valvulitis leaves some valves stenotic and others insufficient.

Mitral Stenosis

Mitral stenosis is the most common disabling lesion in adults with mitral valvular disease. The lesion has economic significance because it is manifested in adulthood when familial obligations are highest.

The valvulitis affects the margins of the cusps by deforming and thickening them. If the cusps fuse at the commissures (sites of junction between adjacent cusps of the valves) where the chordae tendineae insert, the latter become contracted and the valve becomes less mobile as well as narrowed. There is a compensatory enlargement of the left atrium; thereafter, backward failure occurs. The lungs become congested and pulmonary resistance may increase enough to cause right-sided heart failure. Atrial fibrillation is common if not inevitable. The fibrillation increases the risk of thrombus formation, especially in the auricle (the ear-shaped atrial appendage). Arterial emboli may lodge in the brain, kidneys, spleen, or extremities.

The onset of mitral stenosis may be gradual with fatigability, or sudden with acute pulmonary edema. A diastolic click and murmur are heard as the valve opens and blood flows with difficulty into the ventricle. The systolic blood pressure is low. Fluoroscopy during barium swallow shows the bulging atrium as a curve along the esophagus. Any calcification that has occurred can be seen.

The disorder is treated surgically. The operation is termed *commissurotomy.* The valve is made more functional by "fracturing" the commissures. This may be done blindly by the surgeon's finger, which is inserted through the auricle and atrium into the stenotic valve. If the valves do not separate easily, valvulatomes or dilators may be used to accomplish separation. When there is much thrombus formation or a friable mass on the valves is present, open heart surgery may be performed (Fig. 23–11, left).

Mitral Insufficiency

Mitral insufficiency occurs when the leaflets are partially destroyed or the chor-

Figure 23–11
Repair of mitral valve
insufficiency. Left. A,
normal valve; B,
thickened, stenotic
valve; C, mitral
commissurotomy. Right.
Complete replacement of
mitral valve by ball-in-
cage prosthesis.

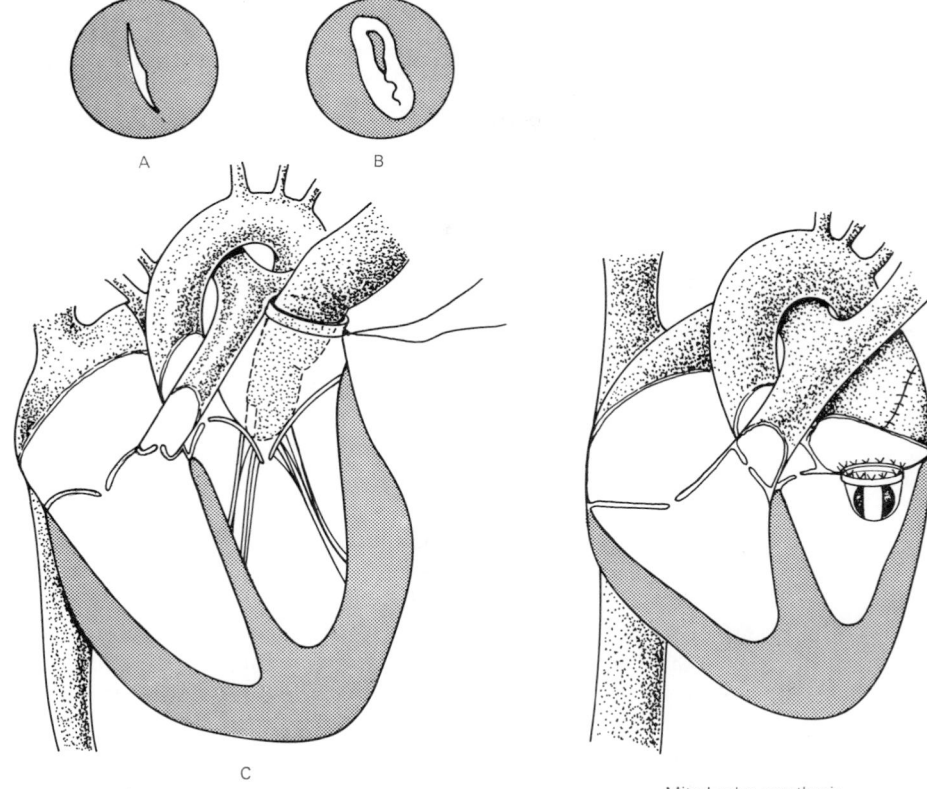

Mitral valve prosthesis

dae tendineae or papillary muscles are ruptured. The cusps no longer meet in systole and blood regurgitates into the atrium. Mitral insufficiency is caused by rheumatic fever but may be secondary to other causes of left ventricular enlargement, e.g., aortic valve disease and hypertension. Bacterial endocarditis associated with the alterations caused by rheumatic fever gives rise to mitral insufficiency in many cases.

Minor degrees of insufficiency are asymptomatic. In other cases there is fatigability and generalized weakness. Stress on the left ventricles causes hypertrophy and dilatation of the ventricles. In time atrial dilatation will develop and pulmonary congestion will supervene. Auscultation will reveal a loud systolic murmur.

Surgical correction offers the only hope of permanent relief. Favorable results have been made possible through the development of the pump-oxygenator for temporary cardiopulmonary bypass. Valvuloplasty is performed. In this plastic repair of the valve, strong silk sutures are tied over trauma-reducing pledgets of Teflon or Ivalon. If valvular destruction is extensive, a prosthesis of the ball-in-cage type can be inserted. It is fitted so that in diastole the ball drops to the bottom of the cage and allows blood to enter the ventricle. In systole, the ball is forced tightly against a Teflon-covered ring sewn into the valve orifice, and regurgitation of blood is prevented (Fig. 23–11, right).

AORTIC VALVULAR DISEASE

Aortic valvular disease occurs about one-fourth to one-third as often as mitral disease. Many times it is found in conjunction with mitral disease. It occurs approximately three times as often in males as in females.

The tricuspid valve is located between the left ventricle and the aorta. It opens in systole to allow blood flow into the systemic circulation and closes in diastole to prevent backward flow. An important anatomical consideration is that the coronary arteries, which supply the heart, fill during diastole by the recoil pressure from the elastic aorta.

Aortic Stenosis

Aortic stenosis may be congenital or acquired. In the congenital form the obstruction may be above, at, or below the valve. In the most common type fibrous thickening and partial fusion of the commissures occurs leaving a small central opening. As years pass, inflammatory processes may arise and produce the characteristic calcium deposits, with the result that the congenital origin is concealed. The valve becomes deformed.

The most common cause of acquired stricture is rheumatic fever. Atherosclerosis has been found in older age groups.

Ten years may pass before symptoms appear because the valve may have been capable of only 10 percent of normal opening before failure began. The left ventricle compensates for the narrowing of the outflow tract by hypertrophying without dilating, and blood is thus forced through. With decompensation (inability of the heart to maintain adequate circulation) blood is retained, so the atrium can never empty completely. Pulmonary congestion with its attendant symptoms appears. Systolic blood pressure is lowered but diastolic is not; thus there is a narrow pulse pressure. The pulse is felt to rise slowly under the examining fingers. The coronary arteries receive less blood because of the short diastole, the decrease in circulation, and the possible partial occlusion by calcific plaques. Angina pectoris develops. A systolic murmur is heard. With the onset of heart failure, life expectancy is less than 2 years unless treatment is initiated. Ventricular fibrillation or coronary occlusion is a frequent cause of sudden death.

The objective of medical care is to relieve the congestive failure. The goal of surgical treatment is to relieve the stenosis through valvulotomy, with removal of the calcific plaques if possible. This procedure may be accomplished by briefly opening the aorta while the patient is under hypothermia or by performing a longer operation with the patient under cardiopulmonary bypass. In many cases it is necessary to replace the valve with a prosthetic valve.

Aortic Insufficiency

Aortic insufficiency may be congenital or acquired. Congenital deformities encourage the development of subacute bacterial endocarditis, which worsens the lesion. Rheumatic fever and syphilis are the primary etiologic factors in the acquired type. Following rheumatic fever, 10 years may pass before symptoms appear;

typically the symptoms develop in the third or fourth decade. Following syphilis, symptoms may develop any time between 5 and 25 years later.

In both the congenital and acquired types, the valve is deformed and widened, and blood regurgitates into the left ventricle. There is hypertrophy of the ventricle with dilatation because the reflux of blood is considerable. There is a wide pulse pressure (difference between systolic and diastolic pressures; i.e., 160/60 blood pressure indicates a pulse pressure of 100), since the systolic pressure is raised in compensation and the diastolic pressure is lowered by regurgitation. The pulse is jerky (strong and full with systole followed by sudden collapse in diastole because the valve cannot close to prevent regurgitation)—a *waterhammer* pulse. The coronary arteries are not well perfused because the diastolic recoil pressure (pressure of blood in the aorta during diastole, a rebound caused by the elasticity of the aorta) is reduced. Though the pathophysiology is different from that of aortic stenosis, the symptoms are the same. In aortic insufficiency there is less time between the onset of heart failure and death.

Open heart surgery is performed to correct the defect. If only one cusp (leaflet) of the valve is deformed it may be removed and a leaflet prosthesis sewn in its place. The leaflet may be artificial or one removed from an animal or a cadaver. In some cases the surgeon may elect to obliterate the space occupied by the deformed cusp; he performs an annuloplasty. He plicates the annulus (fibrous ring in the wall of the heart from which the aortic valve arises) and pulls the remaining two cusps together; the valve becomes bicuspid. If the entire valve is deformed it is usually replaced by a ball-in-cage type, such as the Starr-Edwards valve.

PULMONIC VALVULAR DISEASE

Deformities of the pulmonic valve are usually limited to those caused by stenosis that is primarily congenital. Pulmonic valvular disease has been described in conjunction with tetralogy of Fallot. Incompetency is extremely rare and is usually found with pulmonary hypertension; it is improved with treatment of the underlying disease.

The pulmonic valve, which lies between the right ventricle and the pulmonary artery, opens and closes to promote the forward movement of blood to the lungs. An isolated stenotic lesion causes right ventricular enlargement to force blood through the narrowed opening. The defect may be well compensated into adulthood. When hypertrophy can no longer counterbalance the pulmonic resistance, the ventricle dilates and symptoms of right heart failure appear. During cardiopulmonary bypass, the right ventricle is opened and the stenotic valve is exposed and opened by surgical incision (valvulotomy). Although there will be some regurgitation from the pulmonary artery because the valve now remains open, the amount is usually insignificant and asymptomatic.

TRICUSPID VALVULAR DISEASE

The tricuspid valve may be either stenotic or incompetent. The disease develops in one-third of patients with rheumatic fever and in 40 percent of patients with combined aortic and mitral disease.

The tricuspid valve lies between the right atrium and ventricle. It promotes blood flow into the ventricle and prevents regurgitation. Stenosis may develop but is rarely diagnosed on a clinical basis. It is often associated with mitral stenosis when it does occur. Valvular deformity is most frequently found as a combination of stenosis and regurgitation.

Tricuspid insufficiency causes both atrial strain and ventricular strain. The right heart becomes markedly enlarged and failure ensues. There is a systolic murmur, and a systolic venous pulse may be seen in the neck and felt in the liver. When the patient is lying supine he experiences fatigue rather than dyspnea. Treatment is directed toward relieving the congestive failure rather than toward repairing the lesion. Surgical procedures have been performed in only a few cases. The associated mitral and aortic lesions are usually surgically treated.

CARE OF PATIENTS UNDERGOING CARDIAC SURGERY

A presumptive diagnosis may be made on the basis of the history, the physical examination, and certain tests made in the office or clinic. The electrocardiogram may point to the presence of hypertrophy, predominance of a chamber, heart block, and arrhythmias. Determination of circulation time may be of diagnostic and prognostic value in congenital heart disease and congestive heart failure. (Both right and left circuits are checked by injecting a special medication, such as sodium dehydrocholate, into the antecubital vein and using a stopwatch to mark time until the patient senses a bitter taste. Normally 8 to 14 seconds is required for the drug to move from the arm through the right heart and into the lungs, and to return to the left heart, where it is pumped into the aorta, thence to the tongue where it is tasted.) Fluoroscopic examination demonstrates changes in heart configuration. Nonetheless, the patient must be hospitalized if a conclusive diagnosis is to be made, because the tests required may be followed by complications for treatment of which meticulous nursing care is necessary.

Cardiac Catheterization

One of the most accurate diagnostic methods is cardiac catheterization. A special team of doctors and nurses carries out this test. To examine the right heart and pulmonary artery, a radiopaque catheter is inserted into a peripheral vein, usually the right antecubital. The left side of the heart may be approached retrogradely through the aorta or by direct puncture of the atrium or ventricle and insertion of a catheter. The left side may also be entered by saphenous vein catheterization. In this procedure, a catheter is passed through the system until the tip reaches the foramen ovale in the right atrium. A special needle is then passed through the catheter and the tip plunged through the septum. A finer catheter is then passed through the needle and manipulated into the left atrium and ventricle. The fluoroscopic image intensifier makes this task and the advancement and manipulation of the catheters in other types of catheterization much easier. Special equipment records oxygen saturation and pressure changes as the catheter is advanced or withdrawn. Intracardiac electrocardiography and phonocardiography (heart sounds) is accomplished through special electrodes. Electrocardiography demonstrates the location of the catheter tip by recording characteristic electrical waves of each chamber. Phonocardiography is useful in locating murmurs. The catheter may be manipulated through a septal defect. Angiocardiographic contrast material is used to fill and outline a chamber. Dye may be injected and its dilution curve in the peripheral arterial system recorded to demonstrate the type of existing intracardiac shunt. Refinements in technique and equipment have been made which enable the surgeon to approach the reparative operation with more certainty about the diagnosis. The need for more complete information is weighed against the dangers of cardiac catheterization which include puncturing a thin-walled vessel, stimulating arrhythmias, causing trauma and intracardiac hemorrhage, and dislodging atherosclerotic plaques or thrombi. The patient is well informed by the physician and given supportive explanation by the nurse. He should know that he will be well sedated and the procedure will be relatively painless, although he may feel rather warm when the contrast medium is injected. He should remain calm during the procedure, since restlessness or crying raises oxygen requirements and makes possible false values for oxygen concentrations. If the patient knows what to expect, is well sedated, and is aware of the presence of concerned personnel, this should not be a problem.

After cardiac catheterization, the patient is usually kept in bed for 24 hours. He may be nauseated. Vital signs are checked frequently and sites of puncture are inspected for bleeding, particularly when an artery has been used. Antibiotics are given prophylactically before and after the procedure.

Angiocardiography

Angiocardiography is used to visualize the chambers of the heart and the great vessels around it. Contrast material, usually an organic iodide, is rapidly injected into a vein and serial radiographic films are exposed as the bolus of dye moves through the system. Arch aortography is performed to demonstrate anomalies of the arch. With this procedure, a catheter must be introduced through a peripheral artery and moved to the aortic valve, where the radiopaque material is released. The arch is visualized as the dye is pumped forward by heart action. Both procedures can be dangerous. Again the patient will experience a warm sensation; he should be forewarned. It is important that he remain perfectly still to prevent dislodgment of instruments. After either procedure he is placed on bed rest, and vital signs, sites of puncture, and warmth of extremities are checked.

Ballistocardiogram

A ballistocardiogram will give information about the efficiency and ease with which the heart works. The patient lies on a balanced, suspended board and the heart and arterial pulsations are recorded.

The Preoperative Period

Once the condition is diagnosed, the decision regarding surgery is made based on the maximum benefit offered the patient in relation to the possibility of operative death. The surgical risk is greater in this type of surgery than in most others, excluding organ transplants.

Another salient factor is the cost of surgery. The average length of hospital stay for valve replacement is approximately 2 weeks. With conservative management of accommodations and treatment, the patient's total bill, including physician fees, can be held to approximately $7,000. Comprehensive hospitalization insurance should pay most of the cost except for the blood.

Once the decision to operate is made, the meticulous preparation begins. The patient's physical condition is improved. Congestive heart failure is treated with digitalis, diuretics, and dietary sodium restriction. Many patients have a low cardiac reserve that needs support with digitalis or its derivatives, whether or not obvious failure is present. Arrhythmias are controlled. The lungs are examined radiographically and pulmonary function is studied. Blood and urine are carefully examined; supplemental or replacement therapy is instituted to bring the body to near homeostatic condition. Antibiotics are given prophylactically to ensure that residual or latent infection is eradicated.

The nurse has important functions in the preoperative period. She assists the doctor as necessary and helps the patient meet his fears about the various procedures and the surgery. Many patients and their families feel that surgery represents a gamble between sudden death or a life of increasing debilitation and the outside chance that the patients may get better and resume productive living. The last decade has brought advances in techniques and equipment that have reduced the risks to survival. This should be emphasized. The nurse, by her observations and recording, establishes baselines not only of vital signs, weight, and other physical characteristics but also of psychological and sociological personality components. All are important for evaluation of postoperative reactions.

Preoperative teaching includes a description of customary postoperative procedures. In addition the patient is shown the intensive care unit and much of the equipment that will be used, such as oxygen source, chest suction unit, monitoring devices, and intermittent positive pressure breathing apparatus (IPPB). He is taught to use the IPPB unit so that he will not have to learn its use while under sedation. He should meet the special nurses who will be caring for him. A warm relationship of mutual trust is invaluable.

The immediate preoperative care has been described under thoracotomy preparation. The skin preparation is extended to include the inguinal region if cardiopulmonary bypass is to be used.

The type of surgical incision to be made is dependent upon the condition being treated. A right thoracotomy is used to expose the vena cava and the atria for repair of interatrial defects or mitral and tricuspid lesions. A left thoracotomy is used in carrying out blind manipulations of the mitral and aortic valves and operating on the aorta or ductus. An anterior sternum-splitting incision affords the widest exposure and has largely replaced bilateral thoracotomy because the risk of pulmonary complications and severe postoperative pain is thereby lessened.

One of the major difficulties in open heart surgery was the problem of operating on a continuously pulsating organ filled with vision-obscuring blood. If the heart stopped, the brain immediately became anoxic. A technique utilizing hypothermia (subnormal temperature of the body) was developed to decrease oxygen needs by slowing the rate of metabolism. First the patient is anesthetized, then the body cooling process is begun by application of the hypothermia blanket. The blanket maintains a constant temperature automatically. A thermisto probe is inserted into the rectum or esophagus, the dials are set, and the cooling fluid is circulated through the blanket coils until the body temperature reaches the desired level. The machine responds to temperature changes by automatically shutting off and turning on. Ventricular fibrillation becomes a threat as the body reaches the temperature desired for surgery, 28 to 30° C. The surgery is performed in a relatively quiet bloodless field with the heart stopped for short periods.

With the development of the heart-lung machine, or pump oxygenator, for extracorporeal circulation, even longer periods of cardiac asystole could be tolerated. The machine supplies oxygen and circulates the blood while the patient's cardiopulmonary system is at rest. The machine is primed, i.e., filled with blood or diluent such as 5 percent dextrose in distilled water, as recommended by DeBakey, the chest is opened, and the extracorporeal circuit is instituted. The venae cavae are cannulated and tied off so that no venous blood returns to the heart. A vacuum pump draws blood from the venae cavae into the machine where it is pumped in a fine film over screens or sheets of material designed to remove carbon dioxide and add oxygen. Once oxygenated, the blood is pumped back into one of the large arteries, usually the femoral. It flows in a retrograde fashion through the aorta to supply the body. If the aortic valve is competent, blood does not enter the heart chamber, but does perfuse the coronary arteries. The coronary arteries are cannulated and perfused by a separate circuit during prolonged operations or when surgery is performed in their vicinity. A heat exchanger unit on the pump controls body temperature by warming or cooling the blood. (See Figure 23–12.)

Hypothermia is combined with cardiopulmonary bypass. The blanket is used to cool the patient while the bypass is instituted and to help warm him when bypass is discontinued. Profound hypothermia, 6 to 8° C, may be attained and the entire circulation made motionless. More often, moderate hypothermia is used. After the operation, the heart is restarted by electrical stimulation.

Hyperbaric oxygenation is now being used in some large medical centers. Oxygen is administered to the patient in concentrations up to 100 percent in an environment of increased atmospheric pressure. This is accomplished by placing the patient and the surgical team inside a pressure chamber. The oxygen dissolved in the body fluid is greatly increased in both the patient and the team. The technique presents many problems, e.g., fluids do not flow as they would in a normal atmosphere. The hyperbaric chamber is used primarily for surgery in children with cyanosis who could not tolerate a thoracotomy.

The Immediate Postoperative Period

The first 48 hours postoperative is the critical period for patients who have undergone heart surgery. The nurse plays a vital role during this time. She provides an environment conducive to efficient, calm care. She is alert to significant changes in vital signs that signal arrhythmias, shock, hemorrhage, cardiac tamponade, or other

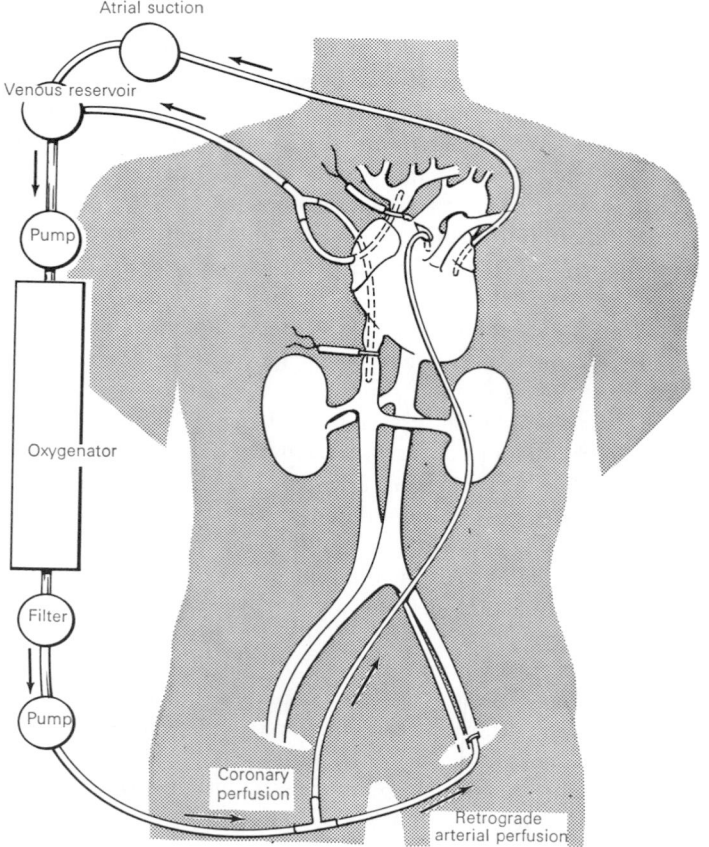

events. She is aware of other possible complications, such as infection, pulmonary congestion, emboli, oliguria. She gives emotional as well as physical support.

So much detailed observation must be made by the nurse that a systematic approach has to be developed. The pattern may be varied but a common method is to start with observation of the head and examine all systems as one proceeds toward examination of the feet. The following should be observed:

Nervous system: Level of consciousness, psychological state, pupil size and equality, ability to move limbs, and body temperature.

Respiratory system: patency of airway, equality of chest excursion, color of skin, character and rate of respirations, chest tube patency and drainage, pain, color of sputum, and function of respirator.

Cardiovascular system: apical-radial heart rate and rhythm, volume and character of pulse at all major points bilaterally (radial, femoral, dorsalis pedis), monitor pattern, color and temperature of skin, pain, arterial pressure, and venous pressure.

Gastrointestinal system: fluid intake, character of gastric secretions, presence of pain, nausea, vomiting, or distention, and color of stools.

Renal system: color, volume, and specific gravity of urine, suprapubic distention.

In order that significant postoperative observations may be made, preoperative baselines are established for each patient, e.g., a blood pressure of 100/60 is insignificant if the baseline is 110/70; the situation is entirely different if the baseline is 180/110.

The postoperative unit is a single room or an intensive care unit. It contains equipment for routine care, such as intravenous solutions, oxygen, and suction. It has emergency equipment for cardiac arrest, such as the defibrillator, pacemaker, laryngoscope, and tracheostomy tray. An intermittent positive pressure breathing apparatus, commonly the Bennett or Bird, is ready for use. A monitoring system is essential. It may be a simple one and monitor only the electrocardiogram with a single lead, or it may monitor temperature, pulse, respiration, venous and arterial blood pressures, electroencephalogram, various electrocardiographic leads, and heart sounds.

When the patient is brought to the unit, all tubes and monitoring attachments should be checked for proper function. Oxygen is administered.

Frequently patients who have a tendency to retain carbon dioxide because of a preexisting pulmonary condition, such as emphysema, are tracheotomized to ensure better ventilation and provide for easier removal of bronchial secretions. Arterial blood gases are studied before and after surgery. Patients who experience respiratory difficulty during surgery may also be tracheotomized. Assisted ventilation with IPPB may be given to decrease respiratory effort. Mucolytic agents are administered periodically to facilitate removal of secretions by coughing or suctioning. The respiratory movements are kept active to prevent accumulation of carbon dioxide which could lead to respiratory acidosis. Reexpansion of the lungs is promoted and atelectasis prevented by having the patient cough and use the IPPB. Optimal respiratory function reduces the work load of the heart.

THE TRACHEAL TOILET

The tracheal toilet must be meticulous. The nurse must be highly skilled in this procedure because it may cause serious consequences in the hands of a novice. There is obvious need for preventing retention of secretions in the bronchi with resultant congestion of the lungs and back pressure on the newly repaired heart. Not so obvious is the fact that prolonged or too-frequent inadequate suctioning leads to decreased intrathoracic pressure with reduction of venous return and lowered cardiac output. Paroxysms of coughing greatly increase the work of the heart. A further consideration is that there is very little ventilation taking place during suctioning. The catheter removes air along with mucus. Persistent, prolonged suctioning can cause atelectasis.

Proper suctioning is a nursing art. The patient is well ventilated before the procedure begins. The flow of oxygen, or its concentration, and depth of respiration are increased. The catheter is introduced, with suction turned off, to a depth of approximately 6 inches from the tracheostomy, for deep suction to clear the bronchi. The head is turned to the left to straighten the right bronchus for suctioning and to the right to straighten the left bronchus. Suction is applied intermittently as the catheter is withdrawn with a rotating movement to allow aspiration in all directions. Suctioning is not continued for more than 15 seconds. If secretions are tenacious, 2 to 5 ml of saline may be instilled prior to suctioning to liquefy them. A rest of 2 to 3 minutes with increased ventilation is provided between and at the end of aspiration. Suctioning is performed at least every hour or as necessary. Noisy respirations, dyspnea, tachycardia, cyanosis, restlessness, or apprehension may indicate a need for suctioning.

CHEST SUCTION

If the pleural cavity has been entered, necessitating reexpansion of the lungs, or if the physician wishes to drain the pericardial sac, chest suction equipment will be utilized. Tubes should be supported with tapes in areas where they are apt to bend and prevent drainage, e.g., at the chest exit, the edge of the bed, and sites of connections with other tubes or the bottles. They should be checked frequently for kinks. It is necessary to milk the tubes (slide thumb and index finger down the tube with one hand and support the tube near the chest exit with the other) to express clots that might cause obstruction.

BLOOD TRANSFUSION

Whole blood is given in exact replacement of blood lost in chest drainage. The amount of drainage is measured carefully and the transfusion rate set to keep the loss balanced by replacement. An hourly record must be maintained. If more blood is lost than the surgeon anticipated would be, he should be notified immediately. Sudden gushes of blood can be expected when the patient is coughed or turned, but sustained hemorrhage (more than a minute) is reported immediately. In a study by Pillsbury, the average amounts of blood loss postoperative to open heart surgery were documented. The overall average for all types of lesions was 18 ml per kg of body weight. The average amount of blood loss for each type of patient not reoperated for excessive hemorrhage, as well as that of those who were reoperated, is shown in Table 23-1. Drainage can be expected to be as high as 300 ml per hour for the first few hours. If the rate has not decreased by the end of 4 hours, emergency reoperation may be necessary. If the drainage does not seem excessive but the venous pressure is low and symptoms of shock appear, there may be

TABLE 23-1
*Average Blood Loss in Patients Not Reoperated and in Patients Reoperated upon for Excessive Hemorrhage**

LESION	BLOOD LOSS IN NONREOPERATED PATIENTS (ML/KG)	BLOOD LOSS IN REOPERATED PATIENTS (ML/KG)
Acquired aortic stenosis	18.2 (6.1–48.7)[1]	43.3 (27.8–69.4)
Aortic insufficiency	21.5 (11.3–43.8)	52.0 (32.6–70.8)
Atrial septal defect	13.5 (4.3–38.4)	38.0 (18.7–44.0)
Combined aortic and mitral stenosis	18.1 (7.5–41.5)	71.8
Fallot's anomaly	25.2 (7.3–46.4)	64.5 (25.7–147.7)
Mitral stenosis	14.3 (3.1–56.4)	42.4 (30.6–60.0)
Ventricular septal defect	14.4 (5.7–98.0)	42.7

* From Pillsbury et al.
[1] Range of blood loss given in parentheses.

other sites of bleeding. The femoral and chest incisions are inspected. There may be greater oozing of blood in patients who have had pump oxygenation as a result of heparinization of the blood in the pump. Bone marrow is exposed in the sternum-splitting incisions and causes further oozing.

VITAL SIGNS

Vital signs are checked frequently, as often as every 15 minutes for 12 hours. The temperature can be expected to rise during the first and second postoperative days; it is thought to be due to retention of blood in the pericardium. The fever is treated with aspirin and cooling measures. For persistent temperature over 101° F, it may be necessary to use the hypothermia blanket.

The apical-radial pulse is checked as well as the monitor. The nurse should become familiar with the normal pattern on the monitor and recognize the changes that herald arrhythmias such as fibrillation and heart block. (See Figure 23–8.)

The blood pressure reading provides a critical tool for evaluation of the patient's status. A significant drop in arterial pressure is serious following open heart surgery. With slowed circulation, clotting may occur at graft sites, shunts, or prosthetic devices. Immediate reversal of shock is imperative. Low blood pressure with a narrow pulse pressure may indicate cardiac tamponade (hemorrhage in pericardium with resultant compression of the heart). Other symptoms of cardiac tamponade include distant heart sounds, a low-volume pulse, restlessness, cyanosis, and increased venous pressure with distention of the neck veins. A wide pulse pressure may indicate insufficiency of an aortic prosthesis.

The venous pressure is monitored continuously. During surgery, a catheter is placed in a vein and advanced to the superior vena cava or right atrium. It is attached to a manometer at the level of the heart. The manometer measures the pressure that indicates the volume of returning blood in relation to cardiac pump action. If there is too much circulating blood or the heart action is ineffective, the venous pressure will be high. If there is hypovolemia, venous pressure will be low. Normal central venous pressure is 8 to 12 cm water.

The treatment of hypotension is based on both arterial pressure and venous pressure, since hypotension may be due to hypovolemia, deficient heart action, or dilatation of the peripheral vascular bed. Simply treating the hypotension with vasoconstrictor drugs may cause an irreversible shock by so decreasing the peripheral blood flow that tissue hypoxia occurs and metabolites (waste products that cause metabolic acidosis) are released. Addition of blood to an adequate volume may overload the system and compromise a failing heart; digitalis is used instead.

FLUID BALANCE

Fluid intake and urinary output are checked carefully. Renal function is dependent upon cardiac function; kidneys cannot filtrate what they do not receive. Post-operative oliguria may be related to hypotension, fluid and acid-base disturbances, and actual kidney damage. With improvement of heart action, return to normotension, and correction of any existing metabolic imbalance, kidney function usually will improve. Occasionally the patient is simply inadequately hydrated and renal function will improve with additional water. A check of renal ability can be made by the intravenous injection of mannitol. If diuresis does not follow, the physician will institute treatment for renal shutdown. Inadequate kidney function is a burden on the heart which is corrected quickly to minimize strain.

RENAL FAILURE

The technique of hemodilution now being used during cardiopulmonary bypass promises to reduce renal damage and postoperative cases of renal shutdown. The pump oxygenator is primed and the blood diluted up to 32 percent with 5 percent dextrose in distilled water, buffered electrolyte solution, dextran, or combinations with heparinized blood. It has been shown that high dilutions, especially if combined with short perfusions, tend to protect the body from renal failure. Hemodilution may protect the gastrointestinal tract from bleeding; a lower incidence of serum hepatitis has occurred with higher degrees of hemodilution. It apparently has many advantages.

EMBOLISM

Another possible danger is embolism from a broken fragment of tissue, blood clots, or disruption of the prosthesis. The peripheral pulses are checked. If absent and there is discoloration of the extremity, pain, and coolness, the incident needs immediate attention. Emboli to the brain result in disturbances of sensorium, muscle weakness, or paralysis. Hematuria may indicate a renal embolus. Chest pain, combined with frothy pink sputum, is indicative of pulmonary embolism.

Antibiotics and some form of digitalis are administered. The digitalis is increased to improve cardiac function if the central venous pressure is high. Pain is controlled with small, frequent doses of narcotics. Too much analgesia will depress respirations and the cough reflex. A lesser amount may be given before bed exercises to help the patient cooperate. Bed exercises include frequent turning, coughing, and deep breathing; complete range of motion is most desirable. All exercises are designed to improve circulation; this is particularly important if the patient has had hypothermia as well as cardiopulmonary bypass. The prolonged period of slowed circulation contributes to an increased incidence of phlebothrombosis.

The Later Postoperative Period

Water is given when the patient is able to tolerate it, which is usually within 12 hours. The diet is advanced from liquids to full regular meals that may be restricted in sodium.

Time and amount of ambulation are planned based upon the surgical procedure. Usually the patient is allowed to dangle his legs on the day of surgery and to sit up in a chair by the second day. By then, the chest tubes are removed and exercise is gradually increased.

The patient needs psychological support during all phases of the recovery period. Postoperative psychoses are not uncommon; the patient may be disoriented, agitated, or frankly delusional. There is controversy about the causes of the mental disturbances, but it is believed that some of the contributory factors are sensory deprivation from prolonged existence in an atmosphere of continual activity affording no change from day to night, depersonalization caused by more attention being paid to the equipment than the patient, excessive fatigue from lack of sleep, and agitation from prolonged fear. The patient must be considered an individual and be addressed by name when personnel approach him. *He* should be observed before the monitors are. The presence of a clock in the room will help to remind him of the progression from day to night, as will dimming of lights at night. The monitor should be placed so that the patient cannot see it and react to the patterns being recorded by it. Nursing care must be so organized that rest periods become a part of the treatment plan. Explanations should be offered about the monitor and other apparatus. If the patient cannot communicate verbally, another means should be provided, such as a "magic slate." The nurse should hold his hand and look directly at him as she does so. A child may be comforted by having a small familiar toy nearby or by being held in the nurse's lap. The family should be allowed to visit the patient, after being instructed about his condition and the appearance of the unit. Courtesies shown the family will give the patient comfort.

Many patients are depressed postoperatively. It may be that they expended so much energy during surgery that they now feel depleted of it. They may find it hard to believe that they are better—suddenly, they must resume or face new responsibilities. They need constant reassurance during their gradual progression toward convalescence.

Doctor, nurse, and family work together to help the patient focus his attention on long-term goals. He may be able to return to his former job or may require a radical change. Possibly he is eligible for retraining through a local vocational rehabilitation agency. If an appreciable degree of restoration has not been possible, he should be referred to the local visiting nurse association to ensure continuity of care.

The patient should be taught the program he is to follow prior to discharge. He should be informed that although he may not experience the maximum benefit of surgery in less than a year, he should be aware of progress. Careful medical supervision and psychological support should be maintained. He may expect a complete cure and return of previous abilities, and will be disappointed unless he has been forewarned.

The nurse who recognizes that the psychological component of heart disease is sometimes more limiting than the disease itself is more likely to be able to help the patient accept his status. He can go home with an understanding of his disease and confidence in his ability to meet whatever problems it imposes.

Bibliography

Abrams, L. D. and W. A. Hudson: The Treatment of Complete Heart Block. *Postgraduate Medical Journal,* 3:240–244, May, 1961.

Allansmith, Robert and Noel P. Thompson: *Thoracic Surgery and Medical Electronics.* Menlo Park: Pacific Coast Publishers, 1962.

Allen, Edgar, et al.: *Peripheral Vascular Disease,* 2d ed. Philadelphia: W. B. Saunders Company, 1959.

Beeson, P. B. and Walsh McDermott (Eds.): *Cecil-Loeb Textbook of Medicine,* 12th ed. Philadelphia: W. B. Saunders Company, 1967.

Bernstein, Harold: Drug Treatment of

Cardiac Arrhythmias. *American Journal of Nursing*, 64:118–120, July, 1964.

Biggs, Louise W.: Nursing Care of the Patient with a Prosthetic Heart Valve. *American Journal of Nursing*, 63:66–70, October, 1963.

Binger, Carl: Psychological Phenomena in Cardiac Patients. *Bulletin of New York Academy of Medicine*, 24:687, November, 1948.

Braun, Harold A., Gerald A. Diettert, and Vera E. Wills: *Coronary Care Unit Nursing, Part II: A Workbook in Clinical Aspects.* Missoula, Montana: Mountain Press, Publishers, 1969.

Cecil, Russell L. and Robert F. Loeb: *A Textbook of Medicine*, 10th ed. Philadelphia: W. B. Saunders Company, 1959.

Chardack, William, et al.: Two Years' Clinical Experience with the Implantable Pacemaker for Complete Heart Block. *Diseases of Chest*, 43:225–239, March, 1963.

Cole, Warren H. and Robert M. Zollinger: *Textbook of Surgery*, 8th ed. New York: Appleton Century Crofts, 1963.

Cooper, Philip: *Ward Procedures and Techniques.* New York: Appleton Century Crofts, 1967.

Dean, Virginia: Measuring Venous Blood Pressure. *American Journal of Nursing*, 63:71–72, October, 1963.

DeBakey, Michael E. *Yearbook of General Surgery.* Chicago: Year Book Medical Publishers, Inc., 1964–65.

DeBakey, Michael E.: *Year Book of General Surgery.* Chicago: Year Book Medical Publishers, Inc., 1968.

deTakats, Geza: *Vascular Surgery.* Philadelphia: W. B. Saunders Company, 1959.

Donmoyer, Theodore L., Roman W. De Sanctis, and W. Gerald Austen: Experiences with Implantable Pacemakers Using Myocardial Electrodes in the Management of Heart Block. *Annals of Thoracic Surgery*, 3:3: March, 1967.

Furman, Seymour, Doris J. W. Escher, and Norman Solomon: Standby Pacing for Multiple Cardiac Arrhythmias. *Annals of Thoracic Surgery*, 3:4:April, 1967.

George, Joyce H.: Electric Monitoring of Vital Signs. *American Journal of Nursing*, 65:68–71, February, 1965.

Gray, Henry: *Anatomy of the Human Body*, 28th ed. Philadelphia: Lea & Febiger, 1966.

Grollman, Arthur: *Pharmacology and Therapeutics*, 4th ed. Philadelphia: Lea & Febiger, 1960.

Gross, Robert E.: *The Surgery of Infancy and Childhood.* Philadelphia: W. B. Saunders Company, 1953.

Guyton, Arthur C.: *Textbook of Medical Physiology*, 3d ed. Philadelphia: W. B. Saunders Company, 1966.

Hardy, James D.: *Pathophysiology in Surgery.* Baltimore: The Williams & Wilkins Company, 1958.

Heller, Anne F.: Nursing the Patient with an Artificial Pacemaker. *American Journal of Nursing*, 64:87–92, April, 1964.

Hickey, Mary C.: Hypothermia. *American Journal of Nursing*, 65:116–122, January, 1965.

Humphreys, George H., II et al.: Immediate Complications of Thoracotomy for Heart Disease. *Surgical Clinics of North America*, 44:2:335–347, April, 1964.

Julian, Ormand C., et al.: *Cardiovascular Surgery.* Chicago: Year Book Medical Publishers, Inc., 1962.

Keown, Kenneth K.: *Anesthesia for Surgery of the Heart*, 2d ed. Springfield, Ill.: Charles C Thomas, Publisher, 1963.

Long, Janet M.: Arch Aortography. *American Journal of Nursing*, 64:97–99, December, 1964.

Modell, Walter, et al.: *Handbook of Cardiology for Nurses*, 5th ed. New York: Springer Publishing Co., Inc., 1966.

Morehead, Robert P.: *Human Pathology.* New York: McGraw-Hill Book Company, 1965.

Neelon, Virginia J.: Hyperbaric Oxygenation Benefits and Hazards. *American Journal of Nursing*, 64:73–78, October, 1964.

Papper, Solomon and Robert Whang: Hyperkalemia and Hypokalemia. *Disease-a-Month,* June, 1964.

Pillsbury, R. C., et al.: Emergency Re-operation following Open Heart Surgery. *Annals of Thoracic Surgery,* 1:50–63, January, 1965.

Pitorak, Elizabeth F., et al.: *Nurse's Guide to Cardiac Surgery and Nursing Care.* New York: McGraw-Hill Book Company, 1969.

Rae, Nancy M.: Caring for Patients following Open Heart Surgery. *American Journal of Nursing,* 63:77–82, November, 1963.

Reiser, M. F.: Emotional Aspects of Cardiac Disease. *American Journal of Psychiatry,* 107:781, April, 1951.

Sessler, Alan D. and Emerson A. Moffitt: Measurement and Interpretation of Venous Pressure during Surgery. *Surgical Clinics of North America,* 45:4:853–862, August, 1965.

Shafer, Kathleen, et al.: *Medical-Surgical Nursing,* 3d ed. St. Louis: The C. V. Mosby Company, 1964.

Starke, Rodman, et al.: Cardiac Arrhythmias—Diagnosis and Clinical Treatment. *Cardiovascular Nursing,* 1:4, Fall, 1965.

Sutton, Audrey L.: *Bedside Nursing Techniques.* Philadelphia: W. B. Saunders Company, 1964.

Whitehouse, Frederick A.: The Psychosocial Aspects of Cardiovascular Disease. Forum, II:2:28–45, 1965.

Wood, Edwin C.: Understanding the Patient with Heart Disease. *Nursing Outlook,* 7:90, February, 1959.

Zoll, Paul, et al.: Long-Term Electrical Stimulation of the Heart for Stokes-Adams Disease. *Annals of Surgery,* 154:330–345, September 1, 1961.

SECTION 2
HYPERTENSION

IRENE E. POLLERT

Epidemiology

Although in recent years a number of important advances have been made in the control of hypertension, the subject remains complex and one of the primary problems facing medicine today. At least 5 percent of the population of the United States is believed to be hypertensive (Perera). In 10 to 15 percent of all persons diagnosed as hypertensive the cause of the hypertension can be determined through various diagnostic tests. The elevated blood pressure in these cases is *secondary* to another condition. In the remaining 85 to 90 percent the cause for the persistent increase in the blood pressure cannot be identified and the diagnosis of *primary* or *essential* hypertension is made by excluding other possible conditions.

There is a high incidence of hypertension among Americans and Europeans as compared with Chinese and Africans. According to Dahl, the salt intake of people in different geographical areas can be correlated very well with the incidence of hypertension.

The onset of hypertension is at an average age of 32 years, and it is asymptomatic at that time. The average course of untreated hypertension is 20 years. It is twice as common among women but is tolerated better by them than by men (Wilkins).

Diastolic Hypertension

A systolic pressure of 140 to 150 mm mercury and a diastolic pressure of 90 to 100 mm mercury are generally regarded as the upper limits of normal. One such reading is of course not indicative of hypertension, and a careful evaluation must be made. In the doctor's office the patient is allowed a period of rest and the pressure in both arms is again measured. When the stress of the examination causes an increase in the blood pressure, it is believed that the individual may "react with vasospasm" to many internal and external stimuli (Schroeder).

Of the factors that normally control the blood pressure—peripheral resistance, blood volume, blood viscosity, and cardiac output—it is peripheral resistance which increases the diastolic pressure (Selkurt) and precipitates damage to the vascular system and the vital areas of the heart, brain, kidney, and eye. Increase in the systolic pressure alone is not related to increased peripheral resistance, but the elevation is due to increased cardiac output caused by a number of conditions known to produce an elevated blood pressure. Systolic hypertension is therefore always secondary (Sodeman).

The factors that initiate an increase in blood pressure are unknown. Increased peripheral resistance is the function of the arterioles that are innervated by the sympathetic nervous system. The basic pathology is a decreased caliber of the arterioles (Selkurt). This decrease in the diameter of the arterioles increases the peripheral resistance to the flow of blood. The peripheral vasoconstriction is caused by vascular reactivity in response to increased sympathetic stimulation and increased levels of vasopressor hormones in the blood, and by hereditary mechanisms (MacBryde).

PRIMARY HYPERTENSION

Repeated findings of a diastolic pressure of 90 mm mercury or above, in the absence of any recognizable condition that can give rise to an elevated blood pressure, is the criterion for the diagnosis of primary hypertension (Perera; Goldring and Chasis). In primary hypertension vasoconstriction always occurs. Many studies are in progress to determine the relationship of genetic factors and family history to the development of primary hypertension; there is little doubt at the present time that there is a genetic basis (Pickering) and a hereditary tendency, but the role which either of these plays in the etiology is not clearly defined. Genetically susceptible people are hyperreactive to both internal and external stimuli. Environmental influences early in life and patterns of eating and resting may accentuate the hyperreactivity and thus produce or aggravate the hypertension (Wilkins).

The arterial blood pressure in both normotensive and hypertensive individuals varies with time of day, exercise, digestion, sleep, and changes in the emotional state. A number of mechanisms identified as responsible for the rise in arterial pressure include neurogenic, renal, adrenal, and vascular factors. As the elevation in blood pressure becomes chronic, the baroceptors in the carotid sinus become reset and lowering the pressure by therapeutic means is more difficult (Page).

Hypertension may be present for many years without giving rise to symptoms and without causing marked changes from one year to another. The course is then referred to as benign in contrast to accelerated or *malignant*. Malignant hypertension is a sudden and severe increase in the arterial pressure accompanied by many symptoms and severe vascular damage (Goldring and Chasis).

SECONDARY HYPERTENSION

A number of renal and endocrine conditions, toxemia of pregnancy, and coarctation of the aorta cause hypertension. Both diastolic and systolic readings or the systolic reading alone may be elevated. Hypertension secondary to a primary condition is curable when the primary disease is remedied.

Primary renal diseases including congenital anomalies, pyelonephritis, acute and chronic glomerulonephritis, and renal artery obstruction may lead to hypertension. When blood flow to the kidney is reduced, an enzyme called *renin* is released into the blood and interacts with a serum protein, an alpha-2-globulin, which is formed in the liver. Angiotensin I, a weak pressor substrate, is formed and is converted by an enzyme in the blood to angiotensin II (Helmer and Judson; Peart). Angiotensin and other humoral agents such as serotonin may have a role in initiating and maintaining increased arterial pressure.

An atherosclerotic plaque is the most common renal artery lesion (Winter). Symptoms of polyuria, albuminuria, and a sudden increase in the blood pressure occur in an individual having no family history of hypertension (Hoobler). Kidney function tests include the phenolsulfonphthalein excretion test, blood urea nitrogen determination, creatinine clearance, urinalysis, and intravenous pyelography. Indications for renal arteriography include an abnormal intravenous pyelogram, a sudden development of the malignant phase, and a negative family history in a patient under 35 years of age.

When an obstructive lesion in the renal arteries is demonstrated by arteriography, the hypertension may be alleviated by means of endarterectomy or bypass graft, or by removal of a severely damaged kidney (Winter; Martin; Zimmerman and Levine; Colby).

Endocrine hypertension may be associated with a pheochromocytoma, a tumor of the medullary portion of the adrenal gland. Large amounts of epinephrine and norepinephrine released from the tumor cause sudden rises in the blood pressure. The finding of abnormal levels of catecholamines in the urine may aid in the diagnosis of a pheochromocytoma. An increase in aldosterone secretion, in tumors of the adrenal cortex, and an excess in adrenocortical steroids, in Cushing's disease, also cause secondary hypertension.

Coarctation of the aorta (stenosis of the aortic arch) increases the resistance to blood flow and thus produces a higher pressure in the upper extremities while an adequate amount of blood is prevented from reaching the lower part of the body. Low or diminished femoral pulses suggest the diagnosis, and aortography aids in confirming it (Sodeman; Zimmerman and Levine).

Primary hypertensive disease of pregnancy is characterized by an elevated blood pressure, edema, and proteinuria occurring during the third trimester, but never before the twentieth week (Schroeder; Pickering). In some patients the blood pressure remains high even after parturition. Some authorities suggest that toxemia during pregnancy has precipitated a primary hypertension that would have developed later anyway (Smirk).

Complications

The elevated diastolic pressure places a strain on the arterial wall. The changes in the arterioles are caused directly by vasoconstriction. According to Thomas' law (Orbison), increase or decrease in the thickness of the vessel wall is dependent on the blood pressure. The tension of the wall is dependent on the diameter of the vessel and the blood pressure. Thickening and calcification of the arterial media narrows the lumen of the blood vessel. The amount of sclerosis which develops depends on the structure of the vessels and their ability to tolerate the strain of increased pressure, and the length of time during which the pressure is heightened. When the blood pressure rise is rapid, the vascular lesions consist of areas of necrosis in the media; when the rise is slower, the lesions are hyaline in appearance; and a very slow rise causes fibrotic lesions. Material from the blood seeps through the endothelium because of the increased mural permeability and is deposited in the intima and the media (Pickering). The hypertension may lead to cerebral ischemia, myocardial ischemia, or renal ischemia.

CARDIOVASCULAR COMPLICATIONS

The work of the heart is increased in proportion to the arterial pressure (Pickering; Selkurt). In hypertension the left ventricle must pump blood into the arterial system against a higher than normal level of pressure. This leads to hypertrophy and eventually failure. Increased diastolic pressure, increased cardiac work load, and increased peripheral resistance promote atherosclerosis (MacBryde). Early signs of cardiovascular involvement include increased carotid pulse, loud atrial sound, accentuation of the second pulmonic sound, and changes in the electrocardiogram and the chest x-ray film.

CEREBROVASCULAR CHANGES

The onset of symptoms and the type of generalized or localized findings are extremely important. In cerebral hemorrhage, cerebral thrombosis, and subarachnoid hemorrhage, the onset occurs in a matter of seconds or hours. Localized findings predominate and remain stationary. These findings are persistent in cerebral thrombosis and in cerebral hemorrhage, but they are transient in subarachnoid hemorrhage.

Cerebrovascular spasm is suspected when neurological symptoms are present in a patient with a very high blood pressure followed by recovery of function within a few hours. Vascular insufficiency syndromes are associated with advanced arteriosclerosis and are rarely seen in younger patients (Pickering).

Cerebral hemorrhage causes an acute rise in cerebrospinal pressure which will lead to papilledema and retinal hemorrhages. The history commonly reveals a previous blood pressure consistently above 200 mm mercury. Headache is prominent in the early stages and examination of the spinal fluid reveals the presence of red blood cells. Hemiplegia usually occurs and the patient lapses into a coma. In acute cerebrovascular thrombosis an atherosclerotic vessel is occluded by a blood clot. The occlusion is preceded by transient limb paresis, aphasia, and tingling sensations (Hoobler).

A subarachnoid hemorrhage is due to rupture of an aneurysm in the circle of Willis, Symptoms include stiffness of the neck, presence of blood cells in the cerebrospinal fluid, and a dilated pupil on the side of the hemorrhage (Hoobler).

Hypertensive encephalopathy refers to the occurrence of mental confusion and disorientation in a patient with a very high arterial pressure. The onset occurs in a matter of days; consciousness is depressed; generalized findings predominate; and the localized findings are migratory and transient. Elevated blood pressure and increased vasospasm are directly related to the development of hypertensive encephalopathy (Harrison).

CHANGES IN THE RETINA

In hypertension the ratio of the diameter of the arterioles to the venules is less than normal. The arterioles are light reflective. The optic disk reveals blurring of disk margins and changes in the contour. Necrotizing arteriolitis results in papilledema. Hemorrhage and hard exudates suggest a poor prognosis.

RENAL COMPLICATIONS

Renal pathology with arteriosclerosis is a complication of hypertension. When there is also a history of urinary infection, chronic pyelonephritis may occur. A history of nephritis and proteinuria preceding the hypertension may suggest the presence of chronic glomerulornephritis. Microscopic hematuria and uremia are rare in the moderate phase of hypertension (Schroeder).

PHASES OF HYPERTENSION

Prehypertensive Phase

In the prehypertensive phase there is a rise in the blood pressure but there are no indications of vascular damage. Such symptoms as do occur are expressions of anxiety: headache, giddiness, sleeplessness, forgetfulness, and irritability. The systolic pressure is below 200 mm mercury and the diastolic is below 100 mm mercury. Except for relief of symptoms treatment is not indicated.

Mild or Early Phase

In the mild established or early phase, the pressure varies little and is still below 200 mm mercury. The diastolic pressure is greater than 90 mm mercury in persons who previously had normal readings. No drugs are necessary, usually, but the patient should have periodic examinations. Some clinicians suggest that a mild anti-hypertensive agent be prescribed for patients under 40 years of age (Hoobler).

Moderately Severe Phase

In the moderately severe phase, the pressure is above 200 mm mercury systolic and above 100 mm mercury diastolic, but there is still no evidence of vascular damage. Repeated review is necessary, and rauwolfia and a thiazide are prescribed. Reduction of weight and salt restriction may also be advised. Prophylactic treatment against cerebral hemorrhage is necessary at this time. With the advent of arteriosclerosis the hypertension advances to the severe stage; the diastolic pressure is persistently elevated and damage is apparent (Moyer and Nodine).

Immediate treatment is required in the presence of convulsive movements, abnormal neurologic signs, severe occipital headache occurring abruptly, and pulmonary edema. The blood pressure is lowered with use of a ganglionic blocking agent. If full hypotensive effects are not immediately necessary, reserpine is administered (Hoobler).

Malignant Phase

During the course of hypertension the blood pressure may increase very abruptly with serious damage to vital organs. With a sharp elevation there are symptoms of visual difficulty, hemorrhages, exudates, and papilledema. Renal blood flow is decreased and vasoconstriction increases. Renal damage follows. Plasma renin activity increases; there is albuminuria, proteinuria, decreased specific gravity, and an increase in the blood urea nitrogen. Epigastric pain may be so severe as to suggest peptic ulcer or cholelithiasis. Left ventricular failure and an increase in such symptoms as morning headache, nausea, and vomiting may also occur. The pressure must be lowered as effectively as possible with use of a ganglionic blocking agent combined with chlorothiazide. The standing blood pressure is reduced to normal levels as promptly as renal function will permit (Goldring and Chasis).

Medical Management

The physician considers the measure of the blood pressure and the amount of vascular damage as the primary factors in determining the type of therapy for the patient with hypertension. The complexity of hypertension was mentioned earlier; there cannot be a simple or single answer to the problem of therapy for all patients. When the etiology is unknown, as it is in primary hypertension, the therapy must be directed toward treating the problems of the individual, rather than toward instituting a standard type of treatment to cure or to modify the disease process.

Repeated reviews of the blood pressure and surveys of the vital organs to detect complications as early as possible are important aspects of the medical management. One of the first steps in deciding on the therapy is to know the patient as an individual and to gain insight into the interaction of his age, sex, personality, environment, and health history in relation to this condition. He must be helped to understand that he has a chronic condition, that excesses in dietary fat and salt intake must be avoided, and that obesity must be combated. He should learn to rest, eat light meals, refrain from running up stairs, and avoid engaging in arguments or worry (Master et al.). Whether or not the patient will be restricted in any way will be determined by the specific factors involved in his condition and by the symptoms.

Modifications in occupation and in living conditions will have to be made if emotional tension is severe. Sympathetic reassurance often relieves disturbing symptoms. Psychotherapy is indicated in the young and may also be very beneficial for older patients. This would help them to gain a more relaxed attitude toward living and to solve some of their problems of interpersonal relationships. Although psychotherapy has not resulted in arresting the progress of the disease, it has helped to improve the patients' comfort and their satisfaction in living (Page).

EVALUATION OF THE PATIENT

A careful evaluation of the patient must be made to determine the phase of hypertension, whether mild, moderately severe, or severe (Goldring and Chasis). The following tests are indicated: blood pressure, electrocardiogram, chest x-ray study, routine urinalysis, blood urea nitrogen, and optic fundus. An electrocardiogram to establish a baseline and chest x-ray examination to determine cardiac size are essential in all patients. Measuring the specific gravity, albumin, and protein in the urine will give some indication of kidney function. The retinas are carefully examined for the presence of edema, spasm, and hemorrhage. Neurological testing is performed to detect cerebral damage.

DRUG THERAPY

In the early phase of hypertension and prior to manifestations of vascular damage, symptoms are treated to relieve anxiety. Therapy with antihypertensive drugs is prescribed on an individual basis, according to the severity of the hypertension, whether or not the blood pressure level fluctuates, and the individual's tolerance for the drug. Drugs do not cure hypertension, but they lower the blood pressure and thus alleviate some of the symptoms and modify the complications.

The rauwolfia alkaloids block epinephrine at the nerve endings and decrease the peripheral resistance. Wilkins and Judson found that hypertension of nervous origin responded best to these drugs. Reserpine depletes certain cells of their catecholamines and releases serotonin from the tissues, with the net effect of parasympathetic overactivity. Reactions to these drugs include nasal stuffiness, diarrhea, increased appetite, and bradycardia, and prolonged use may cause depression. The rauwolfia drugs may be administered alone or in combination with other antihypertensive agents. Included in this group are rauwolfia (Raudixin), reserpine (Serpasil), and rescinnamine (Moderil) (DiPalmer).

Diuretic agents of the chlorothiazide group effect a fall in blood pressure by promoting excretion of salt and water, therefore the volume of circulating fluid is decreased. Combined therapy including a diuretic and an antihypertensive drug has been found to be effective because the amount of the diuretic is decreased and the side effects of the antihypertensive drug are lessened. Use of diuretics may lead to a low serum potassium unless potassium chloride is replaced. Chlorothiazide derivatives include flumethiazide (Ademol), methyclothiazide (Enduron), and chlorthalidone (Hygroton).

The ganglionic blocking agents deplete stores of norepinephrine by acting on both the sympathetic and the parasympathetic nervous systems. Sympathetic blockade results in loss of postural reflexes, producing hypotension due to a reduction in cardiac output which is seen primarily in the erect position (DiPalmer). One of the ganglionic blocking agents, hexamethonium, causes many side effects and has been replaced by mecamylamine (Inversine), which causes fewer side effects, although constipation, postural faintness, and interference with visual accommodation may occur.

Guanethidine (Ismelin) is a potent agent that depletes the sympathetic postganglionic fiber of its effector substance, norepinephrine. Side effects include dizziness, fluid retention, nasal stuffiness, and skin rash. Methyldopa (Aldomet) also interferes with the biosynthesis of norepinephrine (McCombs).

Monoamine oxidase (MAO) inhibitors currently being employed lower the blood pressure by causing the catecholamines and serotonin to accumulate in the tissues. Among these agents are nialamide (Niamid), phenelzine (Nardil), and pargyline (Eutonyl). The MAO inhibitors possess mood-elevating and antianginal effects in addition to antihypertensive activity. Ingestion of cheese and certain other foods is contraindicated when MAO inhibitors are being administered because the tyramine in those foods causes an increase in blood pressure. Side effects of MAO inhibitors include insomnia, agitation, constipation, and dry mouth.

Other antihypertensive drugs include the Veratrum alkaloids, which interfere with the sensory receptors in the myocardium, and hydralazine (Apresoline), which is a peripheral dilator and increases renal blood flow as it blocks pressor response to angiotensin (Modell).

SURGERY

When the patient's blood pressure is not lowered by medical therapy and there is evidence of severe kidney involvement and cerebral dysfunction, a sympathectomy may be indicated.

In this procedure the sympathetic chain from the tenth thoracic ganglion through the first or second lumbar ganglion is resected. Postoperatively, failure of the blood pressure–adjusting role of the sympathetic nervous system may result in orthostatic hypotension. When the patient assumes the standing position abruptly, the blood pressure may fall because there is pooling of blood in the dependent vessels. Sympathectomy is not curative and the long-range effects are not always satisfactory (Zimmerman and Levine).

DIET THERAPY

In addition to restricting excesses of dietary fat and sodium, the physician may prescribe a reduction of sodium to less than 2 g per day. The manner in which salt restriction reduces blood pressure is unknown but it is believed that the decrease in extracellular fluid reduces cardiac output and peripheral resistance (Smirk; Peart). When the blood cholesterol level is elevated, a low-cholesterol diet may be prescribed in hopes of delaying the progress of atherosclerosis.

Prognosis

When the diastolic blood pressure remains elevated and does not return to normal levels, the height of the pressure cannot be used as a reliable indicator of the progress of the underlying disease. The appearance of complications depends on such factors as race, weight, family history, and blood cholesterol. The course of hypertension is usually more rapid and severe when the onset occurs at an early age than when it occurs after the age of 40. With therapy complications may be prevented and the patient's life span increased. As therapy is currently being initiated during the earlier stages of hypertension, it is hoped that life expectancy will be increased and the cause of primary hypertension will be identified.

Nursing the Patient with Hypertension

There is no single basis for the nursing care of a patient with primary hypertension, since many complex factors are involved. Age, sex, race, occupation, and environmental conditions have been identified as influencing the course of the disease. The patient's reaction to therapy and his acceptance of the adjustments he is encouraged to make will affect control of the arterial pressure. His understanding of his condition, his relationship with the physician prior to hospitalization, and his previous hospital experiences will affect the extent of nursing intervention. Nursing care is directed toward enlisting the patient's cooperation in following the physician's suggestions, helping the patient to understand the need for modifying his way of living, and teaching him how to make the necessary adjustments. The nurse's chief contributions include instruction, reassurance, and encouragement.

The nurse's attitude toward the patient and his problems and her understanding of the prescribed therapy will have implications for the patient, not only while he is in the hospital but after he returns home. The nurse recognizes that the presence or absence of observable symptoms differs considerably among patients, even though the levels of blood pressure may be identical. She makes every effort to understand the patient in a personal way, because a lack of such individualized understanding may be detected by him and increase his feelings of insecurity and anxiety. The coordinated efforts of all who deal with the patient are essential so that he is not placed under increased tension. There must be uniformity and agreement about the explanations given to the patient with regard to his activities and to the diagnostic and therapeutic measures.

One objective of nursing care is to prevent an increase in arterial pressure, and one preventive measure is the avoidance of anxiety, anger, and stressful situations. Psychological stress affects physiological function. Alterations in physiological functions such as digestion, sleep, and elimination lead to symptoms that add to the patient's discomfort with a resultant increase in his stress. The nurse can facilitate relief of this stress by providing a favorable environment, relieving discomfort, and giving attention to physical needs. Systolic pressure and pulse pressure increase during exercise but opinions differ regarding diastolic blood pressure. Cardiac output increases with meals and a large volume of fluids may increase blood pressure. Food should therefore be served in small quantities and more frequently rather than in three heavy meals. Rest periods before and after meals or a rest period of 1 full hour during the day is beneficial to many patients.

Straining at stool stimulates reflex sympathetic activity and causes an increase in the blood pressure at the end of the expiratory phase (Zimmerman and Levine). Any activity having the effect of a Valsalva maneuver, e.g., pushing oneself up in bed with the elbows, will also cause an increase in blood pressure.

The nurse should approach the patient in a calm, reassuring, and permissive manner, understanding that he usually finds it difficult to accept the restrictions necessary for control of his pressure. Observation of his behavior, appearance, and demeanor with hospital personnel, visitors, and other patients is essential. Evidence of uneasiness, restlessness, and avoidance of eye contact should be noted. An effort should be made to determine the cause, and measures should be instituted to help the patient.

Satisfying interpersonal relationships aid in reducing the patient's anxiety, contribute to his feeling of security, and help to build his self-confidence. The nurse accepts the patient's complaints and his right to express them, understanding that he must have the opportunity to express his feelings about his chronic condition and the need to adjust to changes in his way of living. Any misconceptions must be corrected. The patient should be encouraged to ask questions about matters he does not understand. The manner in which he accepts or rejects the therapy is related to his previous experience with stressful situations. He must be aided to accept help and to learn to live with hypertension without fearing it. He must learn to accept and enjoy the simple things of life, to live each day at a slower pace by reducing the number of responsibilities he accepts, and to refrain from becoming angry over things he cannot control (Pickering).

Dietary restrictions should be carefully reviewed with the patient, and efforts should be made to determine his food preferences and to satisfy his appetite. A reduction in caloric intake may be prescribed for obese patients (Master et al.).

An important consideration in nursing care following sympathectomy is recognition of increased sensitivity to change in position. Since the vascular system is not adjusted to the low blood pressure, the patient may feel faint when he assumes the standing position. Ambulation must be gradual. A corset that compresses the blood vessels and thus prevents a sudden drop in blood pressure on his arising may be beneficial. Elastic bandages or elastic stockings aid in decreasing pooling of blood in the legs when the patient is sitting (Freis and Lodge).

The nurse must be alert to both physical and behavioral changes that may occur in patients receiving antihypertensive drugs. Many of these drugs are very potent and cause distressing side effects. Each patient responds individually to the drug. The specific prescription of drugs is based on the reaction of the patient, the observations of the nurse, and the judgment of the physician. Improvement is related to reduction of the pressure. The nurse must possess adequate knowledge of the actions, characteristics, and side effects of the drugs. Accuracy in reporting the patient's physical symptoms and behavioral manifestations will facilitate adjustments in the prescribed therapy. Instructions given to the patient before his discharge should include the dosage, frequency, desired effects, and untoward symptoms of the drugs prescribed.

If the patient is required to take his own blood pressure readings at home, he should be instructed in wrapping the cuff, positioning the arm at heart level, recording the time and the arm tested, and detecting systolic and diastolic sounds. The nurse helps the patient to understand why there are variations in these sounds.

Bibliography

Allen, Arthur C.: *The Kidney*, 2d ed. New York: Grune & Stratton, Inc., 1962.

Allen, James H.: *May's Manual of the Diseases of the Eye*. Baltimore: The Williams & Wilkins Company, 1963.

Beeson, Paul B. and Walsh H. McDermott: *Cecil-Loeb Textbook of Medicine*, 11th ed., Philadelphia: W. B. Saunders Company, 1963.

Birshall, Robert and Hugh M. Batson: Diagnosis of Hypertension Due to Renal Arterial Stenosis. *Circulation*, XXIX:6–13, January, 1964.

Brainerd, Henry, Sheldon Margen, and Milton J. Chatton: *Current Diagnosis and Treatment*. Los Altos, California: Lange Medical Publications, 1964.

Brest, Albert N. and John H. Moyer: *Cardiovascular Disease*. Philadelphia: F. A. Davis Company, 1968, pp. 929–1017.

Colby, Fletcher H.: *Pyelonephritis*. Baltimore: The Williams & Wilkins Company, 1958.

Corday, Eliot and David W. Irving: *Disturbances of Heart, Rate, Rhythm and Conduction*. Philadelphia: W. B. Saunders Company, 1962.

Dahl, Lewis K.: Possible Role of Chronic Excess Salt Consumption in the Pathogenesis of Essential Hypertension. *American Journal of Cardiology*, 8:571, 1961.

DiPalmer, Joseph R. (Ed.): *Drill's Pharmacology in Medicine*, 3d ed. New York: McGraw-Hill Book Company, 1965, pp. 636–638.

Evans, William: *Diseases of the Heart and Arteries*. Baltimore: The Williams & Wilkins Company, 1964.

Freis, Edward D.: Office management of the Hypertensive Patient. *Modern Concepts of Cardiovascular Disease*, 32:10, October, 1963.

Freis, Edward D. and Mary Patricia Lodge: Treatment and Nursing Care of Hypertension. *American Journal of Nursing*, 54:11:1336–1339, 1954.

Goldblatt, Harry: Hypertension Due to Renal Ischemia. *Bulletin of New York Academy of Medicine*. 40:10, October, 1964.

Goldring, William and Herbert Chasis: *Hypertension and Hypertensive Disease*. New York: The Commonwealth Fund, 1944.

Griffith, George C.: The General Approach to the Treatment of Patients with Diastolic Hypertension. *American Journal of Cardiology*, IX:6:822–824, June, 1962.

Grollman, Arthur: The Relationship of Salt and Diet to Diastolic Hypertension. *American Journal of Cardiology*, IX:5:700–703, May, 1962.

Harrington, Michael: *Hypotensive Drugs*. New York: Pergamon Press, 1956.

Harrison, T. R. (Ed.): *Principles of Internal Medicine*, 5th ed., New York: McGraw-Hill Book Company, 1966.

Helmer, Oscar M. and Walter E. Judson:

The Quantitative Determination of Renin in the Plasma of Patients with Arterial Hypertension. *Circulation,* XXVII:6:1050–1060, June, 1963.

Hoobler, Sibley: *Hypertensive Disease Diagnosis and Treatment.* New York: Paul B. Hoeber, Inc., 1959.

Lang, Erick K.: A Survey of the Complication of Percutaneous Retrograde Arteriography. *Radiology,* 81:2:257, August, 1963.

MacBryde, Cyril Mitchell: *Signs and Symptoms,* 4th ed. Philadelphia: J. B. Lippincott Company, 1964.

Martin, Peter: *Indications and Techniques in Arterial Surgery.* Baltimore: The Williams & Wilkins Company, 1963.

Master, Arthur M., Charles L. Garfield, and Max B. Walters: *Normal Blood Pressure and Hypertension.* Philadelphia: Lea & Febiger, 1952.

McCombs, Robert Pratt: *Internal Medicine,* 2d ed. Chicago: Year Book Medical Publishers, Inc., 1960.

Modell, Walter: *Drugs of Choice, 1962–1963.* St. Louis: The C. V. Mosby Company, 1962.

Modell, Walter, et al.: *Handbook of Cardiology for Nurses,* 5th ed. New York: Springer Publishing Company, Inc., 1966.

Moyer, John H. and John H. Nodine. *Psychosomatic Medicine.* Philadelphia: Lea & Febiger, 1962.

Orbison, Lowell J.: *The Peripheral Blood Vessels,* Baltimore: The Williams & Wilkins Company, 1963.

Page, Irvine H.: The Changing Outlook for the Hypertensive Patient. *Annals of Internal Medicine,* 57:96–109, 1962.

Peart, W. S.: The Renin-Angiotensin System. *Pharmacological Review,* 17:2:143–172, June, 1965.

Perera, George A.: in R. Cecil and R. Loeb (Eds.): *A Textbook of Internal Medicine,* 10th ed. Philadelphia: W. B. Saunders Company, 1959.

Perera, George A., et al.: The Family of Hypertensive Man: Progress Report of a Long-Range Study Program.

American Journal of Medical Science, 241:18, 1961.

Pickering, George: *The Nature of Essential Hypertension.* New York: Grune & Stratton, Inc., 1961.

Pickering, George, William Ian Cranston, and Michael Andrew Pears: *The Treatment of Hypertension.* Springfield, Ill.: Charles C Thomas, Publisher, 1961.

Report to the President. A National Program to Conquer Heart Disease, Cancer and Stroke. The President's Commission on Heart Disease, Cancer, and Stroke. Vol. II, February, 1965.

Ruskin, Arthur: *Classics in Arterial Hypertension.* Springfield, Ill.: Charles C Thomas, Publisher, 1956.

Schroeder, Henry Alfred: *Mechanisms of Hypertension with a Consideration of Atherosclerosis.* Springfield, Ill.: Charles C Thomas, Publisher, 1957.

Selkurt, Ewald E. (Ed.): *Physiology,* 2d ed. Boston: Little, Brown and Company, 1966.

Selye, Hans: *Stress.* Montreal: ACTA, Inc., Medical Publishers, 1950.

Smirk, Frederick Horace: *High Arterial Pressure.* Springfield, Ill.: Charles C Thomas, Publisher, 1957.

Smith, Edward B., et al.: *Principles of Human Pathology.* New York: Oxford University Press, 1959.

Sodeman, William A. and William A. Sodeman, Jr.: *Pathologic Physiology,* 4th ed. Philadelphia: W. B. Saunders Company, 1967.

Stone, Clement A. and Karl H. Beyer: Pharmacodynamic Action of the Newer Autonomic Drugs Used in the Treatment of Essential Hypertension. *American Journal of Cardiology,* IX:6:830, June, 1962.

Thorek, Philip: *Surgical Diagnosis.* Philadelphia: J. B. Lippincott Company, 1965.

Wall, C. Allen and Thaddeus J. Whalen: Criteria for Screening the Hypertensive Patient with Renal Artery

Occlusion. *Journal of the American Medical Association,* 192:13, 95–99, June 28, 1965.

Wilkins, Robert W.: The Test of Time. *The Boston Medical Quarterly,* 16:2, June, 1965.

Wilson, Clifford: Experimental Observations on the Role of the Kidney in the Etiology of Hypertension. *American Journal of Cardiology,* IX:5:685–691, May, 1962.

Winter, Chester C.: *Correctable Renal Hypertension.* Philadelphia: Lea & Febiger, 1964.

Wood, Edwin and Louis L. Battey: The Natural History of Diastolic Hypertension and the Effects of Blood Pressure Regulation. *American Journal of Cardiology,* IX:5:675–679, May, 1962.

Zimmerman, Leo M. and Rachmiel Levine: *Physiologic Principles of Surgery.* Philadelphia: W. B. Saunders Company, 1964.

SECTION 3
VASCULAR
DISORDERS MAGDALENE FULLER

Terminology related to vascular disorders is extensive and varied; therefore, for the purpose of this text, vascular disorders are defined as structural or functional conditions of the veins or arteries which cause disturbances of blood flow in the peripheral circulatory system.

There are many mechanisms involved in maintaining essential metabolic needs of the tissue and in removing the metabolic end-products, as discussed elsewhere in this textbook. Disturbances in any one or a combination of these mechanisms may lead to tissue ischemia and tissue death. The major problem in vascular disorders is concerned with the hemodynamic disturbance produced by the occlusive process, regardless of the specific disease entity. However, it must be kept in mind that there are distinct diseases with characteristic pathological processes which will produce circulatory disturbances. These include varicose veins, Buerger's and Raynaud's diseases, arteriosclerosis, thrombosis and embolism, aortic aneurysms, and trauma.

Since some terms provide a framework for understanding the description of vascular diseases, it is essential that their definitions be readily available. The following are definitions of selected terms:

Ischemia is a lack of blood supply to meet the normal tissue demands. The condition is acute in arterial embolism and spasm and chronic in arteriosclerosis. It is characterized by numbness, tingling, heaviness, and less frequently by coldness and pallor. Other manifestations are pain, absent or diminished pulsations, and color changes that are dependent on posture, i.e., abnormal pallor on elevation and abnormal redness in the dependent position.

Intermittent claudication is pain that occurs with exercise and is relieved by rest.

Collateral circulation refers to utilization of existing accessory or secondary blood vessels to carry blood to deprived tissue. Collateral circulation is more efficient if the occlusion develops slowly. Sudden occlusion of an artery does not allow time for collateral circulation to develop. Vascular disorders diminish the body's ability to develop collateral circulation.

Vasospasm is a functional disorder causing constriction of blood vessels and characterized by coldness and ischemia.

Functional is the term used to describe disturbances of circulation caused by changes in caliber of the blood vessels which are not structural or pathologic but are transient and reversible.

Paresthesia signifies the manifestation of abnormal sensations such as numbness, tingling, and heightened sensitivity.

Paresis is the term used to denote muscular weakness, or partial or slight paralysis.

Varicose Veins

Varicose veins are large, tortuous (twisted), distended venous channels. The incidence of varicose veins in the lower extremities is common throughout the general population. Both sexes are affected; however, in the younger age group the incidence is higher in females who have had multiple pregnancies than in males. In addition to multiple pregnancies, other predisposing factors are hereditary weakness of the vein walls and valves, abdominal tumors, obesity, occupations involving considerable standing, and degenerative processes resulting from aging.

Pathophysiology

The development of varicosities appears to depend upon a combination of factors, and the presence of any one factor predisposes the individual to the others. These factors are incompetent valves, increased hydrostatic internal pressure in the veins, and inadequate support from the surrounding tissues.

Veins in the upper and lower extremities have numerous sets of valves, which by successive closure keep the blood flowing toward the heart and prevent backward seepage. Incompetent valves lead to dilatation and congestion of the superficial veins due to backflow. (See Figure 23–13.)

Increased internal hydrostatic pressure causes the vein walls to stretch, elongate, and become thin in segments. The thinned segments become dilated and tortuous. The thinned inner coat of the vein protrudes through the thinned outer coat and is manifested by bluish nodule-like masses. Venous stasis and edema are manifestations of hydrostatic pressure becoming equal to, or higher than, capillary pressure.

Figure 23–13
Great saphenous and small saphenous veins, showing the communication system: A, incompetent valve; B, competent valve. (Courtesy Mary Jo Mirlenbrink and Craig C. Gosling.)

There is adequate muscle support and adequate muscle pump action of the deep femoral veins; therefore, these are rarely affected. However, the greater and smaller saphenous veins, being more superficial, are more frequently affected. (See Figure 23–13.) Varicosities are still more commonly found in the veins superior to and at the ankles, because there is less supporting tissue.

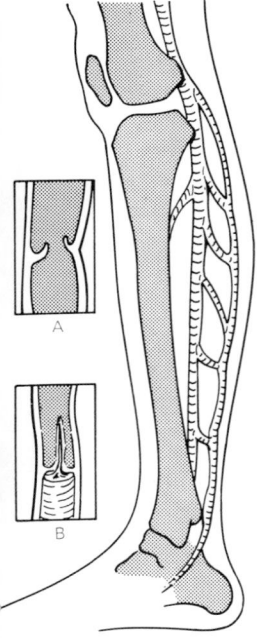

Symptoms

The most frequent symptoms resulting from venous congestion are fatigue of the leg muscles, sensation of fullness, and soreness and congestion of the tissues of the leg and foot, particularly after prolonged standing. This congestion may lead to decreased arterial blood supply, resulting in tissue ischemia. Tissue ischemia may cause cramping pain in the extremities, especially during exercise. Ischemic tissue has a reduced ability to resist and combat infections; therefore, minor injuries may become infected and ulcerated. If the varix ruptures, infiltration of blood into the tissue may occur. Then an eczematous eruption often appears which may be followed by an ulcer; ulceration may precipitate hemorrhage.

Diagnosis

The most commonly used and most accurate diagnostic test is the Trendelenburg test. The patient assumes a recumbent position while the extremity is raised until the vein is emptied and collapses; then the patient rises and the vein is observed. A varicose vein fills from above and a normal vein fills from below. A variation of this test is done by applying a tourniquet above the midthigh after the suspected vein has been drained and before the patient stands. If the greater saphenous fills within ½ minute after he stands, the communicating veins are incompetent. If it requires longer than this, the veins are competent. If the patient walks about for a few minutes, and the foot becomes swollen and cyanotic, the deep veins are incompetent. An angiogram will aid in determining the exact location and extent of venous circulatory involvement.

Treatment

Treatment consists of measures to reduce increased hydrostatic pressure and to aid venous return. Supportive medical measures include the application of elastic bandages or stockings to provide an even pressure from the toes to the midthigh. This external structural support reduces the volume of the venous channels in the legs, thereby increasing the venous flow rate and return. Another supportive measure is to elevate the extremities thereby reducing gravitational pull, which in turn reduces hydrostatic pressure and aids venous return. An additional measure is performance of active or passive exercise to promote muscle pump action in the lower extremities which increases venous return.

Surgical treatment is the most effective measure to reduce increased hydrostatic pressure. This is done by ligating the saphenous vein in the upper thigh and removing the vein and its tributaries by the vein stripping procedure. (An appropriate text-book should be consulted for details of this procedure.) Bleeding is usually controlled by external pressure along the course of the vein through application of elastic bandages from the toes to the upper thigh while the patient is in surgery. Sclerosing solutions are used only for cosmetic purposes to destroy the superficial veins following ligation. Mild analgesics such as aspirin and codeine are prescribed for pain. By the second postoperative day, the patient is usually ambulating every 2 hours.

Nursing Care

The nurse must know how to promote preventive and supportive measures to reduce intravenous hydrostatic pressure and facilitate venous return. She must understand the rationale behind the measures and how to evaluate their effectiveness.

Preventive and supportive measures are based on the cause-effect relationship and are evaluated by the changes in signs and symptoms. Examples of predisposing factors that cause increased hydrostatic venous pressure are pregnancy, abdominal tumors, abdominal obesity, and sitting for long periods of time which compresses the ileofemoral veins and decreases venous return. Additional factors are wearing tight underwear and sitting with the legs crossed at the knees which compresses the popliteal veins. If any symptoms of varicose veins occur during pregnancy, the patient should lie horizontal for periods of time. The patient with an abdominal tumor or obesity would follow the same regimen until the cause is removed. The sitting position should be interrupted at frequent intervals by alternate standing and walking.

Standing decreases venous blood return by gravitational pull. Signs and symptoms of venous stasis develop in persons who must maintain a standing position for long periods; they should take rest periods and elevate their extremities. An additional measure is performing leg exercises, while standing, such as alternate flexion and extension of the toes, ankles, and knees. This promotes muscle pump action and aids in venous return. If the symptoms persist, an occupational change may be indicated. If pregnancy and the complications of abdominal tumors and obesity are added to this factor, the patient would relieve symptoms not only by lying down but also by elevating the extremities.

Measures to increase structural support are indicated if there is a combination of predisposing factors such as heredity, which has a role in the development of weakened vein walls; obesity, which decreases structural muscle support through infiltration of fatty tissue; and the aging process, which brings a decrease in vein wall and muscle tone. Elastic bandages or elastic stockings extending from the toes to the thighs produce an even external pressure. The bandages or stockings may be removed at night when the hydrostatic pressure is reduced by lying down. Walking is beneficial for increasing muscle tone and aids venous return through muscle pump action. If the patient is not ambulatory, the physician may order active or passive leg exercises. Active exercises are performed by the patient alternating flexion and extension of the knees, ankles, and toes. If active exercise is contra-indicated passive exercise in the same form of alternate flexion and extension of the knees, ankles, and toes is provided by the nurse.

Postoperative nursing care of the vein stripping procedure includes elevating the foot of the bed on 6- to 8-inch blocks to facilitate venous return. The legs should not be elevated on pillows as this causes uneven pressure on the veins. The patient should not be placed in the modified Fowler's position with the head and knees elevated; this causes obstruction of the ileofemoral and popliteal veins. The position should be changed frequently to avoid pressure on the thigh and calf of the legs. The elastic bandages that are usually applied in surgery must be observed to ensure even pressure, as a rolled bandage or tight bandage in an area may cause constriction decreasing arterial circulation and venous return. Deep breathing exercises should be done every 2 to 4 hours to increase negative pressure in the thorax which facilitates emptying the large veins.

The extremity must be observed for color and temperature and/or changes in sensation to determine adequacy of circulation.

The patient usually makes a rapid uneventful recovery from surgery and resumes normal activities in a few weeks.

Venous Thrombosis and Embolism

Thrombosis is the formation of a thrombus; the thrombus is the clot itself. An occlusive thrombus causes complete obstruction of the vessel, whereas a mural thrombus causes partial obstruction of the vessel. Embolism is the occlusion of a blood vessel by an embolus—a bit of matter foreign to the bloodstream.

Phlebothrombosis is formation of a thrombus in a vein. *Thrombophlebitis* is the inflammatory reaction of the intima of the vein to the thrombus.

Etiology

Venous thrombosis and embolism is common throughout the general population but is more prevalent in older individuals. Decreased venous circulation as occurs in cardiac failure, obesity, prolonged bed rest, varicose veins, surgery, trauma, and tissue degeneration due to aging are all predisposing factors.

Pathophysiology

Three properties of the blood platelets will be discussed in relation to the pathophysiology of thrombosis. These properties are the release of thrombin by the platelets during degeneration, the platelet, and the negative charge of the normal platelet. Thrombin, which is released from degenerating platelets, is an essential element in clot formation. The platelets become more sticky and adhesive following surgery, childbirth, and during shock. Under normal conditions the flow of blood in the blood vessels is laminar, that is, when blood flows at a continuous rate through a long smooth vessel, the velocity of flow in the center of the vessel is greater than that near the vessel wall. The fluid elements of the blood are near the vessel wall and the cellular elements are in the inner core. Turbulent flow is caused by dilated vessels, projections into the intima, rapid increase in blood flow, sharp turns of the vessel, or rough surfaces of the vessel. These conditions allow the platelets to come into contact with each other and with the intima. The platelets degenerate and release thrombin which causes more platelets to adhere to the ruptured platelets and the intima of the vessel. (See Figures 23–14 and 23–15.) This small mass of intact or ruptured platelets initiates the clotting sequence. Decreased blood flow allows the platelets to come into contact with each other and with the intima of the vessel wall which again initiates the clotting process. Decreased blood flow, or the formation of the mass in a small vessel, permits the thrombin

Figure 23–14 Normal laminar blood flow through long normal blood vessel.

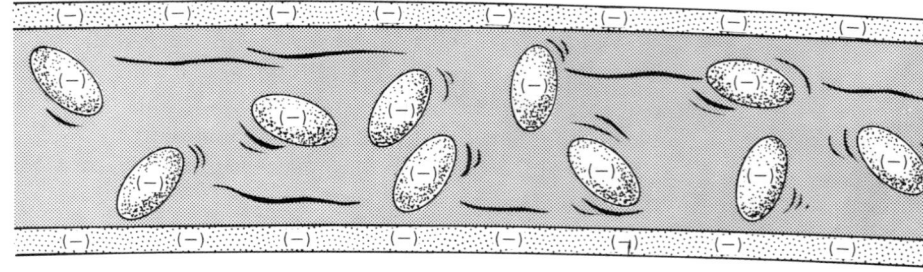

(−) Negative charge

Figure 23–15 Dilated blood vessel, showing turbulence of flow and blood cells beginning to come together.

Dilated vessel

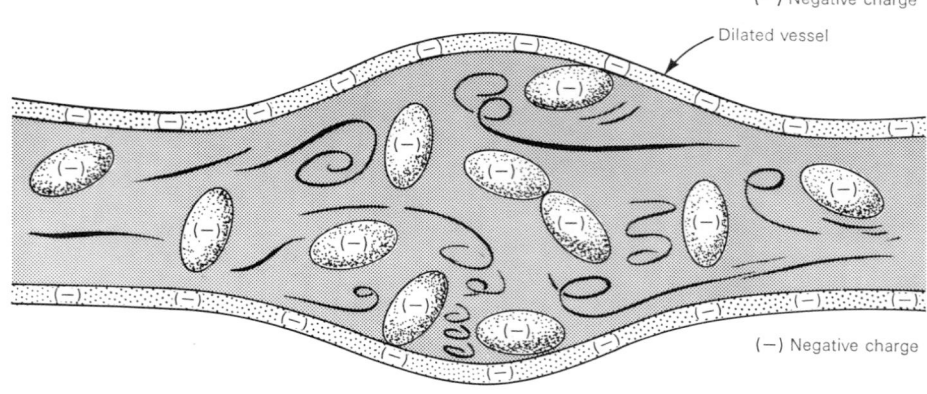

(−) Negative charge

Figure 23-16
Decreased blood flow
with blood cells falling
out of the laminar flow
and massing together.

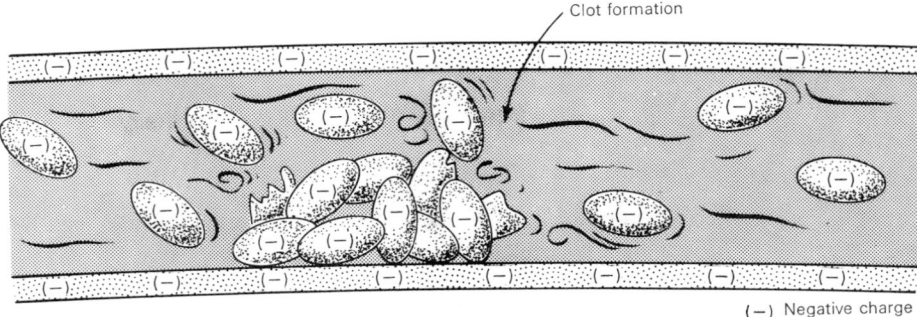

(−) Negative charge

Figure 23-17
Clot formation from
blood cells degenerating
and adhering to vessel
wall. Vessel wall
electrical charge has
changed from negative to
positive.

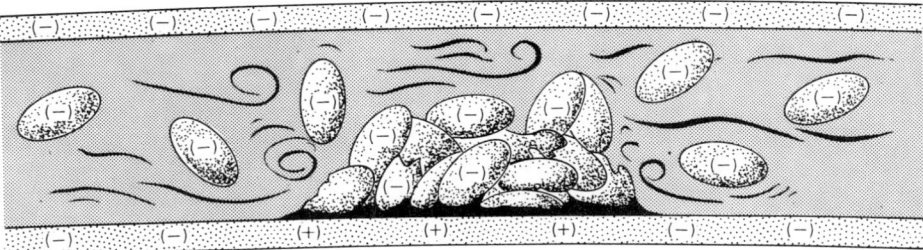

(−) Negative charge
(+) Positive charge

to become concentrated in the mass, which further precipitates clot formation. (See Figure 23–16.) With increased blood flow, or involvement of a larger vessel, the liberated thrombin is removed and clot formation decreased.

The normal endothelial lining of the vessel has a layer of negatively charged protein which repels the negative charged platelets. Once the clotting sequence has been initiated and the clot adheres to the vessel wall, lysis of the thrombosis causes an inflammatory process; this leads to fibrosis, which destroys the negatively charged protein surface and leads to a positive charge of the vessel wall, thus attracting more negatively charged platelets. (See Figure 23–17.)

Thrombophlebitis promotes incompetent venous valves, varicose veins, venous stasis, and pulmonary embolism.

Venous embolism most frequently originates from a thrombus in the deep calf muscles. The embolus flows through progressively larger veins to the right heart. Unless the clot is extremely large, it passes through the right heart chambers and enters the pulmonary arterial circulation. The embolus may occlude a major pulmonary vessel or become impacted at the bifurcation of the main pulmonary artery to create a saddle embolus.

Signs and Symptoms

Signs and symptoms will be discussed in relation to the lower extremities; involvement of other areas is discussed elsewhere. Venous thrombosis usually is occlusive and leads to congestion, stasis, edema, and possibly ischemia. If the deep veins are involved, the superficial veins, which control collateral circulation, become enlarged. Usually there is local pain, tenderness, increased skin temperature, and color changes, i.e., redness, bluish-green, or brown coloration above the affected vessel. Homan's sign is usually present, and pulsations and reflexes are usually normal.

Treatment

The aim of treatment is to prevent pulmonary embolism by a dislodged thrombus, facilitate venous return, and relieve venous stasis. Bed rest is prescribed until the acute symptoms such as fever, congestion, edema, and local tenderness have subsided. Other medical measures include elevation of the extremity to increase venous return, application of warm moist packs to relieve pain and congestion, anticoagulant therapy to prevent propagation of thrombosis, and use of elastic bandages or stockings after the acute phase to increase structural support.

Embolectomy or thrombectomy may be performed to relieve simple noninflammatory thrombosis of a large vein.

Nursing Care

The aim of nursing care is to promote measures to prevent or decrease venous stasis and avert pulmonary embolism through exercise and avoidance of pressure on the extremity veins.

Walking is the most effective form of exercise; patients who are unable to walk should have active or passive leg exercises unless specifically contraindicated. The nonambulatory patient should be taught and assisted in doing active exercises such as full rotation and dorsiflexion of the foot, and flexion and extension of the hips, knees, and plantar digits. Passive exercises are indicated if the patient is unable to carry out active exercises.

Pressure is prevented by proper positioning and frequent turning; pillows should not be placed under the legs. Nursing measures to prevent pressure and to facilitate venous return have been discussed under varicose veins.

During the acute phase of thrombophlebitis exercise of the involved extremity is contraindicated because of the possibility of dislodging the thrombus. Some authorities believe that exercise and massage should be initiated as soon as the acute inflammatory process has subsided which in turn prevents extension of the thrombosis. These measures are specifically prescribed by the physician. Massage is never indicated when thrombosis is suspected.

Another measure to decrease venous stasis is directed toward alleviation of the inflammatory process. Moist packs are applied over the thrombosed vein and kept warm by a thermostatically controlled heat cradle. The cradle maintains constant temperature, which should not exceed 90° F, and prevents pressure on the extremity. After the acute phase elastic bandages are applied to provide support, which facilitates venous return. The bandages are applied from the tips of the toes to the midthigh, and should be changed at least once each day. The skin should be observed for color changes, particularly degrees of redness, and for temperature variations. The skin should be kept scrupulously clean.

Anticoagulant therapy is prescribed to prevent further thrombosis. Until the dosage has been established, daily prothrombin time is taken and recorded. The nurse never administers daily orders of anticoagulants without checking the report of the prothrombin time. The nurse must be aware that spontaneous bleeding may occur anywhere in the body when anticoagulants are given. One of the first danger signs of a hemorrhagic diathesis is bleeding from the kidneys which is detected by the finding of microscopic hematuria on routine urinalysis. Bleeding from the gastrointestinal tract is detected by stool hematest or gross observation. Excessive bleeding may follow a parenteral injection, for example. The physician must be notified when bleeding is observed or suspected by changes in the vital signs.

The prognosis depends upon the predisposing condition. If venous stasis is decreased and there is adequate venous return, the thrombus usually dissolves within a few weeks and the patient is able to return to his usual pattern of living. He should be taught preventive measures, particularly maintaining a balance of walking, sitting, elevating the extremity, and standing. Elastic stockings or bandages may be prescribed by the physician, and the patient should be taught how to apply these to prevent constriction.

Buerger's Disease (Thromboangiitis Obliterans)

The description of Buerger's disease (or *thromboangiitis obliterans,* a frequently used term) is being questioned. There is evidence that it may not be a separate disease entity but either one or a combination of the following conditions: atherosclerosis, embolism, peripheral thrombosis. There seems to be general agreement that it is an inflammatory condition involving segments of the artery lumen and less frequently the veins. The condition leads to occlusion and fibrous encasement of the nerve, artery, and vein.

Etiology

Buerger's disease is a relatively uncommon disorder that is more prevalent in young and middle-aged adults who smoke at least a package of cigarettes a day than in other groups. Some authorities believe the condition is an allergic reaction to nicotine because, if the patient continues to smoke, the condition progresses despite treatment. When smoking is discontinued, new lesions of superficial phlebitis rarely develop and there is little evidence of further arterial occlusion.

Pathophysiology

The lesions may appear in any organ of the body; however, the usual site is in the large and medium-sized arteries of the lower and upper extremities, most frequently the anterior or posterior tibial arteries. The disease may progress to involve one or several arteries, veins, and nerves in the lower or upper extremities. The pathological process begins with inflammation of a segment in the intima of the vessel which decreases the size of the lumen and causes decreased blood flow (Robbins). This in turn encourages thrombosis and occlusion. Lysis of the thrombus causes fibrosis of the vessel which may lead to permanent and complete obstruction. If the occlusive process develops slowly, collateral circulation may be sufficient to minimize tissue damage. A sudden occlusion of a large artery may lead to tissue necrosis and gangrene.

Symptoms

The symptoms are primarily related to ischemia and local venous insufficiency. Symptoms of ischemia are manifested by pain, muscle fatigue, intermittent claudication, and possibly rest pain such as severe cramping or squeezing pain. The ischemic tissue is cold, pale, or blanched and usually is hypersensitive to heat and cold. Vasospasms may be produced by cold environmental temperature. Venous insufficiency, which is chiefly manifested by stasis and edema of the legs and ankles, has been discussed under varicose veins. Ulceration and gangrene may be a presenting complication.

Diagnosis

The diagnosis is based chiefly on the patient's history and signs and symptoms, and ruling out of other types of vascular diseases such as atherosclerosis, embolism, and thrombosis. Diabetes, which affects the vascular system, must also be ruled out. Arteriography may be of value in determining the extent and location of the obstruction.

Treatment and Nursing Care

The aim of treatment is to arrest the progress of the disease, increase the blood supply, and prevent infection of the ischemic tissue. Complete and permanent abstinence from tobacco is considered essential in arresting the progress of this disease. Vasodilating drugs may be beneficial in the development of collateral circulation, but the effect is limited in dilating the fibrotic vessel. Since cold is a vasoconstrictor, the patient should avoid exposure to cold environmental temperature by wearing heat-insulating clothing. He is usually more comfortable in a warm climate, which is conducive to vasodilatation. Exercise such as walking is beneficial in increasing circulation, but if ischemia is marked, intermittent claudication will result from short walks. Buerger-Allen exercises stimulate circulation by alternating gravitational pull. This is achieved by elevating the feet and legs until the feet are blanched, lowering them until they appear red (dangle over side of bed), then resting with legs in a horizontal position. The number of times and the frequency of the exercises are ordered by the physician. Prolonged standing should be avoided as this causes edema, which may lead to a further ischemic condition through compression of the tissues.

Pain is treated conservatively and may be relieved to a degree by alternating the horizontal and slightly dependent position. Narcotics are used discriminately because the condition tends to be chronic, and frequent use may lead to addiction

A sympathectomy may be performed to relieve vasospasm. If the ischemic condition persists and is severe, necrosis and gangrene result and amputation may be necessary.

Raynaud's Disease

Raynaud's disease is a functional vascular disorder characterized by paroxysmal constriction of the arteries of the hands and feet. The occurrence of Raynaud's disease is limited almost entirely to females between the ages of 20 and 40 years. The exact cause of the disorder is unknown, although emotional disturbance, exposure to cold, and familial predisposition are considered predisposing factors.

Pathophysiology

Raynaud's disease is best known as an abnormality of the peripheral sympathetic nervous system due to tonic contraction of the small arterioles on the basis of sympathetic overactivity. The intermittent vasospasms may completely obstruct the arterial blood flow to the digits or to the extremities. The blood flow is changed largely in the digital arterioles of the hands and feet. This causes acute tissue ischemia of the fingers or toes which is manifested by pallor, coldness, pain, or numbness. The capillaries react by becoming dilated, due to an increase in metabolites and manifested by color changes from pale to cyanotic. When the spasm subsides, arterial circulation is reestablished and is manifested by the color changing from cyanosis to rubor then to the normal pink. If the vasospasms are frequent and prolonged, the artery wall reacts by becoming thickened. The size of the lumen is decreased and thrombosis may develop. This may cause complete and permanent occlusion of the vessel which may lead to permanent decreased circulation to the extremity, manifested by continuous cyanosis, coldness, numbness or tingling, atrophy of the digits, and ulceration or gangrene.

Signs and Symptoms

The onset is usually gradual, with pallor of one or two fingers or toes on one hand or foot when exposed to cold. Later all the digits of both hands and feet may become involved. The signs and symptoms are related to the degree of tissue ischemia. The skin temperature may change suddenly from cold to warm due to relaxation of the vasospasm. Nerve involvement causes changes in sensations such as numbness, tingling, throbbing, or a dull ache. Trophic changes may include a taut, white, smooth, shiny appearance with nail deformity. Severe prolonged ischemia may lead to signs and symptoms of ulceration and gangrene such as persistent dull aching pain, malaise, and lassitude.

Treatment

The aim of treatment is to prevent vasospasm by relieving emotional stress and protecting the extremities from cold. Professional psychological counseling may be indicated to assist the patient in identifying and coping with stressful experiences.

Avoidance of cold is essential to prevent vasoconstriction. Smoking is contraindicated as nicotine is a vasoconstrictor.

Medications such as rauwolfia alkaloids, which decrease peripheral vasoconstriction, are indicated. Adrenergic blocking agents such as Dibenamine Hydrochloride and tolazoline (Priscoline Hydrochloride) are valuable in increasing vasodilatation and muscular tone.

A regional sympathectomy to remove vasoconstricting impulses may be indicated if the condition is progressive and fails to respond to medical measures. Amputation of one or more digits may be necessary if gangrene is a complication.

Nursing Care

The aim of nursing care is to assist the patient in identifying and coping with stressful experiences and identifying and instituting measures to reduce exposure to cold. The incidence of vasospasm presents a stressful experience, which in turn precipitates vasospasms. The patient should understand that the symptoms usually do not develop into anything more than an inconvenience. The patient should be encouraged to think about experiences that can be identified as precipitating the condition. For example, what happened to her or what was she doing when the symptoms developed? Can a common experience such as the home or work situation be identified as a cause? Encourage the patient to verbalize the stressful experiences and to think about means of either avoiding or accepting them.

The patient must be able to identify ways to avoid exposure to cold. Clothing must be adapted to meet body temperature demands in relation to environmental temperatures. The effect of clothing on conduction of heat from the body is to increase the insulating effect of the zone of air adjacent to the skin. Clothing entraps additional layers of air next to the skin and in the weave of the cloth, thereby increasing the thickness of the zone of air adjacent to the skin and decreasing the flow of convection currents. Consequently, clothing reduces the rate of heat loss from the body by conduction. Arctic type of clothing with a close thick weave, such as wool socks, fleece-lined footwear, and wool gloves, can decrease heat loss from the hands and feet to as little as one-sixth that of the bare state. Thermal blankets may be indicated as bed covers because of their increased insulating qualities. The patient should avoid handling cold objects such as glasses of iced liquids which produce vasoconstriction.

Immediate relief of vasoconstriction may be brought about by immersion of the hand or foot in warm water, but no warmer than 90° F, to prevent thermal trauma to the ischemic tissue. Moist heat is indicated as water has several thousand times more specific heat than air, so that each unit portion of water adjacent to the skin can absorb far greater quantities of heat than can air; also, the conductivity of heat through water is very marked in comparison with that through air. The vasodilatation in the hands and feet during warming results from a reflex reduction in vasoconstrictor tone.

Arteriosclerosis

Authorities have defined arteriosclerosis in a variety of ways. However, there seems to be common agreement that the muscle and elastic fibers are replaced by fibrous tissue, which impairs the functional elasticity of the blood vessel wall and causes segmental hardening of the arteries.

Arteriosclerosis ranks first as a cause of death in the United States, accounting for over 50 percent of deaths from all causes. Arteriosclerotic hypertension involving the brain, heart, kidneys, and peripheral vascular system is included in this figure. Atherosclerosis is the underlying cause of more than 95 percent of all coronary heart attacks. Individuals of all ages may be affected; however, it occurs chiefly in the age group past the sixth decade. Males are more susceptible than females, but females become more susceptible following the menopause.

Etiology

Many theories have evolved concerning causal factors which lead most authorities to believe that there are multifactors in various combinations causing different degrees of development within each individual. Several authorities have given merit to the following factors. Mechanical stress attributed to the constant pounding of the thrust of blood through the arteries combined with the normal aging process causes senile degeneration. This degeneration is believed to increase arterial permeability to lipid infiltration, thus leading to atheroma plaque formation of the subintima in the arterial wall.

Additional contributing factors with less substantial data include metabolic dysfunctions of insulin, thyroxine, and estrogens. It is known that atherosclerosis and diabetes frequently occur together and that the atherosclerotic lesion is usually more extensive in diabetes. The question is whether or not atherosclerosis is a metabolic disease due to dysfunction of lipid metabolism which may predispose to diabetes or whether diabetes, which tends to cause degeneration of connective tissue, increases proneness to atheroma formation.

The question of diet in atherosclerosis has provoked considerable controversy in recent times. Opinions about diet range from the view that it is insignificant to the belief that diet is the primary cause of atherosclerosis.

Pathology

Arteriosclerosis is considered to consist of three pathological classifications that may occur separately or in combination. They are atherosclerosis, medial calcific sclerosis, and arteriolosclerosis.

Atherosclerosis is characterized by formation of an atheroma or atheromas in the medium- and large-sized arteries. The atheroma plaques may become fibrotic or calcified and ulcerate into the lumen. As the plaques increase in size and number, there is marked deformity, narrowing, and occlusion of the artery. This in turn predisposes to thrombosis, ischemia, atrophy, and infarction of the surrounding tissue. As the arterial walls become weakened, aneurysms may develop.

The second classification is medial calcific sclerosis, characterized by calcifications within the media of medium- to small-sized arteries of the muscular type (Robbins). This condition is found on routine x-ray studies but is not considered of clinical significance, as it does not decrease the size of the lumen and cause vascular occlusions.

The last classification is arteriosclerosis, which is characterized by thickening of the walls and narrowing of the lumens of small arteries and arterioles (Robbins). The predominant cause is prolonged significant elevation of the blood pressure.

Arteriosclerotic disease most frequently involves the following peripheral arteries: the thoracic and abdominal aorta, iliac, and femoral. However, in older individuals and in diabetics, the smaller arteries may also be involved.

Earlier beliefs that arteriosclerosis was a degenerative and diffuse disease have been largely dispelled (DeBakey). It is now believed that the disease often tends to be well localized and segmental in nature, with relatively normal patent channels immediately proximal and distal to the lesion, and that it is slowly progressive, localized, and self-limited.

Signs and Symptoms

The degree and severity of symptoms depend upon the degree of ischemia in the surrounding tissue. If the blood supply is decreased gradually by a slow occlusive process, the tissue reaction is not dramatic. On the other hand, an abrupt occlusion, such as by an embolus, may cause the surrounding tissue to react dramatically (described under arterial thrombosis and embolism).

Intermittent claudication is an early symptom of the occlusive process of arteriosclerosis.

The location of the pain is indicative of the arteries involved. Hip pain denotes abdominal aorta or iliac involvement; thigh pain denotes aortoiliac or common femoral involvement; and calf muscle pain denotes popliteal occlusion. As the disease progresses, the patient may have ischemic neuropathy, signified by moderate to severe pain which radiates down one or more nerve trunks, and by numbness or a burning sensation.

An awareness of predominant observable signs will aid in determining the degree of arterial insufficiency. First, are the pulsations in the tibial or popliteal arteries impaired or absent? Are there signs of redness, blueness, or marked pallor? Does changing the position of the extremity cause color changes, for example, does elevation cause pallor and dependency cause rubor? Trophic skin changes may be noticed such as loss of subcutaneous tissue, loss of hair, and toenail deformity. Edema may be noted after the patient has kept his extremities in a dependent position for a long period of time to relieve pain. The most obvious sign of severe ischemia is ulceration or gangrene of the digits or foot.

Prognosis

The prognosis for survival of the affected extremity depends upon the extent and rapidity of the development of the occlusion, the frequency of the development of other occlusions, and the state of development when treatment is initiated (Allen et al.).

Medical Diagnosis

The medical diagnosis, first of all, is based upon careful evaluation of the presenting signs and symptoms. Angiography, which is the visualization or outlining of a blood vessel (artery or vein) on an x-ray film, permits precise delineation of the location, nature, and effect of involvement. This test provides valuable information concerning the operability of the artery. Authorities agree that the larger the artery and the more localized the occlusive lesion, the greater are the benefits from surgery. To perform this test a radiopaque dye is injected into the vessel and the x-ray film is taken immediately. Fluoroscopy may aid in demonstrating the course of the dye. The specific method used in the performance of this test depends on the location of the vessel under study. The chief complication is damage to the vessel wall at the point of introduction of the contrast medium and the vasoconstrictor effect of the solution on the vessels through which it flows. Another complication may be damage to the organs and structures supplied by the vessels being visualized. Following this test the patient usually remains on bed rest for the first 24 hours. The injection site is checked for signs of swelling, discoloration, and bleeding. If any of these signs occur an ice bag (or a sterile pressure dressing, for active bleeding) is applied and the physician notified. Other nursing measures include observation for signs and symptoms of arterial occlusion as follows: checking the extremity pulses, checking the surface temperature of the extremity for coldness, observing the color for pallor or cyanosis, and checking for sensations of numbness or pain.

Oscillometric readings have proven valuable as a comparative measure of pulse volume in both extremities. The oscillometer is a manometer attached to a cuff used to measure the blood pressure. This reading determines the point of pressure at which circulation through the deep vessels of the lower extremities ceases; digital palpation may provide the same information. Skin temperature studies may aid in providing information as to the degree of arteriospasm present, but these studies are not considered valuable in diagnosis or treatment. As has been mentioned previously, the amount of exercise the patient can tolerate without pain is an extremely important diagnostic system.

Laboratory blood studies usually consist of quantitative determinations of plasma cholesterol, complete blood count, and platelet count. It is believed that in the presence of occlusive arterial disease a concentration of total cholesterol in excess of 250 mg per 100 ml strongly suggests that the lesion is atherosclerotic. A high concentration of platelets and erythrocytes is a predisposing factor to thrombosis.

Treatment

The major problem is concerned with the hemodynamic disturbances of the tissue produced by the occlusive process. The primary objective of treatment is to correct the disturbances by restoration of normal circulation (DeBakey). An additional aim of therapy is to halt the progression of the pathological process and improve circulation by medical measures especially when surgical measures are not indicated.

Surgical therapy designed to restore circulation consists of thromboendarterectomy, patch graft angioplasty, bypass graft, or excision with graft replacement, the procedure depending upon the nature, extent, and site of involvement. A thromboendarterectomy consists of removal of the diseased inner portions of the arterial media and the thickened intima. Most grafts are flexible, seamless, knitted, synthetic tubes. These procedures are described in detail in textbooks of surgery.

The most frequent complication of arterial surgery arises from an acute arterial occlusion in other areas, generally affecting the renovascular, coronary, or cerebrovascular system.

Other surgical procedures are lumbar sympathetic block and regional sympathetic ganglionectomy. These too are described in surgical textbooks.

Ulceration and gangrene are treated conservatively when possible. Boric acid solution dressings are applied and are kept at an even temperature of 90° F by means of a thermostatically controlled heat cradle. Secondary infections are prevented or controlled by the use of antibiotic therapy. Amputation is indicated for extensive gangrene or intractable pain.

A low-cholesterol diet, discussed earlier, and a low-caloric diet (in the case of obesity) may be prescribed. Estrogenic drugs may be prescribed to reduce concentrations of serum cholesterol and increase the concentrations of serum phospholipids in hypercholesteremic men and postmenopausal women (Allen et al.). Circulation may be enhanced by Buerger-Allen exercises (described under Buerger's disease) and by the use of the Saunders oscillating bed, which improves blood flow by alternately raising and lowering the lower extremities above and below the level of the heart, thus decreasing and increasing gravitational pull.

Nursing Care

Nursing care is aimed at promoting medical measures to correct or improve circulation, applying nursing techniques to prevent tissue damage, and initiating a patient education program to facilitate self-care.

Pre- and postoperative nursing measures for patients undergoing reconstructive arterial surgery are essentially the same as for other types of abdominal surgery and general surgery and have been discussed elsewhere. An additional preoperative measure is to mark the sites of the arterial pulses in the operative extremity. (See Figure 23–18.) This measure will assist postoperatively in determining whether the pulses are absent or difficult to detect. The pulse sites may vary as much as 1 inch

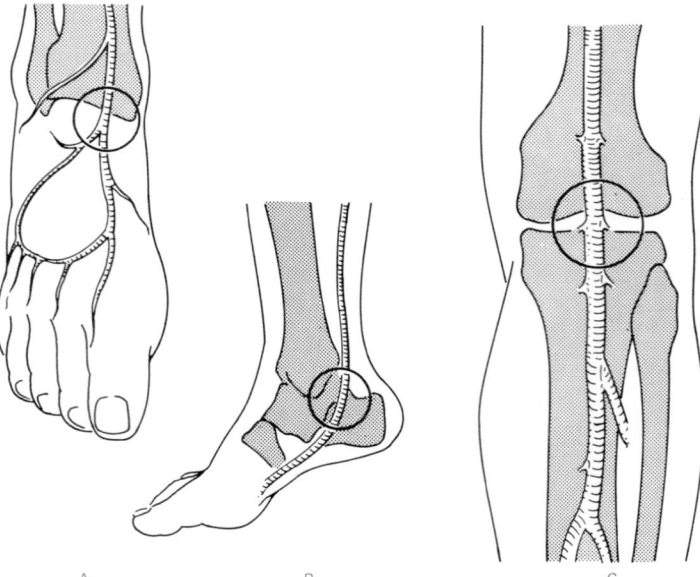

Figure 23–18
Sites for palpating lower extremity pulses: A, dorsalis pedis; B, posterior tibial; C, popliteal. (Courtesy Mary Jo Mirlenbrink and Craig C. Gosling.)

A   B   C

from the usual sites. Close observations should be made of the skin color and temperature. Neurological signs and symptoms such as foot drop, paresis, and paresthesia should be evaluated and recorded. Severe ischemia of a large area of the extremity may be caused by an embolus. Emergency measures are usually indicated, and are discussed under arterial thrombosis and embolism.

Environmental temperatures may improve or impede circulation. Low temperatures cause vasoconstriction, thus decreasing circulation, while high temperatures cause increased body metabolism which increases the demands on an already inadequate circulation. Environmental temperature should be maintained at 80° F. A thermal blanket may be helpful, and bed socks may be indicated for patients who complain of persistent coldness of the feet.

The nurse must appreciate the effect of positioning upon the circulation in the extremities. The patient should be taught to avoid prolonged periods of knee and hip flexion, crossing of the knees and feet, and sitting and standing without changing position. The extremity may be placed in a slightly dependent position by elevating the head of the bed on 6- to 8-inch blocks. Prolonged dependency, as occurs when the patient dangles his legs to relieve pain, should be avoided as this predisposes to edema of the feet and ankles. The patient may not wish to exercise since this causes pain; however, exercise to the point of tolerance should be maintained each day.

To determine the progression of the disease process and the effectiveness of treatment, color and temperature of the extremities should be observed and compared. Other signs and symptoms to be investigated in the same manner are extremity pulse, edema, blisters, traumatic or spontaneous ulceration, and the condition of the nails. Specific observations must be accurately recorded each day to serve as a guide for the recognition of changes.

Proper foot care is essential, since minor breaks or irritations may lead to uncontrollable pathology. The skin should be washed frequently with a mild soap and patted dry. A bland oil will help keep the skin soft.

Arterial Thrombosis and Embolism

Arterial thrombosis and embolism are common in the middle and older age groups and account for 10 to 20 percent of deaths from all causes. The two chief causes are arteriosclerosis and auricular fibrillation. Other causes are surgical procedures, local trauma, and decreased circulation from decompensated heart disease.

Pathophysiology

The pathophysiology is related directly to that described under venous thrombosis and embolism, but there are additional factors relating directly to the artery. The artery wall contributes to thrombosis by its muscular structure. Trauma causes constriction, decreasing the lumen and causing platelet contact and formation of a small mass. This mass sticks to the vessel lumen thus initiating the clotting sequence. Arteriosclerosis causes segmental roughening and thickening of the lumen which decreases blood flow, promoting platelet adhesion, which initiates clot formation.

Embolism is more common in the extremities than thrombosis because of faster blood flow in the arteries. In arterial circulation the embolus frequently originates in the right chamber of the heart and is carried through the larger systemic arteries to the smaller arteries of the extremities. The embolus usually lodges distal to a bifurcation when the artery suddenly diminishes in size.

Signs and Symptoms

Regardless of the cause, complete sudden arterial occlusion, which leads to marked tissue ischemia, may cause necrosis and gangrene within a few hours. A sudden arterial occlusion is manifested by sudden, sharp, excruciating pain; the severity may cause shock. The extremity becomes cold, pale, pulseless, with diminished reflex, paresis, and anesthesia. An additional complication may be severe vasospasm of the surrounding vessels. The superficial veins collapse.

Treatment

The aim of treatment is to restore adequate or normal circulation in order to prevent tissue necrosis and gangrene. Vasospasm may be relieved by such medications as papaverine and a lumbar sympathetic block using a local anesthetic agent. Circulation may be increased to the extremity by external heat such as is provided by a light thermal blanket or absorbent cotton. This improves collateral circulation by dilating the accessory arteries. Direct heat is never applied to ischemic tissue because of possible thermal trauma and resultant acceleration of the necrotic process. Anticoagulant therapy is initiated to prevent further thrombosis.

If the acute signs and symptoms of arterial occlusion are not controlled medically within a few hours, surgery is indicated. The type of surgery depends upon the site and extent of the occlusion. For example, if the embolus is large and embedded at the bifurcation of the aorta into the iliac arteries (saddle block), a bypass graft may be indicated. This procedure has been described under surgical measures for atherosclerosis. In medium- and large-sized extremity arteries, an embolectomy may be indicated. This procedure involves incision above the occlusion, suctioning out the clot, and suturing the vessel. Endarterectomy is indicated when the thrombus or embolus has become firmly attached to the intima causing fibrosis and thickening. In this procedure the vessel is ligated above the occlusion, the occluded section of the intima is removed, and the artery is anastomosed.

Nursing Care

Constant nursing attention is mandatory. The patient's signs and symptoms must be checked every 15 to 20 minutes to detect manifestations of shock which include restlessness and apprehension; pale, cold, moist skin; decreased blood pressure; and increased pulse rate. These signs and symptoms must be reported to the physician immediately. Treatment for shock is essential to prevent extension of the occlusive process, because blood flow is decreased, platelet surface adhesiveness is increased, and there is a tendency toward increased clotting time.

Specific nursing measures are indicated for patients undergoing peripheral vascular surgery. These measures include observations of signs and symptoms that would suggest occlusion from surgical trauma. The pulse below the operative site must be checked frequently. Color changes of the extremity must be noted. Pallor indicates inadequate circulation; cyanosis indicates blood stagnation in the dilated arterioles. Coldness indicates ischemia; the line of temperature change indicates the site of the occlusion. If the patient is on anticoagulant therapy, the operative site must be checked for bleeding, which if it does occur, is usually severe. Pressure is applied on the pressure point immediately above the operative site and directly over the wound and transfusions of whole fresh blood are usually given. Surgical intervention may be necessary.

The prognosis depends upon the precipitating factors. If the patient is older and auricular fibrillation is present, the embolic process may continue with grave effects. If the thrombosis is due to arteriosclerosis, the thrombotic process may or may not continue. The patient may make a complete recovery and follow his usual pattern of living.

Aortic Aneurysm

Aneurysm is a localized, permanent dilatation of an artery caused by weakening and destruction of the arterial media. Several types of aneurysms have been described according to the anatomic pathologic features: (1) fusiform—a uniform, segmental dilatation of the entire circumference of the artery usually in the aortic arch and abdominal aorta; (2) saccular—a segmental dilatation involving one side of the circumference of the artery causing sac-like formation usually in the thoracic and abdominal aorta; and (3) dissecting—resembling a hematoma in the arterial wall caused by seepage of blood between the layers of the intima and media. (See Figure 23-19.)

Pathology

Multiple pathologic processes may be directly involved in the formation of an aneurysm. Arteriosclerotic lesions are chiefly responsible in the late middle and older age groups, and are second to syphilis as a pathological factor. Congenital defects and trauma are occasionally predisposing factors.

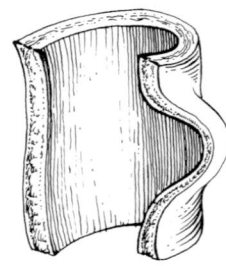 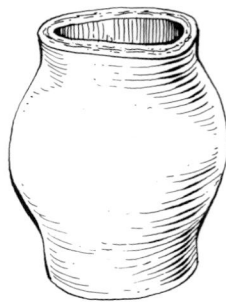 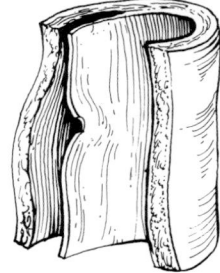

*Figure 23-19
Types of aneurysms: A, saccular; B, fusiform; C, dissecting. (Courtesy Mary Jo Mirlenbrink and Craig C. Gosling.)*

Signs and Symptoms

Signs and symptoms of an aneurysm may not be present until it is large enough to produce pressure on the surrounding structures or becomes palpable. If there is compression of the trachea or bronchus, the patient may display symptoms of dyspnea and hoarseness. Dysphagia may be present if there is esophageal pressure; nausea and vomiting may be caused by pressure on the intestines. Obstruction of the superior vena cava or subclavian vein may cause unequal pulses in the arms. Aneurysms from arteriosclerosis develop slowly and unlike arteriosclerotic obstruction of other arteries, the symptoms of arterial insufficiency are usually minimal. Pain is caused by compression and stretching of the nerves in surrounding tissues. It is usually of long duration and thus can be differentiated from cardiac pain.

Physical findings are of limited value. The diagnosis is made by angiography.

According to DeBakey, the most significant characteristic of an aneurysmal lesion is that once it has formed through weakness and destruction of the media, it tends to progress and ultimately to produce serious and even lethal complications either from compression of surrounding structures or from rupture.

Treatment

The recommended therapy is surgical excision of the diseased segment and replacement with a flexible, seamless, knitted synthetic tube or a bypass graft. If the aneurysm is in the thoracic area, this procedure requires a cardiopulmonary bypass with the use of the artificial heart-lung machine. Prognosis depends upon the age and general condition of the patient and the pathological involvement. The prognosis is good if the aneurysm is not of the advanced dissecting type.

Nursing Care

Nursing care for a patient having excision and graft of a thoracic aortic aneurysm is essentially the same as for open heart surgery. Preoperative care in abdominal aortic aneurysmal repair is similar to that of other types of abdominal surgery. Arterial pulse sites in the lower extremities should be marked prior to surgery as described earlier. Postoperative care includes frequent checking of the extremity pulse, skin temperature, and color as described. The nurse must check for signs and symptoms of bleeding and shock. Bleeding from the operative site requires immediate detection and treatment.

Trauma

Traumatic injuries to the peripheral vascular system continue to be a major health hazard. These are caused chiefly by accidents in the home, industry, and automobiles. Lacerations, contusions, crushing injuries, fractures, and dislocations comprise the traumatic injuries. Bleeding of a small vein usually is of little consequence and can be controlled by direct pressure on the lesion, whereas that of a large vein usually requires suturing or ligation. A delayed complication may be thrombosis, which may cause a pulmonary embolus; this is rare since the thrombus is usually firmly attached to the wall of the vein at the site of injury. If a large artery is severed, the immediate concern is to control hemorrhage by direct compression on the pressure point superior to the lesion until surgical measures can be initiated. Severance of a large artery causes interruption of peripheral blood flow which results in severe ischemia of the surrounding structures. Large ruptured arteries may be excised and replaced by a graft.

Compression by a hematoma or a fragment of a bone, intimal spasm, or local thrombus may cause arterial occlusion. Since this condition usually results as an emergency situation, it is imperative that the nurse recognize the signs and symptoms. Arterial occlusion was discussed earlier.

In the patient with arteriosclerosis of the peripheral arteries, mild trauma may precipitate ulceration in an ischemic limb. This situation could lead to medicolegal implications, and the nurse must understand these implications.

Bibliography

Allen, Edgar V., Nelson W. Barker, and Edgar A. Hines, Jr.: *Peripheral Vascular Disease,* 3d ed. Philadelphia: W. B. Saunders Company, 1962.

Beeson, Paul B. and Walsh McDermott (Eds.): *Cecil-Loeb Textbook of Medicine,* 12th ed. Philadelphia: W. B. Saunders Company, 1967.

Brunner, Lillian Sholtis, et al.: *Textbook of Medical-Surgical Nursing.* Philadelphia: J. B. Lippincott Company, 1964.

Connor, William E.: Medical Approaches to the Control and Prevention of Atherosclerosis. *Journal of Iowa Medical Society,* 53:583–593, September, 1963.

Darling, R. C. et al.: Aortoiliofemoral Endarterectomy for Atherosclerotic Occlusive Disease. *Surgery,* 55:184–194, January, 1964.

DeBakey, Michael E.: Basic Concepts in Arterial Diseases. *Bulletin of New York Academy of Medicine,* 39:707–749, November, 1963.

Denman, F. R., et al.: Sudden Arterial Occlusion. *Texas Journal of Medicine,* 59:1042–1046, November, 1963.

DeTakats, Geza: *Vascular Surgery.* Philadelphia: W. B. Saunders Company, 1959.

Edwards, Edward Allen: *Thrombosis in Arteriosclerosis of Lower Extremities.* Springfield, Ill.: Charles C Thomas, Publisher, 1950.

Fogarty, Thomas J. and John J. Cranley: Catheter Technic for Arterial Embolectomy. *Annals of Surgery,* 161: 325–330, March, 1965.

Fogarty, Thomas J.: Catheter Technic for Acute Venous Thrombosis of the Iliofemoral System. Edwards Laboratory, Inc. Santa Ana, California, July, 1965.

Foote, R. Rowden: *Varicose Veins,* 3d ed. Bristol, England: John Wright & Sons Ltd., 1960.

Hardin, C. A.: Survival and Complications in 134 Surgically Treated Cases of Aortoiliac Thrombosis. *Surgery,* 55:617–620, May, 1964.

Harrison, T. R. (Ed.): *Principles of Internal Medicine,* 5th ed. New York: McGraw-Hill Book Company, 1966.

Hoak, J. C., et al.: Thrombosis Associated with Mobilization of Fatty Acids. *American Journal of Pathology,* 43:987–988, December, 1963.

Johnson, A. J.: Present Status of Thrombolytic Therapy. *American Heart Journal,* 67:418–420, March, 1964.

Juergene, J. L.: Traumatic Occlusive

Disease of Peripheral Arteries. *Heart Bulletin,* 13:31–33, March-April, 1964.

Julian, Ormand C., et al.: *Cardiovascular Surgery.* Chicago: Year Book Medical Publishers, Inc., 1962.

Kagen, Abraham, et al.: The Coronary Profile—Heart Disease Epidemiology Study, Framingham, Mass., and National Institutes of Health. *Annals of New York Academy of Science,* 97:879–960, August, 1963.

Kannel, William B., et al.: Risk Factors in Coronary Heart Disease. An Evaluation of Several Serum Lipids as Predictors of Coronary Heart Disease—The Framingham Study. *Annals of Internal Medicine,* 61: 888–899, November, 1964.

King, R. D.: Evaluation of Lumbar Sympathetic Denervation. *Archives of Surgery,* 88:23–35, January, 1964.

Krause, G. Lynn and Frances C. Vester: Varicose Veins—Diagnosis and Treatment and Nursing Care. *American Journal of Nursing,* 53:70–72, January, 1953.

Krug, Elsie E.: *Pharmacology in Nursing,* 8th ed. St. Louis: The C. V. Mosby Company, 1960.

Marple, Charles D.: *Thromboembolic Conditions and Their Treatment with Anticoagulants.* Springfield, Ill.: Charles C Thomas, Publisher, 1950.

Moffott, W. P., et al.: Lumbar Sympathectomy in Arteriosclerosis Obliterans. *American Journal of Surgery,* 30:409–410, July, 1964.

MonCrief, J. A.: Use of Dextran to Prevent Arterial and Venous Thrombosis. *Annals of Surgery,* 158:553–560, October, 1963.

Morris, G. C., Jr., et al.: Aortic Aneurysms and Occlusive Diseases of the Aorta. *American Journal of Cardiology,* 12:303–308, September, 1963.

Moses, Campbell: *Atherosclerosis, Mechanisms as a Guide to Prevention.* Philadelphia: Lea & Febiger, 1963.

Orbison, J. Lowell and David E. Smith: *The Peripheral Blood Vessels.* Baltimore: The Williams & Wilkins Company, 1963.

Quint, Jeanne C.: Nursing the Patient with Endarterectomy. *American Journal of Nursing,* 58:996–998, July, 1958.

Robbins, Stanley L. *Textbook of Pathology with Clinical Application.* 2d ed. Philadelphia: W. B. Saunders Company, 1962.

Sanders, Howard J.: Heart Disease the Tangled Web of Evidence. *Chemical and Engineering Nurse,* 43:130–158, March, 1965.

Sandler, Maurice: *Atherosclerosis and Its Origin.* New York: Academic Press, Inc., 1963.

Seijffers, M. J., et al.: Systemic Vascular Insufficiency. *American Journal of Medicine,* 36:158–166, January, 1964.

Smith, Dorothy W. and Claudia D. Gips: *Care of the Adult Patient: Medical-Surgical Nursing,* 2d ed. Philadelphia: J. B. Lippincott Company, 1966.

Smith, Dorothy W. and Claudia D. Gips: *Facts on The Major Killing and Crippling Diseases in The United States Today.* New York: The National Health Education Committee Inc., 1964.

Tice, D. A., et al.: Lumbar Sympathectomy: Effect on Vascular Responses in the Lower Extremity of Patients with Arteriosclerosis Obliterans. *Archives of Surgery,* 87:461–463, September, 1963.

Troedsson, B. S.: The Use of Oscillometry on the Lower Extremities to Diagnose and Evaluate Occlusive Vascular Disease of the Aorta and Iliac Arteries. *Archives of Physical Medicine,* 44:651–655, December, 1963.

Winsor, Travis and Burrell O. Raulston: *Peripheral Vascular Diseases.* Springfield, Ill.: Charles C Thomas, Publisher, 1959.

Wohl, Michael G. and Robert S. Goodhart: *Modern Nutrition in Health and Disease,* 3d ed. Philadelphia: Lea & Febiger, 1964.

SECTION 4
LYMPHATIC
DISORDERS
RUTH E. BARSTOW

Lymphangitis
ACUTE LYMPHANGITIS
CHRONIC LYMPHANGITIS
Lymphadenitis
Lymphedema
CHRONIC LYMPHEDEMA
ELEPHANTIASIS

The lymphatic system forms a network that penetrates every tissue of the body supplied by blood with the exception of the brain. Its channels lie in close proximity to the venous system and, like the veins, are well supplied with valves to prevent retrograde flow as fluid is propelled toward the chest. The lymphatic system has both a superficial and a deep layer, but, unlike the channels of the venous system, there is no communication between the two. Because the lymphatics are tiny, translucent, and filled with colorless fluid, they are not visualized until they join to form large trunks in the chest. Dye injected into subcutaneous tissue is absorbed and outlines the network.

The main purpose of the lymphatic system is to drain intercellular fluid and return it and especially plasma protein to the bloodstream. The lymphatic capillaries absorb the fluids and other microscopic particles pressing against them in the interstitial space. Lymph passes through the network to afferent tubular lymphatics that drain into lymph nodes. The lymph nodes, or glands, are scattered in chains and groups along the course of the vessels. The glands return some lymph to the bloodstream and otherwise act as sieves to filter out foreign particles, such as bacteria and cancer cells. In many cases the phagocytes (lymphocytes) are able to contain and engulf the causative organism thereby curing the infection; whereas in other cases the lymph channels actually carry foreign cells, e.g., cancer, to distant areas of the body. The regional groups of glands collect from the deep and superficial lymphatics and move the lymph through efferent channels to the thoracic and right lymphatic ducts, which empty into the venous system at the left and right subclavian veins where they join the internal jugulars.

The lymphatics are subject to many influences, since they comprise an extensive system that receives and transports any matter entering it; thus the system is subject to infection, trauma, obstruction, and tumors. The role of the lymphatics in neoplasia is more appropriately studied under the reticuloendothelial system. This section is primarily concerned with infections and obstruction.

Lymphangitis

Lymphangitis, an inflammation of the vessels, may be caused by a variety of microorganisms and may be acute or chronic. Streptococci and staphylococci are the most frequent causative organisms; tubercle bacilli, spirochetes, fungi, and viruses are less commonly so.

ACUTE LYMPHANGITIS

Red streaks traveling up the extremity toward the lymph node are characteristic. The initial infection may have seemed minor or even gone unobserved. Infection confined to the major lymphatic channels is called *tubular lymphangitis;* that involving a large area or the entire limb is called *diffuse* or *reticular* lymphangitis. Both are frequently accompanied by chills, fever, malaise, and aching; leukocytosis occurs. The nodes become enlarged and tender. The pain may be so exquisite that movement is seriously hampered.

In diffuse lymphangitis there is edema of the entire limb. After treatment, the swelling does not subside entirely because of fibrotic changes and persistence of a chronic mild infection.

Treatment is directed toward eradicating the infection and relieving the symptoms. Antibiotic therapy is based on blood culture and sensitivity tests. Bed rest is indicated. The extremity should be elevated. Hot moist packs are applied to aid healing and relieve pain. Sedatives, analgesics, and antipyretics are usually necessary. Nursing care is generally supportive and typical of that given a bed patient with a systemic infection.

CHRONIC LYMPHANGITIS

Diffuse lymphangitis leads to chronic lymphangitis, but often the chronic form is the result of recurrent infections. The channel becomes firm and cord-like beyond the area of initial infection. Abscesses and ulcers may develop.

The disease is treated similarly to the acute form. Progression is prevented but the fibrotic changes cannot be reversed.

The most important aspect of nursing care is teaching the patient to prevent recurrent infections. Cleanliness, meticulous care of fingernails and toenails, and prompt attention to any injury should be emphasized. Protective devices should be worn when called for, e.g., gloves and suitable shoes for gardeners.

Lymphadenitis

Lymphadenitis is inflammation of lymph nodes caused by an infectious organism, and is secondary to infection of the area of drainage. The nodes mose commonly involved are the cervical, axillary, inguinal, and femoral. The affected gland becomes warm and tender, and with progression other nodes become involved. Frequently they become confluent and the overlying skin becomes inflamed and edematous. Purulent drainage usually remains as a localized abscess. Untreated lymphadenitis can cause septicemia.

Today public awareness of good health practices and the availability of assistance, plus the excruciating pain and immobilizing effects of lymphadenitis, lead most victims to the physician before suppuration occurs. Faith in home remedies, denial of seriousness of the disease, isolation, and deprivation may deter some individuals until the disease has progressed, although, suppuration may occur in spite of treatment when the infection is overwhelming.

Treatment and nursing care in lymphadenitis are essentially those of lymphangitis. The adenitis subsides as the primary infection is treated and cured. The size and tension of the gland should be observed carefully. If the gland becomes large and fluctuant, it is incised and drained. Meticulous care of the wound is important. The patient is usually placed on isolation.

Rarely tuberculous adenitis may occur. A permanent draining sinus is formed due to the irritant calcium deposits. The primary disease is treated and the involved nodes are excised.

Lymphedema

Lymphedema is a localized deposition of lymph particularly in the extremities. It may be acute and transitory or chronic and unremitting.

CHRONIC LYMPHEDEMA

There are primary and secondary forms of chronic lymphedema. The primary type is classified as congenital, thought to be caused by underdevelopment of the lymphatic system, or hereditary; if the latter it is called *Milroy's disease*. Chronic primary lymphedema of unknown cause is called *lymphedema praecox*. The primary type is most often seen in women.

Secondary lymphedema is due to obstruction or destruction of the lymphatics. Chronic lymphangitis with recurrent infections is a primary factor. The consequences of infection can be quite serious when lymph nodes and channel vessels have been removed surgically, affected by neoplastic disease or metastases, or otherwise destroyed.

Differentiation of obstructive causes and visualization of the lymphatics is accomplished through lymphangiogram. Evans blue dye is injected in the webbing of fingers or toes and the largest visible lymphatic is cannulated with a fine needle. A radiopaque substance suspended in oil is slowly infused. The procedure is tedious and tiring for the patient, but is a rewarding diagnostic tool.

The pathophysiology is similar in both types. Infection or increased pressure within the obstructed vessels causes distortion and destruction of the valves. They become incompetent and dilate. Fluid collects in the extremity and pitting edema is seen. The protein-rich fluid and the tight, thin skin are predisposing factors to infection.

A vicious circle ensues and the condition worsens. If treatment is deferred, elephantiasis eventually occurs.

The extremity is elevated to allow lymph drainage, and support is provided during waking hours by the use of elastic bandages. Nursing principles and techniques involved have been described elsewhere. Elastic stockings may be improved to the point where they give adequate support, but at the present time they are worn primarily for "special" occasions to afford cosmetic improvement. It is essential that infections be prevented. Antibiotics are prescribed and the part is put at rest in an elevated position. The patient should be taught to rest the limb whenever possible and particularly at night. She should not wear constrictive clothing, e.g., tight shoulder straps if an arm is affected or roller garters if a leg is affected. Mild exercise is beneficial but prolonged sitting or standing is detrimental. Diet may be restricted in salt and diuretics may be given.

ELEPHANTIASIS

Chronic lymphedema that has progressed unabated with a tremendous, fibrosed extremity covered by leathery rough-textured skin is called *elephantiasis*. This condition can be relieved only by surgery. The Kondoleon operation is the procedure employed. The operation is usually done in four stages. Sections of skin and all of the underlying tissue down to the muscle are removed from the extremity. The remaining skin may be thinned with use of a dermatome to remove the lymphatic capillaries. The skin is then sutured together. In some cases the surgeon removes the skin as well and replaces it with autogenous split thickness grafts. The recovery period is lengthy. There is considerable serosanguinous oozing after each stage. Pressure dressings are applied and the limb is elevated. Antiobiotics are prescribed. Scrupulous dressing technique and protection of the extremity from injury are important nursing measures.

Education concerning prevention and treatment of burns and infections is an essential aspect of nursing care, especially since the superficial lymphatic channels have been removed. The patient needs much emotional support and encouragement throughout his hospitalization, to help him meet the realities of his unsightly condition and the mutilating operation he must face. Hope based on the improvement he will gain through the surgery should be encouraged, yet the nurse should help him to realize that there will be differences in appearance between the two extremities but that carefully chosen clothing will help to hide the scars.

CHAPTER 24
THE PATIENT WITH RENAL DISEASE

DORIS COLEMAN, KATHLEEN MIKAN,
LOIS NUGENT HOUGH, AND GRACE TOEWS*

* Richard Urwiller, M.D., served as medical consultant in the preparation of this chapter.
The assistance of Mathilda C. Frank in the preparation of this chapter is acknowledged.

The disorders discussed in this chapter involve the kidneys and ureters, the bladder, and the urethra. These disorders, by compromising kidney function, may impair renal excretion and produce serious imbalances of the body fluids which sooner or later lead to death unless the process remits or is corrected. The synthetic functions of the kidney may be affected also: (1) ammonia production, if diminished, may contribute to acidosis; (2) erythropoietin manufacture, if decreased, may be a factor in the development of anemia; and (3) the increased renal synthesis of vasopressor material is believed to be one mechanism underlying the onset of arterial hypertension.

Renal dysfunction may be due to a disturbance within the urinary tract itself, such as infection, obstruction, trauma, or congenital anomalies; or it may be secondary to a disturbance in some other organ system, for example, heart failure or diabetes mellitus. Conversely, renal impairment and resulting imbalances of body fluids may affect other organ systems of the body. To fully understand the symptomatology of renal disease, it is necessary to appreciate the interdependence of renal dysfunction and extrarenal disturbances. A thorough review of normal renal function and of the principles of fluid and electrolyte balance is recommended at this time.

Treatment of conditions of the urinary tract is aimed primarily at the preservation of renal function. The treatment may be of a specific or a nonspecific nature. Specific treatment is directed toward the correction of the process underlying the problem, i.e., antibiotic therapy for infection, surgical relief of an obstruction. Unfortunately, not all the underlying problems lend themselves to such direct approaches. In these cases treatment must be of a nonspecific, supportive nature, aimed at maintaining homeostasis. A good example of this kind of therapy is the careful control of fluids and electrolytes. This type of treatment may be life-saving, too, if it keeps the patient alive until natural "healing" occurs, as it may in some cases of renal failure.

To make sound nursing judgments and give intelligent and specific care to the patient, the nurse must know and understand the patient's diagnosis. "Understanding the diagnosis" implies that the nurse possesses a working knowledge of the patient's disorder, of how it produces physiological disturbances of body fluids and renal function, and of how these disturbances are reflected in particular signs and symptoms. Such knowledge is essential if her observations and interpretations are to be of any value to other members of the health team or to herself in planning and adapting care.

Another necessity, obvious but sometimes overlooked, is for the nurse to know the patient. Because illness is such a personal experience, everyone reacts to it in his own individual way. The patient's personality, his life situation, and the severity and duration of his illness are some of the factors that influence his reactions.

Disorders of the renal system are found in all age groups. Because a patient's reaction to illness is partly dependent upon his maturational level, the nurse must call upon her knowledge of growth and development to understand what special threat the illness may have for him. Is it endangering his career plans or affecting family relationships, for example?

Some of the conditions of the renal system are preventable, as are some of the complications. If the nurse is to teach positive health and preventive measures, she must be well informed regarding the causative and predisposing factors peculiar to the various conditions. When such information is nonexistent at the current stage of medical knowledge, this fact should be known also and emphasis placed on prevention of disability and delay in progress of the disease.

Some of the conditions of the renal system require that the patient make some modifications in his pattern of daily living. Such needs must be identified and appropriate measures taken to help him. Families and friends must be supported also to prevent rejection or overprotection of the patient.

Care of the patient at any time goes far beyond that necessitated by particular therapy and requires the intelligent application of physiological, psychological, and sociocultural knowledge.

Evaluation of the Patient

The urinary system possesses a unique capacity for extensive investigation. By means of instrumentation, such structures as the urethra, bladder, and ureteral orifices can be directly visualized. More complicated techniques utilizing contrast media and roentgenography reveal the status of the ureters, kidneys, and associated structures. Laboratory analysis of urine serves as a barometer of the integrity of kidney function and reflects the state of health of the individual as a whole. In the following paragraphs the gamut of urologic diagnostic studies is reviewed so that the student might gain some insight into their variety and significance. Before proceeding the student is advised to read Chapter 7 in which history-taking, the physical examination, and routine laboratory studies are described in detail.

Symptoms of a urinary dysfunction are carefully evaluated as they may be indicative of a urinary tract disorder or may reflect an abnormality elsewhere in the body. Hematuria may suggest kidney disease or a blood dyscrasia such as paroxysmal nocturnal hemoglobinuria. Enuresis, urinary retention, and incontinence are common to urologic, neurologic, and psychologic problems. Polyuria occurs with renal tubular disease or in diabetes mellitus, diabetes insipidus, hyperparathyroidism, aldosteronism, and brain injury, or is psychologically induced by excessive water drinking. Oliguria may also indicate a form of renal tubular disease or may occur following inadequate fluid intake, profuse perspiration, diarrhea, and bleeding. Frequency and urgency may be present in gynecologic as well as urologic conditions. Hesitancy, dribbling, and nocturia can mean prostatism, pregnancy, or a host of congenital obstructive abnormalities. To complicate the situation further the nonspecific complaints of illness and symptoms referable to the other organ systems occur.

COMMON DIAGNOSTIC STUDIES

Probably the most frequently performed urologic test is urinalysis of single specimens obtained by voiding or catheterization. Occasionally it is desirable to obtain fractional specimens. When this is the case the two- or three-glass procedure is used. In the two-glass test, approximately 100 ml of urine is collected in the first container and the balance of the urine in the second. In the three-glass test, prostatic massage is performed by the doctor before the final emptying of the bladder. The purpose of these procedures is not to determine the presence or absence of a specific constituent of the urine, but to note its appearance at the time of voiding. The contents of the first bottle contain washings from the urethra; of the second, from the bladder and kidneys; of the third, from the prostate. The origin of pus formation, sediment, or bleeding can be readily pinpointed.

Hematological tests contribute greatly to evaluation of the urologic patient. Among the significant tests are the complete blood count, sedimentation rate, hematocrit, and determination of levels of specific constituents affected by kidney function. Kidney concentration and dilution tests are being done with less frequency because they are uncomfortable for many patients and are not nearly as informative as the simple phenolsulfonphthalein test. In a concentration test such as the Addis, Mosenthal, or Fishberg, the patient is brought to a certain stage of dehydration and the urine is collected to determine the kidney's ability to concentrate urine. In a dilution test the opposite effect is accomplished, the patient being required to swallow a massive quantity of fluid in a short time, and the amount excreted in a given time span being measured. The simple specific gravity test is a valuable indicator of the kindey's ability to concentrate or dilute urine.

Urea and creatinine are measured by means of clearance tests. These measure the efficiency of glomerular filtration. Samples of urine and blood are collected at intervals from a well-hydrated patient.

The manner in which laboratory tests are done varies slightly from one area to another, and the nurse should acquaint herself with the local procedure.

Cystourethroscopy

Cystourethroscopy affords direct visualization of the lower urinary tract. It is accomplished with the cystoscope, the urologist's most important tool. The procedure is done for both diagnostic and therapeutic reasons. Indications for this procedure include recurrent or persistent urinary tract infection, hematuria, dysuria, frequency, urgency, hesitancy, intermittency, and straining at voiding. Any disease or abnormality of the urinary tract that cannot be identified by more conservative means warrants cystourethroscopy. Some contraindications are general debility, acute urethritis, acute prostatitis, severe urethral stricture, acute unobstructive pyelonephritis, and uncontrolled diabetes.

Cystourethroscopy can be done on an inpatient or outpatient basis. Local anesthesia preceded by light sedation is preferable but general anesthesia is used with young children and nervous or fearful patients, and when extreme pain is anticipated. Better results are obtained if the large bowel is empty during the procedure, so laxatives and enemas may be ordered beforehand. If the patient is well hydrated either by orally administered or by intravenously administered fluids it is easier to locate the ureteral orifices. The presence of urine exuding into the bladder helps differentiate the orifices from creases in the undistended bladder.

Stated very simply, cystourethroscopy consists of passing a lubricated cystoscope through the meatus, urethra, and bladder neck, into the bladder. The bladder is distended with fluid and inspected systematically by means of a series of lenses designed to permit complete visualization. The urethra and prostatic bulges can be

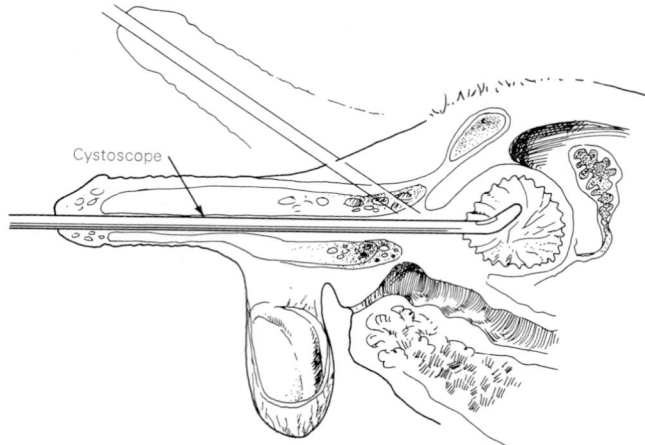

Cystoscope

Figure 24–1
Cystourethroscopy

seen upon withdrawal of the instrument or with the use of the urethroscope. The instrument allows ureteral catheters to be passed into the pelvis of the kidney for procurement of a specimen or if retrograde pyelography is indicated. Stones and foreign bodies can also be obtained. Cystourethroscopy is employed for procuring biopsy specimens.

Following cystourethroscopy the nurse's first responsibility is to ascertain the location and purpose of any catheters that may have been placed. Ureteral catheters may have been placed in the right or left kidney pelvis or in both pelves. A Foley catheter may have been placed in the bladder. Drainage may be collected individually from each catheter or into a single container. Details of catheter care are described in textbooks dealing with fundamentals of nursing.

The major complication following cystourethroscopy is perforation, especially of the bladder. Signs of perforation include sharp abdominal pain and chills and fever, followed by symptoms of peritonitis. The outpatient should be informed in a calm and reassuring manner of what to look for and what action to take in his home.

SPECIAL DIAGNOSTIC STUDIES

The most easily performed x-ray study is known as the *KUB*, or flat plate of the kidneys, ureters, and bladder. No special preparation of the patient is necessary and the study can be done quickly. The KUB generally is the first study in x-ray diagnosis. It is the least informative study and demonstrates only pathology.

Pyelography affords more definitive diagnosis. Intravenous pyelography is a means of studying the outline of the upper urinary tract. It measures the kidneys' ability to excrete an inorganic iodine compound. The dye is concentrated by both glomerular filtration and tubular secretion in varying degrees. The patient is fasted of fluid and food to assure adequate concentration of the dye. The study is greatly facilitated when the bowel is free of gas and feces. There have been instances of sensitivity to the dye and the patient should be skin-tested beforehand. Retrograde pyelography is usually done in conjunction with cystourethroscopy. The dye is injected through ureteral catheters into the pelves of the kidneys and upon with-drawal of the catheters the ureters, bladder, and urethra are outlined. Allergy to the dye is rare because the amount absorbed is negligible. However, air is some-times used as the contrast medium. Nursing care is similar to that following cysto-urethroscopy.

Several angiographic studies provide information about the kidneys. Translumbar aortography, retrograde catheter abdominal aortography, percutaneous brachial aortography, and intravenous abdominal aortography are the procedures most often utilized. The purpose of these studies is to reveal vascular lesions such as arterial occlusions, aneurysms, arteriovenous fistulas, congenital anomalies, and multiple kidneys. The studies help differentiate between cysts and tumors and demonstrate the feasibility of a contemplated surgical procedure.

In retroperitoneal contrast studies air is injected into the retroperitoneal space to afford an outline of the visceral contents. Dimensions and relationships of organs are thereby demonstrated.

In lymphangiography an iodized dye is injected into a lymphatic vessel to afford visualization of the lymphatic channels. The presence or extension of neoplastic processes is thus demonstrated. The dye may be injected into the translumbar area of the vena cava, saphenous vein, and femoral vein with the same object.

Cystometric studies measure intravesical pressure changes during filling and emptying of the bladder. A Foley catheter large enough to completely occlude the urethra is inserted into the bladder and attached to a water manometer. A reading is made of the pressure in relation to the volume of fluid injected into the bladder. The normal bladder shows no significant rise in bladder pressure while filling until the voiding contraction occurs. A flaccid bladder shows little or no increase in pressure, and a spastic bladder shows hyperactivity.

Bacteriologic studies of the urinary tract provide information about the presence and sensitivity of the resident bacteria. Occasionally bladder carcinoma can be detected by cytological methods. Cytologic methods are useful also in determining genetic sex. Needle biopsy provides material for microscopic study.

Disorders of the Kidney

Disorders which primarily affect the kidney are presented first: glomerulonephritis, uremia, acute renal failure, chronic renal insufficiency, nephrosclerosis, and the nephrotic syndrome; the surgical procedure, nephrectomy, is then described. Dis-orders that can affect any part of the urinary tract are then discussed: infections, anomalies, obstructions, diverticula, trauma, and fistulas.

GLOMERULONEPHRITIS

Glomerulonephritis is an acute, subacute, or chronic inflammatory process that predominantly affects the glomeruli. No pathogenic organisms invade the kidney; rather, it appears that the lesions are the result of an autosensitivity or autoantibody reaction against renal tissue following exposure to bacterial or chemical products. By far the commonest cause is a preceding infection of the respiratory tract; less often, of other tissue with beta-hemolytic streptococci. Pneumococcic, staphylococcic, and bacillary infections have also been followed by glomerulonephritis. A disease process, indistinguishable from glomerulonephritis, may be produced by "sensitivity" diseases, such as Rhus dermatitis and reactions to venom or chemical agents.

Pathologically, it appears that the inflammatory process first causes alterations in the glomeruli, a proliferation and swelling of the endothelial cells of the capillary tuft. This is followed by edema of the interstitial tissues and tubular epithelium. The end-effect is the obstruction of circulation through the glomerulus and degenerative changes in the tubules.

Glomerulonephritis is essentially a disease of children and young adults, the acute form being most common in children 3 to 10 years of age. It occurs twice as often in males as in females.

Adequate and early treatment of hemolytic streptococcal infections is the prime consideration in the prevention of glomerulonephritis. Treatment with penicillin should be begun on the first or second day of the streptococcal infection and should be continued until throat cultures are negative.

Acute glomerulonephritis may be very mild; in fact, there may be no reason to suspect renal involvement unless the urine is examined and evidence of glomerulonephritis found. However, in more pronounced cases, signs and symptoms appear, usually 10 days to 4 weeks after an untreated upper respiratory infection. Hypertension, edema, and urinary abnormalities are the important clinical disturbances of acute glomerulonephritis. At the time of onset the patient usually experiences headache, malaise, mild fever, and puffiness about the eyes and face. Tenderness in the costovertebral angle is common. There may be moderate tachycardia and moderate to marked elevation of blood pressure. Hematuria is usually noted as either bloody, or, if the urine is acid, as brown or coffee colored. Laboratory studies reveal hematuria and red cell casts in the urine. Proteinuria is also common, because of increased permeability of the capillary membranes. The serum albumin is decreased as a result of loss of protein in the urine. With decreased glomerular filtration and blood flow, little urine is produced and the blood urea nitrogen (BUN) and creatinine become elevated, the levels of elevation being dependent upon the severity of the lesions. The antistreptolysin titer and the sedimentation rate may be elevated, especially if streptococcal infection has been recent. In early acute glomerulonephritis, because the tubules are not yet affected, phenolsulfonphthalein (PSP) excretion is usually near normal.

In severe cases of acute glomerulonephritis, complications occur all too frequently. Severe hypertension and signs of cardiac failure may appear, with cardiac enlargement, tachycardia, gallop rhythm, pulmonary congestion, pleural fluid, and peripheral edema. Signs and symptoms of hypertensive encephalopathy may occur: severe headache, drowsiness, muscle twitchings, convulsions, vomiting, and at times papilledema and retinal hemorrhage. Any infection occurring in a patient with glomerulonephritis must be regarded as a serious complication.

Because there is no specific treatment for glomerulonephritis, the outcome for these patients is dependent upon the judicious employment of general measures. Penicillin or other suitable antibiotics should be given, to stop the antigen-antibody reaction that will go on if streptococci are present anywhere in the body. Bed rest is necessary until the disease activity subsides. One guide to duration of bed rest is the urinalysis: when protein excretion has diminished to near normal and when white and epithelial cell excretion has decreased and stabilized, activity may be resumed on a graded basis. The sedimentation rate should be near normal before unrestricted activity is allowed.

The provision of adequate nutrition for the patient presents unique and challenging problems. Water, electrolytes, and protein must be limited to quantities that can be disposed of by the poorly functioning kidney. Fluid restriction is indicated if the urine output is below normal or if the patient is gaining weight. The patient should be very carefully weighed each day. To control fluid intake, a renal shutdown regimen may be prescribed; for example, 200 ml plus the amount of the previous 8-hour output may be permitted.

The overall management of the patient often involves dealing with troublesome complications. Heart failure is treated in the usual manner, with diuretics, digitalization, oxygen, and restriction of sodium and/or fluids. Hypertensive encephalopathy has been found to respond to reserpine administered parenterally. Infection, if it occurs, should be treated vigorously with appropriate antibiotics.

Of all patients with acute glomerulonephritis, approximately 80 percent recover completely. Of the remainder, some manifest a progressive course of renal failure and die of chronic glomerulonephritis within several years; others have slowly progressive renal involvement over several decades. The importance of long-term follow-up cannot be overstressed.

The onset and development of chronic glomerulonephritis are still surrounded by much mystery. Several months to several decades after a known case of acute glomerulonephritis, the patient may be found to have chronic glomerulonephritis. Other patients develop the condition apparently *without* earlier illness or infection. It is interesting, too, that the disease may be associated with one of the collagen diseases, e.g., lupus erythematosus, periarteritis nodosa, scleroderma. These diseases can result in a picture of renal failure indistinguishable from chronic glomerulonephritis.

The clinical course varies widely from patient to patient. A patient may be asymptomatic but on examination may be found to have anemia, cardiomegaly, hypertension, or retinal hemorrhages. Such "asymptomatic" cases are often found during routine physical examinations. Other patients present with a history of extended illness that began as acute glomerulonephritis years before. Symptoms tend to be secondary to anemia (e.g., palpitations, weakness, pallor, and dyspnea on exertion) and/or to hypertension (e.g., headaches, visual disturbances, and congestive heart failure).

Serum electrophoresis will usually show decreased serum albumin. Serum electrolyte abnormalities are often present, usually low calcium, high potassium, and decreased sodium. An elevated BUN, creatinine, and uric acid are typical findings as is the anemia previously mentioned. PSP excretion is usually decreased as a result of the tubules having become involved. Although proteinuria is the rule, urinalysis findings are highly variable. Evidence of secondary infection is often seen.

Most of these patients progress to end-stage renal failure and uremia. However, with careful management, this eventual outcome may be delayed. Treatment is as described under "Chronic Renal Insufficiency."

UREMIA, ACUTE RENAL FAILURE, CHRONIC RENAL INSUFFICIENCY

Uremia

By definition, uremia is the *elevation of the blood urea above normal levels.* The term usually is broadly interpreted, however, and indicates significant elevation of nitrogenous substances in the blood with accompanying clinical signs and symptoms. These may be referable to any organ system of the body. Most commonly affected are the nervous, cardiorespiratory, and gastrointestinal systems. Uremia may be of either an acute or a chronic nature. As used here, *acute renal failure* designates the condition having rapid onset, and *chronic renal insufficiency* designates the condition resulting from chronic renal disease. In either case, the kidneys are unable to remove from the blood the constituents of normal urine within the proper time. These constituents, then, accumulate in the blood and are instrumental in producing systemic signs and symptoms.

Acute Renal Failure

Acute renal failure is characterized by a rapid loss of renal excretory function. Urinary output is abruptly reduced. If the patient excretes no urine, he is said to be anuric. Oliguria designates a diminution in output.

Various mechanisms and agents are capable of causing acute renal failure. Any situation that reduces blood flow to the kidney produces ischemia, decreases glomerular filtration, and ultimately damages tubular epithelium. The decrease in blood flow may be due to an obstructing abnormality of the renal artery. It may be the result of decreased cardiac output from any source (e.g., shock, hemorrhage, myocardial infarction). Severe water and electrolyte depletion is also capable of producing a picture of renal failure, as are renal diseases such as glomerulonephritis which damage the vasculature. Among other possible causes of acute renal failure, one must list damage by nephrotoxins such as carbon tetrachloride and effects of postglomerular obstruction. The postglomerular obstruction may occur within the tubular lumen as a result of deposition of hemoglobin following incompatible blood transfusion, or of myoglobin following crushing injuries. Postglomerular obstruction is sometimes due to obstruction of the ureters or to obstruction of the urethra (see section on "Obstruction").

It is frequently possible to reduce the occurrence of renal failure by guarding against exposure to harmful agents and by carefully and constantly observing any patient with a history of any of the previously listed conditions. As soon as oliguria is noted, in order to prevent tubular necrosis, immediate treatment of the cause of oliguria is essential. In shock, for example, measures must be taken to restore normal blood pressure levels to overcome renal ischemia.

Although acute renal failure may be the end-result of many different mechanisms, the common factor in all is the impairment of blood supply to the renal tubule. Renal tubular necrosis is the characteristic finding. With severe damage, a back-diffusion of the glomerular filtrate into the tubular cells and vasculature occurs and gives the net effect of an increased tubular reabsorption with little water and waste products being excreted but rather accumulating in the blood.

Recognition of acute renal failure depends upon alertness to decreased output.

During the first few days, a decreased urinary output may be the only sign of serious renal impairment, i.e., less than 400 to 500 ml in 24 hours. The patient may then begin to complain of lumbar aching or of burning about the bladder. There may be puffiness about the eyes, and his blood pressure may be slightly above normal. Gradually other systemic signs and symptoms appear: malaise, nausea, hiccough, muscular twitching, pallor, stupor, convulsions, and sometimes pericarditis.

The rapidity of the development of this picture varies greatly. The rate of catabolism of protein, both endogenous and exogenous, determines the rate of increase of nitrogenous metabolites in body fluids. In the presence of trauma or of fever, the serum BUN, creatinine, potassium, phosphate, sulfate, and organic acids increase rapidly. The serum sodium and chloride tend to fall. Potassium intoxication, a dreaded complication, may appear at any time. When the serum potassium exceeds 7 to 8 mEq per liter characteristic electrocardiographic (EKG) changes begin to appear. Bradycardia and arrhythmias may appear and finally ventricular tachycardia or fibrillation. Cardiac failure may be the terminal event. Flaccid muscular paralysis may occur when the serum potassium reaches 8 to 12 mEq per liter.

The early, or oliguric, phase of acute renal failure had just been described. The later, or diuretic, phase usually begins during the second week after the renal injury—if the patient survives. At this time, tubule cells begin to regenerate and the volume of urine increases daily. When the daily output exceeds 1 liter for several days, clinical improvement is noted. During diuresis, because of persistent deficiencies in tubular function, large quantities of fluid and electrolytes are excreted, and abnormalities in hydration and in concentration of serum electrolytes may occur. These may cause disturbances of cardiac action, peripheral circulation, cerebral function, or neuromuscular conduction.

Survival of the patient in renal failure is at all times dependent upon maintaining homeostasis until healing occurs. This involves precise management of fluid and caloric needs and of electrolyte balance, reduction of tissue catabolism to the minimum, treatment of coexistent disease, and the prevention of infection.

During the oliguric phase bed rest is indicated. The painstaking regulation of fluids and electrolytes is of utmost importance. Precise records of intake and output are vital; these may be kept on an hour-to-hour basis. A catheter may be required for accuracy. Losses through diarrhea, vomiting, and any other mechanism must also be noted. Pains should be taken to obtain a correct daily weight. Because the patient is consuming his own tissues, he may lose as much as 0.5 kg per day. If he fails to lose, he is receiving too much fluid. A shutdown regimen may be instituted, allowing only for insensible loss plus output, for example 200 ml plus the amount of the previous 8-hour output. Daily measurements of serum electrolytes and electrolytes excreted in the urine and careful observation for signs of electrolyte excesses or deficiences help in regulating electrolytes. Providing adequate nutrition is often a problem. Sodium is often restricted as are foods that have a high potassium content. Protein intake is usually limited. To further reduce protein catabolism and to prevent ketosis, high-carbohydrate foods are favored. If the patient is unable to take food orally, the intravenous administration of glucose is necessary, with attention being paid to the exact amount of fluid given.

Every possible precaution should be taken to guard the patient against infection.

Some authorities recommend that these patients be placed in reverse isolation as a safety measure. If infection does develop, it should be treated promptly with appropriate antibiotics. With these agents, as with any other drugs administered to these patients, it must always be remembered that the excretory ability of the kidney is impaired and therefore toxic reactions to drugs may occur much more readily than in patients with normal kidneys.

It is sometimes necessary to treat the patient for anemia, congestive heart failure, or for convulsions and encephalopathy. Therapy must observe certain considerations; in treating anemia, for example, the patient is usually given packed red cells to prevent fluid overloading. In treating encephalopathy and convulsions, paraldehyde, chlorpromazine, or some of the barbiturates may be used. Barbiturates should be restricted to pentobarbital sodium or amobarbital sodium, both of which are metabolized by the liver.

The care of the patient during the diuretic phase is in many respects the same as that just outlined for the oliguric phase. The patient's ability to take food and fluids orally usually improves and a high-caloric, low-protein diet is given. Careful recording of intake and output must be continued because of the large quantities of fluids and electrolytes lost and the possibility of imbalances occurring. Twenty-four hour urine specimens for electrolyte analysis may be requested as well as daily serum electrolytes. Daily weights are continued also. Infection continues to be a threat.

The patient suffering from acute renal failure may undergo spontaneous healing within 2 to 6 weeks, if severe complications of trauma and infection are not present. Skillful care will often tide the patient over this crucial period. Care includes being heedful of the threat of complications such as water intoxication, congestive heart failure, acute pulmonary edema, encephalopathy, or potassium intoxication. Any one of these is capable of causing the death of the patient. (The treatment of potassium intoxication and dialysis is discussed under "Chronic Renal Insufficiency.")

Complete recovery of the patient may seemingly take a long time. Concentrating power and excretory capacity may not return to a normal range for 3 to 6 months. Good general care and reasonable restriction of activity are advisable during this time.

Chronic Renal Insufficiency

Chronic renal insufficiency means that the patient has chronic disease of the kidneys. He may be in either a compensated stage or a decompensated stage. The compensated stage may last for years with the composition of the body fluids remaining essentially normal, even though some separate renal function, such as glomerular filtration, may not be up to normal standards. In the decompensated stage, renal function is more severely impaired and body fluids become abnormal in composition as a result. This stage tends to be progressive, leading sooner or later to death.

The possibilities of preventing chronic renal disease should always be borne in mind. This can often be accomplished with proper attention to the causes of early kidney disease, the prompt treatment of infections and obstructions, for example.

Chronic pyelonephritis, nephrosclerosis, and chronic glomerulonephritis are among the common types of chronic renal disease. Less frequently chronic renal disease is due to diabetic nephropathy, collagen disease, obstructive uropathy, amyloidosis, or polycystic renal disease.

Pathological findings in chronic renal disease vary with the cause of damage to the kidney, but extensive scarring, hyalinization of glomeruli, and tubular and vascular changes are commonly seen.

Clinically it is often impossible to distinguish between renal insufficiency due to chronic glomerulonephritis and/or other causes. However, chronic renal insufficiency presents symptoms and signs related to the functional disability rather than to the *cause* of the renal damage. This is an important concept because treatment therefore is essentially of a nonspecific supportive kind.

Patients with decompensated renal disease sooner or later manifest fairly characteristic symptoms. These symptoms are generally attributed to the retention of nitrogenous metabolites, but other factors that help create the clinical picture must be considered also. These factors may include hypertension, malnutrition, anemia, acidosis, and water and electrolyte imbalances. Various combinations of these factors produce signs and symptoms referable to any organ system of the body, most commonly the nervous, cardiorespiratory, and gastrointestinal systems.

Many of these patients have anemia, are pale, and suffer from exertional dyspnea, tachycardia, and lethargy. The anemia is generally attributed to hemolytic factors and to decreased erythropoeitin. Hypertension is almost universally found and may cause headache, visual disturbances, congestive heart failure, and convulsions. Many patients are edematous; the edema may be minimal, perhaps confined to the periorbital region, or gross anasarca may be present. Bleeding tendencies are very common. The patient may have only increased bruisability, or he may have frank bleeding from even minor trauma, such as that incurred when brushing his teeth. Nearly all these patients eventually experience a bleeding problem. It is believed to be the result of an antiplatelet factor.

Nausea and vomiting, ulcers of the buccal mucosa, and a foul taste in the mouth cause anorexia and weight loss. These gastrointestinal symptoms are thought to be due to a high ammonia content in body fluids. Gastrointestinal pain, indigestion, and diarrhea may occur. There may be frank bleeding due to uremic gastritis. It is postulated that ammonia may actually be secreted through the bowel wall. In some patients, urea crystallizes out of the sweat and is seen on the skin as uremic frost, a white powdery material. Intense pruritus causing self-excoriation is common.

Urinary symptoms vary widely. The patient may have increased or decreased volume or complete shutdown. The specific gravity is usually low and fixed with mild to moderate proteinuria and few red and white cells. Blood chemistries show elevated levels of BUN, creatinine, and uric acid. Serum albumin is decreased. Secondary infections are common, to a great extent because of the decreased serum protein.

Neuromuscular phenomena, i.e., muscle twitching, irritability, and convulsion, are not uncommon and derive, at least in part, from electrolyte abnormalities such as acidosis, decreased calcium, and increased potassium. Electrolyte disorders, potassium particularly, may also produce EKG changes. Because of an imbalance in calcium and phosphorous metabolism, some patients tend to lose calcium, and x-ray studies then reveal demineralization of bone–renal rickets.

The prognosis in patients with chronic renal insufficiency is variable. It is primarily dependent upon the degree of renal failure present, but many unpredictable individual variations in the course of the illness occur. Also, since World War II, it has become possible to prolong life in what was formerly a hopeless situation. Intensive study of the problems really began at that time, and more about the physiology and management of renal insufficiency is constantly being learned.

As previously stated, because chronic renal insufficiency presents signs and symptoms related to the functional disability rather than to the cause of the renal damage, treatment is essentially of a nonspecific nature. Treatment is aimed first at decreasing the load of metabolites which the kidney must excrete. To accomplish this the patient is given a diet that is rich in calories but low in protein, and he is guarded against physical and mental stresses. The second general aim of treatment is the correction of the abnormal body chemistry. This involves careful regulation of fluids and electrolytes and facilities for treating severe disorders such as hyperkalemia, with medical measures and by dialysis, when necessary.

To outline treatment more specifically: it should include, among many considerations, the provision of adequate nutrition. Protein is usually restricted, perhaps to 2 to 30 g per day, to minimize the accumulation of nitrogenous waste products. Because calories act as protein sparers, high-carbohydrate foods are usually given.

Meticulous attention must be paid to ensuring proper hydration of the patient. Fluids are generally given freely unless oliguria, edema, or congestive heart failure is present. When such problems are present, the shutdown fluid regimen may be necessary. As previously described, such a regimen allows only for insensible loss plus output. This necessitates precise recording of all intake and output. A daily weight is also one of the best guides for fluid regulation.

The correction of electrolyte imbalances is often a matter of urgency. Several measures have been found to be useful in alleviating hyperkalemia (elevated serum potassium); glucose and insulin may be administered intravenously (insulin in the presence of glucose causes potassium to leave the serum and enter the cells). Such a shift in potassium also occurs when acidosis is corrected with soda bicarbonate. Most of these patients are acidotic. When acidosis is corrected, the patient must be observed carefully for tetany, which may occur at that time if serum calcium is low. Ion exchange resins are sometimes used for relieving hyperkalemia. They bind potassium in the bowel so that it can be excreted in the stool. This is a slow process, however, requiring about 12 hours. Also, patients often find the resins difficult to take.

Another electrolyte abnormality, low serum calcium, which may cause tetany and convulsions, responds to calcium chloride or calcium gluconate.

The final outcome for the patient with chronic renal disease is often dependent upon the control of accompanying disorders. Severe anemia must be treated with transfusions; bleeding difficulties usually require whole blood or fresh frozen plasma. Complications arising in patients with renal insufficiency often present unique and perplexing problems. A seemingly minor infection can rapidly assume vast proportions; in patients receiving digitalis for heart failure arrhythmias are likely to develop if hypokalemia occurs; and the lowering of a dangerously elevated blood pressure in the hypertensive patient may result in a decreased glomerular filtration rate and further loss of renal function.

It is quite impossible to predict which patients will experience particular complications and equally difficult to forecast exactly how they will respond to treatment. Therefore the importance of intelligent observation, together with knowledgeable interpretation, cannot be overemphasized.

When the patient's condition deteriorates in spite of conservative medical measures, or when severe fluid and electrolyte problems develop, dialysis is indicated. This may be accomplished by hemodialysis with the artificial kidney or, if a simpler procedure must be employed, by peritoneal dialysis.

Hemodialysis. The accumulation of toxic substances in the body may ultimately result in the patient's death. These substances may accumulate as a consequence of the ingestion of such harmful agents as excessive barbiturates or poisons, or as the result of faulty body processes, of impaired kidney function particularly. In any case, their efficient removal is imperative. To accomplish this feat, various methods of dialysis have been found to be effective. *Dialysis* is the passage of molecules through a semipermeable membrane placed between two solutions. A substance passes from the solution where its concentration is greater into the solution of its lesser concentration. In the artificial kidney, a length of tubing, part of which is coiled in a bath of dialyzing solution, constantly removes blood from one to the patient's arteries and returns it through a vein. While the blood is passing through the section of tubing (made of cellophane) that is submerged in the bath, any substance that is excessive in the blood, potassium perhaps, moves through the pores of the cellophane membrane out into the dialyzing solution. Protein molecules are too large to make this transfer and therefore serum protein is not affected. Time required for the treatment averages about 6 hours.

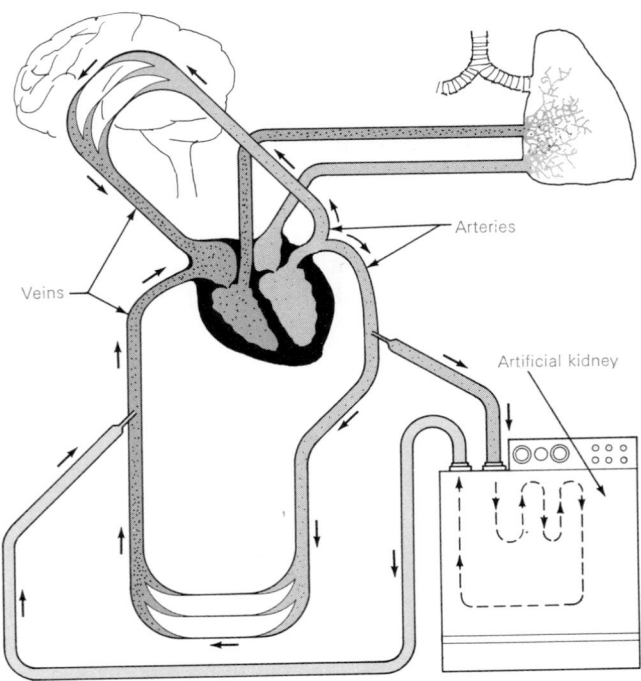

Figure 24–2
Hemodialysis

The treatment, though simple in principle, is complex in its execution. It requires a highly trained team of doctors, nurses, and laboratory technicians. The nurse who is responsible for the care of the patient must be sensitive to the effect that the total treatment has upon the patient and she must be cognizant of unique complications that may arise at any time. Such complications may be related to abrupt changes in blood pressure, arrhythmias, changes in sensorium, and bleeding difficulties.

Peritoneal Dialysis. Although hemodialysis, as accomplished by the artificial kidney, is generally acclaimed to be the most efficient means of dialysis, the complexity of that procedure may preclude its being used in some situations. Peritoneal dialysis, a comparatively simple procedure, is often employed at such times. The principle involved is the same, i.e., the establishment of equilibrium across a membrane, in this case the peritoneum. To illustrate: if potassium is high in the interstitial fluid and a solution containing no potassium is put into the peritoneal cavity, potassium will move from the patient's interstitial fluid into the solution. After 60 to 90 minutes, the solution is drained off. This process takes about 36 hours.

The careful preparation, observation, and support of the patient are largely nursing functions. It is paramount that strict adherence to principles of aseptic technique be maintained, since the procedure carries some risk of infections, the most dreaded of which is peritonitis.

Renal Transplantation. The place of renal transplantation in the treatment of terminal renal disease is not yet clear. The matter is currently receiving a great deal of experimental and clinical attention. The crucial problem is an immunologic one—how to prevent rejection and destruction of the grafted kidney. Current methods of inhibiting the rejection process tend to cause marrow depression and a general impairment of the immune response, rendering the patient more susceptible to infection. In addition to the patient's increased susceptibility to infection, the management of water and electrolyte balance and the use of antibiotic therapy present perplexing problems. The use of antibiotics may foster the development of resistant organisms and the proliferation of fungi. Other problems are related to the unprecedented ethical considerations involved. When is the removal of an organ from a healthy person justified?

At the present time one must say that the employment of renal homografts is essentially in the experimental stage; but the future is not without hope. It would seem likely that as the biological factors of rejection become more clearly understood more satisfactory agents for inhibiting the rejection process will become available.

ARTERIOLAR NEPHROSCLEROSIS

Arteriolar nephrosclerosis is a condition wherein blood vessels of the renal area are affected by hypertensive vascular disease. The result is impaired renal function and the development of signs and symptoms identical to those which characterize chronic glomerulonephritis.

Nephrosclerosis affects the afferent arteriole of the glomeruli primarily. The intima becomes thickened, and this intimal thickening causes severe narrowing or even obliteration of the arteriole, depriving the nephron of its blood supply and producing areas of infarction and scarring. This process eventually leads to renal insufficiency.

Nephrosclerosis may be of a benign nature; that is, for a long period of months or even years, renal function remains adequate. Sooner or later, however, the dreaded picture of chronic renal insufficiency appears. Disturbances in renal function then occur. There may be loss of ability to concentrate, depression of urea clearance and excretion of PSP, and retention of end-products of nitrogen metabolism. Urinary abnormalities including proteinuria, red cells, and cylindruria are marked. Anemia is often found. Eye ground changes and severe headache are present. Signs of cardiac insufficiency may be dominant, i.e., hypertrophy, congestive heart failure, and pulmonary edema.

Because there is no specific therapy for nephrosclerosis, treatment is centered upon the management of hypertension and of chronic kidney disease, both of which are discussed elsewhere.

It is difficult to forecast the outcome for any given patient, but the course is a progressively downhill one. The disease may progress gradually or rapidly. It may change in nature from benign to malignant. Patients eventually die in renal failure unless cardiac insufficiency or cerebral hemorrhage intervenes.

THE NEPHROTIC SYNDROME (NEPHROSIS)

The nephrotic syndrome is a renal functional defect resulting from injury to the glomerulus, causing it to become more permeable to plasma proteins. Cardinal manifestations of the nephrotic syndrome are massive edema, profuse proteinuria, hypoalbuminemia, and hyperlipemia.

Present evidence indicates that this syndrome is the result of diseases that affect the glomerulus, e.g., glomerulonephritis, or of diseases that affect the blood vessels, e.g., syphilis, the collagen diseases, or diabetic nephropathy. The nephrotic syndrome is occasionally associated with allergic reactions to drugs, e.g., nitrogen mustard, penicillin, and 6-mercaptopurine, or to toxins such as bee venom. In children, nephrosis appears to occur without clear proof of any cause.

Regardless of the patient's history, however, biopsy and autopsy studies show a fatty degeneration of tubule epithelium.

The chief symptom of the nephrotic syndrome is edema. It may appear insidiously and increase slowly or suddenly and increase rapidly. Pallor is usually marked, and striae may appear in the stretched skin of the extremities. As fluid accumulates in the serous cavities of the chest and abdomen, anorexia and shortness of breath develop. Hypertension, with changes in the retina and retinal vessels, is common, particularly with collagen disease, diabetes mellitus, or renal insufficiency. Laboratory studies show anemia due to anorexia or renal damage, and decreased plasma protein, especially albumin. The plasma is lipemic. Serum electrolytes may be unaffected or may reflect renal insufficiency. With impaired renal function, the BUN is elevated. The urine tends to be decreased in volume and to contain large amounts of protein and casts.

There is no specific treatment for the nephrotic syndrome, except in those cases caused by syphilis. In such cases penicillin is of great benefit. Otherwise treatment is nonspecific and is aimed at the relief of symptoms and the prevention of complications such as infection. Bed rest is advisable when edema is severe or when infection is present, and suitable antibiotics are in order. Steroid therapy has been found to be helpful in many cases of the nephrotic syndrome in children, and in adults, in some cases due to glomerulonephritis, collagen disease, or idiosyncrasy to toxin or venom. Treatment with steroids may be continued intermittently for a year. Diuretics may be used. Of these diuretic agents the chlorothiazide derivatives appear to be quite effective. Ethacrynic acid and fursemide (Lasix) are two of the more effective newer drugs. A nutritious diet, adequate in calories and normal in protein, should be encouraged. Sodium restriction, usually to 0.5 to 1 g daily, may be indicated. Oncotic agents, such as salt-free albumin, and dextran may be administered but the effects are transient. Planning and care should include stressing the need for follow-up visits to the physician or clinic.

The ultimate fate of the patient with the nephrotic syndrome is determined mainly by the nature of the underlying disease. Generally, adults fare less well than children because the underlying disease is apt to be of an irreversible nature. Remissions may be induced but the presence of hypertension and nitrogen retention are serious signs. In about half the children, the disease runs a rather benign course and leaves insignificant sequelae. Of the others, most are cases of glomerulonephritis which go on to terminal renal failure.

NEPHRECTOMY

Nephrectomy is the removal of a kidney, but the term has come to encompass both total and partial procedures. With conservation of renal tissue as the therapeutic aim, it can be readily understood that the excision of an offending upper or lower pole is preferable to the sacrifice of the entire kidney. Partial procedures are done in cases of nephrocalcinosis, renal tuberculosis, trauma, and renal calculi. Total removal of a kidney is indicated when there is carcinoma, hydronephrosis with marked renal destruction, perinephritis, perinephric extravasation of urine, multicystic disease, advanced unilateral renal tuberculosis, extensive renal infarction, or severe trauma. Some of the indications call for either a total or partial procedure depending upon the degree of disease involvement.

In the preoperative period the aim of the health team is twofold: the establishment of the diagnosis and the mental and physical preparation of the patient for surgery. The diagnosis is confirmed by evaluating the combined results of the history, physical examination, urinalysis, complete blood count, blood urea nitrogen, phenolsulfonphthalein excretion, hematocrit, roentgenologic study of the kidneys, ureters, and bladder, pyelography, and cystoscopy. The more sophisticated diagnostic techniques are used when the diagnosis is too elusive to be detected by ordinary means. At the same time the function of the contralateral kidney is being evaluated. If it cannot be shown that the remaining kidney is capable of sustaining life, the prospect of surgery is abandoned. Throughout this period of testing the patient should be informed as he is capable of comprehending. When his enlightened cooperation is elicited, maximum results can be achieved with a minimum of distress or discomfort to him.

Partial or total nephrectomy is usually done under general anesthesia. With the patient lying in the nephrectomy position, an incision is made in the vicinity of the twelfth rib. The pleura occasionally extends this low and may accidentally be incised. When this occurs it may be necessary to insert chest tubes for control of pneumothorax. The kidney is dissected away from its adjacent structures and the pedicle is exposed. The blood vessels and ureter are ligated and severed. The organ mass is removed and the wound is closed without drainage except in extraordinary circumstances such as the presence of exudate in the retroperitoneal space. When the partial procedure is done, the structures in the renal pedicle are identified so that the renal artery can be located and temporarily occluded to control hemorrhage until adequate hemostasis is obtained. Suturing of the kidney is difficult because of its vascularity and friability. Oozing is a frequent occurrence and for this reason either a Penrose drain or a nephrostomy tube is utilized to remove blood, urine, or any other fluids accumulating in the wound. Finally, the anatomical layers are reapproximated with sutures and a dressing is put in place.

In addition to routine postoperative nursing care as described elsewhere, special attention is directed to the needs of the patient with a flank incision. The location of the incision immediately beneath the ribs deters the patient from responding enthusiastically to the nurse's suggestion to cough or breathe deeply, and less direct procedures such as splinting the wound should be employed. If these are successfully managed, atelectasis and pneumonia can be prevented. At the same time the nurse should observe for signs of pneumothorax which may have developed from a small nick in the pleura that was not detected during surgery. These patients are susceptible to abdominal disturbances. A nasogastric tube is frequently passed preoperatively to either prevent or treat distention and paralytic ileus. The use of a rectal tube with or without neostigmine (Prostigmin) may be ordered to control moderate distention. Patients who have had a partial nephrectomy or a procedure other than total removal of a kidney are highly susceptible to hemorrhage because of the nature of the tissue involved. Careful evaluation of the contents of drainage bottles, dressings, bed linen, and vital signs is necessary for differentiating between harmless oozing and dangerous bleeding. Throughout the recovery period the nurse should be alert for signs of acute renal failure which may occur during the immediate postoperative period or may be delayed. Prior to discharge the patient is instructed in the medical regimen that is established to meet his particular needs. One very important point that should be emphasized is the need for periodic examinations for several years following all surgical procedures other than total nephrectomy. After a period of time has elapsed, pyelonephritis or hydronephrosis may develop or calculi may form in the kidney remnant. Ureteral stricture and urinary fistulas can also develop.

Infections of the Urinary Tract

Bacteria may reach the urinary tract through hematogenous or lymphogenous dissemination or through direct extension from one portion of the urogenital system to another. The majority of urinary tract infections are ascending in nature, traveling upward from the urethra and bladder. These infections generally are associated with gram-negative organisms, particularly *E. coli.* Factors contributing to the likelihood of infection are obstruction, stasis, and lowered general body resistance.

Treatment is determined by the type, source, and site of the infection, and by the character of associated problems.

Numerous factors predispose individuals to kidney infections, including obstructions, instrumentation, and metabolic disorders such as diabetes mellitus. The dehydrated person is quite likely to experience urinary infections, because the scanty, concentrated urine has an irritating effect upon the bladder mucosa. This is especially likely to occur in an individual who has had previous episodes of infection.

Infections tend to occur more frequently in the female than in the male, except that prostatism and the resulting obstruction render older males equally susceptible. The shorter urethra of the female may account in some measure for the higher incidence of infection. Many of the causative organisms are flagellates that are propelled through the urethra into the bladder. Kidney infections are not infrequent during pregnancy, probably because there is some degree of obstruction of the ureters and kidney pelves by the fetus. Hormonal factors also seem to play a part during pregnancy. Early in marriage, infections are quite common in the female, perhaps because new bacteria are introduced during intercourse.

PYELONEPHRITIS

Pyelonephritis may be associated with serious renal impairment. It is therefore extremely important that predisposing factors receive careful attention.

Pyelonephritis is an acute or a chronic infection in which there is invasion of the kidney by pathogenic bacteria. Chief among them is S. *aureus*. The bacteria may be carried by the bloodstream from distant sources (boils, for example). The renal cortex is usually involved.

Diagnosis of Acute and Chronic Pyelonephritis

In acute pyelonephritis, microscopic examination shows acute inflammatory changes with areas of swelling, necrosis, and suppuration in the papillae and pyramids of the medulla. The interstitial tissues also are seen to be affected. In the chronic stage, areas of scar formation as well as patches of acute inflammation are seen. With extensive destruction of kidney tissue, uremia ensues.

In a "typical" attack of acute pyelonephritis, the onset may be sudden or may follow a few days of malaise characterized by chills, temperature of 104 or 105° F, headache, prostration, flank or back pain, and leukocytosis of 20,000 per cu mm or higher. Constitutional symptoms such as tachycardia, headache, nausea and vomiting, dehydration, and abdominal pain may be present. The patient may give a history of preceding "cystitis." Symptoms vary, however, and there may be no manifestations other than albuminuria and pyuria with some frequency or burning on micturition. Renal infection should be suspected when any patient has unexplained fever, chills, malaise, or bladder symptoms such as frequency, burning, and dysuria. Pus and bacteria in an uncontaminated specimen of urine are evidence of possible renal infection.

The onset of chronic pyelonephritis is usually insidious. The patient may be symptomatic or asymptomatic. He may or may not have a history of recurrent urinary tract infections such as cystitis. Urinary frequency and nocturia may be present. Lassitude, headache, or other symptoms related to the presence of anemia or hypertension are not uncommon. Unfortunately, however, symptoms may be so mild that the disease escapes recognition until the terminal stages.

In acute pyelonephritis, laboratory studies reveal leukocytosis and characteristic urinary findings (e.g., large numbers of bacteria—100,000 per ml or more—pyuria, proteinuria, hematuria, and white cell casts particularly). The BUN, creatinine, and intravenous pyelogram (IVP) may or may not show changes. PSP excretion is usually normal.

In chronic pyelonephritis, in addition to bacteriuria, laboratory studies may indicate some degree of renal damage and diminished function. The BUN and creatinine are more likely to be elevated and anemia may be present. The IVP may show small shrunken kidneys or hydronephrosis, if obstruction is present. Urea, creatinine clearance, and PSP excretion are usually decreased.

Treatment of Acute and Chronic Pyelonephritis

The treatment of acute pyelonephritis is aimed at eradicating the infection, relieving pain and other symptoms, conserving the patient's own restorative powers, and finding and correcting any underlying problem, for example, obstruction.

Bed rest is advisable during the acute stage, until the temperature has been normal for 24 hours. A soft diet is usually given. A liberal fluid intake of 3,000 to 4,000 ml daily is of prime importance, to ensure adequate urinary output. The type of organism found to be present determines antibiotic therapy. Usually one of the broad-spectrum antibiotics is required: tetracycline, ampicillin, or a specific agent such as colymycin or kanamycin sulfate, which are active against certain of the gram-negative organisms. Since the infection is in the tissues and not in the lumen of the urinary passages, it is necessary to maintain a high blood level of the drug. The level of concentration in the urine is of less importance. An antipyretic such as salicylamide may be prescribed for fever, and analgesics such as aspirin and codeine for the relief of backache. Pyridium may relieve bladder discomfort.

When obstruction or other underlying difficulty is suspected, procedures such as cystoscopy are frequently necessary for diagnosis and treatment. The patient should be carefully prepared, physically and mentally, and should be given support during the procedure.

Approximately 90 percent of all first attacks of acute pyelonephritis respond to treatment, if no underlying urinary tract problem is present. In the presence of obstruction, stone, or diabetes, infection will persist until such factors are corrected.

It is sometimes difficult to be certain that complete recovery has occurred. When pyelonephritis recurs, it may be impossible to say whether it is due to a new infection or to residual infection from an incompletely healed first attack. Follow-up care is extremely important to ascertain that treatment has been adequate and to prevent further renal damage. At this time agents that suppress bacterial growth are frequently prescribed. Such agents include cranberry juice or ascorbic acid to acidify urine, nitrofurantoin (Furadantin), sulfisoxazole (Gantrisin), and nalidixic acid (NegGram).

In the treatment of chronic pyelonephritis, as in the acute condition, infection must be treated, an adequate urinary output must be ensured with good hydration, and underlying problems must be corrected. In addition to these measures, treatment of symptoms such as hypertension and anemia will probably be necessary. Also, if the BUN is elevated, protein must be restricted in the diet.

The course of chronic pyelonephritis may extend over many years, but with wise management the patient may lead a reasonably comfortable life, even when renal reserve is limited. (See "Chronic Renal Insufficiency" for further discussion of the treatment of chronic renal disease.)

TUBERCULOSIS OF THE URINARY TRACT

Nearly all instances of genitourinary tuberculosis are secondary to pulmonary infection. The bacilli are carried to the urogenital system by the bloodstream. If this event occurs in connection with a primary focus in the lung which heals promptly, the patient may never actually suffer from pulmonary tuberculosis. Tuberculosis of the urinary tract occurs most frequently in persons 20 to 40 years of age and is two to four times as common in males as in females.

The kidney is affected more frequently than any other part of the urogenital system, probably because of the great and constant flow of blood through it. The infection if untreated tends to progress in a descending fashion from the kidney to the ureters and bladder. Involvement of the ureters and bladder, with ulceration and scarring, may eventually produce varying degrees of hydronephrosis. Symptoms of urinary tract tuberculosis are not characteristic or specific. Manifestations of chronic infection with malaise, fever, fatigability, and night sweats may be present. Early symptoms are usually those of any bladder infection, including burning on urination, frequency, and nocturia. Painless hematuria, either microscopic or gross, is commonly the first sign. Pyuria, too, frequently occurs. Secondary infections of the bladder are common and may cause the tuberculosis to be overlooked—with dire results. Tuberculosis should be suspected in every case of chronic cystitis or pyuria. The diagnosis is made when acid-fast bacilli are found in urine, tissue, or discharges.

Treatment of urinary tract tuberculosis must include a search for tuberculosis elsewhere in the body and above all must consider the whole patient. Several months of hospitalization is generally advisable for all patients with tuberculosis, to ensure adequate rest, good nutrition, and good hygiene. Medical treatment also includes chemotherapy with antituberculosis drugs such as para-aminosalicylic acid (PAS), isoniazid (INH), and streptomycin. When renal infection is severe and unilateral, or if bleeding occurs, nephrectomy may be combined with medical treatment. A program of drug administration and supportive therapy is indicated preoperatively and is continued for a year or more after surgery.

The prognosis is dependent upon the extent of renal involvement and damage to renal function. Healing has been satisfactory in patients who have received early treatment. Antimicrobial therapy has improved the outlook considerably.

For all these patients yearly check-ups are important for an indefinite period. Patients should be instructed to continue a program of adequate rest and good nutrition, and should be cautioned to avoid overexposure.

CYSTITIS

Cystitis is an inflammation of the bladder mucosa which is often secondary to an infection or obstruction elsewhere in the urinary tract. It may be acute or chronic, and occurs more frequently in women than men as a primary condition. It is thought that this is because women have a shorter urethra than men and ascending infection seems to be more common.

Acute cystitis may be caused by any of a number of factors: ascent of bacteria up the urethra; development following intercourse; association with renal infection; spread from an infected cervix; or secondary infection to inflammation of the kidney or prostate or the presence of residual urine from bladder neck obstruction or a neurogenic bladder.

The clinical findings include a predominance of urinary complaints: burning on urination, urgency, frequency, nocturia, and sometimes hematuria. Low-grade fever, mild low backache, or suprapubic discomfort may be present. In men the signs of prostatitis may also be present, and women may have urethritis, vaginitis, or a cystocele with residual urine. The white blood count may be elevated; urine will usually show pus and bacteria and occasionally red blood cells. Renal function remains unaffected.

Treatment includes locating and eliminating the infection and correcting the contributing factors. More specifically, the use of antibiotics and chemotherapy is indicated to sterilize the urine. General measures of treatment and nursing care are the same as for the patient with an upper urinary tract infection. In addition they may include sedating the irritable bladder by alkalinizing the urine with use of sodium bicarbonate and fruit juices, antispasmodics, and bladder sedatives, hot sitz baths for relief of severe pain and spasms, forced fluids, and bed rest if there is fever or other systemic infection present.

Although the bladder mucosa may be diffusely reddened and edematous, the infected bladder will tend to heal spontaneously unless constantly insulted. With modern therapy the acute infection usually resolves without causing structural or functional injury. If the infection recurs, the underlying cause must be determined.

Chronic cystitis is often secondary to chronic infection of the upper urinary tract, to residual urine, ureteral reflux, urethral or bladder neck stenosis, or to incomplete treatment of simple acute cystitis.

Clinical findings may include no symptoms or those of mild bladder irritability, renal tenderness or enlargement, a distended bladder, or a chronically inflamed urethra. The blood count is not remarkable and few or no pus cells are found in the urine, although bacteria may be present. Renal function tests are normal. Uncomplicated chronic cystitis will show no abnormality on an excretory urogram, but the passage of a large catheter may reveal a stricture or residual urine, either of which can contribute to infection. Cystoscopy will reveal the degree of obstruction, bladder neck contracture, or the presence of a foreign body. Chronic cystitis needs to be differentiated from other chronic infections such as chronic prostatitis, chronic pyelonephritis, tuberculosis of the urinary tract, interstitial cystitis, irradiation cystitis, and senile urethritis in women.

The aim of therapy is to eradicate the cause of the infection, and specific measures include identifying the offending bacteria and administering antibiotic therapy, which often must be intensive and prolonged. Renal infection may occur if drug therapy fails to eradicate the cause of the infection. Treatment will be unsuccessful unless conditions causing the infection are determined and corrected. Other treatment and nursing care measures include those for acute cystitis, although the bladder is not as irritable.

Chronic interstitial cystitis, also called *submucous fibrosis* or *Hunner's* ulcer, occurs primarily in elderly women; the chief complaints are increasing frequency, urgency, and suprapubic pain on postponement of urination. The bladder capacity is reduced and the patient has increasing pain as the bladder fills, and relief while the bladder is empty. Urinalysis frequently is normal. Diagnosis is established at cystoscopic inspection. The cause is unknown and the condition is uncommon in women and rare in men. (For further discussion see a specialized textbook.)

NONSPECIFIC URETHRITIS

Nonspecific urethritis is an inflammation of the urethra occurring in either sex and at any age. Any trauma to the urethral mucosa makes the area susceptible to bacterial attack; the causative organisms include the staphylococcus, the streptococcus, *Escherichia coli,* and Pseudomonas. Signs and symptoms include burning on urination, itching, soreness, and a urethral discharge. The cause is obscure and the condition is difficult to eliminate. It may become a chronic problem. In men it may result in chronic prostatitis.

Treatment and nursing measures include the use of antibiotics or chemotherapy, hot sitz baths, increased fluid intake, physical rest, decreased sexual activity, and dilatation of the urethra, if necessary, to open the ducts of the periurethral glands. Opening of the ducts followed by instillation of a mild antiseptic such as 1:10,000 silver nitrate solution may be necessary to eradicate an obstinate infection, but this should be done gently and should not be done during the acute phase of the infection.

Congenital Anomalies

Urinary tract anomalies occur with the same frequency as anomalies throughout the body. The mere presence of an anomaly does not necessarily connote the presence of a disease condition or a threat to life. Only when the anomaly is such that it contributes to the development of pathological processes peculiar to the urinary tract does medical intervention become mandatory. Since the urinary tract is composed of a variety of structures, it follows that a variety of abnormalities have been described. The kidney may be anomalous in regard to number, form, location, rotation, pelvis construction, and blood supply. Ureters may be absent, reduplicated, strictured, forked, oversized, or undersized, or may possess an unneeded valve system. There may be absence, multiplicity, exstrophy, or diverticulum of the bladder. It is not uncommon to find vestiges of the fetal communication between the bladder and the unbilical cord in the form of a patent urachus, a urachal cyst, or an umbilical fistula. Finally, the urethra is subject to absence, duplication, hypospadias, epispadias, and a host of other aberrations.

Obstruction

Obstruction, the blocking of the free flow of urine anywhere in the urinary tract, may have far-reaching effects upon the structure and function of the kidney. Stones, congenital anomalies, strictures, prostatic hypertrophy, and tumors are some of the more common causes of obstruction. Every age group is subject to the development of one or more of these problems. Regardless of the type or site of the obstruction, the sequence of events is generally the same. The initial effects are upon the organ immediately above the obstruction—hypertrophy, dilatation, and stasis of urine. The urinary stasis favors infection and stone formation. Some authorities maintain that infection inevitably goes along with obstruction. In the later stages of obstruction the kidney becomes involved. At this time three factors may contribute to renal failure: (1) vascular compression, which compromises renal blood flow; the hypertension of obstructive uropathy may stem from this effect; (2) compression of tubular epithelium, resulting in absorptive and secretory defects; (3) interstitial infection of the kidney; this may or may not occur. This total process is capable of virtually destroying the kidney.

Signs and symptoms produced are those of renal function impairment, infection, and extrarenal manifestations such as hypertension.

In the treatment of obstruction, nephron survival is the goal of utmost importance. If irreversible kidney damage is to be prevented, early recognition and treatment of obstruction is essential. Specific treatment consists mainly of treating the infection and surgically correcting the obstruction. Surgical measures may include nephrectomy, correction of ureteropelvic abnormalities, urethral or bladder neck obstructions, and the correction of anatomic abnormalities.

The situation becomes the more emergent as the pathologic process progresses toward total obstruction. Before definitive surgical measures can be attempted, it is sometimes necessary to tap the urinary stream above the site of the obstruction in order to relieve the pressure within the system. The procedures for urinary diversion provide immediate relief from back pressure. They also permit the urologist to postpone corrective surgery until the patient is in better condition to withstand it. Except in the instance of far-advanced malignant neoplasm, the techniques of urinary diversion are usually of only temporary expediency.

The site of entry into the urinary tract is determined by the location of the obstruction. When the occlusion is in and about the urethra, the bladder is the organ of choice for penetration. For obstructions occurring higher, the renal pelvis is entered. The ureter and urethra are never chosen because of their diameter. In small structures such as these the scarring subsequent to surgical insult creates strictures that encourage obstruction, and the patient would be no better off in the long run.

For obstructions occurring at the termination of the urinary tract, the quickest and simplest technique for achieving immediate decompression is the insertion of a needle into the distended bladder. The needle used for lumbar puncture serves the purpose admirably. The contents of the bladder can be withdrawn either rapidly or slowly according to the preference of the attending physician. In many respects the needle cystotomy resembles a paracentesis. Its use is usually restricted to emergency situations, since the procedure does not provide an avenue for continued drainage, which is frequently required.

More often the surgical procedure of suprapubic cystostomy will be done. A small incision is made through the skin and into the distended bladder, which has risen to a point of easy access. An indwelling catheter is inserted and fixed into position under direct visualization. Occasionally a Penrose drain will be placed in the space of Retzius if it is noted that a watertight seal has not been secured around the catheter. By virtue of its simplicity, suprapubic cystostomy can be performed rapidly with use of only a local anesthetic. This is a boon to the patient with long-standing obstruction and impending kidney complications.

In addition to provision of routine postoperative nursing measures, special attention is directed toward maintaining the newly established drainage system. The cystostomy tube is connected to the collecting bottle; the straight gravity drainage principle is utilized. An adequate length of tubing between the patient and the collecting bottle is necessary to avoid undue tension, which might displace the cystostomy tube. Kinking and vertical looping of the drainage tubing should be prevented, as this impedes the flow of urine and recreates the condition of obstruction. If the cystostomy does not leak around the catheter no special considerations for wound care are indicated. Occasionally leakage does occur, necessitating frequent dressing and linen changes. Meticulous attention to the skin prevents irritation and even breakdown resulting from contact with decomposing urine. The large diameter of the indwelling catheter used reduces the need for irrigations almost entirely. Characteristics of the drainage should be noted and recorded. Fluids are encouraged as long as kidney function permits. It may be advisable for the cystostomy to remain for some time, and for the patient to return home during the interval between operations. The patient or a member of his family can be taught to care for the cystostomy. When this is not feasible the visiting nurse service should be requested to assume management of the home program.

When the cause of an obstruction is located high in the urinary tract, decompression is achieved by inserting a nephrostomy tube directly into the renal pelvis through a flank incision. Penrose drains may also be put in place to provide for escape of urine seeping around the nephrostomy tube.

The postoperative nursing care incorporates all the considerations for any patient having a flank incision, with primary concern directed toward maintaining the patency of the tubing leading from the kidney pelvis. The average renal pelvis has a capacity of about 5 ml. In a relatively short period of time any interference with the outflow of urine, such as a clot within the tube or a kink in it under the patient, permits harmful back-pressure to build up. The purpose of the decompression procedure is defeated unless there is free and continuous egress for the urine. An order for irrigation of the drainage system is the rule. The frequency of irrigation is dictated by the viscosity of the blood and pus that often accompany the

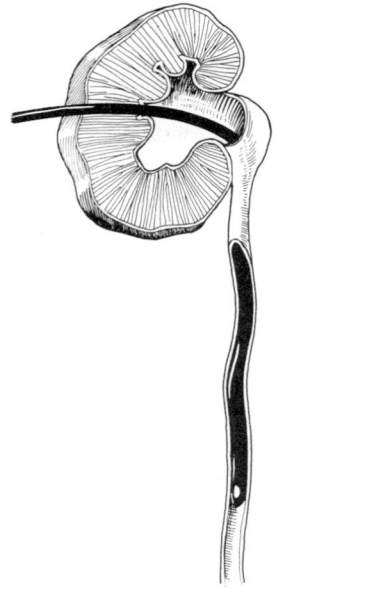
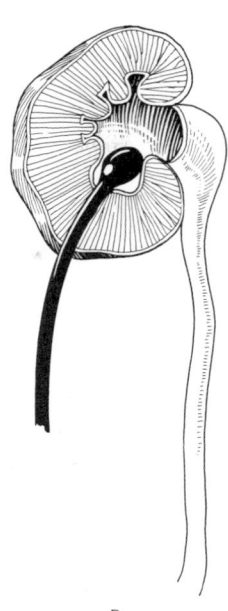

A   B

*Figure 24-3
Foley catheter and
nephrostomy tube in
place. A, Foley
catheter in renal pelvis
is brought out to flank.
B, Nephrostomy tube in
renal pelvis is brought
out to flank through
parenchyma of kidney.*

urine. In the absence of specific orders regarding quantity and type of irrigating solution to be used, no more than 10 ml of sterile normal saline should be inserted at a time, and this should be done at very low pressure to avoid the destructive potential of a forceful stream of fluid. Before the solution is inserted the tube is aspirated to ensure that the pelvis is empty. Return flow must be noted to contain at least the quantity just inserted before additional solution is inserted into the renal pelvis. The wise nurse is absolutely sure of the orders, mechanics of the drainage system, and any unusual circumstances that may modify the procedure before executing it.

Great care is exercised to avoid premature removal of a nephrostomy tube, since its replacement in all probability will involve another surgical procedure. The patient and his family are instructed in safe techniques for sitting, standing, and walking. As a rule patients with nephrostomy tubes in place do not leave the hospital. In all other respects the nursing care of the patient with diversion of the urinary flow through a nephrostomy is the same as for the patient with a cystostomy.

Urinary Calculi

A calculus or stone is a hard concretion formed when there is precipitation within the urinary tract of some of the substances that ordinarily are in solution in the urine. These substances consist of both colloids and crystalloids. The colloids possess a protective action that inhibits precipitation, but in certain conditions this is lost, and they are deposited on the matrix of the crystalloids and precipitate as stones. Infection in the kidney as well as a focus elsewhere in the body may bring about stone formation. Gout, hyperparathyroidism, and cystinuria are some of the more common metabolic disorders that give rise to production of a large quantity of crystalloid substance in the urine and thereby initiate the stone formation process. Vitamin A is believed to contribute to the control of the calcium-phosphate ratio in the blood. When there is a dietary deficiency, large quantities of calcium are excreted through the kidneys. The colloid-crystalloid balance is altered and stones develop. By a similar mechanism, excessive ingestion of calcium and vitamin D can bring about the same results. Stones form more readily in stagnant than in flowing urine and therefore are seen more frequently in immobilized than ambulatory persons. Also, serum calcium is higher in immobilized patients, which situation also contributes and results from mobilization of the calcium from the bones. An obstruction that hinders the free passage of urine gives rise to stone formation in the still pools lying behind it. The presence of a foreign body acts as a core upon which concretions can begin growth.

Stones will develop in either an acid or an alkaline medium. The pH of the urine determines the kind of stone that will grow. An alkaline urine will most likely form a phosphatic type of stone, while an acid urine will produce the common calcium oxalate variety. Stones occur singly or multiply, and range in size from that of a fine grain of sand to enormous dimensions. They are seen most commonly in men in the third to the fifth decade of life. The incidence is highest in Caucasians and is close to zero in Negroes. Stones are found bilaterally in a clinically significant number of cases. Phosphatic stones are more likely to develop in the presence of an infection, grow more rapidly, and take on the configuration of the anatomical structure, calyx, or pelvis in which they are located. Congenital anomalies, especially those possessing obstructing features, are frequently complicated by the presence of stones.

Renal Calculi

When a stone is present in the kidney, interstitial fibrosis develops in the musculature of the wall of the calyx surrounding it. The calyx above the stone dilates at the expense of the parenchyma. If the stone neither migrates out of the kidney nor is removed surgically, it is possible for the entire kidney to be destroyed by compression from trapped urine. This process may be asymptomatic and is then referred to as a *silent* stone. Another individual may complain only of a dull ache in the loin which may vary in intensity but rarely goes away. Or the patient may present the classic picture of kidney colic, which is not a kidney pain at all—it is a ureteral pain resulting from the entry of the stone into the ureter. This pain is described as stabbing, burning, excruciating, and unbearable. As the pain follows the course of the ureter, the patient writhes and his skin becomes pale, cold, and sweaty. The pulse weakens and nausea and vomiting develop. The patient experiences frequency, and passes scant quantities of blood-tinged urine. Such an episode may last for a few minutes during which a small stone passes down into the bladder or drops back into the kidney pelvis, in which case the event may be repeated at another time. Or the episode may last for hours without the stone moving significantly.

The diagnosis of kidney stone is established from the history and physical findings. X-ray studies provide graphic proof of the presence of a radiopaque stone and with contrast techniques, of a nonradiopaque stone. Cystoscopy is carried out to pinpoint the origin of the hematuria and locate the stone in the bladder if it has advanced that far. Passage of the stone through the urethra is unequivocal evidence of the condition.

During an episode of acute renal colic, the patient is given analgesics to help relieve the severe pain. Antispasmodics may be used in conjunction with the narcotic to relax the ureter and facilitate passage of the stone toward the bladder. If nausea is not present fluids may be offered for their flushing effect. Even under heavy doses of narcotics, patients experiencing kidney colic may be restless and should be permitted the position and activity that seem most comfortable and safe for them. When the stone finally passes out of the ureter there is a sudden and dramatic relief of symptoms. If the patient has had unusually high doses of narcotic during this acute phase, he should be observed carefully for signs of central nervous system depression during the period of recovery from physical exhaustion and drug excretion. After the acute episode an attempt is made to determine the etiology of the stone formation and whenever possible to eliminate it.

When stones are lodged in the kidney pelvis surgery is the only recourse. Pyelolithotomy is indicated if the stone is small and unbranched. A partial or heminephrectomy is done when a staghorn calculus is confined to the upper or lower pole. A total nephrectomy is performed when neither of the two preceding procedures is feasible.

Ureteral Calculi

Usually ureteral calculi kidney stones that have become impacted in the ureter, although rarely they may originate in the ureter. The three most common sites for impaction are the ureteropelvic junction, the ureterovesical junction, and the pelvic brim where the ureter crosses the iliac vessels. There is dilatation above the site of impaction producing hydroureter, hydronephrosis, and destruction of parenchyma by compression. Pyelonephritis almost always accompanies this condition. The contralateral kidney undergoes compensatory hypertrophy if it is functional.

The symptoms of kidney colic are seen if the stone shifts its position. Red and white blood cells in the urine, high fever, chills, and sweats occur with the inevitable superimposed infection.

Usually ureteral stones pass spontaneously. They may be dislodged or extracted by cystoscopic manipulation or may be removed through a surgical incision in the ureter. When the ureter has been penetrated surgically, the subsequent scarring in this structure may create a stricture which may produce an obstruction at a later date. To minimize this possibility the ureter is traumatized as little as possible during surgery. A ureteral catheter may be used to splint the defect, and the additional insult of suturing is eliminated. The flow of urine is not impeded nor does it interfere with the healing process in the ureter. When caring for this patient postoperatively the nurse exercises care not to dislodge the ureteral catheter prematurely. If there is far-advanced kidney destruction due to the ureteral calculus, total nephrectomy is the operation of choice.

Vesical Calculi

Vesical calculi have the same etiology and pathology as calculi in other genitourinary organs. In addition, stones can develop on foreign bodies that have been accidentally or deliberately introduced into the bladder. A stone in the bladder causes inflammatory changes in the mucosal wall and can predispose to infection both in the bladder and higher in the urinary tract. Obstruction with its concomitant complications occurs when a stone occludes one of the bladder orifices. The presence of a bladder stone is characterized by pain, hematuria, frequency, and changes in the act of micturition. Some patients can void only in a reclining position when gravity holds the stone away from the urethra. Symptoms of a severe cystitis are seen with an accompanying infection. Occasionally large stones can be palpated suprapubically.

Therapy for vesical calculi includes cystoscopy, in which the stone is flushed out, and use of stone-grasping forceps to remove the stone. Very large calculi are first crushed and then removed. This procedure is known as *litholapaxy*. In instances where these more conservative measures are impractical, perineal or suprapubic cystolithotomy is done and the stone is removed under direct visualization.

When a vesical calculus is first suspected the goal of nursing care is directed toward assisting the patient to pass the stone with a minimum of pain. Fluids are pushed to achieve an internal flushing effect. The urine is strained through some material such as fine gauze so that the passage of stones of any size can be detected. Urinary tract disinfectants and antibiotics are commonly used both to treat and to prevent infections. Analgesics are given to alleviate the pain.

As a result of the teaching efforts by the nurse and their personal experience, some patients who experience repeated episodes of vesical calculi become quite knowledgeable and manage the passage of their stones without medical assistance.

Urethral Calculi

Urethral calculi are rare. During the act of urination small stones may pass into the urethra and lodge there. It is also possible for a stone to form in the urethra in a region where there is stasis of urine due to a lesion such as an urethral stricture or diverticulum. If the stone does not pass spontaneously it will most likely be removed through a cystoscope.

Foreign Bodies

Foreign bodies are objects that are not normally found in the urinary tract. These items are commonly recovered from both the male and female urethra and bladder, and uncommonly from the kidney. They may be introduced into the urinary system by the patient himself, by other humans, or by the process of migration. Self-inserted objects may lodge in the urethra or bladder following abnormal sex practice, inquisitive self-exploration, or utilization of an object as a contraceptive device. Introduction of foreign bodies by other humans usually results from improper medical practice. As a result objects such as surgical sponges, pieces of drainage tubes, parts of urethral instruments, fragments of Foley catheter bags, or other objects are left in the bladder or urethra. Occasionally metallic and non-metallic appliances such as orthopedic nails or screws in the pelvic area migrate to the bladder. The reason for this is unknown, but the process offers no evidence of extravasation of urine nor is the course taken by the objects observable.

The pathological changes that occur with a foreign body are similar to those that result from urinary obstruction. Infection, a frequent companion of urinary obstruction, may also be seen in the presence of a long-standing foreign body. The resulting symptoms are similar to those mentioned in the discussion of urinary obstruction and infection.

Diagnosing the presence of a foreign body is difficult if the object was self-introduced. Embarrassment causes the victim to delay seeking medical help and when he does, he tries to conceal the fact that it was self-inserted. All radiopaque objects can be located through a simple flat plate of the abdomen. Cystoscopy is extremely useful in visualizing and locating other nonradiopaque foreign bodies and also in assessing the associated damage.

The usual treatment for foreign bodies is surgical removal. A cystoscopy is done to remove small objects, whereas larger objects are removed through a suprapubic incision into the bladder.

If the object was self-inserted, the nurse may have to deal with a guilt-laden patient. The nurse should avoid probing into the circumstances surrounding the incident and try to accept the patient as an individual without passing judgment. The patient may want to talk about his feelings, and the nurse should provide ample opportunity for this.

If the implantation resulted from poor medical technique, the nurse should consult with the doctor before revealing this information to the patient, as the incident may have legal implications.

In most cases sound professional practices will avert the introduction of foreign bodies by members of the medical team and will reduce the complications arising from unavoidable equipment failures. These sound practices include careful inspection of instruments, correct surgical sponge counts, and examination of catheter balloons before and after use.

In other respects the nursing care is determined by the surgical method used to remove the foreign body and the extent of damage. This nursing care is presented elsewhere in the chapter.

Neoplasms

CYSTS

In congenital polycystic disease, the normal renal tissue is replaced by numerous cysts of various sizes. Congenital polycystic disease is the most common cystic condition of the kidneys, and is almost always bilateral. The condition is hereditary; symptoms may appear in infancy or between the ages of 40 and 60. The cysts develop because of a failure of resorption of parts of the primitive renal tubule. The kidney is two to three times normal size, and the external surface is roughly and knobby. Most of the renal tissue has been replaced by cysts, the contents of which appear watery, urinous, or hemorrhagic. This disease is often associated with other malformations of the genitourinary tract.

There are no symptoms if the degree of involvement is slight, but with extensive reduction of renal tissue there are symptoms of nephrosclerosis, diminished kidney function, albuminuria, pyuria, anemia, weakness, and gastrointestinal disturbance. Death is usually caused by uremia.

Polycystic disease is fatal in the newborn, but may be latent for years in the adult before progressing rapidly to uremia and causing death. There is no specific surgical or medical treatment for this condition. The patient should be encouraged to continue normal living habits within the limits of his physical ability.

A solitary cyst, which is rare, may be congenital or acquired. The patient may experience a dull dragging sensation and there may be a palpable mass. The cyst is caused by tubular obstruction and ischemia. Treatment consists of complete removal of the cyst or drainage with destruction of the secreting membrane.

TUMORS

Renal Tumors

In the adult kidney tumors are classified as solid tumors of the renal substance and tumors of the renal pelvis. They are usually malignant and usually unilateral. They may grow for some time without causing symptoms; many of them are advanced and incurable when symptoms first appear.

The solid tumor of the renal parenchyma, often called the *hypernephroma*, is the most common malignant tumor of the kidney and occurs more frequently in men. It invades the blood vessels early and metastasizes to the liver, long bones, and lungs.

Primary clinical findings include painless gross hematuria, pain in the lumbar region, and a palpable mass. Because of the bleeding, anemia may be present. Cystoscopy should always be done to determine the source of the bleeding. The presence of the tumor may be established by nephrotomography, excretory or retrograde urography, and by selective arteriography. Urography also helps establish the adequacy of function in the unaffected kidney. X-ray studies may show an enlarged kidney and metastatic lesions of the bone and lung. The diagnosis of tumor must be differentiated from hydronephrosis, polycystic kidney disease, renal cyst, and renal tuberculosis.

The aim of treatment is to excise the tumor before metastases have occurred. Nephrectomy offers the only curative measure. X-ray irradiation has proved of little value because most renal tumors are radioresistant and chemotherapeutic agents have not as yet been found useful. The course of the disease is variable; about 25 percent of patients survive more than 5 years.

Tumors of the renal pelvis are uncommon and comprise 5 to 10 percent of renal growths. They are usually papillary, tend to metastasize along the urinary tract, and may infiltrate the bladder.

The most common clinical finding is painless hematuria; there may be tenderness in the flank and colic may occur due to obstruction of the ureter. Anemia may be present. The urine contains red blood cells, clots, white blood cells, and bacteria when infection is superimposed. The obstruction caused by the tumor can produce the clinical picture of hydronephrosis.

Diagnostic measures include cystoscopy, which reveals bleeding from the involved side, and urography, which reveals the filling defect in the kidney pelvis and shows the obstruction and dilatation of the ureter. Exfoliative cytologic studies may reveal the presence of neoplastic cells.

The goal of therapy is to effect a cure, and specific treatment includes radical removal of the kidney, ureter, and periureteral portion of the bladder unless metastases are extensive. Thereafter cystoscopy every 6 months to 1 year is recommended. The prognosis depends on the type of tumor.

The aim of nursing care of the patient with a kidney tumor is to prevent complications and to assist him and his family in making adjustments to living if metastases are too extensive for curative measures. Responsibilities of the nurse include preparing the patient for diagnostic tests and surgery, providing postoperative nursing care, and assisting the patient and family in planning for the future.

The nurse has important responsibilities in preparing the patient for various diagnostic procedures including physical preparation as indicated for the specific test, as described elsewhere. The patient should understand the purpose of the precedure, since his cooperation is needed. The significance of the test may have to be interpreted for the patient and his family; the nurse should be prepared to answer their questions and encourage them to ask the doctor for clarification. Diversional activities suited to the patient's interests can be helpful during the period of waiting while the diagnosis is being established and therapy is being planned.

Nephrectomy is the treatment of choice if the tumor is operable and the function of the unaffected kidney is satisfactory. In addition to preparing the patient physically for surgery, the nurse should give him an opportunity to express his feelings about himself, his family, his diagnosis and treatment, and whether or not he wishes to include his family in these discussions.

Nephrectomy may be curative. If the tumor is radiosensitive the patient may also undergo a course of radiation therapy. The patient with an inoperable tumor and metastatic disease may have palliative radiation therapy. Nursing care problems are dependent on the degree of involvement of the areas of metastases. The nurse helps the patient and his family to make adjustments according to the symptoms and prognosis and the plan of therapy. Besides knowing the age and physical condition of the patient, the nurse should gain an understanding of the role of the patient in the family, other family relationships, family attitudes and habits of living, interest of the family in having the patient maintain his independence, and economic resources and other resources available or needed in the home. The goal in making any changes or adjustments is to help the patient and family live as normally as possible. If the patient is in the terminal phase of illness the family may need help in accepting the certainty of his death.

Other members of the health team should be available to assist the patient and family in their planning. The family should be made aware of the existence of community agencies such as the local visiting nurse service and The American Cancer Society.

Ureteral Tumors

Primary tumors of the ureter are rare; secondary tumors usually develop from adjacent viscera. Usually hematuria is present. Diagnosis is made following cystoscopy and pyelography. Treatment consists of nephrectomy and ureterectomy including removal of the intramural ureter, followed by a course of radiation therapy. The patient should have frequent follow-up examinations, but the prognosis is poor. The tumors are highly malignant and are discovered late. Nursing care is the same as for a patient with a kidney tumor.

Vesical Tumors

The greatest number of bladder tumors are of the epithelial type. They are papillomas or carcinomas, and all papillomas are potentially malignant. Chronic irritation is thought to be a cause of bladder tumors, which comprise the second most common genitourinary neoplasm. They develop more frequently in men. The tumor grows into the bladder lumen, and as it increases in size it may occlude one or both ureters, causing stasis and infection in the ureter and kidney pelvis.

Clinical findings include painless gross hematuria, although hematuria may not be an early symptom. Late symptoms include frequency and dysuria. If the tumor encroaches on an internal orifice, symptoms of bladder neck obstruction will be present and cystitis will occur if infection supervenes. No abnormalities are found on physical examination in most cases, but signs of metastases may be noted.

Laboratory findings include anemia, severe infection, and uremia; the urine may be bloody and may contain pus and bacteria. Renal function tests are usually normal unless bladder neck obstruction or obstruction of both ureteral orifices is present.

The diagnosis is made on the basis of the findings of cystoscopy, biopsy, and cystography. Conditions that must be ruled out are renal or ureteral neoplasms, acute nonspecific infections, tuberculosis of the urinary tract, urinary calculi, acute hemorrhagic nephritis, and invasion of the bladder by a tumor from an adjacent organ. Complications that may occur are secondary infection of the bladder caused by tumor ulceration, hemorrhage, hydronephrosis due to ureteral occlusion, and uremia.

The prognosis is good in benign tumors. Nonetheless fewer than 25 percent of cancers of the bladder are curable. This is because they are first seen long after the appearance of symptoms and treatment may no longer be effective. Sites of metastases are the pelvic lymph nodes, lungs, lumbar spine, pelvis, and upper third of the femur. The aim of therapy is to prevent failure of the upper urinary tract due to obstruction and infection caused by the tumor. Treatment includes local excision of the tumor before metastases have occurred, radiation therapy, and urinary diversion. Complications are treated and palliation is provided if metastases are too extensive for curative measures. The method of choice for treatment of the tumor depends on its size, type, and location.

Small single or multiple papillomas are best treated by transurethral resection and fulguration unless they have deeply invaded the bladder wall. Cystoscopy should be performed every 6 months for the rest of the patient's life, as papillomas may recur. Radioisotopes inserted into the balloon of a Foley catheter may be used to treat small superficial lesions, and radon seeds, which do not have to be removed, may be implanted around the base of somewhat larger tumors. Partial cystectomy may be done if the tumor does not lie on the base of the bladder, in which event both ureteral orifices must be sacrificed. The patient will be aware of the smaller bladder capacity immediately postoperatively but should be told that with time it will increase to almost normal capacity. Total cystectomy will be done for most malignant and deeply invasive tumors if the disease seems curable. With this procedure the patient will have a permanent urinary diversion. External radiation and chemotherapy utilizing 5-fluorouracil are sometimes administered for palliation.

Specific care depends on the method of treatment of the tumor and includes promotion of urinary drainage by use of catheters and cystostomy tubes or a method of diversion, and treatment of the cystitis which usually develops following radiation therapy.

The object of nursing care is to prevent complications, teach self-care, and assist the patient and family in planning for the future.

In the prevention of complications the nurse is responsible for preparing the patient for diagnostic tests such as cystoscopy and renal function tests, preparing the patient for surgery, and providing care in the postoperative recovery period. Nursing care problems depend on the method of treatment of the tumor, but the following problems are common to most patients undergoing treatment for a bladder tumor: provision for urinary drainage, promotion and maintenance of an adequate fluid intake, symptomatic relief of cystitis, which usually develops following radiation therapy, teaching of self-care to the patient with urinary diversion, and dealing with the fear of metastatic disease.

The nurse should understand the care and management of catheters and cystostomy tubes, and the various methods of urinary diversion, in order to provide satisfactorily for urine drainage. She must recognize the importance of an adequate fluid intake for maintaining hydration, electrolyte balance, secretion, and drainage of urine. The patient with urinary diversion is in need of teaching and support because some adjustment and change of daily living habits are necessary.

Excision of the tumor may be curative, but the patient should be encouraged to have periodic follow-up examinations. Treatment and care of the patient with metastatic disease depend on the location of the metastases and the symptoms produced, the plan of therapy, and the prognosis.

Urethral Tumors

Benign and malignant tumors of the urethra are uncommon. Malignant tumors may present as visible or palpable masses, and symptoms of urinary obstruction may develop. Diagnosis is made on the basis of biopsy. Benign and malignant tumors are cured by transurethral resection and fulguration, and some malignant tumors may be cured by more extensive open surgery and radical inguinal node excision.

Urinary Diversion

Diversion of the urinary stream is necessary following total cystectomy. Other indications for such a procedure are trauma to the bladder, infection causing damage to the lining and muscles of the bladder, birth deformities, and reaction to radiation.

Of the several methods of diverting the urinary stream, none provides a substitute bladder with storage and sphincteral control comparable to the normal bladder. The approaches to urinary drainage are ureterostomy, ureterosigmoidostomy, anal bladder, ileal conduit, and colocystoplasty.

The purpose of any of these procedures is to provide for diversion of the urinary stream in the way most acceptable to the patient and with the least likelihood of complications. The ileal conduit seems to be the most satisfactory procedure at this time.

Ureterostomy

Cutaneous ureterostomy consists of transplanting the ureters to the abdominal wall and providing openings on the skin surface from which the urine drains into a collecting bag. A more recent procedure consists of bringing both ureters out through an opening in the navel, so that just one collecting bag is necessary. Ureteral catheters may be kept in place for about 3 weeks to promote healing of the stoma. These catheters must be kept open to provide for urine drainage and prevent hydronephrosis. The ureteral bud or stoma must be kept moist to promote healing. Normal saline usually is used for this purpose. If the stoma forms properly the patient is able to wear some type of appliance for collection of urine. If ureteral buds do not form the patient must have ureteral catheters placed to provide for urine drainage. He will have to be taught the techniques of inserting and caring for the catheters. Problems of concern to the patient are odor, skin care, stenosis of the ureter, and use of the appliance. To prevent stenosis the ureters may be dilated with ureteral catheters by the doctor.

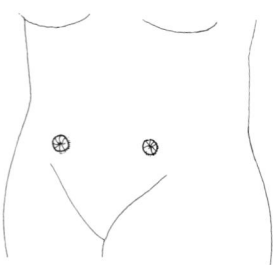

Figure 24-4
Cutaneous ureterostomy

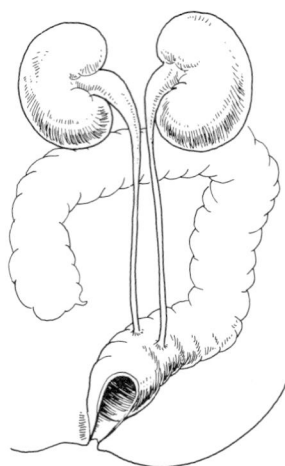

Figure 24–5
Ureterosigmoidoscopy

Ureterosigmoidostomy

Ureterosigmoidostomy is the transplantation of the ureters into the lower portion of the sigmoid colon with the result that urine is excreted through the rectum. The procedure seems to be more socially acceptable, and a collecting bag need not be worn. There are a few disadvantages: the stool is semiliquid, and the lower bowel must be emptied frequently to prevent reflux of urine, ascending infection, and absorption of urinary products. Nausea, vomiting, diarrhea, and lethargy are symptoms of electrolyte imbalance and should be reported. In preparation for the ureterointestinal anastomosis, an attempt is made to sterilize the bowel through administration of cathartics, enemas, and drugs such as phthalylsulfathiazole (Sulfathalidine) or neomycin given orally for a period of 3 to 5 days. Postoperatively a large rectal tube will be in place for about 10 days to allow for urine drainage. Gentle irrigation of the tube may be necessary to keep it open. The urinary output should be very closely observed. Until the drainage tube is removed the patient will be on a low-residue diet. Following removal of the tube the patient should empty the rectum every 2 to 4 hours, but if this procedure is too disturbing at night he may have to insert a rectal tube and attach it to a drainage bottle during sleeping hours. He should not be given enemas or strong laxatives, since either of these may cause contaminated urine to be forced up the ureters.

Anal Bladder

The patient with an anal bladder has a sigmoid colostomy with transplantation of the ureters to a closed loop of the sigmoid. The rectum acts as a reservoir only for urine, and evacuation of urine is controlled by sphincteral action of the anus. Treatment and nursing care are the same as for the patient with a ureterosigmoidostomy, with the addition of the care of the colostomy.

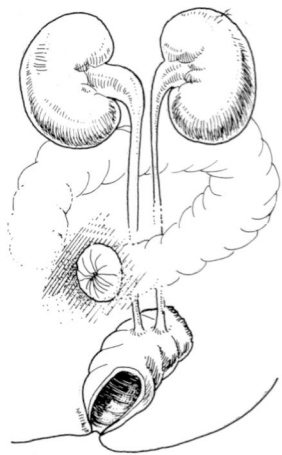

Figure 24–6
Anal bladder

Ileal Conduit

The ileal conduit does not serve as a reservoir for urine, but as a passageway from the ureter to the outside. A short segment of the terminal loop of the ileum is isolated, with maintenance of its blood supply; one end is sutured closed, the other end is brought out through the abdominal wall, the ureters are transplanted into this section of the ileum, and the urine drains out through the ileostomy opening. The remainder of the ileum is anastomosed.

This procedure has several advantages: electrolyte imbalance is less likely, infection is minimal because there is no stool contamination, renal function is adequate, a single opening is necessary, and it is relatively easy to attach a collecting system. Preparation is the same as for a ureterosigmoidostomy. Following surgery, a catheter may be placed in the ileostomy opening, which may require irrigation to keep it open, or a collecting bag may be applied immediately. Several problems may develop in the early postoperative period: distention of the ileal segment by urine may cause back-pressure on the kidneys and rupture of the suture line; swelling about the stoma may prevent emptying of the conduit; abdominal distention may prevent the ureters from emptying; peritonitis may develop if there is leakage of the anastomosis; stenosis of the stoma may develop; and residual

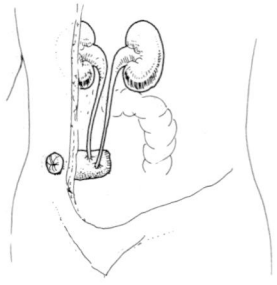

Figure 24–7
Ileal conduit

urine may accumulate in the conduit. The stoma should be dilated daily for a period of time, and the patient should be taught how to do this. He should wear a lubricated finger cot for the purpose. He may also be taught how to measure the amount of residual urine in the conduit periodically with a catheter, and he must learn how to apply and care for the appliance he wears for urine collection.

Colocystoplasty

The procedure of making a new bladder from an isolated portion of the sigmoid colon is called *colocystoplasty*. It can be done only if the urethra and the sphincters are intact. The ureters are transplanted into and the sphincter muscle and urethra are anastomosed to this portion of the sigmoid, which serves as a bladder. There is less psychological adjustment to be made because function is not altered. Care is the same as for the patient with a ureterosigmoidostomy, but in addition the patient should practice control, since the internal sphincter is not always intact. Ureteral and urethral catheters will be kept in place for about 10 days after surgery and they must be kept patent. Follow-up cystometrograms should be done to determine the capacity of the bladder.

POSTOPERATIVE CARE

Preparation for self-care is the most important objective of nursing care of the patient with urinary diversion.

Regardless of the method of diversion, the patient will need much support and encouragement from the nurse and from his family. The individual with a uretero-sigmoidostomy or an anal bladder must exercise good sphincter control because he evacuates urine through the anal opening. The male patient must sit to urinate. Following cutaneous ureterostomy and ileal conduit, some type of collecting bag

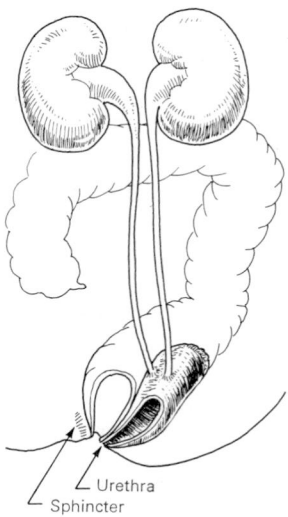

Urethra
Sphincter

Figure 24-8
Colocystoplasty

Colosigmoid bladder
(colocystoplasty)

must be worn. Although one procedure may be preferable to another as far as patient morale or personal convenience is concerned, all of them have the potential of causing complications of fluid and electrolyte imbalance, infection, and changes in self-image; and all raise the question of social acceptability. The appliance can cause skin irritation and may interfere with some activities, but with continued encouragement the individual may finally accept the appliance.

The patient should be encouraged to continue a daily fluid intake of 3,000 ml, eat a regular diet, and continue his normal activities within the limits of his physical ability.

The nurse can gain much useful information from the patient and his family in relation to their attitudes toward the patient and their interest in helping him make a satisfactory adjustment. Resources available to the patient are the local visiting nurse service and The American Cancer Society. Ileostomy clubs in many areas of the country provide information about the purchase, use, and care of appliances. The *Ostomy Quarterly* disseminates information.

Use of Collection Appliances

A collection appliance must be worn following cutaneous ureterostomy and ileal conduit. The simpler the appliance, the better. The basic function of the appliance is to prevent leakage of urine to the skin around the stoma. Leakage results in redness, irritation, and ulceration of the skin, causing the patient much discomfort while wearing the bag.

The appliance may be either a temporary plastic bag which is taped to the skin or a permanent one attached to a plastic Lucite disk which is fitted to the stoma and cemented to the skin. The disk is not custom-made but can be fitted to the individual through an adjustment in its opening. The plastic bag can be removed and emptied as necessary; the disk must be removed and recemented every few days.

Because of the expansion and contraction of the stoma, it is important that the opening in the disk be of the correct size. A clearance of ⅛ inch from the stoma to the opening in the disk should be maintained. An ordinary penknife can be used to enlarge the opening.

Because some individuals have sensitive skins, it is advisable to make a patch test before using a cement. A bit of cement is placed on the skin of the abdomen opposite the side of the stoma. It is allowed to dry and remain on the skin for 24 hours. If there is no irritation, the cement may be used with reasonable safety. It must be applied in a very thin coat to the skin and the disk. A circular motion of the fingers is employed to apply a thin layer of cement to the surface of the disk which makes contact with the skin, and a thin layer is applied to the skin areas where the disk is to be cemented. The cement coating should be dry to the light touch of a clean finger before the disk is placed, since the solvent in the cement is irritating to the skin and must be allowed to evaporate. If itching or burning is felt under the disk it is possible that insufficient time was allowed for the cement to dry. After the disk has been applied to the body, the space between the stoma and the disk opening is filled with a heavy layer of karaya gum powder. A few drops of water are placed on this powder to form a protective coating around the stoma.

Special bags are made to fit on the Lucite disk, and it is important that they fit securely around the disk.

The bag can be removed for emptying and cleaning. It should be washed in hot soapy water, rinsed thoroughly, and dried with a towel. The inside should be dusted with talcum powder or cornstarch to preserve it and prevent it from sticking together. The disk may be removed, cleaned with cold water, and wiped dry. The cement can easily be rolled off the skin with the fingers or a towel and rolled off the disk with a dry towel. If either the disk or the bag becomes stained it should be soaked in vinegar.

If the skin around the stoma becomes irritated it is washed with mild soap and cool water, rinsed with clear cool water, and dried thoroughly. A light coat of Amphogel is applied and allowed to dry, followed by a light application of karaya gum powder on the skin around the stoma; the powder is brushed toward the stoma so that a light film remains on the skin. The space between the stoma and the disk opening is filled with a generous layer of the gum powder (about ⅛ inch in depth). A few drops of water are placed on this powder to form a protective covering around the stoma. Karaya gum powder is not greasy; it aids in healing, absorbs moisture, and permits cement to adhere. It can be used as a protective layer between skin and appliance or as a substitute for cement.

Tincture of benzoin should not be applied to the skin around an ostomy opening if it is to be covered with an appliance or a temporary taped bag, because the skin will blister. The tincture may be applied to irritated skin after it has healed but should not be used each time the disk is removed since it tends to dry the skin. It may be used the first three times the disk is removed, and thereafter every third time the disk is removed. The tincture should be allowed to dry before cement is again applied. Complete instructions for care and use of the bag are included with the purchase.

Strictures

Strictures are abnormal organic narrowings of the ureter, bladder neck, or urethral lumen. Because of the anatomical proximity of the urethra to the bladder neck, strictures of these two areas are discussed together. The most common stricture of the urinary tract is due to an enlarged prostate.

The etiology of strictures is debatable, but most strictures are thought to be acquired rather than congenital in origin. Congenital strictures are due to faulty embryonic development, and acquired strictures result from inflammatory processes or from trauma. The cause of ureteral strictures is unknown but is believed to be closely related to the presence of infection and the occurrence of trauma. Contractions of the urethra are more common in males but they can occur in females who have had prolonged chronic urethritis. Before the advent of potent antibacterial drugs, urethral strictures were frequently seen as sequelae of gonorrheal urethritis. Today urethral strictures are predominantly caused by trauma or injury to the urethra.

A stricture develops similarly to scar tissue. Trauma and inflammation result in proliferation of fibrosis; fibrosis in turn causes contracture of tissue and thus stricture. A stricture may range from a slight narrowing to a complete obstruction of the lumen in cases of severe stricture. The rate of development of a stricture varies with its cause. Inflammatory strictures develop over a period of months to years, whereas traumatic strictures develop rapidly, producing symptoms within weeks to months after injury. Usually the prognosis is good if the obstruction (stricture) has not been present over a long period of time and provided the lumen is dilated regularly.

Strictures can be prevented to some degree. Early and adequate treatment of the traumatized part, adequate chemotherapy for inflammation and infections, gentleness and cleanliness during surgery and instrumentation, and accurate approximation of a laceration or tear are helpful measures.

The history will reveal a gradual onset of signs and symptoms. Strictures form obstructions which contribute to infections; consequently, the same signs and symptoms are present. In general, strictures of the lower urinary tract cause signs and symptoms of disturbances in micturition, while those of the upper tract produce changes in the kidney. These result because of the backing up of urine proximal to the stricture. In the case of stricture of the male urethra, symptoms of sexual aberrations may also be present.

As a diagnostic procedure, the physician may attempt to pass a catheter of average size. If there is a stricture the catheter cannot be passed beyond the site. The presence of residual urine is confirmatory. A complete urological examination is done when a stricture is suspected. The presence of a stricture is confirmed through cystography, urethrography, urethroscopy, or panendoscopy. The doctor decides which x-ray study to utilize based on the history and symptomatology. Urinalysis is the most significant laboratory test; it will reveal the presence of bacteria, pus, and white cells.

Medical Treatment

Treatment of strictures is mainly medical, and its success depends upon skillful manipulation of instruments during diagnosis, control of infection, and cooperation of the patient. The chief objective of treatment is prevention of damage to kidney tissue. This goal is accomplished by dilating the lumen and draining the urine proximal to the stricture. When possible, conservative treatment is carried out with filiforms, bougies, sounds, or catheters. The filiforms, bougies, and sounds provide a means of enlarging the lumen of the vessel and may also serve as a guide for the catheters which are frequently attached to them. The catheter provides relief of urinary stasis above the level of the stricture. Dilators of increasingly larger diameters are employed until a catheter can be inserted beyond the stricture to drain the urine. The catheter is left in place until the inflammation is relieved. After the catheter is removed progressive stretching must be continued periodically, since strictures are likely to recur.

Surgical Treatment

If the doctor is unable to pass a filiform and acute urinary retention is present, surgical intervention is necessary to relieve the back pressure of the urine upon the kidney. In the case of a ureteral stricture, a ureterostomy or a nephrosotmy may be necessary to prevent kidney damage. Incision into the ureter is followed by intubation with a catheter, which is left in place for a period of 2 to 4 weeks. Acute urinary retention following a urethral stricture is relieved by a suprapubic cystostomy. With urinary drainage functional and anatomical improvement can be seen. After the acute urinary retention is relieved, periodic stretching must be continued indefinitely. The need for dilatation varies with the individual and is determined by the rapidity of recurrence of the obstruction. This stretching is done whether or not the patient has symptoms of stricture, since recurrence may be well advanced before symptoms reappear. The intervals between dilatations are lengthened until the optimum interval is reached; this varies from 1 to 12 months. Periodic dilatations are palliative, not curative. The condition is considered cured only when the lumen remains dilated. If stricture recurs so rapidly that the use of sounds is not feasible, surgical intervention is necessary. The strictured portion is incised and intubated with a catheter; suturing of the tube is unnecessary since the catheter serves as a splint over which the tissue is epithelized. With suturing further stricture is likely and for this reason resection generally is avoided. Occasionally plastic repair of the ureter and urethra is performed, but further stricture is likely because of the probability of infection due to use of a catheter and to urine passing near the incision. Surgical treatment is not necessarily curative, and it may be necessary to create a nephrostomy or an ileal loop in order to spare the kidney. Because of associated urinary infection, antibiotics are given, but they will not be effective until urinary stasis is eradicated.

The main nursing problem is prevention of further stricture. The nurse can accomplish this by maintaining asepsis when caring for the catheter, filiform, bougie, or sound. Giving good penile and perineal care, encouraging fluid intake, administering antibiotics according to schedule, and providing hot sitz baths are other beneficial nursing measures.

The nurse should secure the dilator to prevent its becoming dislodged and observe for urinary retention following removal of the catheter. She should help the patient adjust to the chronicity of his condition. Periodic check-ups will be necessary henceforth to prevent chronic urinary tract infections, stone formation, and kidney damage.

Nephroptosis

In nephroptosis the kidney has dropped downward. The normal kidney is not fixed in position but moves with movement of the torso or independently of such movement. Some individuals experience distress because of the downward movement of a kidney, but others have few symptoms. The degree of prolapse and the onset of symptoms are not necessarily correlated.

Nephroptosis occurs five times more frequently in women than in men. The right side is more likely to be affected than the left and bilateral involvement occurs only rarely. The tall slender individual with little perirenal fat, the person with poor musculature, or the person with generalized visceroptosis is likely to be affected. Sudden trauma, excision of abdominal masses, and wasting diseases are other contributing factors.

Classically the patient complains of a dull ache in the loin which is increased by activity and eased by bed rest. Reflex symptoms of epigastric pain, nausea, and vomiting may be noted. The ectopic kidney can usually be felt as a mass in the flank. The extent of prolapse is measured by gauging the portion of kidney that can be palpated and held during an inspiration. From half to all of the kidney may be so palpated. If in addition there is kinking or torsion of the ureter, the symptoms of obstruction will be present.

The diagnosis can be confirmed radiologically in two ways. First, retrograde or intravenous pyelography demonstrates the position of the kidney. Second, the characteristic pain should be reproducible by the overfilling of the kidney pelvis necessitated by the retrograde pyelography. Hematological studies and urinalysis contribute little to the evaluation of uncomplicated nephroptosis, since the kidney continues to function normally.

In the absence of obstruction to the urinary tract, a trial of conservative therapy is warranted. The patient should rest in bed for an extended period of up to 6 weeks, with the foot of the bed elevated. This can be done in the home or hospital. In either case the problem of boredom must be met, and the patient must be encouraged to complete the period of bed rest. If he is extremely slender, efforts should be made to help him gain weight in order to increase the size of the perirenal fat pads. External supports in the form of kidney corsets are helpful in some instances.

If urinary obstruction supervenes or conservative therapy is unsuccessful, surgical treatment is indicated in the form of nephropexy. This is accomplished by surgically creating adhesions that will support the kidney in the desired position. Postoperatively the nursing care differs from that in other flank incisions in one important respect: the patient remains flat in bed for an extended period of time. In the recent past this period was as long as 3 weeks but at this writing is 10 days. When ambulatory the patient may feel more comfortable if a snug abdominal binder is used to support the incision. Physical activities are curtailed until maximum healing has occurred. The prognosis is excellent if the postoperative routine is faithfully maintained.

Diverticula

Diverticula occur in the ureter, bladder, or urethra. The true incidence is unknown but is increasing with better diagnostic methods. It is not known whether diverticula are congenital or acquired. Diverticula of the ureter and bladder are frequently found in association with obstructions and are usually located above the level of the obstruction. Diverticula of the urethra are generally considered to be acquired secondary to infection and trauma associated with obstruction, rather than to arise from the obstruction itself. Because of this association, the pathological changes are typical of changes occurring with obstruction. Initially there is dilatation of the conducting organ with hypertrophy. With obstruction below the level of the bladder, further changes take place in the bladder wall as a result of its anatomical structure. Following hypertrophy, certain muscle bundles enlarge and trabeculations (ridges) are produced. With continued intravesical pressure from the obstruction, the bladder mucosa herniates through the spaces between the hypertrophied ridges, producing the diverticula. Diverticula empty poorly by reason of their formation from weakened muscles, and consequently fill with stagnant urine. Their natural drainage is by gravity and increased intra-abdominal pressure.

Diverticula are symptom-free unless they become infected or greatly enlarged. Onset of symptoms is insidious because of the close association with chronic obstruction, and the symptoms are usually persistent and annoying rather than severe. Common symptoms are urinary obstruction and infection, urinary retention, and hematuria. Pyuria and a purulent discharge are frequently seen. The patient also may complain of pain in the loin if the diverticulum is located in the ureter. If the diverticulum is located in the bladder the patient will complain of voiding large amounts of urine at the second voiding, which occurs a short time after the first voiding (the second voiding contains the urine retained in the diverticulum during the first voiding). The patient with a urethral diverticulum will complain of dribbling after micturition and may experience recurrent infections.

In many instances diverticula are diagnosed as chronic pyelitis, because of the presence of infected urine and because there is no response to drug administration. Diverticula of the ureter can be diagnosed through retrograde urography; diverticula of the bladder, through cystography; and diverticula of the urethra, through urethrography. Masses that disappear on palpation of the abdomen as urine is expelled from the diverticula can be felt in the abdomen or the vaginal wall. Urinary stasis may contribute to stone formation within the diverticula—a not infrequent occurrence. Neoplasms are rarely found.

Treatment of diverticula depends on their size. Small diverticula are left untreated. Larger ones may be treated by relieving the obstruction and eradicating the infection, or by surgically removing the sac. Frequently diverticula become symptom-free upon removal of the obstruction. If the diverticulum is exerting pressure on adjacent structures, it should be removed by diverticulectomy.

Preoperatively the patient must be taught how to empty the diverticula. This can be done by having the patient assume the squatting position during micturition and thereby raise the intra-abdominal pressure. Emptying also can be accomplished manually by applying pressure on the masses, which are present following micturition. Both nurse and patient should check the adequacy and frequency of voiding. The use of antibiotics is futile until the underlying cause of the problem is corrected. Postoperatively the objectives of nursing care are to prevent rupture of the suture line and to promote healing. The catheter should never be clamped. If it comes out, it should not be replaced until the doctor has been consulted, since unnecessary traumatization of the suture line may occur. Catheters are irrigated as ordered. The nurse should observe for and report any loss of urinary control resulting from injury to the urinary sphincters during surgery on the urethra.

Trauma

Trauma to the urinary tract is seen quite frequently in our industrialized and mechanized age. Susceptibility to injury varies with age, sex, and activity. Children, for example, often sustain kidney damage following trauma because their kidneys are low and are not protected by fat. Male urinary organs are more susceptible to trauma than female organs because of their greater exposure and because men are involved in more violent activities.

The extent and type of injury that can occur as a result of trauma anywhere in the urinary system vary from mild contusion to complete dysfunction. Injuries are classified as *penetrating* and *nonpenetrating*. Penetrating or open injury results from perforation by objects. The penetrating object may be a bullet or a knife. Careless instrumentation during surgery may cause penetrating injuries. Non-penetrating or closed injuries result from force directly to the urinary system from a fall or a kick.

Signs and symptoms of urological injury depend on associated injuries, time between injury and institution of treatment, health of the organ at time of insult, and location and extent of injury along the tract. Usually urinary tract injuries are associated with other injuries. Shock may or may not be present depending on the extent of injury to the urinary tract and associated injuries. The onset of signs or symptoms indicating the necessity of treatment may vary from minutes to days, therefore the time of initial treatment varies. Since a diseased organ is more vulnerable to injury than a healthy one, the same degree of trauma will cause greater damage to a diseased organ than to a healthy organ. Hematuria generally is present. It may be intermittent, and gross or microscopic. Pain when present may be constant or intermittent and may vary from mild tenderness upon palpation to severe and excruciating. Pain is a useful indicator of the location of the traumatized part. Extravasation of urine occurs when the collecting portion of the urinary tract is involved, and this may or may not cause tissue reaction. Tissue reaction depends on the amount and rate at which urine enters the tissues and not on whether the urine is sterile or contaminated. Sterile urine can produce a reaction. Leakage of a small amount of urine over a short time may be reabsorbed or may give rise to gangrene and necrosis. Gangrene and necrosis are more common than reabsorption. There are no symptoms if the wound closes spontaneously. The urine may seep into the local perinephric tissue, peritoneal cavity, or retroperitoneal space. Regardless of location, the amount of urinary extravasation influences the extent of tissue reaction.

Early diagnosis of trauma is imperative because of the possibility of extravasation of urine and blood. A careful history concerning the trauma along with a thorough physical examination is necessary. When the extent of damage is out of proportion to the severity of trauma, a preexisting disease is considered. During the physical examination, particular attention is given to the rectum because of its proximity to the urinary tract. Any neurological disorder that may contribute to urinary dysfunction may also be detected at this time. Note is made of the presence of any masses, since they may indicate the area of extravasation or displacement of structures. A valuable diagnostic procedure frequently used following suspected traumatic injuries is catheterization; however, with insult to the conducting portion of the urinary tract this becomes difficult if not impossible. If this happens a urologist should be notified without delay.

Roentgenography is useful in determining the extent and location of urinary tract damage. When trauma to the kidney is suspected and the patient's blood pressure and other vital signs are stable, an excretion study such as an intravenous pyelogram is indicated. It is more definitive than a flat plate, although the flat plate will reveal the fuzzy outline of renal hematoma. Retrograde study demonstrates the presence of extravasation in the kidney, ureter, bladder, and urethra, but the study itself may cause further injury. X-ray studies following traumatic injury also help to demonstrate the condition of the contralateral kidney and ureter.

Laboratory studies include urinalysis, hematocrit, and complete blood count. The urinalysis reveals the presence of hematuria; the hematocrit detects blood loss; and the complete blood count indicates a significant decrease in red cells or an increase in white blood cells. If the former, hemorrhage is likely, and if the latter, infection.

Management of urinary tract injuries may be medical or surgical. The aim of treatment is to repair the injury and return renal function to as near normal as possible. The method of treatment will vary with the extent of damage, location of injury, time lapse between injury and initiation of treatment, and associated damage or injuries. Shock and injuries of greater priority are treated first. Mild injuries such as contusions are treated conservatively. Such treatment includes rest in bed for a few days or weeks in the hope that spontaneous repair will occur. Surgical intervention is usually the treatment of choice when the conducting system is involved, especially if the injury was iatrogenic. These injuries should be recognized and repaired immediately by deligation or anastomosis of the severed parts. Since infection is often associated with trauma, antibiotics are given prophylactically. Tetanus prophylaxis is instituted with contaminated penetrating injuries.

The general nursing care of a patient with a traumatic urinary injury is determined by the medical course and by the presence of nonurologic injuries. Because these injuries are usually associated with other insults to the body, maintenance of life takes priority. If the patient is in a state of shock, this should be treated first and efforts made to determine the cause of the shock. The second nursing responsibility is to assist in the diagnosis and treatment of the patient. The nurse makes provision for rest as ordered, makes observations concerning damage and the treatment thereof, prepares the patient for specific diagnostic procedures, inserts and cares for catheters as ordered, maintains urinary drainage, and takes measures to prevent infection and promote healing. When surgical intervention is carried out, there is the additional care of the flank and abdominal incision. Maintenance of fluid and electrolyte balance is an important nursing responsibility in both medical and surgical management.

The nurse has an important role as teacher when preparing the patient for discharge. The patient may have to be taught self-care of the wound and catheters, and the importance of follow-up examinations over a period of time.

Complications may appear early or late. Early complications are due to extravasation of blood or urine which may be slight or marked according to whether or not the injury occurred close to blood vessels. Extravasation of large amounts of urine leads to local tissue infection; if this is uncontrolled, massive infection ensues which leads to abscess formation, sepsis, and eventually death. Fistulas, strictures, stones, hydronephrosis, or pyelonephritis may also develop.

Renal Trauma

In trauma to the kidney the severity of damage ranges from slight contusion to complete shearing off of the vascular pedicle. Usually the former condition will heal spontaneously, whereas the latter may be fatal. Whenever the collecting system of the kidney is ruptured, extravasation of urine into the retroperitoneal space follows. Whether or not peritonitis ensues depends on the amount of urine extravasated. When the kidney parenchyma is lacerated there is a change in urinary output, depending upon the extent of damage.

Injury to the kidney is accompanied also by pain or tenderness in the costovertebral angle. The pain may be localized to the loin or become colicky; the latter suggests the possibility of clots or kidney fragments passing down the ureter. Oliguria or anuria may be demonstrated. These signs are caused by either extensive damage to the kidney or the use of catheters below the level of the kidney.

Diagnostic procedures are as described in other injuries of the urinary tract. Pyuria noted early in the diagnostic studies suggests a preexisting kidney disease.

Some controversy exists over the place of surgical intervention in renal injury, except that in the presence of severe bleeding or extensive extravasation it is mandatory. The main purpose of surgery would be to conserve renal tissue, provide hemostasis, and drain extravasated blood and urine. A lumbar approach is used when the kidney alone is thought to be involved and a transabdominal approach if other viscera are involved.

Consideration should be give to the possible occurrence of acute tubular necrosis. Conditions associated with trauma to the kidney or other areas which could contribute to tubular necrosis include prolonged hypotension with renal ischemia, prolonged spasms of renal vasculature persisting after blood pressure is stabilized, products of autolysis clogging the tubules, hemolysis from incompatible blood transfusions, and dysfunction in neurogenic control of the urinary system.

Ureteral Trauma

Extensive damage to the ureter is rare, since the ureter is well protected by surrounding structures. Two types of injuries do occur, however. Infrequently the ureter is damaged by penetrating objects following stabbing and gunshot wounds, and by surgical injury. Such injuries should be treated immediately. If recognition and repair are delayed, complications develop. Signs and sysmptoms of complications include anuria with unilateral involvement, pain and tenderness at the costovertebral angle due to hydronephrosis, and infection. The diagnosis is confirmed by x-ray studies.

Treatment for iatrogenic injury is deligation or anastomosis of the ureter at the time of injury. A ureteral catheter may be inserted to serve as both a splint and a means of urinary diversion during healing. In extreme instances, a T tube or nephrostomy drainage may be utilized with drainage of the kidney pelvis through the flank. Retransplantation of the ureters may be necessary when the distal ends are short or cannot be located because of retraction. Permanent urinary diversion is carried out as a last resort.

Nursing responsibilities include care of the ureteral catheter and care of the incision. Gentleness is imperative when catheters are being inserted, and necessary precautions regarding the quantity and sterility of irrigating solutions must be taken to prevent tissue damage. Further damage is likely because of the proximity of the ureteral catheter tip to the kidney pelvis. Precise recording of intake and output is essential. Asepsis should be maintained during handling of the catheter and care of the surgical incision.

Vesical Trauma

The bladder may be damaged by nonpenetrating trauma or penetrating wounds, or it may rupture spontaneously. When the bladder sustains a nonpenetrating injury, the damage that results depends on the state of bladder distention at the time of insult. A full bladder is more vulnerable to damage. It is important to have the patient void prior to surgery or delivery so that the bladder will be less likely to be injured. An inebriated person who was involved in a fight is more likely to sustain bladder damage because the bladder is distended and the abdominal muscles are relaxed.

Penetrating injuries to the bladder are self-inflicted by objects used in masturbating or self-punishment. The bladder can rupture spontaneously, although this rarely happens.

Symptoms of injury to the bladder depend on the area of extravasation of urine which may be intraperitoneal or extraperitoneal. Intraperitoneal extravasation may produce signs and symptoms of peritonitis, inability to void, and pain when the intra-abdominal pressure is increased through such acts as coughing, defecating, voiding, and lifting heavy objects. Extraperitoneal extravasation results in suprapubic induration, swelling of the perivesical tissues, pain and tenderness in the perineum, and urge to void, and the presence of nonhemorrhagic shock. The most significant sign among all these is inability to void. Early diagnosis is important because extravasation can cause infection and electrolyte imbalance. Such imbalance may occur even in the absence of peritonitis by absorption of urine through the peritoneal surface. A cystogram is performed immediately to detect any interruption to the continuity of the bladder wall, for this is the most reliable diagnostic test available.

After shock and hemorrhage are controlled, immediate surgical treatment should be carried out in order to exclude the possibility of a laceration, locate and repair any laceration that is present, and drain the urine from the infiltrated areas. Antibiotics usually are given to prevent infection.

When trauma to the bladder is suspected, the specific nursing care includes observation for signs and symptoms of bladder rupture and urinary retention. The patient's complaint of urgency and inability to void should be reported to the physician at once. Fluids should be withheld until a doctor's order is obtained in order to minimize urinary extravasation if rupture has occurred.

Urethral Trauma

Trauma to the urethra occurs more often in males than in females. The most common cause in males is laceration by an instrument. It can also occur from straddle injuries or self-inflicted foreign bodies. The most common cause in females is laceration by obstetrical forceps.

Symptoms of injury to the urethra are extreme difficulty in voiding and pain upon voiding. In males there will also be swelling and discoloration of the scrotum and penis due to extravasation of urine. In either sex urinary retention may be partial or complete, depending on whether the severance was complete or incomplete. If complete, the patient will be unable to void and will have a distended bladder. If incomplete the patient will be able to void but swelling will follow due to urinary infiltration of the periurethral tissues. In either case, one or more masses caused by tissue infiltration may be felt suprapubically or perineally. Measures are taken to relieve urinary retention and locate the site of injury. In the presence of urinary retention, catheterization is attempted and difficulty or inability to pass a catheter may indicate the extent of urethral injury. A rectal examination is done to detect displaced or boggy masses of blood or urine. Usually urethrography and cystography are performed.

The aims of treatment are to restore continuity of the urethra, divert the urinary stream proximal to the injury, and incise and drain urinary extravasate. Continuity of the urethra may be restored by use of a splinting catheter alone; if the catheter cannot be passed surgical intervention is essential to relieve the pressure of urine upon the kidney. During surgery a suprapubic catheter is inserted to divert the urine proximal to the injury. An end-to-end anastomosis of the urethra may be made at this time. Tissue drainage may be necessary and a drainage tube may remain in place for 7 to 10 days.

Definitive repair of the urethra may not be possible until many weeks after the injury because of the associated injuries. If this is so, the urinary diversion alone will be carried out. The longer definitive treatment is delayed, the more likely will be scar tissue formation at the site of injury and complete recovery will be impossible. With any type of injury, recovery is usually not complete and dilatation of the urethra must be continued throughout the patient's life. Treatment is similar to that of stricture.

Nursing care should be directed at preventing further trauma to the urethra in the form of either injury or infection, and for this good catheter care is mandatory. Care should be taken that catheters and drain tubes are not pulled out, as their reinsertion may necessitate further surgery. Traction may be applied to the catheter to aid in drawing the two ends of the urethra together, and the proper amount of tension must be exerted. The patient should be taught that stricture formation almost inevitably follows trauma to the urethra, so dilatation will always be necessary. He may be taught how to perform this himself. Extensive damage to the male urethra may cause impotence and impaired micturition for the remainder of life, and the nurse may be called upon to help the patient deal with the emotional problems.

Fistulas

Fistulas of the urinary tract are named according to the viscus or organ involved. They may communicate with the skin or intestinal tract or female genital organs.

Fistulas of the urinary tract generally arise secondary to a disease process. Appendiceal abscess, regional enteritis, and cancer of the cervix, uterus, or rectum are examples of diseases of structures adjacent to the urinary tract which may contribute to fistula formation. Fistula formation originating in the urinary tract suggests the presence of an obstruction, a foreign body, tuberculosis, or a neoplasm distal to the site of the fistula. In the presence of these conditions, the involved tissue is traumatized and subjected to perforation, and extravasation of urine usually occurs with rupture. If this urine is not drained, infection develops followed by tissue necrosis, and this eventuates in fistula formation. A fistula may also result from trauma induced physically, surgically, obstetrically, or radiologically.

The signs and symptoms depend on the area of fistulization. If the communication is to the intestinal tract, the urine is infected promptly and a mixture of urine, gas, and feces is passed intermittently or continuously through the urethra or rectum. Frequently the patient complains of changes in bladder and bowel habits. Fistulas that communicate with female genital organs are likely to leak urine into the vagina and this constant leakage is distressing to the patient. Fistulas communicating with the skin produce skin irritation and odors that are very annoying.

X-ray studies are extremely helpful in diagnosing and locating fistulas. A radiopaque substance is injected into one or both sides of the fistula, the reason being that if there is a connection between these two systems the dye will pass through the fistula from one system to the other. Fistulas communicating with the skin are usually located by subcutaneous injection of the dye into the fistula and observation of its excretion.

Treatment of fistulas depends on their size, location, accessibility, and cause. In the case of those originating in the urinary tract, the underlying obstruction must be detected and removed. Seldom will the fistula close permanently unless the obstruction is removed, but once the obstruction has been removed the fistula usually will heal spontaneously. Antibiotic therapy is not curative unless the obstruction is removed. When the fistula develops secondary to diseases of the intestinal or female genital tract, the treatment depends on the extent and cause of the primary disease process. Intestinal and urinary diversion may be necessary, and the diversion may or may not be permanent. When the fistula results from gynecologic disease simple curettage, excision, and repair of the fistulous opening may suffice. Injuries from surgical trauma will heal spontaneously provided there is adequate urinary drainage and the amount of tissue removed or devitalized was not large. The exception to this is injury caused by radiation. Fistulas developing following radiation therapy for cancer do not heal as readily because of the avascularity of the tissue. Urinary diversion may be necessary temporarily to promote healing. Should infection supervene, surgical repair is difficult and often fails. Most fistulas caused by surgical or obstetrical insult necessitate surgical repair, which is usually postponed for several months to allow for some tissue recovery.

Long-standing fistulas usually are treated by one method or a combination of methods, but cure is assured only after the primary disorder is corrected. Cure is difficult because repeated procedures increase local tissue damage, and recurrence is common as is stricture formation at the fistula site.

Because normal patterns of elimination must be altered in the presence of a urinary fistula, many psychological problems arise. These assume great importance in nursing care. Passing gas and feces per urethra is annoying and anxiety-producing to the patient. Uncontrollable leakage of urine from the vagina may be so embarrassing that the patient may withdraw from people and be afraid to socialize. Another factor is the chronicity of the condition. The patient may have to undergo long periods of hospitalization and frequent surgery. Surgical repair of fistulas often fails and leaves the patient discouraged and depressed. The nurse can encourage him to adjust to his condition.

Preoperative care for fistula repair involves surgical preparation of both sides of the communication. Postoperative care involves catheter drainage and administration of antiseptics. Irrigation is not carried out routinely since the suture line may rupture from the pressure of the irrigating solution. Following surgery on a vesical fistula, the catheter should never be clamped because one episode of vesical distention will mean certain failure. Urinary antiseptics are given to control any infection that may be present. Drains and packing may or may not be used, but when they are used proper care should be taken to prevent them from falling out.

Bibliography

Books

A Cancer Source Book for Nurses. American Cancer Society, Inc. New York, 1963.

Beeson, Paul B. and Walsh McDermott (Eds.): Cecil and Loeb's *Textbook of Medicine,* 11th ed. Philadelphia: W. B. Saunders Company, 1963.

Beland, Irene L.: *Clinical Nursing.* New York: The Macmillan Company, 1965.

Campbell, Meridith (Ed.): *Urology,* 2d ed, Vols. I, II, and III. Philadelphia: W. B. Saunders Company, 1963.

Coleman, Doris: A Study to Determine the Understandings and Skills Necessary for Developing a Plan of Comprehensive Nursing Care for the Patient Treated by Hemodialysis with the Artificial Kidney. Unpublished Master's thesis. Boulder: The University of Colorado, 1959.

Creevy, C. D.: *Outline of Urology.* New York: McGraw-Hill Book Company, 1964.

Nosk, Yukihiko: *The Artificial Kidney.* St. Louis: The C. V. Mosby Company, 1969.

Pitts, Robert: *Physiology of the Kidneys and Body Fluids.* Chicago: Year Book Medical Publishers, Inc., 1968.

Sawyer, Janet R.: *Nursing Care of Patients with Urologic Diseases.* St. Louis: The C. V. Mosby Company, 1963.

Schwartz, Seymour: *Principles of Surgery.* New York: McGraw-Hill Book Company, 1969.

Smith, Donald R.: *General Urology.* Los Altos: Lange Medical Publications, 1969.

Straus, Maurice B. and Louis G. Welt (Eds.): *Diseases of the Kidney.* Boston: Little, Brown and Company, 1963.

White, Abraham G.: *Clinical Disturbances of Renal Function.* Philadelphia: W. B. Saunders Company, 1961.

Winter, Chester C.: *Correctable Renal Hypertension.* Philadelphia: Lea and Febiger, 1964.

Articles

Berman, Henry: The Diagnosis of Lower Urinary Tract Obstruction. *Journal-Lancet,* 83:219–226, June, 1963.

Blackard, Clyde E.: Genitourinary Injuries. *Journal-Lancet,* 83:140–152, April, 1963.

Dodson, Austin I.: Urethra Caruncle, Gonorrheal Infection, and Stricture, *Postgraduate Medicine,* 33:423–426, May, 1963.

Farr, Robert C. and David Falk: Traumatic Rupture of the Urinary Bladder. *American Surgeon,* 29:737–739, October, 1963.

Marshall, J. C.: Injuries to the Urinary Tract. *Journal Louisana State Medical Society,* 115:130–135, April, 1963.

Walsh, Michael Adrian, Marion Ebner, and Joseph William Casey: Neo-Bladder. *American Journal of Nursing,* 63:107–110, April, 1963.

CHAPTER 25
THE PATIENT WITH GASTROINTESTINAL DISEASE

SECTION 1
DISORDERS
OF THE
LIVER,
PANCREAS,
AND
GALLBLADDER

GLADYS E. SORENSEN

Disorders of the Liver

Rather than attempt to discuss every disease of the liver, this chapter presents broad groupings that will provide guidelines for the nurse in caring for patients with disorders of the liver. The two major hepatic diseases are hepatitis and cirrhosis. Briefer discussions of neoplasms and vascular conditions are presented. These are representative of the kinds of problems patients have which involve the liver and therefore are the ones the nurse needs to understand. To deal with liver diseases occurring less frequently, the nurse will have to study these as the need arises in her care of patients.

Understanding of the normal function of the liver is vital to recognizing presenting signs and symptoms, understanding patient reaction, understanding and supporting the physician's plan of care, and developing a nursing care plan. Briefly, by way of review of physiology, the liver might be thought of as one of the most important organs of the body. Its functions include, among many, regulation of glucose, manufacture of bile, which is essential for fat digestion, regulation of amino acids, absorption of bilirubin from the blood and its excretion into the bile, detoxification by removal of wastes and poisons, ability to act as a blood reservoir, reduction and conjugation of adrenal and gonadal steroid hormone, and formation of prothrombin to aid in clotting of blood.

Blood coming to the liver from the intestines via the portal vein may contain, after a meal, almost double the normal amount of glucose. The liver removes the excess glucose before it reaches the general circulation and keeps blood glucose from rising above 120 to 130 mg per 100 ml of blood. Glucose is converted to glycogen and stored in the liver. When the blood glucose level falls, glycogen is converted back into glucose and transferred to the blood to meet the needs of the body.

Fat metabolism and utilization are also controlled by the liver. Bile, which is necessary for emulsification of fats in the small intestine so that they can be absorbed, is manufactured in the liver. The liver also stores fat and converts fat into substances that can be used elsewhere in the body.

The liver helps regulate amino acids in much the same fashion as it does glucose. When the concentration of amino acids is high, some of them are absorbed into liver cells and stored until there is a lower than normal concentration in the blood and they pass back into the bloodstream for use where needed. This is possible because the endothelium of the hepatic sinuses is permeable to blood proteins (Guyton).

At times of diminished carbohydrates in the cells and decreased blood sugar, gluconeogenesis occurs. This is the formation of glucose from amino acids and the glycerol portion of fat. Gluconeogenesis occurs in the liver with the aid of glucocorticoids from the adrenal cortex.

Kupffer cells lining the liver sinusoids are a part of the reticuloendothelial system which aids in removal of bacteria and toxins from the bloodstream. Bacteria are picked up from the intestines as blood flows through the intestinal capillaries. The intestinal veins empty into the portal vein and all blood from the intestines passes by the Kupffer cells. Bacteria pass into the Kupffer cells where they are digested. Very few if any bacteria get by these cells into the general circulation. Certain toxins and drugs are also removed from the body as blood flows through the liver.

The ability of the liver to function as a blood reservoir can be of value in times of both excess blood volume and diminished blood volume. The venous sinuses of the liver can expand and contract manyfold. The liver can hold as much as 1,000 ml of blood or as little as a few hundred (Guyton).

Prothrombin and several other clotting factors are formed in the liver and are among the substances essential for clotting of blood. Liver disease that prevents or depresses formation of these substances can lead to bleeding. Vitamin K is essential for blood clotting. If liver disease causes lack of bile in the intestinal tract, the fat-soluble vitamin K cannot be absorbed, since lack of bile prevents fat digestion and absorption. Thus the liver may affect blood clotting in two ways.

The adrenal steroids are deactivated in the liver and are eventually excreted in the feces and urine. Likewise, the gonadal steroid hormone testosterone is converted by the liver and excreted in the urine. Estrogen is also metabolized in the liver and the major portion of it is lost in the urine. In diminished liver function, activity of estrogen in the body is increased.

Disease of the liver may give indication of any or all of these functions being affected, and thus alterations in function provide guidelines for the physician's diagnosis, determining severity of disease, and the progress of the disease as well as guides to nursing care.

VIRAL HEPATITIS

Acute inflammation of the liver is called *hepatitis.* Most commonly thought of is the inflammation caused by viruses. Other organisms (such as streptococci, gonococci, *E. coli,* and salmonellae), drugs, and chemical substances can produce inflammation of the liver.

Etiology

Viral hepatitis may be caused by two viruses—the virus of infectious hepatitis or epidemic hepatitis, known as *IH* or *virus A,* and the virus of serum hepatitis, known as *SH* or *virus B.* The clinical picture produced in the patient is essentially the same for both.

The IH virus has been found in blood, urine, and feces and may be transmitted to man by either the oral or the parenteral route. Its incubation period is 2 to 6 weeks. The SH virus has been found in blood only and is thus transmitted by the parenteral route. The incubation period is 6 weeks to 6 months. Both viruses may be found in asymptomatic carriers. One attack of hepatitis usually confers immunity against the specific virus for a period of about 2 years (Harrison).

Infectious hepatitis may occur sporadically or in epidemic forms. Crowding under unsanitary conditions such as exist during wartime or in summer camps, disasters that contaminate the water supply, and similar conditions lead to infection through the oral route. The virus may also be transmitted by blood transfusions or by improperly cleaned and sterilized syringes, needles, and surgical instruments.

Serum hepatitis is transmitted chiefly by pooled plasma or blood transfusions. As with IH, syringes or needles, dental instruments, or surgical equipment that have been contaminated from previous use may also transmit the virus.

Prevention

Prevention of viral hepatitis may be aided by use of disposable syringes and needles, taking care to avoid anyone's accidentally being pricked by the needle. Laboratory personnel should always be made aware of the patient's diagnosis. Proper cleansing and sterilizing of dental and surgical instruments are also of prime importance.

Specific to IH is the care of patients' excreta. In the hospital situation the patient is frequently on intestinal isolation to protect other patients and personnel. The nurse needs to teach the patient about the presence of virus in his stool and measures of cleanliness to prevent self-reinfection or spread to others. Discarding the patient's excreta in the regular bedpan hopper is a safe method of disposal. Linens as well as bedpans should receive special handling as they may have become contaminated with the patient's stools.

According to Iber (Harrison) the clinical disease will develop in one-tenth of persons living in the same household as a hepatitis patient. Exposed individuals may be passively immunized by gamma globulin in a dose of 0.01 ml per pound of body weight for IH. The gamma globulin only suppresses the clinical manifestations and does not prevent infection or confer subsequent immunity. SH clinical symptoms can also be suppressed with two doses of 10 ml each of gamma globulin given a month apart. There is no evidence that the gamma globulin causes attenuation of the disease once it is present or that it prevents chronic hepatitis.

Pathology

The hepatitis virus causes necrosis of the parenchymal cells throughout the liver. In addition, proliferation and swelling of the reticuloendothelium and infiltration of the sinusoids and portal triads by monocytes, eosinophils, plasma cells, and lymphocytes occur producing hepatomegaly. The reticulum fibers are preserved and regenerating liver cells grow from the reticulum to form new columns of cells. If no regeneration occurs the sinusoids collapse and the reticular fibers fuse to form collagen with a resulting cirrhosis (Boyd).

In acute fulminating cases every parenchymal cell may become necrotic and death of the individual can occur 8 to 10 days after symptoms appear. The liver loses weight and is soft, and the capsule has a wrinkled appearance due to rapid shrinkage. The liver becomes bile-stained and yellow. This condition used to be known as *acute yellow atrophy.*

In uncomplicated viral hepatitis the inflammation eventually subsides. In some patients there may be a residual fibrosis in the portal zone. It may take up to 4 months for the individual to fully recover from viral hepatitis. The mortality for viral hepatitis is low; 0.1 to 0.4 percent of patients succumb in first few months (Boyd).

Clinical Manifestations

Early signs and symptoms may include general malaise and gastrointestinal symptoms for a few days to 2 weeks preceding the appearance of jaundice. In some persons the onset is abrupt with fatigue, anorexia, and remittent fever. In addition, there may be nausea, vomiting, indigestion, dull aching epigastric or upper right quadrant pain, headache, pain on moving the eyes, arthralgia, and myalgia (Harrison). In severe infection fever may be high with chilly sensations. There may be marked abdominal tenderness and spasm. The liver may be slightly enlarged, and splenomegaly and palpable lymph nodes may be present.

Damage to liver cells prevents bilirubin from being absorbed from the blood and jaundice or icterus of skin and sclera results because of large quantities of bilirubin diffusing into the tissues. The excess bilirubin in the plasma is also excreted by the kidneys and the urine is dark amber in color. Fever and other preicteric symptoms may become less severe, though the jaundice increases. Jaundice reaches its maximum in about 2 weeks and gradually clears in 1 to 6 weeks. The intensity of the jaundice gives some evidence of the extent of liver damage, though jaundice may be minimal in severe cases. In a few instances of viral hepatitis the patient never becomes jaundiced. The patient needs to be cautioned that disappearance of jaundice does not mean he is well. The liver may still be enlarged and tender, and the lesions are not completely healed. Too much activity too early may produce a relapse. The posticteric phase may last 2 to 6 weeks, and complete recovery usually occurs within 4 months. Jaundice has been presented in greater detail in Part IV and will not be discussed further in this chapter.

Laboratory studies show bilirubin in the urine and in the serum. The phenolsulfonphthalein test (Bromsulphalein [BSP]) gives evidence of increased retention of the dye with return to normal when healing is complete. Other tests of liver function also are abnormal; these are discussed later. Results of these tests apprise the health team members of the damage still present even though the patient may feel quite well and the jaundice has subsided.

A subacute form of hepatitis can occur. The manifestations vary according to the amount of necrosis and amount of healing and regeneration. Relapses are common. Postnecrotic scarring and cirrhosis develop which can lead to protal hypertension. The subacute form may become progressive, terminating in hepatic failure and death.

TOXIC HEPATITIS

Certain substances, such as carbon tetrachloride, mercury, and phosphorus, as well as some drugs, such as cincophen, arsphenamine, and the sulfonamides, are toxic to the liver. The effects are related to the amount of toxin and length of time over which the toxin acts. These agents damage the liver by causing parenchymal degeneration which may vary from simple swelling to acute necrosis. If the amount of toxin the patient is exposed to is not very great and the drug or toxin is no longer available, healing may occur. In severe cases cirrhosis may result.

The symptoms are similar to those of acute viral hepatitis with anorexia, nausea, and vomiting, as well as hepatomegaly and jaundice. Considerable liver damage may occur without jaundice.

Kidney damage and gastrointestinal irritation may also be present, as may other symptoms of drug hypersensitivity such as rash, fever, lymphadenopathy, and hematopoietic injury. Recovery is usually more rapid than with viral hepatitis.

There is another reaction to drug sensitivity which also occurs in some persons.

This reaction is due to drugs such as chlorpromazine and some of the oral anti-diabetic drugs, and produces bile stasis and bile thrombi but little or no change in parenchymal cells. With the advent of many new drugs it is possible that this type of hepatitis may be seen with increasing frequency.

Determining the exact cause of hepatitis is important to the treatment of the patient. Whether the cause be a virus, bacteria, or a toxic substance, the physician needs to determine the cause, since treatment at least in part is based on cause.

Medical Treatment

The physician's aim of treatment is to remove the cause, minimize the harmful effects to the liver, encourage healing and regeneration, and prevent death of the patient with a minimum number of liver cells (Harrison).

There is no known drug that is specific for the virus causing hepatitis. Adreno-cortical steroids have been known to produce what appears to be dramatic improvement, but they do not actually shorten the course of the disease, and relapse is frequent following their withdrawal. Steroid therapy is not used in uncomplicated cases.

If sedation is needed for restlessness, short-acting barbiturates may be safer to use than long-acting ones, since metabolism of drugs is altered in liver damage.

Rest has been found valuable in minimizing the effects of hepatitis. The patient is kept in bed until symptoms have subsided. Should there be a recurrence of symptoms when more activity is allowed, bed rest should be reinstituted.

Adequate diet is also essential to minimize effects of disease and to encourage healing. Whether or not a diet extremely high in protein is necessary is not known for certain, but studies have shown that 70 to 100 g of protein per day is adequate, and if no contraindication exists protein may be increased to 200 g a day (Harrison). Wohl and Goodhart state that diets containing ample protein often improve the healing tendency in liver disease. They state further that optimal dietary intake has been shown to shorten convalescence slightly. The amount of fat in the diet need not be restricted unless it causes flatulence or other digestive disturbances. One dietary restriction to be observed, however, is in regard to ingestion of alcohol. Alcohol has been shown to cause a relapse or to prolong convalescence. It would appear that the patient benefits most from a regular, well-balanced diet, which should be initiated as early as possible. He may find such a diet easier to tolerate if it is given in frequent small feedings rather than three large meals a day. Some patients complain that large meals tend to make them feel nauseated (Wohl and Goodhart). Patients bothered by anorexia and nausea may be able to tolerate a liquid formula in small amounts. In the early stages, if the patient is nauseated and vomits, intravenous solutions of glucose may be utilized to which sodium, potassium, and chloride may be added. The above measures will support the patient who has a minimum number of functioning liver cells, until regeneration can occur.

In treating patients with toxic hepatitis, attention must also be given to renal complications, which may be more marked than liver damage. In these cases it may be necessary to regulate fluids and electrolytes, restrict protein intake in order to reduce nitrogen retention, and provide sufficient carbohydrates and fats in order to minimize protein catabolism.

Nursing Care

Observation of changes in patient status and reporting these to the physician are a nursing responsibility. This includes noting jaundice, pruritus, color of urine and stool, restlessness, or increase or decrease in any of the other manifestations described earlier.

As in other acute illnesses, the nurse's calmness, gentleness, and understanding contribute to the patient's well-being. In addition to hygiene and comfort measures which are a part of the care of all patients, a few items are specific to the care of the patient with hepatitis.

Disposal of stool and needles and syringes to prevent spread of infection has already been discussed.

The aims of nursing care are based on the physician's aims and relate to minimizing the effects of inflammation. This is achieved through carrying out the orders for bed rest. The patient may not feel the need for rest in later stages of illness and will need explanation of its importance. Studies have shown that activity within the hospital unit for young, previously healthy individuals may not produce exacerbations, whereas greater activity, i.e., activity outside the hospital, may. When the patient is restless because he is restricted to bed the nurse may check with the physician to learn whether activity within the unit may be allowed. However, for most patients bed rest is important in preventing complications of hepatic necrosis. In the chronic phase the physician will probably allow more activity to prevent the problems that can arise from prolonged bed rest. The nurse will need to encourage ambulation as it is allowed.

Diet of the prescribed type is important to recovery. In a few instances tube feedings may be ordered either as the entire diet for a time or as a supplement to meals if the patient is not eating well. The comfort and safety of the patient receiving tube feedings were discussed earlier. According to Wohl and Goodhart, eating hard candy between meals in order to increase the carbohydrate intake is a poor practice because the candy decreases the appetite and provides too many calories of the wrong kind. The nurse should see that small, well-balanced meals are served and can discuss a plan for this with the patient and the dietitian. All the suggestions presented in Chapter 19 regarding nutrition and feeding should be employed by the nurse. Intravenous fluids are administered as ordered and nursing observations and measures taken to assure their continuance and proper timing.

CIRRHOSIS

Cirrhosis is a chronic progressive disease of the liver characterized by extensive degeneration of the liver with disorganized regeneration in relationship to blood and lymph vessels and bile ducts, and with fibrosis that distorts the normal lobular architecture of the liver. The lobules become irregular in size and shape, some being greatly enlarged and others very small.

Because of irregular, disorganized regeneration some parts of the liver do not receive an adequate blood supply. The resulting poor nutrition and hypoxia cause further cell destruction and prevent regeneration.

Authorities have classified cirrhosis in a number of ways. Boyd classifies cirrhosis as portal and biliary, subdividing portal cirrhosis into nutritional, posthepatic, and postnecrotic causes, and subdividing biliary cirrhosis into intrahepatic and extra-hepatic causes. Others classify cirrhosis as (1) alcoholic, nutritional, or Laennec's, (2) postnecrotic, and (3) biliary (Harrison; Beeson and McDermott).

In this discussion cirrhosis will be presented in fairly general terms and major differences among types will be pointed out. Further information may be found in a medical textbook.

In nutritional or Laennec's cirrhosis there may be no clinical manifestations until long after extensive liver damage has occurred. The onset may or may not be insidious. There is a period of fatigue, indigestion, flatulence, diarrhea, anorexia, nausea, vomiting, and abdominal pain. The exact cause of these symptoms is unknown. As the disease progresses, there is evidence of portal hypertension and hepatocellular failure and eventually of hepatic coma.

If the functions of the liver are kept in mind it is fairly easy to see what is happening as failure occurs: jaundice, testicular atrophy, impotence, gynecomastia, loss of body hair, nasal bleeding or bleeding into the skin, ascites, and other dis-turbances in fluids and electrolytes. Fetor hepaticus, a characteristic odor, may be present about the patient and on the breath due to an amine in the urine. This is caused by failure of the liver to deaminate amino acids from the intestine. Spider nevi and palmar erythema may be present. Laboratory tests show BSP retention, decrease in serum albumin, positive cephalin-cholesterol flocculation test, and retention of direct- and indirect-reacting bilirubin. The serum glutamic oxaloacetic transaminase (SGOT) level will be elevated because of release of this enzyme from damaged live cells. Normal SGOT level is 40 units, but it may be increased many times in liver damage. There may be remittent fever due to the inflammatory process.

Portal hypertension is due to compression and destruction of the portal and hepatic veins and sinusoids by irregular nodules. This may produce edema of the lower extremities and splenomegaly. Pressure on the portal veins leads to establish-ment of collateral circulation with the systemic circulation. Varicosities may develop at areas where the two circulations communicate and may result in hemorrhoids, esophageal varices, or a ring of varicosities around the umbilicus known as *caput Medusae*.

Ascites, if present, is due to transudation of fluid through the wall of the mesen-teric vein and is also produced by reduction in serum colloid osmotic pressure and retention of electrolytes because of hormonal imbalance.

In biliary cirrhosis bile stasis causes reabsorption of bile salts in the blood, leading to pruritus and jaundice. Steatorrhea is due to the presence of free fatty acid. Xanthomatosis may be present due to high blood lipids.

Medical Treatment

The prognosis in nutritional cirrhosis is fairly good if treatment is started early. This includes abstinence from alcohol, and an adequate diet. Diet should be high in protein and calories. Supplemental vitamins may be given if the intake has been poor for some time. Sodium may be restricted in the diet if ascites and edema are present. As in hepatitis, rest is a vital part of the treatment.

Because some patients may be sensitive to drugs, the physician is cautious in prescribing any medications that might produce a drug reaction. (See discussion of Toxic Hepatitis.)

If esophageal varices are present and bleeding occurs it must be brought under control. If there is edema and ascites the patient may be placed on a low-sodium diet and given diuretics. Abdominal paracentesis may be done to relieve respiratory and abdominal distress caused by the pressure of the fluid.

Hepatic coma may develop as a complication of liver disease. It is manifested by changes in levels of consciousness ranging from lethargy to deep coma. There may be anxiety, depression or euphoria, irritability, and memory loss. Tremor of outstretched hands often is present, and there may be other motor disturbances such as blinking and grimacing. Hepatic coma is thought to be due to the presence of ammonia in the blood. Low serum potassium, hypoxia, anemia, depressant drugs, and infection are also thought to play a part. If coma is impending, potassium may be given when the potassium blood level is low. Protein is eliminated from the diet to prevent further protein from reaching the bowel, where bacterial action on nitrogenous substances from protein foods is thought to produce the ammonia that is absorbed into the blood and carried thus to the brain. Normally the liver detoxifies or removes the ammonia by formation of urea, but when damaged or diseased it cannot do so. Antibiotics are given to reduce the intestinal bacteria because of their ability to form ammonia, which is then absorbed into the blood. As the coma clears, protein should be gradually added to the diet.

In extrahepatic biliary cirrhosis surgical intervention may be necessary to relieve the obstruction. (See section on gallbladder.)

Nursing Care

As with hepatitis, diet and rest are two important features of treatment which are nursing responsibilities. The patient may feel sufficiently ill that he is ready to rest in the early stages of his illness, but diet may be problematical. Since approximately 75 percent of patients with nutritional cirrhosis have a history of alcoholism, they will probably have poor eating habits, since they have been used to drinking rather than eating. They will need help and understanding in establishing new patterns. Some will not care whether or not they do establish new habits; others will be sufficiently frightened by what is happening to them that they will be receptive to suggestion. The diet will be ordered by the physician as described in the section on Medical Treatment. The nurse's responsibility is to see that the patient receives the proper diet and encourage him to eat, since a nutritionally well-balanced diet is one of the important factors in treatment.

The patient may need psychiatric help in overcoming the problems of alcoholism. The nurse should accept the patient and not censure him because of his history of alcoholism.

As with the hepatitis patient, the patient with cirrhosis may be acutely ill, requiring the utmost in supportive care and hygienic measures. Treatment and care of the patient with jaundice are discussed elsewhere.

Tests which are often done to determine extent of liver damage are depicted in Table 25-1.

TABLE 25-1
*Frequently Performed
Tests of Liver Function*

TEST	BODY FLUID	PATIENT INVOLVEMENT	OUTCOME OR INTERPRETATION
Bromsulphalein (BSP)		Food withheld; blood taken for control. BSP given i.v. (note time); blood withdrawn in 30 min and in 1 hr	BSP ordinarily removed by liver. If liver function normal, less than 5% of dye remains 1 hr after injection. Dye retained in obstructive jaundice.
Transaminase SGOT	Blood	Blood withdrawn from vein	Injury to liver releases enzymes from liver cells into circulation. SGPT blood levels may be higher than SGOT, as liver contains more SGPT.
SGPT	Blood		Normal range—SGOT 10–40 units Normal range—SGPT 5–35 units
			Both may be above 500 units in hepatitis; seldom above 500 units in cancer.
Alkaline phosphatase	Blood	Blood withdrawn from vein	Alkaline phosphatase formed in liver and excreted in bile. In obstructive jaundice it is returned to bloodstream with bile.
			Normal range—2–4 Bodansky units
			In obstructive jaundice more than 10. In viral hepatitis may be elevated but usually not above 10 units.
Cephalin-cholesterol flocculation	Blood	Blood withdrawn from vein	In hepatic cellular damage albumin in serum produces a flocculation when mixed with an emulsion of cephalin-cholesterol and water.
			Normal range-negative to 2+.
			Increased in liver damage.
Thymol turbidity	Blood	Blood drawn from vein	In liver damage plasma proteins precipitate out when blood-serum is added to a solution of thymol. Degree of turbidity may depend on amount of liver damage.
			Normal—1–4 units.
			Increases with damage.

TEST	BODY FLUID	PATIENT INVOLVEMENT	OUTCOME OR INTERPRETATION
Urobilinogen	Urine	Save total urinary output for a 2 hr period in afternoon; maximal urobilinogen excretion occurs midafternoon to early evening	In total obstruction of bile flow no bilirubin reaches intestine to be converted to urobilinogen by bacteria. No urobilinogen to be reabsorbed into blood and thereby excreted by kidneys. Therefore in total obstructive jaundice tests for urobilinogen in urine are negative. (Exposure of urine to air causes urobilinogen to be oxidized to urobilin so specimen should be sent to laboratory as soon as it is obtained.) Normally about 4 mg urobilinogen excreted in urine in 24 hr. If liver unable to clear blood of reabsorbed urobilinogen as in some liver diseases urinary excretion of urobilinogen increases.
van den Bergh	Blood	Blood withdrawn from vein	Used to differentiate between protein-bound and soluble bilirubin in the plasma. In hemolytic jaundice an indirect reaction occurs (increased protein-bound bilirubin) and in obstructive jaundice a direct reaction occurs (increased soluble bilirubin). See section on jaundice for further explanation of this.

In addition to these tests, liver biopsy may be performed. Usually a needle biopsy is done, a special needle being inserted into the liver after the area over the site has been surgically cleansed and draped and a local anesthetic injected. The special needle removes a small piece of liver for study. Care should be taken that the specimen is labeled and sent to the laboratory.

This procedure is usually carried out with the patient in bed in his room. A sedative is ordered to be given 30 minutes before the procedure begins. The nurse is in attendance to assist the physician and to observe and support the patient. Following the procedure the patient is kept in bed and observed closely for 24 hours for signs of hemorrhage, bile peritonitis, or perforation of an abdominal viscus. The observations include being alert to pain in the biopsy area and signs of shock. The nurse reports these to the physician immediately. Blood for transfusion should be available. If any of the three complications occur the patient may be taken to the operating room for surgical repair.

Scintillation scan (*scintiscan*) or *photoscan* are other tests for disorders of the liver. The patient is given ^{131}I or dadioactive colloidal gold labeled rose bengal. Normally the liver takes up these materials homogenously showing its shape and size. In liver disease there are distortions in shape and size, since the cells cannot take up the radioactive material uniformly.

CIRRHOSIS DUE TO CONGESTIVE HEART FAILURE

A number of other conditions can cause cirrhosis, among them congestive heart failure. The increase in central venous pressure causes a persistent increase in the hepatic venous system. The liver is enlarged and tender. Atrophy, degeneration, and necrosis occur. In periods of remission of heart failure, some regeneration of liver cells may occur.

CANCER OF THE LIVER

Cancer of the liver may be either primary, that is, originating in the liver, or secondary as a result of metastasis. Men are affected by primary liver carcinoma more frequently than women. It is found more frequently in persons who have cirrhosis than in those who do not. About 60 percent of persons with cancer of the liver have or have had cirrhosis. Primary tumors may arise from either liver cells or bile ducts.

The cancer cells cause the liver to be enlarged and misshapen. Necrosis and hemorrhage in the liver may occur. The cancer may spread by direct extension to the neighboring bile ducts, peritoneum, and diaphragm and may invade the hepatic and portal veins and spread to the pancreas, lung, and bone.

Cancer is difficult to differentiate from cirrhosis in its early stages, since it too causes hepatomegaly, portal hypertension, ascites, weight loss, and fever. Gastrointestinal bleeding may be present. In some persons the first noticeable signs and symptoms may appear in the lungs or in bone. The cancer usually grows rapidly and the patient succumbs in a short time, dying from cholemia or massive blood loss.

Secondary or metastatic carcinoma of the liver often is carried to the liver by the portal vein, and seeding occurs throughout the liver. The blood supply does not keep up with cell growth. The liver is usually hard and irregular. Enlargement of the liver may be the first indication. There may be right upper quadrant pain, and fever and ascites may develop. Jaundice appears if the biliary tract becomes obstructed. Needle biopsy and scintiscans of the liver may be used as aids to diagnosis.

In both primary and secondary carcinoma the treatment is largely palliative. If the tumor is localized to one portion of the liver surgical excision may be helpful. If the tumor is discovered early and primary tumors from other sites can be removed there may be some regression of the metastatic cancer.

The mortality rate is high and patients succumb rapidly. Nursing care consists chiefly of keeping the patient as comfortable as possible. Both the patient and his family are often aware of the nearness of death, and the nurse can offer understanding and support. The patient may be comatose and unaware during the last few days of life.

TRAUMA TO THE LIVER

With more automobile accidents occurring today than did some years ago, individuals with trauma to the liver are being admitted to emergency rooms. At one time it was felt that nothing could be done for such patients. They are often in shock due to hemorrhage or from the pain caused by release of bile into the peritoneum.

Surgical repair of the liver, if done immediately, may be life-saving. Even so, the mortality rate is between 27 and 30 percent. The surgeon sutures the liver in an attempt to control bleeding and leakage of bile. Drainage to the outside is established to prevent bile from irritating the peritoneal cavity.

Nursing care is as for a patient undergoing abdominal surgery following trauma. Other injuries occurring from the accident would of course compound the nursing care.

Disorders of the Pancreas

Pancreatitis and carcinoma of the pancreas are discussed in this section. A brief review of pancreatic function will help the reader understand these disorders.

Pancreatic juice is vital to normal digestion. It contains enzymes that digest proteins, carbohydrates, and fats, chief among them trypsin and chymotrypsin for protein digestion, amylase for carbohydrate digestion, and pancreatic lipase for fat digestion.

The proteolytic enzymes do not become active until secreted into the small intestine. Here they are activated by enterokinase, an enzyme secreted by the mucosa of the small intestine when chyme comes in contact with the mucosa. Inactivation of trypsin until it reaches the duodenum is a protective mechanism, since if the trypsin were active while still in the pancreas the enzyme would digest the pancreas. Further protection against digestion of the pancreas by trypsin is provided by a trypsin inhibitor secreted by the pancreas.

The secretion from the pancreas contains sodium bicarbonate in addition to the enzymes to aid digestion.

Hydrochloric acid in the chyme causes the mucosa of the small intestine to release secretin. This hormone is absorbed into the bloodstream and carried to the pancreas where it in turn causes the pancreas to secrete quantities of a fluid containing sodium bicarbonate into the duodenum. This tends to neutralize the gastric juices in the duodenum producing two results—protecting the duodenal mucosa from acid and providing a neutral environment for the pancreatic enzymes to enhance their action.

Another hormone, pancreozymin, which also is secreted by intestinal mucosa and passes by way of the bloodstream to act on the pancreas, is secreted as a result of protein in the chyme and to a lesser extent fats and carbohydrates. Pancreozymin stimulates the pancreas to produce the digestive enzymes.

Vagal stimulation is also thought to produce secretion of the pancreas though not to the extent that pancreozymin and secretin do.

A number of factors may cause pancreatitis: infections such as mumps and scarlet fever; alcohol ingestion; obstruction of bile flow with reflux into the pancreas; obstruction of flow of pancreatic juice from pancreas; trauma; autoimmune mechanisms; some drugs (Beeson and McDermott).

Pancreatitis occurs when the enzymes produced by the pancreas escape into the interstitial tissues of the pancreas due to blockage or trauma. Blockage may be due to a stone from the biliary system blocking the ampulla of Vater. Pancreatic enzymes, unable to flow into the duodenum, are blocked in the pancreas and eventually seep into the pancreatic tissue. The trypsin inhibitor is eventually overcome and the trypsin digests the pancreatic tissue. Edema of the pancreas may occur. In a small number of cases there may be hemorrhage and necrosis. Necrotic areas may become fibrous as the inflammation subsides. Adjacent tissues may also be digested, producing a peritonitis. The peritoneal cavity may contain a fluid characteristic in nature and often described as "beef broth." Pseudocysts made up of collections of fluid and cellular debris may form. They may become quite large and cause symptoms of pressure on duodenum, stomach, or diaphragm. These cysts may need to be drained.

The disease may subside in a week or two, and there may be residual fibrosis and dysfunction of the pancreas, or there may be a steady decline due to malnutrition, since fat and protein are poorly digested and absorbed due to lack of sufficient secretion from the pancreas.

Pain and shock are the two most frequently observed symptoms. Pain is usually midline and boring through to the back, though it may be widespread. The patient often finds that sitting with his knees drawn up and his arms clasped around his abdomen offers some relief. Shock in acute hemorrhagic pancreatitis may be so great as to cause death in a few hours. The abdomen may be distended and tender, there may be a slight fever, and blood pressure may be elevated if shock has not occurred. Jaundice appears in about 25 percent of cases due to obstruction of the terminal common bile duct through an edematous pancreas. A frequent complication is pulmonary atelectasis, pneumonia, and pleural effusion. This is thought to be due to pancreatic enzymes reaching pleural fluid from exudate in the peritoneal cavity by passage through transdiaphragmatic lymph channels (Beeson and McDermott). Laboratory studies show an elevated serum amylase early in the disease as amylase passes into the veins following injury to the pancreas. Later there is a rise in serum lipase. The leukocyte count is elevated to 10,000 to 30,000 per cu mm.

Pancreatitis can simulate other acute conditions such as perforated peptic ulcer, bowel obstruction, and cholecystitis.

Medical Treatment

Since pain is an outstanding symptom, its control is of first importance. Meperidine hydrochloride (Demerol), since it does not cause spasm of the sphincter of Oddi as morphine does, is the analgesic of choice. The nurse may find that the physician has left orders for her to administer 100 to 200 mg every 4 to 6 hours. The nurse should observe the patient carefully and give the medication as needed to control pain. In prolonged severe cases sympathetic nerves may be blocked to control pain.

The physician's aim of therapy is to reduce secretions of the pancreas, avoid increase in ductal obstruction, and prevent and treat complications (Harrison). Nothing is given orally. Gastric suction is employed to control distention and the production of secretin and pancreozymin in the small intestinal mucosa. In place of food by mouth, intravenous fluids and electrolytes are given. If shock is present whole blood transfusion may be utilized. Prophylactic antibiotic therapy may be instituted, since infection of necrotic tissue and atelectasis of lungs are complications of pancreatitis. Drugs such as acetazolamide (Diamox) may be administered to interfere with the formation of pancreatic juice at the cellular level, as may anticholinergic drugs to block the parasympathetic innervation of the pancreas.

In efforts to prevent future attacks patients are often advised to eat a low-fat, high-carbohydrate diet, to eat small meals in order to avoid stimulating pancreatic secretion, and to avoid ingestion of alcohol. The exact effect of alcohol is not known, but it does seem to increase pancreatic secretion.

CHRONIC PANCREATITIS

A chronic recurring type of pancreatitis may follow an acute attack or may occur insidiously with no previous history of pancreatic disease. Early the main symptom is pain, but later in the disease metabolic disturbances such as diabetes and steatorrhea are seen.

Nausea, vomiting, chills, and jaundice may occur with the pain. With the metabolic disturbances weight loss in spite of a satisfactory intake occurs due to faulty digestion and absorption of fat. The stools become bulky, frothy, foul-smelling, and greasy-appearing.

As attacks recur and more of the pancreas becomes nonfunctioning there is deficient secretion of pancreatic juice.

Medical Treatment

The treatment is as described for prevention of attacks. The dietary intake of fat is restricted to 50 to 70 g per day, with carbohydrates increased to make up for caloric deficiency due to fat restriction. Oral pancreatic extract as replacement may be taken with meals to aid in digestion. A number of surgical measures have been tried with some degree of success: if stones or other biliary tract abnormalities are a causative factor, surgical measures may be helpful; partial pancreatectomy has been tried as a means of relieving pain if the lesion is localized; vagotomy to reduce gastric secretion; and cutting a spastic sphincter of Oddi, to increase drainage.

CANCER OF THE PANCREAS

Malignant neoplasms of the pancreas are seen more frequently in men than in women and tend to appear in individuals beyond 60 years of age. The head of the pancreas is most frequently involved. Pain and jaundice are the outstanding symptoms. Pain, which may be colicky or dull, may be felt in the upper right quadrant of the abdomen or midepigastrium radiating to the back. Weight loss, extreme distaste for food which is more than anorexia, nausea, and vomiting may occur. Bleeding into the gastrointestinal tract is manifested in bloody stools, especially if the stomach and duodenum have become involved.

Many patients with cancer of the pancreas become anxious and depressed more so than do other types of patients. Cancer of the pancreas is fatal and usually causes death very soon after symptoms appear. Surgical resection of the head of the pancreas, if this or the ampulla of Vater is the tumor site, may prolong life somewhat, but other surgical measures do not usually add to life.

NURSING CARE OF PATIENTS WITH DISORDERS OF THE PANCREAS

Nursing care of patients with diseases of the pancreas is discussed under one heading, since there are many similarities regardless of specific diagnosis. In addition to the usual nursing measures, the nurse pays particular attention to the patient's need for pain medication, since severe pain is one of the outstanding symptoms especially of pancreatitis. A careful record of amount of medication and how long it seems to offer relief will aid in understanding the specific needs of a particular patient so that orders can be adjusted if necessary.

Particular nursing care of patients with jaundice is discussed elsewhere.

As with some hepatitis patients, alcoholism may be a problem; explaining to the patient the need to refrain from alcohol may or may not be successful.

Low-fat diets are not always as palatable as they might be and this, too, represents an area where the patient and his family may need some teaching and suggestion for making diets as palatable as possible. Some authorities believe that a well-balanced normal diet is of more benefit to the patient who can tolerate fat than low-fat diet. However, the patient's diet will be prescribed by the physician.

Replacement therapy with pancreatic enzymes means that the medication must be available to the patient *at mealtimes,* since he takes it along with meals to aid in digestion. The medication may be left at the bedside, and the nurse can remind the patient to take it, if this arrangement is agreeable with the physician. This prepares the patient for continuing the therapy at home.

During the acute phase, the nurse will find that knowledge of signs and symptoms and complications will alert her as to when she should call the physician immediately regarding a patient's condition and when she can report to him at the time he is making his rounds.

Since it is believed that the patient with cancer of the pancreas is more anxious and depressed than patients with many other illnesses, supporting him in his anxiety and depression by listening to him, spending time with him, and seeing that he receives all medications and treatments as he expects them is an important part of nursing care. During this acute phase the nurse will also be involved with observing and maintaining effective gastric suction apparatus and administering and supervising the intravenous therapy.

Disorders of the Gallbladder

Persons with disease of the gallbladder or the ducts leading to and from the gallbladder, namely, the hepatic, cystic, and common ducts, will present a number of signs and symptoms that are fairly typical and will manifest challenging problems in nursing care. In assessing the patient with cholecystitis and/or cholelithiasis the nurse will observe for a number of typical manifestations.

BLOCKAGE OF HEPATIC OR COMMON DUCT

Whenever the hepatic duct or the common duct, especially at the ampulla of Vater, is blocked by a stone or several small stones or by a tumor, the bile which is secreted continuously by the liver is not able to flow into the duodenum; it tends to back up into the liver and produces obstructive jaundice or icterus. The cause of gallstones is not known. Jaundice is due to the reabsorption of bile into the bloodstream in the liver when it is prevented by blockage from reaching the intestine where it is normally excreted in intestinal contents. The bloodstream carries the bile to tissues throughout the body. Jaundice is apt to be observed first in the sclera and can progress to the point where the patient is yellow all over. In addition to the yellow color in the skin, the bile is excreted in the urine, imparting a dark amber color to it. Also, because of lack of bile in the intestinal contents, the patient's stool will be void of pigment and is described as being clay colored.

In addition, there may be an increase in bile acid concentration in tissues which may cause pruritus. Some patients will be extremely uncomfortable due to the itching. One may observe the marks where the patient has scratched himself in an attempt to relieve the itching.

Because of concern in our culture with physical appearance and our desire not to be different, some patients will be sensitive to their jaundiced appearance and will not want others to see them or want even to look at themselves in a mirror.

Bile is necessary in the digestion of fat. As fatty food reaches the duodenum bile is released from the gallbladder into the duodenum by means of a hormone, cholecystokinin, carried by the bloodstream, which is formed by the intestinal mucosa when fat is present in the duodenum. When bile is not able to reach the duodenum because of blockage of hepatic or common ducts, and fatty foods such as gravy, mayonnaise, fat meat, and butter are ingested sensations of fullness, nausea, and anorexia arise, and the patient has an intolerance for fatty foods. His abdomen may be distended; he may belch; flatulence and constipation may be present. Some patients, though still overweight, give a history of weight loss from not eating because of anorexia and nausea.

Another result of blockage of bile to the intestine is faulty absorption or lack of absorption of the fat-soluble vitamins, A, D, E, and K. Bile is needed to emulsify fat in the small intestine and to help in the absorption of fat from the intestinal tract. Without bile much fatty acid is excreted in the stool leading to a loss of fat-soluble vitamins. Vitamins A, D, and E are stored in the body for some time, but vitamin K is synthesized in the intestinal tract by certain bacteria. Since K is fat-soluble and bile salts are necessary in the intestinal tract for emulsification of fats, if this essential vitamin, which contributes to blood clotting, is to be absorbed, bile must be present. Some patients with bile duct obstruction have signs of lack of vitamin K as shown by presence of petechiae, easy bruising, etc.

Obstruction of the common or hepatic duct, if not corrected, eventually produces great damage to the liver. Inflammation of the ductal system of the liver—cholangitis—can involve a large part of the liver. With each episode of cholelithiasis causing blockage of the common or hepatic duct there is inflammation and scarring that could eventually lead to cirrhosis of the liver, as discussed in greater detail in the section on disorders of the liver. Therefore, early treatment of cholecystitis and cholelithiasis is advocated to prevent liver damage.

BLOCKAGE OF CYSTIC DUCT AND CHOLECYSTITIS AND CHOLELITHIASIS

If the block is in the cystic duct or gallbladder, bile does not back up into the liver or fail to reach the duodenum and jaundice and other signs of bile blockage do not occur. When the cystic duct is blocked, or stones block the gallbladder outlet to the cystic duct, or the sphincter of Oddi does not relax, bile present in the gallbladder cannot escape. This stasis of bile can lead to inflammation of the gallbladder. The obstruction also gives rise to further stones. If the stone is lodged in the cystic duct, dilatation of the gallbladder may occur, with inflammation and swelling developing. In 90 percent of cases of cholecystitis gallstones are present, and no bacteria are present in bile removed from the inflamed gallbladder.

When cholecystitis does not involve formation of stones, inflammation is thought to be due to chemical irritants in the bile or to bacterial invasion via the vascular or lymphatic route. The bacterium most commonly isolated from the gallbladder is *Escherichia coli;* streptococci and salmonellae have also been cultured.

Cholecystitis may be acute or chronic. There may be acute recurring attacks in the chronic type. Cholecystitis may exist alone or concomitantly with stones in the ducts (choledocholithiasis); if the latter, not only will there be signs and symptoms as already discussed in blockage of bile from the liver, but also manifestations of spasm and distention of the ducts and gallbladder. When a stone is lodged in the bile system there may be contractions or spasms with efforts to move the stone. If the stone cannot be moved, bile will accumulate behind it and cause distention of the ducts or bladder depending upon the location of the stone. This distention and spasm cause pain. This *colic,* as it is called, is an excruciating kind of pain, which usually appears in the upper right quadrant, and can be quite disabling. The pain is continuous in nature, rather than colicky. The patient often is restless and prostrated and in severe pain for as long as an hour; then the pain gradually abates leaving a residual tenderness in the right upper quadrant. The residual pain may radiate through to the right scapula and occasionally to the left upper quadrant. Biliary colic is not increased by the patient's moving about, but if he raises his right arm he may feel discomfort because of reflex spasm of the upper abdominal and lower intercostal muscles. In some instances the pain may simulate pain of myocardial insufficiency, and the physician must then make a differential diagnosis based on a number of additional factors. In this respect the nurse can be of assistance by making careful observations and keeping records and reports of patient behavior, and by noting the patient's comments both during periods of pain and in relation to his past history.

Chills, fever, and leukocytosis may accompany or precede attacks of pain.

If the nurse possesses knowledge of what is most apt to be expected in a patient who has a dysfunction of the gallbladder or a stone in the bile ducts, she can assess each patient and his problem and plan the nursing care accordingly.

MEDICAL TREATMENT

Nursing plans must dovetail with and be based, at least in part, on the physician's plan of diagnosis and care for the patient. To assist in diagnosing the patient's illness the physician orders x-ray studies. The preparation of the patient consists of the administration of an iodine-containing radiopaque dye such as iopanoic acid (Telepaque) or iodoalphonic acid (Priodax) which is excreted by the bile. The dye is given in tablet form at 2½- to 5-minute intervals with the evening meal or with water. The evening meal is limited to low-fat foods so that there will be no stimulus to gallbladder emptying and it will retain the dye-stained bile. The morning of the x-ray study an enema is given to prevent interference with visualization of the gallbladder. Breakfast is omitted, but a small amount of water, coffee, or tea may be permitted. After a series of films is made the patient is given a fatty meal; this is followed by additional films taken to determine whether or not the gallbladder is functioning, i.e., reacting to the presence of fat in the duodenum. If the gallbladder is functioning it empties the bile containing the dye that had been concentrated in the gallbladder. If the gallbladder is not visualized there has been lack of concentration of dye in the gallbladder. Lack of concentration of dye also may be due to pyloroduodenal obstruction, poor excretory liver function, or intrahepatic gallbladder obscured by liver shadow; or the patient may have vomited the dye. There may be some diarrhea following ingestion of the dye, but this usually does not interfere with absorption of dye.

If the dye cannot be administered orally or if a higher concentration of dye is desired, it can be given intravenously followed by cholangiography to outline the gallbladder and ducts. Intravenous administration of dye is also performed following cholecystectomy to diagnose the presence of stones and dilatation of the ducts. In some instances of difficult diagnosis of obstructive jaundice percutaneous transhepatic cholangiography may be utilized. In this procedure dye is injected directly into the ductal system, usually the gallbladder, with a needle under peritoneoscopic control.

Some of these studies may be done on an outpatient basis. In this case the physician or office or clinic nurse will instruct the patient regarding the taking of the dye, diet, and enema. In either event, the nurse should explain the procedure to the patient in order to reduce his apprehension about this new experience. The nurse can find out if the patient has had x-ray studies previous to this and his reaction to them. She should explain that the present study consists of a series of films taken from several angles and positions. She can explain that he may need to wait if he is an outpatient or to return to the x-ray department if he is an inpatient for a second set of films after he has eaten a meal high in fat. This explanation will help him realize that the procedure is routine and that he is not returning because something has gone wrong.

The physician will take the patient's history and perform a physical examination also, questioning the patient about attacks of gallbladder pain, family history of gallbladder trouble, color of urine and stool, and eating habits and foods that seem to cause digestive disturbances. The dietary history may reveal that greasy or fried foods or others with high fat content, as well as such vegetables as onions, cabbage, and radishes, and highly spiced foods may cause flatulence and discomfort. The physician will palpate the right upper quadrant to elicit tenderness, muscle guarding, or the presence of a mass. A white blood count and icteric index of blood and urine may be ordered. The physician will order that the patient have nothing by mouth. A nasogastric tube is connected to suction apparatus if there is distention and abdominal distress with nausea and vomiting. Medication for pain, usually Demerol, is ordered, since morphine is thought to cause constriction of the sphincter of Oddi. In some instances of severe pain morphine is given if Demerol is ineffective. Nitroglycerin may be taken sublingually to help relax the smooth muscle of the cystic duct. Intravenous fluids are administered as long as the gastric suction is necessary. When distention and nausea have subsided the nasogastric tube is clamped and the patient allowed to have water. If he remains free of distention or nausea and vomiting, the tube is removed and clear liquids are given, until he is able to tolerate a full low-fat diet.

If jaundice with pruritus appears, topical application of lotion such as calamine, or starch baths, may be ordered.

Vitamin K may be administered in the presence of jaundice. Parenteral medication as needed for nausea and vomiting may be ordered.

Surgery for removal of gallbladder or gallstones may be necessary and will be discussed later.

NURSING CARE OF PATIENT WHO DOES NOT HAVE SURGERY

Nursing plans are based on the assessment the nurse has made of the patient situation, including the physician's plan of care, taking the presenting signs and symptoms into consideration. The nursing diagnosis takes into account what was learned during the period of assessment.

Pain and itching may be the most prominent symptoms in some patients; in some nausea and anorexia may be. With others, concern over their jaundiced appearance may be of prime importance. If pain is allowed to become too severe before the analgesic narcotic is administered, more medication may be required than if it had been given earlier, and the patient may experience greater pain than is necessary or than would occur if the nurse had been alert to the beginning of pain and gave the medication early.

Nursing care for the patient receiving nothing by mouth, having nasogastric suction and intravenous fluids, is described elsewhere.

If the patient is allowed food, a dietary history can be elicited and the nurse can inform the dietitian which foods should be avoided within the diet prescribed by the physician. Final checking of trays might be done by the nurse, since frequently the kitchen personnel are not closely supervised by a dietitian in the preparation of each tray. Note is then made of the patient's reaction to his diet. If he is nauseated or anorectic it might be helpful to find out what foods might tempt him and to make the tray as attractive as possible. Diet may need to be limited in the acute phase of the disease to small amounts of carbohydrate such as fruit juices, toast, and crackers. Later solids can be added, including lean meat, fish, and white meat of chicken. The patient should be given as broad a choice as possible in selecting his diet since this may contribute to his willingness to eat. If the patient is nauseated administration of medication for nausea 30 to 60 minutes prior to meals may improve his appetite. Since the majority of patients with gallbladder disorders are overweight, a short period of little food consumption may not be detrimental to health. The nurse should, however, attempt to have the patient take fluids even if he refuses solid food. The physician should be informed if he is refusing food and fluids, in which case intravenous fluids may be ordered.

Daily skin care, especially if jaundice and pruritus are present, will be included in the plan of care. Using a minimum of soap, rinsing well, and applying a lotion such as calamine may help. Even though there is debate as to whether or not it is the deposits of bile salts in the tissues which cause the itching, administration of resins that bind bile salts has been found to relieve the itching, and if these are ordered the nurse will administer them. If antimicrobials and vitamin K have been prescribed they are given as ordered.

If fever is present vital signs should be checked every 4 hours, at least until fever subsides.

Another responsibility of the nurse is to observe the color of urine and stools, save specimens if she thinks it is necessary, and record and report any deviations from normal, or the return to normal if urine has been dark or stools clay-colored.

If the patient expresses concern over any aspect of his condition, such as the jaundice, change in color of stools or urine, or fear of pain, the nurse should be an understanding listener.

SURGICAL TREATMENT OF PATIENT WITH GALLBLADDER AND DUCT DISEASE

In some instances medical management does not suffice. Instead of stones being passed they may block either the common duct or the cystic duct. There may then be gradual and progressive dilatation of the gallbladder. The resulting inflammation of the gallbladder may cause sufficient swelling of tissue to occlude the blood vessels supplying the gallbladder, leading to infarction of the gallbladder, rupture, and bile peritonitis. On occasion very large stones have been known to erode the wall of the gallbladder; an inflammation follows and the gallbladder adheres to a loop of bowel. Surgical intervention may prevent these complications from occurring. It may be necessary to perform surgery to explore the common duct (choledochostomy) to remove stones, or to remove the gallbladder (cholecystectomy).

NURSING CARE OF PATIENT WHO HAS HAD SURGERY

In event that surgery is the treatment of choice, some additional understanding is needed by the nurse. The preoperative care, except for preparing the patient for operation, will be similar to that just described in the preceding paragraphs on nursing care of patients with gallbladder disease and in Chapter 23 on preoperative care. The area to be washed and shaved in preparation for surgery includes the chest region somewhat above the nipples and the entire abdomen down to the pubic region, as described elsewhere. The incision is usually made in the right subcostal region which means that during the early postoperative phase the patient will be reluctant to take deep breaths because of the incisional pain it causes.

In the operating room the patient will be in the supine position with some elevation of the section of the operating table at the costal margin to ensure adequate exposure of the operative site. The usual precautions are taken to protect the patient from pressure points and to maintain him in the desired position. X-ray studies are often done during or toward the end of the procedure to check on the patency of the ducts so that the nurse in the operating room works in conjunction with the x-ray technician to be certain the necessary equipment and arrangements are made.

The type of surgery carried out depends upon the patient's need. If he has cholecystitis or cancer the gallbladder may be removed (cholecystectomy); stones in the gallbladder, known as cholelithiasis, may require an incision into the gallbladder (cholecystostomy) for their removal, usually done when the patient's condition does not allow for more extensive surgery; stones in the bile duct (choledocholithiasis) may require an opening into the common bile duct for their removal (choledochostomy); or there may be a need to establish an anastomosis between the gallbladder and stomach (cholecystogastrostomy) or gallbladder and duodenum (cholecystoduodenostomy) to relieve an obstruction at the distal end of the common duct.

In cholecystectomy a drain, such as a cigarette Penrose drain or catheter, is placed in the area from which the gallbladder was removed (gallbladder bed) to prevent accumulation of fluid in the area. In choledochostomy the common bile duct and hepatic ducts are explored and any stones found are removed. The common duct is irrigated and the duodenum may be opened for visualization of the ampulla of Vater and the sphincter of Oddi. A T tube is inserted to ensure that the bile duct remains patent until the edema due to trauma has subsided in order that bile will be drained off and not back up into the liver. The T tube is fastened to the skin with a suture to keep it from slipping in and out until time for its removal. See Figure 25–1 for placement of T tube.

Postoperative nursing care includes, in addition to the general measures described in the chapter on postoperative care, observing amount and color of drainage from the T tube and/or the drain that was placed in the gallbladder bed; being certain that the tube or drain is not pulled out and does not become kinked when the patient turns or ambulates; and observing for drainage around the T tube. The T tube is not irrigated, aspirated, or clamped unless the physician so orders. Bile can be very irritating to skin tissues so the wound needs to be kept clean and dry by change of dressing as ordered by the physician. Various ointments may be applied to protect the skin. The T tube is connected to a straight drain. Height of the drainage bottle is prescribed by the physician, since height determines the pressure that must be built up in the ducts to cause the bile to drain into the tube

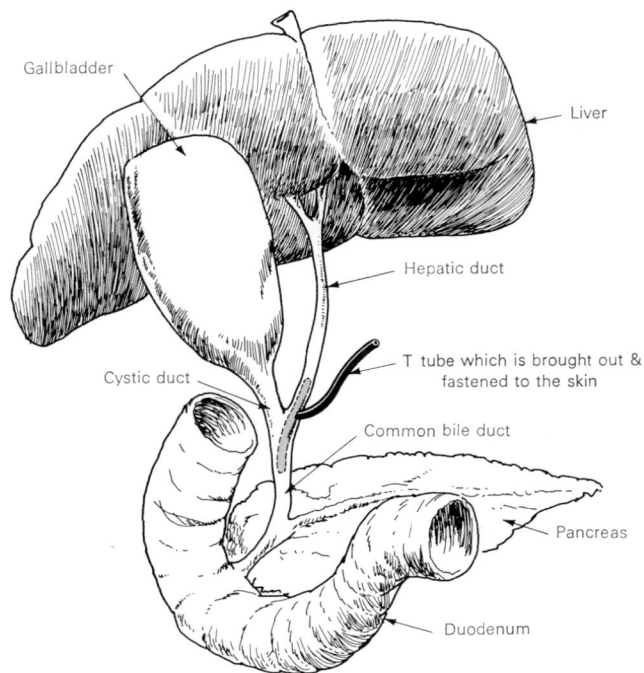

Gallbladder

Liver

Hepatic duct

T tube which is brought out & fastened to the skin

Cystic duct

Common bile duct

Pancreas

Duodenum

Figure 25-1
Placement of T tube in cholecystectomy.

leading to the drainage bottle or to continue through the common duct into the duodenum.

Following cholecystectomy or surgery on the ducts the patient is usually ambulated on the first postoperative day. If he has a T tube in place, the drainage tube and bottle are moved with him as he ambulates. Diet usually consists of clear liquids. However, the patient may have a nasogastric tube in place, in which case he will be given nothing by mouth and the usual mouth care and care of the nares will need to be carried out. In addition, there will probably be an order to irrigate the Levin tube at periodic intervals with normal saline to keep it open. Such a patient will probably be receiving intravenous fluids and the nurse will need to observe and carry out the prescribed orders in relation to the fluids and their additives. The nurse will continue to observe and report the color of stools and urine as she did in the preoperative period.

The nasogastric tube, if present, usually remains in place for approximately 48 hours. Following its removal the patient is offered a full liquid diet. If he tolerates this his diet will gradually be increased. Since bile is secreted from the liver and not the gallbladder the patient is able to function without his gallbladder as far as digestion of foods is concerned. The physician may wish the patient to remain on a low-fat diet for a time, or he may permit the patient to eat whatever he wishes and finds will not cause him any difficulty. If the patient is to remain on a low-fat diet the dietitian and the nurse can discuss the diet with the patient and the person responsible for preparing the food if this is someone other than the patient.

In a week or 10 days, if all goes well, the physician removes the Penrose drain.

There may be a small amount of drainage for a few days so that the dressing should be changed as necessary to protect the skin. The wound from which the drain was withdrawn heals over rapidly. The T tube is also clamped off in a week to 10 days to determine how well the patient tolerates closing of the tube. If no signs of any problem appear the physician withdraws the T tube 48 to 72 hours after it has been clamped.

In summary, it could be said that the factors specific to the patient with disease of the gallbladder or the ducts that would not be seen in other disorders are the specific pain due to spasms and dilatation of the gallbladder and the ducts, abdominal distress and the need for a low-fat diet, jaundice and pruritus with their accompanying problems, and in the postoperative phase the special attention to the drain and skin around it and the T tube. In other respects much of the nursing care is similar to that for patients with many other disturbances and bears out the fact that there are commonalities in patient care regardless of diagnosis.

INCIDENCE OF GALLBLADDER DISEASE

About 500,000 persons are hospitalized in the United States each year for gallbladder disease according to statistics of the Metropolitan Life Insurance Company. About two-thirds of these are treated surgically. Mortality is low—less than 1 percent in surgery for chronic inflammation. It is higher in acute cases—2.7 percent —reflecting the presence of cardiovascular and other complications in acute cases.

Gallbladder and duct disease occurs more frequently in women than in men, with the highest incidence in women 45 to 59 years old. Three-fourths of the deaths occur in persons 65 or over, nearly half of these age 75 and over.

Women who have been pregnant seem more susceptible to the disease than nonparous females.

Cancer of the gallbladder occurs most often in the seventh decade of life and according to Sodeman is rare, being found in 0.35 percent of autopsies in the United States. It usually follows calculous cholecystitis. Since cholelithiasis is rather common and cancer of the gallbladder rare, cholecystectomy in all cases of calculi for prevention of cancer is not generally recommended.

Bibliography

Beeson, Paul B. and Walsh McDermott (Eds.): *Cecil-Loeb Textbook of Medicine,* 12th ed. Philadelphia: W. B. Saunders Company, 1967.

Best, Charles H. and Norman Taylor: *The Physiological Basis of Medical Practice.* Baltimore: The Williams & Wilkins Company, 1966.

Bielski, Mary T. and David W. Molander: Laennec's Cirrhosis. *American Journal of Nursing,* 65:82–86, August, 1965.

Boyd, William: *Textbook of Pathology.* Philadelphia: Lea & Febiger, 1961.

Davis, Loyal (Ed.): *Christopher's Textbook of Surgery,* 9th ed. Philadelphia: W. B. Saunders Company, 1964.

French, Ruth M.: *Nurse's Guide to Diagnostic Procedures.* New York: McGraw-Hill Book Company, 1967.

Ganong, William: *Review of Medical Physiology.* Los Altos: Lange Medical Publications, 1965.

Glenn, Frank: Surgical Treatment of Biliary Tract Disease. *American Journal of Nursing,* 64:88–92, May, 1964.

Glenn, Frank and Charles Frey: Reevaluation of the Treatment of Pancreatitis Associated with Biliary Tract Disease. *Annals of Surgery,* 160:4, 723–736, October, 1964.

Goodman, Louis and Alfred Gilman: *The Pharmacological Basis of Therapeutics,* 3d ed. New York: The Macmillan Company, 1965.

Guyton, Arthur C.: *Textbook of Medical Physiology,* 3d ed. Philadelphia: W. B. Saunders Company, 1966.

Harrison, T. R. (Ed.): *Principles of Internal Medicine,* 5th ed. New York: McGraw-Hill Book Company, 1966.

Henderson, Lillian M.: Nursing Care in Acute Cholecystitis. *American Journal of Nursing,* 64:93–96, May, 1964.

Hinchey, E. J., et al.: Acute Cholecystitis, *Surgery, Gynecology and Obstetrics,* 120:3, 475–480, March, 1965.

Hopps, Howard C.: *Principles of Pathology.* New York: Appleton Century Crofts, 1964.

Kimber, Diana C., et al.: *Anatomy and Physiology.* New York: The Macmillan Company, 1966.

Metropolitan Life Insurance Company: *Gall Bladder Disease Hospitalizes 500,000 a Year.* Statistical Bulletin, Vol. 46. New York, November, 1965.

Ibid.: Increase in Mortality from Cirrhosis of the Liver.

Monge, James, et al.: Radical Pancreatoduodenectomy. *Annals of Surgery,* 160:4, 711–719, October, 1964.

Sodeman, William A.: *Pathologic Physiology.* Philadelphia: W. B. Saunders Company, 1961.

Wohl, Michael G. and Robert S. Goodhart. *Modern Nutrition in Health and Disease.* Philadelphia: Lea and Febiger, 1964.

SECTION 2
OTHER DISORDERS OF THE GASTROINTESTINAL SYSTEM

PATRICIA FELTZ COHEN

Most diseases of the gastrointestinal tract can be classified as infections, neoplasms, injuries, or acquired abnormalities in structure or function. Those selected for consideration here are significant not only for their high morbidity rates or serious consequences for the patient, but also because they present problems to the nurse in either the community or in the hospital. Preventive and rehabilitative aspects of public health nursing practice will continue to grow during the next decade and should not be overlooked.

Disorders of the Mouth and Related Structures

Regardless of age, diagnosis, or severity of illness, the patient's comfort and well-being depend to a large extent upon the state of his oral hygiene. The physiological and psychosociocultural importance of having attractive, odor-free, healthy teeth and gums cannot be overestimated.

Community dental health programs are best supported by a nurse who not only is committed to the prevention, early detection, and correction of dental disease, but who is well enough informed to make a worthwhile contribution. She needs to understand normal appearance, growth, and development of the oral structures as well as pathological. In addition to emphasizing the necessity of regular, periodic dental examinations, she can recognize early signs of dental disease and refer the patient for treatment. She should facilitate the dentist's therapeutic plan by demonstrating and supervising correct dental practices between office visits. She can encourage the patient to cooperate and continue with periodontal treatment once begun.

More than merely stressing the importance of adequate nutrition to dental health, the nurse should help the patient in planning appropriate diets with consideration for his socioeconomic means and cultural preferences as well as his age, weight, and state of dentition. She should realize that persistent efforts are necessary in prophylaxis because of the addition of many refined carbohydrate products to the American diet. Besides dietary deficiencies, fatigue, tension, and injury lower the resistance of oral tissue to exogenous bacteria.

The nurse can reinforce the advice of the dentist by enthusiastically practicing good oral hygiene herself and encouraging her family, friends, and patients she cares for to do so. The most effective dentifrice is one which is used as often as necessary to keep the mouth and teeth clean of food particles and sweetened liquids. Clear water rinsing of the mouth after ingestion of any food or liquids is at least as effective as most commercial preparations. Brushing the tongue and massaging the gums should be encouraged as well as brushing the teeth.

The nurse should be familiar with the proper use and care of artificial dentures. Both partial and complete plates can be removed nightly or left in the mouth. Some people are more comfortable and sleep better with dentures continuously in place. Dentures stored for any period of time should be brushed thoroughly, then placed in a soft unbreakable plastic container filled with cool water and a 5 percent sodium bicarbonate solution to keep them fresh and to prevent warping. Slight staining may be reduced by occasionally soaking them for 20 minutes in a 5 percent solution of chlorine bleach and water. The dentures should be thoroughly rinsed before being reinserted in the mouth. Because dental plates are slippery to hold during brushing and rinsing, and because the more tightly they are held, the more forcefully they move if they fall out of the hands, it is wise to half fill the sink basin with water, which will serve as a cushion. Holding the plates near the surface of the water well below the rim of the basin and away from its sides reduces the danger of striking the faucets, the basin, or nearby objects. Over a period of years, the edges of the plates can become thin and sharp, or a tooth may break. As the thin, sharp dental plates settle down on the receded gum structures, the resulting poor fit causes rubbing which then results in sores. To prevent further difficulties the nurse should refer the patient with loose, ill-fitting, or damaged dentures to his dentist.

CARIES

Dental caries has been known since the beginning of recorded history. With advancing civilization and modern food processing, its incidence has increased to an astonishing degree. Dental caries is one of the leading causes of occupational absenteeism and a major public health problem in the United States. It affects the general health and contributes to many disease processes.

Acid-producing bacteria attack the enamel and then the dentin, but the mechanism of their action and the associated factors which contribute to caries are still incompletely understood. There is a direct and well-established correlation between the frequency and extent of ingestion of refined carbohydrate and the development of caries. Fermenting sugar produces an acid which with the acidogenic lactobacilli is maintained in contact with the tooth by a mucinous film or plaque. Within 15 to 30 minutes enamel destruction begins unless something is done to interfere with the process.

Optimum oral hygiene to reduce the bacterial count and to remove food and plaques is essential. Immediate rinsing of the mouth or brushing of the teeth after meals and all snacks should be emphasized. Teeth formed during periods of balanced and adequate nutritional states are more resistant to decay. By altering the chemical structure of the enamel, topical applications of fluoride to clean teeth surfaces have been helpful in reducing caries in children. A more practical preventive measure is fluoridation of public water supplies. A reduction of up to two-thirds in the decay rate of a given population has been shown to occur with the addition of 1 part fluoride to 1 million parts water.

INFECTIONS AND INFLAMMATIONS

Gingivitis

The most common disease of the oral tissues is gingivitis. In its initial form, only the superficial gingivae and the interdental papillae are inflamed and somewhat swollen. Slight bleeding may occur only during tooth brushing, and the patient may then refrain from frequent and careful cleansing practices, thus fostering a more unhealthy situation. The most important etiological factor in acute inflammatory or chronic degenerative gingivitis is neglected oral hygiene, which results in accumulation around the teeth of food debris, bacterial plaques, and calculus (tartar). Other possible precipitating causes include malocclusion, missing or irregular teeth, faulty dentistry, and the practice of eating soft rather than fibrous foods, which require more vigorous chewing and help to toughen the gums. If untreated, gingivitis develops into a more serious condition called *periodontitis.* As the inflammatory process continues, pockets develop between the gingivae and teeth creating areas for pus and abscess formation. In its later stages, progressive degeneration of the periodontal fibers and supporting bone structures produces loosening or loss of teeth. After age 35, people lose more teeth from periodontal disease than from all other causes. Patients should be urged to see their dentist with the first sign of "pink toothbrush" and to appreciate the necessity of professional teeth cleaning to remove calculus periodically as it develops. Early correction of dental abnormalities, gum massage provided by chewing of raw fruits and vegetables, and conscientious brushing habits can significantly reduce the incidence and development of this highly prevalent disease.

Vincent's Infection

Acute necrotizing ulcerative gingivostomatitis (shortened to ANUG) has been known as Vincent's infection for the man who first described it. Although the lesions of ANUG characteristically reveal predominant numbers of fusiform bacteria and *B. vincentii* spirochetes, these microorganisms are also continuously present in healthy mouths of adults. What is significant is the individual's lowered resistance locally or systemically which allows organisms to multiply in deteriorated gingival tissues with less efficient natural defense mechanisms. Predisposing causes include worry, excessive fatigue, poor oral hygiene, and nutritional deficiencies particularly of the water-soluble vitamins B and C. The patient complains of a sore mouth caused by pressure sensitive gingiva with eroding, necrotic lesions of the interdental papilla. The gray pseudomembranous surface sloughs easily leaving an erythematous ulceration that bleeds spontaneously. The increased saliva has a metallic taste and the mouth has a distinctively fetid odor. Anorexia, fever, and generalized malaise often accompany the above clinical manifestations.

Rest (physical and mental) and avoidance of smoking and alcoholic beverages are recommended during the acute phase. A soft, nutritious diet is important, but no special precautions are needed for the eating utensils because the condition is not easily transmitted except to other debilitated persons. Correct oral hygienic habits must be instituted to prevent recurrence of the disease, permanent destruction of gum and bone tissue, and complications such as Vincent's angina, which involves similar lesions of the tonsils and pharynx. The disease is more common in adolescents than in other age groups. The student health nurse should be alert to this disease because it develops frequently during periods of academic examinations.

Topical applications of antibiotics, such as a mixture of polymyxin, neomycin, and bacitracin, may be used after the mouth has been cleansed of all necrotic debris, calculus, and other surface irritants. Systemic antibiotics may be given. Vigorous mouth irrigations with a tepid solution of hydrogen peroxide and water or saline solutions are frequently ordered until the painful symptoms have disappeared.

Oral Candidiasis

Oral candidiasis, moniliasis, or *thrush,* as it is commonly called, is caused by a yeast-like fungus, *Candida albicans.* The nurse practicing with infants or geriatric patients in the community is most likely to encounter this condition, although it occurs in debilitated persons of all ages. Those undergoing prolonged high-dosage antibiotic regimens or corticosteroid therapy may manifest the disease because normal mouth bacteria which usually prevent fungal overgrowth have been suppressed. Antibiotic-containing troches may promote the condition and produce inflamed, painful areas on the mucosal surface sites of prolonged contact. Contaminated nipples and bottles in the care of infants and poorly cleaned, ill-fitting dentures and faulty aseptic techniques in crowded institutions in the care of the elderly contribute to transmission of candidiasis. Diagnosis is confirmed by a smear and culture of the pearly, bluish-white "milk curd" membranous lesions that dot the mucosa of the mouth and larynx. The erythematous, ulcerated regions are sore, and a yeasty halitosis may be noticed. Nystatin or amphotericin B is the agent of choice. It is given in an oral suspension or buccal tablets several times daily, held in the mouth for several minutes for direct contact with the causative organism.

Viral Infections

Common viral infections of the mouth include herpes simplex and aphthous stomatitis. They are related in that the latter is a recurrent or chronic form secondary to the initial infection of the herpes simplex virus. Incidence of the initial infection is highest in children between 2 and 5 years of age. The disease is so common that it has been estimated that more than 80 percent of 3-year-old children have antibodies in their sera indicating previous exposure. The primary condition varies in severity, is self-limiting, and runs its course in 5 to 14 days. Predisposing conditions include upper respiratory infections, excessive exposure to sunlight, food allergies, and emotional tension such as the onset of menstruation. Lip lesions are usually treated with camphorated tincture of benzoin compound or a corticosteroid cream. The pain of mouth lesions is relieved with mildly antiseptic mouthwashes or applications of viscous lidocaine. No specific antiviral therapy has been developed, but frequent recurrences of the herpetic lesions may possibly be prevented with administration of smallpox vaccine, gamma globulin, or attention to removal of known predisposing factors.

TRAUMA

Injury to the Buccal Mucosa and Tongue

Common but usually minor injuries to the buccal mucosa and tongue include those of mechanical, thermal, chemical, and radiational origin. A tabular classification of these may be studied in Table 25-2. These agents produce lacerations, abrasions, and loss of epithelium resulting in ulcerative lesions that cause inflammation and soreness. Occasionally there is hyperkeratinization or thickening of the affected tissues. White patches may form from the coagulation of protein in the superficial layer of epithelial cells. Except for radiation tissue damage, which takes longer to heal, these injuries heal spontaneously within days if the person is generally healthy and adequately nourished. Otherwise, prevention and control of secondary infection are necessary. All chronic lesions should be subjected to biopsy to detect early carcinoma.

Maxillofacial Fracture and Contusions of Soft Tissues

Of more serious consequence are those injuries to the oral structures produced by falls, fights, seizures, and accidents. Maxillofacial fractures and contusions of the soft tissues require immediate and long-term comprehensive treatment to ensure survival, to prevent complications, and to restore satisfactory function and appearance.

EMERGENCY ROOM CARE

The patient is received in the emergency room in a prone position with chin extended to facilitate breathing. Gauze pressure dressings have usually been applied directly to bleeding sites. The attending physician first examines the patient to detect obstructions to the air passage. He removes dentures, loose teeth, bone fragments, or blood clots from the pharynx and pulls the tongue forward. If the tongue has been severely lacerated, or if trauma and fractures are extensive, a tracheostomy is performed, eliminating an emergency procedure later when severe edema develops. This provides an easy access for anesthetic administration and the aspiration of secretions during critical operative and recovery periods.

Hemorrhage is controlled by direct pressure and by compression of arteries supplying the bleeding area. Blood loss is estimated and replaced as necessary, following required laboratory procedures. Plasma expanders and dextrose (5 percent) in water are administered parenterally to prevent hypovolemic shock. (See Chapters 11 and 21.)

A thorough physical examination is begun to determine the nature and extent of the injuries. Brain damage and abdominal trauma are of major concern as is chest and eye injury. The presence or absence and location of pain helps determine nerve injury. Malocclusion, asymmetry, deformity, unnatural mobility, and a clicking noise (crepitus) with jaw movement are typical clinical features of mandibular fractures, which are more common than maxillary fractures (Farmer and Lawton). Once the type, location, and severity of injuries have been determined, the patient may be medicated to relieve pain and anxiety. Meperidine hydrochloride and hydroxyzine (Vistaril) may be used in sufficient dosage to assure analgesia and relaxation without masking important neurological signs or depressing respiration unduly. Morphine and codeine may produce nausea so are not commonly used. Injuries are repaired in order of priority as judged by the physician in charge. Soft tissue injuries of the face and oral mucosa are cleansed thoroughly and examined for foreign material. Irrigations with copious amounts of normal saline are employed. Some lacerations are debrided and sutured immediately. A pressure dressing is then applied to reduce swelling, thereby preventing undue tension on the sutures which cause scarring. Lacerations of the lips and cheeks are covered with moist antibiotic or saline dressings until after the facial fractures have been reduced. To further prevent infection, the patient is given a tetanus toxoid booster injection or tetanus antitoxin after skin-testing for sensitivity. Systemic antibiotics are commonly ordered. Procaine penicillin 600,000 units and streptomycin 0.5 g intramuscularly every 12 hours have been used. If the patient is allergic to penicillin, a tetracycline is often substituted.

Roentgenograms are then taken in preparation for open or closed reduction and immobilization of facial fractures. It is necessary to have many views from various angles to adequately determine the most suitable type of fixation and appliance to be used. If both the maxilla and the mandible are fractured, the mandible is first reduced and immobilized and then acts as a guide for moving the maxilla into proper position. Teeth are held in occlusion with wires or elastic bands. The technique is called *intermaxillary fixation* and follows immobilization of the jaw bones with arch bars wired to the teeth. If the patient is edentulous, splints resembling denture plates without teeth are used for immobilization and interosseous wiring. Sometimes bone transplants from the iliac crest are used at fracture sites to facilitate healing.

The patient arrives in the recovery room with wire cutters or scissors taped to his head or neck bandage or to his person. These are used to cut the intermaxillary wires or elastic bands if the patient begins to vomit. Aspiration of vomitus and asphyxiation can thereby be prevented. The nurse must ascertain that the cutters are always in clear view and never placed on or in the bed linen or bedside stand. They are usually attached to the head of the bed until the patient is ambulatory. After that, they should be hung in a protective sheath around his neck, and he should be instructed in their use.

RECOVERY ROOM CARE

The nurse monitors the patient's vital signs when ordered and as needed until they have stabilized. She observes and reports indications of increased intracranial pressure or shock. She watches for signs of respiratory distress and has a tracheostomy tray available if needed. She positions the patient so that mouth secretions are easy to suction as necessary. The extent of injury and the nature of repair will be considered in deciding whether oral or nasal suctioning should be used. An ice glove or collar is ordered to reduce edema, bleeding, and discomfort. A nasogastric tube may have been inserted if the oral tissues have been severely injured. It is attached to low suction during the initial (acute) recovery phase in order to keep the stomach empty and to reduce likelihood of vomiting. Usually it is removed as soon as possible to alleviate nasopharyngeal irritation and the possibility of gagging.

Intake and output records kept by the nurse are carefully reviewed by the physician. Dextrose and saline in water are given intravenously with vitamins B and C until nourishment by mouth can be safely taken. Medications are also given parenterally during this time to reduce pain and restlessness and to prevent infection and nausea.

LATER ASPECTS OF CARE

When the patient is fully conscious, he is returned to the standard nursing unit. Speaking presents the first problem and in the beginning it is helpful to provide paper and several sharp pencils or a "magic slate." Soon the patient is able to speak intelligibly, and if one listens carefully there is no need for him to repeat.

It is most reassuring and satisfying to him if the same nursing personnel are re-assigned to care for him because it is then possible to develop a better understanding of his needs.

Mouth care is another extremely important facet of the nursing care plan. The patient is unable to moisten his lips with his tongue, so dryness, cracking, and crusting should be prevented with periodic applications of lubricant. Because the immobilized mouth cannot clear itself effectively, and because high-carbohydrate nutritional supplements are ordered between meals, it is imperative that the mouth be thoroughly rinsed after each feeding throughout the day. Tap water or tepid normal saline is most frequently recommended but well-diluted, mildly antiseptic commercial preparations are sometimes permitted. Irrigations given slowly under low pressure can be introduced through the available space distal to the molars, using a soft rubber catheter and Asepto syringe. Soon the patient can be taught to do this himself over a lavatory basin with a mirror. The importance of conscientious regularity must be emphasized in order to prevent caries and other infections during the long weeks that the jaws are to be kept wired.

A high-protein, high-carbohydrate liquid diet is ordered with sufficient calories to maintain optimal weight for the patient's age, sex, and body build. A patient often loses weight because he does not take the full liquid diet of 2,500 to 3,000 ml scheduled for each day. This happens sometimes because he is embarrassed to suck noisily through a straw or feed himself with a syringe in front of other people. Using a spoon with soft, semiliquid foods is laborious and time-consuming, especially when one's appetite is diminished by the sight of baby foods or other bland-colored puréed concoctions. Never is a steak so desirable! By providing privacy for the patient, by preparing an attractive tray highlighted with a cartoon or flower, by arranging for music or television during mealtime, and by other devices, the creative and considerate nurse may encourage her patient to persist in his dietary regimen.

Constipation and flatus will concern the patient. The low-bulk, high-carbo-hydrate diet along with air ingested by drinking through a straw contribute to this problem. The ambulatory patient should be encouraged to take short walks several times daily. Bulk-forming laxatives may be ordered, and prune juice can be taken as needed.

After the shock phase of his accident and hospitalization passes, the patient may begin to worry about the problems he faces during his convalescence. The memory of the unfortunate cause of his injury may disturb him, especially if family or friends were involved. Financial arrangements for his hospitalization and future treatments may present difficulties, and he may need help with insurance claims, loan applications, or compensation and unemployment benefits. He may be self-conscious and worried about his appearance and the success of treatment. Since the patient cannot readily discuss these and other worries because of his speaking problem, it is often helpful for him to write letters to family and friends. Diver-sional relaxation opportunities and occupational therapy can reduce tensions and shorten boring time lags. Another outlet is the problem-solving, wish-fulfilling effect of dreams, and the patient should not receive sleeping medications nightly which lessen this desirable activity.

Finally, the oral appliances need to be checked for satisfactory position and for potential sites of irritation. The nurse encourages the patient to keep his check-up appointments after his discharge from the hospital. Further orthodontia is sometimes required.

NEOPLASMS

Neoplasms of the oral structure may be benign or malignant.

Benign Tumors

Oral tumors are classified according to the tissue from which they form. The benign lesions most commonly seen in the oral mucosa include papilloma, lipoma, fibroma, and hemangioma (Kerr and Ash). The papilloma is a white firm lesion with little lobules. It arises from the squamous layer of epithelium. The lipoma originates from adipose tissue and in the oral region may be seen as a soft, yellowish swelling in the buccal fat pads of the cheek. The fibroma is composed of fibrous connective tissue and can be recognized as a pale, firm, often pedunculated lesion. Hemangiomas involve vascular structures and are soft reddish or bluish lesions varying in size.

Malignant Tumors

The most common malignant neoplasms are those arising from the epithelium. The squamous cell carcinoma comprises 90 percent of all oral cancer (Burket). A whitish or grayish slightly elevated lesion grows as a keratinized plaque or as a superficial ulcer. It is seen most frequently on the lower lip, but also occurs on the tongue and other oral structures. Basal cell carcinoma is also a squamous layer epithelioma.

TABLE 25–2
Some Causes of Injury to Oral Structures

TYPES OF INJURIES	COMMON CAUSES
Mechanical	Toothbrush with stiff or bent bristles Dentures with rough surfaces or extended flanges Rough teeth due to caries, calculus, or fractures Cheekbiting or gnashing of teeth habitually Food impactions (foreign body reaction) Accidents (vehicles, sports, household, rough play)
Thermal	Hot foods or liquids such as pizza pie and coffee Tobacco smoking
Chemical	Regular use of full-strength antiseptic mouthwashes Aspirin tablets or toothache "drops" and "gums" held in mouth for a period of time Tobacco chewing or smoking Spicy foods and carbonated beverages Fruit-flavored candy drops Silver nitrate or phenol applications Lemon juice in warm water or grapefruit juice
Irradiation	X-ray therapy Radium implants Sunburn
Bacterial	Poor oral hygiene and dietary habits

Its lesion may be flat or slightly elevated, scaly or ulcerated, and white or pinkish red. It is most commonly seen on the face, such as lips or cheeks.

Predisposing causes of buccal cancer include syphilitic lesions, excessive and prolonged use of tobacco—often pipes, cigars, and chewing tobacco—and other forms of irritation described in Table 25-2. For lip cancer there is a direct relationship to sun exposure over a period of years. This is especially true in such occupations as farming and sailing, and for those with fair complexions such as blonds and redheads. Leukoplakia, or "white patch," is a common and serious precancerous condition caused by chronic irritation to the oral mucosa and by some systemic states. In its early stages, the lesion is hard and leathery, but fissuring and ulceration often signal cancerous changes. Developmental factors affect the protection and susceptibility of individuals to oral cancer, because exposure to chronic irritants over a period of years does not always result in malignant neoplasms. Nevertheless, prevention of these obviously depends to a large extent upon removal of the predisposing factors, and the public health nurse can do much to assist toward education and early recognition of precancerous conditions.

Everyone should know the potentially serious danger signals of oral cancer: (1) any pain or soreness with no apparent cause; (2) any numbness or loss of feeling in any part of the mouth; (3) any unusual bleeding in the mouth; (4) any difficulty in swallowing; (5) any lump or swelling of the neck, lips, palate, or gums, whether painful or not; and (6) any sore or white patch on the lip or inside of mouth that does not heal or disappear.[1]

It is important for the nurse to realize that these conditions often exist in individuals who disregard their health and who are indifferent and poorly motivated. Some people minimize the importance of preventive dentistry, especially when the lesion is not painful or when it is one which has been present for a long time. A freshly ulcerated lesion may be attributed to having recently bitten the tongue or to another simple cause so delays before seeking definitive diagnosis and treatment are common. The cure rate for cancer of the lip is 80 to 90 percent because it is one late to metastasize. On the other hand, in cancer of the tongue the cure rate is 30 percent. For this reason, it is essential to help patients obtain medical or dental care promptly for any of the above six signs.

Disorders of the Esophagus

Congenital or acquired abnormalities, neoplasms, and trauma constitute the most common diseases of the esophagus. They are ordinarily diagnosed by endoscopy and roentgenography. Treatment involves removal of the traumatic agent, surgical correction of the defect, or symptomatic and supportive measures. The nurse who is qualified can be very helpful to the patient and physician during these procedures.

Esophagoscopy has been discussed in Chapter 7.

The patient who is to have a barium swallow and x-ray study needs only to be prepared with an explanation of the procedure and a restriction of fluids and food for several hours prior to the test. An empty stomach facilitates visualization of small lesions and reduces the possibility of regurgitation after the barium is

---

[1] American Cancer Society, California Division, and Southern California State Dental Association. *You and Oral Cancer.*

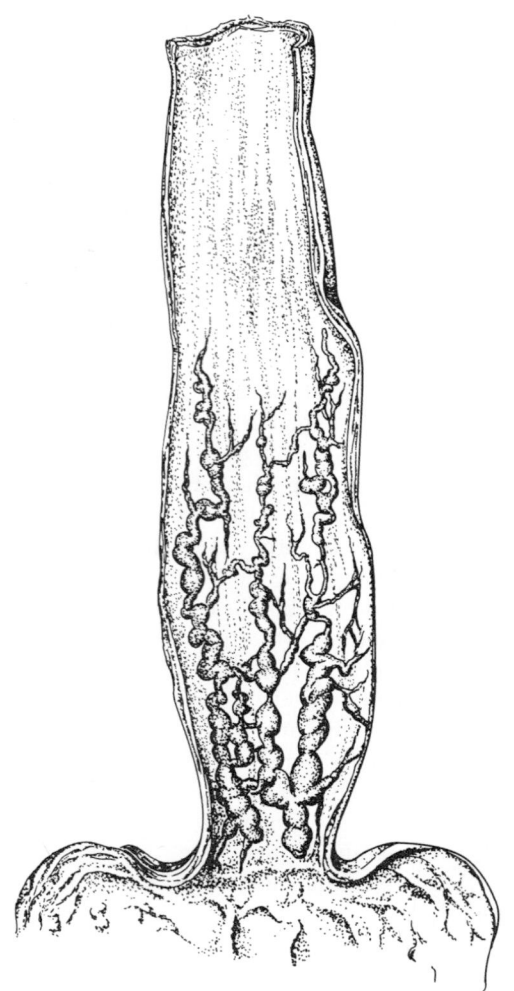

Figure 25–2
Esophageal varices.

swallowed. Following the examination, a laxative is ordered for two consecutive evenings to rid the alimentary tract of the barium. An enema may be necessary on the morning of the third day following x-ray examination.

VARICES

The submucosal veins of the lower half of the esophagus become distended and tortuous when venous obstruction has occurred in the portal system or the liver. Blood from the intestines and spleen seeks an alternate pathway to the right side of the heart. Collateral circulation through the esophageal veins and through the coronary and left gastric veins is developed.

The most frequent cause of esophageal varices is the portal hypertension resulting from Laennec's cirrhosis.

Often the varices go unrecognized until an episode of bleeding occurs, resulting in hematemesis and the passage of tarry feces. A large percentage of patients do not survive the first attack of hemorrhage and a fair portion of those who do will succumb within 5 years from another episode of exsanguination or other complications associated with progressive liver damage.

Diagnosis of esophageal varices may be confirmed in most cases by esophagoscopy, barium swallow, and splenoportography. Varices are suspected in any patient with gastrointestinal bleeding who demonstrates clinical manifestations of liver disease with impaired liver function.

Nursing Responsibilities

The coordinated efforts of a skilled medical and nursing team are required to control serious hemorrhage from ruptured varices. Replacement of blood loss, restoration of blood volume, and control of bleeding are the immediate aims of treatment. If advance notice of an impending admission is possible, the nurse may prepare for expedient and life-saving measures to facilitate patient care. At least three nursing personnel will be needed to carry out the physician's orders. One will be engaged in monitoring the patient's vital signs at least every 10 minutes during the critical first few hours. She can also help comfort the patient with explanations and a calm manner. He will be fearful for his life, alarmed at the sight of so much blood, and anxious because of the amount of equipment and numbers of people around him. Another nurse will be concerned with the administration of medications and the preparation or use of equipment and supplies for care as ordered. Someone should be available to keep the family informed and reassured, to bring additional supplies, and to requisition auxiliary services as indicated. The presence of a clergyman may be requested by the patient or his family. A laboratory technician must be on hand for periodic determinations of the hemoglobin and hematocrit levels, the prothrombin time, and the typing and cross-matching of many units of whole blood.

The patient's unit may be prepared if time permits. Plastic-covered mattresses and pillows should be used and bed linen should be protected with soft paper pads. When blood-soaked, these can be removed easily without unduly disturbing the patient. The patient will be sedated and encouraged not to move more than absolutely necessary in an attempt to stop bleeding. Oxygen via nasal catheter may be administered and ought to be quickly accessible. Venoclysis sets and infusion supplies must be ready for use. Plasma expanders and dextrose in saline or water are given intravenously until whole blood is available. Sometimes simultaneous infusions are started to ensure sufficient blood volume replacement to prevent hypovolemic shock. Vitamin K is frequently administered to patients in whom liver damage has given rise to an increase in clotting time. Sodium luminal, 120 mg, is usually given for the patient's restlessness since this drug is excreted primarily through the kidneys rather than the liver. Diphenhydramine (Benadryl HCl) may be used to control blood transfusion reactions, although this drug is known to be metabolized by the liver. Benadryl has been found to decrease gastric motility and acid secretion, and this effect makes the drug additionally useful for the patient with ruptured varices.

ESOPHAGEAL TAMPONADE

Esophageal tamponade accomplished with a Sengstaken-Blakemore tube is often necessary to control severe bleeding. As shown in Figure 25–3, this tube has two

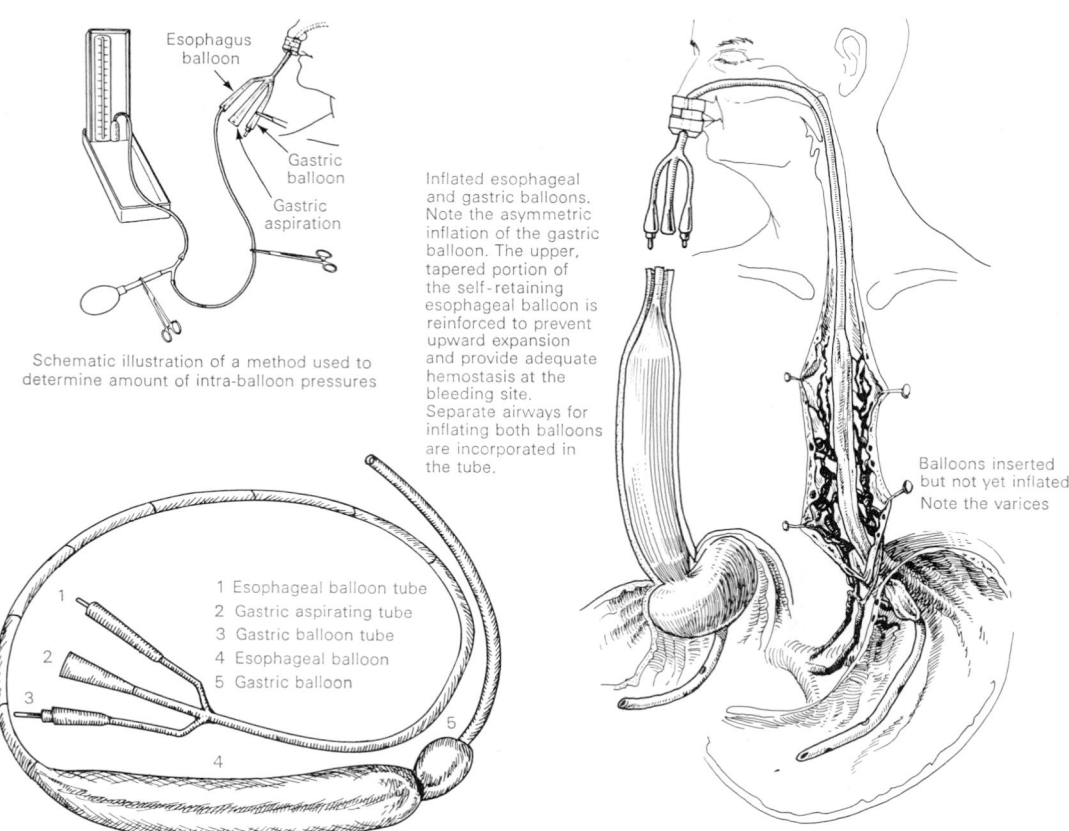

Esophagus
balloon

Gastric
balloon

Gastric
aspiration

Inflated esophageal
and gastric balloons.
Note the asymmetric
inflation of the gastric
balloon. The upper,
tapered portion of
the self-retaining
esophageal balloon is
reinforced to prevent
upward expansion
and provide adequate
hemostasis at the
bleeding site.
Separate airways for
inflating both balloons
are incorporated in
the tube.

Schematic illustration of a method used to
determine amount of intra-balloon pressures

1 Esophageal balloon tube
2 Gastric aspirating tube
3 Gastric balloon tube
4 Esophageal balloon
5 Gastric balloon

Balloons inserted
but not yet inflated
Note the varices

Figure 25-3
Esophageal tamponade
acommplished with
Sengstaken-Blakemore
tube. (By permission of
Davol Rubber Company,
Providence, R.I.)

balloons and three lumens. One lumen transmits gastric contents to a collection bottle with a suction apparatus; the other two lumens lead to gastric and esophageal balloons. These are tested for leakage by the physician or nurse before use. Instructions for passing the tube are carefully reviewed if necessary. A thin coat of water-soluble lubricant is applied to the deflated balloons and lower end of the tube. The physician usually sprays the patient's throat with a topical anesthetic. The tube is then passed through the nostril or mouth until it has reached the stomach. The numbers on the tube should be on the right side of the esophagus (which is the *patient's left* side) so that the gastric balloon will properly engage the cardiac and fundus portions of the stomach. Bleeding may occur at this site as well as from the esophagus. The gastric balloon is inflated and the tube is retracted until resistance is felt. Traction may or may not be applied to the tube in order to hold it more securely in place. The upper end of the tube is encircled with the plastic sponge cuff provided. This is held in place by an adhesive strip at the point where it emerges from the nostril or mouth. The sponge helps to protect the mucosal surfaces from irritation and injury by the tube which is left in place for several days or longer.

The esophageal balloon is then inflated to the pressure determined by the doctor. Both tubes leading to the balloon portions are clearly marked to differentiate them. Each is clamped with a rubber-tipped hemostat. A small Y tube connected to an aneroid gauge and a rubber bulb from a sphygmomanometer is attached to the balloon tubes periodically in order to measure and alter the pressure as necessary. A third rubber-tipped clamp is used to close the connecting tube to either the bulb or the gauge while the other is being used. This helps to prevent air leakage.

Next, the stomach is aspirated of air and fluids. Frequent lavaging with tepid or cool normal saline is performed to prevent clots from forming which may clog the tube. The patient will be unable to swallow saliva and so must be helped to expectorate. Gentle mouth irrigation and suctioning may be done to cleanse the mouth and remove the taste of blood. A careful intake and output record is kept. When bleeding is controlled, medications and bland high-carbohydrate liquids may be fed through the tube. Water to rinse the tube should follow each feeding. Aspiration of stomach contents should be accomplished before feeding is done to note any recurrence of bleeding or undue distention.

The patient is kept in a supine position with head lowered until his condition stabilizes. Then the head of the bed is elevated to reduce gagging and nausea. Passive exercises, changes of position, and deep breathing are instituted as soon as possible to prevent the development of hypostatic pneumonia and thrombophlebitis. Antibiotics may be given to prevent the development of infection. Skin care must take into account any jaundice, dryness, or pruritus which the patient may have as a result of his liver disease. As long as the prothrombin time is abnormal, the nurse must watch for prolonged bleeding at the sites of injections and venepuncture. She should note and report the presence of blood in the urine or feces. She should protect the patient from accidental injury by padding headboards and bed rails, and by instituting other safety measures as indicated.

When the patient's bleeding has been controlled following several days of balloon deflation, the tube is very carefully removed. A soft, bland diet with several small feedings daily is ordered. The patient is discharged with instructions and follow-up appointments to continue the medical management of his condition. Surgical control of bleeding is sometimes necessary, but usually the patient's poor condition makes this very undesirable unless it cannot be postponed. Hemostasis may be accomplished surgically by various resection procedures or by ligatures of the varices. Nursing care measures are similar to those for a patient having thoracic or abdominal surgery.

NEOPLASMS

Benign Tumors

Benign tumors of the esophagus rarely occur. They are usually asymptomatic and present no significant physical findings. Most are discovered at autopsy. If a pedunculated lesion of the upper esophagus is found through barium swallow and fluoroscopy, it is commonly removed with a wire snare and the area is cauterized.

Malignant Tumors

About 95 percent of malignant esophageal neoplasms are of the squamous cell type. Most patients first notice a slight dysphagia with ingestion of solids, because most lesions are of the stenosing type. There may be pain or epigastric distress and regurgitation of food and salivary juices. Often there is a delay between the appearance of symptoms and the diagnosis. The patient voluntarily restricts his diet to foods more easily swallowed and soon shows severe weight loss and near starvation. Perforation and fistulas may develop. The disease is rapidly fatal and the prognosis is poor because it is recognized late in the course.

The tumor may be visualized through fluoroscopy with barium swallow, but definitive diagnosis is made on the basis of a biopsy specimen. The decision regarding surgery will be based on these findings. The physician may decide upon supervoltage irradiation as a palliative measure if the tumor is inoperable. If complete blockage of the esophagus occurs, a gastrostomy may be inserted as a means of feeding the patient. If the tumor is operable, an esophagogastrectomy may be done followed by an esophagogastrostomy to reestablish gastrointestinal continuity. Other procedures may be carried out according to the patient's general status and need for palliation, however temporary.

NURSING CARE

Nursing care of the patient with esophageal cancer involves meeting the biopsycho-social needs of a person who is aged and most probably a male, who has terminal cancer, whose ingestive system is seriously disrupted, and who is having radiation therapy or palliative surgery of the thoracic and abdominal regions. Since nursing measures for most of these conditions may be found elsewhere in this text, only those pertaining to the patient who has had a gastrostomy will be discussed. Of course, the above factors will strongly influence the plan of nursing care. Post-operative orders reflect those for the usual patient with abdominal surgery. The care regimen includes observations for complications of hemorrhage, infection, and electrolyte imbalance; progressive slow ambulation as tolerated; medications as needed for pain, sleep, and elimination; dietary considerations; and the care of the gastrostomy.

Intravenous infusions of whole blood, dextrose, electrolytes, and vitamins maintain the patient's critical nutrition needs until gastrostomy feedings are permitted. Initially the gastrostomy tube is irrigated gently with 20 to 50 ml normal saline at room temperature to assure patency, to remove clots, and to detect fresh bleeding. When bowel function returns and the sites of anastomoses have healed sufficiently, tube feedings are ordered to be given every 2 hours. These may be highly nutritious commercial preparations, a special formula prescribed by the physician, or a selection of soft, bland foods which have been homogenized in a blender and then strained.

The feeding is warmed and tested for temperature before being administered. A small amount of water (30 to 60 ml) is given before and after the food formula to clear the tube. The feeding is allowed to flow in slowly by gravity. The patient should be in a sitting position. He may assist by holding the tube and pinching it as necessary to slow the flow and to prevent intake of air while additional formula is poured into the funnel attached to the tube. The tube is then clamped, after being rinsed, and covered with a gauze dressing to avoid catching on the patient's clothes. If a Martin-Pitou flange has been used at the gastrostomy site instead of a tube, then it is merely uncapped and a soft rubber tube is inserted about 2 inches for the feedings. Gastrostomy feedings will improve the patient's nutrition so at least he will not succumb from starvation. Of course, they are often unsatisfying to the patient who has relished chewing his food. Some nurses have suggested the practice of allowing the patient to chew small amounts of meat or other food and then expectorate these. The patient will prefer to do this in privacy, so he must be warned to take care to avoid accidentally swallowing since the esophagus is usually closed and choking will occur.

The patient is discharged to a convalescent nursing home or is returned to his family who will assist in his care. Visiting nurse services are available in many communities, and the cost of visits may be paid by some local cancer societies if the patient has no funds. Transportation for the patient to have radiation treatments or to be seen by the physician when necessary is also provided by the local cancer society as are dressings and sickroom supplies. Teaching of the patient and family which is begun in the hospital is reviewed and supplemented by the public health nurse. The teaching concerns usually include diet, skin care, and general health measures.

ACHALASIA

This condition, formerly misnamed *cardiospasm, is a narrowing and atrophy of the* mucosa and muscle fibers in the lower esophagus above the cardia. It is believed to be caused by a degeneration of the autonomic nerve plexus supplying the region. As a result of this neuromuscular dysfunction, there is a delayed passage of food, and its retention produces a gradually increasing dilatation of the proximal portion of the esophagus. The abnormality may occur in children, but it is more common in adults past middle age, and it affects men slightly oftener than women.

Dysphagia and epigastric discomfort associated with emotional factors, hurried eating, and bulky foods are the initial complaints. Later there is regurgitation of sour-tasting food and liquids. Diagnosis is made by fluoroscopy and x-ray examination.

Treatment with medications has been unsuccessful although antispasmodics have been tried. A low-bulk, bland diet eaten slowly in several small feedings daily will reduce severity of symptoms. The patient should sleep with his head elevated to reduce the possibility of aspiration. Periodic dilatations of the lower esophagus with bougies have helped a small percentage of patients.

DIVERTICULA

Sac-like protrusions of one or more esophageal layers are known as *diverticula*. They may be congenital or acquired. If caused by pressure from inside the esophagus, they are of the pulsion type. The mucosal sac pushes through weakened muscular layers. If pressure has come from outside the esophagus, all layers are involved and they are of the traction type. Signs and symptoms are the same as for achalasia and carcinoma, that is, difficulty in swallowing and regurgitation. The patient can smell a foul odor and taste sour food. He soon learns how to apply pressure at a point on the neck to empty the pocket of food that has collected. X-ray studies utilizing barium are diagnostic. Esophagoscopy is ordinarily contraindicated because of the danger of perforation. This abnormality is a progressive one and when symptoms become sufficiently disruptive to nutrition, corrective surgery is indicated. The sac is amputated at its junction with the esophagus. Local or general anesthesia is utilized. A gauze pack or Penrose drain may be inserted at the site of closure and

TABLE 25–3
Pathophysiology of Diverticulitis

PATHOLOGY	→ PHYSIOLOGICAL CHANGES	→ SIGNS AND SYMPTOMS
Local inflammation of diverticula	Fibrosis, narrowing of colon	Constipation, narrow stools
Granulation tissue	Bleeding, iron deficiency anemia	Blood in stools, fatigue, weakness
Pericolic abscess	Leukocytosis, development of a mass	Fever, abdominal tenderness
Perforation abscess	Peritonitis	Constant abdominal pain, distention, rigidity, loss of bowel sounds, shock, free intraperitoneal air
Vesicocolic fistula	Contamination of urine, inflammation of bladder	Pyuria, hematuria, dysuria, pneumaturia, frequency

led out through a stab wound in the neck. The nurse reinforces the external dressing to keep it clean and dry in order to prevent infection. A nasogastric tube is passed while the patient is in surgery to keep the surgical site undisturbed, to allow for postoperative decompression of the gastrointestinal tract, and for use in tube feedings before the esophagus has healed.

Esophagitis

Esophagitis, or "heartburn," is a common occurrence resulting from the chemical irritation of regurgitated gastric acid. Reflex activity may be caused by fetal displacement of the stomach during pregnancy, by hiatus hernia, or by reconstructive surgery for total gastrectomy. Ulceration of the sensitive mucosa will eventually develop. Alternate periods of healing and ulceration will result in scarring and stricture. In the later stages, esophagoscopy with biopsy is necessary to definitively differentiate esophagitis from carcinoma, although x-ray studies may be strongly suggestive. Treatment involves administration of antacids and milk. The diet should consist of several small feedings daily of bland, nonirritating foods.

Benign Strictures

Benign strictures of the esophagus are fairly common. Usually they result from ingestion of strong alkalies, acids, or phenol derivatives. Gunshot wounds, ingestion of foreign bodies, and throat lacerations may also cause stricture development. The patient's history and x-ray examination are diagnostic.

Strictures can develop weeks, months, or years after the causative trauma, hence periodic examinations and dilatations are advised. In simple chronic stricture, dilatation is accomplished with bougies passed over a previously passed thread. In severe cases, surgical excision and anastomosis is sometimes performed, or bypass procedures may be carried out. Emergency care of the person who has ingested caustics is described in Chapter 33.

Foreign Bodies

Foreign bodies may be ingested accidentally or intentionally by both children and adults. Meat bones, pins, buttons, coins, and other small objects are items frequently taken by mouth. Denture plates are sometimes dislodged and swallowed. Choking, coughing, gagging, vomiting, dysphagia, and painful discomfort are the most obvious symptoms. Roentgenography performed without barium swallow will demonstrate most opaque objects. Barium is not desirable because a perforation may have occurred and removal with forceps is made more difficult. Speedy removal is desirable, although many smooth objects will pass through the intestinal tract if they have not become lodged in the esophagus.

Spontaneous Esophageal Rupture

Spontaneous esophageal rupture occurs as a result of pressure upon a weakened wall, usually in the last 3 or 4 inches of the esophagus. Overingestion of food or alcohol often precedes the event, which may be associated with vomiting. Middle-aged men are the most frequent victims. Severe pain, shock, subcutaneous emphysema, abdominal rigidity, and pneumo- or hydrothorax mark the acute onset of esophageal perforation. Emergency surgery is carried out to repair the rupture and establish chest drainage. Restoration of blood volume, irrigation of the pleural cavity, and intensive measures to control infection are carried out.

Disorders of the Stomach

Peptic ulcer, carcinoma, and congenital pyloric stenosis constitute the most frequent pathological conditions affecting the stomach. Hiatus hernia and gastritis are troublesome problems also.

HIATUS HERNIA

Diaphragmatic hernias are classified according to two acquired structural defects. The largest proportion are of the sliding type, in which the stomach is displaced upward through an enlarged esophageal hiatus. In the rolling variety, a section of gastric wall rolls up through the diaphragm, forming a pocket alongside the esophagus. A weakening of the muscles in the diaphragm around the esophago-gastric aperture seems to predispose one to this condition. It is found most commonly in the obese and older age groups and affects women more frequently than men. The space-displacing presence of a portion of the stomach in the chest produces a cough, dyspnea, or hiccoughing episodes. Epigastric burning and fullness are commonly experienced as a result of a reflux of gastric acid and contents.

Palliative medical treatment is recommended for the patient with minor symptoms or the one who is a poor surgical risk. Alleviation can sometimes be accomplished with a weight reduction program and the elimination of tight corsets and girdles. Esophagitis may be relieved by administration of alkalies and small frequent bland low-fat feedings to promote more rapid gastric evacuation. The patient needs little reminder to avoid stooping or lying down too soon after meals. It is suggested that he wait for 3 hours. Short walks have been)recommended. Epigastric discomfort due to reflux of gastric contents increases with the size of the meal and often keeps the patient awake late into the night. Ingestion of alcohol, highly spiced, fatty or very rich foods can cause symptoms so severe that they are relieved only by self-induced vomiting. Elevation of the head of the bed helps to prevent accidental tracheal aspiration of regurgitated material while the person sleeps. Additional symptomatic relief may be obtained with prescribed sedatives and antispasmodics.

For some patients, surgical repair of the hernia may be the treatment of choice. If gastric analysis demonstrates hyperacidity, vagotomy may be done to reduce the likelihood of postoperative ulceration at the repair site.

GASTRITIS

This term has been used to describe inflammatory, erosive, atrophic, or hypertrophic tissue changes of the stomach mucosa. In acute gastritis, inflammation with ulceration and bleeding may occur as a result of chemical or mechanical irritation. Chronic gastritis, on the other hand, may cause no gastric distress but elicits symptoms associated with its cause. Treatment of acute or chronic gastritis is directed toward eliminating the cause and correcting its consequences.

CARCINOMA

In the United States, stomach cancer affects men more often than women and is the fourth leading cause of death from cancer. Morbidity rates increase significantly after age 45 and are highest in the sixth decade.

Adenocarcinoma is the most common type of gastric tumor and may occur anywhere in the stomach.

In its earliest stages, gastric carcinoma presents no symptoms. Then a persistent indigestion may be noticed but is usually self-medicated or ignored. According to the type of lesion, there may or may not be ulcer-like symptoms of intermittent epigastric distress initially relieved by ingestion of food. If so, treatment with the typical ulcer regimen produces symptomatic relief for a time. Later this is replaced by a dull, constant aching sensation in the stomach which is often aggravated by ingestion of food. The patient may complain of a distaste for meat or a loss of appetite. The symptoms of gastric hypofunction continue: nausea, vomiting, gaseous distention. Loss of weight and malnutrition follow. Incipient blood loss through slow oozing may go unrecognized by the patient. Occult blood may be found in the feces; anemia, fatigue, and weakness develop. Eventually a mass in the upper abdomen becomes palpable, back pain indicating pancreatic involvement may occur, and the patient may appear jaundiced (from liver metastases), breathless (from spread to lungs), and ascitic (from invasion of the peritoneum).

Fluoroscopy and x-ray studies, from different angles and with the patient in various positions, following ingestion of a barium meal still provide the clinician with his most important evidence. If following diagnostic studies the carcinoma is thought to be operable, the Billroth II procedure will probably be carried out.

In the Billroth II gastric resection, from 80 to 100 percent of the stomach is removed along with the adjacent lymph nodes and the gastrocolic omentum. A thoracic or abdominal approach is used, depending on the site of the lesion in the proximal or distal stomach and on other factors. The primary aim of treatment is, of course, to completely remove all malignant tissue. In those cases in which this can be accomplished and the lesion is smaller than 4 cm and has not metastasized, 5 year cure rates of from 20 to 60 percent are possible. In larger, less easily resectable lesions, the aim of treatment is to prolong life, to assure minimum suffering, and to decrease the probability of complications such as obstruction and hemorrhage.

Nursing Care

The nurse who cares for a patient with cancer of the stomach has the opportunity to help him accept his condition, to assist him toward self-care for as long as possible, and to help him maintain his patterns of living with comfort and dignity whether at home or confined to an institution. Since only half the patients have an operable lesion when first diagnosed, one of the most important things that a community health nurse can do is to increase her case-finding efforts in order to get more patients to see their physicians earlier in the course of the disease. The person over 40 years of age, the one with chronic stomach ailments, the ulcer patient who is not helped by diet and medications, the anemic one who is losing weight: these are the people to whom the nurse must direct her concentrated efforts.

For the patient who is hospitalized, the nurse can be helpful throughout diagnosis and treatment. She will have an opportunity to listen to him and to study his behavior for clues that indicate his needs. Upper and lower gastrointestinal x-ray examinations are time-consuming and exhausting to debilitated individuals and elderly ones. Patients will need repeated explanations of their necessity and of the preparation and follow-up which are required. Atonic constipation is common, so enemas until clear will probably be ordered. Mineral oil or milk of magnesia is usually given the night before x-ray examination. The patient will receive no food and fluids for at least 8 hours prior to examination and throughout the series. Laxatives and enemas following barium series are given to clear the alimentary tract and to prevent obstruction from hardened barium sulfate. If films are unsatisfactory or incomplete, the series may be repeated. The patient's right to feel annoyed and to express himself should not be denied.

Gastroscopy is an even more unpleasant experience. The presence of a sympathetic and understanding nurse can comfort the patient and facilitate his acceptance and cooperation. Usually medications that sedate and reduce secretions are given after the patient has fasted for at least 8 to 12 hours. A topical anesthetic is sprayed onto the pharyngeal membranes and a short waiting period is allowed. If the gastroscope is flexible, the patient may be asked to swallow it from a sitting position. Otherwise, a left lateral reclining position is employed for passage of the more rigid instrument. The nurse assists the patient to remain quiet during the procedure by interpreting what is happening and by telling him what to expect. She assists the physician by ascertaining the ready accessibility of what he will probably need to use. A suction machine should be in operational readiness with a container of water for clearing mucus from the suction tube. When the examination is over, she accompanies the patient to his room and provides for his comfort before carrying out other tasks. She makes sure he takes no fluid until the swallowing reflex, diminished by the local anesthetic, has returned.

Preoperative care is discussed in Chapter 21 and will not be repeated here.

Following gastric surgery, care is directed toward maintaining fluid and electrolyte balance and preventing complications. Monitoring vital signs closely and performing endotracheal suctioning of secretions as needed keeps the nurse busy during the first hour or so until the patient has recovered sufficiently to be returned to his room. She checks the nasogastric tube for patency by periodic irrigations with 30 to 60 ml of normal saline, keeping an accurate record of intake and output. These irrigations are usually ordered for every 2 hours but they may have to be done more often if the tube becomes clogged. The nasogastric tube keeps the stomach empty until peristaltic activity returns, usually by the third or fourth day. Continuous intermittent low-pressure suction helps prevent undue tension on the suture lines and detect bleeding. The nurse regulates the administration of intravenous fluids according to the physician's orders and watches to see that the tubing is not disturbed during the patient's restless movements or while he is being transported. She may administer the initial medication for pain and restlessness, if necessary, as the patient emerges from anesthesia and his vital signs begin to stabilize. The physician may order administration of a phenothiazine antiemetic such as promethazine hydrochloride (Phenergan) to reduce postoperative vomiting.

Because of the age and general condition of patients ordinarily undergoing a gastric resection for carcinoma, a number of measures are necessary to prevent cardiopulmonary complications such as atelectasis, pneumonia, and venous stasis. Frequent turning, coughing, and deep breathing are essential. Elastic bandages from foot to thigh may be ordered by the physician to support circulation in the extremities and promote venous return of the blood to the heart. Correct skin care prevents tissue breakdown and bacterial invasion. Early ambulation is usually prescribed and most patients are assisted in standing by the bed on the first postoperative day. By the third day, the patient should be able to sit in a chair for short periods and to walk in the hallway for short distances with little assistance. Of course the individual practice of the surgeon and the individual tolerance of the patient must be considered and modifications made accordingly. A chest film is usually ordered several days after surgery to detect untoward pulmonary developments.

Intravenous fluids of dextrose in saline and in water are administered for the first few days. Potassium chloride is added to maintain electrolyte balance on the basis of blood chemistry results. Vitamins B and C are added because they are water-soluble and are needed to support nutrition and wound healing, counteracting the catabolic effects of surgery. When bowel sounds can be heard, the naso-gastric tube may be clamped for from 2 to 4 hours, during which time the patient is given an ounce of water hourly. If there is no nausea, vomiting, or distention, and if at the end of the prescribed period the aspirated gastric fluid measures less than 50 ml, the tube is removed. The patient is given clear to full liquids as tolerated and then advanced to soft diet on a daily schedule of six feedings. When he goes home, he is permitted to eat whatever agrees with him as long as he takes it in regular moderate amounts rather than larger meals taken less frequently.

Micturition usually presents no problem except in the aged male with benign prostatic hypertrophy. A Foley catheter may be kept in place for a few days postoperatively, and output is measured for adequacy. A specimen may be obtained for culture and sensitivity studies when the catheter is removed to detect any infection. Urine may be tested for specific gravity a few times daily as an index of renal function and fluid balance. Intestinal flatus may be relieved by administration of an enema during which the container is alternately raised and lowered in relation to the level of the patient's buttocks (Harris flush). In this way gas may be trapped and removed along with small particles of feces. Studies have shown that this procedure may not be helpful until about the fifth postoperative day. A rectal suppository may be inserted in addition to enemas. Bisacodyl (Dulcolax) 10 mg is popular because it acts directly on the bowel mucosa and produces the desired results with little straining. When the patient is eating normally, he may be given dioctyl sodium sulfosuccinate, 120 mg daily, which produces a soft fecal mass that is easily expelled.

Other general postoperative nursing measures are presented in detail in Chapters 20 and 21 and will not be restated here.

GASTRIC ULCER

Most ulcers develop in the duodenum (about four of five) and they are rarely malignant. The stomach ulcer, on the other hand, while less common, is regarded more seriously because it must be differentiated from gastric carcinoma as promptly as possible.

Between 60 and 70 percent of individuals with gastric ulcers are men. Hormonal influences are thought to be associated with a protective mechanism, since there is a lower incidence of ulcers in premenopausal women and pregnant women, and women with ulcers often experience remissions during pregnancy. Gastric ulcers are more common in individuals 40 to 60 years old and in poor people, whereas duodenal ulcers occur more frequently in individuals 25 to 40 years old, businessmen, and executives. Acute gastric ulceration can occur as a result of severe emotional stress or in patients who have been severely burned (the Curling ulcer).

The stomach is a remarkably hardy organ, resistant to trauma to a large extent through continuous secretion of tenacious, viscous, alkaline mucus which protects the gastric lining. Buffering ions present in secretion serve to neutralize gastric acid. The slimy surface of the mucous membrane reduces the frictional irritation due to mechanically abrasive agents. A mucus-supplying layer of cells in the membrane provides a second line of defense. When the protective mechanism is defective or is overwhelmed by a destructive stimulus of sufficient force, tissue erosion quickly occurs. Unless the defense mechanisms are supported from the outside (food or alkalies), ulceration of a localized area of lowered resistance continues unchecked to the point of bleeding and perforation of the stomach wall.

Symptoms vary according to the nature of the ulcer and the person reporting, but the classic picture is one of intermittent pain episodes (periodicity) relieved by ingestion of food, fluids, and alkalies. Increased salivation, nausea, anorexia, and vomiting may be noted if the ulcer is one that involves the pyloric region and thus causes obstructive consequences. The pain usually begins 30 to 90 minutes after ingestion of a meal and may last up to 2 hours. With a duodenal ulcer, the pain does not begin until at least 2 hours after eating or during the middle of the night. Exacerbations and remissions of ulcer symptoms continue for 5 to 25 years in up to three-fourths of patients. Bleeding occurs when the gastric vessels are eroded by the penetrating crater. It may appear as hematemesis (sometimes bright red, but often like "coffee-grounds" because hemoglobin converted into a hydrochloride makes a powdery brown clot) or as tarry feces. Gastric carcinoma is more likely to produce slow, steady oozing that results in a stool with occult blood. An acute and profuse hemorrhage in gastric ulcers will produce signs of shock (pallor, diaphoresis, rapid pulse, drop in blood pressure).

Another complication of ulcers is perforation. Most perforations occur with duodenal ulcers, but can occur in gastric ulcers as well. If located on the lesser curvature of the stomach, the ulcer will open into the peritoneum; if it is a posterior ulcer, it is more likely to penetrate the pancreas. The nurse practicing in industry may see an employee who has a sudden, severe onset of upper abdominal pain. Sometimes there will be pain in the shoulders, indicating subphrenic irritation. The pain is aggravated by movement and the person will want to lie rigidly still, as opposed to the victim of coronary thrombosis who needs to sit straight up and is more restless. The blood pressure, pulse, and temperature are usually normal in the beginning, but the person may have rapid, shallow respirations and break out into a cold sweat. If a physician is not on the premises, one should be called, and an ambulance should be procured so that the individual is transported to the hospital quickly.

Obstruction of the pyloric region or duodenum due to fibrotic scarring is another possible complication. To compensate the stomach will dilate and hypertrophy in order to hold quantities of food for a longer time while the peristaltic waves try to force material past the stenosis. When this mechanism fails, there will be profuse vomiting of foul smelling and stale food ingested 6 or more hours previously. Continued vomiting leads to loss of weight and dehydration, and this produces constipation and electrolyte disturbances.

Medical Care Program

If the ulcer is thought to be benign, surgical intervention will be delayed until a suitable medical regimen has been attempted. The aims of treatment for the ulcer patient include the following: (1) to reduce gastric secretion by providing physical and mental rest, by reducing stress, by controlling tension with sedatives and tranquilizers, and by administering smooth muscle antispasmodics; (2) to eliminate ulcerogenic agents such as tobacco, alcohol, highly spiced and mechanically irritating high bulk foods, carbonated beverages, coffee, aspirin, and others; (3) to neutralize gastric acid as often as necessary with alkalies, milk, and small, frequent, bland feedings; and (4) to correct systemic imbalances, improving the general condition and health of the patient.

If the patient cooperates in an intensive regimen and receives good nursing care, pain is usually relieved within a week as the inflammation and edema around the ulcer lesion subside. Depending on the ulcer's size, healing is usually complete within 2 to 6 weeks. Repeat barium studies should show only a shallow scar. If healing is incomplete after 6 weeks, or if infiltration is seen around the site, the lesion is considered possibly malignant. Exploratory surgery and a gastric resection will probably be performed. Although cancer may not be observable on frozen section at the time of operation later tissue studies may demonstrate it.

Liberalization of the traditional Sippy diet has been encouraged in recent years by physicians and patients who complain that the ulcer diet is fattening and disagreeable, and raises the blood cholesterol. Polyunsaturated fat preparations to reduce lipemia are being used and are becoming more popular. A nonirritating modified bland diet that is nutritionally adequate is most likely to be ordered. Patient comfort is a prime concern, since studies have not demonstrated that a specific dietary regimen will speed healing or prevent recurrences. Vitamin supplements are frequently ordered to correct and prevent deficiencies. Some physicians permit patients to eat anything they desire, as long as it causes no problems.

Probably the most important aspect of treatment is the modification of the patient's life situation and his approach to problems. A balanced program of proper exercise and true relaxation is still one of the most important contributions to optimum health and longevity. Understanding nurses who are well trained in communication and counseling skills can be very helpful to patients not only while they are hospitalized, but also when they return to their work in the community. Patients can help themselves to better physical and mental health through a variety of methods. The restorative value of music, art, and reading should not be underestimated. Periodic reexaminations by physicians to detect complications or early malignant changes are an integral part of the medical care program.

Gastric ulcer recurrence is common and may eventually produce a stenosing obstruction. "C-H-O-P"—C-hronicity, H-emorrhage, O-bstruction, and P-erforation—these are the four primary indications for surgical intervention. The type of operation depends in part on the site of the ulcer and the situation to be corrected. (See Figure 25–4.) Currently recommended is a combination procedure, i.e., vagotomy-antrectomy-pyloroplasty or vagotomy-pyloroplasty. In the vagotomy, a complete transection of all vagal branches to the stomach is performed to reduce gastric secretion by innervation. Because vagotomy produces stomach atonicity, it must be accompanied by a drainage procedure such as pyloroplasty or jejunostomy. An antrectomy is often done to remove that portion of the stomach that produces the antral hormone, gastrin, which is known to stimulate acid secretion. The combined procedure has been successful in its aim of preserving more of the stomach to prevent stasis in the antrum, to prevent later duodenal ulceration, and to reduce the incidence of postoperative complications that occur with more extensive gastric resection. Furthermore, mortality has been reduced in recent years, especially in the poor-risk patient, the aged, and the patient having surgery for massive gastric hemorrhage.

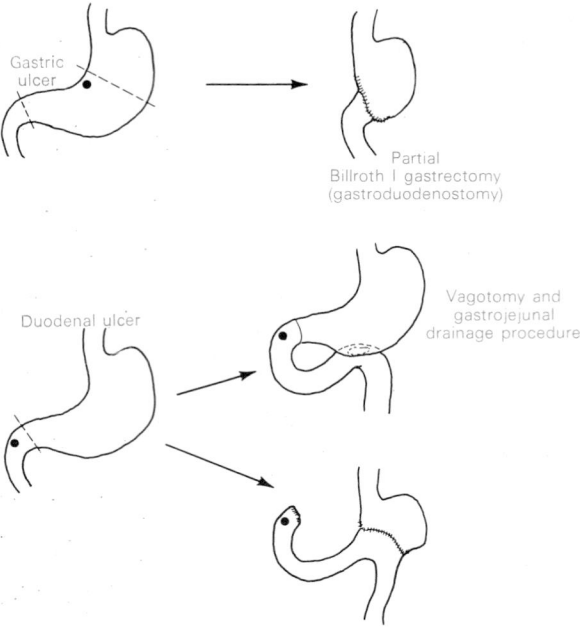

Figure 25–4
Types of operations for
peptic ulcer.

The postoperative course is smooth and uncomplicated in the majority of patients. Bleeding at the site of anastomosis is possible as is a leaking duodenal stump (in a Billroth II gastrojejunostomy). Infections of the skin suture line can develop. Pulmonary embolus, atelectasis, and pneumonia may be complications, particularly if the patient is a heavy smoker with a chronic cough, who is not properly cared for pre- and postoperatively and trained in deep breathing and coughing exercises. After vagotomy, steatorrhea and diarrhea may develop, although the reasons are not clearly understood.

More extensive gastric resection may be necessary, giving rise to nutritional problems. A smaller stomach results in a feeling of fullness after a moderate size meal, and the attending discomfort may produce an impairment of appetite with a developing weight loss. Furthermore, mucosal atrophy with diminished secretion can lead to deficiency of intrinsic factor which causes a poor absorption of vitamin B_{12}. A lowered serum B_{12} can produce megaloblastic anemia. Since hydrochloric acid is needed for iron absorption, an anemia can develop from reduced levels of hydrochloric acid in the stomach. Sometimes a "dumping" syndrome or hypoglycemic type of attack occurs following high carbohydrate meals. The high osmotic fluids pass too quickly into the jejunum, absorbing fluid from the bowel wall and producing an oligemia and hyperthermia. Syncope, vertigo, diaphoresis, and tachycardia are common, and nausea, vomiting, and diarrhea may result.

Nursing Care Program

Because of the varying manifestations and wide range of differences in the clinical picture of patients with peptic ulcer disease, individualization of medical management and nursing care programs is the sine qua non of therapeutic effectiveness.

Some general objectives of a nursing care plan for the ulcer patient include the following: (1) to assist in fulfilling the goals of the medical care program by following the physician's orders in an intelligent, conscientious, and safe manner; (2) to promote rest and relaxation for the patient by giving prompt consideration to his needs and by controlling or eliminating stressful environmental stimuli; (3) to establish and maintain a therapeutic relationship with the patient which conveys a warm understanding and a sincere concern for him as an individual; (4) to promote and maintain the biological, psychological, and sociocultural equilibrium of the patient by preventing complications and reinforcing healthful behavior.

Because the occurrence and continued existence of an ulcer seem to be associated with emotional tension, the nurse needs to try to minimize stress for the patient. The perceptive nurse with an understanding of human behavior will readily identify cues to guide her approach in effectively supporting this patient through a stressful hospitalization. She must watch for evidences of increased tension and restlessness, attempting to eliminate the stressors or reduce their impact. She should take every precaution to avoid the frustrating annoyances of delayed meals, cold food, and unnecessary waiting for treatments, tests, or care procedures. These may be interpreted as a lack of interest and concern for him as a person. A frequent offense is the common, generally accepted nursing practice of placing milk and antacid medications at the patient's bedside to be taken as needed. Even when this is permitted by the physician, the nurse should carefully assess the patient's feelings about this, being sensitive to any feelings of rejection which he may try to conceal. Remember that what he says may not be what he really means by the words. Encouragement and strong reassurance are needed periodically by everyone, and the chronic ulcer patient is certainly one who could benefit from a warm, sympathetic approach to his concerns. Experimental evidence indicating that gastric acid-pepsin secretion is stimulated by emotional stress makes the nursing approach as important as the medication she brings to the patient. Methods of inducing relaxation are valuable additions to the techniques of providing physical and mental rest which the nurse may employ. This is essential for attaining the maximum degree of gastric inactivity.

Since ulcers recur as easily as they heal, the regimen must not be considered lightly by any member of the physician-patient-nurse triad. The rate of recurrences is a more important criterion of therapeutic success than subjective interpretation of symptoms or an x-ray film's "seal of approval" on a healed lesion. One of the persistent problems that health workers face is how to convince patients of the need to remain faithful to a prescribed regimen for 8 weeks or longer following symptomatic relief.

The occupational health nurse has a responsibility in the preventive aspects of this disease. By assisting her patients to realize the necessity of modifying work and living habits, as well as continuing treatment, she can make a major contribution to a prolonged remission.

Disorders of the Intestinal Tract

As with other portions of the alimentary canal, disorders of the intestinal tract may be classified as congenital or acquired and structural or functional disorders.

They may also be categorized according to clinical manifestations or causes. In the section that follows, major emphasis will be given to those infections, neoplasms, injuries, and conditions most likely to be encountered by today's practicing nurse. Because disorders of elimination have important physical and psychosocial consequences, the nurse is likely to draw upon a broad base of knowledge in order to care properly for these patients.

DUODENAL ULCER

The therapeutic regimen and nursing care are essentially the same in both duodenal and gastric ulcers. Duodenal ulcer is more common than gastric ulcer and it afflicts men more often than women. The gastric acidity output is usually higher in patients with duodenal ulcer than with a stomach ulcer.

Barium x-ray studies are diagnostic of duodenal ulcer, but an augmented histamine test and gastric analysis studies are frequently ordered to detect the possibility of the Zollinger-Ellison syndrome. In this condition a noninsulin-secreting islet cell tumor of the pancreas produces a potent gastric-stimulating hormone. As a rusult, ulcers may develop in any location from the esophagus to the ileum, but they are commonly found in the duodenum. In 85 percent of affected individuals 2 liters (2,000 ml) of gastric juice is secreted in a 12-hour overnight period. (Normal secretion is about 350 ml.) A total gastrectomy along with removal of the pancreatic tumor are necessary to correct the condition.

Performance of the augmented histamine test may be delegated to the nurse but is usually the responsibility of the physician. Since interdigestive secretion varies daily in amount and acidity in the same individual, it is important to record the date and time when the test is done and to note any medications or food taken by the patient during the preceding 8 hours. Ordinarily the test is done when the patient has fasted for 6 to 8 hours, but this is not always the case. Histamine acts as a local chemical stimulant of the parietal cells in the gastric glands, and analogues of this drug are known to be more potent activators of gastric secretion than histamine itself. Maximum gastric response is commonly achieved with administration of 1.7 mg betazole (Histalog) per kg body weight. Continuous gastric suction is maintained, and specimens are collected every 15 minutes following a fasting specimen and administration of betazole (Histalog) intramuscularly. Although systemic side effects are lessened when this histamine analogue is employed pyrilamine (Anthisan) or other antihistaminics may be given to prevent unnecessary flushing of the skin due to vasodilation of capillary beds. The nurse may also notice a drop in the patient's blood pressure or his complaint of a headache, but these effects are transient and easily relieved by administration of an antihistamine, as prescribed by the physician. The antihistamine will not interfere with the histamine's local stimulating activity on the gastric mucosa for purposes of the test.

If a gastric analysis is ordered, a 12-hour specimen will probably be ordered to be collected throughout the night, every 1 to 2 hours. This enables the physician to know when acidity and volume are greatest. A baseline specimen is collected to empty the stomach. Throughout the night the nurse is watchful that the nasogastric tubing does not become kinked and that low, continuous suction is maintained. Mouthwashes should not be offered since some liquid may be swallowed and alter the chemistry of gastric contents. The patient should be urged to expectorate all saliva because continued swallowing of throat secretions, produced by the irritating presence of the tube, can alter the volume of aspirated contents.

With the exception of the Zollinger-Ellison syndrome, duodenal ulcer often can be cured by the combined operation of vagotomy-antrectomy-pyloroplasty. This procedure eliminates the cephalic and hormonal phases of acid secretion and provides adequate drainage for the hypotonic stomach.

Medical Management

Rest, diet, and drugs comprise the medical management of the active, uncomplicated duodenal ulcer. Rest has been shown to be far more efficacious than diet in promoting the complete healing desired. Antacids that are insoluble, harmless, palatable, and inexpensive as well as effective neutralizers of gastric acid are recommended. A popular one is aluminum hydroxide gel; it combines chemically with the hydrochloric acid in the stomach producing neutral aluminum chloride and water, and is thought to have a demulcent, adsorptive, and protective action. Dosage varies from 4 to 30 ml. Unfortunately this preparation can cause constipation, so a product which has added magnesium hydroxide (Maalox) or magnesium trisilicate (Gelusil) is frequently substituted. Eight milliliters is the usual dose of these compounds.

Antacids whether in tablet or liquid form do not remain in the stomach long enough to be protective. Unless given hourly, treatment with antacids is considered to be inadequate. To prevent merely coating the esophagus, antacids should be diluted or followed with water. The patient must be warned never to substitute one antacid preparation for another as a practice without the physician's permission. Some antacids are high in sodium content and can produce edema in the cirrhotic or cardiac patient. Some alkalies are more absorbable than others and alkalosis or hypercalcemia has been known to develop. Common offenders include soda bicarbonate and calcium carbonate, when used over a period of time.

Anticholinergic medications that block acetylcholine and inhibit gastric secretion of acid and pepsin are required. These preparations block vagal stimulation of smooth muscle, thus reducing stomach tone and motility and allowing food and antacid medications time to neutralize gastric acid. Troublesome side effects of anticholinergic preparations include dryness of mouth, blurred vision, urinary retention, vertigo, and tachycardia. Dosage must then be reduced to an optimum effective level without producing uncomfortable symptoms.

Prevention of recurrences is a major problem in the treatment of patients with duodenal ulcer disease. Dietary restrictions and antacid regimens are tedious, distasteful, and impractical, and many patients are resistant to following this program faithfully and indefinitely. Spontaneous remissions may continue for a number of months when patients neglect their treatment, so it is difficult to convince them of the necessity of maintaining it. Careful studies on the use of prolonged anticholinergic therapy to reduce the frequency and severity of exacerbations and complications have been conducted; they indicate that "effective" medications used in optimum dosage tailored to each patient have produced gratifying results (Sun).

Nursing Care

In a significant number of patients, complications warranting surgery do develop. Again, emphasis must be placed on the value of an education program that helps the patient to understand his ulcer and those particular factors that produce his symptoms. Teaching begun by the hospital staff can best be reinforced by that of a community health nurse, who may detect problem areas in the home and on the job. Utilizing principles of the teaching-learning process in an atmosphere of warm, encouraging acceptance, the thoughtful nurse can help the patient to maintain his self-esteem and confidence in making a more satisfactory adjustment within his family and circle of business associates.

If the patient must have a vagotomy-antrectomy-pyloroplasty, his preparation and postoperative care will be similar to those of other types of abdominal surgery in the gastrointestinal tract. In emergency situations such as hemorrhage and perforation, an effort is made to stabilize the patient's condition preoperatively. Associated cardiopulmonary conditions are carefully evaluated and treated as necessary as well as other medical problems which the patient may have that will affect the course of his operation for the ulcer.

NASOGASTRIC TUBE

Ordinarily a nasogastric tube is inserted on the morning of the scheduled surgery. Stomach dilatation and intestinal distention are thus prevented, relieving the patient of unnecessary pain due to flatulence. Stress on the suture line in the abdominal incision is reduced; this lessens possibilities of wound dehiscence, evisceration, and respiratory embarrassment. Vomiting is controlled, thereby preventing tracheal aspiration of vomitus and a resultant pneumonia. Healing is facilitated because the stomach and duodenum are kept free of fluid and air.

Usually the patient finds the nasogastric tube very uncomfortable and annoying. The nurse can do much to help him accept and adjust to this temporary distress. Explanations about the purpose of the tube, what it accomplishes, and what happens when it is not used are a good beginning with the patient who can understand and cooperate. Changes of position, frequent mouth rinsing, and application of a soothing cream around the nostril containing the tube may also contribute to a reduction in distress. Proper taping of the tube to the face will eliminate pressure and sites of irritation. If Band-Aids or paper masking tape is used instead of adhesive or Cellophane tape, it will not be necessary to remove adhesive traces on skin and tube. Adherence to skin which becomes oily or moist with perspiration is also enhanced.

In preparation for insertion, rubber tubes are placed in ice for about 20 minutes. This practice facilitates insertion because the slight stiffening reduces likelihood of the tube curling or kinking in the back of the mouth. The cold chills the sensitive nerve endings and makes swallowing less unpleasant for the patient. If the tube is plastic, it should be placed in *warm* water to reduce the force of friction during instillation and to soften the tube, making it more flexible and less likely to damage mucosa. Water-soluble lubricant is placed on the patient's nostrils and along the first 8 inches of the tube to reduce surface friction more effectively than water alone can do. The patient's gown is protected with a towel and he is placed in a sitting position. The length of tube to be inserted may be estimated by measuring from the nose to the ear and then to the xiphoid process of the sternum. During insertion, the patient is repeatedly asked to swallow; this encourages him to concentrate on cooperating with verbal instructions rather than on his fear and the discomfort caused by the tube. Advancing the tube as the patient is in the act of swallowing facilitates its insertion. When a fasting gastric specimen is not needed and in the absence of contraindications, the patient may be asked to drink cool water while the tube is going down. This is frequently more effective than using chips of ice which may either be too large to swallow immediately or may melt so quickly that there is little left to swallow. In some cases the tube's position in the stomach is verified through inserting a very small amount of air which can be heard through a stethoscope and by aspirating the stomach juices. Roentgenography or fluoroscopy may be done to determine the exact location of the tube when gastric secretions must be adequately collected over a period of time for accurate testing procedures.

OTHER MEASURES

Postoperative orders for vagotomy-antrectomy-pyloroplasty include considerations for pain, sleep, activity, elimination, prevention of respiratory and circulatory complications, replacement of fluids and vitamins parenterally, and laboratory tests to determine the presence of infection, occult bleeding, or electrolyte imbalance.

The patient's dressing is changed daily and sutures are removed after 1 week. Sometimes a repeat gastric analysis is performed, insulin being employed to stimulate gastric secretion. If the vagotomy has been successful, no acidity will be produced as a result of giving the insulin. The patient is discharged with instructions to continue a six-meal diet of foods which are well tolerated and to return for a check-up periodically as indicated by his physician.

INFECTIONS AND INFLAMMATIONS

Appendicitis

Appendicitis is still the most common acute inflammatory disease of the abdomen in individuals under 40 years of age. Incidence is highest in teenagers and young adults, but it can occur at any age. Both sexes are equally affected. Unless treatment is given at once, gangrene develops and leads to perforation, bringing about a localized abscess or a generalized peritonitis and causing the patient's death. Occasionally an abscess may drain into the rectum or burst through the skin. A first attack may be mild and can be treated with antibiotics. More severe attacks are likely to follow, however, because after the initial inflammation subsides, constricting adhesions may develop or the lumen may be narrowed. The possibility of perforation and peritonitis is always present in any attack, so early appendectomy is generally advocated.

Contrary to public opinion, the signs and symptoms of appendicitis do not present a uniform pattern in all patients. An unequivocal diagnosis is still very difficult (though at times very simple), depending upon the age and condition of the patient and the position of the appendix. A careful history and physical examination are essential. The first and most prominent symptom is a sudden onset of abdominal pain, usually around the umbilicus (especially in children) and later localizing at the right iliac fossa. Pyrexia is common. The average temperature during an attack ranges from 37.5° to 39° C (100° to 102° F), but often will be slightly lower. Occasionally if an abscess or peritonitis has already developed, the temperature may be normal or subnormal. An increase in pulse rate is usually associated with the acute episode and rises as the disease progresses. The tongue may appear furry and feel dry. Vomiting at the onset of the attack is common and nausea is almost continuous. Constipation is the rule, but diarrhea may occur when there is rectal irritation due to a retroileal position of the appendix. Movement of the abdomen is guarded, and one can notice that the lower and right sides of the abdomen move less with each respiration than the upper and left sections. There is rebound tenderness and pain with palpation and quick release of the hand over the right lower quadrant. An absence of bowel sounds may be detected with a stethoscope over the region of the cecum. The right rectus muscle feels rigid with spasm. If blood counts are done, an increasing leukocytosis of 10,000 to 20,000 may be revealed. Once the diagnosis is made, immediate appendectomy and drainage is recommended. Exceptions may be made in patients with severest complications or those whose peritonitis is unquestionably receding, and in these persons saline and plasma are administered to combat shock and sodium depletion. Vomiting and abdominal distention are controlled with intubation, which also allows the intestinal tract to rest quietly and heal. Vital signs are taken frequently and medications given to manage general systemic complications. When the patient's condition improves and stabilizes, corrective surgery is usually performed to prevent recurrent attacks.

The incidence and mortality rates of appendicitis have decreased appreciably in the past two decades because the symptoms are widely recognized and the danger in using laxatives or hot water bottles for continuing abdominal pain is appreciated. Antibiotics, nasogastric suction, intravenous fluids, and early ambulation have helped to reduce postoperative complications. With prompt diagnosis and surgery most patients are discharged from the hospital within 1 week. Sutures are removed on the fifth to the seventh day, sometimes on the first office visit. If a Penrose drain has been inserted, a dry, sterile dressing is applied as needed until drainage has ceased and healing is complete.

Regional Enteritis

Regional enteritis, or Crohn's disease, is primarily a chronic disease of the small bowel although it may affect the colon as well. The terminal portion of the ileum is most frequently involved, hence the name, *terminal ileitis.* Its cause is unknown, but many physicians believe that a faulty autoimmune mechanism may be involved. Both sexes are about equally affected and most individuals have initial symptoms before the age of 35. There is some familial predisposition to Crohn's disease, and it occurs throughout the world.

Signs and symptoms vary according to the phase of development and the extent of disease. In the acute stage, the symptoms resemble an attack of appendicitis. Diagnosis is made by gross examination during an exploratory laparotomy in conjunction with an appendectomy.

Conservative medical treatment is advised for as long as possible. Symptomatic improvement has been seen with therapy consisting of a low-residue bland diet, vitamin and iron supplements, corticoids and ACTH, and some antibiotics (chloramphenicol, streptomycin, or sulfonamides). Surgery is delayed until medical treatment fails or until definite signs of obstruction or abscess appear. A variety of procedures have been attempted: ileostomy, ileotransverse colostomy, and bypass-anastomosis of healthy segments. None have been remarkably successful in controlling the course of the disease. About half the patients do fairly well for a period of years after surgery while others continue to be aggravated by severe symptoms. Nursing measures in regional enteritis are designed to assist each individual patient to accept his condition and its treatment with the best adjustment possible for him.

Gastroenteritis

Gastroenteritis, the well-known syndrome of sudden diarrhea, vomiting, and colicky pains, has a variety of causes. Organisms responsible for bacterial food poisoning episodes commonly include staphylococci, salmonellae, and occasionally streptococci. Different strains of viruses are believed to initiate the periodic outbreaks of "intestinal flu." Allergies, drug sensitivities, and alcohol intoxication also may instigate an acute attack of these distressing s&mptoms. Normally, recovery can be expected in less than 24 hours for nausea and vomiting of brief duration with treatment consisting of bed rest and nothing by mouth. When tolerated, paregoric (camphorated tincture of opium, 4 to 8 ml) is given as necessary to control diarrhea. Tea, Jell-O, bouillon, and carbonated beverages are offered when the patient feels able to retain them. Dehydration, shock, and prostration may ensue if vomiting and diarrhea are prolonged. The patient may be hospitalized to receive intravenous infusions of 5 percent dextrose in normal saline. Potassium chloride is added for severe cases of electrolyte disturbances. Sodium phenobarbital, 60 to 120 mg by injection, is given for sedation. Dimenhydrinate (Dramamine), prochlorperazine (Compazine), or other preferred antiemetics may be given. Atropine is often administered to relieve the cramp-like spasms. The patient is sedated, and atropine is usually ordered. He is usually discharged the following day, unless the causative organism is a salmonella or other agent necessitating a longer period of treatment.

Nurses who practice in institutional settings such as schools, camps, military reservations, and domiciliaries are likely to encounter a gastroenteritis epidemic sooner or later. Although she may feel greatly taxed by having to care for a large number of very sick patients in a short period of time, it is vital that she provide an accurate record of each patient's output, so that the physician may be quickly directed to those who are most seriously ill. In episodes of suspected food poisoning, the public health epidemiologist will want to interview patients and food handlers. He will also need to have samples of food which were served at the most recent meal to those who became ill. It is the responsibility of the nurse or health officer in charge to ascertain that no leftover food is hastily discarded before it can be examined.

Dysentery

The passage of loose stools containing blood and mucus characterizes *bacillary and amebic dysentery,* also known as *shigellosis* and *amebiasis.* These infectious diseases of the colon are widely found throughout the world, but the pattern of pathogenicity varies from one endemic area to another as well as from patient to patient. Both types are acquired by ingestion of food or water contaminated with feces carrying the causative organisms. Laboratory examination of a fresh, warm stool specimen is diagnostic, although rectal biopsy may demonstrate presence of the disease when the feces is found to be negative. Control of these diseases can be accomplished only with improvement of sanitation and food handling practices and the extermination of flies and roaches. Rest, soft bland diet with vitamin and mineral supplements, parenteral administration of normal saline and potassium chloride, and specific antibiotic drug therapy are needed.

Diverticulitis

Diverticulitis is brought about by the stagnation of bowel contents in diverticula, usually located in the cecum or in the sigmoid region of the large intestine. These herniations or outpouchings of mucosa through the colon musculature become inflamed and edematous. Blockage of the neck of the diverticulum ensues, abscesses develop, and fistulas or perforations to the adjacent organs may occur. Signs and symptoms arising from the altered pathophysiology can be studied in Table 25–3.

Diverticula are most common in those over 40 years of age, especially if they are obese. Although the cause of diverticula is unknown, their development is thought to be acquired in association with weakening of the musculature with aging. Men are more likely to have diverticulosis than women.

Other than a mild, chronic diarrhea, diverticulosis often produces no symptoms. Patients with an inflammatory process may experience a sharp pain in the region of the obstructed diverticulum, often in the left lower abdominal quadrant. Because an alteration of bowel habits and rectal bleeding are common signs, the diagnosis must be established to rule out carcinoma, polyps, ulcerative colitis, or hemorrhoids. Barium x-ray studies often reveal the presence of diverticula.

If the attack is a mild one, the patient is encouraged to rest, to eat a moderately low-residue diet, and to take a prescribed laxative. Sulfonamides or antibiotics are usually ordered to control the infection. The patient is cautioned to avoid episodes of constipation in order to prevent recurrences. Surgery may be indicated for complications such as abscesses, fistulas, perforation, and obstruction. A one-stage colon resection of the diseased segments with end-to-end anastomosis is advocated in some cases. For patients with severe inflammations, fistulas, or obstructions, a temporary colostomy may be advisable. Later, when the situation warrants, the surgeon will close the colostomy, repair the diseased segment, and rejoin the healthy segments of intestine. The nursing care of a patient with a colostomy is described elsewhere in this chapter; otherwise the nursing plan is similar to that for patients having general surgery.

Ulcerative Colitis

Nonspecific idiopathic ulcerative colitis is an intestinal inflammatory disease of serious significance for the physician, the patient, and the nurse. The aggravating symptom complex has depressing psychological concomitants and debilitating physical consequences for its victims. The problems of care are sufficient to challenge the competence and compassion of the most experienced nurse. The sociocultural significance of elimination and the secrecy that shrouds defecation practices made adjustment difficult for the person afflicted with ulcerative colitis. A courageous and determined attitude is needed by the patient and his professional health consultants in order to provide a united approach to the patient's personal and social world.

The etiology of ulcerative colitis remains unknown, although present medical research demonstrates a possible linkage with disorders of the autoimmune mechanism. Evidence is inconclusive but promising. A genetic factor appears likely, yet environmental influences cannot be ruled out. Incidence is higher among Jews than Gentiles, but the reason is not known. Although more women are affected than men according to some studies reported, consistent significant sex differences have not been found. The greatest incidence of ulcerative colitis is found in the young adult group (18 to 35), although it has been found to occur at any age.

Categorization of patients' personality traits is fraught with dangers of overgeneralization, subjectivity, and stereotyping. Ulcerative colitis, nevertheless, has been associated especially with persons who may be more than usually intelligent, sensitive, shy, dependent, conscientious, and anxious. Some researchers have reported that these patients tend to be insecure, passive, emotionally immature, and fastidiously neat. Patients frequently report that the initial colitis symptoms occurred following an acute emotional crisis. Exacerbations often develop during prolonged episodes of certain types of stress, including infection, allergy, and grief.

Attacks may be acute, fulminating episodes with severe symptoms and extensive colon involvement, or they may be intermittent and chronic involving only distal segments of the large intestine and causing milder discomfort. In severe cases, the patient may have fever, anorexia, nausea, vomiting, and abdominal cramp-like pains. Bloody diarrhea is the characteristic sign, with 10 to 20 movements per day. The patient may eliminate bright red blood, mucus, and pus with or without semifluid feces. Loss of weight, weakness, anemia, and electrolyte disturbances ensue. Mortality is high, about 10 percent, for patients with acute attacks (Watts et al.). There is an especially high risk if the patient is over 60 years of age or if there is pathological involvement of the entire colon. For milder cases, spontaneous remissions occur with or without treatment in about 10 to 15 percent of the patients. Steroid therapy and surgical intervention have reduced mortality rates significantly in those having moderately severe episodes of the disease. After the initial attack, the patient must remain under medical supervision indefinitely in order to control exacerbations of recurring symptoms and to prevent or treat complications. Initially there is an edema and hyperemia of the mucous membrane, which bleeds superficially upon contact with passage of the bowel contents. Shallow ulcerations of irregular dimensions form, separated by pseudopolyps of edematous mucosal tags. Small abscesses form in the crypts. The inflamed colon wall is thin and friable, subject to perforation and progressive shortening with continued exacerbations and remissions. This process, which begins usually at the rectum and eventually involves the total colon, results in a loss of the normal haustration (sacculation of wall) causing a characteristic drainpipe appearance on roentgenograms.

COMPLICATIONS

In addition to complications of anemia, dehydration, and perforation, fistulas may develop between the colon and adjacent organs. Perianal abscesses are common. Other disorders associated with the condition include skin rashes (e.g., eczema, urticaria, neurodermatitis), liver disease, renal lesions, inflammations of the oral cavity, and arthritis. This latter condition is frequently known as *colitic arthritis* to distinguish it from rheumatoid arthritis or osteoarthritis. It may take a peripheral form affecting a few joints (often the knees) or it may be a spondylitic form occupying the sacroiliac joint. In most cases these are self-limiting episodes of 4 to 10 weeks which disappear without sequelae until the next recurrence. Relief of painful symptoms is obtained by corticosteroids used to treat the colitis. Sometimes symptoms of the complications gain the attention of the patient before the colitis is noticed.

The most serious complication associated with ulcerative colitis is a malignant disorder. The incidence of intestinal carcinoma is reported to be 20 to 30 times higher in these patients than in the normal population. It is not necessary that the bowel be severely damaged for the cancer to be present, and the cancer may occur after the patient has been in remission for some time. For this reason, continuing medical supervision with regular examinations is mandatory for patients with a history of ulcerative colitis.

MEDICAL CARE PROGRAM

Mild attacks of ulcerative colitis are often controlled with diet and drugs under the supervision of a physician while the patient rests at home. For individuals with moderate or severe symptoms, hospitalization is advocated in order to prevent and control serious complications. The generally accepted aims of treatment are as follows: (1) to establish and maintain the patient's confidence, hope, cooperation, and perseverance with the treatment plan; (2) to reduce the patient's anxiety and tension by removing or alleviating environmental stressors and by assisting him to identify and resolve his emotional conflicts; (3) to relieve physical symptoms of the attack; (4) to replace systemic deficiencies brought about by the disease; (5) to prevent and control secondary infections and complications; (6) to facilitate a remission of the disease as soon as possible by an intensive short-term medical regimen of diet, rest, and drugs, or by surgical intervention when indicated; and (7) to rehabilitate the patient and restore him to a productive life.

The satisfactory accomplishment of these objectives requires the concerted efforts of a team of professionals—physician, nurses, social worker, dietitian—working with the patient and his family. Diagnostic measures (barium enema, sigmoidoscopy, numerous laboratory tests, and roentgenograms) necessary to assess the extensiveness of the disease and possible complications are often tiresome irritations to the patient, sapping his already weakened physical and emotional resources. A major contribution of the nurse to the therapeutic plan is her support of the patient's coping devices and her efforts to achieve the first two objectives in association with the physician. The behavior of the health care team must convincingly demonstrate to the patient a sincere interest in him as a person as well as a patient, a firm optimism regarding the successful outcome of treatment, and a sympathetic understanding of the problems to be faced by the patient and those who care for him. If the patient is to recover and learn to live with his condition in optimum adaptation, then it is the achievement of the first two objectives which must be given thoughtful consideration and devoted energy.

Relief of physical symptoms and replacement of systemic deficiencies will improve the patient's well-being. A complete appraisal including history, physical examination, and tests previously mentioned will determine what needs to be done. The nurse assists the physician by carefully observing and reporting patient complaints and behavior; by monitoring and recording vital signs, intake, output, and responses to treatment; and by consulting with the doctor on problems of care which need his attention. If nausea and vomiting plague the patient, an antiemetic is ordered. Often a preparation is chosen that has antihistaminic and tranquilizing properties to combat tenseness and anxiety that may contribute to the problem. To control diarrhea and to relieve abdominal discomfort or tenesmus, codeine (15 to 30 mg orally or intramuscularly) may be given. Sedative-antispasmodic preparations are sometimes helpful, and mixtures of phenobarbital and belladonna are still popular. Camphorated tincture of opium (paregoric), 4 to 8 ml, has been ordered commonly to reduce peristalsis. Newer preparations such as diphenoxylate and atropine sulfate (Lomotil), 15 to 25 mg daily in divided doses, have been found to be effective without the analgesic and addictive tendencies.

To replace the electrolyte loss in diarrheic stools, oral or parenteral minerals (sodium and potassium chloride) are administered. Iron in the form of ferrous gluconate (given orally) or iron-dextran complex (Imferon, given intramuscularly) is given to restore loss from intestinal bleeding. An occasional transfusion of whole blood may be ordered for anemia. Large amounts of nitrogen are also lost in the frequent elimination of mucus with blood and feces. Hypoproteinemia is common. A diet high in proteins and vitamins is prescribed with between-meal nourishment. Water-soluble vitamin supplements of the B-complex and ascorbic acid are frequently prescribed. To prevent further irritation to the bowels, foods high in coarse residue are avoided.

To bring about a remission of the ulcerative inflammatory process in the colon, steroid therapy is currently advocated. It has been effective in reducing by about half the overall mortality rate and in lessening serious complications. It has been used to prepare patients for surgery by improving their general condition and by alleviating severe symptoms of an acute attack. Operative risk is thereby reduced and one-stage colectomy-ileostomy procedures are safer to perform. Steroid dosage depends on the size of the patient and his needs according to the severity of an attack and the extensiveness of colon involvement. A dosage that is too high or too low may be harmful to the patient and may cause complications.

Because of the serious side effects of steroids (osteoporosis, hypertension, edema, psychotic reactions, and others), other preparations, notably the sulfonamides, have been tried. Salicylazosulfapyridine (Azulfidine), 4 to 8 g daily, has produced successful results, keeping some patients symptom-free for as long as a year. Toxic reactions such as rashes, hemolytic anemia, and agranulocytosis must be watched for on periodic reevaluations during the course of treatment. Antibiotics have not been effective for the management of patients with ulcerative colitis and, because prolonged usage may cause moniliasis or diarrhea, they are not given except to combat episodes of secondary infection which may occur.

NURSING CARE PROGRAM

General Aspects of Nursing Care. In support of the medical care program, the nurse has a number of important objectives to guide her activities. In addition to those previously mentioned, she must observe and report drug reactions and watch for initial complications caused by the disease or arising as a response to treatment. When giving Azulfidine, she is alert to patient complaints of nausea, headaches, or skin rashes. For patients receiving steroids, daily records of intake and output, weight, and blood pressures should be kept. These will be helpful in noting fluid retention and hypertension. The nurse should also watch for signs of muscular weakness, mental depression, nervousness, and insomnia. Because these signs are also seen as a part of the syndrome with ulcerative colitis, they are often overlooked as possible drug reactions to adrenal corticosteroid therapy. Resistance to infection is lower in these patients so nursing plans must include arrangements to maintain a clean, protective environment for the patient. Safeguarding from injury is important because of weakness caused by the disease and because prolonged steroid administration depresses osteoblast activity, thereby leading to osteoporosis and the possibility of pathological fractures.

Bathtime can be a particularly pleasant experience for the ulcerative colitis patient. A gentle, warm, cleansing bath can promote relaxation of the patient's physical and mental tensions. Protective massaging of the skin and bony prominences of thin, emaciated bodies is necessary to prevent tissue breakdown. Stomatitis, gingivitis, and glossitis are common disorders accompanying this disease, so oral hygiene is vital. If the patient is too weak to walk to the bathroom, it is desirable to place the bedpan in a quickly accessible location. Room deodorants should be used freely. Extra bed linens and clothing for the patient should be kept in a convenient place. Personal attractiveness is important to most people, and for the debilitated young adult patient it is especially desirable to encourage good grooming and use of his own toiletries. Pajama pants and long-sleeved robes are welcomed by patients whose limbs chill easily.

The establishment of a therapeutic relationship between a compassionate nurse and her colitis patient is particularly valuable if she is to successfully enable him to cope with his disease and its treatment. He needs to feel free to express both positive and negative feelings; he needs to believe he is understood and respected; he needs to develop self-confidence and independence both personally and interpersonally. The nurse should know the special needs of an adolescent, of an aged person, of a parent, of a spouse, of a person with job or school responsibilities, and should understand a variety of personality dispositions. Her growing understanding of human behavior is as essential as her up-to-date knowledge of the proper care of a patient with ulcerative colitis who may soon have an ileostomy. If her patient is a teenager, for example, he may be more demanding and hostile as a result of this annoying, uncomfortable, restricting disease. It may make him more dependent, more anxious, more depressed, and more immature than the average adolescent, who is already striving to find his way through a confusing period of changing beliefs, relationships, body image, and conflicting emotions. He may be modestly embarrassed by rectal diagnostic measures. He may be even more fearful and discouraged as he worries about his illness and its effect on his plans for school, courtship, marriage, having children, and a career. Sometimes it takes more than a warm, sympathetic ear; guidance in the right amount at the right time in the right way needs to be given when sought.

Dietary considerations for the medically treated colitis patient are another aspect of comprehensive nursing care. Food preferences and dislikes are frequently revealed to the nurse between consultation and teaching visits by the hospital dietitian. In other settings the nurses may still supervise meal planning for patients. Encouragement and reemphasis of savory, nutritious foods that are permitted is more desirable than frequent reminders of food restrictions.

To combat the effects of restless inactivity and boredom through long weeks of hospitalization, the nurse should assess and plan for meeting the patient's needs for recreation and occupational therapy. Substitutions for a thwarted achievement pattern, for mounting sexual frustration, and for increasing tensions as a result of limiting hospitalization and treatment regimens are necessary. They can be found by the thoughtfully creative nurse who takes the time to know her patient's interests and aptitudes. Reading and television viewing are popular diversions if the patient does not have iritis or conjunctivitis (sometimes associated with ulcerative colitis). Music and "talking books" are emotionally and intellectually restorative after visiting hours or meals and at other appropriate times.

Some behavioral and emotional reactions of the patient with ulcerative colitis defy explanation. If in the professional judgment of the nurse the patient needs psychiatric assistance, it is valuable to document her belief with facts and behavioral observations carefully recorded in nurse's notes. Fortified with substantiated data, she should then discuss the patient's problem with his attending physician so that he may, after consideration, order an appropriate consultation.

Once the diarrheic episode has been controlled and the patient has been brought into a period of remission, the nurse helps prepare him for returning to home and social roles. Instructions about drug and diet therapy are reviewed, and the patient is encouraged to increase his activity and interpersonal contacts. More time should be spent with the family of the patient providing them with information and encouragement. If some nursing care is necessary in the home during a convalescent period, the visiting nurse should be called, or arrangements for a private nurse can be made. The hospital nurse should contact the patient's school nurse or occupational health nurse in order to confer on the medical and nursing orders to be followed. Keeping appointments for periodic medical check-ups should be urged because patients are likely to minimize mild episodes of bleeding and diarrhea since they have become so accustomed to these. Early carcinoma may not be detected until too late.

Nursing Care in Surgical Treatment. Surgical intervention is likely to be indicated at some time during the course of the disease. The proposed operation is often a permanent ileostomy with a total proctocolectomy as the initial procedure. Sometimes, because of the patient's condition, a subtotal colectomy may be performed with a second stage abdominoperineal resection necessary a few months later. For the very small percentage of patients who have a rectum free of disease, an ileorectal anastomosis is occasionally done. Since there is an increased incidence of cancer in these patients, ileorectal anastomosis is not favored unless there is extreme resistance to the idea of an ileostomy. If the proposed operation is elective and is accepted by the patient, chances for a successful outcome and a more satisfactory adjustment are heightened. A significant percentage of patients who have surgery for this condition are found to be in better health years later than their counterparts treated medically through recurrent attacks. When their ileostomy is properly fitted with an appliance and its care has been successfully learned, patients who have had surgery are sorry only that they did not have the operation earlier.

If the patient has been given a period of time for preparation to have an ileostomy with colectomy, then it is desirable that he be introduced to the people and services available at his nearest ileostomy association. He will be invited to attend the meetings and to become acquainted with the care of an ileostomy by those who have successfully mastered the challenge. As role models, happily active at home and work, they can convincingly encourage the colitis patient to accept the forthcoming operation as a blessing. Postoperatively they are an invaluable resource of practical suggestions for the various problems accompanying ileostomy management and social adjustment. Every hospital should prepare a list of ileostomates willing to visit new patients. For a complete list of addresses, one may write to United Ostomy Association, Inc., International Office, 1111 Wilshire Boulevard, Los Angeles, California 90017. An information leaflet is available free of charge describing the purposes of the association and supplying a membership application.

True adjustment must be inner as well as outer to be complete. The longer one has held a value, the more difficult it is to change. This is especially true if the change is in conflict with an idea held by one's society. Therefore, in spite of intellectual acceptance of the necessity of surgery, the patient may continue to be resistive at the time of his next hospitalization. It is imperative that the nurse realize this possibility and not assume that her patient has actually incorporated the reality of an ileostomy deep within his psyche. Furthermore it is doubtful that he has yet modified his culturally based values of a "body beautiful" which includes absolute bowel control. The nurse needs to acknowledge her patient's generalized fear of the unknown and his need to undergo the "work of worrying," so that a more adequate postoperative adjustment may be facilitated. Accurate, adequate, yet reassuring information should be provided in small amounts with time allowed for emotional assimilation.

Even though the surgeon has explained the proposed operation, it is often necessary for the nurse to repeat the essential facts, giving the patient time to ask questions and to voice his real concerns. Compared to bizarre fantasies, honest details are a genuine relief to many people. Unless the patient is too sick to care, it is possible to show him diagrams and pictures of an ileostomy and its collection appliance. If for some reason he has not been seen by an ileostomate prior to the hospitalization, he should probably be introduced to one at this time. It is particularly helpful if the ileostomate is of the same age, sex, marital status, and socioeconomic group so that mutual understanding and role identification will be more likely to develop.

Improvement in surgical techniques during the last 15 years has remarkably reduced postoperative complications for the ileostomy patient. After he has been psychologically prepared for the operation and his general condition is sufficiently stabilized, the patient receives the usual physical preparations for general abdominal surgery. In addition to nasogastric intubation and preanesthetic medications, he is given additional doses of corticosteroids to compensate for increased needs due to surgical stress. Neomycin or sulfonamide preparations are often administered to reduce the likelihood of infection by killing pathogenic intestinal microorganisms.

THE ILEOSTOMY

Instead of bulky dressings or indwelling catheters for collection of ileostomy drainage and prevention of excoriation⁺ of periostomal skin which retards healing, immediate placement of a temporary appliance before the patient leaves the operating room can be accomplished. (See Figure 25–5.) The transparent bag permits observation of the color and consistency of ileostomy drainage as well as the stoma and its activity. Healing of the mucocutaneous junction is facilitated with a thin layer of antibiotic ointment containing polymyxin, neomycin, and bacitracin. Additional protection is provided with a mixture of karaya gum powder and a commercial antacid preparation to form a roll around the circumference of the stoma. An appliance face plate is cemented to the patient's skin, which has been painted with a film of tincture of benzoin. The plastic collection bag is placed in a horizontal position while the patient is bedfast, and then it is changed to a vertical plane when he is allowed to be ambulatory. If the appliance does not leak or loosen around the stoma, it may remain in place for as long as 10 days to 2 weeks. Some patients prefer to continue wearing the temporary bag when rehabilitated, while others prefer a one-piece opaque device of rubber or plastic.

The ileostomy will act within 12 to 24 hours and may discharge a profuse amount of liquid fecal material when it does. Sudden loss of minerals and fluids could result in dehydration and shock unless the patient is adequately hydrated with parenteral fluids. In addition to electrolyte laboratory studies, a careful intake and output record is kept. Intravenous fluids are ordered to replace loss by nasogastric tube and by ileostomy.

During the critical postoperative period the nurse is busy helping the physician by attending to measures designed to support respiration, circulation, and electrolyte balance and to prevent complications. Although the patient is relatively passive, he will be sensitive to the attitude and behavior of his caretakers. Their competent manner and consistent approach to details of nursing care will help him to feel safe and reassured. It is often preferable to assign only one or two persons to

Figure 25–5
Types of drainage bags

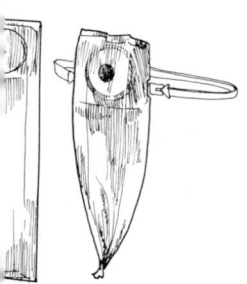

provide meticulous attention to the ileostomy and surrounding skin. Constant vigilance is necessary to detect loosening of the appliance and leakage and to prevent and correct early skin excoriation immediately. Care should be planned according to the patient's reasonable wishes, and appliance changing should ordinarily not be done around mealtimes.

Odor is humiliating to the patient, and it can be readily avoided by frequent emptying and rinsing of the bag, by airing or deodorizing the room after emptying the bag, and by use of various deodorizer preparations. One drop of Nilodor inside the bag and another drop in the rinse water used to clean the appliance will be found to be very effective. Bismuth subgallate, N. F., a tasteless yellow powder, can be taken for internal control of odor. The patient takes 1 teaspoonful three times daily with meals for 24 to 48 hours until deodorization is accomplished. The dosage is then reduced to meet individual requirements. The average dosage is ¼ teaspoonful twice daily. Another advantage of bismuth subgallate is that it tends to thicken the fecal discharge, which otherwise is normally semiliquid. A pound of bismuth subgallate will last for about 6 to 8 months and can be purchased without a prescription, although of course the permission of the physician is initially necessary.

Encouraging Self-care of the Ileostomy. The patient begins to care for his ileostomy as soon as he is physically and emotionally able. The nurse sensitively feels her way, responding to the patient's behavioral cues. His depression, silence, refusal to cooperate, or apathy may conceal feelings of hostility, anger, and grief from the shocking reality of the operation's meaning for him. Establishing visual contact, first with the nurse and then with her hands as she cares for him, is followed by listening to her as she explains what she is doing and why it is necessary. After his eyes and ears are attuned to the procedure, he may be encouraged to ask questions and to help by holding some of the supplies. Helping the nurse is followed by the nurse helping him.

When the patient is able to manage his care alone, the nurse allows him to develop skill through practice under her close supervision. If left without her reassuring guidance, he may regress to previous levels of fear and helplessness the first time he encounters any unforeseen difficulty. Managing his own care coupled with the impact of recovering from major surgery is enough to produce high levels of tension. Any complications in the process may be frustrating enough to cause his behavior to become unpredictable. He may vacillate from quiet passivity to demanding abusiveness. Interpretation to the family, his friends, and the staff may be necessary. Sometimes the patient himself needs to be made aware of what he is doing. Getting him to become more independent in his care regardless of setbacks needs to be gently but firmly promoted yet never pushed.

Diet. Return to normal nutrition is accomplished according to the patient's tolerance. High-residue foods are avoided during the early postoperative and convalescent period to diminish the likelihood of ileal obstruction. Gradually the small intestine takes over the function of the large intestine and the patient is able to eat nearly everything he wishes without adverse effects. Following an ileostomy, the patient eagerly anticipates consuming everything that was previously forbidden. Some patients will eat too many high-residue foods too soon, but more often patients will be overly hesitant and unwilling to take chances. They will unnecessarily restrict themselves for many months. A written plan for gradually increasing the diet to include all foods is frequently advisable. By taking very small amounts (½ to 1 teaspoonful, initially) of each untried food and noting the intestinal reaction, the patient may learn his individual tolerances for such foods as corn, nuts, raw vegetables, cabbage, onions, prunes, chocolate desserts, and highly seasoned dishes. It is important also to remind the patient that thorough mastication is needed to diminish undigested residues in the alimentary tract. Excessive weight gain is often a problem for the ileostomy adult after he has been rehabilitated.

As soon as the patient successfully learns a basic program for the care of his ileostomy and appliance, he is discharged under the continuing follow-up care of his physician. The nurse plays a major role in preparing the patient to be self-sufficient as far as his elimination is concerned, as, in association with the surgeon and the social worker, she assists him to regain a sense of well-being.

Educating the Patient. Whether in public health or private or general practice, the nurse assumes responsibility for keeping abreast of current developments in patient care so that her knowledge and skills remain practical and fresh. She herself, as well as the agency's inservice education department, should maintain up-to-date collections of information, charts, manuals, demonstration models, sample appliances, and other aids for teaching her patients and her auxiliary coworkers.

Patients frequently use ileostomy appliances marketed in their area, although all appliance companies provide mail order service. If one appliance proves unsatisfactory, the patient can learn of another one through a fellow ileostomate. Instead of one-piece rubber appliances, many patients prefer to wear more durable aluminum or Lucite plastic faceplates with detachable polyethylene bags. (Some patients have begun to use food freezing bags because they are thinner, odorproof, and inexpensive and do not rustle.) The patients find them easier to clean, less likely to retain an odor, more comfortable to wear, and lighter in weight and bulk under current clothing styles. Custom-made appliances are available for patients with a protruding abdomen; a hollow or concave abdomen; a stoma of irregular length, width, shape, or location; or excessive scar tissue, double stomas, and other special fitting problems.

COMPLICATIONS

Complications needing to be brought to the attention of a physician should be known by both public health and hospital staff nurses. The patient should be informed of untoward signs that may arise during convalescence. If the ulcerative colitis had progressed to the ileum before surgery, then postcolectomy ileitis is a possibility. The symptoms and signs include pain, fever, abdominal distention, foul watery discharge, fistulas to skin, and retraction of stoma. Abdominal abscesses are an early postoperative complication and are treated with antibiotics and an incision with drainage procedure. Abdominal tenderness, distention, and fever are commonly seen in patients with an abscess. Although relatively infrequent, retraction of the stoma is a third postoperative complication. It may be caused by excessive internal pressure or weight gain. To prevent internal peritoneal soiling and unnecessary problems with appliance fit, prompt surgical correction is advocated. Prolapse, or herniation of the ileum through the stoma, is a frightening sight and requires surgical or medical manipulation by a physician to reduce it.

Ileal obstruction occurs in a large number of patients, often a year or more after surgery. Peritoneal adhesions are sometimes the cause of cramps, vomiting, and cessation of ileostomy drainage. Surgical correction will probably be necessary.

Difficulties with appliances and skin excoriation are the most common problems facing the ileostomy patient during his rehabilitation. Enlightened nursing care and helpful hints from fellow ileostomates can do the most to correct unfortunate situations. Skin excoriation is generally caused by contact with ileal contents due to an ill-fitting appliance or an improperly applied one. If the skin is not dry before the adhesive is applied, or the adhesive is not dry before the appliance is placed, loosening and leakage can be expected. Other causes of skin irritation include the following: pulling off appliance in a rough manner without using solvent; too frequent changes of appliance when unnecessary (except in the case of a new ileostomate in whom an appliance left longer than 5 days can produce irritation); sensitivity reactions to adhesive or appliance; and inadequate protection of the skin with suitable methods and pharmaceutical preparations.

Eliminating causes of skin irritation and establishing better methods of skin protection will solve most problems. Some patients use silicone creams and sprays for coating sensitive skin. These must be used sparingly and according to directions so as not to interfere with appliance adherence. Patch-testing new products will detect sensitivities and reduce incidence of more serious allergic manifestations. Putting waterproof and perspiration-proof tape around the edges of the appliance before swimming, bowling, or other strenuous sports are undertaken will promote holding power, especially if appliance cement extends to the area under the tape.

Vacations away from home and job are important for the ileostomy patient and he need not hesitate about making extensive travel plans. He can carry an extra appliance and all necessary supplies with him in his hand luggage so they will be available at all times. He should carry an identification card stating his medications and ileostomy care as well as other necessary medical information in the language of those countries he intends to visit.

Interpersonal problems, job discrimination, and other psychosocial adjustment problems of the patient may become apparent only after he has been home for a number of weeks. For this reason, referrals for additional guidance, welfare, and vocational assistance are not usually made by the hospital staff nurse. She should instead refer the patient to his local visiting nurse association. State vocational rehabilitation department services and other community resources may then be interpreted to the patient for his consideration at more appropriate times when the need is manifested.

TUMORS

Most tumors of the small intestine are benign, and the ileum is most frequently involved (Moyer et al.). Adenomas, polyps, lipomas, myomas, and fibromas are the most common types, yet these are not seen as often as the inflammatory lesions previously described. Because some benign tumors are considered to be premalignant or potentially malignant growths, they are usually excised when discovered.

Adenomatous Polyps

The incidence of adenomatous polyps increases with age. They are often asymptomatic, but later cause rectal bleeding of varying degrees. Sigmoidoscopy enables visualization of most polypoid adenomas, since about 75 percent of them are found in the last 25 cm of intestinal tract (Nardi and Zuidema). Barium examination with air contrast studies is often diagnostic and helps in differentiation from other intestinal diseases. Because particles of feces may resemble adenomatous polyps of different sizes on x-ray study, it is extremely important that the patient be sufficiently prepared with laxatives and enemas until the colon is clear. The nurse should reposition the patient to a prone or a knee-chest position during the enema to facilitate more adequate cleansing of the transverse and ascending segments of the large intestine.

Multiple Polyposis

In multiple or familial polyposis, an inherited disease, adenomatous polyps are scattered throughout the large bowel. When they begin to develop, sometimes in puberty, sometimes in late middle age, they may cause no symptoms. Later the patient experiences recurrent episodes of bloody diarrhea and cramps eventually resulting in anemia and weight loss, and finally in cancer. Upon diagnosis a total proctocolectomy with a permanent ileostomy is ordinarily advocated to prevent a rapid growth type of carcinoma. The premalignant phase is shorter in those in whom polyposis develops at an early age. Because multiple polyposis is a dominant mendelian trait transmitted through both sexes, it is important that public health nurses be persistent in their case-finding efforts. Usually one-half of the victim's children will inherit the disease; all family members should be examined carefully and regularly by a physician throughout life.

Adenocarcinoma

Adenocarcinoma is the most common malignant tumor of the large intestine and rectum. For those aged 35 to 74 years the colorectal cancer mortality rate is second only to that of lung cancer.

Cancer of the rectum is somewhat more common in men, and cancer of the colon is seen more frequently in women, but no socioeconomic factor like that reported for cancer of the esophagus and stomach has been observed. Although the cause remains unknown, adenocarcinoma of the colon and rectum is somehow related to familial polyposis and to ulcerative colitis.

The most frequent initial sign is rectal bleeding. Many persons also experience constipation, diarrhea, or a change in their bowel habits. About one patient in four with cancer of the rectum will notice an excessive passage of flatus. Sometimes there will be symptoms of bowel obstruction with pencil-caliber stools. This is likely to be seen when the lesion is low on the left side of the colon.

Nearly three-quarters of low-lying lesions can be promptly diagnosed by means of proctosigmoidoscopic examination and biopsy. For high-lying lesions a barium roentgenogram utilizing an air contrast method is normally done. Hemoglobin determinations and eosinophil counts support the findings. Prognosis is poorer in individuals with high eosinophil rates. Sometimes a silicone foam enema is given and the retrieved mold can aid in localizing the tumor.

For the nearly 60 percent of individuals with operable lesions at the time of diagnosis, the prognosis is very good; in those with metastases or acute obstructive symptoms the mortality rate is high. Curative or palliative surgery results in an overall 5-year-arrest rate of more than 50 percent for patients with colorectal carcinoma.

PREOPERATIVE CARE

Initial objectives of treatment for the patient during his preoperative period include the following: (1) to restore nutritional status to the best possible level; (2) to restore total circulating blood volume to normal levels; (3) to correct electrolyte imbalances if present; (4) to evaluate cardiovascular-renal status, and thereafter modify the therapeutic plan as needed; and (5) to prepare the patient psychologically for implications of his diagnosis and the proposed operation. These objectives are accomplished by orders, first of all, for a high-carbohydrate, high-protein diet to interrupt catabolic processes and to fortify depleted liver glycogen and body proteins. Vitamins B-complex, ascorbic acid, and K are given to support metabolism, to promote appetite, and to recover losses from antibiotic therapy, diarrhea, and other causes. Iron and minerals are frequently given. Transfusions may be desirable. Routine and special laboratory tests are done to assess the need for additional measures. An electrocardiogram may be ordered. After the surgeon talks to the patient and his family about his diagnosis and plan for care, he may ask a nurse, a social worker, and a colostomy patient to visit in order to assist with a satisfactory adjustment.

Immediate preparation of the patient for colon surgery includes measures to cleanse and decompress the bowel and to reduce the bacterial flora. A low-residue diet will be ordered for at least 1 or 2 days prior to scheduled surgery. Sometimes a clear liquid diet is prescribed. The patient may receive succinylsulfathiazole (Sulfasuxidine), 12 g daily in divided doses for 5 days, or neomycin sulfate, 1 g every hour for 4 hours followed by 1 g every 4 hours for 24 to 48 hours. Castor oil or another laxative is given 2 days before surgery and repeated if necessary. Saline enemas may be ordered. If obstruction has developed, laxatives will be withheld and a temporary cecostomy or colostomy may be done as a preliminary measure to relieve distention. Sometimes a long tube (Miller-Abbott, Cantor, or other) is inserted for decompression (aspiration of intestinal contents) proximal to the obstruction. Otherwise a nasogastric tube will be placed the day before surgery and low intermittent suction established. On the evening before the operation, the skin from nipple line to the knees will be shaved and cleansed with surgical soap. The anesthetist will visit to assess the cardiopulmonary status and to leave preanesthetic orders (similar to those for other general abdominal surgery) suitable for the patient's age and requirements.

POSTOPERATIVE CARE

Postoperative treatment objectives are the following: to prevent abdominal distention until bowel function returns; to restore physiological balance of urinary elimination; to maintain fluid and electrolyte balance; to reestablish patterns of bowel elimination; and to prevent infections, cardiopulmonary complications, and other postoperative problems. A Foley catheter will be in place for about a week. When it is removed, the patient's voiding ability will be measured, and catheterization will be carried out to remove retained urine. If the residual urine of the bladder exceeds 150 ml, the patient will be carefully observed and recatheterized as necessary to prevent urine bladder distention. Sometimes bethanechol chloride (Urecholine) is prescribed. Later on it is sometimes necessary for male patients to undergo a prostatectomy. Initiation of micturition commonly causes postoperative complications in patients requiring abdominoperineal resections.

A few days after surgery the clamped or intact colostomy will be opened. Soon after that daily irrigations of normal saline will be ordered. Irrigations are not always done on patients with colostomies of the ascending or transverse portions of colon because the stool is soft-formed or semiliquid. Drainage tubes for the pelvic and suprapubic region are shortened periodically and withdrawn when drainage subsides. Skin sutures are removed after 7 to 10 days. When bowel function is reestablished the nasogastric tube is removed and a graduated liquid-to-soft-to-regular diet is ordered. Parenteral fluids are discontinued when oral intake is sufficient to meet nutritional needs.

Early gradual ambulation and self-care are encouraged as tolerated, and other measures including routine chest film to detect pulmonary complications, elastic bandages applied from the feet to the thighs to support circulation, and antibiotics may be ordered. The medical follow-up program is then planned.

NURSING CARE PROGRAM

Nursing care for the patient with cancer of the intestinal tract begins in the community. The public health nurse should be alert for signs of malignant change and urge persons she sees to seek earlier care. A visiting nurse or occupational health nurse can help the patient anticipating surgery to face his fears and anxieties regarding hospitalization and surgery. If homemaking services, child care arrangements, and financial assistance are needed, she can locate appropriate resources and can visit the family while the patient is in the hospital.

In the hospital, the staff nurse continues this care by assessing the new patient's need for additional information and emotional support. Even when it is not the patient's first hospitalization, she realizes that the experience of a serious illness and its implications are fraught with stress. She spends as much time as necessary getting to know her patient so that she may better support his behavior, reduce sources of tension, and help him adjust to his disease and its treatment.

For the patient who is to have a colostomy, being assigned a nurse who knows and cares about him is crucial to a satisfactory recovery.

After a general but thorough physical examination, the patient needs to be prepared for a digital and sigmoidoscopic examination of the anal canal, rectum, and sigmoid. After explanations and reassurances appropriate to this patient, he is given enemas as ordered to cleanse the lower colon. One to three saline enemas may be required until returns are clear. The nurse assembles the necessary equipment as follows: gloves, rubber bulb and tube inflator, sigmoidoscope, biopsy specimen bottle and formalin, sponge forceps, goose-neck floor or overhead lamp, cotton balls and gauze, light bulb, cord, and carrier, water-soluble lubricant, suction tip with rubber connection tube, biopsy forceps, suction machine and pan of water, and other supplies requested by the sigmoidoscopist.

The examining table is jackknifed to facilitate placing the patient in a knee-chest position, unless a side-lying (Sims') position is desired initially for the digital examination. One end of the table is fixed with a vertical support and cushioned with a pillow to hold the patient's head. The other end is placed to support the patient's knees. A sheet is used to cover the patient's back and legs for warmth and comfort as well as privacy. Only the immediate area of the anus and buttocks is exposed.

The sigmoidoscope is usually warmed under running water or with the physician's hands to avoid chilling the patient. After arranging the light for adequate viewing, the nurse moves to the patient's side in order to be readily available for answering his questions and for providing both physical and psychological support as needed. When the physician has finished, the patient's anus is cleansed of lubricant and he is assisted to an upright position. Because his head has been lowered for some time, the patient is supported at all times to prevent falls from dizziness. Even though he may have been able to walk to the examining room, he should be returned to his room by wheel chair or litter and assisted to a comfortable position in bed by the nurse.

To prevent obstruction by retained barium that has hardened, the nurse will give cleansing enemas and laxatives to her patient for 2 days following a barium enema x-ray series. For patients with partial obstructions caused by the tumor, she should take care to give gentle enemas under low pressure. For patients with nearly complete obstructions, a cecostomy may be performed to provide immediate and effective drainage and to decompress the bowel prior to definitive surgery. The nurse takes precautions to secure the drainage catheter from accidental dislodgment. She covers the collection receptacle with a cloth or bag and takes vigorous deodorization measures to prevent nausea in the patient, his roommate, and visitors. She applies tincture of benzoin, karaya powder mixtures, or skin protective creams with each regular and frequent dressing change around the tube, because cecostomy feces is semiliquid and irritating to the skin. She checks the Miller-Abbott tube or the nasogastric tube and the suction machine for effectiveness and corrects leaking connections. Periodically, she may need to irrigate the tube with normal saline to remove semisolid particles that may clog the catheter lumen. Correct measurement of irrigating solution is important for accurate intake and output records.

COLOSTOMY CARE

The most challenging nursing care required during the postoperative phase of treatment is that needed for the patient who returns with a colostomy. The first sight of the swollen, discolored stoma is shocking to patients. There may be only one stoma (single-barreled) if the terminal colon has been removed or two stomas (double-barreled) if the intestinal tract is to be rejoined at some future date. This allows the distal colon to rest, to regain normal tone and size, and to permit the inflammation or bacterial growth to subside. Some double-barreled colostomies are permanent. They are life-saving palliation measures when the tumor is obstructive and unresectable.

The nurse should ascertain and clearly mark the stoma leading to the proximal colon from which the feces will be emitted. This is the stoma that will be irrigated with 500 to 1,500 ml of tepid saline or tap water to promote the establishment of regularity. Only small amounts of saline or antiseptic solution (100 to 200 ml) will be used in the daily irrigations of the distal colon for cleansing purposes. This solution may be absorbed by a dehydrated terminal segment or it may be expelled rectally.

During the immediate postoperative period, the exposed bowel probably will be covered with petroleum jelly gauze and abdominal pads. (Later, temporary postoperative plastic bags can be applied to fit around the stoma and collect fecal discharge.) These are reinforced or changed as necessary. Because of the age and debilitated condition of many patients, the nurse takes special precautions to keep the abdominal suture lines and drain sites clean and dry, thus helping to prevent secondary infections and wound dehiscence. Usually the stoma(s) will be clamped for 1 to 4 days to prevent peritoneal soiling from leakage and to promote healing of the suture lines. Sometimes the colon is brought out to the abdominal surface and fixed over a glass rod sling or a skin flap. After a sufficient time lapse (1 to 3 days) for the wound margins to heal, sealing off the peritoneum, the double-barreled colostomy is created by the surgeon with a diathermy knife or cautery. No anesthetic is required for the insensitive mucosa, but the odor of burning tissue can be quite upsetting to the patient or others in the room. The glass rod will be left in place for 2 to 3 weeks to support the bowel and prevent its retraction below the skin surface. It is removed when the cut mucosal margins shrink and become united to the skin edges. After a few months the edematous stoma will be only a few centimeters in size.

The Emotional Component. It is not necessary that the patient see his colostomy until he is ready to participate in his own care. The sensitive and understanding nurse will not force him to face the realization until he is stronger and more able to cope with his own feelings. The patient's reactions to a great extent will depend upon his previous patterns of adaptation to living before the onset of his illness. Incapacitation, the prospect of colostomy management, the status of his tumor, and the reactions of his family and friends will be extremely worrisome. His basic values regarding his. acceptability to himself and to others and those attitudes that determine his independence and achievement behavior are seriously threatened. Resentment, tears, depression, and anxiety are to be expected as fairly typical postoperative reactions. Refusal of treatment, profound apathy, helplessness, and even suicide attempts may be observed in some patients who were not told (or who could not accept) that they would have a colostomy performed. The nurse's calm, confident, matter-of-fact, yet sympathetic manner will encourage the patient's acceptance of himself with an altered body image and his willingness to cooperate in his convalescence. Many patients can resume normal activities and social obligations just a few months after discharge from the hospital. Others, however, will require continued care by family or professional staff.

Irrigations. A few words about irrigations are in order. Essentially, these are simply enemas of the colostomy given to facilitate a natural evacuation pattern so that the patient may resume his daily schedule of activities without further attention to elimination needs or the bother of wearing a collection pouch. The habit of a bowel movement once or twice daily with or without irrigations some-times is developed in a matter of 6 months. Colostomy irrigations should be viewed therefore as an optional convenience or as a simple method for relief of constipation when needed. It is important that the nurse impress this idea upon the patient so that he does not develop compulsive ritualistic practices with irrigations that are disproportionate to the procedure and its purpose. It is astonishing to find that some patients spend several hours daily for their irrigations using several gallons of water and planning their whole life around this central act.

Elimination regularity depends on several factors: the location of the colostomy, dietary habits, exercise, fluid intake, emotional influences, and the general physical condition, among other things. True, some patients are able to irrigate themselves with 1 or 2 quarts of water, experience an immediate return with feces, and need wear nothing but a tissue or gauze to protect the stoma and absorb its mucus. A significant number of colostomy patients, on the other hand, have little control over the frequency or consistency of stools and the flatus expelled. They will need to wear a bag continuously. They should *not* be made to feel guilty if regularity cannot be established.

For the initial irrigation ordered, less than half a liter of normal saline may be used. The container of solution is held about 12 to 18 inches above the stoma to obtain the desired amount of gravity pressure. The lubricated catheter is inserted gently and slowly about 6 inches while the tepid saline flows into the colon. The expelled fluid is collected in a basin. Fecal return will probably be small but flatus is often relieved and the patient is introduced to the procedure with a minimum of disturbance. Untoward signs of severe pain or blockage are indications for the irrigation to be immediately stopped and reported to the surgeon. Usually there is little difficulty other than mild distention, slight cramping, and a feeling of fullness.

After this gradual introduction to the procedure, it commonly becomes necessary to use 750 ml or more of tepid tap water in order to obtain a good fecal return and satisfactory relief for the patient. No more than 2 liters should ever be used and the solution should *never* be given in its entirety before it is allowed to be expelled. Usually some of the solution returns around the catheter while it is being administered. Gentle massage of the abdomen also facilitates solution return. The procedure should be neither hurried nor unduly prolonged. Ordinarily 45 to 90 minutes is sufficient. A casual relaxed attitude should be encouraged. Music, reading material, or other appropriate diversions may reduce tensions and discourage unnecessary preoccupation with the routine once it is learned. Nevertheless, privacy should be insured and freedom from disturbing interruptions should be provided. The nurse ought to plan her schedule so that this is possible and so that she may be readily available for consultation and assistance.

The daily irrigations are most easily given when the patient is sitting on a toilet, on a commode, or in a chair with a bucket near the feet when toilet facilities are not available, so that the expelled solution flows directly into a large receptacle. If the patient is bedridden it may be necessary to administer the solution to him while he is in a semisitting or side-lying position. Large basins to collect the expelled solution and towels to protect the patient and the bed linen will probably be necessary. Many patients receive commercial irrigation sets during their hospitalization, and these greatly facilitate colostomy care and patient teaching but are not necessary.

The nurse can teach the patient and his family the use of substitutes for irrigating such as an Asepto or bulb syringe and a bowl of water, or an enema can or hot water bottle with tubing, or a funnel and a pitcher for solution. Drainage sleeves can be fashioned from plastic bags by snipping holes for stoma and catheter in the closed end. Petroleum jelly, vegetable shortening, or cooking oil may be used to lubricate the catheter prior to insertion instead of water-soluble surgical lubricant. Low cost or free supplies for colostomy irrigations and management may be obtained by cancer patients through their local cancer association or colostomy club.

Skin Care. Plain soap and water cleansing, drying, and sprinkling with talcum powder or cornstarch will provide adequate care for the peristomal skin of most colostomy patients. Cold cream, hand lotions, or vegetable shortening may be applied by those patients who wear appliances throughout the day, but sometimes nothing is necessary. Skin irritation is less common for the colostomy patient than the ileostomy patient, who must at all times be protected from excoriating, skin-digesting ileal drainage. Facial or toilet tissues can be used instead of costly sterile gauze pads to cover or cleanse the stoma after care. These are adequately held in place by girdles or other abdominal supports and clothing.

Stomal Dilatation. Dilatation of the stoma may or may not be prescribed by the physician. Modern surgical techniques of suturing the mucosa to the skin margins have reduced the incidence of strictures. If necessary the patient can be taught this procedure. Either the index or the little finger is covered with a rubber cot (to prevent irritation by the nail and for esthetic purposes), then lubricated and inserted slowly and gently. The finger is rotated and held in the stoma for about 30 seconds and then carefully removed. Digital dilatations are repeated once daily or as often as the physician deems necessary to keep the orifice open. A small amount of blood and mucus from the sensitive stoma surface may be expected, and the patient should be reassured about this occurrence. Prolapse, wound herniation, retraction of colostomy, hemorrhage, necrosis, and infection are all postoperative complications to be reported, but most of these will occur in the early postoperative weeks and usually need not concern the patient following a few months' convalescence.

Diet. The patient may eat anything that agrees with him, although he will probably prefer to avoid those foods which for him are likely to cause diarrhea, constipation, or gaseous distention. Many patients avoid such foods as onions, beans, prune juice, cabbage, and nuts. Foods should be chewed with lips closed to reduce air swallowing. Chewing gum also can cause flatus. Laxatives should not be taken without a doctor's order. Occasionally stool softening agents will be ordered to facilitate fecal passage. Bismuth subgallate, charcoal, or chlorophyll preparations will be helpful for internal odor control. Odors of appliances or irrigating equipment can be reduced by substituting plastic for rubber supplies, by vigorous cleansing and airing practices, and by use of commercial deodorants.

Education of Patient and Family. One professional nurse should assume responsibility for teaching a given colostomy patient and a family member about his care, irrigations, diet, medications, and referrals to community resources. If additional nursing staff or students are to participate in the process, all should meet together to outline and record a plan that will be consistent yet flexible. Account should be taken of the variations in abilities to learn and to teach by all who are involved. Return demonstrations and written directions should be included in the teaching plan to enhance effective recall after discharge. Patient information leaflets should be appropriately selected and given with ample opportunities to read, digest, discuss, and ask questions before the patient is dismissed from the hospital. Referral forms to visiting nurse associations *should provide a detailed description* of what has been taught the patient and family so that intelligent follow-up reviews by community health nurses can be instituted. As a general rule, once the colostomy management is learned, the patient can return to his former employment and recreational interests. Marital relationships can continue as they were before surgery in many cases, but for extenuating circumstances some patients will need to see a physician or psychiatrist.

TRAUMA

Injuries to the colon may be caused by missiles, blows with sharp or blunt objects, and foreign bodies. Crushing and bruising injuries resulting from vehicular accidents, military skirmishes, natural disasters, and other forms of violence may be responsible for lacerations and hemorrhage of internal organs. Perforation of the bowel also may be caused by instruments, tubes, or enemas as well as an accumulation of fecaliths. When this occurs the bowel wall may have been previously weakened by diverticulosis, regional enteritis, or other pathological conditions.

The patient usually experiences tenderness and pain at the site of the injury. Nausea and vomiting commonly follow. Spillage of fecal contents and the presence of free intraperitoneal air cause abdominal distention, rigidity, and peritonitis. Leukocytosis and fever ensue. The patient often goes into shock. The pulse rises and the blood pressure drops. Death is likely unless adequate treatment is begun promptly.

Blood or plasma transfusions and dextrose in saline and water are administered with large doses of broad-spectrum antibiotics. Exposed bowel should be covered with warm wet saline compresses. After the patient has been treated for shock, hemorrhage, and infection, an exploratory laparotomy probably will be done. Extensive irrigation and debridement may be necessary. The type of operation depends upon the nature of the trauma, the location and extent of injury, and the degree of contamination. Exteriorization of bowel loop on the abdomen, an intestinal resection with anastomosis, or a temporary colostomy may be performed.

Nursing care for these patients is primarily life-saving. Measures are aimed at reestablishing physiological equilibrium and correcting complications such as shock and infection. Careful administration of medications and parenteral fluids as ordered, maintenance of accurate intake and output records, immediate reporting of untoward signs, and support of cardiopulmonary function are essential nursing tasks.

OBSTRUCTION

When the normal passage of bowel contents is impeded, the condition is called *intestinal obstruction*. Causes of this well-known yet grave development may be classified as those arising from outside the bowel, those occurring within the lumen, and those associated with the intestinal wall itself. Hernias and adhesions (which are secondary to surgery, infection, and trauma) are the two most common extrinsic determinants of mechanical obstruction. Intraluminal antecedents include neoplasms, inflammatory lesions, aberrant gallstones, and fecaliths. Adynamic or paralytic ileus precipitated by surgery or injury affects the bowel wall motility. Another example of this third type of cause is an infarction of intestinal mucosa caused by an occlusion of the main mesenteric vessels, arterial or venous.

Diagnosis of an intestinal obstruction is suggested by one or more of these characteristic signs and symptoms: abdominal pain, distention, obstipation, and vomiting. Further differentiation of the type of obstruction, site or level of pathology, and complicating factors, if any, depends on a thorough investigation, including a detailed history, a careful physical examination, a series of abdominal films, and various laboratory studies. Acute attacks are characterized by a sudden onset of severe symptoms. A chronic obstruction is partial or recurrent in nature with an insidious gradual onset.

If symptoms develop rapidly the obstruction is likely to be located high in the intestinal tract. The state of dehydration (due to repeated emesis) is often greater, as the obstructive lesion is higher in the alimentary canal. A later onset of vomiting frequently means that the site of obstruction is lower, and if the ileocecal valve is still functioning there may be no vomiting at all. Thus, abdominal distention is greater when the obstruction is lower in the colon.

Pain may be slight to severe, intermittent or constant. Patients with partial obstructions may have nausea and diarrhea without pain.

For the first few hours of a patient's admission to the hospital with an intestinal obstruction, the medical objectives are to relieve his symptoms, improve his general condition, and establish a definitive diagnosis. Immediate surgical intervention is indicated for acute obstructions associated with strangulation, perforation, vascular occlusion, and other causes not amenable to supportive conservative therapy. Stereoscopic abdominal roentgenograms of the patient in a supine position are the basis for differential diagnosis (Moyer et al.). Cleansing enemas should not be given before x-ray examinations because they could confuse results. Fluid and electrolyte balance is restored and gastrointestinal intubation frequently carried out. When the patient's condition has improved sufficiently (or when conservative treatment fails) an exploratory laparotomy is scheduled. Relief of the obstructive state may be accomplished in various ways depending on the circumstances. Removal of the cause, resection or anastomosis to short-circuit or bypass the obstruction, and a colostomy or ileostomy are among the procedures considered by the surgeon to reestablish intestinal continuity and function.

Nursing Care Program

The patient with an intestinal obstruction is usually a very sick person. Often he is prostrate, anxious, restless, and temporarily disoriented to some degree. If he is dehydrated his tongue and mouth will be dry. The breath will be foul and sordes may be present on his teeth. This is especially true if there is fecal vomiting. The nurse should provide thorough and frequent mouth care as soon as possible. She may assist the physician with preparations for administration of intravenous fluids. She will initiate intake and output records and collect urine specimens for microscopic analysis and for specific gravity determinations.

If an intestinal tube is to be used, the nurse will assemble the necessary equipment and assist the patient to cooperate with its insertion. A single lumen Cantor or Harris tube with a balloon for mercury may be used but a Miller-Abbott double lumen tube is more common. The larger lumen is for aspiration of bowel contents, and the smaller lumen is for inflation of the rubber balloon. The procedure is similar to the passage of a nasogastric tube until it reaches the stomach. Then about 5 ml of mercury is used to inflate the balloon so that it acts as a bolus of food enabling its passage with the peristaltic action of the bowel. To facilitate passage of the tube through the pylorus, the patient is placed on his right side in a flat or Trendelenburg plane for at least 2 hours. When the tube reaches the duodenum the patient is placed in Fowler's position for 1 to 2 hours. The tube is not taped to the patient or restricted in any way, so that it can advance naturally without hindrance. Draping the coils loosely near the top of the bed where the tube is connected to the suction machine tubing will be satisfactory. Tepid normal saline is used to irrigate the tube every hour and as often as needed to keep it open. After the tube reaches the jejunum it will be advanced by the nurse about 2 inches every 30 minutes and the patient's position can be modified as desired. X-ray films will be taken periodically to determine the location of the tube.

The degree of illness, shock, disorientation, and sometimes senility compound the fears, anxiety, and restlessness of the patient. The sight of so many tubes is alarming to him and his family. A typical patient with a severe intestinal obstruction may receive simultaneous intravenous infusions in two sites and at the same time have in place a bladder catheter, a rectal tube, a nasal catheter for oxygen, a gastric or intestinal tube attached to suction, and a cecostomy tube for additional drainage and relief of distention distal to the obstruction. If someone cannot be present at all times with this patient, it may be necessary to restrain him in order to prevent dislodgment of the tubes and accidental injury. Repeated explanations and reassurances are sometimes helpful but may not be sufficient to ensure the patient's safety. In addition to maintaining the patency and correct functioning of all tubes, the nurse will be busy monitoring the patient's vital signs, recording intake and output, and administering medications for pain, infection, restlessness, and sleeplessness. She will change the patient's position, provide skin and mouth care, perform passive exercises with his extremities, encourage deep breathing, and try to maintain his level of awareness. These activities are suitable whether or not surgery is performed, and they are similar to nursing measures indicated for most patients having serious gastrointestinal conditions.

HERNIATION

A protrusion of bowel or omentum through the abdominal wall is a *hernia*. Various types are identified by the anatomical site of weakness: inguinal, femoral, umbilical, ventral, and incisional. Inguinal hernias are by far the most frequent type, comprising about 80 percent of all hernias. Whether they are diagnosed as direct or indirect depends upon their anatomical relationship to the inguinal canal and the direction of presentation.

Hernias are brought about by a combination of two factors: an abdominal wall weakness, which may be due to previous surgery, obesity, muscular wasting, or congenital abnormalities, and second, an intra-abdominal pressure, which may be due to a chronic cough, constipation, and fluid or gaseous distention. If the herniation can be easily and completely manipulated back into place, it is considered reducible. If it will not return to place, usually because of adhesions, the hernia is *irreducible* or *incarcerated*. A *strangulated* hernia is one in which the contents have been cut off from an adequate blood supply. Gangrene is inevitable, and the patient experiences a sudden onset of severe pain, a tense and tender hernial protrusion, and other symptoms of intestinal obstruction previously mentioned.

Surgery is the treatment of choice for all hernias as soon as possible after their discovery to prevent complications of incarceration and strangulation. When this occurs, emergency surgery is necessary and the operative risk is increased. Trusses or abdominal supports are often ill-fitting, uncomfortable, and unsatisfactory for years of continued usage. The danger of strangulation is ever-present. Properly fitted trusses are recommended for patients who refuse surgery or who are in very poor general health making an operation inadvisable. Various techniques for hernia repair are available to surgeons, but the essential objectives are to excise or reduce the herniated sac or omentum and to repair the defective cause. The recurrence rate varies from between 2 and 30 percent of all patients undergoing surgical correction (herniorrhaphy) and is higher for those with direct inguinal hernias.

Preoperative preparations are similar to those for other general surgery. After the patient recovers from the anesthetic and his vital signs are stabilized, he will be returned to his nursing unit. Intermittent positive pressure breathing inhalations with Alevaire and isoproterenol (Isuprel) nebulization may be ordered several times daily to stimulate deep breathing and removal of mucus. Pain and the fear of pulling a tight incision cause the patient to guard his movements, to breathe more shallowly than desired, and to postpone coughing. Medications to relieve pain, support of the incision with hands or a pillow, and strong urging may be necessary to promote adequate coughing to bring up loosened secretions. Sometimes the surgeon orders elixir of terpin hydrate to liquefy tenacious sputum. Early ambulation is also encouraged. Male patients may be allowed to stand at the bedside to void on the day of surgery if they have difficulty in voiding. Use of mirror and coaching by a nurse may be useful in correcting posture. If the patient does not stand up straight, the abdominal muscles will shorten and make later posture correction more difficult. The patient is reminded to lift nothing heavier than a book and to avoid strenuous activity for at least 3 to 6 weeks. Medications to prevent constipation and excessive coughing may be given to the patient to avert unnecessary tension on the healing sutures. He may return to a sedentary job in about 2 weeks and to manual labor in about 6 to 8 weeks. If he is obese, he may be asked to lose weight in order to reduce the probability of recurrence.

Disorders of the Anus

A good knowledge of anatomy and bacteriology will provide the primary basis for understanding most anal disorders. Some conditions are related to pathology of the intestinal tract while others are of a local nature.

Pathological disorders of the anus and perianal region are usually diagnosed by direct visual examination and digital palpation. Possible colon involvement necessitates proctosigmoidoscopy. Biopsy, stool analysis, barium enema x-ray studies, and various laboratory tests are frequently indicated to rule out associated systemic disease. A careful history of the patient's complaint is also important.

The main symptoms experienced by patients with anal disorders are bleeding, pain, prolapse, pruritus, and mucopurulent discharge during defecation or apart from it. The bleeding may be slight or profuse, bright red or dark, with or without clots, and mixed in the stool composition or present on its surface. Usually the pain is localized. Sometimes it is accompanied by swelling and visible inflammation or infection. The consistency and frequency of the stool as well as its gross appearance should be observed and noted. Procidentia, or prolapse, may be constant or may occur only when the patient is straining, coughing, or sitting. The prolapse may involve a small amount of tissue or a large mass. It may retract spontaneously or necessitate manual replacement. Itching may be incessant or may occur only when the patient defecates or urinates, when he is sleeping, or when he is wearing certain undergarments. In female patients itching may occur only during the menstrual period.

Surgery is often indicated for anorectal disease, either as an office procedure or with hospitalization required. The therapeutic goal is to cure the condition without complications and to restore normal function compatible with the best attainable level of comfort and health for the patient.

Operative treatment of anal conditions can correct many situations yet cause additional physiological problems in a small percentage of cases. Anal incontinence may occur following fistulotomy, obstetrical injury, or other resection in this region. Sometimes the condition can be remedied with plastic surgery. For postoperative or post-traumatic anal canal strictures, regular periodic dilatations with instruments or a finger may be necessary. Inflammatory diseases such as lymphogranuloma venereum or granuloma inguinale also can produce strictures of the anorectal region which require corrective measures after the disease has been controlled with tetracylines.

INFECTIONS AND INFLAMMATIONS

Anorectal Abscess

Anorectal abscesses are most common in the perianal or ischiorectal region. Most of them originate in the anal glands or crypts of Morgagni. These infections are usually caused by staphylococci, streptococci, or *Escherichia coli*. Sometimes the cause is not known, or the abscess may be associated with Crohn's disease, ulcerative colitis, tuberculosis, or previous surgery. The reddened, painful swelling at the involved site is usually treated by incision and drainage along with parenteral administration of broad-spectrum antibiotics.

To promote cleanliness, drainage, wound healing, and the relief of pain, the patient often receives sitz baths four times daily and more often if desired. The heat of the water increases the circulation of blood to the area, and the patient's relief is apparent. Electrically heated sitz units should be grounded to control static electricity; the nurse must ascertain that the clips for this purpose are securely fastened to appropriate connections. The patient should be shielded from drafts and covered to prevent chilling and assure privacy. Prolonged sitting is uncomfortable for these patients who also may be weakened from age, previous surgery, or associated disease. The nurse should watch the time carefully and be readily available when the patient has achieved the maximum benefits from the treatment. Ordinarily 15 to 20 minutes is sufficient. Gauze fluffs and perineal pads secured with T binders or elastic belts are applied between sitz baths to absorb drainage.

Sometimes half-strength peroxide solution is ordered for irrigation of the abscessed area prior to sitz baths. This germicide releases oxygen, which destroys anaerobic organisms. To preserve its activity the solution must be kept in a tightly closed dark bottle, and it should be replaced with a fresh solution when it loses ability to effervesce. The nurse uses a straight catheter with multiple openings for wide dispersal of solution inside the tissues. An Asepto syringe, a pitcher or basin of irrigating liquid, provision for adequate protection of bedclothes, and a means of collecting the returned solution are all that is needed for this simple procedure. The old dressing is discarded, and a clean towel is placed over the area until the patient gets into the sitz bath. The nurse is careful, of course, to use aseptic techniques in order to prevent introduction of a new infection and cross-contamination with other patients.

If the abscess covers a wide area, the nurse may be required to make frequent changes of wet dressings. A warm, normal saline solution is soaked into cheese-cloth gauze fluffs after the exposed tissues have been cleansed with a bactericidal soap such as pHisoHex and then rinsed with sterile water. Sometimes 3 percent peroxide solution or a mixture of polymyxin B, neomycin, and bacitracin is applied after the cleansing and before packing in the moist saline dressings. These dressings are covered with thick abdominal pads and sometimes a plastic sheet to contain the moisture and help to keep the patient's clothing and bed dry. If continuing warmth is desired, hot water bottles or electric Aquapads may be placed over the outer dressings.

Fistula-in-Ano

A fistula-in-ano is a granulomatous, fibrous tract between epithelial surfaces. It may be open at both ends or closed at one end (called a *sinus* or a *blind fistula*). Most fistulas-in-ano enter the anal canal at or below the level of the anal valves. They are usually brought about by previous abscesses that were inadequately drained and healed. A seropurulent drainage persists until properly treated. Chronic fistulas may become malignant so surgical extirpation of all tracts is the recommended therapy along with correction of the underlying cause.

Fissure

A break in the anal mucosal lining continuity causing a linear ulcer is known as a *fissure*. A polyp of skin tag may be adjacent to one end of this groove. The patient frequently complains of sharp, localized pain that persists long after defecation. Fear of bringing on the pain may cause him to postpone natural evacuation and lead to problems of constipation. Then bleeding and mucus discharge may occur with passage of hardened feces. Treatment for fissures consists of administering topical anesthetic ointment or sprays to relieve pain; perscribing a low-roughage diet and fecal softener laxatives or rectal suppositories to facilitate passage of feces; and eventually performing a surgical excision of the polyp, skin tag, and ulcerated region. Microscopic examination of excised tissue to rule out other diseases is routinely made. An internal sphincterotomy may have to be performed. Because mineral oil preparations retard the absorption of fat-soluble vitamins and because saline cathartics are considered unnecessarily harsh for the patient with a fissure, the detergent wetting agents like dioctyl sodium sulfosuccinate (Doxinate, Colace) are becoming more popular. Divided doses of from 60 to 240 mg are ordered for adults. A soft-formed bulk stool thus produced exerts a natural stimulus to bowel peristalsis and is therefore safer for older patients.

MALIGNANT NEOPLASMS

Tumors of the anus and anal canal are less common than is cancer of other body structures. Malignant tumors include melanoma, squamous cell carcinoma, basal cell carcinoma, and adenocarcinoma spreading from the rectum. Cancer of the anus is more likely to be seen in men, whereas cancer of the anal canal is more common in women. Slow-growing basal cell lesions can be excised locally. Cancer of the anal canal and melanoma are more serious. Treatment for these consists of a combined abdominoperineal resection with removal of adjacent inguinal glands and other associated standard procedures. Periodic postsurgery check-ups are routinely done. An overall 5-year survival rate of from 35 to 60 percent has been reported. The possibility of cure is greater in malignant tumors of the anus. Early and correct diagnosis and treatment are still the key to cancer control, so the nurse should assist the physician in his case-finding work.

HEMORRHOIDS

Varicosities of the hemorrhoidal veins usually develop at three main locations (right anterior, right posterior, and left lateral) in the anus. They may be caused by hereditary factors, by obstruction in the portal circulation, or by straining with defecation, or in association with pregnancy and delivery. They are likely to develop with increased age and they are more common in men than in women. Hemorrhoids are said to appear in nearly 80 percent of persons 30 to 60 years of age (Howard). Internal hemorrhoids are covered by mucous membrane and are usually painless because there are no sensory nerve endings above the pectinate line (irregular demarcation between the anus and the rectum). External varices of the anus are covered by skin and are very sensitive. Hemorrhoids also are classified by degree of severity: first degree, the mucosa-covered internal variety producing only slight bleeding with defecation; second degree, there is some prolapse exteriorly that will retract spontaneously; and third degree, hemorrhoidal masses which require digital manipulation for reduction.

When the bleeding, itching, pain, or prolapse becomes sufficiently severe to require medical attention, initial diagnosis should be accompanied by other tests to rule out coexisting cancer, ulcerative colitis, liver disease, or other pathology. Most people treat their hemorrhoids with well-advertised patent remedies and put off surgery until it becomes absolutely necessary. This is often because of ignorance, fear, and superstition regarding the excruciating pain and lasting effectiveness of proper treatment. Nurses need to help physicians reeducate the public about hemorrhoidal disorders.

Thrombosis

Thrombosed external hemorrhoids are large, painful, bluish-purple masses, covered on the outer surface with skin and on the inner surface with mucosa. They are caused by a rupture of the involved vein and an accumulation of clotted blood which distends the subcutaneous tissues. The patient is in acute distress with severe throbbing pain and must be promptly treated lest sloughing and necrosis of the mass develop. Sitting and standing are too uncomfortable so the patient is put on bed rest with his feet elevated. Continuous warm moist saline or witch hazel compresses are applied to the area and held in place with binders, supports, or sandbags. When tolerated, sitz baths are prescribed and a hemorrhoidectomy is performed as soon as possible. The masses are excised and allowed to drain freely to prevent infection, abscess, or fistula formation. Postoperatively the area should be kept clean and dry between defecations and sitz bath treatments.

Strangulation

Strangulation occurs when internal hemorrhoids prolapse and become trapped within the anal canal. This causes the sphincter muscle to contract spasmodically in an attempt to close the opening. Since necrosis, hemorrhage, and gangrene can develop in the strangulated tissue it is essential that the mass be replaced within the anus as soon as possible. This can be done most readily with a lubricated, gloved finger using gentle care, by the patient himself or with the help of a nurse or doctor.

Medical Treatment

While the hemorrhoids are mild (first and second degree) treatment may consist of a low-roughage diet, laxatives to aid elimination, and sitz baths or suppositories for symptom relief when necessary. Soothing comfort and lubrication may be achieved with use of rectal suppositories containing cod liver oil, zinc oxide, cocoa butter, or petrolatum, Hydrocortisone preparations alleviate inflammation.

Injection therapy has been recommended for some patients with simple early internal hemorrhoids. No preoperative or postoperative measures are needed because this is an office procedure. The physician injects a sclerosing solution subcutaneously

to cause a fibrosis which effects shrinkage of the hemorrhoidal masses and obliteration of the vessels.

Surgical Treatment and Nursing Care

Surgical correction of hemorrhoids consists of ligature and excision, clamping and
cauterization, or various other procedures. The objective is to completely remove
all internal and external hemorrhoids while leaving a minimum of scar tissue and
sufficient normal tissue to ensure good sphincter control and an adequate anal
aperture for elimination without difficulty. Preoperative care consists of administering
a low-residue diet and tap water cleansing enemas. The perianal area is shaved
and operative consent is obtained. The patient needs to be assured that both his
physician and his nurses will be considerate of his comfort after surgery. The
postoperative course is a painful one for many patients, and repeated injections
of narcotics may be necessary. Ice packs over the dressing give relief. Anesthetic
ointments such as dibucaine (Nupercaine) provide welcome, if only temporary,
relief but can delay wound healing. This is especially likely when they are used
excessively by patients who are permitted to have them as desired and therefore
keep them conveniently within bedside reach. Some surgeons have successfully
injected long-lasting, oil-soluble anesthetic agents subcutaneously during the operation. This has reduced the need for constipating narcotics during the first few
postoperative days.

Mineral oil is given on the second postoperative day followed by a gentle low
retention enema of oil on the third morning. An injection of narcotic is administered
about 30 minutes before the patient attempts to defecate. The nurse should allow
the patient privacy but be readily available in case he should become dizzy from
the pain of defecation or the effects of the medication. Following each evacuation,
the patient takes a warm sitz bath to cleanse the operative area of feces, to
promote healing, and to relieve the pain. A rubber ring or foam cushion with a
center section cut out should be placed in the tub for the patient's comfort. Again
the nurse remains in close attendance should the combination of the heat of the
bath and the patient's weakened condition produce vertigo and syncope. After
the bath a fresh perineal dressing is applied and the patient is assisted to bed for
a rest. Sometimes a gauze plug or spool is placed by the surgeon to ensure hemostasis. This needs to be removed before the patient defecates for the first time.
A sitz bath will loosen it sufficiently for easy removal. The nurse should be certain
the patient knows what to expect so that he will not be alarmed when the plug
or spool is removed.

The patient is placed on a liquid or soft low-residue diet prior to surgery and
immediately following it so that he will not have a bowel movement until some
healing has taken place. After the first successful defecation the patient is offered
a regular diet. Early ambulation helps to prevent impaction and facilitates passage
of flatus. The patient is usually given 4 to 8 g of psyllium hydrophilic mucilloid
(Metamucil) three or four times daily. This bulk-forming colloid preparation
produces a soft, water-retaining gelatinous residue which modifies the consistency
of the stool facilitating easy passage. It is important that the nurse mix the prepara-

tion with sufficient water just before giving it to the patient and that she urge him to drink water following the dose so that sufficient water is provided to prevent absorption of fluids from the bowel.

During the first 24 hours after surgery the patient may complain of bladder distention. Inability to void may be caused by fear of bringing on pain or by the drowsiness produced by postanesthetic sedatives and narcotics. The situation may be remedied in the case of a male patient by having him stand to void, by helping the patient use a bedside commode, by urging fluid intake (coffee and tea are diuretic but do not cause flatulence), by having him take sitz baths, and by asking the patient to void when he feels the urge. Catheterization should be resorted to only if absolutely necessary. Bethanechol (Urecholine), 2.5 to 5 mg, may be given subcutaneously to stimulate the desire to void. Retention with dribbling overflow is not uncommon. The nurse should palpate the suprapubic region to detect bladder distention and should measure urinary output with each micturition.

Occasionally postoperative bleeding may be a problem. It may occur soon after surgery or later (4 to 10 days) because of a slipped suture or wound separation. Continuous bright red bleeding with the passage of clots should be noted by the nurse and reported to the doctor. He may place a ligature, clamp the bleeding source with a hemostat, apply an absorbable cellulose pressure dressing, or return the patient to the operating room for treatment. He may order administration of vitamin K to hasten clotting. While waiting for the physician to arrive, the nurse can postpone giving laxatives and sitz baths, put the patient on bed rest, record his pulse and blood pressure, and apply a local pressure dressing with an ice bag.

Other complications of hemorrhoidectomy include infections, fistulas, fissures, anal incontinence or stenosis, drug reactions, and cardiopulmonary problems. Nevertheless hemorrhoidectomy is a relatively "safe" operation that is usually successful and should be considered as such by the nurse, who is often in a position to encourage people to seek treatment.

Bibliography

Almy, Thomas P. and Andrew G. Plaut: Ulcerative Colitis: A Report of Progress, Based upon the Recent Literature. *Gastroenterology,* 49:3:295–308, September, 1965.

Amshel, Albert L.: Hemorrhoidal Problems Medical and Surgical Treatment. *American Journal of Nursing,* 63:87–89, December, 1963.

Badenoch, John and Bryan N. Brooke: *Recent Advances in Gastroenterology.* London: J & A Churchill Ltd., 1965.

Brindley, George V., Jr.: Surgical Management of Esophageal Hiatal Her-

nia. *Postgraduate Medicine,* 39:5: 463–471, May, 1966.

Burge, Harold: *Vagotomy.* London: Edward Arnold (Publishers) Ltd., 1964.

Burket, Lester W., and S. Gordon Castigliano: *Oral Medicine.* Philadelphia: J. B. Lippincott Company, 1965.

Downs, Howard S.: The Control of Vomiting. *American Journal of Nursing,* 66:76–82, January, 1966.

Ellis, Harold and Roy Y. Calne: *Lecture Notes on General Surgery.* Oxford: Blackwell Scientific Publications, Ltd., 1965.

Ellison, Edwin H., Stanley R. Friesen, and John H. Mulholland (Eds.): *Current Surgical Management III.* Philadelphia: W. B. Saunders Company, 1965.

Farmer, E. Desmond and Frank E. Lawton: *Stones' Oral and Dental Diseases.* Edinburgh and London: E. & S. Livingstone Ltd., 1966.

Fostiropoulos, G. and Th. Doxiades: Systemic Manifestations of Ulcerative Colitis. *American Journal of Proctology,* 17:1:64–69, February, 1966.

Gallagher, J. Roswell: Ulcerative Colitis. In *Medical Care of the Adolescent,* 2d ed. New York: Appleton Century Crofts, 1966, Chap. 15.

Hass, Robert L.: The Case for Fluoridation, *American Journal of Nursing,* 66:2:328–331, February, 1966.

Havener, William H., William H. Saunders, and Betty S. Bergersen: *Nursing Care in Eye, Ear, Nose, and Throat Disorders.* St. Louis: The C. V. Mosby Company, 1964.

Hopping, Richard A.: Common Disorders of Anus, Rectum, and Sigmoid. *Clinical Symposia,* 16:4:103–134, October-November-December, 1964.

Howard, G. Turner: Surgical Management of Hemorrhoids, *American Journal of Proctology,* 17:3:213–220, June, 1966.

Irby, William B. and Kenneth H. Baldwin: *Emergencies and Urgent Complications in Dentistry.* St. Louis: The C. V. Mosby Company, 1965.

Irvine, W. T. (Ed.): *The Scientific Basis of Surgery.* London: J & A Churchill Ltd., 1965.

Kaplan, Murrel H., Edmundo J. Bernheim, and Besse McCoy Flynn: Esophageal Varices. Esophageal Varices: Components of Nursing Care. *American Journal of Nursing,* 64:104–108, June, 1964.

Kerr, Donald A. and Major M. Ash, Jr.: *Oral Pathology.* Philadelphia: Lea & Febiger, 1965.

Kirsner, Joseph B.: Peptic Ulcer: Review of the Literature for 1964. *Gastroenterology,* 49:1:79–100, July, 1965.

Lenneberg, Edith: Facts, Figures and Mutual Aid; Some Findings of the Research and Demonstration Project for Ileostomy Patients. *Ileostomy Quarterly,* 6:2-3-4:30–77, Spring, Summer, Fall, 1962.

Manousos, O. N. and Th. Doxiades: Colitis and Liver Disease. *American Journal of Proctology,* 17:1: 48–51, February, 1966.

Miller, Herman: Postoperative Complications of Hemorrhoidectomy. *American Journal of Proctology,* 17:5:361–370, October, 1966.

Moyer, Carl A., et al.: *Surgery Principles and Practice,* 3d ed. Philadelphia: J. B. Lippincott Company, 1965.

Naish, J. M. and A. E. A. Read: *Basic Gastro-Enterology.* Bristol, England: John Wright & Sons Ltd., 1965.

Nardi, George L. and George D. Zuidema (Eds.): *Surgery: A Concise Guide to Clinical Practice,* 2d ed. Boston: Little, Brown and Company, 1965.

Palmer, Walter L.: Gastric Ulcerations: Differentiation and Treatment. *Postgraduate Medicine,* 39:2:123–131, February, 1966.

Passos, Joyce Y.: Esophageal Perforation: A Case History. *American Journal of Nursing,* 65:73–76, May, 1965.

ReMine, William H., James T. Priestley, and Joseph Berkson: *Cancer of the Stomach.* Philadelphia: W. B. Saunders Company, 1964.

Sachs, David and Wiley Barker: Immediate Postoperative Management of the Ileostomy. *Surgery,* 59:3:373–375, March, 1966.

Schreiber, Frederick C.: Dental Care for Long-Term Patients. *American Journal of Nursing,* 64:84–86, February, 1964.

Scott, Ronald Bodley (Ed.): *Price's Textbook of the Practice of Medicine,* 10th ed. London: Oxford University Press, 1966.

Shapiro, Max (Ed.): *The Scientific Bases*

of Dentistry. Philadelphia: W. B. Saunders Company, 1966.

Sheridan, Brigid A.: After Hemorrhoidectomy; Postoperative Nursing Care. *American Journal of Nursing,* 63:90–91, December, 1963.

Sun, David C. H.: *Chemistry and Therapy of Peptic Ulcer.* Springfield, Ill.: Charles C Thomas, Publisher, 1966.

Usher, Francis C. and Joan Matthews: Surgery: Treatment of Choice for Hernia. *American Journal of Nursing,* 64:85–87, September, 1964.

Watts, J. McK., et al.: Early Course of Ulcerative Colitis. *Gut,* 7:1:16–31, February, 1966.

Weiss, Leonard and Estelle Weiss: Facial Fractures. Facial Fractures: Nursing Care. *American Journal of Nursing,* 65:96–100, February, 1965.

Wolf, Stewart: *The Stomach.* New York: Oxford University Press, 1965.

Wright, V. and G. Watkinson: Articular Complications of Ulcerative Colitis. *American Journal of Proctology,* 17:2:107–115, April, 1966.

CHAPTER 26
THE PATIENT WITH METABOLIC AND ENDOCRINE DISORDERS

SECTION 1
DIABETES
MELLITUS

Diabetes mellitus is an important chronic disease problem in the United States. It affects individuals of all ages, but in the majority the disease is discovered in the fourth decade or later. Diabetes mellitus is commonly referred to as *diabetes* and the person affected, a *diabetic*. The number of female diabetics exceeds the number of male by nearly one-third. In the United States one person in four— nearly 50,000,000 people—is believed to be a carrier of diabetes; he can transmit diabetes to his offspring without necessarily being a diabetic himself.[1] Diabetes now ranks eighth in statistics of mortality by disease although it frequently accompanies diseases that rank higher. Nation wide detection programs have facilitated diagnosis and treatment for thousands of previously undiagnosed cases of diabetes.

Diabetes mellitus is a metabolic disorder that affects the metabolism and is characterized by a relative or absolute lack of secretion or utilization of the hormone, insulin. This disorder was described in Egypt as early as 1500 B.C., yet it was not until the end of the nineteenth century that the relationship of diabetes to the pancreas was proven. The isolation of insulin by Banting and Best in 1921 provided the first known treatment for the disease.

---

* The author acknowledges the editorial assistance of Philip B. Hartley, M.D., in the preparation of this section.

[1] U.S. Department of Health, Education, and Welfare, Public Health Service: Publication No. 100, Series 10, No. 40. Washington, D.C.: U.S. Government Printing Office, August, 1967.

The life span of diabetics has been prolonged not only by insulin administration but more recently by oral medications. These agents usually are used alone in the management of diabetes but may be employed occasionally as adjuvants to insulin therapy.

The clinical characteristics of diabetes vary depending on the age at which the disorder develops or is detected; nonetheless these characteristics remain constant and the disease progresses with time, regardless of the age at onset. Because of this progressive quality, the younger the patient at onset the less favorable the prognosis. With certain exceptions, diabetics generally are categorized into two groups: childhood or juvenile diabetes, and adult onset diabetes. Synonyms commonly used for juvenile diabetes are "insulin-dependent," "severe," "brittle," "labile," "growth-onset," and "unstable." Adult onset diabetes is referred to as "mild," "maturity-onset," "stable," and "senile."

Pathophysiology and Clinical Manifestations

The pathogenesis of diabetes mellitus is unknown. Normally, a rise in the blood glucose concentration triggers the release of insulin from the beta cells, which in turn initiates metabolic activities. Insulin is believed to act on both cellular and endoplasmic membranes by causing a rearrangement in lipoprotein molecular structure of these membranes in which molecules of glucose, phosphate, and potassium move into cells or metabolic sites fixed on the endoplasmic reticulum. Insulin promotes (1) tissue uptake of glucose, (2) storage of glucose in the form of glycogen in the liver and muscles, (3) incorporation of amino acids into muscle protein, and (4) synthesis of fatty acids into fat for storage in adipose tissue. Insulin apparently is not required for glucose transport across red blood cell or neuronal membranes; the latter situation explains why diabetics do not manifest primary central nervous system symptoms.

Blood glucose levels, maintained by the liver under the influence of insulin, are regulated to homeostatic quantities (60 to 100 mg percent). All digested carbohydrates are processed by the liver, which (1) moves them out into various metabolic pathways, (2) releases them for transport to other tissues, (3) converts them into glycogen, or (4) by the acceptance of glucose inhibits the production of glucose (gluconeogenesis) from amino acids. When the blood glucose level rises insulin is secreted; when it falls insulin secretion ceases. The blood glucose is thereby maintained at homeostatic levels through this feedback control.

When insulin quantities are deficient or inefficiently utilized the liver is no longer under feedback control. The sequence of metabolic events is reversed. Liver glycogen is mobilized to provide glucose for the central nervous system, which must at all times have glucose available for fuel. Most other tissues can utilize free fatty acids released from adipose tissue for fuel. Muscle tissue releases amino acids from stored protein which are used as precursors for gluconeogenesis. The energy needs of the liver are met by partial oxidation of fatty acids that are converted to ketone bodies. If gluconeogenesis and the production of ketone bodies occur more rapidly than they can be metabolized, the blood levels rise and hyperglycemia and ketonemia develop. When the renal threshold for reabsorption of glucose from the glomerular filtrate is exceeded, glycosuria results. Glucose, as an osmotically active molecule in the urine, obligates the excretion of water. Ketone bodies also spill into the urine, taking water because of their acidic nature. During diuresis both sodium and potassium are lost in the urine. As this process continues, large quantities of water are required, hence the diabetic consumes large amounts of fluid—polydipsia—and excretes urine in large quantities—polyuria.

Diabetics fail to utilize glucose efficiently despite the presence of hyperglycemia. The voluntary muscles normally consume most of the available glucose; however, without insulin the entry of glucose into muscles is impeded. The excess of glucose in the circulation soon exceeds the capacity of the liver to metabolize it, and hyperglycemia persists. The muscle then must oxidize other fuel sources, namely, tissue fat, to meet energy requirements. The resulting loss of body fat stores is reflected by weight loss. In an effort to compensate for weight loss, which the individual perceives as starvation, a pathologic increase in food consumption—polyphagia—ensues.

Acidosis

Biochemical acidosis may develop if elevated blood ketone levels exceed the blood buffer systems and hence lower the pH. The respiratory centers in the brain respond to acidosis by stimulating increased rate and depth of breathing. This breathing pattern permits loss of plasma carbon dioxide, reducing the plasma concentration of the bicarbonate, an ion, and thus allows the cation, previously bound to the bicarbonate, to neutralize the accumulating acid ketones. This compensatory mechanism for maintaining body pH becomes ineffective if the acidotic state is prolonged.

The acidotic patient subjectively feels ill and has little interest in food or fluid. As a consequence of anorexia, release of fuels from storage depots continues and the poor fluid intake intensifies the dehydration caused by polyuria. Protein catabolism causes depletion of tissue protein and a resulting chemical loss of nitrogen and potassium which contributes to dehydration. Furthermore, hypotension compromises tissue nutrition, and anuria may result from diminished renal blood flow.

If the acidotic state progresses without treatment, the brain is affected and coma develops. Respiratory centers may fail to be stimulated resulting in apnea and death. The above sequence of pathophysiologic processes may occur in a previously undiagnosed patient or one previously under adequate diabetic control. Since diabetes is a chronic disease, a diabetic may eventually experience an episode of acidosis, with or without coma. Hospitalization is imperative to provide medical intervention for the acidotic or comatose state.

Causative Factors in the Development of Diabetes

About 90 percent of diabetic cases are termed *idiopathic,* indicating that a specific cause has not been determined. Although the tendency for diabetes to develop is inherited, those in whom the disorder develops do not necessarily exhibit the same clinical manifestations. Some diabetics produce very little insulin, whereas others produce adequate or even excessive amounts of the hormone but cannot efficiently utilize it because of an inborn metabolic error or active inhibition of the insulin molecule. This has been evidenced by the fact that restoration of high blood glucose to normal levels in most diabetics requires more insulin than in the totally depancreatized person.

Hyperfunction of other endocrine glands, particularly the anterior pituitary and the adrenal cortex, may be the etiologic factor in the development of diabetes. If secreted in excessive amounts, somatotropic hormone (STH) has a diabetogenic effect. Diabetes may develop in patients with hyperplasia or a neoplasm of the adrenal cortex, with concomitant increase in adrenocortical secretion. Of the three important types of adrenocortical hormones, the gluconeogenic, salt-retaining, and virilizing, the first is responsible for production of glucose from amino acids. If the hyperglycemia resulting from gluconeogenesis is attributable to adrenocortical hyperfunction, this blood glucose elevation often is not homeostatically overcome, and diabetes ensues. Other hormones such as epinephrine, glucagon, and thyroxine may have a diabetogenic effect if excessive secretion (endogenous source) or drug administration (exogenous source) occurs. Diabetes precipitated by an exogenous source is termed *iatrogenic*.

Diabetes can be caused by any disease that physiologically interferes with or destroys the activity of insulin-producing islet tissue. Although rare, chronic pancreatitis, cancer of the pancreas, and hemochromatosis may cause diabetes by destruction of the beta cells of the islets of Langerhans.

Juvenile diabetes is characterized by little if any production of insulin, therefore as the disease progresses the total amount of beta cells and pancreatic islet tissue decreases. Patients with adult onset diabetes usually have some insulin production and a normal-appearing pancreas. Histologic alterations in the islet cells seen microscopically are changes consisting of hyalinization or fibrosis. If diabetes is the result of primary destruction of the pancreas, the organ shows changes of chronic inflammation or iron deposition and is scarred, fibrotic, or calcified. Frequently pancreatic tissue is partially replaced by fat when diabetes is accompanied by obesity.

Diagnosis of Diabetes and Assessment of Control

The responsibility for diagnosis of diabetes rests with the physician. The nurse practitioner in public health, hospitals, schools, industry, or the physician's office can actively participate in the detection of diabetes. Nurse interaction with patients may reveal observations and a history that prompt further medical investigation. The more subtle environmental factors affecting the development of the disease, dietary habits, and obesity may come to the attention of the nurse who knows the history of the patient and his family. The nurse may observe overt symptoms of the disease which the patient does not realize are meaningful. If during her observations the nurse finds evidence of unexplained weight loss or weight gain, susceptibility to infections, increased fatigue and weakness, xanthomas, chronic skin ulcerations, intermittent visual disturbances, unexplained pruritus of the female genitalia, insatiable thirst and appetite, or increased urination, she should notify the physician in order to facilitate further study or follow-up. The nurse should also encourage the patient to seek medical assistance.

Certain tests used to assess the degree of control of diabetes are executed and interpreted by the patient or the nurse. Following these, decisions regarding initiation of a therapeutic regimen or changes in an existing treatment program are made by the physician.

Numerous tests are available for use in screening for diabetes as well as assessing control. A selected few will be discussed, since it is not possible to discuss them all. Studies primarily on blood and urine are performed to determine the presence of diabetes or to evaluate the status of management. Differences in methods employed to execute these procedures as well as interpretation of results may exist from one health agency to another. The nurse should explain the prescribed test to the patient as an aid in securing his cooperation. Commonly used blood tests are the following:

Fasting Blood Sugar Level Determination. The normal range for sugar in the venous blood of a fasting person is between 60 and 100 mg percent (Somogyi's method) or 80 and 120 mg percent (Folin-Wu method). Concentrations greater than 120 mg percent are diagnostic of diabetes if analysis on a second occasion confirms the finding. A glucose tolerance test is performed on persons with blood values between 100 and 120 mg percent.

Two-Hour Postprandial Blood Sugar Determination. The blood sugar value is established 2 hours after ingestion of approximately 100 g carbohydrate, usually glucose. The presence of diabetes is shown by values of 140 mg percent or higher. Persons with levels between 110 and 140 mg percent should have administered a glucose tolerance test.

Oral Glucose Tolerance Test. A number of factors influence the results of the test because measurement is made of the balance between absorption of glucose from the intestines, its uptake by tissues, and its excretion in the urine. Preparation for the test includes ingestion of a high-carbohydrate diet for 3 days prior to the test. Then, after an 8- to 10-hour overnight fast, the person drinks 100 g glucose in 400 ml water, usually flavored with lemon juice to increase palatability. Commercial preparations, Glucola and Gel-a-dex, which contain the proper amount of glucose, may be used instead. Usually venous blood and urine samples are obtained at the beginning of the test and every half hour for 3 hours, although occasionally the test is extended to 4 or 5 hours. If diabetes is present, the blood values will reflect the following alterations in the glucose tolerance curve: increased fasting level, increased peak value, and delayed return to normal ranges.

All the urine testing methods described below utilized in detecting sugar or acetone, the principal ketone, may be carried out by the patient or the nurse, with the exception of the last. The others are qualitative in nature, and the last one, a quantitative study, must be performed by a laboratory.

Testape, Clinistix, and Urostix. A paper strip impregnated with enzymatic reagent, glucose oxidase, is dipped into a urine specimen to detect the presence of glucose. The color change is read according to the accompanying scale. Directions for timing and handling the strips should be followed to guarantee maximal accuracy.

Benedict's Solution and Clinitest Tablets. Both these agents utilize copper reduction methods to indicate the presence or absence of sugar in the urine. The degree of positivity is seen in color changes, which are graded on a scale as trace, and 1+ to 4+. Methods depending upon copper reduction are neither specific for glucose alone nor as sensitive as the glucose oxidase tests.

Acetest. The presence or absence of acetone is revealed when a drop of urine placed on the reagent tablet turns lavender or remains colorless. The intensity of color change is compared to a graded chart.

Ketostix. The comparison of color change after an enzymatic paper strip is dipped into a urine specimen permits detection of acetone.

Fractional Urine Collection. To aid the physician in prescribing adequate dosages of antidiabetic medication, urine specimens are checked periodically for the presence or absence of sugar and/or ketones. The specimens are taken at four intervals, usually prior to each meal and at bedtime. However, if the diabetic is hospitalized they may be collected at 6-hour intervals throughout the day to ascertain whether glycosuria or ketonuria exists. To obtain an accurate result, it is wise to have the patient empty the bladder approximately 30 to 60 minutes before a specimen is to be tested and drink water, and obtain another specimen that will show current urinary content of sugar or its lack.

Twenty-four Hour Urine Collection. Quantitative evaluation of the excretion of glucose in grams during a day is accomplished by urine collection and subsequent laboratory analysis.

Classification of Diabetes

To provide a frame of reference for comprehending the intensity of metabolic disturbance present in various diabetics, the following classification is given (Danowski):

Stage I. Prediabetes or prodiabetes is the phase preceding the appearance of obvious diabetes. One inherits the predisposition to the disease or the diabetic tendency through a single recessive gene.

Stage II. Stress diabetes is transient, present only during a period of stress when insulin requirements are increased, and is no longer chemically detectable when the stress no longer exists. When stress is compensated for by overeating, obesity develops with accompanying chemical changes mirroring diabetes. If obesity is not controlled, diabetes may remain permanently.

Stage III. This is an undiagnosed form of diabetes common in the adult but infrequent in children. Blood tests reveal normal fasting glucose levels and hyperglycemia with postprandial or glucose tolerance studies, yet no ketosis is present.

Stage IV. This is the most commonly recognized form of diabetes in both adults and children. An elevated fasting blood glucose is present as are increases in the 2-hour postprandial or glucose tolerance test blood glucose concentrations. The absence of ketosis is significant since it is a characteristic of the subsequent stages.

Stage V. Fasting and postprandial hyperglycemia is present as well as ketonuria, although there is not a significant accumulation of ketone bodies in the plasma. Children with diabetes are usually diagnosed in this stage of the disorder; however, it is not uncommon for them to be in Stage VI or VII when the diagnosis is made.

Stage VI. This stage is referred to as *ketoacidosis* and has these characteristics:

marked ketonuria, ketone accumulation in the plasma, reduction of the serum carbon dioxide content (20 to 10 meq per liter range), decrease in serum pH (7.3 to 7.1), tachypnea, and development of overbreathing.

Stage VII. Diabetic acidosis-coma is demonstrated through clinical studies with marked accumulations of ketone bodies in plasma and urine, diminished serum carbon dioxide (10 meq per liter), reduction of serum pH values (6.8 to 6.9), and the presence of Kussmaul overbreathing.

Clinical Course of Diabetes

The course of diabetes is reflected in pathophysiologic changes that develop as a result of the underlying metabolic disturbance. Most diabetics have pathologic changes in tissues regardless of degree of control. If control is poor, it is reasonable to infer that these processes are accelerated. Angiopathy, neuropathy, retinopathy, and nephropathy are common among diabetics.

Most diabetics have hypercholesterolemia, an elevation above 200 mg percent in the serum. It is believed to be due to defective excretion or metabolism of cholesterol. This retention of fats may be seen as xanthomas and is implicated in atherosclerotic changes in blood vessels. Although atherosclerotic changes are seen in nondiabetics, these lesions develop earlier, progress more rapidly, and cause more disability in the diabetic.

Plaque deposits, proliferation of the intimal layer of the vessel wall, and local dilatation with subsequent weakening of the wall develop. The coronory and common iliac arteries are affected as are smaller peripheral vessels. Occlusion or thrombosis of the smaller arteries and arterioles may result. Thickening of the capillary basement membrane is found in the small vessel lesions of the retina, peripheral nerves, and the glomerulus.

Since arterioles are directly visible in the fundus of the eye, confirmation of the presence of small lesions, called *microaneurysms,* can be made. White patches or exudate may be seen on the fundus resulting from plasma loss from the weakened vessels; or retinal hemorrhages may occur. Cholesterol deposits in the lens can cause opacity or cataract formation. If retinopathy is severe it may lead to blindness.

Clinical manifestations that may arise from arterial compromise, occlusion, thrombosis, or neuropathy include intermittent claudication, extremity pain at rest, gangrene, lack of color change of an extremity with elevation and dependency, skin ulcerations, changes in perception of temperature to the extremity, myocardial infarction, and cerebrovascular accident.

The peripheral neuropathy is thought to be a related pathology of small vessels supplying nutrition to the nerves of the legs. Diminished sensation, pain, and motor weakness are characteristics of peripheral neuropathy. The patient may be indifferent to minor trauma affecting an extremity because of diminished sensation.

Some degree of kidney involvement usually develops. Lesions caused by diffuse or focal deposition of hyaline, an amorphous cellular material composed of polysaccharide and protein, in the renal glomeruli or their intercapillary spaces, or about the tubules cause renal dysfunction, uremia, or renal failure. The Kimmelstiel-Wilson syndrome seen in diabetics consists of hyaline infiltration within the glomerulus or the intercapillary spaces of the glomeruli. Nephrosclerosis with accompanying hypertension may further affect renal function and eventually culminate in renal failure.

Nursing Care and Patient Education

The primary objective in treating diabetes is to enable the patient to live within the limits imposed by the disease and to prevent, insofar as possible, pathologic changes and complications. This objective requires education of the patient.

Once the diagnosis is established the main issue is achievement of control, which usually is more readily attained in adults than in children. What constitutes "good" or "satisfactory" control is a standard usually arbitrarily set by the physician in his evaluation of the individual patient.

Initially the diabetic may have the attitude that he is "different" from other people as a result of his perceptions of restrictions in diet, physical activities, or perhaps his dependence on drugs. Diabetics who have been studied psychologically as well as physically and are educated about the disease can overcome misconceptions and unhealthy attitudes.

With the guidance of the physician, the nurse practitioner can actively participate in educating the patient about his disease. Formal diabetic teaching programs are sponsored by some hospitals or clinics, while informal teaching may be done at the bedside in the hospital, in the physician's office, in the school, or in industry, or in the patient's home by a public health nurse. Visual aids and demonstrations are useful in teaching, and the diabetic should have practice sessions to enable him to make meaningful the factual information he has acquired. Numerous pamphlets, manuals, and books on diabetes are available. The nurse may wish to secure such literature for use in patient teaching or may recommend that the patient seek additional information sources. The American Diabetes Association has prepared several booklets on meal planning, and material is available from other sources as well (Rosenthal and Rosenthal; Schmitt).

The nine-point program outlined by the American Diabetes Association for the management of patients with diabetes (Hamwi and Danowski) includes instruction in each of the areas described below.

DIET

A regimen of diabetic control focuses upon the proper integration of physical activity, diet, and drug therapy. The patient's customary physical activity is considered when the physician prescribes the diet and drug therapy. When diabetes is controlled by diet alone, variations in physical exertion are well tolerated. If, however, drug therapy is employed to effect control, additional food supplements must be taken to offset temporary increases in physical activity which decrease insulin needs. Thus, activity, diet, and insulin are closely interrelated.

The diet prescription for patients is usually explained by a dietitian, but there are circumstances when a dietitian is not available for teaching the diabetic patient, and the nurse becomes responsible for instructing him in planning the diet.

Approximately 50 percent of diabetics can be managed by diet alone, although a large proportion of them are obese. Measures to control or eliminate obesity are sought.

Space does not permit a complete discussion of food classes, essential nutrients, and food values that must be considered in diet planning. Two major types of diet programs are prescribed for the diabetic: qualitative diets in which restrictions are minimal and measurement is unnecessary, and the more rigid quantitative diets in which methods of exchange measuring, fixed weighing, or figured weighing are accomplished with household measures, food scales, or gram weights. These methods ensure greater accuracy in diet therapy. References to nutritional textbooks should be made when the nurse teaches the dietary regimen.

URINE TESTING

The nurse should teach the patient the urine testing method recommended by his physician, and he should test his urine at least once a day. The urine sample should be a second voided specimen. Patients in whom regulation is underway, those whose control is erratic, and those requiring insulin injections are usually expected to perform fractional urine testing before meals and at bedtime. Diabetics may need only to test the urine for ketones when they are ill or if control is erratic. The most commonly used urine testing methods for the detection of sugar and ketones are described under the diagnostic studies.

ACTION OF INSULIN AND OTHER HYPOGLYCEMIC AGENTS

If control of diabetes cannot be achieved by dietary therapy alone, the administration of oral sulfonylureas or insulin may permit effective control. The effects of drug dosage excess are described in relation to hypoglycemic and hyperglycemic states. A pharmacology textbook should be consulted for detailed information about these preparations.

Treatment of diabetes with oral agents became possible with the development of the sulfonylureas, namely, tolbutamide (Orinase), chlorpropamide (Diabinese), acetohexamide (Dymelor), and tolazamide (Tolinase). Their mode of action is to lower blood sugar by stimulating the beta cells of the pancreas to release insulin; thus no beneficial clinical response can be anticipated in patients without endogenous insulin. Phenformin (DBI or DBI-TD) is another oral agent; however, it reduces blood sugar levels in the absence of functioning pancreatic tissue. Dosage for each drug differs from the others.

The individual adult with onset, ketoacidosis resistant, mild diabetes is the ideal candidate for oral hypoglycemic therapy because the beta cells usually are active even if they do not liberate sufficient insulin. Some diabetics who have been receiving 20 units or less of insulin daily may be given an oral agent instead. Patients differ in their responsiveness to the sulfonylureas and phenformin; some experience effective control with one preparation or a combination of agents, while control may not be attainable with another preparation. All the drugs are readily absorbed from the gastrointestinal tract; however, their metabolism varies as is reflected by the duration of action.

The physiologic activity of insulin has been described in relation to the pathology present in the person in whom diabetes develops. The normal person secretes approximately 60 units of insulin daily; in the diabetic, however, the supplemental or replacement dosage of insulin must be adjusted to his metabolic requirements as well as the islet cell activity and the insulin-inhibiting factors that may be present.

Table 26-1 lists information the nurse and patient need to know regarding the type of insulin preparation prescribed. Unmodified insulin is known as *regular* insulin. A more highly purified insulin, crystalline insulin, has a similar duration of action. These two are generally viewed as interchangeable rapid-acting insulins. These insulins may be used to supplement a longer-acting insulin; because of their quick effect, these preparations are often used to reestablish control when the patient is ill or in an acidotic state. Crystalline/regular insulin is the only insulin that can be administered by the intravenous route.

The duration of insulin action has been extended by a change in its solubility in water accomplished by combining substances (zinc, protamine, globin) called *modifiers* in the other insulin preparations. All the modified insulins, except globin, are cloudy, so the vial contents must be gently mixed by being tilted or rolled back and forth to ensure uniform suspension. Semilente is a modified, short-acting insulin used to supplement the activity of lente or ultralente insulins.

Lente, isophane (NPH), and globin insulins are intermediate in their duration of action. Lente and NPH are the two insulins most commonly used in treating diabetes. Supplements of regular insulin with NPH and semilente with lente may be required to meet the needs of the patient.

Long-acting insulins include protamine zinc (PZI) and ultralente. Ultralente is utilized to supplement the activity of lente or semilente insulin. Two types of insulin preparations may be mixed in one syringe to eliminate the need for two injections. When an insulin mixture is prescribed, the unmodified insulin should be drawn into the syringe first, to prevent contamination by the modified insulin.

Insulin is supplied in 10 ml vials containing 40 or 80 units of insulin per ml. Since a U-40 concentration contains 40 units of insulin in 1 ml of solution and U-80 insulin contains 80 units per ml, the nurse must convey to the patient that U-80 is twice as concentrated as U-40 insulin. Her instructions should include reiteration of the differences in concentrations available in relation to the syringe used to measure the insulin.

The nurse should also explain the side effects that may be experienced. Subjective undesirable effects from the oral preparations include gastrointestinal symptoms (anorexia, nausea, vomiting, diarrhea, abdominal discomfort). Other

TABLE 26-1 *Properties of Insulin Preparations*	ACTIVITY	TYPE OF INSULIN	ONSET OF ACTION (IN HOURS)	PEAK ACTION (IN HOURS)	DURATION OF ACTION (IN HOURS)
	Rapid acting	Insulin (unmodified: regular or crystalline)	1–2	2–4	5–7
	Intermediate acting	Semilente	1–2	6–7	10–14
		Isophane (NPH)	2	8–12	24–28
		Lente	2	8–12	24–28
		Globin	2	8–12	22–24
	Long acting	Protamine zinc (PZI)	4–6	16–24	24–36
		Ultralente	6–8	16–24	24–36

symptoms may be drug specific; for example, the sulfonylureas may cause skin rashes. Untoward reactions occasionally occur with insulin use. A hypersensitivity of the skin manifested by erythema, pruritus, and local swelling is usually eliminated by changing the brand or using an insulin obtained from the pancreas of a different animal. Insulin resistance indicates failure of the body to respond to the usual amounts of insulin, and very large insulin dosages must be employed. The cause of resistance has not been fully clarified; fortunately, however, this difficulty does not arise very often.

TECHNIQUE OF INSULIN INJECTION AND INJECTION SITES

Utilizing the principles employed in subcutaneous injection techniques, the nurse should give demonstrations and supervise practice with the diabetic until he can perform the steps confidently and with accuracy and dexterity.

The diabetic must be taught the importance of systematic rotation of injection sites. Areas on the abdomen and thighs should be selected for self-injection of insulin. When another person administers insulin, sites on the arms or buttocks are used. The desirable injection sites should be diagrammatically illustrated to the patient as shown in Figure 26–1. The same site should not be used more than

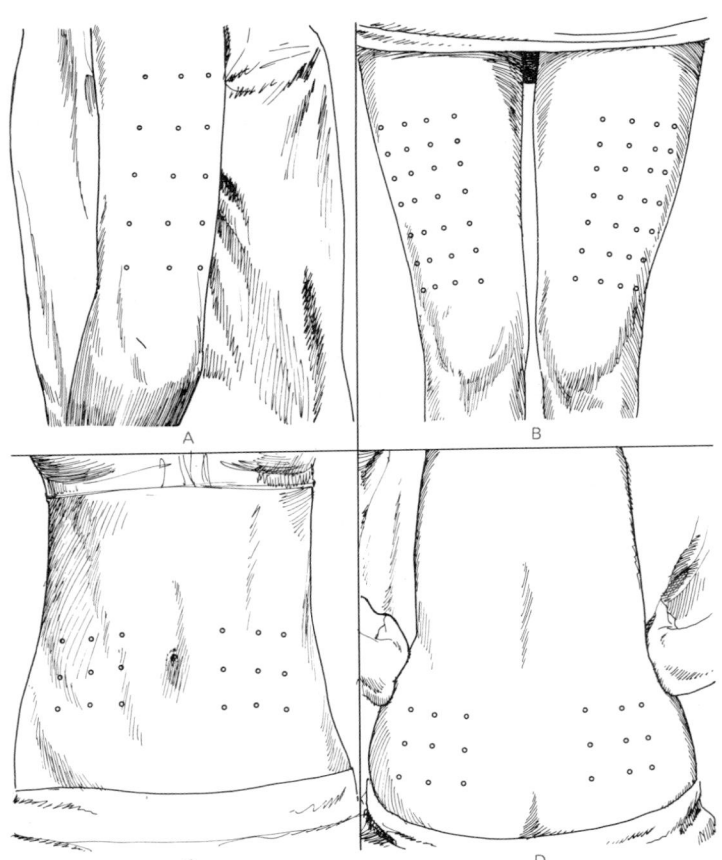

Figure 26–1
Sites for insulin
injection

once a month and a space of 1 inch should be maintained between sites. Repeated injections in the same area give rise to fibrous fatty tumors, termed *insulin lumps*. They cause irregular absorption of insulin and are cosmetically unattractive. An atrophy or loss of fat tissue beneath the skin, with subsequent depression of the area, called *insulin hollows,* may result for the same reason. Subcutaneous tissue changes can be minimized by systematically rotating injection sites, injecting deeply under the skin, and using insulin at room temperature.

CARE OF SYRINGE AND OF INSULIN

To avoid confusion in the measurement of insulin dosage, the use of a single scale syringe has been recommended by the American Diabetes Association. These types are as follows: (1) a syringe used only for U-40 insulin, marked in red enamel at 10, 20, 30, and 40 units and having a total capacity of 1 ml; (2) a syringe used for U-80 insulin, marked in green enamel at 20, 40, 60, and 80 units and having a total capacity of 1 ml; and (3) a syringe used when the single dosage exceeds 80 units. The scale is marked for U-80 insulin with a total capacity of 160 units or 2 ml.

Stainless steel needles, No. 25 or No. 26 gauge, ½ to ¾ inch long, are recommended. Disposable needles are satisfactory, although they are more expensive since they must be discarded after one injection.

Sterilization of the syringe and needle can be accomplished by placing the individual parts in a strainer submerged in water and boiling them for 10 minutes. After cooling, the plunger is taken by the handle and inserted into the barrel of the syringe. The needle can be picked up easily by the shoulder and attached to the syringe, then twisted into place to ascertain that it is secure. The plunger should be moved back and forth to allow removal of any water remaining in the shaft of the needle. After instruction and practice the diabetic should be able to demonstrate his ability to handle the sterile equipment without contamination.

The current supply of insulin should be kept at room temperature, and reserve supplies should be refrigerated but not frozen.

Purchase of a kit with receptacles for syringe, needles, insulin vial(s), alcohol, and cotton may be convenient for travel. When the patient is traveling, the physician may permit alcohol (isopropyl) sterilization of the syringe and needle if the boiling method is not feasible; or the patient may prefer to use disposable needles and syringes. The diabetic should carry insulin supplies on his person and reserve items only in his luggage. It is also advisable that he carry a snack with these supplies in the event a meal is unavoidably delayed.

SYMPTOMS OF HYPOGLYCEMIA

There is no way by which the body can regulate the rate of insulin entry into the bloodstream, since it is given by injection. Thus absorbed insulin will act whether the blood sugar is high, normal, or low. Similarly, the mild diabetic treated with oral preparations responds to their activity following ingestion of them. A hypoglycemic reaction may occur if the diabetic has taken too much medication, has increased his muscular activity or has vomited food or medication, has omitted or delayed eating a meal, or if the metabolism becomes altered and less insulin is

SIGNS AND SYMPTOMS	HYPOGLYCEMIA	DIABETIC ACIDOSIS/KETOACIDOSIS
Behavior	Nervous; confused	Drowsy
Breath	Normal	Fruity odor (acetone)
Breathing	Normal; rapid and shallow	Deep; labored
Hunger	Present	Absent
Skin	Moist; pale	Flushed; dry
Sugar in urine	Absent or slight	Large amounts
Thirst	Absent	Present
Tongue	Moist	Dry
Vomiting	Absent	Present

TABLE 26-2
Clinical Signs and
Symptoms of Acute
Complications

required. The reaction is also referred to as *hypoglycemic shock, insulin reaction, insulin shock,* or *hyperinsulinism.*

Manifestations accompanying the rapid development of low blood sugar levels are shown in Table 26-2. The physiologic basis for symptoms that may be present is the dependence of nervous tissue upon glucose for energy metabolism. Diminished plasma glucose levels, as little as 50 to 100 mg percent, stimulate centers in the central nervous system which respond by increases in sympathetic nervous system activity. The activity of epinephrine accounts for the characteristic symptoms of hypoglycemia—pallor, sweating, and tachycardia. The role of the sympathetic nervous system in elevating blood glucose during emotional stress is discussed elsewhere. Additional symptoms referable to the nervous system are confusion, dizziness, incoordination, slurred speech, stupor, and, with prolonged hypoglycemia, convulsions and coma. Brief hypoglycemic episodes may cause some irreversible brain damage, and if they occur repeatedly progressive neurological damage may result. Irreversible lesions in the brain causing death may develop if hypoglycemia remains uncorrected for longer than 1 or 2 hours.

The release of the hormone glucagon from the alpha cells of the pancreas is stimulated by lowered blood glucose levels. Both glucagon and epinephrine activate phosphorylase in the liver; thus glycogenolysis restores the blood glucose level to a normal range.

Rising blood concentrations of growth hormone and adrenocorticotropin reflect anterior pituitary response to low blood glucose levels. Insulin action is opposed by these hormonal changes, glycogen is mobilized, and gluconeogenesis is accelerated. The role of excesses of growth hormone and adrenocortical secretion as an etiologic basis for diabetes was described earlier.

Not all the symptoms will appear in each individual experiencing hypoglycemia, but the same symptoms will usually recur in each individual.

Hypoglycemia is treated by administering a form of carbohydrate (orange juice, a lump of sugar, candy, or corn syrup) if the diabetic is able to swallow. If he is unconscious, small amounts of granulated sugar or corn syrup may be placed in the cheek and will be absorbed. Because neurological damage may occur if the brain is deprived of glucose, a physician should be summoned if the patient does not respond promptly. An injection of 50 percent glucose or glucagon 0.5 to 1.0 mg may be necessary.

The patient must understand why hypoglycemia occurs, the warning symptoms of lowered blood sugar levels, and what measures he should take if hypoglycemia develops. He should understand that brain function is the first area to be affected, therefore careful consideration must be given to activities requiring mental acuity (e.g., driving a car, operating hazardous machinery, making business decisions, taking examinations) in planning preventive measures.

SYMPTOMS OF UNCONTROLLED DIABETES

Diabetic acidosis or ketoacidosis is the end-result of uncontrolled diabetes. The juvenile or insulin-dependent diabetic is more susceptible to acidosis than the mild diabetic. The biochemical events resulting from the lack of insulin cause acidosis. The nurse should observe the patient for insulin lumps or hollows in the event these problems contributed to poor insulin absorption and subsequent loss of control. An increase in the insulin need arises when an intercurrent stress is present such as injury, infection, surgery performed with or without anesthesia, pregnancy, or emotional disturbances. Since the diabetic has limited or no ability to produce insulin, the available supply cannot meet his metabolic demands, and supplementary doses of his prescribed medication must be administered or acidosis will develop.

The pathophysiologic manifestations of uncontrolled diabetes were described earlier. The clinical manifestations of acidosis shown in Table 26-2 develop gradually; the patient is very ill and requires hospitalization.

Medical therapy is directed toward reestablishment of control which involves the use of insulin, even in the case of diabetics who previously required only an oral agent. Treatment is focused upon repair of cellular losses of fluid, food, and electrolytes. The nurse will assess the status of the patient by closely observing him and studying the laboratory findings. Improved hydration may be revealed by improved skin turgor, cessation of vomiting or diarrhea, lack of diuresis, or elevation of blood pressure. Reversal of metabolic acidosis may be indicated by improved cerebration, diminution or absence of glycosuria and ketonuria, ability to retain ingested food and fluids without vomiting or having diarrhea, elevated serum levels of carbon dioxide, bicarbonate, sodium, potassium, and chloride, and the return of the normal rate and depth of breathing.

Acidosis can be prevented if the diabetic learns to be alert to the precipitating conditions. Careful attention to any illness or injury can obviate this complication. Rapport between the diabetic and the physician or community nurse is helpful in encouraging the patient to seek such help when problems arise.

CARE OF THE FEET

The vascular impairment and peripheral neuropathy that accompany diabetes mellitus, particularly if control is poor, give rise to complications in the lower extremities. With impairment of peripheral sensation there is greater likelihood of trauma or injury to the feet. Minor abrasions, blisters, or cuts heal very slowly because the vascular system cannot provide sufficient circulation for prompt healing. A localized lesion may become secondarily infected. Furthermore, gangrene can result from the poor circulation and may eventuate in amputation of one or more toes, the foot, or the leg.

The nurse can assist the patient by giving close attention to care of the feet and helping him avoid practices that could aggravate the problem. Most sources of injury to the feet can be eliminated by having the patient follow these practices: (1) wash and inspect the feet daily; (2) keep the feet protected by wearing properly fitted shoes or slippers; (3) apply lanolin regularly if the skin or toenails are dry; (4) apply no form of artificial heat (electric heating pad, hot water bottle, electric blanket); (5) when bathing or sitting near a fireplace or radiator, estimate the temperature of the area by first exposing another part of the body; (6) cut toenails straight across; (7) consult the physician or a podiatrist if calluses, corns, or nail problems persist (razor blades, knives or similar devices should not be used to trim calluses or corns); and (8) maintain optimal circulation by avoiding vascular constriction due to tight foundation garments or garters, sitting with legs crossed, smoking, or overexposure to cold arising from inappropriate dress. Buerger's exercises may be done to aid circulation to the extremities.

Any break in the integrity of the skin should be cleansed thoroughly with soap and water, then rinsed under running water. No antiseptics should be used. The area should be dried and covered with a sterile gauze. The physician should be consulted if the affected area becomes inflamed or shows evidence of infection.

MANAGEMENT OF ACUTE COMPLICATIONS

The diabetic's adjustment to his disease involves a comprehension of self-care measures to be carried out when an acute complication arises. Injuries and illnesses (fever, cold, influenza, gastrointestinal upset) increase the body's need for insulin, and the diabetic must be aware of changes in drug and dietary regimens that must be made. The physician prescribes an individualized alternate drug and diet plan for such complications. The patient must adhere to the increase in the dose of insulin or oral medication. Increases in fluid intake are recommended if feasible, and a liquid or soft diet may be substituted for the customary one to ensure ingestion of nutrients. To avoid a decrease in blood sugar due to exercise, bed rest is recommended until the critical period has passed. The urine is tested with greater frequency to assess the effectiveness of control. If fluid loss due to vomiting or diarrhea continues, or glycosuria or ketonuria persists, hospitalization will be necessary so that intravenous therapy may be administered.

Bibliography

A Cookbook for Diabetics; ADA Forecast; Diabetes; Facts about Diabetes; Meal Planning with Exchange Lists. New York: American Diabetes Association, Inc.

Danowski, T. S. (Ed.): *Diabetes Mellitus: Diagnosis and Treatment.* New York: American Diabetes Association, Inc., 1964, pp. 21–22.

Danowski, T. S.: Types of Diabetes Mellitus. *Annals of Internal Medicine,* August, 1962, 321–323.

Donaldson, James: Current Concepts in the Treatment of Diabetes. *Medical Clinics of North America,* September, 1965, 1349–1360.

Goodman, Louis S. and Alfred Gilman: *The Pharmacological Basis of Therapeutics,* 3d ed. New York: The Macmillan Company, 1965, pp. 1579–1604.

Hamwi, George S. and T. S. Danowski (Eds.): *Diabetes Mellitus: Diagnosis and Treatment*, Vol. II. New York: American Diabetes Association, Inc., 1967, p. 233.

Rosenthal, Helen and Joseph Rosenthal: *Diabetic Care in Pictures*, 4th ed. Philadelphia: J. B. Lippincott Company, 1968.

Schmitt, George F.: *Diabetes for Diabetics: A Practical Guide*, 2d ed. Miami: The Diabetes Press of America, 1968.

Traisman, Howard S. and Alvah L. Newcomb: *Management of the Juvenile Diabetic*. St. Louis: The C. V. Mosby Company, 1965, pp. 32–39; 44–45; 125–128.

Williams, Robert H. (Ed.): *A Textbook of Endocrinology*, 4th ed. Philadelphia: W. B. Saunders Company, 1968, pp. 613–789.

SECTION 2
THYROID
GLAND DISORDERS

The thyroid gland manufactures, stores, and secretes thyroid hormone, which acts as a stimulus to the consumption of oxygen by all body cells. The malfunctioning thyroid gland itself may show evidence of disease, may cause disease of major body systems, or may be affected by disorders in other parts of the body. Hypothyroidism, hyperthyroidism, and thyroiditis are thyroid disorders that may threaten life. Goiter, an enlargement of the gland, is a malady recognizable by nonmedical persons throughout the world. Thyrocalcitonin is a hormone produced by thyroid gland tissue. This hormone has no known relation to hypothyroidism or hyperthyroidism. Thyrocalcitonin does affect the action of the parathyroid gland hormone, and will be discussed in Section 3 of this chapter. To be able to understand the composite problems presented by thyroid disorders, the nurse must have knowledge of all body systems and appropriate clinical nursing care.

Hypothyroidism

Hypothyroidism is a systemic disorder resulting from a failure of the thyroid gland to secrete thyroid hormone sufficient to meet the requirements of human metabolic processes. Age and the degree of thyroid hormone deficiency are variables that affect the clinical picture of hypothyroidism. Cretinism, juvenile myxedema, and adult myxedema are classified as clinical entities of hypothyroidism. The term *myxedema* is used to describe severe thyroid hormone deficiency accompanied by visible edema. *Myxedema* and *hypothyroidism* are used synonymously in the literature. The incidence of all degrees of hypothyroidism is not available because of difficulty in diagnosing mild forms of the disorder. Approximately 80 percent of patients with adult myxedema are females.

CRETINISM

Cretinism is severe thyroid hormone deficiency developing in fetal or neonatal life. Most cases of cretinism appear in endemic goiter regions, and these patients frequently have a goiter. The terms *endemic* and *goitrous cretinism* are used to describe this condition. *Sporadic* cretinism occurs in nongoitrous regions. Cretinism may be caused by an iodine deficiency, thyroid tissue deficiency, genetic lack in enzymes that synthesize thyroid hormones, and thyroiditis. All these factors develop and affect the fetus prenatally; as a rule, one parent, usually the mother, has thyroid deficiency. Prevention of cretinism may be achieved in some instances by giving thyroid hormone to mothers who have had cretins. The community nurse working with pregnant women should be alert for a patient's history of previous or existing thyroid disease and should notify the attending physician.

A pre- and postnatal deficiency of thyroid hormone results in pathophysiologic effects involving the entire body. Growth is retarded and the maturation of body tissues is delayed. In the fetal brain, myelin sheath formation is impaired, with resulting irreversible damage. The clinical manifestations of cretinism vary with the age at onset of the disease, the severity of the disease, and the length of time without treatment. Cretinism may not be recognized in the first few postnatal months because sufficient hormone was supplied by the mother. The diagnosis may be suspected if the infant fails to gain weight and height and refuses food. Once the classic clinical picture of frank cretinism is present, the diagnosis is easily recognized. The usual history is one of lethargy, constipation, dry skin, and hoarse cry as well as feeding problems and failure to grow. On examination, the head is large and fontanel closure is delayed. The eyelids are puffy; the nose is broad and thick; the lips and tongue are large and protruding; the neck is short and thick; the skin is dry, cool, pale, and rough; the abdomen is protuberant; and commonly an umbilical hernia is present. The extremities are short. Intellectual and motor development is delayed. The mental level is that of an idiot.

Two laboratory tests, a low-serum protein-bound iodine (PBI) and a high-serum cholesterol, confirm the diagnosis of cretinism. The basal metabolic rate (BMR), which for infants must be done in a special respiratory chamber, is not available in all medical centers but is a useful diagnostic measure. Skeletal roentgenograms show failure of ossification of the epiphyses of the long bones.

The course of cretinism is dependent on the initiation of treatment. If treated early in neonatal life (before 4 months of age), the infant may develop normally and attain sexual maturity. If mental damage has occurred, treatment will minimize but not always eliminate this deficiency. If cretinism manifests itself in the second or third year of life and diagnosis and treatment are prompt, the likelihood of normal physical and mental development is good.

Medical and Nursing Therapy

The aim of medical treatment of the cretin is to restore him to the euthyroid state and reverse the clinical manifestations of the disease. Specific therapy involves the administration of thyroid hormone throughout life. Desiccated thyroid, 30 to 90 mg per day, is the range of dosage for infants. Older children are given 90 to 240 mg per day. Thyroxine or triiodothyronine may be used. Dosage of thyroid hormones is an individual matter and is determined according to the child's response. Height, weight, bone maturation, intellectual development, the PBI, and signs of the euthyroid state are clinical measurements that guide the physician to a physiological dosage.

The aim of nursing therapy of cretins is to assist the physician in evaluating the return to the euthyroid state and to assist the parents in understanding the nature of their child's disease and the care the child requires.

Specific nursing care includes observation of the child's clinical condition and recording of changes in the signs and symptoms indicative of his response to thyroid hormone therapy. Changes expected during the first months of treatment include weight loss; increase in physical activity, growth rate, and appetite; and decrease in constipation, dry skin, and cold intolerance. The nurse teaches the parents the importance of giving the daily dose of thyroid drug and suggests ways the parents may handle specific problems. Slow eaters require time and patience to feed. Only the most nutritious foods should be used. Constipation may be relieved by giving the child warm water before feedings to stimulate the gastrocolic reflex. Leg exercises to strengthen the abdominal muscles may indirectly counteract constipation. Skin care could include the use of water and oil to lubricate the dry, coarse skin. The child should be warmly dressed to prevent exposure to cold. The parents are made aware of the possibility of hyperactive and irrational behavior indicative of excessive thyroid hormone and should be advised to report this state to the physician. The community nurse assists the parents in adjusting their household to a child who requires time and care and who may never achieve the physical and mental development of normal children. If the mother becomes pregnant, she is advised to notify her attending physician of the history of thyroid disease in her family. Administration of thyroid hormone during pregnancy may prevent another child from being born a cretin.

JUVENILE MYXEDEMA

Juvenile myxedema is a hypothyroid disorder that develops due to thyroid hormone deficiency in a previously normal child who has not attained puberty or full growth. Age of onset is after 2 years of age.

The etiology of juvenile myxedema is the same as that of adult myxedema. Pathophysiologically, there is a lack of thyroid hormone to meet the prepubertal growth and developmental requirements. The clinical picture is intermediate between cretinism and adult myxedema. Early growth and development are normal.

After initiation of the disease, skeletal development is delayed with epiphyseal dysgenesis. The child is dwarfed, with an infantile extremity-trunk ratio. Sexual development is also delayed past the average pubertal age. The mentality is normal but cerebration is slow. Anorexia, constipation, dry skin and nails, delayed dentition, increased sensitivity to cold, and slow motor development are signs and symptoms of juvenile myxedema. The idiocy of cretinism and the myxedema accompanying adult hypothyroidism are rarely seen.

Laboratory findings indicate that the protein-bound iodine, the ^{131}I uptake, and the BMR are slightly decreased. The serum cholesterol is elevated. The diagnosis is confirmed by the laboratory findings. Usually the age at onset of the disease may be determined by the stage of skeletal and sexual development which the child has achieved. Untreated juvenile myxedema would result in a sexually and skeletally immature person of adult chronological age.

Medical and Nursing Therapy

Medical therapy of juvenile myxedema is directed at restoring the euthyroid state. Desiccated thyroid, 90 to 240 mg, is administered daily. As in the cretin, changes in the physical signs and laboratory tests provide an index for the therapeutic dosage of thyroid hormone.

Nursing therapy of patients with juvenile myxedema is similar to that for children with cretinism. In addition, the nurse may judge the child's mental capability for learning to administer drugs to himself. Both parents and child must realize that the drug therapy is necessary for life. Community nurses working in homes and schools should be alert to the possibility of case-finding children with juvenile myxedema.

ADULT MYXEDEMA OR HYPOTHYROIDISM

Adult myxedema or hypothyroidism is the disease syndrome resulting from a severe thyroid hormone deficiency occurring in a previously normal postpubertal adult. The disease is also known as *Gull's disease*, after the physician who first recognized it as a clinical entity. Subclinical forms of hypothyroidism occur, particularly in older individuals, in which the clinical and laboratory findings are of less severity than in full-blown myxedema. The degrees of hypothyroidism may range from a life-threatening situation to one very difficult to diagnose. Most cases of hypothyroidism develop in persons between 30 and 60 years of age. The exact incidence is unknown, but the disease is probably more common than is presently recognized.

Etiologic factors that affect the thyroid gland and cause myxedema are (1) a reduction in thyroid tissue due to atrophy or destruction by thyroidectomy, irradiation with ^{131}I or x-ray, or thyroiditis; and (2) a reduction in thyroid tissue function due to impaired synthesis of the thyroid hormone, as in iodine deficiency or following administration of thyroid-inhibiting drugs, or in impaired release of the thyroid hormone as in hypopituitarism.

The pathophysiologic mechanism of myxedema is a decrease in thyroid activity resulting in a decrease in all body metabolism. Effects associated with this decrease occur in many parts of the body. The widespread effect of thyroxine lack is probably due to its stimulation of a "single basic energy-producing reaction" that occurs in most tissues (Williams). Thyroxine stimulates the oxygen consumption of most body tissues, with the exception of the spleen, brain, and testes.

The cardiovascular system in myxedema has reduced demands for blood, probably because of a reduced peripheral oxygen requirement. The heart rate and pulse pressure are decreased. Because the stroke volume is decreased, cardiac output is decreased. Dyspnea on exertion and peripheral edema are found in more than half the patients. Angina pectoris is a complaint of one-quarter of the patients. As fluids accumulate in the tissues, excess sodium is retained and the plasma volume is decreased. Total serum protein is increased because the lack of thyroxine retards protein synthesis. Protein-bound iodine is decreased; serum cholesterol and phospholipids are increased. Serum cholesterol increases as a result of a decrease in its rate of synthesis. Vitamin A level is decreased because the lack of thyroxine prevents the synthesis of vitamin A from carotene. As the blood carotene increases, the skin becomes yellow. Anemia is found in most of the patients and varies directly with the basal metabolic rate. The low hemoglobin and reduced red blood cell mass may be an adaptation to reduced oxygen requirements. The lack of thyroxine retards the rate of glucose entering the cell and the peripheral utilization of glucose.

Although cerebral metabolism is considered independent of thyroid hormone action, there is decreased cerebral blood flow with resultant decrease in available glucose. The slowed mentation, disinclination to engage in physical or mental activity, impaired comprehension, poor memory, decreased perception of all stimuli, and delayed reactions and clumsiness may be explained by the decrease in cerebral glucose. The patient may progress to drowsiness, stupor, and irreversible myxedema coma. All nerve conduction is slowed and deep tendon reflexes are delayed in the relaxation phase. Most patients show few emotional reactions; they are usually pleasant and exhibit a "dry" humor known as "myxedema wit." Some patients are emotionally labile.

The skin in hypothyroidism receives deposits of protein and polysaccharide materials into the connective tissue. These changes are accompanied by increased water in the connective tissue—the *myxedematous state*. The skin is dry, rough, scaly, inelastic, and puffy. The skin is pale due to the anemia; yellow from carotenemia; and cool because of the decreased metabolic rate. The muscles are also swollen with fluid and the result is weakness, fatigue, stiffness, and cramps. Obesity is present in over half the patients and is probably due to the edema and lack of activity. Respiratory capacity is reduced in myxedematous patients who are obese. The muscles of respiration may be affected, causing reduced breathing capacity. Pleural effusions are common.

The gastrointestinal system reflects the lack of thyroid hormone with an anorexia probably due to a lessened need for food concomitant with a general lethargic state. Stimulation of intestinal peristalsis is poor, and anorexia and constipation are the result. Although the renal concentrating mechanism is not affected in myxedema, the kidney is unable to excrete water loads until the thyroid hormone deficiency is corrected.

The clinical manifestations of myxedema may all be traced to the accumulation of protein and water in the body and to decreased anabolism and catabolism of carbohydrate, protein, fat, water, and mineral. The degree of clinical hypothyroidism is determined by the duration and degree of thyroid hormone deficiency. The onset of the disease is usually insidious, so much so that neither the patient nor his family can date the physical and mental changes, which may develop over a period of years. Early in the disease the symptoms are increased sensitivity to cold and decreased perspiration. The patient's face and eyelids are puffy, and physical and mental activity is slowed. The face becomes expressionless. A tendency to gain weight is noticed. The voice is husky and low-pitched. The hair is dry and may fall out. The nails are brittle. The patient complains of easy fatigue, muscular weakness, and lethargy. Speech is slow and concentration inadequate. In the untreated patient the way of life will diminish to an almost vegetative existence with death from myxedema coma the final outcome.

Laboratory findings in full-blown myxedema include a basal metabolic rate between −30 and −40. The protein-bound iodine is below 3.5 μg per 100 ml. The hemoglobin is between 8.5 and 11.5 g, and the red blood cell count is between 3.5 and 4.0 million per cu mm.

The classic history, clinical manifestations, and laboratory findings point to a clear-cut diagnosis of hypothyroidism. The course of the disease is steadily progressive. In the final stages the patient is comatose and hypothermic and may die from failure of the organ systems, infection, or extreme cachexia.

Medical and Nursing Therapy

The medical treatment of myxedema is replacement therapy with the objective of restoring the patient to the euthyroid state. Three thyroid hormone preparations are used in the following dosages: desiccated thyroid, 90 to 240 mg; L-thyroxine, 150 to 400 μg; and L-triiodothyronine, 50 to 150 μg. Qualitatively, all three drugs will reverse the symptoms of myxedema. Quantitatively, the initial effects of thyroxine may be seen in 48 hours, whereas the initial effects of triiodothyronine may be seen after 6 hours. The maximal clinical response to daily thyroid hormone dosage may not be observed for 2 to 3 months, and symptom relief is slow— a matter of days or weeks. The optimum daily dosage is individually determined by each patient's clinical response to the drug.

The nursing therapy of the myxedematous patient has two major objectives: (1) to restore the patient to the euthyroid state, and (2) to alleviate the symptoms of hypothyroidism. Restoration of the patient to the euthyroid state specifically includes the administration of the thyroid hormone drug and the observation and reporting of the signs and symptoms indicating the patient's clinical response. Patients with long-standing myxedema may be particularly sensitive to thyroid hormone drugs. Headache, palpitations, and angina pectoris should be reported because a decreased drug dose may be indicated in order to allow the patient's cardiovascular and nervous systems to adapt to the return to euthyroidism. If congestive heart failure or angina occurs, the nurse gives the specific care described for that disease.

The nurse makes the following clinical measurements and observations in patients receiving the initial dose of thyroid hormone: (1) fluid intake and output to determine the expected fluid diuresis; (2) blood pressure, temperature, and pulse to determine the extent of the expected increase; (3) daily weights to determine the expected weight loss; (4) physical and mental activity to determine the expected increase; and (5) appetite to assess the return of desire for food. These observations are stressed as major guidelines in determining the appropriate drug dosage. The laboratory tests used in diagnosing hypothyroidism are less accurate as early guides. The nurse informs the patient of the changes he may expect in his body systems and explains that these changes occur over a period of days and weeks.

Prior to the initiation of thyroid hormone therapy and until the desired euthyroid response is achieved, the nurse gives symptomatic care to lessen the patient's appreciation of his symptoms. Nursing activities are carried out at a pace consistent with that of the patient. The patient is allowed time to think, speak, and act. When conversing, the nurse gives the patient time to work out his thought processes and to complete his sentences. The teaching of necessary information, such as the importance of daily drug therapy, is conveyed in simple terms and is repeated frequently. The patient is encouraged to engage in physical and mental activity, the successful outcome of which is not dependent on quick reflexes. The nurse may assist the occupational therapist in initiating leather work, knitting, and other activities and thus decrease the patient's sense of inadequacy and relieve his boredom. All activity is spaced with frequent rest periods during the day and unbroken sleep at night in order to allow the muscle fibers and body cells time to recover from fatigue.

Increased sensitivity to cold necessitates a warm environment for hypothyroid patients. A room at 75° with no drafts is comfortable. Extra clothing and bedding will protect the patient from the sensation of cold. The discomfort of dry skin may be alleviated by restricting the use of soap, which removes the available sebaceous gland secretion. The patient may soak in water and then apply lanolin or a skin cream.

The nurse may counteract the poor gastrointestinal function by several means. Anorexia may be diminished by providing small frequent feedings of preferred foods. Elimination of anorexigenic factors such as excessive smoking, fatigue, boredom, and depression are nursing responsibilities. Constipation may be counteracted by providing hot water before the first meal of the day. Hot water passes rapidly through the empty upper gastrointestinal tract and stimulates the gastrocolic reflex to initiate peristalsis. Measures to alleviate constipation include the following: foods high in cellulose and fiber; 6 to 8 glassfuls of water per day; irritant, bulk-forming, emollient, or stool-softening cathartics; and exercises to strengthen the abdominal muscles.

The patient may be disturbed by his physical appearance of obesity, and his baggy eyelids and dull facial expression. The nurse avoids comments that might reflect her observations of the patient's appearance. Emotional instability, delusions, and hallucinations are hypothyroid manifestations that respond slowly to drug therapy and therefore are a long-term nursing responsibility. Behavioral responses and the nursing care are described elsewhere. The psychotic patient is watched for an intensification of psychosis which may be caused by the drug therapy.

When the hypothyroid patient is safely on the way to euthyroidism and is ready to return to community life, the hospital nurse may refer her patient to the community nurse. The community nurse reiterates previous teaching with particular emphasis on the importance of taking the prescribed daily dose of thyroid. A useful comparison for impressing this fact is to tell the patient that his thyroid drug is as important to him as is insulin to a diabetic. Long-term prognosis is excellent when the adult hypothyroid achieves and maintains the euthyroid state.

Hyperthyroidism

Hyperthyroidism is a systemic disorder resulting from the action of excess thyroid hormone causing an accelerated metabolism in most body tissues. The terms *hyperthyroidism* and *thyrotoxicosis* are used interchangeably. The eponym *Graves' disease* is used to signify the classic picture of hyperthyroidism with thyroid enlargement and ophthalmopathy. A multiplicity of eponyms and terminology abounds reflecting the work of various clinicians who described the disease and the various etiologies ascribed to the disease. These terms will be introduced where relevant to the text.

The precise incidence of hyperthyroidism is not known. The disease is not reportable and mortality from it is uncommon, so the usual medical statistics are not helpful. Hyperthyroidism is found throughout the world and in all age groups from infancy to old age. The peak age incidence is in the third and fourth decades. Seven times as many females as males exhibit the disease.

The etiology of hyperthyroidism may be exogenous or endogenous. Exogenous hyperthyroidism is traced to the administration of thyroid or thyroid-stimulating hormones. Overtreatment of hypothyroidism or of hypometabolic states and the administration of iodides are examples. Endogenous hyperthyroidism may be traced to pituitary tumors producing excessive thyrotropin; to thyroiditis or radiation injury followed by release of stored thyroid hormone; and to toxic adenoma and toxic multinodular goiter. Genetic similarities, severe emotional stress, and infection are other factors considered to have an etiologic base in hyperthyroidism. Graves' disease, sometimes designated *diffuse toxic goiter,* is considered the most important and most common cause of hyperthyroidism.

Prevention of hyperthyroidism is not yet possible as the exact etiology is unknown. One exception to this situation is the exogenously induced disease. Precautions in administering thyroid hormone therapy and in observing the clinical response may prevent exogenously induced hyperthyroidism.

The pathophysiologic mechanism of hyperthyroidism is an increase in thyroid activity resulting in increased combustion of food and increased liberation of energy. Goiter and exophthalmos complete the classic picture of Graves' disease, although these two signs are not inevitable nor are they presently attributed to the excess circulating hormone. Recent studies have isolated a thyroid-activating substance (long acting thyroid stimulator [LATS]) present in the serum of patients with Graves' disease (Means et al.). LATS may cause thyroid hyperplasia resulting in excessive production and secretion of thyroid hormone. An exophthalmos-producing substance (EPS) has been identified, and both EPS and LATS are implicated in the production of exophthalmos and the localized (pretibial) myxedema of Graves' disease.

EFFECTS OF HYPERTHYROIDISM UPON BODY SYSTEMS

The increased liberation of energy in hyperthyroidism is reflected in the cardiovascular system. Tachycardia (90 to 110 beats per minute), increased cardiac output, and increased blood volume are indicative of the cardiovascular response to the demand for oxygen made by the increased oxidative metabolism. Systolic blood pressure is usually increased as a result of the increased pulse volume. Diastolic blood pressure is normal. The heart beats with such force that the patient experiences palpitations. Superficial capillaries are dilated. Auricular fibrillation occurs in 1 of 10 patients. Congestive heart failure, particularly in the older age group with prehyperthyroid damaged hearts, is not uncommon. The hemoglobin is low normal or decreased, but this change is relative to the increased blood volume.

The increased energies of hyperthyroidism promote central nervous system irritability. Although the brain does not have an increased rate of oxygen consumption, cerebral blood flow is increased. The irritability may be due to the excess thyroid hormone causing an increased sensitivity to circulating epinephrine. In fact, the clinical response is comparable to that caused by increased autonomic activity. The patient is jittery; his thoughts flash from one subject to another; one or another part of his body is in constant motion; and a fine rhythmical tremor of extended fingers and tongue, and eyelids, is common. Reflex time and reaction time for many activities are accelerated. Mood swings are frequent and are characterized by fits of laughter, crying, talkativeness, and exuberance. The tremendous expenditure of energy results in fatigue. Coexistence of fatigue and compulsion to hyperactivity are not uncommon.

The skin in hyperthyroidism receives increased circulation. As a result the skin temperature is elevated and the skin is smooth and elastic. The skin is thin, presumably to facilitate dissipation of heat from the circulating blood. Flushing of the skin is common in young persons. The increased work of the heat-eliminating mechanisms that require body water and the excessive autonomic nervous system activity cause the skin to be excessively moist. The palms of the hands may be dripping wet. The patient has increased sensitivity to heat and decreased tolerance to warm environments. The hair and nails are dependent on thyroid function but the exact mechanisms are unknown. The hair is fine, soft, and straight and temporary hair loss may occur. The nails are friable and may be grooved and atrophied. Localized myxedema occurs in the pretibial area of many patients with Graves' disease and in some patients following thyroidectomy. This localized edema is not to be confused with the generalized edema of hypothyroidism. Excess mucopolysaccharides are deposited in the pretibial dermis. Because this condition occurs in Graves' disease, it is presumed that LATS or EPS is involved in the etiology. Circulatory stasis and dependent edema may also be causes for this selective deposition in the lower legs. The skin over the tibial aspect of the lower leg is firm, elevated, and thickened. Color may range from pink to brown. The lesions may be present in patches or be confluent. The patient complains only of the unsightly appearance and the difficulty in fitting shoes.

Muscular disturbances in hyperthyroidism are attributed to impaired biochemical reactions. Lack of muscle nutrients and increased activity also account for muscular weakness, easy fatigue, and muscular atrophy. The legs and arms quickly weaken in repetitive activities such as climbing stairs and elevating arms.

The major respiratory symptom of hyperthyroidism is dyspnea. Studies have found decreased vital capacity, decreased pulmonary compliance, weak respiratory muscles, and increased respiratory dead space ventilation. Combined, these abnormalities may cause dyspnea.

The gastrointestinal system reacts to thyroid hyperfunction. Increased metabolic demands for nutrients lead to hyperphagia. Though many patients eat excessively, they tend to lose weight unless their food intake exceeds their metabolic needs. Diarrhea occurs in one-quarter of the patients, and another one-third of the patients have increased bowel movements. Overactivity of the autonomic nervous system with resulting increase in peristaltic activity and decrease in absorption are the pathophysiologic processes underlying the diarrhea. The increased food intake also contributes to the diarrhea. Toxic levels of thyroid hormone may precipitate anorexia, nausea, and vomiting. Abdominal pain in hyperthyroidism has been associated with hypercalcemia.

Polyuria in hyperthyroidism is the result of increased renal blood flow and glomerular filtration rate which, in turn, is the result of increased cardiac output.

The majority of severely hyperthyroid patients have mild eye signs. Overactivity of the cervical sympathetic nerves is considered the cause of spasm and retraction of the eyelids. A staring, frightened, or popeyed expression, jerky movements and tremor of the lid, lid lag on downward movement of the eyeballs, and globe lag on upward gaze are present. The eye appears to be exophthalmic but measurements do not indicate protrusion.

The severe oculopathy of Graves' disease is characterized by an edematous increase in the size of the orbital contents. The globe protrudes, the lids are swollen, and paralysis or paresis of the extraocular muscles may occur. Conjunctival, retinal, and optic nerve damage may result. A sense of pressure and excessive tearing is reported. EPS or LATS may be the factor that increases the mucin and, therefore, the edema in the orbital area. The globe is protruded because its rigid bony frame allows only forward expansion. The eyelids may be unable to appose, and ulceration and infection of the cornea may develop.

The thyroid gland is enlarged. This sign of hyperthyroidism is clinically termed a *goiter*. The goiter may be smooth or diffuse as in Graves' disease, or nodular and unevenly enlarged as in hyperthyroidism in the older age group. In either case, this enlargement is presumed due to overstimulation of the gland. This sign has given rise to the use of such terms as *toxic goiter* and *exophthalmic goiter* to indicate hyperthyroid states.

The most frequent clinical manifestations of hyperthyroidism are representative of increased work of many body systems and are summarized as follows: nervousness, excessive sweating, intolerance to heat, palpitations, fatigue, weight loss, tachycardia, dyspnea, weakness, hyperphagia, eye changes, lower leg swelling, diarrhea, frequent bowel movements, goiter, skin changes, and tremor. These signs and symptoms portray the hyperthyroid clinical picture so frequently that the diagnosis of hyperthyroidism is considered one of the easiest in medicine. The disease is manifested in all degrees of severity and with variation in the symptom pattern. The onset of the disease is usually gradual with symptoms developing over a period of weeks or months. Sudden or prolonged psychic trauma is frequently the activating episode to the development of hyperthyroidism. The course of the disease is now altered by medical therapy, but in the past it was potentially fatal particularly when thyroid storm occurred. Thyroid storm is an intensification of hyperthyroid symptoms with hyperthermia, uncontrolled tachycardia, weakness, and delirium.

Several laboratory findings verify the diagnosis of hyperthyroidism. Basal oxygen consumption measured by the basal metabolic rate is increased. The protein bound iodine is elevated above 8 μg per 100 ml. ^{131}I uptake at 24 hours is elevated above 45 to 50 percent. If the patient has a rapid ^{131}I turnover a 3- or 6-hour test will be indicative. A discriminating test between normal states and mild forms of hyperthyroidism is the triiodothyronine suppression test. In hyperthyroidism the thyroid fails to be suppressed after triiodothyronine administration.

Medical Therapy

The medical therapy of hyperthyroidism is not completely satisfactory because the exact cause of the disease is unknown. Several forms of therapy are in use, all of which are designed to interfere with thyroid hyperfunction. The three common forms of therapy are irradiation, antithyroid drugs, and thyroidectomy. The physician and patient choose the therapy that is economically, emotionally, and physically suitable.

Administration of radioiodine (^{131}I) in doses of 160 μcuries per g of thyroid weight is used to implant destructive radiation in the gland. The total dose may range from 5 to 10 millicuries (5,000 to 10,000 μcuries). Iodine has an affinity for the gland; the isotope is deposited and emits rays as it disintegrates. Early euthyroidism is achieved. Investigators have recently found, however, that a high incidence (30 percent) of hypothyroidism develops several years following the radioiodine. The problems posed by the need for daily thyroid replacement plus the mobility of both the patients and the physicians have led to the suggestion that the radioiodine dose be halved. This, it is hoped, would reduce the risk of late hypothyroidism; however, hyperthyroidism is more likely to recur. Antithyroid drugs are administered following the radioiodine until euthyroid effects are achieved. This method of treatment is advocated for patients over 40 years of age (post childbearing age) and those in whom surgery is contraindicated.

Antithyroid drugs are used as long-term hyperthyroid therapy or in the pre-thyroidectomy period. Iodine, one of the first antithyroid drugs used, lessens hyperthyroidism by decreasing the rate at which thyroid hormone is released and increasing the quantity of stored hormone. Iodine exerts this action only on the hyperfunctioning gland, having little effect on the normal gland. The mechanism of iodine action is obscure. A saturated solution of potassium iodine or Lugol's solution is used as an iodine medication. Iodine as a single therapy is rarely used because of its long-term failure and its interference with other therapy.

Antithyroid drugs in common use are the thiocarbamides. The thiocarbamides suppress hormone synthesis and the binding of iodine to protein. These drugs also interfere with the trapping of iodine by the gland. Carbimazole, methimazole, propylthiouracil, and methylthiouracil are used. The high initial dosage provides complete thyroid blocking. As the patient becomes clinically euthyroid, usually in 4 to 6 weeks, the maintenance dosage is established for a 1-year period. The medication is gradually withdrawn over the next few months. Most exacerbations of hyperthyroidism occur 3 to 6 months following withdrawal of drug therapy. Toxic reactions to the thiocarbamides include fever, rash, jaundice, and agranulocytosis. Forty-five to seventy-five percent of the patients experience prolonged remission of hyperthyroidism after thiocarbamide therapy is withdrawn. This remission is not attributed to the drugs but rather to the disease passing into a latent or inactive phase. Surgery is most frequently chosen for the young adult who decides against or has adverse reactions to the antithyroid drugs.

Subtotal thyroidectomy, in which some thyroid tissue is permanently removed, provides long-lasting relief from hyperthyroidism. The occurrence of hypothyroidism may be as high as 30 percent, however.

Nursing responsibilities in the administration of radioiodine are primarily to teach the patient what to expect of the treatment. The tasteless, colorless radioiodine is administered in water by the physician. Following this procedure no radiation precautions are necessary unless the patient expels excreta such as vomitus, urine, or excess perspiration onto the bedclothes. In these instances the linen and any other object in contact with the excreta must be decontaminated. No other radiation hazards exist, since the radioiodine is concentrated almost entirely in the thyroid gland. The patient may be discharged from hospital and followed by a community nurse while he awaits the return to euthyroidism.

The nurse assists in restoring the patient to the euthyroid state by administering the antithyroid drugs. The nurse is alert to toxic reactions to the thiocarbamides and, when discharging a patient, tells him to report immediately symptoms of sore throat, fever, erythematous rash, and pruritus to his doctor. Explanations of ^{131}I therapy or long-term drug therapy can be reinforced by the nurse. The nurse can explain the time interval required for the regression of clinical manifestations, thereby clarifying the patient's expectations of treatment. If the patient is scheduled for a thyroidectomy, the nurse can teach him what to expect following surgery. The time in the recovery room, the 45-degree angle position in bed, and holding the hands behind the head to elevate the head and prevent strain on the incision are specific points to include in preoperative teaching. Postoperatively the nurse watches the patient closely for the first 24 hours. Hemorrhage into the soft tissues of the throat could cause asphyxiation. The recurrent laryngeal nerve may be damaged resulting in hoarseness—usually a temporary problem. Tetany, from transient hypoparathyroidism due to trauma and interrupted blood supply, may develop. Intravenous calcium should be readily available to counteract the tetany. The general pre- and postoperative care required by the surgical patient is discussed in Part V.

During the diagnostic period and prior to the clinical response to therapy, the hyperthyroid patient requires symptomatic nursing care to lessen his apprehension of the symptoms. The major nursing problem is to counteract the tremendous energy expenditure of all body systems. The overworked cardiovascular system requires rest to reduce its work load. Rest may be an exceedingly difficult achievement for the nervous hyperactive patient. The nurse spaces her nursing activities so that the patient is not expected to take part in a series of events without rest.

Subtotal thyroidectomy is preceded by the administration of the thiocarbamide drug to return the patient to euthyroidism and of iodine to decrease the size of the gland. This preparation allows the patient's nutritional and cardiovascular status to improve, and surgery is performed without the risk of the sympathetic discharge common to thyrotoxic patients. The thyroid storm of poorly prepared patients is rarely seen nowadays.

Adjunctive therapy to the three primary methods of treatment is the use of the sympathetic antagonist drugs. Reserpine, guanethidine, and propranolol antagonize the hyperthyroid signs which are mediated by the sympathetic nervous system. Tremor, tachycardia, lid retraction, and nervousness are decreased. These effects are of greatest value as the patient awaits surgery or the return to euthyroidism.

Nursing Therapy

The nursing therapy of the hyperthyroid patient has similar objectives as that for hypothyroidism—to restore the patient to euthyroidism and to alleviate the symptoms of the disease. The nurse maintains a composed and unrushed appearance in front of the patient to avoid intensifying his own nervousness. Explanations of the cause of disturbing cardiovascular symptoms, such as palpitations and headache, may lessen his fear of the symptoms. The patient should be protected from stress situations of fear and worry which can increase central nervous system irritability. Mood swings are understood as occurring beyond the self-control of the patient and are accepted calmly by the nurse.

A cool environment and the minimal amount of clothing are provided. Frequent changes of clothing are allowed for the patient who is diaphoretic.

Muscular fatigue may be lessened by protecting the patient from repetitive activities involving action of the arms and legs.

The increased appetite of hyperthyroidism should be satisfied by extra feedings. Some patients require six full meals per day. A well-balanced diet of carbohydrate, protein, fat, and vitamins is essential to provide nutrients to the body systems. The patient is weighed daily to determine his nutritional balance. Diarrhea, which contributes to the weight loss and malnutrition, may be counteracted by eliminating fibrous and highly seasoned foods and excessive intake of water, coffee, and alcohol. These ingestants may cause reflex diarrhea. The diarrhea of hyperthyroidism is therefore accentuated because it is due primarily to a quick response to intestinal reflexes. The nurse may be present during the patient's mealtime to ensure slow ingestion of food thereby lessening the peristaltic stimulus of a large food bolus.

When eye changes occur, the features most distressing to the patient are the symptoms of conjunctival or corneal irritation. Shielded and deeply tinted glasses may protect the patient from photophobia. Protective drops, such as methylcellulose, are soothing, cooling, and protective to the exposed cornea. If the eyelids do not close in sleep they may be taped shut. The development of exophthalmos may be lessened by restricting salt and water intake and by elevating the head of the bed. The patient will require some explanation of his eye changes. These changes tend to increase as the hyperthyroidism is reversed. For this reason, regression to hypothyroidism is avoided. The exophthalmos increases, perhaps because of increased water content in the tissues. Nursing care in reduced vision is described in Part V. If the cosmetic appearance of exophthalmos is disturbing to the patient, the nurse avoids comments that reflect her observations of this physical sign. A large goiter may cause dyspnea and dysphagia. Nursing care of a dyspneic and dysphagic patient is described in Part IV.

The hospital nurse may refer the patient to the community nurse, who can observe the patient's clinical response to therapy and report untoward toxic signs and symptoms.

Goiter

Goiter is a general term applied to any noninflammatory or benign enlargement of the thyroid gland. The pathology basic to the enlargement is a functional hyperplasia and hypertrophy of the gland. Other synonymous terminology is *nontoxic goiter, adenomatous goiter,* and *nodular goiter.* The last-named has arisen because nodules or small lumps are the most frequent basis of goiter.

The incidence of goiter, specifically endemic or simple goiter, has ranged from 20 to 100 percent in geographic zones known to have iodine-deficient soil and water. The Midwest, Northwest, and the Great Lakes region of the United States have had a higher incidence of goiter. In nonendemic areas the incidence of goiter in population studies varies from 4 to 8 percent. The incidence of goiter is two to four times higher in females than in males.

Goiter results from the following causes: (1) iodine deficiency, (2) goitrogens of dietary or drug origin, (3) genetic enzyme defects, and (4) increased thyroxine demand. All these factors interfere with the synthesis of thyroxine. The resulting thyroxine deficiency stimulates excess production of thyrotropin, which causes hypertrophy and hyperplasia of thyroid cellular tissue. Goiter and thyroid adenoma are the resulting clinical condition. Increased production of thyroxine is stimulated and, dependent on the hormone level achieved, hypothyroidism or hyperthyroidism develops or euthyroidism is maintained.

Goiter due to iodine lack is usually associated with euthyroidism, sometimes with hypothyroidism. Many persons are aware of the swelling in their throat but have no complaint other than the cosmetic appearance. Diagnosis may be confirmed by the fact that many goiters of iodine-deficient origin take up excessive amounts of ^{131}I. Prevention is relatively simple and consists of intake of a minimum of $50\mu g$ iodine per day; 200 to 300 μg of iodine provide a safe level. Seafood, drinking water, food that takes iodine from the soil, and iodized salt are dietary sources of iodine. Iodized salt has proved most effective in decreasing the incidence of goiter in endemic goiter areas. The average adult salt intake of 6.2 g provides 474 μg of iodine. Once the goiter has passed the early stages of development, the treatment may be administration of desiccated thyroid, thyroxine, triiodothyronine, or purified thyroglobulin in subtoxic doses. This treatment has resulted in regression of the goiter but has the disadvantage that it may produce thyrotoxicosis. Subtotal thyroidectomy is performed when there are serious cosmetic or local pressure symptoms or sudden growth of the goiter.

Goitrogens are ingestible substances that inhibit the synthesis of thyroxine. Turnips and cabbage contain a compound, goitrin, which is a thiocarbamide. As a single cause of goiter, however, a diet consisting exclusively of these foods is unlikely. Long-term therapy in large doses of any of the thiocarbamide drugs can also produce a goiter.

Several thyroid enzymatic defects have been discovered. The fact that several members of one family are afflicted with goiter and other types of thyroid disease (usually hypothyroidism) suggests an inherited metabolic defect. Therapy consists of maintaining the patient on subtoxic doses of thyroid hormone for the remainder of his life. The maximal safe dose is achieved by administering the drugs to the point of hyperthyroid symptoms and then lessening the dosage by a small amount.

Increased thyroxine demand as in pregnancy or during puberty has been known to induce goiter. Increase in dietary iodine during such periods is usually an effective prophylaxis.

Medical and Nursing Therapy

The major objective of the medical therapy of patients with goiter is to reduce the size of the thyroid gland while maintaining the patient in a euthyroid state. Administration of thyroid hormone and subtotal thyroidectomy are the therapeutic measures employed. Nursing therapy for patients receiving these treatments has been described under hypothyroidism and hyperthyroidism.

The community nurse may be concerned with the prophylaxis of goiter in endemic areas. A sufficient daily intake of iodine may be determined by the nurse who questions the dietary habits of families and school children. Asking mothers to show the package of salt they use and checking on its iodine content is a simple measure. When objection to the adulteration of salt with iodide arises, the nurse may advise the family to buy pure salt and consult with the medical health officer or family physician for a suitable iodine supplement. Potassium iodide may be used.

Thyroiditis

The term *thyroiditis* includes a group of inflammatory conditions of the thyroid which appear in acute, subacute, and chronic forms. Acute suppurative thyroiditis is a rare and dangerous condition of bacterial invasion of the thyroid. Acute (subacute) nonsuppurative thyroiditis is an inflammatory febrile disease localized to the thyroid and self-limiting in duration. Chronic thyroiditis, the most common form of which is Hashimoto's disease, is a diffuse long-term inflammation of the thyroid.

As the incidence of acute suppurative thyroiditis is very low, and the clinical manifestations and treatment are those of any infection, this disease will not be discussed.

SUBACUTE THYROIDITIS

The incidence of subacute thyroiditis is low, approximately one-eighth that of Graves' disease. The number of diagnoses made, however, has increased in the last few years.

The cause of subacute thyroiditis is not apparent. The disease tends to follow upper respiratory infections, rheumatic fever, streptococcal infections, and mumps.

These infections, particularly those of viral origin, cause destruction of the thyroid resulting in liberation of thyroglobulin and antigens and an inflammatory reaction. Antibodies are formed and antigen-antibody reactions may take place leading to further thyroid destruction.

Clinically the patient complains of goiter of less than 4 months' duration. The thyroid region is exquisitely tender and the pain may radiate to the jaw and ears. Half of the patients complain of neck pressure symptoms such as dysphagia and dyspnea. Fatigue, malaise, and fever occur. Signs and symptoms of hyperthyroidism may occur in the first week. The laboratory finding is a moderate elevation of the erythrocyte sedimentation rate. Diagnostic tests include thyroid function tests, antibody tests, and serum flocculation tests. The disease has a gradual onset over a 1- to 2-week period. Symptoms continue for 3 to 6 weeks. Subsequent weeks or months may be characterized by remissions or exacerbations. When the symptoms finally subside, thyroid function usually is normal although myxedema may develop in up to 10 percent of the patients.

Medical Therapy

The objective of medical therapy for patients with subacute thyroiditis is to reduce the inflammation and alleviate symptoms. Acetylsalicylic acid, 4 to 5 g per day, provides analgesia and may have an effect in reducing the inflammation. Other analgesics may be used as well as local applications of heat. Desiccated thyroid is given to those patients in whom a tender, enlarged thyroid persists and is continued until the goiter decreases in size or maintains the same size. If these measures do not alleviate the symptoms, prednisone or one of its analogues, in 10 to 20 mg or equivalent doses, is given for 1 week. Reduction of this dosage is made slowly over the next few weeks until the symptoms subside.

CHRONIC THYROIDITIS

The true incidence of chronic thyroiditis, specifically Hashimoto's disease, is not known because many patients are not clinically diagnosed. This thyroiditis is the most common type, occurring half as frequently as Graves' disease. Nine of ten patients are females in the third to the fifth decade of life.

The etiology of chronic thyroiditis is traced to an agent such as surgery, x-ray, or radioiodine, which causes thyroid destruction. As in subacute thyroiditis, antigens are released. These antigens presumably come in contact with the body's immune apparatus and antibodies develop in profusion. Antigen-antibody reactions occur. These autoimmunologic reactions appear to cause the major thyroid damage. A genetic predisposition may also play a part in the etiology of chronic thyroiditis. The disease has been diagnosed in several members of one family.

Clinically, the disease has an insidious onset with the thyroid gradually enlarging. Only rarely does the patient complain of neck pressure symptoms or of thyroidal pain or tenderness or of fever. Hypothyroid symptoms present over a period of several years and myxedema develops in some patients. Antithyroglobulin antibodies are found in the serum of most patients. The cephalin flocculation test or the thymol turbidity test is higher than normal. A needle biopsy of the thyroid revealing a whitish plug of tissue combined with the clinical goiter and signs of hypothyroidism is diagnostic of Hashimoto's disease. The disease runs a slowly progressive course which, if untreated, eventually ends in myxedema.

Medical and Nursing Therapy

The objective of the medical therapy of Hashimoto's disease is to reduce the size of the thyroid gland and prevent the development of myxedema. Thyroid hormone therapy is given with the rationale of reducing thyroid activity and the manufacture of thyroglobulin. Antigen production is decreased and antigen-antibody reactions are diminished. The thyroid gland decreases in size, particularly in young persons who have less fibrosis of thyroid tissue. The thyroid hormone also serves as replacement therapy if hypothyroid symptoms are present. If an enlarged and tender thyroid persists, one of the thiocarbamide drugs may be given. This drug also decreases the manufacture of thyroglobulin. A partial thyroidectomy is performed if pressure symptoms persist. This surgery increases the likelihood of myxedema, and the patient is maintained postoperatively on thyroid hormone therapy.

Nursing therapy of patients with subacute and chronic thyroiditis follows the established medical regimen. Specific nursing care has been discussed under hypothyroidism and hyperthyroidism. Community nurses have a responsibility in case-finding and bringing patients with suspicious symptoms to a doctor's attention.

Laboratory Tests

TESTS TO MEASURE THE RATE OF THYROID HORMONE PRODUCTION

Protein-Bound Iodine. Protein-bound iodine is a measurement of the amount of iodine in the serum protein. The serum protein is precipitated by chemicals that also precipitate the hormone, thyroxine. As iodine is bound to this hormone, a measurement of iodine is also a measurement of the serum thyroxine. The test is inaccurate if the patient has received therapeutic or diagnostic iodine in the preceding 6 months. Normal range is from 3.0 to 8.0 μg per 100 ml of serum.

Butanol-Extractable Iodine. Butanol-extractable iodine is a measurement of the amount of iodine in the serum protein. The tests differs from the PBI in that iodine from food and medications is removed. Iodine from x-ray dyes is not removed and the BEI test is difficult to perform. Normal range is from 3.2 to 6.4 μg per 100 ml of serum.

Radioactive Iodine Uptake. The radioactive isotope of iodine (^{131}I) is taken up by the thyroid gland. The diagnostic tracer dose is 5 μcuries contained in a capsule, which is handed by tongs to the patient. The patient swallows the capsule. The ^{131}I breaks down, releasing gamma rays, which are detected and counted by a scintillation counter. Six and twenty-four hours later the scintillation counter measures radioactivity, which is an indication of ^{131}I uptake. There are no radiation dangers from the tracer dose, and no precautions, other than the use of tongs, are taken. The test is inaccurate if the patient has had iodine in the preceding 30 days. Since the rate of iodine uptake is equal to the rate of iodine output, this test is a measurement of the thyroxine output of the thyroid gland. Normal range is from 10 to 40 percent uptake.

TESTS TO MEASURE THE METABOLIC EFFECTS OF THE THYROID HORMONE

Basal Metabolic Rate. The basal metabolic rate is a measurement of the oxygen consumption per unit time under basal conditions. The rate of heat production is calculated from the oxygen consumption. Because the body's heat production is governed by skeletal and smooth muscle activity as well as by thyroid activity, the test must be performed on a patient who is mentally and physically relaxed and who has fasted from food for 12 hours. Normal range is from −20 to +20 percent.

Achilles Tendon Reflex Time. The reflex recording of the ankle jerk is a measurement of the response time (time for the rise and fall of the foot) following tapping of the Achilles tendon. The response is fast in hyperthyroidism and slow in hypothyroidism.

Serum Cholesterol. Cholesterol may be a substance from which hormones are synthesized. The exact function of cholesterol is unknown. Serum cholesterol is elevated in hypothyroidism because cholesterol is slowly synthesized. Normal range is from 120 to 260 mg per 100 ml of serum.

TESTS INDICATING HOMEOSTATIC RELATIONSHIPS OF THE THYROID GLAND

Triiodothyronine or Thyroid Suppression Test. The triiodothyronine suppression test is preceded by a radioactive iodine uptake test. The patient is given triiodothyronine, 25 μg three times a day for 7 days. The radioactive iodine uptake is repeated. In normals there is a 50 percent suppression of radioactive iodine uptake by the thyroid. In hyperthyroid persons there is little or no suppression and the radioactive iodine uptake remains the same. This test is one of the most accurate in clinical medicine. The suppression is considered due to decreased secretion of thyroid-stimulating hormone (TSH). A normal suppressive response eliminates the possibility of hyperthyroidism.

TSH Stimulation Test. The TSH stimulation test begins with oral administration of radioiodine. After 3 hours the thyroidal iodine uptake is measured and blood for PBI measurement is taken. TSH, either 5 units or 10 units, is then given. Twenty-four hours after the first dose of radioiodine, thyroidal radioactivity is measured and blood for PBI is drawn. A second dose of ^{131}I is given and thyroid radioactivity is measured at 3 and 24 hours. In normals, ^{131}I uptake is approximately doubled and the PBI increased following administration of TSH. This test distinguishes between primary hypothyroidism and pituitary failure and between true primary hypothyroidism and instances of persons receiving but not requiring thyroid replacement therapy.

Bibliography

Books

Ingbar, Sidney H. and Kenneth A. Woeber: The Thyroid Gland. in Robert H. Williams (Ed.): *Textbook of Endocrinology,* 4th ed. Philadelphia: W. B. Saunders Company, 1968.

Means, James Howard, Leslie J. DeGroot, and John B. Stanbury: *The Thyroid and Its Diseases,* 3d ed. New York: McGraw-Hill Book Company, 1963.

Rawson, Rulon W., William L. Money, and Roger L. Greif: Diseases of the Thyroid. in Philip K. Bondy (Ed.): *Duncan's Diseases of Metabolism,* 6th ed. Philadelphia: W. B. Saunders Company, 1969.

Werner, Sidney C. (Ed.): *The Thyroid,* 2d ed. New York: Harper & Row, Publishers, Incorporated, 1962.

Articles

Bernstingl, M.: Subtotal Thyroidectomy. *Nursing Times,* 63:1332–1334, October 6, 1967.

Croft, D. N.: Radioisotopes in Clinical Medicine. 1. The Physics, Thyroid Function and Treatment. *Nursing Times,* 64:1416–1418, October 18, 1969.

Derby, A. C.: Surgical Approach to Disease of the Thyroid Gland. *Canadian Nurse,* 61:878–880, November, 1965.

Ellis, Mary: Assessment of Thyroid Function. *Canadian Nurse,* 61:881, November, 1965.

Garde, Sister Mariana: Cancer of the Thyroid. *American Journal of Nursing,* 65:98–102, November, 1965.

Martin, D: Undetected Hypothyroidism. *Canadian Nurse,* 62:57–58, May, 1966.

Mason, A. S.: The Treatment of Thyrotoxicosis. *Nursing Times,* 65:202–203, February 13, 1969.

Michie, W.: The Complications of Thyroidectomy for Thyrotoxicosis. *Nursing Times,* 64:1689–1692, December 13, 1968.

Nordyke, Robert Allan: The Overactive and the Underactive Thyroid. *American Journal of Nursing,* 63:66–71, May, 1963.

Rawson, Rulon W.: The Thyroid Gland. *Clinical Symposia,* 17:35–63, April-May-June, 1963.

SECTION 3
PARATHYROID
DISORDERS

ROSEMARY PRINCE COOMBS

The parathyroid glands, though anatomically close to the thyroid gland, are neither functionally nor developmentally related to the thyroid. The parathyroid glands synthesize and secrete a parathyroid hormone, parathormone. Parathormone's primary function is to maintain, within narrow limits, the constancy of calcium ion in the serum. Parathormone performs this function by influencing the exchange of calcium in the bone, kidney, gastrointestinal tract, and lactating mammary gland. The serum level of calcium acts as a negative feedback mechanism and thereby controls the amount of parathormone secreted. A low serum calcium stimulates the secretion of parathormone. Parathormone also exerts a phosphaturic effect, the significance of which is unknown. Thyrocalcitonin is a hormone produced by the parafollicular cells of the thyroid gland. A hypercalcemic state stimulates the production of thyrocalcitonin. This hormone inhibits the bone resorption induced by parathormone and thereby prevents a rise in serum calcium.

Disorders of the parathyroid gland are usually accompanied by abnormal serum calcium and phosphorus. Knowledge of the biochemical relationships between the parathyroid gland and calcium and phosphorus metabolism is still incomplete. The multiple effects of parathyroid gland disorders on many body systems are well documented and demand a general symptomatic as well as a specific endocrinologic nursing approach.

Hypoparathyroidism

Hypoparathyroidism is the clinical state resulting from an inadequate secretion of parathormone by the parathyroid gland. The biochemical syndrome that results consists of hypocalcemia, hyperphosphatemia, hypocalciuria, and hypophosphaturia.

Hypoparathyroidism is traced to one of two known etiologies. A rare form of the disease is an idiopathic hypoparathyroidism. Children are most commonly affected, and females are affected twice as frequently as males. When the disease occurs in children of hyperparathyroid mothers, the etiology may be traced to a maternal compensation for the hyperparathyroidism. Several children in one family may be affected. The parathyroid glands are absent or atrophied. A more common form of hypoparathyroidism occurs in 1 to 5 percent of patients postoperative from a thyroidectomy. Patients who have had repeated thyroid surgery or those in whom total thyroidectomy has been performed are most likely to be affected.

The idiopathic form of the disease is not preventable. The serious effects of hypoparathyroidism on the infant may be prevented by early recognition and treatment. Every surgeon is aware of the possibility of unintentional removal of the parathyroids and makes every effort to identify and avoid these glands. Most cases of postoperative hypoparathyroidism are due to disturbance of the blood supply and subsequent infarction of the glands or to fibrous scar tissue with subsequent compression of the glands. In these patients the symptoms of hypoparathyroidism do not develop immediately but may take weeks, months, and even years to make their appearance.

The pathologic physiology that develops as a result of inadequate parathormone is a series of biochemical reactions. Decreased renal excretion of phosphate occurs because parathormone deficiency causes decreased secretion of phosphate by the distal tubules of the kidney. As a result, the serum phosphate increases and increased numbers of phosphate and calcium ions are deposited in bone. As the serum phosphate rises the serum calcium falls. The serum calcium changes are not altogether secondary to serum phosphorus changes. The hypocalcemia is also attributed to inadequate parathormone resulting in decreased intestinal absorption of dietary calcium, decreased resorption of calcium from bone, and decreased renal tubular resorption of calcium. These three mechanisms result in loss of calcium. Because of decreased renal excretion of phosphate, hypophosphaturia occurs. The fall in serum calcium results in hypocalciuria.

The most prominent clinical manifestations of hypoparathyroidism are the result of the hypocalcemia, which causes increased excitability of nerves and muscles. In infantile idiopathic hypoparathyroidism, convulsions are the most common clinical signs. Both adults and children exhibit signs and symptoms of neuromuscular irritability culminating in tetany. Numbness, tingling and cramps of the extremities, sensation of stiffness in the hands, feet, and lips, and twitching of the facial muscles are indicative of latent tetany. Dysphagia, dysarthria, bronchospasm, laryngeal spasm as evidenced by laryngeal stridor, carpopedal spasm (a position of flexion of the elbows, wrists, and carpophalangeal joints), blepharospasm, photophobia, cardiac arrhythmias (due to decreased contractility of the cardiac muscle), and convulsions are the result of spontaneous activity of the nerves and muscles and comprise the clinical syndrome of overt tetany.

Latent tetany may be diagnosed by two signs that elicit muscular contraction. Carpopedal spasm following a restriction of circulation to the arm by the application of a blood pressure cuff is a positive Trousseau sign. The test is negative if there is no sign after 3 minutes of the cuff pressure just above the systolic pressure level. Twitching of the facial muscles of the upper lip and eye following a sharp tapping over the facial nerve anterior to the ear is a positive Chvostek sign. Latent tetany may develop into overt tetany during stressful states such as pregnancy, lactation, menstruation, hyperventilation, and febrile illnesses.

Emotional lability with symptoms of irritability, anxiety, depression, and delirium are psychiatric symptoms of hypoparathyroidism. A frank psychosis may develop.

Ectodermal structures in patients with long-standing and idiopathic hypoparathyroidism show the effects of parathormone lack. The skin is coarse, dry, scaly, and pigmented. The hair is thin and patchy, particularly on the head. The nails are atrophic, ridged, and brittle. In children poor dental development occurs and is indicative of the age of onset of the disease.

The bones in hypoparathyroidism reflect the decreased rate of bone resorption of calcium. On x-ray study the bones show increased density. Calcifications in the lungs, gastric mucosa, and in the basal ganglia of the brain may also be visualized on x-ray film. Calcifications may also be seen in the lens of the eye.

The laboratory findings in hypoparathyroidism reflect the biochemical syndrome. Serum calcium may drop to 4 mg per 100 ml. Tetany occurs when the serum calcium is at 5 to 6 mg per 100 ml. Serum phosphate increases to as high as 12 mg per 100 ml. The serum alkaline phosphatase may be slightly low or normal. Urinary calcium is quantitatively diminished, particularly when the serum calcium is below 8 mg per 100 ml. Urinary phosphate clearance is below 5 ml per minute. In the Ellsworth-Howard test the hypoparathyroid patient's urinary phosphorus excretion increases twice over that of normal subjects. The tubular reabsorption of phosphate (TRP) is increased to above 95 percent. The intravenous calcium tolerance test produces a dramatic phosphaturia.

The diagnosis of acute hypoparathyroidism is made with ease if a complete history is obtained and if the neuromuscular manifestations are present. Chronic hypoparathyroidism presents diagnostic difficulties because the symptoms of cramps, cataracts, and neuroses are vague and attributable to many disorders. In all instances the characteristic biochemical syndrome should be sought by laboratory measurements.

Untreated hypoparathyroidism may result in chronic tetany or convulsions, and the patient may die of asphyxiation. Mental retardation occurs in children, while delusions and psychoses occur in adults. If the disease has produced calcifications of the basal ganglia a parkinsonian-like picture develops. Similarly, calcification of the lens causes diminished visual acuity. Treated hypoparathyroid patients usually have relief of symptoms, although if mental defects, cataracts, or skin changes have occurred these do not regress.

MEDICAL THERAPY

The medical objective in the treatment of hypoparathyroidism is to restore the serum calcium concentration to the normal range. Preparations of parathormone have not provided satisfactory replacement therapy because of the instability of the extract and the need to administer the protein substance parenterally. Tissue transplantation of parathyroid glands has been performed. When the problems associated with tissue transplantation are solved, this method may be the treatment of choice. Meanwhile, restoration of the normal serum calcium and limitation of gastrointestinal phosphate absorption is the specific objective guiding the symptomatic therapy of both acute and chronic hypoparathyroidism.

Acute hypoparathyroidism with tetany may occur in the immediate postoperative period following a thyroidectomy. Intravenous administration of 10 ml of a 10 percent solution of calcium gluconate will rapidly relieve the tetanic syndrome due to hypocalcemia. Chloral hydrate, pentobarbital, or paraldehyde may be administered if the calcium does not immediately relieve convulsive tendencies. When the tetanic crisis is controlled, the medical therapy is administration of oral calcium. Caution is used to prevent the development of hypercalcemia. Hypercalcemia may cause kidney damage and suppression of any possible parathyroid function.

When the state of chronic hypoparathyroidism and permanent impairment of the parathyroid glands is diagnosed, the doctor determines each patient's individual requirement of calcium by serum calcium determinations. The patient is given a high-calcium, low-phosphate diet. Milk and milk products, egg yolks, and cauliflower are restricted because, although their calcium content is high, they also contain high levels of phosphate. Spinach contains oxalate and will form insoluble calcium complexes, therefore it is eliminated from the diet. The high calcium diet is supplemented with oral tablets of calcium gluconate or lactate. A daily dose of 6 to 8 g is divided and given with each meal. An aluminium salt, such as aluminium hydroxide gel or basic aluminium carbonate (Amphogel or Gelusil), in 30 ml doses, is given before each meal to counteract gastrointestinal absorption of phosphate.

If the above measures do not provide a normal serum calcium, two other drugs may be used. Dihydrotachysterol (A.T. 10 or Hytakerol) promotes gastrointestinal absorption of calcium and phosphate diuresis—actions attributed to parathormone itself. The daily dose ranges from 1.25 mg to 3.75 mg (1 to 3 ml) dependent on the individual patient's calcium requirements. Calciferol (vitamin D_2) has proved even more effective and less costly than dihydrotachysterol in promoting calcium absorption. Initial daily doses of 250,000 units may be reduced to 50,000 units per day, once a normal serum calcium is achieved.

The therapeutic measures are aimed at providing a serum calcium level of 10 mg per 100 ml for the chronic hypoparathyroid patient. Measures of the serum calcium are taken every week to 2 weeks during the initiation of therapy. When the patient is free from neuromuscular symptoms and the serum calcium is within the normal range, serum estimations of calcium content may be done three or four times a year or at the return of neuromuscular symptoms. Postsurgical hypoparathyroid patients may also be hypothyroid. Administration of thyroid hormone in these patients has a direct effect on elevating the serum calcium and on increasing their sensitivity to vitamin D as well as maintaining the euthyroid state.

NURSING THERAPY

Nursing therapy of patients with hypoparathyroidism has the same objective as medical therapy—to restore the serum calcium to a normal range. Relief of the neuromuscular disturbances is an objective requiring symptomatic nursing care.

The nurse anticipates the possibility of acute hypoparathyroidism in all postoperative thyroidectomy and parathyroidectomy patients. Observations for tetany, convulsions, and respiratory difficulties are made. Intravenous calcium gluconate with equipment for intravenous injection is available at the patient's bedside. If the patient has been receiving a cardiac glycoside (digitalis) or is subject to cardiac arrhythmias, calcium gluconate is administered by slow infusion. Calcium is essential for contraction of the cardiac muscle. Digitalis and calcium both increase systolic contraction. An excess of calcium, however, seems to potentiate the action of the digitalis. The cardiac depressant effect is expressed initially by bradycardia and later by cardiac standstill. The nurse should be present continually with patients who have cardiac problems and who are receiving intravenous calcium. Nursing observations or cardiac developments are greatly facilitated if the patient is on continuous cardiac monitoring until the calcium and cardiac statuses are stable.

The nurse administers the prescribed p.r.n. sedation when the patient's convulsive tendencies persist. Specific nursing care of the patient with neuromuscular irritability includes provision of an environment free from stimuli such as noise, sudden light, sudden temperature change, movement, and pain. Nursing care of a patient with convulsions is described elsewhere.

The respiratory difficulties of tetany may be unrelieved by the first dose of intravenous calcium. The nurse administers the prescribed bronchodilator drugs or assists with the insertion of an endotracheal or tracheotomy tube. The patient's respiration may be assisted with positive pressure respirators; other nursing measures are presented in Chapter 22.

Once the tetanic crisis of acute hypoparathyroidism has subsided and the doctor has determined the patient's daily calcium and vitamin D requirement, the nurse is directly responsible for providing the prescribed calcium intake. At this time the nurse can explain to the patient the rationale of the drug and diet therapy. The necessity and means of maintaining a high calcium and low phosphate intake are emphasized. The nurse observes the patient for symptoms indicating hypocalcemia such as awkward gait, stiffness, muscle spasm, and behavior changes. Observations indicating hypercalcemia are also made (Kupperman). The nurse teaches the patient and his family the signs and symptoms of hypocalcemia and hypercalcemia and suggests they report to their doctor if these clinical changes occur. The nurse reiterates the doctor's plan for estimations of the serum calcium concentration and assists the patient in making appointments for these visits. As the patient becomes familiar with the symptoms indicating a serum calcium outside the normal range, the nurse may assist the doctor in teaching the patient to adjust his daily dose of calcium and/or vitamin D_2 according to the Sulkowitch test for urinary calcium.

Hypercalciuria may develop in patients receiving vitamin D_2 even though hypocalcemia is present. As continued hypercalciuria may cause renal damage, the nurse saves and reports all urine containing "sand" and collects urinary specimens for calcium determinations.

Hyperparathyroidism

Hyperparathyroidism is the clinical state resulting from an excessive production of parathormone by the parathyroid gland. The accompanying classic biochemical syndrome is the exact opposite of that in hypoparathyroidism—hypercalcemia, hypophosphatemia, hypercalciuria, and hyperphosphaturia. This biochemical syndrome is not complete in many of the patients. Hypercalcemia is the one consistent finding. Blood chemistry estimations often vary just slightly from the normal range. Secondary hyperparathyroidism occurs when the amount of parathormone produced is independent of the body's need. Hyperparathyroidism may be manifested by diverse clinical syndromes reflecting involvement of many body systems. Terminology specific to each clinical syndrome will be introduced where relevant.

The exact incidence of hyperparathyroidism, the most common disorder of the parathyroids, is not known. The first diagnosed case was reported in the 1930s. Since 1945 the diagnosis has been made with increasing frequency, presumably as a result of greater use of diagnostic techniques and a high index of suspicion for patients who present renal or bone disorders. Women in the fourth decade of life are most commonly afflicted with the disease.

The etiology of primary hyperparathyroidism is unknown. An adenoma of a single parathyroid gland occurs in 90 percent of the cases. Multiple parathyroid adenomas occur in 3 to 5 percent of the cases. Hypertrophy and hyperplasia of the parathyroid with cells distinct from the chief cell of the adenoma comprise the remaining 5 percent. Carcinoma of the parathyroid is very rare.

Prevention of primary hyperparathyroidism is not yet a clinical possibility. Prevention might be achieved if the stimulus that results in a parathyroid adenoma was identified.

The pathophysiology underlying primary hyperparathyroidism results from an excess of parathormone affecting the renal tubules, the bone cells, and the gastrointestinal mucosal cells. Parathormone causes the renal tubules to readily excrete phosphate. Hyperphosphaturia and hypophosphatemia result. Excess parathormone increases the tubular reabsorption of calcium, the gastrointestinal absorption of calcium, and the resorption of bone releasing phosphate and calcium ions. The phosphate from osteolytic activity is excreted, but calcium from the kidneys, gastrointestinal tract, and bones is retained. Hypercalcemia results. Once the limit of the parathormone action to increase tubular reabsorption of calcium is reached and hypercalcemia is present, calcium begins to spill over into the urine. Hypercalciuria results in about one-half of hyperparathyroid patients.

Excess parathormone causes increased osteolytic activity of the bone cells. Osteoblastic activity, resulting in building up of new bone cells and establishment of a new balance, increases. This formation of new bone is partially dependent on the phosphate supply. The phosphate supplied in a normal diet is quickly excreted in hyperparathyroidism. Bone resorption, therefore, exceeds bone build-up. Early bone disease and eventually osteitis fibrosa generalisata develop.

As the hypercalciuria and hyperphosphaturia increase, the concentration of calcium and phosphate ions in the urine increases beyond their solubility. The ions precipitate in the kidney parenchyma causing nephrocalcinosis. The ions also precipitate in the renal tubules, collecting ducts, kidney pelvis, and ureters causing calculi. The resulting renal failure is considered a complication of primary hyperparathyroidism.

The clinical manifestations of primary hyperparathyroidism reflect involvement of many body systems. The bones, kidneys, gastrointestinal tract, and central nervous system may be affected. Hypercalcemia with its associated symptoms always accompanies the disease and may be the presenting sign.

The hypercalcemic syndrome includes mental changes ranging from apathy, severe fatigue, depression, confusion, insomnia, and irritability to severe headaches. The gastrointestinal tract in severe hypercalcemia is disturbed by dysphagia, anorexia, nausea, vomiting, constipation, and weight loss. Calcium phosphate crystals have been found in many body organs including the gastrointestinal and respiratory tracts, the kidneys, the blood vessel walls, the myocardium, the meninges, the cornea, and the ear drums. The amount of calcium deposited varies directly with the degree of decreased function in each organ. The nerves show decreased excitability and the muscles are hypotonic.

Bony involvement, in some degree, is found in all patients with primary hyperparathyroidism. The bone lesions were first described by von Recklinghausen and still bear his name. The disease is also known as *osteitis fibrosa generalisata* or *osteitis fibrosa cystica*. The patient may complain of long-standing skeletal pains. Generalized bony decalcification (bone resorption), bone cysts, and giant cell tumors are noted on x-ray and histologic examination. Bone deformities of the vertebrae and pelvis, bending of the long bones, spontaneous pathological fractures, decreased stature, and pigeon-breast deformity may occur.

Renal disease occurs in approximately 80 percent of patients with primary hyperparathyroidism. The patient complains of low back pain. Hematuria, passing of "sand," and renal colic are manifestations of nephrocalcinosis (calcium deposits in the collecting tubules) or nephrolithiasis (calcium deposits forming kidney stones). Urinary tract infection may result. Nephrocalcinosis may also be manifested by marked polyuria and polydipsia. These symptoms occur because of functional damage to the renal tubules.

The most common gastrointestinal occurrence in hyperparathyroidism, apart from the symptoms associated with hypercalcemia, is ulcer. Gastric ulcer may occur in 8 to 25 percent of hyperparathyroid patients as compared to 5 to 10 percent in the general population. Gastric ulcer in hyperparathyroidism may develop from the hypercalcemia, which causes increased gastric secretion.

The above signs and symptoms of primary hyperparathyroidism are primarily chronic manifestations of the complications of the disease. An acute form of hyperparathyroidism, parathyroid crisis, may occur. Pathophysiologically, large amounts of parathormone are secreted into the system producing severe hypercalcemia. The symptoms of the "hypercalcemic syndrome" are accentuated. Profound weakness, lethargy, and intractable nausea and vomiting occur. Calcium deposits in the renal tubules may result in infarction and necrosis with uremia. Coma and sudden death is the outcome. Widespread metastatic calcifications of the lung, heart, stomach, brain, and kidneys are found at autopsy.

The classic laboratory findings in primary hyperparathyroidism are a serum calcium ranging above 11 mg per 100 ml, a serum phosphate level below 3 mg per 100 ml, and a urinary calcium output of 250 to 500 mg in 24 hours. These values are not consistently obtained, since they tend to vary with the dietary intake and the parathyroid adenoma activity. In borderline cases the tests may be repeated several times and additional laboratory tests may be performed. An elevated plasma ionized calcium, a urinary phosphate clearance above 15 ml per minute, a tubular reabsorption of phosphate (TRP) below 85 percent, and a phosphate deprivation test resulting in a fall in the serum phosphate and a rise in the serum calcium are positive results for hyperparathyroidism.

All laboratory tests are indirect measurements of parathormone activity, which possibly explains the number of tests used and the difficulties in diagnosing early hyperparathyroidism. No direct measurement of serum or urinary parathormone is yet available.

The plasma alkaline phosphatase level increases directly with the degree of loss of bone calcium in hyperparathyroidism.

Radiological examinations are useful diagnostic tools when hyperparathyroidism has progressed to the stage of bone, kidney, or gastric disease. Skeletal x-ray surveys will, by demonstrating changes in bone density, illustrate bony decalcification. This evidence is seen only when 25 to 40 percent of the bony calcium has been reabsorbed. Abdominal flat plate x-ray films will demonstrate calcium oxalate or calcium phosphate stones, which give an opaque shadow. A gastric ulcer will be demonstrated by x-ray film following ingestion of barium.

The diagnosis of primary hyperparathyroidism is difficult. The early signs of the disease are nonspecific, and the diagnosis of an emotional disorder may be made. Biochemical signs are inconclusive. Many patients have had symptoms for several years before a correct diagnosis is made. Bone and kidney lesions frequently comprise the presenting complaint; yet, in fact, these lesions are actually complications of hyperparathyroidism. Primary hyperparathyroidism, because of its multiple system involvement, may be confused with and must be differentiated from several other diseases, e.g., hypervitaminosis D, sarcoidosis, malignant neoplasms, and Addison's disease.

The course of primary hyperparathyroidism is that of a slowly progressive disease except in a few instances in which excess parathormone production occurs rapidly. As the hypercalcemia increases, calcium phosphate is precipitated in the tissues, renal failure ensues, and a chemical death due to hypercalcemia, hyperphosphaturia, and a high nonprotein nitrogen occurs.

The prognosis of treated hyperparathyroidism is primarily dependent on the degree of existing complications. In patients with no overt bone disease or renal disease, the blood chemistry returns to normal in 1 to 4 days. In patients with overt bone disease, the removal of all pathologic parathyroid tissue does not result in prompt return to normal body chemistry. Increased formation of the bony matrix requires all the available plasma minerals. This "bone hunger" continues until the bony matrix lost during the disease is replaced. In patients with severe renal disease, the long-term prognosis is poor. In many patients the renal changes may be irreversible and may even progress following treatment.

MEDICAL THERAPY

The objective of the medical treatment of primary hyperparathyroidism is to decrease the amount of circulating parathormone, thereby restoring chemical balance and reversing the development of osseous and renal complications.

Medical treatment for primary hyperparathyroidism, such as the administration of high-calcium, high-phosphate diets, does cause reossification of the bony lesions. The renal complications of this treatment, however, contraindicate its use. Surgical removal of the parathyroid adenoma(s) is the only treatment of choice. Specific preoperative care involves placing the patient on a low-calcium, low-phosphate diet. Aluminium salts may be given to decrease gastrointestinal absorption of phosphate. Inositol sodium hexophosphate may be given to decrease gastrointestinal absorption of calcium. Water and noncalcium-containing beverages are encouraged in large amounts. X-ray examination of the neck, esophagus, and mediastinum may be performed in an attempt to locate the parathyroid adenoma. The surgeon identifies all four parathyroids. He removes a single adenoma or, if all four glands are hyperplastic, leaves from 100 to 200 mg of the fourth gland.

Postoperatively serum and urinary calcium and phosphate measurements are made to determine the effects of the operation. If hypercalcemia persists, a second adenoma or malignant metastases from a parathyroid cancer are suspected. In either case a repeat parathyroidectomy may be performed. Radiation may be employed if a malignant neoplasm is diagnosed. In postoperative patients with overt bone disease a high-calcium, low-phosphate diet is provided to ensure sufficient calcium for bone formation and to prevent tetany from hypocalcemia. Calcium gluconate or lactate may be infused intravenously and vitamin D supplements may be given if severe calcium deficit is anticipated.

In parathyroid crisis, emergency removal of the parathyroid adenoma may be performed. Administration of phosphate intravenously or orally may bring the serum calcium to safer levels below 17 mg per 100 ml. Metastatic calcifications are more common and severe with intravenous than with oral therapy. Phosphate, EDTA (ethylenediaminetetraacetic acid), sodium sulfate, and sodium citrate have been prescribed for hyperparathyroid patients because of their calcium lowering effects. Complications with the former two drugs may be severe; the latter two drugs have not, as yet, been widely used. Thyrocalcitonin is being investigated for use as drug therapy in hyperparathyroidism and other hypercalcemic states. This hormone, which blocks bone resorption of calcium, would act to control hypercalcemia.

NURSING THERAPY

The objectives of nursing therapy of patients with hyperparathyroidism are to assist the doctor in restoring the normal level of circulating parathormone and to relieve symptoms that accompany the complications of the disease.

The relatively great number of diagnostic tests for hyperparathyroidism, the necessity for frequent repetition of tests, and the medical consideration of many differential diagnoses may cause the patient considerable anxiety and worry. The nurse may explain the pathophysiology of hyperparathyroidism, the reasons for difficulty in establishing the exact diagnosis, and the reasons for the repetition of diagnostic tests.

Symptomatic nursing care of a patient with the hypercalcemic syndrome includes planning frequent rest periods to combat fatigue, advising against excessive exercise because of muscle hypotonia, observing for cardiac arrhythmias, providing small frequent feedings of the low-calcium diet to counteract anorexia, and administering prescribed analgesics to relieve headaches and bone pain.

Once the diagnosis of primary hyperparathyroidism has been established, the nurse prepares the patient for surgery. Specific preparation includes reiterating the surgeon's explanation of the location of the neck and, possibly, sternal incision (parathyroid glands may be located behind or in front of the mediastinum). The nurse shows the patient how to use his hands to lift his head postoperatively to prevent strain on and pain from the incision. The rationale of the milk- and milk-product-free diet is explained as providing the lowest possible level of calcium in the patient's body. The patient is told of the need for extra fluids both for their diuretic effect and to limit further calculi formation. The patient may be asked to keep a measurement of his own fluid intake. This activity not only gives the patient the sense of cooperating in his therapeutic regimen but it may provide the stimulus to drinking more fluids.

Specific nursing care of a patient postoperative from a parathyroidectomy is dependent on the preoperative condition and complications. The nurse observes for the clinical manifestations of hypocalcemia, particularly in the patient who has overt bone disease. The tetany that occurs when overt bone disease is present is almost intractable. The nurse ensures that the patient receives and ingests a high-calcium diet. Intravenous calcium gluconate or oral calcium lactate may be administered as an additional source of calcium. The nurse immediately reports if the patient has received less than the medically prescribed intake of calcium. The nurse observes for changes in bone pain and tenderness and reports their disappearance, which is expected 3 to 4 days postoperatively. The nurse observes for clinical manifestations of hypercalcemia, which may continue 7 or more days postoperatively or may recur following the establishment of a normal serum calcium.

The specific nursing care of the renal, bone, gastrointestinal, and central nervous system complications of hyperparathyroidism is planned according to the patient's symptoms and is discussed in other chapters.

Laboratory Tests

TEST TO MEASURE CIRCULATING PARATHYROID HORMONE

Radioimmunoassay. The radioimmunoassay test was developed in the latter 1960s and should be in general use in the next few years. This test is a measurement of circulating levels of human parathormone. The normal concentration of human hormone is less than 0.6 mμg per ml. Hyperparathyroid patients have values ranging from 2 to 10 mμg per ml (Potts and Deftos). This test will establish an accurate diagnosis of hyperparathyroidism. The test will also demonstrate that excess parathormone arises from a parathyroid adenoma with no feedback mechanism involved. Levels of serum calcium can be altered by administration of calcium or EDTA. A subsequent radioimmunoassay test would indicate no change in the circulating parathormone.

TESTS TO MEASURE CHEMICAL MANIFESTATIONS OF PARATHYROID HORMONE ACTIVITY

Changes in Body Calcium

Total Serum Calcium. The total serum calcium test is a measurement of the amount of ionized and nonionized calcium in the serum. Only ionized calcium is essential to the body processes of muscular contraction and transmission of nerve impulses. Approximately 50 percent of total serum calcium represents calcium ions. Normal range is from 9.0 to 11.0 mg per 100 ml of serum. (Limits of the normal range vary in different laboratories.)

Plasma Ionized Calcium Fraction. The plasma ionized calcium fraction test measures the amount of ionized calcium in the serum. The values of ionized calcium have been found to be elevated in patients with symptoms of hyperparathyroidism and normal total serum calcium. This test has not been widely used. Normal range is 5.9 to 6.5 mg per 100 ml of serum.

Urinary Calcium (Qualitative). The qualitative urinary calcium or Sulkowitch test is a rough estimate of the amount of calcium in the urine. The calcium in the urine precipitates with oxalate from a buffered oxalate solution. Normal range is a fine white precipitate. An increase or decrease in the density of the precipitate indicates an increase or decrease in urinary calcium.

Urinary Calcium (Quantitative) or Calcium Deprivation. The quantitative urinary calcium test is an exact estimate of the amount of calcium in a 24-hour urine specimen following administration of a calcium-deprived diet. The patient receives a low-calcium diet (containing approximately 0.137 g of calcium) for 3 to 6 days before the test. Normal range is 75 to 175 mg of calcium per 24 hours.

Corticosteroid Therapeutic Test. The corticosteroid therapeutic test is a daily measurement of the serum calcium during a 5- to 6-day administration of 100 to 200 mg of cortisone per day. The test is used to evaluate hypercalcemia in any patient. If the hypercalcemia is suppressed to normal levels, hyperparathyroidism may be ruled out. If the hypercalcemia is not suppressed, hyperparathyroidism and other conditions with hypercalcemia must still be considered.

Changes in Body Phosphorus

Serum Phosphorus. The serum phosphorus test is a measurement of the amount of inorganic phosphate in the serum. Normal range is 3 to 4 mg per 100 ml.

Phosphate Deprivation. The phosphate deprivation test consists of administration of a diet low in phosphate (less than 350 mg per day) and normal in calcium and calories for 3 days. The patient may be given aluminium salts to decrease gastrointestinal absorption of phosphate. Serum phosphorus, total calcium, and total protein are measured daily. Normal range is a maintenance of normal blood chemistry. In hyperparathyroid patients the serum phosphorus falls below the normal range and the total calcium has a compensatory rise.

Tubular Reabsorption of Phosphate. The tubular reabsorption of phosphate (TRP) test is a 24-hour measurement of the amount of phosphate excreted in the urine minus the amount of phosphate filtered by the renal glomeruli. The patient receives a diet adequate in phosphorus. Accuracy of the test depends on normal kidney function. Measurements of urine phosphate and creatinine and serum phosphorus and creatinine are taken. Normal range is from 82 to 97 percent.

TEST TO EVALUATE BONE ACTIVITY

Serum Alkaline Phosphatase. The serum alkaline phosphatase test is a measurement of the amount of the enzyme, alkaline phosphatase, in the serum. The level increases directly with increased bone formation. Normal range is 1 to 4 Bodansky units or 3 to 13 King-Armstrong units.

TEST TO DETERMINE PARATHYROID TISSUE RESPONSE

Intravenous Calcium Tolerance. The intravenous calcium tolerance test is a measure of the serum phosphorus and urinary phosphate following intravenous administration of calcium gluconate. Calcium gluconate, 15 mg per kg of body weight, is given in 1,000 ml of normal saline over a 3- to 4-hour period. A 24-hour urine collection is begun at the same time and repeated the following day. The patient eats exactly the same diet on each of the 2 days. Normal patients show a rise in the serum phosphorus and a 50 percent reduction in urinary phosphate. This finding indicates that the normal parathyroid gland responds to hypercalcemia by decreasing the production of parathormone. Hyperactive parathyroid glands do not respond to the hypercalcemic stimulus, and the serum phosphorus and urinary phosphate are not altered significantly. Hypoparathyroid patients show a marked phosphate diuresis.

TEST TO DETERMINE PARATHYROID HORMONE RESISTANCE

Ellsworth-Howard Test. The Ellsworth-Howard test is a measurement of urinary phosphate once every hour for 3 to 5 hours following intravenous administration of parathormone. Normal response is an increase in urinary phosphate five to six times above the normal range. Hypoparathyroid patients show a tenfold increase. Pseudohypoparathyroid patients show a twofold increase.

TEST TO DETERMINE TUBULAR RESPONSE
TO PARATHYROID HORMONE

Parathyroid Hormone Infusion Test. The parathyroid hormone infusion test measures the TRP before and after the intravenous administration of 200 units of parathyroid extract. Hyperparathyroid patients show a difference in the two

TRP measurements of between 2 and 7 percent. Patients with hypercalcemia not caused by hyperparathyroidism show a difference of 12 to 30 percent.

Bibliography

Books

Gaillard, P. J., et al. (Eds.): *The Parathyroid Glands.* Chicago: The University of Chicago Press, 1965.

Kupperman, Herbert S.: *Human Endocrinology,* Vol. 3. Philadelphia: F. A. Davis Company, 1963, pp. 1038–1085.

Potts, John T., Jr. and Leonard J. Deftos: Parathyroid Hormone, Thyrocalcitonin, Vitamin D, Bone and Bone Mineral Metabolism. in Philip K. Bondy (Ed.): *Duncan's Diseases of Metabolism,* 6th ed. Philadelphia: W. B. Saunders Company, 1964.

Rasmussen, Howard: The Parathyroids. in Robert H. Williams (Ed.): *Textbook of Endocrinology,* 4th ed. Philadelphia: W. B. Saunders Company, 1968.

Articles

Edwards, P. A.: Parathyroid Adenoma. *Nursing Times,* 65:1162–1165, September 11, 1969.

Moffatt, E. P.: Hyperparathyroidism with Renal Failure: Nursing Care Study. *Nursing Times,* 65:9–11, January 2, 1969.

SECTION 4 PITUITARY DISORDERS

MARY ALICE CHELGREN

The pituitary gland, or hypophysis, is sometimes referred to as the *master gland* because hormones released by it have widespread influence upon many other glands and body processes. The anterior lobe of the pituitary (adenohypophysis) is composed primarily of glandular tissue; the posterior lobe (neurohypophysis), of nervous tissue. The optic chiasm lies directly over the pituitary gland. Secretions from the pituitary are mediated by the hypothalamus under control of the nervous system. The hypothalamus is connected to the pituitary via the hypophyseal stalk.

The pituitary produces growth hormone, adrenocorticotropic hormone, thyroid-stimulating hormone, and gonadotropic hormone. All except growth hormone act primarily on "target glands" and are effective only if the target glands are intact and functioning. Changes in the release of these hormones cause changes in the activity and secretion of the target glands. Hormones from the anterior pituitary are regulated by hormonal blood levels and respond negatively to feedback from secretions of the target glands.

Vasopressin (antidiuretic hormone [ADH]) and oxytocin comprise the identified posterior pituitary hormones. The rate of ADH secretion is influenced directly by the concentration of body fluids. A positive water balance causes cessation of ADH release and excretion of hypotonic urine; a negative water balance causes release of ADH and excretion of hypertonic urine.

Deficiency of Hormones Produced by the Anterior Lobe

The anterior lobe of the pituitary may produce insufficient hormones as a consequence of disease or surgical removal of the gland. Clinical manifestations of hypopituitarism are usually absent until about 75 percent of the gland has been destroyed. Manifestations of deficiency are primarily due to insufficient stimulation of the adrenals by corticotropin and insufficient stimulation of the thyroid by thyrotropin. Laboratory tests that reflect corticotropin production include the measurement of urinary excretion of 17-ketosteroids and 17-hydrocorticosteroids.

With decreased corticotropin, both measurements are very low, less than 3 mg each, and there is a subnormal response to a single intravenous injection of corticotropin because of adrenal atrophy. Decreased thyrotropin production is reflected in a decrease of protein-bound iodine and decreased thyroidal iodine accumulation. Measurable gonadal pituitary hormones are diminished also.

The treatment of anterior lobe deficiency centers about replacement of target organ hormones. (Tropic hormones are expensive and tend to lose their effectiveness when used over long periods of time.) Cortisone acetate may be used as replacement for corticotropic hormone. The maintenance dose may range from 12.5 to 37.5 mg daily; the dose may be increased in the presence of unusual stress. Thyroid hormone may be replaced gradually with desiccated thyroid. Estrogens and androgens are useful in replacement therapy for both women and men.

Signs and symptoms of anterior pituitary deficiency include those caused by corticoid withdrawal. These are nausea and vomiting, severe asthenia and eventual collapse, hyperthermia above 104° F, and moderate to severe hypotension. Hypothyroidism may be evidenced by torpor, intolerance to cold, dryness of the skin, and myxedema.

Persons receiving corticosteroid replacement therapy have decreased ability to combat infection. They should be instructed to recognize and promptly report any infection, and should make efforts to avoid infection and to carry out preventive measures. The dosage of medication may vary according to the situation, as indicated above. Hypoglycemia is a potentially catastrophic development because the absence of glucosteroids prevents gluconeogenesis. Diabetics who have had a hypophysectomy are particularly susceptible to hypoglycemia. Hunger, weakness, nervousness, and fatigue indicate impending hypoglycemia and may warn the patient of his need for food. Persons receiving replacement therapy should carry an identification card indicating the type and dosage of medication they receive, the need for prompt attention if injured, and the need for sugar if found uninjured but unconscious. A patient newly admitted to a hospital should be questioned about corticosteroid administration; this may avert an addisonian crisis arising from a failure to continue the medication. The patient should be helped to understand his need for replacement therapy. It would seem wise that a family member also be instructed about the rationale of treatment and prevention of complications.

Deficiency or Overproduction of Growth Hormone

Pituitary dwarfism, a primary deficit of the growth hormone, is manifested when the child is 2 to 4 years of age. Growth is severely retarded, although body proportions are normal and the child is of normal intelligence. Symptoms of corticoid insufficiency and hypothyroidism may accompany dwarfism. Treatment with growth hormone from nonprimate sources has not been successful. Androgenic steroids have been used to induce growth, but this growth is achieved through acceleration in bone maturation and the amount of growth is therefore limited.

Excessive activity of certain cells of the anterior lobe of the pituitary causes an increase in the production of the growth hormone and probably, to a lesser extent, other hormones. Giantism results from this rapid tissue growth if the cellular activity occurs before puberty and before the epiphyseal plates of the long bones have closed. There may be a 20 percent increase in the basal metabolic rate in persons with giantism, and there is an increased tendency toward hyperglycemia and ketosis. If the excessive secretion occurs after closure of the epiphyseal plate, the resulting condition is *acromegaly*. Tissue growth is limited chiefly to soft tissue, the small bones of the hands and feet, and the membranous bones such as those of the nose and forehead. Enlargement of the thyroid, increased metabolic rate, and impaired glucose tolerance may also occur.

Giantism and acromegaly lead to observable changes such as increase in pulse rate, headache, visual changes (due to pressure on the optic chiasm), increased pigmentation of the skin, and weight gain. Affected persons may experience psychological disturbances, and almost always exhibit emotional instability. The changes in body image perceived by the patient also influence the reaction of family and friends to him. Early recognition and treatment of this disorder are important, since bony or soft tissue changes that occur before treatment has been given remain unchanged by treatment. Treatment frequently involves surgical removal of the pituitary or destruction by radiation and subsequent replacement therapy.

Deficiency of Hormones Produced by the Posterior Lobe (ADH and Oxytocin)

The principal effect of ADH is to enhance the reabsorption of water by the renal tubules, although it is thought also to cause a rise in blood pressure in anesthetized mammals. Oxytocin causes stimulation of uterine contractions and promotes secretion of milk from the lactating mammary gland. The reader is referred to textbooks on obstetrics for further discussion of oxytocin.

In the absence of ADH, the renal tubules are rendered practically impermeable to water, and diabetes insipidus develops. In this disease there is an extreme loss of water and an increased salt loss into the urine. The volume of urine excreted in a 24-hour period may be 7 to 11 liters, or as much as 17 liters (polyuria). This urine is hypotonic (when compared to body fluids) and has a specific gravity of 1.001 to 1.005. The osmolarity of body serum becomes elevated and this causes inordinate thirst (polydipsia). The patient drinks large quantities of water in order to satisfy this thirst. If he is deprived of adequate quantities of water, signs and symptoms of severe dehydration may develop, including thirst, fatigue, mental clouding or confusion, dry skin and mucous membrane, loss of tissue turgor, soft eyeballs, and low blood pressure; finally coma may supervene. The volume of urinary output may be within "normal range," but is far less than the individual's output when he is well hydrated. The specific gravity of the urine may fail to rise much above 1.010. During the diagnosis of diabetes insipidus, water may be restricted in order that changes in urine volume, specific gravity, and concentration may be observed. At this time the individual must be observed carefully lest too much fluid be lost from the body and circulatory collapse ensue. Careful note should be made of changes in weight accompanying restriction of water. Water restriction should be discontinued if weight loss reaches 3 to 5 percent of the patient's normal weight.

Vasopressin tannate salt may be given to control the polyuria. Control of polyuria and reduction in serum osmolarity will bring about control of the polydipsia as well. Vasopressin tannate must be carefully mixed before being administered, since the salt is suspended in oil and suspension is difficult to achieve. A preparation of posterior pituitary powder suitable for insufflation is available, but this is irritating to the nose and cannot be used in the presence of sinusitis.

The patient should be allowed fluids as desired; in this regard particular care must be taken if because of general anesthesia, or head injury or other causes of unconsciousness, the patient is deprived of water. A measure that will help avert water intoxication and hyponatremia is to include salt with the fluid.

Temporary or permanent deficiency of ADH production may be caused by primary disease of the posterior pituitary, inadequate blood supply to the pituitary, or hypophysectomy. Certain drugs also affect ADH production. Alcohol causes a decrease in ADH release, and morphine, nicotine, certain tranquilizers, and certain anesthetics cause an increase. Severe anxiety, fright, depression, and tension apparently cause an increase in ADH production, which may partially explain the occurrence of edema in persons experiencing certain types of stress. It is clear that the central nervous system exerts a definite effect upon ADH production.

Tumors of the Pituitary

Clinical manifestations of tumors are both local, from extension of the tumor, and hormonal, from altered hormone secretion. Local signs may include loss of vision from pressure on the optic nerve; intermittent headaches, usually of moderate severity; disturbance of appetite, sleep, and temperature regulation from invasion of the hypothalamus; and hemorrhage if blood vessels are invaded. Hormonal changes usually are similar to those occurring from hypophysectomy but rarely of equal severity. In other instances there may be hypersecretion of pituitary hormones, causing giantism or acromegaly, persistent lactation, Cushing's syndrome, and hyperthyroidism with exophthalmos. Pituitary tumors are treated symptomatically and through radiotherapy and surgical procedures.

Nursing Therapy

Primary pathology of the pituitary is rare, although the number of surgically induced alterations has increased in recent years. In caring for the patient the nurse should give attention to the target organs as well as to the gland itself.

Localized tenderness, slight temperature elevation, and change in the character of respiration may be premonitory signs of an infection. Fatigue, nervousness, hunger, trembling of the extremities, and mental clouding may indicate impending hypoglycemic reaction. Visual changes including those in the visual fields change in the character and type of eye movement, decreased vision, or diplopia may be brought to the nurse's attention. The patient who consistently bumps into objects when walking or who misjudges distances when using his hands may be unaware that visual changes are occurring.

The nurse carefully records fluid intake and output in order to ensure maintenance of adequate hydration. The quantity of fluid excreted in the urine can easily be measured; the specific gravity should be measured and recorded. An abrupt change in either volume of urinary output or in the specific gravity of the urine should be noted. The quantity of fluid lost should be replaced through administration of fluids containing sodium and potassium. Fluid replacement should be carried out at regular intervals during each 24-hour period. Loss of inordinate amounts of fluid through the gastrointestinal tract, respiratory tree, or skin deserves special attention and may necessitate an increase in fluid intake.

The nurse has an important teaching function. The patient and a family member should understand the nature of the illness and the rationale of treatment. They should learn to recognize signs and symptoms of complications and be instructed about appropriate actions when complications arise. The psychological impact of a pituitary disorder is strong; the patient and his family need time to react to the illness before they are ready to learn to live with it. The need for taking medication regularly must be stressed, and a method of record keeping (medication, amount, time, response) must be maintained. The cost of prolonged medical supervision and medications may impose a hardship on the patient, and an appropriate referral for assistance should be made.

Finally, the patient must avoid undue emotional stress, as mentioned earlier. Helping the patient to achieve this goal poses a challenge to the nurse who seeks creative innovation in her care of the patient.

Bibliography

Astwood, E. B.: Anterior Pituitary Hormones and Related Substances. in Louis S. Goodman and Alfred Gilman (Eds.): *The Pharmacological Basis of Therapeutics,* 3d ed. New York: The Macmillan Company, 1965, pp. 1515–1539.

Brazean, Paul: Agents Affecting the Renal Conservation of Water. in Louis S. Goodman and Alfred Gilman (Eds.): *The Pharmacological Basis of Therapeutics,* 3d ed. New York: The Macmillan Company, 1965, pp. 859–870.

Dingman, Joseph F. and George W. Thorn: Diseases of the Neurohypophysis. in T. R. Harrison (Ed.): *Principles of Internal Medicine,* 5th ed. New York: McGraw-Hill Book Company, 1966, pp. 412–421.

Hawken, Patty: Hypophysectomy with Yttrium 90. *American Journal of Nursing,* 65:122–125, October, 1965.

Nelson, Don H. and George W. Thorn: Diseases of the Anterior Lobe of the Pituitary. in T. R. Harrison (Ed.): *Principles of Internal Medicine,* 5th ed. New York: McGraw-Hill Book Company, 1966, pp. 403–412.

Pearson, O. H.: Treatment of Patients after Therapeutic Ablation of the Pituitary. *Modern Treatment,* 3:205–214, January, 1966.

Travis, Randall H. and George Sayers: Adrenocorticotropic Hormone: Adrenocortical Steroids and their Synthetic Analogs. in Louis S. Goodman and Alfred Gilman (Eds.): *The Pharmacological Basis of Therapeutics,* 3d ed. New York: The Macmillan Company, 1965, pp. 1608–1648.

SECTION 5
ADRENAL
DISORDERS
LOUISE FULTON WORSTER

In considering disorders of the adrenal glands, it is well to consider the adrenal medulla and the adrenal cortex separately, since they are derived from two embryologically distinct tissues and function relatively independently of one another. Disorders of the adrenals are manifest by an excess or a deficiency of one or more of the hormones normally elaborated by the gland.

Adrenal Medulla

The medullary portion of the adrenal gland arises embryologically from the ectoderm of the neural crest and is a modified postganglionic neuron. The hormones produced by the medulla are epinephrine (adrenalin) and norepinephrine (noradrenalin or arterenol). These hormones are classified as catecholamines, since they are amino derivatives of pyrocatechol—$C_6H_4(OH)_2$. Although other compounds are classified chemically as catecholamines, in common medical usage the term *catecholamines* refers only to epinephrine and norepinephrine.

The adrenal medulla is rarely the site of clinical disorders. No clinical syndrome due to medullary deficiency has been identified, but abnormalities due to hyperfunction of the adrenal medulla do occur. Each of the four types of cells that comprise the medulla may give rise to a tumor, but only chromaffin cell tumors are of clinical significance in adults. Consequently this is the only disorder of the adrenal medulla that will be considered.

PHEOCHROMOCYTOMAS

Chromaffin cell tumors are most frequently called *pheochromocytomas* and originate from the adrenal medulla in 90 percent of cases and from extra-adrenal chromaffin tissue in 10 percent of cases. Extra-adrenal pheochromocytomas may be located along the aorta, in the spleen, ovaries, or testes, in the bladder wall, along the thoracic sympathetic chain, or anywhere that chromaffin tissue is located. Usually a single, unilateral, benign tumor in the adrenal medulla is responsible for the clinical manifestations that are seen, but multiple, bilateral, and/or malignant tumors may be responsible. The tumors occur with equal frequency in males and females, and a familial tendency has been noted. The incidence is highest between the ages of 20 and 50.

The clinical manifestations of pheochromocytomas are due to excess secretion of catecholamines by the tumors. The variability of manifestations is very great; this results from the variation in the rate of secretion of hormones and the variation in the relative amounts of epinephrine and norepinephrine secreted. The most frequent manifestation is hypertension, which may be paroxysmal or persistent in nature depending upon whether the tumor releases its hormones intermittently or continuously.

Patients with paroxysmal hypertension due to pheochromocytomas have attacks of increased blood pressure which may occur as frequently as every few hours or as seldom as every 2 or 3 months. The attacks may last a few minutes, several hours, or even days. In addition to a sharp rise in blood pressure, symptoms of a severe classic attack of paroxysmal hypertension include severe headache, palpitations, nausea, occasional vomiting, epigastric or substernal pain, blanching of the skin, profuse perspiration, dyspnea, difficulty in focusing the eyes, paresthesias, and fear of death. Following a severe attack there is flushing of the skin, diaphoresis, and a feeling of extreme fatigue and muscular weakness. Only one-fourth to one-third of patients with pheochromocytomas have these severe classic attacks. Other patients experience intermittent hypertension without other symptoms, intermittent hypertension associated with a few symptoms of the severe classic attack, or persistent hypertension.

Patients who have persistent rather than intermittent hypertension may also experience attacks during which the blood pressure rises even higher. During these attacks, the patient may have headache, palpitation, evidence of vasoconstriction, such as coldness and numbness of the extremities, blanching of the fingers or face, and bluish-red discoloration of the extremities.

Other symptoms that should raise the suspicion of pheochromocytoma in patients with either intermittent or persistent hypertension include hyperglycemia and glycosuria without ketosis, and symptoms of hypermetabolism, such as tachycardia, excessive perspiration, tremor, and an increase in basal metabolic rate. Epinephrine stimulates the conversion of liver and muscle glycogen to glucose and is responsible for the hyperglycemia. The basis for the hypermetabolism is not understood. Protein-bound iodine and radioactive iodine uptake are normal in these patients.

Although pheochromocytomas are responsible for only a small percentage of cases of hypertension, they cause a form of hypertension which is curable if surgery is done before vascular changes have become irreversible. Nurses in community settings can help detect hypertension and help people with hypertension obtain careful medical evaluation and therapy for their condition. Unless every person with hypertension receives careful medical evaluation, many people with hypertension that could be cured will not receive proper treatment.

Most nurses will see few, if any, patients with pheochromocytomas, but they will see many patients with hypertension being evaluated to rule out this condition as a cause of their hypertension. During this evaluative period the nurse should observe the patient carefully for any symptoms that may be indicative of pheochromocytoma. If the patient experiences attacks of paroxysmal hypertension, the attacks should be carefully observed and described. The level of the blood pressure should be documented during the attack and, if possible, precipitating factors should be identified. The patient should not be left alone during attacks of paroxysmal hypertension, since a feeling of fright and impending doom may be caused by large amounts of epinephrine.

Diagnostic Procedures

A variety of diagnostic procedures are used to determine if a pheochromocytoma is present. Two types of pharmacologic tests are available—one designed to provoke an increase in blood pressure by giving a drug to stimulate secretion of the tumor and the other designed to markedly lower the blood pressure in persons with pheochromocytomas by giving a drug to block the action of the catecholamines. The nurse should be present to support the patient during these tests and to protect the patient by helping recognize untoward reactions and by helping initiate appropriate therapy, since both types of tests are associated with potential dangers. (The pharmacologic tests are becoming outmoded as better diagnostic tests are becoming available.)

The provocative tests are rarely used, but they may be performed when patients who have a history suggestive of intermittent hypertension are being evaluated during a period when their blood pressure is within normal limits. Histamine is the drug most frequently used in provocative tests. Results indicative of a pheochromocytoma are marked increases in both systolic and diastolic blood pressures within 1 to 4 minutes after the intravenous administration of histamine. In normotensive people without pheochromocytomas, intravenous administration of histamine produces a flush, headache, and usually a slight fall in blood pressure. Although not common, a danger associated with this test is an excessive rise in blood pressure which may precipitate an acute myocardial infarction or a cerebrovascular accident. Phentolamine (Regitine) should be available for administration in the event of a dangerous rise in blood pressure.

The blocking tests are used only if the patient has a sustained elevation of blood pressure. The drug most frequently used to block the action of the catecholamines is phentolamine. This drug is administered intravenously and a reduction of blood pressure exceeding 35 mm mercury systolic and 25 mm mercury diastolic and lasting 3 to 5 minutes is strongly suggestive of a pheochromocytoma. Persons without pheochromocytomas usually show an increase in blood pressure or occasionally a mild hypotensive response. No narcotics, sedatives, or antihypertensive drugs should be given for at least 3 days prior to the test, since they tend to cause false-positive reactions. Undue lowering of the blood pressure and precipitation of shock is an infrequent, but potential, danger with this test. This can usually be counteracted by placing the patient in the Trendelenburg position, but it may require administration of vasopressor drugs.

Hormonal assays are also valuable diagnostic procedures. As less complex and more reliable laboratory methods are becoming available, the assays are replacing the pharmacologic tests, since they are more definitive and are not potentially dangerous for the patient. The chemical studies most frequently utilized at the present time are determination of catecholamines in urine or blood and of vanillyl mandelic acid (VMA) in urine. Vanillyl mandelic acid is the major metabolite of the catecholamines, and more than a normal amount is excreted in the urine during times when the pheochromocytoma is secreting hormones. Careful collection of specimens for these tests is essential for accurate diagnosis. The collection period may eed to be carefully timed, all urine must be collected without contamination of feces, and precautions designated by the laboratory must be taken to preserve the specimen during the collection period and until the analyses can be done. This may involve collection in special containers, acidification of the specimen, addition of a perservative, and/or refrigeration of the specimens. Certain foods and drugs, for example, bananas, vanilla, reserpine, insulin, nicotine, and morphine, alter the amount of VMA excreted. Some laboratories require omission of certain foods and drugs for 2 days prior to the collection of the specimens and others do not. This and the methods of analysis utilized will influence what the particular laboratory considers a normal range of values for these tests.

Treatment

The treatment of pheochromocytoma is surgical removal of the tumor. During the immediate postoperative period the nurse will be responsible for observing the blood pressure carefully, since hypotension is usually present during this time. The hypotension results from the sudden decrease in the level of catecholamines in the blood and may last 24 to 48 hours and occasionally even longer. The nurse must be very conscientious about regulating the rate of administration of intravenous fluids and sympathomimetic drugs, for example norepinephrine, metaraminol (Aramine), or phenylephrine (Neo-Synephrine), according to the instructions of the physician. In other respects the postoperative care is similar to the care given after major abdominal surgery.

Adrenal Cortex

The adrenal cortex is formed embryologically from mesodermal tissue and secretes a number of steroid hormones. Steroids are a group of compounds that have as a common nucleus four carbon rings fused together; there are three 6-carbon rings and one 5-carbon ring with a total of 17 carbon atoms involved. In addition two other carbon atoms are usually attached to the tenth and thirteenth carbon atoms of the rings. Most adrenocortical steroids also have a side chain of two carbon

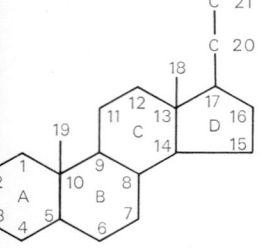

Figure 26–2
Basic structure of
adrenocortical steroids
and numbering of the
carbon atoms

atoms attached to the seventeenth carbon of the ring structure. (See Figure 26–2.) The adrenocortical hormones that are most significant clinically can be grouped as glucocorticoids, mineralocorticoids, and androgens. Minute amounts of progestins and estrogens are also produced.

The most important glucocorticoid in man is cortisol; corticosterone is the second most important. These hormones are necessary for the regulation of protein, carbohydrate, and fat metabolism. The major metabolic action of the glucocorticoids is promotion of gluconeogenesis. This action enables the blood sugar to be maintained at a normal level during periods of fasting. If this metabolic action were not possible, a person could not skip a meal without symptoms of hypoglycemia and could not survive longer periods of fasting, for example, following surgery. The glucocorticoids also have a mild electrolyte-regulating effect; they increase sodium reabsorption in the kidney and are necessary for excretion of a water load. Although many effects are noted when abnormal amounts of glucocorticoids are present, the physiological bases for these effects are not understood.

The most potent mineralocorticoid in man is aldosterone. This is complemented by a very small amount of 11-desoxycorticosterone. These hormones control sodium and potassium levels in the body and secondarily affect water balance. The mineralocorticoids exert their major action on the distal convoluted tubules of the kidney where they promote active reabsorption of sodium and decrease reabsorption of potassium from the tubular urine.

The adrenal androgens may exert an anabolic, androgenic, or pyrogenic effect. The anabolic effect is due to promotion of the synthesis of protein from amino acids and is important in recovery from injury. Some of the adrenal androgens are dehydroepiandrosterone, Δ4-androstenedione, and 11β-hydroxyandrostenedione. (See Figure 26–3 for the biosynthetic pathways of the adrenocortical hormones.)

EVALUATION OF ADRENOCORTICAL FUNCTION

Many diagnostic procedures are available for evaluation of adrenocortical function. Most of the tests used currently are based on determination of the levels of hormones present in the blood and the excretion of hormones or their metabolites in the urine. The 17-hydroxycorticosteroids (17-OH, 17-OHST, or 17-OHCS) can be measured in the urine and reflect primarily production of glucocorticoids. The determination of 17-ketosteroids (17-KS) in the urine reflects primarily the pro-

Figure 26–3
Biosynthesis of
adrenocortical hormones

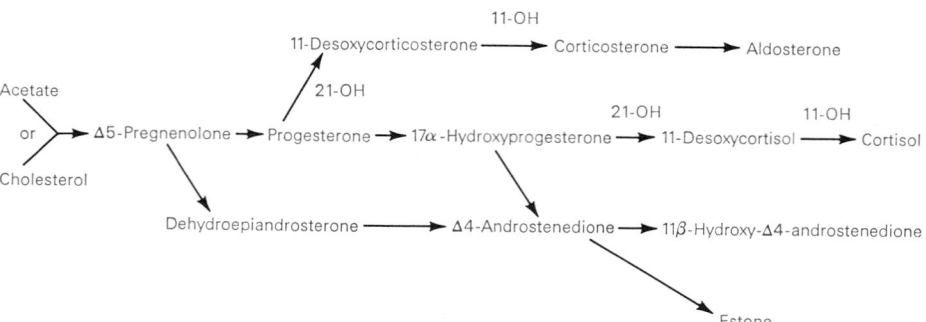

duction of androgens. In the female, 17-ketosteroids are normally derived entirely from the adrenals. In the normal adult male, approximately two-thirds of the urinary 17-ketosteroids are derived from the adrenals and one-third is from testicular hormones. Plasma levels of cortisol are useful in determining whether the normal diurnal variation in secretion of cortisol is present. The lowest level of plasma cortisol normally occurs shortly after midnight and the maximum level normally occurs at about 8 A.M. This variation is not influenced by sleep patterns. Aldosterone levels can be measured in the urine and aldosterone secretion rates can be measured in plasma. Determination of the rate of cortisol secretion by the use of radioactive carbon or tritium-labeled steroids is helpful in ambiguous cases. More precise methods for chemical assay of adrenocortical hormones will undoubtedly be available in the future.

The other diagnostic approach used for evaluation of adrenocortical function is to evaluate the response of the adrenal cortex to the administration of various drugs. The responses to the administration of ACTH and dexamethasone are useful in differentiating hyperplasia, adenoma, and carcinoma in persons with Cushing's syndrome, a clinical condition resulting from one type of hyperfunction of the adrenal cortex. Responses to ACTH and metyrapone help in the diagnosis of adrenocortical insufficiency. (See Table 26-3.) When these tests are to be done, a control level of 17-hydroxycorticosteroids in the urine is determined by collecting and analyzing at least one 24-hour urine specimen and usually several 24-hour urine specimens. It is very important that the total amount of urine excreted during the 24-hour period be collected. A check on the completeness of the collection

TABLE 26-3
Interpretation of Tests for Evaluation of Adrenocortical Function

TEST	RESPONSE					
	NORMAL	CUSHING'S SYNDROME			ADRENOCORTICAL INSUFFICIENCY	
		HYPERPLASIA	ADENOMA	ADENOCARCINOMA	PRIMARY	SECONDARY
ACTH	Increase in urinary 17-OH	Increase in urinary 17-OH	Increase in urinary 17-OH	No response	No response	Gradual but sustained increase in urinary 17-OH on successive days of ACTH
Metyrapone (Metopirone)	Increase in urinary 17-OH	Increase in urinary 17-OH	No response	No response	No response	No response
Dexamethasone suppression 2 mg daily	Urinary 17-OH less than 4 mg/24 hr	Urinary 17-OH more than 4 mg/24 hr	No suppression	No suppression		
8 mg daily	Urinary 17-OH less than 4 mg/24 hr	At least 50% suppression of urinary 17-OH	No suppression	No suppression		

of the 24-hour urine specimen can be made by determining the creatinine in each specimen. An individual excretes about the same amount of creatinine each day; if varying amounts of creatinine are reported in the specimens, it indicates that an incomplete collection of the urine specimens is being made.

In the intravenous ACTH test for adults, 25 international units (IU) of ACTH is added to 500 ml of normal saline and given intravenously over a period of *exactly* 8 hours. The nurse will be responsible for regulating the rate of the infusion and for collecting a 24-hour urine specimen for 17-hydroxycorticosteroids so that the response to the drug can be evaluated. The intramuscular ACTH test is being used frequently now; in this test 80 units of ACTH gel is given intramuscularly and the response is evaluated in the same manner as in the intravenous test. Following the administration of ACTH, the urinary 17-hydroxycorticosteroids will increase in persons with hyperfunction of the adrenal cortex due to hyperplasia or adenoma. In persons with hyperfunction of the adrenal cortex due to adenocarcinoma, there will be no change in the level of urinary 17-hydroxycorticosteroids following ACTH administration. In persons with secondary adrenocortical insufficiency, there will be a gradual but sustained increase in urinary 17-hydroxycorticosteroids if ACTH is administered on successive days, but there is no response in persons with primary adrenocortical insufficiency. (See Table 26-3.)

Metyrapone (Metopirone) is a compound that blocks 11β-hydroxylation and therefore, prevents formation of cortisol. (See Figure 26-3.) When it is given to a normal individual the resulting decrease in plasma cortisol would stimulate secretion of ACTH. The ACTH would increase production of cortisol precursors, which would be measured as 17-hydroxycorticosteroids in the urine. In adults, the metyrapone is usually administered orally in a dosage of 750 mg every 4 hours for six doses. A 24-hour urine specimen for 17-hydroxycorticosteroids must be collected on the day following the administration of the metyrapone. The metyrapone may be administered intravenously in 500 to 1,000 ml of saline over a 4-hour period. If so, a dosage of 30 mg per kg of body weight is given and a 24-hour urine specimen is collected on the day the drug is administered. After the administration of metyrapone, the urinary 17-hydroxycorticosteroids will increase in persons with normal adrenocortical function and in persons with hyperfunction of the adrenal cortex due to hyperplasia. There is no change in urinary 17-hydroxycorticosteroids in other types of adrenocortical dysfunction. (See Table 26-3.)

Normally, the level of cortisol in the blood acts via a feedback mechanism to regulate secretion of ACTH from the pituitary. Dexamethasone is a potent synthetic glucocorticoid that acts like cortisol in regard to regulating ACTH secretion, but it is not excreted in the urine as a hydroxysteroid, as cortisol is. Consequently, any change in urinary 17-hydroxycorticosteroid excretion following administration of dexamethasone would represent a change in the amount of endogenous glucocorticoids secreted and not the dose of exogenous glucocorticoid. During the first 2 days of the dexamethasone suppression test, 0.5 mg of the drug is given orally every 6 hours. Over the next 2 days 2 mg is given orally every 6 hours. Again the results of the test are determined by measuring 17-hydroxycorticosteroids in the urine. In persons with normal adrenocortical function, administration of either

2 mg or 8 mg of dexamethasone daily will result in a suppression of urinary 17-hydroxycorticosteroid level to less than 4 mg per 24 hours. In persons with hyperfunction of the adrenal cortex due to hyperplasia, 2 mg of dexamethasone daily will not suppress urinary 17-hydroxycorticosteroids below 4 mg per 24 hours; 8 mg of dexamethasone daily, however, will suppress urinary 17-hydroxycorticosteroids at least 50 percent of the control level. Dexamethasone does not suppress urinary 17-hydroxycorticosteroids in individuals with hyperfunction of the adrenal cortex due to adenomas or adenocarcinomas. (See Table 26-3.)

HYPOFUNCTION OF THE ADRENAL CORTEX

The more important disorders that result from a deficiency of adrenocortical hormones are chronic primary adrenocortical insufficiency, secondary adrenocortical insufficiency, acute adrenocortical insufficiency, and hypoaldosteronism.

Chronic Primary Adrenocortical Insufficiency

Chronic primary adrenocortical insufficiency, or Addison's disease, is caused by progressive destruction of the adrenal cortex. The destructive process is most frequently caused by idiopathic atrophy (which, according to Prunty, may represent an autoimmune reaction) or infections, such as tuberculosis and histoplasmosis.

The death rate from Addison's disease is only four per 100,000, but many deaths actually due to adrenocortical insufficiency are probably attributed to another disorder that has placed extra demands on the adrenals, thereby precipitating acute adrenal insufficiency and death. The majority of cases of Addison's disease occur in persons between the ages of 20 and 50.

The clinical manifestations of Addison's disease are usually insidious in onset and include weakness, fatigue, weight loss, dehydration, anorexia, nausea, vomiting, diarrhea, hypotension, hypoglycemic manifestations, nervous irritability, apathy, and brown or bronze pigmentation of the skin and mucous membranes due to deposition of abnormal amounts of melanin. The pigmentation is more marked in areas that are normally pigmented and in areas exposed to light and friction. These symptoms are the results of inadequate production of glucocorticoids, mineralocorticoids, and androgens. (See Table 26-4.) The reason for the pigmentation is not well understood, but it may be due to increased plasma levels of melanocyte-stimulating hormone or to the high plasma level of ACTH, which has a chemical structure similar to melanocyte-stimulating hormone. The secretion of ACTH is regulated by the amount of cortisol in the blood; since the cortisol level is chronically low in individuals with untreated Addison's disease, the blood level of ACTH stays high.

The availability of hormones for replacement therapy has made successful treatment of Addison's disease possible. The glucocorticoids most frequently used are cortisol (hydrocortisone) and cortisone, which are usually given orally two to four times daily with meals or with antacids to decrease gastric irritation. A larger dose may be given in the morning than in the late afternoon in order to simulate normal diurnal variation. Mineralocorticoid replacement is often necessary as is 9α-fluorohydrocortisone (Florinef) administered orally two to three times a week;

EXCESSIVE GLUCOCORTICOIDS	DEFICIENCY OF GLUCOCORTICOIDS
Catabolism of protein; muscle wasting and weakness; striae; easy bruisability; osteoporosis	Anorexia; nausea and vomiting; diarrhea
Decreased glucose tolerance	Muscular weakness
Centripetal fat distribution with moon face, buffalo hump, supraclavicular fat pads, pendulous abdomen	Extreme lassitude and constant fatigue
Hyperlipemia; hypercholesterolemia	Weight loss
Metabolic acidosis	Depression or irritability
Mental and motor excitability with lability of mood	Hypoglycemic episodes
Hypertension	Poor vasomotor tone of arterioles
Leukocytosis, relative lymphopenia, eosinophilia	Pigmentation of skin and mucous membranes
	Leukopenia, relative lymphocytosis, eosinophilia
	Hyperplasia of lymphoid tissue
	Anemia

EXCESSIVE MINERALOCORTICOIDS	DEFICIENCY OF MINERALOCORTICOIDS
Sodium retention	Sodium, chloride, and water loss
Potassium depletion	Potassium retention
Hypertension	Dehydration
Muscle weakness	Metabolic acidosis
Metabolic alkalosis	Hypotension
Tetany	Circulatory collapse

EXCESSIVE ADRENAL ANDROGENS	DEFICIENCY OF ADRENAL ANDROGENS
Hirsutism; receding hairline; baldness	Decreased pubic and axillary hair in females
Acne	Loss of libido
Deepening of voice	Loss of muscle substance
Menstrual disorders; amenorrhea	
Atrophy of breasts	
Enlargement of clitoris	
Marked increase in musculature	

TABLE 26-4
Symptoms Due to Abnormal Amounts of Adrenocortical Hormones

a salt intake of about 10 g daily, which can be supplied by the diet, is usually satisfactory. Desoxycorticosterone can also be used, but it must be given intramuscularly to be most successful and is seldom used for this reason. In females, since the adrenals are the only source of androgens, small doses of oral androgens may be helpful to increase their strength and sense of well-being, but the androgens are not essential for life.

The diagnosis of Addison's disease can often be overlooked early in the course of the disease unless someone's suspicions are aroused and careful evaluation of adrenocortical function is done. Nurses in public health and industrial settings are in positions to recognize individuals who have the vague, nonspecific symptoms associated with adrenocortical insufficiency and can help them find a reliable source of medical evaluation and treatment for whatever condition underlies their symptoms.

The early symptoms of Addison's disease are very similar to symptoms associated with psychoneuroses. A person with Addison's disease may not have sought medical evaluation for a long period of time because of the nonspecific nature of the symptoms or may have been previously diagnosed as having a psychoneurosis. Consequently during the diagnostic period the nurse may be the person the patient tests to see if anyone believes he is sick—if anyone really believes how he feels, and cares. The nurse in this position needs to find out by careful listening, questioning, and observation how the patient does, in fact, feel. Then she will have information that can be used to convey understanding and caring to the patient, used to help arrive at a diagnosis, and used to help the patient adjust to whatever diagnosis is made. It is important to remember that lack of glucocorticoids can affect the central nervous system and be manifest by apathy, listlessness, depression, and irritability.

When a person does have adrenocortical insufficiency, the nurse's observations for symptoms indicative of glucocorticoid or mineralocorticoid excess or deficiency are important in helping regulate the dosage of replacement therapy. (See Table 26-4.) The teaching role of the nurse should also be utilized. It is very important that the patients understand their replacement therapy and that they have sufficient financial resources or assistance to ensure that medication will always be available. They should be helped to make a realistic plan for adequate medical supervision. They should always carry information regarding their medical condition and wear an identification bracelet that will quickly call attention to their condition in emergency situations. They need to know the types of situations, such as extreme emotional shocks, illness, and trauma, that are likely to increase their need for glucocorticoids and what to do if these situations occur. For events such as dental extractions, mild viral upper respiratory infections, and emotional upsets, the dosage of oral glucocorticoids may need to be increased for 2 or 3 days. If nausea, vomiting, or diarrhea occurs, intramuscular glucocorticoids will need to be used. During very hot weather or during episodes of great physical exertion, the dosage of mineralocorticoid may need to be increased and additional salt should be added to the food or salt tablets should be taken.

Secondary Adrenocortical Insufficiency

Atrophy of the adrenal cortex from lack of adrenocorticotropic hormone from the anterior pituitary is called *secondary adrenocortical insufficiency*. This may be due to pituitary disease or to suppression by exogenous adrenocortical steroids of the corticotropin-releasing factor of the hypothalamus, which is responsible for release of ACTH from the anterior pituitary. In the latter case insufficiency would be manifest only if the steroids were discontinued too rapidly or if extra stress were encountered which was not covered by additional medication. This is the most common cause of adrenal insufficiency today and is manifested by the symptoms of adrenal crisis which are discussed in the next section.

Adrenal insufficiency secondary to pituitary disease can be differentiated from primary insufficiency by the ACTH test. This drug will not stimulate production of glucocorticoids in persons with primary adrenal insufficiency. In individuals with adrenal insufficiency secondary to pituitary dysfunction, a gradual but sustained increase in production of glucocorticoids will be stimulated by ACTH. The delay in response will be proportional to the degree of secondary adrenocortical atrophy. A normal response to the ACTH test but a failure to respond to metyrapone is indicative of a defect in the hypothalamic-pituitary mechanism, which normally regulates ACTH secretion. The clinical manifestations of secondary adrenocortical insufficiency result from insufficient glucocorticoids and androgens (see Table 26-4); mineralocorticoids are usually adequate since they are primarily independent of pituitary control. Replacement of glucocorticoids is necessary for these patients.

Acute Adrenocortical Insufficiency

Persons with chronic primary or secondary adrenocortical insufficiency can also have episodes of acute adrenocortical insufficiency, called *adrenal crises,* when severe stress such as surgery, trauma, or infection is superimposed. Acute adreno-cortical insufficiency may also be due to adrenal hemorrhage associated with trauma or with a fulminating hemorrhagic infection, such as acute meningococcal septicemia. Symptoms usually develop over a period of 8 to 12 hours and include lassitude, apathy, irritability, headache, diffuse abdominal pain, nausea, vomiting, diarrhea, hyperpyrexia, circulatory collapse, and loss of consciousness. The most important symptoms to watch for are extreme lassitude and apathy, since they are the earliest and most consistent indications of adrenocortical insufficiency.

When caring for patients with a known adrenocortical insufficiency (and this would include any patient who is having long-term steroid therapy or who has had such therapy within the last year), the nurse should observe carefully for symptoms that might be indicative of impending adrenal crises during periods of acute illness, after traumatic injuries, and after surgery. She should also remember that an adrenal crisis can occur under these circumstances in persons without a previous history of adrenocortical insufficiency. Any such indications should be reported to the physician promptly, since adrenal crisis is an emergency situation and demands prompt treatment. Treatment consists of intravenous administration of large doses of glucocorticoids, glucose, saline, and sometimes vasopressor agents. Large doses of glucocorticoids exert sufficient effect on salt and water balance that mineralocorticoids need not be administered during this time. Treatment must also be directed toward the precipitating factor.

Hypoaldosteronism

A few cases of isolated hypoaldosteronism have been reported. These persons have symptoms of hyperkalemia and hyponatremia secondary to a deficiency of aldosterone without other evidence of adrenocortical insufficiency. The specific symptoms reported have included cardiac arrhythmias and complete heart block, muscle weakness of severe degree, dizziness, and postural hypotension. Studies by Jacobs and Posner suggest that a defect in the 18-aldolase enzyme system may be responsible for inadequate formation of aldosterone. Replacement of mineralo-corticoids is the basis of treatment.

HYPERFUNCTION OF THE ADRENAL CORTEX

The three most important clinical conditions that result from hyperfunction of the adrenal cortex are Cushing's syndrome, hyperaldosteronism, and the adreno-genital syndrome. On rare occasions a feminizing syndrome due to excess production of adrenal estrogens may be seen in individuals with adrenal carcinoma.

Cushing's Syndrome

Cushing's syndrome is primarily the result of an excess of glucocorticoids, although increased androgens may contribute to the symptoms in some cases. The syndrome may be the result of endogenous hormones or may be induced by the administration of large doses of glucocorticoids for the treatment of other diseases. The latter is the most frequent cause of Cushing's syndrome currently. Increased endogenous production of glucocorticoids may be caused by adrenocortical hyperplasia, adrenal tumors, adrenal-like tumors of the ovaries, ACTH-producing tumors of the pituitary, or carcinomas of other organs (for example, the lungs, thymus, and pancreas) which produce an ACTH-like substance. In adults with endogenous Cushing's syndrome, approximately 60 percent have bilateral adrenocortical hyperplasia, 30 percent have adrenal tumors (one-half adenomas and one-half adenocarcinomas), and 10 percent have no discernible pathology in the adrenals. Adrenocortical hyperplasia occurs secondary to increased ACTH from the pituitary in some cases, but in many cases the cause of the hyperplasia remains in doubt, although many hypotheses have been offered.

The full-blown clinical picture of Cushing's syndrome is easily recognized, but a wide variation of symptoms may occur. The common symptoms due to excess cortisol include trunkal obesity with normal extremities (usually without weight gain); fat pads in the supraclavicular areas, on the back of the neck (buffalo hump), and in the cheeks (moon face); thinning of the skin with facial plethora, capillary fragility, and purple striae on the abdomen; muscle wasting, fatigability, and weakness; osteoporosis; atherosclerotic vascular changes; alteration in utilization of glucose which may develop into diabetes; hypokalemic alkalosis; changes in mood and mental activity such as depression or euphoria, anxiety, irritability, apathy, and occasionally acute psychosis. Many of the above are due to excessive protein catabolism, and some of them can be avoided or minimized by a high-protein, low-carbohydrate, low-sodium diet with potassium supplementation. Supplemental androgens may be useful for their anabolic effect on protein metabolism.

Clinical manifestations due to excess androgens include hirsutism, baldness, deepening of the voice, acne, menstrual irregularities, amenorrhea, and enlargement of the clitoris. All these symptoms, except deepening of the voice and enlargement of the clitoris, may occur with administration of large doses of glucocorticoids; this appears to be due to an increased conversion of glucocorticoids to substances with androgenic activity in the metabolic breakdown of the glucocorticoids.

Appropriate laboratory tests help establish a definite diagnosis and can help determine the underlying pathology. (See Table 26–3.) Often these tests involve collection of 24-hour urine specimens for several consecutive days. Loss of a single urine specimen during this time can invalidate the results of the tests or prolong the diagnostic period and hospitalization of the patient for many days. It seems impossible to overemphasize the responsibility of the nurse in this aspect of the diagnostic endeavor. She will need to gain an understanding of the patient and his emotional responses (due to physiological and psychological factors) in order to find ways to enlist his cooperation in this endeavor also. Often this period of time seems long, lonely, and useless to the patient, and unless the nurse helps meet his interpersonal needs, he is likely to feel that he has no importance and that no one cares about him.

Persons with Cushing's syndrome are often deeply concerned about their physical appearance and their altered sexual functions. The alterations in body contour, the changes in secondary sex characteristics, and the weakness and fatigue may be very apparent to the patient and to others. Other alterations, such as amenorrhea, are not so apparent to others but may be of concern to the patient. Significant family members may react to these alterations in a variety of ways. If they are accepting and understanding of the changes that occur, they can be very helpful to the patient in his adjustment to these changes. If they are frightened or repelled by the alterations, they may reject the patient and deprive the patient of an important source of emotional support. Social, cultural, and religious factors will influence the manner in which these alterations will affect the patient's body image. Emotional reactions are a natural consequence of a disturbance in body image and may include anxiety, depression, hostility, denial, and guilt. The nurse will need to collect information about the factors that influence the particular patient's body image concept, his perception of the alterations that have occurred, and his responses to these alterations. This information can be used as a basis for planning nursing intervention that will be useful in helping the patient achieve a healthy adaptation to the disturbance of body image which may be temporary or permanent depending on the cause of the Cushing's syndrome.

Treatment of Cushing's syndrome depends upon the underlying cause. In cases due to exogenous corticoids, it may be possible to gradually decrease the dosage to a level that alleviates some of the symptoms. At other times the benefits of the corticoid therapy must be weighed against the disadvantages of the manifestations of the disorder and a choice made. Patients will need to be helped to adjust to the choice that is made; the nurse is frequently in a position to supply this help, since she cares for persons with chronic illnesses.

In cases due to pituitary disorders, surgical hypophysectomy or pituitary irradiation is frequently utilized. Cushing's syndrome due to adrenal adenoma or carcinoma is treated by removal of the tumor. Treatment of that due to adrenal hyperplasia is more of a problem, since the underlying stimulus for the hyperplasia is not well understood as yet. Pituitary irradiation is sometimes useful, but total bilateral adrenalectomy is probably the most effective form of treatment for bilateral adrenal hyperplasia currently.

Persons who are to have adrenal surgery should be in as good a nutritional state as possible before surgery. This may necessitate control of hyperglycemia by diet and possibly insulin and correction of potassium deficiency. Administration of an androgen, such as testosterone, is useful to promote protein anabolism in persons with protein depletion. Total adrenalectomy will necessitate permanent replacement therapy similar to that given individuals with Addison's disease, and the nurse will have the same responsibilities as have been discussed previously.

Postoperatively the nurse must be very alert for indications of inadequate replacement therapy (see Table 26-4) and must act promptly to prevent episodes of acute adrenal insufficiency. The dosage of glucocorticoids administered during this period is adjusted frequently and gradually decreased to a maintenance level.

The level of the blood pressure and character of the pulse should be observed carefully not only to detect adrenal crisis but also to detect postoperative hemorrhage. Intake and output should be carefully recorded to help evaluate and regulate fluid balance.

Particular care should be taken to prevent conditions that add more stress than already exists during the postoperative period. The nurse can help alleviate environmental stress by giving careful attention to comfort measures, gentle physical care, simple explanations, careful determination of priority of care, and provision for rest. Nursing measures should also be utilized to prevent postoperative complications such as atelectasis, hypostatic pneumonia, and thrombophlebitis which would increase the requirements for glucocorticoids.

Hyperaldosteronism

Hyperaldosteronism is a clinical syndrome that results from the excessive production of aldosterone, a mineralocorticoid, by the adrenal cortex. The term *primary aldosteronism* (Conn's syndrome) is used for those cases in which the excessive aldosterone is produced by a functioning tumor of the adrenal cortex. Other cases of hyperaldosteronism, with an identical clinical syndrome, have been described in which the patient had bilateral adrenal hyperplasia or normal appearing adrenal glands. These cases have been designated as cases of congenital aldosteronism and are believed by Conn to be secondary to some abnormality of the mechanism that normally regulates production of aldosterone rather than a defect in the adrenals per se. Other instances of secondary hyperaldosteronism are associated with a variety of clinical conditions in which there is fluid retention, for example, cirrhosis of the liver, congestive heart failure, and nephrosis.

Primary aldosteronism has only been recognized since 1955 and an accurate assessment of its incidence is not available. The symptoms include the following: hypertension, which may be very mild or severe; episodes of muscle weakness and occasionally paralysis; muscular tetanic manifestations; polydipsia, polyuria, and nocturia; headache; paresthesias. Laboratory findings include hypokalemia, mild hypernatremia, alkalosis, increased urinary aldosterone, normal urinary 17-hydroxycorticosteroids, and normal urinary 17-ketosteroids. Although administration of aldosterone to normal subjects initially leads to sodium and water retention, after retention of 2 to 3 kg of fluid the kidneys begin to "escape" from the salt-retaining effects of the hormone. An equilibrium is attained, and more retention of sodium and water does not occur even though the level of aldosterone remains high. This "renal escape" mechanism would account for the fact that edema is rarely a symptom of primary aldosteronism and the elevation of serum sodium is slight.

As with the other adrenal abnormalities, the "typical" case is easy to recognize and diagnose, but patients may have benign hypertension and borderline kypokalemia as their only clinical abnormalities. In these patients metabolic balance studies with careful regulation of sodium and potassium intake may be necessary. The diagnosis is finally based on the finding of an elevated level of aldosterone secretion, but the measurement of aldosterone in blood or urine is accurately and reliably performed in relatively few laboratories at present. There also seem to be fluctuations in the secretory activity of the tumors, so multiple determinations of aldosterone level may need to be made in order to arrive at an accurate evaluation of aldosterone production.

Treatment of primary aldosteronism is surgical excision of the tumor, which, in 90 percent of cases, is a single adenoma; occasionally multiple adenomas may be found. Surgical removal usually leads to disappearance of most of the clinical symptoms by the third postoperative week. The blood pressure gradually returns to a normal or near normal level in about 3 months in the majority of patients.

Treatment of congenital aldosteronism consists of total adrenalectomy, and replacement therapy is necessary for these patients. They are often very sensitive to mineralocorticoids, and regulation of replacement dosage may be rather difficult. The replacement dosage of mineralocorticoids may be smaller than one for patients who have had adrenalectomies for other reasons.

The nurse's responsibilities would be similar to those discussed in previous sections related to evaluation of adrenal function and nursing care after adrenal surgery.

Adrenogenital Syndrome

The adrenogenital syndrome characterizes the clinical entities related to excessive production of androgens due to metabolic defects or tumors. These disorders are infrequent. In most cases the adrenogenital syndrome is a result of an inborn error of metabolism due to an autosomal recessive genetic factor. In these cases, which are called *prenatal adrenogenital syndrome,* there are deficiencies of the enzymes needed for synthesis of cortisol. The deficiency of cortisol leads to an excess of ACTH and consequently an accumulation of intermediate steroid metabolites, some of which are converted into androgenic hormones. The enzyme most frequently lacking is 21-hydroxylase, but in other cases there is a deficiency of 11β-hydroxylase or other enzymes. (See Figure 26–3 for the sites of action of these enzymes in the synthesis of adrenocortical hormones.) Prenatal adrenogenital syndrome occurs in infants, and the adrenogenital syndrome may occur in children due to metabolic defects or to adenomas or adenocarcinomas of the adrenal cortex. Readers are referred to books on endocrinology and special articles listed in the bibliography for additional information on this syndrome in children.

The adrenogenital syndrome in adult females is characterized by hirsutism, amenorrhea, and variable degrees of virilization. Virilization may be manifest by receding hairline, atrophy of the breasts, enlargement of the clitoris, masculine distribution of fat, and development of heavy musculature and a thickened skin. In adult males indications of adrenogenital syndrome include an unusually well-developed, large penis; well-developed scrotum; small, soft testes; few or no sperm.

The pathogenesis of this syndrome in adults (except in cases due to tumors) is not as clearly understood as in the prenatal syndrome; however, recently cases first manifested in adult women due to 11β-hydroxylase deficiency have been reported by Gabrilove. It is thought that these patients may have been born with only a mild enzymatic deficiency, and that with increasing age, the deficiency became great enough to lead to the development of symptoms.

The syndrome is more often diagnosed in women than in men, since increased virilization is often not as apparent nor as psychologically traumatizing for men. Diagnosis is established by assay of hormones and their intermediary metabolites. Differentiation of adrenogenital syndrome from androgenic disorders of the ovary may be difficult and time-consuming.

Treatment consists of surgical removal of tumors when they are responsible for the increased production of androgens. A medical therapeutic approach is indicated for cases due to enzyme deficiencies or to unknown pathology; this involves administration of glucocorticoids to depress the production of ACTH to normal levels and consequently to decrease the production of androgens. This type of suppression therapy will usually decrease some of the symptoms of virilization and return the menses and spermatogenesis to normal. The hirsutism will usually decrease somewhat, but persistence of some of the extra hair growth is usual. Deepening of the voice is usually not reversible.

These patients will be faced with the psychological problems and nursing needs associated with alterations in body image that were discussed in the section on Cushing's syndrome. The hirsutism may be a problem even with adequate treatment. Depilatories can be used to remove some of the excess hair. Hairy areas may be bleached by daily bathing of the area with a 50 percent solution of hydrogen peroxide in water.

These patients may need extra glucocorticoid therapy in the event of injury or surgery and should wear suitable identification and carry adequate instructions to ensure this in emergency situations.

Bibliography

Books

Cope, Cuthbert L.: *Adrenal Steroids and Disease.* Philadelphia: J. B. Lippincott Company, 1964.

Grollman, Arthur: *Clinical Endocrinology and Its Physiological Basis.* Philadelphia: J. B. Lippincott Company, 1964.

Kupperman, Herbert S.: *Human Endocrinology,* 2d ed. Philadelphia: F. A. Davis Company, 1963.

Prunty, F. T. G.: *Chemistry and Treatment of Adrenocortical Diseases.* Springfield: Charles C Thomas, Publisher, 1964.

Williams, Robert H. (Ed.): *Textbook of Endocrinology,* 4th ed. Philadelphia: W. B. Saunders Company, 1968.

Articles

August, J. Thomas, Don H. Nelson, and George W. Thorn: Response of Normal Subjects to Large Amounts of Aldosterone. *Journal of Clinical Investigation,* 37:1549–1555, November, 1958.

Bass, Allan D.: Drugs Affecting Adrenocortical Function. *Postgraduate Medicine,* 37:82–86, January, 1965.

Bongiovanni, Alfred M. and Allen W. Root: The Adrenogenital Syndrome. *New England Journal of Medicine,* 268:1283–1342, June 6, 1963; 1342–1350, June 13, 1963; 1391–1399, June 20, 1963.

Carr, Herman E., George W. Curtis, and George W. Thorn: A Clinical-Biochemical-Histologic Correlation in Hyperadrenocorticism Caused by Acquired Adrenocortical Hyperplasia. *American Journal of Surgery,* 107:123–135, January, 1964.

Conn, Jerome W.: Evolution of Primary Aldosteronism as a Highly Specific Clinical Entity. *Journal of American Medical Association,* 172:1650–1653, April 9, 1960.

Conn, Jerome W., Ralph F. Knopf, and

Reed M. Nesbit: Clinical Characteristics of Primary Aldosteronism from an Analysis of 145 Cases. *American Journal of Surgery,* 107: 159–172, January, 1964.

Cope, C. L. and J. Pearson: Clinical Value of the Cortisol Secretion Rate. *Journal of Clinical Pathology,* 18:82–87, January, 1965.

Ferriman, D.: Toxicity of the Corticosteroids. *Practitioner,* 194: 43–50, January, 1965.

Gabrilove, J. L.: Diseases Associated with Some Enzymic Defects in the Gonads and Adrenal Cortex: A Classification Based on a Theory of the Biogenesis of the Feminizing and Virilizing Syndromes. *Journal of Mount Sinai Hospital (New York),* 31:449–456, November-December, 1964.

Gabrilove, J. L., D. C. Sharma, and R. I. Dorfman: Adrenocortical 11β-Hydroxylase Deficiency and Virilism First Manifest in the Adult Woman. *New England Journal of Medicine,* 272:1189–1194, June 10, 1965.

Graber, Alan L., et al.: Natural History of Pituitary-Adrenal Recovery following Long-Term Suppression with Corticosteroids. *Journal of Clinical Endocrinology and Metabolism,* 25:11–16, January, 1965.

Greenblatt, Robert B. and Virendra B. Mahesh: Clinical Evaluation and Treatment of the Hirsute Female. *Clinical Obstetrics and Gynecology,* 7:1109–1119, December, 1964.

Greer, William E. R., Charles W. Robertson, and Reginald H. Smithwick: Pheochromocytoma. Diagnosis, Operative Experiences and Clinical Results. *American Journal of Surgery,* 107:192–201, January, 1964.

Herrera, M. G., G. F. Cahill, Jr., and George W. Thorn: Cushing's Syndrome. Diagnosis and Treatment. *American Journal of Surgery,* 107: 144–152, January, 1964.

Jacobs, David R. and Jerome B. Posner: Isolated Analdosteronism. II. The Nature of the Adrenal Cortical Enzymatic Defect, and the Influence of Diet and Various Agents on Electrolyte Balance. *Metabolism,* 13:522–531, June, 1964.

Migeon, Claude J., et al.: The Diurnal Variation of Plasma Levels and Urinary Excretion of 17-Hydroxycorticosteroids in Normal Subjects, Night Workers and Blind Subjects. *Journal of Clinical Endocrinology and Metabolism,* 16:622–633, May, 1956.

Posner, Jerome B. and David R. Jacobs: Isolated Analdosteronism. I. Clinical Entity with Manifestations of Persistent Hyperkalemia, Periodic Paralysis, Salt Losing Tendency, and Acidosis. *Metabolism,* 13:513–521, June, 1964.

Priestly, James T., Walter F. Kvale, and Ray W. Gifford, Jr.: Pheochromocytoma: Clinical Aspects and Surgical Treatment. *Archives of Surgery,* 86:778–790, May, 1963.

Relman, Arnold S.: Diagnosis of Primary Aldosteronism. *American Journal of Surgery,* 107:173–177, January, 1964.

Rovner, D. R., et al.: Nature of Renal Escape from the Sodium-Retaining Effect of Aldosterone in Primary Aldosteronism and in Normal Subjects. *Journal of Clinical Endocrinology and Metabolism,* 25:53–64, January, 1965.

Smithwick, Reginald H., et al.: Surgical Treatment of Aldosteronism, Combined Experiences at the Massachusetts Memorial and the Peter Bent Brigham Hospitals. *American Journal of Surgery,* 107:178–191, January, 1964.

Sunderman, F. William, Jr.: Measurements of Vanilmandelic Acid for the Diagnosis of Pheochromocytoma and Neuroblastoma. *American Journal of Clinical Pathology,* 42:481–497, November, 1964.

CHAPTER 27
THE PATIENT WITH DISEASE OF BONE, JOINT, MUSCLE, OR SUPPORTING STRUCTURES

GERALDINE SKINNER

Socioeconomic considerations in the care of the patient who has disease of the bones and joints frequently are far more critical than in most other disorders largely because of the long recovery period necessary before the patient can return to home, family, and work. The toll in wages lost, pain suffered, and hardship endured by these patients and their families is enormous, and the resulting disability often requires a change in occupation. To be able to deal with the many problems imposed by such diseases, the nurse must have a sound knowledge of all the implications of long-term illness and must be prepared to offer the psychological and emotional support that both patient and family will need.

Normal Process of Bone Repair

Bones have a relatively poor blood supply compared with soft tissue, particularly long bones. Since portions of these bones are firm, healing following disease or trauma takes place at a slower rate than in any other body tissue.

The sequence of events occurring at the tissue level following fracture of a bone provides a clear picture of the process of bone healing. After a bone injury, the ends of the bones and the surrounding soft tissues are bound together by an interlacing mesh of fibrin from clotted blood, lymph, and inflammatory exudate, which are present at the injury site. A certain amount of swelling or edema is always present. Granulation tissue forms within a few hours with the appearance of fibroblasts. If immobilization of the injured part can be maintained, tissue organization proceeds uninterrupted within the first 48 hours.

The cells forming the newly organized tissue are derived from the bone layers, namely, endosteum, marrow reticulum, and periosteum, from the soft tissues around the bone, and from the lymphocytes that infiltrate the injury site as a result of the inflammatory reaction. By 72 to 96 hours the new mass of cells becomes organized tissue uniting the bone ends. It is loosely meshed and very friable. Interposition of tissue, e.g., torn muscle fibers, at the injury site will, of course, prevent formation of the newly organized tissue and inadequate immobilization will interfere with organization.

New bone formation is called *bone callus*. Early callus formation comes about when calcium is deposited in the new tissue. Some deposition of calcium may occur as early as 72 hours after a fracture. Bone connective tissue is made up of matrix, which is composed of an organic material, chiefly collagen (a protein) and an inorganic substance, of which calcium is the major component. From this point on calcium is progressively laid down in a denser concentration until the callus eventually becomes hard bone. With use of the body part resulting in normal stress and strain over a period of months, the bone develops new lines and channels. The total healing process may take a year or more. The success of the process depends to a large extent upon the circulation to the injured or diseased parts.

Retarded calcium deposition in an injured area may cause delayed union, and absence of calcium deposition causes a nonunion fracture. Some fracture sites, e.g., the neck of the femur, are characterized by a prolonged healing time. A non-weight-bearing bone may become functional earlier than a weight-bearing one, since it is not subjected to stress and strain. A limited amount of stress and strain will, however, speed healing in accordance with Wolff's Law, which states: *Every change in the form and the function of bones, or in their function alone, is followed by certain definite changes in their interval architecture, and equally definite changes in their external conformation, in accordance with mathematical laws.* Stating Wolff's Law more simply: Bones form according to the stresses and strains placed upon them.

Soft tissue healing occurs simultaneously with bone healing, i.e., skin, muscles, ligaments, and tendons.

Care of the Immobilized Patient

A lengthy period of immobilization follows bone and joint surgery. This immobilization may include care in a cast, in traction, or on an orthopedic frame such as the CircOlectric bed, the Stryker frame, or the Foster reversible bed. The physician will select the method of therapy depending upon the injury, the age of the patient, and the availability of skilled nursing care and orthopedic equipment, and may consult with the patient and his family, since immobilization will influence the length of hospitalization, the cost of care, and the nursing to be given at home during the convalescent period.

CARE OF THE PATIENT IN A CAST

Although immobilization is the main purpose of cast application, it may also be used when it is desired to support a body part, to prevent deformities, and to correct them. To illustrate the second and third of these purposes, casts are frequently applied to joints for the patient with rheumatoid arthritis, both to correct existing deformities and to prevent further joint damage from the disease. Casts are commonly applied following fractures and following bone and joint surgery, e.g., after a spinal fusion in which the parts must be stabilized to permit bone and tissue healing. Plaster of Paris is used for this purpose. It is available in a dry powder form enmeshed in crinoline.

The plaster of Paris bandage is immersed vertically in tepid water. When bubbling stops the bandage is removed and the excess water is gently compressed from it. The wet roll of plaster is applied to the body part, which has been covered with a layer of stockinet or a thin layer of sheet wadding. This covering is placed next to the patient's skin so that the plaster of Paris will not irritate it. In rare instances, when complete immobilization is necessary, a skin-tight cast may be applied directly to the skin. The bony prominences may be protected with pieces of felt or sponge rubber cut to fit. This padding helps to protect nerves and blood vessels close to the bony surfaces from undue pressure that would hinder circulation and nerve action. The wet bandages are applied evenly and rubbed to make a smooth cast surface, on both the inner and outer aspects of the cast.

Casts applied to protect or immobilize the hip or shoulder joints are called *spica casts*. The bandages are applied in a spiral fashion between the trunk and one extremity. The hip spica usually covers the patient up to his midtrunk and the entire leg, and often the foot, on the involved side. The shoulder spica includes the shoulder joint, the elbow, and the lower arm. It extends to the midtrunk. A

TYPES OF CASTS

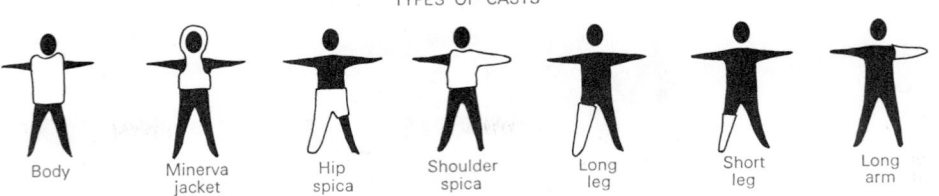

Figure 27-1
Types of casts

| Body | Minerva jacket | Hip spica | Shoulder spica | Long leg | Short leg | Long arm |

body cast is applied to the trunk, and a *minerva jacket* encases the trunk and head. A *short leg cast* covers only the lower leg, ankle, and foot. It frequently is equipped with a bar or a heel on the sole so that it can be used as a *walking cast*. The *long leg cast* includes the foot and lower leg and up to the midthigh. This cast immobilizes both the ankle and the knee. *Short* and *long arm casts* may be applied. In fractures the joint above the injury and the one below it are included in the cast.

Precast Care

Whenever possible the nurse should discuss the application of the cast with the patient and his family, to ensure that the patient is accepting this form of therapy without undue concern. Giving him an opportunity to discuss any fears and concerns will aid in securing his fullest cooperation.

The nurse should carefully examine the patient's skin prior to cast application and record her observations on the chart. The skin should be clean and free from abrasions. It will not be shaved unless bone surgery is to be carried out. It should be cleansed with a hexachlorophene solution such as pHisoHex or another cleansing agent as ordered. Rubbing the skin gently with alcohol just prior to cast application will increase skin tone.

The physician may order an analgesic to be administered prior to cast application. If the cast is to be a body jacket or spica the patient is frequently transported to the cast room in his bed to minimize movement. Casts are most often applied in the emergency room, a special cast room, or in the operating room. The application of a body jacket or hip spica usually requires the use of a special orthopedic cast table (Fig. 27-2). The patient is carefully moved from his bed or the operating table onto the cast table. Mobilization of a fracture site can be minimized by personnel applying manual traction or a strong steady pull on each side of the fracture site as the patient is being moved.

The patient's bed should be prepared. The mattress should be firm and level; hinged bed boards may be placed under it. A sagging mattress can cause a new cast to crack, flatten, or assume a different shape producing underlying pressure on soft tissues, and can change the position of the encased body part. Four or five medium-sized pillows should be placed in the bed and protected with plastic cases placed under the cotton ones.

Cast Application

The nurse may prepare the plaster bandages for wetting and make available the other needed supplies, such as sheet wadding and stockinet. She may also assist in positioning the patient for cast application as directed by the physician. When

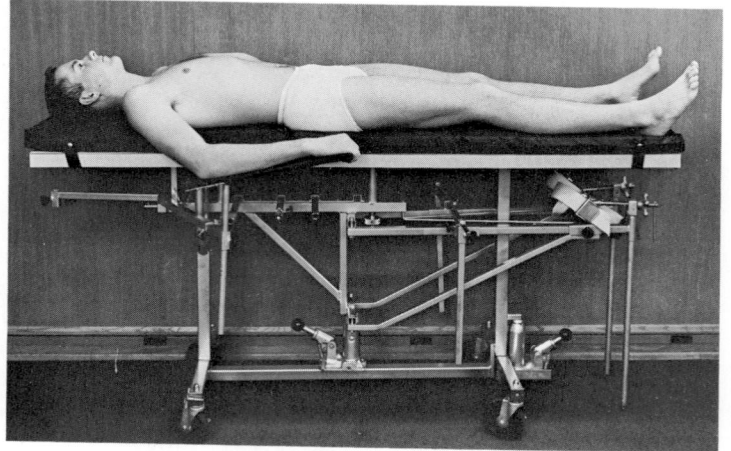

*Figure 27–2
Orthopedic table. (Courtesy Orthopedic Frame Company, Kalamazoo, Mich.)*

holding a new cast she should hold the part with the palms of the hands and not with the fingers. Indentations made by the fingers can produce pressure areas in the soft tissues under the cast. The application of a large cast, e.g., a hip spica, takes teamwork by orthopedist, nurse, and other assistants.

When casting is nearly completed, the orthopedist trims the edges. With a body cast he cuts an opening in the abdominal region to facilitate breathing and permit normal distention, and trims the perineal area of the cast to facilitate use of the bedpan. He pulls the cast lining, stockinet, or sheet wadding out beyond the cast edge and secures it in place with an extra plaster bandage. The toes or fingers are always left free so that circulation in the extremities can be observed.

If a shoulder or hip spica was applied the physician may place additional plaster bandages between the legs or between the arm and the trunk and wind these with more plaster to form a brace. *Nursing personnel should never use these braces as hand-holds when moving or turning the patient.* This bracing strengthens the cast so that proper positioning can be maintained but is not strong enough to be used as a handle for lifting the heavy cast.

Drying the Cast

When the cast is partly set the patient is carefully lifted onto his bed by as many persons as are needed to support him. The pillows already in the bed are placed in areas of body curvatures, if needed, to maintain the shape of the cast and provide comfort. When lifting a patient in a damp cast the fingers should be cupped together, and the main weight of the cast should be held in the palms of the hands to prevent indentation of the soft plaster by the fingers.

Next, the exposed parts of the patient's body are covered, if indicated, to keep him comfortably warm. The damp cast should be left exposed to the air to permit complete drying and top bedding eliminated until the cast is dry. It is preferable for the cast to dry from the inside out. Drying usually takes from 12 to 24 hours according to cast size and local humidity. A cast dryer may be used to speed drying.

Excess plaster should be removed by washing with clear water or a weak solution of vinegar. As soon as the cast is thoroughly dry, the nurse should bind any rough edges with adhesive tape, being careful to keep all tape to the outside of the cast. In curved areas of the cast, such as around the perineal opening, short strips or petals are used to bind the cast edges. The stockinet is pulled over the edge of the dry cast and the adhesive tape petals secure it smoothly to the cast by being overlapped.

During the first 24 hours the patient in the large body or hip spica cast should be turned every 2 hours from front to back and vice versa, to permit uniform drying and maintenance of cast contours. If pillows are used the cases should be changed when the patient is turned.

Daily Care of the Patient

If the cast was applied following surgery or an injury that involved soft tissue trauma, it must be observed for signs of bleeding. A new blood spot should be carefully circled with a pencil mark and the time of observation recorded on the circle. If bleeding continues the spot should be circled at intervals to indicate the rate of hemorrhage. Blood or drainage may appear along the inside planes of the cast. If hemorrhage is excessive it may be necessary to remove the cast.

The leg or arm is usually elevated with the fingers or toes at the highest level by means of slings, ropes, pulleys, and weights, or use of pillows. Elevation facilitates drainage thus stimulating circulation and decreasing edema in dependent parts. If edema is excessive the cast may have to be split or removed in order to restore circulation and prevent destruction of soft tissues.

Signs and symptoms that point to complications are as follows: (1) excessive pressure on soft tissues causing interference with innervation, indicated by persistent *smarting* or *burning* sensation under the cast, or increasing *pain*, sensation of deep *pressure*, and *numbness* of the part; (2) developing ischemia of soft tissues due to pressure that reduces circulation and venous return, indicated by *swelling* of exposed fingers and toes, marked *blanching* of exposed fingers and toes, abnormal *coldness* of exposed fingers and toes, or *bluish discoloration* of exposed fingers and toes; (3) death and necrosis of tissue, indicated by increasing musty or foul *odor* about the cast or *drainage* through the cast or out of an opening.

To detect early mustiness the nurse may need to sniff very close to the cast. This odor may indicate the development of a decubitus ulcer. The nurse should observe the patient every 10 to 15 minutes for the first 6 to 12 hours and promptly report to the physician should any of the sensory or circulatory changes mentioned develop. Odor or drainage will not arise for a few days, but paralysis and necrosis can occur within the first 24 hours of cast application. Any complaints made by the patient must be investigated.

The patient's fingers and toes, which must always be exposed from the end of the cast, must feel warm, and capillary refill should be rapid with release of pressure on the exposed area. Compression of thumbnail or toenail should cause blanching, and with release the part should turn pink rapidly. *Bluish discoloration may be a very late symptom.* With continued satisfactory circulation the nurse can lengthen the interval between observations.

The physician may have cut an opening in an arm cast whereby the radial pulse can be taken in order to measure the circulation in the extremity rather than the patient's general circulation.

The patient in an immobilizing cast needs much psychological support during his therapy period. His call bell or intercommunications system should be working and within easy reach at all times. Nursing personnel should be most receptive to his requests and listen carefully to complaints. He should be taught not to push pencils or other objects under his cast to scratch his skin. Such a foreign object could cause a decubitus ulcer if it produces a skin abrasion or breaks off and remains under the cast.

The nurse should anticipate the patient's fear of falling out of bed during turning. She plans her moves carefully in advance and advises him of each step as she proceeds. Usually it is best to turn the patient on his unaffected side, since there may be slight movement within the cast. While a hip spica is damp, she pulls him on his pillows to one side of the bed. Fresh pillows are then arranged on the far side of the bed. His arms can be positioned over his head during turning, to avoid injury to them. The patient is then gently rolled onto the freshly covered pillows and pulled back to the center of the bed. When the cast is completely dry the pillows can be removed.

An overhead frame having a trapeze bar attached to it allows the patient to use his arms or free arm to readjust his position in bed.

He should be taught deep breathing exercises, abdominal tightening, gluteal setting, and quadriceps setting. These exercises will speed recovery and shorten the rehabilitation period. The nurse should teach the patient in a hip spica how to do quadriceps setting exercises with his good leg and then encourage him to do the same with the immobilized leg. While bathing him, nursing personnel should assist him in putting all free joints through a normal range of motion.

The patient in a hip spica may be dependent upon nursing personnel for his perineal care. He must be kept clean, for both physical and psychological reasons. Irritated skin areas may easily break down into decubitus ulcers, especially where there are skin folds.

The patient should be encouraged to ambulate insofar as possible, as this helps prevent complications, stimulates circulation, and promotes healing. Such devices as rubber heels or walking irons may be utilized on a leg cast to facilitate ambulation.

The length of time the patient will remain in his cast will depend upon many factors, including the type of fracture, extent of disease or injury, and rate of healing. If it is necessary that the cast be worn for a long period, a coat or two of shellac can be applied to keep it clean.

Removing the Cast

The cast can be removed with either a manual cast cutter or a Stryker cast cutter (Fig. 27–3). To overcome the patient's fears about cast removal, the nurse should carefully explain the procedure. In the Stryker cast cutter, the sawtooth blade moves back and forth rapidly; the teeth stop moving when they meet sheet wadding or stockinet.

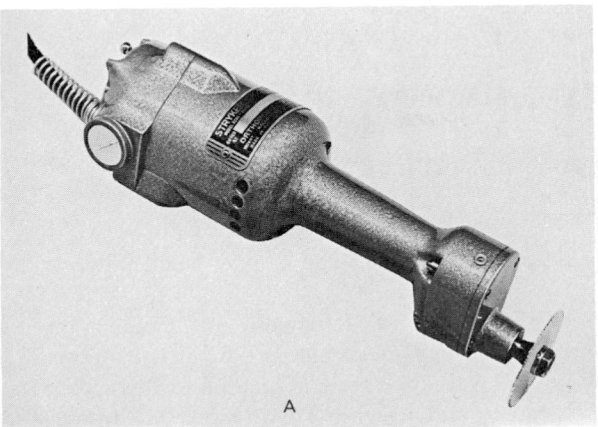

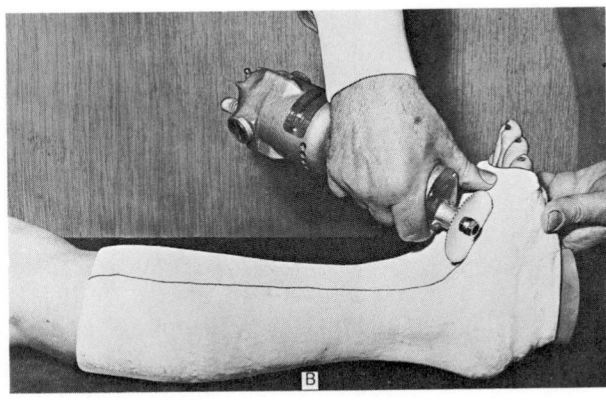

Figure 27-3
Stryker cast cutter, and
cutter in use. (Courtesy
Orthopedic Frame
Company, Kalamazoo,
Mich.)

Postcast Care

A patient who is immobilized for a prolonged period requires good nursing care because changes have occurred in the skin, muscles, ligaments, and tendons, and disuse atrophy will be present. There may be several layers of dead skin covering the part which should be softened with skin oil first and removed gently and gradually. The underlying tender skin may be irritated if it is exposed immediately.

A second important point for the nurse to remember is to *support the part.* The lower shell of the cast may be saved and the edges bound, and the shell used to provide support until strength is regained, or a brace or splint can be prepared to replace it. A body cast can be replaced by a back brace or corset. Pillows can be used to support the involved part temporarily.

CARE OF THE PATIENT IN TRACTION

Immobilization in traction may be the treatment of choice, rather than a cast. The freedom of movement which traction provides may help to avert the development of pneumonia and circulatory disorders, especially in elderly patients.

Traction serves several functions in disorders of the musculoskeletal system: (1) to reduce muscle spasm and fractures, (2) to immobilize bones, joints, and muscles, (3) to maintain correct alignment for prolonged periods, and (4) to correct and prevent deformities. It may be exerted on extremities, neck, or pelvis.

Traction may be continuous or intermittent. Continuous traction is most often used with fractures or dislocations of a bone or joint, whereas intermittent traction is often used in rheumatoid arthritis to reduce flexion contractures or in back disorders to reduce muscle spasm and pain. In an emergency situation manual traction may be applied to either reduce a fracture or to immobilize the part while the patient is being moved.

There are basically two types of traction: skin and skeletal. In skin traction the pull is exerted indirectly on muscle and bones by traction to the skin and underlying soft tissues through the application of strips of moleskin tape or foam rubber. The latter are bound onto the extremity by elastic bandages. The tapes are

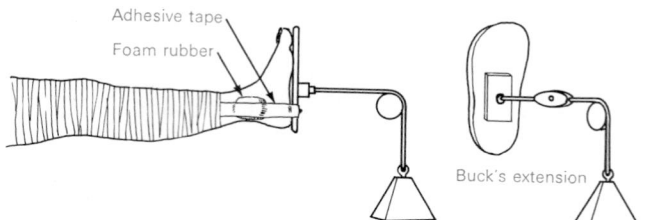

Figure 27–4
Buck's extension

attached to a rope leading over a pulley to a weight. The canvas head halter is another form of skin traction.

Skeletal traction exerts pull directly on bones. A Steinmann pin or Kirschner wire is inserted directly through the involved bones. A traction bow or U clamp is attached to the end of the pin or wire and a traction rope is secured to the vertex of the bow. The rope passes over a pulley and weights are attached to the end of the rope. For skeletal head traction, special tongs, such as Crutchfield tongs, are applied to the outer table of the skull and attached to the rope and weights so that direct pull can be exerted on the head, producing the desired pull on the injured cervical vertebrae. A form of traction in which there is a straight pull on the involved part is running or straight traction. The simplest form is Buck's extension (Fig. 27–4). Surface traction and Bryant traction are forms of straight traction.

For traction to be effective, countertraction—a pull in the opposite direction—is necessary. When traction and countertraction are equal the patient is immobilized. The patient's weight and the friction between his body or skin and the lower surface of the bed create much of the countertraction, but if this is insufficient elevating the bed under the part that is in traction will increase the countertraction. If it is necessary to keep the patient flat in bed, countertraction can be increased through the use of weights, ropes, and pulleys drawing in the opposite direction. The goal is to maintain continuous and effective pull on the injured part while keeping the patient well centered in the bed.

The Traction Bed and Equipment

The patient is placed in a hospital bed equipped with an overhead frame. The Balkan frame, an overhead quadrilateral supported by uprights fastened to the bedposts, is frequently used (Fig. 27–5). Cross bars can be attached to the overhead frame to which pulleys, clamps, or other devices may be attached. The traction bed must have a firm, level mattress. A bed board is often used to ensure a firm surface. Central service units in most hospitals are equipped with traction carts that can be wheeled to the patient's bedside or to the operating room where the physician is going to establish the traction. This cart holds small items such as moleskin tape, foam rubber, rope, weights, foot plates, and spreaders. Although the physician generally prepares the traction initially, the nurse has the responsibility to see that it is functioning properly at all times. She will make no major adjustments in the traction but will report to the doctor when adjustments need to be made.

The bed is usually equipped with a trapeze bar, which the patient will use to

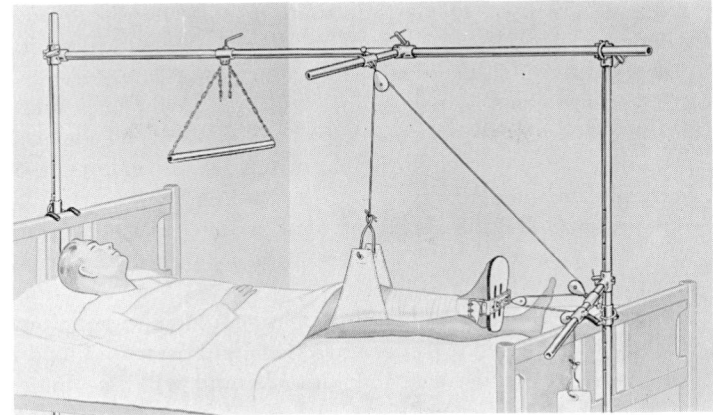

*Figure 27-5
Overhead orthopedic
frame with Russell's
traction. (Courtesy
Orthopedic Frame
Company, Kalamazoo,
Mich.)*

raise himself up or change his position slightly. He should be encouraged to use his muscles and move about as much as possible. He should be taught active bed exercises and should put his unaffected joints through a normal range of motion at least once daily.

Suspension equipment may be utilized in conjunction with traction to permit the patient to move with relative ease and without disturbing the line of pull on the affected extremity. It consists of special splints that keep the extremity off the bed surface. Obviously nursing care is made easier. Suspension equipment combined with traction provides balanced traction. Russell traction, employed in fractures of the femoral shaft, is an example of balanced traction; as the patient moves up off the surface of the bed, the weights attached to the traction equipment move down thus maintaining the original line of pull.

In general, the patient can assume only back-lying positions, although the physician may permit some flexibility in placement of the back rest during the day. The prone position cannot be utilized unless a reversible bed or frame is being used, and the side-lying position is not permitted because it might disrupt the alignment of the traction. Nonetheless traction therapy allows greater freedom of movement than the body cast.

The nurse must understand why the patient is in traction, the position that is to be maintained, the line of pull of the traction, the amount and kind of movement the patient is allowed, and which adjustments of traction equipment she can make.

An explanation of the purpose of the traction and its advantages will do much to reassure the patient and his family of its benefits. She can explain that the patient will begin to feel comfortable as his muscles relax as the result of traction for a few hours. There are several self-care measures that the nurse can explain and that will encourage the patient to participate in his own care.

Pointers for the Patient in Self-care

You will have to remain on your back unless you are advised otherwise by your physician.

Since you will be maintaining this position for some time, the care of your back and buttocks is of special importance, and you should accept special back care whenever a member of the nursing team offers to give it. The development of pressure areas can decidedly slow your convalescence.

If you are given a sheepskin to use under your back and buttocks it should be left in place unless it becomes soiled. The oil in the sheepskin and the padding it provides will do much to help prevent the development of pressure areas over bony prominences.

A pressure area or decubitus ulcer is much easier to prevent than to cure and is mainly caused by lack of circulation to a part. Excessive pressure may be exerted on the coccyx and heels.

With your doctor's permission, you should raise your buttocks off the bed frequently by using your trapeze bar. This will promote blood flow into the skin and soft tissues of your back and buttocks and will also maintain arm strength for later use when you must use crutches.

Report to me the presence of any wrinkles in your undersheet, or any food crumbs in your bed, as these can irritate your skin.

The skin areas around your Thomas ring, your pelvic sling, or your head halter should be washed thoroughly at least once daily and inspected for signs of irritation.

Always lie flat in bed part of the day even though the doctor has permitted you to use your back rest. This will maintain muscle length and ensure good posture later on.

If you are in leg traction inspect your "good" heel carefully for any signs of irritation, redness, or numbness.

Try to remain in the center of the bed at all times. Do not slide down in bed so that the foot in traction is resting against the foot of the bed, as this would negate the effect of the traction.

Ask your doctor about exercising your involved arm or leg.

If you are in skeletal traction do not touch the skin areas around the pins, wires, or tongs—infection can develop at these points.

Your traction weights should swing free of the bed and should not rest on the floor or be lifted up and placed on the bed at any time.

In order to speed your recovery, do the following bed exercises several times daily as you have been taught by me or your doctor: deep breathing exercises with emphasis on exhalation; abdominal and gluteal tightening; quadriceps setting in both legs; ankle exercises—foot circling, bringing your forefoot up toward your knee; flexion and extension exercises of your good knee; range of motion exercises of your uninvolved joints; push-up exercises with your arms when you are able to sit up.

Pointers in Nursing Care

In addition to instructing the patient in self-help measures, the nurse should bear in mind the following:

Be sure that there is a sufficient amount of countertraction to keep the patient centered in his bed. For example, if he is permitted to have his back rest elevated, it may be necessary to elevate the foot of the bed to provide additional countertraction.

Give special back care at least *twice daily*. Look at the skin of the shoulders, back, and coccygeal areas frequently to be sure redness and decubitus ulcers are not forming.

Discourage the use of air rings for the buttocks or "donuts" for the heel areas as these merely create pressure and further interfere with circulation to the part.

Encourage the use of real sheepskin or synthetic sheepskin materials as they distribute the body weight without creating pressure points.

An alternating pressure mattress may be helpful.

When placing and removing the bedpan handle the patient's skin with care. It may be helpful to powder the bedpan.

When working with a patient in skin traction remove the elastic bandages at least daily. Carefully examine the skin areas around the tape or foam rubber. Keep the skin clean and dry. Rewind the elastic bandages smoothly and snugly but not so tight as to interfere with circulation.

Observe the skin areas around the skeletal wires, pins, and tongs for redness, odor, or drainage. Small dry dressings should cover the insertion points.

The ends of skeletal pins should be covered with corks.

A firm and smooth foundation for the lower bedding is one key to prevention of skin irritations. Check frequently to see that it is wrinkle free and free of crumbs.

All movement should be smooth and gentle, and any jarring of bed or equipment should be avoided.

Be sure the bedding is not interfering with the ropes and pulleys.

Be sure the traction ropes are in the pulley grooves and are riding freely to permit maximum traction.

Be sure knots do not limit the action of the ropes over the pulley grooves.

Ropes should be tied securely to weights to prevent interference of traction and jarring of the patient. Knots should be taped after they are tied.

The patient should be encouraged to do as much for himself as he can within the limitations imposed by traction.

The patient's "good" foot should have a support placed so that he is able to brace himself against it to help maintain himself in the desired bed position.

Weights should never be lifted or removed when the patient is in continuous traction.

Weights should never rest directly over the patient where they might fall upon him in the event that a knot became untied.

Be sure the patient's extremity in traction is kept warm with a light covering that will not interfere with the traction equipment.

When making a traction bed it is usually best to change the foundation bedding by starting on the patient's unaffected side. He usually must be raised off the bed to remove the soiled sheet as he can turn only very slightly from side to side. Encourage him to assist himself through the use of the trapeze bar.

CARE OF THE PATIENT ON AN ORTHOPEDIC FRAME OR BED

An orthopedic frame is a supportive rectangular frame, made with heavy metal piping and covered with canvas, and used to support a patient in the supine or prone position. The Stryker frame was the first turning frame developed;

modifications include the CircOlectric bed, and the wedge frame. The objectives in utilizing orthopedic frames include the following: to facilitate nursing care of helpless and incontinent patients, including quadriplegics, paraplegics, and children in plaster casts; to facilitate nursing care of patients with second- and third-degree burns, permitting frequent change of position, stimulation of circulation, and increased comfort; to maintain spinal hypertension in spinal fractures, tuberculosis, and rheumatoid (Marie-Strümpell) arthritis; to facilitate nursing care of the patient with marked edema of the extremities or spinal paralysis due to malignant spinal neaplasms; to provide a form of restraint that renders certain types of traction care more effective; to immobilize the spine during healing of fractures, tuberculosis, osteomyelitis, or malignant disorders of the vertebral column; and to facilitate the care of the patient not permitted to be turned or elevated onto a bedpan in the conventional manner.

Rotating frames such as the Stryker frames, the Foster reversible bed, and the CircOlectric bed are made in matching pairs, a prone-lying or anterior frame and a supine or posterior frame. The canvas coverings are padded with foam rubber pads covered with matching tailored sheets. Directions for use of the equipment are supplied by the manufacturers.

Placing the Patient on the Frame

While both frames are attached to the frame standard, the nurse should check to see that the coverings on both frames match exactly at the perineal area. The anterior frame is removed. If a perineal strap is to be used with the posterior frame it should be in place before the patient is moved onto the frame.

In preparation, the patient's bed or stretcher can be moved parallel to the posterior frame. In the case of a cervical fracture patient, his head should be held

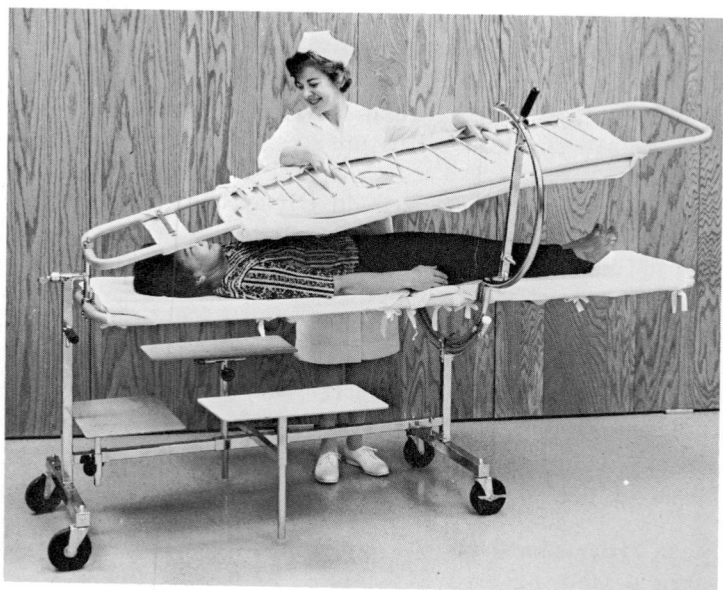

Figure 27–6
Stryker wedge frame.
(Courtesy Orthopedic Frame Company, Kalamazoo, Mich.)

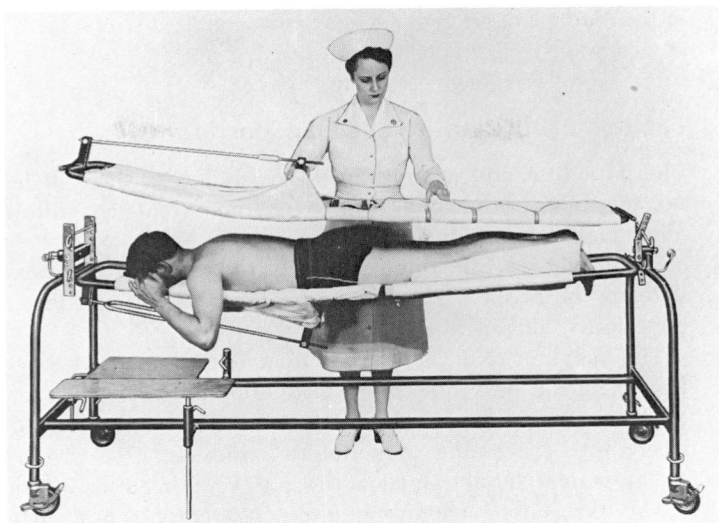

Figure 27–7
Patient on Foster
reversible bed.

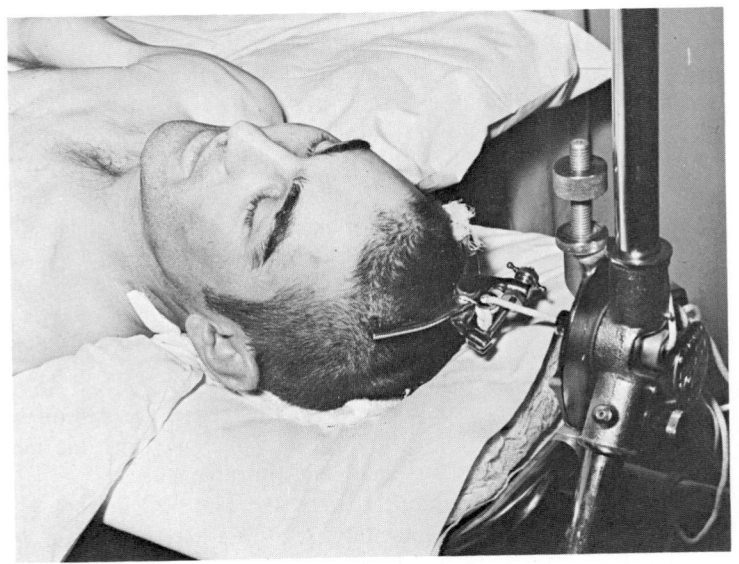

Figure 27–8
Patient on Stryker frame,
with cervical traction
being applied by Crutch-
field tongs. (Courtesy
Orthopedic Frame Com-
pany, Kalamazoo, Mich.)

firmly by one person and his hips by another, each applying enough traction to produce spinal immobility during moving. Adequate help should be secured so that the patient can be lifted carefully onto the posterior frame. Next, the patient's body should be centered on the frame so that his coccyx rests at the edge of the perineal opening but not on the perineal strap or in the opening. This will eliminate the need to move the patient up or down on the frame when he is turned.

Once the patient is correctly placed on the frame, traction equipment can be attached as needed (Figs. 27–6 to 27–8). The patient with a cervical fracture can be turned readily and safely with maintenance of continuous traction to his head or extremities. This reduces discomfort and provides for a much-needed change of position.

Pointers about Care on the Posterior Frame

The patient should not need a pillow under his head. If he desires one and it is not contraindicated, it is best to use an infant-size pillow so that good spinal alignment is maintained.

The perineal strap should be kept in place at all times except when the patient is using the bedpan. Sagging of the buttocks through this opening can make for poor spinal alignment.

The bedpan should be placed under the frame, not between the patient and his frame. He can best defecate in the supine position.

The arm supports should be used to allow the patient to abduct his shoulders freely, thus preventing adduction deformities.

The patient should be encouraged to keep his arms off his chest.

The foot support should be used consistently to prevent foot drop.

The patient should be encouraged to do bed exercises that do not require movement of the spine or the affected part such as deep breathing, gluteal and abdominal tightening, and dorsiflexion of the ankles.

The patient should be encouraged to promptly report the presence of any wrinkles in his frame covers or pads.

The patient should be bathed, with the exception of his back, while in the supine position.

The patient may prefer to sleep on the posterior frame, and will feel more secure if a webbed strap is placed around him and the frame in the region of the hips. This will be especially important until the patient becomes fully adjusted to being on the frame.

Turning the Patient on the Frame

The first time the patient is turned the procedure should be carefully explained to him and his family, if the latter are present. Until he becomes adjusted to this new program he may be somewhat apprehensive.

The upper bedding should be removed and the patient's gown or pajamas placed smoothly over his anterior body. A pillow may be placed across his *lower legs* to furnish padding between the frames during the turning process. The anterior frame can then be secured to the turning device so that the patient is now placed between the two frames, anterior and posterior. Heavy webbed straps should be placed around the two frames with the enclosed patient, in the region of his shoulders, hips, and knees. Next the pivot or turning device should be released and the frame held steady. Then the nurse will count aloud: one, two, three, and turn. Turning should be done moderately fast so that the patient will not slide sideways as he turns. An effort should be made not to jar him as he turns.

A headpiece may be used to support the patient's head when he is in the prone position. He usually prefers to have his chin, face, and neck free.

The upper section (canvas) of the anterior frame should end just below the patient's shoulder girdle so as not to cause pressure on his shoulders. His pubis should rest on the lower edge of the upper anterior canvas. A 4-inch perineal opening, which need not be covered, is usually provided on the anterior frame. The lower anterior canvas should end at the level of the external malleoli so that the forefeet and toes can extend through the lower frame opening. Plantar flexion of the ankle *must not* be permitted in the prone position, as this can lead to injury to the peroneal nerve with resultant foot drop.

While on the anterior frame the patient may not wish to use the arm supports if he can use his arms to feed himself, turn pages, or work with his hands. A good reading light should be provided. Many patients prefer to spend most of the daylight hours in the prone position since they can perform more activities when in this position. Women frequently are more comfortable in this position if a small pad or pillow is placed in the abdominal area so that pressure is decreased on the breasts and breathing is facilitated. This small pad or pillow should be placed across the upper abdomen prior to turning from the posterior frame to avoid raising the patient's trunk off the frame.

Preventing Complications

Special consideration must be given to the maintenance of normal range of motion of the joints and maintenance of muscle strength.

Frequent turning in the frame equipment can do much to prevent the development of decubitus ulcers, circulatory stasis, pulmonary stasis resulting in pneumonia or emboli, and urinary calculi. The frequency with which the patient should be turned will depend upon the reasons for his being on the frame. He might be turned every 15 minutes postoperatively, e.g., following a spinal fusion. It is desirable to turn the patient every 2 hours, although many patients, after becoming adjusted to the frame, may prefer to remain in one position for as long as 4 hours. The CircOlectric bed is most advantageous because of its ease of turning by electrical power. It also turns vertically and can be placed in a variety of positions, including one that maintains the patient in an upright position.

Home Care of the Patient on a Frame

The patient needing long-term care may be sent home positioned on a frame. The nurse must teach the patient and his family the care he will need at home. A practical nurse or aide may come to the hospital to learn this care, and this is a good plan to ensure adequate learning and safe home care. In explaining this care, the nurse should consider how the procedures already discussed can be adapted for use in the home.

MOBILIZATION OF THE PATIENT WITH BONE AND JOINT DISORDERS

Support of the Patient in a Wheel Chair

Mobilization is an early goal for the patient who has been either acutely or chronically ill. One of the first steps toward this goal is to get the patient out of bed

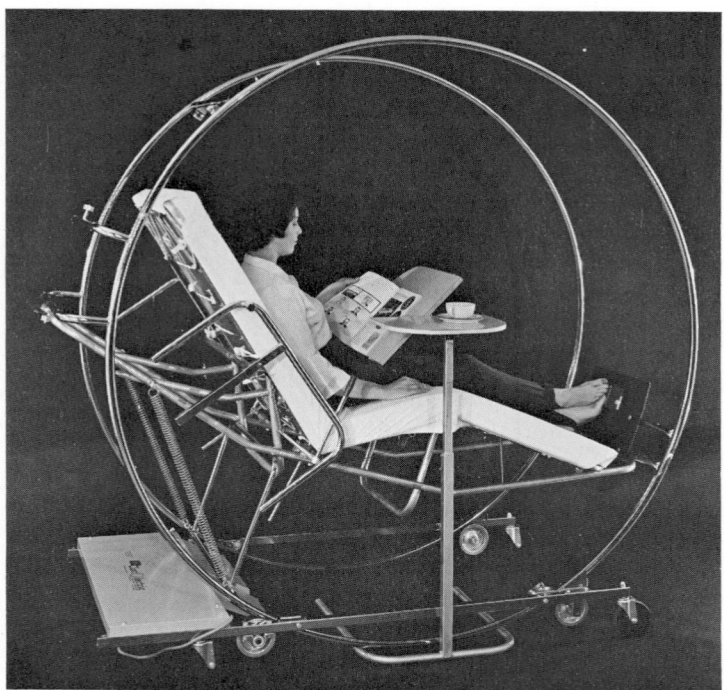

Figure 27–9 CircOlectric bed. (Courtesy Orthopedic Frame Company, Kalamazoo, Mich.)

and into a wheel chair. Early in his convalescent period, while he is still weak, he may need the chair principally to provide support in the sitting or semisitting position. The wheel chair chosen to give the best support may differ markedly from the one used to facilitate the best locomotion.

The patient who is weak, elderly, or immobilized in a cast or brace may greatly benefit by sitting up. In this position deep breathing is facilitated, circulation is improved, and alertness may be enhanced. It is a position of rest after prolonged recumbency.

The large wooden or wicker type of wheel chair provides maximum support. The high back gives full spinal and head support, especially to the weak or paralyzed patient; it is usually adjustable, permitting either a reclining or a sitting position. Pillow supports can be placed underneath, behind, and at the sides of the patient, if needed. The long hard seat provides support for the entire thigh, eliminating strain on the hips and knees and providing a firm foundation for the patient's buttocks, and thus gives firm spinal support. The wide arm rests provide needed support, which reduces fatigue by eliminating pull on the shoulder joints and encourages the patient to keep his arms off his chest. The adjustable foot and leg rests help to maintain the lower extremities in normal alignment. Elevation of the leg or legs may be desirable to promote good circulation or to support a leg cast. When the chair leg extensions are elevated the nurse should be sure that the wheel chair is well balanced. If it tends to tip forward weights should be placed on the posterior lower framework of the chair to compensate for overweight from elevated leg supports. If the patient's head drops back too far he may

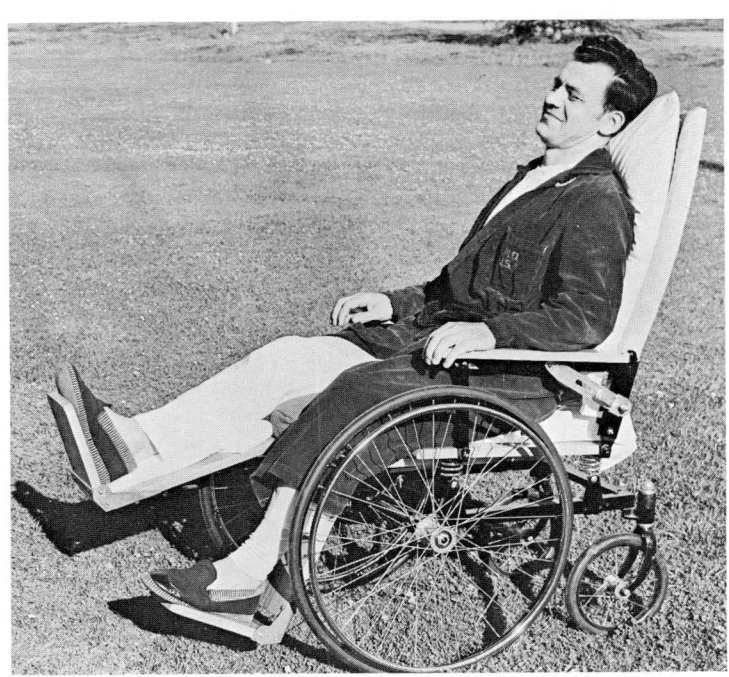

*Figure 27–10
Supportive wheel chair.
(Courtesy Veterans
Administration Center,
Los Angeles, Calif.)*

need a small roll or pad behind his head or neck. His chin should be high, not resting on his chest. His chest should be up and forward. He may need a small pad for support in the region of his lumbar spine. If his wrists are weak they should be cocked up in a hyperextended position with a roll or ball in his hand to keep his thumbs in opposition. His thumb should not rest adjacent to his forefinger.

The collapsible type of wheel chair is most commonly used today. This was designed essentially for the patient who has progressed to the stage of recovery where transportation is of concern. Since support of the body cannot usually be given in this chair to the same degree as in the more cumbersome wooden wheel chair, the patient needs strength and stability to use it. This chair is provided for home care and is available with many variations. Equipment such as brakes, arm rests, and leg supports is specially ordered according to the patient's specific needs, and the cost thereof is added to the basic price of the wheel chair.

Every wheel chair should be equipped with hand brakes, 3-inch arm rests, foot supports, hand rims, and skirt guards. The paralyzed patient may greatly benefit by the provision of swinging foot rests, a removable armrest, 20-inch wheels (to permit him to move sideways without lifting himself over the wheel), a zipper in the back rest, and leg rest panels.

The patient who sits for long periods in a chair should be taught to develop the habit of periodically (every 10 to 15 minutes), raising his buttocks off the chair by means of push-up exercises. Releasing the pressure of body weight on the buttocks will increase circulation to the soft tissues and help prevent the development of decubitus ulcers. Air rings should not be used under the buttocks as they form

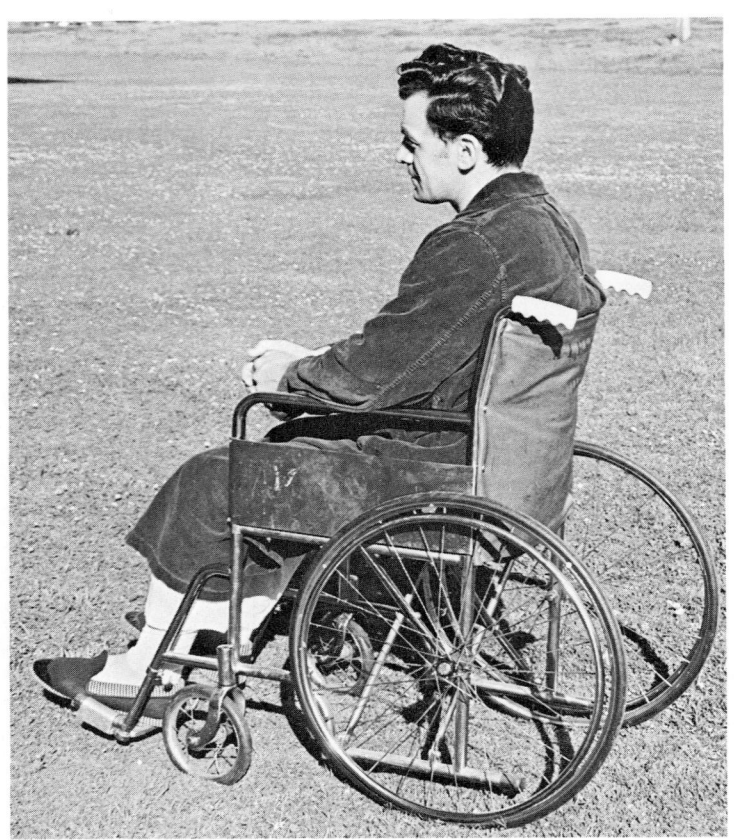

Figure 27–11
Collapsible wheel chair.
(Courtesy Veterans
Administration Center,
Los Angeles, Calif.)

a ring of pressure which decreases circulation and encourages hemorrhoid formation. The use of a thick foam rubber pillow and/or a sheepskin is advantageous
for the paralyzed or debilitated patient.

Walkers, Crutches, and Canes

Preparation for ambulation should start immediately after the onset of the illness.
Bed exercises are vital to early ambulation. Deep breathing aids circulation and
gluteal and abdominal muscle tightening increases trunk stability and promotes
good standing posture. Quadriceps setting helps stabilize the knees. Dorsiflexion
exercises increase ankle strength. Push-up arm exercises done while the patient
is bedfast increase strength in the triceps muscles. Pull-up and lifting exercises increase biceps muscle strength. The patient should be encouraged to carry out
active range of motion for all uninvolved joints, and passive exercises must be done
at least daily for all joints he cannot move, to maintain free joint motion.

Many patients today undergo hip surgery for fractured hips or hip arthroplasty to
increase mobilization of the hip. Prior to ambulation the patient may have been
treated in roller skate traction in bed to increase his range of hip joint motion.

He may be given stationary bicycle exercises. These increase hip and knee joint action and strengthen his muscles.

WALKERS

Several types of walkers are used for early ambulation. For the patient who is quite unstable a small light-weight walker with rubber-tipped feet is preferred.

The larger walker is equipped with wheels and often underarm supports to aid him in learning a normal walking gait. This may be equipped with a seat and a sling to support his back, and should be equipped with hand brakes. The principles of ambulating with a walker are essentially the same as in crutch walking.

Prior to using a walker the patient may be taught to balance between parallel bars, and may be taught a normal walking gait and weight-bearing on his hands.

CRUTCHES AND CRUTCH WALKING

In some hospitals the nurse is responsible for instructing the patient in crutch walking, and she may have to measure the patient for crutches. He should lie supine with his arms at his sides. The shoes he will wear while walking should be placed on his feet. These shoes should be supportive oxfords with a fairly broad heel. With a tape measure she should measure from his axilla to a point about 6 to 8 inches laterally from his foot and on a level with the bottom of the heel of his shoe. If he must be measured in the standing position this may be done by subtracting 16 inches from his total height. The hand bars on the crutches should be positioned to permit nearly complete extension of the elbows without having the axillary bar press into the axilla. The patient will rest his weight on the palms of his hands with his wrists in hyperextension if he is using his crutches correctly.

Many crutches can be adjusted to fit the patient, both as to placement of the hand bar and length of the crutch. Body weight should rest on the palms of the hands at the hand bars—not on the axillary bars. Some physicians prefer to have the crutches short enough so that the axillary bar rests on the lateral chest wall well below the axillae. It should be impressed upon the patient that too much pressure in the axillae may result in damage to the radial nerves and cause "crutch paralysis."

Crutches are made of wood or metal. Wood crutches are most commonly used. The crutch should have a suction tip made of pure rubber, for safety.

The nurse should instruct the patient as follows:

Stand with head up and feet 6 to 8 inches apart. This gives a wide base of support.

Place crutches about 4 inches to the side and 4 inches in front.

Crutches should always be ahead of you or at your side, never behind you.

Flex your elbows slightly and fully extend them as you move forward, bearing your weight on your hands.

Look straight ahead—not at your feet.

When walking contract or tighten your abdominal and gluteal muscles.

Take steps no longer than the length of your own feet, to maintain maximum stability.

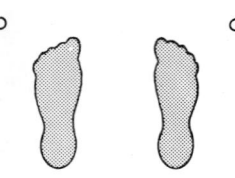

Figure 27–12
Good standing balance:
four point.

Figure 27–13
Four point crutch
walking.

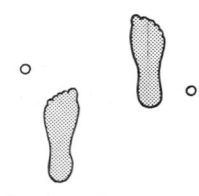

4. Right foot forward

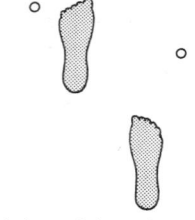

3. Left crutch forward

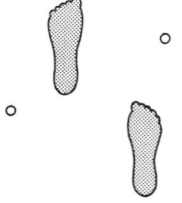

2. Left foot forward

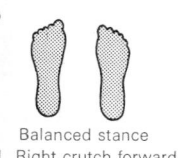

Balanced stance
1. Right crutch forward

If you start to fall learn to throw your crutches to the side, away from you so that you do not fall upon them.

If you start to fall try to relax or go limp so that you will not injure yourself.

When you sit down or go to bed get in the habit of placing your crutches within easy reach at all times.

Crutch-walking Stance. It is well worth the effort to teach a patient correct stance before teaching crutch gait. Before assisting him out of bed be sure that the bed wheels are locked so that the bed does not slip away from him as he leans against it. Assist the patient out of bed, have him lean against it, and place his crutches under his axillae. Encourage him to stand up straight, looking ahead of him and not at his feet. Discourage him from flexing his hips. His feet should be held slightly apart and the crutches to his sides and slightly ahead of him. He should practice balance and maintenance of correct posture in the erect position, resting his weight on his arms and hands before he attempts to walk using his supports.

Crutch-walking Gaits. The most stable gait is the four point walking gait. The points are the two crutches and the patient's two feet. Three points are always resting on the floor while the fourth point is being moved. The sequence is as shown in Figure 27–13. As the patient learns to use this gait he can repeat: right foot, left crutch, left foot, right crutch; this may assist him to develop a rhythm of moving. This gait simulates normal walking motion of arms and legs, but can be employed only if all extremities can be used at least to some extent. When balance is excellent, he may wish to progress to the two point gait. It is a faster gait, one crutch and the opposite leg moving at the same time.

A third walking gait is the three point gait, used when no weight or only partial weight can be borne on one leg. The body is balanced on two crutches and both the weak leg and the normal leg are advanced simultaneously.

A fourth gait is the swing-through crutch gait, used when paralysis is present in both legs. The legs are braced and the patient swings his body through the crutches alternately. The patient should wear slacks while learning crutch walking. The nurse can often assist the patient best by walking behind him, grasping him lightly at the belt if he is very unstable.

USING THE CANE

The patient must be fairly stable on his feet before he can use a cane. The length of the cane must be such that he can extend his elbow to bear weight on his hand on the handle of the cane. The cane should be held on the side of the strong leg, so it is opposite the leg needing support. Balance is maintained by use of the cane and the weak leg while the good leg is being moved. The cane should have a curved handle and a comfortable, firm grip, and be equipped with a pure rubber suction tip.

PRE- AND POSTOPERATIVE NURSING CONSIDERATIONS

Preoperative Nursing Care

In general, preparation of the patient who is to undergo orthopedic surgery is similar to that of most types of surgery, with one important difference. Bone being a dense tissue, it is more susceptible to infection than soft tissue; joint sepsis causes restriction of motion and eventual crippling. Hence certain measures must be taken to reduce the likelihood of infection, i.e., meticulous skin preparation and improvement of general health.

The skin preparation is more extensive than that for most other surgical procedures. Skin preparation for hip and shoulder operations includes the hip or shoulder, the next distal joint, and the area to the midline of the trunk. For knee and elbow operations both the distal and proximal joints should be included. For hand and foot operations one-half to two-thirds of the extremity should be included. The nurse will carry out the skin preparation in accordance with the surgeon's directions. Meticulous bathing, scrubbing, and shaving are necessary. The area is then covered with dry sterile towels. If surgery is to be performed on a part that had been immobilized in a cast, the cast is removed 2 to 3 days preoperatively so that the skin can be oiled and cleaned.

Because bone and joint surgery is usually lengthy, the total muscle relaxation during the period of anesthesia can cause severe back pain postoperatively. Therefore the lumbar spine should be supported with a firm smooth pad and full attention should be given to proper alignment and support of all parts during surgery.

Postoperative Nursing Care

Postoperatively, nursing observations and patient care are similar to those of any surgical patient, as described elsewhere. An important goal of postoperative care is early ambulation, which is promoted by having the patient exercise early in the postoperative period.

Care of the Patient with an Amputation

Amputation is surgical severance of an extremity with loss of continuity of bone and soft tissue. When an extremity is removed in a joint area the procedure is a disarticulation. Amputation may be performed for one of several reasons: loss of blood supply due to blockage of a major blood vessel in the extremity; removal of a part in which a malignant tumor has developed; removal of a persistently infected portion of an extremity; complications of diabetes; war-incurred injuries; and industrial and automotive accidents.

Open or guillotine amputation is most frequently done when the surgeon deems it advisable for the stump to drain freely because of persistent infection. The blood vessels have been tied off but the surface of the stump has not been closed with a skin flap. Antibiotics are ordered and strict asepsis is maintained. Open amputation is always followed by stump revision or closure, the time when this is done depending upon the patient's general condition and clearing of infection.

In a closed amputation the incisions are made by cutting skin and tissue flaps to cover the stump. These are sutured over the end of the stump with the suture line away from the end of the stump where it might be subjected to pressure from the artificial limb. Small drains to prevent accumulation of blood and serous fluid are inserted at the time of closure. These are usually removed at the end of

24 hours. Closed amputation may be done initially if infection is not present even when a later stump revision is necessary, as, for example, following a crushing injury or in the presence of gangrene in the fingers or toes. If a stump revision is to be done the level of amputation is determined by the type of artificial limb to be applied, and the surgical procedure itself will also be determined on that basis.

Preoperative Nursing Care

Preoperatively the skin preparation is similar to that for any orthopedic surgery, meticulous care being given the area of amputation. Psychological preparation of the patient is critical, since he has tremendous adjustments to make. In her efforts to help him, the nurse should stress his remaining capabilities, rather than dwell on his loss. Helping him understand the usefulness of the artificial limb may do much to motivate him to work toward recovery and rehabilitation, and the attitude of his family will greatly influence his willingness to do this. The nurse should find ways to encourage the family to support the patient.

Postoperative Nursing Care

Postoperatively the stump should be elevated to reduce edema, prevent hemorrhage, and improve circulation. A pillow or pillows should be used only for 24 to 48 hours, since prolonged stump elevation can give rise to hip flexion contracture.

Immediately after surgery and during the early healing period, bedclothing should not cover or rest on the stump. The dressed stump should rest freely on an elevated support to maintain good circulation and permit nursing personnel to observe it for signs of hemorrhage. Later in the postoperative period it may be desirable to use an overbed cradle or foot board to elevate the bedding.

A large stump tourniquet should always be placed in the immediate area of the new amputee, tied to his bed or wheel chair in such a manner that it will come free with a single motion for instant application in the event of hemorrhage. Dressings should be continually checked for bleeding for several days postoperatively.

The surgeon may have applied a pressure dressing over the stump, and he will want to change this dressing himself the first time so that he can remove the drain or drains and examine the wound. The nurse should assist him, since aseptic technique is essential.

Following open amputation the stump may have been placed in Buck's extension traction. This traction holds the skin and superficial tissue on the leg or arm so that it cannot retract, and prevents flexion deformities. Principles of simple traction care should be carried out.

A special bandage may be used over the stump dressings to hold the dressings in place, support the soft tissues, and maintain the proximal joint in a functional position. Elastic bandages are commonly used. They should be applied evenly, smoothly, with moderate tension, and obliquely to help maintain circulation. Bony prominences should be well padded.

If the stump is conical, bandaging may be ordered to mold and shrink it by reducing the amount of subcutaneous tissue. The patient may be taught to apply this pressure bandage but the nurse should be familiar with it and should check the patient's work (Slocum). The patient may have to wear a stump sock inside his prosthesis socket later on to reduce friction, absorb perspiration, and keep the socket clean. The sock is pulled out over the edge of the socket, and should fit the stump snugly and smoothly. Even if the limb shrinks, the patient should never wear more than two socks at one time. If the socket is too large as a result of stump shrinkage it should be relined.

Postoperatively the patient will have considerable pain. Narcotics will be ordered but such nursing measures as special back care and proper positioning will contribute greatly to comfort.

From the beginning of the postoperative period the patient should be put on a bed routine wherein he is turned to the prone position at specific hours of the day. This will put the hip or shoulder in a position of extension to counteract the many hours in flexion. Placement in a position of abduction is also desirable. Rotation exercises of the hip or shoulder should be done. When the patient is in the prone position he can be taught to exercise the stump by bringing it into a position of hyperextension. The nurse should explain that these exercises will do much to help him when he is ready to use his artificial limb. After the wound has healed physical therapy will be prescribed. All too often too little attention is paid by nursing personnel to the maintenance of muscle power and joint motion during the first few postoperative days, but if the nurse fails to carry out her important responsibilities at this time, rehabilitation may be a painful, prolonged experience.

PHANTOM LIMB

Phantom limb is the perception of the presence of all or part of the lost part of the body. Most amputees experience this sensation, which is believed to be due to the patient's memory of the lost part. Psychologically it is viewed as the adaptive process of mourning following loss of a needed object. As he adapts to a change in body image there is a progressive disappearance of the phantom.

Some patients experience painful phantom limb, the pain appearing simultaneously with the phantom.

The pain is commonly described as a burning or throbbing sensation, a dull ache rather than an acute or a sharp pain. It may occur without obvious reason but possible stimuli are palpation of the stump, warming or cooling of the stump, and dependent position of the limb. Examination for probable causes is careful and detailed. The stump is examined carefully and an investigation is carried out to detect possible irritating lesions in the muscles and connective tissue of the extremity, observe the circulation in the extremity, and assess the patient's psychological make-up. Treatment is instituted according to the findings.

PROSTHESES

Physicians hold different opinions as to when prosthetic devices should be applied. According to Nardi and Zuidema, it is advisable to fit the new limb as early as 3 weeks after wound healing. This may encourage the patient and allow less time for complications or contractures to develop.

A lower extremity prosthesis will carry the patient's body weight. Three types of prostheses are available. In one weight is borne on the upper part of the socket, with pressure falling on bony prominences, e.g., the ischial tuberosity in a thigh amputation. In this case the patient may use the stump sock. The second type of prosthesis places the body weight on the bottom of the socket, the end of the stump bearing the pressure. The third type, a suction limb, distributes weight throughout the socket.

When the patient has been fitted he should be transferred to a rehabilitation unit where he can have the benefit of the services of a physiatrist, a prosthetist, a physical therapist, and other personnel. Fitting a limb and teaching the patient to use it correctly is a specialty in itself. The patient must be taught to give himself good stump care so that the skin will be in the best possible condition. He should use a hand mirror, if necessary, to carefully inspect the entire stump daily in order to detect any signs of impending skin breakdown from abrasions, blisters, or ingrown hairs. Skin breakdown is of great significance to the diabetic patient. In the presence of a skin irritation he should discontinue wearing the prosthesis until the skin is intact.

The stump skin should be washed daily with a mild soap containing hexachlorophene, then dried carefully; powder if used should be applied sparingly and be of the finest grade. Stump socks should be made of soft, 100 percent virgin wool. These should be washed by hand in a solution such as Woolite and cool water, squeezed gently, and dried thoroughly. The socks should be absorbent and soft. During warm weather frequent change may be necessary. The sock should fit the stump smoothly and should not be mended; wrinkles also can produce pressure and skin breakdown.

If socks are not worn the sockets must be washed daily. They should be dry and smooth.

The patient should be instructed about the need to keep his clinic appointments, since periodic adjustments will be necessary and the stump must be examined. Wearing more than two stump socks simultaneously may indicate tissue shrinkage requiring socket adjustment. By following all the instructions given him, the patient will be able to make the necessary adjustments to his condition.

The nurse caring for an amputee on a general surgical or orthopedic nursing unit can render her most valuable service by giving him psychological support, preventing joint stiffness through maintaining a program of regular exercises, maintaining muscle strength, and preparing him for crutch walking. Triceps muscle strengthening is especially important.

Burgess and coworkers have described a new method of providing an immediate temporary prosthesis. With the patient under anesthesia, a plaster of Paris bandage is applied over a rigid stump dressing. Suspension straps for the prosthesis are inserted in the outer layers of the bandage. An artificial leg and foot of metal, the *pylon,* is attached to the plaster socket by the suspension straps. Weight-bearing can begin after the first 24 hours postoperatively and walking with weight supported on parallel bars can begin in about 5 days. Weight-bearing gait training is continued daily, and in about 25 days a permanent prosthesis is provided. At the same time a light plaster cast (socket) is provided to be worn whenever the permanent prosthesis is not worn. This early ambulation promotes mental acuity, stimulates circulation, prevents hypostatic pneumonia, and helps ensure adequate kidney and bowel function. A revision of the stump can be accomplished later when the patient's condition warrants.

Care of the Patient with Bone and Joint Injuries

STRAINS, SPRAINS, AND DISLOCATIONS

The high-speed forms of transportation currently utilized give rise to many accidents resulting in multiple bone and joint injuries. The average individual's lack of physical exercise makes him susceptible to muscle and ligamentous strain. Strains, sprains, and dislocations are commonly treated in the doctor's office or hospital clinic.

Strains

A strain is a simple injury caused by overstretching or pulling muscles and/or tendons. Back strain resulting from poor body mechanics is common and patients with this disorder are frequently treated in hospitals. The patient may feel a sudden "stitch" or sharp pain in his back with a certain movement. A strain may also occur during a fall. Following the fall there is the gradual development of stiffness, soreness, and pain on movement. The patient with severe back strain should be examined promptly by his physician.

Treatment consists of putting the injured part at rest. Heat in any form, elevation of the part to reduce edema, and gentle massage as pain and swelling subside are helpful. Taping the injured part provides support and reduces pain and swelling.

Sprains

A more severe soft tissue injury is a sprain, in which ligaments are torn and muscles and tendons are stretched. Sprain may or may not be accompanied by fracture. It is frequently difficult to differentiate between sprain and fracture and x-ray examination may be necessary. The symptoms of a sprain are pain increasing with movement of the joint or extremity, tenderness to touch, and rapidly developing edema. Ecchymosis may occur almost immediately or several hours later, depending upon the area involved.

Prompt splinting of the injured area is essential to relieve pain, immobilize the part, and prevent further injury. An extremity, such as the ankle or wrist, should be elevated to minimize edema. Cold compresses should be applied to relieve pain and further reduce edema. Heat in the form of hot compresses should not be applied until at least 48 hours after the injury.

Application of adhesive straps or a cast may be necessary. Not infrequently a severe sprain is as painful and incapacitating as a fracture.

Dislocations

A dislocation is loss of continuity of structures within a joint usually resulting from a blow to the region of a joint. The joint capsule and ligaments may be torn. In the knee, the internal cartilages may be displaced or torn. The articulating surfaces of the bones are no longer in contact and muscle spasm soon develops in the surrounding musculature. This is nature's way of splinting the injured part. A dislocation of the hip or shoulder is a major injury.

Treatment involves replacement of the bones in normal anatomical alignment within the joint as soon as possible. The bones may slip back into place rather easily in some cases; in other cases an anesthetic may be required to produce muscle relaxation and permit the manipulation to be carried out. The physician often is able to reduce the dislocation through use of manual traction. When large joints are dislocated and severe muscle spasm of large muscles is present, e.g., around the hip or shoulder joint, he will apply skin or skeletal traction to accomplish reduction. The steady pull will gradually relax the muscle and at the same time cause the bone ends to move back into normal joint articulation.

Subluxation is partial displacement or partial dislocation of a bone. It can often be reduced by manipulation. Generally injury to the joint capsule and the ligaments is not as severe as complete dislocation.

FRACTURES

A fracture is a loss of continuity of a bone. It is most frequently caused by injury due to a fall or a blow, although it may be due to pathology such as a tumor or osteoporosis. Fractures are classified variously. Figure 27-14 illustrates some common fractures.

An infraction occurs when a bone has broken within its periosteal sheath, e.g., a hairline fracture or a greenstick fracture in a child, in which the bone bends but does not break through the periosteal sheath. In an overriding fracture one bone fragment has slipped over another. An impacted fracture occurs when the bone is broken and the ends are driven together forcefully. Shortening of the limb occurs with impaction and overriding.

The most common fracture is the Colles fracture, a break in the distal end of the radius following a fall upon the outstretched hand. In Pott's fracture there is a break in the lower end of the fibula and the internal malleolus.

Fractures are treated according to their location and severity. Prompt reduction is essential to minimize muscle spasm and pain and promote healing. Efforts should be made to prevent improper bone alignment, movement of bone ends or fragments at the fracture site, introduction of bacteria into bone during surgery or into bone from skeletal wires or pins, interposition of tissue between bone ends, malnutrition, and overpulling with excessive traction, since any of these can cause delayed healing or nonunion. Should this happen, surgical intervention would be necessary to accomplish internal fixation. In this procedure the bone fragments are fixed in place. Elderly women, in particular, may have osteoporosis, which leads to a break in the neck of the femur followed by a fall. Surgical pinning, plating, or implantation of a plastic prosthesis to replace the head and neck of

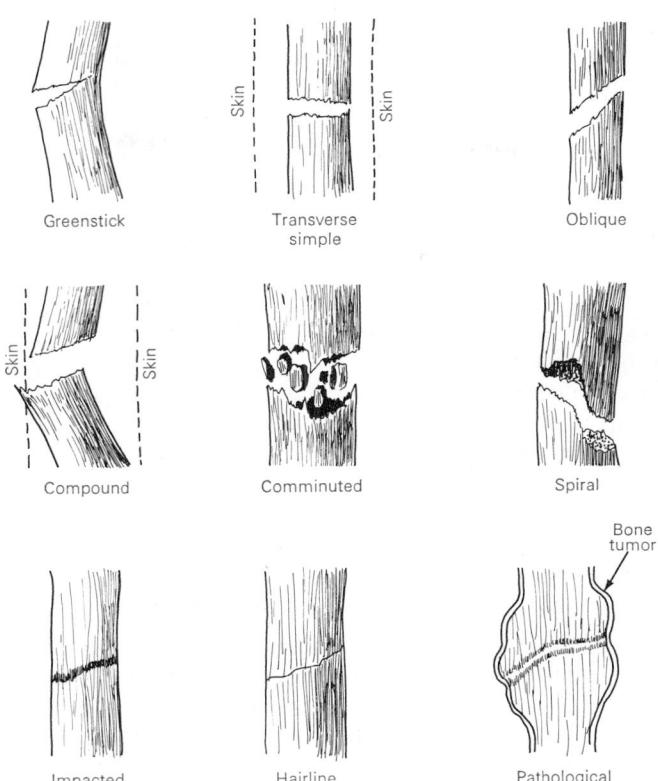

Figure 27-14
Common fractures

the femur is usually performed. Simple traction may be necessary for a short period.

Care of the Patient with a Laminectomy

Compression fracture of the spine is being seen with increasing frequency in acute hospitals as a result of ʌutomobile accidents in which the vertebral bodies are

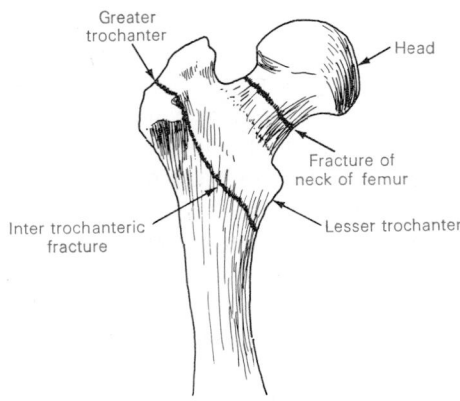

Figure 27-15
Proximal femoral
fractures

crushed, with impingment of bone upon the spinal nerves. Hemorrhage and congestion in the injured area also create pressure on the nerves, giving rise to complete or partial paralysis below the level of injury. A patient so injured may be cared for on an orthopedic frame. If the fracture is in the region of the cervical spine, cervical or head traction is applied while he is on the frame.

Laminectomy (decompression of the cord) generally is performed shortly after admission to hospital. A portion of lamina of one or more vertebrae is removed so that the emerging nerves may be exposed and tissue impinging on the involved nerves may be removed. Needless to say, an extensive neurological study will have been made prior to laminectomy in an attempt to identify the involved spinal nerves. If complete paralysis occurs at the time of the injury laminectomy may not be indicated since the spinal cord may have been severed. In this case the patient would be a quadriplegic or paraplegic, depending upon the level of the injury. Laminectomy frequently is performed for a ruptured nucleus pulposus in order to relieve impingement on the emerging spinal nerves.

Postoperatively, the patient is placed on a firm bed with a turning sheet under him. For the first 24 hours he will be maintained in the supine position as pressure on the operative site will help to prevent the development of hemorrhage and hematoma. Even though he cannot turn or be turned during these first 24 hours the nurse should encourage him to exercise his legs frequently, and record his ability to do this. The patient's back is well supported by adhesive taping; after the first 24 hours an order may be written to turn him every 2 hours or so. He should be turned in a log rolling manner, with his back supported by the turning sheet. Plastic-covered pillows should be placed between his legs before he is turned to prevent the upper leg from falling into a position of adduction. This support will also reduce the strain on his back muscles. The patient's hips should not be twisted when he is being turned. He can cooperate by tensing or splinting his back, pinching his buttocks together, and tightening his abdominal muscles to provide a supportive muscular "corset." The pillows should remain between his legs while he is in the side-lying position and his back should be supported with additional pillows. Normal spinal alignment in all positions should be maintained at all times as long as he is on bed rest to ensure muscle balance and comfort.

Ambulation is encouraged within 1 to 4 days after laminectomy, since this will help prevent hypostatic pneumonia, urinary retention, and circulatory problems. The patient should keep his back quite straight while getting out of bed and ambulating.

Spinal fusion may be done along with laminectomy, as in severe injury or for removal of a spinal tumor. In this event nursing care is more complex. The patient must be immobilized on an orthopedic frame, in a firm bed, or in a body cast for a prolonged period while healing takes place.

A full discussion of nursing care following spinal fusion is available in orthopedic and neurosurgical nursing textbooks.

Following simple laminectomy or laminectomy combined with spinal fusion, a back brace may be worn during ambulation. The patient may be more comfortable if he wears a simple cotton knit shirt under the brace which will absorb body moisture and help prevent the leather or elastic of the brace from rubbing against the skin. Care should be taken to prevent wrinkles under the brace. A woman's cotton knit shirt is not suitable for wear under an open-neck dress because of the high neckline. A suitable substitute is an inexpensive cotton slip of loose fit from which the skirt is cut off approximately 4 inches below the lower edge of the brace. In warm weather, talcum powder sprinkled on the skin under the brace is soothing.

The nurse should teach the patient how to apply his brace by having him roll into it while lying in bed and tighten and tie the laces or buckle the straps securely. The brace thus supports his back as he arises. It maintains proper back alignment and prevents pain.

Orthopedic braces are prescribed to fit the individual patient. The brace should be applied carefully so that it is fastened in place according to the physician's prescription. Bony prominences must be observed by the nurse, the patient, or a member of the patient's family for evidence of excessive pressure and breakdown of tissue, which would necessitate immediate adjustment. A loss or gain in weight may necessitate brace adjustment.

Care of the Patient with Bone and Joint Disease

RHEUMATIC DISEASE AFFECTING THE MUSCULOSKELETAL SYSTEM

The term *arthritis* means *inflammation of a joint* but both *arthritis* and *rheumatism* are "umbrella" terms that refer to a number of musculoskeletal disorders. In this text attention will be focused upon chronic arthritis, including rhematoid arthritis, ankylosing spondylitis, osteoarthritis, and gout. For a detailed discussion of pathology and medical treatment the reader is referred to appropriate textbooks.

Arthritis

About 13 million Americans suffer from some form of arthritis, and more than 3 million of these persons report that the disease limits their ability to carry on customary activity.[1] Arthritis affects more persons and causes more crippling than any other chronic disease.[2] It is the cause of well over 1 million days of hospitalization yearly and 2 billion dollars in medical costs per year.[3] The increasing number of elderly persons in the population will aggravate these problems.

RHEUMATOID ARTHRITIS

Although rheumatoid arthritis accounts for two-thirds of the deaths due to arthritis, it is of greatest significance because of the disability it causes. All too frequently the patient and his family do not recognize that much can be done to prevent severe deformities. Although individuals in all socioeconomic levels are affected, there is a greater incidence among those in lower socioeconomic levels. Rheumatoid arthritis is seen throughout the world, is most frequent in temperate climates, and is three times more common in women than in men. Onset is generally between the ages of 30 and 40 years.

[1] U.S. Department of Health, Education and Welfare: *Arthritis Source Book.* Washington D.C.: U.S. Government Printing Office, 1966, p. 3.
[2] *Ibid.,* p. 1.
[3] *Ibid.,* p. 29.

Still's disease is the juvenile form of rheumatoid arthritis. It causes severe crippling if the cervical spine is involved along with other joints. The epiphyseal cartilages of the long bones may be destroyed, with arrest of longitudinal bone growth. The systemic effects are usually more severe than those of adult forms of arthritis.

Rheumatoid arthritis is a systemic disease of the connective tissue having an acute or insidious onset. Manifestations include lassitude, generalized fatigue, muscular atrophy and weakness, loss of body weight, and in the most severe cases, exhaustion. Secondary anemia is frequently associated, and the sedimentation rate is usually elevated, especially during an acute attack. The sedimentaton rate is followed closely during the course of therapy since it provides an index of disease activity.

An acute attack frequently starts with swelling and stiffness in one or more joints. This stiffness may be especially noticeable when the individual arises in the morning. The involved joints may loosen up as the patient moves about and performs his customary activities. These early manifestations may be followed by an acute episode in which joints become enlarged, red, warm, and very painful. Muscular aching, pain, weakness, and fatigability are early complaints. Multiple joints may be involved, especially the knees, ankles, elbows, wrists, and proximal joints of the phalanges. The hallmark of rheumatoid arthritis is fusiform joints, i.e., the proximal phalangeal joints and the enlarged metacarpophalangeal joints of the hands.

Inflammation of the synovial membrane results in roughening of the smooth articular surfaces and pain upon motion. There is a narrowing of joint spaces. In severe cases there is complete joint destruction and partial or complete ankylosis of the involved joints. Formation of excess synovial fluid formation is stimulated, the joint capsule may become thickened and distended, and the ligaments and joint cartilages are damaged. The joints become enlarged due to thickening of the capsules, accumulation of fluid, and muscle atrophy. Acute attacks may occur periodically, lasting several weeks or months and followed by remissions.

Since the etiology of rheumatoid arthritis is not known, treatment is largely symptomatic according to the stages of disease. During the acute stage it is treated medically and by supportive nursing care. In the chronic phases of the disease surgery may be performed to correct deformities and improve function. Physiological rest is a cardinal principle of treatment in the acute stages. Chemical and hormonal therapy may be second in importance. The provision of a nutritious diet high in vitamins is paramount. The most effective means of preventing or minimizing crippling is provided by having the patient maintain correct posture both while at rest and while ambulating, and perform the prescribed exercises. This is especially important during remissions.

A firm mattress and a foot board should be provided. The exercises should be carried out under the supervision of the doctor and the physical therapist. Special splints or molds may be prepared to protect involved joints during acute episodes. These must be employed as ordered if maximum recovery is to be made. For example, a special wrist and hand mold may be ordered for night use to prevent ulnar deviation and to maintain thumb opposition and finger extension. This support may be alternated with passive movement and active exercises carried out under the direction of the physical therapist, the nurse, and/or the physician. Such treatment should in every case prevent the development of a nonfunctioning hand and wrist.

Many arthritics have to be constantly urged to breathe deeply. The arthritic tends to breathe shallowly, keeping his shoulders adducted and his arms on his chest. This leads to a narrow, rounded chest; the patient has difficulty in abducting his shoulders. The nurse should encourage him to practice deep breathing, exhaling fully and slowly, several times each day. The patient will greatly benefit by resting in the prone position in bed for at least part of each day, with his arms abducted. A small pillow or pad should be placed under his abdomen to allow adequate chest expansion.

All uninvolved joints should be put through a normal range of motion daily, and the patient should be encouraged to do this for himself. Since muscle atrophy is intrinsic to rheumatoid arthritis, he should be taught correct exercises to help alleviate this. Abdominal tightening, gluteal setting, quadriceps setting, foot circling, and deep breathing exercises are helpful.

The nurse should remember that the patient is the key figure in the recovery program. Although she can assess his needs and, in cooperation with other therapists, make elaborate plans for his rehabilitation, these may not succeed if he is not made an integral part of the team.

Considerable understanding of the dynamics of human behavior is needed to deal with the arthritic, who is often very demanding and quite inflexible. Empathy, consistent care, and noncritical objectivity are needed to render good nursing care. With the patient whose motivational level is low, the nurse plays a key role as confidante and supporter. She further serves as coordinator for the many therapists who are concerned with various aspects of care.

The nurse is responsible for observing reactions to drugs and accurately reporting these. The most widely used drugs are the salicylates, which have an analgesic effect and in high dosages also appear to exert an antirheumatic effect. The dosage may vary from 40 to 100 g per day according to the patient's tolerance. Salicylates are usually given to the point of toxicity, e.g., the development of tinnitus.

Phenylbutazone is an anti-inflammatory, analgesic, and antipyretic drug that may be used on a short-term basis in a dosage of 400 to 600 mg per day. It is poorly tolerated by some patients (Goodman and Gilman), and should be given with meals. Blood studies should be done frequently to detect possible untoward effects, such as decrease in the white blood cell count and bone marrow depression. Gastric intolerance and generalized edema may develop.

The antimalarial compound, chloroquine, has been used in some cases, but it is now administered less frequently because it causes visual defects. Hydroxychloroquine has not been associated with visual difficulties, as far as is known.

Gold compounds, i.e., gold sodium thiomalate and gold sodium thiosulfate, have been used for approximately 30 years in the treatment of rheumatoid arthritis. Their action is not definitely understood, but they do modify the disease in many cases, and some physicians believe gold salts to be the most effective therapeutic agents available (Goodman and Gilman), although they do not appear to modify the natural history of the disease (Goodman and Gilman). The physician's orders must be scrupulously followed and the nurse must observe the patient closely for signs of toxicity. Skin reactions may appear varying from simple erythema to severe exfoliative dermatitis. Pruritus often precedes the skin reaction and may occur when the tolerance level has been exceeded. Lesions of the mucous membranes may develop, e.g., stomatitis, gastritis, colitis, and glossitis. Severe blood dyscrasias may result, hence blood studies must be done repeatedly. Renal complications such as albuminuria and microscopic hematuria may occur.

Adrenocorticosteroids are used in selected cases. They have a potent anti-inflammatory effect, but do not alter the course of the disease. Here again, the patient must be closely followed for signs of undesirable effects including osteoporosis, peptic ulcers, diabetes, susceptibility to infections, psychoses, and Cushing's syndrome. Prednisone or prednisolone TBH is often prescribed for joint injections.

If proper body alignment is maintained so that all joints are kept in functional positions, flexion contractures of the muscles of the hips, knees, elbows, and shoulders will be prevented. During the acute phases of the disease the patient is more comfortable in a position of flexion and may place pillows under his knees, and bend his hips, elbows, and fingers. Prolonged maintenance of these positions can only lead to deformity. Hence the patient should change his position frequently. This will also relieve pressure and help prevent decubitus ulcers. Nursing personnel should put all uninvolved joints through a full range of motion at least once daily. *This can be done without a physician's written order, and should be as much a part of daily care as is the bath.* In an affected joint, the nurse carries the range of motion only to the point of pain; the physical therapist has responsibility for carrying out stretching and strengthening exercises.

Occasionally traction is used to reduce contractures, correct deformities, and maintain functional position. Since the sense of touch probably has been affected, pressure points on splints, braces, and cast molds should be observed for development of decubitus ulcers.

ANKYLOSING SPONDYLITIS (MARIE-STRÜMPELL SPONDYLITIS)

Ankylosing spondylitis is a progressive disease of the joints of the spine occurring chiefly in men between the ages of 20 and 40 years and of unknown etiology.

The disease is manifested initially in stiffness and low back pain. In the early stage it may involve the sacroiliac joints, then progress until the entire spine and the hips become ankylosed. The long spinal ligaments become calcified and frequently the costovertebral joints become ankylosed. This impairs chest expansion by inhibiting rib movement. Ankylosis of the cervical spine markedly restricts or prevents rotation of the head and neck. Marked deformities, such as flexion of the cervical spine, kyphosis, and flattening of the chest, may develop, unless preventive measures are promptly undertaken.

Treatment is aimed at keeping the spine erect in order to prevent ankylosis in a position of deformity. There is no therapy presently available that will arrest the disease process; spontaneous arrest may occur at any stage or the disease may progress until the entire spine becomes ankylosed. The process "burns itself out" in time, but takes a great toll of its victims.

The nurse should teach the patient to maintain good body alignment at all times, including periods of bed rest. He will be more comfortable during the acute stages if he assumes a position of flexion, but he should be taught the dangers of maintaining this position and be given a program of spinal hyperextension exercises.

The physical therapist will prescribe the exercises but the nurse should be familiar with this program and implement it; the therapist can spend only a short period each day with the patient, whereas the nurse supervises his care over many hours of the day and night.

In some cases ankylosis of the hip develops and an arthroplasty may be performed. If the arthroplasty involves placement of a vitallium cup, the usual skin preparation for hip surgery will be necessary (Crenshaw). The patient should be encouraged to ambulate as much as possible before surgery. Postoperatively he will be placed in hip traction with the hip held in a position of adduction, so that the head of the femur is held in the acetabulum and tissue healing takes place. When tissue healing is complete roller skate traction may be utilized followed by bicycle exercises and ambulation between parallel bars and on crutches. Exercises that can be done in bed are of great value during the recovery period.

OSTEOARTHRITIS

Most individuals over the age of 50 years show some degenerative cartilaginous changes. When degeneration is evident on radiological examination, the condition is osteoarthritis. This disorder is also called *degenerative* and *hypertrophic* arthritis. The etiology is unknown but it appears to be associated with the aging process. A high percentage of individuals do not complain of symptoms although x-ray studies reveal pathological changes. Unlike rheumatoid arthritis, osteoarthritis is not a systemic disease, being limited to specific joints, most commonly the weight-bearing joints of the hips, knees, and spine. The joint cartilage gradually becomes thin and may eventually disappear, thus markedly impairing the smooth gliding surface of the involved joints. The process does not cause pain as does rheumatoid arthritis, since cartilage contains no pain receptors. Pain develops when the process is far advanced as a consequence of the rubbing together of the rough bony surfaces.

Osteoarthritis may occur as a result of chronic trauma to joints; obesity may contribute to this. There may be malformation of the joint due to overgrowth of underlying bone, spur formation, and loss of cartilage. Gross deformity does not develop nor does joint fusion occur except when rheumatoid arthritis is present also.

Heberden's nodes develop in many patients. These bony enlargements of the distal phalangeal joints of the fingers occur most frequently in women but do not significantly affect hand and finger function. There may be aching in affected joints.

In most cases of osteoarthritis there is aching, pain and stiffness in the involved joints, but not acute inflammation. Pain characteristically is relieved by rest and subsequent increased physical activity. Pain is most severe in weight-bearing joints such as the hips and knees. Some limitation of joint motion may occur due to contracture of the joint capsule. Spinal involvement may be complicated by spur formation and pressure on nerve roots which may cause limitation of motion of the spine. Hospitalization is seldom necessary.

Older patients commonly are afflicted with several chronic diseases, degenerative arthritis being one of them. Reduction of weight may decrease strain on the spine, hips, and knees, and efforts to improve posture and strengthen muscles may be helpful. Periods of physical activity should be followed by periods of rest. Local application of heat and ingestion of analgesics may relieve the pain, but because of the chronicity of osteoarthritis, narcotics are not recommended. Occasionally the physician will inject a steroid, such as hydrocortisone, directly into the involved joint to relieve pain and stiffness. A brace may be prescribed to stabilize the spine or the knees and to relieve pain. Therapeutic efforts are aimed largely at reducing strain and pain in the involved joints. Residence in a warm, dry climate is beneficial for some patients.

GOUT

It is estimated that 800,000 to 1 million persons in the United States have gout, and that 100,000 to 120,000 new cases are found each year. Approximately 95 percent of the patients are males and they are usually past 30 years of age (Shands).

Gout is caused by a defect in purine metabolism giving rise to a marked increase in serum uric acid concentration. Renal excretion of uric acid is impaired and urate crystals are deposited in the joint cartilage, synovium, and capsule. These tophi often appear in the skin of the ear lobes.

Gout usually is monarticular. The involved joint abruptly becomes very painful, reddened, and swollen, and the overlying veins may become distended. An acute attack lasts from 3 to 10 days and is most likely to occur in the joints of the foot, especially in the first metatarsophalangeal joint. Any joint may be involved, but the spine, shoulders, and hips rarely are.

Both acute and chronic forms are seen. An acute attack may incapacitate the patient. Colchicine is administered orally to relieve the pain in an acute attack. A new drug, allopurinol, may be prescribed. Phenylbutazone (Butazolidin), ACTH, and probenecid (Benemid) are other agents sometimes prescribed. All these agents must be administered under the close supervision of a physician because near-toxic amounts are given which may cause skin rash, fever, and other undesirable side effects. Dosage must be carefully regulated and blood studies must be done routinely.

Nursing care may involve application of wet packs or ice packs to the affected joint and protection of the joint from injury. The part usually is elevated, if possible, to stimulate circulation. Fluids should be forced to at least 2,500 ml daily in efforts to flush the uric acid salts from the kidneys and bladder. Deformities rarely arise; they are treated similarly to other joint deformities.

TUMORS OF BONE

Bone tumors may be primary or secondary.

Primary tumors may be either benign or malignant. The benign form of primary bone tumor is usually slow growing and well circumscribed, and rarely metastasizes or spreads. Benign tumors include osteochondroma, osteoid osteoma, and bone cyst. These tumors seldom cause marked symptoms, and rarely are the cause of death. Bone fracture develops occasionally because of weakening of the supporting structure.

Primary malignant tumors, although rather rare, are highly malignant, metastasizing early. Lung metastases are most likely to occur. Osteogenic sarcoma is seen most frequently in young males. The usual site is the area of the epiphyseal line of the long bones. Early in the course there may be enlargement of the bone and the extremity. Some aching may be felt and a fracture may occur.

Cartilaginous tumors develop in both benign and malignant forms. Enchondroma and benign chondroblastoma are benign forms; chondrosarcoma is a primary malignant form.

Preoperatively the nurse carries out the customary preparations for bone surgery, and postoperatively provides the customary care of the amputee. Her psychological support of the patient is extremely important, since he will have many fears including fear of major surgery, fear of loss of an extremity, and fear of a recurrence of the neoplasm or a metastasis. The reader is referred to orthopedic textbooks for a detailed discussion of these tumors.

INFECTION OF BONE: OSTEOMYELITIS

Prior to the development of the antibiotic drugs, osteomyelitis was a severe orthopedic disease. It is caused most frequently by either beta hemolytic streptococci or *Staphylococcus aureus*. Septicemia is the initiating factor in many cases as a consequence of bacterial invasion of the terminal loops of the capillaries in the ends of the long bones.

If the infection is untreated, marked pyrexia (102 to 104° F) develops. There is extreme tenderness around the joint and jarring of the extremity may cause excruciating pain. With increased production of pus the periosteum may be elevated causing severe pain. Finally rupture of the periosteum may occur with spread of pus throughout the soft tissues. An abscess develops; there is redness and swelling and possibly rupture giving rise to a chronic draining sinus that is difficult to heal. Scarring and disfigurement may be the end-result.

Osteomyelitis may develop from infection about the site of a bone pin or wire or skeletal head tongs. Thus it is most important that the nurse maintain surgical asepsis in bone wounds. Compound fractures and gunshot wounds may be contributory factors. Every possible precaution must be taken by all members of the surgical team to prevent sepsis during bone surgery of osteomyelitis.

Osteomyelitis may become chronic as in development of draining sinuses. With suppuration bone is destroyed. The dead pieces, called *sequestra,* are extruded through the draining sinuses, and a wide excision, or saucerization, may be packed with gauze. If the bone has been markedly weakened by the excision it may be immobilized in a cast.

It is worth repeating that *prevention* of osteomyelitis is all-important, and that as a team leader the nurse should teach all team workers to employ the approved technique in handling wounds and skeletal traction equipment.

Bibliography

Books

Baker, Louise: *Out on a Limb.* New York: McGraw-Hill Book Company, 1946.

Burgess, Ernst M., Joseph E. Traub, and A. Bennett Wilson, Jr.: *Immediate Postsurgical Prosthetics in Management of Lower Extremity Amputees.* Washington, D.C.: Veterans Administration.

Covalt, Nila K.: *Bed Exercises for Con-*

valescent Patients. Springfield, Ill.: Charles C Thomas, Publisher, 1968.

Crenshaw, A. H. (Ed.): *Campbell's Operative Orthopaedics,* Vols. I and II. St. Louis: The C. V. Mosby Company, 1963.

de Gutierrez-Mahoney, C. G. and Esta Carini: *Neurological and Neurosurgical Nursing,* 4th ed. St. Louis: The C. V. Mosby Company, 1965.

Gartland, John J.: *Fundamentals of Orthopedics.* Philadelphia: W. B. Saunders Company, 1965.

Goodman, Louis S. and Alfred Gilman: *The Pharmacological Basis of Therapeutics.* New York: The Macmillan Company, 1966.

Hartung, Edward F., et al. (Eds.): *Arthritis. Manual for Nurses, Physical Therapists and Medical Social Workers.* New York: Arthritis and Rheumatism Foundation.

Larson, Carrol B. and Marjorie Gould: *Calderwood's Orthopedic Nursing,* 7th ed. St. Louis: The C. V. Mosby Company, 1970.

Lowman, Edward W. *Rehabilitation Monograph VI: Self Help Devices for the Arthritic.* New York: The Institute of Physical Medicine and Rehabilitation, 1954.

Nardi, George L. and George D. Zuidema (Eds.): *Surgery. A Concise Guide to Clinical Practice,* 2d ed. Boston: Little, Brown and Company, 1965.

Shands, Alfred R. and Richard B. Raney: *Handbook of Orthopaedic Surgery,* 6th ed. St. Louis: The C. V. Mosby Company, 1963.

Slocum, Donald B.: *An Atlas of Amputations.* St. Louis: The C. V. Mosby Company, 1949.

Strike Back at Arthritis. U.S. Public Health Service Publication No. 747. Washington, D.C.: U.S. Government Printing Office, 1960.

Tuttle, W. W. and Byron A. Schottelius: *Textbook of Physiology,* 15th ed. St. Louis: The C. V. Mosby Company, 1965.

Williams, Marian and Catherine Worthingham: *Therapeutic Exercise for Body Alignment and Function.* Philadelphia: W. B. Saunders Company, 1957.

Winters, Margaret C.: *Protective Body Mechanics in Daily Life and in Nursing.* Philadelphia: W. B. Saunders Company, 1952.

Articles

Bartels, Elmer C.: Allopurinol (Xanthine Oxidase Inhibitor) in the Treatment of Resistant Gout. *Journal of American Medical Association,* 198: 7:708–712, November 14, 1966.

Gibbs, Gertrude E.: Perineal Care of the Incapacitated Patient. *American Journal of Nursing.* 69:1:124–125, January, 1969.

Glover, John R.: The Major Amputations. *American Journal of Nursing* 50:9: 544–550, September, 1950.

Herman, Irwin F. and Richard T. Smith: Gout and Gouty Arthritis. *American Journal of Nursing,* 64:12:111–113, December, 1964.

Jordan, Victoria, Yoshie L. Ohara, Marilyn Smith, and Jo-Ann D. Townsley: Halo Body Cast and Spinal Fusion. *American Journal of Nursing,* 63:8:77–80, August, 1963.

Kelly, Mary: Exercises for Bedfast Patients. *American Journal of Nursing,* 66:10:2209–2213, October, 1966.

Kottke, Frederic and Russell Blanchard: Bedrest Begets Bedrest. *Nursing Forum* III: 3:56–72, November 3, 1964.

Madden, Barbara and John Affeldt: To Prevent Helplessness and Deformities. *American Journal of Nursing,* 62:12:59–61, December, 1962.

Marmor, Leonard, Barbara C. Walike, and Mary Jane Upshaw: Rheumatoid Arthritis. Surgical Intervention. *American Journal of Nursing,* 67:7: 1430–1433, July, 1967.

Monteiro, Lois A.: Hip Fracture, a Sociologist's Viewpoint. *American Journal of Nursing,* 67:6:1207–1210, June, 1967.

Moskopp, Mary Elizabeth and Jane Sloan: Nursing Care of the Amputee. *American Journal of Nursing,* 50:9: 550–555, September, 1950.

Olson, Edith V. and Ruth E. Edmonds: The Hazards of Immobility. Effects on Motor Function. *American Journal of Nursing,* 67:4:788–790, April, 1967.

Senf, Harriet R.: Caring for the Patient in the CircOlectric Bed. *American Journal of Nursing,* 60:2:227–230, February, 1960.

Skinner, Geraldine: Head Traction and the Stryker Frame. *American Journal of Nursing,* 52:6:694–697, June, 1952.

Skinner, Geraldine: The Nurse—Key Figure in Preventive and Restorative Care. *Hospitals,* 35:1:52; 55–56, January 1, 1961.

Skinner, Geraldine: The Wheel Chair Patient. *Nursing World,* 128:6:28–29, July, 1954.

Walike, Barbara C.: Rheumatoid Arthritis—Personality Factors. *American Journal of Nursing,* 67:7:1427–1430, July, 1967.

Walike, Barbara C., Leonard Marmor, and Mary Jane Upshaw: Rheumatoid Arthritis. *American Journal of Nursing,* 67:7:1420–1426, July, 1967.

Instant Limbs for Amputees at Surgery. *Medical World News,* 7:28:35–38, July 29, 1966.

CHAPTER 28
THE PATIENT
WITH DISEASE
OF THE
SKIN AND
SUBCUTANEOUS
TISSUE

SECTION 1
DISORDERS
OF THE
SKIN

HONOR B. DUFOUR

The nurse often assumes a unique role in dermatologic practice. It is interesting that individuals who would not hesitate to consult a physician concerning medical problems in general think nothing of asking a nurse, a pharmacist, or even a friend how to treat a variety of skin disturbances. In most of these instances, the individual is really seeking relief of symptoms such as itching and rash. There is really no way of determining how much self-medication and treatment are practiced in skin conditions. In addition to this tendency on the part of the public to seek advice where they may find it is the fact that the nurse is often employed in jobs such as school nursing, public health nursing, or industrial nursing where she is charged with making certain initial decisions concerning diseases of the skin. Consequently, it is necessary for the nurse to know certain basic information concerning the common skin diseases. She should be able to describe skin lesions accurately and in detail. Included in this description are the shape, size, and color of a lesion as well as its distribution, e.g., whether it is localized to some specific area or generalized. She should attempt to elicit a history through careful questioning of the patient. Her questions should concern such items as (1) date of onset, (2) manner of progression of the lesion(s), (3) change in appearance of the lesion, (4) itching, (5) presence of pain, redness, or swelling, (6) possibility that the dermatosis is associated with certain food, drugs, or cosmetics, (7) any treatment the patient has been receiving. With this information, the nurse should be able to make a sound clinical judgment as to the kind of medical care the patient should seek.

Structure and Function of the Skin

The skin is more than just a covering for the body. It is a complex structure serving three principal functions: protection, sensation, and temperature regulation.

The intact horny surface of the skin, its normally slightly acid reaction, and certain chemical constituents of the sebum and sweat are important factors in protection against infection. As the largest sensory organ of the body, it acts as a barrier between the internal organs and the external environment. Not only is the skin subjected to noxious external agents, it is also a sensitive reflector of internal disease. It is necessary to understand the structure of the skin in order to comprehend the cause and effect of this complex interplay.

The skin is divided into three layers. The outer layer of the skin is the *epidermis*. This is the most superficial layer and it performs a number of complicated functions. The two distinct types of cells in the epidermis are the keratin-forming cells and the melanin-forming cells. The latter cells synthesize melanin, the principal pigment of the epidermis. The cells in the lower portion of the epidermis are constantly reproducing. The new cells are pushed outward and gradually age and change through several stages, finally dying. These cornified or horny flakes are constantly being shed from the surface of the body.

The dermis or corium is the second layer of the skin; it is a firm, fibrous, elastic connective tissue network containing the blood vessels, lymphatics, nerves, and glands. The sebaceous glands and the shorter hair follicles originate in the corium. The ground substance of the corium is of great physiological importance since it contains proteins, electrolytes, tissue fluid, and hyaluronic acid.

Beneath the dermis is the subcutaneous tissue, which is composed of a looser type of connective tissue. It varies greatly in extent in different parts of the body. This layer acts as a depot for the storage of fat and it supports the blood vessels and nerves that pass from the tissues beneath to the corium above. The deeper hair follicles and the sweat glands originate in this layer.

The skin is richly supplied with sensory and motor nerves and contains several types of specialized end-organs. Some are sensitive to touch; others to pain, pressure, heat, cold. Itching of the skin is an important presenting symptom in a large group of patients.

Hair, nails, and glands (both sebaceous glands and sweat glands) are appendages of the skin. Each hair consists of a cylindrical shaft and a root, which is contained in a hair follicle in the corium and subcutaneous tissue.

The nails are closely packed, cornified epidermal cells produced by specialized cells on the dorsa of the terminal phalanges of the fingers and toes. Unlike hair growth, which is periodic, nail growth is continuous. Nail growth may be altered by such factors as old age, serious illness, systemic disease, occupational injury, or dermatoses of the hands.

The two principal types of glands in the skin are situated in the dermis or subcutaneous tissue and are produced by invagination of specialized cells from the epidermis. Sebaceous glands are present over the whole body except the palms and the soles. They produce the oily material (sebum) that keeps the skin and hair soft and pliable. Sweat glands consist of coiled tubes situated in the subcutaneous tissue opening by a duct on the surface of the skin. The eccrine (exocrine) glands are present over the entire surface of the body, being especially numerous on the palms and soles. They produce a watery secretion which by wetting the body surface causes evaporation; this mechanism serves to maintain body temperature. The secretory rate is under the control of the autonomic nervous system. Salt and small amounts of waste products are present in the sweat. The apocrine sweat glands are larger than the eccrine and their ducts usually open into a hair follicle. They occur chiefly in the armpits, the genital and oral areas, and the nipples and areolae.

General Principles of Diagnosis and Treatment

The physician will attempt to establish a diagnosis, but if an exact diagnosis cannot be made, then the nature and causes of the eruption will be determined as far as possible. The physician will consider the history, location, and configuration of the eruption as well as its character. Is the cause primarily internal or external? If external in origin, is it due to an external irritant (physical, chemical, or allergic) or an infectious agent (bacterium, fungus, virus, or animal parasite)? If internal, is it due to a specific infection, drug sensitization, or other allergic phenomenon? Although no two skin diseases look alike, it is important to recognize and describe the primary changes produced in the skin by the disease as well as secondary changes subsequently produced by such factors as rubbing or scratching, medication, and involution and healing.

Primary Lesions

The *macule* is a circumscribed flat spot on the skin. The *papule* is a circumscribed, solid elevation of the skin, no larger than a pea. The *nodule* (a tubercle or a tumor) is a larger solid circumscribed elevation of the skin. The *wheal* or *hive* is an elevation of the skin due to edema of the dermis. It may be whitish or pink and tends to change in shape and to appear intermittently. The *vesicle* is a circumscribed

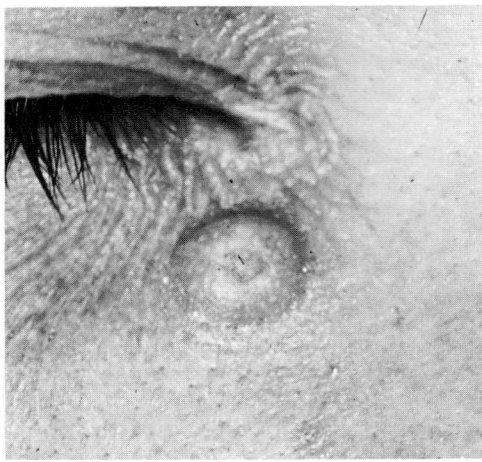

Figure 28-1 Nodule. Note size in relation to patient's eye and eyelid. (Courtesy of Victor A. Newcomer, Professor of Dermatology, School of Medicine, UCLA.)

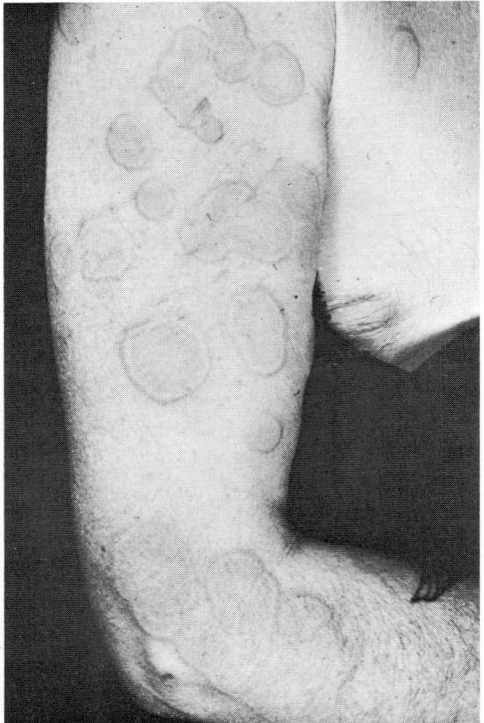

Figure 28-2 Wheal. (Courtesy of Victor A. Newcomer, Professor of Dermatology, School of Medicine, UCLA.)

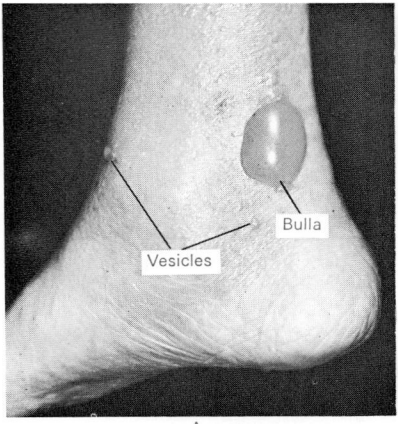
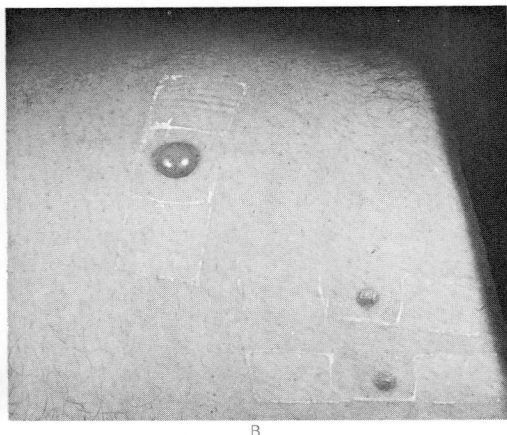

Figure 28–3
A, Bulla and vesicles on heel and ankle. Note difference in size. B, Vesicles on outer aspect of knee and thigh. (Courtesy of Victor A. Newcomer, Professor of Dermatology, School of Medicine, UCLA.)

elevation containing fluid and is no larger than a pea. The *bulla* is similar to the vesicle but is larger. The *pustule* is similar to the vesicle but contains pus.

Secondary Lesions

A *scale* is a thin, compacted plate-like structure composed of dead cornified cells, which are shed by the skin. A *crust* is a dried mass of serum, pus, dead skin, medication, and debris. An *excoriation* is a superficial loss of substance produced by rubbing, scratching, or other injury. A *fissure* is a linear break in the skin which is sharply defined. An *ulcer* is a loss of skin substance of irregular size and shape extending into the corium. A *scar* is the connective tissue that forms to replace tissue lost through injury or disease. A *keloid* is a hypertrophic scar. *Lichenifica-*

Figure 28–4
Pustule. (Greatly enlarged from actual size.) (Courtesy of Victor A. Newcomer, Professor of Dermatology, School of Medicine, UCLA.)

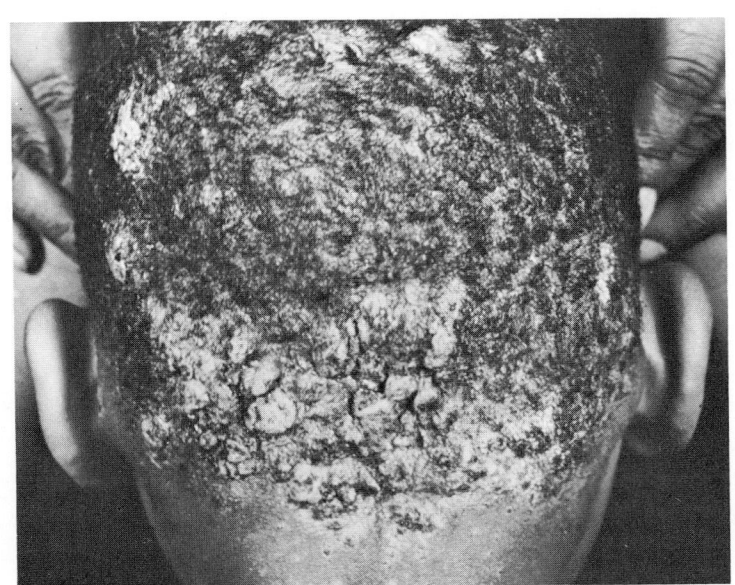

Figure 28–5
Crusts. (Courtesy of Victor A. Newcomer, Professor of Dermatology, School of Medicine, UCLA.)

tion refers to diffuse thickening and scaling with resultant increase in the skin lines and markings.

ESTABLISHING THE DIAGNOSIS AND PLANNING THE TREATMENT

The nurse plays an important role in the diagnosis of skin disease. Often it is she who sees and talks to the patient both before and after the physician has taken the history and examined him. It is essential that the nurse be a keen observer and an intelligent listener and interviewer. Frequently the patient will talk more freely with the nurse than with the physician in the mistaken idea that the physician is "too busy" to listen to a long story. Many patients are anxious and a little frightened

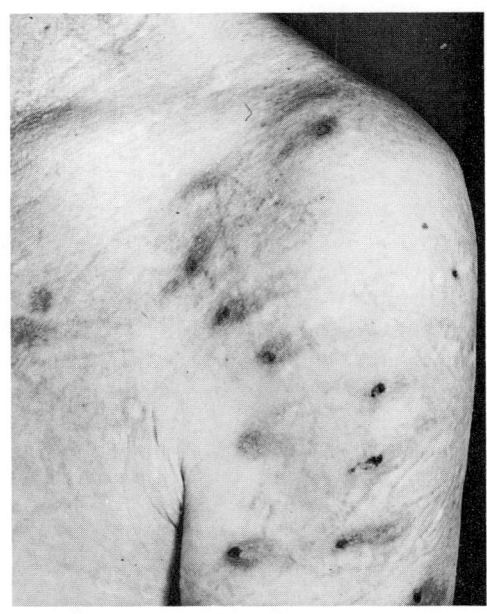

Figure 28-6
Excoriations on shoulder and upper arm. (Courtesy of Victor A. Newcomer, Professor of Dermatology, School of Medicine, UCLA.)

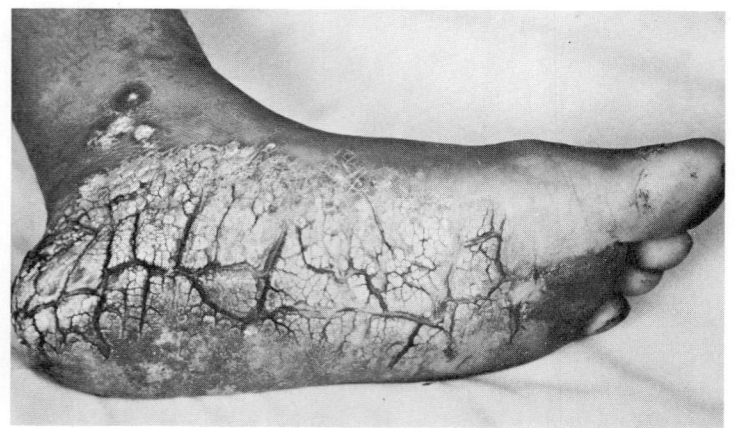

Figure 28-7
Fissures. (Courtesy of Victor A. Newcomer, Professor of Dermatology, School of Medicine, UCLA.)

when the physician is examining them and remember answers to questions only after the physician has left. The nurse can fill in these gaps, and can assure the patient that the information will be given to the physician.

Having established the diagnosis, the physician will determine what treatment, if any, is called for. In assisting the physician with treatment and procedures, the nurse must learn to handle her own feelings. Although the patient with a skin disorder may have a repulsive appearance, he may feel a need for emotional support. If the nurse communicates her feeling of distaste or revulsion, this can only compound the problems already present. The nurse should remember that the patient's self-image is largely colored by his reflection.

The plan of therapy may consist of topical and/or systemic measures. The demands upon the nurse's patience and ingenuity are endless and often require her to adapt procedures to meet the specific patient's needs. Thus the nurse must have an understanding of the principles upon which the therapy is based. The treatment selected should be the one best suited to the particular need and the *least likely to cause irritation.*

TOPICAL TREATMENT AND SYSTEMIC TREATMENT

Topical treatment generally includes baths, soaks, and wet dressings. These solutions are employed for the following purposes: (1) relief of itching, (2) disinfecting and deodorizing, (3) soothing irritated and inflamed skin, (4) softening crusts and scales, and (5) softening and lubricating dry lichenified skin. Warm compresses and heating pads aid by increasing circulation and thereby combating infection.

Starch (1 to 2 cupfuls) or oatmeal (2 to 3 cupfuls poured into a cheesecloth bag)

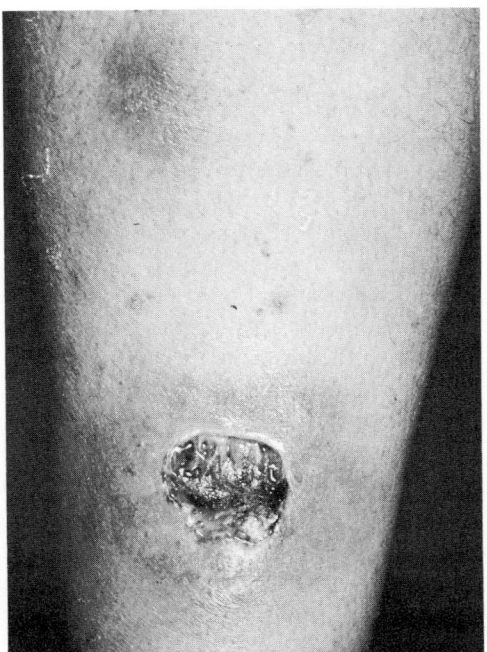

*Figure 28-8
Ulcer. (Courtesy of
Victor A. Newcomer,
Professor of Dermatology,
School of Medicine,
UCLA.)*

may be used in acute irritative eruptions. Potassium permanganate (10 g in 30 gallons of water, 1:12,000 dilution) is disinfecting and deodorizing. Household bleach (5 percent hypochlorite solution, 2 ounces) combined with sodium bicarbonate (2 ounces) in a half-tubful of water may be used for the same purpose and does not stain. Several oils are available for this use also. The temperature of the solution should be about 99° F unless otherwise ordered. The complete therapeutic tub bath provides the greatest relief from irritation due to temperature change, bedclothes, and other aggravating factors. The skin should be patted dry, *never* rubbed.

Wet dressings are widely used for acute, swollen, vesicular, and eroded eruptions. The following dressings are in general use: physiologic salt solution, boric acid (saturated solution), aluminum acetate solution U.S.P. (Burow's solution, approximately 1:16), potassium permanganate solution (1:5,000 to 1:10,000), silver nitrate solution (1:5,000 to 1:10,000).

The dressing should not be applied heavily. It should not be covered with rubber or plastic but should keep the part cool through evaporation. It should be kept sopping wet and should be changed two or three times daily. It is not safe practice to keep applying solution to the same dressing, because the evaporative process causes the solution to become concentrated and this higher concentration might be irritating. The nurse must painstakingly remove and replace dressings several times a day. Normal skin areas adjacent to the treated area can be protected from maceration through the application of a protective bland substance such as petrolatum.

Usually after the acute condition has been treated as described, the physician will prescribe a specific kind of therapy.

The nurse also needs to have some knowledge about application of lotions and pastes. In general, no substance is applied to the skin for cleansing or any other purpose without a specific order and none is applied until the previous medication has been removed. It is not uncommon to encounter lesions so thickly covered with a topical medication as to be completely obscured; the lesions must be thoroughly cleansed before any ordered medications is applied.

The nurse should explain every procedure beforehand and allow the patient to ask questions. She should not hesitate to tell the patient that a certain procedure will be painful. Often it is the patient who provides support to the nurse during a debridement procedure, because she has previously explained it to him. In this way, the patient is actively participating in his care and treatment.

If the lesion is covered by a crust that must be removed by forceps, the physician may order that it first be soaked with normal saline, hydrogen peroxide, or a similar substance. Another method is to gently scrub the involved area with sponges soaked in a hexachlorophene solution. All debris and materials used for cleaning should be collected in a paper bag or other receptacle for disposal.

The nurse should take necessary measures to protect the bed linens against soil and moisture, as a matter of both patient comfort and institutional operation. This may pose a problem, because most waterproof substances retain heat when in contact with the body surface; therefore, plastic sheets and similar materials are not recommended. Disposable bed protectors (Chux) may be useful in certain cases, but in severely weeping lesions it may be necessary to change bed linen frequently.

If the disorder is communicable, customary isolation procedures must be observed.

In certain cases, these substances act as a vehicle for other medications, e.g., an antipruritic or bacteriostatic agent may be added. In general, local anesthetic agents ("caines") are used with caution because of their tendency to cause allergic dermatitis. Bacitracin, polymyxin, and neomycin are effective against a wide variety of bacteria and rarely cause irritation.

Systemic treatment is necessary in many cases in addition to local treatment. Any underlying metabolic or endocrine disorder, blood dyscrasia, or nutritional deficiency should be corrected if possible. Appropriate antibiotics given either orally or by injection will quickly cure many infections of the skin and subcutaneous tissues.

Since any skin lesion is usually noticeable and often distasteful to the average person, the tendency to self-treat is great. It is difficult to educate the public to the fact that such self-treatment usually is worse than none at all. Dermatologists and members of the health team frequently are required to treat the disagreeable complications of overzealous or misdirected therapeutic efforts.

The clinical pictures presented in this section are divided into etiological grouping and limited to the major or common examples of each group. Systemic diseases that may manifest cutaneous lesions are not covered in this section. Principles of treatment and nursing care are presented rather than specific procedures, since there is little standardization in dermatologic therapy.

Bacterial Infections

Bacteria exist on the skin as both normal nonpathogenic flora or as pathogenic organisms. The most common pyodermas are caused by either streptococcal or staphylococcal organisms.

Impetigo Contagiosa (Streptococci or Staphylococci)

The infection begins as a reddish macule that becomes vesicular or vesiculopustular. It ruptures easily, leaving a superficial moist erosion. It tends to spread peripherally producing sharply marginated lesions that may be ringed or bizarre in outline. The exudate dries to form heavy, honey-colored crusts (the color may be altered in the presence of bleeding, medication, or debris). It tends to heal without scarring, and usually involves the exposed parts, especially the face. It is autoinoculable and contagious.

The condition is seen most often in children, and usually the burden of treatment falls upon the mother, who thus must understand the principles of therapy. The nurse is responsible for teaching the parent how to perform the necessary tasks even though most dermatologists and skin clinics provide printed instructions for this. General principles of treatment and nursing care include these points:

1. Prevention of spread of the disease through extreme cleanliness and careful disposal of waste materials. The patient should have a separate towel and wash-cloth and his bedding should be changed frequently and washed immediately.

2. Careful removal of undermined skin, crusts, and debris is necessary. This removal is accomplished by softening the crusts with hydrogen peroxide or an antiseptic soap solution and then gently pulling them free with forceps. This process is often referred to as *tweezing* and is a form of debridement.

3. After removal of crusts, bacitracin, polymyxin, neomycin, iodochlorhydroxy-quin (Vioform), or an ammoniated mercury ointment is applied.

4. Children may *not* attend school as long as the disease is active. Usually, treatment is continued for 3 days after the lesions have disappeared.

5. Antibiotics are administered orally or parenterally only in severe or extensive eruptions.

Folliculitis, Furuncle, Carbuncle (Usually Staphylococcus aureus)

These infections involve the hair follicles or occasionally the duct of a gland, varying primarily in the extent of the involvement. The lesion of staphylococcal folliculitis is a small, red, raised "pimple" in a single hair follicle; there may be one or many lesions. The patient usually does not seek medical advice unless there is widespread involvement of such areas as the scalp, beard, axilla, or genital region with recurrent and chronic pustular lesions. The *furuncle* (boil) is a larger lesion, deeper red and causing more swelling, but still confined to a single hair follicle; it frequently extends into the subcutaneous tissue. Localization of the infection produces hardening in the involved area, and with tissue destruction the lesion "points." In the case of a single furuncle, the patient may derive great relief from the use of hot moist compresses, and the drainage will be hastened. No effort should be made to force drainage prematurely by either squeezing or pricking the lesion since this may lead to deeper, more widespread tissue involvement. If the furuncle does not drain spontaneously, or if the pain is very severe, then the physician may incise and drain the area of infection. Following incision and drainage, it is usual to irrigate the wound with antibiotic solutions and apply neomycin or other appropriate bacteriostatic ointments to prevent the spread of infection. If the infection is not adequately controlled by the above measures and shows signs of spreading, the lesion should be cultured and sensitivity tests performed before appropriate systemic antibiotic therapy is started.

A *carbuncle* is a more extensive lesion than a furuncle; it is characterized by widespread inflammation of skin and subcutaneous tissue and "pointing" at several follicular orifices. Predisposing factors include general debility and metabolic disorders such as diabetes mellitus. In the older patient it is routine to rule out diabetes. This condition can occur in any location but appears most commonly on the posterior neck region. Carbuncles may be associated with systemic symptoms such as general malaise, fever, leukocytosis, and even septicemia. Before the advent of antibiotics, fatal cases were not uncommon. Carbuncles do not tend to localize as do furuncles, therefore the treatment of choice is systemic administration of the antibiotic to which the invading organism is sensitive. Incision and drainage also are carried out when the condition is fluctuant. In severe cases there may be extensive cellulitis, lymphangitis, lymphadenitis, or general toxic symptoms.

Paronychia (Staphylococci, Streptococci)

This infection is characterized by redness and swelling of the tissues about the fingernails. The invading organisms gain entry at the side of the nail through a break in the cuticle or at the site of a hangnail. This condition is found most commonly in individuals who must wash their hands frequently or whose occupation

DISEASE	CAUSATIVE FACTOR	TYPE OF LESION	USUAL LOCATION	MEDICAL TREATMENT
Erysipelas	Beta hemolytic streptococcus	Angry, red inflammation of skin and subcutaneous tissue; often irregular blisters	Face, corner of mouth, beneath ear	Isolation; antibiotics, cold compresses; general symptomatic and supportive measures
Tuberculosis of skin (lupus vulgaris)	Tubercle bacillus	Nodules, ulcers, plaques	Face	Antituberculosis chemotherapy; general symptomatic and supportive measures
Leprosy (Hansen's disease) Lepromatous form	*Mycobacterium leprae* (Hansen's bacillus)	Inflammatory granulomatous lesions	May occur anywhere; most common on extremities	May be isolated; sulfones (Diasone, Promin, Promizole)
Tuberculoid form		Less pronounced lesions; reddish macule with indefinite border		
Tularemia	*Pasteurella tularensis*	Nodule or ulcer; regional lymph node involvement	Site of inoculation	Antibiotics (streptomycin, tetracycline); general supportive measures

TABLE 28-1
Uncommon Bacterial Infections

entails "wet work." Boggy redness and swelling of the paronychial tissues occurs with separation of the nail folds from the nail plate. If ignored, this process may extend beneath the cuticle and lead to dystrophy of the nail. As pus collects, the area becomes swollen, hot, and painful. The treatment is usually conservative, involving the use of hot soaks to encourage drainage. In some instances, it is necessary to incise the soft tissues at the side of the nail to relieve pressure and allow for drainage of pus. Topical or systemic antibiotics are usually not necessary. Successful treatment requires that the involved finger or fingers be kept clean and dry except for prescribed treatments.

A description of less common bacterial infections is given in Table 28-1.

Viral Infections

Warts

Warts (verrucae) are benign epithelial tumors caused by a filtrable virus. They are autoinoculable and transmissible. They occur in several forms according to location: common wart (verruca vulgaris), juvenile wart (verruca plana juvenilis), plantar wart (verruca plantaris), and venereal wart (verruca acuminata). All these warts are formed through hypertrophy of the papillae, and they may be found singly or in numbers. The nurse will encounter the so-called common wart most often in children and must be prepared to educate parents concerning treatment. Warts may disappear spontaneously; this makes treatment difficult to evaluate. There is no specific therapy; however, local destructive measures are most likely to be successful although regardless of the method employed scars will probably result. The modality chosen depends on the type, location, size, and number encountered. Local destructive methods include curettage or excision, freezing, electrodesiccation, use of caustics, and x-ray treatment, among others. Systemic measures include administration of bismuth salicylate in oil, 1 cc intramuscularly, or bismuth orally, wart vaccine injections, and smallpox vaccination every 2 weeks for eight to 10 times.

Herpes Simplex

Herpes simplex is caused by a filtrable virus producing grouped burning, itching vesicles on an inflammatory base usually on or near mucocutaneous junctions (lips, nose, face, or genitalia) though no area of skin is immune to attack. Unless herpes is complicated by secondary infection, the vesicles dry, forming a crust, followed by exfoliation and spontaneous healing in 8 to 10 days. In many cases the physical resistance is lowered due to illness, fatigue, or exposure to irritants such as sun and wind, before the lesions appear. In some cases there appears to be an association with menstrual periods or gastrointestinal upsets.

Treatment is designed to promote comfort and prevent secondary infection. Boric acid or Burow's solution compresses are applied through the acute weeping stage, followed by ointments (boric acid, bacitracin, or neomycin) once the lesions are dry and crusted. In recurrent cases, smallpox vaccinations once every 2 weeks for eight to 10 times may be effective.

Herpes Zoster

Herpes zoster is caused by a filtrable virus that attacks the posterior root ganglia and posterior horn of the spinal cord and skin. It is sometimes associated with leukemia, Hodgkin's disease, trauma, or lowered physical resistance, and undoubtedly is associated with varicella. The dermatitis is usually preceded by neuralgic pain, hyperesthesias, or itching, and at times by constitutional symptoms. Following the development of erythema, grouped vesicles appear in crops along the course of the affected nerve. Herpes zoster varies in severity from mild cases in which vesiculation does not occur to gangrenous forms that leave permanent scars. When the ophthalmic branch of the trigeminal nerve is involved there may be such complications as corneal ulceration, iritis, cyclitis, and scleritis.

At present there is no systemic treatment; local treatment is directed toward relieving pain and preventing neuritis. Analgesics, compresses, and lotions are administered through the acute stage followed by mild ointments or pastes after the lesions have dried. Eye lesions should be treated by an ophthalmologist from the onset. Useful measures include intramuscular injections of thiamine chloride and posterior pituitary injection (Pituitrin). Although tetracycline is not specific, it is thought that complications may be prevented thereby.

Fungal Diseases

DEEP MYCOSES

Actinomycosis

Actinomycosis (lumpy jaw, nocardiasis) is caused by *Actinomyces bovis* and several species of Nocardia. The majority of cases follow dental extraction or trauma to the lower jaw. In some cases there is antecedent local trauma to other areas. The lungs may be involved through inhalation of the organism; the abdomen, through swallowing or formation of metastases. Indolent dark purple granulomatous abscesses develop usually followed by draining sinuses. The surface of the affected area is lumpy.

Tetracycline, sulfadiazine, and penicillin are effective (listed in declining order of efficiency). Surgical excision is of value if osteomylitis occurs and in small superficial lesions. X-ray therapy often is used as adjunctive therapy.

North American Blastomycosis

The causative organism is *Blastomyces dermatitidis*. The infection begins as a papule or papulopustule and spreads by peripheral extension, assuming a serpiginous or arciform shape. The edges are wart-like crusts containing tiny abscesses. The organism is found in cultures and demonstrated on microscopic examination of tissue.

Blastomycosis is treated by both local and systemic methods, including excision, debridement, administration of specific antibiotics, and use of vaccine. X-ray therapy is of value.

Coccidioidomycosis

In coccidioidomycosis (San Joaquin Fever, Valley Fever) the initial infection produces fever and chest symptoms often misdiagnosed as pneumonia or influenza. Skin lesions appear similar to those of erythema nodosum. With dissemination to bones, joints, lungs, and meninges, subcutaneous abscesses, ulcers, and sinuses develop. Death is not uncommon if the infection is widely disseminated.

Complete bed rest is ordered and supportive measures are given. A blood transfusion and intramuscular injections of amphotericin B or vaccine may be of value. Thymol given locally and orally has been recommended.

SUPERFICIAL MYCOSES

Fungus Infection of Scalp (Tinea Capitis)

The infection is caused in over 90 percent of cases by *microsporum lanosum* or *microsporum audouini,* both of which fluoresce green under the Wood light. The former produces greater inflammation than the latter in general, although infection with either can produce bald patches in prepubertal children. Inflammation may vary from a gray scaling patch to deep pustulation resembling a carbuncle (kerion). Rarer types that are nonfluorescent or poorly fluorescent may infect adults also. The diagnosis in all cases is proved by microscopic examination of the hairs and by culture.

The hair must be clipped weekly. A daily shampoo is given followed by manual epilation of the patches and application of a fungicide. A stocking cap must be worn and epilated hairs must be collected and burned after each treatment session. Common use of combs and caps must be avoided. Floors and furniture must be vacuum-cleaned frequently. X-ray epilation is necessary if the above measures fail after 1 to 2 months of trial or if the patient or parent fails to cooperate in carrying out the treatment. If topical treatment is unsuccessful after a reasonable length of time an antifungal drug such as griseofulvin may be administered orally.

Fungus Infection of Body (Tinea Corporis)

The infection is characterized by the formation of well-circumscribed circular, ring-like lesions. In the early stage they are often acutely red, but soon fade centrally with peripheral extension. The lesions are caused by various species of Trichophyton and Microsporum.

The infection is successfully eradicated by fungicides such as sulfur, iodine, mercury, and certain newer proprietary preparations (e.g., Asteral, Sopronol, Desenex).

Fungus Infection of Extremities (Epidermophytosis)

The infection is chiefly caused by two species, *Trichophyton gypseum,* which causes an inflammatory infection, and *Trichophyton purpureum,* which causes a chronic noninflammatory infection. The inflammatory type in the acute state is vesicular, appearing usually between and about the toes, with fissuring and maceration.

In the acute stage, the treatment consists of mild compresses (boric acid, Burow's solution or potassium permanganate solution) and debridement. In the subacute and chronic stages, compresses for shorter periods combined with one-half strength Whitfield's ointment, Desenex ointment, Sopronol ointment, sulfur, or ammoniated mercury ointments and pastes may be used. Post-treatment eczematization and "id" involvement of hands or body are treated as eczema.

The noninflammatory type is most difficult to treat and exists as dull red, scaling patches often involving the nails as well as adjacent skin of palms and soles. Stronger preparations are often necessary. Asterol ointment has been reported to be curative.

Fungus Infection of Nails (Onychomycosis)

Involvement usually begins at the distal or lateral border of the nails producing whitish patches with heaping of scale under the nail. The involved nail is friable and dull.

Treatment is difficult, often extending through years, and necessitates continual debridement of diseased nail tissue followed by use of 5 percent thymol in chloroform or 5 percent chrysarobin in chloroform applied after the nail has been scraped. Some success has been achieved with the systemic use of griseofulvin (Fulvicin).

Fungus Infection of Ear (Otomycosis)

The infection occurs in all degrees of activity from erosion and weeping to chronic infiltration and scaling and is caused by several species of fungi, but true cases are extremely uncommon. Most cases diagnosed as such are due, rather, to eczema or bacteria. It is well to prove the presence of a fungus before instituting specific therapy.

Fungus Infection of Beard (Tinea Barbae)

The infection is usually caused by *M. lanosum* or *T. gypseum*, producing inflammatory lesions, which at times are kerionic, as in tinea capitis of animal origin.

The treatment is similar to that of tinea capitis, including manual epilation.

Eruptions Due to Animal Parasites

Arachnidism (Spider Bites)

The most serious bite is that of the black widow spider. The bite produces severe pain and serious systemic symptoms: chills, vomiting, cramps, delirium, partial paralysis. Intense reaction usually occurs at the site of the bite.

Calcium gluconate is administered intravenously. A specific antiserum is available and is recommended. Morphine, atropine, and epinephrine are used to combat shock.

Bee Stings (Wasps, Ants)

The common symptoms are urticaria-like eruptions with local swelling and pain. However, in persons highly allergic to the venom, severe systemic reactions including shock can occur, and death may follow.

Antihistamines in the form of ointments and tablets are given to block systemic reactions. In severe cases, injections of caffeine or epinephrine may be necessary.

Flea Bites

Flea bites occur commonly in beach and coastal urban areas and are characterized by grouped, itching, papular, or papulovesicular lesions varying with the sensitivity of the individual. In hypersensitive individuals hives may result secondary to absorption of flea antigen from the primary bites. Itching papular lesions may develop in children particularly on the extremities (papular urticaria). Excoriation and secondary pyoderma often result. Diagnosis is confirmed by the presence of grouped wheal-like lesions with central puncta. Flea bites are more frequent during warm weather.

Antipruritics are applied locally; antihistamines and thiamine chloride are administered orally as repellents. Prophylactically, DDT 5 to 10 percent in powder may be applied to clothing and sprayed in breeding places. A series of injections of flea antigen may hasten desensitization, which usually develops spontaneously in time.

Pediculosis

Pediculosis is due to bites of the head (pediculosis capitis), body (pediculosis corporis), and pubic areas (pediculosis pubis) by crab lice. Intense itching results. Excoriations with secondary impetiginization or cellulitis and regional adenitis are often present. Head and pubic lice live on the skin and leave their eggs or nits attached to hair. The body louse lives in and lays its eggs in clothing and goes onto the body to feed. One should look for it in the clothing when diagnosis is suspected.

Lindane (Kwell) or benzyl benzoate is effective in head and pubic infestations. In body lice infestations, all clothing should be sterilized. Secondary dermatitis and infections should be appropriately treated.

Scabies

Scabies is due to infestation by *Sarcoptes scabiei* var. hominis (a mite), which causes itching and eruption on the extremities and trunk manifested usually by minute excoriated papules. The elementary lesion is the burrow which usually is seen most clearly on the sides of the fingers or about the wrists; the mite or its eggs can thereby be demonstrated microscopically. In infants, it is often manifested by vesiculopustules on the fingers, palms, and soles. Secondary pyoderma is common.

With the availability of Kwell ointment or lotion and benzyl benzoate emulsion, the treatment has been greatly simplified. The whole body must be treated, and the entire family and personal contacts must be treated at the same time to prevent cross-transmission. Clothing and bedding must be sterilized.

Treatment of secondary dermatitis and pyoderma, if they occur, will be determined by the causative organism.

Eczema, including Allergic Contact Dermatitis

The term *eczema* describes a type of eruption rather than a specific disease. Eczema may be due to widely differing causes. Mild eczematous eruptions may consist of erythema and papules or papulovesicular lesions. More severe eruptions are edematous, frankly vesicular, eroded, weeping, and crusted. In chronic forms the skin may be markedly thickened, scaling, and fissured. Itching is present in all forms. Eczema is an allergic response to exogenous or endogenous allergens.

Contact Eczema

In contact eczema the eruption is localized to the area in contact with the offending agent.

In contact dermatitis caused by poison ivy, poison oak, primrose, and other plants, the eruption is often asymmetrical, streaked, patchy, and bizarre in outline.

Nearly all cases of contact dermatitis are due to chemical agents. Physical agents play a minor role. Most causative chemicals are either *primary irritants* or *sensitizers*. Occasionally, primary irritants may also be sensitizers. Primary irritants cause dermatitis by direct contact if present in sufficient intensity or quantity for a sufficient length of time, e.g., sulfuric acid, soaps, solvents, cutting oils.

Cutaneous sensitizers do not necessarily cause demonstrable cutaneous change on first contact, but sensitize the skin so that after 5 to 7 days or more further contact anywhere on the body will cause dermatitis, e.g., poison oak, benzocaine, perfumes, cosmetics, dusts, feathers, and wool.

In allergic individuals a persistent dermatitis may remain after the precipitating allergen apparently has been removed.

Cross-sensitization can occur when an allergen is present in two or more chemicals, e.g., a sulfonamide and procaine and paraphenylenediamine.

THE PATCH TEST

If correctly understood and employed, the patch test is frequently very helpful in establishing the causative agent. The proper concentration of the suspected antigen found in the patient's environment is employed so as to avoid the occurrence of false positive irritant reactions. The suspected substance is applied to an area of normal skin. It is covered by an innocuous impermeable material, which is then covered with adhesive plaster. The test is read after 24 to 48 hours to detect immediate reactions, and then preferably daily for at least 5 days after the patch is removed to detect delayed reactions. Reactions are graded 1 to 4 plus, depending on the degree (e.g., erythema, edema, vesiculation).

Atopic Eczema

This form of eczema is genetically transmitted and gives rise to abnormal cutaneous responses and vascular reactions. Such substances as inhaled dusts, pollens, animal danders, and ingested foods and drugs are often contributory factors. The eruption tends to be more widespread and symmetrical. Frequently the neck, elbow flexures, wrist, popliteal spaces, and ankles are involved initially. In severe cases the eruption may be generalized. The skin is reddened and infiltrated and the normal lines or "cross-hatching" of the skin are exaggerated (lichenification). Vesiculation does not occur but excoriation and erosion may be present.

Atopic eczema is often associated with emotional disturbances and tension; it is sometimes called *disseminated neurodermatitis*. In testing to determine the causative agent, an extract of the suspected substance is scratched or injected into the skin; if the reaction is positive a wheal develops at the site.

Infectious Eczematoid Dermatitis

This term is applied to an eczematous eruption due to bacterial infection of the skin in which the products and toxins produced by the bacteria act as the antigen. The primary infection may be a chronic abscess, an infected draining sinus, or a folliculitis, or there may be a secondary infection complicating a minor abrasion, burn, or laceration. Many skin eruptions caused by *fungi* are eczematous in character and cannot be differentiated from eczema without laboratory study.

Nummular Eczema

The cause of nummular eczema is unknown; multiple factors probably are present. Food allergy, contact dermatitis, bacteria, molds, neurogenic disturbances, and vitamin A deficiency may be involved.

The eczema appears as discrete, coin-shaped, erythematous patches studded with vesicles or papulovesicles that go on to form crusts. The lesions may heal centrally but spread peripherally. Areas of greatest involvement are the hands, fingers, and extensors of the forearms, arms, legs, and thighs, the back of the feet, and the shoulders.

Stasis eczema develops on the ankles and legs as a complication of chronic edema usually secondary to varicose veins or phlebitis. The edema causes alterations in skin metabolism thereby decreasing its resistance to such factors as minor injuries, chapping due to soap and hot water, and infection. In severe cases, ulceration may result.

Eczema of the hands commonly develops in industrial workers and housewives, and multiple causes usually are present. Detergents, bleaches, solvents, chemicals, foods, plants, and other commonly used products usually play an important role. Mechanical injury, physical agents, and local infection frequently are contributory factors, and allergy to foods or drugs may occasionally play some part.

Autosensitization Dermatitis (Absorption Dermatitis)

In autosensitization dermatitis the primary eruption is a stasis eczema, a contact dermatitis, or infectious eczematoid dermatitis; after a variable period, the skin in another area becomes sensitive to products absorbed from the original eruption. The eruption usually is symmetrical; it may be widespread and in some cases is generalized.

Seborrheic Dermatitis

In this dermatitis the sebaceous glands are hyperactive, secreting an excessive amount of sebum, which causes the skin and hair to be shiny and oily or greasy. Seborrheic dermatitis is an inflammatory reaction superimposed on a seborrheic skin. The areas most commonly involved include the scalp, ears, eyebrows and eyelid margins, nasolabial folds, external and interscapular areas, armpits, and pubic, genitocrural, and intergluteal areas. Varying degrees of erythema, scaling, crusting, erosion, and weeping occur depending on the severity of the process. The oiliness, crusting, and scaling usually present in the scalp constitute *dandruff*.

Multiple factors apparently combine to cause seborrheic dermatitis. Disturbances in carbohydrate or fat metabolism, endocrine disorders, and nutritional factors may be involved. Low-grade infection probably plays an important part.

TREATMENT

Treatment varies with the acuteness of the dermatitis.

ACUTE FORM

In acute eczema only the mildest treatment should be applied in the form of *open* wet dressings or therapeutic baths prepared with dilute Burow's solution or normal saline.

SUBACUTE FORM

In subacute eczema in which there is no oozing or vesiculation, mild, soothing "shake" lotions such as calamine lotion N.F. or calamine liniment N.F. may be applied. As healing progresses, bland pastes or ointments may be ordered. During this stage, the skin is still irritable and lotions must be applied carefully.

CHRONIC LICHENIFIED FORM

Initially the chronic lichenified form is treated with pastes or ointments. Tar is effective but it must be utilized in low concentrations and increased as tolerated. Colloidal baths and fractional doses of x-ray and ultraviolet ray may be of value. Specific or known allergens must be removed or avoided; if the allergen is not known, efforts must be made to identify it in order to ensure control and cure.

General supportive care may include the use of sedatives, tranquilizers, or antihistamines to assist in the relief of severe itching. It may be necessary in the case of a child to have him wear some device, such as mitts, to prevent scratching. Psychologic counseling may help the patient develop an understanding concerning the interrelatedness between emotional tension and exacerbation of eczema.

Drug Eruptions

Drugs can cause many eruptions. In the majority of cases, the eruption is not specific to a particular drug.

In general, drug eruptions tend to develop abruptly and are symmetrical and widespread. They may be generalized. The latent period between administration of the drug and appearance of the eruption varies greatly and may be prolonged.

Occasionally a localized or fixed drug eruption occurs in which the eruption reappears in the same area or areas each time the drug is taken.

Drug eruptions are common. They must be suspected whenever an eruption develops during the course of administration of any topical or internal medication.

The eruption may be severe and may be accompanied by such symptoms as fever, joint pain or swelling, gastrointestinal disturbance, hemorrhage, and shock. Death occasionally may occur due to drug sensitivity.

Urticaria

Urticaria is characterized by the development of wheals that vary in size and shape, tend to spread irregularly, and tend to disappear and reappear so that the eruption presents a changing picture. The eruption tends to be widely distributed. In associated angioneurotic edema there is involvement of the lips, eyelids, entire face, head, and feet. Involvement of the structures of the larynx and trachea may lead to respiratory difficulty and death. Itching is marked and tensely swollen areas may be tender.

Urticaria is usually an allergic response. Foods, drugs, bacterial products, intestinal parasites, insect bites, and even heat, cold, or light may act as allergens. Urticaria is the most common eruption caused by penicillin. Psychic disturbances may be aggravating or precipitating factors. In some cases the cause may be difficult to find and correct.

Treatment includes the use of local soothing and antipruritic lotions. Antihistamine drugs may be helpful. In severe cases ephedrine or epinephrine may be required, as may cortisone or corticotropin.

Toxic Erythemas

Erythema Multiforme

This eruption tends to be widespread and symmetrical. The dorsa of the hands, the feet, and the face are usually involved initially, and the mucous membranes are often affected. The lesions usually begin as macules or maculopapular lesions but may go on to vesiculation, erosion, and hemorrhage. Itching is usually absent.

The disease is caused by many factors. It may be an accompanying symptom in an infectious disease such as rheumatic fever, and often is a manifestation of drug sensitivity.

Erythema Nodosum

The lesions of erythema nodosum are smooth, dome-shaped, firm, red, tender nodules usually occurring on the shins. The extensor surfaces of the legs, buttocks, and arms may be involved. The disorder is due to many causes and often accompanies the onset of such diseases as rheumatic fever, tuberculosis, coccidioides, and streptococcal sore throat. Erythema nodosum may be due to drug sensitivity.

Miscellaneous Dermatoses of Nonspecific Origin

Acne Vulgaris

Acne vulgaris, or "pimples," develops during adolescence and early adult life. The face, chest, and back are usually involved and in most cases the skin is seborrheic. Although the cause is unknown, the acne is manifested in plugging of the duct with the formation of a comedone (blackhead). Varying degrees of inflammation and secondary infection develop resulting in papules, pustules, or abscesses. Endocrine, dietary, metabolic, and emotional disturbances may contribute to the condition, and hereditary factors and individual skin types play a part.

Treatment should include attention to the factors mentioned. Local cleanliness and the use of bacteriostatic and drying local medications are helpful. Careful removal of comedones and incision and drainage of abscesses may be indicated. Exposure to ultraviolet light or the sun is usually helpful. A daily shampoo containing selenium disulfide (Selsun) may be given. In severe infections antibiotics orally or by injection may be administered and x-ray treatment may be indicated.

Rosacea

In rosacea there is exaggreated and persistent flushing of the normal blush areas of the face. The upper anterior chest may also be involved. The skin is usually seborrheic, and acne-like papules and pustules are often present. In long-standing cases there may be telangiectasia and irregular hypertrophy of the tissues, especially the nose (rhinophyma).

There are multiple causes in this disease of middle age. Emotional disturbances and intolerance to stimulants may be contributory. There may be a deficiency of vitamin B complex, gastrointestinal disturbances, or a secondary infection.

Psoriasis

The cause of psoriasis is unknown. There may be a hereditary factor, or fat metabolism may be abnormal. The disorder occurs in both sexes and at all ages. The lesions are chronic and red, and covered with a silvery or mica-like scale. In many cases psoriasis is limited to the scalp, elbows, knees, and shins, but it may be widespread or generalized. Irregularity, pitting, separation, and thickening of the nail bed frequently occur. The individual's health is rarely affected, but there is an association with arthritis, fever, and general debility in a small percentage of cases. Itching is usually absent.

The treatment is not specific. Often a low-fat diet and vitamin B complex are prescribed. Local medications and sunbathing or ultraviolet light treatment usually afford relief.

Lichen Planus

This dermatosis of unknown cause is characterized by itching, dry, flat-topped, polygonal, violaceous papular lesions. The volar surfaces of the forearms, the ankles, and the lumbar area, and the mucous membranes of the cheeks and genitalia are often involved, but the general health is not affected.

The treatment is empiric. Antipruritic agents, x-ray therapy, and injection of bismuth are used.

Pityriasis Rosea

The cause of pityriasis rosea is unknown. It usually begins with a single erythematous and scaling lesion, often confused with tinea corporis (ringworm). After several days, a widespread symmetrical eruption of similar lesions appears. These tend to fade and scale in the center so that oval lesions result. They are present mainly on the trunk and covered parts of the extremities. The long axis of the oval lesions tends to parallel the lines of cleavage of the skin. Itching is usually not marked.

The disease is self-limited. It may last 6 weeks or more. Ultraviolet light and sunbathing are beneficial.

Lupus Erythematosus

Lupus erythematosus is of unknown cause. It occurs chiefly in two forms. In *chronic discoid lupus erythematosus* the general health is unaffected. There are localized red, scaly, infiltrated lesions occurring usually on areas exposed to sunlight, especially the face. Older lesions may show atrophy, depigmentation, and telangiectasia. There is no specific treatment. General supportive care with special attention to nutrition and rest is important.

The second form, *disseminated lupus erythematosus,* is a serious systemic disorder. It is discussed elsewhere.

Pemphigus

The cause of pemphigus is not known. The outstanding manifestation is the presence of large, superficial bullae. Although three variations of this disease exist, for practical purposes they may be considered together. The early lesions are small vesicles or bullae appearing on apparently normal or slightly reddened skin. These may be seen in widely scattered areas of the skin and mucous membranes. The bullae rupture easily leaving large areas of painful, denuded skin. Large amounts of tissue fluid are lost from these areas. Secondary infection is a dreaded complication and is difficult to treat. With spread, the entire body surface may be involved with production of redness, weeping, edema, and an offensive odor. The condition is characterized by exacerbations and remissions that may vary from weeks to years.

The treatment of pemphigus embodies all the skills of the health team. There is no cure for pemphigus; however, the disease may be controlled by the use of steroids. All other measures are supportive and symptomatic. Of prime importance is the maintenance of body nutrition with a high-caloric and high-protein diet. Antibiotics and chemotherapeutic agents are employed to prevent or control secondary infection. Fluid and electrolyte balance, with the loss of sodium, is much the same as for any other condition in which large amounts of tissue fluid are lost; it may also be necessary to maintain plasma proteins and blood volume with whole blood or plasma transfusions. Anemia should be combated through diet and iron and vitamin supplements.

The nurse will be challenged to give or supervise the most expert hygienic care. She must ensure that the miserable, odoriferous, and debilitated pemphigus patient is not ignored by the hospital personnel; good nursing care including control of secondary infection will make this task easier.

Alopecia Areata

The cause of alopecia areata is unknown. It may follow emotional shock or acute infectious disease and may be associated with reflex nerve irritation from defective teeth or an otolaryngological disorder. The hair falls out, usually rapidly and cleanly, leaving shiny bald areas of scalp which appear otherwise normal. The beard and other hairy areas may be involved. The fall is usually of limited extent and spontaneous regrowth usually occurs. Usually the regrowth is fine, white, and lanugo-like at first; later, it gradually becomes normal in color and texture. Treatment consists in correcting any associated defect or disease together with massage and stimulating local applications.

Neoplastic Disorders

BENIGN EPIDERMAL PROCESSES

Sebaceous Cyst

These are caused by occlusion of a hair follicle or sebaceous gland duct with retention of sebaceous gland secretion producing a sac-like tumor. The size of the cyst is determined by its age and rate of secretion. The cyst becomes infected and abscessed. Treatment usually is excision.

Milium

A milium is a small cyst containing desquamated cornified epithelial cells that usually arise from lanugo hair follicles or sebaceous glands. It may follow trauma (burns, incision, abrasion) or may arise spontaneously. It is treated by incision and expression and healing usually takes place without scar formation.

Mucous Cyst

A mucous cyst may develop on mucous membranes due to occlusion of a mucous gland duct. In most cases it is semitranslucent and about the size of a pea. The inner surface of the lip is the usual site. Treatment consists of removal or destruction of the entire sac.

NEVI (MOLES)

The common mole is an intradermal nevus consisting of collections of abnormal cells in the upper portion of the cutis. It may occur on any portion of the body but is most frequently seen on the face. The mole may be flat or elevated, nonpigmented or pigmented, smooth or irregular, and hairy or nonhairy.

Aside from cosmetic considerations, the question of potential danger and need for removal of a mole is often difficult to determine. Even biopsy and microscopic examination may not be decisive. In general, changes in color, in size, or in character of a mole, or the development of ulceration, inflammation, bleeding, crusting, or tenderness in a mole suggests malignant change. Location in an area subject to repeated injury is an important consideration. If treated at all, complete removal by excision or electrodesiccation is indicated.

Junctional Nevus

The junctional nevus usually is flat or only slightly elevated, smooth, nonhairy, light to dark brown or black. There may be multiple nevi. Progression to nevocarcinoma or malignant melanoma is a fairly frequent occurrence.

Blue Nevus

The blue nevus is a smooth, flat or only slightly elevated, bluish-black mole that develops most often on the back. Usually it is present from infancy or early childhood and rarely shows malignant change.

SEBORRHEIC KERATOSIS

These superficial warty lesions, fawn colored or brown or darker, develop in middle-aged or older individuals, often those having a seborrheic skin. The lesions tend to be multiple and often develop on the face, especially on the forehead about the hairline, and on the upper trunk. They rarely become cancerous. Treatment is not always necessary; when it is, freezing with liquid nitrogen or solid carbon dioxide, or electrodesiccation and curettage is the preferred treatment.

PRECANCEROUS DERMATOSES

Senile Keratosis (Actinic Keratosis)

The condition occurs usually in those with fair skin. Exposure to sunlight over the years is an aggravating factor. It appears on exposed surfaces as reddish patches covered by hard adherent scales. It is a precursor to squamous cell carcinoma. Treatment is by destruction with liquid nitrogen or electrodesiccation depending on size and location.

Cutaneous Horn

The horn appears as a projection often spiral or conical, arising from a reddened base, that usually is small, but may be 1 to 2 cm in diameter. The base is often an early carcinoma. Curettage and desiccation, or excision, is the usual treatment.

MALIGNANT EPIDERMAL TUMORS

Before the specific types of skin cancer are discussed, some general facts should be stated. The nurse must never forget her responsibility in the fields of preventive medicine and health education.

Cancer of the skin is the commonest cancer and fortunately is the most curable. Several factors contribute to the high rate of cure (over 90 percent, with expert treatment). (1) Skin cancer can be seen readily even in its early stages. (2) The most frequent type does not metastasize; most skin cancers grow slowly, and many remain localized. (3) The accessibility of the lesion and the therapy available make treatment relatively simple and effective. Even though a lesion remains localized, it has the invasive properties of all cancers. Histologic examination is necessary for diagnosis. The informed nurse is often in a position to educate individuals concerning skin cancer and refer them for appropriate diagnosis and treatment.

Basal Cell Epithelioma (Rodent Ulcer)

This is the most common malignant tumor of the skin. Over 90 percent occur on the head, neck, and/or face; a very small number occur on the trunk. The tumor often grows on hornified skin areas and appears as an infiltrative papule or plaque, often with a semitranslucent appearance, a pearly border, and telengiectatic surface. Epithelioma tends to be slow-growing; however, during periods of rapid growth it may produce extensive ulceration. It can invade skin, cartilage, bone, and blood vessels. It is malignant, but does not metastasize. The treatment is destruction through surgical means, electrodesiccation, chemosurgery, or x-ray. More than one modality may be utilized.

Squamous (Prickle Cell) Epithelioma

The tumor may occur on any part of the body or mucous membranes; however, the face, lower lip, ears, tongue, and backs of the hands are the most common sites. It usually appears as an infiltrating nodule or papule with a central ulcer, raised border, and some surrounding redness. The tumor grows rapidly and has invasive tendencies, often destroying bone and cartilage. The grade of malignancy and metastasizing ability vary from very low to very high. Diagnosis is confirmed by biopsy, and treatment is the same as for basal cell carcinoma.

Melanoma (Nevocarcinoma)

Melanoma may begin as a blue-black nodule in an apparently normal skin or may develop from a preexisting nevus. It demonstrates growth and color changes often described as "spilling color." Rarely is this type of tumor nonpigmented. Often the lesion rapidly ulcerates, bleeds, and then crusts. Unfortunately, melanomas metastasize early via the lymphatics and the bloodstream, and they are often diagnosed by the presence of enlarged adjacent glands or the appearance of distant skin metastases. Radical surgical excision of the tumor, including the regional glands, is the only effective treatment, since melanomas are highly resistant to x-ray and radium therapy. The nursing care is as for any radical surgical procedure.

Every effort should be made to inform the public concerning the danger signs of this disease. All forms of skin or mucous membrane irritation should be removed. Attention should be given to broken teeth or dentures, to moles in areas subjected to friction, and to any skin lesion that does not heal or disappear within 3 weeks.

BENIGN CONNECTIVE TISSUE TUMORS

Hemangioma (Hemangioma Simplex and Cavernous Hemangioma)

The hemangioma is a congenital deformity due to growth of capillaries and veins. It appears as a dark to bright red, flat, slightly elevated, or fluctuant mass (when cavernous). This birthmark can be treated satisfactorily with solid carbon dioxide, electrodesiccation, excision, sclerosing agents, or radiation with x-ray or radium.

Nevus Flammeus (Port Wine Nevus)

This variety of hemangioma is deep purple-red, and flat; it may cover large areas of skin and mucous membranes. Usually it is unilateral in distribution and follows a nerve pattern. There is no satisfactory treatment, but many people benefit from the use of covering cosmetics.

Keloids

A keloid is an area of hypertrophic scar tissue that arises following burns or other trauma to the skin. It is found most commonly in darkly pigmented races. The scar becomes raised and lumpy in appearance. The only treatment presently available that may be of early value is x-ray, solid carbon dioxide, or liquid nitrogen.

Bibliography

Andriole, V. T. and H. M. Kravetz: The Use of Amphotericin B in Man. *Journal of American Medical Association,* 180:269–272, April 28, 1962.

Ariel, Irving M.: *Progress in Clinical Cancer.* New York: Grune & Stratton, Inc., 1965.

Chase, M. W.: The Mechanism of Sensitization. *Journal of Allergy,* 28:30–38, 1957.

Kopf, Alfred W. and R. Andrade: Follow-up Study of Combined Treatment of Onychomycosis: Nail Extraction and Griseofulvin. *Yearbook of Dermatology.* Chicago: The Year Book Medical Publishers, Inc., 1967–1968, pp. 67–68.

Montagna, William: *The Structure and Function of Skin.* New York: Academic Press, Inc., 1962.

Sanders, S. H., et al.: Contact Dermatitis Due to Poison Ivy, Oak, and Sumac. *Eye, Ear, Nose, Throat Monthly,* 44:99–100, October, 1965.

Sulzberger, M. B., et al.: Dermatology—Diagnosis and Treatment. Chicago: Year Book Medical Publishers, Inc., 1961.

A Topical Agent for the Treatment of Superficial Fungal Infections of the Skin. *Journal of American Medical Association,* 196:1145, June, 1966.

Vilanova, X., J. P. Agnade, and L. A. Rueda: The Cytologic Aspects of Basal Cell Carcinoma. *Journal of Investigative Dermatology,* 39:123–131, August, 1962.

Zacarian, Setrag A.: *Cryosurgery of Skin Cancer and Cryogenic Techniques in Dermatology.* Springfield, Illinois: Charles C Thomas, Publisher, 1969. pp. 79–80.

SECTION 2
BURNS
MARTHA C. PEAKE

Large numbers of people in all walks of life become victims of burn injury. Burns occur in the home, on the job, in play, as a result of plane, car, and boat accidents, and as a result of military action and natural disasters.

Although a burn manifests itself conspicuously in damage to the skin, every other organ system of the body can become seriously involved as a result of the injury itself or of necessary therapy (Fig. 28–9).

The nursing care of a severely burned patient is intensive, highly individualized, and prolonged and calls on all the skills and knowledge of the nurse. It is "total" patient care in the full sense of the term.

The following represents an outline of those aspects of burn injury which are important to the nurse's understanding in planning for and providing nursing care for burn patients.

945

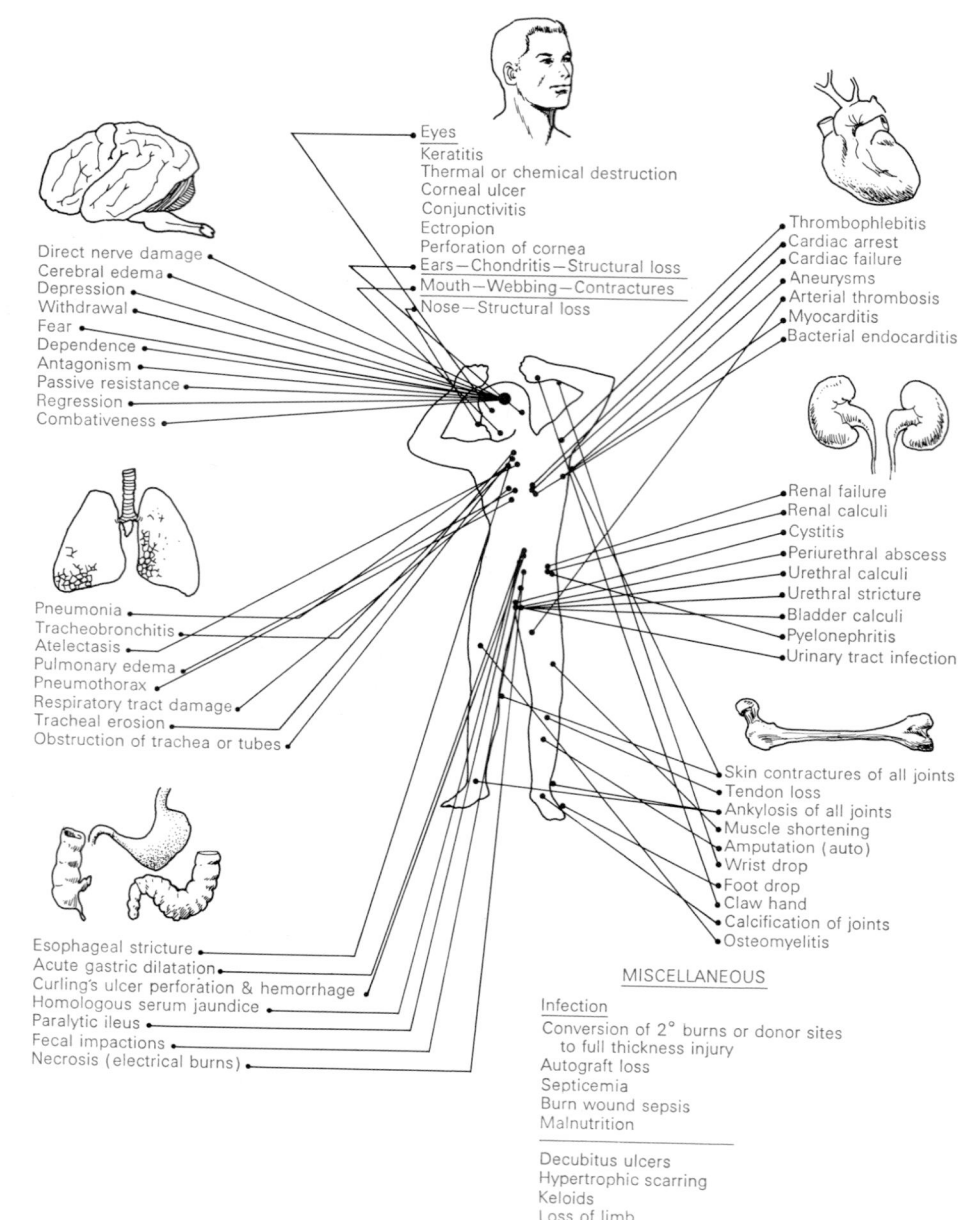

Eyes
Keratitis
Thermal or chemical destruction
Corneal ulcer
Conjunctivitis
Ectropion
Perforation of cornea
Ears—Chondritis—Structural loss
Mouth—Webbing—Contractures
Nose—Structural loss

Direct nerve damage
Cerebral edema
Depression
Withdrawal
Fear
Dependence
Antagonism
Passive resistance
Regression
Combativeness

Thrombophlebitis
Cardiac arrest
Cardiac failure
Aneurysms
Arterial thrombosis
Myocarditis
Bacterial endocarditis

Renal failure
Renal calculi
Cystitis
Periurethral abscess
Urethral calculi
Urethral stricture
Bladder calculi
Pyelonephritis
Urinary tract infection

Pneumonia
Tracheobronchitis
Atelectasis
Pulmonary edema
Pneumothorax
Respiratory tract damage
Tracheal erosion
Obstruction of trachea or tubes

Skin contractures of all joints
Tendon loss
Ankylosis of all joints
Muscle shortening
Amputation (auto)
Wrist drop
Foot drop
Claw hand
Calcification of joints
Osteomyelitis

Esophageal stricture
Acute gastric dilatation
Curling's ulcer perforation & hemorrhage
Homologous serum jaundice
Paralytic ileus
Fecal impactions
Necrosis (electrical burns)

MISCELLANEOUS

Infection
Conversion of 2° burns or donor sites
  to full thickness injury
Autograft loss
Septicemia
Burn wound sepsis
Malnutrition

Decubitus ulcers
Hypertrophic scarring
Keloids
Loss of limb

*Figure 28-9
Complications of burns
and burn therapy.*

Factors Determining the Seriousness of Burn Injury

There are several factors that determine the seriousness of a burn and have a direct bearing upon therapy. These are the extent or percent of total body surface involved, the depth of injury, the patient's age, his general health, the site of burn, the presence of associated injury, and the agent causing the burn.

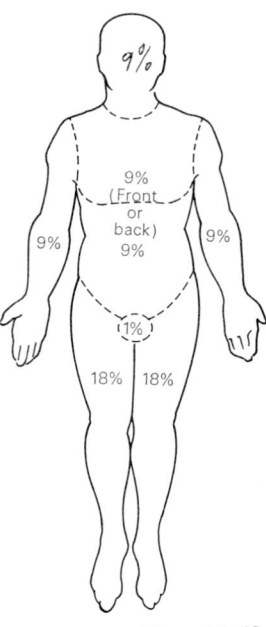

*Figure 28–10
Rule of nines: a con-
venient method of
determining percent of
total body surface injury.*

EXTENT OR PERCENT OF TOTAL BODY SURFACE BURN

Several methods of determining the area or percent of total body surface have been described (Artz and Reiss). The Rule of Nines, by which the body area is divided into nine or multiples of nine (e.g., 18) percent, provides a satisfactory and convenient method (Fig. 28–10).

DEPTH OF BURN INJURY

When a burn occurs, tissue cells are destroyed. The deeper the cell destruction extends, the more pronounced are resultant local and physiologic changes. To indicate depth of injury, burns are commonly divided into three categories: (1) first-degree, (2) second-degree, and (3) third-degree.

First-Degree Burns

First-degree burns involve only the superficial layers of the epidermis and are characterized by erythema, slight localized edema, muscular discomfort, and exquisite tenderness.

First-degree burns commonly result from exposure to natural sunlight or sun-lamps.

Treatment of first-degree burns is usually palliative. Topically applied powders or cooling lotions provide a soothing effect; and a mild analgesic, taken orally, is generally all that is needed to control discomfort. As a rule, a first-degree burn is uncomplicated and heals without scarring, within a few days following injury. Patients who have sustained first-degree burns, unless extensive, generally do not require hospital treatment.

Second-Degree Burns

Second-degree burns vary in depth of injury. A burn is classified as second-degree as long as any epithelial elements remain.

Second-degree burns are characterized by a bright pink, mottled red, or blanched appearance. Blisters are usually present, and the wound is moist and extremely sensitive to external stimuli, particularly to the movement of air, and upon contact with water. This sensitivity remains until exposed nerve endings are covered. Marked edema is a prominent feature of second-degree burn injury; it becomes evident in the first 3 to 6 hours following injury and reaches its peak in from 48 to 72 hours, after which time it begins to resolve.

Second-degree burns usually occur as a result of brief exposure to heat regardless of the source.

If uncomplicated by infection or trauma, second-degree burns will epithelize.

Third-Degree Burns

Third-degree burns involve the full thickness of the skin, and may involve underlying muscles, tendons, or bones. Third-degree burns are often referred to as *full-thickness* burns. By definition, all epithelial elements are destroyed.

Third-degree burns vary in appearance. A third-degree burn may appear blanched or charred, or the involved area may appear semitranslucent with a visible network of thrombosed superficial vessels present.

A third-degree burn is characteristically anesthetic, and is further typified by marked edema that becomes evident during the first few hours following injury. A distinguishing feature of third-degree burn injury is the dry, tough, inelastic eschar that forms as a result of dehydration of the burned skin.

Third-degree burns usually result from contact with hot metal (such as an iron), open flame, steam, chemicals, electricity, or prolonged exposure to hot liquids.

AGE AND GENERAL HEALTH

A burn injury is more serious in the very young and the elderly. In both age groups the skin is more easily damaged because of its thinness.

In the very young, a burn represents a greater area per unit of weight than in an adult, and as a result, physiological derangements are more acute. In the elderly, degenerative changes are taking place, and these, together with the local and physiological derangements caused by the burn, increase the severity of the injury.

It could be expected that the presence of preexisting renal, cardiovascular, pulmonary, or gastrointestinal disease would contribute to the seriousness of a burn injury when one considers that renal failure, cardiovascular problems, pulmonary problems, and gastrointestinal disturbances are frequent complications of severe burn injury.

SITE OF BURN AND PRESENCE OF ASSOCIATED INJURY

Burns that are not severe from the standpoint of percent of body area involved are often quite serious from the standpoint of disfigurement or loss of function. Face burns, burns over major joints, and burns of the hands, feet, and external genitalia fall into this category.

As one might suppose, when a burn injury is complicated by an associated traumatic injury such as a severe fracture, head injury, or crush injury, treatment is considerably more difficult, and the threat to survival is greatly increased.

AGENT CAUSING THE BURN

The characteristics of the agent causing a burn are of importance from the standpoint of the depth of injury, treatment, and complications. Electricity is a case in point. Electrical burns usually involve the full thickness of the skin, and more often than not extensive vascular thrombosis and nerve degeneration occur far beyond the burn area, since current travels along these structures. Electrical burns are extremely difficult to treat as a result of the magnitude of tissue destruction, and often require surgical intervention. Electrical burns are frequently complicated by infection, and even though surface inspection of an electrical burn indicates satisfactory response to treatment, serious hemorrhage resulting from erosion of deep vessels can occur several weeks postburn.

Immediate Care of the Patient

A severely burned patient is characteristically extremely apprehensive, will probably have severe pain, and may be in shock. The manner in which he is received on arrival for admission to the emergency room and/or ward has a decided influence upon his emotional state and his ability to cooperate in his care. If he is received calmly and confidently in an atmosphere free of unnecessary noise and confusion, his apprehension will be considerably lessened and he will be better able to cooperate with personnel concerned with his care.

A number of procedures must be accomplished upon the admission of the patient to the hospital. Depending upon the severity of the situation, there may be several members of the health team performing different activities with the patient simultaneously, but if the team members act smoothly and efficiently and demonstrate consideration for the patient, heightening of his apprehension can be avoided. The order in which the procedures are accomplished is determined by the particular aspect of the patient's injury which presents the greatest threat to his survival. The immediate problems are maintenance of respiratory function, control of fluid and electrolyte balance, and care of the injury.

Airway obstruction is relieved if indicated. Replacement of fluids is administered via an intravenous cutdown. The patient's clothing and first aid dressings are removed in order to observe and estimate the amount and degree of burn. The patient is weighed to obtain a baseline weight by which to judge at later intervals the amount of edema formation and fluid loss and to calculate the amount of fluid replacement. A history is obtained of the time and circumstances of the injury and of any preexisting illness. The examination of the patient includes an overall estimate of the burn injury, determination of the presence of associated injury, appraisal of his general condition including vital signs, and evaluation of the patient's need for medication to relieve discomfort, pain, or apprehension. An indwelling urinary catheter is inserted so that exact urinary output can be measured. Urine and blood samples are drawn for laboratory determinations and chest x-ray examination and electrocardiograph tracing are obtained not only to establish the patient's current physiological state but also for use in judging the significance of later physiological changes. Tetanus prophylaxis is given if indicated. The burn wounds are cleaned and debrided, escharotomy is accomplished if necessary, and cultures are taken of affected areas. The local treatment of the burn wound is initiated.

Suggested supplies and equipment to have in readiness upon the patient's admission are listed below.

Routine Supplies and Equipment

1. Standard hospital bed, rotating frame, or crib made up with fresh, clean linens
2. Venous cutdown tray
3. Intravenous administration equipment with fluids (5 percent Dextrose in water, Ringer's lactated solution, dextran)
4. Catheterization tray and equipment for urine specimen collection and for indwelling catheter drainage
5. Burn pads

6. Sterile clean-up tray on Mayo stand containing the following: 4 × 8 gauze sponges, 25; sponge basins (used for surgical soap and normal saline); Asepto syringe, 1; sterile towels, 4 to 6; rubber gloves, 2 pairs; dressing forceps, 1; straight hemostats, 2; one-point sharp scissors, 1
7. Sterile normal saline (irrigating), 2,000 to 4,000 ml
8. Liquid surgical soap (nonirritating)
9. Blood sampling equipment
10. Stethoscope
11. Sphygmomanometer
12. Clinical thermometer (rectal)
13. Medications: tetanus toxoid and/or tetanus antitoxin, morphine sulfate or meperidine (Demerol), sodium pentobarbital
14. Face masks and surgically clean gowns
15. Scale (in-bed type)
16. Electrocardiograph

Emergency Supplies and Equipment

1. Oxygen and equipment required for administration
2. Suction and equipment required for use
3. Tracheostomy tray
4. Laryngoscopic equipment
5. Emergency drug tray
6. Cardiac arrest tray
7. Venous pressure tray
8. Escharotomy tray

Care of the Patient during the Acute Period

CARE OF THE TRACHEOSTOMIZED PATIENT

Burn patients who are likely to require tracheostomy to relieve airway obstruction are those who have sustained severe head and neck burns caused by flame or steam, and those who have been burned in a confined area where they have been subjected to smoke inhalation (Epstein et al.).

Essential factors involved in the nursing care of the tracheostomized burn patient do not differ from those involved in the care of other patients with tracheostomy. However, certain aspects of their care require special emphasis, and are discussed below.

Following establishment of tracheostomy, the patient must be carefully observed for cyanosis, tachypnea, persistent coughing, expiratory wheezing, depressed respiratory movement of one side of the chest, and increased restlessness and apprehension. Such signs and symptoms must be reported to the physician immediately since they may be indicative of improper placement of the tracheostomy cannula, dislodgment of the cannula, obstructed cannula, pneumothorax, atelectasis, or bleeding from the tracheostomy wound.

Severely burned patients are usually cared for on turning frames, and are turned at prescribed intervals from supine to prone position and vice versa. When the patient is being turned down, dislodgment of the tracheostomy cannula can readily occur. Indications of cannula dislodgment are observed in changes in the rate and quality of respirations. Therefore, prior to and following turning, the patient's respirations should be carefully noted. If respiratory alterations appear, the cannula should be checked and repositioned if necessary.

When tracheostomy toilet is being carried out, aseptic precautions should be practiced insofar as is possible to avoid introducing pathogenic microorganisms from the contaminated burn wound or from the oral or nasal passages into the tracheobronchial tree.

BODY FLUID IMBALANCE FOLLOWING BURN INJURY

In the absence of respiratory obstruction, the imbalance of body fluids which occurs following severe burn injury presents the most serious threat to the patient's survival.

The mechanism of fluid imbalance following burn injury is quite complex, and there are numerous references on the subject. These should be consulted by readers wishing to cover this particular aspect of the burn problem in detail. That which follows is an attempt to present a simplified explanation of fluid imbalance so that the nurse will be better prepared to understand the rationale of fluid resuscitative therapy.

It is convenient to describe fluid imbalance as internal and external fluid losses. Internal losses include losses from the vascular compartment into the burn area of water, red cells, protein, and electrolytes (i.e., sodium, potassium, and chlorides). Internal losses account for the edema, both visible and hidden, that characteristically forms following second-degree and third-degree burn injury. Approximately 3 to 5 days postinjury, the situation is reversed, and fluids return to the vascular compartment from the tissues of the burn area (Moncrief and Mason). Visible evidence of this phenomenon may be seen in increased hourly urinary output, and in reduced local edema.

External fluid losses are both sensible and insensible. Included among sensible losses are wound weeping, urine, stool, gastric drainage, and vomitus. Insensible fluid losses include water lost in respiration, and in the evaporation of large quantities of water through the burn wounds. This evaporative loss contributes significantly to the burn patient's requirements for tremendous volumes of resuscitative fluids.

In large burns, during the early part of the resuscitation period, as a precaution against aspiration of gastric contents, and because of such complications as paralytic ileus and water intoxication, oral fluids are withheld and resuscitative fluids are given intravenously.

Assisting the physician with the administration of intravenous resuscitative fluids in the correction of body fluid imbalance following burn injury is one of the most important responsibilities the nurse has in the care of the burn patient.

The physician establishes the intravenous route, usually a venous cutdown, and prescribes the kinds and amounts of fluids to be administered within a given period of time. Daily weighing of the patient is usually requested so that estimates of fluid loss can be made and used to assist in calculating the amount of fluid to be replaced.

The nurse is responsible for administering the fluids in the sequence specified, adjusting the rate of administration according to the physician's directions and as indicated by the patient's signs and symptoms, maintaining the patency of the intravenous route, and recording the amounts and kinds of fluids administered.

Of these several responsibilities, the responsibility of maintaining the patency of the intravenous route requires special emphasis, because of the sparsity of available veins in severely burned patients, and because of the difficulty of re-establishing an intravenous route when the procedure is complicated by circulatory insufficiency and generalized edema.

In order to fully meet the responsibilities outlined above, and thus provide the best service to the patient, the nurse must have a knowledge of the following:

1. The seriousness of the patient's condition.

2. The nature and action of the kinds of solutions commonly used in the resuscitation of the burn patient. Solutions commonly used are as follows: electrolytes (lactated Ringer's solution, 5 percent dextrose in normal saline); colloids (heat-treated plasma, whole blood, packed cells, dextran, plasma); water (5 percent dextrose in distilled water).

3. The nature and action of medications commonly prescribed by the physician to be added to one or more of the intravenous solutions. Medications commonly prescribed include the following: vitamin preparations, antibiotics, potassium chloride, sodium bicarbonate, sodium pentobarbital, aminophylline.

4. The effects of introducing into the bloodstream solutions of varying osmotic pressures, i.e., isotonic, hypertonic, and hypotonic solutions.

5. The tolerance of patients of different age levels to varying volumes of intravenous fluids administered at varying rates.

6. Unfavorable reactions occurring from intravenous therapy, e.g., chilling, dyspnea, headache, flushing.

7. Common causes of cessation of intravenous flow, including a kink in tubing obscured by dressing, very slow rate of infusion, backup of blood into tubing from negative pressure in flask, failure to establish flask airway when changing flasks, exhaustion of fluid in flask (usually occurs when the rate of flow increases upon patient's change in position), flask of solution not high enough.

8. The signs and symptoms of fluid deficiency and fluid overload. *Signs and symptoms of fluid deficiency:* increasing restlessness, increasing disorientation, thirst unrelieved by fluid administration, decreasing hourly urinary output, sharp increase in pulse rate, sudden decrease in blood pressure. *Signs and symptoms of fluid overload:* increasing hourly urinary output, weakening in pulse volume, chest rales, moist sound to breathing, feeling of fullness in chest, feeling of anxiety or apprehension, frequent coughing, increased sputum that may appear frothy and blood tinged, extreme restlessness.

URINARY OUTPUT

A serious complication for the burn patient is pulmonary edema or renal failure due to fluid and/or electrolyte imbalance. The urinary output is one of the principal indices used in determining the adequacy of fluid resuscitative therapy. To assure accurate hourly monitoring of urinary volume, an indwelling catheter is inserted into the bladder, and the catheter is connected to a bedside collection unit.

As a rule, the nurse is directed to regulate the flow of intravenous fluids in accordance with the hourly volume of urine output. Unless otherwise specified by the physician, the hourly flow of urine should be maintained at from 30 to 50 ml for adults, and from 10 to 30 ml for children.

Hourly urine volume in excess of specified amounts usually indicates excessive fluid administration, which if not corrected can lead to pulmonary edema. On the other hand, a diminished hourly urine output usually indicates the need for increased fluid administration, which if not accomplished can lead to serious complications such as renal failure or hypernatremia, the early signs of which can be detected by urine volume, specific gravity, and constituents.

The importance of giving conscientious attention to hourly monitoring and recording of urinary volume and of reporting discrepancies to the physician cannot be overemphasized. And as one might suppose, it is equally important that the physician's attention be called to changes in the character of the urine such as the presence of blood or sediment, an unusual odor or color, and a sharp increase or decrease in specific gravity reading. Specific gravity readings above 1.025 or below 1.010 should be reported to the physician.

Conscientious attention must also be given to care of the indwelling catheter, which usually remains in place until the patient has been adequately resuscitated. The catheter must be anchored in a manner permitting freedom of movement of the patient without resulting in tension or drag on the urethrovesical segment. Equal care must be taken to keep the meatus free of accumulated material, which not only causes the patient discomfort, but also invites infection. Cleansing of the meatus should be accomplished at routine intervals throughout a 24-hour period.

Most physicians prefer that a retention catheter not be irrigated or changed at routine intervals because of the danger of contamination of the urinary tract by pathogens from the burn wound; therefore, an indwelling catheter is irrigated or changed only upon direction of the physician. When a catheter is irrigated, the amount of solution used must be noted on the patient's intake record.

In the treatment of a burn patient, it is the exception, rather than the rule, that an indwelling catheter need be left in place for such an extended length of time that it presents a problem. Usually, the patient is adequately resuscitated within the first 2 to 5 days following the initiation of fluid resuscitative therapy; and the catheter is removed.

Hourly monitoring of urinary volume is greatly facilitated by connecting an indwelling catheter to a length of clear plastic tubing, which drains into a rigid, finely calibrated, tubular bedside urine collection unit equipped at its base with an outlet valve. The urine measurement can be read in the same container in which the urine is collected, thereby eliminating the necessity of transferring the urine from one container to another in order to measure it.

NUTRITION

One of the most challenging responsibilities the nurse has in the care of the severely burned patient is assisting the physician in his efforts to prevent the patient's nutritional status from deteriorating.

In order that the nurse may fully appreciate the necessity of maintaining a proper nutritional program for the severely burned patient, it is mandatory that she have a knowledge of how related metabolic responses occurring following burn injury influence the patient's nutritional requirements and affect his chances of survival. This information is readily available in textbooks and current literature, and such sources should be consulted by the reader. That which follows is confined to a discussion of the patient's nutritional requirements, related problems, and measures to improve intake.

The nutritional problem is caused by the great loss of protein nitrogen in the early postburn period due to nitrogen catabolism as a result of endocrine response to stress mediated by adrenal corticosteroids and to loss of protein derived from plasma and interstitial fluid in exudate from the burn surface (Harper). The ingestion of high-protein and high-caloric nutrients as soon as possible is essential. Curling's ulcer, an acute gastrointestinal ulceration following burns, is believed to be a type of "stress ulcer" associated with the increased production of adrenocortical hormone, which acts to increase gastric secretion. With severe burns it is likely to develop in the first or second postburn week and with less severe burns after the second or third postburn week. There is little indication that it has developed until a massive hemorrhage occurs. When the patient has extensive burns, antacids may be given prophylactically during the first 2 to 3 weeks (Hummel et al.).

As soon as nausea and vomiting cease, and active bowel sounds can be heard, oral feedings are given—cautiously at first—and then in increasing amounts. When it becomes evident that oral feedings are well tolerated, the patient is started on a high-protein, high-caloric diet with between-meal high-energy nutrients given around the clock. Vitamin supplements are given at regular meal hours.

Few severely burned patients eat voluntarily until their wounds are nearly healed or closed with autograft. In addition to the general factors such as food dislikes, weakness or fatigue, environmental disturbances, and emotional responses that may affect the desire to eat, the burned patient may have other conditions that contribute to his poor intake of necessary nutriments. He may have moderate to severe pain or discomfort resulting from exposure of sensitive nerve endings to air currents, feeling chilled, maintaining a fixed position, or the use of body parts that have been injured, such as movement of the affected hand or arm or chewing using affected face and neck. Face dressings, hand or arm dressings, or splints obviously will affect both the desire and the ability to eat or feed oneself. Contractures of the neck and/or about the mouth will interfere with chewing and swallowing. Unpleasant odors and poorly timed treatments, especially cleaning and dressing of the burn wounds, are environmental conditions that can affect the appetite of the burned patient. Since the recovery from burns is a slow process, it is common for patients to become depressed and lose interest in recovery or become discouraged or frustrated over obvious weight loss and the seemingly slow progress in efforts toward self-help or in the healing of the wounds.

Though the elimination of some of these deterrents to the patient's intake of adequate nutriments cannot be accomplished by the nurse alone, awareness of their existence gives her a better understanding of the patient's problems. This understanding, in turn, increases her capacity for patience, and strengthens her resolve to persist in her efforts to help the patient.

Inducements to Eating

There are some practical inducements the nurse can use to attempt to improve the severely burned patient's intake of necessary nutriments. As soon as the patient is fully oriented, reasons for the stress placed upon his eating should be explained to him. If he is prepared for such eventualities as loss of appetite and noticeable weight loss, he will be less likely to feel that he is fighting a losing battle. It is not uncommon for severly burned patients to lose from 20 to 30 pounds during the course of their hospitalization.

Painful or unpleasant treatments should be scheduled well in advance of meal times. If the patient has difficulty chewing solid foods, these should be chopped, or ground in the kitchen prior to serving. "Fussing" with the preparation of food before the patient is to be avoided.

If the patient is to be out of bed for meals, he should be gotten up in sufficient time prior to eating to permit his adjusting to the position change, and to overcome anxiety and discomfort experienced in the process of being moved. Further, he should be protected, insofar as is possible, from unpleasant sights and from air currents.

If the patient is to be fed, the person feeding him should not appear hurried or overanxious if he fails to eat all the food served him. The burned patient's intake may be better when he is fed by a family member who cares "about" him, rather than nursing personnel who care "for" him. The nurse should be alert to the possibility that an overindulgent or oversolicitous relative may find it difficult to resist helping the patient to the point of discouraging his efforts toward self-help. If this becomes apparent, the nurse can explain to the relative the importance of encouraging the patient to help himself. If the relative's indulgent behavior persists the nurse must then weigh the value of the patient's food intake when he is fed by a relative against the effects of delayed development of self-help in deciding whether or not to restrict visiting during meal hours.

Patients often eat better when they can feed themselves. Self-help eating devices similar to those used in the rehabilitation of patients with nervous system diseases are equally useful for patients with burns of the hands and/or arms.

A favorite television or radio program often serves to take the patient's mind off the emphasis on his eating, and the process of eating then becomes mechanical. And, too, a meal served away from the narrow confines of his unit is usually conducive to improved intake. Eating with other patients at a common table or in a wheel chair circle often inspires a desirable competitive attitude resulting in improved intake. And seeing other patients really enjoying their food provides an additional incentive.

Since nutrition is vital for the severely burned patient, if he is unable to eat adequately it may be necessary to utilize tube feedings. The tube is left in place and the patient is given high-protein, high-caloric liquids as directed by the physician. With the tube in place, the patient is served a tray at regular meal hours and between meal nutriments are offered. As soon as he eats an adequate amount the tube feeding can be discontinued.

LOCAL MANAGEMENT OF BURN INJURY

Contrary to popular belief the burned skin is not sterilized at the time of burning. Although large numbers of surface microorganisms are destroyed, those lying deep in the hair follicles and sweat glands survive, and multiply in the damaged tissue deprived of its natural inflammatory response to trauma; and bacterial colonization of the wound occurs within from 3 to 5 days following injury (Teplitz et al.).

Local therapeutic efforts are directed toward suppressing progressive bacterial colonization of the burn wound to permit early spontaneous healing of second-degree burns and successful closure of third-degree burns. Early wound closure is the best assurance against fatal burn wound sepsis, which is the principal cause of mortality following severe burn injury.

Various methods of local management of the burn wound are practiced, many of which have been described by Artz and Reiss and more recently by Order and Moncrief. Such sources should be consulted for a comprehensive coverage of this aspect of burn therapy. The approach to local management of the burn wound which is described here is the approach currently used at the U.S. Army Surgical Research Unit.

Initial care of the burn wound includes thorough cleansing with pHisoHex and normal saline, the breaking of blisters, and the removal of all loose epithelium. This is generally accomplished in the intensive care area of the ward. However, if the patient is several days postburn upon admission, and the condition of his wounds is such as to require a more aggressive approach, cleansing and debriding of the wounds is accomplished in the physical therapy section in a whirlpool unit or in the Hubbard tank. Morphine or meperidine (Demerol) is given intravenously

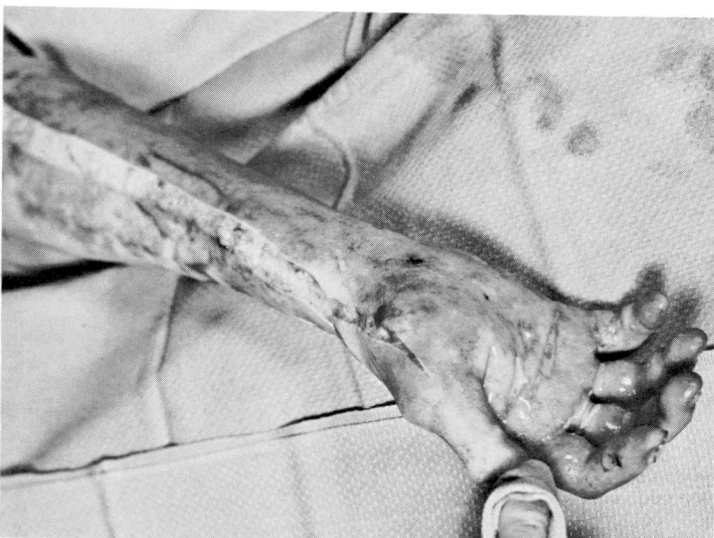

Figure 28-11 Escharotomy of lower arm accomplished to relieve tourniquet effect following circumferential third-degree burn injury.

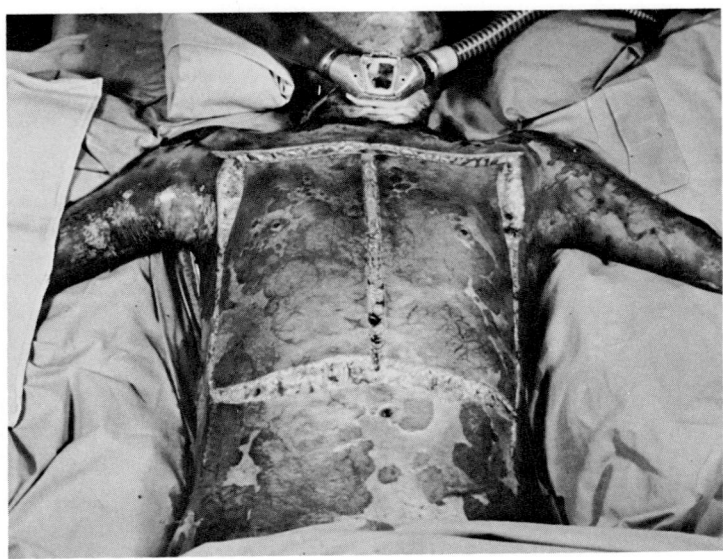

*Figure 28-12
Escharotomy of chest
accomplished to permit
greater ease of move-
ment of rib cage
and improve
respiration.*

for discomfort if required. If indicated, escharotomy is performed to relieve circulatory impairment in circumferential burns of an extremity (Fig. 28–11) or to permit greater ease of movement of the rib cage, and improve respirations in third-degree burns of the chest (Fig. 28–12).

Following cleansing and debridement of the wounds, the areas involved are cultured and a 10 percent water-soluble mafenide (Sulfamylon) preparation is applied to all second-degree and third-degree burned areas (Lindberg et al.).

The patient is placed in a bed, in a position permitting maximum exposure of his wounds. This may be a crib (about 30 percent of the patients are children), in a regular bed, on a rotating frame, or on a Nylon netting stretched tautly over a modified Bradford frame. The patient is turned from the prone to the supine position and vice versa as associated injuries or pulmonary status permits. In the absence of elevated body temperature, warming lights or a lightly covered bed cradle is used to provide protection from chilling and to promote drying of the wound. Sterile linens are not used. Sterile burn pads are placed under open wounds (Figs. 28–13 and 28–14). These pads have excellent absorptive qualities, and because of their tensile strength facilitate lifting an extremity of an adult or turning a small child thereby avoiding direct contact with open wounds, grafted areas, or donor sites.

Each day the patient's wounds are carefully examined by the physician. Examination is followed, when indicated, by gentle debridement and mechanical cleansing of the wounds. This is accomplished at the patient's bedside or in a hydrotherapy unit. Sulfamylon cream is applied to the wound following daily cleansing, and may again be applied at bedtime. The nurse should wear sterile gloves when applying Sulfamylon.

Second-degree burn wounds are treated with Sulfamylon until visible, abundant islets of epithelial tissue are present. Homograft is frequently used as a biologic dressing to stimulate complete epithelialization.

Third-degree wounds are treated with Sulfamylon to suppress bacterial pro-

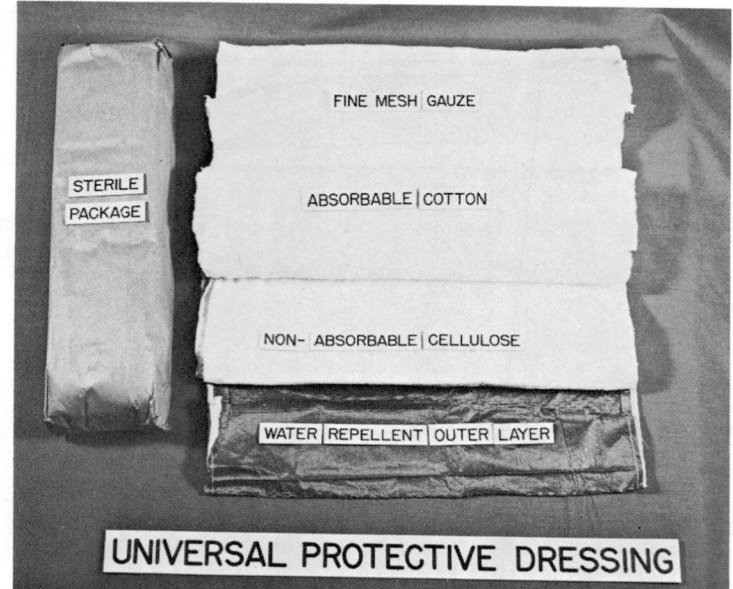

FINE MESH GAUZE

STERILE
PACKAGE

ABSORBABLE | COTTON

NON- | ABSORBABLE | CELLULOSE

WATER | REPELLENT | OUTER LAYER

UNIVERSAL PROTECTIVE DRESSING

*Figure 28–13
Universal protective
dressing used under open
burn wounds and freshly
grafted areas; this
dressing is also used
under extremities from
which autograft is taken.*

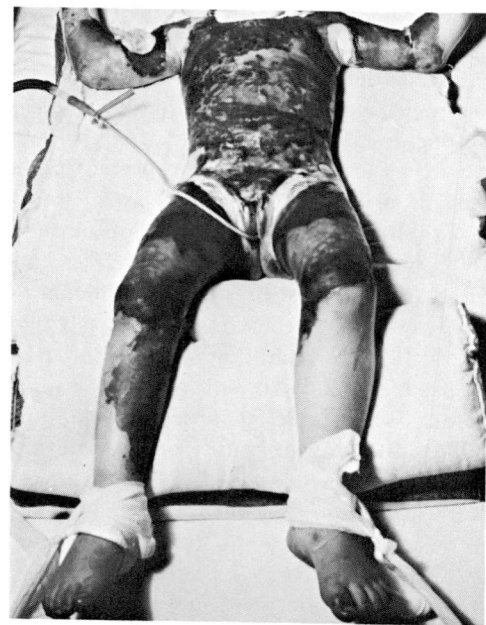

*Figure 28–14
Child with third-degree
burns of trunk and lower
extremities lying on
opened universal pro-
tective dressings.*

liferation while allowing granulation tissue to form. When granulation tissue becomes exposed, Sulfamylon is discontinued and homograft is applied. When donor sites are available, and when homograft testing reveals a viable graft bed, autograft is applied for permanent wound closure. In third-degree burn wounds, Sulfamylon is often applied to the eschar while adjacent granulating areas are covered with homograft.

Since Sulfamylon suppresses bacterial activity in the burn wound, separation of the eschar—a phenomenon dependent upon bacterial activity—is often delayed. When eschar separation is delayed, the physician, in order to encourage eschar separation, may temporarily discontinue treatment with Sulfamylon and apply wet or dry dressings to the area involved.

Nurses are often concerned about odor control in the care of the burned patient. Experience has shown that odor is related to the condition of the burn wound. When burn wounds are cleansed and debrided frequently, there is little odor problem.

INFECTION CONTROL

Infection of the burn wound is a common and often severe complication that can result in conversion of second-degree burns to full-thickness skin loss, failure of skin grafts to take, malnutrition, or fatal burn wound sepsis. Sources of contamination may be air, dust, or personnel and visitors via organisms on skin and clothing or from the respiratory tract.

To what extent the practice of employing aseptic precautions in the care of burn patients has a positive effect upon infection control has not been satisfactorily demonstrated. Until this question can be answered authoritatively, attempts are made to minimize transfer of organisms to and from the patient through aseptic technique in accordance with the practices of the particular hospital.

Irrespective of the presence or absence of special facilities or provisions for infection control, thorough hand washing with soap under running water is the most effective single measure that can be employed in preventing cross-contamination (Lindberg et al.; LaVerne). The importance of careful hand washing cannot be overemphasized, particularly if gloves are not available for use to prevent direct contamination of the hands. The hands should be washed thoroughly before and after treating each patient, and after handling contaminated objects.

Frequently aseptic precautions are severe, requiring that all equipment to be used for the patient, bed linens, bedpans, and the like be sterile, though in some instances only clean equipment is considered necessary. As a precaution against the possibility of contamination by indirect contact, all articles of equipment used in the care of burn patients must be disinfected or sterilized after use. This includes such equipment as parts of respirators, thermal blankets, electrocardiograph attachments, and otoscopes.

Bath basins, emesis basins, urinals, bedpans, and other such articles, whether or not they are kept at the patient's bedside, should be sterilized after each use.

A multitude of prepackaged, sterile, disposable items such as catheterization sets, irrigation sets, gastric feeding sets, enema sets, drainage tubing, plastic gloves, and various catheters are available at reasonable costs through medical supply companies. As an added means of preventing contamination by indirect contact resulting from improper cleaning and sterilization of nondisposable items, it is strongly recommended that disposable items be utilized.

It is desirable that personnel caring for burn patients wear scrub suits or dresses similar to those used in operating rooms. However, if these are not available, a gown should be worn over the hospital uniform. Suits, dresses, and/or gowns should be changed as necessity seems to dictate.

During the critical resuscitation period, while the patient requires constant observation and frequent attention must be given to intravenous therapy, monitoring of urinary output, oxygen therapy, tracheostomy toilet, and the like, it is recommended that face masks be worn by all personnel concerned with direct care of the patient. Following the resuscitation period, masks should be worn when wounds are cleansed and debrided, when dressings are changed, and when grafts are being applied. When masks are worn, they should be changed frequently.

BEDS USED FOR SEVERELY BURNED PATIENTS

The type of bed used for the severely burned patient is determined by the extent and site of his injury, and by his age or size. Several beds are described here.

Rotating Frames

Rotating beds such as the Stryker frame, Foster bed, and CircOlectric bed are well suited to the care of the burn patient. Of the three mentioned, the CircOlectric bed offers the advantage of having a wider posterior frame, which adds to the patient's comfort and sense of security. In addition, the patient's position can be changed more gradually from the supine to the prone and vice versa.

When planning for and providing care for a severely burned patient, the nurse will find that certain requirements for his care can be met more conveniently and effectively when coordinated with the patient's "up" or "down" burns (see Table 28-2). It should be remembered, when using patient's turns as a guide to planning nursing care, that it is advisable to further coordinate plans for his care with the physician and physical therapist.

TABLE 28-2 *Patient Care Requirements Coordinated with Up Turns (Supine Position) and Down Turns (Prone Position)*

REQUIREMENTS TO BE MET on Up Turns	REQUIREMENTS TO BE MET on Down Turns
Tracheostomy toilet	Mouth care if patient is unable to cooperate
Eye care	Giving an enema; turning for expulsion
Tube feeding	Taking rectal temperature
Care of indwelling urinary catheter	Self-feeding
Care of hair (cutting, combing, shampooing)	Bathing unaffected areas of posterior body
Care of fingernails and toenails	Inducing bowel elimination
Intramuscular injections (anterior thigh muscles when buttocks are burned)	Changing leg splints
Feeding helpless patient	Changing dressings, posterior body
Bathing unaffected areas of anterior body	
Changing hand splints	
Whirlpool (hands or arms)	
Changing dressings, anterior body	
Shaving	
Mouth care, including attention to lips	
Care of nose	

Crib with Mattress-upon-Mattress Arrangement

Standard rotating frames are not well suited to the care of very small children. However, many advantages afforded by the use of turning frames for adults can be realized for small children when a crib with a mattress-upon-mattress arrangement is used (Fig. 28–15). The upper mattress, which is made of synthetic foam rubber, is approximately 12 inches shorter than the lower mattress, and has a through-and-through circular cutout measuring approximately 6 inches in diameter. The cutout portion accommodates a disposable container for trapping urine and/or feces. Both mattresses are covered with protective rubber sheeting. Additional advantages afforded by the mattress-upon-mattress arrangement are described below.

1. When a child is in prone position with the shoulders even with the top end of the mattress and the head supported on a small foam rubber pad (Fig. 28–16), requirements for care such as tracheostomy toilet, mouth care, and taking of rectal temperature can be readily met.

2. Hyperextension of the neck to avoid maceration of tissues about the chin or neck, or to permit maximum graft take, is a frequent requirement in the care of the burned child. This can easily be achieved by placing the child in supine position with the shoulders even with the top end of the mattress. The head rests on the lower mattress or on a foam rubber pad, the thickness of which is determined by the degree of hyperextension desired.

3. The greater width provided by the two mattresses permits the use of a wider variety of sandbags, foot boards, splints, and other devices used to maintain a position of function and prevent musculoskeletal disorders and/or the formation of pressure sores.

Although the mattress-upon-mattress arrangement does not permit turning of the child without his being physically lifted, a small child can be easily turned without

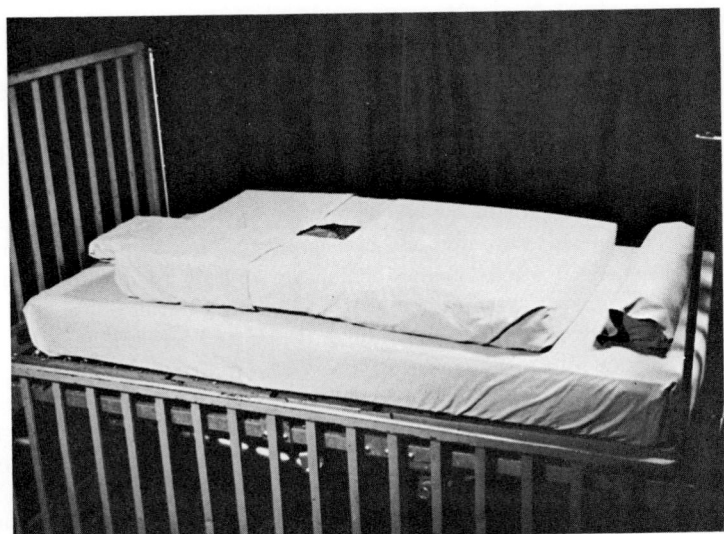

Figure 28–15
Crib with mattress-on-mattress arrangement used to facilitate care of severely burned child.

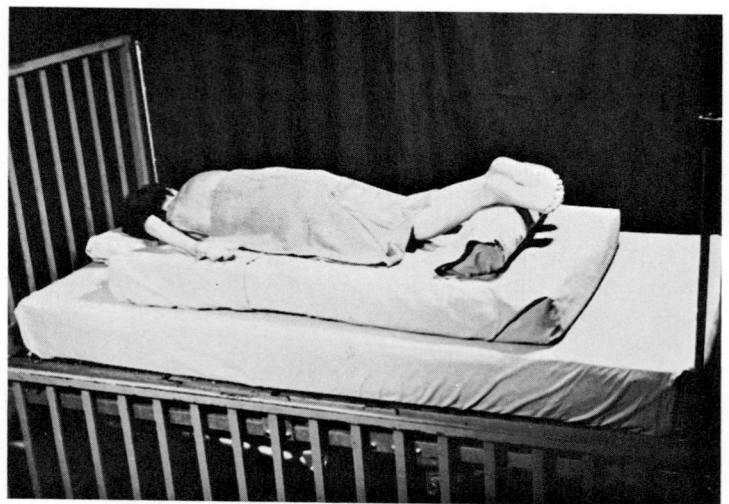

Figure 28–16
Child lying in prone
position in crib with
mattress-on-mattress
arrangement.

trauma to local wounds. This can be accomplished by simply sandwiching him between two burn pads, lifting him and turning him over.

Modified Bradford Frame

A modified Bradford frame with a Nylon mesh netting stretched tautly over the frame provides an excellent means of achieving maximum exposure of burn wounds in circumferential burns of the trunk and/or the lower extremities for either adults or children (Figs. 28–17 and 28–18). It is also used to advantage when large body areas are grafted and to facilitate drying of the donor site.

POSITIONING AND EXERCISE

Complications that frequently result from the necessary treatment when the trunk or an extremity must be immobilized are muscle shortening, loss of muscle mass and tone, and ankylosis. In addition, fecal impaction, decubitus ulcers, and pneumonia are frequent complications of immobilization. Contractures such as those preventing complete closure of the eyes or mouth or those interfering with joint motion and structural loss of an ear, extremity, or part of an extremity may occur as a result of the burn injury.

The nursing care involves consistent practice of preventive measures to minimize these complications. General principles of body positioning and exercise as discussed in Chapter 14 are applicable to the burned patient. The patient should be turned frequently and positioned not only for comfort but also to prevent contractures. The site and seriousness of the burn injury and the method of treatment will influence the selection of body positions that can be utilized. When the burned area involves or is near joints of the extremities, splints may be applied or correct positioning may be utilized to minimize contractures. The unaffected body parts can be exercised by the patient performing those activities within his capacity. The nurse often assumes the responsibility for finding methods to motivate the

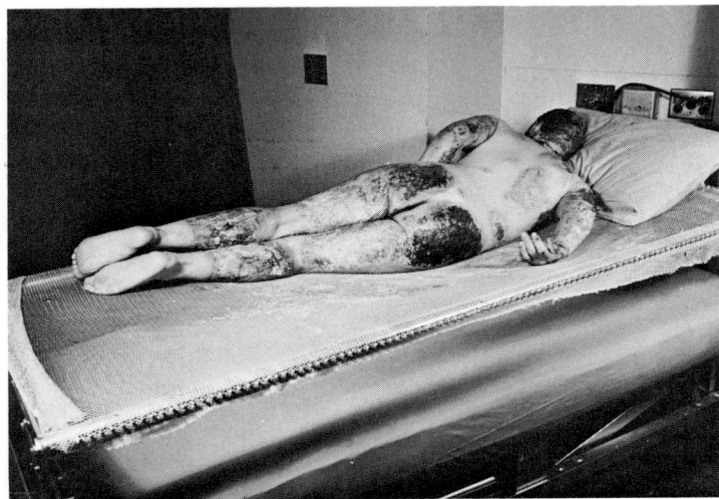

*Figure 28–17
Modified Bradford frame
with Nylon netting used
to permit maximum
exposure of burn wounds.*

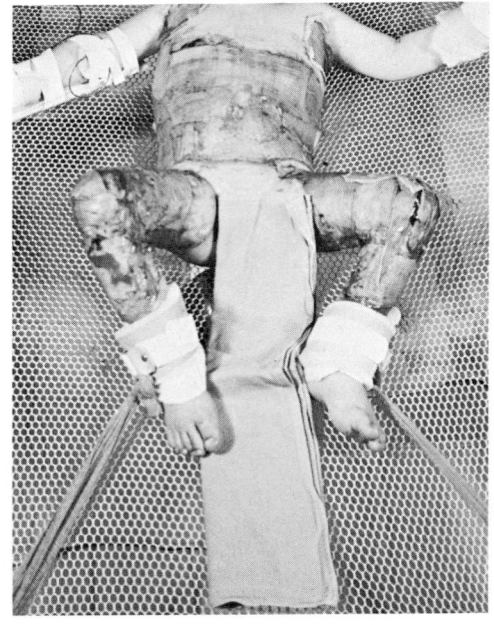

*Figure 28–18
Child with extensive
third-degree burns of
trunk and lower
extremities on modified
Bradford frame with
Nylon netting which
permits maximum
exposure of burn wound.*

patient to perform these activities. In other circumstances, the nurse may give passive exercise and range of motion exercise to the patient.

NURSING CARE OF PATIENTS WITH BURNS OF THE HEAD, FACE, AND NECK

Hair

Whether the patient is male or female, the hair should be clipped or closely cut if the hair or scalp is involved. Whatever the condition of the shorn hair, it is advisable that it be put in safekeeping should it be wanted for cosmetic purposes in the event of the patient's death.

Although a shorn head undoubtedly makes nursing care easier, particularly of female patients, the hair should not be cut because of its value as a morale factor if it does not interfere with medical treatment. Having the hair combed, shampooed, curled, beribboned, or otherwise groomed gives the patient a sense of being cared "about"; and, too, the hair often helps provide the incentive a patient needs to become interested in personal appearance or to use an arm that needs to be exercised.

Eyes

Special attention to the eyes is a frequent requirement in the care of patients who have sustained deep second-degree or third-degree burns of the face. Although the eyes themselves are rarely burned, serious eye damage secondary to burns of the eyelids and tissues surrounding the eyes can readily occur.

The chief dangers are from infection, resulting in a chronic conjunctivitis, and from corneal ulceration, resulting in permanent visual damage. A less common danger, but one to be considered, is the presence in the eye of a broken or embedded contact lens.

Infection is caused by the constant entrance into the eye of bacteria from contaminated burned tissues adjacent to the eye. Corneal ulceration occurs indirectly as healing of the eyelids and surrounding tissues takes place, and scar tissue contracture, causing eversion, or ectropion, of the upper or lower eyelid prevents complete closure of the eyes (Fig. 28–19). The cornea is then exposed to drying as tears spill out over the margin of the everted eyelid. Drying of the cornea, in turn, leads to corneal ulceration.

The nursing care of patients who have sustained burns involving the eyes is extremely important. It includes the following:

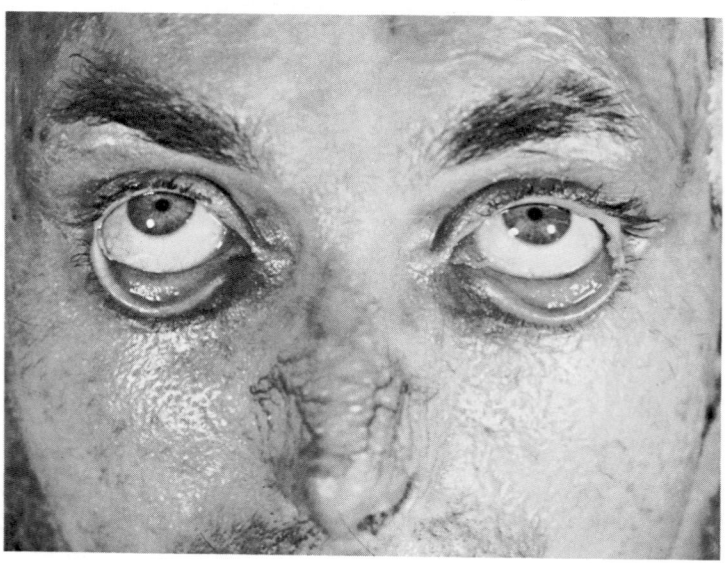

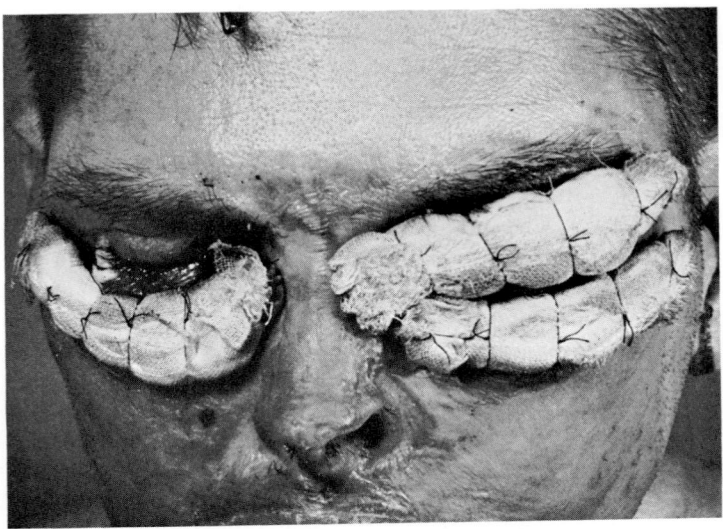

*Figure 28–20
Adult male following
corrective surgery for
ectropion of eyelids, with
dressings in place.*

1. Recognizing and reporting significant signs and symptoms, among which are the presence in the eye of exudate and/or adherent specks, redness and/or congestion of the eye, sleeping with the eyes partly open, and blurring of vision, burning or stinging, scratchiness and dryness.

2. Giving emotional support to the anxious patient, and to his equally anxious relatives, during the early postburn period when his eyes are temporarily closed from edema, and later when his eyes are bandaged or sutured following reparative surgery (Fig. 28–20), and remembering to always address the patient before approaching him for any reason.

3. Protecting the patient from acts of his own which might interfere with treatment or cause further injury. Examples include rubbing his eyes, removing his dressings or disturbing eye sutures, displacing an intravenous or a urethral catheter, and attempting to get out of bed.

4. Faithfully carrying out eye irrigations, applications, and instillations as directed by the physician.

When irrigating the eyes of a patient with burns about the face, the nurse may find the following suggestions helpful: (1) Several thicknesses of folded 4 x 4 gauze squares held gently but firmly against the face at the outer angle of the eye may be used to receive the return flow of irrigating solution in lieu of a curved basin, the use of which may cause further trauma to tissues of the face. (2) When the patient has face dressings, eye irrigations may be coordinated with dressing changes, to prevent, insofar as is possible, the return flow of solution from escaping into the dressings. At frequent intervals between dressing changes, cotton pledgets well saturated with irrigating solution are used to remove exudate from about the eyes.

Nose

The burn patient's nostrils often become obstructed as a result of edema, the accumulation of dried secretions, and/or destruction of nasal tissue. Although he may be able to breathe through his mouth, or by way of a tracheostomy, nasal obstruction adds to his general discomfort and increases his anxiety.

If nasal obstruction is unrelieved following resolution of edema, a few drops of normal saline applied to the nostrils at frequent intervals will generally soften obstructive material permitting removal with cotton-tipped applicators. If this measure fails, the physician may remove obstructive material with nasal forceps.

When attempting to clear the nostrils of a patient with burns involving the nose, the nurse must proceed cautiously to avoid precipitating bleeding.

Occasionally full-thickness burns of the face may result in destruction of portions of the nose. When this occurs, it can be anticipated that separation of devitalized nasal tissue may occur simultaneously with the nurse's efforts to relieve nasal obstruction, or upon change of face dressings. The nurse who is prepared for such a disquieting eventuality is better able to maintain her composure should this occur while she is caring for the patient.

Mouth

The patient who has sustained burns of the face, neck, and hands, and whose hands are burned so that he cannot use them, requires careful and persistent mouth care, often over a prolonged period of time. Contributing to these requirements are edema of the face, neck, or hands; burn eschar and burn crusts; total or partial loss of the hand or fingers; face and/or hand dressings; hand splints; operative procedures; pain; contractures of the neck, axilla, and/or elbow; poor nutritional status; disorientation; and emotional reactions such as apathy.

When the patient is unable to open or close his mouth normally, to handle his oral secretions, or is disoriented, care of the mouth is more easily and effectively accomplished if measures used are similar to those commonly practiced in the care of an unconscious patient. The use of a child-size rather than an adult-size toothbrush or an electric toothbrush is a further aid to effective mouth care.

When giving mouth care, in addition to seeing that the patient's mouth is clean, the nurse must be alert to detect and report dental problems that require the attention of the physician or a dentist. Older patients, those who are malnourished, and young children often have loose teeth. A loosened tooth can easily be aspirated while the patient is under anesthesia.

Measures must also be taken to keep the patient's lips free of oral secretions and loosened crusts. Crusts are kept softened with appropriate emollients. When cleaning the patient's lips, the nurse must be careful to avoid precipitating bleeding.

Whatever procedure is used to accomplish mouth care for a burn patient, it is important that it be suited to the patient's needs and that it be employed at frequent intervals for as long a period of time as the patient is unable to care for himself.

PSYCHOLOGICAL REACTIONS

Depending on the severity and extent of the damage from burn and the impact of this event upon the patient, various concerns and psychological reactions of the patient may occur.

Initially, concern for survival and freedom from pain may be of primary importance to the individual. Some concerns are related to the patient's concept of his body (body image) such as the observability and extent of the scar and the amount of disfigurement and/or functional disability this will cause. The actual loss or loss of usefulness of a body part can be a threat to the patient. Some concerns are related to the expense and loss of income associated with the long and expensive hospitalization and recovery. With severe burns there is the prospect of long, tiring, repetitive and expensive treatment of defects such as physical therapy for improvement of muscle and joint action or plastic surgery for contractures, disfigurement, or structural loss.

Common psychological reactions are depression, regression, withdrawal, dependence, passive resistance, and antagonism. When such concerns and reactions occur the nurse is presented with a serious challenge to select the appropriate supportive and motivational interventions in order to help the patient cope with the distress of the illness experience.

Bibliography

Artz, Curtis P. and Eric Reiss: *The Treatment of Burns.* Philadelphia: W. B. Saunders Company, 1957.

Epstein, B. S., L. R. Ross, C. Teplitz, and J. A. Moncrief: Experiences with Low Tracheostomy in the Burn Patient. *Journal of American Medical Association,* 183:966–968, 1963.

Harper, H. A.: The Nutritional Problem. In L. Goldman and R. E. Gardner (Eds.): *Burns: A Symposium.* Springfield, Ill.: Charles C Thomas, Publisher, 1965, pp. 28–33.

Hummel, R. P., B. Balikov, and C. P. Artz: Studies in Curling's Ulcers. *Surgical Forum,* 6:306–312, 1955.

LaVerne, Ruth T.: *Microbiology and Epidemiology.* Philadelphia: W. B. Saunders Company, 1962.

Lindberg, R. B., J. A. Moncrief, W. E. Switzer, S. E. Order, and W. Mills, Jr.: The Successful Control of Burn Wound Sepsis. *Journal of Trauma,* 5:601–161, 1965.

Moncrief, J. A. and A. D. Mason, Jr.: Evaporative Water Loss in the Burned Patient. *Journal of Trauma,* 4:180–185, 1964.

Order, Stanley E. and J. A. Moncrief: *The Burn Wound.* Springfield, Ill.: Charles C Thomas, Publisher, 1965.

Teplitz, C., D. Davis, A. D. Mason, Jr., and J. A. Moncrief: Pseudomonas Burn Wound Sepsis. Pathogenesis of Experimental Pseudomonas Burn Wound Sepsis. *Journal of Surgical Research,* 4:200–216, 1964.

Teplitz, C., D. Davis, A. D. Mason, Jr., and J. A. Moncrief: Pseudomonas Burn Wound Sepsis. II Hematogenous Infection at the Junction of the Burn Wound and the Unburned Hypodermis. *Journal of Surgical Research,* 4:1964.

Suggested Readings

Adams, R. H. and L. MacToggert: Physical Therapy in the Treatment of Burns. *Physical Therapy Review,* 38:481–482, 1958.

Artz, Curtis P. (Ed.): *Research in Burns.* Philadelphia: F. A. Davis Company, 1956.

Blocker, T. G., Jr., S. R. Lewis, D. A. Grant, V. Blocker, and J. E. Bennett: Experiences in the Management of the Burn Wound. *Plastic and Reconstructive Surgery,* 26:579–589, 1960.

Harmer, Bertha and Virginia Henderson: *Textbook of the Principles and Practice of Nursing.* New York: The Macmillan Company, 1957.

Larson, D. L.: Closure of the Burn Wound. *Journal of Trauma,* 5:254–266, 1965.

Lewis, S. R., H. A. Goolishiam, C. W. Wolf, J. B. Lynch, and T. G. Blocker, Jr.: Psychological Studies in Burn Patients. *Plastic and Reconstructive Surgery,* 31:323–332, 1963.

Long, R. T. and O. Cope: Emotional Problems of Burned Children. *New England Journal of Medicine,* 264:1121–1127, 1961.

Moncrief, J. A.: Tracheostomy in Burns. *Archives of Surgery,* 79:45–48, 1959.

Moncrief, J. A.: Burns of Specific Areas. *Journal of Trauma,* 5:278–291, 1965.

Moncrief, J. A., L. R. Rose, and W. E. Switzer: Burn Therapy—A Requirement for Team Effort. *Southern Medical Journal,* 56:1063–1067, 1963.

Moncrief, J. A., W. E. Switzer, and C. Teplitz: Curling's Ulcer. *Journal of Trauma,* 4:481–494, 1964.

Order, S. E., A. D. Mason, Jr., H. L. Walker, R. B. Lindberg, W. E. Switzer, and J. A. Moncrief: Vascular Destructive Effects of Thermal Injury and Its Relationship to Burn Wound Sepsis. *Journal of Trauma,* 5:62–71, 1965.

Order, S. E., A. D. Mason, Jr., W. E. Switzer, and J. A. Moncrief: Arterial Vascular Occlusion and Devitalization of Burn Wounds. *Annals of Surgery,* 161:502–508, 1965.

Sutton, Audrey L.: *Bedside Nursing Techniques in Medicine and Surgery.* Philadelphia: W. B. Saunders Company, 1964.

Switzer, W. E., J. W. Jones, and J. A. Moncrief: Evaluation of Early Excision of Burns in Children. *Journal of Trauma,* 5:540–544, 1965.

Teplitz, C., B. S. Epstine, L. R. Rose, and J. A. Moncrief: Necrotizing Tracheitis Induced by Tracheostomy Tube. *Archives of Pathology,* 77:6–19, 1964.

Teplitz, C., B. S. Epstine, L. R. Rose, W. E. Switzer, and J. A. Moncrief: Pathology of Low Tracheostomy in Children. *American Journal of Clinical Pathology,* 42:56–63, 1964.

SECTION 3
PLASTIC AND RECONSTRUCTIVE SURGERY EM OLIVIA BEVIS

Plastic surgery is the repair, restoration, or alteration of either damaged or normal tissue in order to improve function, comfort, or esthetic appearance. It may be accomplished by the removal of tissue or the grafting of tissue or tissue substitute. Grafting is the most common form of plastic surgery and is the form that will be dealt with in this section.

Types of Grafts

A graft is a tissue or a noninflammatory tissue substitute placed in the body and incorporated by the body into the existing tissues and functions as substitution for, in addition to, or in coordination with the body's own tissue. Thus any material, natural or synthetic, used as described is a graft.

The four major types of grafts are substitute grafts, homografts, isografts, and autografts. The interested student is referred to a basic textbook on plastic surgery for information about other types.

SUBSTITUTE GRAFTS

Substitute grafts are commonly used for orthopedic and vascular repair. Non-pyogenic plastic and Nylon mesh tubes are used in vascular surgery. When mesh

969

vessel substitutes are used, fibrous tissue is laid down in the mesh and creates a fibrous tissue canal through which blood can flow. Plastics that can be molded and formed during surgery are used extensively for plastic repair of the cranium, and nonreactive metals are used for repair of fractured hips.

HOMOGRAFTS

Although there is wide popular interest in homografts, they are presently of limited value and highly specific use. Homografts are grafts from an immunologically distinct donor to an immunologically distinct recipient. Without adequate control most homografts set up an antigen-antibody reaction characterized by a nonsuppurative inflammation. At the graft site there is edema, fibroblastic reaction, leukocyte infiltration, and ultimate dissolution of and/or rejection of the graft. Blood transfusions are the most common and most successfully used homografts. Corneal implants have had some success, although immunological inflammatory response with chronic inflammation, clouding of implanted cornea, or rejection of the grafted cornea is not uncommon.

Organ transplantation is still in the investigative stage. Kidney and heart transplantation is under intensive study, but few conclusions have been reached about the use of transplants of these organs as feasible alternatives in patients whose own organs have ceased to be adequately functional.

Homografts are used in vascular surgery. They are used widely in the treatment of severely burned individuals, in whom they are often life-saving.

ISOGRAFTS

An isograft is a graft taken from one identical twin and given to the other. Since antigen-antibody reactions do not occur, the isografts often are life-saving when one identical twin has been extensively burned or has suffered bilateral renal failure.

AUTOGRAFTS

An autograft is a graft taken from, and used in, the patient himself. The autograft is the most frequently used and the most successful of all grafts. Almost any part of the human body can be autografted; only a few of the more common types will be discussed here.

Tissues Useful as Autografts

ARTERY AND VEIN

These autografts revascularize rapidly; however, despite this great advantage, their usefulness is limited by the scarcity of large arteries for replacement. Small segments of large arteries may be used, but long segments cannot be reanastomosed. Veins cannot be used as replacements for arteries except in segments subjected to low pressure.

FASCIA

Fascia is used to replace destroyed joint capsules or weakened supporting structures in inguinal and umbilical hernias. Fascia is usually obtained from the fascia lata of the thigh.

TENDONS

Tendon grafts are extremely useful in plastic surgery of the hand. Tendons revascularize slowly but heal well.

NERVES

No large nerves can be sacrificed; however, some small nerves may be used as grafts, for example in facial and digital nerves.

BONES

Bone grafting is a highly successful form of plastic surgery which is performed frequently. The graft serves as a foundation for new bone formation.

SKIN

Autografts of the skin may be split-thickness or full-thickness, attached or free. An *attached* graft is partially attached to the donor site and derives its blood supply from the intact vessels attached to the donor site. A *free* graft is severed from the donor site and obtains its nutrition from the recipient site by means of diffusion until an adequate blood supply is established.

Skin Autografts

SPLIT-THICKNESS GRAFTS

Split-thickness grafts are of two types, thin split-thickness grafts and thick split-thickness grafts. Thin split-thickness grafts are composed of epidermis and very small amounts of dermis. The chief disadvantage of these grafts is that they do not possess a sufficient amount of dermis (corium) to be functionally stable. Skin grafts contract in direct relationship to their thickness; therefore, thin split-thickness grafts contract the most. Thick split-thickness skin grafts are composed of epidermis plus one-half to two-thirds dermis. The large amount of dermis is necessary to produce tough, resilient skin. They provide good cover and function; however, they are not practical in patients who have extensive skin areas to be covered since a single donor site must provide skin several times. These grafts are used most frequently in large denuded areas, such as those resulting from burns or radical mastectomy.

Pinch grafts—or postage stamp grafts—are small split-thickness grafts that are used on large denuded areas. These grafts take fairly well. Grafted sites healed in this manner have a checkerboard or hobnailed appearance. A large number of the grafted cells survive; epithelization takes place by outward spread from the implanted skin. Reinnervation occurs within 3 to 6 months.

FULL-THICKNESS GRAFTS

A full-thickness graft may be attached or free, and includes the epidermis and the dermis down to but not including the subcutaneous fat. Revascularization occurs within 5 to 7 days. This graft is tough and its contraction is less than that of the split-thickness graft. It is often used over joints or in areas subjected to pressure, stress, or friction. Donor sites will not regenerate; they must be sutured closed or split-thickness grafts must be placed over them.

PEDICLE FLAP

The pedicle flap is a full-thickness graft that maintains an intact blood supply from the donor site. A flap is raised, sometimes the denuded sites are sutured together, and one end is detached and sutured to the recipient site or a carrier site. When a blood supply has been established from the recipient end, the donor site end can be detached. If the recipient site is distant from the donor site, the skin flap may be sutured to an intermediate site between the donor and the recipient sites and left there until an adequate blood supply has been established. This may be done several times; each time the distant end of the pedicle flap is detached and reattached nearer the desired position. This process is called "walking" a graft. Thus, a pedicle flap from the abdomen can be "walked" to replace a constricting scar over the patella or tibia or to cover a denuded plantar surface. Disfigured or deformed parts of the body can be reconstructed with the use of pedicle flaps which serve as tissue mass, and bone, tendon, and cartilage. Pedicle flaps are used extensively following radical surgery for cancer of the face and neck.

Reconstructive Surgery Utilizing Pedicle Flaps. Reconstructive surgery utilizing large pedicle flaps is done in several stages over a protracted period. The patient should be fully prepared for the length of time required, the discomfort involved, and his unpleasant appearance. He may expect immediate repair. Encouragement is difficult to give without sounding unrealistic, and platitudes only add to the patient's burden. There are several "rules of thumb" the nurse can follow to promote optimal mental and physical health. The first is to promote and encourage good physical hygiene. A mild alkaline mouthwash several times a day will diminish mouth odor and give the mouth a more pleasant taste. In the case of a male patient, his beard should be shaved every day if this does not endanger the wound. Tissue wipes should be kept within easy reach of the drooling patient; a disposable bag for used wipes must be kept within his reach at all times. The nurse should maximize the esthetic value of the undamaged tissue by encouraging the patient to be coiffed and manicured. The family should be requested to bring simple clothing that is easily laundered and is not pulled on over the head; getting dressed every day enables the patient to walk around freely and helps him to feel that perhaps his goal is achievable. Good nutrition is essential to good body repair yet is difficult to achieve for the patient who has had radical neck or mouth surgery. A liquid or soft diet usually must be given and the patient often lacks an appetite. Exercise and fresh air will increase his appetite, but precautions must be taken to protect the patient who is susceptible to upper respiratory infections. He must not become exhausted, chilled, or overheated. Food likes and dislikes should be catered to, and the family should be encouraged to bring favorite foods.

Nursing Care

THE DONOR SITE

Epithelium regenerates at the donor site of split-thickness grafts from the hair follicles, sweat glands, and sebaceous glands left in the deep portions of the dermis. A nonirritating, light, thin single layer of sterile mesh is laid over the donor site and a pressure dressing is applied until hemostasis is complete. The pressure dressing is then removed and the mesh remains in place; the donor site heals exposed to air. No ointments, dressings, or external medications can hasten the healing of the donor site. However, since burns and grafts being treated with silver nitrate may adjoin donor site areas, donor sites may be included in the silver nitrate treatment. Good results have been obtained with this treatment. Donor sites being treated by the open method should be kept clean and dry. Bedclothes, gowns, and pajamas should not adhere to the open wound. Air should circulate freely. The surrounding tissue should be washed and dried. Seepage may be a problem, and the sight of the wound may be upsetting to the patient. Preparation should be given the patient prior to surgery regarding the location, appearance, and care of the donor site. Pain at the donor site may be experienced because surface nerves are damaged. As the wound heals, severe itching will occur. It can be diminished by salicylates and antihistamines given orally; in persistent cases, an anesthetic may be administered. Under normal conditions, reepithelization is usually complete in 10 to 12 days, and the mesh covering the wound then falls off.

THE RECIPIENT SITE

For optimal graft survival, the recipient site must meet all the requirements for good wound healing, including intact blood supply; absence of foreign materials, old blood, dead skin, and infection; raw or denuded contact areas; stability.

A free graft does not have a direct intact blood supply; it receives fluids and nutrients through diffusion until capillaries in the granulation tissue are formed in the recipient site. This capillary generation must occur quickly, for skin survival is probably limited to 48 hours at normal body temperature. The absence of any factor promoting wound healing lessens tissue survival.

The failure of a skin graft to survive may be due to either local or systemic causes. In addition to those local conditions previously mentioned, there are several matters that should be attended to so as to promote optimal take of grafted tissue. Graft sites should be prepared by vigorous removal of eschar and treatment of infection. This is done by means of repeated changes of dry dressings, wet soaks, and/or surgical excision as described for burns. Chemical agents and enzymes have been used to remove eschar, dead tissue, and islands of granulation, but none have proved more effective than saline tub baths. Nonetheless, vigorous and thorough removal of devitalized eschar is the first step in healing and preparation for grafting.

Thermal burns comprise the largest category of burns necessitating skin grafts, although chemical burns and injuries or surgical procedures that cause destruction of dermal layers call for similar nursing measures to promote graft survival.

Infection

Infection is the most serious problem and grafting is not undertaken until infection is controlled. The one exception to this general rule is the pinch graft described earlier. Infection may result in destruction of deeper layers of tissue which had been undamaged by the original trauma, as well as the graft itself; if the infection is unchecked septicemia may ensue and may be fatal.

The application of occlusive dressings saturated with 0.5 percent aqueous silver nitrate has significantly reduced the frequency of wound sepsis and thus has improved skin graft survival. One important advantage of this treatment is that in the absence of infection reepithelization of deep partial-thickness injuries will take place without grafting. Another is that sites on which grafts are necessary can be more readily identified.

If the patient's injury is not being treated with silver nitrate, strict reverse isolation and aseptic technique must be followed; if the injury is being treated with silver nitrate this treatment is continued, in most cases, after grafting and after both donor and recipient sites have been treated. Meticulous cleanliness, but not strict reverse isolation, is required for these patients. The patient's room should be damp-dusted with antiseptics daily, irrespective of the type of treatment.

If the area of injury is a large one, grafting is done in stages and the injury and the graft area are treated concurrently.

Wet soaks on the ungrafted injury (silver nitrate, saline, and acetic acid are most commonly used) cause considerable discomfort, so the nurse must provide a warm, comfortable, clean environment. At the same time there should be no interference with the evaporative process that is necessary for precipitation of the silver nitrate. Cotton blankets provide warmth; they should be changed several times a day. The physician may advise the use of a light cradle; in this event extreme caution is necesssry because the cradle can hasten drying or cause burns.

Fever

A high fever will markedly decrease the survival time of grafts, so the nurse should observe the patient closely for postoperative fever and should report its development to the physician immediately. The patient should never be exposed to drafts. Cooling can be achieved through proper ventilation, by regulating the heat in the winter and the air conditioning in the summer. Covers can be removed in order to allow free circulation of air; if the patient's dressings are wet, this reduces body temperature quickly. The patient may be given cold fluids, and his face, neck, and hands may be rinsed with cool water.

Pruritus

Pruritus may be intense both at the donor site and at the healing graft site. Itching at the graft site is an important symptom and should be observed, described, and reported to the physician in full detail. If severe, it may signal the formation of keloid tissue at the site of the graft. These keloids can cause contractures or mar the appearance of the healed wound. Scratching the healing graft site can damage the new friable dermal layers. Mild itching and scratching are controlled with salicylates, which the nurse should administer according to the physician's order before the itching becomes intense. Tranquilizers and barbiturates are moderately successful in controlling more severe itching, while intractable or intense itching is often treated with steroids, which are injected at the site of the wound by the physician. Occasionally a local anesthetic is used.

The nurse can do many things beyond administering ordered medication to alleviate itching and prevent scratching. Soaps and detergents dry the skin oils and should not be used. Cool tap water decreases itching and warm or hot water tends to increase it. An explanation of the damage scratching can do to grafts should be made but the nurse should not depend upon such an explanation to deter the patient from scratching. It is difficult for the patient to ignore the itching, and scratching is a natural response. With very young patients mittens may be used but these are not suggested for adult patients unless the patients request them, because such restraints leave alert patients feeling vulnerable and helpless. The fingernails should be trimmed close and kept clean.

Contractures

Contractures are a constant problem and may necessitate further plastic surgery. The nurse should do everything possible to minimize the inevitable contraction of the scar tissue. Splinting of joints may be accomplished with plaster casts or splint boards; half casts have the advantage of being molded to the part. The splint should be removed daily so that the nurse can cleanse the area and observe for pressure points. She should exercise the part only when the doctor determines that healing has progressed to a satisfactory stage. At this time the nurse should help the patient to move the affected part slowly yet consistently, with the goal of steadily increasing the range of activity.

General Supportive Measures

Most principles governing the nursing care of the patient with a surgical wound are applicable to the care of the patient receiving skin grafts. The central problem in the care of patients with skin grafts is the revascularization of the grafted tissue, and the nurse must devote her energy to the promotion of this process. Locally, the promotion of revascularization involves prevention of infection as previously discussed and positioning of the body so as to prevent pressure on the vascular supply. The nurse must also institute measures to support venous return, prevent edema, and promote immobilization of the graft. An example of the kind of problem the nurse might encounter is the case of a patient who has had reconstructive surgery of the right hand and is receiving intravenous infusions in the left arm. Postoperatively, blood pressure taken in the right arm would cause venous congestion and rupture of newly formed capillaries. The nurse can deal with this problem by placing the cuff on the upper thigh and palpating the popliteal artery. If this, too, is impossible, she could determine whether or not the blood pressure is adequate by observing the patient's pulse rate, skin color, and kidney output.

Revascularization is promoted through adequate hydration, correct environmental temperature, and good nutrition. Patients who have extensive injuries are anemic. A hemoglobin count below 9 g per 100 ml markedly decreases the take of a skin graft, and it is preferable for the count to be at least 12 g. Hypoproteinemia and hypovitaminosis can severely inhibit revascularization. Appetizing meals served at the proper temperature will improve the patient's appetite. Food preferences should be followed whenever possible, and the family should be encouraged to bring the patient's favorite dishes from home. Exercise and socialization help boost the appetite and should be encouraged. The importance of vitamin C in healing is well recognized and the nurse should encourage the patient to eat foods high in this vitamin.

Patients undergoing necessary plastic or reconstructive surgery are damaged, both physically and psychically. Nurses gnerally accept these patients more readily than those undergoing elective plastic surgery. Yet the woman with large, pendulous breasts or the man with a hooked nose may be just as severely damaged as the woman with a contracture or the man with a cut tendon. They need compassion and understanding, not sympathy, and their problems should not be ignored. As soon as the doctor feels that the patient is physically able, he should be encouraged to venture into public places, since his dread of meeting outsiders will be aggravated by procrastination. His mental health will be promoted through open and clear communication.

Bibliography

Books

Arieti, Silvano (Ed.): *American Handbook of Psychiatry*, Vol. I. New York: Basic Books, Inc., Publishers, 1959.

Davis, Loyal (Ed.): *Christopher's Textbook of Surgery*, 9th ed. Philadelphia: W. B. Saunders Company, 1968.

Jourard, Sidney M.: *The Transparent Self*. Princeton: D. Van Nostrand Company, Inc., 1964.

MacGregor, Frances Cooke: Some Psychological Hazards of Plastic Surgery of the Face. in D. Apple (Ed.): *Sociological Studies of Health and Sickness*. New York: McGraw-Hill Book Company, 1960.

Mosley, H. F. (Ed.): *Textbook of Surgery*, 3d ed. St. Louis: The C. V. Mosby Company, 1959.

Warren, Richard: *Surgery*. Philadelphia: W. B. Saunders Company, 1963.

Articles

Cohn, Roy: Transplantation in Humans. *Stanford Today*, Winter 1967, Series I, No. 18.

Edwards, Benjamin: Endoprostheses in Plastic Surgery. *American Journal of Nursing*, 64:5:123–125, May, 1964.

Polk, Hiram C.: Treatment of Severe Burns with Aqueous Silver Nitrate (0.5%). *Annals of Surgery*, 164:4, 753–767, October, 1966.

CHAPTER 29
THE PATIENT WITH DISEASE OF THE NERVOUS SYSTEM

SECTION 1 DISORDERS OF THE BRAIN

PAMELA HOLSCLAW MITCHELL*

* The author acknowledges the assistance of George A. Ojemann, M.D., and Donald W. Mitchell, M.D.,
in reviewing the manuscript of this section.

Because of the structure of the nervous system, care of the neurological patient is determined not so much by the nature of the disease as by the location of it. In this section, therefore, emphasis is given primarily to types of dysfunction produced by disease, rather than to specific disease entities. A basic knowledge of the functional anatomy of the nervous system is essential for planning nursing care; for this, the student's own basic anatomy and physiology textbook, supplemented by a specialized neurology textbook, should be sufficient. Details concerning specific disorders can be found in medical and neurology textbooks.

There are four principles which, in the author's experience, serve as a frame of reference for care of any neurological patient, whether his disorder is in the brain, spinal cord, or peripheral nerves. These principles will be referred to throughout the chapter.

1. *The nervous system is an electrical conducting system. Any break in conduction will produce dysfunction distal to that break. The kind and degree of dysfunction depend on the location, nature, and size of the lesion.* For example, a stroke involving the motor cortex will prevent nerve impules from initiating movement anywhere from the cortex to the hand; a tumor in the same place will have the same effect. Knowledge of the site and nature of the lesion will enable the nurse to predict and understand the patient's abilities and disabilities, to estimate his rehabilitation potential, and to determine which observations are especially pertinent.

2. *The central nervous system is a closed system with little room for expansion; unrelieved pressure in it will eventually be transmitted downward.* This will be discussed further under "Increased Intracranial Pressure."

3. *Cells of the central nervous system can regain function, even after considerable edema, if no cell death occurs, but dead cells do not regenerate. The axons of peripheral nerves can regenerate.* (See Section 3 of this chapter.) This principle becomes important in the assessment of the potential for return of function, and in understanding why return of function may vary in similar disorders.

4. *The individual's reaction to neurologic dysfunction depends upon his pattern of reaction to stress, the extent and location of the lesion, and the effects of changes in body image.* This is discussed under "Emotional Reactions."

Locating the Lesion

Locating the lesion and diagnosing its nature is one of the physician's concerns, and is the purpose of the neurological examination, a specialized physical and mental examination. The physician uses his knowledge of normal neurologic function to pinpoint the site of dysfunction. Through the use of specific tests designed to detect abnormalities of general nervous functioning and of the functioning of individual nerves and nerve tracts, possible sites are successively excluded until one site appears most probable. Other diagnostic studies are then used to determine the cause of the dysfunction.

The nurse's role in the examination is primarily to prepare the patient for the various diagnostic tests and for the lengthiness of the physical examination itself. Neurologic evaluation may require many days, depending upon the complexity of the problem. Often the physical and mental components of the examination are performed on separate occasions to avoid tiring the patient. Details of such examinations may be found in appropriate textbooks.

DIAGNOSTIC TESTS

Blood tests will be performed to exclude systemic disease as the cause of the neurologic symptoms (renal, endocrine disorders). A good laboratory manual will aid the nurse in understanding the purpose of such tests. A number of tests are specific to neurological evaluation; the more common of these tests are discussed below.

Cerebrospinal Fluid Examination

The cerebrospinal fluid is examined to detect the presence of subarachnoid bleeding, increased intracranial pressure, infection, and other diagnostic abnormalities. (Section 2 of this chapter discusses the value of cerebrospinal fluid examination in spinal cord disorders.) Normal cerebrospinal fluid has the following characteristics: pressure of 80 to 180 mm water; clear and colorless; no red blood cells, fewer than five lymphocytes per cu mm; varying amounts of protein, depending upon the laboratory; and presence of sodium chloride, urea, and glucose.

Cerebrospinal fluid is usually obtained by lumbar puncture, a safe procedure which is nevertheless frightening to many patients. The nurse can assure the patient that there will be only brief discomfort, when the needle passes through the dura. If the patient expresses fear of paralysis, the nurse can assure him that there is no danger of this, because the spinal cord ends at the level of the second lumbar vertebra, a few inches above the site of puncture (fourth to fifth lumbar interspace).

The nurse can use the information about the cerebrospinal fluid to determine the need for frequent observations in patients with rapidly changing conditions. For example, if the opening pressure (pressure at which the cerebrospinal fluid flows into the manometer) is greatly increased and if any of the fluid is removed for testing, there is some danger of brain displacement into the foramen magnum following the reduction in pressure. For this reason, the nurse should take frequent neurologic vital signs (includes pupil reaction; see "Increased Intracranial Pressure") for several hours after the procedure. Particular attention should be paid to the level of consciousness, since a decreasing level of consciousness is an early sign of this displacement.

Cerebrospinal fluid can be obtained through a cisternal puncture; the fluid is taken from the cisterna magna, at the base of the medulla. It can be risky because of the proximity of the needle to the medulla. There is the danger of impaction of the brain stem into the foramen magnum if cerebrospinal fluid under increased pressure is removed. Particularly close observation is thus warranted.

Angiography

Angiography is a general term referring to radiographic studies of blood vessels. The studies are used to determine the patency of cerebral and extracerebral vessels, and to determine the presence of aneurysms, vascular anomalies, and vascular tumors. The latter three often displace major vessels in the brain, a situation which is detected by angiography. Radiopaque dye is injected intra-arterially (hence these studies are called *arteriograms*) using the carotid, vertebral, or brachial artery, and serial radiograms are taken to determine the course and speed of dye flow. Both the puncture and injection of the dye can be uncomfortable, the dye causing a warm flush and perhaps an unpleasant taste. The apparatus that changes the film plates is under the patient's head and is quite noisy. This can frighten the patient if he is not forewarned, and may cause him to struggle enough to necessitate repeating the test.

There is a small chance of neurological deficit resulting from arteriography; this may be due to vascular spasm or to inadvertent injection of dye into the vessel wall (intramurally) with subsequent dissection of the vessel. The nurse should notify the physician immediately upon observing any neurological deterioration following arteriography.

Because this procedure involves arterial puncture, specific care is required afterward. For brachial puncture, pressure dressings are applied over the puncture site and left in place for several hours. The nurse is responsible for ascertaining that circulation is adequate below the dressing. The limb distal to the dressing may become red, because of interference with venous return, but should not become dusky; a radial pulse should always be palpable. The doctor should be summoned immediately if any signs of vascular insufficiency occur.

A pressure dressing cannot be applied to the carotid area to reduce swelling; ice bags, however, are effective in most cases. A carotid artery hematoma is apt to displace the trachea, particularly if the hematoma forms medial to the vessel. For this reason, frequent and careful observations of the position of the trachea (note position *before* the procedure, as a baseline), presence of visible or palpable hematoma, and the character of the respirations are essential. The hematoma can become quite large before it is visible externally.

Pneumoencephalography

In a pneumoencephalogram the ventricular system and basal cisternal system are outlined; air is used as the contrast medium. It is performed to detect ventricular obstruction, cerebral atrophy (in which large ventricles, with no evidence of distortion, are seen) and hemispheric and ventricular or cisternal distortion due to tumor or intracerebral hematoma. The patient often sits in a chair, which may be rotated like a CircOlectric bed, and varying amounts of air are injected by lumbar puncture. The patient is then rotated to promote distribution of the air throughout the ventricular system while serial radiograms are taken. Severe headache can result from the procedure, particularly if the air enters the subarachnoid space; hence codeine is usually given as a premedication. The headache is apt to be more severe if equivalent amounts of cerebrospinal fluid are removed as the air is injected.

Close observations of vital signs and level of consciousness are necessary for the first few hours following a pneumoencephalogram. Headache may continue for 1 to 3 days and is aggravated by sitting; therefore, most doctors do not allow early ambulation. However, the patient should be encouraged to move about in bed, which will aid in the distribution and absorption of the air. As with any patient with suspected cerebral pathology, no narcotic stronger than codeine is ordered; the analgesic ordered should be administered frequently until the headache subsides.

Additional Diagnostic Tests

Other tests commonly performed are as follows: the *electroencephalogram,* which records the electrical activity in the brain; the *electromyogram,* which records electrical activity in the muscles; radioisotope *brain scan,* which is employed to detect brain tumors (tumors selectively take up certain radioactive heavy metals; this can be detected by an apparatus similar to a Geiger counter); and the *echogram,* in which reflected sound waves are used to detect tumors (the difference in density of normal and abnormal tissue is measured).

Nursing Evaluation

The basic principles of nursing evaluation are discussed in Part IV; therefore only those aspects specific to brain disorders are included here. It cannot be emphasized too strongly that assessment must be purposeful, not merely casual observations made in contacts with the patient. Observations will be needed to judge the acuteness of symptoms and thereby to determine priority of nursing action (e.g., maintaining the airway in the acute phase of a cerebrovascular accident versus rehabilitation in later phases), to determine changes in condition (for example, impending tentorial herniation), and to determine the extent of disability and the patient's residual abilities. The last is important in helping the person utilize his remaining abilities to cope with problems of daily living. The nurse will also need to assess the patient's mental status in order to determine his ability to participate in his care and to detect early signs of deteriorating condition.

COMPONENTS OF NURSING EVALUATION

Mental Status

Change in mental status is one of the prime gauges of increasing intracranial pressure and therefore a most important observation. Initially, the nurse should observe the patient's level of consciousness: is he awake and alert to what is happening, or responsive only to certain stimuli? Terms such as *alert, semiconscious,* and *comatose* are of little value unless qualified. It is more meaningful to describe someone as "responding appropriately to verbal stimuli," "alert but disoriented to place," "stuporous but arousable by light shaking," "arousable only upon painful stimulation," or "responding reflexly to deep pain." The nurse needs also to determine the patient's orientation to time, to place, and to person. Does he know the date, where he is, who he and others are? Are his replies appropriate or does he use jargon and nonsense words? Can he follow directions? Observations of mental status need to be made in order to determine the baselines for future observation and to assess how well the person can communicate with others.

Motor Function

The nurse should determine if the patient can move all four limbs and if the strength in them is equal and symmetrical. This can be tested by having the patient squeeze two fingers of each of the nurse's hands and comparing strength, and by having him raise his leg against resistance. She should also determine if there is any evidence of weakness in speaking or swallowing. If the patient is ambulatory, the nurse should note if his gait is normal and if he can perform coordinated movements.

Sensory Function

Important questions to consider are these: Does the patient feel touch and pain in affected areas; are abnormal sensations present and, if so, what are they; does he know the position of a limb without looking at it (proprioception)? Can he taste, smell, hear, and see? Is one field of vision lost? Most of this testing will have been done by the doctor, and the information can be found in the record, but the nurse must have some idea of which aspects of this information about the patient's sensory abilities she needs to know.

Autonomic Function

The nurse needs to determine if the patient is continent, or if he is incapable of controlling elimination or of making his need for the bedpan or urinal known. When there is increased intracranial pressure she must be cognizant of the trends of vital signs and pupillary responses (see "Increased Intracranial Pressure").

The nursing evaluation should not only include observations of the patient's present state regarding the above factors, but should be designed to determine how well the patient will be able to carry out activities of daily living. It is helpful to analyze various activities in order to determine what functions a patient needs in order to perform them. For example, buttoning one's shirt requires certain coordinated movements of both hands. Any disorder that interferes with fine coordination or motor power in one arm or hand will make it difficult for the patient to perform this activity, and the nurse will need to make plans to help him compensate for this. Brushing one's teeth requires similar fine, coordinated movement but requires only one hand, and therefore should pose no problem for a person with motor loss in one hand. However, further analysis will demonstrate that thorough oral cleaning depends upon the sensations of the brush and the water on the gums and the cheek. Therefore, the person whose motor disability also produces one-sided sensory loss (as in many cerebrovascular accidents) will not be aware that he has not cleaned one-half of his mouth.

Classification of Lesions

A classification of pathology is included to help acquaint the student with common terminology. The specific aspects of nursing care are related to the location of the lesion more than to the type and will be discussed later.

Trauma occurs in lacerating, penetrating, and crushing injuries. Blows to the head may produce direct injury from bone fragments (laceration), or concussion or contusion even without fracture of the skull. Details on care after head injuries may be found in Chapter 33.

Concussion

Concussion is a transient disorder due to head injury in which there is transient paralysis of nervous function. There is instantaneous loss of consciousness, usually followed by total recovery of function; however, occasionally death may occur, presumably due to medullary paralysis. There is no observable neuropathology. The severity of symptoms is not always proportional to the severity of the blow to the head. Furthermore, recovery of consciousness after concussion does not preclude the possibility of additional injury. For this reason, any person who loses consciousness, even briefly, after a blow on the head, should be seen by a doctor and kept under observation for a time.

Contusion

Contusion is an actual "bruising," without tearing, of the brain tissue, probably resulting from the brain hitting the skull. The contusion may be at the site of the blow or on the opposite side, and the symptoms will depend upon the area of the cortex injured as well as upon the presence of other injury. Subcortical structures can also be displaced by a contusing blow, and this will cause additional symptoms, depending on the structure affected.

Laceration

Laceration of the brain and tearing of cerebral vessels may be caused by bony fragments or foreign objects, as well as by the shearing force of a blow to the head. Laceration of the brain is most apt to cause intracerebral hematoma and subdural hematoma, while tearing of the vessels in the meninges may result in epidural hematoma. Permanent disability or death may result from either subdural or epidural hematoma and can often be prevented by good nursing observation. Therefore, these disorders will be discussed briefly.

SUBDURAL HEMATOMA

Subdural hematoma occurs when the veins lying between the dura and the surface of the brain are torn. Since the bleeding is at venous pressure, the blood accumulates slowly and symptoms may not occur for several hours or even days or weeks. The hematoma acts as an external mass and displaces the brain. Focal symptoms, determined by the location of the mass, develop, and if the hematoma is not evacuated, generalized signs of increased intracranial pressure wi' become evident. If the hematoma accumulated rapidly, general and focal sig' may occur simultaneously. Unrelieved hematoma may cause death due to d' placement of brain tissue and increased intracranial pressure. Pertinent nur' observations are discussed under "Increased Intracranial Pressure." If detected early enough, the hematoma can be surgically evacuated and full recovery will ensue. If, however, the hematoma is sufficiently long-standing to have caused cell death from ischemia, some disability may be permanent.

EPIDURAL HEMATOMA

Epidural hematoma forms after tearing of the meningeal arteries; blood accumulates between the dura and the skull. Because this bleeding is at arterial pressure, the accumulation is much more rapid than in subdural hematoma and will rapidly cause death unless the hematoma is evacuated and the bleeding is stopped. The most common site of bleeding is the middle meningeal artery, either at the base of the brain or as the vessel passes over the cortex in the inferior temporal area (Mullen). Fractures of either the basal or temporal area of the skull are very apt to tear this artery; for this reason, the nurse should be especially watchful of any patient with these fractures.

NEOPLASMS

Brain tumors can be classified as malignant or benign, but, in reality, any central nervous system tumor will eventually be fatal when it displaces or compresses vital structures. Encapsulated, noninvasive tumors such as meningiomas and acoustic neuromas are slow-growing and excisable. The most common primary brain tumors are categorically called *gliomas* and include glioblastomas and astrocytomas. Because these are infiltrative tumors, complete excision is often impossible. Some are radiosensitive and may be treated palliatively. Tumors in other parts of the body may metastasize to the brain; such tumors account for a significant proportion of all brain tumors. Metastatic brain tumors are frequently multiple and therefore not excisable. However, a single metastatic tumor is often removed as a palliative measure.

Focal symptoms resulting from a tumor depend upon its location. For example, a meningioma compressing the motor cortex may cause hemiplegia, whereas a brain stem tumor may produce symptoms of cranial nerve dysfunction. Many tumors will cause convulsions due to irritation of the cortex. This may be the first sign of a tumor. Symptoms due to increased intracranial pressure may also be seen with brain tumors. The increased pressure may be caused by such factors as the presence of a growing mass in a closed space, edema surrounding the tumor, and hemorrhage within the tumor.

VASCULAR DISTURBANCES

Cerebrovascular disorders will be discussed in somewhat more detail than the other pathological categories because of the importance of cerebrovascular disease as a major cause of death and disability in the United States. The 1964 report of the President's Commission on Heart Disease, Cancer and Stroke reported that in 1963 there were 201,000 deaths due to stroke (cerebral hemorrhage, embolism, or thrombosis). Stroke was the third leading cause of death, representing 11 percent of all deaths and 20 percent of cardiovascular-renal deaths. An estimated 80 percent

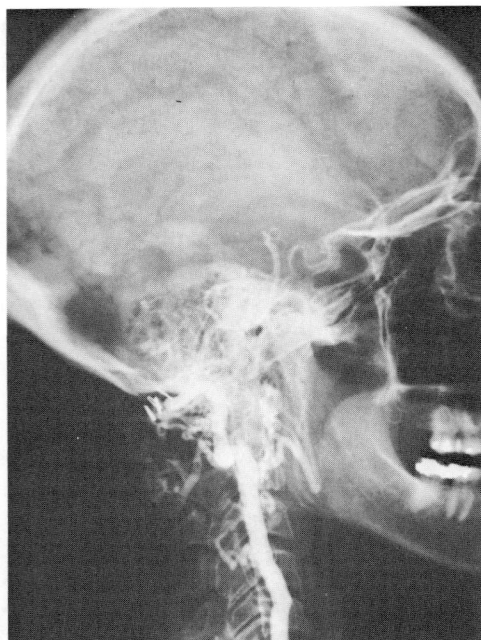

*Figure 29–1
Arteriogram. Left
vertebral angiogram,
showing many abnormal
vessels at the base of
the skull. A tumor of the
glomus jugulare has
invaded the base of the
skull.*

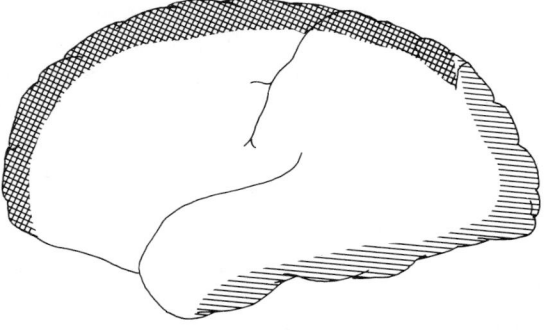

*Figure 29–2
Major blood supply to
the cortex. The arteries
are branches of the
circle of Willis, which is
supplied by the internal
carotid artery and the
basilar artery.*

Anterior cerebral artery

Middle cerebral artery

Posterior cerebral artery

of persons survived the first attack; however, many of this group of over 2 million people were disabled to some extent.

The most common site of defect is in the anterior cerebral circulation (internal carotid, middle cerebral, anterior communicating, and anterior cerebral arteries). These vessels comprise the system that supplies the frontoparietal area of the brain (see Figures 29–1 and 29–2). Because of the functions served by this area, disturbances within it may result in common clinical manifestations such as hemiplegia, aphasia, and sensory changes. This is true whether the disturbance is due to thrombosis, embolism, or hemorrhage. Therefore, many aspects of nursing care will be determined primarily by these clinical manifestations, irrespective of the nature of the vascular disturbance. An understanding of the differences in pathological sequelae will help the nurse to plan pertinent observations and to understand differing rates of recovery of function.

Hemorrhage produces rapid brain swelling secondary to the hematoma mass (when there is bleeding into cerebral tissue) or to external pressure from blood collecting in the subarachnoid space. Vascular occlusion produces a more localized swelling, around the ischemic or infarcted area. The symptoms of hemorrhage, particularly if entirely subarachnoid, will be more generalized, whereas those from occlusion are apt to be localized to the affected area.

Cerebral Hemorrhage

Cerebral hemorrhage may be caused by intracranial aneurysms or hypertension. Aneurysms are most apt to be found in younger persons and are thought to be due to a congenital weakness of the vessels. The most common sites of aneurysms are the anterior communicating, internal carotid, and middle cerebral arteries (Ojemann). Cerebral aneurysms usually bleed into the subarachnoid space, producing signs of increased intracranial pressure including a generalized decrease in the level of consciousness. In addition, there may be hemorrhage into cerebral tissue, with consequent focal symptoms. Bleeding often stops spontaneously but can resume. Increases in arterial blood pressure may be responsible for bleeding, and hence straining, coughing, or agitation of the patient should be prevented. McKissock's study of 772 patients demonstrated the value of surgical repair of the ruptured vessel after the initial acute brain swelling, but before rebleeding occurs. Surgical techniques include occlusion of the carotid artery, coating of the aneurysmal sac with acrylic plastics, gauze, or occasionally muscle. The blood supply to the aneurysm may also be occluded. Nursing observations after surgery vary to some extent with the procedure performed and will be specified in the surgeon's orders.

Hypertensive hemorrhage, involving arteriosclerotic vessels, occurs most frequently in older persons. The hemorrhage is usually into brain substance, although subarachnoid hemorrhage may also occur (Wechsler). There will be focal symptoms as well as acute increased intracranial pressure. The dysfunction will decrease to some degree as surrounding edema subsides, but the resolving blood clot will leave a cystic cavity that may permanently disrupt function in that area. The common sites for this type of hemorrhage are the middle cerebral artery branches supplying the internal capsule, basal ganglia, and thalamus (Wechsler). Thus, fairly severe motor and sensory defects may occur.

Cerebral Embolism

Cerebral emboli arise most often from vegetative plaques in the heart. An embolus frequently produces sudden and complete anoxia, with subsequent infarction. The resolving infarct leaves a cystic cavity or a scar, which may serve as a focus for later seizures. Subsidence of edema that initially surrounds the infarct will allow some recovery from the initial degree of dysfunction. However, disability resulting from the infarct itself will be permanent. In general, the clinical picture is less severe and recovery is faster in embolization than in cerebral hemorrhage or thrombosis.

Cerebral Thrombosis

Cerebral thrombosis is the most common cause of stroke in older persons (Fawcett and Smith). It usually occurs in the middle cerebral, basilar, and carotid arteries. Because a thrombus produces ischemia at a slower rate than does an embolus, clinical manifestations evolve more slowly. Massive occlusion will produce infarction and subsequent disability. As with cerebral embolism, an area of edema forms around the infarct, producing greater dysfunction than that due to the infarct alone. The slow resolution of this edema accounts for the delayed improvement, seen over a period of time.

Recent studies indicate that some strokes may be prevented, particularly those caused by atherosclerotic narrowing of the extracranial vessels (carotid and vertebral arteries) (Ostfield). Disease in these vessels may give warning signs of transient ischemia—dizziness, transient hemiplegia, aphasia. Carotid endarterectomy, by improving blood flow, has been moderately successful in alleviating transient ischemic attacks and preventing stroke. Anticoagulants are also used, with variable efficacy (Javid and Julian). The nurse can encourage the patient with transient ischemia to seek medical help before a major stroke has occurred.

INFECTION AND INFLAMMATORY DISEASES

Infection and inflammatory diseases include brain abscess, meningitis, and encephalitis. These may be due to primary bacterial or viral infections, secondary spread from chronic ear or sinus infections, or irritation of the meninges by aseptic irritants. Nursing care centers around acute increased intracranial pressure, specific focal signs, and measures to combat the infection.

DEGENERATIVE DISORDERS

Degenerative disorders are generally of unknown etiology although some are thought to be of autoimmune or postinfectious origin. These include multiple sclerosis, Parkinson's syndrome (paralysis agitans), cerebral atrophy, and arteriosclerotic cerebral degeneration. There are few acute problems due directly to the degenerative process. Major problems of nursing care reflect the chronic, disabling nature of these disorders and include preventing deformities, coping with emotional and behavioral lability, and preventing complicating conditions (especially respiratory infection and decubitus ulcers). Nursing care of persons with multiple sclerosis is discussed with the degenerative disorders of the spinal cord in Section 2.

Nursing Problems Basic to Many Lesions

INCREASED INTRACRANIAL PRESSURE

Because the brain is contained in a rigid box (the skull), expansion of the intracranial contents will be limited by the skull. Intracranial pressure will increase, resulting in a group of generalized signs. Because the pressure is exerted throughout the brain, nervous system dysfunction will be widespread. This will be superimposed on any focal signs that are a direct result of the primary lesion.

Increased intracranial pressure may develop rapidly or slowly, depending upon such factors as the rate of growth of the primary lesion and the degree of obstruction of the ventricular system. The general manifestations will be the same but the number and rapidity of appearance of signs will vary; this, in turn, will dictate medical and nursing management.

Mechanism of Increased Intracranial Pressure

The mechanism of increased intracranial pressure is related to the fact that the central nervous system is composed of blood vessels, cerebrospinal fluid, and cells, enclosed in an inexpandable skull. An increase in any of these components will increase pressure in the total compartment. Increase in the vascular compartment occurs with vasodilatation resulting from increased carbon dioxide content in the blood (hypercapnia). It is of significance only if it is superimposed on preexisting increased intracranial pressure.

Increase in the amount of cerebrospinal fluid may be generalized, due to overproduction or inadequate absorption by the arachnoid villi, or localized, due to blockage of the ventricles or aqueducts. This condition of an excessive amount of cerebrospinal fluid is called *hydrocephalus*.

Increase in the cerebral content may be the result of an increase in the cell mass, as in tumors, or an increase in the fluid content, i.e., edema. Cerebral edema may be associated with many lesions of the central nervous system and may be interstitial or intracellular. Edema, particularly if intracellular, may resolve slowly and this may account for the slow resolution of symptoms after relief of increased intracranial pressure. Interstitial edema is significant because the interstitial fluid comprises an estimated 14 to 35 percent of the weight of the brain (Bakay and Lee).

The manifestations of increased intracranial pressure are produced both by direct pressure on cerebral structures and by distortion of tissue secondary to the pressure. Outward expansion of the brain, in response to pressure, is limited by the skull and hence the pressure is eventually transmitted downward (see Principle 2). With increasing pressure a portion of the temporal lobe will be pushed through the incisural notch (the space between the tentorium—the portion of the dura separating the temporal and occipital lobes from the cerebellum—and the brain stem, see Figure 29–3). As long as the pressure can be relieved by this herniation of the temporal lobe, the process is *compensated*, that is, pressure on the medulla has not reached a critical state. When further herniation is prevented by the limited space at the incisural notch, pressure increases on the brain stem and the stage of *decompensation* occurs. The medulla herniates into the foramen magnum and death ensues from paralysis of the cardiac and respiratory centers.

Manifestations of increased intracranial pressure are decreased visual acuity, papilledema, decreased level of consciousness, changes in the equality of the pupils and pupillary reaction to light, increased systolic blood pressure, decreased pulse

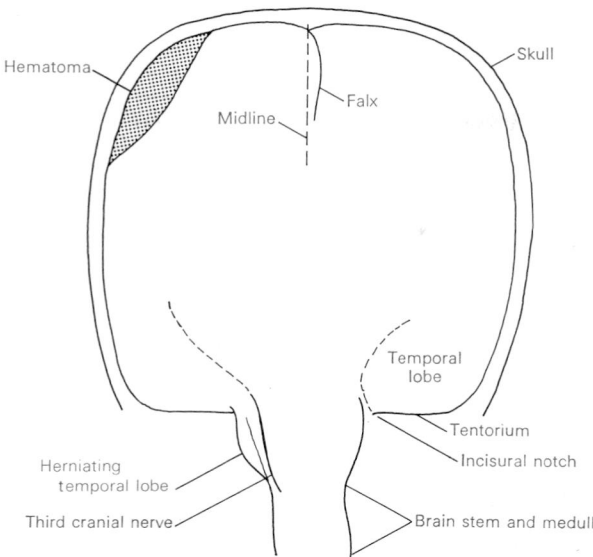

Figure 29–3
Schematic representation
of the anatomical
boundaries of the brain.
Note displacement of
falx cerebri by the
hematoma mass.
Herniation of temporal
lobe and stretching of
third cranial nerve are
shown on the left.

rate, and decreased respiratory rate. Other manifestations that are variably present include headache, vomiting (with or without nausea), elevated temperature, seizures associated with transtentorial herniation, and worsening of focal neurologic signs. These are classified in Table 29-1, in the stages in which they may be seen. The mechanisms by which these manifestations are produced will be discussed in order that the nurse may understand the significance of the observations she makes.

An early sign, rarely noticed by the patient, is an increase in the normal blind spot. (The area on the retina where the optic nerve leaves the eye has no visual receptors and thus produces a blind spot in the field of vision.) Increased intracranial pressure will be exerted upon the optic nerve because the dura, covering the central nervous system, extends to ensheath the optic nerve. The pressure on the optic nerve causes the increase in the blind spot. This pressure is also the cause of papilledema, the swelling of the optic disk which can be seen through an ophthalmoscope. By the time that papilledema is present, the patient may notice a decrease in visual acuity. Although papilledema will not be observed by the nurse, her knowledge that it is present will make her aware of the need to observe for other signs of increasing intracranial pressure.

As pressure increases, structures in the brain stem become compressed and ischemic. The level of consciousness decreases as the reticular activating system is affected. Subtle decreases in the level of consciousness are the earliest sign of increasing pressure and transtentorial herniation. Therefore purposeful observations of the patient's mental status and level of consciousness are of major importance in nursing care of these patients. Hemiplegia may occur when the corticospinal tract is compressed against the incisural notch by the herniating temporal lobe. Generalized or focal seizures may occur as cortical and subcortical areas are irritated.

COMPENSATION			DECOMPENSATION
EARLY	VARIABLE	LATER	VERY LATE
Increase in normal blind spot	Headache	Decreased level of consciousness	
Papilledema	Vomiting	↘	
Decreased visual acuity	Elevated temperature	Stupor → Coma	
	Focal signs	Change in pupil size, equality, reactivity	
	Seizures	oo → o · → ··	
			Dilated and fixed
		Increased systolic blood pressure	Decreased systolic blood pressure
		Decreased pulse rate	Increased pulse rate
		Labored respirations → decreased respiratory rate	
			Respiratory arrest
		Rigidity; decerebrate posture	Bilateral decerebrate posturing

o = Pupil reactive to light
• = Pupil nonreactive to light

TABLE 29-1
The Symptoms of
Increased Intracranial
Pressure, Classified by
Stage of Appearance

Changes in pupillary size, equality, and reactivity to light occur as the third cranial nerve is stretched by the descending brain stem, or actually compressed by the herniating temporal lobe. The pupil becomes dilated and fixed (nonreactive to light) when the nerve is completely paralyzed. This occurs at a late stage of herniation and indicates impending decompensation. Bilaterally dilated and fixed pupils generally indicate irreversible herniation. Inequality of pupil size is as important as the absolute sizes. For example, one pupil might be of normal size but the other very small, thus indicating irritation of the third cranial nerve to the smaller pupil. The speed of reaction to light is also indicative of third nerve function; extremely slow reaction, in particular, suggests dysfunction of this nerve.

As pressure increases on the brain stem, hypoxia of the vasomotor and cardio-inhibitory centers may stimulate a rise in systolic blood pressure, with or without decrease in the diastolic pressure, and a decreased pulse rate. Absolute values are important to some extent, but *trends* in blood pressure and pulse rates are most important. For this reason a graphic recording of frequent vital signs and pupillary reaction (every 15 to 30 minutes) is essential for persons with rapidly increasing intracranial pressure. When pressure is exerted on the medulla, the resulting hypoxia to the respiratory center causes decreased rate and force of respiration. Respirations should be counted for a full minute, and a slowly decreasing respiratory rate or a rate of less than 12 respirations per minute should be considered significant. However, blood pressure and respiratory rates cannot be relied upon to gauge the progress of herniation, for they change quite late in the process.

Decerebrate posturing may occur when increasing pressure has effectively cut off motor inhibitory impulses from the cerebrum. It is thought that pressure on the pyramidal and extrapyramidal tracts eliminates normal inhibition to the muscles, resulting in muscular rigidity, palmar and plantar flexion, and extension of the arm and leg (Bakay and Lee; Mullen). This muscular reaction is initially on the side opposite the lesion, but eventually occurs bilaterally. Initially decerebrate posturing occurs in response to noxious stimuli, but finally is constant.

When decompensation occurs, the respiratory rate becomes markedly decreased, the previous rise in blood pressure may give way to an abrupt fall in blood pressure, and the pulse rate increases; respiratory arrest is then imminent.

Nursing Observations

The consequences of increasing intracranial pressure are often reversible, until the phase of decompensation (although occasionally even then, particularly in children); it is thus imperative that nursing care be planned to prevent decompensation; Observation is of prime importance. It can be concluded from the preceding discussion that certain observations must be made in any patient with increasing intracranial pressure. Baselines must be recorded initially in order to provide a basis for comparison for further observations. These observations are as follows:

Decrease in the Level of Consciousness. Observations of the level of consciousness are the most important ones the nurse can make, for changes appear early in tentorial herniation, at a potentially reversible stage in the process. As noted in "Nursing Evaluation," such terms as *semiconscious* and *comatose* are not very meaningful unless qualified by a description of the patient's response to stimuli. The nurse needs to ask herself if the patient is oriented and if he is easily aroused. If the patient is obtunded, the nurse must determine if he is more or less obtunded than he was an hour ago and make definite attempts to arouse him. Changes in level of consciousness can be quite subtle and not readily observed by a person who has not been with the patient for a period of time. This emphasizes the importance of one nurse being responsible for these observations.

Changes in Pupil Size, Equality, and Reactivity to Light. Pupillary reaction to light can be determined by shining a flashlight on the eye. Normal pupils will constrict when stimulated by light. It is wise to remember that bright room light may have already caused pupillary constriction; in such cases, darkening the room will facilitate determining if the pupil reacts to light. Since pupillary changes also occur relatively early, any change in them must be brought immediately to the physician's attention.

Trends in Vital Signs. As discussed above, an increase in systolic blood pressure, a decrease in pulse rate, with or without increased force of pulse beat, and decreased respirations are all suggestive of increasing intracranial pressure. These are late changes, however, and waiting for them, in the presence of level of consciousness and pupillary changes, before contacting a physician is waiting too long.

Worsening of Focal Neurologic Signs. For example, weakened grasp may be present in one hand; increased weakness or complete loss of motor power may indicate increasing pressure due to worsening of the underlying brain disorder. The appearance of new neurologic signs such as focal or generalized convulsions, hemiplegia, and aphasia will also signify worsening of the underlying disorder.

Intracranial pressure can increase slowly (days to weeks) or rapidly (minutes to hours); the rate at which manifestations change will enable the nurse to determine the frequency with which observations must be made. She will be guided to some extent by the physician's orders; however, any indication of rapidly increasing pressure must be brought to the physician's attention immediately.

Nursing Measures

Nursing care should be planned to prevent sudden increases in pressure in persons in whom the intracranial pressure is already elevated. Straining upon defecation and vigorous coughing increase both intra-abdominal and intrathoracic pressures. Since this in turn increases intracranial pressure, it must be prevented. The use of stool softeners and mild laxatives will prevent constipation. Nasotracheal suctioning, if required, must be done gently in order to minimize the coughing that attends this procedure.

Emotional and physical agitation can be prevented by placing the patient in a quiet room, allowing short visiting periods, and counseling families in preventing emotional upsets. Agitation can also be produced by vigorous and rough turning of the patient and can be prevented by using turning sheets and sufficient personnel to turn the patient smoothly. When there is a ruptured aneurysm, where rebleeding is a major danger, or when there is active cerebral hemorrhage, the physician may request that the patient have all activity (such as feeding and bathing) done for him in order to decrease the probability of further hemorrhage.

Since hypoxia can cause brain swelling, which may accentuate already elevated intracranial pressure, it must be avoided in these patients (Bakay and Lee). This primarily involves maintaining a clear airway. Positioning of the patient to prevent airway obstruction and use of nasopharyngeal and nasotracheal suctioning, when indicated, are important in accomplishing this. Hypoxia during suctioning can be minimized by limiting the suctioning to 15-second periods, allowing the patient breathing intervals between each period.

Medical Measures

The ideal treatment of increased intracranial pressure is the removal of the cause, and this is often feasible in slowly progressing lesions. When pressure is increasing very rapidly, removal of the cause may not be feasible or even possible (e.g., an infiltrating tumor or an active intracerebral hemorrhage); nevertheless the pressure must be relieved to prevent deterioration of the patient's condition or even death. This can be achieved by mechanical decompression or by the use of certain drugs.

Cerebrospinal fluid can be removed to decrease pressure. In situations of rapidly increasing pressure, this is usually accomplished by ventricular puncture (insertion of the needle directly into the lateral ventricle) because of the danger of cerebral herniation after lumbar puncture in such conditions. Mechanical decompression may also be effected by removing a piece of the skull to allow the brain to expand; postoperative positioning of the patient upon the operated side is contraindicated.

Osmotic diuresis is frequently promoted in an attempt to decrease cerebral edema; *mannitol* and *urea* are the agents most commonly used (Matson). The large urinary output necessitates accurate measurement in order to allow the physician to maintain electrolyte balance.

The use of corticosteroids to reduce cerebral edema is a recent development. The mechanism by which these agents act is unknown, but there is some suggestion that they alter the cell membrane and promote diuresis (French and Galicich).

Dexamethasone (Decadron) and *methylprednisolone* (Solu-Medrol) are most commonly used, as side effects are fewer with these forms than with other steroids. However, gastrointestinal bleeding and fluid retention are potential complications, indicating the need to be alert for blood in the stools and for peripheral edema.

In conjunction with these therapeutic measures, fluid intake is frequently limited to obligatory losses in order to minimize interstitial fluid. This intake will be about 1,500 ml per day and may be administered intravenously in patients with rapidly increasing pressure. The nurse has an important responsibility to regulate the intravenous infusion so that the rate of flow is even; it is detrimental to the patient if most of the daily allotment is administered during the last 3 hours.

NEUROSURGERY

Neurosurgery is most commonly performed to remove a tumor mass or hematoma, or to repair ruptured vessels. It may also be employed to create specific lesions in the treatment of such entities as Parkinson's syndrome, intractable pain, and trigeminal neuralgia. Much of the preoperative and postoperative nursing care of these patients is similar to that of any surgical patient.

It is important to be aware that the patient about to undergo neurosurgery is under a great deal of emotional stress, similar to that experienced by patients undergoing cardiac surgery. For most people, the brain is viewed as essential for meaningful existence; therefore, any intrusion into it may be seen as potentially destructive to one's existence. Although this fear may be unspoken, many patients who are anticipating brain surgery fear being "left a vegetable." The nurse should recognize that this fear is common and should allow the patient to express it. It may also help him to meet a postoperative patient who is doing well.

Some neurosurgical patients are stuporous or comatose preoperatively. However, their families are highly alert to the dangers of surgery and need much support from the nurse. They should be prepared for the patient's postoperative condition including the appearance of head dressings and swollen eyes (if a frontal craniotomy was done), and the presence of special mechanical equipment, such as that for hypothermia and positive pressure breathing. It is essential that the nurse communicate with the surgeon to determine what information he has given the patient and family, in order that she may reinforce this information.

Postoperative Care and Nursing Observations

Manipulation of the brain and surgical trauma to it will often cause some cerebral edema and consequent increased intracranial pressure. Therefore, there is the potential for postoperative temporal lobe herniation, particularly if bleeding occurs, and the nurse's observations are as important as they were preoperatively. Corticosteroids are frequently employed to decrease this postoperative cerebral edema.

The postoperative patient is usually positioned with his head elevated 15 to 45 degrees to promote venous return and thereby decrease possible increased intracranial pressure. The Trendelenburg position is contraindicated in these patients, because it may aggravate increased intracranial pressure. It may be necessary to place a sign on the head of the bed indicating the degree of elevation desired, so that well-meaning relatives or auxiliary personnel will not change the position. If a large mass has been removed from the brain, there is the potential for shifting of the brain to the operative side; therefore, positioning of the patient on this side may be contraindicated. This will be specified in the surgeon's orders.

Postoperative headache may be severe. Since brain tissue itself is insensitive to painful stimuli, this pain is thought to be due to traction exerted upon blood vessels and irritation of the dura during surgery. The headache is constant and difficult to relieve. Codeine is the strongest narcotic that should be given. Stronger narcotics, such as morphine or meperidine (Demerol) can mask pupillary evidence of increased intracranial pressure (the parasympathetic action of narcotics causes constriction of the pupils), can produce mental obtundation, and can cause respiratory depression.

A craniotomy above the level of the tentorium is called a *supratentorial craniotomy* and that done in the posterior fossa, below the tentorium, is called an *infratentorial craniotomy*. Some aspects of postoperative care differ in these surgical procedures. Infratentorial incisions expose structures very near the medulla and often involve cutting neck muscles that prevent excessive flexion of the head. Consequently, heavy supportive dressings are applied and any flexion of the neck is contraindicated. These patients must be turned by at least three people—two to manipulate the turning sheet and the third to support the head. When the patient is lying on his side, a small, firm pillow should be used to keep the head in the midline position, in order to prevent lateral flexion of the head.

Since postoperative edema in the posterior fossa and upper brain stem may exert pressure on the medulla, observation for respiratory distress must be made frequently for the first few days. The number of respirations should be counted for a full minute, and any decreases should be quickly reported to the physician. The patient may have difficulty in swallowing his secretions and may require gentle nasopharyngeal suctioning. Following infratentorial neurosurgical procedures there is usually some degree of brain stem edema; this renders the brain stem more vulnerable to even slight degrees of increased intracranial pressure. Since vigorous or deep suctioning will cause coughing and subsequent increased intracranial pressure it is contraindicated unless absolutely necessary. For this same reason postoperative coughing in general is discouraged. Deep breathing is therefore even more important to prevent atelectasis. Coughing is less critical following supratentorial surgery because there is not apt to be postoperative brain stem edema. However, vigorous coughing should be avoided because of the generally deleterious effects of increased intracranial pressure. Similarly, vigorous suctioning may produce hypoxia and spasmodic coughing and should not be employed without first consulting the physician.

A frontal craniotomy will produce ecchymosis and edema around the eyes; conjunctivitis and ulceration may occur if proper eye care is not given at least every 4 hours for the first few days. Normal saline and methylcellulose are adequate to cleanse and soothe the eyes.

EMOTIONAL REACTIONS

Emotional manifestations associated with neurological disability are due to a combination of organic changes and psychological reactions. Behavioral changes may be produced by some cortical lesions, for example, the distractibility and loss of social inhibitions seen in frontal lobe lesions. These are further discussed elsewhere. In addition, there are common psychological reactions to organic dysfunction which are related to alterations in the body image.

Body Image

The body image, that is, a person's concept of his physical body and its capabilities, is determined by a combination of his sensory experiences and his interpretation of how others view him (Schilder). His previous experiences will demonstrate to him what his body is capable of doing, and his conception of the expectations of others acts as feedback to influence his expectations of himself. In neurological disturbance, the person cannot immediately assess his changed capabilities. Consequently, the reactions of others will assume a major role in his modification of his body image.

Any neurological disorder will affect the experiential component of the body image. For example, paralysis and anesthesia may make a person feel as if he has no arm or leg, even though he can see it. In a disorder that produces anosognosia, the person loses awareness of one-half of his body. He also visualizes only one-half of the external world; for example, he draws a picture of only one-half of an object. Accentuated sensation, such as pain, may increase the person's awareness of one part of the body to the extent that his body image is dominated by that area.

These changed perceptions of body image will be a factor in the precipitation of a characteristic sequence of reactions to disability: shock, depression, regression, denial, withdrawal (Wright). The intensity of these reactions depends upon the person's own reaction to disturbed function and the reactions of others. Ultimately, all these factors influence the formation of a new body image.

The person's reaction to disability depends, in part, upon the importance of the lost function to his concept of self. The loss of fine finger motion may be viewed as more devastating by the pianist than by the heavy laborer. The degree to which that function is necessary in order for the person to feel worthwhile is also a factor in his reaction. For example, motor aphasia may make a person feel that he is stupid.

The attitude of a disabled person may be either positive or negative. He may strive to do as much as he can for himself with his remaining function, or he may assume an attitude of complete helplessness because of his lost function. These attitudes will be determined to a large degree by his new body image but can be significantly modified by the attitudes of those about him.

Nursing Measures

The nurse can be instrumental in promoting positive attitudes by encouraging his remaining abilities while recognizing his disability. The latter is important in order to avoid reinforcing the denial that so frequently occurs and that may impede rehabilitation. Not infrequently, the staff expects a patient to perform poorly and thereby reinforces his attitude of helplessness. It is also common to expect a person who is disabled in one sphere to be disabled in many spheres. As this may be erroneous, it should be guarded against so that intact function can be reinforced. Lastly, the nurse must examine her own values concerning persons with physical defects. She may be repelled by such a patient or may become angry with his inability to help himself; only if she acknowledges these feelings will she be able to change them and thereby avoid reinforcing the patient's low estimate of himself.

The nurse cannot prevent the possible reaction of disgust by a patient's family, but she can aid them in accepting his disability. Families of neurological patients are often termed "difficult." In reality, they are no more difficult than any other family but are often more frightened and bewildered because of the abrupt changes in behavior and in appearance of their relative. Strange behavior, previously associated only with mental illness, may be seen in their own family member and may repel them. The helplessness of the hemiplegic person may produce anger or overprotectiveness in the family. This is particularly apt to occur if there was significant ambivalence in the relationship before the illness; the subsequent disability may engender guilt within the family. Families need to be aided in recognizing the frequent occurrence of ambivalent feelings, in expressing these feelings, and in then accepting the patient's disability. They must allow the patient to do what he can, but must not push him beyond his abilities.

The importance of understanding the patient's view of his situation is clearly described by Eric Hodgins. This individual, who writes about his experiences with hemiplegia following a stroke, discusses such aspects as the importance of compassion and understanding, the frustration of having helplessness reinforced by the staff, the emphasis of the hospital personnel on motor ability without considering the disabling effect of perceptual difficulties, and the significance of disabilities to everyday living.

Nursing Problems Related to Location of Lesion

This discussion is by no means exhaustive of problems associated with specific sites of lesions, but describes those more commonly encountered. Neurological textbooks should be consulted for specific disorders, from which discussions nursing care can be anticipated.

CEREBRAL CORTEX

The cerebral cortex is the most highly developed part of the brain. It is concerned with intellect and the ability to reason, with memory, with speech, with the initiation of voluntary movement, and with the appreciation of and reaction to discrete sensation. Therefore, injury to the cortex will result in interrelated physical and behavioral manifestations.

Experiments with humans and lower primates show fairly specific sites for certain cortical functions, although these are by no means discretely localized (Wechsler). From these studies, it has been determined that each lobe of the cortex performs specific functions. It is also known that a dominant cerebral hemisphere develops in humans in which handedness and the language centers are more highly developed. Intellectual functions and emotion are not so easily localized.

Frontal Lobe Lesions

The frontal lobe is important in intellectual and emotional processes: judgment, the ability to think abstractly, social control, and the appreciation of pain and emotion. Lesions in this area may cause a release of social inhibitions, which may result in aggressive tendencies in a previously passive person or in blandness in an active one. Inability to make decisions, short attention span, inability to learn from experience, and lack of concern over ordinarily upsetting events also characterize patients with frontal lesions. The person with a frontal lobe lesion may also be incontinent of urine and stool; this may be due to lack of concern or to actual damage to medial frontal areas concerned with bowel and bladder function. Frontal lobe lesions may be made surgically in order to destroy pain appreciation in patients with intractable pain. This procedure is designed to interrupt connections with the thalamus (where pain sensations are integrated) and does not interfere with intellectual processes.

From the common manifestations of frontal lobe disorders one can anticipate the need to structure the environment for the patient: to present one decision at a time, and to ask him to do tasks requiring little time and minimal concentrated attention. Since people are accustomed to using abstractions frequently in everyday speech, the nurse must make a conscious effort to be concrete in her conversations with such a patient. For example, "Dinner will be here in a while," may mean nothing to him, whereas "Your meat and potatoes will be here in five minutes" may. Persons with frontal lobe lesions are not incapable of being frustrated and may display their emotions in very disruptive behavior. Anticipating their difficulties and providing a more highly structured environment for them can prevent many problems on a busy ward.

The area of Broca is located in the inferior portion of the frontal lobe, just anterior to the motor area for the head and face muscles. This area is concerned with the initiation of speech and is most apt to be affected by a local tumor or by a vascular disturbance of the middle cerebral artery system. The person with a disturbance of Broca's area has an expressive aphasia, that is, he can understand language, but cannot initiate intelligible speech. The subject of aphasia is discussed later.

The motor cortex is located along the anterior aspect of the central sulcus (see Figure 29-4) and contains the cell bodies of the corticospinal (pyramidal) tracts. This area lies in the distribution of the middle cerebral artery and its branches. The neurons of the motor cortex (the upper motor neurons) initiate innervation of muscles throughout the body. Those serving the muscles of the lower extremities are located at the uppermost portion of the motor strip, while those serving the muscles of the face are most inferior. Thus the body is represented along the motor strip in an upside-down fashion. In addition, the muscles of fine movement, especially those of the face and hands, are represented in disproportionately large areas, thereby rendering them more vulnerable to lesions.

Figure 29-4
*Localization of cortical
function. A, motor
language; B, auditory
language; C, visual
cortex—primary visual
sensory area; D,
secondary visual sensory
areas—visual perception;
E, angular gyrus—sensory
interpretation; F, body
awareness; G, motor
cortex; H, sensory
cortex.*

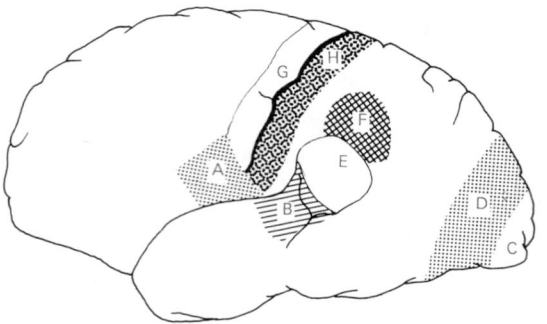

HEMIPLEGIA AND MONOPLEGIA

Lesions may affect the whole motor strip or one part of it, producing *hemiplegia* or *hemiparesis* (paralysis or weakness, respectively, of one side of the body), or *monoplegia* or *monoparesis* (paralysis or weakness of a single extremity). Vascular disorders are more apt to disrupt function in the whole motor area, while tumor masses affect localized parts. Since the corticospinal paths cross in the medulla, the side opposite (contralateral) to the lesion will be affected. Therefore, the nurse caring for a patient with disruption of the frontoparietal cortex can expect weakness or paralysis on the side opposite the lesion and should look for some degree of aphasia.

Nursing care of the patient with hemiplegia and hemiparesis is initially supportive, aiming to preserve remaining function and to prevent complicating conditions and deformities. The problems encountered will depend upon the extent of motor weakness.

If innervation of the facial musculature is involved, one side of the face will be flaccid, with flattened nasolabial fold, a drooping of the corner of the mouth, and a blowing out of the affected cheek during exhalation. Weakness of the tongue and the muscles of swallowing should be anticipated; such weakness may allow the tongue to fall back and occlude the airway. In addition, the patient may not be able to swallow his secretions and may aspirate them. The nurse must place the patient on his side or in a prone position so that his tongue will not fall backward and so that secretions will drain out of the mouth. Nasopharyngeal suctioning may be necessary if secretions become copious. Once food and fluids are allowed to the patient, careful assessment needs to be made of his ability to swallow them safely. This may be done with small amounts of water, which, if aspirated, will not be so harmful as solid foods. Once the patient has demonstrated that he can swallow safely, he should be allowed thick foods, such as cereal, ice cream, and Jell-O, which are more easily manipulated by a weakened tongue than are nonviscous fluids. Other foods can be added to the degree that he patient can swallow them. Food may accumulate in the affected cheek, and the patient needs to learn to clean this after each meal.

Injury in the motor cortex produces upper motor neuron paralysis (lower motor neuron paralysis is discussed in Sections 2 and 3). As mentioned above, the cell bodies of the upper motor neurons form the motor cortex; their axons form the descending corticospinal tracts, eventually synapsing with the lower motor neurons

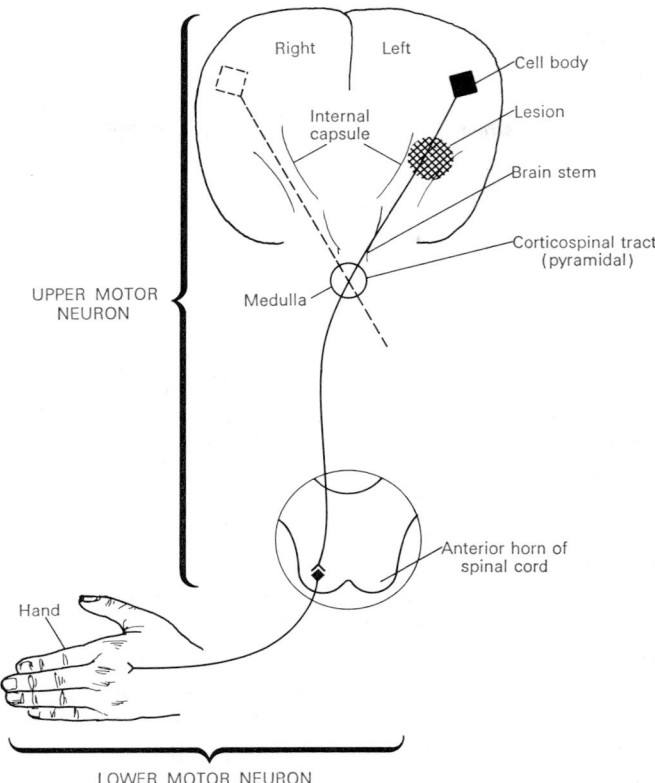

*Figure 29-5
Schematic representation
of an upper motor
neuron lesion. Note
crossing of the cortico-
spinal (pyramidal) tract
in the medulla.*

in the anterior horn of the spinal cord (see Figure 29-5). Upper motor neuron paralysis characteristically produces spasticity. This may be immediate, as in midbrain and brain stem lesions, or it may follow a period of initial flaccidity, such as that seen in cortical lesions. The spasticity is believed to be due to release of cortical inhibition to flexor muscles. Flexion contractures are therefore apt to occur, but can be prevented by passive range of motion exercises to the affected limbs and by positioning the limbs in neutral position. Range of motion exercises need to be instituted early but are contraindicated during active cerebral hemorrhage, as this activity increases the danger of further bleeding.

A number of measures will help to prevent the flexion contractures characteristic of upper motor neuron paralysis. A paralyzed arm should not be placed across the chest. Rather, the arm should be elevated with each joint higher than the one proximal to it. A hand roll may be used to maintain normal finger position. Foot drop may be prevented by using a box or a small firm support to maintain the feet at right angles to the leg when the patient is in any position. Trochanter rolls placed along the trochanter and thigh will prevent external rotation of the hip. Compare this positioning with that discussed in Section 2, which deals with lower motor neuron paralysis.

The paralyzed side is susceptible to edema and to skin breakdown, because of both loss of muscle tone and actual circulatory changes. Elevation of the limbs,

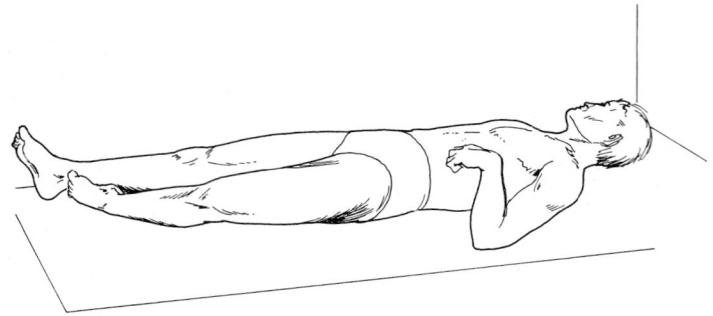

*Figure 29–6
Typical flexion con-
tractures in hemiplegia
due to upper motor
neuron lesion. Left arm
is adducted; forearm is
flexed; hand is flexed
and pronated. Left hip
is externally rotated;
knee is flexed; foot is in
plantar flexion.*

as discussed above, will help decrease the edema. Because of the changes in muscle tone and circulation, the affected side cannot tolerate body weight for any length of time; therefore one should avoid positioning the patient on that side. Skin breakdown on the nonparalyzed side may necessitate some turning onto the affected side; this should be for periods of 1 hour or less. The nurse can utilize the prone and three-quarter prone positions to provide a greater number of positions; this distributes the body weight over a greater surface and also promotes drainage of secretions.

Rehabilitation of the person with hemiplegia is a lengthy process, and it cannot be emphasized too often that poor care in the initial stages will lengthen and hamper efforts. A defeatist attitude is often taken, particularly concerning patients who have had a stroke; this attitude is not justified. The National Heart Institute has estimated that 90 percent of people who have had strokes should be able to walk again and that 30 percent should be able to return to work. However, a study of such patients in Connecticut indicated that only 18 percent of them had been even partially rehabilitated after 4 years (Conant et al.).

Techniques of rehabilitation are similar no matter what the cause of hemiplegia. If there has been an initial period of increased intracranial pressure, active re-

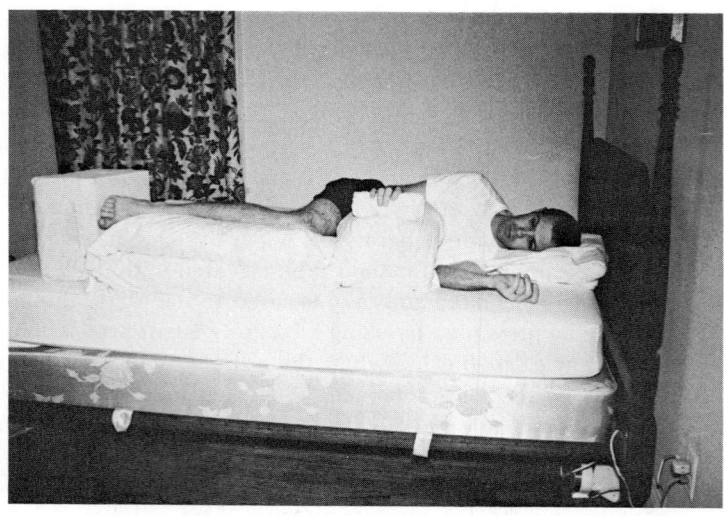

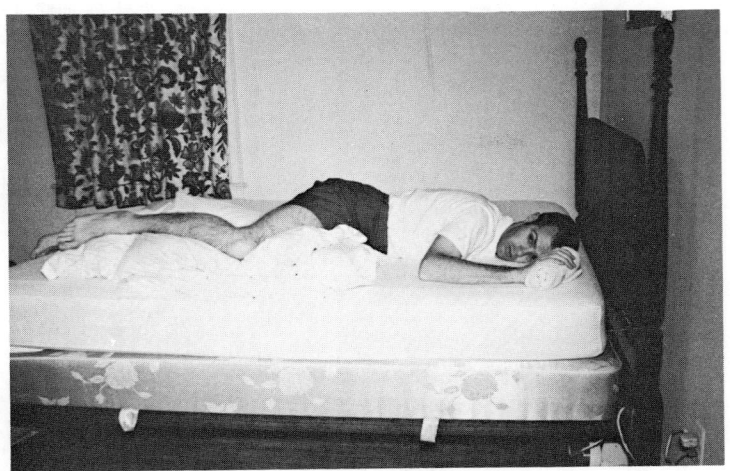

*Figure 29–8
Proper three-quarter
prone position. This
position facilitates
drainage of secretion and
distributes body weight
over a large surface
area. Note that pillows
are placed under the
leg to prevent internal
rotation of hip.*

habilitation must be delayed until this subsides. The degree of recovery possible will depend upon the amount of actual cell death (see Principle 3). Infarction, tumor, or other mass will cause surrounding edema, which will compress nerve pathways and cause more extensive symptoms than the lesion alone. Dysfunction secondary to edema is reversible so long as there is no cell death secondary to ischemia. Hence there will be some functional return as edema diminishes, which, however, may take 6 months to 1 year.

Activities of everyday living are great problems for the patient, and an active program to teach these activities needs to be planned and carried out by medical, nursing, and physical and occupational therapy personnel. If extensive rehabilitation facilities are not available, patients and their families can, with physician approval, use literature published by the American Heart Association. The nurse will find that these publications also contain valuable techniques for hospital and home care. The material describes such activities as how the patient can move about in bed and can transfer to a wheel chair unaided. Such simple things as lowering the hospital bed to the height of a conventional bed, or taking off the wheels, will enable most patients to move from bed to chair unaided. There are very few persons with hemiplegia who need to be lifted in and out of bed, yet this is common practice in many hospitals and nursing homes.

APHASIA

Aphasia is a general term connoting several forms of disordered language expression and perception and is seen in disorders affecting the dominant cerebral hemisphere. Language centers are found in all of the lobes of the dominant hemisphere.

Motor language (the ability to initiate speech) is located primarily in the frontal lobe, auditory language (the ability to recognize and recall the spoken word) in the temporal lobe, and visual language (the ability to recognize and recall the printed word) in parietal and anterior occipital lobes (see Figure 29–2). All but the occipital area are supplied by branches of the middle cerebral artery, the most common site of involvement in cerebrovascular accident; this may account for the

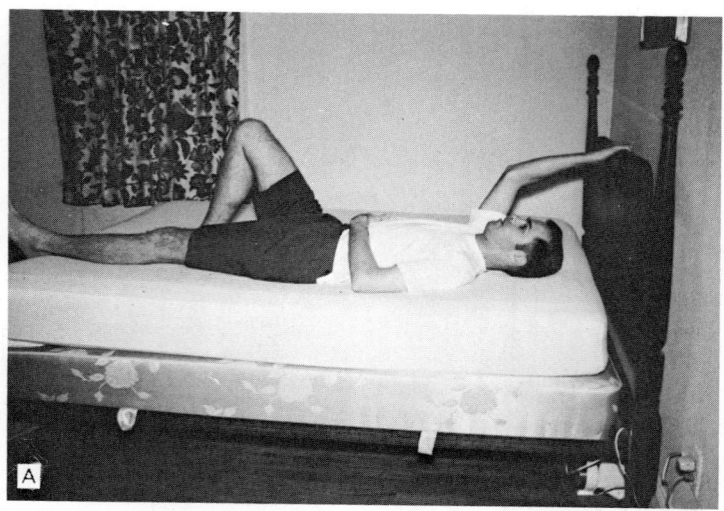

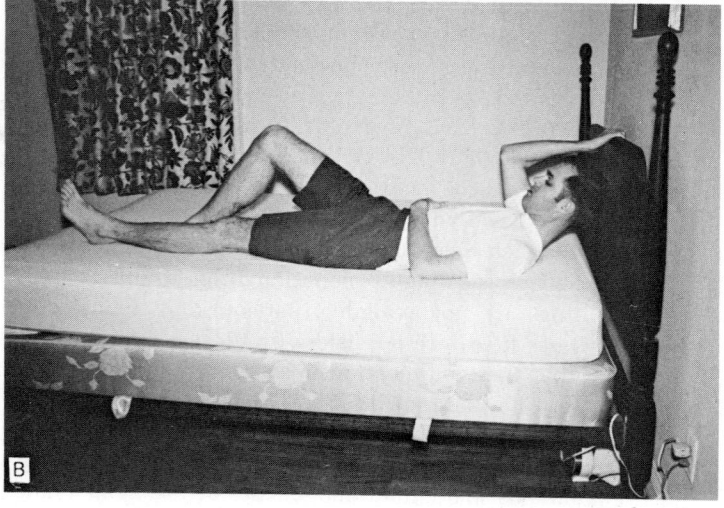

Figure 29-9
Activities of daily living:
moving up in bed un-
assisted. A, Patient grasps
the head board with his
unaffected arm and
flexes the unaffected
knee. B, He then pushes
with his foot and
simultaneously pulls
against the head board.

mixed aphasia often seen in this condition. Common terms are as follows: *motor (expressive) aphasia*—inability to initiate spontaneous speech in the absence of damage to muscles of speech; *sensory (receptive) aphasia*—inability to perceive meaning of spoken or written words; however, the person can speak; *global aphasia* —comparatively rare loss of both utterance and understanding.

It should be emphasized that one rarely sees pure motor or sensory aphasia, but rather degrees of both. There are other intellectual deficits closely related to aphasia, such as *alexia* (word blindness and inability to read) and *agraphia* (inability to write); these are discussed in specialized textbooks.

The nurse should realize that such aphasias are frequently partial. For example, a patient with motor aphasia may nevertheless be able to initiate some speech. Furthermore, many partial aphasias are not obvious, and the nurse will need to evaluate the patient's useful language ability. This cannot be based solely on

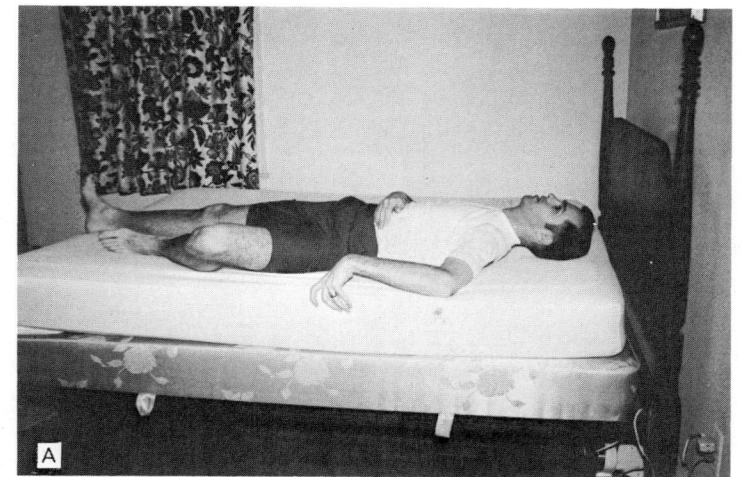

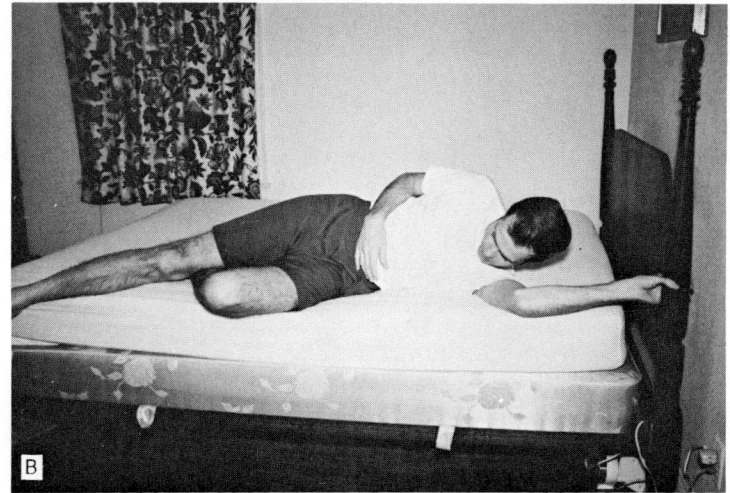

Figure 29–10
Activities of daily living:
sitting up unassisted.
A, Patient works himself
to the side of the bed
with his unaffected leg
while grasping edge of
the mattress with his
hand. B, After placing
the paralyzed arm across
his chest, he begins to
turn to the unaffected
side, still grasping the
mattress or the head
post. C, The unaffected
leg is utilized to move
the affected leg
off the edge of the bed.
This maneuver is
accomplished by hooking
the unaffected foot under
the knee of the other leg;
the strong arm acts as
a lever to move the body
into sitting position.

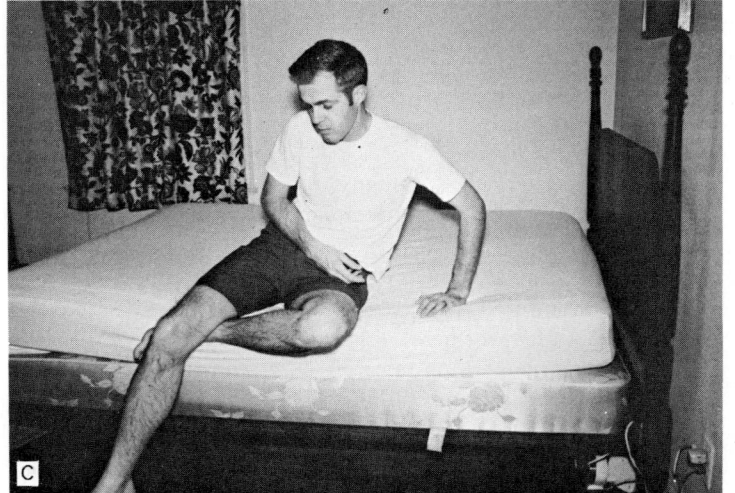

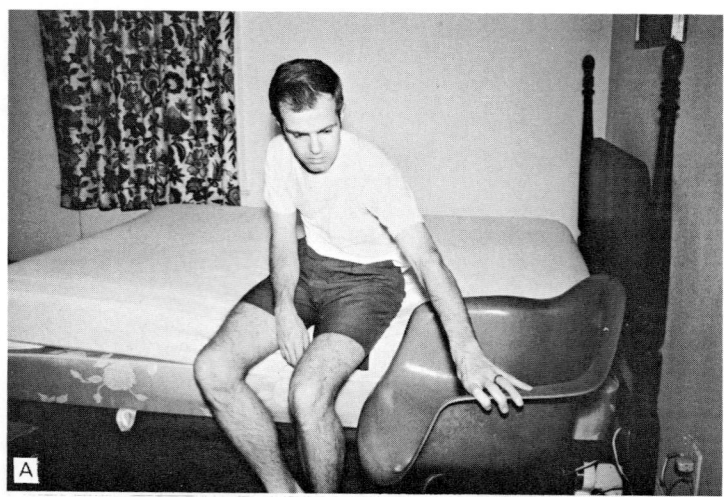

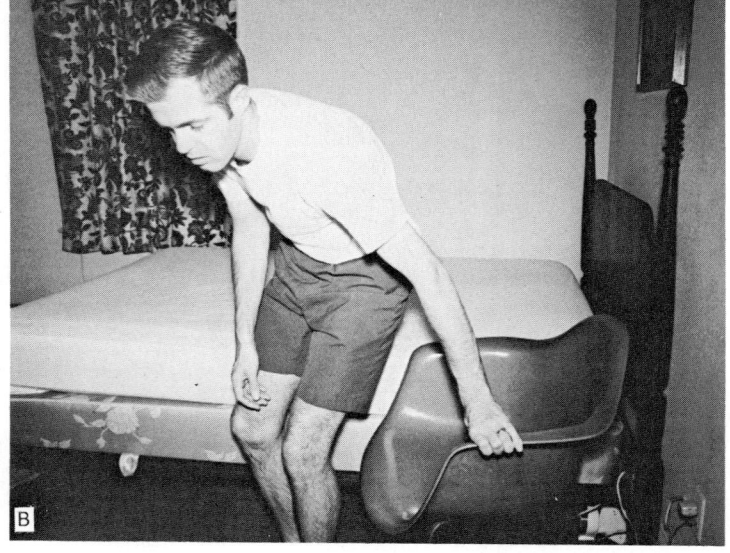

*Figure 29–11
Activities of daily
living: transferring to
chair. A, Patient sits
on the edge of the low
bed. Chair is at right
angles to bed. B, He
grasps far arm of the
chair with his
unaffected arm,
stands on the unaffected
leg, and pivots himself
into the chair.*

casual conversation, for many aphasic persons retain some automatic words or phrases. An example of how aphasia may be missed is shown in the case of Mr. B.

Mr. B. was a 53-year-old man hospitalized for evaluation of carotid stenosis. He had suffered a right middle cerebral artery stenosis 5 years previously. Mr. B. was a pleasant man, always said "Good morning," answered "yes" or "no" to questions concerning morning care, and thanked the staff for services. Since he was ambulatory and without significant motor deficits, he required little nursing help with physical needs. He had been on the unit for 1 week before any of the nursing staff realized that this patient had severe motor aphasia, and was able to say no more than the automatic pleasantries noted.

The nurse can utilize the physician's assessment of language function as a baseline, but will want to make her own evaluation of the effect of the disorder on everyday living. Important questions for the nurse to ask herself are these:

1. Can the patient understand spoken directions? Ask him to *do* some act; questions that can be answered "yes" or "no" indicate little.

2. Can he follow written directions?

3. Is his spontaneous speech relevant? Are there unintelligible or inappropriate phrases? Subcortical or less extensive cortical lesions can produce fluctuating inability to express the proper word, which can be very frustrating to the patient.

4. Does he understand the meaning of a picture? This, and his ability to comprehend a spoken idea, will help to determine the level at which he understands abstraction. If this ability is limited, one needs to speak to the patient in concrete terms.

5. Can he name an object shown him? Many persons with motor aphasia can describe the object but not name it.

The answers to these questions will assist the nurse in determining the patient's ability to participate in his own care, i.e., his ability to comply with requests and his ability to make his needs known. The nurse must communicate to the nursing staff the nature of the patient's specific language difficulties, in order to prevent frustrating him with requests he is not capable of carrying out.

It is important to remember that the person may not be disabled in all sensory spheres and, in particular, can hear. Even though he may not answer, shouting as though he were deaf will not help. He will benefit from language stimulation and thus should be talked to. The person who intersperses occasional nonsense words into otherwise intelligible sentences can be helped by having the appropriate word repeated to him. This word can often be surmised from context, and the patient can be asked if this is the word that he means. The nurse and the family should not be too quick to supply words with which the patient is having difficulty; however, they should assist him when he is obviously becoming frustrated. Emotional stress and frustration markedly decrease his performance.

Persons with mild aphasia soon learn to compensate and not to use the complex sentence or multisyllabic words that cause difficulty. Speech therapy is frequently beneficial and may be suggested to the family. Publications of the American Heart Association and the Institute of Physical Medicine and Rehabilitation are available which may aid the family in helping the aphasic person.[1]

Parietal Lobe Lesions

The sensory cortex lies in the parietal lobe along the central sulcus, with the same somatic representation as in the motor cortex. Lesions here can produce variable sensory deficits on the contralateral side of the body; these may include hypesthesia and diminished perception of pain, loss of discrimination for touch, and loss of proprioception (the ability to determine the position of a part of the body without looking at it). Other deficits resulting from parietal lobe lesions may include the loss of ability to judge the quality of sensation (astereognosis), the loss

---

[1] Reference to these publications in the bibliography is preceded by an asterisk.

of ability to differentiate degrees of pressure, and lack of recognition of identity (self versus others). In addition, because the optic tract runs through the parietal lobe, visual defects may also result. In general, parietal lobe lesions tend to produce deficits in discriminatory sensation rather than sensory modality deficits.

ASTEREOGNOSIS

Astereognosis refers to the inability to discriminate the shape, texture, size, and weight of an object. For example, the person can name an object shown him, but if it is placed in his hand he has no idea what it is. Consideration of the number of things one does each day by touch alone, such as finding change for the bus and locating objects in a purse, makes it apparent that astereognosis is a significant handicap. Astereognosis is particularly important in children as they learn the nature of the world.

Impairment of the ability to judge intensity of pressure also presents practical problems for the patient. Many everyday activities, such as writing with a pencil and cutting with a knife, require knowing how much pressure one is applying. In similar fashion, loss of proprioception requires that the patient watch his arm, for example, in order to perform a skilled act with it. It is important that the nurse realize that these deficits can exist without significant motor loss, and therefore she should modify her expectations of the patient's abilities when such deficits are present.

ANOSOGNOSIA

Anosognosia is the impairment in the ability to recognize parts of one's own body and to recognize the difference between oneself and others. This disorder is seen primarily in nondominant hemisphere lesions, and these lesions frequently produce concomitant hemiplegia. It is possible that the aphasia of a dominant hemisphere lesion precludes the expression of an anosognosia associated with that lesion. In anosognosia, the person does not recognize the contralateral side of the body as a part of himself. When the involved arm is pointed to, he may reply, "I don't know whose arm that is; someone must have put it there." There is also a lack of insight into one's own role in daily events; for example, an incontinent person may say, "The bed is wet; someone has wet my bed." When asked where he is, the patient might reply that he is in a hotel. Likewise, he might identify the nurse as a waitress. As is implied in these examples, a major characteristic of anosognosia is not only a denial of any neurologic deficit on the involved side but also a failure of the patient to appreciate his entire situation.

One aims to increase the patient's awareness of his affected side. This cannot be done by persuasion or logic, however, for he will honestly deny the existence of the side; eventually both nurse and patient become exasperated. "Going along" with the denial will only reinforce it. However, one can try to selectively reinforce the patient's attention to that side. This can be accomplished by directing his attention to that side frequently, by referring to it as his, and by praising him whenever he acknowledges that side. Techniques of operant conditioning to aid in this are described by Pigott and Brickett.

Visual fibers of the optic tract pass through the parietal and temporal lobes en route to the occipital cortex. Therefore, lesions such as tumors or infarcts in these

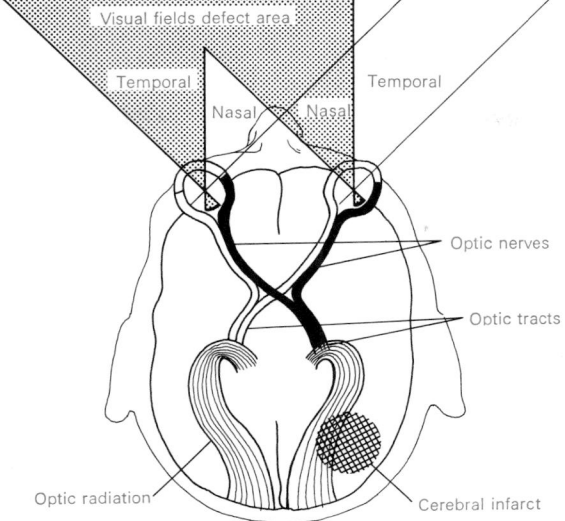

*Figure 29–12
Left homonymous
hemianopsia associated
with right posterior
parietal infarction.
Visual loss is indicated
by shaded area. (By
permission from Richard
Pigott and Florence
Brickett: Visual Neglect.
American Journal of
Nursing, 66:101–105,
January, 1966.)*

lobes may interrupt these fibers and produce visual defects. Because of the neuroanatomy of the optic system, a lesion on one side of the brain will produce a
defect in the opposite half of the visual field of each eye (see Figure 29–5). Total interruption of an optic tract will produce a complete *homonymous hemianopsia*
—loss of one-half of each visual field. As a result, the patient cannot see past the
midline toward the side opposite the lesion unless he actually moves his eyes to
that side; he sees only one-half of what the normal person sees in any position.
Homonymous hemianopsia is not confined to parietal lobe lesions but will occur
with tumors or vascular disorders anywhere along the course of these fibers.

This disability is not uncommon, particularly after strokes, but is often missed
by the nursing staff. The patient himself, particularly if he has an anosognosia,
may be unaware of the visual defect; he knows only that he bumps into things,
and that people "sneak up" on him from the affected side. The physician's notes
will almost always mention the presence of homonymous hemianopsia or other
visual field defects. This can also be assessed by the nurse by using such techniques as asking the patient to describe an object or count fingers shown him on
the side of the suspected deficit. It is most important that his gaze be fixed at the
midline for this test to be accurate. More detailed evaluative procedures than can
be discussed here are outlined by Pigott and Brickett.

The patient needs to learn to compensate for this deficit. He may be helped initially by having the hospital environment rearranged for him: the bedside stand
should be placed on his "good" visual side, food trays should be placed within
his intact field of vision, and he should be approached from his good side. He can
be taught to scan widely (to turn his head to include the blocked visual field) and
to read the line of print until he sees the edge of his book or paper. If anosognosia complicates the picture, techniques of operant conditioning and reinforcement
are helpful. These are too detailed for discussion in this text, but are fully described by Pigott and Brickett.

Temporal Lobe Lesions

The temporal lobe is concerned with auditory perception, memory, and smell. Disturbances in auditory language perception have been discussed under the topic of aphasia. As noted above, fibers from the optic tracts pass through the temporal as well as the parietal lobe. Optic tract involvement by temporal lobe lesions will produce visual deficits; however, these are more apt to consist of visual block in the medial and lateral aspects of the upper visual quadrant, rather than the half-field defects described before.

For unknown reasons, recent memory is most affected in memory disturbances. Since recent memory is important in learning, the patient with a memory defect will have difficulty in this sphere. This has implications not only in intellectual pursuits but in adaptation to any new situation. For pragmatic reasons, the nurse must assess the patient's capacity for remembering recent events in order to determine the extent of his ability to learn to care for himself. Simple assessment can be made by asking the patient to remember progressively more complex sentences and to repeat them later. Expecting persons with memory damage to retain directions or explanations for any length of time may lead to frustration of both patient and staff, and the staff must plan to repeat explanations if there is much memory loss. However, there is obvious danger in assuming that all patients with temporal lobe lesions have memory loss.

Some lesions, particularly tumors, may cause temporal lobe seizures. These are more commonly manifested in the psychic form, with strange odors, visual memory phenomena (*déjà vu,* the sense of having been through the present event before), or auditory hallucinations. These can be very frightening to the patient and to others. The patient may act upon his hallucination; this should be handled in the same way as any hallucination. The nurse must appreciate the reality of the hallucination to the person, but she must not positively reinforce that perception by agreeing that it is real. Statements such as, "I don't hear a band playing, but it must be disturbing to you to hear one," point out reality and yet acknowledge to the patient that the nurse believes him.

Occipital Lobe Lesions

The occipital lobe is supplied by the posterior cerebral artery and is not so commonly involved in cerebrovascular accidents as are the other lobes. This lobe is concerned with receiving visual stimuli and simple visual images and, to some extent, interpreting their shapes, sizes, and meaning. However, the angular gyrus, where the temporal, parietal, and occipital lobes meet, has the more important visual interpretive functions. Lesions at the occipital pole may produce homonymous hemianopsia, cortical blindness, and some visual interpretive defects. In cortical blindness, the patient receives or "sees" visual stimuli (this is determined by the presence of intact pupillary responses) but perceives no meaningful visual image (Guyton; Wechsler). Nursing problems arise when the patient denies his blindness, insisting that he can see. He is apt to incur physical harm when he attempts to engage even in everyday activities but fails to recognize his visual limitations. Community resources for rehabilitation of the blind may be suggested to the family.

ALEXIA

A patient with occipital lobe lesions situated more anteriorly, in the secondary visual sensory areas, may suffer from alexia or "word blindness." He can actually see and often can pronounce or spell the word, but he cannot recognize its meaning. Unless auditory sensory areas are also damaged, he will be able to understand the same word if it is spoken to him.

Lesions of the angular gyrus cause difficulty in coordinating visual images with appropriate motor acts. The patient may see a glass of water and yet be unable to use the visual information to direct his hand to the glass and pick it up. He can be taught to compensate for this defect by feeling objects before him and using his stereognostic sense to determine the nature of the object. This will be effective only if the angular gyrus is not so fully involved as to produce a global aphasia.

THALAMUS

The thalamus is concerned with integrating incoming sensory information before such sensory stimuli are interpreted by the cortex. Lesions in this area may produce aberrant sensations. Initially there may be anesthesia on the opposite side of the body. This may be followed, after some time, by the presence of painful sensations in response to stimuli. The pain is frequently "primitive," i.e., diffuse and of a persistent, burning nature; it is made worse by superficial stimuli, such as light touch or the pressure of bedclothes. Nursing measures such as using a foot board or cradle to keep the covers off affected limbs and avoiding the handling of paresthetic portions of limbs can be helpful. Cerebrovascular accidents in this area may be followed by this type of pain, as well as concomitant motor deficits.

BASAL GANGLIA

The basal ganglia are lateral and slightly superior to the thalamus and are part of the extrapyramidal motor system. This system is important in the mediation of posture and the integration of coordinated movement. With lesions in the basal ganglia the clinical manifestations are largely those of excessive motor activity. This is in contrast to the clinical picture of motor deficits seen in lesions in other parts of the brain.

Parkinson's Syndrome   (Basal Ganglia)

The classic disorder of this area is Parkinson's syndrome or paralysis agitans. The cause is unknown, although some feel that it is the result of postencephalitic degeneration. Degeneration of basal ganglion cells is seen, with replacement by connective tissue cells (Wechsler). In this syndrome there is postural rigidity and difficulty in performing movements smoothly. Clinical manifestations include muscular rigidity with a paucity of spontaneous movement, stooped posture, shuffling gait, and intention tremor (tremor occurring upon initiation of movement). Lack of spontaneous movement often manifests itself in the mask-like appearance of the face, in which there is little change of expression. The person's speech and chewing are both affected as movement of the jaw becomes restricted. There is gradual decrease in general voluntary movement and concomitant stiffening of muscles and joints from disuse. Many patients will benefit from active physical therapy; Doshay outlines a series of exercises designed to prevent the early disability so often seen. The nurse can assist the patient and his family in planning daily activities to promote the use of muscles and to avoid the emotional crises that seem to accentuate symptoms. The syndrome is slowly progressive; the patient's condition may remain stationary for many years or the patient may become bedridden after a few years.

Medical treatment is primarily symptomatic, and anticholinergic drugs are employed to decrease rigidity. The drugs used are of the hyoscine–strabonium–atropine family (Artane, Pagitane, Parsidol) and as such may produce the same side effects (i.e., those of the parasympatholytic agents). A dry mouth is a common complaint of patients and is related to the secretion-drying effects of the drugs. Such side effects as blurred vision, tachycardia, urinary retention, constipation, and increased intraocular pressure can be particularly harmful in older patients, and the nurse should be alert for these effects. Although its use is still restricted, L-DOPA (levodihydroxyphenylalanine) appears to offer more effective relief from rigidity and tremor than any drug currently in use. According to *The Medical Letter,* major side effects from this drug include transitory nausea and vomiting, orthostatic hypotension, and, rarely, depression of granulocytes.

Stereotactic surgical procedures are performed to destroy areas in the thalamus (nucleus ventralis lateralis) or putamen and thereby reduce rigidity. Special apparatus are used to localize the area, and cautery or chemical agents are used to destroy that area. Since the procedure is performed under local anesthesia and only small holes are made to enter the skull, there is no specialized nursing care required after surgery.

Chorea; Athetosis

Chorea (irregular, rapid, involuntary movements) and athetosis (involuntary but smooth and blended movements) are other manifestations of thalamic-basal ganglion disorders. They are frequently found in persons with cerebral palsy. Nursing problems are posed because of the random motions, which may predispose the patient to trauma from falling or from hitting objects. The ambulatory patient needs some protection but should not be overly restricted, for he can learn to adapt to his involuntary movements to some degree. Bed rails can prevent the patient confined to bed from falling; however, such bed rails may need to be padded to prevent constant abrasion.

THE BRAIN STEM: MIDBRAIN, PONS, AND MEDULLA

The brain stem contains cranial nerve nuclei, nerve tracts interconnecting the spinal cord and higher centers, and the controlling centers for the vital functions of the body. The critical role of the brain stem is evidenced by the fact that a person may completely lose cortical function and yet still exist so long as the brain stem is intact; this existence will be at a primitive level, with only vital functions persisting.

The nuclei of all the cranial nerves except the olfactory and optic nerves are located in the brain stem. Because of the compact nature of this region, a lesion within it may involve multiple cranial nerves. The common types of lesions are infarction, hemorrhage, and tumor. The symptoms seen may be produced not only from direct nervous tissue involvement by the lesion but also from secondary pressure on the respiratory and circulatory centers.

Difficult nursing problems arise when the nuclei of the ninth, tenth, and twelfth cranial nerves (located in the medulla) are involved, for these nerves innervate structures necessary for swallowing, speaking, and effective coughing. Resultant dysfunction is called *bulbar palsy* ("bulbar" referring to the medulla and "palsy" referring to paralysis) and is usually the result of hemorrhage, thrombosis, or degeneration (e.g., multiple sclerosis) in the region. This disruption of medullary cranial nerve function produces flaccid paralysis of the palate, pharynx, and tongue, all on the same side as the lesion; therefore, the patient may have a hoarse or whispering voice, may choke easily when swallowing, and may have an ineffective cough because of inability to close the glottis completely.

A major concern in patients with bulbar palsy is the prevention of aspiration. The patient may aspirate his own secretions (particularly during the acute phase) or food and fluids. Dizziness and vomiting may also be present in brain stem lesions, complicating the problem of aspiration. Nasopharyngeal and endotracheal suctioning are necessary if the patient cannot cough effectively or if he aspirates food or vomitus. Once food and fluids are permitted to the patient, he must learn to eat slowly and in small portions. Viscous foods and fluids are most easily swallowed, but the patient can learn to tolerate thin liquids by taking small sips. Patients with any degree of swallowing difficulty should not be fed by minimally trained personnel, and any increase in the difficulty should be brought to the physician's attention for reevaluation of oral feeding.

The compact neuroanatomy of the brain stem which is a predisposing factor to multiple cranial nerve involvement by a single lesion also is the source of predisposition to simultaneous involvement of the nerve tracts that run through the brain stem. These include the ascending sensory and the descending motor tracts. The motor tracts include not only the corticospinal or pyramidal tract (voluntary motor) but also the extrapyramidal system. This system emanates from the cerebellum and from subcortical centers and mediates muscle tone, posture, and coordination. Hence brain stem disorders may produce hemiplegia, ataxia, and sensory disturbances, in addition to cranial nerve dysfunction.

CEREBELLUM

The cerebellum coordinates motor activities. It makes possible the smooth, accurate movements we take for granted; it is also important for the equilibrium necessary in standing and walking. Persons with cerebellar dysfunction are unable to maintain stable posture with the eyes closed, to move a finger from one object to another with precision, or to walk in a straight line.

Ataxia

Lack of coordinated movement is called *ataxia*. Gross movement is possible, but there is much difficulty with fine, coordinated action. Normally, a voluntary action is balanced by a "checking" mechanism, which limits the action to its intended range. In cerebellar lesions, this check (synergia) is lost and movement overreaches the target.

Extent of the dysfunction will vary with the extent of the lesion, but the nurse needs to note what coordinated movements can be performed in order to avoid making impossible demands on the patient. For example, the patient may be able to put on his shirt and pants but may be unable to button the shirt. The need for assistance should be anticipated, rather than allowing the patient to struggle in vain. Feeding oneself may be a major problem to some patients with ataxia; the use of utensils with padded handles, in order to facilitate grasp, may aid the patient whose predominant problem is with fine movements of the hand.

SEIZURES

Seizures are the manifestation of abnormal and excessive neuronal discharge in the brain. The term *seizure* is often used synonymously with *convulsion;* the latter term, however, refers only to the muscular contractions that may be one component of a seizure. The neuronal mechanisms of the brain are such that anyone, given appropriate stimuli and predisposing factors, may have a seizure. Predisposing factors may include genetic predisposition, lesions of the brain which produce an irritable focus (such as brain tumors or scar tissue from old trauma), cerebral ischemia (such as that caused by heart block), and metabolic disturbances (hypoglycemia, acidosis, uremia). However, the majority of seizures occur in persons with "seizure disorders" or epilepsy. This is a condition in which the seizure is the primary manifestation, rather than one in which the seizure is secondary to another disease process.

Although there are no accurate statistics on the incidence of seizure disorders, they are generally estimated to occur in about 0.5 percent of the population (Beeson and McDermott; Lennox). The incidence is evenly distributed between males and females, and most persons having multiple seizures have their first before the age of 20. (Indeed, onset of seizures after age 20 is strongly suggestive of a brain tumor or other pathology.) A small number of persons have "acquired" or "symptomatic" epilepsy—a seizure disorder due to verifiable organic lesion or brain trauma at or after birth. The majority, however, have no history of such organic etiology. It is felt that these persons have genetic factors in the etiology of their seizures. Investigations of family history and family electroencephalograms suggest that there is an inherited brain dysrhythmia that predisposes a person to seizures (Lennox; Rodin and Gonzolaz). The presence of these dysrhythmias in family members without clinical symptoms suggests that only the tendency to epilepsy, but not the clinical state, is inherited.

Seizures are commonly classified as *grand mal, petit mal, psychomotor,* and *autonomic.* The first two terms are of little descriptive value, simply meaning "big sickness" and "little sickness," but they are so widely used that they will be used in this discussion.

In any seizure, there is (1) some disturbance in consciousness, and (2) involuntary motor activity (or cessation of motor function). A relatively rare type of epilepsy is manifested by autonomic symptoms (such as abdominal pains, tachycardia, diaphoresis, hypertension), rather than the foregoing characteristics. It can be diagnosed only by history and an electroencephalogram suggestive of seizure dysrhythmia.

An *aura* may precede some seizures, particularly grand mal episodes. It may consist of such phenomena as strange odors, visual disturbances, irritability, and a sense of foreboding. The character of the aura can be helpful in localizing the focus of seizure discharge. It can also warn the patient of the impending seizure in time to seek a safe place.

Grand Mal Seizures

The grand mal convulsion is believed to originate in the reticular activating system in the brain stem, and to spread to the cortex. It may be preceded by a loud cry; the patient immediately loses consciousness and convulses. His muscles become rigid, and he falls if not supported. This is the *tonic* stage of the convulsion and is a momentary state of decerebrate rigidity. All limbs are rigid and extended; the pupils are dilated and nonreactive to light; the blood pressure rises; and respirations have ceased. The face and neck become red and turgid, and then cyanotic. The jaws are clamped shut, and if the tongue was between the teeth at the onset of the seizure, it is bitten. This stage lasts less than a minute and is followed by the *clonic* stage. At this point the muscles alternately contract and relax, causing the head and limbs to thrash about. This sometimes occurs with enough force to cause fractures, particularly if well-meaning bystanders attempt to restrain the limbs. Breathing resumes, and the saliva that has collected in the mouth may be blown out with each respiration; this gives the appearance of "foaming at the mouth." Incontinence of urine and feces may occur at this time.

The entire seizure is usually over in about 3 minutes; the clonic movements cease; the person opens his eyes and may make aimless motions. The pupils are reactive to light and of normal size; the sclerae are injected or "blood-shot." The person will be very tired; he may have a headache, and he may be stuporous for an hour or even a day after the episode. The stuporous and disoriented behavior is referred to as the *postictal state* (ictus referring to convulsion).

During the apneic period, it appears as though the patient will die of asphyxiation. This period is relatively short, however, and of no real danger unless the patient is in *status epilepticus*—prolonged seizures, or continuous seizures that follow one upon another. The major danger is that the patient may be injured during the initial fall or if his head or limbs strike objects during the clonic phase.

Petit Mal Seizures

Petit mal seizures are seen most commonly in children, and may take the form of absence, myoclonic, or akinetic episodes. Absence seizures are the most common and consist of short (5 to 10 seconds) periods in which consciousness is lost. There is no change in muscle tone. The person has no awareness of the episode; indeed, he may stop in the middle of a sentence, stare for a few seconds, and then resume the sentence as if nothing had happened. Absence seizures may markedly interfere with children's progress in school if they occur frequently.

Myoclonic seizures are relatively rare. They are also of short duration and are characterized by clonic jerking of head or limbs, with a concurrent lapse in consciousness. Akinetic or "drop" seizures consist of sudden, brief loss of motor tone, causing the person to fall or drop whatever he is holding. Concurrent loss of consciousness seems to vary with individuals.

Psychomotor Seizures

Psychomotor seizures or *epileptic equivalents* are characterized by brief amnesia (with or without apparent awareness of the environment) or lapses of consciousness, accompanied by purposeful motor activity. This type of seizure may also take the form of psychic phenomena, such as auditory or olfactory hallucinations, feelings of unreality or *déjà vu* phenomena (the sense of having been through the present event before). The motor activity may be simple acts, such as repeated chewing or swallowing, or more complicated activity known as *automatisms*. The latter may include moving about a room, or undressing. The actions are purposeful, but they are done unconsciously and without relevance to the situation at hand. Occasionally, aimless running or violent behavior may accompany the amnesia. Since restraint tends to increase the violence, it is better in such cases to attempt to protect the bystanders, rather than to restrain the patient.

Although the majority of seizures are *idiopathic* or of unknown cause, some are symptomatic of underlying brain lesions, such as a tumor or scar tissue from an old trauma. If a tumor is causing the seizures, it must be removed or death will eventually occur. Some cortical scars can be removed surgically and thus be of benefit in relieving the seizure disorder. Tumors often produce seizures that start in one area of the body, such as a hand or one side of the face, and progress to a generalized grand mal episode. These are called *jacksonian* convulsions (after John Hughlings Jackson, who first described them), and are helpful in localizing the seizure focus. For this reason, a detailed description of the seizure is essential.

Nursing Measures

The nurse's role during any type of seizure is the same as that of any bystander: to prevent injury to the person having the seizure. This is particularly important in grand mal seizures; the character of petit mal and psychomotor seizures is such that the danger of self-injury is small.

If a grand mal seizure is preceded by an aura, the person may have time to sit or lie down. Usually, however, there is no warning, and bystanders may not be able to prevent the initial fall. If the jaws are not yet clenched, a wad of fabric or a well-padded tongue blade may be placed between the molars to prevent biting of the tongue. However, such materials should never be forced between clenched teeth, nor should anything hard, such as a spoon or a pencil, be used.

Once the grand mal seizure has begun, little can be done except to place a pillow, folded jacket, or such beneath the head, to prevent it from hitting the floor during the clonic phase. Limbs must not be restrained, since this predisposes them to fractures; if the person is in danger of hitting furniture, it is better to move the furniture than to hold the person's limbs. The hospitalized patient who has frequent seizures, or the patient in status epilepticus, needs to have his bed rails padded well to prevent injury. If commercially made pads are not available, firm pillows taped to the bed rails will suffice.

The patient in status epilepticus is in danger of aspirating his saliva and should be suctioned during the clonic phase or in the interim between seizures. Phenobarbital, paraldehyde, and intravenous sodium amobarbital are often used in an attempt to control these episodes. More recently, intravenous diazepam (Valium) has been used with success (Premsky et al.).

A second important nursing role in the care of patients with seizures is to make accurate observations of the episodes. Careful observations and recording are essential in aiding the physician to diagnose the disorder and then assess the efficacy of the drug control program. Such information as where the seizure started, the nature of any aura, the nature of motor activity, and after effects of the episode can aid the physician in diagnosing the kind of seizure and in determining if it is "idiopathic" epilepsy or a remedial brain disorder. Pertinent observations should include the following:

1. Duration of the seizure; the time it began and ended should be recorded.

2. Description of an aura if present.

3. State of consciousness. It should be noted if there was an immediate loss of consciousness (as in grand mal), or if the person was responsive to verbal stimuli during the activity (in describing petit mal and psychomotor episodes).

4. Motor activity. Important points to include are these: where the motor activity started; presence or absence of tonic and clonic movements in grand mal episodes; any deviation of eyes, tongue, etc.; and the nature of any automatisms in psychomotor seizures.

5. Presence or absence of incontinence in grand mal seizures.

6. State of consciousness after the epidode; the patient's awareness of, or memory for, the event.

7. Frequency and number of seizures. This is particularly important in gauging drug control.

Several drugs have been found to be efficacious in seizure control. It is estimated that 70 to 80 percent of persons with seizure disorders are well controlled by medication. Only the more common drugs will be listed here; a pharmacology textbook should be consulted for a more complete listing and for details of action and side effects.

The drugs most commonly used in grand mal and psychomotor seizures are diphenylhydantoin (Dilantin), phenobarbital, methylphenylhydantoin (Mesantoin), and primidone (Mysoline). These drugs tend to be more effective in controlling grand mal seizures than psychomotor seizures. A later drug, carbamazepine (Tegretol), appears to hold promise in controlling the latter (Livingston et al.). Drugs used commonly in petit mal epilepsy include trimethadione (Tridione), dimethylethyloxazolidinedione (Paradione) and methylphenylsuccinamide (Milontin). Many patients with "idiopathic" epilepsy have both grand and petit mal seizures and will be taking a combination of drugs.

Public and patient education is a third important nursing function. The patient and his family need to learn what to do during a seizure, to assume responsibility for drug therapy, and to seek medical care if side effects occur. Rash, ataxia, and drowsiness are seen with several of the drugs, and blood dyscrasias have occurred with a few. The latter can be detected only by blood studies; therefore the nurse can help stress the importance to the patients taking these few drugs of complying with the physician's request that they appear regularly for blood tests. Hyperplasia of the gum is often a problem in children receiving Dilantin and may require surgical treatment.

Even though drug control is effective in the majority of persons with seizure disorders, public misinformation and fear influence many aspects of daily living for the epileptic. Such aspects include choice of a job, ability to obtain a driver's license, and the right to marry and to have children. Both physician and nurse can help the patient and his family to cope with these problems and can educate the public to understand epilepsy.

Driving an automobile is obviously hazardous in anyone whose seizures are not completely controlled by drugs; however, a few states prohibit *anyone* with epilepsy from obtaining a driver's license, no matter what his state of medical control. Patients whose seizures are not fully controlled should not work at jobs involving driving mechanical equipment or those involving heights, or in any situation where they or others might be injured were they to have a seizure. Unfortunately, many employers will not hire a fully controlled person for these jobs, or for any position, regardless of the type of work. The misinformed attitude of much of the public is exemplified in the laws of a few states, which classify the epileptic with "idiots and the insane." This is despite the fact that many studies have been made of epileptic persons showing that their intelligence is distributed in the same way as that of the general population (Lennox). Decisions about marriage and children need to be made by the individual, based on his physician's advice.

It is not uncommon for parents of school age children to deny that the child has seizures, because of their fear of the stigma and fear for the child's future if he is labeled "epileptic." This, unfortunately, denies him treatment and the possibility that he can be seizure-free with medication. Public health nurses and school nurses have a major role in aiding these parents to overcome their fears and seek help for their children. School nurses can also aid in acceptance of these children by educating the school personnel about epilepsy, by aiding them in recognizing the "inattentive" child who really has petit mal seizures, and by teaching them what to do in the event a child has a convulsion in their classroom.

Nurses, with the other health professionals, have a responsibility in educating the public about epilepsy and in encouraging legislators to update outmoded laws relating to epileptics. Several voluntary organizations such as the National Epilepsy League and the National Association to Control Epilepsy have literature available and carry out local programs for public education.

Decisions about marriage and having children need to be made by the individual, based on his physician's advice. Unless the disorder is so severe as to be a burden to the spouse, there is no reason a person with a seizure disorder should not marry. If his seizures appear to be genetically based, his offspring have about three times greater chance of having more than two seizures in their lifetime than do the children of "normal" individuals. It is well to note, however, that this is much less than the chance of a diabetic having diabetic children (Beeson and McDermott; Lennox). In a few states there are laws prohibiting epileptics from marrying, or requiring them to have certification that they are seizure-free with drug therapy. Three states still enforce sterilization of epileptics.

Bibliography

Aphasia and the Family. American Heart Association, New York, 1965.

Bakay, Louis and Joseph C. Lee. *Cerebral Edema.* Springfield, Ill.: Charles C Thomas, Publishers, 1965.

Beeson, P. B. and Walsh McDermott (Eds.): *Cecil-Loeb Textbook of Medicine,* 12th ed. Philadelphia: W. B. Saunders Co., 1967, p. 1508.

Cerebral Vascular Disease and Strokes. National Heart Institute. U. S. Public Health Service Publication 513. Washington, D.C.: U. S. Government Printing Office, 1964.

Conant, R. G., J. A. Perkins, and A. B. Ainley: Stroke, Morbidity, Mortality and Rehabilitation Potential. *Journal of Chronic Diseases,* 18:347–403, April, 1965.

Do It Yourself Again: Self-help Devices for the Stroke Patient. American Heart Association. New York, 1965.

Doshay, Lewis: Method and Value of Exercise in Parkinson's Disease. *New England Journal of Medicine,* 267:297–299, August 9, 1962.

Fawcett, F. Q. and W. T. Smith: Current Views on the Pathogenesis of Common Strokes. *Postgraduate Medical Journal,* 42:5:5–15, January, 1966.

French, L. A. and J. H. Galicich: The Use of Steroids for Control of Cerebral Edema. *Clinical Neurosurgery* (Proceedings of Congress of Neurological Surgeons), 10:212, 1962.

de Gutierrez-Mahoney, C. G. and Esta Carini: *Neurological and Neurosurgical Nursing,* 5th ed. St. Louis: The C. V. Mosby Company, 1970.

Guyton, Arthur: *Textbook of Medical Physiology,* 3d ed. Philadelphia: W. B. Saunders Company, 1966, pp. 746–752.

Hodgins, Eric: Listen: The Patient. *New England Journal of Medicine,* 274:657–661, March 24, 1966.

Javid, H. and O. C. Julian: Prevention of Strokes by Carotid and Vertebral Surgery. *Medical Clinics of North America,* 51:113–122, January, 1967.

Lennox, William G.: *Epilepsy and Related Disorders,* Vol. I. Boston: Little, Brown and Company, 1960.

Livingston, S., et al.: Use of Carbamazepine in Epilepsy. *Journal of American Medical Association,* 200:204–208, April 17, 1967.

Matson, Donald: Treatment of Cerebral Swelling. *New England Journal of Medicine,* 272:626–628, March 25, 1965.

McKissock, W., K. W. E. Paine, and L. S. Walsh: An Analysis of Results of Treatment of Ruptured Intracranial Aneurysms; Report of 772 Consecutive Cases. *Journal of Neurosurgery,* 19:762–776, 1960.

Mullen, Sean: *Essentials of Neurosurgery.* New York: Springer Publishing Co., Inc., 1961.

A National Program to Conquer Heart Disease, Cancer and Stroke, Vol. I. Report of the President's Commission. Washington, D. C.: U.S. Government Printing Office, December, 1964.

New and Old Drugs for Parkinsonism. *Medical Letter,* 10:18:68–70, September 6, 1968.

Ojemann, Robert: The Surgical Treatment of Cerebrovascular Disease. *New England Journal of Medicine,* 274:440–448, February 24, 1966.

Ostfield, A. M.: Are Strokes Preventable? *Medical Clinics of North America,* 51:105–111, January, 1967.

Pigott, Richard and Florence Brickett: Visual Neglect. *American Journal of Nursing,* 66:101–105, January, 1966.

Prensky, A. L., et al.: Intravenous Diazepan in the Treatment of Prolonged Seizure Activity. *New England Journal of Medicine,* 276:779–784, April 6, 1967.

Rodin, Ernst and Gonzolaz Salvador: Hereditary Components in Epileptic Patients; Electroencephalographic Family Studies. *Journal of American Medical Association,* 198:221–225, October 17, 1966.

Schilder, Paul: *The Image and Appearance of the Human Body.* Science Editions. New York: International Universities Press, Inc., 1950.

Strike Back at Stroke. American Heart Association. New York, 1961.

Strokes—A Guide for the Family. American Heart Association. New York, 1964.

*Taylor, Margeret: *Understanding Aphasia: A Guide for Family and Friends.* Institute of Physical Medicine and Rehabilitation, New York University Medical Center, New York.

Ullman, Montague: Disorders of Body Image after Stroke. *American Journal of Nursing,* 64:84–91, October, 1964.

Up and Around. American Heart Association, New York.

Wechsler, Israel: *Clinical Neurology,* 9th ed. Philadelphia: W. B. Saunders Company, 1963, pp. 295–560.

Wright, Beatrice: *Physical Disability—A Psychological Approach.* New York: Paul B. Hoeber, Inc., 1960.

Suggested Reading for Students

Boshes, Louis: Epilepsy and the Law. *Diseases of Nervous System,* 26:569–573, September, 1965.

Goda, Sidney: Communicating with the Aphasic or Dysarthric Patient. *American Journal of Nursing,* 63:80–84, July, 1963.

Martin, M. Arlene: Care of a Patient with Cerebral Aneurysm. *American Journal of Nursing,* 65:90–95, April, 1965.

Merritt, Hiram H.: *A Textbook of Neurology,* 4th ed. Philadelphia: Lea & Febiger, 1967.

SECTION 2
DISORDERS OF THE SPINAL CORD

M. ARLENE GARDNER

Nature has provided the spinal cord with elaborate structural protection against invading forces. This delicate organ, which with the brain makes up the central nervous system, is housed within the firm, bony protection of the vertebrae. The cord is surrounded by circulating cerebrospinal fluid, which further protects it by serving as a shock absorber. No doubt the elaborate protection provided is due in part to the fact that spinal cord tissue does not spontaneously regenerate, for once it is injured, a lasting deficit ensues. Reports of current research in spinal cord regeneration in the laboratory appear promising, and although there is no proof that human neurons lack a growth potential, neither is there proof that effective spontaneous regeneration has occurred (Windle).

The function of the spinal cord is to integrate information received from the skin and muscles to nerve cells. This constitutes a very complex system. Within the cord are located long conducting pathways as well as cell bodies from which nerve fibers going to the periphery originate. Essentially, disturbances of function of the cord are created by deficits in motor, sensory, autonomic, and reflex activity.

The structure and function of the spinal cord are well adapted to correlating clinical manifestations of deficit and locating the disorder within the cord. Thus, an understanding of normal anatomy and physiology is prerequisite to scientifically based planning and predicting of nursing management for patients with cord disorders.

Disorders of the spinal cord generally are entirely unrelated to age, sex, or socioeconomic status. Some may develop slowly with hardly perceptible symptoms, such as a slowly growing extramedullary neoplasm, whereas others may be abrupt in onset with permanent damage, as seen in a traumatic complete transection. Although some disorders can be treated, and complete or nearly complete restoration of function is possible, the course of many cord disorders is a progressively deteriorating one. The loss of any degree of motor function may necessitate a modification and adjustment in the patient's total life pattern. Inability to ambulate could necessitate change of employment, change in role relationships with family and friends, and increased dependency upon others.

The rehabilitation concept must be utilized throughout the illness. Rehabilitation is aimed toward assisting the patient to adjust to his limitations and work toward his maximum potential. Concomitant with this is the understanding and reinforcement of the individual's actual potential. The patient and his family should be encouraged to maintain hope, but not to strive to attain unrealistic goals. The kind and enthusiastic nurse who encourages the patient with a complete cord transection to believe that he is regaining voluntary motor ability when she observes the phenomenom of hyperreflexia may do more harm than good. The profession of nursing can ill afford this kind of care.

The clinical picture depends upon the location of the lesion, regardless of whether the cause be trauma, neoplasm, infection, or another. The practitioner of nursing should possess a working knowledge of the nervous system, an understanding of the pathophysiology responsible for the presenting symptoms, the typical progression pattern of the disorder, the therapies frequently employed and their desired results, and the medical care goals. From these data she can begin to formulate short- and long-term nursing care objectives.

This section will deal with the nursing care of patients with commonly encountered disorders of the spinal cord. No attempt will be made to present a comprehensive picture of all disorders of the cord. The reader is referred to basic textbooks in neurology for this information. Rather, by providing the reader with a detailed plan of care for patients with the cord deficits commonly seen, these same principles of care can be applied to other cord conditions with similar symptom manifestations.

Trauma, neoplasms, infections, and degenerative diseases are discussed. Special attention is given to the care of the patient with spinal cord injury with resultant extensive motor–sensory–autonomic deficit as seen in quadriplegia and paraplegia. The same underlying physiological principles related to skin care in denervated areas are applicable whether the cause be cord transection, demyelinization, or infection of the cord. The deficit manifestation remains the same. The reader will be referred again to this presentation as it is appropriate throughout the discussion of other disorders.

Trauma

Incidence

Spinal cord injuries with resulting paraplegia and quadriplegia have become increasingly common during the past few decades, the large number of casualty victims with spinal cord injury in World War II being primarily responsible for the initial focusing of attention upon this problem. Improved means of travel and increased leisure time are two factors that have contributed to this increased incidence. Better understanding among the laity in the appropriate handling of individuals with potential cord injury and advanced medical techniques have helped to save the lives of victims of spinal cord injury who might have succumbed in a less advanced age.

Mechanism of Injury

Injury to the spinal cord is rarely a result of direct violence except in the form of missile wounds. Generally, damage to the cord occurs indirectly from fracture, dislocation, or fracture-dislocation of the vertebral bodies or their processes with resulting flexion or extension of the cord. This type of indirect trauma occurs as the result of falls, automobile accidents, or diving into shallow water. In flexion injuries, a compression fracture is the most common type produced. The mechanism of injury is frequently a forward displacement of an upper vertebra upon a lower one with resulting laceration to or compression of the cord itself caused by acute hyperflexion. Bleeding into the subarachnoid space may occur at this time. Hyperextension injuries occur more frequently when mobility of the spine is impaired, as in the arthritic spine. These injuries are usually the result of forward fall accidents, as in falling down a flight of stairs.

Cervical cord injury without fracture or dislocation usually results from forcible extension rather than flexion.

Pathology

Injury to the cord may be of a concussion type. Although this mechanism is not well understood, it is known to result in transient neurological symptoms. It is felt that there may be edema in or surrounding the cord brought about by transmission of pressure waves to the substance of the cord and that this situation is responsible for the temporary deficit (Merritt).

Direct laceration, or compression of the cord or its blood supply, produces a variable clinical picture. Hematomyelia, although very rare, may occur as result of compression of the cord or from a tear by vertebral bone fragments with bleeding spreading to the surrounding cord substance. More common is ischemia of the cord produced by compression upon the cord's blood supply. The deficit produced indicates the area of the cord damaged. The most common site of hemorrhage is in the lower cervical region of the cord.

A complete cord transection results in permanent loss of motor, sensory, and autonomic activity below the affected segment. An incomplete transection may initially produce a similar picture but the deficit will depend upon the pathways and cellular structures severed. Partial division of the spinal cord presents a clinical picture known as Brown-Séquard syndrome. If one side of the cord is severed, the signs are loss below the lesion level, loss of voluntary motion and the sensations of touch, vibration, proprioception, and passive motion on the ipsilateral side, and loss of pain and temperature perception on the contralateral side. The anatomical explanation for this situation is as follows: The *posterior* tract, which conducts sensation, and the *lateral* tract, which conducts motor impulses, carry fibers that cross in the medulla oblongata; the *anterolateral* tract, which controls pain and temperature perception, is an ascending tract that carries fibers crossing at the level of entry into the cord before they ascend toward the cerebrum.

Levels of Injury

Although injuries to the cord may occur at any level, the most common sites are the fifth and sixth cervical vertebrae and the eleventh and twelfth thoracic vertebrae.

Cervical Cord Injury. This is usually the result of a forward displacement of the head and the upper portion of the cervical spine over the lower portion. This area is especially vulnerable because of the weight of the head and the mobility of the cervical spine. Injuries at the level of the first four cervical vertebrae are usually incompatible with life. The phrenic nerve leaves the cord at this level; death results from respiratory embarrassment. In transecting cervical cord injuries there is immediate flaccid paralysis of all extremities, loss of sensation and reflexes below the level of transection, urinary retention, priapism, and absence of perspiration in the affected parts. This picture varies with the level of involvement. In general, cord severance in the upper cervical region results in *complete quadriplegia.* If the injury is at a lower level and greater upper extremity function is preserved, the condition is termed *incomplete quadriplegia.*

Thoracic Area. Injury to the cord in the thoracic region occurs only after violent trauma, for the thoracic spinal column provides a strong protective defense. Paraplegia occurs after cord damage in this area with bladder and bowel involvement.

Lumbar Spinal Cord and Cauda Equina Injury. Cord injury in the lumbar region is sustained in most cases as a result of compression fracture of the vertebral body with forward displacement. The spinal cord terminates at the level of the first lumbar vertebra and the cauda equina occupies the spinal canal below that level. Injuries to the lumbar spine result in injury to the cauda equina (lumbar and sacral spinal roots) which presents a symptom picture of flaccid paralysis of the lower extremities, loss of deep tendon reflexes, loss of sensation in the area of distribution of the lumbar and sacral segments, urinary retention, fecal incontinence, and severe back pain radiating anteriorly and along the thighs.

Spinal Shock

A complete and immediate loss of motor, sensory, autonomic, and reflex activity below the lesion level is termed *spinal shock*. This reaction is present in complete cord transections but an incomplete lesion may be accompanied by some degree of spinal shock, thereby mimicking complete transection. The reasons for this state are not fully understood. It has been observed, however, that when transection occurs slowly over days or weeks, as might be seen in compression from a neoplasm, the picture of shock may not appear; this might occur, it is thought, because in addition to loss of functions normally performed by the cord, there are abnormal phenomena due to hyperactivity of the area which is normally held in check by various mechanisms (Gardner). Spinal shock may subside in a few weeks to a few months following cord injury. The initial indication is minimal reflex activity, i.e., muscles have been severed at the level of the transection itself so that the reflex arcs are intact. The flaccid paralysis initially present may then become spastic. Because all motor and sensory tracts are severed, the reflex arcs react only to cutaneous stimulation such as touch, the weight of bed linen, or a gentle breeze blowing over the extremities. The first signs of this movement usually occur in the lower part of the limbs, and consist of mild contractions of flexor muscles following cutaneous stimulation (Gardner). This activity increases and a generalized reflex follows in which involuntary contractions of the flexors, extensors, abductors, and adductors may by initiated by merely touching the foot. This hyperreflexia should not be interpreted as a return of voluntary motor power.

The autonomic functions lost during spinal shock are restored as the shock clears. Return of sympathetic activity is evidenced by constriction of cutaneous vessels and sweating during a mass reflex state. Sweating, which may be reflexly induced, follows the distribution of loss of function on the body surface. Parasympathetic control is restored gradually; eventually, as cells in the sacral cord resume function by exerting influence on smooth muscle, the urinary bladder begins to contract reflexly. With proper training automatic control of bladder and bowel can be developed in almost all patients.

The nurse needs an understanding of spinal shock so that she can explain the involuntary movements to the patient and his family. By recognizing the symptom clues of the changing stages of spinal shock she can assist the patient toward self-help in the activities of daily living, especially bowel and bladder training.

Clinical Manifestations

CARE AT ACCIDENT SCENE

Transporting the Patient. Patients with suspected spinal cord injury require expert care at the scene of the accident, since inept management can turn a relatively minor injury into an irreparable one. Cord injury is a possibility in automobile accidents or those involving falls, as from a diving board. An injured person who is unable to move his arms or legs or who complains of neck pain should not be moved until trained personnel arrive.

The aims of care in the immediate stage of injury are to preserve life and to prevent further injury. The greatest danger in moving the patient is the possibility that bony fragments of fractured vertebrae will damage the cord when his body or extremities are moved. Flexion and rotation of the spine must be avoided. He may also have sustained head injury, so the possibility of hemorrhage should be avoided. The victim should be kept flat, covered, and quiet until an ambulance arrives.

The patient with suspected fracture-dislocations of the cervical spine should be maintained in a face-up, neutral plane on a firm stretcher or board. Support should be provided to each side of the head to prevent lateral movement. Covered bricks, folded blankets, or small sandbags can be used for this purpose. If it is necessary to move the victim from a prone to a supine position, at least three assistants are needed. The extremities should be handled with great care. Continuous gentle traction should be maintained by one assistant who grasps the patient's chin and occiput and applies steady traction along the body axis, while a second assistant exerts countertraction along the same plane by grasping the ankles. Simultaneously the third assistant gently brings the patient's trunk toward him into a supine position.

Possible cord injuries at other levels of the spine are handled similarly. Some degree of extension may be desirable in thoracic or lumbar spinal injuries, and may be accomplished by placing the patient in a prone position or, if supine, placing a small 2-inch support under the thoracolumbar spine. Extension should not be employed if it increases pain or necessitates undue movement and manipulation.

EMERGENCY ROOM CARE

Knowledge that a patient with suspected cord injury is en route to the hospital enables the emergency room nurse to expedite care by anticipating problems.

Respiratory Needs. The phrenic nerve is innervated at C3 to C5. Thus, if the cord injury is high cervical, respiratory difficulty would be anticipated; in a lower cervical injury there may be symptoms of dyspnea because of ascending cord edema. Tracheostomy, mechanical aids to respiration, and suctioning equipment should be at hand.

Bladder Distention. Initially, the bladder becomes paralyzed and atonic with resulting distention. If the lesion is above the sacral level the reflex arc is intact and automatic evacuation can be established later. The immediate goal is to prevent overdistention and stretching of the bladder with resultant bladder sepsis. A retention catheter is usually inserted immediately.

Autonomic Nervous System Disturbances. Disturbances in the autonomic nervous system can be anticipated because of loss of vasomotor control in the extremities including orthostatic hypotension, disturbances of sweating, periodic hypertension with filling of the rectum or bladder, and abdominal distention. The patient will not perspire below the level of the lesion during the period of spinal shock so that one means of heat regulation is lost. An elevated temperature must be assessed in light of this factor as well as the degree of hydration, and the presence of sepsis. Some hypotension on admission thus accounted for may necessitate an intravenous infusion to which is added an adrenergic agent such as ephedrine or phenylephrine. Abdominal distention is treated by a nasogastric tube connected to continuous suction. With paraplegia or quadriplegia paralytic ileus may occur and will necessitate immediate treatment, particularly in cervical and high thoracic cord injuries. A nasogastric tube and a rectal tube are inserted. Neostigmine methylsulfate (Prostigmin Methylsulfate) is administered. Prostigmin stimulates the parasympathetic nerve endings thereby causing contraction of the smooth muscles of the intestine and increasing peristalsis.

Nursing Assessment. The nurse should make an early assessment of vital signs, pupillary response to light, and degree of responsiveness. This assessment will serve as a baseline for later comparison and may provide evidence of intracranial involvement. A detailed neurological examination will be made by the physician and portions of these data may be available. A Horner's syndrome (paralysis of the sympathetic system of the cervical portion of the spinal cord due to a lesion of the stellate ganglion) is usually present in cervical cord injuries and should be kept in mind. The syndrome is manifested by constriction of the pupil on the side of cord injury, mild ptosis of the eyelid with retention of voluntary opening and closing, and absence of sweating with vasodilatation on the affected side, especially the forehead, lending a flushed, warm, dry appearance to the face and neck on that side.

Injuries to other parts of the body are common following automobile accidents, and careful observation of the entire body should be made for wounds and fractures, and prophylaxis instituted against tetanus and gas gangrene.

Neck pain, common initially in cervical injury, may result from compression upon a nerve root or from fracture and tearing of ligaments. Codeine or meperidine hydrochloride (Demerol) may be given, but morphine is contraindicated because of its depressant action. Chest pain is common in thoracic injuries and leg pain in lumbar injuries.

Diagnosis

The diagnosis of cord injury is made on the basis of trauma sustained and the neurological examination. The level of injury is confirmed by roentgenograms. Subarachnoid block on lumbar puncture indicates cord compression, and a positive Queckenstedt test is confirmatory. In this test the jugular veins are compressed; a prompt rise in intraspinal pressure occurs in normal persons, but little or no rise occurs with blockage. Myelography will confirm the location. Great care should be taken to protect the patient from further injury during this procedure. Bloody cerebrospinal fluid indicates rupture of the vessels of the cord or of the meninges and the protein content will be elevated.

Understandably, the patient will be quite apprehensive about what is happening to him and about the implications of a "broken" neck or back. All procedures should be explained to him carefully and tactfully; the calm self-assured manner of the patient care team will help him to feel more secure. If family and friends are present they will need corresponding support.

Medical Treatment

There is a direct relationship between the level of cord injury and mortality. The higher the level of injury the higher the mortality, and the more severe the damage to the cord the higher the mortality (Davis and Davis).

Laminectomy may be performed in the presence of demonstrated subarachnoid block with cord compression; the nature of the lesion, the degree of disability, the progression of neurological deficit, and the general condition of the patient must be taken into account.

Fracture dislocations of the cervical spine are best treated by skeletal traction with Crutchfield or Vinke tongs. Up to 40 pounds of weight may be attached to promote satisfactory realignment of the cervical vertebrae, and the treatment may be necessary for 6 to 12 weeks (see Figure 29–13).

Malalignment due to fracture dislocations of the thoracic spine cannot be satisfactorily corrected, but laminectomy may be performed to relieve pressure on the cord. Hyperextension usually is successful in compression fractures of the lumbar vertebrae; surgical treatment is not necessary.

Nursing Care of Patients with Extensive Motor and Sensory Deficit: Paraplegia and Quadriplegia

SKIN CARE

Circulation in denervated tissue is poor because of decreased muscle activity. The presence of this pathologic state combined with physiological changes due to prolonged immobilization explains the increased potential for tissue breakdown in patients with extensive sensory and motor deficit. The normal restless movements that protect against pressure injuries to the skin and superficial nerves are absent.

Pressure areas develop most frequently as the result of local ischemia caused by constant pressure upon soft tissue. Bony prominences are the most frequent sites of breakdown. Body protein may be lost as a result of drainage of these ulcers and a negative nitrogen balance created. Vulnerability to ulceration is increased by hypoproteinemia and anemia. Correction of the patient's nutritional state is imperative.

Prevention, by means of the following measures, is the crux of treatment: frequent inspection of the total body surface for early evidence of breakdown; cleanliness; frequent change of position; improvement of circulation; and maintenance of an

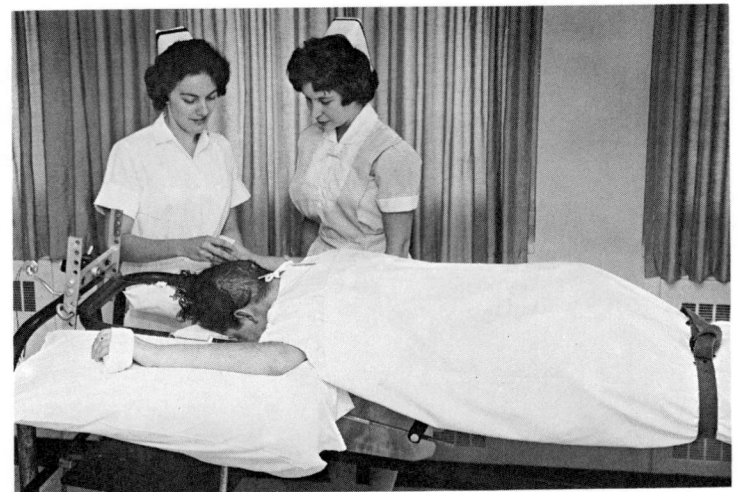

Figure 29–13 Patient lies face down on Foster frame. Vinke skull tongs with weights attached provide skeletal traction. Note that arm wings are placed at shoulder level, hand rolls are utilized to prevent contractures, and webbed restraining strap placed at mid-thigh protects the patient during muscle spasms. (By permission from M. Arlene Martin: Nursing Care in Cervical Cord Injury. American Journal of Nursing, 63:60–66, March, 1963.)

adequate dietary state. Range of motion exercises should be carried out several times daily, unless contraindicated, as a means of improving circulation and preventing contractures and atrophy of muscle groups. Elastic stockings may improve the circulation in the lower extremities. If the patient is being maintained on a frame he should be turned according to a schedule alternating supine and prone positions. Gentle total body massage and inspection should be done at this time.

Impairment of circulation, especially at the capillary and precapillary level, should be considered when administering injectable medications. Whenever possible this should be done above the level of deficit to ensure adequate absorption.

In sensory loss the warning signal of pain is lost and the tissue is thus vulnerable to any form of heat. Extreme care should be used whenever heat is applied to the skin, as with a heat lamp or hot water bottle.

POSITIONING

When a lengthy hospitalization with prolonged immobilization seems indicated, a CircOlectric bed or a Stryker or Foster frame may be preferable, since continuous cervical traction can be maintained on these frames. The CircOlectric bed has a range of horizontal, vertical, and sitting positions and when the patient's condition permits, the bed provides for gradual advancement to a standing position. The Stryker and Foster frames are manually operated and permit only face-up and face-down positions. These frames should be adjusted to correspond to the individual patient's measurements; ill-fitting frames can aggravate deformities and prolong hospitalization. The Foster frame has a hyperextension regulating bar that provides hyperextension or flexion, if desired. The regulating bar should not be used as a handle while turning the frame since this might result in an unordered or undesirable degree of flexion or hyperextension.

A regular bed can be modified by use of fracture boards and variations in

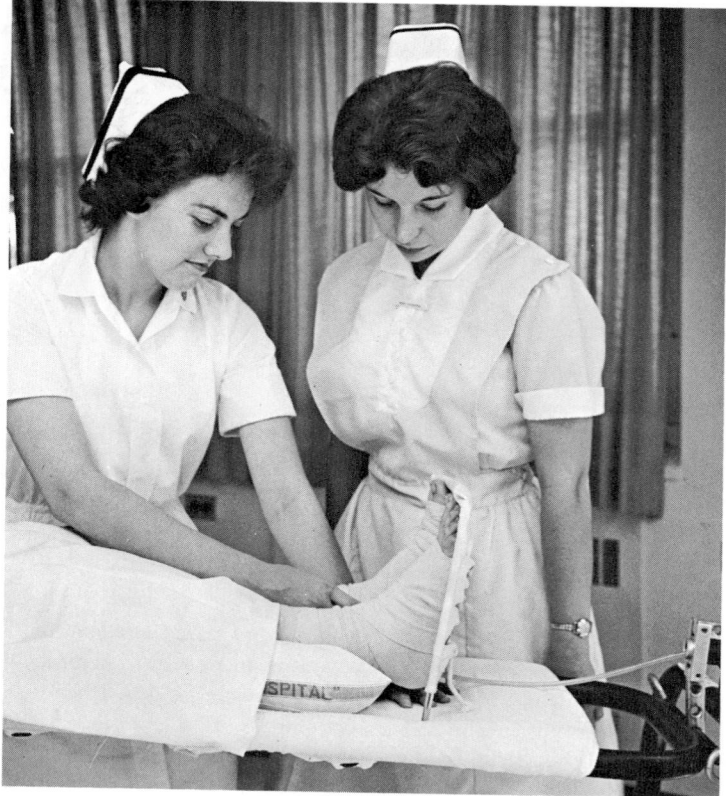

Figure 29–14
Proper positioning of
foot support. Patient's
heels are suspended
above canvas of frame
and placed at 90 degree
angle against foot sup-
port. Elastic stockings
applied to both lower
extremities improve
circulation. Drainage
tube from retention
catheter rests between
patient's legs and feet.
(By permission from M.
Arlene Martin: Nursing
Care in Cervical Cord
Injury. American Journal
of Nursing. 63:60–66,
March, 1963.)

gatching. An alternating pressure mattress will help to prevent development of decubitus ulcers by alternating the points of pressure at regular intervals.

Extreme care should be exercised to maintain the patient in proper body alignment in order to prevent contractures and deformities. If a frame is used the arm rest wings must be at shoulder level to prevent undue strain on the shoulder girdle. Foot boards should be used to keep the feet at a 90-degree angle with the heels suspended free from the canvas (Fig. 29–14). Small hand rolls can be placed in the patient's grip to prevent contractures and become fixation of the hand in a nonfunctional state of marked flexion.

Wrist Drop. The forearms should be kept slightly elevated with the elbows slightly flexed to help prevent wrist drop. This elevated position also helps to prevent dependent edema (Fig. 29–13). When the patient is in the supine position, his elbows and wrists should be slightly flexed, with the hands lying across the chest or abdomen. It may be necessary to employ aluminum or plastic wrist splints if additional support seems indicated. Periodic full range of joint motion is routinely employed unless contraindicated.

The patient should begin to perform suitable exercises as early as possible in preparation for use of braces and crutches, and weight-bearing should be begun early so as to counteract the osteoporosis resulting from prolonged immobilization. By stimulating osteoblastic activity demineralization of bone is decreased. Standing boards and tilt tables are usually employed for this purpose.

NUTRITIONAL NEEDS

The anorexia usually present in these patients leads to excessive weight loss eventuating in negative nitrogen balance. Gastric atony, commonly seen, retards stomach emptying; a feeling of fullness results from distention and partially accounts for the loss of appetite. Lean tissue and fat are catabolized, protein intake being rapidly excreted through urine, and large amounts of nitrogen and potassium are lost. This condition may persist for a week or two. In the acute period forced feedings are discouraged since they cause nausea and vomiting, which further increases the electrolyte imbalance. Plasma given intravenously is the only form of protein which can be adequately metabolized during this early stage. Fluid intake of 3,000 ml daily should be encouraged.

Because of protein loss during the early stage of catabolism with resultant negative nitrogen balance, an increased protein intake is indicated. A positive nitrogen balance is achieved only after a prolonged period of high protein intake. A deficiency of B vitamins is frequently seen with inadequate protein intake since these vitamins occur in protein-rich foods. Protein loss over a period of time can lead to malnutrition, weight loss, lowered resistance to infection, and lowered tissue resistance to pressure which is predisposing to formation of decubitus ulcers. Thus, it is essential that an average daily intake of protein be maintained at 150 to 300 g in a diet high in calories and vitamins. Fluid intake of 3,000 ml daily should be encouraged to ensure adequate hydration and urinary tract function. In planning menus and supplemental feedings, consideration must be given to the total response to the injury: (1) excessive calcium loss due to osteoporosis, (2) alkalinization of urine by citrus fruits contributing to the formation of urinary calculi and urinary sepsis, and (3) formation of decubitus ulcers contributing to hypoproteinemia.

ELIMINATION

Urinary Bladder. The nursing goals in this aspect of care are to prevent urinary tract infection and to help the patient achieve normal urination insofar as possible. According to Breithaupt, genitourinary sepsis is the leading cause of death in paraplegic patients, accounting for approximately 50 percent of deaths.

Cord injury results immediately in an atonic bladder. A retention catheter is employed to relieve distention and usually must be maintained until spinal shock subsides and the bladder functions reflexively. This initial stage may persist for weeks to months. Strict aseptic technique in catheter irrigations helps to prevent infection, but prolonged use of catheter drainage is a predisposing factor in infection. Early indications of possible urinary infection include a cloudy appearance of the urine on gross examination, a foul smell of the urine, and a highly concentrated urine. Such changes, coupled with the presence of a febrile state, may indicate a need to increase the fluid intake or to begin therapy with, for example, sulfisoxazole (Gantrisin). Attention should be given to dietary and fluid intake by avoiding foodstuffs and juices that tend to alkalinize the urine and create a suitable culture medium for bacteria and to foster formation of urinary calculi. Prune juice, cranberry juice, grape juice, and other noncitrus juices should be offered.

With recovery from spinal shock and the return of the reflex arc the bladder may become *automatic.* Management is based on the state of reflex activity in the sacral segments governed by the pelvic and the internal pudendal nerves. A return of near-normal bladder function may be possible following spinal cord injury except when the bladder is completely denervated below the level of the first lumbar vertebra. In the automatic state, the bladder detrusor muscle responds to pressure from the accumulating urine and contracts reflexly in response to this stretching. Although the automatic voiding reflex present when the bladder is distended may be weaker than the normal voiding reflex, the reflex may be increased by stimulation from below the level of the cord lesion. Reflex voiding may also be stimulated by stroking the lower abdomen or inner aspects of the thighs, or by exerting gentle pressure over the bladder. Spontaneous contractions of the detrusor muscle occur in the functioning reflex bladder.

Many patients with cord injury have subjective symptoms indicating that the bladder is about to empty, for example, a feeling of pressure or tightening in the head and the abdomen, sudden diaphoresis in the face and neck, and piloerection. When observed objectively or experienced subjectively, it may allow time for provision of a bedpan or urinal or use of a toilet.

Although more definitive evaluation of bladder status is made by urological investigation, an assessment may be begun on the nursing unit by intermittent clamping and opening of the patient's catheter to observe capacity tolerance.

Care should be given to prevent overdistention of the bladder which results in stretching and fissure formation predisposing to infection. Because the patient may not experience the sensation of fullness or distinguish it from pain, it is advisable that the urologist carry out a bladder capacity study.

Much patience and guidance must be given during efforts to reestablish urinary continence, and participation by the patient is necessary for achieving this. A carefully scheduled program of fluid intake must be followed. The achievement of bladder continence provides a great psychological boost to the patient as he progresses toward independence. Knowledge of the patient's predeficit micturition routine will serve as a guide to planning for his current needs. The schedule must be planned with consideration of the patient's overall program, including such activities as physiotherapy and occupational therapy.

Suprapubic drainage may become necessary if urinary tract infection is imminent. However, patients who initially had suprapubic drainage do less well in recovering bladder function later because of the prolonged period of bladder imbalance.

Exercises for conditioning the voiding reflex, chemotherapy, and such procedures as nerve block, neurectomy, and transurethral resection are described in specialized textbooks.

Bowel. Bowel continence can be maintained through reflex defecation. The defecation reflex is stimulated by a full rectum, which produces rectal contraction and relaxation of the sphincter. Dependency upon enemas can be averted if the stool is kept soft and rectal impaction is avoided. Attention to dietary intake, with provision for adequate roughage and nonconstipating foods, and adequate fluid intake can help establish a normal routine. Hypomotility consequent to immobilization may contribute to difficulty in establishing a routine.

A mild cathartic containing a wetting agent that draws fluid into the stool by lowering surface tension, such as dioctyl sodium sulfosuccinate (Colase), may be helpful. The application of gentle pressure to the abdominal wall by pressing one's palms against it may aid in initiating the defecation reflex.

Much will be gained by establishing an effective program of elimination. The ability to manage one's own toileting needs is a basic desire in most individuals. The patient will be able to participate in other rehabilitation activities earlier and usually with greater ease. His active participation is an important part of his overall program.

MUSCLE SPASMS

As described earlier, with subsidence of spinal shock and reactivation of the lower motor neuron reflex arc the flaccid paralysis changes to spastic paralysis. This occurs in both complete and partial lesions and usually occurs as spasticity in extension.

In the healthy paraplegic patient spasticity may be somewhat annoying but is usually not serious unless other complications of paraplegia develop. Spastic movements may be produced by applying various stimuli to the skin, such as stroking, pinching, and tickling. Laughing, crying, anger, and apprehension may give rise to spastic movement. The patient should be encouraged to recognize the "triggering mechanism" of these movements, since these may be utilized in his daily activities such as emptying his bladder, shifting to a chair, and dressing. The patient should be tactfully and honestly informed of the basis for these spasms so that he does not interpret their occurrence as a return of voluntary movement. The problem with spasticity is that repeated stimulation of the spinal reflex centers as occurs with urinary infections, decubitus ulcers, fever, emotional disturbances, and physical factors such as ill-fitting braces may cause interference with the patient's daily activities.

The violent spontaneous flexion spasms thus produced result in severe flexor contractions in which the anterior thighs rest against the chest wall and the heels against the buttocks—"paraplegia in flexion." It is generally held that paraplegia in flexion is a consequence of poor care and causes extensive decubitus ulcer formation and malnutrition.

Spasms may vary from mild twitching to violent mass reflex states according to the patient's posture at the moment. A violent spasm can throw the patient out of his bed or frame. It is essential that the patient be protected by restraining straps loosely tied around his body while he is lying on the frame or by side rails on his bed.

Special care should be taken with hot foods and fluids to avoid spillage if placed close to the patient during a period of hyperreflexia. Flexor spasticity is a greater problem in nursing care than extensor spasticity, since it is difficult to maintain proper alignment when the body is in a flexion state.

Mild spasms may be relieved by meprobamate, chlordiazepoxide hydrochloride, or methocarbamol. Some patients find their side effects of muscle weakness and drowsiness very unpleasant and discontinue their use. Warm tub baths and stretching exercises may be helpful.

If the spasms are so extreme as to interfere with the patient's rehabilitation and well-being and are not relieved by medical treatment, anterior rhizotomy, cordotomy, subarachnoid alcohol block, or peripheral neuromyotomy may be indicated.

PAIN

Pain may occur with spasticity and it may be difficult to distinguish the pain from the spasticity itself. Sedatives, opiates, antispasmodics, ataractics, or anticonvulsants may be prescribed. When the threat of addiction is imminent, neurosurgical intervention as discussed above may be indicated. The individual with cord injury may complain of sharp shooting pains in the area of nerve root distribution. This pain may develop from scar tissue formation or irritation upon a nerve root. Deep visceral pain may also be a complaint. The magnitude of such pain may be exaggerated if it is the only physical discomfort experienced. If mild analgesics do not give relief, a neurectomy or a cordotomy may be indicated. Narcotics must be administered with great caution.

OTHER PROBLEMS

Respiratory Difficulties. Hypostatic pneumonia is a threat to all patients with cord injuries during the early period, but particularly to patients with cervical cord injury. The patient with a fracture dislocation of the lumbar area is highly susceptible also, because drugs are needed in large quantity for relief of pain attendant to positioning in a hyperextension plane; there is consequent respiratory depression. Oxygen and antibiotics must be administered, and this therapy has first priority. Deep breathing exercises should be encouraged to promote lung expansion.

Communication. The patient with cord injury may be literally unable to "move a muscle." He is totally dependent upon others for many aspects of daily living and hygiene. He may be frightened about his future and may be experiencing a grief reaction. He needs to be able to communicate with and to trust at least one person. The nurse should be able to fulfill this role if the patient so chooses. He may fear that new personnel are not as competent to handle his needs as more familiar ones; thus it is helpful if a staff member whom he knows is present with the new one for a few times.

If skull tongs are attached obviously there will be few sources of environmental stimulation available. If a hearing dysfunction is present as well his world will be narrow indeed. The sensory deprivation thus engendered may cause hallucinations, illusions, and delusions. By such measures as conversing with him, adjusting the lights, and arranging the flowers, the nurse can convey her appreciation of his situation at the same time that she is acting to increase his sensory input.

Because swings in mood are frequent, hostility and bitterness may be directed toward the hospital staff and family. These may be the patient's only means of expressing his depression and disappointment, and the behavior is often directed toward the person with whom the patient feels most comfortable and least fearful. The family need to be understanding about such behavior so that they can provide a stable, supportive, and accepting background when he returns home.

The patient also needs time to be alone, knowing that assistance is available if needed. A microswitch, which is supersensitive to the slightest touch, should be placed near his shoulders for use (Fig. 29–15). Shrugging the shoulders is accomplished via the spinal accessory cranial nerve (preserved in quadriplegia) innervating the trapezius and sternomastoid muscle. When the patient is in a face-down position the switch can be placed next to his cheek, and the movement of tongue to cheek will be sufficient to trigger the switch. Such equipment as the extra-long flexible straws (Fig. 29–16) and prism glasses for viewing television programs can be utilized.

Depersonalization. It is not unusual that the patient feels detached from parts of his body which have been denervated. He may even deny that they belong to him. The nurse should continue to refer to such parts in a normal manner and to speak to and about him as a whole person.

Sexual Function. The male patient has disturbances in sexual function varying according to the level of the lesion. Reflex erection is usually possible but in most complete lesions ejaculation is not. As a rule male patients are unable to procreate, whereas female patients are able to do so. If marriage is planned the advice of a neurologist should be sought.

LONG-TERM GOALS

Throughout the hospitalization period one of the goals should be to teach the pa-

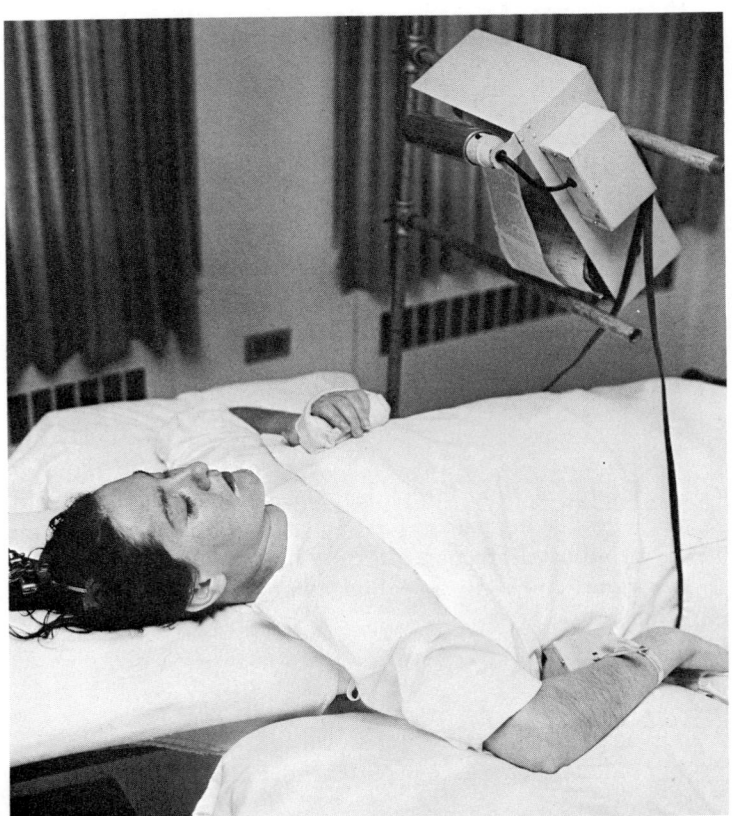

Figure 29–15 Jack Martin reader in use. Reader is controlled by microswitch which is next to patient's right hand. Minute movement of switch causes roller to make one full turn.

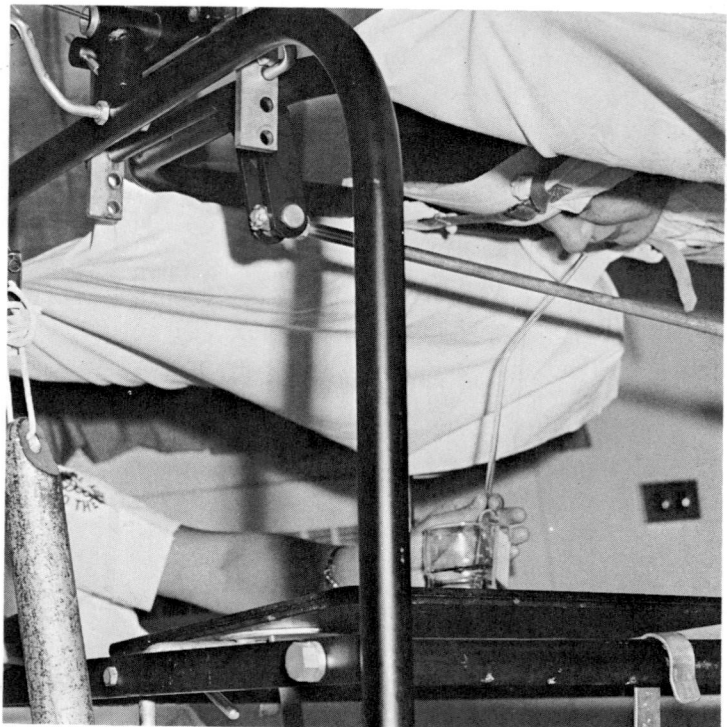

*Figure 29–16
Long plastic straw is
measured and adjusted
to patient's needs, Plastic
clip attached to side of
glass holds straw
securely. This device
allows patient to drink
fluids without assistance
while in face-down
position. (Photograph
taken from head of
frame.)*

tient to do for himself as much as he is capable of doing and to understand the meaning of his symptoms and how they can be relieved. Some patients will be faced with "living in a wheel chair," some will be able to ambulate with the aid of crutches, braces, or other devices, and some will have full return of function without residual neurological deficit.

Before the patient can return to society as a contributing, economically capable person, he should have achieved bowel and bladder control, should be able to sit upright for extended periods, and—most essential—should have made a psychological adjustment to his disability. Grief over the loss, the depressive reaction, and other manifestations should have been expressed and resolved in large measure.

Optimum care during the rehabilitation period is provided in an intensive rehabilitation center in which trained personnel and specialized equipment are available.

It is obvious that the patient with permanent motor and sensory deficits must modify his living patterns and must always be alert to evidence of symptoms that might indicate infection, pressure areas, or extension of the disorder. The aim in long-term care is to help him attain and maintain the greatest degree of independence possible.

Prognosis

It is usually impossible to prognosticate within the first few days after injury. The outlook depends not only on the extent of permanent cord injury but upon age, general health, accompanying injuries, and the patient's own motivation toward realizing his maximal abilities. It is generally agreed that in patients with complete motor and sensory loss lasting longer than 24 to 48 hours no significant recovery of voluntary motor function is encountered (Suwanwela et al.).

Neoplasms

Definition, Classification, and Epidemiology

Neoplasms of the spinal cord develop less commonly than intracranial neoplasms. Cord neoplasms are classified according to location within the spinal canal as *extradural* (outside the dura mater). Intradural neoplasms are either *extramedullary* (developing outside the spinal cord and arising in nerve roots, blood vessels, or meninges) or *intramedullary* (originating in glial tissue of the cord itself).

Extradural tumors, which comprise about one-fourth of all cord tumors, are generally malignant, invading from an adjacent vertebra or metastasizing from a remote source. Tumors of the breast and lung spread mainly to the thoracic vertebrae; tumors of the kidney, to the upper lumbar area.

Among intradural tumors, the extramedullary ones are the most common, which is fortunate since they are usually benign. Neurofibromas and meningiomas, the common extramedullary tumors, are operable, but less common intramedullary tumors infiltrate the cord tissue and may be adequately excised only at the sacrifice of cord function.

Meningiomas are more common in females, but otherwise the sex distribution is equal. Spinal tumors develop far more frequently in adults than in children.

Clinical Features

Symptoms of cord tumor reflect its level and location. Because the cord is smaller than the canal that surrounds it, there is space in which an expanding lesion can grow, especially posteriorly. In extramedullary neoplasm the symptoms reflect the area of cord compression. There is interference with vascular supply due to compression on arteries and ischemia within the cord. As the tumor expands and the cord swells, a subarachnoid block ensues.

Pain is the earliest symptom in the majority of cord tumors, and it may be present for some time before other symptoms of compression become evident. The pain may be aggravated by coughing, sneezing, and exertion. Burning, tingling, and numbness are other early clues. Gradual progressive motor symptoms usually follow, although in some instances paraplegia may develop rapidly as a result of a sudden shift in the position of the tumor or in the presence of metastasis, hematoma, or epidural abscess. The clinical picture may be similar to that of transverse myelitis.

Diagnosis

Diagnosis is established on the basis of the history, neurological examination, roentgenograms, lumbar puncture, and possibly myelography. In the presence of tumor, x-ray films may reveal localized vertebral destruction, enlargement of the canal, and calcification of tumor mass. Myelography will help to localize the level of the lesion. The Queckenstedt sign may be positive on lumbar puncture. The protein content in the cerebrospinal fluid is increased. Differentiation must be made from other conditions giving rise to similar symptoms, such as syphilis, multiple sclerosis, amyotrophic lateral sclerosis, and syringomyelia.

Course and Medical Treatment

If untreated, most cord tumors grow slowly but progressively with resulting spastic paraplegia and symptoms of complete cord transection. Rapid onset of symptoms of transection may occur if there is compression upon the spinal blood vessels as is seen in metastatic tumors and Hodgkin's disease.

The treatment of cord tumors is surgery or irradiation. Laminectomy is done to relieve the compression upon the cord or its roots. Removal of an encapsulated tumor such as a meningioma or a neurofibroma is generally successfully done. Little improvement can be anticipated in the presence of cord necrosis from compression or interference with circulation. Only partial removal or decompression is possible with infiltratingintramedullary glial tumors. Irradiation following this procedure may give further relief. In general, surgical success is related to the accessibility of the tumor and the degree of irreversible neurological deficit at the time of surgery.

Nursing Care

The care of patients with cord tumors is dictated by the degree of sensorimotor deficit and is based on the same principles as care of the patient following cord injury.

Pain may be severe, necessitating use of narcotics. In an attempt to avoid discomfort the patient may guard the area to the point of being afraid to move for fear of having more pain. Activity within realistic limits should be encouraged in efforts to prevent complications of immobilization. Contractures and deformities must be prevented through appropriate measures, although relief may be achieved in some cases by constant walking or by standing or leaning in various positions throughout the day and night.

Cord tumor may be secondary to a primary malignant lesion elsewhere, so nursing attention must be directed to the primary disorder.

Postoperative complications peculiar to surgery for spinal cord tumor include edema and hemorrhage which is grossly undetected and may be manifested in progressively increasing motor and/or sensory deficit. If a comparison made to the patient's preoperative deficit status reveals an increase in deficit, this should be called to the neurosurgeon's attention immediately.

Infections

Infections of the spinal cord usually are widespread throughout the central nervous system. Bacteria, viruses, spirochetes, fungi, and other organisms may *directly* invade the cord. Sepsis introduced during spinal punctures, direct invasion from a deep decubitus ulcer, or a penetrating gunshot or stab wound into the spinal cord may be the cause. *Indirect* causes of infection are carried hematogenously as in pneumonia and influenza.

Spinal epidural abscess may be secondary to remote infection, e.g., in the head or neck region, causing characteristic symptoms of a space-occupying extramedullary lesion, with the deficit dependent upon the area of the cord compressed.

Generalized central nervous system infections cause hyperpyrexia, increased pulse and respiration, headache, nuchal rigidity, and typical reflex responses. The underlying infection is treated with appropriate antibiotics.

Myelitis develops with acute infectious diseases such as pneumonia, measles, and influenza. There is elevated temperature and sudden flaccid paralysis of the extremities, with pain occurring usually at the level of the disease in the cord. Sensory disturbances arise and sphincter control is lost. The infection may involve any level but is most common in the midthoracic region. The prognosis depends on the severity of infection and the area involved. Slow recovery may be followed by partial paralysis, or death may occur within a few days if the process extends upward to the muscles of respiration. Treatment and nursing care are determined by the symptoms and are directed toward limiting the disorder and preventing complications.

Some infections may be widespread yet attack specific areas of the spinal cord. Poliomyelitis, which frequently attacks the motor cells of the anterior horn, and tabes dorsalis, or spinal neurosyphilis, are two such conditions. Neither is widely prevalent any longer, because chemotherapy and immunotherapy have drastically lowered their frequency and improved the prognosis. The practitioner may complete her career without ever caring for a patient having a primary diagnosis of either condition. Thus, these conditions will be briefly discussed, and the focus will be on prevention and early treatment. The reader is referred to the wealth of literature available for more detailed coverage.

POLIOMYELITIS

Definition and Epidemiology

Anterior poliomyelitis (infantile spinal paralysis) is an acute inflammatory infection caused by a filtrable virus that invades chiefly the anterior horn cells of the cord. It has been a disease of infants and children under 10 years rather than of adults, although it can develop at any age. It is slightly more frequent in males than females and less frequent among colored races than white (Merritt). The incidence is higher during summer and early fall, and it is more common among rural families than urban families.

The advent of the Salk vaccine in 1955 and the Sabin oral vaccine more recently has resulted in a remarkable gain in control of poliomyelitis. In the period between 1950 and 1954 about 30,000 cases were reported per year in the United States; approximately 58,000 cases were reported in 1952 alone. In 1962, 910 cases were reported and the number has continued to fall. Currently, about 85 percent of all reported cases involve paralysis. The mortality has fallen dramatically since the introduction of mass immunization programs.

Etiology

Poliomyelitis is a highly contagious, infectious disease due to one of three virus strains. The virus is believed to be insect-borne and to enter the body through the gastrointestinal system. Investigation of poliomyelitis led to the identification of the ECHO and Coxsackie viruses, which cause an illness very similar to a mild, nonparalytic attack of poliomyelitis and thus must be considered in the differential diagnosis.

Pathology

Invasion takes place principally along the lumbar and cervical enlargements of the anterior horn of the cord, causing an inflammatory reaction with resulting necrosis. The motor cells of the brain and brain stem may also be invaded, but the sensory pathways are seldom involved. The three types of poliomyelitis— bulbar, encephalitic, and spinal—are distinguished by the location of the cells affected.

Clinical Manifestations and Course

In the prodromal stage there is a mild infection characterized by malaise, irritability, gastrointestinal upset (especially diarrhea), headache, and fever. The incubation period is up to 3 weeks. In an abortive case these symptoms subside and full recovery ensues. In a paralytic case the symptoms are followed in a few days by the paralytic stage, which is characterized by hyperpyrexia and resulting motor paralysis of a flaccid nature, pain of the muscles of the trunk and extremities, stiff neck, and possibly coma. Respiratory paralysis may occur with involvement of the diaphragm and intercostal muscles.

Maximum recovery may take place within the first few months after onset or may continue for as long as 2 years, being dictated by the degree of the motor cell destruction.

Diagnosis

Characteristic clinical symptoms and changes in cerebrospinal fluid are aids to diagnosis. The cerebrospinal fluid has an elevated protein and white cell content. Poliomyelitis may be difficult to diagnose in the preparalytic stage and cannot be confirmed unless acute asymmetrical flaccid paralysis develops or the virus is recovered in blood or stool, or from the nasopharynx. Differential diagnosis may include meningitis, ECHO or Coxsackie viral infections, and similar conditions.

Medical Treatment and Nursing Care

Care during the preparalytic stage encompasses rest, symptom relief, prevention of deformities, and prevention of spread of disease through strict isolation; care is similar during the paralytic stage. Since the sensory tracts have not been invaded, the ability to feel pain is retained; this must be considered in positioning the patient and in all other aspects of care. Application of moist heat is helpful in relieving muscle pain and spasms.

The acute paralytic stage gives rise to severe pain on movement. Proper body alignment of the bed patient with support to joints during turning and use of appliances such as foot boards and knee rolls will help prevent contractures. Antibiotics may be administered in intercurrent infections.

The patient must be closely observed for symptoms of respiratory difficulty and bulbar involvement. In bulbar poliomyelitis there is insufficient air exchange causing carbon dioxide to be retained in the blood and leading to respiratory acidosis. The patient then must be transferred to a respirator, and it may be necessary to perform a tracheostomy.

Weakness or paralysis of muscles of the face and neck causes difficulty swallowing. Excessive saliva will form because of inability to coordinate deglutition and respiration. Oral suctioning or a side-lying position may be necessary to promote gravity drainage. The danger of aspiration is ever-present; if fluids are to be given orally during this acute stage, they must be given slowly and in small amounts. Attention must be given to fluid and electrolyte balance and to adequate nutrition during this period.

The nurse's most important function is to help educate the public about immunization. It has been recommended that all persons under 50 years of age be immunized and that infants receive initial vaccination at 2 months of age. The local medical society or health department should be consulted for specific recommendations and mass immunization programs.

NEUROSYPHILIS: TABES DORSALIS (LOCOMOTOR ATAXIA)

Untreated, syphilis spreads to the nervous system, after a period ranging from 4 to 30 years, resulting in tabes dorsalis (locomotor ataxia).

Etiology and Epidemiology

Tabes dorsalis is chronic and progressive. It results from degeneration of the posterior roots and columns of the spinal cord and brain stem. It is four times more frequent in men than women and is more common in the white race than the colored. The earliest symptoms develop over a range from 5 to 50 years after initial infection. The age of onset is usually in the fifth to sixth decades.

Pathology

Tabes dorsalis is the late or chronic stage of syphilis. There is atrophy of spinal roots, particularly in the lower thoracic and lumbosacral regions. There is deterioration of position sense, coordination, touch, and pressure.

Clinical Manifestations and Course

The onset is usually insidious. The symptoms reflect the site of pathology. Sensory symptoms predominate in the form of pain, paresthesias, and ataxia. Sphincter disturbances and impotence develop. Intense paroxysmal pain is felt, particularly in the legs and arms. Paresthesias of the feet are common. A gastric crisis may occur suddenly in which acute abdominal pains are accompanied by nausea and vomiting over a period of several hours to days. There may be similar painful crises in the bladder, rectal, or laryngeal area. There are visual changes due to optic atrophy and a characteristic ataxia. The individual must stand and walk on a wide base requiring him to walk in a foot-slapping fashion. Later in the course Charcot joints develop and add to the difficulties of ambulation.

The course of tabes is variable but usually progressive, with death resulting from genitourinary infection or cardiovascular disease.

Diagnosis

Diagnosis is based on the clinical findings and patient's history. Cerebrospinal fluid evidence of syphilis is not a reliable index since the fluid frequently reverts to normal with or without treatment of the disease.

Medical Treatment and Nursing Care

Treatment of tabes dorsalis is as in other forms of neurosyphilis; results depend upon the stage of illness. Cordotomy may become necessary to relieve the intense pain of gastric crisis. The patient should empty his bladder frequently in order to help prevent urinary infection. Interruption of afferent fibers in the posterior roots may result in bladder hypotonicity. The pain of gastric crisis should be differentiated from that due to gastric ulcer, neoplasm, and other causes. Recognition of these possibilities should be inherent in the assessment of the symptoms.

In the presence of other characteristics pointing to tabes dorsalis one might anticipate a heightened potential for gastric crisis, being mindful of secondary or unrelated acute abdominal problems. The nurse should observe the frequency and characteristics of the attack to establish the existence of a pattern similar to that of gastric ulcer (with pain related to eating) or another disorder that might be reflected in leukopenia or anemia, for example. Gastric pain in tabes dorsalis does feature abdominal wall tenderness, but rigidity is absent. In advanced tabes the abdominal disease may not manifest pain and rigidity. This may serve to further cloud the interpretation of symptoms. Prophylaxis is the best treatment. The nurse should utilize every opportunity to educate patients she deals with in the prevention of syphilis.

Degenerative Diseases

MULTIPLE SCLEROSIS

Degenerative diseases of the spinal cord are usually of unknown cause and of a progressive nature. Multiple sclerosis, characterized by degeneration of the myelin sheath, will serve to exemplify these disorders. Demyelinization occurs also in

Schilder's disease (diffuse sclerosis), Devic's disease (neuromyelitis optica), and acute disseminated encephalomyelitis, among others. Pathologic changes may take place in any component of the nervous system; in multiple sclerosis, the spinal cord is most frequently affected.

Definition and Epidemiology

Multiple sclerosis (disseminated sclerosis) is a progressive central nervous system disorder characterized by myelin destruction in the white matter of the spinal cord and brain with accompanying cellular proliferation. Studies of Kurland and other investigators indicate a significant geographic incidence with the highest prevalence and mortality in relatively cold and damp areas of the temperate zones of both hemispheres. There is a slightly higher incidence in females than in males (Kurland et al.). Symptoms usually appear in young adults between 20 and 35 years of age, and onset before age 18 or after age 45 is rare.

Pathology

Areas of demyelinization are scattered throughout the white matter of the brain and spinal cord and are replaced by scar tissue. These scattered plaques of scar tissue give the disease its name. Initially only the sheath is destroyed, and impulses continue to travel along the fibers even though function may be impaired. If the condition of the sheath improves, function is restored, thereby accounting for the possibility of remission. When the nerve fibers themselves are replaced by scar tissue so that they can no longer carry impulses, the loss becomes permanent. The various locations and degree of invasion are reflected in its changing symptomatology.

Clinical Manifestations

The onset is frequently insidious, with symptoms so mild that the individual may not seek medical attention. This attack may be followed by a period of customary well-being only to give place later to further symptoms of increased severity.

Clinical features of early motor system involvement include weakness and clumsiness with a tendency to drop things, or marked weakness in the extremities at the end of the day. These may be transient or may progress to cause marked impairment. Intention tremor and cerebellar ataxia may develop along with loss of abdominal reflexes. As the disease progresses weakness and spasticity increase, and a spastic paralysis develops.

Sensory manifestations include paresthesias and numbness. Loss of perception of pain and temperature is usually mild, if present. Pain is not a common symptom.

Disorders of speech in the form of dysarthria are common and may be related to cerebellar ataxia and bilateral corticobulbar tract involvement. Dysarthria is characterized by "scanning" i.e., breaking words into syllables and pausing between syllables.

Visual disturbances are common in the form of nystagmus, due to brain stem or cerebellar involvement, and diplopia and scotoma (central vision loss); partial to complete blindness may develop because of disturbances in ocular movement and involvement of the optic nerve.

Bowel and bladder disturbances are not common in the early stages and if present are limited to hesitancy or frequency in urination. Involvement of the sacral cord leads to retention overflow incontinence in late stages. Sexual impotence is not uncommon.

Vestibular or brain stem invasion may be manifested by vertigo and often is accompanied by vomiting, possibly explained by autonomic nervous system disturbances. Mental disturbances ranging from euphoria to depression and a mild degree of intellectual deterioration may also occur. Early symptoms of multiple sclerosis are frequently ill-defined and bizarre and when accompanied by an emotional disturbance may be wrongly interpreted by friends and family as a psychoneurotic or hysterical condition. The nurse may be influential in helping the individual seek appropriate medical attention and helping him and his family understand the meaning and significance of his symptoms.

Since this disease does not follow a distinct distribution pattern, the symptoms are varied in duration and character and run the gamut from mildly blurred vision and clumsiness to paralysis and total dependency.

Diagnosis

There is no laboratory test that is specific for multiple sclerosis. The spinal fluid frequently has an elevated gamma globulin content as is common in most neurological disorders, except neurosyphilis. The disease is diagnosed on the basis of its clinical features and careful history-taking. Initially multiple sclerosis may frequently masquerade as numerous other neurological disorders such as cord tumor, general paresis, and encephalomyelitis.

Course

Multiple sclerosis is generally characterized by periods of remissions and exacerbations. Typically the symptoms may disappear completely or partially, only to reappear in greater severity later. In some patients the disease may progress rapidly without remission, whereas in others the symptoms may occur suddenly and persist without improvement or progression; thus it is difficult to foretell the course of multiple sclerosis.

Multiple sclerosis is rarely fatal and death is usually due to an intercurrent infection. A near-average life expectancy is possible for the majority of patients through following a prescribed therapeutic regimen.

Although the reason for exacerbation is not clear, there are certain potential precipitating causes of relapse which have been identified. A lowered status of health which would increase vulnerability to upper respiratory infection, undue fatigue, poor nutritional state, allergic disease, injuries to head or spine, emotional upsets, surgery, and pregnancy may be contributing factors.

Medical Management

Treatment is aimed toward minimizing distressing symptoms and halting disease progression, if possible. Because remissions occur spontaneously, false interpretation of the value of a specific therapy may result if a remission occurs simultaneously with the therapy.

DRUGS

Vitamins may be given since there is a feeling that avitaminosis may play a role. Histamine and vasodilating drugs are administered in an effort to improve circulation and reduce arterial spasm.

Steroid therapy has given some evidence of usefulness during acute exacerbations. The anti-inflammatory action of ACTH may be responsible for reducing swelling and therefore reducing pressure on nerve fibers during exacerbations. This may be why acute visual symptoms are relieved by steroid therapy. If side effects of such therapy are severe, however, it may be necessary to discontinue this treatment.

An antispasmodic drug may be ordered to relieve spasticity. Intrathecal injection of alcohol or anterior root rhizotomy is rarely indicated for the relief of spasticity.

PHYSIOTHERAPY

Physiotherapy in the form of active and passive exercises, massage, and warm baths is ordered to relieve spasticity, increase coordination, and improve utilization of muscle groups.

OTHER CONSIDERATIONS

Avoidance of infections and adequate treatment with antibiotics when they do occur is essential.

A program that promotes rest, builds general resistance, maintains a good nutritional status, and avoids undue fatigue and lowered resistance is the keynote of therapeutic planning.

Nursing Care

The adjustment to a condition of a chronic and progressive nature is surely a difficult one to make. The characteristics of remission in multiple sclerosis, when the patient may return to a normal or near-normal health status only to be followed by a more severe and permanent deficit later, unfortunately may serve to increase his denial of his disease. The lay interpretation of this condition is frequently one of distinct pessimism, and a cloud of hopelessness may prevail over the patient and his family when learning of his diagnosis. The occurrence of this disease in the young adult, possibly at the beginning or height of his productive period, frequently creates an astronomical financial burden through modification or loss of earning power coupled with increased medical expenses. The patient may seek a variety of medical sources to confirm or refute the diagnosis. He is especially vulnerable to the unethical who promote quick and sure cures. A program of educacation is essential to help the individual learn about his condition and understand its symptom meaning and possible course, to enable him to formulate realistic personal and career goals. In some instances the physician may make the decision to withhold the diagnosis from the patient if he feels the patient cannot handle the information. The nursing staff can best serve this patient by reinforcing this medical judgment.

Generally the patient with multiple sclerosis is hospitalized only during a period of exacerbation or in a later stage of heightened physical dependency. At all other times it is hoped that he will be able to maintain himself in his home with a fair degree of independence. The role of health teaching is of special importance during this time and every opportunity should be utilized to help the patient plan a home care regimen. Although the etiology and thus prevention are yet unknown factors, certain prophylactic measures can be instituted to help minimize exacerbations. A highly routinized life should become the pattern of living for these patients. To avoid undue fatigue, generous sleeping and rest periods should be established. The false security of a remission period may encourage the patient to "test out" staying up later or greatly increasing his activities; this should be discouraged. Excessive fatigue must be avoided. It is felt that stressful emotional states may trigger exacerbations. Certainly a life free of stress would be most unnatural, but a fairly stable and crisis-free emotional environment seems helpful. A sound nutritional state should be maintained. Dietary fads are no cure and should be avoided.

Conscious effort should be directed toward preventing the diagnosis of multiple sclerosis from dominating the patient's life. Efforts toward becoming involved in useful outer-directed activities can help to take the focus off one's own limitations after the initial reaction to loss and subsequent grieving has occurred.

Helping the patient adjust to the disturbing symptoms of the disease constitutes another focus for teaching and care. As the disease progresses, care is directed toward the neurological deficit, as was discussed in the earlier section under care of the paraplegic patient.

A disturbing symptom specific to this patient is the intention tremor, which may become severe enough to interfere with the manual dexterity essential for such activities as eating and dressing. Although he should be allowed to do as much as possible for himself, he should not be subjected to needless frustration because he cannot accomplish these activities.

A visual disturbance may further limit the patient's activities. Covering one eye with a patch may help relieve the visual problem created by diplopia. Alterations in gait coupled with decrease in visual acuity increase hazards in ambulation. Accident prevention and the anticipation of the potential for accidents from a fall, a burning cigarette, spilling hot food or drink, and so forth should be included in the care and teaching program.

Later states of progression in multiple sclerosis may lead to urinary incontinence. Catheter dependency is not uncommon. An uninhibited neurogenic bladder, which is a purely reflex bladder causing sudden uncontrolled voiding without residual, may develop. All the dangers inherent in urinary tract infection are common and of particular significance, thus every effort should be made to prevent an intercurrent infection. Fecal incontinence, though rare, can usually be managed by means of diet, fluids, and activity, or use of cathartics and enemas.

The emotional lability, ranging from uncontrolled, inappropriate laughter to crying, can be a source of great embarrassment to both patient and family. Reprimanding may only serve to increase this response, but calm acceptance and possibly distraction may help to decrease or stop the outburst.

The patient should avoid chilling, dress appropriately for the weather, and avoid individuals with colds. Some patients may inquire if it is recommended that they move to a warmer climate where the incidence of multiple sclerosis is lower and temperature changes are moderate. There is no evidence that moving to a warm climate will control or cure multiple sclerosis once it has occurred, and the economic and social factors would make this move prohibitive in many instances.

A helpful resource is the National Multiple Sclerosis Society, which stimulates, coordinates, and finances research in multiple sclerosis and provides the public with pertinent information. Local chapters develop and conduct service programs at the community level.

OTHER DEGENERATIVE DISORDERS

Amyotrophic lateral sclerosis, sometimes referred to as "Lou Gehrig's disease," is characterized by progressive degeneration of the anterior horn cells of the spinal cord, the motor nuclei of the lower cranial nerves, and the corticobulbar and corticospinal tracts. It develops predominantly among males in the age range of 40 to 70 years. The cause is unknown. Early symptoms include muscle weakness and wasting, especially in the hands, with extension to muscle groups of the forearms; other muscle groups, however, may be initially involved, such as muscles of respiration and muscle groups of the lower extremities. Objective sensory changes usually do not occur, and the mind usually remains clear throughout the course. Bulbar palsy is usually present in later stages, with progressive difficulties in speech articulation, mastication, and swallowing. The course of amyotrophic lateral sclerosis is inevitably fatal, usually within 1 to 4 years. There is no specific treatment, and therapy is directed toward providing comfort measures and preventing complications. Care must be exercised to prevent aspiration of food. Use of a respirator may be indicated in the presence of respiratory difficulties.

Syringomyelia is a chronic and progressive disorder of the spinal cord, believed to be congenital, which causes cavitation of the central canal of the cord. Progressive gliosis of the central canal is usually most marked in the cervical cord but may extend into the thoracic segments. With transverse extension, damage occurs to the anterolateral pathway. There is loss of pain and temperature with preservation of touch and pressure in the lower cervical dermatomes. The loss of pain and temperature is frequently described as having a "shawl-like" distribution. Although syringomyelia may occur in childhood and later adult life, it is most frequent in young adults between 20 and 40 years of age.

The patient must exercise great care to avoid burning his hands. Muscle weakness and atrophy may occur later in the course. The disease progresses slowly over many years, although the onset may be rapid. Accompanying congenital skeletal defects lend support to the belief that syringomyelia is a developmental disease.

Brain stem involvement, *syringobulbia,* may occur alone or in association with syringomyelia. The symptoms of syringobulbia include progressive dysphagia, dysarthria, weakness of one side of the tongue, loss of pain and temperature unilaterally, and other symptoms reflective of disease involvement. Precautions to prevent aspiration while maintaining adequate nutrition become self-evident nursing measures. Treatment may include deep x-ray therapy, which seems of questionable value; in some instances decompression laminectomy may be indicated. Patient education is focused upon preventing accidental injury to areas of analgesia.

Spinal Cord Surgery for Relief of Pain

Rhizotomy

Rhizotomy is resection of a spinal nerve root just before it enters the spinal cord. This therapeutic measure may be performed through laminectomy in the low cervical or high thoracic region. The posterior (sensory) roots are divided to abolish pain perception in the upper trunk. Because proprioception is also lost this procedure is contraindicated for relief of extremity pain. Posterior rhizotomy may be combined with cervical cordotomy for the relief of incisional neck pain.

Anterior rhizotomy, in which the anterior (motor) roots are severed, affords relief in cases of marked spasticity as is seen in spastic paraplegia.

Nursing care is similar to that for laminectomy and dictated by the specific deficit created.

Cordotomy

Cordotomy for the relief of intractable pain is approached through one of two methods: open-surgical or closed-percutaneous.

OPEN—SURGICAL

Cordotomy (surgical [open technique] severance of the spinothalamic [anterolateral] tract) is performed at the level of C2 or C3 unilaterally to relieve pain in the upper extremities and chest. Bilateral cervical cordotomy is seldom performed because of the proximity of the phrenic nerves and the potential for respiratory failure. Dorsal (thoracic) cordotomy, at the level of the first and second thoracic vertebrae, is performed most frequently for pain due to malignant pelvic tumor or intractable pain of the lower trunk and lower extremities. Bilateral dorsal cordotomy may be a one-stage or a two-stage procedure. Because of the proximity of the anterior spinal artery, an incision made too far anterior may result in paraplegia, while an incision made too far posterior could cause disturbance of the pyramidal tract with resulting paresis in the contralateral leg. Bowel anl bladder disturbances may also develop if the incision is not precisely placed. Urinary distention caused by retention may be transitory and relieved by placement of a retention catheter for a few days postoperatively. Constipation may develop because of decreased peristalsis and intestinal tone, and enemas may be necessary to induce initial evacuation postoperatively. These symptoms, which are more common in bilateral cordotomy, will remain permanently. They may develop postoperatively, because of cord edema, then subside temporarily. Laminectomy may be necessary.

CLOSED—PERCUTANEOUS

Percutaneous cordotomy may be accomplished by inserting a spinal needle into a cervical interspace. In the lateral approach interspace C1 to C2 is usually utilized; in the anterior approach C5 to C6 or C6 to C7 interspace is the site. An electrode is then precisely directed into the cord and a lesion is created by coagulation and destruction of the sensory fibers of the lateral spinothalamic tract. The patient is presedated but awake during this procedure and his cooperation is necessary to ensure accuracy in placement of the electrode. This procedure may be unilateral or bilateral. The complications of cord edema and hemorrhage as well as a misplaced lesion may be manifested in extremity weakness on testing. Respiratory difficulty is not usually encountered with the unilateral approach but may be with the bilateral approach. These difficulties may be mild and transitory, or may progress to apnea during sleep, so close observation of respirations at all times is necessary. Awareness of this possibility is essential for at least the first 24 hours and thereafter at the hours of sleep.

Bowel and/or bladder dysfunction may occur. Urinary retention is commonly seen. Discomfort at the operative site and headache are not uncommon complaints and are usually relieved by mild analgesics and local ice compresses.

The patient must be instructed to take all necessary precautions, since his inability to feel pain and recognize temperature changes may give rise to undetected injury. Both patient and staff should be cautioned regarding temperature of too hot bath water, heating pad, and hot water bottle. The patient should be observed carefully daily so that tissue irritation or infection can be treated at once.

Bibliography

Books

Chusid, Joseph G. and J. McDonald: *Correlative Neuroanatomy and Functional Neurology,* 12th ed. Los Altos, Calif.: Lange Medical Publications, 1964.

Davis, Loyal and Richard A. Davis: *Principles of Neurological Surgery.* Philadelphia: W. B. Saunders Company, 1963.

deGutierrez-Mahoney, C. G. and Esta Carini: *Neurological and Neurosurgical Nursing,* 4th ed. St. Louis: The C. V. Mosby Co., 1965.

DeJong, Russell N.: *The Neurologic Examination,* 2d ed. New York: Paul B. Hoeber, Inc., 1958.

Elliott, Frank A.: *Clinical Neurology.* Philadelphia: W. B. Saunders Company, 1964.

French, John D. and Robert W. Porter (Eds.): *Basic Research in Paraplegia.* Springfield, Ill.: Charles C Thomas, Publisher, 1962.

Gardner, Ernest: *Fundamentals of Neurology,* 4th ed. Philadelphia: W. B. Saunders Company, 1963.

Harrison, T. R. (Ed.): *Principles of In-*

ternal Medicine, 4th ed. New York: McGraw-Hill Book Company, 1962.

Kahn, Edgar A., et al.: *Correlative Neurosurgery.* Springfield, Ill.: Charles C Thomas, Publisher, 1955.

Merritt, H. Houston: *A Textbook of Neurology,* 3d ed. Philadelphia: Lea & Febiger, 1963.

Mullen, Sean: *Essentials of Neurosurgery.* New York: Springer Publishing Co., Inc., 1961.

U.S. Department of Health, Education, and Welfare, 5. Public Health Series: *Syphilis: Modern Diagnosis and Management.* Washington: U.S. Government Printing Office, 1960.

Wechsler, Israel S.: *Clinical Neurology,* 9th ed. Philadelphia: W. B. Saunders Company, 1963.

Windle, W. F.: Regeneration in the Central Nervous System. in John D. French and Robert W. Porter (Eds.): *Basic Research in Paraplegia.* Springfield, Ill: Charles C Thomas, Publisher, 1962, p. 6.

Articles

Barnes, Roland: Paraplegia in Cervical Spine Injuries. *Proceedings of Royal Society of Medicine,* 54:365–367, May, 1961. Abridged.

Barron, Kevin D., Lewis P. Rowland, and H. M. Zimmerman: Neuropathy with Malignant Tumor Metastases, *Journal of Nervous and Mental Disease,* 131:10–31, July, 1960.

Bertrand, Gilles: Management of Spinal Injuries with Associated Cord Damage. *Postgraduate Medicine,* 37:249–262, March, 1965.

Boyce, Helen E.: Rehabilitation in Multiple Sclerosis. *Nursing Outlook,* 3:549–551, October, 1955.

Comarr, A. Estin: Neurogenic Bladder. *Paraplegia,* 2:125–131, August, 1964.

Covalt, Donald A., et al.: Early Management of Patients with Spinal Cord Injury. *Journal of American Medical Association,* 151:89–94, January 10, 1953.

DeJong, Russell N.: Multiple Sclerosis: Crippler of Young Adults. *Today's Health,* 42:36–37, November, 1964.

Drake, Charles: Cervical Spinal Cord Injury. *Journal of Neurosurgery,* 19:487–494, 1962.

Hahn, Richard: Some Remarks on the Management of Neurosyphilis. *Journal of Chronic Diseases,* 13:1–5, 1961.

Hyland, H. H.: Prognosis and Treatment of Multiple Sclerosis. *Postgraduate Medicine,* 37:241–248, March, 1965.

Kaplan, Lawrence I., B. B. Grynbaum, K. E. Lloyd, and H. A. Rusk: Pain and Spasticity in Patients with Spinal Cord Dysfunction. *Journal of American Medical Association,* 182:918–925, 1962.

Kurland, L. T. and H. J. Dodge: Multiple Sclerosis: Its Frequency and Distribution with Special Reference to Denver, Colorado. *Neurology,* 3:577, 1953.

Kurland, L. T. and H. W. Newman: Multiple Sclerosis: Its Frequency and Distribution with Special Reference to San Francisco, California. *California Medicine,* 79:381, 1953.

Kurland, L. T. and Dwayne Reed. Geographic and Climatic Aspects of Multiple Sclerosis. *American Journal of Public Health,* 54:588–597, April, 1964.

Kurland, L. T., Antonio Stazio, and Dwayne Reed. An Appraisal of Population Studies of Multiple Sclerosis. *Annals of New York Academy of Sciences,* 122:521–541, March 31, 1965.

Martin, M. Arlene: Nursing Care in Cervical Cord Injury. *American Journal of Nursing,* 63:60–66, March, 1963.

Massy, Shirley: Treatment of a Patient with a Complete Cervical Cord Lesion When Nursed on a Stryker Frame. *Physiotherapy,* February, 1962, 26–29.

Multiple Sclerosis. Neurology Conference. *Minnesota Medicine,* 48:221–230, February, 1965.

Remvig, Ole: Rehabilitation of Patients with Spinal Cord Injuries. *Acta Psychiatrica et Neurologica* Suppl. 1961, pp. 282–294.

Schneider, Richard C.: Surgical Indications and Contraindications in Spine and Spinal Cord Trauma. *Clinical Neurosurgery No. 8.* Baltimore: The Williams & Wilkins Company, 1962, pp. 157–184.

Schumacher, George A. and Mary Ellen Palmer: Multiple Sclerosis and Nursing the Patient with Multiple Sclerosis. *American Journal of Nursing,* 57:751–755, June, 1957.

Schumacher, George A., et al.: Problems of Experimental Trials of Therapy in Multiple Sclerosis: Report by the Panel on the Evaluation of Experimental Trials of Therapy in Multiple Sclerosis. *Annals of New York Academy of Sciences,* 122:552–567, March 31, 1965.

Schwartz, Henry G.: High Cervical Cordotomy—Technique and Results. *Clinical Neurosurgery No. 8.* Baltimore: The Williams & Wilkins Company, 1962, pp. 282–293.

Shepherd, Gwendolyn: Significant Trends in the Control of Poliomyelitis and its Sequelae. *Journal of Chronic Diseases,* 13:190–199, January, 1961.

Sibley, William A. and Joseph M. Foley: Infection and Immunization in Multiple Sclerosis. *Annals of New York Academy of Sciences,* 122:457–468, March 31, 1965.

Skinner, Geraldine: Nursing Care of a Patient on a Stryker Frame. *American Journal of Nursing,* 46:288–293, May, 1946.

Stazio, Antonia and Leonard Kurland: Multiple Sclerosis: Its Frequency and Distribution with Special Reference to Washington, D.C. *Neurology,* 12:445–452, 1962.

Steele, William L.: Spinal Cord Injuries and Paraplegia. *Journal of Arkansas Medical Society,* 58:102–105, August, 1961.

Stickle, Gabriel: Observed and Expected Poliomyelitis in the United States 1958–1961. *American Journal of Public Health,* 54:1222–1229, August, 1964.

Suwanwela, Charas, Eben Alexander, Jr., and Courtland H. Davis, Jr.: Prognosis in Spinal Cord Injury with Special Reference to Patients with Motor Paralysis and Sensory Preservation. *Journal of Neurosurgery,* 19:220–227, 1962.

Taren, James A. and Edgar A. Kahn: The Surgical Relief of Intractable Pain. *Surgical Clinics of North America,* 41:1159–1167, October, 1961.

Wachs, Hirsh and Misha S. Zahs: Studies of Body Image in Men with Spinal Cord Injury. *Journal of Nervous and Mental Disease,* 131:121–127, August, 1960.

SECTION 3 DISORDERS OF THE PERIPHERAL NERVES

PAMELA HOLSCLAW MITCHELL*

The peripheral nerves are the structures of the nervous system which lie outside the brain and spinal cord; these consist of the cranial nerves and the spinal nerves and their peripheral branches (including the plexuses). Nursing problems arising from peripheral nerve disorders are not markedly different from those of brain and spinal cord disorders, for the disabilities produced are similar. However, nursing care in peripheral nerve disorders is discussed separately for the sake of clarity.

Peripheral nerve disorders are discussed primarily in relation to cause of dysfunction rather than specific disease entities. The latter are too numerous for the scope of this section, and the basic principles of nursing care relate to the type of dysfunction more closely than to the disease itself. Nursing care specific

* The author acknowledges the assistance of George A. Ojemann, M.D., and Donald W. Mitchell, M.D., in reviewing the manuscript of this section.

for the disease can be inferred by the student. Knowledge of the function of the nerve and location of the lesion will enable her to anticipate the disability, and observation of the patient will allow further definition of the nursing problems. It is suggested that the student consult an anatomy textbook for details of the innervation of specific nerves and a neurology textbook for details of specific disorders.

Disorders of the autonomic nervous system are not included in this chapter. Such disorders, as they affect the cardiovascular, pulmonary, gastrointestinal, and genitourinary systems, are discussed in the appropriate chapters.

Peripheral Nerve Function

The basic functions of the peripheral nerves are (1) to transmit sensory stimuli from the periphery to the spinal cord and brain, and (2) to transmit motor impulses from the brain to the periphery. Peripheral nerves are generally composed of both motor and sensory fibers; most of the cranial nerves, however, are pure motor or sensory.

Peripheral nerve fibers are capable of regenerating when injured, provided that the ends of the nerve do not become widely separated (see Principle 3, in Section 1 of this chapter). Injury to the nerve may be due to trauma, ischemia, inflammation, or degenerative disorders, but the changes occurring in the nerves are similar.

PROCESS OF DEGENERATION

Initially the myelin sheath breaks up, and the axon splits and disintegrates, leaving an empty axis cylinder. Subsequently, the neurilemmal cells (Schwann cells) proliferate and fill the empty cylinder, forming a tract that occupies the place of the nerve fibers. This degeneration may occur proximal as well as distal to the injury and may occasionally move in a retrograde fashion as far as the cell body. This process, occurring immediately after injury, is called *secondary* or *Wallerian degeneration*. In an inflammatory process there is hyperemia, swelling, and exudation. This neuritis initiates the degenerative process.

PROCESS OF REGENERATION

An understanding of the mechanism of regeneration is based on studies of severed axons (Ruch and Patton). Some of the axon fibers extend from the end of the nerve "stump" and find their way through the connective tissue tract to the distal nerve sheath. The fibers grow down the sheath to the end-organ, forming an intact, but unmyelinated, nerve fiber. As it matures, it acquires a myelin sheath, and the Schwann cells eventually assume their normal position. It is estimated that regeneration occurs at the rate of 0.5 to 4.5 mm per day (Ruch and Patton; Guyton). If the continuity of the nerve sheath has not been interrupted, regeneration will proceed at a somewhat faster rate. In this situation, it is also more likely that not all fibers are injured and hence some conduction remains. If the injury is a traumatic severing and muscles have pulled the nerve stumps apart, the new fibers may branch off in all directions and form a *neuroma*, a painful mass of axons. This process begins even in injury to the central nervous system; however, the axons fail to make effective connections within the brain. This leads to the irreversible effects of trauma within the central nervous system.

The foregoing is important so that the nurse may understand how potential for recovery following peripheral nerve injury differs from that following injury to the central nervous system. This will also help her to interpret to the patient his slow recovery of function.

Symptoms of Peripheral Nerve Disorders

As in the central nervous system, the symptoms of a peripheral nerve disorder depend on the location of the lesion and the function of the nerve. Just as with the brain and spinal cord lesions, function will be disrupted distal to the lesion (see Principle 1 in Section 1). Since most nerves are mixed motor and sensory, the symptoms will also be mixed. However, there are exceptions: for example, lead toxicity affects primarily sensory components, and arsenic toxicity affects primarily the motor fibers.

SENSORY DISTURBANCES

Sensory disturbances are common and are often the reason that the person seeks medical attention. These disturbances include anesthetic areas, loss of position and vibratory sense, and changes in perception of touch, temperature, and pain. Such disturbances are localized to the areas innervated by the affected nerve or nerves. Knowledge of the location and nature of the sensory changes is necessary for the nurse to plan specific care. This care may include (1) protecting anesthetic areas, (2) avoiding the stimulation of paresthetic areas, and (3) teaching the patient to compensate for losses of position or vibratory sense.

Pain

Pain is a common symptom, particularly with inflammatory or irritative lesions. (See Chapter 15 for a more detailed discussion of the nature of pain and unusual sensations.) Inflammation often produces hypersensitivity in the affected areas, causing burning or prickling pain. There may be the sensation of constant burning in areas that are relatively insensitive to sharp touch. Superficial stimuli, such as light touch or the brushing of bedclothes, can trigger a prolonged increase in this pain. If the pain is localized, simple measures, such as using a cradle to keep the weight of the covers off the legs and avoiding contact with affected areas, can do much to increase the patient's comfort. Analgesics are frequently ordered but are of limited help in this type of pain. Some physicians utilize hyperstimulation of these areas, e.g., the patient is instructed to pound on the area with a rubber mallet or to rub it with a washcloth.

Most of us have not had to live with this diffuse, "primitive" pain and are not aware of how distressing it can be. Patients who suffer from it are often irritable and withdrawn and may be labeled "complainers." They may not display their pain so overtly as does someone suffering acute postoperative pain, but it is nevertheless real. The inability of the patient to communicate this pain and the failure of the hospital staff to appreciate it may combine to isolate him. The understanding nurse can do much to break this cycle of mutual withdrawal, which otherwise serves to increase tensions, and thus pain.

Anesthesia

Complete functional interruption of a nerve, due to severing or to degenerative processes, will produce anesthesia distal to the injury. The person will not feel warnings of injury to the denervated area, for example, when his hand is against a hot radiator, or when he bumps into something. The nurse needs to protect him from such injury and to teach him to protect himself. In addition, there may be unusual and disturbing sensations in the area if the cause of the anesthesia is nontraumatic.

Proprioception, Stereognosis, and other Sensory Discriminations

Proprioception, stereognosis, and other sensory discriminations may be lost in peripheral nerve lesions, just as they are with cortical lesions (see Section 1), although in the former there is more discrete localization (Wechsler). As with cortical lesions, one cannot assume that the person can do tasks involving delicate movement even though strength is intact.

MOTOR IMPAIRMENT

Motor impairment ranges from mild weakness to complete paralysis, depending on the nature of the lesion. Severing of the nerve will cause a *flaccid paralysis*, with rapid wasting of muscles. This is typical of lower motor neuron lesions since the reflex arc, which maintains muscle tone, is interrupted at the periphery (Wechsler). Severe compression will have the same effect as transection, but lesser compression and irritative lesions (inflammation, toxicity) will cause incomplete paralysis with varying degrees of weakness, plus the concomitant changes in sensation.

Even though the paralysis is flaccid, deformities can occur. These may include wrist and foot drop, hyperextension of the knee, internal rotation of the hip, and specific contractures depending on the nerve or nerves involved. Normally, muscle groups oppose one another and maintain flexible motion. When there is denervation of a specific muscle group, the tone in the unaffected muscles is no longer opposed and the limb is pulled into a contracted position. The contracture is permanently maintained if the associated tendons shorten. Methods of preventing deformity are discussed elsewhere.

Loss of innervation results in muscle wasting; this is illustrated by the atrophied thenar pad of a person with loss of innervation to the hand. No amount of passive exercise will restore muscle tone.

VASOMOTOR CHANGES

Vasomotor changes are likely to occur in peripheral nerve disorders, as a result of loss of sympathetic stimulation to the vessels. These changes may result in keratitis, glossy and swollen or wrinkled skin, cold extremities, and impaired resistance of the skin to injury. Vasomotor phenomena, such as Raynaud's phenomenon, are also believed to be due to disturbances in sympathetic function. If the person has some degree of anesthesia in addition to these changes, he should be cautioned against the use of hot water bottles and heating pads "to warm up my cold feet," for serious burns could occur before he would be aware of them.

Neuropathies and Associated Nursing Problems

AIMS OF CARE

There are basic aims of both medical and nursing care which are applicable to any peripheral nerve disorder. These should be kept in mind during the following discussion of general classifications of neuropathies.

The aims of medical care are (1) to diagnose and, if possible, reverse the cause of dysfunction, (2) to restore continuity of severed nerve fibers, (3) to maintain the patient's general health and prevent complicating factors, thus promoting maximal recovery, and (4) to preserve and improve upon remaining function.

The aims of nursing care are (1) to observe for, and to assist the physician in prevention of, complicating illness, (2) to maintain remaining function and to prevent deformities, (3) to protect the patient from further injury to the affected parts, and (4), in conjunction with the physician, to teach the patient and his family how to deal with changes in living patterns necessitated by disability. Rehabilitative nursing assumes the same primary importance as discussed in the care of patients with brain and spinal cord disorders. It is apparent that the goals of nursing care complement those of medical care; the difference is primarily in the method of implementation.

Disorders of peripheral nerves can be classified as *mononeuropathies,* (those involving single nerves) and *polyneuropathies* (those involving multiple nerves). They may also be classified as *localized* and *generalized* disorders.

LOCALIZED NEUROPATHY

The localized disorders generally involve one nerve or, at most, a few nerves. Causes include trauma, compression, and degeneration.

Trauma

Trauma to peripheral nerves occurs with tearing or severing injuries, such as those seen in gunshot wounds, knife injuries, amputation (traumatic or surgical), fractures, and therapeutic transections (e.g., for relief of pain). Treatment of these injuries is primarily surgical and is intended to restore continuity of the nerve and to prevent infection and resultant scarring (the new fibers cannot grow through scar tissue). If the nerve union is successful, it may take 6 months or longer before functional results are seen (Wechsler).

Nursing care after surgery on peripheral nerves involves maintenance of nerve continuity, by careful positioning of the limb, and prevention of infection. Careful dressing technique is important in the latter, and reverse isolation procedures may also be employed. The operating room nurse, along with the surgeon, has a responsibility in preventing the introduction of pathogens at the time of surgery.

The limb should be positioned to prevent kinking or stretching of the repaired nerve, and the neutral position of function should be maintained. In addition, limb position may be used to gain additional length of the nerve sheath and thereby to facilitate repair. In such a case, it is imperative that the nurse maintain this position to prevent disruption of the sutured nerve sheath. The surgeon will usually specify the exact position to be used and he should be consulted if there is any question in the nurse's mind. Range of motion exercises are begun at the discretion of the surgeon.

Compression

Compression of peripheral nerves may result from fractures, tumors, tight bandaging or casts, and prolonged external pressure on the nerve. Arthritic cervical spurs and herniated intervertebral disks may exert pressure on spinal nerves.

Compression produces nerve injury by direct pressure or by causing local ischemia. Nerve dysfunction is reversible if the pressure or ischemia is of short duration. However, with prolonged ischemia the changes within the nerve eventually become irreversible and there will be no return of function. Treatment, therefore, is directed toward the early relief of pressure.

The nurse can be instrumental in preventing many compression injuries in hospitalized persons and can teach preventive measures to those in home and in industry. Orthopedic patients are prime candidates for experiencing nerve compression, and observation of the casted extremities is quite important in these patients. For example, foot drop may occur if the common peroneal nerve is compressed between cast and bone in its course around the neck of the fibula. It is difficult to detect this if the cast immobilizes the foot, but the patient who has a portion of the foot exposed can be asked to dorsiflex his toes (not just wiggle, but actually lift them). As dorsiflexion of the toes is served by this nerve, inability to do this may indicate common peroneal nerve injury and should be called to the attention of the doctor. Peroneal nerve compression may also occur in thin, older persons who sit for long periods with their legs crossed. Such persons should be encouraged to change position and move about often.

The dangers of radial and ulnar nerve damage in crutch walking are discussed in Chapter 27. Radial nerve damage can also occur during sleep or unconsciousness if the person assumes an abnormal position in which the nerve is compressed for a prolonged time (for example, sleeping with the arm over the hard edge of a cot). Movements during sleep ordinarily prevent continued pressure on any nerve; however, an unconscious individual or one in a stuporous state (perhaps due to alcohol) may remain in the same position and may be found the next morning with wrist drop. Obviously the nurse cannot prevent the alcoholic from sleeping on his arm, but she can avoid positioning the unconscious patient so that his body weight lies on his arm, and she can change his position frequently. Compression paralysis of the radial nerve usually subsides within 1 to 4 months; however, contractures will occur, unless the wrist is extended by a splint and kept supple by range of motion exercises (Wechsler).

Compression of the third cranial nerve in temporal lobe herniation associated with increased intracranial pressure is another example of compression injury. This is fully discussed in Section 1.

Degeneration

Localized degeneration may follow ischemia or use of toxic agents. Paralysis of the sixth cranial nerve, occasionally seen in diabetes, is thought to be due to vascular changes leading to localized ischemia of the nerve; generalized diabetic neuropathy (affecting mainly the extremities) is felt to be primarily metabolic in origin (Locke). Streptomycin toxicity, specific for the eighth cranial nerve, is an example of a localized toxic degeneration. Deafness can be prevented if the physician is notified and the drug discontinued at the first sign of hearing loss. Lead toxicity affects primarily the radial nerve and occasionally the peroneal nerves. It may produce symptoms of generalized peripheral neuropathy or dysfunction of the central nervous system, in addition to these localized neuropathies.

GENERALIZED NEUROPATHY

Generalized neuropathies (polyneuropathies) may be associated with infection and inflammation, metabolic disorders, and toxic agents. The student may see the terms *neuropathy* and *neuritis* used interchangeably; however, neuritis is more properly applied only to inflammatory processes, whereas neuropathy refers to peripheral nerve disorders in general. The latter term will be used in this section.

Infection and Inflammation

Polyneuropathy may be seen in infectious diseases such as diphtheria, mumps, influenza, tuberculosis, meningitis, syphilis, gonorrhea, and malaria. The dysfunction is thought to be due to bacterial toxins rather than actual infection of the nerve (Beeson and McDermott). The neuropathy of acute idiopathic polyneuritis is felt to be an inflammatory process.

Metabolic Disorders

Polyneuropathy may be associated with diabetes, vitamin deficiencies (particularly the vitamin B complex, e.g., beriberi and pellagra), and porphyria. In both metabolic and infectious neuropathies, medical therapy includes treatment of the underlying disorder, as well as supportive treatment of the polyneuropathy.

Toxic Degeneration

Toxic neuropathies are caused by arsenic, heavy metals, carbon monoxide, benzene (a common ingredient in drycleaning fluids) and other organic compounds, mercury, and drugs, such as antibiotics and antitoxins. The medical therapy is aimed at removing the cause of, or preventing exposure to, the toxic agent. Prognosis varies with the severity of the intoxication and the duration and frequency of exposure. Much work is being done in industry to identify and remove harmful agents, and industrial nurses may have a part in such epidemiological studies. Public health nurses can also help by counseling families to use caution in handling dangerous substances (such as lead paint and cleaning fluid) and to keep them away from children.

Nursing Problems

Patients with generalized neuropathies, regardless of the cause, present similar problems and nursing needs. Therefore, certain basic principles are applicable. Some aspects will vary, depending upon the extent of disability (e.g., involvement of only the lower limbs versus all extremities) and the causative agent (e.g., the need for isolation in an infectious disease, or needs resulting from systemic disease). The prognosis will depend upon the cause of the disorder (e.g., full recovery is probable with acute idiopathic polyneuritis, but is less likely in generalized alcoholic neuropathy).

The basic nursing problems encountered in polyneuropathies include the following: (1) prevention of deformity; (2) protection from injury in the area of disturbed function; (3) prevention of directly related complicating illness (such as respiratory infection); (4) provision of emotional support, both during the acute anxiety engendered by loss of function, and during the long rehabilitative stage; (5) provision for physical comfort if sensation is disturbed; and (6) promotion of maximum rehabilitation which includes helping the patient and the family to accept disability and to set realistic goals, making the best use of remaining function, and teaching adaptation to limitations imposed by the disability.

These aspects of nursing care will be illustrated by the following discussion of acute idiopathic polyneuritis (also called *Guillain-Barré syndrome, infectious polyneuritis,* and *Landry's paralysis*). This syndrome is used for illustration not because it is a common disorder (the incidence is relatively low) but because it encompasses most of the above aspects of nursing care in generalized neuropathies. Information about other neuropathies may be found in neurology textbooks.

Acute idiopathic polyneuritis often follows upper respiratory infections; however, the etiology of the disorder is unknown. The term *infectious polyneuritis* is a misnomer, for epidemiologic evidence does not demonstrate that the disease is transmitted to others in the environment (Beeson and McDermott).

The disease is characterized by ascending motor and sensory loss, usually preceded by a burning and prickling sensation in the extremities. There may be gradually or rapidly progressing weakness, with variable loss of sensation. However, the motor loss is generally greater than is the sensory loss. The disease may be limited to the lower extremities or may ascend to the cranial nerves; it is characteristically self-limited and rarely ascends above the seventh cranial nerve. Spinal fluid analysis shows albuminocytologic dissociation (increase in protein without an increase in cells), and pathologic study of affected nerves demonstrates infiltration of the axis cylinders and the cell bodies with lymphocytes. There is no specific cure for the syndrome; therefore, the medical therapy is purely supportive and is directed toward preventing life-threatening complications, such as pneumonia and bladder infections, and promoting maximum rehabilitation. Full recovery can be expected, if deformities have been prevented, although it may take a year or more. Hence the nursing care is concerned with supporting the medical plan, preventing complicating illness and deformities, and supporting the patient emotionally through a long illness. In severe cases, the survival of the patient depends largely on intelligent nursing care.

SUPPORT OF THE MEDICAL PLAN

Of initial importance are the nurse's observations. Knowing that the disorder proceeds in an ascending manner, the nurse can anticipate possible involvement of the intercostal and phrenic nerves and, therefore, should watch for respiratory weakness. Signs of respiratory involvement include the use of accessory muscles of respiration, flaring nostrils, difficulty in speaking a full sentence without stopping for breath, increased apprehension, restlessness, headache, and decreased vital capacity. An early indication of respiratory involvement is the patient's reluctance to sleep, for fear that he will stop breathing. It cannot be emphasized enough that cyanosis is a very late sign of hypoxia. The nurse's observations of respiratory weakness may prompt the physician to begin serial vital capacity measurements; tracheotomy may be required if the vital capacity reaches 30 to 50 percent of the expected normal (Eiben and Gersony).

Nursing care in the acute stage of the syndrome includes maintaining the airway and maintaining adequate ventilation. When the respiratory musculature is involved, the patient's ability to exchange air is markedly decreased, and he may require assisted ventilation, usually with an intermittent positive pressure apparatus. Occasionally a tank respirator is used, without tracheotomy. It is essential that the attending nurse understand the mechanics of the respirator used, or she will not be able to evaluate the effectiveness of its performance. Such information can be obtained from the manufacturer's manual, which should be kept with the machine, or from the hospital oxygen therapy department.

Most positive pressure respirators have "apneic" settings, which automatically initiate positive pressure after a set period of apnea. The weak patient is thereby freed from the inspiratory effort needed to start the flow of air. A frightened patient with some inspiratory ability may fight the respirator and not breathe in harmony with the machine, thus tiring himself further. Occasionally narcotics have to be given to depress the individual enough to allow the machine to take over the breathing. This is obviously quite hazardous and may be avoided by having a nurse whom the patient trusts stay with him and calmly and slowly instruct him when to breathe in and out, until he is synchronized with the respirator.

Since mechanical respirators do not provide the deep breaths which we take periodically (about once each hour), the nurse must accomplish this for the patient, by either using a hand ventilating bag or by increasing the positive pressure by 5 cm water for a few breaths. This may require a physician's order in some institutions.

PREVENTION OF COMPLICATING ILLNESS

Patients on long-term assisted ventilation, as these patients frequently are, tend to lose the normal compliance of the lungs and thereby become more prone to respiratory infection. Hence the prevention of such infection is an important nursing problem. In addition to the periodic deep breathing discussed above, deep tracheal suctioning is necessary. (See the references for material on the principles of deep tracheal suctioning.) Nurses should learn to auscultate the chest for rales, to determine if their suctioning endeavors have been adequate. The services of a pulmonary physiotherapist are invaluable in loosening and raising thick secretions. If one is not available, the nurse can, with physician approval, utilize the techniques described by Kurihara.

With bulbar involvement, there is weakness of the swallowing muscles. In addition to the danger of aspiration of food and fluids, this presents the problem of providing sufficient nourishment for the patient. Therefore intravenous fluids are given initially, but eventually nasogastric tube feeding may be necessary. Aspiration continues to be a danger during initial oral feedings, and for this reason such feedings should not be entrusted to inexperienced personnel. Assessment of the patient's ability to swallow safely is similar to that made of the person with central nervous system bulbar involvement. His swallowing ability must first be ascertained with a small amount of water or saline; if choking or coughing occurs he is not ready for oral feeding. Sitting the patient upright will aid in proper swallowing. Once swallowing is adequate, thick foods, such as gruel and cooked cereal, should be introduced since these are more easily managed than thin liquids. Other foods can be added as tolerated. A suction machine should be at the bedside during initial oral feeding, in the event the patient aspirates.

In the acute stage, autonomic involvement may impair bladder function. Urethral catheterization is performed if bladder distention occurs; measures for preventing urinary infection apply. During recovery, bladder function will return; therefore, extensive bladder training will not be necessary. However, reestablishment of tone may be necessary. Laxatives and daily glycerin suppositories may be required in later stages of recovery to combat constipation associated with inactivity.

Decubitus ulceration is a potential problem, particularly if there is widespread paralysis. The combination of loss of sensation, loss of motor power, and vasomotor changes leading to decreased circulation makes skin breakdown a problem in any degree of polyneuropathy. Nursing measures to prevent this are presented in detail in other chapters.

PREVENTION OF DEFORMITY

In severe motor involvement, the person may become quadriplegic, with only the upper cranial nerves functioning, or he may have only loss of innervation to the lower legs. The prevention of deformities will involve the same care as that of a person with a flaccid paralysis of any extent.

Contractures can develop, even with flaccid paralysis, due to the pull of unopposed muscle groups; this is particularly so in less severe polyneuropathies or during the stage of returning function. Function in some muscles may return faster than in others. Contractures associated with foot drop, wrist drop, and hyperextension of the knee can develop because the flexor muscles that maintain normal position are no longer functioning. Passive range of motion exercises and careful positioning will prevent these deformities.

PHYSICAL COMFORT

Although during the period of maximum involvement sensation may be diminished or even lost, at the onset of the syndrome and during recovery there may be burning and other paresthetic sensations. The muscles in particular may become quite hypersensitive. Therefore, the nurse can increase comfort by handling limbs at the joints, keeping covers off the legs, and administering the pain medication ordered.

EMOTIONAL SUPPORT

A major problem is maintenance of the patient's emotional stability. The gradual loss of sensation and ability to move is extremely frightening. As the paralysis ascends, the patient knows, although not always consciously, that his breathing is in danger; this concern is accentuated when there is any degree of actual respiratory difficulty. As indicated earlier, this increasing apprehension is an early sign of hypoxia and should be brought to the physician's attention. The patient may not voice his fear, in the almost magical dread that saying it will make it so. The fear is nevertheless there and may make itself known by "excessive demands" on the nursing staff, such as frequent requests for "little" things, just to make sure that someone will come. The opposite occasionally occurs: there are few requests, even for major needs, in the fear that the service available to him will be "used up" and will not be available when he "really" needs it. The patient may be frightened by the frequent assessments of motor and sensory function, and some attention to other things (such as bringing in extra juices and magazines, or simply sitting and talking) will help reduce the patient's preoccupation with his physical function.

The importance of having the same nurse or few nurses for the patient with acute idiopathic polyneuritis cannot be overemphasized. His anxiety is characteristically expressed by extreme attention to detail and ritual; frequent changes of nurses, who are not aware of these details, will only increase his anxiety and create a "problem patient." The anxiety demonstrated by patients with any polyneuropathy may be out of proportion to the objective functional loss. If loss of sensation and motor power has come on gradually, he has no idea when it will stop progressing or if he will recover. It is important that the nurse realize this so that she may better understand the patient's reactions.

REHABILITATION

The person recovering from the Guillain-Barré syndrome or any widespread neuropathy faces a long rehabilitative period and may become discouraged frequently. The favorable prognosis for full return of function in acute idiopathic polyneuritis can be used honestly to bolster the person, but this prospect is not true for all persons with extensive neuropathies, especially those associated with chronic disorders (diabetes, alcoholism). In the Guillain-Barré syndrome, function returns in descending progression. This necessitates a long-term sedentary existence, challenging the nurse and family to help the patient to find satisfying diversions. Despite reassurances that function will return, many patients seriously doubt it and find the routine of exercises and physical therapy more than they can bear. The patient often does not realize how well he is progressing because changes are not dramatic in his minute-to-minute existence. Since this depression is common and understandable, the nurse should allow the patient to express it and should not make light of it; however, she needs to continue to move him toward recovery by setting short-term, achievable goals with him. The long road to complete recovery may seem overwhelming to the patient, but the ability to feed himself half of his meal "tomorrow" may be quite easily imagined.

Nurses often have difficulty in working with these patients, for they too may become discouraged with the slow progress. Setting short-term, accomplishable goals and looking for satisfaction in these can help the nurse as well as the patient.

Specific problems of rehabilitation in generalized neuropathies will depend on the location of dysfunction, its extent, and its permanance. The major rehabilitative task in acute idiopathic polyneuritis is to prevent deformities and skin breakdown so that the person will be able to use his limbs once motor power has returned. Wrist drop, foot drop, and hyperextension of the knee are the most usual deformities seen. During the stage of recovery, physical therapy is essential to strengthen muscles that have become atrophied due to loss of tone.

In any generalized neuropathy resulting in permanent dysfunction, the patient and his family will need help in learning to live within limitations imposed by the disability. This may involve learning to use braces, crutches, a cane, or other mechanical devices, or learning simple daily activities such as getting in and out of bed unassisted.

Cranial Nerve Disorders

Specific cranial nerve disorders will not be outlined for the reasons stated at the beginning of the section. If the student studies the function of the cranial nerves, she can anticipate problems that are apt to arise from their dysfunction, and verify the existence of these problems by her observations, thus forming the basis for planning care. An example of this methodology can be demonstrated in the following discussion of trigeminal neuralgia.

Trigeminal neuralgia

Trigeminal neuralgia (tic douloureux) is a disorder characterized by intermittent shooting or burning pain in the sensory distribution of the fifth cranial nerve (trigeminal nerve). The three branches of the nerve are the ophthalmic branch, which transmits sensation from the cornea, forehead, eyelid, and a portion of the nose; the maxillary branch, which mediates sensation from the nose, cheek, and midface; and the mandibular branch, which supplies sensation to the cheek, jaw, lip, and temple. The latter two are the most commonly affected branches in this disorder.

The pain is often triggered by a local superficial stimulus (such as a breeze) or motor activity (such as chewing, shaving, or talking). The pain becomes severe and may last minutes to hours. Analgesic medication is usually of little benefit, particularly when the pain is of short duration. Diphenylhydantoin (Dilantin), nicotinic acid in large doses, trichloroethylene, and mephenesin carbamate are currently used in medical management of the disorder. They provide variable long-term relief. Carbamazepine (Tegretol) is a recent drug, felt by some investigators to be sufficiently effective to preclude the need for surgery in a large percentage of cases (Lutz). Carbamazepine has occasionally been reported to cause serious blood dyscrasias, including agranulocytosis, thrombocytopenia, and rarely aplastic anemia. For this reason, patients taking the drug must be encouraged to remain under close medical supervision, and to promptly report symptoms of such disorders, such as easy bruising, mouth ulceration, petechial hemorrhage, and fever.

Surgery may be required in those patients who do not respond to medical therapy. Some surgeons inject the affected branch with alcohol, as a temporary measure. Relief from this procedure may last from 6 months to 3 years. The supra- and infraorbital branches may be sectioned peripherally or avulsed (pulled out) at the Gasserian ganglion (the point of division of the branches, just inside the skull). These procedures also provide temporary relief since the branches regenerate, but are of value in older patients. Both Gasserian ganglion percussion and rubbing are currently popular procedures because the patient has relief from pain without sensory loss. However, relief is often not permanent and a second surgical procedure may be needed. The most successful procedure is partial transection of the sensory root inside the skull, proximal to the Gasserian ganglion; the motor root remains intact (Fager).

From the preceding information, general nursing problems can be outlined. Specifics of care will depend upon the pattern of the individual's pain and his reaction to it. Initially, the nurse will want to prevent triggering of the pain; this may entail eliminating breezes or not insisting that a man shave during a series of attacks. It is important to understand that he may exhibit withdrawal during the interlude between attacks in his attempt to prevent further attacks. She will also understand that the pain is not constant, and hence her observation of his complete comfort between attacks will not lead her to question the authenticity of his pain.

Surgical treatment indicates other nursing care. Transection of ophthalmic fibers may produce corneal anesthesia; this will necessitate an eye shield, taping of the eyelid, and flushing of the eye with a saline solution every 4 hours. In any procedure except ganglion percussion, areas of numbness are to be expected. These may be quite disagreeable to the patient, and the nurse can help the physician prepare the patient for this outcome.

Bibliography

Beeson, P. B. and Walsh McDermott (Eds.): *Cecil Loeb Textbook of Medicine,* 11th ed. Philadelphia: W. B. Saunders Company, 1963, pp. 1501–1505; 1580–1584; 12th ed., 1967, pp. 1654–1656.

Carbamazepine (Tegretol). *Medical Letter,* 40:13:49–50, June 28, 1968.

Eiben, Robert and Welton Gersony. Recognition, Diagnosis and Treatment of Guillain-Barré Syndrome (Acute Idiopathic Polyneuritis). *Medical Clinics of North America,* 47:1375. September, 1963.

Fager, Charles A.: Trigeminal Neuralgia. *Geriatrics,* 20:425–480, June, 1965.

Guyton, Arthur C.: *Textbook of Medical Physiology,* 2d ed. Philadelphia: W. B. Saunders Company, 1961, p. 241.

Kronsnick, A.: Diabotic Neuropathy. *American Journal of Nursing,* 65: 90–95, April, 1965.

Kurihara, M.: Postural Drainage, Clapping and Vibrating. *American Journal of Nursing,* 65:76, November, 1965.

Locke, Simeon: Diabetes and the Nervous System. *Medical Clinics of North America,* 49:1081–1092, July, 1965.

Lutz, Elmar H.: Treatment of Tic Douloureux with G-32883 (Carbamazepine). *Disease of Nervous System,* 27:600–603, September, 1966.

Mulder, D. W., J. K. Calverly, and R. H. Miller: Autogenous Mononeuropathy; Diagnosis, Treatment and Clinical Significance. *Medical Clinics of North America,* 44:989, July, 1960.

Respiratory Tract Aspiration (Programmed Instruction). *American Journal of Nursing,* 66:2483–2510, November, 1966.

Ruch, Theodore C. and Harry D. Patton (Eds.): *Physiology and Biophysics,* 19th ed. Philadelphia: W. B. Saunders Company, 1965, p. 84.

Stanton, J. H., F. L. Hendrickson, and D. Wagner: Care of the Patient with Infectious Neuronitis. *Nursing Clinics of North America,* 1:503–510, September, 1966.

Wechsler, Israel S.: The Peripheral Nerves. in Israel S. Wechsler (Ed.): *Clinical Neurology,* 9th ed. Philadelphia: W. B. Saunders Company, 1963, pp. 195–292.

Suggested Reading for Students

Merritt, Hiram H.: *A Textbook of Neurology,* 4th ed. Philadelphia: Lea & Febiger, 1967.

SECTION 4
MYASTHENIA
GRAVIS

PAMELA HOLSCLAW MITCHELL*

Pathophysiology
Medical therapy
DRUGS USED
Surgical therapy
Nursing care
ACUTE CRISES
THYMECTOMY

Myasthenia gravis is a comparatively rare disease; the incidence is estimated as 0.3 to 1.0 case per 10,000 persons. It affects people of all ages, but more commonly occurs in the third and fourth decades; the disease is more frequent in women than in men. Although myasthenia gravis is a rare disease, there are nevertheless about 20,000 persons affected with it in the United States, and many nurses will come into contact with such patients. Furthermore, the nursing care is based on specialized physiological and pharmacological principles that are difficult to find in current nursing references.

Myasthenia gravis is not strictly a disease of the nervous system, nor of the muscular system, but of the juncture between the two. However, since effective transmission of nervous impulses to the muscles is impaired, the disease is commonly considered with neurologic disorders.

The disease is manifested by increased fatigability of voluntary muscles. The fatigue increases as the day goes on; symptoms may increase during the premenstrual period and in emotional stress and are worsened by concurrent illness. Muscles of the face, particularly those of the eyelids, are often affected first. Ptosis, drooping of the lid, is common, as is nasal speech and difficulty in swallowing food. The latter two are the result of weakness of the bulbar muscles. Regurgitation of food and fluid through the nose is frequently the symptom prompting the person to seek medical attention. The disease may progress to involve the extremities; in some patients, the symptoms begin there.

Prognosis is variable; the disease may remain at a fairly mild level or may progress to cause total helplessness. A small percentage of patients (Schwab estimates these as 5 percent) appear to have spontaneous remissions, but, without medical treatment, the majority of patients worsen.

The physician makes the diagnosis on the basis of the history, particularly the pattern of muscle fatigue, and the response to neostigmine or edrophonium chloride

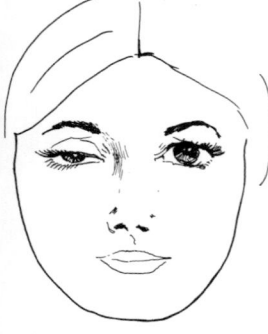

Symp.

Figure 29–17
*Unilateral ptosis in
myasthenia gravis.*

* The author acknowledges the assistance of George A. Ojemann, M.D., and Donald W. Mitchell, M.D., in reviewing the manuscript of this section.

1066

(Tensilon). Electromyography (the electrical recording of the response to muscle stimulation) may be performed to demonstrate the rapid muscle fatigue and to exclude other disorders with similar symptoms.

Pathophysiology

The conduction defect in myasthenia gravis is thought to occur at the myoneural junction. Normally, acetylcholine is released from the nerve ending, transmitting the nerve impulse to the motor end-plate of the muscle fiber. The muscle fiber is then depolarized, which produces a muscle contraction. The acetylcholine is present for only a fraction of a second; cholinesterase rapidly hydrolyzes it to acetate and choline, thus removing it from the end-plate. (See Figures 29–18 and 29–19.)

In myasthenia gravis, three possible abnormalities in this sequence are suggested: (1) too little acetylcholine is released; (2) too much cholinesterase is present, destroying the acetylcholine before it reaches the end-plate; (3) the end-plate no longer responds to acetylcholine.

The first is thought by many investigators to be the most likely (Beeson and McDermott; Guyton). An autoimmune factor may play a role in this abnormality. This has been suggested in view of the increased incidence of thymoma in myas-

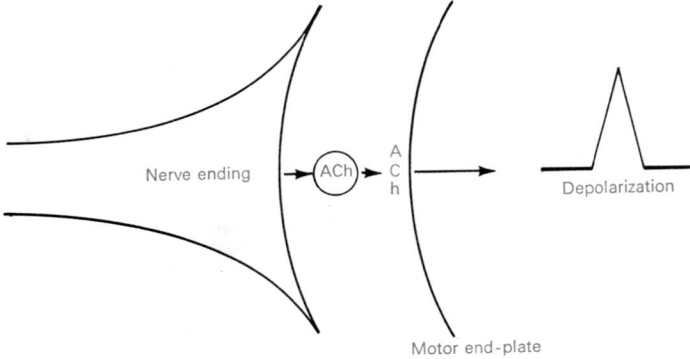

Figure 29–18
Schematic representation of muscle depolarization. Acetylcholine (ACh) transmits nerve impulses to motor end-plate.

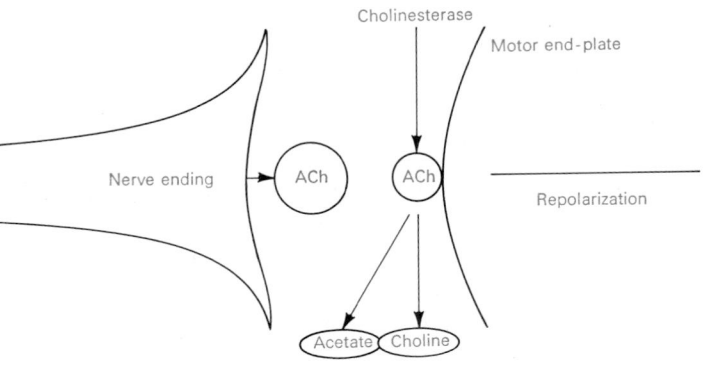

Figure 29–19
Schematic representation of hydrolysis of acetylcholine (ACh) and repolarization of muscle fiber.

thenic patients and the apparent involvement of the thymus in the establishment of the immune reaction (Adner; Kornfield).

Medical Therapy

It was found that certain cholinesterase-inactivating drugs improved muscle function in myasthenic patients. This suggested that the drugs inactivated that enzyme, allowing a smaller amount of acetylcholine to work or eliminating excess cholinesterase. Therefore anticholinergic drugs are used to maintain and improve muscle function. As with insulin in the treatment of diabetes, the drugs do not cure the disease but only supplement the body's store; hence they must be supplied at regular intervals.

DRUGS USED

The anticholinergics most commonly used are the following:

Generic Name	Trade Name
Neostigmine methylsulfate (parenteral)	Prostigmin
Neostigmine bromide (oral)	Prostigmin
Pyridostigmine bromide (tablets or syrup)	Mestinon
Ambenonium chloride (tablets)	Mytelase
Edrophonium chloride (intravenous)	Tensilon

These drugs vary in potency, in route of administration, and in duration of action. As with insulin, the regimen must be adapted to the needs of the individual. Detailed information about the drugs may be found in pharmacology textbooks.

The first four drugs are used in therapy; they vary in length of action (2 to 8 hours) and severity of side effects. Most commonly, one of the intermediate-acting drugs (for example, Mestinon, lasting 4 to 6 hours) is used during the day, and a sustained-release form (Timespan Mestinon, lasting 6 to 8 hours) is taken to last the night. Since the long-acting form is not available in parenteral or liquid form, the patient who is unable to swallow tablets must be awakened for doses of another drug.

Edrophonium (Tensilon) is used only as a diagnostic test, for its maximum duration of action is 5 to 10 minutes. It is injected intravenously, and, if marked improvement is noted, the diagnosis is probably myasthenia. Intramuscular neostigmine is also used for this test. Tensilon may also be used to determine whether weakness in a person under treatment is due to overdosage or underdosage of the anticholinergic agent. Because Tensilon is very short-acting, its cumulative effect in an overdosed patient will last only a few minutes. A nurse assisting in such a trial should be certain that pralidoxime (Protopam) and atropine are at the bedside. Pralidoxime is an anticholinergic blocking agent and may be necessary to counteract the extensive muscular weakness that can occur with overdose.

Atropine is useful in ameliorating the excessive autonomic effects of anticholinergic overdose.

Side effects of all the drugs are related to their anticholinergic effects on the autonomic nervous system. The parasympathetic system is mediated by acetylcholine; hence any agent (for example, an anticholinesterase) that prolongs acetylcholine activity will produce signs of excessive parasympathetic stimulation. These signs include diarrhea, abdominal cramping, increased salivation, and small pupils. These side effects are of some protective value, for their continued presence can warn the patient of impending overdosage.

Overdosage occurs when too much cholinesterase is blocked; acetylcholine accumulates to the extent that depolarization at the motor end-plate is prolonged. This, in turn, produces continuous muscle stimulation, with subsequent fatigue and paralysis. The acetylcholine accumulation will also accentuate parasympathetic side effects. This state can be detected by noting, in addition to the aforementioned side effects, increased weakness *after* medication, fine muscle twitching (fasciculations), cold sweat, and difficulty in breathing, coughing, or swallowing. Undermedication presents a similar picture but can be differentiated by the presence of normal pupils, absence of cramps and diarrhea, increased ptosis, and absence of fasciculations. Although dosage regulation is not the nurse's responsibility, it is important that she be able to recognize over- and undermedication so that the physician may be notified. If overdosage is suspected, the physician must be contacted immediately, *before* the next dose is given. Continued overmedication can result in severe respiratory weakness and inability to handle secretions. This life-threatening situation is often called *cholinergic crisis*.

Surgical Therapy

Several studies have shown thymectomy to be a valuable procedure in selected patients, particularly young women with a short history of myasthenia (Schwab; Beeson and McDermott; Kornfield). The reason for the effectiveness of this procedure is not understood. Radiation to the thymus is sometimes of value and may be given before surgery is attempted.

Nursing Care

Myasthenia gravis is a chronic disease, requiring for control responsible and informed participation by the patient. The nurse is in a prime position to reinforce the doctor's teaching of the patient, and to help the person cope with a life-long illness.

In the newly diagnosed patient, drug regulation will require some time. The nurse can use this time to help him and his family understand the nature of the drugs and their side effects. If the patient has been instructed to regulate the drug dosage on the basis of his symptoms, he will need help in interpreting these symptoms. As he may need to take the medications for life, he should be allowed and encouraged to begin self-medication as soon as possible. Hospital policies that forbid the keeping of medications at the bedside need to be discussed and adapted to the needs of these patients. If for any reason the patient cannot administer his own medication, it is very important that the nurse give these drugs on time, not within arbitrary half-hour leeways, for the patient may become too weak to swallow a tablet that comes late. It is not uncommon for "experienced" patients to become very apprehensive if their dose is even 5 minutes late. Parenteral and liquid preparations of the drugs being used should be available in the hospital unit in the event that the patient experiences swallowing difficulties.

Nurses can also help patients with myasthenia plan for changes in their physical activities which are consistent with their abilities. Services of vocational rehabilitation and social workers may be needed if increasing weakness will prevent the person from continuing his occupation.

Most patients quickly learn their limitations and live within them. However, myasthenics are not immune from the use of denial and may exhaust themselves in an attempt to prove that they are not really different. Teenagers find acceptance of the diagnosis particularly difficult and need much help from both hospital and community nurses in learning to conserve energy so that they can participate in school and social activities. The scheduling of activities to fall within the peak action of medication can be a help. The aggravating effect of other illness and of emotional stress on the myasthenic symptoms should be anticipated for the new patient. The importance of seeking medical care promptly, particularly for respiratory ailments, should be stressed to him.

The family must be included in this teaching for they need to be able to recognize drug overdosage or other crises. They should be made aware of symptoms of increasing muscular fatigue, i.e., increased nasality in speaking, difficulty in swallowing, use of the accessory muscles of respiration, and generalized weakness. In addition to recognition of symptoms, the family may need to learn how to arrange some activities (such as active sports, household chores, family outings) to coincide with the peak activity of the drug used. Both patient and family need to know the symptoms of over- and underdosage and the importance of seeking medical evaluation if they occur.

ACUTE CRISES

Intercurrent illness, cholinergic crisis, and surgical treatment of the disease all may induce acute crises; these require similar nursing care. Since myasthenic weakness commonly affects muscles of chewing, swallowing, and respiration, increased weakness is apt to cause a respiratory crisis. Increasing respiratory distress is the major manifestation of the patient in acute crisis. The person is dyspneic, is using the accessory muscles of respiration, is having difficulty in swallowing. The nostrils flare and respirations are apt to be noisy due to difficulty in swallowing secretions. Hypoxia is probably present to some degree and may be reflected earliest by increasing apprehension and vague or specific fears. The rapid collection of oral secretions indicates the need for frequent nasopharyngeal suctioning to prevent aspiration. The patient should be positioned on his side in order to prevent his tongue from occluding the airway and in order to promote drainage of secretions. Increasing respiratory distress may necessitate tracheotomy and assisted ventilation. Detailed information about the care of persons with assisted respiration may be found in other chapters.

Upper respiratory infections are more serious in these patients than in most people because myasthenia limits the strength available to raise secretions. Therefore, the nurse must assist the patient to raise and clear secretions. The former can be accomplished by placing one's hands on the patient's rib cage and manually compressing and vibrating the chest as the patient exhales. Additional techniques are described by Kurihara. Nasopharyngeal suctioning will aid in clearing the secretions thus raised. Nasotracheal suction may be necessary for those who cannot raise the secretions to the pharynx. Tracheotomy may eventually be necessary in such instances.

The patient will still be receiving medication but will probably be too ill to medicate himself. It is wise to remember that he is susceptible to becoming hypoxic. An early sign of hypoxia is clouded judgment; therefore, the patient cannot be relied upon to judge his own symptoms of overdosage.

THYMECTOMY

Nursing care of a person after thymectomy requires much technical skill plus the ability to care for a very apprehensive person. The patient's drug requirements change after surgery and must be reassessed; therefore, all anticholinergics are initially discontinued. Consequently, he is usually on assisted respiration, since the intercostal muscles are too weak to maintain effective inspiration. Tracheotomy and positive pressure respiration are used for this assistance.

Although the patient is able to move about in bed, he is quite weak and requires much assistance. The same needs for prevention of deformity exist as with any person with muscle weakness.

If anticholinergics are reinstituted (even if the surgery is successful, the ability to go without medication may not occur for several months), it is very important that the nurse recognize the difference between under- and overdosage and contact the physician if there is any question in her mind.

Bibliography

Adner, M. M., et al.: An Immunologic Survey of 48 Patients with Myasthenia Gravis. *New England Journal of Medicine,* 271:1327–1333, December 24, 1964.

Beeson, P. B. and Walsh McDermott (Eds.): *Cecil-Loeb Textbook of Medicine,* 12th ed. Philadelphia: W. B. Saunders Company, 1967, pp. 1675–1676.

Guyton, Arthur C.: *Textbook of Medical Physiology,* 3d ed. Philadelphia: W. B. Saunders Company, 1966, p. 85.

Kornfield, Peter, et al.: Studies in Myasthenia Gravis: Immunologic Response in Thymectomized and Nonthymectomized Patients. *Annals of Internal Medicine,* 63:416–428, September, 1965.

Kurihara, M.: Postural Drainage, Clapping and Vibrating. *American Journal of Nursing,* 65:76, November, 1965.

Schwab, R. S.: Problems in the Diagnosis and Treatment of Myasthenia Gravis. *Medical Clinics of North America,* 47:1511–1524, November, 1963.

Schwab, R. S.: Management of Myasthenia Gravis. *New England Journal of Medicine,* 268:717–719, March 28, 1963.

CHAPTER 30
THE PATIENT WITH DISEASE OF THE EYE AND EAR

SECTION 1
DISEASES
OF THE
EYE

ELIZABETH FORD PITORAK*

* Charles I. Thomas, M.D., Professor of Ophthalmology, Edward W. Purnell, M.D., Assistant Professor of Ophthalmology, and Philip Kazdan, M.D., Clinical Instructor in Ophthalmology, all of Case Western Reserve University, served as consultants in the preparation of this manuscript.

Vision is something most individuals take for granted. To be sure, the percentage of individuals who have normal sight is far greater than that of those who are partially sighted or blind. Nonetheless, the prevention of the loss of sight is of utmost importance as, in most instances, once vision is lost it cannot be regained. The nurse's role is all-encompassing, including not only that of teacher in the prevention of loss of sight in the community and hospital setting, but that of practitioner in the therapy of ophthalmological conditions. This role is not always an easy one to assume, as patients are frequently quite apprehensive because of fear of pain when any procedure is done to the eye and fear of loss of sight.

As with any specialty in medicine, there is wide variation in the treatment of diseases of the eye depending upon the ophthalmologist, the institution, and the geographical location. For that reason, the following discussion is written with emphasis upon general principles that apply to various ophthalmological conditions and the indicated therapy, rather than upon specific procedures or routines. The disease conditions discussed are those most commonly seen in the community and hospital setting. Both intraocular and extraocular conditions of a surgical and medical nature are considered, along with the nursing care which pertains thereto.

Because there is considerable variation in even the most commonly used opthalmological terminology, there is included an anatomical drawing of the eye bearing the descriptive terms used (Fig. 30–1). The reader should refer to an ophthalmology textbook for a detailed explanation of the anatomy and physiology of the eye.

Blindness

It is estimated that 399,000 persons in the United States are legally blind. Such persons demonstrate 20/200 or less vision in the better eye with corrective lenses,

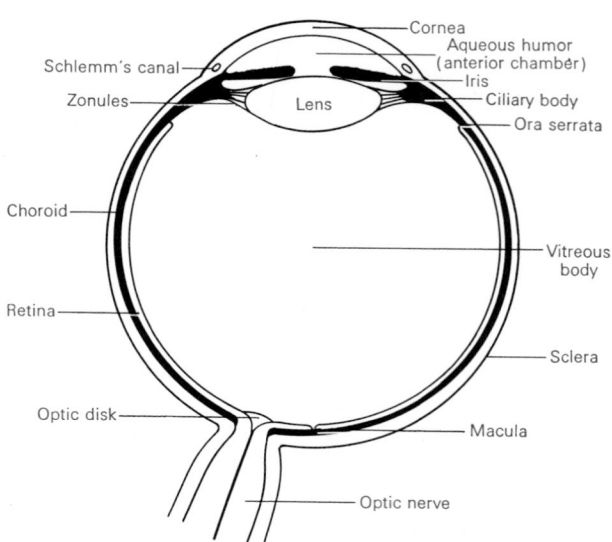

Figure 30–1
Anatomy of the eye.

or have a visual field subtending an angular distance no greater than 20 degrees at its widest diameter.

Much blindness has been prevented through research and medical therapy. Examples of this are retrolental fibroplasia, caused by overoxygenation of the premature infant, and ophthalmia neonatorum, caused by the gonococcus (*Neisseria gonorrhoeae*). Despite diligent research in prevention, there continue to be several thousand people blinded each year from diseases such as glaucoma and cataracts, diseases of unknown etiology which affect the ever-increasing older age group. It is hoped that continued, world-wide efforts in medical research, health education, and safety precautions will substantially reduce the incidence of blindness in forthcoming generations.

SOCIETAL CONSIDERATIONS

It is not the loss of sight which causes maladjustments in the blind but rather the resultant deprivation of love and respect which each individual deserves. Society has great difficulty in controlling its feelings and attitudes about the blind. For centuries, society has held a multitude of fixed ideas about the blind. They have been stereotyped as one class without considering individual differences, intellect, ambition, education, or personality. Historically there has been the connotation that blindness is a punishment for sins, particularly of a sexual nature. Also of a historical nature is the association between begging and blindness. At one time this was the only way the blind could possibly survive, as they were not educated or trained in any vocation. This is not true today; unfortunately, however, begging still exists. As a result of the many preconceived ideas that have persisted through the years, the blind individual has many fears and anxieties to cope with in addition to the fear of physical injury accompanying the loss of sight. Society seems to have ambivalent feelings about these individuals. One person will pity the blind person and expect him to be very dependent, whereas the next person will expect him to be completely independent. In general, people try to impose dependency upon the newly blind person instead of helping him work toward gradual independence.

Before the nurse can give therapeutic nursing care to a blind person, she must explore her own feelings about blindness. If the nurse is unable to govern her own emotions about the loss of sight, she will have difficulty in working with the sightless person. One main problem is having the same expectations for the blind person as she has for the sighted patient. This can result in having higher or lower expectations for the patient which is unrealistic. This problem can be solved by evaluating the patient more objectively, and reevaluating her own feelings.

It is easy to think of blindness as just a loss of sight; however, far more is involved than just the loss of one sense. There is a marked change in total body image and self-concept. Body image is the mental picture each of us has of his own body; self-concept includes the psychological self in addition to the physical self. This is not necessarily an accurate picture, but rather the individual's own interpretation. Body image and self-concept begin developing at the time of birth and continue to develop throughout life. It is through different sensory experiences and interactions with others that these concepts develop. How well an individual adjusts to a change in body image depends upon several factors, namely, his age, his usual reaction to stress, the significance of the lost part, how it interferes with interpersonal relationships, and society's attitude toward the disability.

THE REHABILITATION PROCESS

The rehabilitation process for a blind person is generally the same as for any person with a physical defect. The stage of shock is followed by the stage of depression. During the stage of shock lasting from days to weeks, the individual is unable to think or feel anything emotionally. It has been discovered through rehabilitation work that the longer this stage lasts, the more difficult it is for the individual to adjust to blindness. As the individual begins to experience emotions again, he feels depressed. There are different degrees of depression varying from mild to severe which could include thoughts of a suicidal nature. The patient goes through a period of mourning for his eyes, the same as an individual might mourn the loss of a loved one. The period of mourning is extremely important because it is during this period that the patient reorganizes his body image and self-concept. Without sight, he is a different person. Frequently friends, family, and medical personnel try to prevent the mourning period by giving the patient false hope of recovery. This stage should not be prevented as it has been demonstrated that the patient cannot be successfully rehabilitated until he has gone through this state of depression. Resolution of depression may be hastened by judicious use of activities at which the patient can succeed. One activity might be something as simple as successfully finding his way to the next room. To be sure, if the chosen task is too complex, it may prolong the stage of depression (Cholden, 1954).

Many principles utilized in guiding a blind person apply to a patient who is temporarily without sight because both eyes are covered by patches. If the sighted person would close his eyes for just a few minutes and try to orient himself to his environment and the people who enter it, he would soon become aware of some of the problems and feelings a sightless person encounters.

Whenever the nurse enters a sightless patient's room she should always introduce herself by name and relationship to the patient. Remember, a sightless person cannot identify people by their dress or face. After the nurse has spoken, it is thoughtful of her to touch the sightless person's arm or hand so that he can orient himself to her location in the room. This is particularly important for the person who is just beginning to adjust to a loss of sight. The nurse should also indicate her purpose in being there. Whenever a procedure is performed, it should be explained in detail. There have been anecdotes about sightless patients receiving intramuscular injections without any previous indication that this was going to happen. It seems impossible that any professional person could be so thoughtless. When leaving the room, the nurse should indicate that she is leaving and when she will return, as a sightless person finds it extremely annoying and embarrassing to continue the conversation thinking that someone is still in the room, and later realize that he has been talking to the wall.

When orienting the sightless person to his immediate environment, the nurse should show him exactly where the furniture and windows are located by touring the room with him, placing his hand on each object, and indicating its spatial relationship to the surrounding objects. The patient should also be oriented to the entire ward through indications of such things as the location of the nurses' station and the public telephone and their relationship to his room. One should explain the different hospital sounds he is likely to hear, as unfamiliar noises can be upsetting to the sightless person.

When guiding a sightless person, the nurse should always offer her arm for him to grasp rather than grasping his arm, as the latter places the sightless person in front of his guide and gives him the feeling that he is being pushed. The sightless person can feel the movements of his guide as he steps left or right, or up or down. One should always hesitate before ascending or descending stairs. When helping a sightless person to a chair, place his hand on either the arm or the back of the chair. When introduced to a sightless person, one should always speak and shake hands, as this helps him judge age, personality, character, physical strength, and the direction in which to turn. Also, touch helps to establish rapport.

Frequently people try to avoid using any words that give reference to sight in their conversation with blind persons. This is inadvisable. These words should be used in their usual context. For example, "Look at this material." The blind person can "see" it with his sensitive fingers determining the texture of the material, while the sighted person indicates the color and/or design. One should not be apologetic in a conversation when it gives references to sight. For example, "I am sorry you are unable to see the beautiful sunset today."

Have you ever watched a sightless person walk within a few inches of a wall and suddenly stop? This is because of the change in the pitch of sound. Also, changes in air currents are helpful in indicating the location of windows and doors.

The environment should never be changed in any way unless the sightless person realizes the change is taking place. For example, if the patient's comb is moved from the top of the bedside table and put in the dresser drawer, it might take hours for him to find it. Doors should be either completely opened or completely closed. If a door is left partially opened, he might walk directly into it, injuring himself.

Further rehabilitation outside the hospital is usually done by a local agency for the blind which may be affiliated with a national or philanthropic organization. The two main national organizations are The American Foundation for the Blind and The National Society for the Prevention of Blindness, both of which are located in New York City. These organizations provide information on problems of the blind including all types of literature and carry on research.

In addition to becoming independent in the tasks of daily living, the blind person must learn to travel independently. He is assisted in this learning through the use of a guide dog, a cane, or a sighted person.

Through government legislation many provisions have been made for the blind person. An example is the Pratt-Smoot Act, which authorizes the federal government to coordinate and expand library services for the blind on a national and regional basis. The program includes Braille books, Talking Books (literature that has been recorded), the machines on which these records are played, and a variety of other services. These services are available only to the legally blind.

Through the centuries, much progress has been made in the total area of blindness. Both society's attitude and the total rehabilitation of the blind have improved markedly; nonetheless, the future must demonstrate continued progress in these areas.

Refractive Errors

Few people go through life without having eye refraction done at one time or another. To understand refractive errors, it is important to understand the mechanism of accommodation, that is, the adjustment of the eye for seeing at different distances. As the object is brought closer to the eye, the ciliary muscle contracts, causing the lens to become more convex; thus the image is focused clearly on the retina.

The types of refractive errors are farsightedness (hyperopia), nearsightedness (myopia), distorted vision (astigmatism), and loss of accommodation (presbyopia). A collective term for these refractive errors is *ametropia*. *Emmetropia* refers to normal vision.

In addition to a decrease in visual acuity, there are other nonvisual signs and symptoms indicative of refractive errors. Because of the increased effort of accommodation, the patient complains of eye pain and headache, symptoms of "eye strain."

Hyperopia

In hyperopia, a hereditary disease, the rays of light entering the eye focus behind the retina. At birth most infants are hyperopic, but as the eyes grow, the condition disappears unless the person is destined to be hyperopic. Near vision is affected, but vision beyond a distance of 20 feet is usually normal. A second condition, which may be caused by hyperopia, is convergent strabismus, commonly known as *cross eyes*. The treatment for hyperopia is the use of corrective convex lenses.

Myopia

In myopia, also a hereditary disease, light rays focus in front of the retina because of an excessive refractive power. Obviously, there is no mechanism in the eye which can decrease the power of refraction. The myopic eye continues to grow at an abnormally fast rate throughout the "growing" years and to decrease in rate of growth after the early twenties. The main symptom is defective distant vision with normal near vision. In myopia, the retina, formed from neuroectoderm, does not grow at the same rate as the sclera, formed from mesoderm. As a result, the retinal tissue has to be stretched to grow at the same rate as the sclera; the resulting effect is degeneration of the retina. Secondary to the degenerative changes of the retina, tears and holes may occur, precipitating a retinal detachment. If these degenerative changes are detected with an ophthalmoscope, the patient is cautioned to limit vigorous physical activity, as trauma could predispose the patient to a retinal detachment (Saunders et al.). Myopia is corrected with use of concave lenses, which cause the light rays to diverge onto the retina.

Astigmatism

With an astigmatism, distorted vision results from unequal curvatures of the cornea, causing differences in the refractive power. This condition is also hereditary and may occur alone or in association with myopia or hyperopia. To treat an astigmatism, cylinder lenses are prescribed.

Presbyopia

Presbyopia is a decrease in the power of accommodation resulting from the gradual hardening of the nucleus of the crystalline lens. Because of this, people in the middle forties begin having difficulty in focusing on near objects, and experience blurring and discomfort when doing close work. Persons with presbyopia must hold reading material at an arm's length to focus well enough to read. Since the presbyopic eye is unable to focus from far to near vision, corrective bifocal lenses for both far and near vision are usually prescribed.

Refraction

A cycloplegic preparation such as Cyclogyl, atropine, homatropine is instilled into the cul-de-sac of the eyelid. The cycloplegic temporarily paralyzes the ciliary muscles thus blocking accommodation and dilating the pupil.

Refraction may be done through both subjective and objective methods. The subjective method involves having the patient try different lenses and distinguishing the effects these lenses have on the clarity of the letters on the Snellen chart. This method tests only distant vision. In vision screening with the Snellen chart, the patient usually stands 20 feet from it. The large E is scaled so that it can be read at a distance of 200 feet, and the following rows of letters are scaled to a size that can be read at various distances. The visual acuity is expressed in a fraction with the numerator indicating the distance in feet from the chart at which the patient is standing, and the denominator indicating the distance in feet of the lowest line of letters which the patient can read. For example, if the person tests 20/200, this means that at 20 feet the person is able to read a letter that should be visible at a distance of 200 feet. If the patient is unable to see the big E, the examiner holds up fingers for the patient to count, for example, C F 3 feet (able to count fingers at 3 feet). When the patient is unable to count fingers a light is shined into his eye, and if he can see the light it is recorded as L P (light perception). Individuals who are unable to perceive light are blind.

The objective methods involve the use of an ophthalmoscope and a retinoscope. In a retinoscopic examination a beam of light is directed through the pupil of the eye and the focus of rays of light is observed as they are reflected from the retina. Since each refractive error has a characteristic pattern of light movement when visualized with a retinoscope, corrective lenses can be prescribed by this method of examination. There is great confusion among the public about the names given the specialists who treat eye conditions. In the nurse's contact with the public she is frequently requested to explain what these differences are. An *optician* grinds and fits lenses; an *optometrist* is a nonmedical person who measures refractive errors and prescribes lenses; and an *ophthalmologist* or *oculist* (terms used interchangeably) is a medical doctor who diagnoses and treats ophthalmological conditions.

Contact Lenses

Corneal contact lenses, worn on the anterior surface of the cornea, are thin plastic disks with the optical correction ground into the front surface. The visual correction is usually good with these lenses. They are indicated for the following reasons: extreme myopia, hyperopia, keratoconus, and aphakia and for cosmetic reasons. Corneal contact lenses are worn more widely for severe myopia than for any other refractive error. This may be attributed to the fact that myopes are usually young people who would find the thick lenses necessary to correct their errors unsightly. It is advantageous for a person with hyperopia to wear contact lenses, as the size of the image is reduced, the visual field is larger, and near vision is increased. The prime ophthalmological indication for contact lenses is keratoconus, in which spectacles cannot adequately correct the marked astigmatism. In most cases of early keratoconus, contact lenses will restore vision by substituting a smooth surface for the irregular-shaped cornea. If contact lenses are worn in unilateral aphakia, binocular vision results because there is no discrepancy in the size of the image as occurs with spectacles. In bilateral aphakia, there is less distortion of the image and the image is reduced in size with an increase in the visual field. Also the ability to judge distance is improved over that with spectacles. Over 75 percent of individuals who wear contact lenses do so for cosmetic reasons. The contraindications to wearing contact lenses include both physical reasons, i.e., active inflammatory lesions of the eye and decreased lacrimation, and a psychological reason, i.e., poor motivation.

There are definite metabolic changes which occur in the cornea when adjustment is made to corneal contact lenses. Chief among these is corneal edema, the signs of which are tearing, burning, blurred vision, and decreased corneal sensitivity (Girard). Until the corneal edema subsides, it is necessary to wear the lenses for short periods of time with frequent rest periods and to gradually increase the wearing time each day. Before the lenses are inserted they should be cleaned well, and under no circumstances should saliva be used as the wetting agent as it has a high bacterial count. At times it may be necessary to use lemon juice to remove oil and makeup from the lenses.

The care and storage of the contact lenses are most important. Studies have indicated that a high degree of contamination that may lead to secondary bacterial infection of the cornea may be the direct result of improperly storing these lenses. The preferred method of storage is to clean the lenses of lid secretions and to store them in a dry, well-ventilated case, as a moist container acts as a culture medium for pathogenic bacteria. The lens case should be sterilized at least once a week by boiling. The common complication from wearing contact lenses is a corneal abrasion. There are relatively few cases of permanent eye damage resulting from wearing corneal contact lenses in relation to the large number of people who wear them (Dixon).

Trauma and Inflammatory Conditions

Any injury of the eye, either penetrating or nonpenetrating, is potentially dangerous. An injury of the same magnitude affecting any other part of the body might be insignificant, but in the eye it could lead to blindness. Even with broader public education about the need for safety glasses in industry, there continues to be a high incidence of injury. Children frequently sustain injuries to the eye from accidents with such articles as pointed toys and air rifles.

For the nurse it is important that the first aid measures used in case of injury be understood, as emergency treatment may save someone's sight. Whenever she is working with an injured eye, her hands should be washed well and all medications used in the eye should be sterile. For example, fluorescein, a dye used to stain the cornea in detection of corneal abrasions, can easily become contaminated with *Pseudomonas aeruginosa,* an organism highly pathogenic to corneal tissue. The cornea can be destroyed in a matter of several hours by this organism. Everyone has experienced having a foreign body, such as a piece of dirt or a tiny insect, in his eye at one time or another. Most foreign bodies, such as these, can be removed with a piece of twisted cotton. If the foreign body is on the cornea, it should be removed by an ophthalmologist, as the delicate epithelium of the cornea can be easily damaged. The cornea is less resistant to infection than the conjunctiva and scarring can easily occur impairing vision. Commonly, foreign bodies lodge on the inner surface of the upper lid and upon eversion of the upper lid they can be removed.

With any kind of chemical burn of the eye, regardless of the cause, the emergency treatment is always the same. Immediately open the eyelids and wash out the eye with copious amounts of tap water. Continue washing out the eye for 15 to 20 minutes before consulting an ophthalmologist (Saunders). Never take time to go to a hospital before washing out the eye, as the chemical will do damage as long as it is in contact with the cornea.

When working with a penetrating injury, the most important principle is to prevent the exertion of pressure upon the injured eye which might drive the object further into the eye causing additional damage. Apply a metal shield if available, or do nothing to the eye. Do not attempt to remove the foreign body or wipe the eye as this could cause more damage. The patient should not engage in any activity that might increase the intraocular pressure such as coughing, bending, or lifting, as this could result in the loss of intraocular contents.

An ophthalmologist should remove the foreign body if it is still present and treat the eye. Massive doses of antibiotics are given to control infection and steroids are administered for their anti-inflammatory effect.

With a penetrating injury the most feared complication is sympathetic opthalmia, the exact cause of which is unknown. The most accepted theory as to the cause is that it is the result of an allergic reaction to the uveal pigment. Sympathetic opthalmia is a severe uveitis in one eye resulting from a similar inflammation in the other eye which initially was caused by a penetrating injury into the uveal tissue. Less than 2 percent of perforating eye injuries result in this condition. The incubation period is 2 weeks to several years. If the injured eye is enucleated within 2 weeks after the injury, sympathetic ophthalmia will not develop. Since the advent of corticosteroids, most patients are treated with ACTH at the first sign of uveitis rather than sacrificing the eye. Once the uveitis has appeared in the second eye, an enucleation is not effective. If the patient is left untreated and sympathetic ophthalmia develops, the disease process will result in complete bilateral blindness. The second complication of a penetrating injury is the loss of the contents of the eye. If this should happen, it would be necessary to enucleate the eye.

Blepharitis

Blepharitis is an inflammatory condition of the lid margins which generally occurs bilaterally. Frequently it is a disease of long standing. The two main causes are the *Staphylococcus aureus* and a seborrheic condition of the scalp and brows.

The patient will have crusting with scale formation and irritation of the lid margins. As the disease progresses, ulcers may develop on the lid margins causing a loss of eye lashes. The symptoms are burning and itching of the eyes and lacrimation.

For treatment to be effective, the lid margins must be thoroughly cleansed of all crusts and scales. Warm compresses are applied for about 15 minutes three times a day to soften the crusts, which are then mechanically removed. Antibiotic ointments are applied to the lid margins and conjunctival sac. If the blepharitis is caused by a seborrhic condition, the scalp condition must be treated first.

Hordeolum

A hordeolum (stye) is one of the most common inflammatory conditions of the lid margin involving one of the hair follicles (glands of Zeis and Moll). In most cases, it is caused by a staphylococcal infection. A localized redness with swelling and tenderness appears at the site of infection. There are many pain fibers near the lid margin, so the pain will be commensurate with the degree of swelling. Warm moist compresses are applied for 15 minutes three or four times a day followed by the application of antibiotic ointments. Recurrent hordeolum may be an early sign of diabetes.

Chalazion

A chalazion is a granulomatous inflammation of the meibomian gland, a sebaceous gland of the eyelid. It frequently appears during pregnancy. In the acute stage the symptoms may be similar to those of a hordeolum. During this stage, warm moist compresses and antibiotic ointments are used. In the chronic stage a hard painless lump, or cyst, appears on the inner aspect of the eyelid. The cyst is excised by an ophthalmologist in his office or clinic setting.

Conjunctivitis

Conjunctivitis is an inflammatory condition of the conjunctiva commonly known as *pink eye*. Since the conjunctiva is commonly in contact with many microorganisms, it is susceptible to infection. There are many causes of conjunctivitis, the more common ones being of viral, bacterial, or allergic nature. Sometimes mechanical trauma, such as a sunburn to the conjunctiva, may be the cause.

The conjunctiva contains many blood vessels and few pain fibers; this accounts for the main symptoms of redness without pain. Tearing is always present with conjunctivitis. When the lids are closed the temperature of the conjunctival sac increases thus providing a favorable environment in which the organisms can grow and produce pus. This causes the eyelids to adhere when one awakens in the morning. Treatment depends upon the specific cause. Usually antibiotics, sulfonamides, or steroids are utilized as therapeutic measures. Most forms of conjunctivitis are contagious, so hygienic measures should be utilized to prevent contamination of the other eye or of other people. Recommended practices are frequent hand washing, using a separate towel and washcloth for the infected eye, and use of individual towels and washcloths by other family members.

The public health nurse has an important role in teaching preventive measures of general hygiene to be used in the home and school setting, as conjunctivitis frequently occurs in school-age children.

Trachoma

Trachoma is a bilateral granular conjunctivitis caused by a virus. It affects approximately 15 percent of the world population causing more cases of blindness than any other known condition. All races are affected. There is a definite and direct relationship between the incidence of trachoma and impoverished socioeconomic conditions. In the United States, the disease is well controlled with some cases occurring among the mountain people of West Virginia and Tennessee, Indian Americans, and Mexican Americans.

Follicles form on the palpebral surfaces of both eyelids causing the sensation of a foreign body and accompanied by mild itching and irritation. The symptoms are much more severe in the superior than the inferior conjunctiva. Gradually the upper position of the cornea is invaded with development of white spots and a network of blood vessels known as pannus. Ulcers of the cornea may form leading to clouding and eventual scarring of the cornea. The usual treatment is the use of antibiotics. Personal hygiene is important in both prevention and spread of the disease. Since trachoma is a disease generated by filthy living conditions, health education about the proper use of individual towels and washcloths including frequent laundering and hand washing before and after touching the eyes must be emphasized (Vaughan et al.).

Keratitis

An inflammation of the cornea is called *keratitis*. There are two types: superficial keratitis is caused by infection from the outside, and deep keratitis is caused by spread of the etiologic agent by the blood or from neighboring structures. The cornea has many pain fibers giving rise to the symptom of pain. The circumcorneal blood vessels dilate causing ciliary injection, and the involved cornea usually becomes cloudy. The patient complains of photophobia, lacrimation, and impaired vision.

Cultures are done to determine the nature of the organism and treatment is instituted. Topical steroids are used except in herpes simplex and dendritic keratitis in which they are contraindicated.

Corneal Ulcers

Corneal ulcer is an ulcerated area on the surface of the cornea with definite loss of epithelium. Frequently the ulcer is caused by actual trauma to the cornea or infection of the conjunctiva which involves the cornea. The offending organisms are usually bacterial, viral, or fungal in nature.

Corneal ulcers are treated with wide-spectrum antimicrobial agents and topical and systemic steroids. Steroids are contraindicated if herpes simplex or fungal involvement is present. Even with treatment, scarring causing opacification and eventual blindness may result.

Uveitis

Uveitis is an inflammatory condition of the uveal tract, the pigmented vascular layer of the eye (iris, ciliary body, and choroid). If just the iris and ciliary body are involved, it is referred to as *iridocyclitis*. When the choroid is involved the retina will be involved also because of the proximity of the two structures; this condition is known as *chorioretinitis*. Uveitis is usually a unilateral disease affecting the young middle-age group.

The etiology is unknown in the majority of cases. The agents responsible are classified as exogenous or endogenous infections and allergic manifestations. Exogenous infections indicate a direct entrance of bacteria or virus into the eye resulting from a puncture wound. Cases of uveitis resulting from organisms in the bloodstream, focal infections, tuberculosis, brucellosis, or toxoplasmosis are classified as endogenous infections. Allergic manifestations are nonpurulent infections caused by an antigen-antibody reaction. An example of an allergic manifestation is arthritis.

The signs and symptoms of uveitis depend upon which part of the uveal tract is involved. If the iris is involved, pain and photophobia will be present, as the iris has many pain fibers. Because of dilatation of the iris blood vessels, there is a sluggish movement to the iris. Adhesions (synechiae) may form between the posterior surface of the iris and the lens resulting in an irregular-shaped pupil. Associated with iris involvement is ciliary injection caused by dilatation of the limbal blood vessels. The iris forms a white exudate which is deposited on the endothelial surface of the cornea. The patient may complain of blurred vision if the aqueous humor in the anterior chamber is cloudy due to the presence of fibrin.

With choroidal involvement, yellowish-white lesions appear on the retina and the resulting visual loss in the peripheral areas of the retina corresponds with the location of these lesions. If there is a lesion on the macula, a decrease in central acute vision results. Also, decreased visual acuity may be caused by clouding of the vitreous.

In the diagnosis of uveitis, skin tests are given to rule out tuberculosis, histoplasmosis, and toxoplasmosis. In addition, it is important to rule out other diseases such as conjunctivitis and glaucoma, which can cause similar symptoms.

The course of the disease varies greatly depending upon the etiology. Uveitis caused by an allergic manifestation will last for a few weeks and recurrences are common; however, if the etiologic agent is of an endogenous type, such as tuberculosis or toxoplasmosis, it may last from months to years with frequent remissions and exacerbations. Visual loss occurs more frequently with the endogenous type.

In treatment the pupils of the eyes are dilated with a mydriatic, atropine, to keep the iris at rest and to prevent the formation of posterior synechiae. If posterior synechiae form, the normal pathway for the aqueous humor would be blocked resulting in an increase in intraocular pressure and secondary glaucoma. Symptomatic treatment includes the use of warm compresses, codeine and aspirin to relieve pain, and dark glasses to relieve photophobia. Corticosteroids are used widely for their antiallergic and anti-inflammatory effects. Topical steroids, examples being dexamethasome (Decadron) and prednisolone phosphate sodium (Hydeltrasol), are indicated when the anterior segments of the uveal tract are involved. In treating the posterior segments of the uveal tract, systemic forms of corticosteroids, such as prednisolone and ACTH, are used. When ACTH is given intravenously the initial dose may be as high as 80 to 120 units in 1,000 ml of fluid. Each day the dose is gradually decreased. As a last resort fever therapy may be used. A temperature elevation of 103° to 104° F is considered desirable, and this is usually achieved by the intramuscular or intravenous injection of typhoid vaccine. The treatment is given every day or several times a week. Possible complications secondary to uveitis are the following: glaucoma, caused by synechiae; cataract, caused by poor metabolism of the lens; and detached retina, caused by vitreous strands resulting from the inflammatory process (Shafer et al.).

The aims of nursing care are to prevent cross-infection and to foster healing by accomplishing hygienic measures, administering the anti-inflammatory medications and mydriatics, and making pertinent observations about the disease and side effects of the medications. With large doses of corticosteroids the patient may experience symptoms of Cushing's syndrome. To make safe nursing judgments, the nurse must be cognizant of these symptoms.

The patient and family need much reassurance from the medical team, as the patient may have frequent exacerbations requiring prolonged therapy. During an acute attack the therapy may be prolonged with a slow change in the condition of the eye. In addition, the patient may lose his sight despite medical therapy. Considering all these facts, it is obvious how very depressed the patient and his family may become. They need to be shown much psychological support and handled with patience throughout the stormy course of the disease.

Disorders Necessitating Surgery

NURSING CONSIDERATIONS

Preoperative Care

Some conditions of the eyes such as cataract, glaucoma, and detached retina may necessitate surgery. Certain preoperative preparations apply to both intraocular and extraocular surgery. The patient is usually quite fearful because of the extreme importance of the eyes, and the possibility of a complication occurring and leading to loss of sight is frequently uppermost in his mind. He should be given sufficient opportunity to verbalize his fear and to discuss his needs.

The patient should be thoroughly oriented to the environment of the ward and to the personnel. This orientation includes familiarizing him with such things as the physical arrangement of his room and the location of the telephone, the lavatory, and the nurses' station. Even though only one eye may be covered postoperatively, the patient may have poor visual acuity in the unoperated eye which inhibits his ability to walk about in the unfamiliar environment. The majority of these patients are elderly, and at times they become disoriented. Sometimes this disorientation will clear as soon as they return home to familiar surroundings, which suggests that the more familiar the patient is with his surroundings, the less likely is there to be a problem with disorientation.

Preoperative teaching should cover the essential aspects of postoperative care, including the patient's position in bed, permissible activity, and restrictions according to the principles involved. Most hospitals have established routines dealing with eye surgery generally, with additional orders varying according to individual patient needs. Routines in preoperative care vary with the institutions, the geographic location, and the individual ophthalmologist; however, there are certain common aspects in preoperative care. Some of these procedures may be performed in either the patient's room or the operating room. As in any patient undergoing surgery, the operative area has to be carefully cleansed. The area must be shaved or closely clipped prior to surgery. The eyelashes are cut with tiny scissors coated with petrolatum, which makes the lashes adhere to the scissors and prevents them from getting into the eye. This procedure may be performed by either the doctor or the nurse depending upon the hospital routine. A hexachlorophene solution such as pHisoHex is used for scrubbing the brows, including the area surrounding the eyes. Normal saline irrigations of the eye may be carried out.

In most cases of intraocular surgery, cycloplegics, mydriatics, and local anesthetics are instilled into the cul-de-sac of the lower lid to obtain maximum dilatation and to anesthesize the eye locally. Since this type of surgery is performed under a local nerve block, the patient usually is not given a cleansing enema preoperatively. Male patients must be shaved preoperatively since shaving is not permitted during the first postoperative days. Since a shampoo may not be allowed for several weeks postoperatively, the patient should have a shampoo before the day of operation. If the patient's hair is long, it should be combed and braided since only gentle hair combing is permitted postoperatively.

The morning of the day of surgery an analgesic and a sedative are given in preparation for the local anesthetic. Local anesthetics are preferred in intraocular surgery because of the possibility that the patient will become nauseated under general anesthesia and vomit, thereby increasing the intraocular pressure. Further, the majority of the patients are of the older age group and are poor surgical risks.

When a local anesthetic is administered, a retrobulbar infiltration is made into the muscle cone producing akinesia of the rectus muscles innervated by cranial nerves III and VI and blocking the ciliary ganglion, a branch of cranial nerve

V, which is the sensory innervation of the cornea, iris, and sclera. In addition a facial infiltration is performed to block cranial nerve VII producing akinesia of the eyelids. Extraocular surgery including muscle surgery, enucleation, and retinal detachment surgery is usually done with the patient under a general anesthetic.

Postoperative Care

Intraocular surgery is classified as any surgery in which the eye is opened, i.e., cataract extraction, keratoplasty, iridectomy, and filtering procedures for glaucoma. Certain types of surgery for detached retina would also be considered intraocular surgery as needles are inserted through the choroidal coat to drain subretinal fluid. The major aims of nursing care are to prevent an increase in intraocular pressure, to prevent stress on the suture line, and to prevent hemorrhage.

To prevent an increase in the intraocular pressure, any activity that increases the venous pressure in the area of the head must be avoided. When the venous return from the head is blocked, the blood vessels in the eye dilate from the increase in venous blood, thus potentially increasing the intraocular pressure to pathologic levels. With an increase in the venous pressure, arterial pressure, or both, a change in the blood flow through the uvea will occur simultaneously. This increases the intraocular pressure, as the amount of aqueous humor secreted is increased. An increase in intraocular pressure would put additional stress on the suture line. Examples of these activities are vomiting, straining at bowel movements, bending over, lifting heavy objects, and coughing. If the patient becomes nauseated, an antiemetic should be given immediately, without waiting until the patient vomits. The patient should not move any object weighing more than 2 to 3 pounds, and then only from waist level. If he feels he has to cough, he should be instructed to keep his mouth open to prevent any repercussion in the head. The nurse's role is to help the patient realize the necessity for restricted activity, as most patients feel fine and think they can resume normal activity. During the first few hours after surgery the head of the bed is usually elevated to 30 degrees with position of choice used thereafter. The furniture in the room should be arranged so that the bedside stand is on the patient's unoperated side and he can reach everything on it without straining. In most institutions, a complete bed bath is given on the first postoperative day and thereafter he can do the parts of his bath which do not cause any straining. The activity permitted the patient will vary depending upon the individual ophthalmologist and institution; the trend is to permit the patient to be out of bed on the first postoperative day with a gradual increase in time each day.

The second aim in nursing care is to prevent stress on the suture line. The patient should be cautioned not to squeeze his eyelids as this could force the wound open. To prevent putting pressure on the eye, the patient is instructed to turn to the unoperated side only. A soft diet is ordered at first to avoid the stress of mastication. Male patients should not shave until the doctor so orders. Gentle hair combing is not contraindicated.

The third aim is to prevent hemorrhage. Forceful squeezing of the eyelids is contraindicated as this may cause hyphema (hemorrhage into the anterior chamber). General overactivity is another factor that may cause hemorrhage.

In addition to specific principles, there are general measures to be considered. Some patients have hallucinations of a visual or auditory nature postoperatively. Although it is unquestionable that there are patients wearing eye patches who are or become psychotic, it is a mistake to think that all patients whose eyes are covered and who experience hallucinations are psychotic. Many investigators believe that these hallucinations are caused by sensory deprivation, although proof for this is lacking. At present the many uncontrolled variables make it impossible to infer a correlation between the two.

Sometimes an elderly patient will become disoriented when both eyes are covered, especially at night when other environmental stimuli are decreased. With the removal of one eye patch, the patient can usually reorient himself.

Providing appropriate diversional activity can be quite a challenge, since many patients have poor visual acuity in the unoperated eye. The use of Talking Books can be quite helpful. Information about them can be obtained from the Division for the Blind, Library of Congress, Washington, D.C. There is a regional agency in every state which lends Talking Book machines, and each state has regional public libraries that lend Talking Book records. The nurse or a family member can read to the patient. Since many patients tend to keep to themselves and not venture out of their rooms, it is important for the nurse to introduce them to other patients if they seem to desire company.

Some time should be spent with the family members in instructing them about permitted activity, including those restrictions necessary to ensure an uncomplicated recovery. The family can be made to feel that they are important to the patient's recovery. For example, if the patient has poor visual acuity in the unoperated eye, it will be necessary to feed him—an activity in which the family can participate. Since the family will not be present for all meals, a member of the health team will be feeding the patient the majority of his meals. That person should always explain the contents of the tray before feeding the patient and should learn the order in which the patient likes his food presented. Mealtime should be made pleasant and unhurried—most people dislike being fed even under the best of circumstances. Consideration should be given to teaching the patient who has poor visual acuity this activity. The easiest approach is through the "clock" method. The nurse might say, for example, "The meat is at nine o'clock, the potato is at three o'clock, and the beets are at six o'clock. Your coffee is to the right of your plate." It is a rare patient who cannot be taught to feed himself.

There are various opinions about the need for side rails. In some institutions side rails are kept raised during both waking hours and the hour of sleep; in others the side rails are raised at the hour of sleep only and are kept lowered during the daytime unless the patient is disoriented or very debilitated. Usually, if both eyes are covered, both side rails are raised and if only one eye is covered, the side rail on the ipsilateral side is raised.

Cataract

Any opacification of the lens is classified as a cataract. Since this is not a reportable disease, there are no reliable figures as to incidence. Cataracts may occur at any age; however, the majority occur in the older age group as a result of aging and degeneration, and they are present to some degree in most persons over the age of 60.

There are several types of cataracts, depending upon the cause. The most common are senile cataracts. Traumatic cataracts, caused by intraocular foreign bodies penetrating the lens, infrared light, radioactive materials, poisons, or x-rays, represent a second type of lens opacification. The third type is the congenital cataract, which may result from maternal rubella during the first trimester of pregnancy. In some instances cataract is associated with systemic diseases among which are diabetes mellitus and hypoparathyroidism, or is secondary to an intraocular disease such as uveitis. At present the exact etiology of this disease entity is unknown.

Measures can be taken to prevent the development of traumatic cataracts, e.g., wearing safety glasses wherever necessary in industrial installations to prevent the entrance of an intraocular foreign body into the lens.

Pathological changes occur in the lens whenever there is a disturbance of its transparency, specifically lens edema, opacification, necrosis, and interruption to the continuity of the lens fibers.

The onset is usually gradual and it is impossible to determine how rapidly the process will progress, as it varies from individual to individual. Usually the only symptom is progressive blurred vision or a hazy appearance to objects. The effect on visual acuity will be determined by the area of opacification. A peripheral opacification of the lens will not affect the visual acuity as quickly as a central opacification. Also, there is some change in color perception especially of yellow and blue. As has been previously stated, the course of the disease varies; in some cases, if the cataract is not extracted, vision will be reduced to light perception and ultimately blindness will ensue.

SURGICAL TREATMENT

The aim of therapy is to restore visual acuity. At present, there is no known medical therapy, and surgical treatment is indicated at that time when visual impairment interferes with the patient's ability to pursue normal daily activities. The method of intracapsular lens extraction does not necessitate waiting for the lens to "ripen" and in most cases is currently the method of choice. In this method, alpha-chymotrypsin, an enzyme that dissolves the zonular fibers, is usually instilled into the anterior chamber of the eye if the person is under 50 years of age. After this age, the zonules lose some of their elasticity and break more readily, and administration of the enzyme is usually not necessary. Slight traction on the lens and countertraction at the corneal scleral junction (limbus) causes the lens within its capsule to tumble from the eye. At the time of surgery, a prophylactic iridectomy is done to prevent the vitreous from moving forward, blocking the pupil, and causing secondary glaucoma.

The second surgical method of treatment is through extracapsular lens extraction, consisting of removal of the anterior capsule and lens and leaving the posterior capsule in place. This method is used in patients up to the age of 20 years and also in cases of extreme myopia. Up to the age of 20 the posterior capsule is adherent to the vitreous which prevents the use of the intracapsular method. In approximately one-third of patients having an extracapsular lens extraction, a secondary membrane forms requiring a discission, or needling, of the membrane. The principles applying to intraocular surgery are utilized in post-operative nursing care.

Visual acuity is improved in 90 percent or more of patients following a lens extraction. As with any surgical procedure, certain complications are possible. An infection may develop. Hyphema may develop within 48 to 72 hours after surgery. In the latter case the patient usually experiences a sudden pain in the eye. Hyphema may develop without apparent cause, or the patient feeling dis-comfort may inadvertently squeeze the eye and thereby cause the hyphema. Secondary glaucoma can result from the presence of peripheral anterior synechiae. Finally, a serious complication is retinal detachment, occurring in the eye with degenerative changes in the retina. If vitreous is lost at the time of surgery, a vitreous band may form and pull off the retina (Fasanella).

POSTOPERATIVE MEASURES

The patient who has undergone a lens extraction must make many adjustments when he receives his spectacles. Following a unilateral lens extraction the person cannot wear spectacles and have binocular vision, because cataract spectacles magnify everything seen by one-third. As a result, vision in the unoperated eye would be normal, whereas that in the operated eye would magnify all objects seen by one-third, with consequent diplopia. If a contact lens is worn there is about 5 percent magnification, because the closer the corrective lens is to the retina the less magnification there will be. Therefore if a patient who has had a unilateral lens extraction wears a contact lens on that eye he will have binocu-lar vision. A major problem is that many of these patients are in the older age group and they have difficulty in learning how to insert and remove contact lenses.

With bilateral lens extractions, either corneal contact lenses or heavy spectacle glasses may be worn. The majority of patients wear the spectacles and find that many adjustments must be made. Because of the magnification produced the wearer may misjudge spatial relationships. For example, when pouring coffee, he may miss the cup because it appears to be closer than it actually is. Then too, optical illusions may develop. For example, a door frame may appear to be curved. To help the patient correct the problem, the nurse might suggest that he learn to fix his gaze through the center of the correcting lens and move his head slowly when looking to the side rather than move his eyes only. To improve his manual coordination he should be encouraged to practice tasks requiring fine coordinated movements. In the periphery of the visual field there is a ring of a blind area; thus the patient constantly hits objects, and when he is in a group of people faces keep appearing and disappearing as they enter the blind area. Crossing the street could be hazardous, since a car turning into the patient's path would not be seen if it was in the area of blind vision. Then too, if the heavy spectacles are dropped, they are no longer properly adjusted. For proper focusing the spectacles must be at the correct distance from the eye (Woods).

Upon his discharge from the hospital the patient will follow the same restric-tions of activity for an additional 6 weeks. Probably the most helpful instruction the nurse might offer is that he use normal common sense—eye tissue heals more slowly than tissue elsewhere in the body. The hair should not be washed at home for 6 weeks. It can be washed in 3 weeks if it is done in a beauty parlor equipped with a tray arrangement for shampoos, and the operator should be instructed to be gentle and not scrub. Sponge baths are taken during the first month; the patient may not shower or get into and out of a bathtub. Cooking and light housework are permitted during the first 6 weeks. After 5 to 6 weeks the patient's vision is tested in preparation for his wearing spectacles. He should be instructed to hold his glasses by the tips when putting them on to avoid touching the eye, and to wear sun glasses when in sunlight to avoid photophobia.

Eye care is minimal. Mild discomfort, ache, and pain are to be expected, but if the pain is persistent the doctor should be notified. Tap water boiled for at least 10 minutes is used to cleanse the edge of the lower lid. For 3 to 4 weeks a patch is worn over the eye at night to prevent the patient from rubbing it and to prevent pressure on it.

Glaucoma

There are several types of glaucoma, as will be described. Glaucoma is a condition of the eye characterized by increased intraocular pressure leading to cupping and degeneration of the optic disk and changes in the visual field. Thirteen percent of verified cases of blindness in the United States are caused by primary glaucoma, and 2 percent of the population aged 40 or above have glaucoma. Primary glaucoma, a bilateral disease usually affecting one eye earlier than the other, is probably genetically determined.

For the nurse to understand the pathology of glaucoma, the normal physiology of intraocular pressure must be reviewed. The intraocular pressure expresses the relationship between the rate of aqueous humor production by the ciliary body and the resistance to outflow of aqueous humor. Aqueous humor diffuses through the pupil into the anterior chamber, where it passes through the angle of the eye and trabecular meshwork into Schlemm's canal. In Schlemm's canal there are collecting canals which lead into the venous system.

OPEN ANGLE GLAUCOMA

The most common type of glaucoma is open angle glaucoma, also classified as chronic, simple, or wide angle glaucoma. It is hereditary. There is an obstruction to the outflow of aqueous humor caused by degenerative changes in the trabeculum, Schlemm's canal, and adjacent channels that collect the aqueous, but the angle of the eye appears normal. The constant increased intraocular pressure results in damage to the nerve fibers of the retina and optic nerve, and the optic nerve undergoes degeneration with cupping of the disk giving a "bean pot" appearance.

Although open angle glaucoma cannot be prevented it can be controlled medically and blindness can be prevented. The condition must be detected early. All persons over 40 years of age, but particularly those with a familial history of open angle glaucoma, should have tonometry readings done to determine whether there is an increase in intraocular pressure.

The onset is insidious, and loss of vision occurs in the absence of symptoms. There is a gradual loss of peripheral vision which the patient may become aware of only accidentally. One example is that of an excellent tennis player who began to consistently miss the ball when it entered the area of his peripheral vision; upon examination he was diagnosed as having advanced glaucoma. In the absence of headache, pain, or redness of the eye, the patient usually does not seek medical treatment until there is a loss of central acute vision, by which time the disease is far advanced.

One method utilized in diagnosis is tonometry, which measures intraocular pressure. A topical anesthetic is placed on the eye and the tonometer is placed on the cornea. (The patient should be cautioned to protect the eyes following the test since the cornea may be anesthetized for a period of time and he will be unaware should foreign objects enter the eye.) A reading of 20 mm mercury indicates an increase in intraocular pressure. Cupping of the optic disk and changes in the visual fields are significant findings.

The water provocative test may be carried out. In this test the patient drinks 1 quart of water after fasting for at least 8 hours. The intraocular pressure is then recorded at 15-minute intervals. In normal individuals there will be a slight rise in intraocular pressure; a rise of 10 mm mercury or more is positive for open angle glaucoma.

The course of the disease is variable and the prognosis is usually guarded. If it is not treated, absolute glaucoma and blindness will result, but if it is treated with miotics the prognosis is fairly good provided that extensive damage has not occurred prior to initiation of therapy.

The aims of medical therapy are to control the intraocular pressure and to prevent visual field loss with miotics, which constrict the pupil. Most commonly pilocarpine is used in a strength of 1 to 6 percent. Cholinesterase inhibitors, such as eserine, isoflurophate (DFP, Floropryl), and demecarium bromide (Humorsol) may be used; they are more potent than pilocarpine. Acetazolamide (Diamox) is given to inhibit the enzyme, carbonic anhydrase, which appears to be necessary to aqueous production, so that the volume of aqueous humor is decreased.

The patient must understand that miotics will not cure the glaucoma but will control the intraocular pressure. He must follow the prescribed therapy for the rest of his life and must not skip a dose.

If the intraocular pressure cannot be controlled with medical therapy, a surgical procedure must be performed. In open angle glaucoma a filtering procedure is performed in which an opening is created in the subconjunctival space for diffusion of aqueous humor, thus bypassing the trabecular meshwork. Examples of filtering procedures are the Scheie procedure, corneal scleral trephination, and iridencleisis. In some cases cyclodiathermy may be necessary to reduce the formation of aqueous humor by partially destroying the ciliary body.

The aims of nursing care are to educate the patient about the nature of glaucoma, to administer the medication as ordered, and to give the correct nursing care postoperatively. Probably the nurse's most important role is that of teacher. Among nurses there seem to be many misconceptions about necessary restrictions for the glaucoma patient, and by imposing unnecessary restrictions the nurses merely aggravate matters. A frequent cause of treatment failure is the patient's lack of understanding of his disease and its therapy (Schwartz).

Use of the eyes is not harmful and the patient's reading need not be restricted.

Drinking a normal amount of fluids will not increase the intraocular pressure. Ingestion of a cupful or two of coffee at one time is not contraindicated. There are rare cases where the patient's intraocular pressure rises due to caffeine. Ingestion of alcohol per se is not contraindicated, but it imposes two problems: it transiently lowers the intraocular pressure which could cause an error in management if the patient had consumed alcohol just before tonometry was done; and if the patient consumes excessive amounts of alcohol and becomes intoxicated he cannot follow the prescribed therapy (Saunders; Schwartz).

Since with miotic therapy the pupils will remain constricted regardless of the presence of light or darkness, the patient should be allowed to sit in theaters and other darkened places. The effect of emotional states on intraocular pressure is controversial. In general, emotional tension does not greatly affect the intraocular pressure although a few cases have been reported wherein emotional tension initiated an acute attack of narrow angle glaucoma.

It is extremely important that the patient understand that the lost vision cannot be regained, but that further loss will be largely preventable through the correct use of eye drops. Each patient should be taught to administer his own eye drops. The nurse might instruct him as follows: Put pressure on the bony orbit to pull down the lower eyelid. Drop the medication into the pocket of the lower lid (cul-de-sac), where it is absorbed, and not on the cornea, which is highly sensitive.

If he is using a potent medication such as DFP, he should be instructed to wipe the excess from the inner corner of the eyelid so that it will not be absorbed systemically. The nurse must be certain that the patient understands how and when to use the drops. Since intraocular pressure is slightly higher in the early morning hours, miotics are usually prescribed for use upon arising and at bedtime as well as at intervals between. Many systemic side effects can occur and the patient should be aware of the specific effects of the miotic prescribed and taught to notify the doctor should they arise.

The family must understand the nature of the disease and the need for lifetime therapy. Glaucoma is like diabetes mellitus in that it can be controlled but not cured. Even if a filtering procedure is performed, it is still necessary for the patient to visit the doctor regularly as the procedure sometimes is not successful.

Several problems are associated with the use of miotics. The patient has difficulty seeing in dark places because mydriasis does not occur, and extra lighting must be provided. Night driving demands extra precautions. Leisure-time activities are impaired by the loss of accommodation; it is difficult to read for long periods of time, and impossible to play games in which there are fast-moving objects. Even with good lighting it is difficult to descend stairs.

Most patients with open angle glaucoma whom the nurse sees in the hospital are admitted for reasons other than glaucoma unless they are to undergo a surgical procedure for glaucoma. For this reason it is very easy for the doctor to forget to order the necessary miotics. If the patient states that he uses miotics, the nurse should follow through in procuring the necessary order, as it is very risky for him to miss a dose. The miotic should be administered according to the patient's normal schedule, rather than trying to make his schedule conform to the hospital routine.

The postoperative nursing care is the same as for other intraocular surgery except that the patient's activity is not restricted for as long a period of time.

ANGLE CLOSURE GLAUCOMA

The second type of glaucoma is angle closure glaucoma (narrow or closed angle). This type is much less frequent than open angle glaucoma. There is a sudden rise in intraocular pressure caused by closure or blockage of the angle of the anterior chamber of the eye. The root of the iris blocks the angle thus preventing outflow of aqueous humor. Any of several predisposing factors may be present: (1) Hyperopia, in which the anterior chamber is narrow. (2) Pupillary block may precipitate an acute attack of glaucoma. With pupillary block, synechiae form between the lens and iris obstructing the normal pathway of aqueous from the posterior chamber. Consequently, aqueous accumulates in the posterior chamber and forces the root of the iris forward to block the chamber angle. (3) Increased thickness of the iris caused by mydriasis.

The pathology of angle closure glaucoma is different from that of open angle glaucoma. In angle closure glaucoma, the trabecular meshwork and Schlemm's canal are normal, whereas in open angle there is degeneration of these two structures. The only abnormality in angle closure glaucoma is a narrowed chamber angle that may be blocked by the root of the iris (Fig. 30–2). The pathological changes occurring in an acute attack are edema and congestion of the ciliary processes and iris. There is damage to the nerves of the retina, which undergoes degeneration in the same manner as in advanced open angle glaucoma.

With angle closure glaucoma, the patient experiences excruciating pain in the eye which radiates to adjacent areas. This pain is caused by the very high intraocular pressure, which may be as high as 80 to 100 mm mercury (normal, not above 20 mm). The corneal edema causes blurring of vision and the impression of halos around lights. If the corneal edema is severe, low visual acuity permitting light perception only or temporary blindness may result. The eye is severely injected. Frequently the patient is nauseated and vomits, but unfortunately these symptoms may be mistaken for signs of an acute abdomen.

An acute attack is diagnosed on the basis of the signs and symptoms, tonom-

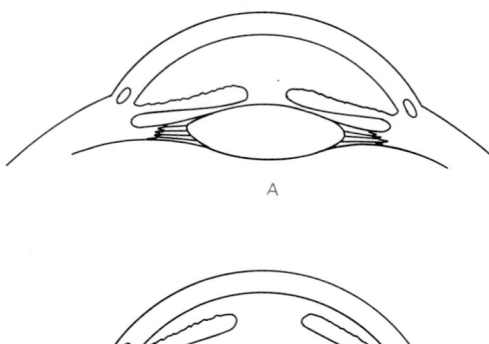

Figure 30–2 A, Normal chamber angle. B, Chamber angle blocked by iris root.

A

B

etry readings, and gonioscopy (visualization of the angle of the eye). A narrow and blocked angle indicates acute angle closure glaucoma. If the acute attack is not treated, it is possible for absolute glaucoma to develop within a few days. In this condition the eye becomes hard and sightless and may be painful, and enucleation is necessary. Between acute attacks, the eye is normal, but after repeated attacks there is permanent damage in the form of synechiae at the chamber angle, cupping of the disk, and field changes. In 50 percent of cases there will be an acute attack in the other eye even though miotic therapy has been initiated.

The aims of medical therapy are to decrease the intraocular pressure and to relieve the pain and nausea. A miotic such as pilocarpine is administered every 15 minutes for a few hours to decrease the intraocular pressure by pulling the iris away from the angle of the eye and thus permit drainage of aqueous. In addition to topical medications, either urea or mannitol is administered intravenously to reduce intraocular pressure.

If these measures do not produce a decrease in the intraocular pressure within 6 hours, surgery is indicated. An iridectomy, which is the removal of a wedge of iris, is done to provide an opening of the angle, and a prophylactic iridectomy is usually done on the other eye. If synechiae have formed at the angle, a filtering procedure may be necessary.

During the acute attack the patient experiences excruciating pain, and either morphine or meperidine (Demerol) is administered. Nothing should be given by mouth as the patient is usually nauseated and may be vomiting.

ABSOLUTE GLAUCOMA

In absolute glaucoma the eye is stony hard, painful, and blind. Alcohol is injected into the retrobulbar area to relieve the pain, but the pain is usually so severe and annoying that the eye is enucleated.

Retinal Detachment

A retinal detachment is the separation of the layer of rods and cones of the retina from the pigmented layer. Detachment is most likely to occur in elderly individuals, but can occur at any age. In many cases there are predisposing factors such as aphakia, extreme myopia, or both. Other predisposing factors are chorioretinitis and cystic degeneration of the retina.

The etiology of retinal detachments varies. That all detachments are caused by trauma is a popular misconception. Trauma may be a cause particularly if any of the previously mentioned factors are present, as in myopia, in which the retina does not stretch at the same rate as the scleral coat and a retinal hole forms. About 60 percent of patients with retinal detachments are extremely myopic. A second factor is formation of vitreous strands secondary to intraocular inflammatory processes, as in chorioretinitis. As these strands contract, the retina is pulled off and a hole forms. Degenerative conditions of the retina can lead to tears. A neoplasm of the choroid, i.e., malignant melanoma, may grow and elevate the retina because of the additional subretinal content. Finally, there is the idiopathic retinal detachment.

In order to understand the principles of therapy and nursing care in this condition, the nurse must be cognizant of the underlying pathology. Usually a tear is present unless there is a choroidal tumor. In the majority of cases, the tears occur at the ora serrata, the peripheral attachment of the retina. As a result, a subretinal fluid, which is probably an exudate, accumulates behind the retina and causes its detachment from the underlying coat. Normally the retina is firmly attached at the ora serrata and at the optic disk. Also the retina is held in contact with the choroid by the intraocular pressure of the vitreous. In approximately 20 percent of cases there is an underlying weakness in both eyes and a detachment may occur in the other eye at a later date.

The onset may be either gradual or sudden. The area of loss of vision corresponds to the area of detachment. Normally the pigmented layer traps the light for the rods and cones, but with subretinal fluid present between these two layers, this cannot occur. If the upper portion of the retina is detached, the force of gravity strips off the retina so that the patient has the sensation that a curtain has fallen before his eye. There is a decrease in visual acuity if the macula, which controls central acute vision, is detached. The individual may see black spots and flashes of light, caused by blood cells or pigment floating in the vitreous.

Retinal detachment can be diagnosed through visualization with an indirect ophthalmoscope. The blood vessels in the area of the detachment appear black instead of red; the retina is gray; and the tear is horseshoe-shaped with red choroid visible (Fig. 30-3). Usually the tear is in the extreme periphery of the retina. A disinsertion—a tear with separation of the ora serrata where it joins the ciliary

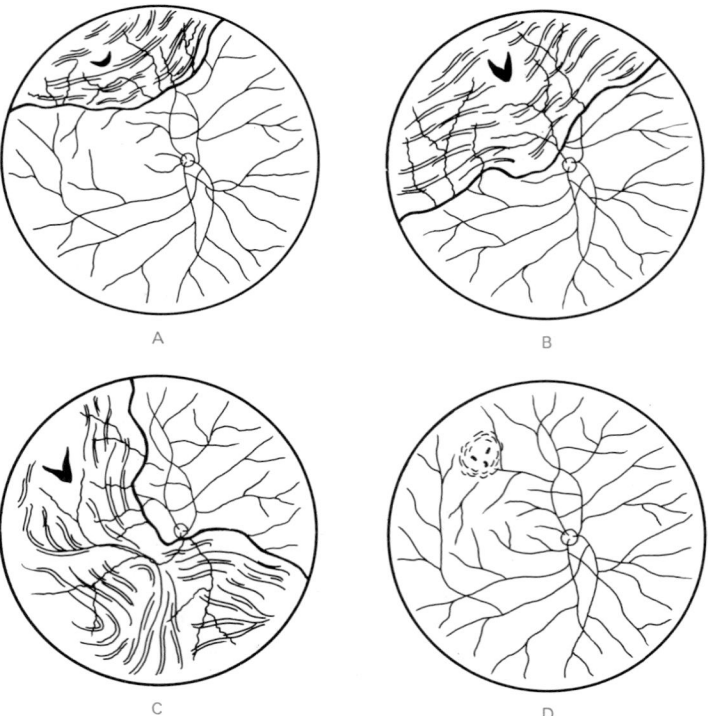

Figure 30–3 A, B, C, Retinal detachment showing a horseshoe tear and gradual enlargement of detachment as volume of subretinal fluid increases. D, Appearance of retina following surgical repair.

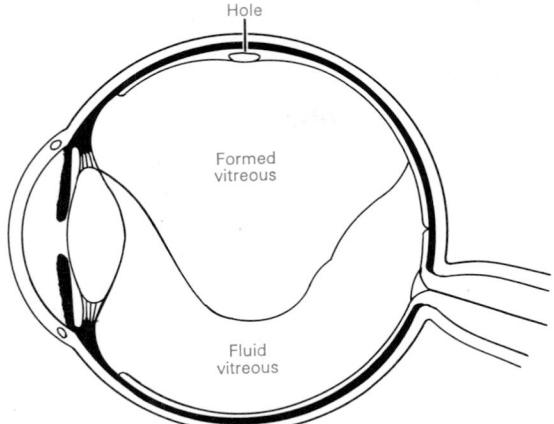

Figure 30–4
*Rise of solid vitreous
and sinking of fluid
vitreous which occurs
in mechanism of
tamponade.*

body—may be present also. The patient's peripheral field is constricted. Upon arising from a night's rest, the patient finds his vision improved because the retina has settled back onto the pigmented layer.

The course of retina detachment is varied. If untreated, it will lead to a complete detachment within a few months and the eye will be blind. If the retina remains attached for 6 months after surgical treatment, there is little likelihood of its detaching again.

The aim of treatment of a detachment with a tear is to reattach the retina by shortening the eyeball. The only treatment in detachment caused by a malignant melanoma is immediate enucleation.

Preoperatively both eyes are covered to prevent movement of them. This is probably more important than the patient's position in bed. The patient is positioned in one of two ways: with the area of the tear in the dependent position, so that the force of gravity helps the retina to settle against the choroid, or with the tear uppermost, so that the vitreous acts as a tamponade. The mechanism of this tamponade is that formed vitreous rises and fluid vitreous sinks (Fig. 30–4). The pupils are widely dilated by administration of a mydriatic, phenylephrine (Neo-Synephrine), and a cycloplegic (Cyclogyl), to facilitate visualization of the retina and to decrease movement of the intraocular structures.

SURGICAL TREATMENT

In surgery the retina is repaired with the patient under general anesthesia. Several types of surgery can be done, but all utilize one or all of three principles. First the tear is sealed by application of diathermy to the sclera directly around the tear, thus creating a choroidal exudate. In the case of a flat detachment, i.e., a detachment without subretinal fluid, photocoagulation may be utilized. In photocoagulation a beam of intense zenon light from a carbon arc source is directed through the pupil onto the retina and produces the same effect as diathermy. The laser, also a form of photocoagulation, may be used. A newer method is cryosurgery, in which a supercooled probe is applied to the sclera, causing a chorioretinal scar (Vaughan).

Next the subretinal fluid is drained. This is accomplished by inserting several needles or electrodes through the scleral and choroidal coats into the space where the subretinal fluid has collected and then withdrawing them. The subretinal fluid must be drained so that the retina can settle against the choroid.

Finally the eyeball is shortened. This may be accomplished through a lamellar scleral resection in which a layer of the sclera is removed and the opposing sides of the sclera are sutured together. A second method of shortening is scleral buckling. With this method, a 360 degree encircling tube of fascia or similar materials is used to push the outer layers of the eye into contact with the retina. Should a higher buckle be desired, pieces of silicone are inserted between the sclera and the encircling tube. A third method of shortening is to inject air, saline, or vitreous into the posterior chamber, thereby creating mechanical pressure to push the retina into contact with the choroid.

NURSING CARE

Essentially, nursing care consists of minimizing movement of the patient's eyes and head, and preventing an increase in the venous pressure in the area of the head. Both eyes are covered to minimize the movement of the eyes. The patient's position in bed is determined by the location of the tear, the extent of the detachment, and the doctor's preference; the principles of gravity and tamponade are again employed, as described. The patient must be instructed to keep his head still and not to turn from side to side or raise his head.

To keep head movement at a minimum, it is imperative that complete nursing care be given. If the patient must be rolled onto his side for a back rub or a linen change, the log rolling technique from the neck down is used; the patient lies with his eyes pointed toward the ceiling and turns on either side from the neck down. Thus the head is kept still. To give mouth care without having the patient move the head to the side, mouthwash should be sucked up through a straw and blown back through the straw into an emesis basin. To prevent phlebitis, the patient should be encouraged to exercise his lower extremities, especially the calf muscles, by pushing the ball of the foot against the foot of the bed. His position should be changed frequently to prevent skin breakdown and pulmonary complications. A well-balanced diet with sufficient roughage is ordered to prevent constipation due to inactivity. Fluids are offered frequently to prevent dehydration.

The patient may unknowingly remove his eye patches during periods of decreased awareness, as during hours of sleep. Although the nurse may think that the act is intentional, Ziskind's research suggests that the patient is entirely unaware of his act.

Diversional therapy is an extremely important aspect of nursing care. If one can imagine himself with both eyes covered, flat in bed, and totally dependent for every need from personal hygiene to being fed, then he can appreciate some of the problems the patient will experience. The use of Talking Books, as described earlier, can be invaluable. The patient's need for verbal stimulation must be evaluated beforehand.

Finally, precautions must be taken to prevent an increase in the venous pressure in the head area which in turn would increase the intraocular pressure. Coughing, vomiting, and straining at stool are to be avoided. If the patient becomes nauseated, an antiemetic should be given since vomiting would increase the likelihood of hemorrhage.

The patient's activity depends upon the procedure done and the physician's preference. Some patients may be permitted to be out of bed on the first post-operative day, but the majority will remain flat in bed for 10 to 14 days. After the patient is permitted to be out of bed and the eye patches are removed, pinhole glasses are worn. These are dark glasses with a very small opening in the center of each glass and blinders on each side. These glasses require the patient to look straight ahead and not to move his eyes. This is another method that minimizes eye movement.

In about 90 percent of cases the retina will be reattached successfully with the first surgical procedure, but good visual acuity returns in only 50 to 60 percent. If the macula has been detached from the choroid for any length of time, the central acute vision will be impaired, because the macula receives its entire blood supply from the choroid. The remainder of the retina receives blood from the retinal artery also. There is a direct relationship between the cure rate and the length of time the retina has been detached, and obviously the retina may be successfully reattached without improvement of visual acuity.

In general, the convalescent period is very similar to that of a patient who has had intraocular surgery. Physical activity that would increase the intraocular pressure is restricted for at least 3 to 4 weeks. Usually the patient is not permitted to return to work for about 6 months unless the work is sedentary. If he has suffered loss of vision, this would probably necessitate a change of occupation.

Keratoplasty

Corneal graft (keratoplasty) is performed for corneal scars and keratoconus. Keratoconus offers the most favorable prognosis, with improved vision in up to 80 percent of cases. The prognosis is less favorable in keratoplasty performed in cases of corneal scarring.

Donor grafts are obtained from cadavers and from enucleated eyes, provided that the cornea is not diseased. The eye should be enucleated as soon as possible following death, as the cornea becomes soft after death. The Eye Bank for Sight Restoration recommends that the eye be removed within 12 hours but most ophthalmologists prefer to remove the eye within 2 to 4 hours following death. Following enucleation the eye is preserved in an upright position on a piece of gauze that has been soaked in normal saline, and placed in a closed glass jar. If the eye is not to be used immediately, it is stored at a temperature of 4° C (Fasanella).

The type of graft depends upon the size and depth of the diseased area of the cornea. A penetrating graft is one involving all five layers of the cornea. For this procedure, a fresh cornea from an eye enucleated within the previous 24-hour period must be used. A trephine is used to remove the cornea from the donor eye, and the same trephine is then used to remove the diseased cornea from the recipient eye. It is important to use the same trephine to insure an exact fit. The donor cornea is then sutured in place with at least eight sutures.

A second type of corneal graft is a lamellar graft, one involving only some of the five layers of the cornea. The age of the cornea is not as important in a lamellar as in a penetrating graft. The endothelium, the innermost layer of the cornea, disintegrates after 3 days in an enucleated eye that is preserved in a moisture chamber. Since this layer is not used in a lamellar graft, the time element is not critical. The cornea of a preserved eye may be used as late as 72 hours after enucleation. In recent years, lamellar grafts have been performed that utilized eyes preserved in a frozen state for months. With this method there have been fewer instances of rejection as the protein molecules causing the antigenic effect are in an inert state. In some cases, both methods may be combined. In addition to the penetrating and lamellar grafts, there can be a combination of the two (Rizzuti).

Care following a penetrating graft is the same as in any intraocular procedure in which the eye has been incised, except that the patient may have both eyes covered and may be kept flat in bed for approximately 48 hours. In most cases the patient will be hospitalized for approximately 3 weeks, after which time the sutures may be removed.

Following a lamellar graft the patient's activity is less restricted and only the operated eye is covered. In general the principles used to guide nursing care are similar to those for intraocular surgery.

From 4 to 6 weeks are required for a corneal graft to flatten. During this time the patient will experience moderate photophobia because the constant movement of the eyelids over the edge of the donor cornea will be irritating (Paton et al.).

The most common complication of keratoplasty is vascularization. Normally the cornea is avascular; with vascularization the cornea becomes cloudy. This clouding is believed to be a manifestation of rejection of the graft. Steroids may be administered 1 week postoperatively to prevent vascularization. The use of steroids results in delayed healing, so they are contraindicated before this time. Once vascularization is underway, however, beta irradiation may be administered to induce sclerosis. It is possible to perform a second grafting procedure in most cases if the donor graft becomes cloudy.

For humanitarian reasons it seems important that the general public be made aware of the need for eyes from which the cornea is to be donated at the time of death. If the patient's eyes are going to be donated at the time of death, it is important that the cornea be preserved. The eyelid should be closed over the cornea and pieces of gauze, moistened with normal saline, should be put on the lids to prevent further drying. Nothing should be placed directly on the corneal tissue as this would damage its delicate epithelium.

Neoplasms

Retinoblastomas and malignant melanomas compose the most common tumors of the eye. Retinoblastoma, the most common intraocular tumor of childhood, is a malignant tumor of the retina which is clinically apparent between 2 and 4 years of age. In 25 to 30 percent of cases it is bilateral and one eye is usually more deeply involved.

Pathologically the lesion is nodular with numerous seeding nodules in the posterior part of the retina. The first clinical manifestation is a peculiar yellowish-white reflex from the pupil replacing the normal black color. Frequently there is deviation of the eye because of lack of vision. The neoplasm metastasizes rapidly, involving the optic nerve and brain and eventually causing death.

If the disease is unilateral, the eye and a long segment of the optic nerve are removed. If the disease is bilateral, the more severely diseased eye is enucleated and massive irradiation is given the other eye. Photocoagulation has been carried out, but the number of cases is very small and its effectiveness is not known at present. In this procedure the tumor is isolated from its blood supply and destroyed by direct coagulation (Boniuk). Recurrences have been successfully treated by photocoagulation. Chemotherapy and x-ray therapy may also be utilized.

MALIGNANT MELANOMA

Malignant melanoma is the most common malignant intraocular tumor. It develops in the uveal tract, most commonly in the choroid. Individuals 50 to 60 years of age are affected as a rule. Most melanomas are unilateral. The symptoms vary according to the area of the uveal tract involved. With involvement of the iris, both the color of the involved portion and the size of the pupil may be altered. Melanomas of the choroid will eventually give rise to a solid retinal detachment. The sudden or gradual loss of vision caused by the detachment will make the patient seek medical advice. Pain will be present if the tumor is large enough to cause an increase in intraocular pressure (glaucoma). Involvement of the macula will cause blurring of the central acute vision.

Melanoma is treated by enucleation of the eye. Fifty percent of patients survive 5 years or more. Iridectomy is performed in tumors confined to a small area of the iris.

ORBITAL TUMORS

Tumors or other space-occupying lesions of the orbit cause symptoms of exophthalmia, proptosis, decreased mobility, and diplopia due to asymmetrical movements of the eyes.

Diagnosis is established through x-ray examination of the orbit which demonstrates erosion of the bone and associated bony defects. Biopsy may be necessary, since frequently orbital tumors are resistant to x-rays.

Enucleation

Enucleation is removal of the eye. Following the surgery a gold ball or one composed of fat, glass, bone, or other substances is implanted in the fascia of the eyeball (Tenon's capsule). The rectus muscles are attached to the implant to provide motility of the artificial eye. Evisceration is removal of the contents of the eye, the scleral coat remaining. Exenteration is removal of the eye and surrounding tissue.

Enucleation is performed because of severe trauma, absolute glaucoma, malignant tumors, as prophylaxis in imminent sympathetic ophthalmia, and for cosmetic reasons in the case of a blind eye.

Following surgery, possible early complications are hemorrhage, edema, and acute infection. A pressure dressing is applied to prevent hemorrhage and the formation of a hematoma. Another possible complication is meningitis; headache or pain on the operated side of the head is suggestive.

Most patients are permitted up on the first postoperative day with no limitation of activity or diet.

The patient usually is not fitted for a prosthesis until edema has subsided; this period may vary from a few days to weeks. Until that time a plastic conformer resembling the shape of the prosthesis is worn. Prostheses are made from either glass or plastic. The plastic prosthesis has a more natural-appearing iris and is nonbreakable, and permits modifications to be made more readily. The glass prosthesis may break in very hot weather as a result of the expansion of gases within it. The surface of either type of prosthesis may become roughened, and should this occur the prosthesis must be polished before being worn again (Fasanella).

Both stock and custom made prostheses are available. A stock eye, matching the natural eye in color, is less expensive than a custom made eye, which is made to match the natural eye as closely as possible in color, shape, size, and other qualities.

The ophthalmologist will instruct the patient as to whether the prosthesis is to be removed or worn throughout the night. A normal saline irrigation should be used to cleanse the socket. When the artificial eye is not in use, it should be stored as follows: The plastic eye should be cleansed with soap and water (never with alcohol) and stored in plain tap water, which aids in maintaining luster; the glass eye should be stored in its case. The hands should be washed with soap and water before touching the prosthesis or the eye socket, since the socket is easily infected. As a rule it is necessary to wipe the socket area four to five times a day to remove the teary discharge. If this becomes necessary oftener than five times daily an infection may be present. The patient should be instructed to wipe the eye with tissues from a packet rather than use a handkerchief or boxed tissues, since these might be contaminated (Fasanella).

The nurse must provide psychological support to the patient during the immediate postoperative period, which is similar to that of the newly blinded person. Eye enucleation brings about a change in body image. The patient experiences a period of depression, often referred to as the "mourning period," during which he mourns the loss of his eye. This mourning may be manifested in, for example, refusal to eat, depression, and physical complaints such as gastrointestinal upsets.

Instructions should be given about the care of the remaining eye. Safety glasses should be worn even if sight in the remaining eye is normal. The patient should be instructed to consult an ophthalmologist with any sign of irritation or infection or following an eye injury.

Disorders Resulting from Systemic Diseases

The retina is the only structure in which blood vessels are directly visualized. Thus many systemic diseases can be diagnosed through visualization of the retinal arterioles. Arteriosclerosis, for example, is demonstrated through visualization of retinal arteriovenous nicking, deviation of the vein to the right at the arteriolar-venous crossing.

Hypertensive and Renal Retinopathy

With hypertension there is narrowing of the retinal arterioles resulting in a decreased blood supply to the retina causing anoxia. There is an increase in capillary permeability, and this causes retinal edema, exudates, hemorrhage, and papilledema. These changes are reversible if the underlying cause of the hypertension is treated. There is no ophthalmologic treatment for hypertensive retinopathy. Renal retinopathy, also caused by hypertension, is in many cases indistinguishable from hypertensive retinopathy. It develops with subacute or chronic glomerulonephritis.

Rheumatoid Arthritis

Iritis and iridocyclitis, often bilateral, frequently develop with rheumatoid arthritis, and relapses are common. A less common complication is scleromalacia perforans (scleritis), for which no satisfactory treatment is presently available.

Lupus Erythematosus

Ocular complications of lupus erythematosus include retinopathy with exudates and hemorrhage, nystagmus, and occlusion of the central retinal artery with possible loss of all vision.

Anemia

Retinal hemorrhage develops in the vicinity of the blood vessels when the red blood cell count decreases to less than 50 percent of normal. It occurs with all anemias except anemia subsequent to a sudden or massive hemorrhage. Visual loss occurs only if the hemorrhage involves the macula, but since most hemorrhages follow the distribution of the blood vessels and the macula is avascular, this would seldom happen.

Diabetes

Any structure of the eye may be affected by diabetes. Sudden variations in blood sugar levels result in changes in refractive errors, e.g., with a sudden decrease in blood sugar, there is a reduction in myopia and an increase in hyperopia. A patient in diabetic acidosis will have soft eyes because of low intraocular pressure, possibly due to dehydration. Senile cataracts develop at an earlier age and progress more rapidly than in the normal individual.

Probably the most serious ocular change associated with diabetes is retinopathy. Microaneurysms develop at the venous end of the capillaries in the inner nuclear layer of the retina situated near the optic disk and macula. White or yellowish waxy exudates and punctate hemorrhages are present. With hemorrhage into the vitreous, scar tissue forms and new blood vessels appear; with contraction of this fibrous scar tissue a retinal detachment may occur with total visual loss.

The development of retinopathy seems to be related more closely to the duration of diabetes than to its severity. Retinopathy, once established, is not influenced by the course of diabetes, although good control seems to delay the onset.

Senile Macular Degeneration

In this bilateral condition there is degeneration of the macula with pigmentary changes and reduced visual acuity, and only rarely is there any other visual loss. The patient must forego any activity requiring central acute vision. There is no known treatment.

Bibliography

Adler, Francis Heed: *Physiology of the Eye,* 4th ed. Saint Louis: The C. V. Mosby Company, 1965.

Adler, Francis Heed: *Textbook of Ophthalmology,* 7th ed. Philadelphia: W. B. Saunders Company, 1962.

Arruga, H.: *Ocular Surgery.* New York: McGraw-Hill Book Company, 1962.

Berens, Conrad and John Harry King: *An Atlas of Ophthalmic Surgery.* Philadelphia: J. B. Lippincott Company, 1961.

Bindt, Juliet: *A Handbook for the Blind.* New York: The Macmillan Company, 1952.

Blodi, Frederick C. and Ruth C. Honn: Tumors of the Eye—Medical and Nursing Care. *American Journal of Nursing,* 56:1152–1156, September, 1956.

Blodi, Frederick C.: Glaucoma. *American Journal of Nursing,* 63:78–83, March, 1963.

Boniuk, Milton (Ed.): *Ocular and Adnexal Tumors—New and Controversial Aspects.* Saint Louis: The C. V. Mosby Company, 1964.

Bosanko, Lydia: Nursing Care of the Patient with a Cataract Extraction. *American Journal of Nursing,* 60: 1435–1437, October, 1960.

Boyd, T. A. S.: Glaucoma. *Canadian Nurse,* 57:236–240, March, 1961.

Branson, Helen K.: Caring for the Blind Patient. *American Journal of Nursing,* 63:98–100, October, 1963.

Bridgemon, G. F. O.: The Management of Cataracts. *Nursing Times,* 60: 238–240, February 21, 1964.

Calhoun, F. P., et al.: Detachment of the Retina. *American Journal of Nursing,* 53:1316–1318, November, 1953.

Cebis, P. A., et al.: Symposium: Photocoagulation. *Transactions American Academy of Ophthalmology and Otolaryngology,* 66:57–87, January-February, 1962.

Cecil, Russell L. and Howard F. Conn (Eds.): *The Specialties in General Practice.* Philadelphia: W. B. Saunders Company, 1964.

Cholden, Louis S.: *A Psychiatrist Works with Blindness.* New York: The William Byrd Press, Inc., 1958.

Cholden, Louis: Some Psychiatric Problems in the Rehabilitation of the Blind. *Bulletin of Menninger Clinic,* 18:107–112, May, 1954.

Clark, Graham and Cora L. Shaw: The Patient with Retinal Detachment. *American Journal of Nursing,* 57: 868–871, July, 1957.

Cockerill, Eleanor E.: Reflections on My Nursing Care. *American Journal of Nursing,* 65:83–85, May, 1965.

Dixon, Joseph M.: Ocular Changes Due to Contact Lenses. *American Journal of Ophthalmology,* 58:424–443, September, 1964.

Facts on the Major Killing and Crippling Disease in the United States Today. The National Health Education Committee, Inc. New York, 1964.

Fasanella, R. M.: *Complications in Eye Surgery,* 2d ed. Philadelphia: W. B. Saunders Company, 1965.

Flynn, William R.: Visual Hallucinations in Sensory Deprivation. *Psychiatric Quarterly,* 36:55–65, January, 1962.

Galin, Miles A. and Philip Zweifach: Glaucoma. *New England Journal of Medicine,* 267:237–242; 291–295, August, 1962.

Garrett, James F. and Edna S. Levine: *Psychological Practices with the Physically Disabled.* New York: Columbia University Press, 1962.

Girard, Louis J. (Ed.): *Corneal Contact Lenses.* Saint Louis: The C. V. Mosby Company, 1964.

Gordon, Dan M.: The Inflamed Eye. *American Journal of Nursing,* 64: 113–117, November, 1964.

Jones, Ira S.: The Cataract Extraction Operation. *American Journal of Nursing,* 60:1433–1435, October, 1960.

Leopold, Irving H.: Anti-inflammatory Agents in Ophthalmology. *American Journal of Nursing,* 63:84–87, March, 1963.

Manhattan Eye, Ear, and Throat Hospital: Nursing in Diseases of the Eye, Ear, Nose, and Throat, 10th ed. Philadelphia: W. B. Saunders Company, 1958.

The Miotic Life. *British Journal of Ophthalmology,* 48:354–356, 1964.

Okamura, I. D. and C. L. Schepens: Retinal Detachment. *Sight Saving Review,* 25:138–146, Fall, 1955.

Paton, R. Townley, et al.: *Atlas of Eye Surgery.* New York: McGraw-Hill Book Company, 1962.

Peczon, J. D. and W. M. Grant: Glaucoma, Alcohol and Intraocular Pressure. *Archives of Ophthalmology,* 73:495–501, April, 1965.

Pischel, D. K.: Symposium: Present Status of Retinal Detachment Surgery. *Transactions of American Academy of Ophthalmology and Otolaryngology,* 68:919–1008, November-December, 1964.

Rizzuti, A. Benedict: Corneal Surgery. *New York State Journal of Medicine,* 63:1508–1510, May 15, 1963.

Ruben, Montague: The Contact Lens in Current Practice. *Nursing Times,* 59:1449–1453, November 15, 1963.

Saunders, William H., et al.: *Nursing Care in Eye, Ear, Nose, and Throat Disorders,* 2d ed. Saint Louis: The C. V. Mosby Company, 1968.

Scheie, Harold G.: Filtering Operations for Glaucoma: A Comparative Study. *American Journal of Ophthalmology,* 53:571–590, April, 1962.

Schwartz, Ariah: Medical Management of Glaucoma. *International Ophthalmology Clinics,* 3:63–84, March, 1963.

Shafer, Kathleen Newton, et al.: *Medical-Surgical Nursing.* Saint Louis: The C. V. Mosby Company, 1964.

Stocker, Frederick W. and Ruth Bell: Corneal Transplantation and Nursing the Patient with a Corneal Transplant. *American Journal of Nursing,* 62:65–70, May, 1962.

Vaughan, Daniel, Robert Clark, and Taylor Asbury: *General Ophthalmology,* 5th ed. Los Altos, Calif.: Lange Medical Publications, 1968.

Ward, Roy J.: Some Psychological and Psychiatric Implications in the Readjustment and Rehabilitation of Newly Blinded Adults. *Virginia Medical Monthly,* 89:506–509, September, 1962.

Woods, Alan C.: The Adjustment of Aphakia. *American Journal of Ophthalmology,* 55:1268–1272, June, 1963.

Ziskind, E., et al.: Observations on Mental Symptoms in Eye Patched Patients: Hypnogogic Symptoms in Sensory Deprivation. *American Journal of Psychiatry,* 116:893–900, 1960.

SECTION 2
DISEASES
OF THE
EAR BETSY EELLS RAY

Hearing Impairment

Although differences in methods of reporting and classifying hearing impairment in the United States make it difficult to give an accurate estimate of its incidence, it is known that at least 4 million persons have some degree of hearing impairment. Since this problem is so prevalent, the present discussion of diseases of the ear will be confined to those disorders that cause or contribute to hearing loss.

Causes

Causes of hearing impairment include congenital factors, hereditary factors, trauma, incorrect or excessive nose blowing, disease states, infections, ototoxicity, tumors of the ear or auditory pathways, and aging. Few conditions of the external ear cause permanent hearing impairment, although temporary impairment may result from swelling due to infection or impacted cerumen.

Types and Degrees

There are several types of hearing loss. *Conduction* deafness occurs when there is a failure of the sound waves to be conducted from the tympanic membrane through the ossicular system into the cochlea. *Nerve deafness,* also known as sensorineural hearing loss, neurosensory hearing loss, and perceptive deafness, is a failure of the sound impulses to reach the auditory cortex because there has been damage to the cochlea or to the neurogenic transmission system for sound. *Combined* hearing loss is, as its name suggests, both conductive and sensorineural. It is also called *mixed* loss. *Central* hearing loss results from a disturbance of the auditory mechanism, rather than from a disturbance of the ear itself. *Functional* hearing loss has a neurogenic basis, for example conversion deafness in hysteria states.

Since there are many degrees of hearing impairment, the criteria suggested by the National Center for Health Statistics are useful in classifying impairment according to the degree of speech comprehension as follows: (1) ability to hear and understand spoken words, (2) ability to hear and understand a few spoken words, and (3) ability to hear and understand most spoken words.

Diagnosis

The physician obtains a detailed medical history, including drug ingestion, family history, and occupational history. The complete physical examination may include an audiogram and screening tests for hearing, such as the ability to appreciate vibrations from a tuning fork and observation of the patient for evidence of lip reading during conversation. Signs and symptoms of disorders of the ear are often slow in onset and circumstances at the time of examination may not suggest a relationship between the symptom and an ear disorder. Consequently great skill in interviewing is essential. The patient with transient dizziness may have considered it merely annoying and therefore fail to mention this as a symptom. The initial attack of vertigo in Meniere's disease may be preceded by tinnitus, yet often this clue has not been reported.

The nurse has an important role in the diagnosis of a hearing loss. She should accurately report such observations as tilt of the head, loudness or softness of speech, and awareness of sounds. She may note unsteadiness of gait or other evidence of dizziness and/or vertigo. The patient's own description of his feeling at the time of the attack is important; in vertigo the hallucinatory movement involves movement of self or of surrounding objects.

If the patient does not have an established hearing loss or is receiving an ototoxic drug, the nurse may be the first person to note early signs of hearing impairment.

Treatment

Otitis media, otosclerosis, and ototoxicity are among the most common causes of hearing impairment.

OTITIS MEDIA

Infections of the upper respiratory tract must be treated promptly and thoroughly in order to prevent spread of the infection from the throat to the middle ear through the eustachian tube. Although the need for adequate treatment in children has been stressed, it is equally important in the care of the adult patient. Foreign material in the middle ear may lead to the formation of scar tissue, with consequent impairment of hearing. The primary goal of treatment is to maintain eustachian tube patency by treating the underlying cause of the infection.

Purulent (acute suppurative) otitis media is a complication of acute infections of the upper respiratory tract or of allergy. It is treated with antibiotics, analgesics as needed, heat applications, and sometimes myringotomy.

Serous (acute nonsuppurative) otitis media results from obstruction of the eustachian tube due to allergy, tumor, infection, or unknown cause. The middle ear is not involved with an infective process, but the eustachian tube blockage causes a serous accumulation. The underlying cause must be treated. Myringotomy may be useful.

Air travel is usually contraindicated when blockage of the eustachian tube is a possibility, as a change in altitude causes increased pressure.

OTOSCLEROSIS

It has been estimated that a least 5 million persons in the United States have otosclerosis. In approximately 10 percent of cases there is ankylosis of the stapes which interferes with vibration of the stapes and transmission of sound to the inner ear. The disorder is seen with greatest frequency in young women, and there is a definite hereditary factor. Progressive loss of hearing is the most characteristic symptom. The patient finds that he has greatest difficulty in hearing low, soft tones. As the disease progresses, tinnitus frequently develops.

The hearing loss in many cases is corrected by surgery, and in others by the wearing of a hearing aid. It is often advised that the patient have a trial period using a hearing aid, before considering surgery. Should it be decided that surgery is to be performed, one of three operations will be done.

Fenestration. In the fenestration operation, a new window is created through which vibrations pass from the external auditory canal to the inner ear. The operation is extensive and complicated. The patient probably will be extremely dizzy and nauseated postoperatively, and will require considerable assistance from the nurse in meeting his personal needs. For the first few days he will have to remain at bed rest, and side rails will have to be raised if the dizziness is severe. A fluid diet generally is ordered. Jarring of the bed must be avoided, as should any activity that may disturb the operated side, such as sneezing or coughing. The nurse should try to anticipate the patient's needs during this period, and should make certain that he receives an adequate diet and sufficient fluids, since the postoperative pain may greatly lessen his appetite and interest in food.

Stapes Mobilization. A second operation frequently performed in otosclerotic patients is the stapes mobilization. In the operation, the footplate of the stapes is loosened, with the patient under local anesthesia, in the hope that the stapes will remain free to vibrate. Vertigo is a frequent postoperative complaint, so the nurse must caution the patient about this.

Stapedectomy. In recent years stapedectomy has become the procedure of choice, because it offers superior hearing improvement to either of the others, and the procedure is much easier on the patient, both during the operation and postoperatively. In this operation, the entire stapes is removed and replaced with a prosthesis composed of bone, fat, or Teflon. Vertigo is a frequent postoperative complaint, and the nurse should instruct the patient accordingly.

OTOTOXICITY

Drugs known to cause ototoxicity include kanamycin, neomycin, streptomycin, dihydrostreptomycin, nitrofurantoin, and acetylsalicylic acid. The symptoms may range from tinnitus to hearing loss. With some of these drugs there is a predictable response; with others the response is highly individual. In some studies it has been reported that 87 percent of persons who received parenteral doses of kanamycin were left with some degree of hearing loss. There is damage to the cochlear and vestibular portions of the auditory nerve, causing vertigo. The damage is halted with discontinuance of the drug. Neomycin administered in high dosages causes nerve damage and this damage progresses even after drug administration is discontinued. Streptomycin may cause permanent labyrinthine damage.

The nurse must have sufficient knowledge of ototoxic drugs to be able to observe the patient for side effects. This requires constant alertness on her part, since, with the current proliferation of drugs, their ototoxic capacity may not be recognized early in treatment. Further, she should instruct the patient to seek medical attention if changes in hearing ability or vertigo occur.

The Patient with a Hearing Loss

Normal hearing gives the individual countless clues about his environment, and this knowledge is of course not available to the person with a hearing loss. He may hear many sounds or few sounds, and these sounds may or may not be distorted. It is important for the nurse to keep these facts in mind when dealing with individuals who have a hearing loss. She should also remember that the patient's total adjustment to his loss is related to the age at which he first experienced the loss. The congenitally deaf adult, as an example, has not had the benefits of establishing a language pattern, attaining an education, and having the many experiences that would be available to the individual whose hearing loss occurred in later life. The congenitally deaf person, or the one whose hearing impairment developed during childhood, must have special education and training. Then too, the older adult would also have the advantage of having established friendships and probably established a family of his own, whereas the younger adult, who may not have had the opportunity to do any of these things, would have greater problems of adjustment.

With the increase in our aged population, the nurse will see and care for many older individuals who have a hearing loss. These individuals may not be able to cope with the problem of hearing loss, when it is added to all the other problems they must face.

The nurse should never assume that because the patient does not hear normally, he is lacking in intelligence or understanding. Some of these individuals may appear to be neurotic or introverted because they think that others are talking about them. It is also true that individuals classified as retarded are more likely to have a hearing loss than normal individuals.

It has been said that no disability is as difficult to manage as impairment of hearing. Often the person attempts to hide the impairment or to try to correct it without telling others about it. Thus he may not seek adequate medical evaluation of the problem, and may become the victim of frauds or quacks. Then too, impaired hearing is frequently accompanied or followed by loss of another sense, such as vision, or loss of a limb.

The nurse can practice, and can urge others to practice, certain measures that will help the person with impaired hearing to communicate adequately with others. The following aids will probably suggest other means for improving communication.

When talking to the hard-of-hearing person, the speaker should always face him directly. There should be adequate light on the speaker's face. Speaking in a normal tone, and enunciating each word slowly and clearly without dropping the voice at the end of a statement, help to eliminate distortions of voice and tone. The speaker should always acknowledge the presence of the hard-of-hearing person in his conversation with others. If the impairment is such that the person must lip read, or speech read, as it is correctly called, the speaker should remember that this is fatiguing.

In rehabilitation activities, the first need is for complete evaluation of the patient's overall physical and mental capacities. The nurse can help in this regard by urging the patient to visit an otologist in private practice or in a clinic, or by directing him to an agency through which he can be taught lip reading or to read sign language. Speech problems resulting from the hearing impairment must receive attention. The correct hearing aid can be prescribed to improve whatever hearing ability is present. In many cases it is possible for the patient to gain the benefit of higher education, either in a special facility such as Gallaudet College in Washington, D.C., or in another setting.

The nurse is often in a position to assist in efforts to prevent hearing disability. She should remember that many respiratory disorders can lead to complications that will cause partial or total loss of hearing; therefore she should help to educate all patients she cares for about the need for early diagnosis and treatment of such disorders. The nurse can also stress that the patient should never insert any foreign body, such as a hairpin (often used for "cleaning") into the ear. Should a foreign body enter the ear, only a physician should remove it. She can also teach patients to blow the nose correctly, that is, with the mouth and both nostrils open, in order to prevent entry of microorganisms into the eustachian tube.

National and Local Agencies That Provide Services to Persons with a Hearing Loss

A number of agencies and organizations provide various services for persons with impaired hearing. Among them are the following:

American Hearing Society, Washington, D.C.: social activities; educational literature; employment bureau; in some areas maintains classes in lip reading and in correct use of hearing aids.

Alexander Graham Bell Association for the Deaf, Washington, D.C.: serves as an information center for persons working with the deaf; maintains a library on all aspects of deafness.

American Speech and Hearing Association, Washington, D.C.: composed of professional workers who train individuals with speech and hearing disorders.

National Society for Crippled Children and Adults, Chicago, Ill.: a variety of programs in many areas.

National Association of the Deaf, Berkeley, Calif.: deals with legislative matters pertaining to the deaf and the welfare of the deaf in employment and educational opportunities.

The Deafness Research Foundation, New York, N.Y.: research into hearing impairment.

The John Tracy Clinic, Los Angeles, Calif.: information services; correspondence courses for children.

Veterans Administration Regional Offices: provide information on hearing rehabilitation to eligible veterans.

State Office of Vocational Rehabilitation: advises on rehabilitation and employment.

U.S. Office of Education, Washington, D.C.: training of teachers of the deaf through training grants; school consultation services.

U.S. Public Health Service, Department of Health, Education, and Welfare, National Institute of Neurological Diseases and Blindness, Bethesda, Md.: research support; training grants; information.

Communication Information Center, Johns Hopkins University, Baltimore, Md. (supported by NINDB): reviews and evaluates published reports.

Bibliography

Bender, Ruth E.: Communication with the Deaf. *American Journal of Nursing,* 66:757–760, April, 1966.

Brown, Lester A.: Newer Types of Ear Surgery. *Nursing Forum,* 4:3:95–98, 1965.

Brown, Robert Alex: Noise and Urban Man. *American Journal of Public Health,* 68:2061–2066, November, 1968.

Canfield, Norton: *Hearing: A Handbook for Laymen.* Garden City, New York: Doubleday & Company, Inc., 1959.

Davis, Hallowell and S. Richard Silverman (Eds.): *Hearing and Deafness.* New York: Holt, Rinehart and Winston, Inc., 1964.

DiBiasco, A. G.: Postoperative Care of Patients Having Ear Surgery. *Nursing Forum,* 4:3:104–108, 1965.

Downs, Marion P.: Hunt to Catch a Handicap. *Today's Health,* 47:46–51, January, 1968.

Goodman, Louis S. and Alfred Gilman: *The Pharmacological Basis of Therapeutics,* 3d ed. New York: The Macmillan Company, 1965.

Guyton, Arthur C.: *Textbook of Medical Physiology,* 3d ed. Philadelphia: W. B. Saunders Company, 1966.

Havener, William H., William H. Saunders, and Betty S. Bergersen: *Nursing Care in Eye, Ear, Nose and Throat Disorders.* St. Louis: The C. V. Mosby Company, 1964.

Littler, T. S.: *The Physics of the Ear.* New York: The Macmillan Company, 1965.

McCurdy, Harry W.: Preoperative Care of Patients Having Ear Surgery. *Nursing Forum,* 4:3:99–103, 1965.

Meyler, L. (Ed.): *Side Effects of Drugs.* New York: Excerpta Medica Foundation, 1966.

Myklebust, Helmer R.: *The Psychology of Deafness,* 2d ed. New York: Grune & Stratton, Inc., 1964.

Noise Exposure Control Guidelines. *American Association of Industrial Nurses Journal,* 16:17–21, May, 1968.

Rainer, John D. and Kenneth Z. Altshuler: *Comprehensive Mental Health Services for the Deaf.* New York: Columbia University, Department of Medical Genetics, New York State Psychiatric Institute, 1966.

Reger, Scott N. Audiology: Yesterday, Today and Tomorrow. *New York State Journal of Medicine,* 68:1431–1434, June 1, 1968.

U.S. Department of Health, Education, and Welfare, Public Health Service, National Center for Health Statistics: *Characteristics of Persons with Impaired Hearing.* Series 19, No. 35. Vital Statistics of the United States, 1963. Washington, D.C.: U.S. Government Printing Office, 1967.

---: *Hearing Levels of Adults by Education, Income, and Occupation.* United States 1960–1962. Series 11, No. 31. Vital Statistics of the United States. Washington, D.C.: U.S. Government Printing Office, 1968.

Van Itallie, Philip H.: *How to Live with a Hearing Handicap.* New York: Paul S. Eriksson, Inc., 1963.

Wolfson, Robert J., Woodrow D. Schlosser, and Richard A. Winchester: Vertigo. *Clinical Symposia,* 17:99–133, October-November-December, 1965.

CHAPTER 31

THE PATIENT WITH DISEASE OF THE REPRODUCTIVE SYSTEM

SECTION 1
DISEASES OF THE MALE REPRODUCTIVE SYSTEM

MARY S. KLEINKNECHT*

Infections of the genitourinary tract
Epididymitis
Acute orchitis
Phimosis
Paraphimosis
Urethral strictures
Neoplasms of the genitourinary tract
Benign prostatic hyperplasia (or hypertrophy)
Carcinoma of the prostate
Disorders of the spermatic cord
Hydrocele
Spermatocele
Varicocele

The disorders of the male reproductive system discussed in this section have been limited to selected conditions resulting from infections, neoplasms, and disorders of the spermatic cord, for two compelling reasons. First, these diseases exert a profound psychosocial impact on the patient because of the implications for reproduction and sexuality that are associated with the male reproductive organs. Second, many men have a profound fear that diseases of these organs will cause severe pain and might result in impotence or penile amputation.

Infections of the Genitourinary Tract

In the healthy person the urinary tract is sterile. However, bacteria may be found along several centimeters of the distal urethra. According to Davis, bacteria may be introduced into a normal urinary tract but will spontaneously be phagocytosed in a

* The author acknowledges the assistance of Matlock M. Mims, M.D., in the preparation of this section.

few days by means of a potent antibacterial action due to either a property of the epithelial cells lining the urinary tract or to substances in the urine. According to Hinman and Cox, the bacterial population is markedly reduced by washing the organisms out of the urinary tract through adequate hydration and frequent voiding. Persistent infection of the urinary tract is due to one or more of the following causes: (1) stasis and obstruction; (2) presence of a foreign body; (3) a decrease in general body resistance. Bacteria introduced into an obstructed urinary tract will remain and multiply until the obstruction is relieved.

Nonspecific infectious organisms, gram-negative rods (e.g., *Escherichia coli* and *Proteus vulgaris*) and gram-positive cocci (staphylococci and streptococci), most commonly infect the genitourinary tract. These are distinguished from specific infectious organisms that cause clinically distinctive diseases (e.g., tuberculosis, gonorrhea, syphilis).

An infection can involve any of the genital organs and can spread from a given locus to any organ. Complications resulting from infection of the kidneys are of the greatest importance because of the parenchymal destruction caused by them.

Bacteria enter the urinary tract through four main pathways: (1) ascending infection, involving the bladder; (2) lymphogenous spread, a migration of infection to the urinary tract through the lymph nodes; (3) hematogenous spread, a common pathway of bacterial invasion of the kidneys, prostate, and testes; or (4) direct extension from other organs, e.g., an intraperitoneal abscess that may infect the bladder.

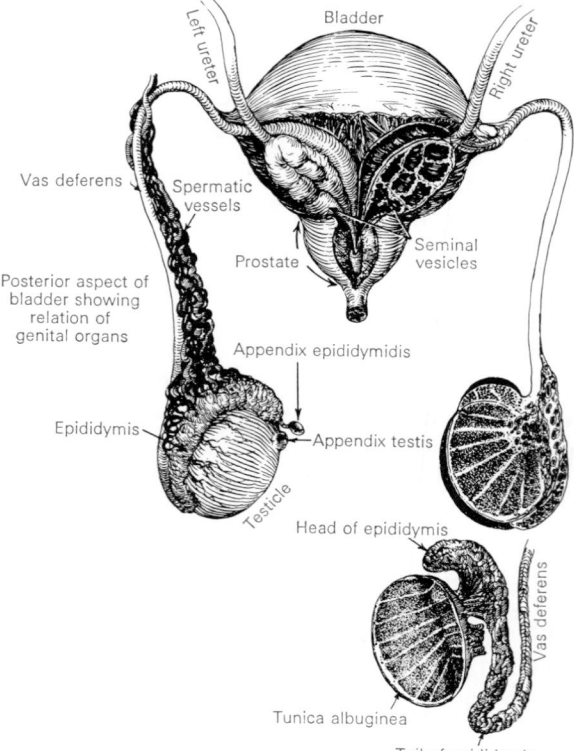

Figure 31-1
Posterior aspect of bladder showing relation of genital organs. (Courtesy of Donald R. Smith: General Urology, 5th ed. Los Altos, Calif: Lange Medical Publications, 1966.)

Epididymitis

Epididymitis is the most common intrascrotal inflammation. It is mainly a disease of adults, although all forms have been seen in children.

Epididymitis may occur as a result of invasion by nonspecific pyogenic organisms, such as colon bacilli, staphylococci, and occasionally streptococci, and by the specific organisms of gonorrhea, syphilis, and tuberculosis. The disease may be seen in association with urethral strictures, cystitis, and prostatitis. It may be a complication of instrumentation, prostatectomy, and urethral catheterization. The organisms frequently enter the epididymis through the lumen of the vas from previously established infections. Straining, which may force urine or infection material into the lumen of the vas, may be a precipitating factor.

Pathologically, in the early stages epididymitis is a cellular inflammation of the vas deferens. It descends to the lower pole of the epididymis. In the acute stage the epididymis is swollen, and induration spreads from the lower pole to the upper pole of the organ. Small abscesses may be seen on tissue cross section.

Symptoms and signs often appear following trauma, urethral instrumentation, and severe physical exercise, such as lifting heavy objects; they may also develop after prolonged sexual activity. Severe pain develops suddenly in the scrotum and radiates along the thickened spermatic cord. The epididymis becomes swollen and exquisitely sensitive. The organ may swell to twice its normal size within 3 to 4 hours, causing the patient to walk with a characteristic "duck waddle." The temperature may reach 104° F and a urethral discharge may be noted. If an abscess is present, the skin may become erythematous, flaky, dry, and thinned.

Potential complications include abscess formation, usually associated with urethral instrumentation or prostatic massage. The abscess may drain spontaneously through the scrotum or may require surgical drainage. Sterility may ensue if the disease is bilateral.

Medical treatment consists of anesthetizing the spermatic cord by infiltrating it with 20 ml of 1 percent procaine hydrochloride, and administering antibiotics. The latter are not curative in every case. With medical therapy the fever usually falls abruptly, the pain is alleviated, and the inflammatory mass resolves in a few days.

Nursing measures include the following: (1) bed rest for 3 to 4 days during the acute stage of the disease; (2) support for the enlarged testicle with a roomy athletic supporter lined with cotton (the usual scrotal supporter is too small); (3) ice bag to the early acutely inflamed and swollen epididymis, then heat to the prostate and epididymis by means of sitz baths. These measures usually afford comfort and probably hasten resolution of the inflammatory process. The nurse should also (4) observe for possible abscess formation; and (5) caution the patient against sexual excitement or physical strain (e.g., defecation), which may cause exacerbation of the infection.

Acute Orchitis

Acute orchitis is infection and inflammation of a testicle. It may be either bilateral or unilateral and may occur with any infectious process, e.g., Coxsackie virus infection. Individuals with mumps parotitis excrete the virus in urine and mumps epididymo-orchitis may develop. The ensuing edema probably leads to death of the spermatogenic cells from ischemia.

Pathologically the testis is greatly enlarged, congested, bluish, and tense. Small abscesses may be noted on section.

Symptoms of acute orchitis begin with sudden pain and swelling of one or both testes, which become tense and exquisitely tender. The scrotum may be red and edematous; the patient's fever may reach 104° F causing marked prostration. Pain radiates to the inguinal canal and is usually accompanied by nausea and vomiting.

Complications of the disease are significant. In one-third to one-fourth of patients, the involved testis becomes sterile due to irreversible damage to spermatogenic cells caused by destruction of the tubules and ductal system. Androgenic function is usually maintained, however.

Antibiotics are helpful in treating bacterial orchitis, but are of no value in treating mumps orchitis. Infiltration of the spermatic cord just above the involved testis with 20 ml of procaine hydrochloride 1 percent will in some cases cause rapid reduction of the swelling and thus relieve the pain. The patient is placed on bed rest and hot or cold compresses are applied to the testicle to relieve pain, and an athletic supporter containing cotton padding is used to support the organ, even when the patient is in bed.

If mumps is the underlying cause, gamma globulin given after the onset of the parotitis may prevent orchitis. The surgical treatment of severe mumps orchitis consists of tapping the hydrocele to reduce the pressure in the tunica albuginea. If abscess occurs, as it does in rare cases, an orchidectomy may be necessary.

Orchitis may lead to infertility because of the destruction of the spermatogenic cells, especially if the disease is bilateral.

Phimosis

Phimosis is a contracture of the prepuce of the penis sufficient to prevent its retraction over the glans. It may be congenital, acquired, or secondary to infection beneath a redundant foreskin. Poor hygiene frequently contributes to the infection, which causes tissue injury. As healing by fibrosis takes place, the foreskin cannot be retracted over the glans and the preputial opening becomes contracted and pinpoint in size permitting only a slow discharge of urine; this condition perpetuates the infectious process. When the preputial orifice is small, urination may be accompanied by ballooning of the subpreputial cavity. The patient may complain of inability to retract the foreskin, but more frequently he is disturbed by symptoms and signs of infection, such as redness and swelling of the foreskin, purulent discharge, and local pain.

Treatment consists of controlling the infection by use of hot soaks and administering antibiotics. If the infection is marked, a dorsal incision of the foreskin will relieve the constriction. Subsequent circumcision will be followed by a permanent cure.

Paraphimosis

Paraphimosis, also known as "Spanish collar," is caused by compression or strangulation of the glans penis by the prepuce. The foreskin retracts behind the glans and cannot be replaced in its normal position. Retraction is due to traumatic swelling or inflammatory swelling of the foreskin or contracture of the preputial skin ring. This ring of skin, caught behind the glans, causes venous occlusion, which leads to edema of the glans and further distortion of the glans. If the condition is neglected, arterial occlusion and preputial gangrene may develop.

The objective of treatment is to reduce the edema which may be accomplished by squeezing the glans for at least 5 minutes, thus reducing its size, and by subcutaneous injections of hyaluronidase into the edematous foreskin. If manual reduction fails, incision of the main constricting bands is necessary, followed later by circumcision.

Urethral Strictures

Strictures of the urethra continue to be a major urological problem, although penicillin, sulfonamides, and other antibiotics have greatly reduced the frequency of postgonorrheal stricture. They occur chiefly in males who have undergone transurethral surgical procedures or have sustained urethral injury.

Injuries to the pendulous urethra occur most often from traumatic instrumentation. The urethra may be injured by the passage of a size 28 French resectoscope, used for transurethral prostatectomy, and injury of the urethral mucosa may occur when a metal sound of small caliber is passed to dilate a stricture.

Trauma to the urethra, as described by Smith, includes injuries to the membranous urethra, usually seen in pelvic fractures. In these injuries the fascia may be torn, shearing off the prostate from the membranous urethra, and the bony splinters may perforate the urethra and bladder.

Trauma to the bulbous urethra, which lies inferior to the urogenital diaphragm, may result from instrumentation but most frequently is caused by forcibly falling astride an object. Contusion or laceration of the urethra may result from injury to the urethra between the symphysis pubis and the straddled object.

The most frequent symptom is gradual diminution of the caliber and force of the urinary stream. Sudden urinary retention may occur if an infection is exacerbated at the stricture site. Cystitis, prostatitis, or pyelonephritis may be present. A history of severe untreated gonorrhea or urethral injury can usually be obtained.

Pathologically, urethral strictures cause severe damage to the urinary tract and produce changes in the urethra which may result in dilatation of the urethra proximal to the stenosis, compensatory changes in the bladder wall, and ureterovesical reflux with hydronephrosis and hydroureter. Stasis of urine in the bladder provides a culture medium for multiplication of bacteria and this may result in prostatitis, cystitis, periurethral abscess, and pyelonephritis.

X-ray findings following a urethrogram will reveal the site and degree of the stricture, and instrumental examination will pinpoint the stricture. A catheter or sound of average size passed into the urethra will be arrested at the site of stricture, and if a cystoscope can be passed, it will demonstrate hypertrophy of the bladder muscle.

Complications of urethral strictures are cystitis, prostatitis, and pyelonephritis. Periurethral abscess may occur at the stricture site; it may resolve with treatment, or may erode through the skin, causing a urethrocutaneous fistula. Urinary stones may form secondary to infection and stasis of urine.

The treatment consists of passing sounds, filiforms, and followers through the stricture and subsequently dilating the urethra. If a filiform cannot be passed and the patient is experiencing urinary retention, a suprapubic cystostomy must be done.

Neoplasms of the Genitourinary Tract

Prostatic hyperplasia, undoubtedly the most common symptomatic new growth in the human male, occurs with high frequency in the presenile and senile periods —an age group the nurse will treat increasingly because of the increase in the number of elderly men in our population. Prostatic cancer, which is often fatal, continues to be one of the major problems in urology and is the most common malignant neoplasm in men over 60 years of age.

Benign Prostatic Hyperplasia (or Hypertrophy)

The majority of men have benign prostatic hyperplasia by the age of 60.

The prostate in the young adult has a thin capsule and is closely attached to the underlying secretory tissue. The pathologically enlarged gland, on the other hand, is composed of a thick true and false capsule, the latter containing compressed adenomatous tissue loosely connected to the underlying tissues.

It is the obstruction of the bladder neck, rather than the enlargement itself, that is harmful. The bladder, like the heart, reacts to an increasing work load by going through successive phases of compensation and decompensation. Normally, urine is expelled through contracture of the detrusor muscle, which pulls the bladder neck open and forms a funnel, and intravesical pressure, which varies between 20 and 40 cm of water, further opens the bladder neck.

In bladder neck obstruction, hypertrophy of the vesical musculature develops and intravesical pressure rises to 50 to 100 cm or more of water in order to overcome the greater urethral resistance. The enlarging prostate seems to interfere with the mechanism that opens the internal orifice. Muscle exhaustion may occur prematurely when the contraction does not last long enough for all the urine to be expelled.

Early in the compensation phase, the vesical musculature begins to hypertrophy, and contraction of the detrusor is so strong that it goes into spasms, producing symptoms of an irritable bladder. The earliest symptoms of bladder neck obstruction are urgency, incontinence, and frequency, both day and night. During the later stages of compensation, as the obstruction increases, further hypertrophy of the muscle fibers of the bladder occurs even though the power to empty the bladder is maintained. Symptoms include hesitation in initiating the flow as the bladder develops contractions strong enough to overcome resistance at the bladder neck, and a marked loss in the force and size of the stream, caused by the obstruction.

Some degree of decompensation begins to occur if the vesical tone becomes impaired or if urethral resistance exceeds detrusor muscle power. The contraction phase of the vesical muscle becomes too short to allow complete expulsion of urine. Symptoms of acute decompensation are a marked hesitancy and a need for straining to initiate urination followed by a weak, small stream and termination of the stream before the bladder completely empties. Acute and sudden complete urinary retention may result. With absolute inability to urinate, there is suprapubic pain with severe urgency; small amounts of urine may be dribbled.

Chronic decompensation occurs as the degree of obstruction increases and a progressive imbalance develops between the power of the bladder musculature and urethral resistance. With increasing difficulty in expelling all the urine, there is increased frequency of urination, and with loss of contraction, overflow (paradoxical) incontinence results. False diverticula develop as the mucosal layer is forced between the muscle fibers, and the diverticula finally balloon into the perivesical fat. These diverticula, having no muscular wall, are readily infected by the contained urine. Dilatation of the ureter and renal pelvis with secondary infection ultimately leads to renal insufficiency and hypertension.

Cystitis is an early complication; renal infection may occur due to stagnation of urine. Frequently the invading organisms are urea-splitting (Proteus, staphylococci) causing the urine to become alkaline, and this results in precipitation of calcium salts and formation of stones in the kidneys and bladder. When the ureterovesical junction fails, reflux into the kidneys occurs, pyelonephritis develops, and the renal damage from back pressure and infection can be fatal.

Conservative therapy may be adequate. Prostatitis is treated with antimicrobials, prostatic massage, and sitz baths. If pyuria is present, antibiotics or sulfonamides are used.

Nursing measures include instructing the patient to void as soon as he feels the urge to do so. The nurse should also caution the patient against excessive intake of fluids within a short period of time. With acute retention, accompanied by complete inability to void and agonizing pain, catheterization is mandatory. A permanent indwelling catheter or a suprapubic cystostomy may be necessary in the debilitated patient.

Surgery may be indicated if there is bladder damage, if renal function is impaired because of the obstruction, or if the degree of symptoms is so annoying to the patient that he requests help. One of four surgical procedures will be employed as described below.

TRANSURETHRAL PROSTATECTOMY

Transurethral resection of the prostate is performed by inserting a resectoscope through the urethra and into the bladder. Under direct endoscopic vision small pieces of the abnormal prostatic tissue are excised until adequate patency of the prostatic urethra has been established and the hypertrophied tissue entirely removed. The mortality is about 1 to 2 percent; the urinary results are generally satisfactory; potency is maintained; and hospitalization is relatively short.

The urinary bladder is drained by a catheter for 3 to 4 days postoperatively. A Foley catheter with a large bag is the most commonly used catheter since it has a large balloon and a large lumen to permit the passage of clots, and it can be used with a closed drainage system, which prevents bacterial contamination of the surgical area.

In rare instances, when postoperative bleeding is severe, a three-way urethral catheter is employed. It permits a through-and-through flow of sterile normal saline to wash out clots. This catheter has three arms. One arm is for drainage; one is connected to a channel within the catheter through which the bladder can be irrigated; and one is connected to the inflation tube of the balloon. This apparatus is frequently employed when continuous irrigation of the bladder is necessary.

Postoperatively, the nurse is responsible for maintaining drainage. If clots obstruct the flow of urine, they must be irrigated out before the bladder becomes distended. Strict aseptic technique is employed when giving catheter care through closed urinary drainage.

As a rule the catheter is removed the morning of the third postoperative day.

SUPRAPUBIC PROSTATECTOMY

A low midline incision is made directly over the bladder. The bladder is opened, and the prostatic tissue is enucleated through an incision into the urethral mucosa. To promote adequate drainage, a Penrose rubber drain is inserted deep into the incision and a Foley catheter is placed in the bladder through the urethra. Mortality is 2 to 4 percent; urinary result is excellent; and potency is maintained.

Postoperatively, in addition to the measures already mentioned, the nurse observes for symptoms of hemorrhage, shock, and clogging of the catheter with blood clots. The Penrose drain is removed within the first 24 hours and the Foley catheter is removed in 4 days.

RETROPUBIC PROSTATECTOMY

In retropubic prostatectomy, a low abdominal incision is used similar to that used for a suprapubic prostatectomy, but the bladder is not opened. The bladder is retracted and the hypertrophied tissue removed through an incision into the anterior prostatic capsule. A Penrose drain is inserted deep into the incision and a Foley catheter in the bladder. The mortality rate is 2 to 4 percent; urinary result is excellent; and potency is maintained.

Postoperatively, the nurse's responsibilities are as discussed for suprapubic prostatectomy. The Penrose drain is removed usually during the first postoperative day and the Foley catheter is removed the fourth day after surgery.

PERINEAL PROSTATECTOMY

Enucleation of the hypertrophied tissue is accomplished through a perineal incision made between the scrotum and the rectum. The posterior capsule of the prostate gland is incised and tissue removed. A Penrose drain is inserted deep into the wound and a Foley catheter in the bladder via the urethra. The mortality rate is 2 to 3 percent; impotency usually occurs; and there may be some delay in regaining perfect urethral sphincter control.

Postoperatively, nursing care measures are as already discussed. The perineal dressings are removed the first postoperative day and perineal care is accomplished with heat lamps to promote healing.

GENERAL NURSING CARE CONSIDERATIONS

Nursing care of the patient with a prostatectomy is centered upon close observation for hemorrhage and meticulous catheter care. Early ambulation is a necessary measure to avert cardiovascular and pulmonary complications and prevent formation of renal and bladder stones, which could injure the mucosal lining of the urinary tract and make it more susceptible to infection. Prolonged use of catheters is discouraged, nor should they be used for the convenience of the attending physician and nurses. The decision to employ the catheter should be made with the knowledge that it involves a risk of causing serious infection. Most patients subjected to urethral catheterization are elderly and many are debilitated, and this makes gram-negative sepsis an even greater hazard.

NURSING CARE MEASURES REGARDING CATHETERIZATION

Specific precautions regarding catheterization: (1) Aseptic technique should be rigorously observed during insertion of the catheter. (2) A sterile, plastic, disposable, closed drainage system must be employed with the collecting tube fixed to the upper portion of the bag and with a spigot attachment at the bottom with a cap that permits continued long-term use of the bag (Fig. 31-2). (3) The junction between the catheter and the closed drainage system must not be broken once the connection is made. (4) Drainage bags may be hung on the side of the bed, a chair, or a stretcher, but must never be inverted. The drainage tube must be secured to avoid low-hanging (redundant) loops that would force urine to run uphill to enter the bag. (5) Drainage bags are drained at 8-hour intervals, care being taken to avoid contamination of the mouth of the spigot. (6) All indwelling catheters must routinely be attached to the closed drainage system. (7) To prevent stasis of urine in the bladder, catheters should not be clamped. (8) Nursing care must include perineal care and thorough washing away of accumulated exudate by cleansing thoroughly around the external meatus and the external portion of the catheter for approximately 4 inches with a disinfectant or hydrogen peroxide. Neomycin hydrocortisone ointment may be placed about 1 inch along the catheter distal to the urethral opening. The penis and foreskin are momentarily pulled gently over the ointment on the catheter. This will aid in preventing urinary tract infection and help prevent urethral strictures. (9) Physicians, nurses, and ward personnel must thoroughly understand the system of closed urinary drainage. (10) Catheters

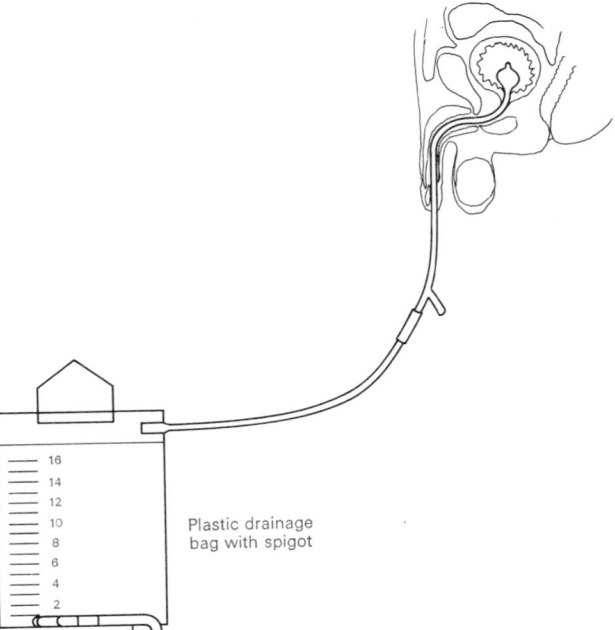

Figure 31-2
Closed drainage system.
(By permission from J. S. Ansell: Journal of Urology, 89:942, 943. © 1963, The Williams & Wilkins Company, Baltimore.)

16
14
12
10
8
6
4
2

Plastic drainage
bag with spigot

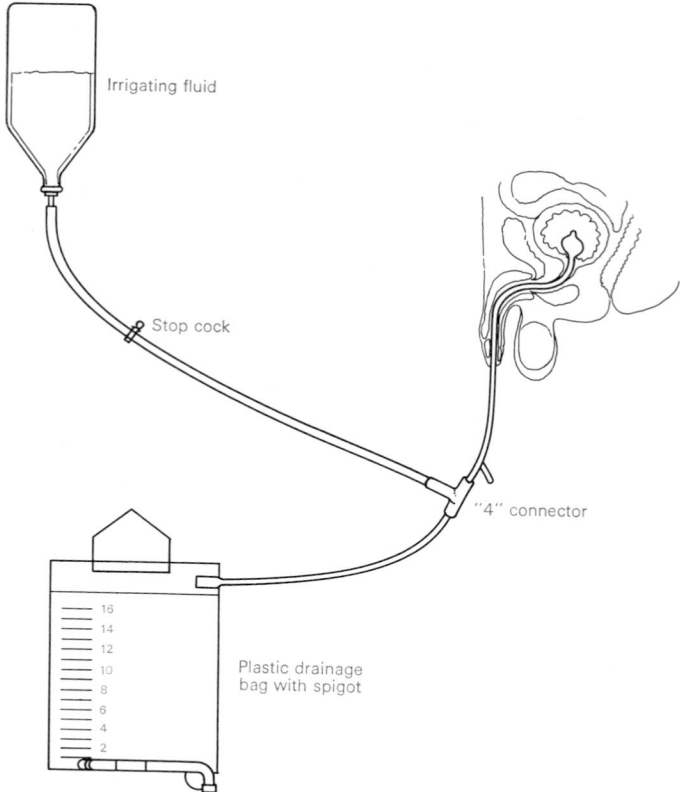

Irrigating fluid

Stop cock

"4" connector

Plastic drainage
bag with spigot

16
14
12
10
8
6
4
2

*Figure 31–3
Intermittent closed ir-
rigation system. (By
permission from J. S.
Ansell: Journal of
Urology, 89:942, 943. ©
1963, The Williams &
Wilkins Company,
Baltimore.)*

are not irrigated unless the physician suspects that obstruction is present.

All catheter care given by physicians, nurses, and ward personnel must be carried out with diligence. Great care must be taken to prevent instillation of bacteria into the bladder during catheterization. Individual sterile catheter trays must be utilized, and plenty of soap and water must be applied to the hands and arms before and after instrumentation.

If a bladder must be irrigated at intervals throughout the day, a closed intermittent bladder irrigating system (Fig. 31–3) is utilized. If a single or occasional bladder irrigation is indicated, manual irrigation maintaining aseptic technique is recommended (Fig. 31–4).

Carcinoma of the Prostate

Carcinoma of the prostate is rare in men under 60 years of age, but increases in frequency thereafter, and probably afflicts 25 percent of men in the eighth decade.

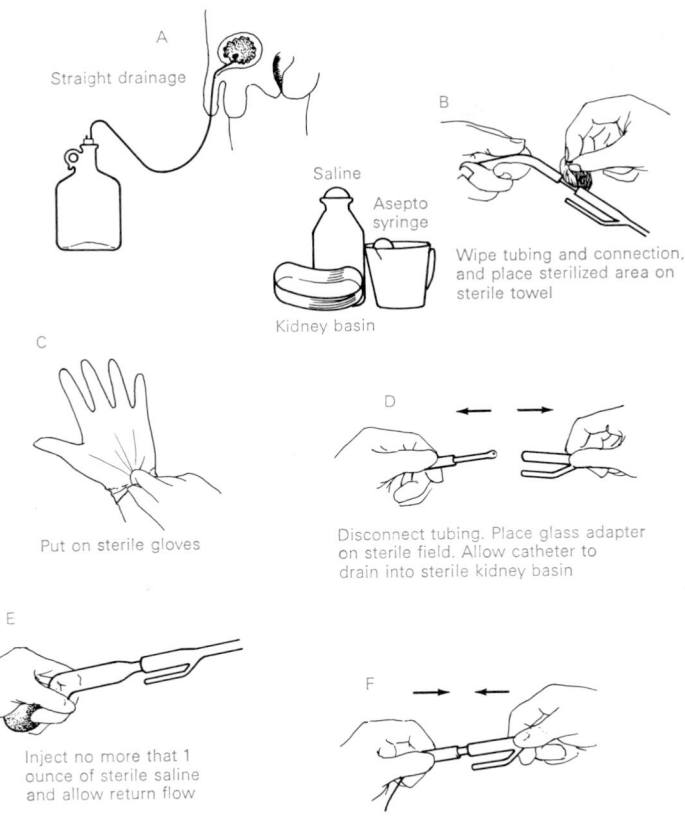

A

Straight drainage

B

Saline

Asepto syringe

Kidney basin

Wipe tubing and connection, and place sterilized area on sterile towel

C

Put on sterile gloves

D

Disconnect tubing. Place glass adapter on sterile field. Allow catheter to drain into sterile kidney basin

Figure 31–4 Manual irrigation maintaining aspectic technique. (By permission from J.S. Ansell: Journal of Urology, 89:942, 943. © 1963, The Williams & Wilkins Company, Baltimore.)

E

Inject no more that 1 ounce of sterile saline and allow return flow

F

Replace glass connector in catheter

Metastasis occurs primarily to the bones of the pelvis and may damage the kidneys because of the vesical obstruction that occurs.

The tumor spreads to the seminal vesicles and may penetrate the urethral mucosa or bladder wall and invade the external sphincter. With extension, the vesical, sacral, external iliac, and lumbar lymph nodes become involved, and finally there will be cancerous extension into the pelvic lymph nodes in 80 percent of patients. Metastases progress by way of the veins, particularly through the paravertebral veins surrounding the spine. Thus, bony metastases in the spine are common.

Clinically, the presenting symptoms in 95 percent of men with prostatic carcinoma are from urinary obstruction, infection, or both. In one of 20 patients the earliest symptoms are due to metastases. Pain in the lumbosacral region which may radiate into the hips or down the legs and a mass may be present in the right upper abdominal quadrant. Loss of appetite, loss of weight, and decline in strength may occur.

Obstruction of the prostatic urethra may promote formation of vesical diverticula or stones with resulting infection. Renal damage may be due to incompetency of the ureterovesical valves. Late in the disease, progressive edema, particularly of the scrotum and lower extremities, may occur from pressure of involved iliac nodes and lymphatics upon the great vessels. Pain in the lumbosacral region radiating into the hips or down the legs indicates osseous metastases to the lumbosacral spine and pelvis, and late in the disease pathological fractures may develop. Metastases have been reported to virtually all organs. Sudden spinal cord compression is not uncommon as a late complication. The most frequent signs and symptoms are low back pain with or without radiation to the lower extremities and weakness of the lower extremities.

The treatment is radical or palliative, according to the individual situation. If surgical cure is possible, a total perineal prostatectomy or a total retropubic prostatectomy is the operation of choice. The entire prostate, including its capsule, the seminal vesicles, and a portion of the bladder neck, is surgically removed. Urinary control is usually normal after the operation, but impotence is to be expected.

If the local lesion is extensive, the prostate is fixed; if there is x-ray evidence of metastases, the preferred therapy includes orchidectomy and administration of estrogen. If the degree of obstruction is severe or if estrogen therapy fails to afford relief, transurethral resection of the prostate will be necessary.

The nursing measures are similar to those of the patient with benign prostatic hyperplasia, although the patient and his family need a greater measure of support and understanding from the entire health team.

Disorders of the Spermatic Cord

The spermatic cord suspends the testicle in the scrotum, protects it from trauma, and thereby preserves optimum spermatogenesis. Anomalies of the spermatic cord which interfere with spermatogenesis are particularly damaging as they may cause impotence.

Hydrocele

A hydrocele is an accumulation of fluid within the tunica vaginalis or processus vaginalis most often surrounding the testicle.

Ninety percent of hydroceles occur in men above the age of 21. The etiology is generally unknown although they may develop rapidly secondary to local injury, acute nonspecific or tuberculous epididymitis, or orchitis, or slowly as fluid collects about the testis and forms a mass. In the newborn, hydrocele of the tunica vaginalis is common and probably results from late closure of the processus vaginalis. In most cases the hydrocele subsides spontaneously during the first few weeks of life. Complications include compression of the blood supply of the testicle which leads to atrophy, hemorrhage into the hydrocele sac following trauma (hematocele), and infection complicating aspiration.

Diagnosis is made by the finding of a cystic intrascrotal mass that transilluminates and is not tender unless there is an underlying inflammatory disease.

The treatment may include aspiration or surgical removal of the sac. Indications for therapy are the presence of a very tense hydrocele that might constrict circulation to the testicle, or a large unsightly and uncomfortable mass. In acute hydrocele aspiration is performed to relieve pain, procure fluid, or clarify the diagnosis by allowing palpation of scrotal contents. The patient is placed at bed rest and the scrotum elevated.

Spermatocele

This painless cystic mass usually occurs after puberty, developing just above and posterior to the testis. Most spermatoceles are less than 1 cm in diameter, but some are quite large and may be mistaken for hydroceles.

Spermatocele is distinguished from hydrocele of the tunica vaginalis in that the latter covers the entire anterior surface of the testis. In most cases spermatocele is asymptomatic, but many patients seek help because of cancerophobia.

The etiology is not known. No therapy is required unless the spermatocele is large enough to cause complaints. In this event a small incision is made in the scrotum and the spermatocele is excised.

Varicocele

A dilatation of the pampiniform plexus within the scrotum leads to a varicocele. It is seen in about 10 percent of young men. The left internal spermatic vein is particularly susceptible and is likely to have incompetent valves. This together with gravity may lead to poor drainage of the pampiniform plexus, the veins of which gradually undergo dilatation and elongation—hence the term often applied is "a bag of worms." At times varicocele is painful, particularly in the sexually aggressive male. There may be testicular atrophy from impaired drainage. The main complaint is of a constant pulling, dragging, or dull pain in the area of the scrotum and occasionally in the testis.

No treatment is required unless the varicocele is thought to contribute to infertility or is painful or large. A scrotal support will often relieve discomfort; otherwise ligation of the pampiniform veins of the spermatic cord above the internal ring is indicated.

Bibliography

Works of General Interest

Bagshaw, Malcolm A., Henry S. Kaplan, and Robert H. Sagerman: Linear Accelerator Supervoltage Radiotherapy. VII. Carcinoma of the Prostate. *Radiology,* 85:128, 1965.

Campbell, Meredith F. (Ed.): *Urology,* 3d ed. Philadelphia: W. B. Saunders Company, 1970.

Davis, David M.: *Mechanisms of Urologic Disease.* Philadelphia: W. B. Saunders Company, 1953.

Gartman, Edward: Epididymitis. *American Journal of Surgery,* 101:736–741, June, 1961.

Jordan, Willis Pope: Hydroceles and Varicoceles. *Surgical Clinics of North America,* 45:1535–1545, 1965.

Marshall, Sumner, Frank H. Tavel, and John W. Schulte: Spinal Cord Compression Secondary to Metastatic Carcinoma of the Prostate Treated by Decompression Laminectomy. *Journal of Urology,* 88:667–673, November, 1962.

Nesbit, Reed M.: Transurethral Prostatic Resection. in Meredith F. Campbell (Ed.): *Urology.* Philadelphia: W. B. Saunders Company, 1970, pp. 2479–2502.

Sawyer, Janet R.: *Nursing Care of Patients with Urologic Diseases,* 2d ed. Saint Louis: The C. V. Mosby Company, 1968.

Smith, Donald R.: *General Urology,* 6th ed. Los Altos, Calif.: Lange Medical Publications, 1969.

Utz, John P., et al.: Clinical and Laboratory Studies of Mumps IV. Viruria and Abnormal Renal Function. *New England Journal of Medicine,* 270:1283–1286, June, 1964.

Suggested Reading List for Students

Ansell, J. S.: Catheter Care. *Journal of Urology,* 89:940–944, June, 1963.

Beeson, Paul B.: The Case against the Catheter. *American Journal of Medicine,* 24:1–3, January, 1958.

Creevy, C. D.: The Care of the Urological Patient before and after Operation. in Meredith F. Campbell (Ed.): *Urology.* Philadelphia: W. B. Saunders Company, 1970, pp. 2055–2083.

Desautels, Robert E.: Aseptic Management of Catheter Drainage. *New England Journal of Medicine,* 263:189–191, July, 1960.

Desautels, Robert E., Carl W. Walters, Roger C. Graves, and J. Hartwell Harrison: Technical Advances in the Prevention of Urinary Tract Infection. *Journal of Urology,* 87:487–490, March, 1962.

Hinman, Frank, Jr., and Clare E. Cox: The Voiding Vesical Defense Mechanism: The Mathematical Effect of Residual Urine, Voiding Interval and Volume on Bacteriuria. *Journal of Urology,* 96:491–498, October, 1966.

Kass, Edward H. and Lawrence J. Schneiderman: Entry of Bacteria into the Urinary Tracts of Patients with Inlying Catheters. *New England Journal of Medicine,* 256:556–557, 1957.

Kasselman, Mary Jo: Nursing Care of the Patient with Benign Prostatic Hypertrophy. *American Journal of Nursing,* 66:1026–1030, May, 1966.

Kunin, Calvin M. and Regina C. McCormack: Prevention of Catheter-Induced Urinary-Tract Infections by Sterile Closed Drainage. *New England Journal of Medicine,* 274:1155–1161, May, 1966.

Leader, Abel J. and C. Eugene Carlton, Jr.: Urologic Diagnosis and the Urologic Examination, in Meredith F. Campbell (Ed.): *Urology.* Philadelphia: W. B. Saunders Company, 1970, pp. 197–276.

Morel, Alice: The Urologic Nurse Specialist. *Nursing Clinics of North America,* 4:475–482, 1969.

Mossholder, Irene B.: When the Patient Has a Radical Retropubic Prostatectomy. *American Journal of Nursing,* 62:101–104, July, 1962.

Olsen, Edith and Lois M. Schroeder: The Hazards of Immobility: Effects on Urinary Function. *American Journal of Nursing,* 67:790–792, April, 1967.

Rubin, Philip, et al.: Cancer of the Urogenital Tract: Bladder Cancer. *Journal of the American Medical Association,* 206:2719–2728, December, 1968.

Rubin, Philip, et al.: Cancer of the Urogenital Tract: Prostatic Cancer. *Journal of the American Medical Association,* 209:1695–1705, September, 1969.

Scott, William W. and Horst K. A. Schirmer: Carcinoma of the Prostate. in Meredith F. Campbell (Ed.): *Urology.* Philadelphia: W. B. Saunders Company, 1970, pp. 1143–1185.

SECTION 2
VENEREAL
DISEASES

MARY S. KLEINKNECHT*

Gonorrhea
Syphilis
CLINICAL MANIFESTATIONS OF EARLY ACQUIRED SYPHILIS
DIAGNOSIS OF SYPHILIS
Primary stage
Secondary stage
Latent syphilis
CONGENITAL SYPHILIS
SYPHILIS IN PREGNANCY
Treatment
Nursing considerations in care of the patient with
venereal disease

This discussion of venereal diseases has been limited to syphilis and gonorrhea in order to focus attention on the momentous public health problem created by them.

Despite widespread efforts at every community level—local, state, and national—to eradicate gonorrhea and syphilis in the United States, these diseases continue to be prevalent. A few statistics will indicate the magnitude of the problem. In 1947 the reported incidence of gonorrhea was 284.2 cases per 100,000 population; in 1950 the rate fell to 204.0; and by 1958 it had fallen to 129.3 per 100,000 population.[1] At that time an increase in the number of reported cases of gonorrhea began to be noted, and by 1966 the rate had climbed to 173.6. The number of reported cases of syphilis, which had reached an all-time high of 75.6 per 100,000 population in 1947, began to fall; by 1950 the rate was 21.6; and by 1957 it was 3.8 per 100,000 population. But in 1958 the rate of reported cases of syphilis, like that of gonorrhea, began to climb, and by 1964 it reached 12.1 per 100,000 population—more than 3.5 times the 1957 rate.[2]

There are complex reasons for the increase in prevalence of these social diseases, including greater sexual freedom among teenagers, public complacency, and an increase in homosexual practices. Thus, even though a powerful tool—chemotherapy in the form of penicillin and other antibiotics—is available which could eradicate these diseases, they remain a serious public health problem. The nurse therefore should take advantage of all the opportunities open to her to help educate the public about the seriousness of these diseases and to help in case-finding efforts.

* The author acknowledges the assistance of Matlock M. Mims, M.D., in the preparation of this section.

[1] VD Fact Sheet, p. 9.

[2] Ibid.

Gonorrhea

Gonorrhea is a purulent inflammation of the mucosa of the genital tract caused by the gonococcus, *Neisseria gonorrhoeae*, a gram-negative coccus.

The disease is almost always acquired through sexual contact, the chief exception being ophthalmia neonatorum, in which it is acquired from the mother at parturition. In rare instances it is acquired from toilet seats, instruments, or fomites, but this is unusual because gonococci die rapidly outside the body. Homosexual transmission may result in urethritis, proctitis, and pharyngitis.

Pathologically, the gonococci multiply on columnar epithelium, spread throughout the mucosa, and proliferate. Decomposition of the organism, which is destroyed by body defenses, creates a toxin. The irritative effect of the toxin causes the outpouring of a purulent discharge representing acute urethritis. In tortuous passages, where drainage is poor, copious amounts of purulent exudate will accumulate.

Diagnosis can be difficult, and demonstration of the gonococcus by laboratory methods is inconsistent. Fluorescent antibody examination (FAT) of material taken from the urethra and cervix probably provides the most reliable identification. This technique involves the microscopic visualization of a specific antigen under ultraviolet illumination. The specific antibody is tagged with a fluorescent dye, so that when an antigen-antibody reaction takes place, the pathogen can be identified (Shapiro and Lentz). Diagnosis may also be established by demonstration of *N. gonorrhoeae* in smears or cultures of exudate from the urethra, cervix, eye, serous cavity, or blood. Endocervical curettage is a newer technique that improves the reliability of cultures of gonococci in the female. In this procedure, the cervix is exposed and the endocervix gently curetted. The endocervical glands are believed to provide a favorable environment for the gonococci, which are located deep in the glands. With curettage, the sealed-over openings of the glands are removed and the trapped material escapes. This technique has increased the number of positive cultures by 13 percent.

Acute gonorrhea in either sex may be asymptomatic for months or years without disappearance of the bacteria, and immunity to reinfection is negligible (Bennett).

Gonorrhea tends to heal by dense scarring, with residuals of urethral stricture, closure of fallopian tubes, or sterility following epididymitis.

Manifestations of gonorrhea ("clap" or "strain") in the male are many. The incubation period is 3 to 7 days. Urethritis becomes established with involvement of the urethral glands; the inflammation spreads to the prostate, seminal vesicles, Cowper's glands, epididymis, and sometimes to the testicle. Copious purulent urethral discharge and severe burning on urination are followed by retention, perineal pain, hematuria, chordee, and local spread. Acute epididymitis complicates 5 to 10 percent of untreated cases. Within 6 weeks the untreated disease subsides and the gonococci disappear, or a chronic carrier state develops with the organism persisting in the prostate. Urethral strictures are a common complication, especially with repeated infections.

In the female, gonorrhea often causes transient urethritis probably because of the absence of urethral glands where the infectious process could localize. The vagina in the adult female does not become infected; however, vaginitis is frequently seen in children. Medical advice is usually sought for cervicitis, manifested by copious, irritating leukorrhea, acute salpingitis with or without tubal abscess, pelvic or generalized peritonitis with abdominal pain and fever, or more rarely proctitis, manifested by bloody, mucoid stools. The disease may be completely without symptoms although the cervix, vagina, and Skene's and Bartholin's glands as well as the urethra are infected (Conger). Complications are more serious in women than in men, and include pelvic inflammatory disease. The end-result of the infection in females is likely to be sterility.

Treatment

Most strains of *N. gonorrhoeae* are resistant to sulfonamides, but are susceptible to penicillin, the tetracyclines, and a few other antibiotics. For gonorrhea in males, a single injection of 600,000 to 1.2 million units of depot penicillin is given. In females, two weekly injections of 1.2 million units are sufficient. A repetition of this treatment will result in a cure in nearly all recurrences. A tetracycline may be substituted if the patient is hypersensitive to penicillin.

Syphilis

Syphilis is a chronic systemic infectious disease caused by *Treponema pallidum*, an anaerobe requiring moisture and tissue for survival and usually transmitted through sexual contact. It is capable of causing tissue destruction and chronic inflammation in most organs of the body and can give rise to many clinical manifestations. *T. pallidum* is able to grow and survive body defenses, but dies quickly when removed from a favorable environment. The blood may contain the organism in abundance; thus the organism may be discharged into the fetal circulation during the early stages of pregnancy or into the vaginal tract in menstrual blood.

The organism is probably transmitted through direct and intimate contact with moist infectious lesions of the mucous membranes and skin, as occurs in sexual contact; but it can be transmitted through kissing, biting, or in blood during a transfusion. *T. pallidum* apparently is capable of penetrating the mucous membranes, but an abrasion is necessary for inoculation to occur through the skin. After the spirochete has penetrated the epithelium, it enters the lymphatics and regional lymph nodes, whence it spreads throughout the body via the bloodstream. This spirochetemia may occur weeks before the appearance of the primary lesion at the site of inoculation. The early dissemination of the spirochete throughout body tissues is the basis for many of the later manifestations of syphilis.

Primary lesions are found on or near the genitalia in 95 percent of patients. In the male, the chancre usually appears on the prepuce or on the coronal sulcus, but any portion of the genitalia may be involved. The primary lesion in the female usually appears on the labia and in the fourchette, but again any portion of the genitalia may be involved. About 5 percent of primary lesions occur on the lips, female breasts, or in the mouth.

DIAGNOSIS OF SYPHILIS

In the early stages, dark-field examination will demonstrate *T. pallidum.* This examination is most useful and should be employed routinely on every genital, cutaneous, and mucosal lesion suspected of being syphilitic. The dark-field examination is reliable and establishes without doubt the diagnosis and stage of the disease.

The serologic tests for syphilis (STS) are the most commonly used diagnostic procedures. These are based upon the finding of an antibody-like substance, sometimes called *reagin,* which appears in the patient's serum shortly after infection from the spirochete. Syphilitic serum interacts with a lipoidal antigen made from an alcoholic extract of beef heart. A number of modifications of the flocculation tests for syphilis have been named after their originators, e.g., Kahn, Kline, and Hinton. The complement fixation technique or Wassermann test employs the same type of antigen; the Kolmer modification is most commonly used in the United States. The VDRL (Venereal Disease Research Laboratory) test is a rapid slide technique utilizing cardiolipin antigen. Because of its high degree of sensitivity and specificity it has become the flocculation test of choice in most state laboratories and hospitals.

The rapid plasma reagin (RPR) test is a very rapid serologic procedure which utilizes unheated plasma or serum. It is more sensitive than the standard serologic tests and is used as a routine screening technique in laboratories performing large numbers of tests or in tests requiring immediate results.

The *T. pallidum* immobilizing test of Nelson (TPI) and other treponemal tests are of considerable value in the diagnosis of false positive reactions. A negative treponemal test is therefore of value in excluding a diagnosis of syphilis. A positive test indicates the existence of a syphilitic infection even if the standard serologic tests are negative.

A spinal fluid examination must be performed in every patient with a diagnosis of syphilis, since it provides the only method of determining whether the central nervous system is involved during the asymptomatic stage, and of determining the efficacy of treatment. Biopsy is valuable in diagnosis, particularly in cutaneous lesions, and it is indispensable in late syphilis to demonstrate involvement of lymph nodes, testes, or larynx.

CLINICAL MANIFESTATIONS OF EARLY ACQUIRED SYPHILIS

Primary Stage

The period of incubation is usually from 10 to 90 days. The chancre is a solitary, indurated, nonpainful ulceration that heals slowly with scar formation. Many times it is accompanied by painless enlargement of the regional lymph nodes. Primary syphilis may also be manifested by small, multiple lesions, or painful lesions that may resemble many other conditions. Because of the frequent atypical appearance of the chancre, every genital lesion should be subjected to a dark-field examination.

Secondary Stage

This stage generally develops about 6 weeks after appearance of the primary lesion and is manifested by systemic symptoms and generalized skin eruptions. The patient may exhibit secondary lesions without ever having a primary lesion; or he may never show secondary manifestations and have the latent stage directly following healing of the primary lesion (Heyman).

The eruptions are macular, papular, papulosquamous, grouped follicular, rarely pustular or nodular. The eruptions are usually widespread and frequently involve the palms, soles, oral cavity, anogenital area, and the trunk and extremities.

Eruptions covered with epithelium are not infectious; infectiousness develops when the eruptions are eroded as occurs in the anogenital area because of the constant presence of moisture. Secondary syphilis is extremely contagious because it spreads from many lesions. Lesions of the mouth are painless, superficial erosions on the buccal surfaces, on the tongue, or inside the lip. Oral lesions covered with a thin, grayish exudate are called *mucous patches;* similar lesions of the genital areas are called *condylomata lata.* They are broad, flat, and wart-like and are found on the labia majora, perineum, and anal region. They are highly infectious. Lesions of the tonsillar area and palate cause a persistent sore throat. Many patients have constitutional symptoms such as malaise, lassitude, headaches, fever, and myalgia; these may also be generalized lymphadenopathy.

Early acquired syphilis is highly infectious. Some secretions such as saliva and semen are frequently in contact with infectious mucosal lesions and may therefore contain *T. pallidum.* Patients with early syphilis should not donate blood for transfusions.

Latent Syphilis

Latent syphilis is that stage of the disease in which there are no symptoms or clinical evidence of the disease. This is by far the most frequent type of syphilis, and although the syphilitic infection is not clinically evident during the latent period it may produce profound changes in the body.

The more time that passes between the primary and secondary lesions of syphilis and the appearance of the clinical manifestations of latent syphilis, the more destructive the lesions become. The localized gummatous lesion of latent syphilis may appear in any organ, affecting the skin and mucous membranes, skeletal system, stomach, kidney, genitourinary tract, and the cardiovascular and central nervous system. The gumma is a dense, firm growth that varies in stages of activity over a period of months or years. Often it causes abscesses and tissue breakdown; healing is slow and characterized by the presence of scar tissue. Latent syphilis is often diagnosed when damage to the aorta causes an aneurysm or when central nervous system damage causes optic atrophy, tabes dorsalis, and general paresis.

CONGENITAL SYPHILIS

The infant is malnourished, dehydrated, and severely ill. Manifestations may include persistent rhinitis, condylomata, fissures, skin lesions, tenderness over the long bones, and pseudoparalysis.

Late congenital syphilis frequently manifests itself in the second decade with evidence of central nervous system involvement, such as eighth nerve deafness, optic atrophy, and interstitial keratitis. The prognosis in congenital neurosyphilis is poor and the patient responds poorly to treatment. Late congenital syphilis often causes hypoplasia, wide spacing and notching of the central incisors (Hutchinson teeth), frontal bossing, a highly arched palate, and saber shins. Occasionally hydrarthrosis of the knee joint (Clutton's synovitis) is associated with interstitial keratitis.

SYPHILIS IN PREGNANCY

Syphilis in pregnancy is a special problem because the fetus becomes infected after the fifth month of pregnancy by the passage of *T. pallidum* through the placenta (Heyman). This is seen in women with untreated early syphilis and sometimes in those with late syphilis. Pregnancy complicated by infectious syphilis may terminate in a spontaneous abortion, a still birth, or a premature or full-term infected syphilitic infant. The early recognition of syphilis in the mother and proper treatment will prevent congenital syphilis in almost every instance.

Treatment

Treatment of early and secondary syphilis consists of giving benzathine penicillin G, 2.4 million units as an initial dose, followed by the same dosage 3 to 4 days later.

In the patient who is sensitive to penicillin or in whom sensitivity to it develops, 30 g of either erythromycin or tetracycline may be given orally over a period of 15 days.

After completing the treatment, the patient should return to his physician monthly during the first year so that quantitative serologic tests can be done and an examination can be made for recurring syphilitic lesions. A spinal fluid examination should be carried out 6 months after treatment for early syphilis.

In latent syphilis or in the clinically asymptomatic stage of the disease which appears after the secondary stage, treatment consists of administration of benzathine penicillin G, 2.4 million units, given at one time, or aqueous suspension of penicillin G, 600,000 units given daily for 8 days to a total of 4.8 million units. If the patient is sensitive to penicillin, either tetracycline or erythromycin, 30 g in doses of 2 g per day, may be substituted.

Nursing Considerations in Care of the Patient with Venereal Disease

The physician will prescribe and supervise a program of treatment with penicillin. If the patient is sensitive to penicillin, erythromycin or a tetracycline will be substituted.

The nurse as a member of the medical team contributes to the health education of the public regarding all aspects of venereal disease and plays a significant role in case-finding by interview-investigation of patients and contacts.

In all areas of nursing, particularly in the community, schools, industry, and hospitals, the nurse uses education as a powerful tool of preventive medicine and has the responsibility to actively participate in satisfying the public's need for health teaching.

The school nurse teaches sex education to the teenager, stressing the spread of venereal disease, preventive measures, and the relationship between promiscuity and venereal disease.

The nurse actively participates in treating the patient with venereal disease whether in the hospital, outpatient clinic, doctor's office, or the community. Although infectious organisms from gonorrhea or syphilis are almost without exception transmitted through coital contact, freshly discharged organisms can be transferred from contaminated clothing to hands and carried by hands to eyes or to a cut in the skin. Modified isolation principles are employed to prevent the spread of infection. Gloves are used to protect personnel with cuts or abrasions on the hands from coming in contact with infectious lesions of the skin or mucous membrane as seen in early syphilis or from materials such as bed linens, clothing, or towels which may have been in contact with the infectious lesions.

The patient with infectious syphilis must be taught how to care for himself, thereby assisting in the prevention of the spread of infection. All cutaneous and mucosal lesions of early syphilis contain *T. pallidum* in great numbers and hence are potentially infectious. The most dangerous lesions from the standpoint of transmission are the innocuous-appearing ulcerated lesions on the skin and about the lips or in the mouth. Anything that comes in contact with discharges from these areas or from the urethra may become infected. Special precautions must be taken to prevent the discharge from accidentally contacting and infecting the eyes. The patient is taught the need for meticulous care and washing of clothing and linen as well as thorough hand washing. He is cautioned to refrain from coitus until the disease has been controlled. The patient should also know that no immunity occurs after infection and that reinfection is possible.

The psychosocial implications of venereal disease may have a profound impact on the patient, who may feel guilty because of the moral-sexual connotations and who may be reluctant or refuse to reveal contacts. In order to be successful the nurse must examine her own attitudes and emotional reactions so that she can accept these patients and help them to feel free to discuss any aspect of their problems. The nurse must not be judgmental but must take time and patience in helping the patient to understand the reason why the public health departments which are responsible for epidemiological control must know the name of the patient's sexual contacts so that treatment can be provided and venereal disease can be eradicated.

Bibliography

AMA National Symposium on Venereal Disease Control. Archives of Environmental Health, 13:351–409, July-December, 1966.

Bennett, Ivan L., Jr.: Gonococcal Infections. in T. R. Harrison (Ed.): *Principles of Internal Medicine,* 5th ed. New York: McGraw-Hill Book Company, 1966, p. 1537.

Brown, William J.: Public Health Aspects of Syphilis. *Southern Medical Journal,* 59:639–642, June, 1966.

Conger, Kyril B.: Gonorrhea and Nonspecific Urethritis. *Medical Clinics of North America,* 48:767, May, 1964.

Heyman, Albert: Syphilis. in T. R. Harrison (Ed.): *Principles of Internal Medicine,* 5th ed. New York: McGraw-Hill Book Company, 1966, p. 1628.

Kampmeier, R. H.: The Rise in Venereal Disease: Epidemiology and Prevention. *Medical Clinics of North America,* 51:735–751, May, 1967.

Kaye, Donald: Gonococcal Disease. in P. B. Beeson and Walsh McDermott (Eds.): *Cecil-Loeb Textbook of Medicine,* 12th ed. Philadelphia: W. B. Saunders Company, 1967.

McDermott, Walsh: Spirochetal Infections. in P. B. Beeson and Walsh McDermott (Eds.): *Cecil-Loeb Textbook of Medicine,* 12th ed. Philadelphia: W. B. Saunders Company, 1967, pp. 318–331.

McDermott, Walsh: Syphilis. in P. B. Beeson and Walsh McDermott (Eds.): *Cecil-Loeb Textbook of Medicine,* 12th ed. Philadelphia: W. B. Saunders Company, 1967.

Shapiro, Leonard H. and John W. Lentz: Gonorrhea. in Howard F. Conn and Rex B. Conn, Jr. (Eds.): *Current Diagnosis.* Philadelphia: W. B. Saunders Company, 1970, pp. 492–495.

U.S. Department of Health, Education, and Welfare, U.S. Public Health Service: *The Eradication of Syphilis. A Task Force Report to the Surgeon General.* Publication No. 918, Washington, D.C.: U.S. Government Printing Office, 1962.

U.S. Department of Health, Education, and Welfare, Public Health Service: *VD Fact Sheet,* 23d rev. Atlanta: Bureau of Disease Prevention and Environmental Control, National Communicable Disease Center, 1966, p. 9.

World Forum on Syphilis. *Public Health Reports,* 78:295–316, April, 1963.

Youmans, John B. (Ed.): Syphilis and Other Venereal Diseases. *Medical Clinics of North America,* 48:573–841, May, 1964.

SECTION 3
DISEASES OF THE FEMALE REPRODUCTIVE SYSTEM
ANNETTE EZELL*

* Mrs. Mary Lou Jones, R.N., of the Washoe County Health Department, Reno, Nevada, assisted in the preparation of portions of this section.

Many women tend to seek more adequate health care for members of their families than for themselves. This occurs for many reasons—cultural, economic, and social —and perhaps because of preoccupation with other matters of interest. The nurse who is aware of the psychological needs of women and who understands their physiological functioning can impart a vast amount of knowledge and emotional support to them. Her relatively intimate ministrations to the woman patient, the sameness of sex, and the assumption by many women that she is a knowledgeable source of medical information contribute to her ability to assume a major responsibility in maintaining the health status of the female patient, regardless of the patient's specific health situation. Not the least important aspect of her care is to assist in clarifying folklore and mystique about the functioning of the female reproductive organs.

Great emphasis is being placed upon adequate diagnosis, treatment, and care of the female patient, especially in relationship to the possibility of neoplasia. Even though much time, energy, and money are expended to promote early detection of pathology, hesitation and delay are constant problems. Therefore this section will attempt to delineate those areas of reproductive pathology which are most frequent and with which nurses may be involved in patient care. For present purposes the female reproductive system is considered to include the vagina, cervix, uterus, ovaries, fallopian tubes, and the mammary glands.

Menstruation

Mammary and endometrial tissues undergo physiological and anatomical changes throughout the female's life, and also are affected by such external factors as drugs and diet. Puberty, menstruation, pregnancy, lactation, and menopause account for the normal changes in these tissues. Nonetheless, the female patient is subject to psychological and physiological discomforts arising from normal changes. The discomfort may range from minor tingling to severe psychological disturbances from repressed sexuality. Fortunately, the incidence of minor discomforts has no bearing upon their seriousness, although in some instances seemingly insignificant symptoms of menstrual irregularity, intermenstrual bleeding, and unusual discharge from the vagina or breast are disregarded. The most serious disorders of the female reproductive organs are those due to neoplasia of the mammary gland or uterus. Delays in diagnosis due to hesitancy and fear contribute to the predominant place of carcinoma of the breast and uterus in statistical surveys.

Hypophyseal hormones and gonadal hormones control function of the uterus and the endometrial lining in cyclic pattern. The menstrual cycle, endometrial proliferation and degeneration, is divided into proliferative, secretory, and menstrual stages or phases (Figure 31–5).

NORMAL MENSTRUAL CYCLE

Proliferative Phase

At completion of the menstrual flow, the endometrium is very thin and the estrogen-progesterone level in the blood is low. The anterior pituitary then stimulates

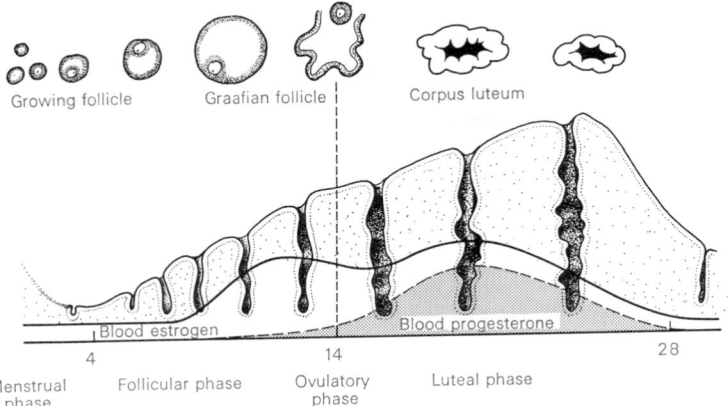

*Figure 31–5
Diagram showing
changes in the
endometrium, the
ovaries, and the circu-
lating ovarian hormones
during the menstrual
cycle. (By permission
from C. Donnell Turner:
General Endocrinology,
3d ed. Philadelphia: W.
B. Saunders Company,
1963.)*

secretion of follicle-stimulating hormone (FSH). *Proliferation* takes place from the fifth to the fourteenth day of the cycle. As the estrogen level begins to rise there is vascularization of breast tissue and proliferation of endometrial tissue. The endometrium increases six to eight times in thickness. This remarkable increase is due to lengthening of the tubular glands, thickening of the stroma, and coiling of the arterioles.

Secretory Phase

The period from the fourteenth to the twenty-fifth day is termed the *secretory phase*. During this time the glands of the endometrium lengthen and become tortuous, glycogen is stored within the cells, and epithelial cells begin to elongate. Endometrial hyperplasia and vascularization occur at the height of proliferation in preparation for the fertilized ovum. If the ovum is not fertilized, the corpus luteum atrophies and inhibits production of progesterone at about the twenty-fifth day, and the endometrium desquamates.

Menstrual Phase

With endometrial desquamation, approximately 5 days before menstruation, there is infarction and necrosis of the involved blood vessels, and the necrotic endometrial tissue is exuded, i.e., menstruation occurs. The *menstrual phase* usually takes place after the twenty-eighth day and results in a blood loss of 150 to 300 ml. The first day of menstruation is counted as day 1 of the cycle. The discharge is heaviest on the first 2 days; it consists of the blood, fragments of endometrium, and mucin from the endometrial glands. The average time for this cyclic pattern is 28 days, but most women do not have such rigid regularity. The normal cycle may range from 21 days to 35 days. The flow generally lasts for 3 to 5 days, but a period of 6 or 7 days is not abnormal.

Ovulation may not occur in the presence of an abnormality of the genital tract. Although menstruation can occur without ovulation, the reverse does not commonly occur. Estrogen replacement therapy may be prescribed and other possible causes (tumor, infection) will be sought.

MENSTRUAL ABNORMALITIES

Amenorrhea

Amenorrhea may result from normal causes, as during pregnancy and lactation, or pathological ones, as from a disturbance in endocrine function or a disorder of the reproductive tract. The term *primary amenorrhea* applies to absence of menstrual periods after puberty. A pituitary disturbance may cause suppression of normal ovarian function, and because of the interrelatedness of all the endocrines, their malfunction can cause amenorrhea. In *secondary* amenorrhea, a normal menstrual cycle has been established, but stops sometime before menopause. The most common causes are surgical removal of the ovaries, destruction of the ovaries by x-rays, chronic debilitating diseases such as tuberculosis and anemia, and severe emotional stress.

Diagnosis is made by a careful history supplemented with physical examinations and laboratory studies. Cytological examination of the vagina, endometrium, and cervix should be done to demonstrate any abnormalities that may exist.

Oligomenorrhea, Polymenorrhea, Hypomenorrhea

In oligomenorrhea the interval between menstrual periods is prolonged, i.e., less than one period per month, whereas in polymenorrhea the opposite situation occurs, i.e., the interval between periods may be as short as 2 weeks.

Oligomenorrhea in the absence of chronic debilitating disease is evidence of ovarian deficiency and is treated accordingly. Polymenorrhea may be due to hormonal imbalance, disease, or pelvic infection. The patient must be convinced of the need for prompt medical attention, since there is a strong possibility that pelvic neoplasm is the cause, especially in the older woman. The presence of tumors can be detected by pelvic examination and biopsy.

Untreated polymenorrhea may give rise to anemia, because the blood loss is beyond the body's replacement ability. The dangers of ignoring neoplasms are obvious.

Hypomenorrhea, or scanty menstrual flow, often is associated with oligomenorrhea or other ovarian disorders. Hormonal dysfunction, chronic infection, and disease of other body systems are possible causes.

Hypermenorrhea

Hypermenorrhea, or excessive menstrual flow, frequently is associated with polymenorrhea, since they have the same causation. Menstrual periods can be of normal length with excessive flow or of prolonged length with normal or excessive flow. In any case, the amount of blood lost is greater than normal and in many patients leads to anemia. Endocrine disturbance is the most frequent cause of hypermenorrhea in younger women. In older women, local pelvic diseases, including polyps of the cervix and endometrium, uterine fibromas, cancer, and pelvic inflammatory disease, are the most frequent causes. Pelvic examination, including curettage (scraping of the uterus), aids in diagnosis.

Metrorrhagia

Metrorrhagia is bleeding or spotting between periods. Spotting occurring regularly near the middle of the cycle, provided that all other causes have been excluded, is probably due to ovulatory bleeding. Nonetheless, metrorrhagia may be a symptom of a serious disorder such as cancer, threatened abortion, or endometriosis, or of a less serious disease such as cervical polyps or cervical erosion.

Dysmenorrhea

Dysmenorrhea, or menstrual pain, includes a wide variety of symptoms and is one of the most common complaints seen by the gynecologist. Primary or intrinsic dysmenorrhea is more difficult to relieve than secondary dysmenorrhea.

Secondary Dysmenorrhea. Secondary dysmenorrhea results from a disorder such as uterine displacement, pelvic inflammatory disease, or neoplasm, and may also be associated with genitourinary or sacroiliac disease. The pain differs from the sharp cramps of primary dysmenorrhea, being usually dull and aching. Although the pain can easily be controlled with rest, analgesics, and local applications of heat, again it is important to treat the cause.

Primary Dysmenorrhea. Menstrual pain in the absence of any pelvic lesion is called *primary* or *intrinsic* dysmenorrhea. The reason for it is not fully understood, although many theories have been advanced. Psychogenic, constitutional, and obstructive causes have been suggested. Many women with neuroses about sex and menstruation suffer from dysmenorrhea, but many such women have no menstrual discomfort whatever. The psychogenic element generally is believed to contribute to dysmenorrhea, but it is not the entire answer. Constitutional factors such as acute and chronic diseases of other body systems, anemia, and fatigue are thought to have some part. Endocrine disturbances are believed to play a large role. Until all the factors have been identified and brought under control, analgesics like codeine and aspirin and application of heat remain the most reliable therapies for dysmenorrhea.

MENOPAUSE

Menopause is cessation of the menstrual cycle. As a rule it occurs between the forty-fifth and fiftieth years. Unfortunately, for many women it is not without problems. The changes occurring at this time have been lumped together as "change of life" for so long that their psychological impact upon the woman often is great. Other than not having menstrual periods and being unable to bear children, the woman has no profound alteration in her living pattern. The woman of 45 usually does not want more children and certainly will not greatly miss the menstrual period. However, for many women menopause has been linked to loss of sexual function, loss of attractiveness and femininity, and rapid aging. Actually, ovarian function has little to do with libido, but these subjective fears can cause much of the nervousness, irritability, and tension that are attributed to menopause. Furthermore, many women relax and enjoy sexual intercourse more after the danger of pregnancy has passed (the aging process has been going on for years and will not accelerate because of menopause).

One of the most common complaints is of "hot flashes." The flushing is noticed most often in the face and neck but may be generalized and may be accompanied by excessive perspiration. In all but about 15 percent of menopausal women, these hot flashes diminish in frequency and intensity without treatment, usually within 12 to 18 months after the first symptoms. During this time, the intervals between menstrual periods increase and the discharge becomes scantier until it stops altogether.

In the small group of women who suffer disturbances of a greater degree, estrogen therapy is helpful. Most gynecologists prescribe oral estrogens for short-term use to tide the woman over the most troublesome months. This therapy tends to lengthen the menopause; therefore vaginal bleeding at this time could be considered normal while a physical disorder actually was present. Women receiving estrogen therapy must be under close medical supervision and have frequent cell studies performed until the therapy is discontinued. Androgen therapy, e.g., stilbestrol, sometimes is administered. Often it causes postmenopausal bleeding, and its side effects of masculinization disturb many women.

Psychological support from family, friends, doctor, nurse, and all with whom the woman comes in contact is a great asset during this time. Women who are busy and who lead active lives seem to adjust to menopause with little or no change in routine. On the other hand, emotionally unstable women often have severe reactions and may become psychotic. The blame should not be placed on menopause, but on the tensions, fears, and misconceptions present. Estrogen therapy alone will not relieve those women who need psychological help.

Pathology of the Female Genital Tract

The most common disorders of the female genital tract will be summarized in this section. The reader is referred to a gynecology textbook for a more extensive presentation.

VAGINAL EXAMINATION

Since examination of the genital tract is essential to diagnosis of all gynecological conditions, it is important for the nurse to have as complete an understanding as possible of the procedures involved. The examination enables the physician to visualize the external genitalia directly and the vagina and cervix by means of a speculum. It also allows for palpation of the uterus and ovaries to determine whether or not any abnormalities are present. In addition, at this time cervical and vaginal secretions can be studied in the laboratory.

In almost every case, whether in the physician's office or the hospital, the nurse has an opportunity to be alone with the patient before the examination. If the patient is told what sorts of questions the physician is likely to ask concerning her menstrual periods, pregnancies, and deliveries, she may be more at ease and may try to give complete answers, knowing that this is important to her diagnosis. This is also the time for the nurse to assume her responsibilities of teaching and explaining the procedures that will be done, especially if the patient has never had such an examination before. Of great assurance to the patient is the nurse's presence throughout the procedure. (It is a legal requirement that she be present.)

In the physician's office, each examination room contains the needed equipment and the nurse quickly becomes familiar with the routine. In the hospital, the nurse may have to assemble the necessary items for pelvic examination in the patient's room. These items are as follows: light-head mirror, gooseneck light, vaginal specula, sterile lubricating jelly, sterile gloves, and sterile applicators and cotton balls. If the physician is to do a biopsy, cauterize the cervix, or take a smear of the vaginal or cervical mucosa, these procedures are usually done in the examination or treatment room.

Before positioning the patient for examination, the nurse should instruct her to void and, if a urine specimen is needed, to save it. An empty bladder makes palpation of the abdomen more comfortable for the patient, eliminates any incontinence during the examination, and enables the physician to palpate the pelvic organs.

The lithotomy position (dorsal recumbent) is the position most frequently used. The nurse assists the patient by having her approach the foot of the table, step on a foot stool, and sit on the edge of the table. The lower panel of the table has already been dropped if the patient is to have only a pelvic examination; otherwise, she is assisted to the side of the table and lies down as for any examination. The nurse then helps her to lie back and place her heels into the stirrups. The height of the stirrups is adjusted so that the buttocks remain flat on the table and there is no strain on the legs. The buttocks should be even with the edge of the foot of the table. A drape, usually triangular, is placed over the patient so that only the perineal area is exposed. A corner of the drape can then be placed over the area so exposed. *The nurse should never place the patient in the lithotomy position until the doctor is ready to examine her, and the patient should never be left alone while in this position.* It can be a frightening experience; many serious injuries have occurred to patients who tried to move and fell off the table. Added embarrassment results from the nurse's walking in and out of the room, opening the door more than is necessary, or leaving the door open at any time while the patient is in the room.

During the examination, the nurse assists the physician as necessary and mainly helps the patient by instructing her when to take deep breaths to help relax the abdominal muscles. After examining the external genitalia, the physician inserts the lubricated speculum into the vagina to visualize the vaginal walls and cervix. Smears are taken at this time, if necessary, and the nurse assists with these.

Next, a digital examination is performed. Gloves and lubricating jelly are utilized. The doctor inserts two fingers into the vagina and palpates the abdoman, locating and noting any abnormalities of the uterus, ovaries, or fallopian tubes. He may then do a rectal examination. (He should be informed before the examination if the patient has complained of hemorrhoids, since a rectal examination in which the ovaries, tubes, and uterus are palpated is rather vigorous and may cause hemorrhoidal bleeding.)

After the examination, the nurse should gently wipe away any secretions or jelly on the genitalia and assist the patient from the table by lowering both her legs at once and bringing her to a sitting position. The patient may wish to rest for a moment and regain her equilibrium before getting down. The nurse must remember to stay with her until she is off the table and has been helped to a chair, if necessary. Perineal pads should be available in the event bleeding has occurred or may occur. At this time the nurse has a good opportunity to clarify anything that the physician may not have explained clearly. The patient is again encouraged to discuss any questions she may have with the physician.

If the nurse has established good rapport with the patient, the latter may speak more freely to her than to the doctor. The emotional aspect of the examination should be kept in mind, as should the emotional overtones of any gynecological disorder, since the patient may be more concerned about the effect of the illness upon her femininity, her marriage, and possibly her ability to have children than upon her physical health. Perhaps the growing practice of including pelvic and breast examinations in every physical examination will help to familiarize the patient with the procedures and make her less reluctant to seek early treatment.

BENIGN DISORDERS OF THE FEMALE GENITAL TRACT

Vaginal Infections

LEUKORRHEA

Leukorrhea, a white vaginal discharge, is normal just prior to menstruation or at the time of ovulation, but a purulent or profuse vaginal discharge is abnormal. The complaint of vaginal pruritus often accompanies this type of discharge. Some of the more common causative organisms are *Escherichia coli, Candida albicans,* and *Trichomonas vaginalis.*

Diagnosis is made by the presence of the organisms in the vaginal secretions or on microscopic examination. The vaginal discharge characteristically is white, membranous, watery, and cheesy, if a monilial infection is present. Verification by laboratory studies is necessary because mixed infections are not uncommon.

Vaginal jellies are usually prescribed. The nurse instructs the patient in their application. The vaginal jelly is dispensed in a tube having an attached applicator. The filled applicator is inserted into the vagina, and the plunger is slowly pushed. After the medication has been expressed into the vagina, the applicator is withdrawn.

If the patient is to continue using the medication at home, the nurse should instruct her in its usage and watch her carry out the procedure, if possible. The medication is applied before the patient retires and after douching. If it is used when the patient is ambulatory, much of the medication will be lost and douching will, of course, remove it completely.

SIMPLE VAGINITIS

In simple vaginitis cause by *E. coli,* the sulfonamide creams are employed vaginally. The nurse carefully inserts the filled applicator into the vagina and pushes the plunger slowly. If the patient is to continue this medication at home, the nurse instructs her in proper usage and watches her do this once, if possible. Vaginal medication is applied before the patient retires and after douching.

MONILIAL VAGINITIS

Monilial vaginitis is fairly common in pregnant women and diabetics. Antifungal agents generally are effective locally and systemically.

TRICHOMONIASIS

Trichomoniasis or trichomonas vaginitis often is associated with other infections. It is resistant to treatment.

GENERAL MEASURES

General treatment for all forms of vaginitis is directed toward improving the patient's overall health through diet, rest, and treatment of any underlying disease. Cleanliness is essential to prevent secondary infection and promote healing. The patient should be instructed to cleanse the perineum with water after voiding or defecating, refrain from touching the area with her hands, and take two or three warm (100° F) sitz baths daily unless the physician orders otherwise. The sitz baths will also reduce pruritus and promote healing by stimulating circulation and washing away irritating secretions. Douches should be used only if prescribed by the physician, since they can be harmful in some cases. If douching is prescribed, a solution of 1 quart of water with 1 tablespoonful of vinegar usually is ordered. The temperature of the solution should be no higher than 100° F because the vaginal mucosa is sensitive and easily injured when inflamed. The nurse should make certain that the patient understands how and when to douche, how to mix the solution, and how to use the other prescribed medications.

Many women confuse vaginal infections with venereal disease, and a careful explanation by the nurse can clarify the difference and relieve the patients' fears. Some vaginal infections can be transmitted through sexual intercourse, but they are not commonly acquired in this way. A patient may be discouraged because of the length of time needed for treatment and uncertainty of cure, and the nurse can encourage her to complete the course of treatment.

Vaginal Tumors

Solid tumors of the vagina include polyps, fibromas, and fibromyomas. They are uncommon. These growths usually are small but some become pedunculated and protrude from the vagina necessitating surgical removal. Papillomas and condylomata acuminata are treated by electrocautery.

Vulvar Disorders

BARTHOLINITIS

Blockage of the Bartholin glands by gonococci or *Trichomonas vaginalis* may cause inflammatory cysts of the Bartholin glands. These cysts usually are asymptomatic, but must be excised should they become large or cause symptoms. With abscess formation there is pain, redness, heat, and edema.

KRAUROSIS VULVAE

Kraurosis vulvae is progressive atrophy and fibrosis of the vulva which may occur following menopause or after radium therapy for cancer of the cervix. Some post-menopausal atrophy is normal, but in kraurosis vulvae there is considerable shrinkage, the subcutaneous fat disappears, and the vulva appears thin and reddened. There is marked narrowing of the introitus and dyspareunia. The patient is highly susceptible to chronic inflammation and abscess formation because organisms easily enter through breaks and fissures in the skin.

LEUKOPLAKIA

Leukoplakia is an opaque, whitish, plaque-like thickening of the vulvar epithelium which is due to increased surface keratinization. The tissue is scaly, wrinkled, and fissured. Leukoplakia is of importance because there is a strong likelihood that carcinoma of the vulva will follow.

Cervical Inflammation

Inflammations of the cervix are extremely common, particularly in the multiparous patient. They are caused by bacteria many of which are normal vaginal flora. The most frequently observed organisms are *E. coli,* alpha- and beta-hemolytic strepto-cocci, and certain staphylococci. Trauma during childbirth, hyper- and hypoestrinism, excessive secretion of the cervical glands, high alkalinity of the cervical mucus, and sexual intercourse are causative factors. The resulting cervicitis is classified into acute and chronic types. Most cases of acute cervicitis are due to gonococci, streptococci, and staphylococci. The lesion usually is limited to the cervical os or the immediate adjacent area. The etiology of chronic cervicitis is similar. The area is red and edematous, with granularity at the margins of the external cervical os spreading in ring-like fashion. Scarring occurs, and eventually the woman becomes sterile if the lesions remain untreated. Most cases of leukorrhea are due to cervicitis.

Cervicitis often remains undetected until it is extensive. As there are no symptoms, the woman is unaware of any abnormality until it is revealed by pelvic examination. Inflammation and infection of the cervix occur for several reasons. Small lacerations after childbirth can cause chronic cervicitis resulting from tissue inability to heal due to constant irritation. In fact, a chief reason for the "6 week check-up" is that these lacerations are thereby visualized and can be cauterized. If they remain untreated, chronic cervicitis occurs with extension into the deeper tissues. There is evidence that untreated chronic cervicitis and inflammation may precede malignant neoplasia.

A less common cause of cervicitis is bacterial invasion after abortion or delivery. The ensuing acute cervicitis must be treated with antibiotics administered locally and parenterally. An untreated or inadequately treated infection spreads rapidly to the endometrium (endometritis) and may result in peritonitis or pelvic inflammatory disease.

Cervical Tumors

The most common benign cervical growth is the polyp. In general, polyps are asymptomatic. Polyps that are pedunculated, bright red, very vascular, fragile, and often sessile may be associated with leukorrhea, intermenstrual bleeding, or postcoital bleeding. Such polyps arise singly or in groups from the endocervical tissue and protrude through the external cervical os. Most are removed because of their potentiality for cancerous change and because they frequently are the site of infection and ulceration. A Papanicolaou smear should be done at regular intervals in the case of small asymptomatic polyps that are allowed to remain.

Pelvic Inflammatory Disease

PATHOLOGY

Pelvic inflammatory disease refers generally to an acute or chronic infection of the upper genital tract, i.e., uterus, tubes, ovaries, pelvic peritoneum, and supporting tissues. The most common sequelae are sterility and the possibility of ectopic (tubal) pregnancy, which is attributed to adhesions and strictures of the fallopian tubes.

The patient complains of severe pain in the lower abdomen not unlike the cramps of appendicitis. Nausea and vomiting may also be present. There is usually a moderate to high temperature elevation (103° F), and the blood studies show increased leukocytes. A foul-smelling vaginal discharge is often present and is significant in the differential diagnosis. If the causative agent is a streptococcus, as following childbirth or abortion, the symptoms are pronounced and the patient is usually prostrate. The course of the disease is long, running weeks or even months.

In pelvic inflammatory disease due to a gonococcus—about 60 percent of all cases—the patient appears less sick, but has more pain and the involved area is more tender. The vulvovaginal glands and urethra are affected also. Even after treatment, chronic infection often remains in the form of pelvic abscesses or chronic inflammatory disease.

TREATMENT AND NURSING CARE

A patient admitted to hospital is acutely ill and in pain. Bed rest is ordered. She is placed in mid-Fowler's position, which helps to localize infection and relieve pain by allowing drainage and relaxation of the abdominal muscles. The amount and character of the vaginal discharge often indicate the progress of the disease, so the nurse must carefully chart any changes. Either an ice pack or a hot water bag may be ordered to be applied to the abdomen, to relieve pain. If liquids cannot be tolerated because of nausea and vomiting, 5 percent glucose in water is administered intravenously for a day or two until liquids can be tolerated by mouth. With control of fever and subjective improvement a soft diet is given. Blood loss due to puerperal infection may necessitate frequent blood transfusion. The patient can ambulate as soon as the acute symptoms are relieved.

Constipation often is a problem. After the first 2 or 3 days, a saline enema can be given. The patient may fear this, but the nurse should explain that the enema will be given very gently and that relief of pain will result when the pressure due to the feces is relieved. Harsh laxatives are contraindicated, since excessive peristalsis may aggravate the infection and cause rupture of abscesses. Warm (100° F) vaginal douches usually are ordered twice a day; this may be an antibiotic solution, but more frequently 1,000 to 1,500 ml of sterile water is used. Needless to say, sterile gloves, equipment, and solution are indicated when the nurse administers the douche. Special precautions must be taken to prevent spread of infection by equipment, bed clothing, or perineal pads. Most hospitals insist upon isolation of these patients, at least until the causative organism is identified.

Daily intramuscular injection of 300,000 units of procaine penicillin is given for 3 days in conjunction with a sulfonamide drug.

Many factors other than the physical symptoms enter into the picture. The patient usually understands the diagnosis and has deep feelings of guilt and embarrassment. Unfortunately, hospital personnel may have added to her discomfort by their obviously disapproving attitudes. Then too, if gonorrhea is the cause or criminal abortion is suspected, the patient is subjected to extensive questioning. Thus the nurse may be dealing with a withdrawn, depressed, anxious patient, who is also very sick. If the nurse can show this patient the same degree of acceptance, interest, and understanding that she would any other patient, the patient's physical and emotional progress will be greatly aided.

A very few cases of pelvic inflammatory disease are caused by puerperal infection and tuberculosis. The patient will have anxiety about the small baby at home and the other family members; in the case of tuberculosis, she will be concerned about the long, depressing convalescent period with extended separation from home and family.

Urethrocele, Cystocele, Rectocele

These are commonly associated with injuries during childbirth. The supportive musculofibrous tissue becomes weakened through stretching and separation. They may occur directly after childbirth, but more commonly appear a decade or more later.

Urethrocele is a downward protrusion of the urethra from its attachment beneath the symphysis pubis. It causes dribbling stress incontinence during coughing, laughter, and other activities producing increased intra-abdominal pressure. Occasionally there is complete incontinence when the individual stands. Cystocele is bladder herniation into the anterior vesicovaginal septum. It is associated with burning painful urination and urgency. Large cystoceles cause urinary stasis and a consequent predisposition to superimposed infections and cystitis. Rectocele is rectal herniation into the rectovaginal septum. It may interfere with bowel evacuation and cause constipation and finally hemorrhoids.

Each of these conditions may cause interference with normal elimination. With any of them, the patient may complain of "dragging" backache or pelvic pain, which often is worse on standing or walking.

Uterine Disorders

BENIGN TUMORS

Benign tumors of the uterus usually are grouped together as fibroids, a category including myoma, leiomyoma, fibromyoma, and fibroleiomyoma. Leiomyoma is the most common of these. It develops more often in Negro women than in white ones, and it tends to develop earlier in Negro women. Leiomyomas frequently are multiple, and range in size from nearly microscopic to 50 pounds or even more. They do not appear before puberty and atrophy in most cases following menopause. Leiomyomas are classified into three types: (1) subserous, appearing under the peritoneal membrane; (2) intermural or interstitial, within the wall of the uterus; (3) submucous or subendometrial, on the inner surface of the uterus.

Leiomyomas can become infected as when torsion causes tissue devascularization and necrosis. Rarely (about 1 percent of cases) they become sarcomatous, usually in the postmenopausal years. There is rapid enlargement of the tumor and bleeding.

Many leiomyomas are small and asymptomatic and require no treatment, while others produce symptoms dependent upon their location and size. These symptoms include hypermenorrhea, abdominal or pelvic discomfort, pressure on surrounding structures, and abdominal enlargement.

General Measures. The relationship of fibroids to infertility is not clear, although there is an established association between them and problems of repeated abortion and premature birth.

Before treatment is instituted, differential diagnosis is undertaken to determine the presence of other conditions such as pregnancy, endometrial hyperplasia, ovarian dysfunction, incomplete abortion, carcinoma, or extrauterine neoplasms. Diagnostic measures include uterine curettage, tests for pregnancy, and x-ray study of the colon. Treatment depends upon the severity of symptoms and the age and condition of the patient. Hysterectomy is generally the treatment of choice, but under favorable circumstances myomectomy is performed in women under 35 years who wish to retain their child-bearing capacity.

The physician may decide that a total or subtotal hysterectomy is necessary.

ENDOMETRIOSIS

Endometriosis is the presence of endometrial tissue in abnormal sites, such as the broad ligaments, ovaries, cul-de-sac of Douglas, cervix, or vulva. The two chief types are internal and external endometriosis.

Internal endometriosis is also known as *adenomyosis*. It occurs most frequently during the fourth and fifth decades of life and often is associated with leiomyomas. The normal endometrial glands penetrate the myometrium and form a diffuse pattern and give rise to small accumulations of blood within the myometrium in response to hormonal activity. The patient complains of menorrhagia, dysmenorrhea, dyspareunia, and pelvic or back pain.

External endometriosis is also called *pelvic endometriosis*. It is most common in women age 20 to 40 years and is seen frequently in women who marry late in life and have few children. It is often seen in sterile women and is associated with ovulatory problems.

These clumps of ectopic tissue are under hormonal control in almost every case, and therefore undergo cyclic changes with menstrual bleeding. With accumulation of blood in these tissues, they become red-brown and are often termed "chocolate cysts." With degeneration, dense fibrotic scars develop that contain much pigment and lipid material.

Laparotomy must be performed to establish the diagnosis. If the endometriosis exists on one or both ovaries, it is seen as large cysts. When efforts are made to free these cysts, they generally rupture and the reddish-brown fluid pours out.

In many cases this endometriosis is asymptomatic; in others there is severe dysmenorrhea, pelvic pain, dyspareunia, and intermenstrual bleeding. Severe pain is associated with involvement of other abdominal structures, e.g., pain on defecation from rectal wall involvement and dysuria from bladder wall involvement.

Diffuse internal endometriosis may necessitate hysterectomy. In other cases it may be possible to remove the endometriosis taking precautions to preserve normal structures. X-ray castration may be undertaken which, of course, bars the possibility of the woman's bearing children.

Hormonal therapy is prescribed in some cases in the form of progestational agents which may induce long periods of amenorrhea and thereby be beneficial.

UTERINE DISPLACEMENT

The uterus may assume various malpositions. Of these, retrodisplacement and downward displacement, or prolapse, are of the greatest clinical significance. The causes, symptoms, diagnoses, and treatment of these malpositions are summarized in Table 31-1.

Ovarian Disorders

CYSTS

Cysts and tumors of the ovaries are quite common, but the ovaries appear to be extremely resistant to other diseases and to inflammation. Ovarian neoplasms account for approximately one-fifth of malignant tumors of the female reproductive system.

Follicular cysts are rarely more than 4 cm in size, are frequently multiple and bilateral, and contain a pale fluid that may have a high estrogen content. These cysts usually cause no symptoms and disappear within 60 days. Any discomfort that does arise may be treated with warm douches, pelvic diathermy, or medication to reestablish ovulation.

Corpus luteum cysts develop when there is a failure of normal retrogression following ovulation. They have a yellowish epithelium filled with pale yellow fluid. They remain quite small (4 to 6 cm) and resolve within about 2 months, and delayed menstruation with increased bleeding usually follows. The corpus luteum cyst may be symptom-free or cause local pain and tenderness. There will be severe pain if the cyst causes ovarian torsion. If torsion or rupture of the cyst and peritoneal bleeding occur, laparotomy is indicated; otherwise symptomatic therapy is adequate.

MALIGNANT DISORDERS OF THE FEMALE GENITAL TRACT

Vaginal Carcinoma

The site of the carcinoma usually is the posterior wall near the cervix, and metastasis to the cervix, urethra, urinary bladder, and rectum occurs rapidly.

Uterine Displacements

DISPLACEMENT	CAUSE	SYMPTOMS	DIAGNOSIS	TREATMENT
Anterior				
Anteversion: forward tilting or tipping	Tumor or effusion in pouch of Douglas: may push uterus forward	Usually none per se	Palpation	Elimination of cause or none required
Anteflexion: acute forward flexion	Retention of infantile characteristics of uterus	Usually no symptoms. Occasionally mild to crampy menstrual discomfort. Occasionally a factor in infertility	Palpation	Usually none; with early underdevelopment may try general building up of body and hormones
Elevation	Retained menstrual blood in vagina (e.g., imperforate hymen). Intrapelvic neoplasia (e.g., cyst, fibroid)	Usually none per se; may show signs of causal condition	Palpation	Elimination of cause
Lateral	Associated abnormality: inflammation, swelling, neoplasia	Usually none per se	Palpation	Elimination of cause
Retrodisplacements				
Retroversion: posterior rotation; may be complete or incomplete	Both may result from: congenital origin; relaxation of supporting structures; trauma, pressure within abdomen (e.g., neoplasia, full bladder or rectum)	May be none. May include: low backache (increasing at time of menstruation or with long standing), bearing down abdominal pain; menstrual disturbance, especially dysmenorrhea, infertility, dyspareunia	Palpation	When displacement is mobile and asymptomatic, no treatment may be necessary
Retroflexion: backward bending	Pelvic tilt			Vaginal pessary. Uterine suspension
Downward (prolapse) may be associated with cystocele; less often, rectocele	Childbirth injury; weakness of supporting structures; congenital weakness; increased abdominal pressure (e.g., tumors, ascites, etc.); association with retrodisplacements	May be: none or minor; sense of dropping; bearing down sensation; backache; pulling pain in groin; appearance of a vaginal mass	Inspection. Palpation	Prevention: by muscle exercises. Pessary (less frequently used). Surgery: uterine suspension; partial or total hysterectomy
First degree: cervix does not protrude through introitus				
Second degree: uterus is within vagina; cervix protrudes through introitus				
Third degree (procidentia): entire uterus including fundus protrudes through introitus				

Carcinoma of the lower vagina tends to metastasize to the regional iliac lymph nodes and to be disseminated via lymphohematogenous routes. The most frequent symptoms are irregular spotting, dyspareunia, and leukorrhea, but in many cases there are no symptoms until metastasis to distant organs is detected. Vaginal carcinosarcoma and sarcoma botryoides, both of which are quite rare, may be found in all groups, including children.

Cervical Carcinoma

Cervical carcinoma is the second most common type of cancer in women and accounts for more than half of all malignant neoplasms of the female genital tract. By far the largest numbers of cervical cancers are of the squamous cell type; adenocarcinoma is less common. The cause of cervical cancer is unknown but it seems to be related to injury and chronic irritation. Chronic cervicitis, if untreated, is thought to be a contributing factor.

There are two types of carcinoma of the cervix, fungating and infiltrative. In the fungating type, which is generally observed in squamous cell carcinoma, the epithelium thickens near the cervical os, and nodularity follows. There is a mass of friable, granular, firm, and irregular neoplastic tissue that may infiltrate surrounding organs or upward to the endometrial cavity. In the infiltrative type, the mucosa thickens and becomes diffusely enlarged and firm. The area soon ulcerates and the cancer penetrates the pericervical tissues. Metastasis to contiguous organs is common if the lesion is not detected early.

Carcinoma of the cervix is more frequent in women who have had children than those who have not. Poor penile hygiene and lack of circumcision are other possible factors. Smegma is a known carcinogenic agent in animals, and many physicians believe that poor penile hygiene contributes to the higher incidence among women whose sexual partners are not circumcised. They think that the improved hygiene, rather than circumcision itself, is the reason for the lower rate of cervical cancer among Jewish women. The stages are classified as follows:

Stage O: preinvasive, or carcinoma in situ; confined to the superficial lining of the cervix.

Stage I: carcinoma confined to the cervix.

Stage II: carcinoma extending beyond the cervix and involving the upper vagina or the paramentrium but not the pelvic wall.

Stage III: carcinoma extending to the pelvic wall on one or both sides and to the lower third of the vagina (this vaginal extension may be considered a part of Stage IV carcinoma).

Stage IV: carcinoma involving the bladder and/or rectum and extending beyond the pelvis by metastasis.

The symptoms of carcinoma of the cervix vary according to stage. In carcinoma or early invasive carcinoma there may be no symptoms, so that an annual or semi-annual pelvic examination after the age of 30 is of great importance. The nurse can help to impress upon the many female patients she cares for the need to have this examination regularly. Carcinoma of the cervix rarely occurs before age 20 or after age 80 and is most frequent during the middle years. The earliest symptom is bleeding, which may occur initially as occasional spotting and finally become a daily occurrence. During this period, when they should seek medical advice, many women postpone examination because of fear or procrastination, or because they attribute the bloody discharge to a menstrual abnormality. A second fairly common symptom is a serous discharge that characteristically becomes malodorous, but this may go unnoticed for weeks, even months. Later, with invasion, there may be vague pelvic discomfort. Pain is a late symptom that usually begins unilaterally. It results from invasion of the pelvic wall and peripheral nerves, obstruction of the urinary tract, and bony metastasis. Weight loss, anorexia, and cachexia are other late symptoms.

The diagnostic modalities for detecting cancer of the cervix are summarized in Table 31-2 and are used in conjunction with or in addition to basic pelvic and rectal examinations.

The two chief therapeutic approaches to carcinoma of the cervix are surgery and radiation. Many gynecologists carry out total hysterectomy, with excision of a vaginal cuff, although conization is sometimes employed in stage O, particularly

TABLE 31-2
*Diagnostic Modalities in
Cervical Carcinoma*

MODALITY	PROCEDURE	FINDINGS
Cytologic examination (Papanicolaou)	Smear of exfoliated cells from cervix or posterior fornix	Negative: normal epithelial cells Suspicious and positive: atypical cells; cells strongly or definitely suggestive of malignant neoplasm Positive results require further diagnostic follow-up Produces a small percentage of false positive and false negative results
Schiller test	Staining of cervix and vaginal vault with aqueous solution of iodine (Lugol's or Schiller's)	Normal mucosa stains mahogany, due to glycogen content If cancer is present the treated area turns white or yellow Areas of erosion or eversion will not stain but remain reddish Positive results indicate need for biopsy
Colposcopic and colpomicroscopic examination	Instrument examination of cervix under high magnification; microscopic examination of superficial layers of cervical mucosa	Permits differentiation of cells of erosion and eversion from those of carcinoma
Cervical biopsy	Tissue sample from lesion or suspected sites	Normal and abnormal cell structures are differentiated Paraffin sections may be utilized for fine histological differentiations
Cone biopsy	Removal of a cone of tissue from cervix including squamocolumnar junction and superficial endocervix	Done in positive smear without visible lesion

during the childbearing years. Some physicians utilize radiation therapy in the early stages, rather than surgery.

Uterine Carcinoma

The primary malignant neoplasm of the uterus is adenocarcinoma arising in the endometrium. Sarcoma infrequently develops directly in the myometrium or in a leiomyoma.

With progress in educational programs for detection of uterine cancer and wider use of the Papanicolaou smear, the death rate from carcinoma of the uterus has fallen sharply within the last 30 years, but it still accounts for approximately 16 percent of deaths from cancer in females. Here again, the nurse in the community setting and in the hospital setting can participate actively in educating female patients to the need for regular pelvic examinations.

The highest incidence of uterine (cervix) cancer occurs in the 30- to 50-year-old group, although 30 to 35 percent of cases are detected in women under the age of 40 years. There are more cases in the lower socioeconomic groups, perhaps because these women generally do not seek medical assistance for diagnostic purposes. Early marriage, childbearing, and frequent sexual intercourse are factors also.

Adenocarcinoma is seen most often in menopausal and postmenopausal women. Leiomyomas are frequently found concurrently but are thought to be incidental. Endometrial carcinoma is increased in frequency in obesity, hypertension, diabetes mellitus, and nulliparity (Robbins). Close to 85 percent of uterine cancers are adenocarcinomas.

Early adenocarcinoma may present no signs or symptoms, particularly if the lesion is well within the uterine cavity. In postmenopausal women uterine bleeding is the usual presenting complaint, and in premenopausal women there may be intermenstrual bleeding or hyper- or polymenorrhea. In some women leukorrhea may be the initial symptom. In most cases pain is not the initial complaint unless the carcinoma has already become invasive and metastatic.

Confirmation of the diagnosis is accomplished through tissue examination obtained by smear, section biopsy, or curettage, and the carcinoma is treated surgically, by radiation, or by both methods, according to the grade, history of symptoms, clinical picture, and age and condition of the patient.

Ovarian Carcinoma

These carcinomas may be cystic or solid, primary or metastatic. The cystic carcinoma may be a papilloma or a cystadenocarcinoma. The solid carcinoma may be bilateral and the less frequent sarcoma usually is unilateral. The carcinoma may be asymptomatic and therefore go undetected, but as it enlarges examination may disclose a palpable mass, and abdominal distention, abdominal pain and pressure, some vaginal bleeding, weight loss, digestive disturbances, dysuria, and possible ascites may be found.

The treatment consists of complete extirpation of both ovaries and the uterus, generally followed by irradiation, and in advanced cases deep x-ray therapy and chemotherapy may be utilized.

NURSING CONSIDERATIONS IN DISORDERS OF THE FEMALE GENITAL TRACT

Surgery of the female reproductive tract places at least some degree of manipulative stress on the urinary bladder and the urethra, because of the proximity of these organs to the organs of reproduction. As a result, some degree of bladder atony and/or urethral edema often occurs.

Although the care of the gynecologic patient is basically similar to that of all patients, the nurse's own attitudes have an important bearing on the adequacy and quality of her care. She must, for example, utilize all her powers of observation, understanding, interpreting of signs and symptoms, and skills of listening and interviewing, if she is to give the ready support that this patient will need. She must be prepared to give her patient sufficient time throughout the course so that the patient never feels that she is being hurried through routines or that her emotional needs are being ignored—this might have a devastating effect on the patient's ability to come through all the stresses of her illness successfully. The woman's age, personality, life style, desires for the future; the circumstances surrounding the disease and its treatment; her relationship with her husband or another significant person will all be involved in her behavioral responses. Obviously this nursing function is not a hit or miss activity based on guesswork or a quick impression derived from a single remark or gesture.

The nurse should be familiar with the routines of the particular hospital and the preferences of the individual physician so that she can give satisfactory explanations to the patient. For example, many surgeons no longer require that the pubic area be shaved for a dilatation and curettage; but shaving is still necessary for any procedure involving an incision.

Nursing Measures

If an indwelling catheter has been inserted, the nurse's responsibility in catheter care is to maintain sterility, perineal cleanliness, and continuous drainage.

Whether or not a catheter was inserted, there may be some difficulty in voiding, and accurate recording of intake and output is essential to be certain that the bladder is not becoming overdistended. Fluid intake should be adequate, yet distention must be avoided. A dehydrated patient may utilize fluid rather than excrete it; another patient may produce urine at a rapid rate, especially with additional fluid intake, and feel bladder distention within 2 to 3 hours or even less. Restlessness, subjective discomfort, and the appearance of fullness in the suprapubic area alert the nurse to this possibility.

It is preferable to have the patient void, if she is able to do so, rather than to catheterize her, because catheterization can contribute to infection. Voiding is accomplished more easily before the bladder becomes overdistended. Many nursing measures are available to help the patient who is having difficulty in voiding.

Privacy, a comfortable environment, and proper positioning all help. The patient should use the bathroom if possible; a calibrated container can be placed upon the toilet in such a way that she does not have to struggle to hold it. It may help to let the tap water run, to put a few drops of oil of peppermint in the bedpan, or to stroke her abdomen. The nurse should try to determine the source of the patient's discomfort or pain. Incisional pain may be mistaken for "gas pains." The physician may prescribe a heat pad to the abdomen or a rectal tube. Ambulation probably gives the greatest relief although it may be uncomfortable. Pressure of feces may be mistaken for incisional pain, hence it is helpful for the patient to resume a normal diet and to ambulate as quickly as possible. Perineal care should be given at least twice a day and after defecation if an indwelling catheter was inserted or perineal surgery was performed. A sterile procedure is necessary if perineal surgery was done.

If vaginal repair was done, applications of heat or cold may relieve discomfort. A perineal heat lamp will dry the skin, increase peripheral circulation, and prevent sloughing of tissue. The patient can take sitz baths after the sutures have been removed. An ice bag applied to the perineum may relieve discomfort.

The physician may order douches to be given both preoperatively and postoperatively, and this procedure must be sterile if performed postoperatively. The nurse should observe any discharge, odor, or pain at this time.

Early ambulation is encouraged to avoid venous stasis. Elevating the legs periodically and exercising in bed are helpful measures, and an elastic bandage or elastic stocking may be applied both pre- and postoperatively to provide venous support.

In the postoperative period, at perhaps the second to the fourth day, the patient may become quite upset and depressed, possibly crying, moving about aimlessly, and refusing to undertake any activity. Such a reaction may last for perhaps a day. This reaction is by no means always the case, but should it occur, the patient needs understanding and support. If a degree of emotional control is lost, the nurse may consider it necessary to interrupt an emotional spiral by word or touch. If such an intervention is used, it is the *professional* nurse who should use it. The nurse should plan adequate time to be with the patient and to allow her to express her feelings as well as she can at the moment.

Special Preoperative Considerations in Particular Surgical Sites

If the need for surgery is anticipated in the area of the vagina or if a hysterectomy is to be performed via the vaginal approach, special cleansing measures are instituted. Usually cleansing douches and perineal care are given in the evening and morning preceding surgery. One or both of these measures may be ordered for as many as several days preceding surgery. In the physical preparation of the patient, particular attention is paid to the condition of the bowel so that it is free of fecal matter and is undistended. The physician may order cathartics and/or enemas. The bladder must be emptied at the time of surgery, either by immediate preoperative voiding or by placement of an indwelling catheter. Either bowel or bladder, if distended, can interfere with the internal operative site and may be subjected to unnecessary trauma from accidental incision during surgery.

Special Postoperative Considerations in Particular Surgical Sites

DILATATION AND CURETTAGE

Following dilatation and curettage, the patient returns from the operating room with vaginal packing and wearing a perineal pad as a dressing. Very little drainage is anticipated; however, the pad should be observed regularly. While the patient is wearing the pad, she should be given perineal care or be taught to give it herself. This care is often carried out under clean rather than sterile technique. With the packing in place, the patient may note some difficulty in voiding as a result of pressure from the packing against the urethra, and she should be informed of this possibility. She may also have cramps due to the packing. This discomfort is readily managed by administration of an analgesic. The patient generally is discharged on the first or second postoperative day. Before discharge, the packing is removed, and she should be instructed to observe for any increase in discharge beyond the minimal amount she may expect. She should also avoid heavy exercise and sexual intercourse until the physician approves, usually at the time of the postoperative office check-up.

HYSTERECTOMY

Hysterectomy may be performed by either the abdominal or the vaginal approach. With the vaginal approach the patient's dressing will be a sterile perineal pad. Her care will include sterile perineal irrigations to insure cleanliness and comfort. As with all surgical dressings, the perineal pad should be observed for drainage on a scheduled basis.

The patient who has had an abdominal hysterectomy will have an abdominal dressing and also, usually, a perineal dressing. Little drainage is expected on the perineal pad as the seepage from the upper vaginal stump suture line is minimal. The pad may be needed for only 1 day. Both perineal pad and abdominal dressing should, however, be observed regularly and carefully for excessive drainage. The abdominal dressing after hysterectomy is usually not large. The patient may require additional support to the incised abdominal musculature, particularly during ambulation and especially if her abdomen is large or its musculature weak. The physician may order or the nurse may choose to employ a scultetus binder to provide additional support during the healing process.

Two complications against which the nurse needs to guard are abdominal distention and thrombophlebitis, particularly of the pelvis and upper thigh. These may occur as a result of manipulation of the abdominal contents and interference with circulation. General measures for dealing with these circumstances have been described above. A further measure for the alleviation of severe distention may be the insertion, on physician's order, of a nasogastric tube. Prophylactic measures for thrombophlebitis include keeping the legs flat, exercise of the legs and feet, placing the head flat periodically during the day, and avoiding a Fowler's position greater than a 45 degree angle. Elastic bandages may be applied to the legs to aid the venous return flow.

An uncommon complication of hysterectomy, but one for which the nurse must observe, is trauma to or (rarely) accidental ligation of a ureter. Symptoms such as low back pain and/or low urine output should be noted and reported with dispatch as they may be indicative of problems with the ureter.

Reparative surgery such as anterior colporrhaphy for cystocele, posterior colporrhaphy for rectocele, and perineorrhaphy for disorders of the pelvic floor are delicate operations that require special attention to reduce strain on the incision and avoid pelvic pressure. An indwelling catheter is utilized postoperatively, particularly with the anterior colporrhaphy. Continuous drainage of the catheter must be assured and measures need to be taken so that the tubing does not pull on the urethra and exert tension on suture lines. The catheter may, on a physician's order, be clamped, as during ambulation, to allow the bladder to regain tone, but no more than 150 ml should be allowed to accumulate in the bladder. The catheter may be removed 2 to 4 days postoperatively, following which the patient should void at least every 4 hours. She must be observed for adequate voiding, and measurement of output is essential. Voidings of small amounts (e.g., 50 ml) should be reported to the physician.

The degree of difficulty in reestablishing natural voiding varies with patients. Some women have considerable difficulty and need support from the nurse both to void naturally and for emotional support, as tension inhibits the ability to void. In the event that recatheterization is necessary, great care and gentleness must be utilized to avoid trauma to the surgical site.

When a posterior colporrhaphy has been performed the prevention of bowel movements is desirable; the patient may be kept on a liquid diet for a few days and when defecation is resumed she may be given mineral oil to ensure a soft stool.

With all surgery in the perineal area perineal care is important, whether or not a perineal pad is utilized as a dressing. Postsurgical perineal care should be a sterile procedure and be repeated several times a day, and should be done after urination or defecation. This gives the nurse an excellent opportunity to observe the pelvic area, and to note the progression of healing or any incipient complications. Later in the postoperative period, when the patient may take over the perineal care herself as a clean procedure, the nurse should continue to observe the area at least once daily so that she is constantly aware of the progress in healing.

Special Considerations in Radiation Therapy

The major modes of radiation therapy the nurse will encounter are (1) external beam therapy, such as deep x-ray or teletherapy with ^{60}cobalt, ^{137}cesium, or another radioactive isotope, (2) intracavitary application of radium by means of various carriers such as ovoids and tandums, or needles, and (3) implants, which may be temporary and removed upon completion of the specified dosage of radiation, or placed permanently. The latter are usually small sources (seeds or grains) of short-lived isotopes such as radon, which has a half-life of 3.85 days. The nurse needs to know which form of therapy is being utilized for a particular patient because the care requirements vary with the type.

X-RAY AND TELETHERAPY[1]

External beam radiation therapy may be done on either an inpatient or outpatient basis. The patient receiving external radiation does not have a source of radio-activity within her body and no precautions are needed from this standpoint. When the patient is able, and no special preparation is required, she may have all or part of her therapy on an outpatient basis, thereby reducing the interruption of living patterns and reducing expense as well.

Modern radiological techniques have greatly reduced the severity of skin reactions but have not eliminated them. Severe reactions are rare. But whether the reaction is mild or severe, it should be referred to as a reaction and not as a burn. The term *burn* implies carelessness when carelessness is not a factor. The professional nurse should be particularly careful to instruct ancillary nursing personnel about the use of the word since it is a familiar and descriptive one, and the term *skin reaction* is not an intrinsic part of their vocabularies.

Reactions to radiation do not begin with the first treatment but occur days to weeks later, depending on dosage and skin sensitivity. The skin may show nothing more than a pinkish color and a temporary loss of hair. In a more extensive reaction the skin may become bright red and this may be accompanied by a decrease in sweat gland activity, loss of hair which may be permanent, and loss of some superficial epithelium. If the reaction is severe the color becomes purplish, blisters form, and fluid exudes with the epithelial loss. Skin structures such as hair follicles and sweat glands are destroyed.

Skin reactions will persist for varying periods after completion of therapy. Following their resolution the skin is apt to remain pigmented. Late skin reactions may also occur, months to years following treatment. Telangiectasias may appear; the skin may become atrophic and subject to easy breakdown and necrosis.

Skin affected by radiation is easily injured and heals very slowly. Therefore a nursing goal is prevention through the elimination of irritants and protection of the skin surface. Modes of skin care vary widely among radiologists and may range from almost no restrictions to detailed instructions for care. However, a general guiding principle to care of the skin during radiation is the avoidance of any irritant, chemical or mechanical. The use of water is not restricted but use of soap may be. Also to be avoided are applications of ointments, alcohol, powders and the like unless they are approved by the physician. Friction should be eliminated whether by rubbing as with a towel, irritation such as may result from constrictive clothing, the pulling of adhesive tape, or by scraping as with a razor and blade. Applications of heat are eliminated, both in its dry form (e.g., heating pads) and in moist form (e.g., compresses) to avoid burning. The skin needs to be kept dry and free of perspiration, and protected from sunlight.

Itching and tenderness are likely to occur. The physician may order a mild emollient, calamine lotion (without phenol), or another anti-irritant.

Other systems and tissues of the body are also affected by radiation. Symptoms

---

[1] X-ray differs from teletherapy in that the x-ray machine can be turned off, whereas the teletherapy unit continues to emit radiation and requires shielding and restriction of personnel time in the therapy room even when the equipment is not in use.

of radiation sickness may arise and cause gastrointestinal irritability, with nausea and vomiting. Small, frequent feedings attractively prepared and served in pleasant surroundings should replace the regular mealtime routine in an effort to maintain nutrition and avoid debilitation.

Radiation in the pelvic area may cause an unpleasant vaginal discharge and possibly some bleeding. Douching may be ordered to control the discharge, but it must be carried out with great care as the vaginal tissues are very friable. The bladder may be affected by radiation, as indicated by irritability and urinary frequency.

General malaise, lassitude, and depression may develop. With a fall in the white blood cell count, the patient is more susceptible to infection. Extra periods of rest, balancing of activities to avoid fatigue, protection against infection, and interest and understanding are important parts of nursing care. There is considerable difference of opinion regarding how much the patient should be told and at what point in time. An effective course of action seems to be one that deals with the various reactions only as they commence to occur. Thus one avoids creating an expectation of problems which could hasten or initiate their appearance.

RADIUM APPLICATION

Radium therapy may be used alone or in combination with external radiation and may be accomplished in one or two applications.

Preparation of the patient for intracavitary radium application is directed toward providing a clean field and an empty bowel and bladder. Therefore, a surgical "prep" is done, an enema is given to clear the bowel, a cleansing vaginal douche is given, a Foley catheter is inserted, and a low-residue diet is ordered to reduce bowel irritation and movements during the period of radium insertion.

Radium application may be accomplished by several techniques utilizing different kinds of carriers (ovoids, capsules, needles) depending upon the area to be radiated, i.e., uterine fundus, fornices, vaginal vault. The carriers are secured in place by vaginal packing, with some portion (string, wire, or handle) projecting through the introitus so that the position and continued presence of the radium applicators can be noted at regular intervals. With some insertion methods the radium within its applicator is placed while the patient is in the operating room. A more recent technique is afterloading, in which the tandems, ovoids, and vaginal packing are placed while the patient is in the operating room. The loading with the radium is done after the patient has left the operating and recovery rooms and has been returned to the clinical unit. The radium is brought in in its protective housing and quickly inserted, thus eliminating radiation exposure to locations other than the patient's room.

Postoperatively, a properly prepared patient already knows the nature of the treatment and what kinds of activities she may or may not undertake, and knows that she will receive good care even though the personnel will remain in the room only short periods.

The patient is, if at all possible, placed in a single room with the bed positioned away from the door. If a double room must be used, a separation distance of 7 feet between the patient and other patients should be established. The patient will be confined to bed for the entire time the radium is in place. She should remain in a dorsal recumbent position, with opportunity to turn the upper trunk somewhat to eat; elevation of the head of the bed to 15 degrees and turning is accomplished by the log-rolling maneuver. The legs may be moved, but should remain extended. Bathing and linen change are not restricted but are done with care not to dislodge the radium. The presence and position of the applicators must be checked not just during morning care but regularly every 4 hours, for the total time of insertion, which may be as long as 72 hours. Any change in location of the applicators should be reported at once.

Intracavitary application of radium may generate some vaginal discharge. For this an absorbent pad placed beneath the patient is preferable to the use of a perineal pad if there are protruding applicator handles that might be disturbed by the presence of the pad. Where strings or wires are used the perineal pad may be satisfactory as long as the strings or wires are not pulled when the pad is removed.

Elimination during radium application is reduced to a minimum. The Foley catheter inserted at the time of surgery provides urinary drainage. The preoperative enema and low-residue diet, sometimes supplemented by daily administration of paregoric, are designed to delay bowel movement. If bowel evacuation is necessary the patient is turned to the side and an emesis basin is used. A bedpan is not utilized because in placing the patient on it the position of the radium could be changed.

Medication for pain, for nausea, and for sedation is ordered according to patient need. Vital signs, particularly the temperature, are taken every 4 hours. A temperature elevation could be an indication of infection and should be reported immediately.

After completion of the required time for radium application the radium is carefully removed. The removal must be done at the *specified time* to avoid overdose. It can be accomplished in the patient's room or in a treatment room. The radiation source is transferred quickly from the patient to a lead-lined container. The patient is then given a cleansing enema and antiseptic douche. Once the radium curator has determined that all radium has been accounted for, the patient may be discharged immediately, as she is no longer a source of radioactivity.

Personnel protection and management of the environment are the second facet of nursing care of patients with radium application. If nurses are on a unit where appreciable radiation therapy takes place they may be assigned film badges, which are monitored for radiation exposure monthly, or pocket monitors for shorter exposures. These provide more rapid exposure information. On units housing only an occasional patient having radium therapy monitors may not be utilized.

Protection from radiation is achieved by limiting the number of contacts with a patient and limiting any given time span of contact to 30 minutes. Similarly, visiting time is limited to 30 minutes. Personnel are encouraged to maintain a distance of 3 feet from the patient except when giving direct care. Personnel may be rotated so that no one individual has a long number of consecutive contact days. Children and any pregnant woman are restricted from the patient's room. Areas in which radiation is present are marked appropriately.

After the therapy has been completed and the radium removed, the patient's linens and her immediate environment are monitored. If the radiation level is high enough to be of concern, decontamination procedures can then be instituted.

RADIOISOTOPE IMPLANTATION

Implants of radioisotopes are similar to intracavitary application of radium in relation to radiation precautions, precautions against dislodgment, maintenance of cleanliness, and avoidance of infection at the implant site; however, generally they permit the patient more freedom of activity.

Implants, whether temporary or permanent, are used less frequently in gynecologic therapy than in other therapies. ^{192}Iridium, which is prepared as seeds contained in a nylon ribbon, is used in the pelvic area. The implants are inserted while the patient is in the operating room, or by means of the afterloading technique. Permanent implants need not be removed; temporary implants are left in place for the specified time and removed similarly to radium.

Pathology of the Female Breast

The nurse plays an important role in assisting with the detection of breast pathology. She is available to countless people while occupying various roles within our society, and therefore can be the ideal person to whom women around her could look for answers to questions, confidence, understanding, and knowledge of her profession.

EPIDEMIOLOGY

As with most chronic disease processes, prevention and early detection are of ultimate concern. Beland states that the nurse's role in prevention is of two basic types: primary and secondary. In primary prevention, the objective is to eliminate or educate others to those known factors that may contribute to the causation of their illness. In relating this concept to the pathology of the breast, the discussion will first consider the benign states and then the malignant.

Little has been written about benign pathological conditions of the breast which might indicate modes of prevention. Many investigators feel that the chief factor in benign breast disease is the alteration of the normal hormonal balance. An area that is perhaps directly related to altered hormonal function and in which much study is being done is that of the long-term effects of hormone utilization for contraception. Thus the nurse can caution women of childbearing age that the accepted limit for contraceptive therapy is approximately 3 to 5 years. Contraceptives keep the breast in a state of prolific activity. This continuous and prolonged activity may be a factor underlying the development of cystic and cancerous growths. Then too, both men and women should be reminded to guard against trauma to the breast because inflammatory processes resulting from trauma often lead to obscure benign pathology. Lastly, certain drugs (phenothiazines) may affect the breasts by causing nipple secretion. Other causative factors of disease such as carcinogenic chemicals, ionizing radiation, toxic gases, poor health habits, psychological factors, and the effects of heredity have been discussed in previous chapters.

In the second type of chronic disease prevention, the goal is prompt identification of the disease process. For this phase to be accomplished, the public must be educated and made aware of the problems that chronic disease might impose. Education through programs in newspapers, television and radio, and distribution of professional pamphlets, films, and filmstrips will go far toward helping the public to identify disease processes.

In the prompt identification of benign or malignant breast pathology, the medical check-up is of utmost importance. Occasionally, regardless of how soon physiological changes are reported, the treatment and prognosis are not favorable, but most frequently, the end-results are rewarding.

Since the breast tissue is readily accessible to observation and sensory perception by the patient, she is usually the first person to notice an abnormality of concern—something that was not there before. The most common complaint is of a painless nodule or thickening in the upper outer quadrant of the breast. Occasionally there may be tenderness, edema, heat, redness (signs of inflammation), skin or nipple retraction, puckering, asymmetrical breast appearance, erosion of the nipple or breast tissue, and nipple drainage (serous or bloody). It is estimated that it takes 6 to 12 months for a breast cancer to grow from a 1 cm size, at which it can be detected by careful palpation, to the 5 cm size at which it is usually found (Haagensen).

PHYSICAL EXAMINATION

The nurse must understand the kind of medical examination that is essential in obtaining the data that will lead to the formation of a medical diagnosis. With this knowledge, she can better prepare the patient to understand her interview and examination and elicit her cooperation by explaining what is expected of her. She can also explain to the patient why seemingly unrelated information might have a bearing on the diagnosis, and why, therefore, it is so important that the patient provide as much information as she can.

PATHOLOGY OF THE MAMMARY GLANDS

Present evidence points to a definite relationship between benign and malignant breast disease. The following sections will discuss first the problems related to benign breast disease, then those of chronic breast diseases (including malignant neoplasms).

ACUTE PATHOLOGY OF THE FEMALE BREAST

Acute pathology of the breast indicates that the symptoms may or may not be severe but that the course of the illness or pathological state is of short duration. Although benign breast pathology is very common its etiology is not definitely known. Many studies indicate that benign breast disease occurs simultaneously with hormonal imbalances, but the manner in which these abnormalities arise remains obscure. It has been repeatedly determined that breast tissue responds readily to hormonal fluctuations and this is also true of various tissues within the same breast. The terminology of breast pathology tends to be elaborate and redundant, and synonymous terms will be indicated in those cases that are the subject of much confusion.

Benign Tumors

FIBROADENOMA

The fibroadenoma is composed of fibrous and glandular tissue. It is the most frequently observed benign tumor of the female breast, and develops mainly after the onset of menstruation, specifically ovulation, and usually before the age of 30. Fibroadenomas are generally asymptomatic and are usually discovered during the monthly breast self-examination or a routine gynecological examination. They are solid, discrete, and freely movable, usually 2 to 4 cm in diameter, but they may be as large as 6 to 10 cm. An increase in size is usually noted at the end of the menstrual cycle or during pregnancy. Fibroadenomas may be located in any area of the breast, but the most frequent location is in the upper outer quadrant.

Surgical removal is carried out after the diagnosis is established. This is usually accomplished with minimal scarring and retention of mammary function, although in some instances, such as giant fibroadenoma, simple mastectomy may be necessary to ensure excision of the ulcerated area and an adequate margin of tissue.

PAPILLOMA

Papilloma is encountered most often in women who are approaching menopause or are menopausal. These tumors may be benign or malignant; their delicate structure and high vascularity make them especially vulnerable to trauma. Papillomas are observed predominantly in women with a history of cystic hyperplasia. Local excision is carried out in benign lesions and radical mastectomy in those having malignant features.

CYSTIC HYPERPLASIA

Cystic hyperplasia, also called *mammary dysplasia* and *fibrocystic disease,* is characterized by numerous cellular changes with an abnormal amount of epithelial hyperplasia and cystic formation within the mammary duct system. Normally, the increase in mammary epithelial hyperplasia is counterbalanced by an equal proportion of atrophy during each menstrual cycle.

Fibrosis of the breast, or mastodynia, develops in young women between the ages of 30 and 35 years. There is tenderness and pain on palpation preceding menstruation, and this tends to regress after the menstrual cycle. The fibrosis may be bilateral or unilateral.

Cystic disease of the breast must be differentiated from cancer. As a rule, the individual with cystic disease is advised to see her physician every 6 months or once a year.

The treatment of cystic hyperplasia depends upon whether it is benign or malignant. Its relationship to malignant neoplasms is still being studied, and a cause-and-effect relationship seems to exist. Because of the evident close association of cystic hyperplasia and estrogen production, many physicians are opposed to estrogen therapy for women with cystic hyperplasia.

Hypertrophy and Atrophy

Hypertrophy of the breasts may occur unilaterally or bilaterally, and is chiefly seen when the breast tissue is excessively sensitive to normal amounts of hormones or when it is stimulated by excessively high levels of hormones. When the condition is unilateral, it is presumed that the tissue of that breast is ultrasensitive. Some causative factors are ovarian tumors, choriocarcinomas, adrenal cortical tumors, and pituitary tumors; in these instances, when the foci of hormone production are removed, the breasts regress to their normal size. Physiological atrophy of the female breasts occurs as a part of the normal aging processes, being seen near the menopause and characterized by an accumulation of interstitial fat within the stromal connective tissue as the remaining breast tissue shrinks in volume.

Inflammations

Acute mastitis is an acute bacterial infection usually caused by *Staphylococcus aureus* or streptococci. It is most often observed during lactation and late pregnancy, although dermatologic conditions or abrasions of the nipple can favor development of cracks and fissures that provide ready entrance of the organisms.

Comedomastitis tends to develop in women 40 to 50 years old, and is more common in women who have had children and in those who have had problems of inverted nipples, cracked nipples, and difficulty in nursing their babies. A focal area of *fat necrosis* may occur from a traumatic blow to the breast or following an inflammatory reaction with subsequent abscess formation. This disorder is unilateral and benign in its original state, and most frequently occurs in obese women. *Galactocele* is difficult to categorize. It tends to present a picture of cystic dilatation and inflammatory reaction.

Other Benign Disorders

Fissures of the breast are narrow slits or cracks that occur near the base of the nipple where it joins the areola. These open areas may become portals of entry for many pathogenic organisms.

Nipple discharge may indicate an inflammatory reaction, duct stasis, or benign and/or malignant tumors of the breast. Most causes of bloody nipple discharge are due to benign intraductal papillomas, although with increasing age, a bloody nipple discharge may more often indicate the presence of intraductal papillary carcinoma.

CHRONIC BREAST PATHOLOGY

Chronic breast pathology includes disorders that will be life-limiting (immediately or in the near future), create varying degrees of incapacitation and limitation of activity, or bring about feelings of grief at the loss of a body part.

Malignant Tumors

In the United States, breast carcinoma is the most common form of malignant neoplasm of women. Mortality has remained unchanged for many years, even though great amounts of time and money have been spent in educating women about the need for routine physical examinations and monthly breast self-examination. Breast cancer is rare before puberty and rather infrequent in women under 40 years, but the rate rises sharply with the increase in age over 40 years.

Among the numerous possible causative factors that have been mentioned are viral agents and stress phenomena. Regardless of etiological factors, however, cancer is the second leading cause of death in the United States, and breast cancer is the leading cause of death in women.

Breast carcinoma usually occurs unilaterally from a single primary focus, although bilateral simultaneous breast carcinomas have been found. Undetected or delayed detection of breast cancer goes on to metastasis either by direct invasion or lymphatic or hematogenous spread. Common breast malignancies are papillary carcinoma, Paget's disease, comedocarcinoma, scirrhous carcinoma, and medullary carcinoma.

SIGNS AND SYMPTOMS

Objective and subjective signs and symptoms of neoplastic changes in the breast are often obscure. The following signs and symptoms are described so that the nurse will be aware of them throughout her care of female patients. These signs and symptoms may also be taught to the patient as she learns the practice of thorough and regular breast self-examination.

The upper outer quadrant and the central subareolar region are the most frequent sites of breast neoplasia. These tumor masses may be detected at specific phases of the menstrual cycle or without reference to cyclic changes. The mass may be freely movable and sharply delineated or fixed within a specified area and delimited with difficulty. If such a mass is noted for a period of 2 weeks, the patient should be urged to see her physician for a definitive diagnosis. The palpable masses are painless in many instances, or may cause slight discomfort, when pressure is applied, during the regular menstrual cycle. Retraction of skin and nipple often is observed in the later stages of carcinoma. It occurs as the tumor begins to attach to and invade the peripheral breast tissue and intraductal tissue, respectively. The overlying tissues then tend to dimple. Occasionally, there is an observable change in the appearance of the skin overlying the breast. As an example, an eczematous allergic response or simple inflammation of the nipple and areola may be ignored or treated symptomatically yet may be the distinctive symptom of Paget's disease or duct carcinoma. If metastases involve the lymphatics, their normal function of draining the breast tissue may be interrupted and lymphedema may result. This lymphedema is often accompanied by local thickening of the skin, often called "orange peel." Any spontaneous nipple discharge not associated with lactation should be thoroughly investigated, as in many cases serosanguineous nipple discharge is a significant sign of a benign or malignant breast tumor.

METASTATIC PATTERNS

Neoplastic cells are spread by lymphohematogenous routes. If lymphatic, the cells

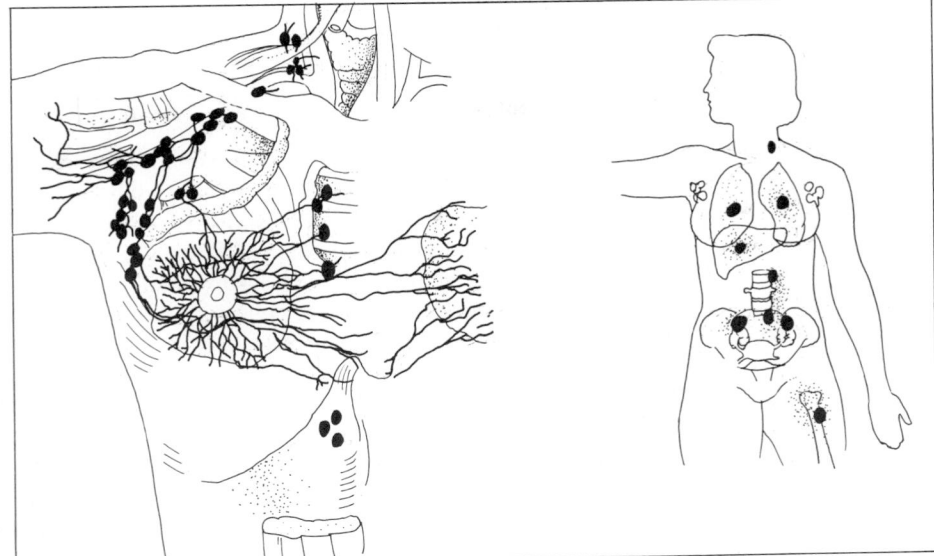

Figure 31–6
Lymphatic spread of
breast cancer and distant
metastases of breast can-
cer. (By permission from
American Cancer
Society: A Cancer Source
Book for Nurses. *New*
York, 1968.)

are carried to tissues closely proximal to the breast tissue. Laterally, extension occurs to the axillary nodes, and superiorly to the cervicoclavicular region. Metastasis occurs inferiorly to the abdominal viscera and lymph nodes and medially to the contralateral breast. Another frequent site (other than axillary metastasis) is that beneath the tumorous area to the lymph nodes near the internal mammary artery, the internal mammary chain. In over 60 percent of diagnosed cases of breast cancer there is metastasis to either of these sites. Lymphatic spread is depicted in Figure 31–6.

Breast cancer is highly invasive and rapidly disseminates throughout the body, but particularly to the lungs, bones, liver, and brain. It is relatively uncommon during pregnancy and lactation, but if diagnosed during this time, the prognosis is extremely grave. Mammary engorgement is so common during pregnancy that it is very easy for potentially malignant changes to go undetected.

DETECTION OF BREAST NEOPLASIA

Detection of breast disorders in the very early stages is most difficult, but once it is accomplished, the neoplasm can then be classified as benign or malignant. With early detection therapy can be started while the disease is localized, whereas a protracted delay is very risky. It is thought that cure is more likely with the smaller, slowly developing cancers than with those that are rapidly fulminant.

Many authorities suggest that more than one diagnostic study be carried out. Besides self-examination of the breasts and routine pelvic examination, these procedures include mammography, cytologic study, transillumination, thermography, xerography, and ultrasound and scintillation scanning.

Mammography. Mammography, or soft tissue radiography, demonstrates grossly whether the tissue is normal or abnormal. It is safe, simple, and generally reliable. With mammography, breast cancer may be detected before other signs and symptoms are present, although the tumor must be of sufficient size to be clearly differentiated from the surrounding tissue. Secondary clinical signs of carcinoma that may be observed include dimpling, skin thickening, nipple retraction, nipple erosion, enlarged axillary lymph nodes, hyperplastic fibrosis, and increased vascularity. Mammography is useful as an adjunct to the physical examination and history, before the tentative diagnosis is attempted. Only after carcinoma cells are actually detected can the physician conclude that a malignant neoplasm is present.

Cytologic Study. Cytologic study of breast tissue can be done on material expressed from the nipple or material aspirated by needle; cell differentiation can be made only after surgical biopsy of the tissue is done. Such studies will reveal the presence of malignant cells or possibly malignant cells. The chief difficulty is obtaining an adequate sample of cells for analysis. Gentle massage or use of a breast pump designed for the purpose may be employed. If this sample can be obtained, it may be extremely helpful in diagnosis, since it often is representative of the entire epithelial lining. Malignant lesions of the larger ducts are more easily detected by this method.

Thermography. Thermography is a recent diagnostic technique, and one that appears to have great potential. It is based on the finding that the area surrounding cancer cells is warmer than the normal areas of the skin. Thus the thermogram is a visual representation of the warm, hot, and cool areas of tissue. Other pathologies, however, and even some normal breast tissue may demonstrate some localized temperature elevation, so careful analysis must be carried out in those cases where "hot spots" have been demonstrated.

Xerography. This method is another recent tool in diagnosis. It utilizes an x-ray image on a selenium-coated metal plate. At the present time xerography is not perfected, but it is believed to give superior results to mammography. With xerography all mammary tissues are demonstrated in a single exposure.

Transillumination. Transillumination does not differentiate benign tumors from malignant ones, but may be useful in localizing hematomas after traumatic injuries. In some cases it permits detection of solid tumors and clear fluid cysts. It is not frequently utilized.

Scintillation Studies and Ultrasound. The modalities are mentioned as a matter of record. At the present writing they are not fully developed and have only limited application.

Excisional Biopsy. An excisional biopsy is the diagnostic procedure of choice in a solid tumor. The tumor is removed in its entirety along with sufficient surrounding tissue to avoid incising the tumor itself and thereby risking the implantation of tumor cells at another site. Biopsy should be performed under general anesthesia so that if the tissue, when examined by frozen section, demonstrates carcinoma a radical mastectomy can be performed immediately. Frozen sections are histologic sections cut from the biopsy tissue which have been rapidly frozen while the patient remains in the operating room. These frozen sections are examined immediately so that the surgeon may know whether or not to proceed with a radical operation. If the frozen section does not reveal a malignant neoplasm the patient is returned to the clinical unit. Further and more detailed histologic studies are then carried out in the next 24 to 48 hours as an additional precaution against the presence of undetected malignant cells.

METHODS OF THERAPY

Hormones may be prescribed after surgical treatment and radiotherapy. The object is to relieve pain, rather than to prolong survival, since only advanced cases are so treated. Survival is increased by a few months in about one-third of the patients.

Chemotherapy appears to offer the most helpful palliation in widely disseminated cancers. The chief problem with these agents is that their action is less selective than that of some other agents, that is, they act upon normal cells as well as cancerous ones, and this may lead to serious side effects (e.g., thrombocytopenia, anemia, reduced resistance to infection).

Simple mastectomy usually is performed for persistent cystic hyperplasia or intraductal adenosis when carcinoma has been found in the contralateral breast. It is considered a prophylactic measure against further carcinoma.

Radical mastectomy is the treatment of choice in patients with cancer of the breast. It is utilized when the cancer is believed to be curable, i.e., a 5-year survival is anticipated. The regional lymph nodes are removed in continuity (en bloc) with the primary tumor and invaded contiguous structures, even if these lymph nodes do not clinically demonstrate invasion.

The decision to perform palliative surgery is not necessarily based on the possibility of prolonging life, but may be done to relieve the patient's distress and suffering. Among the measures employed are bilateral oophorectomy, bilateral adrenalectomy, and hypophysectomy. *Bilateral oophorectomy* is utilized in the treatment of advanced breast cancer in premenopausal women to effect a reduction in the estrogen level. It is especially helpful in reducing bony metastases. *Bilateral adrenalectomy* is effective in improving the patient's general condition. It reportedly causes osseous lesions to heal, ascites to resolve, tumor size to decrease, and appetite to increase. Bilateral adrenalectomy is often combined with oophorectomy to bring about complete cessation of estrogen activity. With *destruction of the hypophysis* via yttrium implantation or implantation of radon seeds, the production of prolactin, growth-stimulating hormone, thyroid-stimulating hormone, and gonadotrophic stimulating hormone is abolished. This result may also be accomplished by *hypophysectomy*. Replacement therapy with cortisone and desiccated thyroid is needed after hypophysectomy.

NURSING CONSIDERATIONS IN DISORDERS OF THE FEMALE BREAST

The responsibilities of nursing regarding the biopsychosocial dimensions of patient care and breast pathology have their true beginnings, not with the patient in the hospital, but with the client in the community, with women of all ages wherever they are or can be contacted by a professional nurse. Interpretation of the nature and behavior of the breast as a tissue and the education of women in the importance of techniques of observation and examination by the physician are probably the most important preventive measures now available.

Women of all ages need to be involved in the health care of their breasts. Assessment of a woman's knowledge about and involvement in her own breast care and the institution of education appropriate to her particular teaching-learning needs becomes an inherent health-team care responsibility in which the nurse has an important role. This role falls not just to the public health nurse but to the hospital nurse as well. It involves all women patients, not just those hospitalized for breast problems. It could even, directly or indirectly, include the male since pathological conditions of the male breast do occur, although rarely. The design, extent, and timing of health teaching of breast observation and care arise from the assessment, planning, and judgment of the professional nurse. It is also the nurse's responsibility to weave health care and teaching into a logical whole with the nursing management of illness and health supervision.

The primary technique of breast observation by the individual herself is the procedure of breat self-examination—a monthly, systematic investigation designed to reveal incipient breast problems. The patient should be told of the physiological behavior of the normal breast so that she will know where to expect ridges

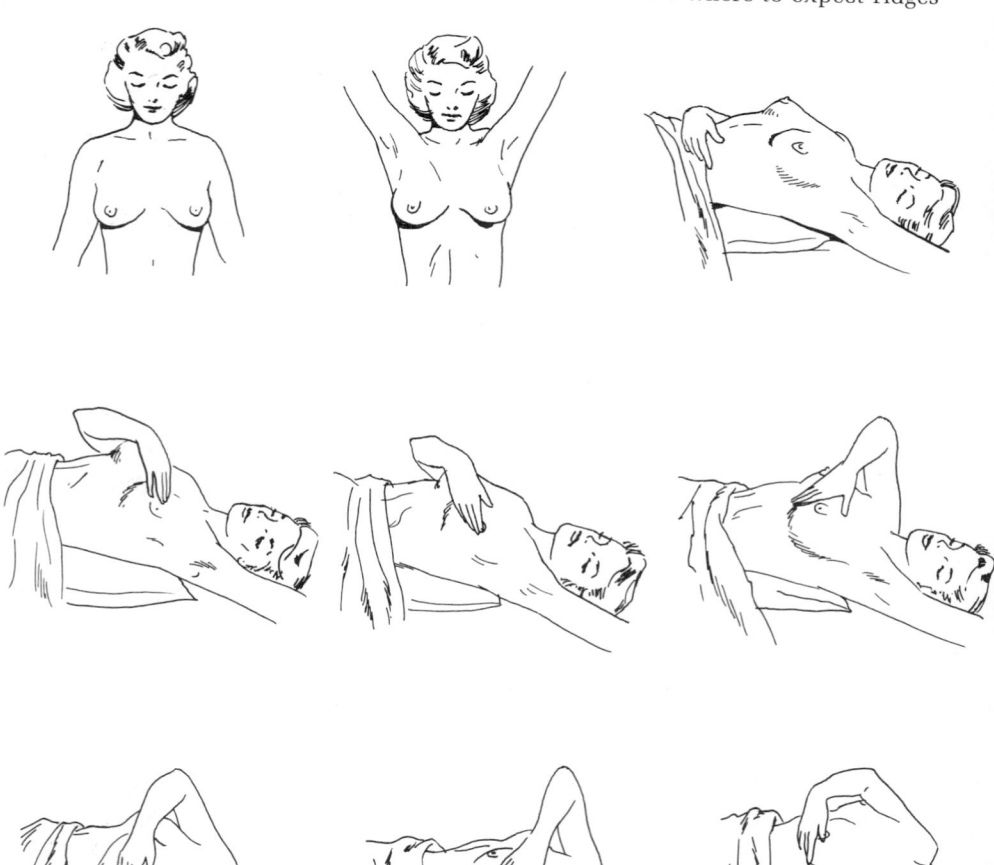

Figure 31–7
Breast self-examination.
(By permission from
American Cancer
Society: The Nurse and
Breast Self-Examination.
Bulletin No. 3408–PE.
New York, 1967.)

of tissue, and when and where she might expect some pain or nodular-like firmness resulting from normal hormonal influences. Because the hormonal influences occur characteristically in the midmenstrual and premenstrual periods, the best time to institute breast self-examination is shortly after cessation of the menses. Establishment of the examination as a regular monthly procedure, even after menopause, provides a woman with an ongoing knowledge of the characteristics of her own breasts so that she will be alerted immediately should any change occur. She can then seek immediate medical advice.

Breast Self-Examination

The breast self-examination procedure is not difficult. The American Cancer Society has developed an outstanding educational program to teach women both the method of breast examination and the importance of its regular utilization. A woman who is used to examining her breasts will probably be less likely to experience the same degree of panic in finding a "lump" than will one who finds a lump by accident, and she will also be more likely to seek medical attention quickly.

Nursing Measures in Benign Disorders of the Female Breast

Although the physician provides the necessary medical treatment in benign disorders of the breast, many times it is the patient herself who must discover the simple comfort measures that mean so much to her general well-being. The nurse can make some very helpful suggestions in this area of care. For example, she might suggest that the patient wear a well-fitting substantial brassiere while she is up and about, and a soft brassiere at night or during periods of bed rest. A brassiere also should be worn following breast biopsy or any other procedure in which a minor surgical excision was carried out. Trauma following needle biopsy of the breast may be relieved in this way. The brassiere can be worn as soon as the surgical dressing is small enough to allow this or as soon as it is removed. The more pendulous the breasts the more important it is that they be supported by a brassiere.

Nursing Measures in Chronic Breast Diseases

Cancer of the breast is a fearsome prospect for any woman. Unless the disease is so advanced that only grossly involved tissue is to be removed by simple mastectomy, the surgical procedure employed is radical mastectomy. Comprehensive nursing care should find full expression in the care of the patient who has had a radical mastectomy.

PREOPERATIVE CARE

Frequently, and unfortunately, the preoperative nursing contact with the patient is brief and the patient is nearly immobilized by anxiety.

The surgeon will have discussed with the patient the nature of the surgical preparation and the reasons for its extensiveness. The nurse may have to reinforce this explanation, and to deal with expressed or unexpressed fears. Preoperative care of the patient facing breast biopsy, whether or not radical mastectomy is probable, is a professional responsibility and should not be delegated to a licensed practical nurse or other nonprofessional personnel. Exceptionally, some routine matters may be delegated if the situation is an unusually favorable one. The emotional tension and the fears of the woman facing possible cancer and mutilating surgery are too often ignored, and she is forced to face this surgery virtually alone.

The nurse should be ready to deal with a wide range of emerging emotional realities and fantasies. She should be ready to handle outbursts of crying, demands of or abuse of the staff, rejection of the family, and the like. These emotional events should be handled without forcing the patient to deal with emotional concerns in a manner that would only increase their destructive dimensions or actually generate a situation that would jeopardize the person's ability or willingness to survive anesthesia and surgery.

POSTOPERATIVE CARE AND REHABILITATION

Postmastectomy care follows a number of sound general principles; but it also is highly individualized. The dimensions of physical care, particularly those referable to the surgical site, need to be discussed thoroughly with the surgeon to ascertain the nature and security of the closure, the presence and location of drains, if and where any skin grafting was done, and particularly how much arm motion the patient may have initially and when a program of arm exercises may be initiated. The nurse needs to know what the doctor considers as the possibilities for prognosis—not that she will discuss this with the patient initially, but because it will help her in planning her approaches to both patient and family and in determining the components of the long-range nursing plans.

The patient will be positioned following surgery according to the physician's preference. The arm on the operated side may be placed across the chest and enclosed in the dressing in order to reduce tension on the wound and promote healing. Other arm positions are as follows: (1) Abducted at the shoulder. (2) Rotated internally. (3) The forearm flexed at the elbow. (4) Elevated with support carried the full length of the arm, the hand slightly higher than the elbow, and the elbow slightly higher than the shoulder. This position supports venous return. (5) The shoulder abducted, the forearm flexed at the elbow and elevated, the hand placed above the head. This position also supports venous return. The position of the arm should be changed and finger and elbow flexion and extension should be ensured in order to maintain joint mobility, encourage venous drainage in the arm, and provide for comfort. Care is taken to avoid pull on the muscles during positioning.

The surgical procedure of a radical mastectomy is extensive and may result in sizable amounts of drainage. The dressing is therefore large and of a pressure-exerting type. One or more drains may be placed in the wound and attached to suction to permit the surgeon to reduce the bulk of the dressing and to allow the patient greater freedom of movement. The drainage catheters are most frequently attached to a Hemovac pump, which is composed of a plastic disk-shaped chamber about 6 inches in diameter and containing springs. It is compressed manually, attached to the drainage tubes, and then released, thereby accomplishing suction. The clear sides allow observation of the drainage. The pump must be emptied regularly and then recompressed to maintain the suction. It is sterile equipment and must be handled accordingly. The potential for infection in a wound exuding serosanguineous drainage is high; and infection interferes with healing, increases the size of the scar, and delays rehabilitative arm exercises for many days.

The nurse must observe for drainage in the dressing. If Penrose drains have been placed within the axilla or chest well, there may be a considerable amount of drainage. She must be aware of the possibility of hemorrhage, which may first be detected under the patient, between her body and the bedclothes, since the downward flow is assisted by gravity. A mastectomy dressing should never be removed; if saturated it should be *reinforced* with sterile dressings. Hemorrhage should be recorded without delay and reported to the physician.

The nature of the mastectomy dressing, in that it snuggly, even tightly, encircles the chest, places additional responsibility on both nurse and patient to see that the lungs are adequately and frequently aerated and that secretions are coughed up. A combination of fear of tearing the incision and discomfort attendant upon the operation itself may further limit the patient's chest excursion and willingness to cough. Frequent turning and support in coughing then become increasingly important.

Ambulation is frequently started on the day of surgery if the postanesthesia recovery is adequate. The affected side is supported at all times. Movement of the arm is begun within 24 hours, and an exercise program is initiated as soon as possible. The physician must be consulted regarding arm motion and exercise programs, since a fragile suture line or a skin graft could be damaged by early active motion.

Exercises are designed to restore full motion and usefulness to the arm and shoulder. The best exercises are those related to activities of daily living and resulting in the accomplishment of something useful in addition to exercise of the arm. For example, combing the hair with the affected arm is begun by giving the elbow some support, as from the overbed table, and advanced until the patient can reach the back as well as the front parts of her head.

When the patient goes home, and some strength is regained in the arm, many such activities can be instituted, for example, cooking, bedmaking, ironing, or window washing. Swimming is an excellent activity for muscle retraining because it fosters maximum usage of the arm and assists the deltoid and other muscles in taking over the functions of the excised pectorals.

Exercises most often recommended include those shown in Figure 31–8.

Arm exercises should be done 10 to 12 times, alternating activity with rest; the procedure should be repeated three to four times daily. The patient should be helped by the nurse and then by the family in order to sustain her motivation to continue the exercises until full use of the arm is regained and/or the normal household and living activities have replaced the exercises. The American Cancer Society booklet, *Help Yourself to Recovery,* is an excellent guide to arm exercises. It contains helpful suggestions regarding clothing, amounts of activity, and the like.

The matter of appearance is important to the postmastectomy patient. With modern prosthetic devices and ingeniousness in the design of clothes (ranging

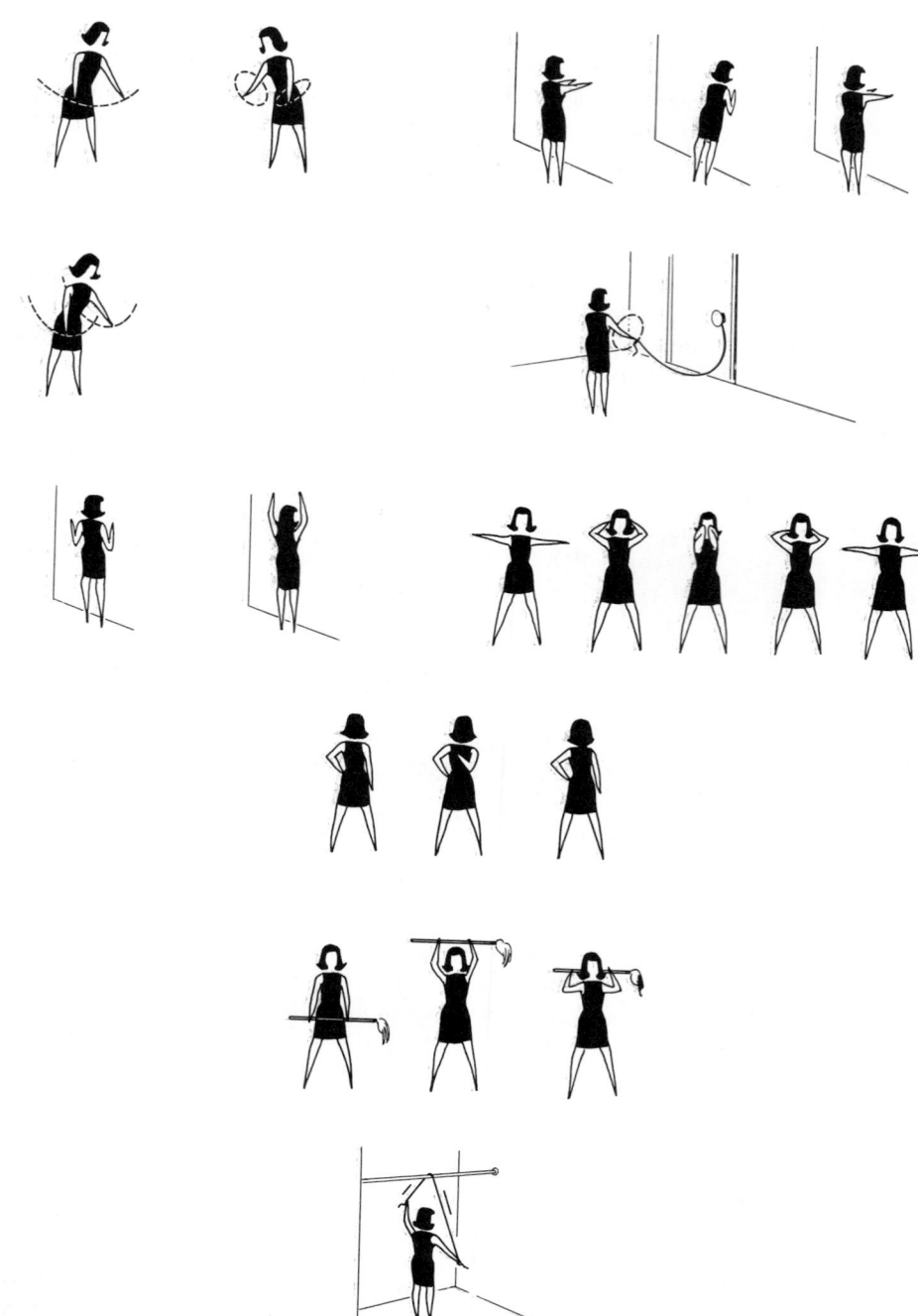

Figure 31–8
Postmastectomy arm
exercises.

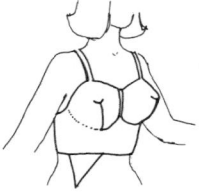

Figure 31-9
Postmastectomy
brassiere.

from the swimming suit to the formal gown) the outward dimensions of the problem of social appearance can be solved. As soon as she is able to wear a brassiere she can stuff it with something soft and clean (e.g., cotton batting, Nylon hose) to improve her appearance while awaiting her physician's approval to begin wearing a prosthesis.

A properly fitted brassiere is essential to the successful use of a prosthesis. It may include some padding of the shoulder strap to avoid undue pressure on the affected shoulder; a V-shaped piece of elastic may be added which can be pinned to the girdle to prevent its riding up on the affected side; it may have a pocket into which the prosthesis is inserted for stability. Prostheses may be foam rubber pads shaped like the natural breast. They may be inflatable plastic pouches, or may be filled with a thick plastic fluid, to approximate the other breast in both size and weight. This type changes shape as does a normal breast when the patient changes her position. Most types of clothing can be worn with the prosthesis remaining unnoticed.

POSTOPERATIVE COMPLICATIONS

The postsurgical complications to which the mastectomy patient may be subject are the same as for other types of surgery, with the addition of lymphedema. This may result from lymphatic blockage or excisional interruption of the lymphatic drainage system, but in either case there is interruption to the interstitial fluid and protein elimination in that limb, with subsequent edema. Lymphedema does not always occur, and much of it is transitory, disappearing as arm function is regained. Occasionally it may be severe and disabling. This form may occur immediately postoperatively or years later, being frequently initiated by a slight infection that impedes or increases the burden on the lymphatic drainage. Thus the patient needs to learn to prevent infections, cellulitis, and other conditions that might cause the skin to become dry or to crack. Any incipient infection or inflammation should be referred to the physician. Elevation of the arm may assist in reducing the edema in obese persons, and weight loss is also quite helpful. In severe cases, a circulator may be employed. This equipment utilizes an inflatable sleeve covering the length of the arm. The circulator exerts an alternating pressure, set at approximately 5 mm below the diastolic pressure, which runs distal to proximal. The device is placed on the arm for several hours daily and may be used for a number of months.

Radical mastectomy is sometimes followed immediately by a course of x-ray therapy to the lymph nodes in the area. When metastases are known to be present or arise at a later date, radiation, chemotherapy, or castration may be employed to reduce the spread, induce regression, and/or increase patient comfort. The nursing management thereby involved is similar to that needed when therapy is given for carcinoma of another site, but is tailored to the individual situation. Gastrointestinal symptoms are less likely with irradiation for breast carcinoma than for carcinoma of the cervix, since radiation does not pass through the intestinal tract. Postsurgical care for oophorectomy, adrenalectomy, and hypophysectomy follows the principles of surgical care, with observations for the effects of hormone level changes.

The chemotherapeutic agents 5-fluorouracil and 5-fluoro-2-deoxyuridine are particularly beneficial in metastatic cancer of the breast, but they increase susceptibility to infection by lowering the hemoglobin, platelets, and white blood cells. Reverse isolation may be ordered. There may also be some soreness or bleeding of the mouth which calls for gentle and frequent mouth care. The appetite may be impaired, increasing the importance of small, more frequent, attractive meals, with attention given to the vitamin, electrolyte, and protein content to provide as much nourishment as possible.

PSYCHOSOCIAL COMPONENT OF MASTECTOMY

The state of the incision or the condition of the arm may appear to be the thing which seems to drive the patient into a shell, but far more often, it is the psychosocial impact of carcinoma and of radical mastectomy which thwarts rehabilitation.

Radical mastectomy represents a classic example of body image threat with all its attendant problems. But although it is classic in nature, the effect upon any given person is individual, arising out of the particular nature of the person and the complexities of her experiences, values, relationships, expectations, indeed her total life experience. Some women, whom one might expect to have a stormy course, move smoothly into adjustment; while others, for whom all factors look favorable, may have considerable emotional upheaval. It behooves the nurse to ascertain what the dimensions of the patient's responses are or what they may be. This kind of assessment must be done in a way that will not be overly stress-generating to the patient nor be interpreted as prying. The great skill of professional assessment lies in the ability to determine *what to, how to, when to,* and *when not to.* Patients who are able to and who prefer to handle the psychological dimensions of the situation themselves and with their families and friends should be granted this freedom. On the other hand, the nurse should not use the concepts of patient independence and privacy as excuses to avoid her professional responsibilities.

Psychosocial rehabilitation is not a nurse-patient project alone; it is a nurse-patient-physician enterprise and a family affair. Postmastectomy patients generally have numerous questions, explicit and implicit, which may or may not be verbally expressed. Nurse and physician need to plan together for the role of each in answering and anticipating questions, in offering information, and, perhaps, in not offering certain information (knowledge of cancer) to both patient and family.

The patient, following mastectomy, to a greater or lesser degree *always* faces the fear of death—perhaps protracted, perhaps painful—and also faces the fear of loss of sexuality and of attractiveness or self-worth. This small section cannot hope to explore this complex, multidimensional situation in any degree of comprehensiveness, but a few key points will be considered. However, the nurse should never forget that the fear of death and dying is a constant factor underlying the entire situation.

The thing a woman needs perhaps the most is loving care and support which is clearly demonstrated whether or not she can, at the moment, respond to it from those who are most important to her: husband, children, family members, and significant friends. Friends may be of particular importance in the case of a single woman. Most families want to give this kind of support, but they are often too frightened and upset; and sometimes, they do not know how. A time to talk, to ask questions, to express feelings needs to be provided for family members as well as for patients. A husband may need to talk about how to show his love for his wife, especially if she seems to reject him. He needs to know what he might expect in terms of his reactions just as she may need to talk out her feelings and expectations about him.

Through all aspects of care, the nurse must weave information to clarify, give more data, and provide for continuity within the patient's hospital stay. The husband and family need to be aware that it is quite possible that the patient may experience a period of depression after her return home. She will need a great deal of support and interest shown in her as a person, but overprotection and dependence should not be fostered.

Communication is another very important aspect of psychosocial adjustment. It must be therapeutic in nature, not punitive or hostile in its tone, whether it comes from the physician, the nurse, or a family member. Often one person who can be most helpful to a postmastectomy patient is a woman who has made a successful recovery and adjustment to her own radical mastectomy. She can give clues from experience; she may also explore feelings with the patient which the patient knows are approached from a true understanding. The American Cancer Society in each particular community usually knows how to contact women who will gladly make visits to hospital patients. These women do so out of true concern for the well-being of another.

Whereas most families welcome back the patient from the hospital, occasionally the nurse is faced with providing support for a patient whose husband, or family, cannot accept the situation; who does, in fact, abandon his wife emotionally and/or physically by leaving the home. In such a circumstance, through efforts of the nurse and probably mobilization of other resources as well, the patient may be guided toward the finding of a new meaning in living and toward finding a new set of important relationships.

Bibliography

Books

A Cancer Source Book for Nurses. American Cancer Society. New York, 1966.

Arey, L. B.: *Developmental Anatomy.* Philadelphia: W. B. Saunders Company, 1962.

Behrman, Samuel J. and John R. G. Gosling: *Fundamentals of Gynecology.* New York: Oxford University Press, 1959.

Best, Charles and Norman Taylor: *The Physiological Basis of Medical Practice.* Baltimore: The Williams & Wilkins Company, 1961.

Bourne, Aleck W. and J. M. Holmes: *A Synopsis of Obstetrics and Gynaecology.* Baltimore: The Williams & Wilkins Company, 1965.

Graber, Edward A.: *Gynecologic Endocrinology.* Philadelphia: J. B. Lippincott Company, 1961.

Greenhill, J. P. (Ed.): *Yearbook of Obstetrics and Gynecology, 1965-66.* Chicago: Year Book Medical Publishers, Inc., 1966.

Guyton, Arthur C.: *Textbook of Medical Physiology.* Philadelphia: W. B. Saunders Company, 1966.

Haagensen, C. D.: *Carcinoma of the Breast.* New York: American Cancer Society, 1954.

Harkins, H., C. Meyer, J. Rhoads, and J. G. Allen: *Surgery: Principles and Practices.* Philadelphia: J. B. Lippincott Company, 1961.

Harper, H. A.: *Physiological Chemistry.* Los Altos, Calif.: Lange Medical Publications, 1967.

Help Yourself to Recovery. American Cancer Society. New York, 1957.

Martin, Laurence: *Clinical Endocrinology.* Boston: Little, Brown and Company, 1964.

Masters, William and Virginia Johnson: *Human Sexual Response.* Boston: Little, Brown and Company, 1966.

Miller, N. F. and Hazel Avery: *Gynecology and Gynecologic Nursing.* Philadelphia: W. B. Saunders Company, 1965.

Novak, Emil and Edmund Novak: *Gynecologic and Obstetric Pathology with Clinical and Endocrine Relations.* Philadelphia: W. B. Saunders Company, 1958.

Quint, Jeanne C.: Mastectomy—Symbol of Cure or Warning Sign? in Jeannette Folta and Edith Deck (Eds.): *A Sociological Framework for Patient Care.* New York: John Wiley & Sons, Inc., 1966.

Robbins, Stanley: *Pathology with Clinical Application.* Philadelphia: W. B. Saunders Company, 1964.

Rogers, Joseph: *Endocrine and Metabolic Aspects of Gynecology.* Philadelphia: W. B. Saunders Company, 1963.

Ruch, Theodore and Harry Patton: *Physiology and Biophysics.* Philadelphia: W. B. Saunders Company, 1965.

Te Linde, Richard W.: *Operative Gynecology.* Philadelphia: J. B. Lippincott Company, 1962.

Turner, C. Donnell: *General Endocrinology,* Philadelphia: W. B. Saunders Company, 1963.

Zimmerman, Lee and Rachmiel Levine: *Physiologic Principles of Surgery.* Philadelphia: W. B. Saunders Company, 1965.

Articles

Bensen, Ralph: Cancer of the Cervix Uteri. Part I. *Ca,* 17:4:173, July-August, 1967.

Bensen, Ralph: Cancer of the Ovary. *Ca,* 18:3:122, May-June, 1968.

Bergel, F.: Current Advances in Cancer Research. *Nursing Times,* 63:12:1609–1611, December 1, 1967.

Boeker, E. H.: Radiation Safety. *American Journal of Nursing,* 65:4:111–116.

Botsford, Thomas: The Early Diagnosis of Breast Cancer. *Ca,* 16:4:161–164, July-August, 1966.

Carpenter, Charles: Host Factors Related to Immunity in Cancer. *Rocky Mountain Medical Journal,* 63:1:51, January, 1966.

Danese, C. and J. M. Howard: Postmastectomy Lymphedema. *Surgery, Gynecology and Obstetrics,* 120:4:797–802, April, 1965.

Farrow, Joseph: Gross Mammary Cysts. *Ca,* 9:5:163, September-October, 1959.

Farrow, Joseph: Fibroadenoma of the Breast. *Ca,* 11:5:182, September-October, 1961.

Haagensen, C. D.: Cancer of the Breast. *Ca,* 11:5:197, September-October, 1961.

Holleb, Arthur I. and Joseph Farrow: The Significance of Nipple Discharge. *Ca,* 16:5:182, September-October, 1966.

Holleb, Arthur I. and Joseph Farrow: Inadequate Simple Mastectomy. *Ca,* 17:4:160–162, July-August, 1967.

Kess, Leopold: The Present Status of Cytology in Uterine Cancer. *Ca,* 16:5:198, September-October, 1966.

Lewison, Edward: Relationship between Benign and Malignant Breast Disease. *Ca,* 9:5:155, September-October, 1959.

Moore, Francis D., et al.: Carcinoma of the Breast. *New England Journal of Medicine,* 277:6, 1967.

Papanicolaou, George: The Value of Exfoliative Cytology in the Diagnosis and Control of Neoplastic Disease of the Breast. *Ca,* 4:6:191–197, November-December, 1954.

Park, Ann: Trends in Treating Breast Cancer. *Nursing Times,* 63:1:70, January 20, 1967.

Quint, Jeanne C.: Mastectomy: Signpost in Time. *Journal of Nursing Education,* 2:3:3, September, 1963.

Quint, Jeanne C.: The Impact of Mastectomy. *American Journal of Nursing,* 63:11:88–92, 1963.

Smith, Ann: The Menace of Breast Cancer. *Nursing Times,* 63:1:73, January 20, 1967.

Sutherland, Arthur: Psychological Impact of Cancer Surgery. *Public Health Reports,* 67:1139–1143, November, 1952.

Symposium of Nursing in Cancer. *Nursing Clinics of North America,* 2:4:585–690, December, 1967.

Symposium on Radiation Uses and Hazards. *Nursing Clinics of North America,* 2:1:1–113, March, 1967.

Symposium on the Woman Patient. *Nursing Clinics of North America,* 3:2:193–273, June, 1968.

Trimble, Frances: The Management of Patients with Advanced Breast Cancer. *Ca,* 9:5:170, September-October, 1959.

Zippin C., D. Wood, and D. Lum: Study of the Joint Committee Recommendations for Clinical Staging of Cancer of the Breast. *Ca,* 12:5:194–199, 1962.

CHAPTER 32
THE PATIENT WITH DISEASE OF THE HEMATOPOIETIC SYSTEM

MARGARET AASTERUD WILLIAMS

The last two to three decades have been a time of remarkable increase in knowledge concerning the blood and blood-forming organs. Before this period Rh blood groups, vitamin B_{12}, antimetabolites, and Christmas disease, to cite only a few examples, were unknown. The rapid proliferation of knowledge about the hematopoietic system has made formerly fatal diseases such as pernicious anemia now controllable. Refined techniques of blood fractionation have enabled the replacement of specific deficient factors of blood rather than voluminous transfusions of whole blood. The use of corticosteroids can now tide patients over hemolytic crises that formerly carried high mortality rates.

The patient afflicted with a blood dyscrasia has been given a great deal of help and hope from medical research and has much to hope for from future research—a valid assurance that can be made even to patients suffering from acute distressful disorders. The care of patients with such diseases as acute leukemia requires the utmost skill and knowledge that the health team possesses. The nurse will find her personal resources and her professional skills taxed to the utmost in many instances.

Not all the hematopoietic disorders are of intense severity, of course. Many are mild and primarily "nuisances" whereas others are moderately incapacitating and require life-long medical supervision. Some require alterations in living patterns; persons with hemorrhagic disorders, for example, may not participate in body-contact athletic activities without danger or work in jobs where cuts or bruises may be a frequent occurrence. Individuals who are carriers of certain disease strains must consider whether or not to marry and to have children.

Through the ages, blood has been considered synonymous with life itself and has been the focus of much superstition, speculation, and folklore. Allusions to blood are legion in our everyday language. "Bad blood" may mean an inherited moral taint to some, or angry feelings between two persons. A pact "sealed in blood" has been deemed irrevocable by primitive tribes and by present-day adolescent gangs. Becoming a "healthy, red-blooded American" is the hope of countless schoolboys.

The ascribed mystery surrounding blood can often be demonstrated in the actions of persons who are ill. Bleeding will usually cause a person to seek medical attention, whereas an equally serious symptom such as fatigue or loss of weight may not. The frequent taking of blood samples, so often necessary for diagnosis and follow-up, can be a source of considerable concern to some individuals. Receiving another person's blood via transfusion has emotional overtones for many persons which may or may not be expressed. The basis for some of these feelings may seem irrational to the scientifically oriented but should not be lightly dismissed. Members of certain religious faiths may refuse altogether to have blood transfusions even though medical opinion might be that such treatment would be life-saving.

Some of the disorders of the blood and blood-forming organs can be quite obscure and necessitate numerous diagnostic tests. The nurse can be a positive source of support to patients during this time, for anxiety is generated simply by a lack of diagnosis. She can acknowledge to the patient that she recognizes the uncertainty and concern he feels, although she may not be able to do anything about the source of anxiety. Her observations may often speed up the process of diagnosis; she may note that the patient's urine was pink-tinged on a voiding, that ecchymoses were apparent which had not previously been seen, or that the patient mentioned a medication he was taking at home which he had forgotten to tell the doctor about.

The nurse may also be a source of accurate information concerning so-called cures for blood problems of family and friends in the community. Many persons attempt to "build up their blood" by taking quantities of vitamins, minerals, syrups, and tonics that are readily available over the counter. This practice, encouraged by ubiquitous advertising, may do most persons none other than monetary harm, but others may spend fruitless weeks or months in self-medication when they should be under medical supervision.

The Hematopoietic System and Associated Laboratory Tests

The hematopoietic system includes the circulating blood, the bone marrow, the spleen, and the lymph nodes supplemented by reticuloendothelial cells scattered throughout the body. The liver, although not usually considered a part of this system, has an important function in blood formation and destruction.

The erythrocytes constitute the greatest part of the cellular elements in the circulating blood; their chief function is to transport oxygen to all tissues of the body. The oxygen is bound loosely to the iron portion of the hemoglobin within the cell. Any decrease in the number of red corpuscles or their hemoglobin will thus affect all organs. When the iron supply is deficient, the concentration of hemoglobin falls markedly.

Red cell formation is regulated largely by the need of tissues for oxygen; when there is increased need as in exercise or from residence in high altitudes, erythrocyte production is stimulated. Lack of exercise will contribute to a low red cell count which is often exemplified in bedridden patients. If the bedfast patient is also elderly, the process is augmented by the normal reduction in red cell formation that occurs with increasing age and produces mild degrees of anemia in most older persons.

The normal red cell count is approximately 4.5 to 5 million per cu mm of blood, with women averaging the lower figure. The hemoglobin content is also normally lower for women, i.e., 14 g per 100 ml of blood as compared to 15 to 16 g per 100 ml of blood for men.

The number of white blood cells is approximately one-five-hundredth of the total number of red blood cells. The most important function of the white cells is defense against infection, primarily through phagocytosis of foreign bodies and detoxification of harmful substances. The total leukocyte count is comprised of granulocytes (myelocytes), lymphocytes, and monocytes. The granulocytes, which are produced in the bone marrow, are further subdivided according to cytoplasmic staining characteristics into neutrophils, eosinophils, and basophils. The lymphocytes are produced for the most part in the lymph nodes but also in other lymphoid tissue distributed throughout the body. The site of monocyte formation is uncertain, but it is generally believed also to be in lymphoid tissue.

A differential white count is done to determine the percent of each type of white cell. Normally, 65 percent will be granulocytes, of which 62 percent will be neutrophils, 2 percent, eosinophils, and 1 percent, basophils. The proportion of lymphocytes will be approximately 30 percent, and of monocytes, 5 percent. The differential count changes in different conditions; in acute infections the proportion of neutrophils is increased; during convalescence the proportion of lymphocytes increases. A high percentage of monocytes is suggestive of chronic infections such as tuberculosis. High eosinophil counts are typical of allergic conditions.

The platelets, or thrombocytes, are small fragments of a large white cell called the *megakaryocyte,* which is produced in the bone marrow. Platelets maintain the integrity of the vascular endothelium and are necessary to blood coagulation. Normally, they number 200,000 to 400,000 per cu mm of blood. Persons with decreased platelet counts are subject to bleeding.

The spleen is an important part of the hematopoietic, portal, and reticuloendothelial systems. It serves as a blood reservoir, plays a part in the final disposal of red blood cells, has phagocytic activity, produces antibodies, manufactures lymphocytes, and performs some function during the life of platelets. Although considered an important internal organ, its removal is not incompatible with life.

Some physiologists also consider the white blood cells to be part of the reticuloendothelial system. The function of this system is to combat infection by means of phagocytosis and by formation of antibodies. The reticuloendothelial system comprises the Kupffer cells in the liver, reticulum cells in the lymph nodes, phagocytic cells in the spleen, bone marrow and lymphoid tissue of the gastrointestinal tract, and histiocyte cells throughout most body tissue.

The lymph nodes are highly efficient filters for bacteria and as such are important defensive structures. As part of the body's general mass of lymphoid tissue, they also assist in the production of lymphocytes.

Because of the varied structures involved and the numerous functions of the hematopoietic system, it is evident that disorders of the system may be manifested in many ways. In general, however, the disorders are characterized by pallor, cyanosis, jaundice, bleeding, or enlargement of the lymph nodes or spleen.

In addition to the laboratory tests measuring values of erythrocytes, hemoglobin, leukocytes, and platelets, other common tests are as follows:

1. The *hematocrit* measures the relative volume of packed red blood cells to plasma. The normal value is approximately 42 to 47 percent, with the higher figure found in men. When a patient is dehydrated or has lost plasma fluid for any reason, the hematocrit is increased. In anemia it is decreased.

2. *Red cell morphology* is useful in distinguishing types of anemia through closer examination of the red cell. The values will include the mean corpuscular volume (MCV), mean corpuscular hemoglobin (MCH), mean corpuscular hemoglobin concentration (MCHC), and mean corpuscular diameter (MCD). Red cells containing less hemoglobin than normal are referred to as being *hypochromic;* those containing more hemoglobin than normal, as *hyperchromic.* A microcytic cell is smaller than normal and a macrocytic cell is larger than normal. Two other terms encountered are *anisocytosis* (variation is size), and *poikilocytosis* (variation is shape).

3. The *bleeding time* measures the time required for effective hemostasis after a standardized wound is inflicted. A prick of the finger or ear lobe (Duke method) will cause bleeding that normally stops in 2 to 5 minutes. The most accurate method is the Ivy technique, in which a blood pressure cuff is kept inflated on the upper arm at 40 mm mercury while a puncture wound is made on the upper

forearm. The bleeding is blotted every 30 seconds and will normally cease in ½ to 6½ minutes.

4. The *clotting time* determines how well the person's blood coagulates without the help of tissue factors, which are present in calculating the bleeding time. A careful venepuncture is done to obtain the sample. Normally the clotting time is about 6 minutes.

5. A *bone marrow biopsy* is done to determine the morphology of formed elements in the blood. It is a tool of major diagnostic value. The specimen is usually obtained from the sternum, although the iliac crest is occasionally used. The patient may anticipate pain with this procedure and become quite apprehensive. A frank explanation that there will be a feeling of pressure when the needle is inserted into the sternum, and that there may also be slight discomfort when the specimen is withdrawn, will be helpful in allaying fears of greater discomfort. The explanation should include the information that the area will be locally anesthetized. The patient will appreciate the nurse's presence throughout this procedure. Afterward, he should know that there may be slight discomfort over the puncture site for a few days.

6. The *tourniquet test* (cuff test) is a useful though crude index of capillary fragility as measured by the ability of the capillaries to withstand stress. It is done by inflating a blood pressure cuff wrapped on the person's upper arm to a point midway between the systolic and diastolic pressures and leaving it in place for 10 to 15 minutes. Five minutes after removal of the cuff the number of petechiae in a previously marked circular area on the forearm are counted. The appearance of a few petechiae is normal, but a "shower" or many confluent petechiae is a positive test. The test is nearly always positive when the platelets are qualitatively or quantitatively abnormal, although the relation of platelets to capillary integrity is unclear.

The Anemias

Anemia, which in itself is a symptom, is characterized by a decrease in the number of circulating red blood cells and a reduction in total hemoglobin. It is a common source of ill health, especially chronic ill health. The actual incidence in communities has not been widely studied but it is believed to be high. Anemia may be caused by loss of blood, impaired blood production, or excessive blood destruction. Since the amount of oxygen available to tissues is reduced by the decrease in its transporting agents, tissue hypoxia is the source of the signs and symptoms of anemia. Systems with high oxygen requirements are those most affected and include the skeletal musculature, the cardiovascular system, and the central nervous system.

Compensatory mechanisms such as increased cardiac output and expansion of plasma volume may allow the person to be symptom-free at rest, but exertion, by increasing the oxygen requirements, promptly causes symptoms.

Fatigue is often the earliest symptom ("I feel tired all the time"). Pallor, especially of the mucous membranes, nailbeds, palms of the hands, and conjunctiva, is characteristic. Skin pallor alone is not a reliable guide since pigmentation, the amount of subcutaneous fluid, and the state of skin vessels all influence skin color. Cardiovascular symptoms may include dyspnea on exertion, palpitation, and tachycardia. When compensatory adjustments fail, the clinical picture of congestive heart failure ensues. Symptoms referable to the central nervous system are common in severe anemia, particularly in older patients with some degree of cerebral arteriosclerosis, and include faintness, giddiness, and headache.

The nurse needs to determine how much activity the patient is able to handle without undue fatigue and shortness of breath. It is often easy to overestimate how much he is able to do, since fatigue is primarily subjective. However, such things as struggling through taking his own bath, walking down a long hall to the bathroom, or climbing steps all may be inordinately tiring. Older patients should be attended when up if there is any history of fainting or falling.

Anemic patients nearly always complain of feeling cold, probably because their chronic fatigue tends to preclude muscular exercise as a heat-producing mechanism, and because a degree of vasoconstriction is thought to accompany decreased peripheral blood flow. Soft cotton blankets on the bed rather than sheets are often welcome. Cotton socks, slippers with "uppers," bed jackets, woolen robes, flannel gowns or pajamas are all items of clothing that will be more comfortable than the usual skimpy hospital gowns, cotton robes, and thin scuff slippers.

The patient with anemia should not be placed in a room with someone who feels warm most of the time and is most comfortable with the windows wide open, as for example, a patient with hyperthyroidism. Both will be unhappy under these circumstances.

In long-standing cases the skin may become dry and the nails and hair, brittle. Measures described in fundamentals of nursing texts may help relieve the dryness and itching of skin and scalp.

ANEMIA DUE TO LOSS OF BLOOD

Blood loss may be either acute or chronic. In acute hemorrhage the loss is usually obvious, and if the total loss is large, peripheral circulatory failure will occur. This is characterized by the signs of shock and constitutes a medical emergency. Blood transfusion is required, but plasma or a plasma volume expander such as dextran can be used when necessary to tide the patient over until blood becomes available.

Marked hemorrhage from any source is frightening to the patient. If at all possible he should not be left unattended while the necessary actions such as telephoning the physician and gathering dressings, linens, and infusion equipment are carried out.

Chronic blood loss may go unrecognized for a long period of time. The cause may be excessive menstrual flow, a bleeding peptic ulcer, bleeding hemorrhoids, or a malignant gastrointestinal neoplasm. The iron stores of the body are gradually exhausted with a chronic loss of blood, and the blood picture becomes one of typical hypochromic microcytic iron-deficiency anemia.

ANEMIA DUE TO IMPAIRED BLOOD PRODUCTION

Iron-Deficiency Anemia

Iron-deficiency anemia results when the supply of iron to the bone marrow is insufficient for hemoglobin synthesis. This type of anemia was first mentioned in the sixteenth century as "the sickness of virgins," probably because of the inadequate diet of adolescent girls and the increased requirements of menstruation and growth. Later the condition was known as *chlorosis*—the "green sickness."

Normally, the body carefully conserves its iron and reuses that which is derived from the daily breakdown of red cells. There is in addition a store of iron in the tissues which can be utilized when an iron deficit occurs by blood loss, increased requirements, or impaired absorption.

The chronic loss of blood is the most important factor in the development of an iron-deficiency anemia. Women are subject to loss through heavy menstruation and by having many pregnancies in rapid succession. Bleeding from the gastrointestinal tract is a common cause in men over middle age.

A nutritional deficiency of iron is not as common as is popularly assumed. However, improper feeding is of major importance in infants and young children, and may occur in adults because of diets restricted by economic reasons, fads, or anorexia. Nutritional deficiency also may occur when there is impaired absorption from the gastrointestinal tract, as in sprue.

Lean meat and organ meats are excellent sources of iron; other good sources include eggs, potatoes, green leafy vegetables such as kale, fruits such as apricots, raisins, and prunes, and enriched cereals and breads. Among shellfish, oysters provide a good source of iron.

Once an iron deficit has occurred, the replenishment of iron from dietary sources is an exceedingly prolonged process, so use of iron supplements is justified for even mild degrees of deficiency. The most commonly used supplements are oral ferrous sulfate and ferrous gluconate tablets. Although iron is better absorbed in a fasting state, the tablets are usually given after meals to reduce the possibility of gastric irritation. Both preparations are available in liquid form; if taken in this way a glass drinking tube or straw should be used to avoid discoloration of the teeth. The patient should know that iron will cause his stools to be black. The housewife will also appreciate knowing that iron will stain silver spoons. Iron tablets should be kept well out of reach of small children, as fatal iron toxicity has occurred in children who accidentally ingested large doses.

Parenteral iron may be given when a person is intolerant of oral iron or a gastrointestinal disorder exists which impairs absorption or is aggravated by oral iron, such as peptic ulcer, ulcerative colitis, or chronic diarrhea. The most common preparation is an iron dextran complex (Imferon), which requires careful deep intramuscular administration. If the solution is deposited in subcutaneous tissue, pain and staining of the tissues result. It is best given using the Z track technique, that is, pushing the subcutaneous tissue aside before inserting the needle. Intravenous iron preparations are available but are seldom used because of the the high incidence of toxic reactions.

Once the cause of the iron deficiency is corrected and the patient's blood picture shows a return to normal (a process requiring anywhere from 1 month to 1 year), dietary sources should be adequate for maintenance, provided of course that the diet is well balanced and that there is no longer a prolonged increased physiological demand for iron.

PERNICIOUS ANEMIA

Pernicious anemia is now seldom seen in the hospital in its advanced stages, since if diagnosis is made early it responds very well to treatment. Without treatment the disease is fatal. It develops in late adult life primarily among individuals of northern European and British ancestry. There is a progressive decrease in the capacity of the gastric mucosa to secrete *intrinsic factor*. The terms *intrinsic factor* and *extrinsic factor* are those used in Castle's original hypothesis in 1926. This hypothesis states that the gastric juice of normal individuals contains a substance called *intrinsic factor* which acts on a substance found in certain foods—*extrinsic factor*—to yield a hematopoietic factor which is essential for red cell production. It is now known that the extrinsic factor is vitamin B_{12} and that it is also the hematopoietic factor. The intrinsic factor is known to facilitate the absorption of vitamin B_{12} through the intestinal wall, but the exact mechanism is unclear. When the extrinsic factor cannot be absorbed abnormal changes take place gradually in the bone marrow which result in anemia and the formation of abnormal macrocytic red cells.

The symptoms common to all forms of anemia, i.e., weakness, lassitude, fatigue, dyspnea on exertion, and palpitation, are present along with the features of vitamin B_{12} deficiency, i.e., macrocytic anemia, mucosal atrophy, and nervous system involvement. The mucosal atrophy is general but the most marked changes involve the tongue and stomach. The tongue becomes smooth and usually there is glossitis with accompanying burning and soreness. Atrophy of the gastric mucosa results in achlorhydria, an invariable finding upon gastric analysis.

Initial complaints stemming from the nervous system involvement are commonly those of numbness, tingling, or "pins and needles" in the toes and feet due to degeneration of the sensory fibers of the peripheral nerves. This may progress to lower limb weakness and an unsteady gait as degeneration progresses to the posterior and lateral tracts of the spinal cord. Mental disturbances are common but usually mild and include loss of memory, irritability, and restlessness. Occasionally there may be more severe disturbances.

The prognosis with early diagnosis is excellent. When degenerative nervous system changes have occurred, reversal is not possible, but the symptoms may be arrested. (Only myelin is lost in the early stages, but nerve fibers themselves are involved during the later stages.) After vitamin B_{12} injections are started, subjective improvement is noted within 2 to 3 days with a return of appetite and a sense of well-being. The soreness and redness of the tongue are rapidly relieved and gastrointestinal symptoms such as nausea and diarrhea disappear within a few weeks.

The nursing care given before treatment is begun depends upon the severity of symptoms. The patient may need help in selecting foods that are nonirritating and easily swallowed. Providing facilities for frequent gentle mouth care will be welcome. If there is neurological involvement, the patient needs the safety of having someone nearby to assist as needed in getting in and out of bed to a chair or to the bathroom, since his unsteadiness or lower limb weakness is conducive to falling. Range of motion exercises are valuable for improving muscle tone. Irritability and impatience, if present, can be understood as symptoms that will disappear; in the meantime the nurse may anticipate many actions as being irritating to the person and avert these if possible. These may include such annoyances as bumping the bed, leaving overhead lights glaring into the patient's eyes, or allowing tepid water to stay in his water pitcher.

There is no special diet to be followed, except that of a varied and nutritious one. Either the patient or a member of the family may be instructed in giving intramuscular vitamin B_{12} injections. The solution (cyanacobalamin) is nonirritating and after the initial doses are given, maintenance is usually attained by injections given weekly or twice monthly.

ANEMIA DUE TO DESTRUCTION OF RED BLOOD CELLS

Anemia may be caused by too-rapid destruction of red blood cells—*hemolysis*. The life span of normal red cells is between 100 and 120 days; in the hemolytic anemias it is shortened by varying degrees and in severe cases may be only a few days.

Hemolysis may be caused by drug therapy; in sensitive individuals large doses of antimalarials, aspirin, phenacetin, nitrofurantoin (Furadantin), and sulfisoxazole (gantrisin) have all at one time or another been causative agents. Benzene, a common solvent in industry, can be an offender. Acute hemolytic anemias have been seen in young children who have swallowed mothballs containing naphthalene, or furniture polish containing nitrobenzene. A mild hemolytic anemia is often associated for unknown reasons with uremia and cancer. Malaria is the classic example of a parasite hemolyzing red cells, and occasionally streptococcal infections will also cause hemolysis.

Since bilirubin is an end-product of hemoglobin breakdown, the patient with hemolytic anemia usually has jaundice of mild to moderate intensity. This type of jaundice is not accompanied by pruritus. In the chronic mild forms of hemolytic anemia, the person suffers the usual symptoms of anemia. In acute forms, however, there usually is fever with chills, headache, and pain in the lumbar area, chest, or abdomen. Urine output decreases, and in extreme cases profound shock and death may result. The nurse will recognize these as the symptoms of incompatible blood replacement in which the cells agglutinate, then hemolyze rapidly, releasing hemoglobin into the circulation which can occlude kidney tubules and cause renal shutdown.

Various hemolytic anemias arise from basic defects within the red cell itself. These are not common, although one type is seen with more or less regularity in areas with a high Negro population. This disorder is characterized by an abnormal hemoglobin-S, as contrasted to normal hemoglobin-A. Approximately 10 percent of American Negroes possesss the hemoglobin-S or sickle cell trait, of whom only about 2 percent experience sickle cell disease with its many manifestations. (Sickle cell disease has been compared with syphilis as one of the great masqueraders of medicine.) In Africa, the incidence for the trait in many populations is over 40 percent. For unknown reasons, possession of the trait seems to confer resistance to malaria.

The sickle cell trait, which is the heterozygous state for the hemoglobin-S gene, does not cause anemia and in general is asymptomatic. However, if both parents possess the trait, the children will be homozygous for the hemoglobin-S gene, and will manifest sickle cell anemia. Many of these children die in the first decade from multiple thromboses and infarcts of many organs. If they survive to adulthood they are usually slender with long, thin extremities and narrow hips and shoulders, and show a greenish-yellow icterus of the sclerae. Gallstones often develop from the excessive bile pigment metabolism that occurs with increased red cell destruction. Ulcers of the legs are also common. The generally sickly course of these individuals is punctuated by crises in which a variety of acute abdominal emergencies may be simulated, or pain in the extremities may be predominant.

Treatment is symptomatic; if anemia becomes extreme, blood transfusions are given. Adequate hydration is important, since dehydration and loss of fluid are associated with the development of crises. During crises, sedatives and analgesics are given as needed. Persons known to carry the sickle cell trait may be advised against high-altitude plane flights, since splenic infarctions have been known to occur during such trips.

APLASTIC ANEMIA

Aplastic anemia is a serious condition resulting from bone marrow depression. The term *pancytopenia* is used to describe the combination of anemia, leukopenia, and thrombocytopenia, which is the usual picture resulting from aplasia of the bone marrow.

The most common cause of aplastic anemia is drug administration. Compounds containing the benzene ring are particularly likely to cause marrow depression. Drugs used in the treatment of malignant lymphomas and leukemias, such as nitrogen mustard, related cytotoxics, and antimetabolites, will in sufficient doses always cause marrow depression. Other drugs that occasionally are offenders are antiepileptics such as mephenytoin (Mesantoin) and trimethadione (Tridione), and antibacterials such as chloramphenicol (Chloromycetin). A major factor with the use of any drug is the individual's reaction to it; some persons become rapidly sensitized to a drug while others may not. A rash, sore throat or mouth, malaise, bruises, fever, epistaxis, or petechiae may all be signs of a developing toxicity.

Excessive exposure to radiation is a cause of bone marrow depression. Certain chemicals, in addition to drugs, may affect the marrow. The incidence of aplastic anemia due to industrial chemicals is decreasing but is still a hazard where large quantities of benzene are used as a solvent. Some insecticides have been implicated.

There is no curative treatment for aplastic anemia. Apart from removal of any possible toxic agent, the aim of therapy is to support the patient in the hope that bone marrow function will improve or return to normal. Blood transfusions and antibiotics are given, and corticosteroids and testosterone are sometimes employed as possible marrow stimulants.

All precautions should be taken to prevent infection, and the nurse plays a key role in this activity. A reverse isolation is usually instituted in which all equipment used in the patient's care is kept as clean as possible. Personnel and visitors wear clean gowns when with the patient, and anyone with an infectious process is not allowed in his room. Meticulous hand washing is, of course, essential.

Because of the relationship between drugs and aplastic anemia, anyone who has had a severe reaction to a specific drug should carry an identification card with him at all times. This card will state that the person should not receive the particular drug or any closely related ones.

Hemorrhagic Disorders

The hemorrhagic disorders are due to defects in the mechanism of hemostasis. In some disorders the bleeding may be mild and limited to the skin; in other disorders uncontrollable bleeding may threaten life.

The mechanism of blood coagulation is an exceedingly complicated one, and still not well understood. The classic theory put forth by Morawitz in 1905 has been expanded to include newly discovered factors in addition to the basic four he saw as necessary, that is, thromboplastin, calcium, prothrombin, and fibrinogen. A much different schema, or enzymatic theory, has been proposed in recent years, so researchers tend to favor either the classic theory or the enzymatic theory. In general, however, both groups see the coagulation process as a dynamic one, in which substances favoring coagulation (procoagulants) briefly overbalance substances that inhibit coagulation (anticoagulants). In broad outline, the process is also seen as including at least three phases: the first phase, initiated with blood vessel damage, is the formation of activated blood thromboplastin, followed by the phase of formation of thrombin from prothrombin, and finally the formation of fibrin from the catalytic action of thrombin on fibrinogen. The end-result of coagulation is the formation of fibrin threads that form a reticulum entrapping red blood cells, white blood cells, and platelets to form a clot.

As researchers discovered factors previously unknown in the coagulation process, the number of terms also grew. These have now been simplified by an international nomenclature, shown in Table 32-1. Deficiency in any of the factors shown in the table will cause faulty hemostasis.

TABLE 32-1
Blood Clotting Factors

INTERNATIONAL NOMENCLATURE	SYNONYMS
Factor I	Fibrinogen
Factor II	Prothrombin
Factor III	Thromboplastin
Factor IV	Calcium
Factor V	Proaccelerin, labile factor, accelerator globulin (Ac-G)
Factor VII	Proconvertin, serum prothrombin conversion accelerator (SPCA), autoprothrombin I
Factor VIII	Antihemophilic factor (AHF), antihemophilic globulin (AHG)
Factor IX	Plasma thromboplastin component (PTC), Christmas factor (CF), autoprothrombin II
Factor X	Stuart factor, Stuart-Prower factor, Prower factor, autoprothrombin C
Factor XI	Plasma thromboplastin antecedent (PTA)
Factor XII	Hageman factor
Factor XIII	Fibrin stabilizing factor

THE PURPURAS

Purpura refers to extravasation of blood into the skin or mucous membrane in the form of tiny petechiae or larger ecchymoses. Many purpuras are accompanied by a thrombocytopenia, which results in a prolonged bleeding time, impaired clot retraction, and a positive tourniquet test. Thrombocytopenia may be drug-induced or occur with other disorders such as leukemia, aplastic anemia, or lupus erythematosus. There is increasing evidence that some forms may be on an autoimmune basis. If no cause for the thrombocytopenia can be found, it is termed *idiopathic thrombocytopenic purpura.*

This disorder is most common in children and young adults and affects females more often than males. The bleeding occurs spontaneously as well as after surgical or dental procedures or trauma. The skin is the most common site of hemorrhage which results in petechiae, ecchymoses, or both. Severe bleeding may occur into vital areas such as the cranium and diaphragm. Bleeding of the gums is frequent and menorrhagia and melena are also seen.

The treatment varies with different schools of thought. Some physicians rely heavily on splenectomy early in the course; it is not understood why this procedure is helpful but it does result in remission of the disease in many patients. One theory holds that antibodies may develop against the individual's own platelets and the spleen removes these "sensitized" platelets; splenectomy would thus reduce the amount of platelet destruction. Another postulation is that the spleen may exert an inhibitory effect on platelet formation in the bone marrow and splenectomy would remove this inhibitory factor.

Other physicians prefer initial conservative management with corticosteroids augmented by transfusions of whole fresh blood or platelet-rich plasma. (Plastic bags are used instead of bottles so platelet "sticking" is reduced.) Remissions have been obtained through this regimen; spontaneous remissions without treatment are often seen in children but less commonly in adults.

The patient should be protected from trauma; trips to the bathroom at night when lighting is inadequate make it easy for him to bump into chairs, stools, or bed cranks. Injections should be given with as small a needle as possible and gentle pressure applied to the injection site for a few minutes afterward. If spontaneous bleeding occurs internally the patient may become pale or may faint, or tachycardia and hypotension may develop. The bleeding may also be evident as epistaxis, tarry stools, or hematuria.

If the disorder is quite severe bed rest is indicated, since it lessens the risk of cerebral hemorrhage. The nurse should be alert to and help prevent upper respiratory infections and constipation, since coughing and straining at stool increase intracranial pressure, which in turn increases the possibility of intracranial bleeding.

THE HEMOPHILIAS

The hemophilias have been known since Biblical times and were probably the disorders referred to in the Talmud by Hebraic writers who described unusual bleeding after circumcision. This group of diseases is now known to be caused by the lack of specific factors in the blood coagulation process. The best known and most common is hemophilia A, which is a congenital deficiency of Factor VIII or antihemophilic globulin (AHG). Hemophilia B occurs from a deficiency of Factor IX, plasma thromboplastin component (PTC), and is known as *Christmas disease*. Hemophilia C, caused by a deficiency of plasma thromboplastin antecedent (PTA), differs from hemophilias A and B in that it is a dominant trait and affects males and females equally.

Hemophilias A and B, inherited as sex-linked recessive traits, are transmitted to males by their mothers, whereas a hemophilic father cannot transmit this disease to his sons. The female transmitter, being heterozygous for the trait, does not exhibit the disease. However, a female can have hemophilia provided that she is born to a hemophilic father and a transmitter mother.

The prognosis for survival, although always guarded, has greatly improved in the last two decades with better use of blood and plasma transfusions with the result that more patients survive into adulthood. It has been said that if the patient does survive into adult life the signs and symptoms become less severe, but this may be on the basis that he has learned to live with his disease and consequently avoids trauma.

In severely afflicted persons the bleeding occurs spontaneously, often as articular hemorrhages. The joints affected, in order of frequency, are the knees, ankles, elbows, wrists, fingers, hips, and shoulders. When this type of bleeding occurs there is sudden pain, swelling, change in color, and limitation of movement. Other episodes of spontaneous bleeding may take the form of epistaxis, hematuria, and gastrointestinal bleeding.

In milder cases there may be no spontaneous bleeding, but it will occur as persistent slow oozing upon trauma or with minor surgery. Hematomas and ecchymoses are common.

The bleeding time, clot retraction, and prothrombin time are normal, whereas the clotting time is prolonged. More specific tests are the prothrombin consumption test (PCT) and the thromboplastin generation test (TGT), which will detect which factor is deficient. Factor VIII (AHF) is unstable, deteriorating rapidly in storage; if whole blood is used in treatment it should be not more than a few hours old. Lyophilized plasma is preferable to freshly frozen plasma, in which Factor VIII deteriorates more rapidly. Concentrates of Factor VIII are also available. Stored blood or plasma is effective in treating hemophilias B and C.

The person with hemophilia will often know at least as much about management of his disease as professional persons whose contact with the disorder may be only occasional. Doctors and nurses are well advised to pay close attention to the patient's suggestions. Only the person most skilled in venepuncture should ever attempt to draw blood or start fresh blood or plasma infusions on hemophilic patients. Venepuncture when skillfully done does not cause fresh bleeding, since the elasticity of the vessel wall suffices to close the puncture wound. When acute joint bleeding occurs prompt efforts are necessary to avoid permanent disability. Bed rest or at least rest of the affected part, transfusions, and local ice applications are immediate steps. Corticosteroids are often used in an effort to prevent loss of joint function. Local bleeding is treated by any or a combination of the following: gentle pressure, application of topical thrombin, epinephrine-soaked dressings, coagulating snake venoms, and cold compresses. Intramuscular injections are given only if necessary and with care.

Any person with hemophilia should carry an identifying card stating his name, his doctor's name, his blood type, and the fact that he has hemophilia.

Polycythemia Vera

Polycythemia vera, or true polycythemia, is characterized by an abnormal increase in the number of circulating red blood cells. It is a specific, chronic, and progressive disease of unknown cause, and is to be distinguished from relative polycythemia, which results from loss of body fluids or decreased fluid intake. It is also to be distinguished from the secondary polycythemia associated with lung or cardiovascular diseases causing decreased arterial oxygen saturation, which is a stimulus to erythropoiesis.

The disease usually occurs in persons over middle age, with the higher incidence being among men. There may be complaints of gradually developing dyspnea, weakness, and headache, or there may be a multiplicity of symptoms. The most striking part of the physical appearance is often the ruddy cyanosis of the face, especially apparent on the lips, ears, tip of the nose, cheeks, and neck. Color changes may also be apparent in the distal portions of the extremities. The degree of deep reddish-blue color depends upon the absolute amount of reduced hemoglobin in the capillaries. The deepest coloration is apparent where there is peripheral vascular dilatation along with the sluggish circulation.

The number of red cells may vary from 6 to 10 million per cu mm of blood. The increased viscosity makes the patient a ready candidate for thromboses, and cerebrovascular accidents are common. Paradoxically, epistaxis, gum bleeding, and larger hemorrhages are frequent in spite of the fact that the number of thrombocytes is usually also increased.

Phlebotomy, chemotherapy, and radioactive phosphorus are the treatments most commonly employed. Phlebotomy, or venesection (historically, "bloodletting"), affords symptomatic relief by reducing the total blood volume; usually 350 to 500 ml of blood is removed via an arm vein at intervals according to the blood picture. The phlebotomy procedure is essentially the same as that employed with donors at blood banks.

Depression of bone marrow activity is attempted through the use of chemotherapeutic drugs such as chlorambucil (Leukeran), cyclophosphamide (Cytoxan), and busulfan (Myleran). These are all alkylating agents and require frequent supervision of their use, but have been shown to be effective (Guyton; Wasserman and Gilbert). Triethylenemelamine (TEM) has also been used.

Radioactive phosphorus (^{32}P) is considered by some as the treatment of choice, since long remissions can be obtained. Others consider the danger of inducing acute leukemia by even slight overcalculation of dose to be too great, and do not employ it. It may be given by either the oral or the intravenous route. It has a half life of 14 days and emits only beta rays, so isolation precautions are not necessary. Urine may be discarded into the general sewage system in the usual manner; careful hand washing is advised after handling of the bedpan, or disposable gloves may be used.

Nursing care is primarily symptomatic, with careful observations for bleeding, as from hemorrhoids, and for signs of thromboses occurring in leg veins or as cerebrovascular accidents. Fluid intake is encouraged because of the high blood viscosity and the need to excrete urates, which are increased because of the nucleoprotein degradation of the large numbers of hematic cells (Wasserman and Gilbert). Pruritus is frequent, and probably associated with increased levels of whole blood histamine; it may be especially intense after a hot bath, so cool water is preferable. The avoidance of foods high in iron content, such as liver, oysters, and legumes, is often urged, though it should be remembered that if frequent phlebotomies are being done, the total iron stores are depleted and iron deficiency may result.

The Leukemias

Leukemia is generally regarded as a neoplastic process of the hematopoietic system causing widespread proliferation of leukocytes and their precursors. It is a fatal disease that affects all age groups; although it has been considered primarily a disease of children, it actually strikes many more adults and at an increasing rate. Deaths from leukemia comprise about 4 percent of all those due to cancer.

The unrestrained production of immature leukocytes leads to suppression of erythrocyte, platelet, and normal leukocyte formation in the bone marrow. The patient with leukemia will thus have anemia, a bleeding tendency, and lack of resistance to infection. There may in addition be leukemic infiltration of the central nervous system, kidney, liver, or spleen.

The various types of leukemia take their names from the predominant abnormal cell present and are termed *myelocytic, lymphocytic,* or *monocytic* leukemia. *Subleukemic leukemia* refers to cases in which the total white cell count may be normal but the cells are abnormal.

The cause of leukemia is unknown, although the theory that it is a neoplastic process is the most widely accepted. Many research findings advance the virus theory and it has been shown that viruses can produce leukemia in experimental animals, cause human tissue cultures to undergo malignant transformation, and shatter chromosomes (Miller). However, it has not been possible to produce leukemia in laboratory animals with any organism isolated from a leukemic patient; neither is the disease transmissible from man to man. Its development may well be the outcome of the interaction of a number of host, agent, and environmental factors.

Proof that radiation could cause leukemia was well established in the early 1950s when studies were made of survivors of the atomic bombings in Japan. Roentgenologists have shown a higher incidence of leukemia than persons in other medical fields, although increased precautions in x-ray departments are rapidly reducing this difference.

Leukemia occurs in both acute and chronic forms. The clinical manifestations of the acute and chronic forms differ markedly; however, all chronic forms produce essentially the same symptoms, and all acute forms are also essentially alike. Acute leukemias reach a peak incidence at 3 to 4 years of age but may be found in all ages. Chronic leukemias are extremely rare below the age of 15 and show a progressive rise in incidence with age. The incidence of chronic myelocytic leukemia reaches its peak in middle life, while chronic lymphocytic leukemia reaches its peak in more advanced years. The chronic forms are perhaps twice as common as the acute forms and affect more males.

Without treatment, the duration of life in acute leukemia is a matter of months; in chronic leukemia it is a matter of years. With treatment, temporary remission in symptoms may be obtained and although these remissions may be short, the fact that they do occur offers one of the more encouraging aspects of this otherwise distressing disease.

ACUTE LEUKEMIA

Acute leukemia may have as sudden an onset in adults as it does in children or it may be more insidious. When the onset is abrupt, there is frequently a sore throat, cough, and petechiae or ecchymoses in the skin, or the first evidence may be excessive bleeding following a tooth extraction. Fever, headache, and malaise follow. The gums may be swollen and purplish.

Anemia is always present and may be severe. The thrombocytopenia may contribute to bleeding from such slight causes as brushing the teeth. The leukocyte count may vary from below normal to levels as high as 100,000 per cu mm of blood. The predominant immature cells in the adult type are usually myelocytes; in children they are usually lymphocytes. Bone marrow aspiration is usually done to confirm the morphologic cell type.

The response to treatment in adult acute leukemia is poor as contrasted to adult chronic leukemia and acute leukemia in children. Eventually death is due to widespread hemorrhage or to infections such as pneumonia.

Treatment is directed toward obtaining as much relief of symptoms as possible. General supportive measures include the use of blood transfusions and antibiotics to combat any infection. Specific measures in chemotherapy include the use of drugs that interfere with cell metabolism, notably purine antagonists and folic acid antagonists. The drug of choice in adult acute leukemia is usually 6-mercaptopurine (6-MP), which interrupts the synthesis of purines essential to the structure of nucleic acids. In well-calculated doses it rarely produces the toxic effect of anorexia, nausea, or vomiting.

The folic acid antagonist, methotrexate (amethopterin), is less effective than 6-MP but may be used when resistance has developed to the latter. During its use the patient should be observed carefully for oral ulcerations. Nausea, vomiting, and diarrhea may also be part of the toxic symptomatology.

Radiation therapy is considered to be contraindicated in acute leukemia except when necessary to control local leukemoid lesions in the central nervous system or kidney. ACTH and cortisone, which are often so effective in producing remissions in children, become less effective with increasing age. They will, however, help to control bleeding and will also suppress high fever. The latter action may be helpful in some cases, but may also obscure the presence of an underlying infection.

CHRONIC LEUKEMIA

The chronic form of leukemia in adults may be either myelocytic or lymphocytic. In either case, symptoms may not develop until the disease has been in progress for a year or more. Complaints may then be those of general weakness, tiredness, and a heavy abdominal sensation with swelling in the left side due to splenic enlargement. (The splenomegaly is more common in the myelocytic form.) As the disease progresses, there may be loss of weight, fever, and bleeding. Enlargement of lymph nodes in the neck, axilla, or groin may be the predominating initial symptom in chronic lymphocytic leukemia.

In the myelogenous form the leukocyte count may be exceedingly high, often over 500,000 per cu mm of blood. In the lymphocytic form the total count is usually under 250,000 per cu mm of blood. The degree of anemia is often an index of the severity of the disease.

Treatment of the chronic leukemias is aimed at making the patient more comfortable and includes the use of x-ray therapy or radioactive phosphorus (^{32}P), the choice usually depending upon availability and convenience. X-ray therapy is nearly always used when there is marked adenopathy or splenomegaly.

Chemotherapeutic agents differ from those used in acute leukemia. Most of the ones in current use are alkylating or cytotoxic agents related pharmacologically to nitrogen mustard. They exert a selective action on rapidly growing cells; however, the margin of safety is narrow before they significantly affect normal cells. Dosage is calculated carefully, and the patient's clinical reaction and blood picture are watched closely. In general, toxic effects include nausea, vomiting, diarrhea, and bone marrow depression. At this time, busulfan (Myleran) is the drug of choice in chronic myelocytic leukemia and chlorambucil (Leukeran) the drug of choice in chronic lymphocytic leukemia. The corticosteroids are helpful in controlling complications such as hemolysis of red cells and platelet depression. (See Table 32–2.)

NURSING CARE OF THE PATIENT WITH LEUKEMIA

The diagnosis of leukemia may literally panic those to whom it must be given. Although the physician bears the responsibility of imparting this knowledge to the patient or his family, the nurse's own personal philosophy will have a great deal to do with how much support she is able to give to the person with leukemia and to his family. Reinforcing the physician's explanation that the disease is neither hereditary nor contagious may, when appropriate, relieve some anxiety and guilt. A genuine interest in the person and his activities will be more helpful than dwelling on his physical state.

Normal pursuits are often possible during remissions and it is possible that life may be more meaningful when there is knowledge of how tenuous that life is. However, false reassurances should never be given, and only the patient and his

	CHRONIC LEUKEMIA		ACUTE LEUKEMIA			HODGKIN'S DISEASE	LYMPHOSARCOMA
	Myelocytic	Lymphocytic	Myeloblastic	Monoblastic	Lymphoblastic		
Irradiation:							
Roentgen ray	+ + + +	+ + + +	0	0	0	+ + + +	+ + + +
Radioactive phosphorus	+ + + +	+ + + +	0	0	0	+	+ +
Chemotherapy:							
Nitrogen mustard	+	+	0	0	0	+ + + +	+ +
Triethylenemelamine	+	+ +	0	0	0	+ +	+
Chlorambucil	+	+ + +	0	0	0	+ + +	+ +
Cyclophosphamide	0	0	0	0	0	+ + +	+ +
Vinblastine	0	0	0	+	0	+ +	+
Vincristine	0	0	+	+	+	0	0
Busulfan	+ + + +	+	0	0	0	0	0
Demecolcin	+ +	0	0	0	0	0	0
Antifolic acid compounds	0	0	+ +	+	+ + +	0	0
6-Mercaptopurine	+	0	+ + +	+ +	+ + +	0	0
Prednisone et al.	0	+ +	0	0	+ + + +	+	+

(From M. M. Wintrobe in T. R. Harrison (Ed.): *Principles of Internal Medicine,* 5th ed. New York: McGraw-Hill Book Company, 1966.)

TABLE 32-2
Relative Value of Different Agents in Treatment of Leukemias and Lymphomas

family can make the decisions regarding how the time remaining will be spent. Sometimes the guideline, "What is the most important thing to do next?" can be helpful. When knowledge about the disease is truthfully and completely given, the persons concerned are better equipped to make decisions and will not be seduced by false claims of those who profess to have found a miraculous cure for leukemia.

Startling changes, such as are evident in remissions, are not as common in chronic leukemia as they may be in the acute form. There is a longer period of life ahead for the person with chronic leukemia, and he may be able to do useful work for several years before weakness and other symptoms force him to stop. This does not mean, however, that the diagnosis of leukemia has any less impact for him.

The physical care given to the gravely ill person will take into account the fact that he has severe anemia and will feel weak, often be chilly, and will tire easily. He will need assistance in personal care and movement; reaching for a glass of water or changing his position in bed may become simply too much effort. When blood transfusions are given it is important that the venepuncture be done skillfully and that especial caution be taken that the needle is not dislodged, as any extravasation of fluid or blood into the tissues can be painful and cause hematomas or tissue breakdown.

The immature white blood cells, even in large numbers, furnish no defense against infection. The patient should have no contact with persons with a cold or other infectious process. Careful hand washing, use of scrupulously clean equipment, and wearing clean gowns over one's uniform are all part of necessary protection. It is important to note any premonitory signs of infection. These signs might include a cough, runny nose, chills, or a small open draining skin lesion.

Since the patient may run a consistent degree of temperature elevation, this cannot always be relied upon as a sign of infection, although a sudden rise is usually indicative.

Observation of all vital signs is important; internal bleeding may be manifested by tachycardia and a fall in blood pressure. Respiratory changes may indicate obstruction from pressure of enlarged lymph nodes on the trachea or bronchi.

The thrombocytopenia makes care with hypodermic and intramuscular injections mandatory. All stools and urine should be observed for the presence of blood; the stool may often consist almost entirely of blood, and the amount should be measured if possible. If the patient is incontinent, a careful estimate should be made. Epistaxis occurs frequently and can be very distressing. Blood clots in the nares should not be removed as this may precipitate further bleeding. Excessive bleeding from any source can of course lead to shock, and accurate reporting of blood loss and vital signs is important to the physican in ordering blood replacement.

The gums will bleed easily and there may be oozing from the oral mucosa. This, often combined with epistaxis, will leave the patient with a constant and disagreeable taste of old blood in his mouth. It also adds to his already considerable anorexia. Development of ulcers about the mouth compounds the discomfort and the problems of eating. Shaving may become unfeasible for men. Problems of mouth care may assume major proportions and become uncommonly distressing. Whatever methods are used in oral care, it is important that the care be frequent and that it be gentle. Dilute hydrogen peroxide (1 percent) is often an effective agent in removing old blood from the mouth, and this may be varied with other mild rinses. Soft cotton applicators can be used to swab the teeth and gums. The patient, if able, may wish to gently "scrub" his teeth with gauze wrapped about his index finger. Various lip creams may be tried depending upon the patient's preference.

Itching and burning of the skin are common in chronic lymphocytic leukemia and infection and bleeding may be induced by involuntary scratching. Fingernails should be kept clean and trimmed; soft cotton gloves may be worn at night, and liberal use of lotions may be helpful.

Any food or fluid the patient desires should be obtained if at all possible. Spiced or very hot foods will usually be intolerable because of the tenderness of the oral mucosa. Such items as carbonated beverages and ice cream are frequently welcome. Most antileukemic drugs are eliminated through the kidney, and oral fluid intake should be encouraged as long as possible.

Mental confusion is often apparent when the patient is terminally ill. He should be protected from falling by use of padded side rails, and if his bed is one that can be raised and lowered to variable heights, it should be kept in "low" position except when up for nursing care. Even minor falls may be a cause of internal or external bleeding.

Although the physical care of the terminally ill patient with leukemia is highly important and frequently taxing, perhaps the nurse's greatest contribution is her effort toward helping the patient die with dignity and not alone. She may gain a measure of satisfaction in knowing that she has done what she could to assure this, and that she has helped in assuring that the family was not excluded from the patient during the last weeks and days of his life.

Multiple Myeloma

Multiple myeloma is an uncommon, painful, and fatal disease involving the bone marrow. The cause is unknown but is generally regarded as a malignant proliferation of plasma cells. It occurs most often in men after the age of 45.

In this disease, multiple tumors of myeloma cells, or abnormal plasma cells, arise in bone marrow. Structures involved include the vertebrae, ribs, cranium, pelvis, and the ends of long bones. Bone destruction and demineralization occur in some way from the process and spontaneous fractures are common. The infiltration of the bone marrow is the probable cause of the accompanying anemia, platelet abnormalities, and leukopenia. The pain experienced may be a dull migratory bone pain, or severe pain from a pathological fracture, or pain in varying severity from frequent muscle spasms.

Plasma proteins are both quantitatively and qualitatively abnormal. Abnormalities in the globulins probably contribute to the decreased resistance to infection. An abnormal protein, called *Bence Jones protein,* is frequently found in the urine.

A hypercalcemia is usually present due to the bone destruction. When this condition is severe it results in nausea, vomiting, and increased weakness, and contributes to kidney stone formation. Altered calcium metabolism may also be related in some way to the problem of muscle spasms because of its influence on neuromuscular irritability.

The course of the disease is distressingly dismal, and medical care at present can be supportive only. Temporary relief of pain has been obtained through irradiation, urethan, corticosteroids, and alkylating agents such as melphalan (Alkeran) and cyclophosphamide (Cytoxan). Blood transfusions are also given as necessary.

It is important in nursing care to assist myeloma patients to maintain activity as long as possible in order to retain independence and prevent increased bone demineralization and hypostatic infections. At the same time, activity may be accompanied by discomfort, muscle spasm, and an increase in the possibility of fractures. The patient will know how he can move with the least discomfort and he will tend to make each movement slowly and cautiously. The nurse's assistance should be as he directs. Turning sheets, fracture bedpans, walkers, and braces are all items of equipment that may be employed in care.

Since the myeloma patient cannot adequately defend himself against infection, visitors and personnel with colds or infections should not come in contact with him. Hypostatic pneumonia easily develops as activities become more restricted and coughing becomes increasingly painful. The possibility of urinary tract infection is decreased by high fluid intake and avoidance of unnecessary catheterization. Adequate fluids also promote calcium excretion.

Analgesics are given as necessary and most physicians will not limit them as the disease progresses. However, anything that the nurse may do to prevent painful muscle spasm and bone pain (gentleness, avoidance of quick movements and jarring, support of extremities when turning) will help decrease early use of potent narcotics which, though they offer relief of pain, may unpleasantly blur cerebral functions.

Agranulocytosis

Agranulocytosis is characterized by an extreme reduction in white blood cells, especially the granulocytes. The most common cause today is the administration of various drugs that depress leukopoiesis.

Many of the offending drugs contain the benzene ring in their structure, as is true of those causing aplastic anemia. Specific drugs known to primarily depress the granulocytes are the cytotoxic drugs, antimetabolites, sulfonamides, streptomycin, thiouracil, and chlorpromazine. Many other drugs may give rise to leukopenia in persons who become sensitized to them.

Another cause may be therapeutic or accidental overexposure to x-rays. Sometimes, an overwhelming infection may so exhaust the defensive processes that a leukopenia results instead of the expected leukocytosis.

The development of agranulocytosis may be heralded by extreme weakness and fatigue, followed by chills, high fever, prostration, and the development of ulcers on the oral mucosa and oropharynx. Especially unfavorable prognostic signs are severe prostration, jaundice, necrotic ulcer, and a leukocyte count below 1,000 per cu mm of blood.

The immediate treatment is of course to withdraw the offending drug when it is known. The person with agranulocytosis lacks one of his principal defenses against infection and may succumb readily to what would normally be a mild infectious process. Gram-positive cocci are common offenders, so penicillin is the antibiotic usually given in large doses in an effort to combat the infection. Measures to prevent infections from reaching the person are a prime nursing responsibility. Scrupulous medical asepsis, as described earlier, must be followed in caring for these patients.

If the condition has not progressed too far before the offending agent is stopped, and if a supervening infection is controlled, the patient will recover. If not, death may occur rapidly from septic bronchopneumonia and exhaustion.

Indiscriminate use of drugs without medical supervision cannot be cautioned against too strongly since in some persons sensitivities readily develop to drugs usually considered innocuous.

Hodgkin's Disease

Hodgkin's disease is one of a group of conditions that affect lymphoid tissue. This disease, along with lymphosarcoma, giant follicular lymphoblastoma (lymphoma), and reticulum cell sarcoma, causes painless, progressive enlargement of the lymph nodes and frequently the spleen; and later, cachexia, anemia, and fever. However, the conditions differ histologically in the mode of onset and in severity.

Hodgkin's disease forms about one-third to one-half of all cases of this group and affects a younger age group. When untreated it is considered to be a fatal disease and fortunately is rare. Perhaps, as one physician states. "The interest in Hodgkin's disease is much greater than its incidence warrants, because of its predominance in young adults. . . ." (Rubin). It is most common in the second and third decades and although more males are affected the proportion of affected females is increasing. The cause continues to be unknown, with the neoplastic and infectious theories being the two most generally accepted.

Cervical lymph node enlargement is usually the first sign, followed by enlargement of axillary and inguinal nodes. These are not painful unless nerves are impinged upon. When mediastinal nodes are enlarged, cough and dyspnea may develop. When the retroperitoneal nodes are the primary ones involved, diagnosis is difficult, since the symptoms may be nonspecific and include fever, loss of weight, and abdominal discomfort.

The technique of lymphangiography, in which a radiopaque iodized oil is injected into the peripheral lymphatics and outlines otherwise visually inaccessible regions, is used by some physicians. Biopsy of accessible lymph nodes will show histologic changes, with the giant Reed-Sternberg cell typically being seen.

The proliferating cells may invade almost any region, e.g., lungs, digestive tract, genitourinary tract, bones, and cause widely different symptoms. Pruritus is common, as is fever with or without chills, loss of weight, splenomegaly, and symptoms of anemia. The classic fever pattern (which is actually uncommon) is known as *Pel-Ebstein fever* and consists of days or weeks of high fever alternating with periods in which there is no fever.

The manifestations of the disease may range from rapid and progressively fatal forms to stable forms that run a chronic course over many years. The survival rate varies greatly, according to the stage of the disease when treatment was begun, but with better diagnosis, the aggressive use of high-voltage radiotherapy in the early stages, and the judicious use of chemotherapy, the outlook has become much brighter, leading some to cautiously use the term *cure* in some instances. However, this is contingent upon early diagnosis and whether the disease is still localized at time of diagnosis. Prognosis in later middle age and beyond is not as good as that in younger patients, probably because in older persons the disease is more widespread.

Irradiation and chemotherapy are the chief agents used in the treatment of Hodgkin's disease and the other conditions of the group. Surgical excision of a single involved lymph node followed by radiotherapy can be, and is, done but the practice is being increasingly supplanted by the use of high-voltage radiotherapy only. When node involvement becomes regional and when there are constitutional symptoms, chemotherapy is usually the method of choice.

Nitrogen mustard is one of the oldest and most useful drugs used in Hodgkin's disease. It is an alkylating agent, destructive to rapidly dividing cells, and in larger doses to normal cells so that dosage is carefully regulated and the patient's blood picture watched closely for any signs of excessive hematopoietic depression. It is administered intravenously, and to prevent thrombosis, is usually injected into the tubing of a normal saline infusion that is already running. The physician may wish to mix the solution himself; rubber gloves should be available for his use in doing this as the drug is highly irritating to skin surfaces. The drug also causes severe nausea and vomiting, probably by direct stimulation of the vomiting center; it is often given in the early evening after the late meal has been withheld, and an antinauseant and sedative are administered so that the patient may sleep through the night and avoid the period of greatest side effects.

Other drugs in use, whose action is similar to that of nitrogen mustard, include triethylenemelamine (TEM), chlorambucil (Leukeran), cyclophosphamide (Cytoxan), and vinblastine sulfate (Velban). The first three may be given orally or intravenously; vinblastine sulfate is given only intravenously. Corticosteroids, though nonspecific in their action, are useful in decreasing the severity of constitutional symptoms. (See Table 32-2.)

Nursing care will take into account the type of treatment being received. Special attention to diet, fluids, use of antinauseants, and control of unpleasant sights, sounds, and odors will help relieve some of the side effects of the chemotherapeutic drugs. The nurse, by careful observation, may also detect early signs of toxicity to these drugs.

When the patient has advanced Hodgkin's disease, he should be watched carefully for any signs of respiratory obstruction; a tracheostomy tray is usually kept in the room. He may have periodic drenching sweats; at this time, prompt tepid sponging and dry linens are welcome. An adequate fluid intake must be encouraged. Occasionally, enlarged lymph nodes may ulcerate and drain, necessitating the use of sterile dressings for both aseptic and aesthetic reasons.

Patients with Hodgkin's disease will often be close to the nurse's own age, in the prime of life, and she may find her own emotional resources taxed in witnessing their struggle with the illness. However, the outlook is not quite so pessimistic as formerly, and advances in diagnosis and treatment may now justify what at least two physicians call a mood of "tempered optimism" (Kaplan and Rosenberg).

Infectious Mononucleosis

Infectious mononucleosis is a relatively common and benign disease seen primarily in young people who spend much of their time within institutions such as high schools, colleges, dormitories, and army camps. Its occurrence in anyone over 35 is rare and it is most frequent in the spring and fall. The disease is a hyperplasia of the reticuloendothelial system and as such gives rise to enlargement of lymphatic glands, spleen, tonsils, and lymphocytosis with abnormal lymphocytes. Because reticuloendothelial tissue is so widespread, individual patients may show much clinical variation and sometimes obscure and puzzling features.

It is sometimes euphemistically called *kissing disease* as well as *students' disease,* since it is commonly believed to be transmitted by kissing or by immediately eating or drinking from a utensil just used by someone with the disease. The causative agent has not been isolated, but it is believed to be a virus. The incubation period has been variously estimated at from 5 days to 6 weeks.

The usual pattern of the disorder consists of a period of malaise and sleepiness (often attributed to curricular or extracurricular causes), followed in 3 to 5 days by complaints of sore throat and fever. Examination of the throat will show a process varying from simple hyperemia to an exudative tonsillitis. If the posterior cervical lymph nodes are enlarged, the diagnosis of mononucleosis is almost a certainty (Hoagland). Enlargement of the anterior cervical lymph nodes is not significant, since this occurs with many types of mouth lesions.

Some patients (about 10 percent) have a painless jaundice with fever. Mild hepatitis occurs from inflammation of the reticuloendothelial cells of the liver; the resulting jaundice usually clears in 2 to 3 weeks.

Two laboratory tests are important: the differential leukocyte count and the heterophil antibody reaction. The differential count will show an increase in mononuclear cells, with about 10 percent of these being atypical. The total white blood cell count is usually 10,000 to 20,000 per cu mm of blood, of which 50 to 70 percent will be lymphocytes. A positive heterophil antibody reaction is required for diagnosis, but in itself is not diagnostic since it is positive in some other diseases. The test is based on Paul and Bunnell's discovery in 1932 that the serum of patients with infectious mononucleosis contains antibodies that agglutinate sheep erythrocytes.

The treatment is usually symptomatic, although corticosteroids given in small amounts and for a short time are employed by some physicians. If the infrequent complication of hemolytic anemia occurs, corticosteroids are routinely used. Penicillin is given if pharyngeal infection is present.

Patients will rarely object to bedrest, since the lassitude and fatigue will make any effort difficult. The length of bedrest will vary with the severity of the illness. Nursing care will be predicated upon the degree of fatigue and weakness, and in addition may include helping the patient with warm saline throat irrigations and administering analgesics such as codeine if necessary. Isolation is not necessary, since mononucleosis is not an air-borne infection. Dishes can be handled in the usual way.

The rate of recovery varies according to the individual and the severity of the disease. Convalescence is sometimes prolonged, but a gradual increase in physical activity can usually be started when the temperature has remained normal for several days. Relapses are said to occur in about 6 percent of cases, but complete recovery is the rule. Complications are rare but have included rupture of the spleen.

Splenic Disorders

Splenic injuries are fairly common, especially in this "age of the automobile." Physicians consider the possibility of *splenic rupture* in most automobile accidents, particularly when the abdomen or left thorax is involved. The rupture may occur at the time of impact or at any time from 1 to 30 days afterward. The later time of rupture may be due to a progressive increase in size of a subcapsular hematoma.

The symptoms of splenic rupture are those of blood loss into the peritoneal cavity causing weakness, abdominal pain and muscle spasm, and diminished abdominal breathing. It is often difficult to tell, after an accident, whether a splenic rupture has been the cause of shock and pain, or whether the other injuries are the cause.

Rupture may also occur spontaneously without any history of trauma. It has been reported to occur with malaria, typhoid fever, lymphomas, and infectious mononucleosis.

An x-ray study will usually confirm the clinical diagnosis, and if a peritoneal tap is bloody, further evidence is afforded. An immediate splenectomy is performed after the diagnosis.

HYPERSPLENISM

Hypersplenism, or splenic overactivity, is thought to be the cause of depression of one or more formed elements of the blood. As indicated earlier, it is not known whether the spleen acts directly on certain elements or affects bone marrow productivity. If platelets are depressed, idiopathic thrombocytopenic purpura results; if the red cells are affected, hemolytic anemia results; and if the white blood cells are affected, a splenic neutropenia results.

SPLENOMEGALY

Splenomegaly accompanies many diseases, notably malaria, typhoid fever, chronic leukemias, Hodgkin's disease, and lymphosarcoma. Banti's disease is a syndrome resulting from vascular congestion of the spleen; in addition to splenic enlargement there is also anemia, leukopenia, and a tendency to gastric hemorrhage.

OTHER DISORDERS

It is not necessary for the nurse to know about all the uncommon disorders of the spleen. However, what is important is her prompt recognition of symptoms that can spell a surgical emergency, i.e., sudden agonizing abdominal or left scapular pain, with signs of impending shock. These may well mean a splenic rupture, and the patient will be taken almost immediately to surgery. A whole blood or plasma infusion may be started before the patient leaves his room. The patient will be exceedingly apprehensive if such an emergency occurs, and as in all such situations, should not be left alone.

Bibliography

Atamer, M. A.: *Blood Diseases.* New York: Grune & Stratton, Inc., 1963.

Beland, Irene L.: *Clinical Nursing,* 2d ed. New York: The Macmillan Company, 1970.

Burchenal, Joseph H.: Chemotherapy and Radiotherapy—Competitors or Partners? *Cancer* 22:790–795, October, 1968.

Dameshek, William and Frederick Gunz: *Leukemia,* 2d ed. London: Grune & Stratton, Inc., 1964.

Desforges, Jane F. and May Y. F. W. Wang: Sickle Cell Anemia. *Medical Clinics of North America,* 50:1519–1532, November, 1966.

Finkel, Harvey E., et al.: Current Concepts in the Therapy of Multiple

Myeloma. *Medical Clinics of North America,* 50:1569–1590, November, 1966.

Ganong, William F.: *Review of Medical Physiology,* 4th ed. Los Altos, California: Lange Medical Publications, 1969.

Gilbert, Harriet S.: Problems Relating to Control of Polycythemia Vera: The Use of Alkylating Agents. *Blood,* 32:500–505, September, 1968.

Guyton, Arthur C.: *Textbook of Medical Physiology,* 3d ed. Philadelphia: W. B. Saunders Company, 1966.

Harrison, T. R. (Ed.): *Principles of Internal Medicine,* 5th ed. New York: McGraw-Hill Book Company, 1966.

Hatch, F. E. and L. W. Diggs: Fluid Balance in Sickle-Cell Disease, *Archives of Internal Medicine,* 116:10–17, July, 1965.

Hoagland, Robert: Infectious Mononucleosis. *American Journal of Nursing,* 64:125–127, October, 1964.

Kaplan, Henry S. and Saul A. Rosenberg: The Treatment of Hodgkin's Disease. *Medical Clinics of North America,* 50:1591–1610, November, 1966.

Livingston, Barbara M.: How Clinical Progress Is Made in Cancer Chemotherapy Research. *American Journal of Nursing,* 67:2547–2554, December, 1967.

Lyman, Margaret and Joseph Burchenal: Acute Leukemia. *American Journal of Nursing,* 63:82–86, April, 1963.

Mann, W. N. (Ed.): *Conybeare's Textbook of Medicine.* Edinburgh: E. and S. Livingstone, Ltd., 1964.

McKinnie, Carol: Multiple Myeloma. *American Journal of Nursing,* 63:99–120, June, 1963.

Miale, John B.: *Laboratory Medicine Hematology,* 3d ed. St. Louis: The C. V. Mosby Company, 1967.

Miller, Robert: The Role of Epidemiology in the Etiology of Leukemia. *CA,* 14:130–134, July-August, 1964.

O'Kell, Richard: Understanding the Hemophilias—A,B, and C. *American Journal of Nursing,* 62:101–102, June, 1962.

Osgood, Edwin E.: Treatment of Chronic Leukemia. *Journal of Nuclear Medicine,* 5:139–153, February, 1964.

Page, Lot and Perry Culver (Eds.): *A Syllabus of Laboratory Examinations in Clinical Diagnosis.* Cambridge: Harvard University Press, 1960.

Petrakis, Nicholas: The Leukemias. *California Medicine,* 101:33–41, July, 1964.

Roxburgh, R. A.: Splenectomy and the Indications for It. *Nursing Times,* 64:1227–1229, September 13, 1968.

Rubin, Philip: Hodgkin's Disease. *Journal of American Medical Association,* 190:910, December 7, 1964.

Smith, Dorothy and Claudia Gips: *Care of the Adult Patient,* 2d ed. Philadelphia: J. B. Lippincott Company, 1966.

Wasserman, Louis and Harriet S. Gilbert: The Treatment of Polycythemia Vera. *Medical Clinics of North America,* 50:1501–1518, November, 1966.

Weinstein, Irwin and Ernest Beutler (Eds.): *Mechanisms of Anemia.* New York: McGraw-Hill Book Company, 1962.

Wintrobe, Maxwell: *Clinical Hematology,* 6th ed. Philadelphia: Lea & Febiger, 1967.

CHAPTER 33
NURSING IN URGENT SITUATIONS

ARLENE M. PUTT

What Is an Emergency? A Disaster?

By dictionary definition an emergency is an unforeseen occurrence or a sudden urgent occasion, an exigency or pressing situation making a demand for action or aid. A disaster is defined as a mischance or possibly fatal mishap or calamity, either manmade or naturally occurring. By American Red Cross definition, a disaster exists in a situation in which five or more families are rendered helpless, suffering, or in need of medical care, food, shelter, clothing, or other necessities of life.

Emergencies occur at all times and in all places. Natural disasters, such as tornadoes, hurricanes, floods, major wrecks, or fires, occur in the United States at the rate of approximately 200 to 300 per year, although in some years, the number and the severity of natural disasters are far greater than in others.

According to the National Safety Council, in 1966 there were 113,000 deaths from accidents, an increase of 5 percent over 1965. In 1966 accidents caused disabling injuries to 10,800,000 individuals. Motor vehicles caused 53,000 deaths in the same year, and work-related deaths were 14,500, with 2,200,000 disabling injuries. Fires killed 7,900 persons, and firearms killed 2,600 persons. All these figures represent increases over previous years. At the same time, the National Safety Council points out that the accidental death rate per 100,000 population has fallen from 89 in 1912 to 58 in 1966. Thus accident prevention and improved medical care account for a saving of 1,200,000 lives.

Reactions to Emergencies

Reactions to emergencies and disasters differ among individuals and in the same individual according to the given circumstances. The reactions may be as follows:

1. A normal response in which the individual displays some sign of disturbance but promptly regains self-control.

2. Individual panic, which may be expressed in flight uncontrolled by reason. A contagious reaction, individual panic can spread rapidly to others, thus magnifying problems and creating further damage. A panicky person must be restrained away from the group for his own protection and the protection of others.

3. Depression to the point of mental numbness in which the individual cannot initiate action on his own. Firm positive direction and even physical guidance may be necessary to overcome the response.

4. Hysteria manifested by overaction with poor or little direction, the individual being unable to concentrate or to focus on any activity. A calm approach with positive direction from another individual can help redirect diffuse activity to purposeful behavior.

5. Disturbances of body function evident by at least one sign or symptom such as nausea, vomiting, diarrhea, or hyperventilation. Removing the patient to quiet surroundings may help reduce the hyperfunctioning.

Certain principles of mental health are useful and may help the nurse in coping with the reactions described. They are as follows:

1. Every person has a right to his own feelings. He needs opportunities to ex-

press his feelings and to have someone listen attentively without censuring him. Expression of emotions is basic to the maintenance of emotional and physical equilibrium.

2. Recognize limitations imposed by casualties as real limitations. Only as a person recognizes and works through his own feelings is he able to focus objectively on the feelings of others. Also, only as an individual achieves satisfaction in his basic needs, such as safety, is he free to function on a higher level.

3. Utilize the potentialities of others. Set the pace with your own calm reassurance and sense of direction. The climate thus created will assist others to return to normal functioning as promptly as possible. Growth in mental health occurs when an individual moves through a positive experience rather than bypasses or withdraws from it.

4. Recognize one's own limitations and utilize the skills of other persons to complement one's own abilities. An individual grows through the realistic evaluation of his personal capabilities with acceptance of his own limitations.

Principles Useful in All Emergencies

Practice and foresight do much to increase the effectiveness of most individuals when confronted with urgent situations. Foresight eliminates fear of the unknown, which is frequently expressed by the question, "What will I do?" Planning gives opportunities for practice or at least thought as to what action would be appropriate. When faced with urgent and chaotic situations, individuals tend to call upon previous thinking, because the time for lengthy rationalization is not then available. A preconceived plan may be put into action immediately with minor changes.

Following are a number of principles that are useful in all emergencies.

1. Reassure the patient by your own calmness and by explaining what can be done to control the situation.

2. Prevent further injury. Do not move the victim unless his life is endangered where he is lying.

3. Examine and evaluate the patient's injuries, giving priority to the most urgent needs. These are listed in order of need:

    a. Maintain a patent airway and adequate ventilation of the lungs.

    b. Control bleeding and maintain heart function.

    c. If intestines are exposed, keep area covered and moist.

    d. Keep patient lying at rest and moderately warm.

    e. Splint fractures as they lie, immobilizing the joint above and the joint below. If vertebrae are injured, *do not* bend, extend, or twist the spinal column. If uncertain whether the back and spinal column are injured, assume they may be.

4. Transport the patient carefully to a hospital, maintaining appropriate measures en route, or call a qualified agency to transport him.

Emergency Techniques

Knowledge of how to maintain body function and how to prevent further damage to the body is needed.

MAINTENANCE OF RESPIRATION

The techniques for maintaining respiration in the order they should be used:

1. Clear the mouth of debris and obstructions.
2. Ensure gravity drainage of the respiratory tract.
3. Hold the jaw forward or insert S-shaped plastic airway, called S *tube.*
4. Suction patient. Use your mouth if no suction equipment is available.
5. If the patient ceases to breathe, only 4 minutes are available before permanent brain damage occurs, so mouth-to-mouth resuscitation must be started immediately. *Procedure:*
   a. Clear mouth of obstructions.
   b. Hyperextend head.
   c. Lift neck and hyperextend head and raise jaw by pushing forward.
   d. Pinch nose closed with your fingers and maintain.
   e. Seal your mouth over patient's mouth.
   f. Exhale into patient until his chest starts to rise. Your exhaled air still contains approximately 16 percent oxygen, since only 4 percent of oxygen is extracted by the lungs during one respiration.
   g. When patient's chest starts to rise, stop exhalation into patient, release your mouth, and permit patient's chest to fall.
   h. Repeat procedure 12 to 20 times per minute until patient resumes his own respirations or until he is declared dead.
   Mouth-to-mouth resuscitation is the most practical method of manual oxygenation.
6. If the patient's larynx is obstructed a cricothyroidotomy is required. *Procedure:*
   a. Place patient on his back with his head and neck straight and hyperextended.
   b. Locate the niche just below the thyroid cartilage (Adam's apple) and above the cricoid cartilage.
   c. Make a small incision over the niche and through the skin only.
   d. Check location of the area between the two cartilages. At this point only a thin membrane covers the trachea.
   e. Puncture the membrane, thus creating an opening into the trachea.
   f. Maintain the opening with a hollow object or a wedge.
   g. Transport patient to a hospital, where standard tracheotomy will have to be performed.
   If maintained for a short period only, cricothyroidotomy will not endanger the larynx.

MAINTENANCE OF CIRCULATION

Techniques for maintaining circulation are as follows:

1. Control bleeding. *Procedure:*
   a. Apply a pad or dressing over the wound and hold it in place by firm pressure or bandage.
   b. Apply firm pressure over the artery proximal to the wound. Pressure points are shown in Table 33–1.
   c. Elevate the bleeding part.

ARTERY	LOCATION	AREA OF BLEEDING CONTROLLED
Carotid	Lateral neck	Face and head
Facial	Angle of jaw	Nose and mouth
Temporal	Anterior to upper ear	Scalp
Subclavian	Clavicosternal junction	Shoulder and arm
Brachial	Medial aspect of upper arm	Forearm
Femoral	Midgroin	Entire leg
Popliteal	Posterior aspect of knee	Lower leg

TABLE 33-1
Pressure Points

d. As a last resort, apply a tourniquet proximal to the wound tightly enough to occlude the pulse. Continue to maintain pressure over the wound. The tourniquet must be applied with great caution, since a limb may be lost if it is maintained for too long a time. Once a tourniquet is applied, usually it is not removed until definitive care is immediately available.

e. Treat patient for shock by keeping him quiet and warm enough to prevent shivering, which would increase the need for oxygen and the metabolic rate. Excessive warmth will cause peripheral vasodilatation, which is undesirable for a patient in shock.

f. Transport patient to a hospital promptly.

2. Administer external cardiac compression in cardiac arrest. *Procedure:*

If cardiac arrest is of less than 5 minutes' duration or if the period is unknown—

a. Place patient on a firm surface, such as the floor, and hyperextend his head.

b. Place heels of the palms one on top of the other over the *lower* half of the sternum, avoiding the xiphoid process. Keep your fingers up and off the patient.

c. Push firmly and release, repeating up to 60 times per minute.

d. This procedure must be done along with mouth-to-mouth resuscitation without interruption. If both measures are being done by one person, then the cardiac compression must be interrupted long enough to inflate the lungs twice after every 15 compressions. It is much easier and more effective to have two persons, one performing cardiac compression, the other, resuscitation. They coordinate their actions to achieve the ratio of five cardiac compressions to one ventilation interjected between compressions. It is important that compression and ventilation be continued without interruptions of more than 5 seconds.

e. When the heart beat is restored, the heart will probably fibrillate; therefore, cardiac compression must be continued until the patient is transported to a hospital where an external defibrillator bearing 400 watt seconds is available.

f. These measures are continued until the patient resumes normal function or he is declared dead.

The hazards of external cardiac compression are several. Ribs may be fractured leading to a flail chest. This is especially true in infants and small children and debilitated adults. To prevent fracture of ribs, the fingers are kept up and off the chest, with only the heel of the palm used. In the average adult, compression at the lower half of the sternum causes only bending of the costosternal cartilages, with possible dislocation of a cartilage which is not serious. If pressure is exerted too high on the sternum, the sternum cannot move without spontaneously fracturing. Therefore, pressure should be applied to the lower half of the sternum.

Pressure over the xiphoid process can cause laceration of the liver. Too much pressure can cause rupture of the heart, damage to lungs, intercostal hemorrhage, bone marrow emboli, and, especially in small children, liver hematoma. Hemopericardium and hemothorax are very rare. *The likelihood of complications secondary to properly applied external heart-lung resuscitation is minimal and acceptable in comparison with the alternative of death.*[1]

The above procedures are the responsibility of the physician, but if no physician is available, the nurse must be prepared to begin or continue cardiopulmonary support.[2]

HLRU, or Heart Lung Rescue Unit, is a portable device that accomplishes both resuscitation and ventilation when connected to a tank of oxygen or compressed air. It is useful in children 12 years of age and older. HLRU facilitates rescue methods while the patient is being transported and conserves the energy of the rescue workers.

If need for HLRU arises in the hospital setting, the nurse then has the responsibility for procuring the necessary equipment: emergency cardiac drug tray including epinephrine, 1:1,000; electrocardiograph; external defibrillator with 400 watt seconds discharge; laryngoscope with endotracheal tubes; venous cutdown tray; suction equipment and aspiration catheters; dependable oxygen source; tracheostomy set; and mask and bag for manual ventilation.

Splinting and Transportation

The nurse should understand the techniques of splinting and transportation. More harm probably is done through improper transportation of the injured person than through any other measure of emergency assistance. The danger of causing paralysis or death by improperly moving the patient with head, neck, and back injuries is considerable. Therefore, the nurse should not be in a hurry to move an injured person unless his life is immediately imperiled where he is. To assess the degree of injury and damage, the patient is asked to move each extremity, and to squeeze both of the nurse's hands simultaneously, thus testing for mobility and equality of strength of the grip. Each pupil should be checked for size and prompt reaction to strong light. Unequal or fixed dilated or sluggishly responding pupils indicate severe trauma to the brain.

Fractures of the extremities should be splinted in the position in which they occur. By tying the extremity to a straight firm object, the joint above and the joint below the fracture are also immobilized. Because the extent of injury to the back, neck, and head cannot always be ascertained, it should be assumed that injuries exist. The cardinal principle to remember is that damage to the spinal cord is increased by flexion, extension, and twisting of the spinal column. Therefore the head, neck, and spine must be kept absolutely straight and supported evenly along the patient's entire length.

For transportation to a hospital the patient is very gently and carefully lifted onto a firm surface, his entire body being evenly aligned, with the coordinated

[1] Heart Association of Maryland.
[2] *Ibid.*

lifting of three or more persons, thereby providing firm support for the entire length of his body. When on a firm surface, the patient needs to be secured against sliding or rolling. Safety belts can be used for this purpose.

Common Threats to Body Function

THREATS TO CARDIOPULMONARY FUNCTION

The greatest threats to the body are those that impair cardiopulmonary function. These have been divided into threats to respiration and threats to circulation. It is understood that because of the interdependence of these two systems, some factors threaten both respiration and circulation.

Threats to Respiration

A nonpatent airway means that the patient is unable to exchange air because of mechanical obstruction of the respiratory tree. The most common cause of respiratory obstruction is sagging of the tongue, which occurs when the patient is lying flat on his back and is unconscious. In this position, the jaw falls backward and the base of the tongue occludes the pharynx. To prevent this, the jaw must be maintained in a forward position. Turning the head to the side or turning the patient on his side may assist in clearing the airway, but to ensure full patency, a plastic airway should be inserted. Unless the jaw is securely maintained in the forward position, the air passageways are partially occluded. (See Figure 33–1.)

Foreign bodies in the mouth are easily aspirated and are frequently lodged at the level of the larynx. A sharp slap on the back may force the obstacle to be expectorated. Inverting the patient so that gravity can assist with ejection is frequently adequate treatment. Attempts to remove the object by using one's fingers may succeed only in wedging the object more tightly. If the airway is partially obstructed, a loud crowing sound, called *stridor,* is heard. Because of developing edema around the foreign object, the partial obstruction tends to increase and a cricothyroidotomy may be required to prevent asphyxiation.

Edema of the larynx is also a common allergic response manifested by swelling, developing stridor, and progressive dyspnea. Epinephrine, 1:1,000, 0.5 ml injected subcutaneously may afford relief or, again, a cricothyroidotomy may be needed.

Asphyxia, or suffocation, occurs when substances other than air are inhaled. In drowning, the victim aspirates water instead of air, loses consciousness, and sinks. When the victim is hauled from the water, his mouth should be cleared of debris and his chest raised higher than his head to allow gravity drainage of some water from the dead air spaces of the respiratory tract. Mouth-to-mouth resuscitation must be initiated and continued until the patient responds or is declared dead.

If the source of asphyxia is noxious fumes from a fire or carbon monoxide from a gasoline motor, the patient should be moved outdoors immediately and mouth-to-mouth resuscitation begun and continued until a mechanical resuscitator with

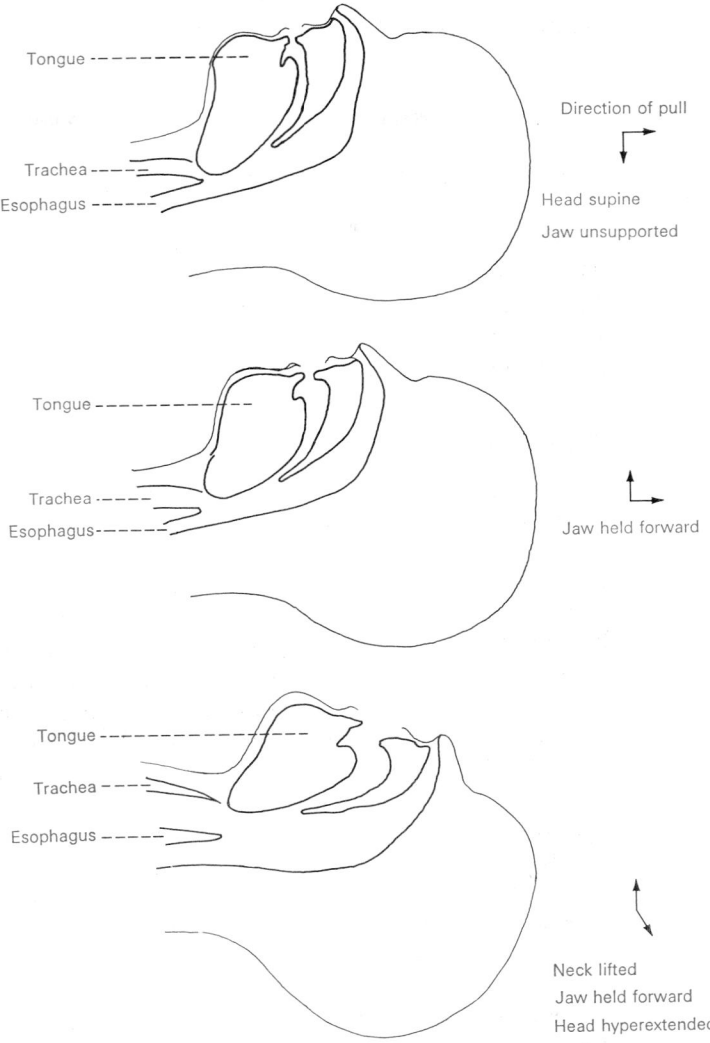

Tongue

Direction of pull

Head supine
Jaw unsupported

Trachea
Esophagus

Tongue

Jaw held forward

Trachea
Esophagus

Tongue

Trachea

Esophagus

Neck lifted
Jaw held forward
Head hyperextended

Figure 33–1
Effects of position on
patency of airway.

oxygen is available. Carbon monoxide combines firmly with hemoglobin, preventing subsequent union with oxygen and necessitating prolonged supportive measures.

Anaphylactoid shock is the rapid development of vasodilatation and urticaria with bronchospasm manifesting hypersensitivity to an antigen such as food, drugs, pollen, or insect sting. Laryngeal obstruction frequently results from laryngeal edema, leading to restlessness, coughing, choking, cyanosis, and unconsciousness unless the obstruction is relieved promptly. Severe gastrointestinal symptoms may appear also.

There is no time to lose if anaphylactoid shock is to be treated effectively and the patient is to survive. Epinephrine, 1:1,000, 0.5 ml is given subcutaneously at once; the dose may have to be repeated at less frequent intervals for continuing

*Figure 33–2
Location of cricothyroid-
otomy and external
cardiac compression.
(Adapted with per-
mission from Robert F.
Mahoney: Emergency
and Disaster Nursing.
New York: The
Macmillan Company,
1965. Copyright ©
Robert Francis
Mahoney, 1965.)*

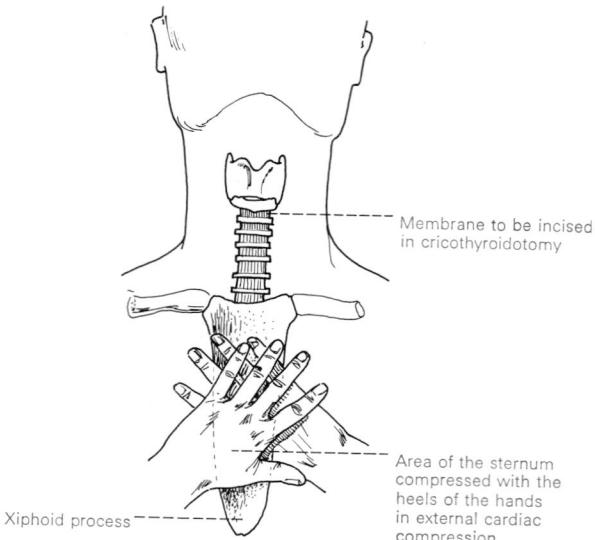

Membrane to be incised
in cricothyroidotomy

Area of the sternum
compressed with the
heels of the hands
in external cardiac
compression

Xiphoid process

relief. If the source of the antigen was an insect sting on the extremities, then a tourniquet placed proximal to the sting may help retard absorption of the antigen by restricting venous return. If laryngeal edema results in a severe reduction in ventilation, then a cricothyroidotomy must be performed to bypass the occluded larynx. Closed chest cardiac compression is initiated if cardiac arrest develops. Hospital care should be sought immediately for treatment of anaphylactoid shock.

To prevent anaphylactoid shock, the patient should either avoid substances to which he knows he is allergic or try to accomplish hyposensitization through a carefully planned program in which minute amounts of highly diluted antigen are injected periodically. The patient also is advised to carry syringettes of epinephrine and an identifying medical tag on his person at all times.

Poisoning can result from many substances, but concern here is with those substances that pose a threat to respiration. The most frequent problem in this respect is overdose of barbiturates, and less frequently, overdose of curare drugs, or poisonous snake bites. An overdose of barbiturates produces slow shallow respirations so that an adequate supply of oxygen to the brain cannot be maintained. Curare paralyzes the muscles of respiration, as may large amounts of certain venoms such as those of pit vipers.

Respiratory poisoning must be treated at once by means of positive pressure oxygen and the specific antidote, if the cause is known. Supportive measures may need to be continued for a period of time; hospital care should be sought.

A sucking wound of the chest (open pneumothorax) is one in which an opening extends from the outside through the chest wall into the chest cavity, producing the characteristic sucking sound on inspiration. Air enters through the opening from the outside into the pleural space, between the lung and chest wall. The lung collapses on the affected side and the function of the opposite lung is also impaired. Shock may supervene requiring immediate treatment. The wound should be covered with petrolatum gauze and a pressure dressing applied. Tight closure should be maintained until the patient is removed to a hospital for further treatment. If oxygen is available it should be administered to alleviate difficulty in breathing.

A flail chest is caused by parallel fractures of the ribs in which the fractured ribs move in paradoxical or reverse movement on respiration. Prompt, but usually not urgent, treatment is required. The fractured ribs are strapped with adhesive tape so that normal movement can take place. The patient should be moved to a hospital for further treatment.

The inspiratory wheezing characteristic of asthma is due to constriction of the bronchiolar musculature which makes breathing exhausting and difficult. Rarely, the condition becomes life-threatening. The nurse should reassure the patient that he will be able to get his breath and that she will help him, by positioning him in a forward-leaning position with his arms supported, and by giving him broncho-dilating medications, as ordered by a physician, such as epinephrine, 1:1,000, 0.3 to 0.5 mg subcutaneously, or aminophylline intravenously, rectally, or by inhalation. Only if the patient is cyanotic or the attack prolonged or exceptionally severe should oxygen be used, because he may come to look upon oxygen as a psychological crutch.

Pulmonary edema develops when the heart is unable to maintain adequate circulation as a result of either inherent weakness or overloading of the circulatory volume. The pulse is bounding, generalized venous distention develops, there is marked dyspnea, and rales and rhonchi appear with pulmonary congestion. The alveoli fill with fluid, which pours from the capillaries, and gaseous exchange is reduced sharply. Immediate medical attention is required. Rotating tourniquets applied to three extremities aid pooling of blood in the arms and legs, thus relieving the burden on the heart. A phlebotomy of 200 to 500 ml further reduces the cardiac burden. The sitting position aids pooling of blood in the lower extremities, and digitalis drugs increase cardiac contractility. Morphine or an allied drug may be ordered by the physician to depress respiration. Positive pressure oxygen forces the fluid back across the alveoli, allowing the membrane to resume function in gas exchange. Treatment is continued until a state of cardiac compensation is reached and then is tapered off slowly.

In convulsions, the muscles of respiration may go into spasm and become paralyzed. The causes of convulsion include epilepsy, high fever, drugs, and cerebral irritation. The patient needs to be protected against self-injury from falling or biting his tongue. He should be closely observed for signs of respiratory embarrassment from either aspiration of vomitus or pulmonary paralysis. Suctioning the gastric contents can eliminate the aspiration hazard. Resuscitation may be required to relieve respiratory paralysis.

Threats to Circulation

Threats to circulation result from three sources: inadequate blood volume, disturbances in the cardiac pumping mechanism, and vasodilatation.

Inadequate blood volume may be caused by blood or fluid loss which may be either external or internal, trauma, burns, rupture of blood vessels (e.g., esophageal varices), or a clotting deficiency (e.g., blood dyscrasias or allergy to pit viper venom). The loss of blood or fluid may be grossly evident, or it may be manifested by a rapid pulse of weak amplitude, restlessness, hematemesis or melena, distention of the abdomen, and pallor. The urgency of treatment depends upon the severity and rapidity of loss. Treatment consists of identifying the source of loss and controlling it by means of externally applied pressure and fluid replacement until definitive measures can be instituted.

Interference with the cardiac pumping function may result from (1) impaired coronary circulation from myocardial infarction, (2) impaired conduction of impulses as in heart block, (3) inadequate force of contraction as in congestive failure or fibrillation, (4) aberrant blood flow as in congenital defects, or (5) cardiac arrest.

With coronary insufficiency with or without myocardial infarction, the patient frequently has angina and may complain of "indigestion" or a crushing or heavy sensation in the chest. In infarction, the signs of shock appear and the patient becomes apprehensive. There is an urgent need to put the patient at complete rest in a low Fowler's position. Tight clothing should be loosened, vasodilators given if ordered by a physician, and oxygen administered if possible. Reassurance of the patient and family, and hospital care to permit evaluation of the problem, are needed.

With impaired impulse conduction, the pulse may be variously rapid or slow,

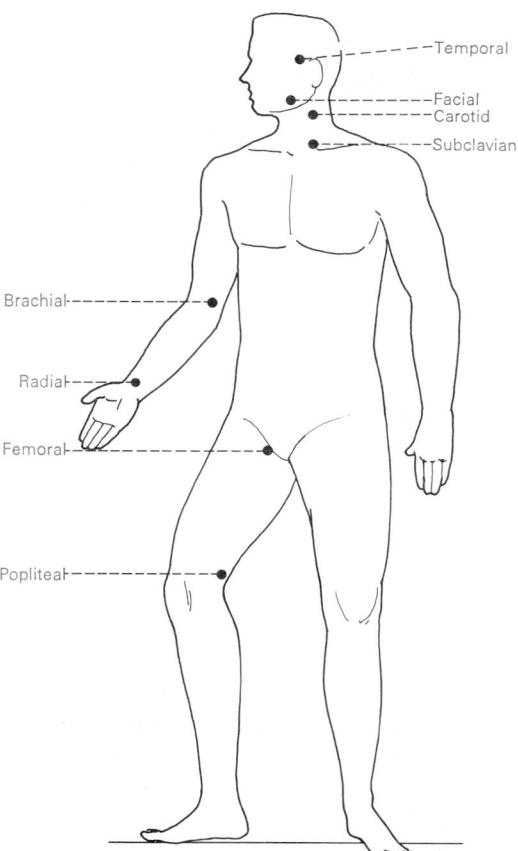

*Figure 33–3
Pressure points for
control of arterial
bleeding.*

regular or irregular. Close observation of the rate and rhythm of the pulse is important, since sudden alterations may necessitate urgent changes in treatment. Complete bed rest is indicated. The physician may prescribe a specific drug, such as isoproterenol, or use of a pacemaker.

Inadequate force of contraction of the heart as in congestive failure or fibrillation results in a reduced supply of blood to nourish the tissues. The venous system becomes engorged and pulmonary congestion may also develop. If the problem suddenly increases in severity urgent treatment is necessary; otherwise there is more time available to aid the patient. Treatment is directed at resting the heart through administration of cardiotonic drugs, which increase the force of contraction and slow the rate, until a state of compensation is reached. Oxygen is administered to increase tissue oxygenation.

Aberrant blood flow due to congenital defects cannot be treated with first aid measures other than positioning and administering oxygen. Cardiac surgery is necessary to correct the condition.

Cardiac arrest has been discussed previously.

The third threat to the integrity of the body's circulation is extreme vasodilatation and loss of vasomotor control, as is found in adrenal insufficiency, anaphylactoid shock, and heat exhaustion.

The threat of acute adrenal insufficiency must be considered whenever prolonged or severe stress is imposed upon a patient who has received or is receiving systemic steroid therapy and in the patient with impaired adrenal function resulting from disease, surgery, or previous prolonged use of steroids. The developing insufficiency produces signs of dehydration and sodium loss, vasodilatation with falling blood pressure and decreasing pulse pressure, weakness, lassitude, apathy, gastrointestinal disturbances, and possibly high fever. Intravenous administration of glucocorticoids and saline fluids must be carried out immediately. The patient must be observed very closely, since the condition may become critical abruptly.

Anaphylactoid shock has been discussed under threats to respiration.

Heat exhaustion results from a combination of dehydration and sodium loss. High temperature, weakness, and weak rapid pulse are evident. Urgent treatment is called for. The patient should be removed to a cool environment and fluids, salt, and vasoconstrictors administered to increase blood volume.

THREAT OF CEREBRAL DAMAGE

The threat of cerebral damage can result from several sources, such as closed head injuries causing increasing intracranial pressure, high fever, open skull fractures, and anoxia. The signs of increasing intracranial pressure are slowed pulse, rising systolic pressure and pulse pressure, deep stertorous respirations, possible unilateral pupillary dilatation, and progressive unconsciousness. Finally the pupils are bilaterally dilated and fixed, the blood pressure falls moderately, and the pulse is rapid and irregular. Cheyne-Stokes respirations appear and the temperature is highly elevated. Observation should include the degree of headache and whether or not it is intensified with movement or straining, and the development of projectile vomiting. Changes in consciousness vary from alertness to stupor to coma. Treatment may be urgent or expectant, according to the individual situation.

The aims of therapy are to reduce the rate of metabolism by cooling the patient and to reduce the intracranial pressure by removing fluid and thus reducing the cerebral edema. The patient needs to be kept quiet and under very close observation. Convulsions may occur and all supplies and equipment necessary for treatment, including padded tongue blades and bed side rails, should be in readiness. Resuscitation may be necessary. After the patient has been moved to a hospital, increased intracranial pressure may be reduced by trephination.

THREATS TO LOCOMOTION

Threats to locomotion arise from injuries to bones, ligaments, or muscle, or their innervation. The simplest sort of impairment is a sprain, in which a ligament or joint capsule is damaged. Sprains can be painful and disabling. Therapy, which is nonurgent, involves limitation of motion and limitation of weight-bearing. Efforts are made to reduce the swelling and provide support to the sprained tissue.

Dislocation occurs when the articulating surfaces of ball and socket or hinge joint are pulled or pushed out of normal alignment. The surrounding tissue may be damaged, and the joint immediately becomes nonfunctional and painful. Treatment is urgent and should be carried out in a hospital, since anesthesia may be required in reducing the dislocation. Support to the injured area should be provided and the patient moved to a hospital. It is important to keep in mind that efforts to reduce the dislocation should be carried out by qualified personnel only.

The severity of fracture varies depending on the location, the extent of injury to bone and surrounding tissue, and whether or not the skin is intact. Fracture is suggested by pain, dysfunction, and abnormal contour, but occasionally diagnosis is possible only through x-ray examination. Usually fractures result from gross trauma, but spontaneous fracture can occur in osteoporosis. Unless there is associated injury to nerves and blood vessels resulting in hemorrhage or loss of sensation, treatment is not urgent. The part should be immobilized without disturbing the fracture, and the patient moved to a hospital.

Spinal cord injuries resulting from pinching or severing of the spinal cord present an immediate threat of permanent impairment to locomotion. Numbness and paralysis develop, and the need for skillful definitive attention is very urgent. Nonetheless, the patient must be moved *only* by an adequate number of skilled attendants and moved with extreme caution to prevent further injury or possible permanent paralysis. The technique for moving patients with spinal cord injuries was outlined early in the chapter. The physician may order that the spinal column be hyperextended in efforts to prevent further pinching, and this is accomplished by means of traction. Traction must be supervised by the physician, and cannot be discontinued except upon his orders.

THREATS TO SKIN AND SUBCUTANEOUS TISSUE

Threats to the skin and subcutaneous tissue are imposed by trauma resulting in abrasions, lacerations, burns, frostbite, or irritation from poisonous contactants.

Abrasion involves the epidermis and sometimes the dermis. While the area becomes painful and subject to superficial infection, urgent treatment is not needed. Simply cleansing with soap or a hexachlorophene solution such as pHisoHex, followed by air drying or a simple dry sterile dressing, is all that is needed.

Laceration involves the muscles, tendons, blood vessels, and nerves. If tendons or blood vessels are lacerated the urgency of treatment is increased. Medical attention usually is promptly sought if bleeding is profuse, although the severity of bleeding is not a reliable indicator of the severity of injury. If tendons have been severed prompt meticulous repair is necessary to prevent disability. The lacerated area must be carefully cleansed, debrided, and sutured.

Puncture wounds, e.g., animal bites and stab wounds, result from perforation of the skin and underlying tissues by a sharp object or impact from a blunt narrow object. Although the skin may show only a minute point of entry, the injury may be dangerous because of the possibility that organisms of *Clostridium tetani,* the causative organism of tetanus, may be introduced. This is a potentially very critical situation, because tetanus is fatal in 60 percent of cases. The wound should be thoroughly cleaned and the bleeding identified. The patient's immunization status must be ascertained. If active immunization has been established within 3 years prior to injury, a booster injection of tetanus toxoid 0.5 ml is given. If no immunity has been acquired or if the interval since the last immunization is unknown or more than 3 years, the doctor must decide whether administration of horse serum tetanus antitoxin is warranted. Tetanus antitoxin is a very toxic substance and the patient must be tested for sensitivity to horse serum before it is administered. To test for sensitivity, 0.1 ml of 1:10 dilution of antitoxin is injected intradermally. If the patient is sensitive to the horse serum, a wheal will develop at the site within 15 to 30 minutes. If sensitivity is present, then the antitoxin can be administered only in very small doses highly diluted. Epinephrine, 1:1,000, 0.5 ml should be available for immediate injection should untoward reactions occur. After the injection the patient should remain quiet and under observation for at least 30 minutes before being released.

If puncture results from an animal bite all precautions and measures pertaining to rabies must be carried out, and this should be done in accordance with the recommendations of the World Health Organization.

Gas gangrene is an acute, very severe inflammation caused by the organism *Clostridium welchii,* which is normally present in the soil and intestinal tract of man and animals. Gas gangrene may follow a traumatic wound in which muscle tissue is damaged, thereby permitting the entrance of the organism. Incineration or autoclaving of all materials that have been in contact with the wound is necessary, and additional measures such as antibiotic therapy, debridement, and possibly employment of hyperbaric oxygen are carried out.

Burns pose a severe threat to the body. Burns can occur from thermal, electrical, mechanical, or chemical contact. In first-degree burns, only superficial erythema develops and no special treatment is needed. In second-degree burns, the skin usually is blistered but heals without scarring in about 10 days without treatment. In third-degree burns, the full thickness of the skin has been destroyed and healing is prolonged until scar tissue forms, unless skin is grafted onto the denuded area. In third-degree burns, the burned area may appear red, brown, white, or gray, but the perception of painful sensations is lost because the nerve endings have been destroyed. The urgency of treatment depends upon the extent and depth of the burn. First-degree burns are not urgent and require only simple cleansing and avoidance of further irritation. With second-degree burns, the part must be removed at once from the source of the burn, carefully cleaned, and protected from further irritation. The vesicles should not be ruptured. In third-degree burns, the urgency of treatment increases with the extent of the burn. When 15 percent or more of the body surface is severely burned, a generalized response of shock may be expected and hospitalization is required. Small children, infants, and older people tolerate burns poorly and are more likely to go into shock.

The patient should be moved from the source of the burn and the tissue cooled, if possible, to prevent further destruction. His clothing should not be removed if it adheres to the burned surface. He should be covered with a coat or other garment to prevent loss of body heat. Salves and ointments should not be applied to large burns. The patient should receive nothing by mouth because peristalsis is absent. He should be transported immediately to a hospital experienced in caring for burns, preferably one with a burn unit. In the hospital, an indwelling catheter is placed in the bladder to permit hourly observation of the amount and character of the urine. A venous cutdown is made for rapid administration of large amounts of fluids. Careful evaluation of the extent of burn is made, the area is thoroughly cleansed, and either open or closed treatment is initiated to promote escharosis. Tetanus immunization is accomplished if necessary. If medication is given for pain relief the intravenous route is used, and only a small amount is given so as not to cloud the patient's perception. Observation of vital signs, fluid administration, and urine output is continued throughout the critical phase of care. Skin grafting is undertaken only after the patient's condition is stabilized.

Contact with the phenolic irritants found in such roadside shrubs as poison ivy, poison oak, and poison sumac may cause various dermatoses. The toxins are present in the leaves and roots of the plants, and may be carried by the wind. Individuals who are sensitive to the toxins manifest erythema, irritation, itching, burning, edema, and vesicle formation from even remote contact. Hyposensitization is only partially successful. One effective prophylactic measure is to cover exposed parts with a paste made of brown naphtha laundry soap and water, and then, following exposure, wash off the soap and irritants. Treatment consists of applying calamine lotion or wet dressings of potassium permanganate, 1:5,000. (Potassium permanganate stains the skin brown temporarily and stains clothing permanently.) Usually the vesicle dries up after 10 or more days. If the reaction was severe the continuing attention of a physician is necessary to prevent secondary infection.

Frostbite, the freezing of superficial tissues, is a constant hazard where temperatures are below 32° F. Prevention is best accomplished through protection from extreme cold and exposure of the skin to cold. A feeling of cold, aching numbness progresses to freezing of tissue followed by tissue breakdown in the affected areas. The part should be rewarmed rapidly by immersion in warm water (90 to 100° F). Vasodilation is also encouraged, frequently by the ingestion of some alcohol. The affected part *should not* be rubbed, because crystallized tissue will undergo further damage if pressure is placed upon it and friction is applied. Any vasoconstriction, such as that resulting from smoking, should be avoided.

THREATS TO DIGESTION

Threats to digestion may arise from ingestion of toxic substances including drugs, swallowed foreign bodies, infection, mechanical obstruction of the digestive tract, trauma, and hemorrhage from peptic ulcer or ruptured esophageal varices.

Overdosage of drugs whether intentional or accidental is a frequent problem. Drugs commonly ingested in large amounts include aspirin, barbiturates, and recently birth control pills ingested by children. Poisons may threaten digestion in various ways. Caustic substances such as lye and strong acids will burn and scar the esophagus if swallowed. Pain, inability to swallow, and prostration following ingestion are noted; the nearest poison control center should be telephoned immediately for advice (further described later in this chapter). Efforts should be made at once to dilute the poison by giving large amounts of water, neutralizing the poison by administering its antagonist, or giving a demulcent. The patient should be moved to a hospital immediately.

Certain foods may be poisonous: some species of mushrooms, contaminated shellfish, and food contaminated with botulin bacilli, salmonellae, or staphylococci. Frequent sources of food poisoning are foods that have been inadequately refrigerated or contaminated in handling. The symptoms vary according to the toxicity of the offending agent, the amount that was ingested, and the patient's general condition. Poisonings of groups of people at gatherings where food is served occur quite often, which indicates the public health aspect of this problem. Restaurants are regularly inspected by local public health departments in a continuing effort to reduce poisoning from this cause. When the patient arrives for treatment, he should be asked, "What did you eat? Where did you eat it?"

Botulism is caused by the toxin produced by growth of *Clostridium botulinum* in improperly canned or preserved food. The toxin affects the nervous system, causing headache, weakness, muscular incoordination, and inability to talk or swallow. Death is due to peripheral respiratory paralysis. Mouth-to-mouth resuscitation is needed to maintain respiration until antitoxin can be obtained. In infants and debilitated individuals the pronounced loss of fluids and electrolytes may cause severe gastrointestinal disturbances. Vomiting and diarrhea with abdominal cramping occur shortly after ingestion of the contaminated food. Treatment focuses upon identifying the cause and eliminating it, and restoring fluids and electrolytes while putting the gastrointestinal tract at rest. Fluid and electrolyte balance can be restored by administration of 1 teaspoonful of salt and one-half teaspoonful of baking soda dissolved in 1 quart of water.

Swallowed foreign bodies pose another threat to digestion. If the swallowed object is sharp, the gastrointestinal tract may be perforated or torn; if large, mechanical obstruction may result. There are few first aid measures for these situations. Bread and potatoes can be eaten in the hope that they will adhere to the swallowed object and serve as a cushion. The patient may also be kept flat on his back with his knees raised to relax abdominal muscles and prevent pressure over the stomach and intestines. Small round objects probably will pass through the tract and be expelled rectally without difficulty, but prompt medical attention is needed if the object is sharp or large. Fluoroscopy will be done and an endoscopic procedure may be necessary. In some cases exploratory surgery must be performed.

Intestinal obstruction is another threat to digestion and may result from incarcerated hernia, intussusception, adhesions, foreign bodies, gallstones, or paralytic ileus. The signs and symptoms include abdominal distention, nausea, vomiting of fecal material, abdominal cramping, and possibly diarrhea of very narrow caliber. The most urgent concern is for the maintenance of an adequate blood supply to the entire intestinal tract, for if the blood supply to any part is impaired, infarction of that segment of the bowel with resulting gangrene will occur. First aid consists of withholding fluids and laxatives or enemas, and moving the patient to a hospital for intestinal intubation and correction of fluid and electrolyte imbalance. If the blood supply remains impaired, surgical intervention is urgently needed.

Appendicitis is the result of inflammation and possibly infection of the vermiform appendix. Peristalsis is halted and the patient has abdominal tenderness which is generalized at first and later localized over the appendix in the lower right quadrant. There may be fever, elevated leukocyte count, dehydration, nausea, and vomiting. First aid measures consist of recognizing the possibility of appendicitis if the patient's appendix had not been removed, and withholding laxatives and enemas, since intestinal stimulating would increase the danger of perforation of the bowel.

Intestinal perforation in itself is a threat to the integrity of the intestinal tract. It can be caused by rupture of an inflamed appendix, a peptic ulcer, a diverticulum, or abdominal wounds resulting from trauma. Perforation of the intestines is a surgical emergency because the patient is likely to go into shock, and peritonitis from contamination of the peritoneal cavity may develop. He must be hospitalized immediately. If the intestines have been exposed, the tissues must be kept covered with a moist compress until the patient is brought to the hospital.

Gastrointestinal hemorrhage is a threat also. Ruptured esophageal varices, bleeding peptic ulcer, carcinoma, or ulceration of the large intestine may be the cause.

Rupture of esophageal varices is an emergency situation that must be treated immediately in a hospital. A Blakemore tube is utilized to maintain pressure against the varices in the terminal third of the esophagus.

Gastric hemorrhage also necessitates hospitalization, in order that attempts to control the bleeding may be made. In the hospital, a hypothermia procedure is carried out.

THREATS TO BODY TEMPERATURE

Threats to body temperature arise from high fever, heat stroke, and freezing.

High fever accompanies many diseases and conditions and increases the metabolism and thus the demand for oxygen. First aid consists of giving fluids and antipyretics such as aspirin, and sponging the patient with alcohol or applying an ice pack to the axilla and groin.

Sunstroke (heat stroke) is an acute threat due to the interference with the normal mechanism of perspiration. The patient becomes confused, dizzy, and weak; his skin is hot and dry and he has a high fever. Urgent need exists for immediate reduction of body temperature and for this, the methods just described can be utilized. Wearing a hat to protect the head from direct sunlight is an aid in preventing sunstroke.

Freezing poses a threat not only to the exposed and superficial areas of the body, but to all tissues, though individual tolerance to cold varies greatly. The person who is in danger of freezing complains of sleepiness and wants to lie down and go to sleep. He must be kept moving, for if he stops he will sink into a stupor from which he cannot be aroused. First aid consists of removing the victim to a warmer environment so that rewarming can take place gradually; he should be offered warm drinks and covered with blankets. His body should not be rubbed, since this would cause damage to the crystallized tissues.

THREATS TO PERCEPTION

Threats to perception involve injuries that interfere with sight, hearing, and consciousness.

Threats to vision arising from urgent situations involve mainly trauma to the eye. Cinders, sawdust, and other small particles should be flushed out with a sterile saline solution or tap water. At times the threat to vision arises from a disorder within the eye, such as a retinal hemorrhage, glaucoma, or a retinal detachment. First aid measures include keeping the patient quiet and covering the eye loosely with a dressing to help prevent eye strain. An ophthalmologist must be consulted. No attempt should be made to remove imbedded foreign bodies.

Chemicals splashed into the eye can be a threat to vision. Large amounts of water are used to flush out the irritant, and this effort should be continued for 15 to 20 minutes. Again, there is urgent need for the care of an ophthalmologist.

Sudden loss of hearing is an emergency that may be caused by infection, a bolus of wax, or an imbedded insect. No attempt should be made to probe the ear canal or remove the foreign object, since this can result in rupture of the ear drum. An otologist should be consulted at once.

THREATS TO CONSCIOUSNESS

Loss of consciousness is another threat to the body's integrity. The loss may be momentary as in fainting, or prolonged as in coma. Fainting is a compensatory mechanism to overcome the inadequacy in circulation; the horizontal position promotes circulation to the brain and consciousness thus is restored promptly. Hence, in first aid measures, this mechanism is recognized—the patient is placed in a horizontal position with his feet elevated.

Prolonged unconsciousness, or coma, can result from many causes including disorders of metabolism, e.g., uncontrolled diabetes mellitus, alcoholism, drug toxicity, trauma to the head, heat stroke, or severe infection. It is a serious development that calls for prompt medical evaluation. Observation of the patient to determine the level of consciousness and maintenance of respiration and circulation are the only measures that can be followed until the cause has been identified. If body temperature is high, attempts at cooling must be made.

THREATS TO RATIONALITY

Rationality may be threatened by an overwhelming emotional shock or prolonged severe emotional stress. Each individual has his own level of tolerance to these stresses and his own techniques for coping, which may vary according to the given circumstances. Ingestion of alcohol or drugs threatens rationality. Signs of disorganization become evident with efforts to carry out an action or to converse. The section on "Reactions to Emergencies" should be consulted.

In first aid, efforts are made to reestablish a rational relationship. Prompt removal from the source of difficulty, constant attendance, and reassurance are needed. It is helpful to bring the patient to his family or to familiar surroundings. A judgment may have to be made about whether the patient will benefit more from quiet isolation or from positive direction within the group, and if he remains irrational, medical care should be sought without delay.

THREAT OF RADIATION

The threat of radiation is present constantly in our environment. To the naturally present radioactivity man has caused to be added radioactivity from a number of sources. Radiation interferes with cellular reproduction and increases the possibility of mutant cell development. Radiation is known to be one cause of leukemia. The effects of radiation are cumulative.

Shielding, time, and distance are considered in calculating safe practices. When an individual is unwittingly exposed to radiation, he must take advantage of whatever protection is offered by the immediate circumstances. The source of the contamination and the individual must be monitored; the individual must undergo decontamination, and he must be kept under surveillance for evidence of radiation sickness.

THREAT OF MASS DISASTER

Mass disaster may be a natural occurrence, e.g., flood or earthquake, or manmade, e.g., dropping an atomic bomb, or chemical or biological warfare. In the United States, basic responsibilities for coping with such catastrophes rest with the American Red Cross and local civil defense agencies. The immediate need is to follow the established system of triage, i.e., selection for care. The person in charge directs all activities and the identification and assignment of priority of care. Priority is assigned as follows: Priority I, individuals requiring outpatient care only, who then can assume a helping role; Priority II, individuals requiring immediate treatment whose chance for recovery is optimal (e.g., airway obstruction); Priority III, individuals whose chance for recovery is not jeopardized by delay in treatment (e.g., fracture); Priority IV, critically injured individuals, those for whom there is no possibility of recovery, and those who will require lengthy medical care (e.g., severe burns).

Resources and personnel are organized to give care on the basis of these priorities. Emergency first aid is provided and the victims are transported to available hospitals. If hospital facilities are inadequate, the civil defense agency has access to 200-bed hospitals which are stored in trailer trucks and are available to nearby areas within a few hours. These portable hospitals are equipped with x-ray equipment, operating room equipment, pharmaceutical supplies, central service facilities and supplies, a portable generator, and an ample water supply tank equipped with a pump and provision for chlorination.

Each existing hospital has its own disaster plan and is responsible for testing it periodically. Municipal, state, and federal agencies have responsibilities for overseeing transportation, communication, police, fire, and shelter services.

In disasters confined to a small area (e.g., a house fire) local police, firemen, and rescue squads may be sufficient. The threats posed by such fires are so well known that they need not be repeated here. First aid measures include removal of persons in the immediate area of the fire. They should be instructed to crawl along the floor or run with the head held low. A wet handkerchief held over the nose will help to filter out the hot ash particles to some extent. Resuscitation and oxygenation may become necessary.

Functions of the Nurse in Disasters

The American Nurses' Association and the American Medical Association recognize the role of the nurse in mass disasters. In its Summary Report on National Emergency Care, February, 1962, the American Medical Association listed the following functions as appropriate for nurses:

1. First aid, including but not limited to artificial respiration; emergency treatment of open chest wounds; relief of pain; treatment of shock; and preparation of casualties for transportation.

2. Control of hemorrhage.

3. Attainment and maintenance of a patent airway, including intratracheal catheterization and emergency tracheotomy.

4. Proper and adequate cleansing and treatment of wounds.

5. Bandaging and splinting.

6. Administration of anesthetics under medical supervision.

7. Assisting in surgical procedures.

8. Insertion of nasogastric tubes to include lavage and gavage as directed.

9. Administration of whole blood and intravenous solutions, as directed.

10. Administration of parenteral medications as directed.

11. Catheterization of males and females.

12. Administration of immunizing agents as directed.

13. Management of psychologically disturbed individuals.

14. Management of normal obstetrical deliveries.

15. Operation of treatment and aid stations in reception areas and in communities where physicians are inadequate in number, including the diagnosis and treatment of minor illness and injuries, institution of life-saving measures, and referral of more serious cases to physicians.

MEDICOLEGAL ASPECTS

While the laws governing the administration of first aid differ from state to state and are redefined from time to time, there are a few principles to guide the nurse in her actions. In some states any person first upon the scene of an accident is required by law to stop and to administer aid. In giving aid the nurse is held to the standard of care expected of a professional person with her professional understanding and professional level of skill. In being judged by this standard she could be cited for either acts of omission (things she should have done but did not do) or acts of commission (things she did but should not have done). The nurse must be aware of the consequences of her actions. In some states "good samaritan" laws protect the nurse from liability while rendering aid.

In each state in which the nurse practices she should familiarize herself with the particular nurse practice act and the laws governing first aid in that state. Further clarification of the law as it may be interpreted may be obtained from the state nurses' association through its attorney.

Poison Control Centers

Poison control centers have been established in medical centers and colleges of pharmacy throughout the United States. Because of the myriad of chemical products available to the general population, the possibility of ingestion or misuse of chemicals—especially by exploring children—is very great. The local poison control center makes available by telephone detailed information as to the content of the product, its toxicity, and a guide for treatment. This service is available free of charge to hospitals, physicians, and occasionally to the lay public directly. In some areas the poison control center also serves as a first aid center for prompt treatment of poisoning.

To reduce the hazards of misuse each manufacturer of poisonous products is required to list the applicable precautions and to include a warning to keep the product out of the reach of children.

Suicide Control Centers

Because the number of suicides continues to increase, suicide control centers have been established in many metropolitan areas. A professional counselor with training in either religion or medicine can be reached at all times, and his telephone number is well publicized. These individuals volunteer their assistance as needed. When the acute threat has been met, the center guides the individual toward further care, and provides follow-up attention.

Prevention of Accidents and Emergencies

The prevention of accidents, emergencies, and disasters is everyone's business. Safety for self and others is a concept that should be emphasized from early youth throughout life. The National Safety Council conducts an extensive educational program whose purpose is to alert the public to certain hazards and to provide instruction in safe practices. Nonetheless, the accident toll continues to rise, with huge costs in life, well-being, and economic earning.

The nurse, both as a member of society and as a professional person, has an important role in teaching and practicing safety for herself, her family, and all persons with whom she deals professionally. Numerous accidents can be prevented, and the nurse should be active in such efforts.

Bibliography

Accident Facts, 1967 Edition. National Safety Council. Chicago, 1967.

American Heart Association: Closed Chest Method of Cardiopulmonary Resuscitation. *American Journal of Nursing,* 65:105, May, 1965.

Antivenin: North American Antisnake-bite Serum. Philadelphia: Wyeth Laboratories.

Ayres, Stephen M. and Stanley Gianelli, Jr.: *Care of the Critically Ill.* New York: Appleton Century Crofts, 1967.

Clarifying Gray Areas of Practice. *American Journal of Nursing,* 64:84, January, 1964.

Clinical Symposium on Poisoning. CIBA, 12:1, January-February, 1960.

Dolman, C. E.: Botulism. *American Journal of Nursing,* 64:119–124, July, 1964.

Emergency Intervention by the Nurse, Monograph No.1. American Nurses' Association. New York, 1962.

Henley, Nellie: Sulfamylon for Burns. *American Journal of Nursing,* 69:2122–2123, October, 1969.

Mahoney, Robert F.: *Emergency and Disaster Nursing.* New York: The Macmillan Company, 1965.

Morris, Ena M.: In Case of Fire Emergencies. *American Journal of Nursing,* 68:1496–1497, July, 1968.

Nelson, Thomas G., George F. Rumer, and Theodore H. Nicholas: Crico-thyroidotomy. *American Journal of Nursing,* 61:74–76, November, 1961.

Radioisotopes in Medicine: A General Guide for Physicians and Hospital Personnel. Oak Ridge, Tenn.: Abbott Laboratories, 1962.

Shneidman, Edwin: Preventing Suicide. *American Journal of Nursing,* 65:111–116, May, 1965.

Staudenmaier, Herbert and Doris Mac-Namarra: Rehabilitation after Frostbite. *American Journal of Nursing,* 64:93–96, December, 1964.

U.S. Department of Defense and U.S. Department of Health, Education, and Welfare, Public Health Service: *Family Guide Emergency Health Care.* Publication No.–0-665–199. Washington, D.C.: U.S. Government Printing Office, 1963.

INDEX

BASIC SET AND MAPPING SYMBOLISM

NOTATION	MEANING
$\varnothing$	The empty set; that is, the set with no elements.
$x \in S$	The object x is an element of the set S.
$S = \{s_1, s_2, \ldots, s_n\}$	The distinct objects of the set S are $s_1, s_2, \ldots, s_n$.
$A \neq B$	A is not equal to B.
$A \subseteq B$	A is a subset of B; that is, each element of A is also in B.
$A \subset B$	A is a proper subset of B; that is, $A \subseteq B$ but $A \neq B$.
$\{x : P(x)\}$	The set of all x for which the assertion $P(x)$ is true.
$f : X \to Y; x \mapsto f(x)$	The mapping f has X as its domain and Y as its codomain and sends x to $f(x)$.

For a list of the other symbolism used in this text, see the inside back cover and its facing page.

SYMBOLISM FOR STRUCTURES

SYMBOL	STRUCTURE	LOCATION OF DEFINITION
$(X, \preceq)$	Partially ordered set	Definition 1 of Section 1.6
$(X, \square)$	Semigroup	Definition 2 of Section 2.2
$[X, \square, e]$	Monoid	Definition 4 of Section 2.2
$[X, \bar{}, \wedge, 1, \vee, 0]$	Boolean algebra	Definition 2 of Section 2.3
$[X, \wedge, \vee]$	Lattice	Definition 2 of Section 2.6
$\langle V, E \rangle$	Digraph	Definition 1 of Section 6.1
$[V, E, r]$	Rooted tree	Definition 1 of Section 6.2
(V, E)	Graph	Definition 1 of Section 6.5
$\langle X, \square, e \rangle$	Group	Definition 1 of Section 7.1
$\langle X, +, 0 \rangle$	Additive group	Notation 1 of Section 7.1
$(X, +, 0, \cdot)$	Ring	Definition 1 of Section 7.6
$[X, +, 0, \cdot, 1]$	Ring with unity	Definition 2 of Section 7.6
$\langle X, +, 0, \cdot, 1 \rangle$	Field	Definition 2 of Section 7.6

DISCRETE AND
COMBINATORIAL
MATHEMATICS

DISCRETE AND COMBINATORIAL MATHEMATICS

ABRAHAM P. HILLMAN
University of New Mexico

GERALD L. ALEXANDERSON
Santa Clara University

RICHARD M. GRASSL
University of New Mexico

DELLEN PUBLISHING COMPANY
San Francisco, California

COLLIER MACMILLAN PUBLISHERS
London

divisions of
Macmillan, Inc.

© Copyright 1987 by Dellen Publishing Company, a division of Macmillan, Inc.

Printed in the United States of America

Permissions: Dellen Publishing Company
            400 Pacific Avenue
            San Francisco, California 94133

Orders: Dellen Publishing Company
            c/o Macmillan Publishing Company
            Front and Brown Streets
            Riverside, New Jersey 08075

Collier Macmillan Canada, Inc.

LIBRARY OF CONGRESS CATALOGING-IN-PUBLICATION DATA

Hillman, Abraham P.
  Discrete and combinatorial mathematics.

  Bibliography: p.
  Includes index.
  1. Mathematics—1961–   . 2. Electronic data
processing—Mathematics.   3. Combinatorial analysis.
I. Alexanderson, Gerald L.   II. Grassl, Richard M.
III. Title.
QA39.2.H555   1986   510   86-9037
ISBN 0-02-354580-1

Printing: 1 2 3 4 5 6 7 8   *Year:* 6 7 8 9 0
ISBN 0-02-354580-1

CONTENTS

1

SETS AND RELATIONS   1

2

ALGEBRAIC STRUCTURES   76

3

LOGIC   147

4

INDUCTION   178

5

COMBINATORIAL PRINCIPLES   210

6

DIGRAPHS AND GRAPHS   293

7
GROUPS   **351**

8
POLYNOMIALS, PARTIAL FRACTIONS   **426**

9
GENERATING FUNCTIONS AND RECURSIONS   **465**

10

COMBINATORIAL ANALYSIS OF ALGORITHMS   555

11

INTRODUCTION TO CODING   587

12

FINITE STATE MACHINES AND LANGUAGES   600

PREFACE

This text provides mathematical foundations for students preparing to use or design computers and for students interested in combinatorial theory and its applications. Some choices of sections for possible courses are listed in charts below. These selections of topics have been successfully class tested, using preliminary editions.

The success of the students in mastering and retaining desired material is attributed to a number of features built into the text. Most important are the well organized graded problem sets consisting of more than 2100 problems. The early problems on each topic help the students to become familiar with the new terms and symbols and to build confidence for later work. Some problems are broken into "bite size" parts; such parts are labeled (i), (ii), and so on. Parts that can be assigned separately are labeled (a), (b), etc. Occasionally a hint, such as a reference to earlier material, is given. Some problem sets contain a series of related problems leading the student through concrete examples to a more general result. Answers or solutions are given to almost all odd-numbered problems.

Several recurrent themes in this text help to unify material presented as unrelated in other sources. For example, bit strings are introduced in the first section and are used in the development of binomial coefficients, subsets of a finite set, algebraic structures, boolean functions, induction, combinatorics and probability, binary codes, languages, and finite state machines. This text also provides a gradual approach to important topics by the foreshadowing of concepts to be discussed more fully in later sections.

The diversity of topics in a course on discrete mathematics requires an above average amount of new vocabulary and symbolism. The format of the text helps to cope with this difficulty by making it easy to find any definition or notation. Every definition, notation, algorithm, and theorem has a name. Each chapter has a summary of terms introduced in the chapter followed by a set of review problems and a set of supplementary and challenging problems.

The examples and worked out solutions to many odd-numbered problems provide illustrations of all the basic techniques. It is not assumed that the readers are already familiar with binomial coefficients, factorials, sum and product notation, arithmetic and geometric progressions, and so on. No previous knowledge of calculus is required.

Biographical notes are given on some of the people who have made special contributions to the fields discussed in this text. An annotated bibliography is furnished for those seeking more advanced material or additional applications of discrete and combinatorial mathematics.

This text contains enough material for a full year course, and there are many ways of selecting sections for a coherent quarter or semester course. The following table indicates some possible choices of 24 sections for a course.

COURSE	SUGGESTED SECTIONS
Discrete and Combinatorial Mathematics	1.1–1.4, 1.8, 2.1, 2.2, 3.1, 3.2, 4.1, 4.2, 5.1, 5.2, 6.1–6.3, 7.1, 7.2, 8.1, 8.3, 9.1–9.3, 10.1
Combinatorial Theory	1.1–1.4, 1.8, 4.1, 4.2, 5.1–5.8, 8.1, 8.3, 9.1–9.6, 10.1
Discrete Structures	1.1–1.8, 2.1–2.5, 3.1–3.3, 4.1, 4.2, 6.1–6.3, 7.1–7.3

The material can also be selected so as to achieve a particular main objective, as illustrated in the following chart.

OBJECTIVE	SUGGESTED SECTIONS
Solving Recursions	1.1–1.4, 1.8, 4.1, 4.2, 5.1, 5.2, 8.1, 8.3, 9.1–9.6
Complexity of Algorithms	1.1–1.4, 1.8, 4.1, 4.2, 5.1, 5.2, 8.1, 8.3, 9.1–9.3, 9.6, 10.1–10.3
Finite State Machines	1.1–1.4, 1.8, 2.1, 2.2, 2.5, 4.1, 6.1, 6.2, 11.1, 12.1, 12.2
Planar Graphs	1.1–1.8, 4.1, 4.2, 5.1, 5.2, 6.1–6.6
Graphs and Their Applications	1.1–1.8, 2.1, 2.2, 4.1, 4.2, 5.1, 5.2, 7.1–7.7, 11.1, 11.2

Flexibility in the selection of topics to be covered is enhanced by the explicit recalling of concepts from previous sections, together with the citations of earlier usage. Other aids are the material on the inside front and back covers, the index at the end of the book, and the summaries of terms for each chapter.

An instructors' manual is available.

ACKNOWLEDGMENTS

The authors are grateful for the valuable suggestions of the following mathematicians, each of whom reviewed one or more of the chapters of a preliminary edition: Don Alton, University of Iowa; Robert Beezer, University of Puget Sound; James Calhoun, Sangamon State University; Philip Feinsilver, Southern Illinois University; David Gale, University of California, Berkeley; Glenn Hopkins, University of Mississippi; Gordon Hughes, California State University, Chico; Takayuki D. Kimura, Washington University; Kenneth D. Lane, Colby College; Zane Motteler, California Polytechnic State University, San Luis Obispo; Peter O'Neil, University of Alabama, Birmingham; Robert Patenaude, College of the Canyons; K. Brooks Reid, Louisiana State University; Karen J. Schroeder, Bentley College; Karen Sharp, C. S. Mott Community College; and Ronald D. Whittekin, Metropolitan State College.

We also express our deepest appreciation to Josephine Hillman who helped in too many ways to mention. Sandra Yeary and Gloria Padilla are thanked for their assistance with the manuscript.

We also recognize with special gratitude the invaluable assistance from Dellen Publishing Company and its editorial and production staffs, including Don Dellen, Luana Morimoto, Phyllis Niklas, and Elliot Simon.

Abraham P. Hillman
Gerald L. Alexanderson
Richard M. Grassl

INTRODUCTION FOR STUDENTS

Students are encouraged to take advantage of several features of this text. The inside front cover has the Greek alphabet to aid in pronouncing these letters and a list of symbols that have fixed meaning when appearing in boldface type. Its facing page has some fundamental symbolism together with the symbolism for structures developed in this book. The inside back cover and its facing page have the other symbolism of the text.

There are answers or solutions near the end of the book for all odd-numbered problems except some "show that" or "prove that" problems. When the parts of a problem are labeled (i), (ii), and so on, this indicates that the problem has been broken into "bite size" parts which should be tackled in the given order. If an even-numbered problem seems difficult, it may be helpful to look at the previous odd-numbered problem and its answer or solution.

Each chapter ends with a summary of the terms introduced and is followed by a set of review problems. Readers desiring a greater test of their knowledge, ability, and perseverance may tackle the supplementary and challenging problems. Also, the annotated bibliography might provide other doors to knowledge.

The chapter summaries are merged in the index at the end of the text.

1

SETS AND RELATIONS

This chapter introduces and develops some important tools for studying the mathematics needed in computer science and computer engineering. Operations on sets are fundamental in all of mathematics. They are presented here as a concrete example of a boolean algebra, the type of algebra involved in the working of electronic circuits and symbolic logic. The study of relations on sets helps in the construction of efficient relational databases, which provide easy access to the accumulated knowledge and techniques of our complicated civilization. The chapter concludes with the study of mappings from a set X to a set Y. This concept is used in many of the topics that follow and is developed in a way that also helps in the combinatorial aspects, which can be applied to appraising the cost in space, time, or money of various procedures.

1.1

BINARY STRINGS

Binary strings are useful in situations that feature dichotomy, that is, separation into two categories. In electrical circuits the dichotomy is that of a switch being either in the "on" or in the "off" position. In logic it involves an assertion's being "true" or "false." In set theory, elements are either "in" or "out" of a set.

In computer science, the symbols used most frequently to represent the two categories of any such dichotomy are the digits 0 and 1. In the applications just mentioned, we may be dealing with several switches, or assertions, or elements of a set; this motivates us to introduce the following definition.

DEFINITION 1   **SET B_n OF BINARY STRINGS**

The digits 0 and 1 are called *bits* or *binary digits*. A string $b_1b_2 \ldots b_n$ with each b_i either 0 or 1 is an *n-bit string* or an *n-digit binary string*. We use B_n to denote the set of all n-bit strings.

For example, there are two 1-bit strings: 0 and 1; and there are four 2-digit binary strings: 00, 01, 10, and 11.

In certain algebraic expressions, braces { } have the same meaning as parentheses ( ), however there are contexts in which this is not true. In a *listing* for a finite set, the elements should be enclosed within braces and no element should be listed more than once. Thus $B_1 = \{0, 1\}$ is the set of 1-digit binary strings, and in this text $\{0, 1, 0\}$ is *not* an allowable use of set notation. Changing the order in which the elements appear creates a new listing but not a new set. For example,

$$\{1, 2, 3\} = \{1, 3, 2\} = \{2, 1, 3\} = \{2, 3, 1\} = \{3, 1, 2\} = \{3, 2, 1\}$$

gives six different listings for the same set. In general, $S = \{s_1, s_2, \ldots, s_n\}$ means that $s_1, s_2, \ldots, s_n$ are the n distinct elements of the set S. We have noted that $B_1 = \{0, 1\}$ and that

$$B_2 = \{00, 01, 10, 11\}. \tag{1}$$

The following notation is used in our systematic procedure for obtaining the strings of B_{n+1} from those of B_n.

NOTATION 1   **PREFIXING A DIGIT**

Let $\beta = b_1b_2 \ldots b_n$ be in the set B_n. Then 0β and 1β denote the $(n+1)$-digit strings $0b_1b_2 \ldots b_n$ and $1b_1b_2 \ldots b_n$, respectively.

For example, if the four strings of B_2 are $\beta_1 = 00$, $\beta_2 = 01$, $\beta_3 = 10$, and $\beta_4 = 11$, then $\{0\beta_1, 0\beta_2, 0\beta_3, 0\beta_4, 1\beta_1, 1\beta_2, 1\beta_3, 1\beta_4\}$ is the set of all 3-digit binary strings

$$B_3 = \{000, 001, 010, 011, 100, 101, 110, 111\}. \tag{2}$$

When listing the strings of B_3, how could one guard against omitting a string? It helps to know that there are eight strings in B_3, as can be seen from Display (2). But suppose one repeated a string and left out another one; this could make it seem that there were the right number of strings. Having an agreed-upon order in which to list the strings lessens the probability of such errors and helps in checking the work of certain applications, such as the case table proofs to be introduced in Section 1.3. A standard order also makes it easier to find a given item in a listing stored in a computer memory.

For these reasons, we introduce a standard way of listing the elements of certain sets, including the sets B_1, B_2, ... Since 0 precedes 1 in the usual numerical order, we adopt $\{0, 1\}$ as the standard listing for B_1. For the same reason, we begin our standard listing of B_2 with the strings that have 0 as the leftmost digit, 00 and 01, and then write the strings that start with 1, namely 10 and 11. Thus our standard listing for B_2 is $\{00, 01, 10, 11\}$. We can then use this listing for B_2 to define the standard listing for B_3, and so on.

The following algorithm states the procedure formally. It is an example of a "recursive procedure," or an "inductive definition," because it gives the desired result for the first set B_1 and then tells how to use the desired listing for a set B_k in the sequence B_1, B_2, ... to obtain the chosen listing for the next set B_{k+1}. Such procedures are discussed further in Section 4.1.

ALGORITHM 1   **STANDARD LISTING FOR B_n**

The standard listing for B_1 is $\{0, 1\}$. Given the standard listing $\{\beta_1, \beta_2, \ldots, \beta_r\}$ for B_k, then the standard listing for B_{k+1} is

$$\{0\beta_1, 0\beta_2, \ldots, 0\beta_r, 1\beta_1, 1\beta_2, \ldots, 1\beta_r\}.$$

We note that Algorithm 1 produces the standard listing $B_2 = \{00, 01, 10, 11\}$ of Display (1) from the standard listing $B_1 = \{0, 1\}$ and also produces Display (2) from Display (1). Hence Display (2) is the standard listing for B_3. As it turns out, the strings of B_n are the base-2 numerals for the numbers $0, 1, 2, \ldots, 2^n - 1$, and the order of appearance in the standard listing is the appropriate order for this application.

NOTATION 2   **NUMBER OF ELEMENTS IN A SET S**

If S is a finite set, $\#S$ stands for the number of elements in S. (One reads "$\#S$" as "the *size* of S" or as "the *cardinal number* of S.")

Thus, if $S = \{s_1, s_2, \ldots, s_n\}$, then $\#S = n$. If $\#S = 1$, the set S is called a *singleton*. If $\#S = 2$, S is called a *pair* or a *doubleton*. If $\#S = 3$, S is a *triple*.

Since $B_1 = \{0, 1\}$ and $B_2 = \{00, 01, 10, 11\}$, we have $\#B_1 = 2$ and $\#B_2 = 4$. We next give $\#B_n$ for n in $\{1, 2, 3, \ldots\}$.

THEOREM 1

FORMULA FOR $\#B_n$

For all positive integers n, $\#B_n = 2^n$.

INFORMAL PROOF

Every string $\beta = b_1 b_2 \ldots b_{n+1}$ in B_{n+1} has as its leftmost digit b_1 either 0 or 1; that is, β is either of the form 0α or of the form 1α, with $\alpha = b_2 \ldots b_{n+1}$ in B_n. The number of β's in B_{n+1} with $b_1 = 0$ is $\#B_n$, as is the number of β's in B_{n+1} with $b_1 = 1$. Hence

$$\#B_{n+1} = \#B_n + \#B_n = 2(\#B_n).$$

This and $\#B_1 = 2$ imply that $\#B_2 = 2 \cdot 2 = 2^2$, $\#B_3 = 2 \cdot 2^2 = 2^3$, and so on. Thus $\#B_n = 2^n$.

We call this proof "informal" because, for many mathematicians, a formal proof of this result requires the steps of "mathematical induction" (which will be discussed in Section 4.2). □

It is important not only to produce the objects of certain sets, such as the strings of a desired B_n, preferably in an easily recognized order, but also to know how many objects are in these sets. One reason for knowing the size of a set is that it helps us estimate the time and space needed for its listing, an important cost consideration when using computers. For example, it follows from Theorem 1 that $\#B_{20} = 2^{20} = 1,048,576$ and hence that a listing for B_{20} using four strings per line and sixty-six lines per page would require 3972 pages.

DEFINITION 2

LENGTH AND WEIGHT

A binary string $\beta = b_1 b_2 \ldots b_n$ with n bits has **length** n. The number of 1's in the string β is the **weight** of β and is denoted by wgt β.

For example, 11001 and 00110 have length 5 with wgt $11001 = 3$ and wgt $00110 = 2$. The weight of β is the sum of its binary digits; that is,

$$\text{wgt}(b_1 b_2 \ldots b_n) = b_1 + b_2 + \cdots + b_n. \tag{3}$$

Also, if β is in B_n, wgt β must be in the set $\{0, 1, \ldots, n\}$.

NOTATION 3

SUBSET $B_{n,k}$ OF B_n

The set of all binary strings of length n and weight k is denoted as $B_{n,k}$.

For example, the sets of 3-bit strings of weight 0, 1, 2, and 3, respectively, are

$$B_{3,0} = \{000\}, \qquad\qquad B_{3,1} = \{001, 010, 100\},$$
$$B_{3,2} = \{011, 101, 110\}, \qquad B_{3,3} = \{111\}. \tag{4}$$

In each of these listings, the strings appear in the same relative order as in the standard listing for B_3.

LEMMA 1 **WEIGHT OF 0β AND 1β**

$$\text{wgt}(0\beta) = \text{wgt }\beta \qquad \text{and} \qquad \text{wgt}(1\beta) = 1 + \text{wgt }\beta.$$

PROOF   Let $\beta = b_1 b_2 \ldots b_n$. Since the weight of a binary string is the sum of its digits,

$$\text{wgt}(0\beta) = 0 + b_1 + b_2 + \cdots + b_n = \text{wgt }\beta,$$
$$\text{wgt}(1\beta) = 1 + b_1 + b_2 + \cdots + b_n = 1 + \text{wgt }\beta. \qquad\square$$

Example 1   Here we use Lemma 1 and listings for $B_{3,3}$ and $B_{3,2}$ to obtain a listing for $B_{4,3}$. Let $\beta = b_1 b_2 b_3 b_4 \in B_{4,3}$. (The notation "$\alpha \in S$" means "$\alpha$ is an element of the set S.") Since b_1 is either 0 or 1, β is of the form 0α or the form 1α, where $\alpha = b_2 b_3 b_4$. If $b_1 = 0$, then wgt $\alpha = 3$ (by Lemma 1) and so $\alpha \in B_{3,3}$. If $b_1 = 1$, then wgt $\alpha = 2$ and $\alpha \in B_{3,2}$. Thus we prefix a 0 to 111, the only string in $B_{3,3}$, to obtain the only β in $B_{4,3}$ with 0 as the leftmost digit, and we prefix a 1 to each of the three strings of $B_{3,2} = \{011, 101, 110\}$ to get the three strings of $B_{4,3}$ with 1 as the leftmost digit. Together these give the listing

$$B_{4,3} = \{0111, 1011, 1101, 1110\} \tag{5}$$

for the set of all 4-digit binary strings of weight 3. $\square$

It is easy to see that

$$B_{1,0} = \{0\}, \qquad B_{2,0} = \{00\}, \qquad B_{3,0} = \{000\}, \qquad \ldots \tag{6}$$

and

$$B_{1,1} = \{1\}, \qquad B_{2,2} = \{11\}, \qquad B_{3,3} = \{111\}, \qquad \ldots. \tag{7}$$

That is, the only string in $B_{n,0}$ is the n-digit string $00\ldots0$, with each digit a 0, and the only string in $B_{n,n}$ is the n-digit string $11\ldots1$, with each digit a 1. Since $B_{n,0}$ is a singleton and $B_{n,n}$ is a singleton for every n in $Z^+ = \{1, 2, \ldots\}$, each of these sets has a unique listing. Hence we adopt the listings of Displays (6) and (7) as the standard listings.

We next give a recursive procedure for obtaining the standard listings for the other $B_{n,k}$, that is, those with $0 < k < n$.

ALGORITHM 2   **STANDARD LISTING FOR $B_{n,k}$**

Let n and k be integers with $0 < k < n$. Let the standard listings for $B_{n-1,k}$ and $B_{n-1,k-1}$ be

$$B_{n-1,k} = \{\alpha_1, \alpha_2, \ldots, \alpha_s\}$$

and

$$B_{n-1,k-1} = \{\gamma_1, \gamma_2, \ldots, \gamma_t\}.$$

Then the standard listing for $B_{n,k}$ is

$$\{0\alpha_1, 0\alpha_2, \ldots, 0\alpha_s, 1\gamma_1, 1\gamma_2, \ldots, 1\gamma_t\}.$$

Using this algorithm and the standard listings $B_{1,1} = \{1\}$ and $B_{1,0} = \{0\}$, we obtain the standard listing $B_{2,1} = \{01, 10\}$. The algorithm together with the standard listings $B_{2,2} = \{11\}$ and $B_{2,1} = \{01, 10\}$ give us the standard listing $B_{3,2} = \{011, 101, 110\}$.

The numbers that give the sizes of the sets $B_{n,k}$ appear frequently in mathematics. The following definition introduces the usual notation for these integers.

DEFINITION 3   **BINOMIAL COEFFICIENT $\binom{n}{k}$**

For n in $\{1, 2, 3, \ldots\}$ and k in $\{0, 1, \ldots, n\}$, let $\binom{n}{k}$ denote the number of n-digit binary strings of weight k; that is, $\binom{n}{k} = \# B_{n,k}$. Also let $\binom{0}{0} = 1$. [One reads $\binom{n}{k}$ as "n choose k" or as "***binomial coefficient*** n choose k."]

For example, the number of binary strings of length 8 and weight 6 is denoted as $\binom{8}{6}$. One obtains a string $\beta = b_1 b_2 \ldots b_n$ in $B_{n,k}$ by choosing k of the n integers of $\{1, 2, \ldots, n\}$ as the subscripts i for which $b_i = 1$ (and letting $b_j = 0$ for the other $n - k$ subscripts j). This indicates why $\binom{n}{k}$ is read as "n choose k." In Theorem 2(b) of Section 1.2, it is shown that $\binom{n}{k}$ is the number of ways of choosing k elements from any set of size n. In Section 5.2, we will see why the $\binom{n}{k}$ are called "binomial coefficients."

We note from Display (4) that $\binom{3}{0} = 1 = \binom{3}{3}$ and $\binom{3}{1} = 3 = \binom{3}{2}$. Example 1 shows that $\binom{4}{3} = \binom{3}{3} + \binom{3}{2} = 1 + 3 = 4$. These illustrate the following formulas.

THEOREM 2   **BORDERS, RECURSION, AND SYMMETRY FORMULAS**

(a) $\binom{n}{0} = 1 = \binom{n}{n}$ for $n = 0, 1, 2, \ldots$.   (*Borders Formula*)

(b) $\binom{n}{k} = \binom{n-1}{k} + \binom{n-1}{k-1}$ for $0 < k < n$.   (*Recursion Formula*)

(c) $\binom{n}{k} = \binom{n}{n-k}$ for $0 \leq k \leq n$.   (*Symmetry Formula*)

PROOF Part (a) follows from Displays (6) and (7) and the definition of $\binom{n}{k}$. For Part (b), let $0 < k < n$ and $\beta = b_1 b_2 \ldots b_n$ be in $\boldsymbol{B}_{n,k}$. Let $\alpha = b_2 \ldots b_n$ result from the deletion of the leftmost digit b_1 of β. If $b_1 = 0$, it follows from Lemma 1 that α is in $\boldsymbol{B}_{n-1,k}$. Clearly $\binom{n-1}{k} = \#\boldsymbol{B}_{n-1,k}$ is the number of such strings β in $\boldsymbol{B}_{n,k}$ with $b_1 = 0$. The remaining strings β in $\boldsymbol{B}_{n,k}$ have $b_1 = 1$ and hence α in $\boldsymbol{B}_{n-1,k-1}$; the number of these strings is $\binom{n-1}{k-1} = \#\boldsymbol{B}_{n-1,k-1}$. Thus the total number of strings in $\boldsymbol{B}_{n,k}$ is given by $\binom{n-1}{k} + \binom{n-1}{k-1}$. Part (c) follows because interchanging 0's and 1's in the digits b_i of the strings $b_1 b_2 \ldots b_n$ of $\boldsymbol{B}_{n,k}$ gives us the strings of $\boldsymbol{B}_{n,n-k}$. [Also see Theorem 4(d) ("Complements of Strings") of Section 1.2.] □

Additional combinatorial properties of the numbers $\binom{n}{k}$ are developed in Chapter 4, "Induction," and Chapter 5, "Combinatorial Principles."

PROBLEMS FOR SECTION 1.1

1. Use Display (2) and Algorithm 1 to give the standard listing for $\boldsymbol{B}_4$.

2. Determine the following.
   (a) $\#\boldsymbol{B}_4$;   (b) $\#\boldsymbol{B}_5$;   (c) $\#\boldsymbol{B}_6$;   (d) $\#\boldsymbol{B}_{10}$.

3. Give the weight of each of the following strings.
   (a) 10100;   (b) 010111;   (c) 0101010;   (d) 10101010.

4. For each of the following strings, find n and k such that the string is in $\boldsymbol{B}_{n,k}$.
   (a) 111;   (b) 0000;   (c) 11010;   (d) 1100110.

5. (i) Use Algorithm 2 with the standard listings $\boldsymbol{B}_{2,1} = \{01, 10\}$ and $\boldsymbol{B}_{2,0} = \{00\}$ to obtain the standard listing for $\boldsymbol{B}_{3,1}$.
   (ii) Use Part (i) and $\boldsymbol{B}_{3,0} = \{000\}$ to obtain the standard listing for $\boldsymbol{B}_{4,1}$.
   (iii) Give the values of $\binom{2}{1}$, $\binom{2}{0}$, $\binom{3}{1}$, $\binom{3}{0}$, and $\binom{4}{1}$.

6. (i) Use the standard listings $\boldsymbol{B}_{3,1} = \{001, 010, 100\}$ and $\boldsymbol{B}_{3,0} = \{000\}$ to give the standard listing for $\boldsymbol{B}_{4,1}$.
   (ii) Use Part (i) and $\boldsymbol{B}_{4,0} = \{0000\}$ to give the standard listing for $\boldsymbol{B}_{5,1}$.
   (iii) Give the values of $\binom{3}{0}$, $\binom{3}{1}$, $\binom{4}{0}$, $\binom{4}{1}$, and $\binom{5}{1}$.

7. (i) Use the standard listings $\boldsymbol{B}_{3,2} = \{011, 101, 110\}$ and $\boldsymbol{B}_{3,1} = \{001, 010, 100\}$ to give the standard listing for $\boldsymbol{B}_{4,2}$.
   (ii) Give the values of $\binom{3}{2}$, $\binom{3}{1}$, and $\binom{4}{2}$.

8. (a) Give the standard listing for $\boldsymbol{B}_{6,1}$ and the value of $\binom{6}{1}$.
   (b) Give the standard listing for $\boldsymbol{B}_{6,5}$ and the value of $\binom{6}{5}$.

9. Given that $\binom{7}{3} = 35$ and $\binom{7}{2} = 21$, use Theorem 2(b), "Recursion Formula," to find $\binom{8}{3}$.

10. Given that $\binom{7}{4} = 35 = \binom{7}{3}$, find $\binom{8}{4}$.

11. Give the values of each of the following.
    (a) $\binom{15}{0}$;   (b) $\binom{15}{15}$.

12. Give the values of:
(a) $\binom{20}{0}$;   (b) $\binom{20}{20}$.

13. Explain why $\binom{n}{0} = 1$ for $n = 0, 1, 2, \ldots$.

14. Does $\binom{n}{n} = 1$ for all positive integers n? Explain.

15. Does $\binom{n}{1} = n$ for all positive integers n? Explain.

16. Does $\binom{n}{n-1} = n$ for all positive integers n? Explain.

17. Explain why $\binom{100}{2} = \binom{99}{2} + 99 = \binom{98}{2} + 98 + 99 = \binom{97}{2} + 97 + 98 + 99$.

18. Explain why $\binom{100}{98} = \binom{99}{97} + 99 = \binom{98}{96} + 98 + 99 = \binom{97}{95} + 97 + 98 + 99$.

19. Explain why $\binom{100}{2} = 1 + 2 + 3 + \cdots + 99 = \binom{100}{98}$.

20. Does $\binom{n+1}{2} = 1 + 2 + 3 + \cdots + n = \binom{n+1}{n-1}$ for $n = 1, 2, \ldots$?

1.2

POWER SETS

In discussing power sets we will provide concrete examples of some algebraic structures that have applications in computer science. These structures are presented in Chapter 2.

| DEFINITION 1 | SUBSET, PROPER SUBSET |

Let A and B be sets. If each element of A is an element of B, then A is a **subset** of B; this may be written as $A \subseteq B$. If $A \subseteq B$ and B has at least one element that is not in A, then A is a **proper subset** of B; this is denoted as $A \subset B$.

Example 1   Let $A = \{0, 1, 4, 9\}$, $D = \{0, 1, 2, 3, 4, 5, 6, 7, 8, 9\}$, and Q consist of the perfect squares in D. Then $A \subseteq D$ and $Q \subseteq D$, since each integer of A, or of Q, is in D. Also, A is a proper subset of D, and we can write the stronger statement $A \subset D$ because D has integers that are not in A, such as 2. It turns out that $A = Q$, so $A \subseteq Q$ is true but A is not a proper subset of Q.   ☐

Clearly $S \subseteq S$ for all sets S. Also, $A \subseteq B$ means that either $A \subset B$ or $A = B$, but not both. Similarly, $A \subset B$ means that both $A \subseteq B$ and $A \neq B$. One way to prove that $A = B$ is to show that both $A \subseteq B$ and $B \subseteq A$.

| NOTATION 1 | EMPTY SET ∅, ELEMENT OF A SET |

The empty set has no elements and is denoted as $\varnothing$. Also, "$x \in S$" means that "x is an element of the set S." (One can read "$x \in S$" as "x belongs to S.")

We agree that $\varnothing \subseteq S$ for all sets S.

DEFINITION 2   **COLLECTION, MEMBER**

A set Γ whose elements are themselves sets will be called a ***collection*** of sets, and an element of Γ will be called a ***member*** of the collection.

DEFINITION 3   **POWER SET FOR A UNIVERSE**

Let S be a set. The collection of all sets A such that $A \subseteq S$ is the ***power set*** for S and is denoted as $P(S)$. Also, S is called the ***universe*** for $P(S)$.

Thus the collection $P(S)$ consists of all the subsets of S. Since the only subset of the empty set $\varnothing$ is $\varnothing$ itself, $P(\varnothing) = \{\varnothing\}$. Also, if $S = \{s\}$ is a singleton, the only subsets of S are $\varnothing$ and S, and so $P(\{s\}) = \{\varnothing, \{s\}\}$. Hence $\#P(S) = 1$ when $\#S = 0$, and $\#P(S) = 2$ when $\#S = 1$.

Example 2   Let $T = \{y, z\}$ and $S = \{x, y, z\}$. The power set for T is

$$P(T) = \{\varnothing, \{z\}, \{y\}, \{y, z\}\}. \tag{1}$$

Since S is the result of adjoining the single element x to T, there is an easy algorithm for obtaining a listing of $P(S)$ from the listing (1) for $P(T)$. First we note that the members A of $P(S)$ for which x is not in A are precisely the members of $P(T)$. The remaining members of $P(S)$, those that contain x, are obtained by adjoining x to each member of $P(T)$. Together, the members of both types give us

$$P(S) = \{\varnothing, \{z\}, \{y\}, \{y, z\}, \{x\}, \{x, z\}, \{x, y\}, \{x, y, z\}\}.$$

We associate a 3-digit binary string $\alpha = a_1 a_2 a_3$ with each member A of $P(S)$ as follows: If x is in A, we let $a_1 = 1$; otherwise we let $a_1 = 0$. We let a_2 be 1 or 0 depending on whether or not y is in A. Similarly, a_3 is 1 or 0 depending on whether or not z is in A. This rule associates the string 110 to the subset $\{x, y\}$ and the string 001 to the subset $\{z\}$.   □

Such characterizations of subsets by binary strings are convenient for computers. We next extend this to any finite set S specified by a given listing.

NOTATION 2   **SUBSET S_α**

For a given listing $S = \{s_1, s_2, \ldots, s_n\}$ of a set of size n and a given binary string $\alpha = a_1 a_2 \ldots a_n$ in $\boldsymbol{B_n}$, the symbol S_α stands for the subset of S consisting of those s_i for which $a_i = 1$.

Using the listing $S = \{s_1, s_2, s_3, s_4\}$ for the universe, we have $S_{0000} = \emptyset$, $S_{0001} = \{s_4\}$, $S_{1010} = \{s_1, s_3\}$, $S_{1110} = \{s_1, s_2, s_3\}$, and $S_{1111} = S$. We note that S_α depends not only on the string α and the set S but also on the order of appearance of the elements of S in the given listing.

THEOREM 1 **CORRESPONDENCE BETWEEN $P(S)$ AND B_n**

Let $S = \{s_1, s_2, \ldots, s_n\}$.

(a) For distinct α and β in B_n, $S_\alpha \neq S_\beta$.
(b) Every member A of $P(S)$ is an S_α for some α in B_n.
(c) $\#S_\alpha = \text{wgt } \alpha$ for each α in B_n.

PROOF (a) Let $\alpha = a_1 a_2 \ldots a_n$ and $\beta = b_1 b_2 \ldots b_n$. If $\alpha \neq \beta$, then α and β differ in some position; that is, $a_i \neq b_i$ for some i in $\{1, 2, \ldots, n\}$. It follows that the element s_i of S is in S_α or in S_β but not in both. Hence $S_\alpha \neq S_\beta$.

(b) Let $A \in P(S)$, that is, let $A \subseteq S$. Define the string $\alpha = a_1 a_2 \ldots a_n$ so that $a_i = 1$ when s_i is in A and $a_i = 0$ when s_i is not in A. Then $A = S_\alpha$.

(c) $\#S_\alpha$ is the number of elements (from S) in S_α. Also, Notation 2 tells us that $\#S_\alpha$ is the number of 1's among the bits a_i of $\alpha = a_1 a_2 \ldots a_n$; that is, $\#S_\alpha = \text{wgt } \alpha$. □

Example 3 Let $S = \{s_1, s_2, s_3\}$. The following table gives wgt α and the member S_α of $P(S)$ for each α in B_3.

α	000	001	010	011	100	101	110	111
wgt α	0	1	1	2	1	2	2	3
S_α	$\emptyset$	$\{s_3\}$	$\{s_2\}$	$\{s_2, s_3\}$	$\{s_1\}$	$\{s_1, s_3\}$	$\{s_1, s_2\}$	S

We note that $\#S_\alpha = \text{wgt } \alpha$ for each α, as stated in Theorem 1(c). □

Next we indicate why $P(S)$ is called "the power set" for S and $\binom{n}{k}$ is read as "n choose k."

THEOREM 2 **NUMBER OF SUBSETS (OF SIZE k) FROM A SET OF SIZE n**

Let $\#S = n$ and k be in $\{0, 1, \ldots, n\}$. Then:

(a) $\#P(S) = 2^{\#S} = 2^n$.
(b) There are $\binom{n}{k}$ ways to choose k elements from the n elements of S, that is, to choose a subset of size k.

PROOF Theorem 1 of Section 1.1 tells us that there are 2^n strings α in B_n. Since there is one and only one member S_α in $P(S)$ for each α in B_n, $\#P(S) = 2^n$. Since $\#S_\alpha = \text{wgt } \alpha$, the number of members A of size k in $P(S)$ is the number $\binom{n}{k}$ of strings of weight k in B_n. □

Example 4 Let $S = \{s_1, s_2, s_3, s_4, s_5\}$. Since $\#S = 5$, then by Theorem 2, $\#P(S) = 2^5 = 32$; that is, there are 32 subsets of S, including $\varnothing$ and S. Also, for each k in $\{0, 1, 2, 3, 4, 5\}$, there are $\binom{5}{k}$ subsets A of S with $\#A = k$. In particular, there is 1 empty subset of S, there are $\binom{5}{1} = 5$ singleton subsets of S, and $\binom{5}{2} = 10$ doubleton subsets of S. □

DEFINITION 4 **RELATIVE COMPLEMENT FOR SETS**

If A and B are any sets, the ***complement of A in B*** is the set consisting of the elements of B that are not in A and is denoted as $B - A$.

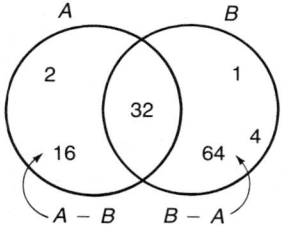

FIGURE 1.2.1

For example, if $A = \{2, 16, 32\}$ and $B = \{1, 4, 32, 64\}$, then $B - A = \{1, 4, 64\}$. Since 16 (or 2) is not in B, it is not in $B - A$. (Whether or not it is in A makes no difference.) The relative complement in the other order is $A - B = \{2, 16\}$. These relative complements are depicted in Figure 1.2.1.

The next two definitions introduce related concepts that use the word *complement*.

DEFINITION 5 **COMPLEMENT OF A SUBSET**

If $A \subseteq S$, that is, if A is in the power set $P(S)$, and the universe S is known from the context, the complement of A in S is called the ***complement*** of A and is written as $\bar{A}$.

For example, if $S = \{+, -, *, \div, \triangle, \square\}$ and $A = \{-, \square\}$, then $\bar{A} = \{+, *, \div, \triangle\}$.

DEFINITION 6 **COMPLEMENT OF A BINARY STRING**

The ***complement*** of a binary string $\alpha = a_1 a_2 \ldots a_n$ is the string $\bar{\alpha} = c_1 c_2 \ldots c_n$ with $c_i = 1 - a_i$ for $i = 1, 2, \ldots, n$.

For example, the complement of $\alpha = 11001$ is $\bar{\alpha} = 00110$. (Replacing 0's by 1's and 1's by 0's in α gives us $\bar{\alpha}$.) Here $\text{wgt } \alpha + \text{wgt } \bar{\alpha} = 3 + 2 = 5$, which is the length of α (or of $\bar{\alpha}$). The connection between complements of members of $P(S)$ and complements of strings will be discussed in Example 7 below.

THEOREM 3   **WEIGHT OF A COMPLEMENT**

If α is in $\boldsymbol{B_n}$, wgt $\bar{\alpha} = n - $ wgt α.

PROOF   Let $\alpha = a_1 a_2 \ldots a_n$ and $\bar{\alpha} = c_1 c_2 \ldots c_n$. Then

$$\begin{aligned}
\text{wgt } \bar{\alpha} &= c_1 + c_2 + \cdots + c_n \\
&= (1 - a_1) + (1 - a_2) + \cdots + (1 - a_n) \\
&= (1 + 1 + \cdots + 1) - (a_1 + a_2 + \cdots + a_n) \\
&= n - \text{wgt } \alpha.
\end{aligned}$$
$\square$

COROLLARY   If α is in $\boldsymbol{B_{n,k}}$, its complement $\bar{\alpha}$ is in $\boldsymbol{B_{n,n-k}}$.

For example, $\alpha = 00110$ is a string of weight 2 in $\boldsymbol{B_5}$ (that is, $\alpha \in \boldsymbol{B_{5,2}}$), and its complement $\bar{\alpha} = 11001$ has weight $5 - 2 = 3$ and so is in $\boldsymbol{B_{5,3}}$.

THEOREM 4   **COMPLEMENTS OF STRINGS, SYMMETRY FORMULA FOR $\binom{n}{k}$**

(a) $\bar{\bar{\alpha}} = \alpha$ for all binary strings α.
(b) If α and β are in $\boldsymbol{B_n}$ and $\alpha \neq \beta$, then $\bar{\alpha} \neq \bar{\beta}$.
(c) Each string in $\boldsymbol{B_{n,n-k}}$ is the complement $\bar{\alpha}$ of a string α in $\boldsymbol{B_{n,k}}$.
(d) $\binom{n}{n-k} = \binom{n}{k}$ for all integers n and k, with $0 \leq k \leq n$. (This is the **symmetry formula** for the binomial coefficients.)

PROOF   (a) Let $\alpha = a_1 a_2 \ldots a_n$ and $\beta = b_1 b_2 \ldots b_n$ be in $\boldsymbol{B_n}$. Then $\bar{\alpha}$ is the string $\gamma = c_1 c_2 \ldots c_n$, with $c_i = 1 - a_i$, and $\bar{\bar{\alpha}} = \bar{\gamma}$ is the string whose ith digit is $1 - (1 - a_i) = 1 - 1 + a_i = a_i$. Hence $\bar{\bar{\alpha}} = \alpha$ and (a) is proved.
(b) If $\alpha \neq \beta$, then $a_i \neq b_i$ for some i. It follows that $1 - a_i \neq 1 - b_i$ for this i, and so $\bar{\alpha} \neq \bar{\beta}$. This proves (b).
(c) Let δ be in $\boldsymbol{B_{n,n-k}}$. Then $\bar{\delta}$ is in $\boldsymbol{B_{n,k}}$ by the corollary to Theorem 3, since $n - (n - k) = k$. Since $\bar{\bar{\delta}} = \delta$ by (a), δ is the complement of the string $\bar{\delta}$ in $\boldsymbol{B_{n,k}}$ and thus (c) is proved.
(d) Parts (b) and (c) imply that there are exactly the same number of strings in $\boldsymbol{B_{n,n-k}}$ as in $\boldsymbol{B_{n,k}}$. This means that $\#\boldsymbol{B_{n,n-k}} = \#\boldsymbol{B_{n,k}}$. Since $\binom{n}{k}$ is defined to be $\#\boldsymbol{B_{n,k}}$, we have $\binom{n}{n-k} = \binom{n}{k}$ and the proof is complete.
$\square$

DEFINITION 7 **INTERSECTION OF THE SETS OF A COLLECTION**

The *intersection* of the sets of a nonempty collection Γ is the set consisting of the objects common to all the sets of Γ and is denoted as

$$\bigcap_{A \in \Gamma} A$$

If $\Gamma = \{A_1, A_2, \ldots, A_n\}$, this intersection is written as $A_1 \cap A_2 \cap \cdots \cap A_n$. Also, one generally drops the braces and uses "intersection of $A_1, A_2, \ldots, A_n$" instead of "intersection of $\{A_1, A_2, \ldots, A_n\}$."

For example if $D = \{0, 1, 2, 3, 4, 5, 6, 7, 8, 9\}$, $P = \{2, 3, 5, 7, 11, 13\}$, and $E = \{2, 4, 6, 8, 10, \ldots\}$ is the set of positive even integers, then $D \cap P = \{2, 3, 5, 7\}$ and $D \cap P \cap E = \{2\}$.

DEFINITION 8 **UNION OF THE SETS OF A COLLECTION**

Let Γ be a nonempty collection of sets. The *union* of the sets of Γ is the set consisting of those objects that are in at least one of the sets A of Γ and is denoted as

$$\bigcup_{A \in \Gamma} A$$

If Γ is a finite collection $\{A_1, A_2, \ldots, A_n\}$, this union is written as $A_1 \cup A_2 \cup \cdots \cup A_n$. Also, one generally drops the braces and uses "union of $A_1, A_2, \ldots, A_n$" instead of "union of $\{A_1, A_2, \ldots, A_n\}$."

For example, if $A = \{<, >, \subseteq, \supseteq\}$, $B = \{<, \leq\}$, and $C = \{\Rightarrow, \Leftrightarrow\}$, then $A \cup B = \{<, \leq, >, \subseteq, \supseteq\}$ and $A \cup B \cup C = \{<, \leq, >, \subseteq, \supseteq, \Rightarrow, \Leftrightarrow\}$. Also, if $\Gamma = \{B_1, B_2, B_3, \ldots\}$, then the union of the members of Γ is the set of binary strings of all positive lengths.

Example 5 Let $A = \{1, 2, 3\}$ and $B = \{3, 4\}$. Then $A \cup B = \{1, 2, 3, 4\}$ and $A \cap B = \{3\}$. Also

$$\#(A \cup B) = \#A + \#B - \#(A \cap B), \tag{2}$$

since $\#(A \cup B) = 4$, $\#A = 3$, $\#B = 2$, and $\#(A \cap B) = 1$. In Problem 19 below, the reader is asked to show that the formula in (2) holds for all finite sets A and B.   □

DEFINITION 9 **DISJOINT SETS**

Sets A and B are *disjoint* if $A \cap B = \varnothing$.

This simply means that A and B are disjoint if and only if they have no element in common. For example, $\{1, 2, 3\}$ and $\{5, 7\}$ are disjoint sets. Also, the set $\{\ldots, -2, 0, 2, \ldots\}$ of even integers and the set $\{\ldots, -3, -1, 1, 3, \ldots\}$ of odd integers are disjoint.

Example 6   If S is a singleton $\{s_1\}$, then $P(S) = \{\varnothing, S\}$ and the complements, unions, and intersections in $P(S)$ are as given in the following tables:

A	$\varnothing$	S
$\bar{A}$	S	$\varnothing$

$\cup$	$\varnothing$	S
$\varnothing$	$\varnothing$	S
S	S	S

$\cap$	$\varnothing$	S
$\varnothing$	$\varnothing$	$\varnothing$
S	$\varnothing$	S

If A and B each represent a member of $P(S)$, then $A \cup B$ would appear as the entry on the row for A and the column for B in the middle table; such a table is called a **matrix table**. The rightmost table is also of matrix type.   □

Example 7   Let $S = \{s_1, s_2\}$ and hence $P(S) = \{S_{00}, S_{01}, S_{10}, S_{11}\} = \{\varnothing, \{s_2\}, \{s_1\}, S\}$. Table 1.2.1 shows, for each A in $P(S)$, the complement $\bar{A}$ of A in S. Table 1.2.2 gives the complement $\bar{\alpha}$ of each binary string α in $\mathbf{B_2}$. Note that S_β is the complement of S_α in S if and only if β is the complement of the string α. In Table 1.2.3 the entry on the row for a subset A of S and the column for a subset B is the union of A and B, and in Table 1.2.4 the entry γ on the row for a string α and the column for a string β denotes the fact that $S_\alpha \cup S_\beta = S_\gamma$. We call Table 1.2.4 the **binary form** of Table 1.2.3; note that in Table 1.2.4 the row labels and column labels appear in the order of the standard listing for $\mathbf{B_2}$.

TABLE 1.2.1

A	$\varnothing$	$\{s_2\}$	$\{s_1\}$	S
$\bar{A}$	S	$\{s_1\}$	$\{s_2\}$	$\varnothing$

TABLE 1.2.2

α	00	01	10	11
$\bar{\alpha}$	11	10	01	00

TABLE 1.2.3

$\cup$	$\varnothing$	$\{s_2\}$	$\{s_1\}$	S
$\varnothing$	$\varnothing$	$\{s_2\}$	$\{s_1\}$	S
$\{s_2\}$	$\{s_2\}$	$\{s_2\}$	S	S
$\{s_1\}$	$\{s_1\}$	S	$\{s_1\}$	S
S	S	S	S	S

TABLE 1.2.4

$\cup$	00	01	10	11
00	00	01	10	11
01	01	01	11	11
10	10	11	10	11
11	11	11	11	11

□

PROBLEMS FOR SECTION 1.2

1. Let $A = \{1, 2, 16\}$ and $S = \{1, 2, 4, 8, 16\}$.
   (i) Find the complement $\bar{A}$ of A in S.
   (ii) Does $\# A + \# \bar{A} = \# S$?
   (iii) Find the complement $\bar{\alpha}$ of $\alpha = 11001$ in B_5.
   (iv) Find wgt α + wgt $\bar{\alpha}$ for the α of Part (iii).

2. Let $S = \{1, 3, 5, 7, 9, 11\}$.
   (i) Copy and fill in the table:

S_α	$\varnothing$	$\{3\}$	$\{1, 7\}$	$\{3, 5, 7, 9\}$	S
α					
$\bar{\alpha}$					
$\bar{S}_\alpha$					

   (ii) Does $\# A + \# \bar{A} = \# S$ for each subset A in the table of Part (i)?
   (iii) Does wgt α + wgt $\bar{\alpha} = 6$ for each α in the table?

3. Let A and B be members of a power set $P(S)$. If $\bar{A} = B$, must $\bar{B} = A$?

4. Let α and β be in B_n. If $\bar{\alpha} = \beta$, must $\bar{\beta} = \alpha$? Explain.

5. Make a table showing the complement $\bar{A}$ of each A in $P(S)$ for the universe $S = \{s_1, s_2, s_3\}$. (This is similar to Table 1.2.1 in Example 7.)

6. (i) Show with a table the complement $\bar{\alpha}$ of each string α in B_3.
   (ii) Does $B_{3,2}$ consist of the complements of the strings in $B_{3,1}$?
   (iii) Does $B_{3,3}$ consist of the complement of the one string in $B_{3,0}$?

7. Let $A = \{1, 3, 5, 7, 9\}$ and $B = \{2, 3, 5, 7\}$.
   (i) Find $A \cup B$.   (ii) Find $A \cap B$.
   (iii) Does $\#(A \cup B) = \# A + \# B - \#(A \cap B)$?

8. Repeat Problem 7, but for $A = \{1, 3, 6, 10, 15\}$ and $B = \{3, 6, 9, 12\}$.

9. Let $S = \{s_1, s_2\}$. Construct a matrix table showing all intersections in $P(S)$. (This should be similar to Table 1.2.3 in Example 7, but with $A \cup B$ replaced by $A \cap B$.)

10. Construct the binary form for the intersection table of Problem 9. (The entry γ on the row for a string α and the column for a string β should denote that $S_\alpha \cap S_\beta = S_\gamma$.)

11. Let $S = \{s_1, s_2, s_3\}$.
   (i) Construct a matrix table showing all intersections in $P(S)$. (This should have 8 rows and 8 columns.)
   (ii) Is there a member E of $P(S)$ such that $A \cap E = A = E \cap A$ for all A in $P(S)$?

12. Repeat Problem 11, but with intersections replaced by unions.

13. (i) Give the binary form for the table of Problem 11(i).
(ii) For what string σ does S_σ equal the set E of Problem 11(ii)?

14. (i) Give the binary form for the table of Problem 12(i).
(ii) Give the string ρ such that $S_\alpha \cup S_\rho = S_\alpha = S_\rho \cup S_\alpha$ for all α in B_3.

15. For $S = \{s_1, s_2, s_3, s_4, s_5\}$, find strings α, β, and γ such that $S_{00101} \cap S_{01100} = S_\alpha$, $S_{00101} \cup S_{01100} = S_\beta$, and $\bar{S}_{00101} = S_\gamma$.

16. For $S = \{s_1, s_2, s_3, s_4, s_5\}$, find strings α, β, and γ such that $S_{11010} \cap S_{10011} = S_\alpha$, $S_{11010} \cup S_{10011} = S_\beta$, and $\bar{S}_{10011} = S_\gamma$.

17. Let $\alpha = a_1 a_2 \ldots a_n$ and $\beta = b_1 b_2 \ldots b_n$ be binary strings in B_n. Describe how to obtain strings $\gamma = c_1 c_2 \ldots c_n$ and $\delta = d_1 d_2 \ldots d_n$ in B_n such that $S_\alpha \cup S_\beta = S_\gamma$ and $S_\alpha \cap S_\beta = S_\delta$.

18. (i) For which strings α in B_3 is $S_\alpha \subseteq S_{011}$?
(ii) For which strings β in B_3 is $S_{100} \subseteq S_\beta$?
(iii) Let $\alpha = a_1 a_2 \ldots a_n$ and $\beta = b_1 b_2 \ldots b_n$ be in B_n. What relationship is needed between the a_i and the b_i to have $S_\alpha \subseteq S_\beta$?

19. Let A and B be finite sets. Explain why:
(i) $\#(A \cup B) = \#A + \#B - \#(A \cap B)$.
(ii) $\#(A \cup B) = \#A + \#B$ if and only if A and B are disjoint.
(iii) $\#(A \cup B) \le \#A + \#B$.

20. Let A, B, and C be finite sets. Explain why:
(i) $\#(A \cup B \cup C) = \#A + \#B + \#C - \#(A \cap B) - \#(A \cap C) - \#(B \cap C) + \#(A \cap B \cap C)$.
(ii) $\#(A \cup B \cup C) \le \#(A \cup B) + \#C \le \#A + \#B + \#C$.
(iii) $\#(A \cup B \cup C) < \#A + \#B + \#C$ if $A \cap B \ne \emptyset$.
(iv) $\#(A \cup B \cup C) = \#A + \#B + \#C$ if each pair of sets from $\{A, B, C\}$ is disjoint.

21. (i) Are any two sets chosen from $B_{3,0}, B_{3,1}, B_{3,2}, B_{3,3}$ disjoint?
(ii) Does $B_{3,0} \cup B_{3,1} \cup B_{3,2} \cup B_{3,3} = B_3$?
(iii) Does $\#B_{3,0} + \#B_{3,1} + \#B_{3,2} + \#B_{3,3} = \#B_3$?
(iv) Does $\binom{3}{0} + \binom{3}{1} + \binom{3}{2} + \binom{3}{3} = 2^3$?

22. (i) Are any two sets chosen from $B_{4,0}, B_{4,1}, B_{4,2}, B_{4,3}, B_{4,4}$ disjoint?
(ii) Does $B_{4,0} \cup B_{4,1} \cup B_{4,2} \cup B_{4,3} \cup B_{4,4} = B_4$?
(iii) Does $\binom{4}{0} + \binom{4}{1} + \binom{4}{2} + \binom{4}{3} + \binom{4}{4} = 2^4$?

23. (a) Is $S \subseteq S$ for all sets S?
(b) Do $A \subseteq B$ and $B \subseteq A$ together imply that $A = B$?
(c) Do $A \subseteq B$ and $B \subseteq C$ together imply that $A \subseteq C$?

24. (a) Does there exist a set S such that $S \subset S$?
(b) Do there exist sets A and B such that both $A \subset B$ and $B \subset A$?
(c) Do $A \subset B$ and $B \subset C$ together imply that $A \subset C$?

25. Let A and B be in $P(S)$ and let $\bar{A}$ be the complement of A in S.

(a) Are A and $\bar{A}$ disjoint?   (b) Does $A \cup \bar{A} = S$?

(c) If $A \cup B = B$, must $A \subseteq B$?   (d) If $A \subseteq B$, must $A \cup B = B$?

26. Let A and B be in $P(S)$ and let $\bar{A}$ be the complement of A in S.
    (a) If $A \cap B = A$, must $A \subseteq B$?
    (b) If $A \subseteq B$, must $A \cap B = A$?
    (c) If $A \cap B = \varnothing$ and $A \cup B = S$, must $B = \bar{A}$?

27. Let U be the union of the sets of a collection Γ. Is $A \subseteq U$ for all A in Γ?

28. Let I be the intersection of the sets of a collection Γ. Is $I \subseteq A$ for all A in Γ?

29. Let S be a nonempty set. Let Γ consist of the nonempty subsets of S; that is, Γ is the complement of $\{\varnothing\}$ in $P(S)$. What must be true of $\#S$ for Γ to have a member L such that $L \subseteq A$ for all A in Γ?

30. Let S be a nonempty set. Let Γ consist of the proper subsets of S; that is, Γ is the complement of $\{S\}$ in $P(S)$. What must be true of $\#S$ for Γ to have a member M such that $A \subseteq M$ for all A in Γ?

31. (a) Is $A \cap B \subseteq A$ and $A \cap B \subseteq B$?
    (b) If $C \subseteq A$ and $C \subseteq B$, is $C \subseteq A \cap B$?

32. (a) Is $A \subseteq A \cup B$ and $B \subseteq A \cup B$?
    (b) If $A \subseteq D$ and $B \subseteq D$, is $A \cup B \subseteq D$?

33. Let $\#A = a$, $\#B = b$, and $\#(A \cup B) = u$.
    (i) What is $\#(A \cap B)$?
    (ii) How many sets C are there with both $C \subseteq A$ and $C \subseteq B$?

34. If $\#A = a$, $\#B = b$, $\#(A \cap B) = c$, and $\#S = s$, then how many sets D satisfy both $A \subseteq D \subseteq S$ and $B \subseteq D \subseteq S$? Explain.

1.3

BASIC SET IDENTITIES

Let A, B, and C be any sets. Then there exists a set S in which each of A, B, and C is a subset; for example, S could be $A \cup B \cup C$. For any subset T of S, let $\bar{T}$ denote the complement of T in S.

Table 1.3.1 presents, for ready reference, twelve properties of complements, unions, and intersections that are basic in set theory and have analogues of similar importance in boolean algebra and symbolic logic. Properties (1) through (10) follow readily from the definitions of complement, union, and intersection (Section 1.2). We assume these properties are true without further proof. Theorem 2 below gives the proof of Property (11). We leave the proof of Property (12) to be worked out in Problem 8 of this section. First we tackle another important result, which has valuable analogues that will be discussed in Chapters 2 and 3. The technique of "proof by case table" will be used frequently in this text.

TABLE 1.3.1

Complement of a Complement	If $\bar{A} = B$, then $\bar{B} = A$, i.e., $\bar{\bar{A}} = A$	(1)
Complements of $\varnothing$ and S	$\bar{\varnothing} = S, \bar{S} = \varnothing$	(2)
Union of Complements	$A \cup \bar{A} = S$	(3)
Intersection of Complements	$A \cap \bar{A} = \varnothing$	(4)
Commutativity for $\cup$	$A \cup B = B \cup A$	(5)
Associativity for $\cup$	$A \cup (B \cup C) = (A \cup B) \cup C$	(6)
Identity for $\cup$	$A \cup \varnothing = A$	(7)
Commutativity for $\cap$	$A \cap B = B \cap A$	(8)
Associativity for $\cap$	$A \cap (B \cap C) = (A \cap B) \cap C$	(9)
Identity for $\cap$	$A \cap S = A$	(10)
Distributivity of $\cap$ over $\cup$	$A \cap (B \cup C) = (A \cap B) \cup (A \cap C)$	(11)
Distributivity of $\cup$ over $\cap$	$A \cup (B \cap C) = (A \cup B) \cap (A \cup C)$	(12)

The following result and its proof mention De Morgan and Venn. Biographical notes on these two mathematicians can be found just before the problem set for this section.

THEOREM 1   DE MORGAN'S LAWS

For any subsets A and B of S,

(a) $\overline{A \cup B} = \bar{A} \cap \bar{B}$,
(b) $\overline{A \cap B} = \bar{A} \cup \bar{B}$.

PROOF   We will prove (a) and leave the proof of (b) to be worked out in Problem 7 below. To prove that $\overline{A \cup B}$ and $\bar{A} \cap \bar{B}$ are equal members of $P(S)$, we have to show that an element s of S is in one of these members if and only if it is in the other member. We do this using four cases, in which the following notation is helpful. Let

$$M_{00} = \bar{A} \cap \bar{B}, \qquad M_{01} = \bar{A} \cap B, \qquad M_{10} = A \cap \bar{B}, \qquad M_{11} = A \cap B.$$

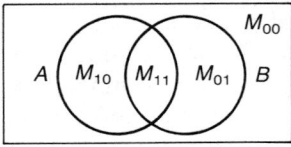

FIGURE 1.3.1

These sets are shown in the **_Venn Diagram_** of Figure 1.3.1, in which the universe S is represented by the inside of the rectangle and A and B are represented by the insides of circles. The four cases are:

(i) s is not in A and is not in B; that is, $s \in M_{00}$.
(ii) s is not in A but is in B; that is, $s \in M_{01}$.
(iii) s is in A but is not in B; that is, $s \in M_{10}$.
(iv) s is in both A and B; that is, $s \in M_{11}$.

Each case has its own row in Table 1.3.2. On a given row, the entry 0 in a column headed by a set T indicates that s is not in T for the case of that row, and an entry 1 indicates that s is in T. The two columns headed A and B are enclosed within vertical lines. On each row, together the two entries in these columns form a 2-digit binary string α; the row has the data for the case in which $s \in M_\alpha$. The order of appearance of these strings α is that of the standard listing for $\mathbf{B_2}$. The column headed $A \cup B$ is obtained from those headed A and B by using the definition of union. The columns headed $\bar{A}$, $\bar{B}$, and $\overline{A \cup B}$ are obtained from those headed A, B, and $A \cup B$, respectively, by using the definition of complement. Finally, the column headed $\bar{A} \cap \bar{B}$ is obtained from the columns headed $\bar{A}$ and $\bar{B}$ by using the definition of intersection. Since the last two columns are identical, an object s is in $\overline{A \cup B}$ if and only if s is in $\bar{A} \cap \bar{B}$. Hence $\overline{A \cup B} = \bar{A} \cap \bar{B}$ for all sets A and B in $P(S)$.

TABLE 1.3.2

Case	A	B	$A \cup B$	$\bar{A}$	$\bar{B}$	$\overline{A \cup B}$	$\bar{A} \cap \bar{B}$
(i)	0	0	0	1	1	1	1
(ii)	0	1	1	1	0	0	0
(iii)	1	0	1	0	1	0	0
(iv)	1	1	1	0	0	0	0

The following concept will help us generalize the case technique of Theorem 1.

DEFINITION 1   **MINISETS**

Let $A_i \subseteq S$ and $\bar{A}_i$ be the complement of A_i in S for $i = 1, 2, \ldots, n$. For each n-digit binary string $\beta = b_1 b_2 \ldots b_n$ let M_β be the intersection $H_1 \cap H_2 \cap \cdots \cap H_n$ in which $H_i = A_i$ if $b_i = 1$ and $H_i = \bar{A}_i$ if $b_i = 0$. Then the M_β are the **minisets** for the members $A_1, A_2, \ldots, A_n$ of $P(S)$.

To obtain the minisets for a finite sequence $A, B, \ldots, K$ of sets, we think of A as A_1, B as A_2, and so on.

Example 1   The eight minisets for a sequence A, B, C of subsets of S are

$$M_{000} = \bar{A} \cap \bar{B} \cap \bar{C}, \qquad M_{001} = \bar{A} \cap \bar{B} \cap C,$$
$$M_{010} = \bar{A} \cap B \cap \bar{C}, \qquad M_{011} = \bar{A} \cap B \cap C,$$
$$M_{100} = A \cap \bar{B} \cap \bar{C}, \qquad M_{101} = A \cap \bar{B} \cap C,$$
$$M_{110} = A \cap B \cap \bar{C}, \qquad M_{111} = A \cap B \cap C.$$

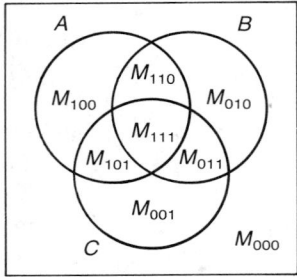

FIGURE 1.3.2

These minisets are depicted in the Venn Diagram of Figure 1.3.2, in which the universe S is represented by the inside of the rectangle and each of A, B, C is represented by the inside of a circle. Any two distinct minisets are disjoint. For example, $M_{100} \cap M_{010} = \varnothing$ because an element of M_{100} is in A and hence is not in $\bar{A}$ or in $M_{010} = \bar{A} \cap B \cap \bar{C}$. Set S is the union of the eight minisets. Also, $A = M_{100} \cup M_{101} \cup M_{110} \cup M_{111}$ is the union of the four minisets M_β, with β of the form $1b_2b_3$, and $A \cap B = M_{110} \cup M_{111}$ is the union of the two minisets M_β, with β of the form $11b_3$. ☐

THEOREM 2   **DISTRIBUTIVITY**

For all sets A, B, and C,

(a) $A \cap (B \cup C) = (A \cap B) \cup (A \cap C)$;

(b) $A \cup (B \cap C) = (A \cup B) \cap (A \cup C)$.

PROOF   In Table 1.3.3 the fact that the column headed $A \cap (B \cup C)$ is identical to the column headed $(A \cap B) \cup (A \cap C)$ proves (a); the proof of (b) is left to the reader as Problem 8 below. In Table 1.3.3 the first three binary digits on a row (i.e., the digits before the vertical line) form a binary string α, and the data on the row is for the case in which an element s of the universe is in the miniset M_α. An entry 1 in a column headed by a set T indicates that s is in T for the case of the entry's row, and an entry 0 means that s is not in T. The strings α that characterize the rows appear in the order of the standard listing for B_3.

TABLE 1.3.3

A	B	C	$B \cup C$	$A \cap (B \cup C)$	$A \cap B$	$A \cap C$	$(A \cap B) \cup (A \cap C)$
0	0	0	0	0	0	0	0
0	0	1	1	0	0	0	0
0	1	0	1	0	0	0	0
0	1	1	1	0	0	0	0
1	0	0	0	0	0	0	0
1	0	1	1	1	0	1	1
1	1	0	1	1	1	0	1
1	1	1	1	1	1	1	1

☐

It greatly facilitates the work of checking a case table (by a human grader or by a machine) if all the people constructing a given table use the same order of appearance for the rows. For this reason, we make the following requirement.

REQUIREMENT 1   **ORDER OF APPEARANCE OF ROWS OF A CASE TABLE**

The binary strings of a B_n that characterize the rows of a case table must appear in the order of the standard listing for B_n.

Example 2   The formula $(B \cap C) \cup A = (B \cup A) \cap (C \cup A)$ could be proved using a case table with 8 rows, but instead we see that

$$(B \cap C) \cup A = A \cup (B \cap C) = (A \cup B) \cap (A \cup C)$$
$$= (B \cup A) \cap (C \cup A)$$

using Properties (5), (12), and (5), respectively, from Table 1.3.1.   □

Example 3   Property (10) can be reworded to state that $A \cap S = A$ whenever $A \subseteq S$. Since $A \subseteq A$ for all sets A, this means that $A \cap A = A$ for all sets A.   □

Example 4   We see that

$$A = A \cup \varnothing = A \cup (A \cap \bar{A}) = (A \cup A) \cap (A \cup \bar{A})$$
$$= (A \cup A) \cap S = A \cup A$$

using Properties (7), (4), (12), (3), and (10), respectively. Hence $A = A \cup A$.   □

Augustus De Morgan,   *an English mathematician, was born in India in 1806. He studied at Trinity College, Cambridge, which has been famous since before the time of Newton for its mathematicians and scientists. Unwilling to agree to the religious test necessary for an appointment at Oxford or Cambridge, he took a chair at the University of London at the age of 22 and remained there almost continuously until 1866. Founder and first president of the London Mathematical Society, he also helped found the British Association for the Advancement of Science. He collected amusing stories and anecdotes, many of them published in his Budget of Paradoxes. De Morgan was a pioneer in the development of abstract ideas in algebra. He died in 1871.*

John Venn,   *an English mathematician interested in probability and logic, was born in 1834. His highly regarded Symbolic Logic was published in 1881. The diagrams named for him and known to every student of set theory and logic appeared in 1876 in his paper on Boole (although such diagrams had been used much earlier, by Euler). Venn died in 1923.*

PROBLEMS FOR SECTION 1.3

1. Use Property (7) of Table 1.3.1, with $A = \varnothing$, to find $\varnothing \cup \varnothing$. Check using Example 4.

2. Use Property (10) of Table 1.3.1, with $A = S$, to find $S \cap S$. Check using Example 3.

3. Draw a Venn Diagram for subsets A, B, C of S that shows M_{011} to be empty and the seven other minisets as nonempty.

4. Repeat Problem 3, but with M_{011} replaced by M_{100}.

5. Prove with a case table that $A \cap (A \cup B) = A$.

6. (a) Use Properties (8) and (11) of Table 1.3.1 to prove that

$$(B \cup C) \cap A = (B \cap A) \cup (C \cap A).$$

   (b) Prove with a case table that $A \cup (A \cap B) = A$.

7. Prove with a case table that $\overline{A \cap B} = \bar{A} \cup \bar{B}$. [This is Theorem 1(b), which was earlier left unproved.]

8. Prove with a case table that $A \cup (B \cap C) = (A \cup B) \cap (A \cup C)$. [This is Property (12) of Table 1.3.1, which was earlier left unproved.]

9. Using the notations of Example 1, express each of the following as a union of minisets.
   (a) B;   (b) $\bar{A} \cap B$;   (c) $B \cup C$.

10. Repeat Problem 9 for the following.
   (a) C;   (b) $\bar{B} \cup C$;   (c) $B \cap C$;   (d) $\bar{B} \cap C$;
   (e) $(B \cap C) \cup (\bar{B} \cap C)$.

11. Using the notations of Example 1, explain why $A \subseteq B$ if and only if $M_{100} = \varnothing = M_{101}$; that is, do both of the following.
   (i) Given that $M_{100} = \varnothing = M_{101}$, explain why $A \subseteq B$.
   (ii) Given that $A \subseteq B$, explain why $M_{100} = \varnothing = M_{101}$.

12. Using the notations of Example 1, explain why $A \subseteq \bar{B}$ if and only if $M_{110} = \varnothing = M_{111}$; that is, explain why:
   (i) if $M_{110} = \varnothing = M_{111}$, then $A \subseteq \bar{B}$.
   (ii) if $A \subseteq \bar{B}$, then $M_{110} = \varnothing = M_{111}$.

13. The *dual* of any of the basic identities listed in Table 1.3.1 is obtained by interchanging $\cup$ and $\cap$ while simultaneously interchanging $\varnothing$ and the universe S. For example, the dual of Property (3) is Property (4).
   (a) Which property is the dual of Property (5)?
   (b) Which property is the dual of Property (9)?

14. (a) Which property is the dual (as defined in Problem 13) of Property (7)?
   (b) Is the dual of each of Properties (1) through (12) also one of these properties?

15. Let A and B be subsets of S and let $\bar{A}$ be the complement of A in S. Use the notation and Venn Diagram of Theorem 1 to tell whether or not each of the following is true.
  (i) $\bar{A} \cup B = M_{00} \cup M_{01} \cup M_{11}$.
  (ii) $A \subseteq B$ if and only if $M_{10} = \emptyset$.
  (iii) $\bar{A} \cup B = S$ if and only if $A \subseteq B$.
  (iv) $A - B = \bar{B} - \bar{A}$.

16. Repeat Problem 15 for the following parts.
  (a) $\bar{A} \cup \bar{B} = M_{10} \cup M_{01} \cup M_{00}$.   (b) $\bar{A} \cap \bar{B} = M_{00}$.

17. Let A and B be sets with $A \cap B = \emptyset$ and $A \neq \emptyset$. Can $A = B$? Explain.

18. What is the only possibility for sets A and B if $A \cap B = \emptyset$ and $A = B$?

19. Give an example of sets A, B, C such that $A \neq B$, $C \neq \emptyset$, and $A \cap C = B \cap C$.

20. (a) Give an example of sets A, B, C such that $A \neq B$ and $A \cup C = B \cup C$.
  *(b) Prove that $A \cup C = B \cup C$ and $A \cap C = B \cap C$ together imply that $A = B$. (The asterisk here indicates that this part is a difficult problem. In general, asterisks are applied to optional material.)

*21. Draw a Venn Diagram in which $M_{1010} = \emptyset = M_{0101}$ and in which the other 14 minisets for subsets A, B, C, D of S are shown as nonempty.

1.4
CARTESIAN PRODUCTS AND RELATIONS

Present-day civilization is very complicated and is getting more so. To cope with our complex problems, we need maximum benefit from the accumulated knowledge from previous years and this requires efficient methods for filing information and retrieving desired information from files. Large collections of data are now stored in computer memories; we search in them with the help of computers. The theory of efficient organization of such databanks uses the concepts of this section and of the rest of this chapter. Examples 8 and 9 below are indications of these applications.

The n terms a_i of a **finite sequence** $a_1, a_2, \ldots, a_n$ do not have to be distinct. An **ordered n-tuple** $(a_1, a_2, \ldots, a_n)$ is a sequence of n terms enclosed within parentheses. Interchanging terms a_i and a_j, with $a_i \neq a_j$, creates a new ordered n-tuple. An ordered 2-tuple (a, b) is called an **ordered pair**; an ordered 3-tuple (a, b, c) is an **ordered triple**.

For example, $(1, 1)$ is an ordered pair. Also, $(1, 2)$ and $(2, 1)$ are two different ordered pairs. Similarly, $(4, 4, 4)$ is an ordered triple, and $(1, 1, 2)$,

(1, 2, 1), (2, 1, 1) are the three distinct ordered triples made using different orderings of the terms 1, 1, and 2.

We note that $(a_1, a_2, \ldots, a_n) = (b_1, b_2, \ldots, b_n)$ if and only if $a_i = b_i$ for $i = 1, 2, \ldots, n$, that is, if and only if $a_1 = b_1, a_2 = b_2, \ldots, a_n = b_n$.

DEFINITION 1   **CARTESIAN PRODUCT**

The *cartesian product* $S_1 \times S_2 \times \cdots \times S_n$ of a sequence $S_1, S_2, \ldots, S_n$ of sets consists of all ordered n-tuples $(s_1, s_2, \ldots, s_n)$ having s_i in S_i for $i = 1, 2, \ldots, n$. When $S_i = S$ for all i, $S_1 \times S_2 \times \cdots \times S_n$ is denoted as S^n.

The adjective "cartesian" derives from the name of René Descartes; see the biographical note just before the problems for this section.

Example 1   Let $S = \{1, 2, 3\}$ and $T = \{a, b, c, d\}$. We display the ordered pairs (s, t) of $S \times T$ in matrix form using s as the row label and t as the column label:

s \ t	a	b	c	d
1	$(1, a)$	$(1, b)$	$(1, c)$	$(1, d)$
2	$(2, a)$	$(2, b)$	$(2, c)$	$(2, d)$
3	$(3, a)$	$(3, b)$	$(3, c)$	$(3, d)$

We see that $\#(S \times T) = (\#S)(\#T) = 3 \cdot 4 = 12$. Also, $S \times T \neq T \times S$ because $(1, a)$ is in $S \times T$ but is not in $T \times S$. It can be shown that $S \times T \neq T \times S$ unless $S = T$ or $S = \varnothing$ or $T = \varnothing$ (see Problems 5 and 6 below).   □

Example 2   Let $A = \{a, b, c\}$ and $B = \{0, 1\}$. Then

$A \times B = \{(a, 0), (a, 1), (b, 0), (b, 1), (c, 0), (c, 1)\}$,

$B \times A = \{(0, a), (1, a), (0, b), (1, b), (0, c), (1, c)\}$,

$\quad B^3 = \{(0, 0, 0), (0, 0, 1), (0, 1, 0), (0, 1, 1), (1, 0, 0), (1, 0, 1), (1, 1, 0), (1, 1, 1)\}$.

We note that $A \times B$ and $B \times A$ are different sets, each with six ordered pairs. Also, if the parentheses and commas are deleted from the ordered triples of B^3, we obtain the 3-digit binary strings of $\boldsymbol{B_3}$.   □

Example 3   Let $A = \{a, b\}$, $B = \{+, -, *, \div\}$, and $C = \{1, 2, 3\}$. Then $A \times B \times C$ consists of 24 ordered triples, including

$\quad (a, +, 1), \quad (a, -, 1), \quad (a, *, 1), \quad (a, \div, 1),$

$\quad (b, +, 1), \quad (b, -, 1), \quad (b, *, 1), \quad (b, \div, 1),$

together with eight more obtained from these by replacing 1 with 2, plus the final eight obtained by replacing 1 with 3. □

Now we use cartesian products to formalize the concept of relations.

DEFINITION 2 **RELATION FOR $S_1, S_2, \ldots, S_n$**

A *relation* for a sequence $S_1, S_2, \ldots, S_n$ of sets is a subset of the cartesian product $S_1 \times S_2 \times \cdots \times S_n$. A relation for a sequence A, B of two sets is a *relation from A to B*.

For example, $R = \{(1, a), (1, b), (2, d)\}$ is a relation from $X = \{1, 2, 3\}$ to $Y = \{a, b, c, d\}$.

DEFINITION 3 **n-ARY RELATION ON S**

An *n-ary relation* on a nonempty set S is a subset of the cartesian product $S^n = S \times S \times \cdots \times S$ of n copies of S. A 2-ary relation is called a *binary relation*.

We see that an n-ary relation on S is a member of $P(S^n)$, and hence a binary relation on S is a member of $P(S \times S)$.

Example 4 Let A be the set of all living people, B be the subset of females in A, and C be the subset of males in A. Let R be the set of ordered triples (a, b, c) in $A \times B \times C$ such that b is the mother of a and c is the father. Then R is a relation for A, B, C.

The "is a square root of" binary relation on the set $S = \{-2, -1, 0, 1, 2, 3, 4\}$ is the subset

$$R = \{(-2, 4), (-1, 1), (0, 0), (1, 1), (2, 4)\}$$

of $S \times S$ consisting of all ordered pairs (a, b) satisfying the simultaneous conditions

$$a \in S, \qquad b \in S, \qquad \text{and} \qquad a^2 = b. \qquad \square$$

DEFINITION 4 **RELATION MATRIX**

Let R be a relation from A to B. If A and B are finite, the *(relation) matrix* for R is the table with a row for each a in A and a column for each b in B in which the entry on the row for a and column for b is 1 if (a, b) is in R and is 0 if (a, b) is not in R.

In the relation matrix for a binary relation R on a finite set S, the roles of A and B in Definition 4 are each taken by S.

In the two following examples, we illustrate first a relation from a set A to a set B and then a binary relation on a set [which happens to be a power set $P(S)$].

Example 5   The "less than" relation from $A = \{2, 4\}$ to $B = \{1, 3, 5\}$ is the subset $R = \{(2, 3), (2, 5), (4, 5)\}$ of $A \times B$. The matrix for R is

R	1	3	5
2	0	1	1
4	0	0	1

$\square$

Example 6   The "is a proper subset of" binary relation on a power set $P(S)$ consists of all ordered pairs (A, B) in $P(S) \times P(S)$, with $A \subset B$. When $S = \{s_1, s_2\}$, we can write $P(S)$ as $\{S_{00}, S_{01}, S_{10}, S_{11}\}$; the matrix for this relation is as follows:

$\subset$	S_{00}	S_{01}	S_{10}	S_{11}
S_{00}	0	1	1	1
S_{01}	0	0	0	1
S_{10}	0	0	0	1
S_{11}	0	0	0	0

$\square$

NOTATION 1   *aRb*

Let R be a relation from A to B. Then aRb denotes that (a, b) is in the subset R of $A \times B$. One reads aRb as "a is related to b (under R)." In specific examples R may be replaced by another letter or by an appropriate symbol, such as $<, \leq, >, \geq, \subset, \subseteq, \supset,$ or $\supseteq$.

In Example 5, aRb would usually be written as $a < b$. Also, in the notation $A \subset B$ for the proper inclusion relation of Example 6, the symbol $\subset$ plays the role of R.

Since a binary relation R on a set S is a subset of the cartesian product $S \times S$, the complement $\bar{R}$ of R in $S \times S$ is also a binary relation on S.

NOTATION 2 *a$\bar{R}$b*, COMPLEMENTARY RELATION

The notation $a\bar{R}b$ means that (a, b) is not in R or, equivalently, that (a, b) is in the **complementary relation** $\bar{R}$. [One may read $a\bar{R}b$ as "a is not related to b (under R)."]

For example, if $S = \{1, 2, 3\}$ and R is the binary relation

$$R = \{(1, 1), (1, 2), (2, 2), (2, 3), (3, 1)\}$$

on S, then the complementary relation is

$$\bar{R} = \{(1, 3), (2, 1), (3, 2), (3, 3)\},$$

and hence we have $1\bar{R}3$, $2\bar{R}1$, $3\bar{R}2$, and $3\bar{R}3$. Clearly, this R and $\bar{R}$ satisfy $R \cap \bar{R} = \emptyset$ and $R \cup \bar{R} = S \times S$.

Also, if R represents $=$, then $\bar{R}$ denotes $\neq$.

DEFINITION 5 REVERSE OF A RELATION

The **reverse** of a binary relation R on a set S is the binary relation V on S such that $(a, b) \in V$ if and only if $(b, a) \in R$; that is, aVb if and only if bRa.

Example 7 On the set $N = \{0, 1, 2, \ldots\}$, the "less than" relation $<$ and the "greater than" relation $>$ are reverses of each other; also, $\leq$ and $\geq$ are reverses of each other. The reverse of the binary relation $R = \{(n, n + 1) : n \in N\} = \{(0, 1), (1, 2), (2, 3), \ldots\}$ on N is $V = \{(n + 1, n) : n \in N\} = \{(1, 0), (2, 1), (3, 2), \ldots\}$. On a power set $P(S)$, $\subseteq$ and $\supseteq$ are reverses of each other, as are $\subset$ and $\supset$. □

Example 8 Let P be the set of people employed by a large organization and T be a set of specialized tasks that might have to be performed at some future time. Let R be the relation from P to T in which pRt means that p has the talent and knowledge needed for successful performance of task t. It may be very valuable to store all the ordered pairs (p, t) of R in a computer's memory and to have a program that, for any given task t_0, prints the set of all p such that pRt_0. □

Example 9 Let X be a set of key phrases such as "data storage" or "database search." Let Y be the set of books and reprints of research papers available in some large library. Let R be the relation from X to Y in which xRy means that reference work y has information concerning the topic of key phrase x. Many university libraries store the ordered pairs (x, y) of such an R in a file and have computer programs for listing, for a given x in X, all the books or papers y such that xRy.   □

René Descartes   *was born in la Haye, France, in 1596. He first studied to be a lawyer and later studied mathematics with Mersenne in Paris. In 1617 he joined the first of several armies he was to be attached to, and in 1628 he moved to Holland. It was about this time that Descartes had his idea for analytic geometry, published as part of his Discours de la Méthode in 1637. Descartes was as much philosopher as · mathematician, but his mathematical work extends beyond just analytic geometry. His work on tangents was an early precursor of the calculus. In 1649 Descartes went to Stockholm at the request of Queen Christina, but the Swedish winter turned out to be too much for him and he died of pneumonia the following year.*

PROBLEMS FOR SECTION 1.4

1. For each of the following, tell whether it is a pair, an ordered pair, a triple, or an ordered triple.
   (a) $\{x_1, x_2\}$;   (b) (x, y, z);   (c) (x, y);   (d) $\{x_1, x_2, x_3\}$.

2. Repeat Problem 1 for the following:
   (a) $(1, 1)$;   (b) $(1, 2, 3)$;   (c) $\{1, 2\}$;   (d) $\{1, 2, 3\}$.

3. (a) Does $\{1, 2, 3, 4\} = \{4, 3, 2, 1\}$?
   (b) Does $(1, 2, 3, 4) = (4, 3, 2, 1)$?

4. (a) Is $\{1, 3, 5, 7, 9\}$ the same set as $\{1, 5, 9, 3, 7\}$?
   (b) Is $(1, 1, 1, 2, 2)$ the same ordered 5-tuple as $(1, 2, 1, 2, 1)$?

5. Let $A = \{1, 2\}$ and $B = \{1, 2, 3\}$.
   (i) List the six ordered pairs of $A \times B$.
   (ii) List the six ordered pairs of $B \times A$.
   (iii) Which ordered pairs are common to $A \times B$ and $B \times A$?
   (iv) Are there ordered pairs of $A \times B$ that are not in $B \times A$?
   (v) Are $A \times B$ and $B \times A$ equal for these sets A and B?

6. Let A and B be nonempty sets. Explain why $A \times B = B \times A$ if and only if $A = B$.

7. Let $S = \{1, 2, 3\}$ and let R be the binary relation on S with

   $$R = \{(1, 2), (2, 3), (3, 1)\}.$$

   (a) Give the ordered pairs of the complementary relation $\bar{R}$.
   (b) Give the ordered pairs of the reverse V of R.
   (c) Give the relation matrices for R, $\bar{R}$, and V.

8. Let $S = \{s_1, s_2\}$ and $P(S) = \{S_{00}, S_{01}, S_{10}, S_{11}\}$. Give the relation matrices for the following binary relations on $P(S)$:
   (a) the "is a subset of" relation $\subseteq$;
   (b) the complementary relation of $\subseteq$;
   (c) the reverse $\supseteq$ of $\subseteq$.

9. Let $B_2 = \{00, 01, 10, 11\}$ and R be the binary relation on B_2, with
   $$R = \{(00, 00), (00, 11), (11, 00), (11, 11)\}.$$
   (a) Write $\alpha \bar{R} \beta$ for each (α, β) in $\bar{R}$.
   (b) List the ordered pairs (α, β) of the reverse V of R.

10. Give the relation matrices for the R, $\bar{R}$, and V of Problem 9.

11. Let R be a binary relation on a nonempty set S.
    (i) How does one obtain the matrix for the complementary relation $\bar{R}$ from the matrix for R?
    (ii) Can $\bar{R} = R$? Explain.

12. Repeat Problem 11, but with $\bar{R}$ replaced by the reverse V of R.

13. Let $S = \{1, 2, 3\}$. For each of the following binary relations R on S, tell which of the symbols $<, \leq, >, \geq$ is an appropriate replacement for the letter R in the aRb notation:
    (a) $R = \{(1, 2), (1, 3), (2, 3)\}$.
    (b) $R = \{(1, 1), (2, 1), (2, 2), (3, 1), (3, 2), (3, 3)\}$.

14. Repeat Problem 13, but for the following R's:
    (a) $R = \{(2, 1), (3, 1), (3, 2)\}$.
    (b) $R = \{(1, 1), (1, 2), (1, 3), (2, 2), (2, 3), (3, 3)\}$.

15. Let $A = \{a\}$, $B = \{b\}$, $S = \{a, b\}$, $X = \{\varnothing, A, B, S\}$, and
    $$R = \{(\varnothing, A), (\varnothing, B), (\varnothing, S), (A, S), (B, S)\}.$$
    Which one of the symbols $\subset, \subseteq, \supset, \supseteq$ is appropriate for the binary relation R on X?

16. Repeat Problem 15 for:
    $$R = \{(A, \varnothing), (B, \varnothing), (S, \varnothing), (S, A), (S, B)\}.$$

17. Let N be the set $\{0, 1, 2, \ldots\}$ of natural numbers and $T = \{0, 1, 3\}$. List the ordered triples (n, t_1, t_2) of the relation R for N, T, T specified by the condition $n = t_1 + t_2$.

18. Repeat Problem 17, but with $\{0, 1, 3\}$ replaced by $\{0, 1, 3, 6\}$.

19. Let $S = \{1, 2, 3, \ldots, 20\}$. List the ordered triples (a, b, c) of the ternary relation R on S specified by $a^2 + b^2 = c^2$.

20. Which of the ordered triples (a, b, c) of Problem 19 have $a < b$?

21. Let $A = \{0, 1\}$, $B = \{a, b, c\}$, and $C = \{d, e\}$. Find:
    (i) $A \times B$;   (ii) $A \times C$;   (iii) $(A \times B) \cup (A \times C)$;
    (iv) $B \cup C$;   (v) $A \times (B \cup C)$.

22.   (a) Let $A = \{0, 1\}$, $B = \{a, b, c\}$, and $C = \{c, d\}$. Find $A \times (B \cup C)$ and $(A \times B) \cup (A \times C)$.
  (b) Does $A \times (B \cup C) = (A \times B) \cup (A \times C)$ for all sets A, B, C? Explain.

23.   Let $A = \{1, 2, 3\}$ and $B = \{a, b, c, d, e\}$.
  (i) How many of the ordered pairs (x, y) of $A \times B$ have $x = 1$?
  (ii) How many (x, y) in $A \times B$ have $x = 2$?
  (iii) What is $\#(A \times B)$; that is, how many (x, y) are there in $A \times B$?
  (iv) What is $\#P(A \times B)$; that is, how many subsets does $A \times B$ have?

24.   Let $\#A = m$ and $\#B = n$. Give:
  (i) $\#(A \times B)$;   (ii) $\#P(A \times B)$.

25.   Let $A = \{1, 2, 3\}$, $\#B = 4$, $\#C = 8$, and $D = A \times B \times C$.
  (i) How many of the ordered triples (a, b, c) of D have $a = 1$?
  (ii) How many (a, b, c) of D have $a = 2$?
  (iii) How many (a, b, c) of D have $a = 3$?
  (iv) What is $\#(A \times B \times C)$?
  (v) What is $\#P(A \times B \times C)$?

26.   Given that $\#A = r$, $\#B = s$, and $\#C = t$, write the values of:
  (i) $\#(A \times B \times C)$;   (ii) $\#P(A \times B \times C)$.

27.   If S and T are finite, does $\#(S \times T) = \#(T \times S)$? Explain.

28.   Let A, B, and C be sets. When does $A \times B \times C = B \times A \times C$? When does $\#(A \times B \times C) = \#(B \times A \times C)$?

29.   Given that $\#A_i = r_i$ for $i = 1, 2, \ldots, n$, find $\#(A_1 \times A_2 \times \cdots \times A_n)$.

30.   Given that $\#A_i = r_i$ for $i = 1, 2, \ldots, n$, find $\#P(A_1 \times A_2 \times \cdots \times A_n)$.

31.   A store stocks shirts of 13 different neck sizes. Each neck size is available in 5 sleeve sizes. Each neck and sleeve size is available in 7 colors. How many different shirts are stocked?

1.5

SPECIAL PROPERTIES OF BINARY RELATIONS

Definition 1 below lists five properties that a binary relation R on a set S may or may not have. Various combinations of these properties characterize important types of relations. For example, Properties (i), (iv), and (v) of Definition 1 are possessed by the order relations involved in computer sorting and filing of data that the next section will develop. Each relation in this section is a binary relation on some set.

The matrix for a binary relation R on a finite set S is a *square matrix*; that is, it has as many rows as columns. The *main diagonal* of a square matrix is the diagonal from the top left to the bottom right. A square matrix is *symmetric* (about its main diagonal) if its ith row is identical with its ith column for all values of i; that is, the matrix is symmetric if it goes into itself when flipped about the main diagonal.

DEFINITION 1   SPECIAL BINARY RELATIONS

Let R be a binary relation on a set S. Then:

(i) R is ***reflexive*** if sRs for all s in S.
(ii) R is ***irreflexive*** if $s\bar{R}s$ for all s in S, that is, if and only if sRs for no s in S.
(iii) R is ***symmetric*** if bRa whenever aRb.
(iv) R is ***antisymmetric*** if aRb and bRa together imply that $a = b$.
(v) R is ***transitive*** if aRb and bRc together imply that aRc.

For each of the first three properties of Definition 1, we next illustrate the use of the relation matrix to see whether R has the property. The other properties of Definition 1 are illustrated in Examples 2 and 3 below.

Example 1   Let $S = \{a, b, c\}$ and let U, V, and W be the binary relations on S having the matrices of Table 1.5.1. The relation U is reflexive, since its incidence matrix has a main diagonal consisting solely of 1's. Relation V is irreflexive, since its main diagonal has just 0's. Finally, relation W is neither reflexive nor irreflexive, since its main diagonal has at least one 0 and at least one 1. Thus "irreflexive" does not mean "not reflexive." The only matrix of Table 1.5.1 that is symmetric about its main diagonal is the matrix for W. Hence W is a symmetric binary relation on S, but neither U nor V is symmetric.

TABLE 1.5.1

U	a	b	c
a	1	1	1
b	0	1	1
c	0	0	1

V	a	b	c
a	0	1	0
b	0	0	1
c	0	0	0

W	a	b	c
a	1	0	0
b	0	1	0
c	0	0	0

We next formalize, for a general binary relation R on a set S, the observations of Example 1.

THEOREM 1   PROPERTIES SEEN FROM A RELATION MATRIX

Let Δ be the main diagonal of the matrix M for a binary relation R on a finite set S. Then R is reflexive if and only if Δ consists solely of 1's; R is irreflexive if and only if Δ consists solely of 0's. Relation R is symmetric if and only if its relation matrix M is symmetric (about Δ).

PROOF   This is just a restatement of Definition 1(i), (ii), and (iii) in terms of the matrix. $\square$

Problem 14(b) below will ask how one can tell whether a binary relation R on S is antisymmetric from the matrix for R.

Example 2   Let $S = \{1, 2\}$ and R be the binary relation $\{(1, 1), (1, 2)\}$ on S. Since sRs holds for $s = 1$ but not for $s = 2$, the relation R is neither reflexive nor irreflexive. Relation R is not symmetric, since $(1, 2)$ is in R but its reverse $(2, 1)$ is not in R. Also, R is antisymmetric, since aRb and bRa hold simultaneously only when $a = 1 = b$; then $1R1$ and $1R1$ together do imply that $1 = 1$. Similarly R is transitive, since aRb and bRc hold simultaneously only when $a = 1 = b$ and then $1R1$ and $1Rc$ together imply $1Rc$ for each c in S.   □

Example 3   Let S be a nonempty set. The "is a subset of" binary relation $\subseteq$ on the power set $P(S)$ is reflexive, since $A \subseteq A$ for all A in $P(S)$; this also shows that $\subseteq$ is not irreflexive. Since $\varnothing$ is a subset of S but S is not a subset of $\varnothing$, the relation $\subseteq$ is not symmetric. Since $A \subseteq B$ and $B \subseteq A$ together imply that $A = B$, the relation $\subseteq$ is antisymmetric. Since $A \subseteq B$ and $B \subseteq C$ together imply that $A \subseteq C$, this relation is transitive.

Let S still be a nonempty set and now let γ be the relation on $P(S)$ for which $A\gamma B$ means that A is the complement $\bar{B}$ of B in S. Since S is nonempty, no A in $P(S)$ is its own complement; hence γ is irreflexive and is not reflexive. Since $A = \bar{B}$ implies that $B = \bar{A}$, γ is symmetric. Since $\varnothing\gamma S$ and $S\gamma\varnothing$ but $\varnothing \neq S$, γ is not antisymmetric. Also, γ is not transitive, since $S\gamma\varnothing$ and $\varnothing\gamma S$ but $S\bar{\gamma}S$.   □

DEFINITION 2   **PICTURE FOR A BINARY RELATION**

A *picture* for a binary relation R on S is a figure whose *vertices* are points representing the elements of S and with an *arc from* vertex v *to* vertex w (having an arrowhead pointing toward w) if and only if vRw. A *loop* at vertex v is an arc from v to itself. Each loop is assumed to have an arrowhead, though it is not always shown.

Example 4   The picture for the binary relation

$$R = \{(1, 1), (1, 2), (2, 1), (2, 2), (3, 2)\}$$

on $S = \{1, 2, 3\}$ has loops at some vertices but not all (see Figure 1.5.1). Hence R is neither irreflexive nor reflexive. This shows that "irreflexive" is not equivalent to "not reflexive." Since there is an arc from 3 to 2 but no arc from 2 to 3, R is not symmetric. Also, R is not antisymmetric, since there are arcs both from 1 to 2 and from 2 to 1 (but $1 \neq 2$). Hence "antisymmetric" is not equivalent to "not symmetric." The fact that there is an arc from 3 to 2 and an arc from 2 to 1 but no arc from 3 to 1 shows that R is not transitive.   □

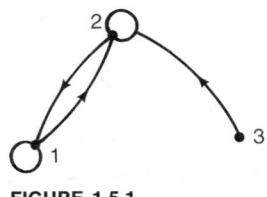

FIGURE 1.5.1

DEFINITION 3   PATH IN A RELATION

A *path* of *length* n in a binary relation R on S is an ordered $(n + 1)$-tuple $(s_0, s_1, \ldots, s_n)$ such that $s_{i-1}Rs_i$ for $i = 1, 2, \ldots, n$. This path is *from* s_0, the *initial vertex*, *to* s_n, the *final vertex*.

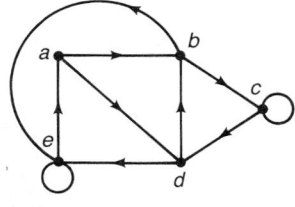

FIGURE 1.5.2

For example, in Figure 1.5.2, some of the paths from a to e are (a, d, e), (a, b, e), (a, b, e, e), (a, b, c, d, e), (a, b, c, c, d, e), (a, d, b, c, c, d, e), and $(a, b, e, a, d, b, c, d, e)$. These paths have lengths 2, 2, 3, 4, 5, 6, and 8, respectively. The last of these paths uses each of the arcs exactly once, and several of the paths go through each of the five vertices. We also note that vertices and arcs may be repeated in a path.

The relation R depicted in Figure 1.5.2 is not transitive, since there is a path of length 2 from a to c but no path of length 1 from a to c; that is, aRb and bRc but $a\bar{R}c$.

Example 5   Let S be any set. Since $S \times S$ is a subset of itself, $S \times S$ is a binary relation on S. Also, the set D of all ordered pairs (s, s) with s in S is a binary relation on S.   □

DEFINITION 4   COMPLETE RELATION, DIAGONAL RELATION

The *complete relation* on a set S is $K = S \times S$. The *diagonal relation* on S is the relation D on S such that xDy if and only if $x = y$; that is, "the diagonal relation" on S is another name for "equality."

Example 6   For $S = \{1, 2\}$, the diagonal relation is $D = \{(1, 1), (2, 2)\}$ and the complete relation is $K = \{(1, 1), (1, 2), (2, 1), (2, 2)\}$.   □

PROBLEMS FOR SECTION 1.5

1. Let $S = \{s_1, s_2\}$, $P(S) = \{S_{00}, S_{01}, S_{10}, S_{11}\}$ and $\subset$ be the "is a proper subset of" binary relation on $P(S)$.
   (a) Give the set of ordered pairs (A, B) such that $A \subset B$.
   (b) Give the matrix for this relation.
   (c) Draw a picture for this relation.
   (d) How should the picture of (c) be augmented to become the picture for $\subseteq$ on $P(S)$?

2. Let R be the relation on $S = \{1, 2, 3, 4\}$ pictured in the figure.
   (a) Give R as a subset of $S \times S$.
   (b) Give the matrix for R.
   (c) Is R reflexive? Is it irreflexive? Symmetric? Antisymmetric? Transitive?

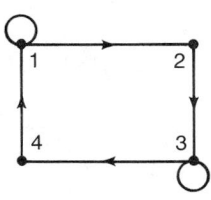

3. For the relation R of Problem 2, give all paths that are:
    (a) of length three with initial vertex 1.
    (b) of length three with final vertex 1.
    (c) of length four from vertex 2 to vertex 4.

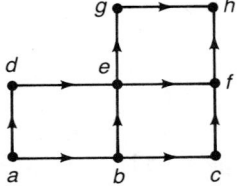

4. For the relation of the figure, give five different paths of length four from vertex a to vertex h.

5. Let $S = \{1, 2, 3\}$ and R be the binary relation on S with
    $$R = \{(1, 1), (1, 2), (2, 3), (3, 1), (3, 2), (3, 3)\}.$$
    Is R reflexive? Is R symmetric? Is R transitive?

6. Let $S = \{1, 2, 3\}$ and R be the binary relation on S with
    $$R = \{(1, 1), (1, 3), (2, 2), (2, 3), (3, 1), (3, 3)\}.$$
    Is R reflexive? Is R symmetric? Is R transitive?

7. (a) Draw a picture for the diagonal relation D on $S = \{1, 2, 3\}$.
    (b) Is D reflexive? Is it irreflexive? Symmetric? Antisymmetric? Transitive?

8. Repeat Problem 7, but with D replaced by the complete relation K on S.

9. Let X be a set of real numbers and let $\leq$ be the "less than or equal" binary relation on X. Is $\leq$ reflexive? Is $\leq$ irreflexive? Is $\leq$ symmetric? Is $\leq$ antisymmetric? Is $\leq$ transitive?

10. Repeat Problem 9, but with $\leq$ replaced by $\geq$.

11. What must be true of a picture for a binary relation R on S for R to be:
    (a) symmetric?   (b) antisymmetric?

12. What property of a picture for a binary relation R guarantees that R is:
    (a) reflexive?   (b) irreflexive?

13. Let R be a binary relation on S. How can one tell from the relation matrix for R whether R is:
    (a) reflexive?   (b) irreflexive?

14. Let R be a binary relation on S. How can one tell from the relation matrix for R whether R is:
    (a) symmetric?   (b) antisymmetric?

15. Let R be a binary relation on a nonempty set S.
    (a) Can R be both reflexive and irreflexive? Explain.
    (b) Can R be neither reflexive nor irreflexive? Explain.

16. Repeat Problem 15, but with *reflexive* and *irreflexive* respectively replaced by *symmetric* and *antisymmetric*.

17. How should one change the picture of Problem 2 to make it the picture for the reverse V of the relation R (as in Definition 5 of Section 1.4)?

18. Let V be the reverse of a binary relation R on S.
    (a) How can one obtain the picture for V from that for R?
    (b) How can one obtain the relation matrix for V from that for R?

19. What is the reverse of the diagonal relation $D = \{(s, s) : s \in S\}$ on a set S?

20. What is the reverse of the complete relation $K = S^2$ on a set S?

21. What relationship between a binary relation R and its reverse V occurs if and only if R is symmetric?

22. Let R be a binary relation on S and $D = \{(s, s) : s \in S\}$ be the diagonal relation on S. What relationship exists between R and D if and only if R is reflexive?

23. Repeat Problem 22, but with *reflexive* replaced by *irreflexive*.

24. Let V be the reverse of a binary relation R on S and $D = \{(s, s) : s \in S\}$ be the diagonal relation on S. What relationship involving R, V, and D occurs if and only if R is antisymmetric?

25. If R is a symmetric binary relation, must its reverse V also be symmetric? Explain.

26. Repeat Problem 25, but with *symmetric* replaced by each of the following:
(a) antisymmetric;   (b) reflexive;
(c) irreflexive;   (d) transitive.

27. Let R be a binary relation on S. Also let aRc whenever there is a path (a, b, c) in R of length 2 from vertex a to vertex c. Is R transitive? Explain.

28. Let R be a binary relation on S. Also let aRd whenever there is a path (a, b, c, d) in R of length three from a to d. Is R transitive? Explain.

29. Let A be the binary relation on the set $\mathbf{B_n}$ of n-digit binary strings for which $\alpha A \beta$ means that $\alpha = a_1 a_2 \ldots a_n$ and $\beta = b_1 b_2 \ldots b_n$ differ in exactly one position; that is, $a_i = b_i$ for all but one i. For example, $00A01$ but $00\bar{A}00$ and $00\bar{A}11$.
(a) Draw a picture for A in the case $n = 2$.
(b) Is A reflexive? Is A symmetric? Is A transitive?

30. Draw a picture for the A of Problem 29 in the case $n = 3$.

31. For each of the following binary relations R on $S = \{1, 2, 3\}$ find the smallest transitive binary relation T on S such that $T \supseteq R$. (This T is called the **transitive closure** of R.)
(a) $R = \{(1, 2), (2, 3)\}$.
(b) $R = \{(1, 2), (2, 3), (3, 1)\}$.
(c) $R = \{(1, 2)\}$.

32. For each of the following binary relations R on $S = \{1, 2, 3, 4\}$ find the smallest transitive binary relation T on S such that $T \supseteq R$.
(a) $R = \{(1, 2), (2, 3), (3, 4)\}$.
(b) $R = \{(1, 2), (2, 3), (3, 1), (3, 4)\}$.
(c) $R = \{(1, 2), (3, 4)\}$.

33. For each R of Problem 31, find the smallest symmetric binary relation U on S such that $U \supseteq R$. (This U is called the **symmetric closure** of R.)

34. For each R of Problem 32 find the smallest symmetric binary relation U on S such that $U \supseteq R$.

35. How many $n \times n$ matrices are there with each entry in $\{0, 1\}$? That is, how many binary relations R are there on a set $S = \{s_1, s_2, \ldots, s_n\}$ of size n?

36. Of the binary relations R of Problem 35, how many are:
(a) reflexive?   (b) irreflexive?   (c) symmetric?

37. Let R be a binary relation on S. Define a new binary relation P on S so that aPb means that there is a path from a to b in R. What is the connection between P and the transitive closure of R? (See Problem 31.)

1.6

ORDER RELATIONS, POSETS

Binary relations that share certain properties with the "is a subset of" relation $\subseteq$ on a power set $P(S)$ are involved in the important tasks of sorting and filing data in computer memories. The following definition indicates the properties that these relations have in common and helps us to study all such relations simultaneously.

DEFINITION 1   PARTIAL ORDERING, POSET

Let R be an antisymmetric, reflexive, and transitive binary relation on a set X. Then P is a *partial ordering* on X, and the ordered pair (X, R) is a *partially ordered set* or (for short) *poset*.

If we use A for "antisymmetric," R for "reflexive," and T for "transitive," the word ART becomes an acronym to aid us in remembering the three properties of a binary relation that make it a partial ordering.

Example 1   Let X be any set of real numbers. We saw in Problem 9 of Section 1.5 that the binary relation $\leq$ on X is antisymmetric, reflexive, and transitive. Hence $(X, \leq)$ is a poset.   □

Example 2   Let S be any set and $P(S)$ be its power set. In Example 3 of Section 1.5 we saw that the binary relation $\subseteq$ on $P(S)$ is antisymmetric, reflexive, and transitive. Hence $(P(S), \subseteq)$ is a poset.   □

Example 3

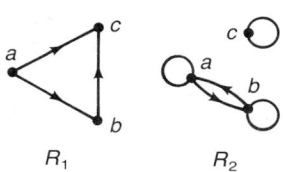

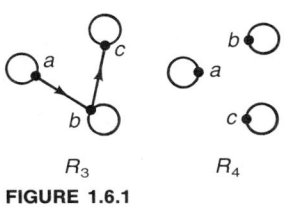

R_3 R_4

FIGURE 1.6.1

Let $X = \{a, b, c\}$. In Figure 1.6.1, we give pictures for binary relations

$$R_1 = \{(a, b), (b, c), (a, c)\},$$
$$R_2 = \{(a, a), (b, b), (c, c), (a, b), (b, a)\},$$
$$R_3 = \{(a, a), (b, b), (c, c), (a, b), (b, c)\},$$

and

$$R_4 = \{(a, a), (b, b), (c, c)\}.$$

We see that R_1 is not reflexive, since, for example, (a, a) is not in R_1. Also R_2 is not antisymmetric, since (a, b) and (b, a) are in R_2 but $a \neq b$. The relation R_3 is not transitive, since (a, b) and (b, c) are in R_3 but (a, c) is not. Hence no one of $(X, R_1), (X, R_2), (X, R_3)$ is a poset. But (X, R_4) is a poset, since R_4 is antisymmetric, reflexive, and transitive. □

DEFINITION 2   **POSET DIAGRAM**

A *poset diagram* (or **Hasse Diagram**) for a poset (X, R) is a figure in which:

1. The vertices are points representing the elements of X.
2. There is an upward sloping line or broken line from x to y whenever $x \neq y$ and xRy.
3. The figure has the least number of segments that accomplish the property in (2).

Example 4

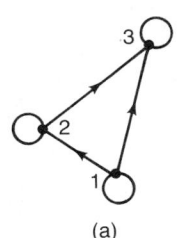

(a)

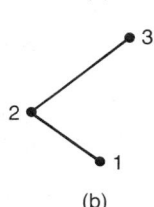

(b)

FIGURE 1.6.2

Let $X = \{1, 2, 3\}$. A picture (as defined in Definition 2 of Section 1.5) for the binary relation $\leq$ on X is given in Figure 1.6.2(a), and a poset diagram for $(X, \leq)$ is given in Figure 1.6.2(b). □

Let (X, R) be a poset. The poset diagram for (X, R) differs from the ordinary picture for the binary relation R in the following respects:

(a) The poset diagram has no loops. Loops are not drawn but are assumed to be present at each vertex because the R for a poset is reflexive.
(b) The poset diagram has no arrowheads. Arrowheads are not needed because each segment is understood to be pointed upward.
(c) A segment for aRc is omitted in the poset diagram when there is an element b in X such that $a \neq b, b \neq c, aRb$, and bRc. The undrawn segment for aRc is implied by the transitivity of R.

As an illustration of (c), there is no segment from 1 to 3 in Figure 1.6.2(b), since $1 \leq 2, 2 \leq 3$, and transitivity of $\leq$ imply that $1 \leq 3$.

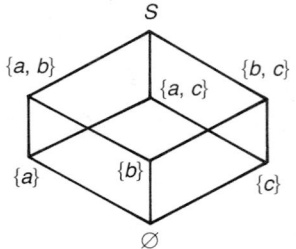

FIGURE 1.6.3

Each of these ways in which a poset diagram can differ from an ordinary picture for a binary relation makes the poset diagram less cluttered.

We noted in Example 2 that $(P(S), \subseteq)$ is a poset for all sets S. Figure 1.6.3 is a poset diagram for $(P(S), \subseteq)$ in the special case of $S = \{a, b, c\}$.

Since $(X, \leq)$ is a poset for every subset X of Z and $(P(S), \subseteq)$ is a poset for every power set $P(S)$, we will use (especially in Section 2.6) the symbol $\preceq$ to represent a general partial ordering.

NOTATION 1 $\preceq$, $\prec$, $\succeq$

In the notation $(X, \preceq)$, the symbol $\preceq$ denotes a partial order relation on X, so $(X, \preceq)$ always represents a poset. For a and b in X, $a \prec b$ means that $a \preceq b$ and $a \neq b$. Also, $b \succeq a$ means that $a \preceq b$.

DEFINITION 3   **LEAST AND GREATEST ELEMENTS FOR A POSET**

Let $(X, \preceq)$ be a poset and S be a subset of X. If $a \in S$ and $a \preceq s$ for all s in S, the element a is a **least** element in S. If $b \in S$ and $s \preceq b$ for all s in S, b is a **greatest** element in S.

Example 5   Let $N = \{0, 1, 2, \ldots\}$ be the set of natural numbers. For the poset $(N, \leq)$, every nonempty subset S of N has a least element. A nonempty subset T of N has a greatest element if and only if T is finite.   □

Example 6   Let $Z = \{\ldots, -2, -1, 0, 1, 2, \ldots\}$ be the set of integers. For the poset $(Z, \leq)$, the subset N of Z has 0 as its least element and has no greatest element. The subset $\{-1, -2, -3, \ldots\}$ has -1 as its greatest element and has no least element. The set Z itself has neither a least nor a greatest element.   □

THEOREM 1   **UNIQUENESS OF LEAST OR GREATEST ELEMENT**

Let $(X, \preceq)$ be a poset and S be a subset of X. Then S has no more than one least element and no more than one greatest element.

PROOF   We prove uniqueness of the least element and leave the proof for the greatest element to be worked out in Problem 26 below. If S has no least element, there is nothing to prove. Suppose that each of a and b is a least element of S. Then $a \preceq s$ and $b \preceq s$ for all s in S. Replacing s by b in $a \preceq s$ and replacing s by a in $b \preceq s$, one has $a \preceq b$ and $b \preceq a$. Since the partial ordering $\preceq$ is antisymmetric, $a \preceq b$ and $b \preceq a$ imply that $a = b$. Thus there is at most one least element of S. □

DEFINITION 4   **MINIMAL ELEMENT, MAXIMAL ELEMENT**

Let $(X, \preceq)$ be a poset and S be a subset of X. A ***minimal element*** of S is an element m in S for which there is no s in S with $s \prec m$. A ***maximal element*** of S is an element q in S for which there is no s in S with $q \prec s$.

Example 7   Let $X = \{a, b, c, d, e\}$ and $(X, \preceq)$ be the poset whose poset diagram is Figure 1.6.4. Let S be the set of all x in X such that both $x \preceq d$ and $x \preceq e$. Clearly, $S = \{a, b, c\}$. The elements b and c are maximal in S. The set S has no greatest element because there is no s in S simultaneously satisfying $a \preceq s$, $b \preceq s$, and $c \preceq s$. In the universe X itself, d and e are maximal elements and there is no greatest element. In X, a is the only minimal element and is also the least element, since $a \preceq x$ for all x in X. □

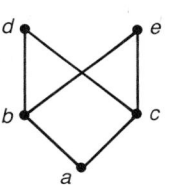

FIGURE 1.6.4

DEFINITION 5   **COMPARABILITY, LINEAR ORDERING**

Let $(X, \preceq)$ be a poset. Elements a and b of X are ***comparable*** if either $a \preceq b$ or $b \preceq a$. If x and y are comparable for all x and y in X, then $\preceq$ is a ***linear ordering*** of X and $(X, \preceq)$ is a ***linearly ordered set*** (or a ***chain***). The word *noncomparable* means "not comparable."

Example 8   Let $S = \{s_1, s_2, \ldots, s_n\}$. If $n \geq 2$, the poset $(P(S), \subseteq)$ is not a linearly ordered set, since, for example, the members $\{s_1\}$ and $\{s_2\}$ of $P(S)$ are not comparable. (Figure 1.6.3 has the diagram for this poset in the case $n = 3$.)

If X is any set of real numbers, the poset $(X, \leq)$ is linearly ordered, since, for any real numbers x and y, either $x \leq y$ or $y \leq x$ (or both). In particular, the posets $(N, \leq)$ and $(Z, \leq)$ of Examples 5 and 6 are linearly ordered sets. □

If X is finite and $(X, \preceq)$ is a linearly ordered set, its poset diagram looks like a chain, as illustrated in Figure 1.6.5 for $(\{2, 3, 5, 8, 13\}, \leq)$.

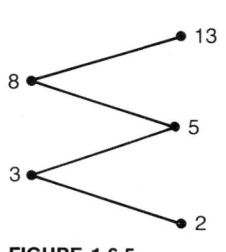

FIGURE 1.6.5

DEFINITION 6   **WELL ORDERING**

Let $(X, \preceq)$ be a linearly ordered set. If every nonempty subset S of X has a least element, $\preceq$ is a ***well ordering*** of X and $(X, \preceq)$ is a ***well-ordered set***.

Example 9   The statements in Examples 5 and 6 tell us that $(N, \leq)$ is a well-ordered set and that $(Z, \leq)$ is not a well-ordered set. However, there exist well orderings of Z, as we now show. Let us relist the integers in the form

$$Z = \{0, 1, -1, 2, -2, 3, -3, \ldots\}. \tag{1}$$

Let W be the relation on Z for which aWb means that either $a = b$ or a appears to the left of b in the listing (1). Then W is a well ordering of Z, and (Z, W) is a well-ordered set.   □

Example 10   Let $N = \{0, 1, 2, \ldots\}$ and $C = N \times N$. Let L be the relation on C for which $(a, b)L(c, d)$ means that

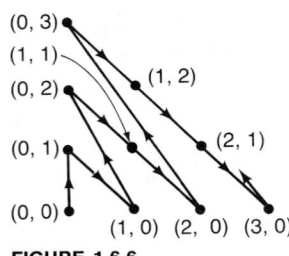

(i) $a + b < c + d$, or
(ii) $a + b = c + d$ and $a \leq c$.

It can be shown that $(a, b)L(c, d)$ if and only if either $(a, b) = (c, d)$ or (a, b) appears to the left of (c, d) in the listing

$$C = \{(0, 0), (0, 1), (1, 0), (0, 2), (1, 1), (2, 0), (0, 3), \ldots\}.$$

This helps us see that L is a well ordering of C. (Also see Figure 1.6.6.)   □

FIGURE 1.6.6

Example 11   Let I consist of all the real numbers x satisfying $0 \leq x \leq 1$. Then $(I, \leq)$ is not a well-ordered set, since the subset $A = \{1, 1/2, 1/3, \ldots\} = \{1/n : n \in Z^+\}$ of I has no least element with respect to $\leq$.   □

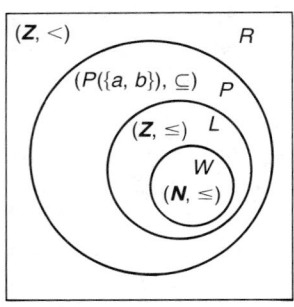

Figure 1.6.7 is intended to indicate that every well-ordered set is linearly ordered and that every linearly ordered set is partially ordered. It also has the example of a binary relation $<$ on Z that is not a partial ordering, a poset $(P(\{a, b\}), \subseteq)$ that is not linearly ordered, a linearly ordered set $(Z, \leq)$ that is not well ordered, and a well-ordered set $(N, \leq)$.

FIGURE 1.6.7

PROBLEMS FOR SECTION 1.6

1.   Let $X = \{1, 2, 3, 6\}$ and

$$R = \{(1, 1), (1, 2), (1, 3), (1, 6), (2, 2), (2, 6), (3, 3), (3, 6), (6, 6)\}.$$

(i) Draw a picture for the relation R.
(ii) Is (X, R) a poset? If so, draw its poset diagram.
(iii) Is (X, R) a linearly ordered set? Explain.
(iv) Is (X, R) a well-ordered set? Explain.

2. Let $S = \{s_1, s_2\}$ and P be its power set $\{S_{00}, S_{01}, S_{10}, S_{11}\}$.
   (i) Draw a picture for the relation $\subseteq$ on P.
   (ii) Draw a poset diagram for $(P, \subseteq)$.
   (iii) In the poset $(P, \subseteq)$, find noncomparable members A and B.
   (iv) Is $(P, \subseteq)$ a linearly ordered set? Explain.
   (v) Is $(P, \subseteq)$ a well-ordered set? Explain.

3. Let S be a singleton $\{s_1\}$. Is $(P(S), \subseteq)$ a well-ordered set? Explain.

4. Let S be a nonempty set. What is the condition on $\#S$ for $(P(S), \subseteq)$ to be a linearly ordered set?

5. Let $(X, \preceq)$ be a poset. Does $x \preceq x$ for all x in X? Explain.

6. Let $(X, \preceq)$ be a poset and $a, b, c \in X$.
   (a) If $a \preceq b$ and $b \preceq a$, what must be true of a and b?
   (b) If $a \preceq b$ and $b \preceq c$, must $a \preceq c$? Explain.

7. Let $A = \{a\}$, $B = \{b\}$, $C = \{c\}$, $D = \{d\}$, $E = \{a, b, c\}$, $F = \{b, c, d\}$, and $X = \{\varnothing, A, B, C, D, E, F\}$. The figure shows a poset diagram for $(X, \subseteq)$. [We see in Problem 11 that $(X, \subseteq)$ is a poset.]

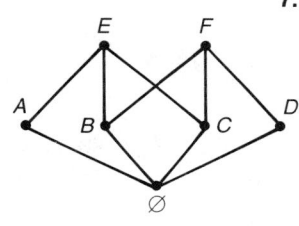

   (i) Find the collection Γ of all members T of X such that $T \subseteq E$.
   (ii) Find the collection Δ of all members V of X such that $V \subseteq F$.
   (iii) Find $\Gamma \cap \Delta$.
   (iv) Does $\Gamma \cap \Delta$ have a greatest member? That is, is there a G in $\Gamma \cap \Delta$ such that $U \subseteq G$ for every U in $\Gamma \cap \Delta$?
   (v) List the maximal elements of $\Gamma \cap \Delta$.
   (vi) Is $\subseteq$ a linear ordering of X? Explain. Is $\subseteq$ a well ordering of X? Explain.

8. Let $H = \{d\}$, $I = \{a\}$, $J = \{b, c, d\}$, $K = \{a, c, d\}$, $L = \{a, b, d\}$, $M = \{a, b, c\}$, and $X = \{\varnothing, H, I, J, K, L, M\}$.
   (i) Draw a poset diagram for $(X, \subseteq)$.
   (ii) Find the collection Γ of all members T of X such that $H \subseteq T$, the collection Δ of all V of X such that $I \subseteq V$, and $\Gamma \cap \Delta$.
   (iii) Does $\Gamma \cap \Delta$ have a least member? That is, is there a W in $\Gamma \cap \Delta$ such that $W \subseteq U$ for all U in $\Gamma \cap \Delta$?
   (iv) Does $\Gamma \cap \Delta$ have a greatest element?
   (v) List the minimal elements of $\Gamma \cap \Delta$.
   (vi) List the maximal elements of $\Gamma \cap \Delta$.
   (vii) Is $\subseteq$ a linear ordering of X? Explain. Is $\subseteq$ a well ordering of X? Explain.

9. Let A and B be in a power set $P(S)$. Let Γ consist of all the subsets C of S such that both $C \subseteq A$ and $C \subseteq B$. Does the subcollection Γ of $P(S)$ have a greatest member? That is, is there a set G in Γ such that $C \subseteq G$ for every C in Γ? Explain.

10. Let A and B be in a power set $P(S)$. Let Δ consist of all the subsets D of S such that both $A \subseteq D$ and $B \subseteq D$. Does the subcollection Δ of $P(S)$ have

a least member? That is, is there a set L in Δ with $L \subseteq D$ for all D in Δ? Explain.

11.   Let (X, R) be a poset, let $S \subseteq X$, and let $R' = R \cap (S \times S)$. (The binary relation R' on S is the *restriction* of R to the universe S.) Prove that R' is reflexive, antisymmetric, and transitive and hence that (S, R') is a poset. (If R is written as $\leqslant$, $\leq$, or $\subseteq$, one would use the same symbol for R' as for R.)

12.   Let X, R, S, and R' be as in Problem 11.
   (a) If R is a linear ordering of X, must R' be a linear ordering of S? Explain.
   (b) Repeat Part (a), but with "linear ordering" replaced by "well ordering."

13.   (i) List the ordered pairs of the reverse V of the relation R of Problem 1. (Relation V is as in Definition 5 of Section 1.4.)
   (ii) For this V and the X of Problem 1, is (X, V) a poset? If so, draw its poset diagram.

14.   Let $\supseteq$ be the reverse of the binary relation $\subseteq$ on a power set $P(S)$.
   (a) Explain why $(P(S), \supseteq)$ is a poset.
   (b) Draw a poset diagram for $(P, \supseteq)$, where P is as in Problem 2.

15.   Let $P(S)$ be the power set for S and let X be a collection of subsets of S; that is, let $X \subseteq P(S)$. Is $(X, \subseteq)$ a poset? Explain.

16.   Let X be as in Problem 15. Is $(X, \supseteq)$ a poset? Explain.

17.   Let $\geq$ be the reverse of the binary relation $\leq$ on $N = \{0, 1, 2, \ldots\}$.
   (i) Is $(N, \leq)$ a poset? Explain.
   (ii) Is $(N, \geq)$ a poset? Explain.
   (iii) In $(N, \leq)$, does N have a least element? Does N have a greatest element?
   (iv) In $(N, \geq)$, does N have a least element? That is, is there an a in N such that $a \geq n$ for all n in N? If so, what is a?
   (v) In $(N, \geq)$, does N have a greatest element? That is, is there an integer b in N such that $n \geq b$ for all n in N? If so, what is b?

18.   Let Z be the set $\{\ldots, -2, -1, 0, 1, 2, \ldots\}$ of integers and let S be a subset of Z. If S has a least element in the poset $(Z, \leq)$, must S have a greatest element in $(Z, \geq)$? Explain. If S has a greatest element in $(Z, \leq)$, does S have a least element in $(Z, \geq)$?

19.   Let $\supseteq$ be the reverse of the binary relation $\subseteq$ on a power set $P(S)$.
   (i) Is $(P(S), \supseteq)$ a poset?
   (ii) In $(P(S), \subseteq)$, what are the least and greatest elements of $P(S)$?
   (iii) In $(P(S), \supseteq)$, what are the least and greatest elements of $P(S)$?

20.   Let V be the reverse of a binary relation R on S. If (S, R) is a poset, must (S, V) be a poset? Explain.

21.   Let m be the least element and g the greatest element of X in a poset

(X, R). What are the least and the greatest elements of X in (X, V), where V is the reverse of R?

22. Let V be the reverse of a binary relation R on S. If (S, R) is a linearly ordered set, must (S, V) be a linearly ordered set?

23. Let $N = \{0, 1, \ldots\}$. The poset $(N, \leq)$ is a well-ordered set. Is $(N, \geq)$ a well-ordered set? Explain.

24. Let (S, R) be a well-ordered set and V be the reverse of R. In each part, give an example to show that:
(a) (S, V) may be a well-ordered set.
(b) (S, V) need not be a well-ordered set.

25. Use a different listing for the set $E = \{\ldots, -4, -2, 0, 2, 4, \ldots\}$ of even integers to characterize a well-ordering relation W on E.

26. Let $(X, \preceq)$ be a poset and let $S \subseteq X$. Given that S has a greatest element, prove that the greatest element of S is unique. (This is the part of Theorem 1 earlier left unproved.)

27. Let $(X, \preceq)$ be a poset and let S be a subset of X. Let m and m' be distinct maximal elements of S. Prove that S has no greatest element.

28. Repeat Problem 27, but with *maximal* and *greatest* replaced respectively by *minimal* and *least*.

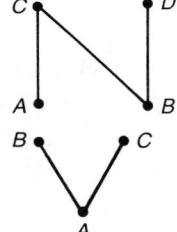

29. Let $S = \{1, 2, 3\}$ and P be its power set. How many ordered 4-tuples (A, B, C, D) are there in $P \times P \times P \times P$ such that the poset $(\{A, B, C, D\}, \subseteq)$ has the figure shown here as its poset diagram?

30. Let $S = \{1, 2, 3\}$. How many ordered triples (A, B, C) are there in $[P(S)]^3$ such that $(\{A, B, C\}, \subseteq)$ is a poset with the figure shown here as its poset diagram?

*31. Use Example 10 of this section to characterize a well-ordering relation W on the set $Q^+ = \{r/s : r, s \in Z^+\}$ of positive rational numbers.

1.7

PARTITIONS OF SETS, EQUIVALENCE RELATIONS

Let S be a set of programs stored in a computer's memory banks. Assume that each program p in S can be called up by just one user in a set $\{U_1, U_2, \ldots, U_n\}$ of n users. Then let R be the binary relation on S for which pRq means that p and q are programs callable by the same user. It can be shown that this R is reflexive, symmetric, and transitive. Also, for each i in $\{1, 2, \ldots, n\}$, let A_i consist of the programs in S that can be called up by user U_i. Then the collection

$$\Gamma = \{A_1, A_2, \ldots, A_n\}$$

of subsets of S has the following two properties:

(i) $A_i \cap A_j = \emptyset$ whenever $i \neq j$.
(ii) $A_1 \cup A_2 \cup \cdots \cup A_n = S$.

This section deals with collections $\Gamma = \{A_1, A_2, \ldots, A_n\}$ of subsets of any set S such that the A_i have these two properties. It also considers the related topic of binary relations that are simultaneously reflexive, symmetric, and transitive.

DEFINITION 1   **PAIRWISE DISJOINT COLLECTION**

The members of a collection Γ of sets are **pairwise disjoint** if any two distinct members of Γ are disjoint.

In other words, the members of Γ are pairwise disjoint if and only if $A \in \Gamma$, $B \in \Gamma$, and $A \neq B$ together imply that $A \cap B = \emptyset$.

DEFINITION 2   **PARTITION OF A SET, RANK**

A collection Γ of subsets of X is a **partition** of X if the two following conditions are met:

(a) X is the union of the members of Γ.
(b) the members of Γ are pairwise disjoint.

The **rank** of the partition is the number of members of Γ.

Example 1   Let $X = \{a, b, c, d, e, f, g\}$, $A = \{a, c, e\}$, $B = \{b, d\}$, and $C = \{f, g\}$. Then $\Gamma = \{A, B, C\}$ is a partition of X, since

(a) $A \cup B \cup C = X$; and
(b) $A \cap B = \emptyset$, $A \cap C = \emptyset$, $B \cap C = \emptyset$.   □

Example 2   Let $X = \{1, 2, 3, 4, 5, 6, 7\}$, $A = \{1, 2, 3\}$, $B = \{4, 5, 6\}$, and $C = \{6, 7\}$. Although $A \cup B \cup C = X$, $\{A, B, C\}$ is not a partition of X, since $B \cap C = \{6\}$, and so B and C are not disjoint.   □

Example 3   Let $\Gamma = \{M_\alpha : \alpha \in B_n\}$ be the collection of minisets M_α for a sequence $A_1, A_2, \ldots, A_n$ of subsets of S where M_α is empty for at most one α in B_n. As illustrated in Example 1 of Section 1.3, Γ is a partition of S with rank 2^n.   □

THEOREM 1	**SIZE OF A UNION OF PAIRWISE DISJOINT FINITE SETS**

Let $\Gamma = \{A_1, A_2, \ldots, A_n\}$ be a partition of X. Then

$$\#X = \#A_1 + \#A_2 + \cdots + \#A_n$$

PROOF This follows from the fact that each element x of X is in one and only one of the members A_i of the partition Γ. □

Example 4 Let B be the set of all binary strings (of all lengths) and B_n be the subset of all strings of length n. Then $\Gamma = \{B_1, B_2, \ldots\}$ is a partition of B with infinite rank. The collection Γ' of the $B_{n,k}$ for $n = 1, 2, \ldots$ and $k = 0, 1, \ldots, n$ is another partition of B with infinite rank.

For every positive integer n, $\{B_{n,0}, B_{n,1}, \ldots, B_{n,n}\}$ is a partition of B_n with rank $n + 1$. Hence it follows from Theorem 1 that

$$(\#B_{n,0}) + (\#B_{n,1}) + \cdots + (\#B_{n,n}) = \#B_n.$$

Since $\#B_{n,k} = \binom{n}{k}$ and $\#B_n = 2^n$, this gives us

$$\binom{n}{0} + \binom{n}{1} + \binom{n}{2} + \cdots + \binom{n}{n} = 2^n.$$

□

DEFINITION 3	**REFINEMENT OF A PARTITION**

Let each of Γ and Γ' be a partition of X. Then Γ' is a ***refinement*** of Γ if each member of Γ' is a subset of some member of Γ.

In Example 4, each member $B_{n,k}$ of Γ' is a subset of the member B_n of Γ; thus Γ' is a refinement of Γ.

Example 5 Let $X = \{a, b, c\}$. Then each of the collections

$$A = \{\{a\}, \{b\}, \{c\}\}, \qquad B = \{\{a, b\}, \{c\}\}, \qquad C = \{\{a, c\}, \{b\}\},$$
$$D = \{\{b, c\}, \{a\}\}, \qquad \text{and} \qquad E = \{X\}$$

is a partition of X. Let ρ be the binary relation on $\{A, B, C, D, E\}$ in which $\Gamma'\rho\Gamma$ means that Γ' is a refinement of Γ. Then $(\{A, B, C, D, E\}, \rho)$ is a poset whose diagram is Figure 1.7.1. The ranks of these partitions are given by

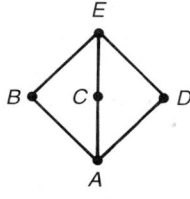

FIGURE 1.7.1

Γ	A	B	C	D	E
Rank of Γ	3	2	2	2	1

□

Next we introduce notation helpful in dealing with certain important partitions of sets of integers.

NOTATION 1   **SETS Z, Z⁺, N**

Z denotes the set $\{\ldots, -2, -1, 0, 1, 2, 3, \ldots\}$ of *integers*;

Z^+ denotes the set $\{1, 2, 3, \ldots\}$ of *positive integers*; and

N denotes the set $\{0, 1, 2, \ldots\}$ of *natural numbers*.

NOTATION 2   **SET** $a + bT$

For a and b in Z and T a subset of Z, $a + bT$ denotes the set $\{a + bt : t \in T\}$. In particular, bT denotes the set $\{bt : t \in T\}$ of multiples of b by integers in T.

Example 6   We can see that $2Z = \{\ldots, -4, -2, 0, 2, 4, 6, \ldots\}$ is the set of all *even integers* and that $1 + 2Z = \{\ldots, -3, -1, 1, 3, 5, \ldots\}$ is the set of *odd integers*. Thus $\{2Z, 1 + 2Z\}$ is a partition of Z with rank 2. Similarly, $3N = \{0, 3, 6, \ldots\}$, $1 + 3N = \{1, 4, 7, \ldots\}$, and $2 + 3N = \{2, 5, 8, \ldots\}$; we see that $\{3N, 1 + 3N, 2 + 3N\}$ is a partition of N with rank 3.   □

Example 7   It should be clear that

$$6Z = \{\ldots, -12, -6, 0, 6, 12, 18, \ldots\},$$
$$1 + 6Z = \{\ldots, -11, -5, 1, 7, 13, 19, \ldots\},$$
$$2 + 6Z = \{\ldots, -10, -4, 2, 8, 14, 20, \ldots\},$$
$$3 + 6Z = \{\ldots, -9, -3, 3, 9, 15, 21, \ldots\},$$
$$4 + 6Z = \{\ldots, -8, -2, 4, 10, 16, 22, \ldots\},$$
$$5 + 6Z = \{\ldots, -7, -1, 5, 11, 17, 23, \ldots\}.$$

In which of these subsets of Z is the integer 52? We answer that question by constructing the sequence

52, 46, 40, 34, 28, 22, 16, 10, 4

in which the first term is 52, each succeeding term is 6 less than the term it follows, and the last term is in $\{0, 1, 2, 3, 4, 5\}$. This sequence shows that $52 = 4 + 6 \cdot 8$ and hence that 52 is in $4 + 6Z$.

We find the member of this collection of subsets that contains -23 by constructing the sequence

$-23, -17, -11, -5, 1$

in which the first term is -23, each succeeding term is 6 more than the term it follows, and the sequence stops when we reach an integer in $\{0, 1, 2, 3, 4, 5\}$. Thus we see that $-23 = 1 + 6(-4)$ and hence that -23 is in $1 + 6\mathbf{Z}$.

Similarly we would find that every integer n is in one and only one of these six subsets. Hence the collection of six subsets

$$\{6\mathbf{Z}, 1 + 6\mathbf{Z}, 2 + 6\mathbf{Z}, 3 + 6\mathbf{Z}, 4 + 6\mathbf{Z}, 5 + 6\mathbf{Z}\}$$

is a partition of $\mathbf{Z}$ with rank 6. The following algorithm formalizes a technique of this example. □

ALGORITHM 1 **DIVISION ALGORITHM**

Let a and b be integers, with b positive. If a is positive, we stop the sequence

$$a, a - b, a - 2b, \ldots, a - qb$$

when we first reach a term r in the set $\{0, 1, \ldots, b - 1\}$. If a is negative, we stop the sequence

$$a, a + b, a + 2b, \ldots, a + hb$$

when a term r in $\{0, 1, \ldots, b - 1\}$ is reached. Either way, integers q and r are found (with $q = -h$ in the case of negative a) such that $a = qb + r$ and $r \in \{0, 1, \ldots, b - 1\}$. (It can be shown that the q and r with those properties are unique for a fixed a and b.)

DEFINITION 4 **QUOTIENT, REMAINDER**

Let a and b be integers, with b positive. The integers q and r such that

$$a = qb + r \qquad \text{and} \qquad r \in \{0, 1, 2, \ldots, b - 1\}$$

found using Algorithm 1 are the **quotient** and **remainder**, respectively, in the division of a by b.

Looking at Example 7, one sees that $4 + 6\mathbf{Z}$ consists of all integers n having a remainder of 4 when divided by 6. In general, if b is a positive integer and r is in the set $\{0, 1, \ldots, b - 1\}$, the set $r + b\mathbf{Z}$ consists of all integers n having a remainder of r when divided by b.

NOTATION 3   *d|m*, **INTEGRAL DIVISOR, INTEGRAL MULTIPLE**

Let d and m be integers. Then $d|m$ means that there is an integer c such that $m = cd$. (One reads $d|m$ as "d is an *integral divisor* of m" or as "d is an exact divisor of m" or, for short, as "d goes into m." One can also read $d|m$ as "m is an *integral multiple* of d.")

For example $(-4)|12$, since $12 = (-3)(-4)$ and 12, -3, and -4 are all integers. We note that $d|m$ if and only if $m \in dZ$ and that $|$ is a binary relation on Z, or on any subset X of Z. Some properties of this relation are discussed in Problem 33 below.

Example 8   In Example 4, we noted that

$$\{B_{n,0}, B_{n,1}, \ldots, B_{n,n}\}$$

FIGURE 1.7.2

is a partition of B_n. In the special case with $n = 3$, this gives us the partition $\Gamma = \{B_{3,0}, B_{3,1}, B_{3,2}, B_{3,3}\}$ of B_3 displayed in Figure 1.7.2. Let W be the binary relation on B_3 in which $\alpha W \beta$ means that α and β are in the same member of Γ; that is, $\alpha W \beta$ means that wgt α = wgt β. In the following theorem we show that a binary relation obtained in this way from a partition of a set is reflexive, symmetric, and transitive.   □

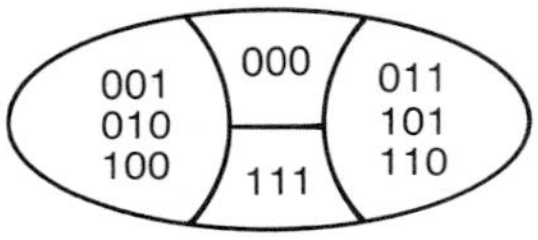

THEOREM 2   **COMEMBERSHIP IN A PARTITION**

Let Γ be a collection of subsets forming a partition of a nonempty set X. Let E be the binary relation on X for which aEb means that a and b are in the same member of Γ. Then E is reflexive, symmetric, and transitive.

PROOF   Relation E is reflexive, since x and x are in the same member of Γ; that is, xEx for all x in X. Also, E is symmetric, since b and a are in the same member of Γ whenever a and b are in the same member; that is, aEb implies bEa. Finally, let aEb and bEc. This means that a and b are in the same member of Γ, as is also true of b and c; these statements imply that a and c are in the unique member of Γ containing b. Thus aEb and bEc imply aEc, and hence E is transitive.   □

We next define the type of binary relation that has the properties proved for the binary relation E of Theorem 2.

DEFINITION 5   **EQUIVALENCE RELATION**

An *equivalence relation* on a set X is a reflexive, symmetric, and transitive binary relation on X.

We can use *RST* (reflexive, symmetric, transitive) as a mnemonic device to aid in remembering the properties of a binary relation that make it an equivalence relation.

Now we can sum up the statements in Theorem 2 by saying that the binary relation defined there is an equivalence relation on X. Note that "=" is an equivalence relation on any set X.

DEFINITION 6 **INDUCED EQUIVALENCE RELATION**

Let Γ be a partition of X. The equivalence relation E determined from Γ as in Theorem 2 is called the equivalence relation on X ***induced*** by the partition Γ of X.

As an illustration of Theorem 2 and Definition 6, the equivalence relation E induced by the partition

$$\{B_{3,0}, B_{3,1}, B_{3,2}, B_{3,3}\}$$

of B_3 in Example 8 is the binary relation on B_3 with $\alpha E \beta$ if and only if wgt $\alpha =$ wgt β.

Example 9 Let $\{6Z, 1 + 6Z, 2 + 6Z, 3 + 6Z, 4 + 6Z, 5 + 6Z\}$ be the partition of Z discussed in Example 7. Then the induced equivalence relation for this partition is the binary relation E on Z for which mEn means that m and n are integers with the same remainder when divided by 6. In texts on the Theory of Numbers, mEn is usually written as "$m \equiv n \pmod 6$" and read as "m is congruent to n modulo 6." □

THEOREM 3 **INDUCED PARTITION**

Let E be an equivalence relation on X. For each a in X, let $C(a)$ be the subset of all x in X such that aEx. Then the collection Γ of the distinct subsets $C(a)$ is a partition of X. [The collection Γ is called the partition of X ***induced*** by E and the $C(a)$ are called the ***equivalence classes*** for E.] Also, E is the equivalence relation on X induced by Γ.

The proof of Theorem 3 is left to be worked out in Problems 29 and 30 below.

Our next example illustrates a technique that is useful in applications of partitions of the integers Z such as those in Examples 6 and 7.

Example 10 Here we show that the product ab is in $4 + 6Z$ whenever a is in $2 + 6Z$ and b is in $5 + 6Z$. For such a and b there exist integers h and k such that $a = 2 + 6h$ and $b = 5 + 6k$. Then

$$ab = (2 + 6h)(5 + 6k) = 10 + 30h + 12k + 36hk$$
$$= 4 + 6(1 + 5h + 2k + 6hk).$$

Since ab is of the form $4 + 6q$ with q in Z, ab is in $4 + 6Z$. ☐

Example 11 Let $Z = \{\ldots, -1, 0, 1, \ldots\}$ and $T = Z - \{0\}$. Let E be the relation on $Z \times T$ for which

$(a, b)E(c, d)$ means that $ad = bc$.

It can be shown that E is an equivalence relation. Under this equivalence relation, the equivalence class containing $(2, 3)$ is

$$\{(2, 3), (-2, -3), (4, 6), (-4, -6), (6, 9), (-6, -9), \ldots\}.$$

Thus an ordered pair (a, b) is in this class if and only if the fractions $2/3$ and a/b are equal. Similarly, each equivalence class for E consists of the ordered pairs (a, b) such that a/b is a representation for a fixed rational number. ☐

PROBLEMS FOR SECTION 1.7

1. Let $X = \{1, 2, 3, 4, 5, 6\}$. For each of the following listings of subsets A, B, and C of X, tell whether or not $\Gamma = \{A, B, C\}$ is a partition of X and explain your answer.
   (a) $A = \{1, 2\}, B = \{3, 4\}, C = \{5\}$.
   (b) $A = \{1, 2\}, B = \{3, 4, 5\}, C = \{5, 6\}$.
   (c) $A = \{1, 2, 3\}, B = \{4, 5, 6\}, C = \varnothing$.

2. Continue Problem 1 for the following parts.
   (a) $A = \{1, 2, 3\}, B = \{3, 4, 5\}, C = \{5, 6\}$.
   (b) $A = \{1, 2, 3\}, B = \{4, 5\}, C = \{6\}$.
   (c) $A = \{1, 3, 5\}, B = \{2, 6\}, C = \varnothing$.

3. Let $S = \{a, b, c\}$. For each of the following binary relations R on S, tell whether R is an equivalence relation and explain your answer.
   (a) $R = \{(a, a), (a, b), (b, a), (b, b), (c, c)\}$.
   (b) $R = \{(a, a), (b, b), (c, c), (a, b), (b, a), (b, c), (c, b)\}$.
   (c) $R = \{(a, b), (b, a)\}$.
   (d) $R = \{(a, a), (b, b), (c, c), (a, b)\}$.

4. Continue Problem 3 for the following parts.
   (a) $R = \{(a, a), (a, b), (b, a)\}$.
   (b) $R = \{(a, a), (b, b), (c, c), (a, b), (b, c), (c, a)\}$.
   (c) $R = \{(a, a), (b, b), (c, c)\}$.
   (d) $R = \{(a, a), (b, b), (c, c), (a, b), (b, c), (a, c)\}$.

5. Let B be the set of all binary strings (of all lengths). Let R be the relation on B for which $\alpha R \beta$ means that α and β have the same length.
   (i) Is R an equivalence relation on B?
   (ii) If so, what are the members of the induced partition of B?
   (iii) What is the rank of this partition?

6. Let $\#S = n$ and let σ be the binary relation on $P(S)$ in which $A \sigma B$ means that $\#A = \#B$.
   (i) Is σ an equivalence relation on $P(S)$?
   (ii) If so, what is the rank of the induced partition of $P(S)$?

7. An integer p greater than 1 is a *prime* if $d \mid p$ and $d \in \mathbf{Z}^{+}$ together imply that $d \in \{1, p\}$. The ability to use computers to find large primes is important in applications such as public-key encryption, a technique in which the method for encoding can be published but decoding is practically impossible because it involves large unknown primes. The first twenty primes are

   2, 3, 5, 7, 11, 13, 17, 19, 23, 29, 31,
   37, 41, 43, 47, 53, 59, 61, 67, 71.

   (i) How many of these primes are in $1 + 6\mathbf{Z}$?
   (ii) How many are in $2 + 6\mathbf{Z}$?
   (iii) How many are in $3 + 6\mathbf{Z}$?
   (iv) How many are in $5 + 6\mathbf{Z}$?
   (v) Are any of these primes in $6\mathbf{Z}$ or in $4 + 6\mathbf{Z}$?
   (vi) Use Theorem 1 to check the answers to the previous parts.

8. The first fifteen squares of integers are

   0, 1, 4, 9, 16, 25, 36, 49,
   64, 81, 100, 121, 144, 169, 196.

   (i) How many of these squares are in $3N$?
   (ii) How many are in $1 + 3N$?
   (iii) How many are in $2 + 3N$?
   (iv) Use Theorem 1 to check the answers to the previous parts.

9. Let $X = \{a, b, c, d, e, f, g\}$, $A = \{a, b, c,\}$, $B = \{d, e\}$, $C = \{f, g\}$, $D = \{a\}$, and $E = \{b, c\}$.
   (i) Is $\Gamma = \{A, B, C\}$ a partition of X?
   (ii) Is $\Gamma' = \{B, C, D, E\}$ a partition of X?
   (iii) Is Γ' a refinement of Γ?

10. Let $X = \{0, 1, 2, 3, 4, 5, 6, 7, 8, 9, 10, 11\}$, $A = \{0, 2, 4, 6, 8, 10\}$, $B = \{1, 5, 9\}$, $C = \{3, 7, 11\}$, $D = \{0, 4, 8\}$, and $E = \{2, 6, 10\}$.
   (i) Is $\Gamma = \{A, B, C\}$ a partition of X?
   (ii) Is $\Gamma' = \{B, C, D, E\}$ a partition of X?
   (iii) Is Γ' a refinement of Γ?

11. Let X be the set of all straight lines in a plane. Let σ be the binary relation on X in which $L\sigma L'$ means that L and L' have the same slope, that is, L and L' are either parallel or identical. Is σ an equivalence relation on X? Explain.

12. Let $\bar{R}$ be the complement of a binary relation R on a nonempty set S. Is $\{R, \bar{R}\}$ a partition of $S \times S$? Explain.

13. Let p be the binary relation on the set X of straight lines in a plane for which LpL' means that L and L' are perpendicular. Is p an equivalence relation on X? Explain.

14. The *parity* relation P on the set $\mathbf{Z}$ of integers has mPn if and only if $m - n$ is an even integer. Is P an equivalence relation on $\mathbf{Z}$? If so, what is the induced partition of $\mathbf{Z}$?

15. (a) Is the partition $\{3\mathbf{Z}, 1 + 3\mathbf{Z}, 2 + 3\mathbf{Z}\}$ of $\mathbf{Z}$ a refinement of the partition $\{2\mathbf{Z}, 1 + 2\mathbf{Z}\}$ of $\mathbf{Z}$? Explain.
    (b) Is the partition $\Gamma' = \{4\mathbf{Z}, 1 + 4\mathbf{Z}, 2 + 4\mathbf{Z}, 3 + 4\mathbf{Z}\}$ of $\mathbf{Z}$ a refinement of the partition $\Gamma = \{2\mathbf{Z}, 1 + 2\mathbf{Z}\}$ of $\mathbf{Z}$? Explain.

16. (a) Is $\{2\mathbf{Z}, 1 + 4\mathbf{Z}, 3 + 4\mathbf{Z}\}$ a partition of $\mathbf{Z}$?
    (b) Is $\Gamma' = \{2\mathbf{Z}, 1 + 4\mathbf{Z}, 3 + 4\mathbf{Z}\}$ a refinement of the partition $\Gamma = \{2\mathbf{Z}, 1 + 2\mathbf{Z}\}$ of $\mathbf{Z}$?
    (c) Is $\{1 + 3\mathbf{Z}, 2 + 3\mathbf{Z}, 6\mathbf{Z}, 3 + 6\mathbf{Z}\}$ a partition of $\mathbf{Z}$? Is it a refinement of the partition $\{3\mathbf{Z}, 1 + 3\mathbf{Z}, 2 + 3\mathbf{Z}\}$?

17. (i) Is 0 in $n\mathbf{Z}$ for all n in $\mathbf{Z}$? Explain.
    (ii) Is 0 an even integer? That is, is 0 in $2\mathbf{Z}$?
   (iii) Does $n|0$ for all n in $\mathbf{Z}$? Explain.
    (iv) List all integers in $0\mathbf{Z}$, that is, $d\mathbf{Z}$ with $d = 0$.
     (v) Find the only integer m such that $0|m$.
    (vi) Is n in $n\mathbf{Z}$ for all n in $\mathbf{Z}$? Explain.
   (vii) Does $n|n$ for all n in $\mathbf{Z}$? Explain.
  (viii) Is $2\mathbf{Z} \subseteq 6\mathbf{Z}$? Explain.

18. (i) Is $1\mathbf{Z} = \mathbf{Z}$? Explain.
    (ii) Does $1|n$ for all n in $\mathbf{Z}$? Explain.
   (iii) Find the two integers d such that $d|1$.
    (iv) Does $(-n)\mathbf{Z} = n\mathbf{Z}$ for all n in $\mathbf{Z}$? Explain.
     (v) Does $n|(-n)$ for all n in $\mathbf{Z}$? Explain.
    (vi) If $a|b$ and $b|c$, does $a|c$? Explain.
   (vii) Is $12\mathbf{Z} \subset 3\mathbf{Z}$? Explain.

19. (a) Find the four integers d such that $d|7$.
    (b) Find the six integral divisors of 25.
    (c) Find the eight integral divisors of 35.
    (d) Find all the integral divisors of -35.
    (e) Find all the positive integral divisors of 70.

20. In each of the following parts, find all integers d with the given property:
(a) $d|5$;   (b) $d|49$;   (c) $d|10$;   (d) $d|30$;   (e) $d|(-30)$.

21. Let E be the equivalence relation on $X = \{-3, -2, -1, 0, 1, 2, 3\}$ for which aEb means that either $a = b$ or $a = -b$.
(i) Give the members of the induced partition of X.
(ii) Check Part (i) using Theorem 1.
(iii) Give the rank of this partition of X.

22. Repeat Problem 21, but with E now the equivalence relation on X for which aEb means that $a^2 = b^2$.

23. Let $A = \{1, 2\}$, $B = \{3, 4\}$, and $C = \{5\}$. List the 9 ordered pairs of the equivalence relation E induced by the partition $\{A, B, C\}$ of $X = \{1, 2, 3, 4, 5\}$.

24. Let $A = \{1, 2, 3\}$, $B = \{4, 5\}$, and $X = A \cup B$. How many ordered pairs are there in the equivalence relation induced by the partition $\{A, B\}$ of X?

25. Let $\{A_1, A_2, A_3, A_4\}$ be a partition of X and let $\# A_i = n_i$ for $i = 1, 2, 3, 4$. How many ordered pairs are there in the equivalence relation on X induced by this partition?

26. Generalize the results in Problems 23, 24, and 25.

27. Show the following:
(i) If n is in $3\mathbf{Z}$, then n^2 is in $3\mathbf{Z}$.
(ii) If n is in $1 + 3\mathbf{Z}$ or is in $2 + 3\mathbf{Z}$, then n^2 is in $1 + 3\mathbf{Z}$.
(iii) There are no squares in $2 + 3\mathbf{Z}$.

28. Show the following:
(i) If n is in $4\mathbf{Z}$ or in $2 + 4\mathbf{Z}$, then n^2 is in $4\mathbf{Z}$.
(ii) If n is in $1 + 4\mathbf{Z}$ or $3 + 4\mathbf{Z}$, then n^2 is in $1 + 4\mathbf{Z}$.
(iii) There are no squares in $(2 + 4\mathbf{Z}) \cup (3 + 4\mathbf{Z})$.

29. Let E be an equivalence relation on X. For each a in X, let $C(a)$ be the subset of all x in X such that aEx. Prove Theorem 3 (left to the reader) by showing the following:
(i) $x \in C(x)$ for each x in X.
(ii) If $c \in C(a)$ and $c \in C(b)$, then $b \in C(a)$.
(iii) If $b \in C(a)$ and $x \in C(b)$, then $x \in C(a)$.
(iv) If $C(a) \cap C(b) \neq \varnothing$, then $C(a) = C(b)$.
(v) The collection Γ of the distinct subsets $C(a)$ is a partition of X.

30. Let E and Γ be as described in Theorem 3. Prove that E is the equivalence relation induced by Γ. (This is the rest of the proof of Theorem 3.)

31. (a) If $d|m$, must $d|(-m)$? Explain.
(b) If $a|b$ and $b|a$, must $b = \pm a$?
(c) If $a|b$, what is the relationship between $a\mathbf{Z}$ and $b\mathbf{Z}$?

32. (a) If $d|m$, must $(-d)|m$? Explain.
(b) If $a|b$ and $b|a$, with a and b both positive integers, must $a = b$?
(c) Does $a|b$ if and only if $b\mathbf{Z} \subseteq a\mathbf{Z}$?

33. Let P be a set of positive integers; that is, let $P \subseteq \mathbf{Z}^+$. Prove that $(P, |)$ is a poset. That is, prove that the binary relation $|$ on P is reflexive, transitive, and antisymmetric.

34. (i) Is the binary relation $|$ on $\mathbf{Z}$ antisymmetric? Explain.
(ii) Is $(\mathbf{Z}, |)$ a poset? Explain.

35. Let $X = \{1, 2, 11, 22\}$. Draw the poset diagrams for:
(a) $(X, |)$;   (b) $(X, \leq)$;   (c) $(X, =)$.

36. Let $X = \{1, 3, 9, 27, 81\}$. Draw the poset diagrams for:
(a) $(X, |)$;   (b) $(X, \geq)$;   (c) $(X, =)$.

37. For n in $\mathbf{Z}^+$, let D_n be the set of all positive integral divisors of n. For example, $D_{24} = \{1, 2, 3, 4, 6, 8, 12, 24\}$. Give the poset diagrams for:
(a) $(D_{24}, |)$;   (b) $(D_{36}, |)$.

38. Repeat Problem 37 for:
(a) $(D_{54}, |)$;   (b) $(D_{100}, |)$.

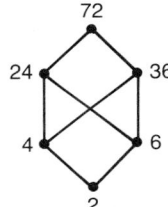

39. Let $X = \{2, 4, 6, 24, 36, 72\}$. The figure shows a poset diagram for $(X, |)$.
(i) Find the set A of all x in X with $4|x$.
(ii) Find the set B of all x in X with $6|x$.
(iii) Find the intersection $I = A \cap B$.
(iv) List the minimal elements of I. (See Definition 4 of Section 1.6.)
(v) Does I have a least element with respect to the partial ordering $|$? That is, is there an m in I such that $m|x$ for all x in I? If so, what is m?

40. Let $Y = \{2, 4, 6, 12, 24, 36, 72\}$. Draw the poset diagram for $(Y, |)$ and repeat Problem 39, but with X replaced by Y.

41. Let $(X, |)$ be as in Problem 39.
(i) Find the set C of all x in X with $x|24$.
(ii) Find the set D of all x in X with $x|36$.
(iii) Find the intersection $J = C \cap D$.
(iv) List the maximal elements of J. (See Definition 4 of Section 1.6.)
(v) Does J have a greatest element? That is, is there an element g in J with $x|g$ for all x in J? If so, what is g?

42. Repeat Problem 41, but with X replaced by $Y = \{2, 4, 6, 12, 24, 36, 72\}$.

43. Let $X = \{1, 2, 3, 5, 6, 10, 15, 30\}$.
(i) Draw a poset diagram for $(X, |)$.
(ii) Find the set A of all x in X with $x|10$ and the set B of all y in X with $y|15$. Also find $I = A \cap B$.
(iii) Does I have a greatest element with respect to the relation $|$? That is, is there an integer g in I with $x|g$ for all x in I? If so, what is g?
(iv) List the maximal elements of I.

44. Let $(X, |)$ be as in Problem 43.
   (i) Find the set C of all x in X with $2|x$ and the set D of all y in X with $3|y$. Also find $J = C \cap D$.
   (ii) Does J have a least element? That is, is there an m in J with $m|x$ for all x in J? If so, what is m?
   (iii) List the minimal elements of J.

45. Let D be the set of all positive integers d such that both 66 and 154 are in $d\mathbf{Z}$.
   (i) List D.
   (ii) Is there an integer g in D with $d|g$ for all d in D? If so, what is g?
   (iii) Does D have a greatest element in the poset $(\mathbf{Z}^+, |)$? If so, what is it?

46. Let M be the intersection $(4\mathbf{Z}^+) \cap (6\mathbf{Z}^+)$.
   (i) Is there an integer b in M with $b|m$ for all m in M? If so, what is b?
   (ii) Does M have a least element in the poset $(\mathbf{Z}^+, |)$? If so, what is it?

47. Let $S_1, S_2, \ldots, S_m$ be a partition Γ of a set X and let $T_1, T_2, \ldots, T_n$ be a ***proper refinement*** Γ' of Γ, that is, a refinement Γ' such that Γ is not a refinement of Γ'. Must Γ' have larger rank than Γ? Explain.

1.8

MAPPINGS

Here we extend to arbitrary sets the concept of a function from a set of real numbers to a set of real numbers.

DEFINITION 1 **MAPPING, IMAGE, EQUALITY OF MAPPINGS**

A ***mapping*** f from a set X to a set Y is an assignment to each element x in X of a unique element y in Y. The y assigned to a specific x is the ***image*** of x under f and is denoted as $f(x)$ (read it as "f of x"). If f and g are mappings from X to Y, and if $f(x) = g(x)$ for all x in X, then $f = g$.

DEFINITION 2 **DOMAIN, CODOMAIN, IMAGE SET**

For a mapping f from X to Y, the set X is the ***domain***, the set Y is the ***codomain***, and the set $\{f(x) : x \in X\}$ of images $y = f(x)$ for all x in X is the ***image set***.

In calculus texts the word *range* is used sometimes to mean "codomain" and other times to mean "image set." Because of this ambiguity, we will avoid using the word *range*.

Example 1   Let f be the mapping from $X = \{1, 2, 3, 4\}$ to $Y = \{a, b, c\}$ for which the assignment to each x in X of an image in Y is given by

$$f(1) = a, \qquad f(2) = c, \qquad f(3) = a, \qquad f(4) = a$$

or equivalently by Figure 1.8.1 or by the table

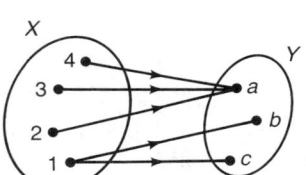

FIGURE 1.8.1

x	1	2	3	4
$f(x)$	a	c	a	a

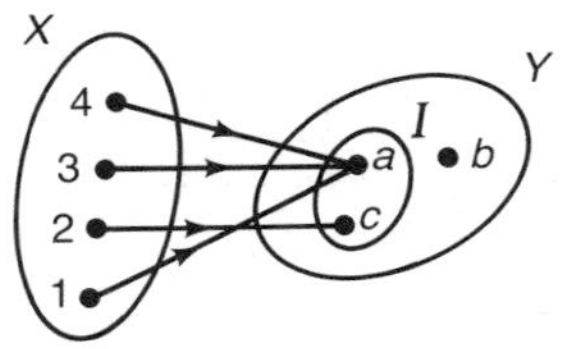

One sees that the image set is the proper subset $I = \{a, c\}$ of the codomain Y.

Figure 1.8.2, on the other hand, does not characterize a mapping from $X = \{1, 2, 3, 4\}$ to $Y = \{a, b, c\}$, since the assignment to the element 1 of X of an element in Y is not unique. The figure assigns both b and c to 1. ☐

FIGURE 1.8.2

Let a relation R from X to Y have the property that for each x in X there is one and only one y in Y with $(x, y) \in R$. Such an R determines the mapping f_R from X to Y defined by

$$f_R(x) = y \qquad \text{if and only if} \qquad (x, y) \in R. \tag{1}$$

The relation $R = \{(1, a), (2, c), (3, a), (4, a)\}$ from $X = \{1, 2, 3, 4\}$ to $Y = \{a, b, c\}$ has this property and determines, using (1), the mapping f of Example 1.

Example 2   Let B_5 be the set of 5-digit binary strings and let $Y = \{0, 1, 2, 3, 4, 5\}$. The mapping f from B_5 to Y, with $f(\alpha) = \text{wgt } \alpha$, has the entire codomain Y as its image set. ☐

Two kinds of arrows are used in dealing with mappings.

NOTATION 1   MAPPING ARROWS

The notation $f: X \to Y$ means that f is a mapping from X to Y. Also, $f: x \mapsto y$ indicates that the mapping f sends x to y, that is, $f(x) = y$.

One can also read "$f: x \mapsto y$" as "y is the image of x under the mapping f." The $\to$ goes from the domain to the codomain, and $\mapsto$ goes from an element of the domain to its image in the codomain.

Thus the mapping of Example 2 can be written as

$$f: B_5 \to \{0, 1, 2, 3, 4, 5\}; \qquad \alpha \mapsto \text{wgt } \alpha.$$

Example 3 Let $B_{n,k}$ be the set of n-digit binary strings of weight k. The mapping

$$f: B_{5,2} \to B_5; \qquad \alpha \mapsto \bar{\alpha}$$

where $\bar{\alpha}$ is the complement of α, has the proper subset $B_{5,3}$ of the codomain B_5 as its image set. Figure 1.8.3 illustrates the mapping f of this example.

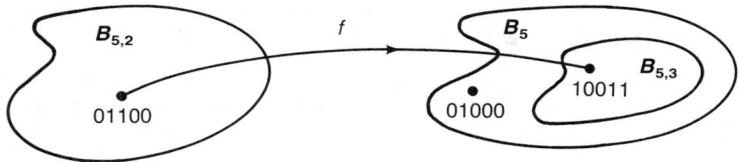

FIGURE 1.8.3

Example 4 Let $f: B_n \to B_n; \alpha \mapsto \bar{\alpha}$. Part (b) of Theorem 4 ("String Complements") of Section 1.2 tells us that $f(\alpha) \neq f(\beta)$ when $\alpha \neq \beta$; that is, distinct strings in the domain have distinct images. Also, Part (c) of that theorem implies that the image set for f is the entire codomain B_n. $\square$

Example 5 Let $S = \{s_1, s_2, \ldots, s_n\}$. For α in B_n, let

$$f: B_n \to P(S); \qquad \alpha \mapsto S_\alpha,$$

where $P(S)$ is the power set for S and S_α is as in Notation 2 ("Subsets") of Section 1.2. Then the image set for f is the entire codomain $P(S)$. $\square$

DEFINITION 3   SURJECTION

A mapping for which the image set is the entire codomain is a **surjection** (or a **surjective mapping**).

The mapping of Example 1 is not surjective, since the element b of the codomain is not in the image set. The mapping of Example 3 is not a surjection, since, for example, the string 00000 of the codomain B_5 is not in the image set $B_{5,3}$. The mappings of Examples 2, 4, and 5 are surjections.

DEFINITION 4   INJECTION

A mapping f from X to Y such that $f(x_1) = f(x_2)$ implies that $x_1 = x_2$ is an **injection** (or an **injective mapping**).

One can prove that f is injective by showing that $x_1 \neq x_2$ always implies that $f(x_1) \neq f(x_2)$. One can show that f is not injective by finding specific unequal elements x_1 and x_2 for which $f(x_1) = f(x_2)$. The mapping f of Example 1 is not injective, since $1 \neq 3$ but $f(1) = f(3)$. The mapping f of Example 2 is not an injection, since $10000 \neq 01000$ but wgt $10000 =$ wgt 01000. The mappings of Examples 3, 4, and 5 are injections, since, for these mappings f, $f(x_1) \neq f(x_2)$ whenever $x_1 \neq x_2$.

DEFINITION 5   **BIJECTION, PERMUTATION**

A mapping f from X to Y is a *bijection* (or is *bijective*) if it is both surjective and injective. A bijection from X to itself is a *permutation* on X.

The mappings of Examples 4 and 5 are bijections. The f of Example 4 is a permutation on B_n.

SYNONYMS   **FUNCTION, ONE-TO-ONE, ONTO**

Mappings frequently are called *functions* and sometimes are called *correspondences*. An injection may be called a *one-to-one mapping*. A surjection from X to Y may be called a *mapping* from X *onto* Y.

Example 6   Let $Z = \{\ldots, -2, -1, 0, 1, 2, \ldots\}$ and $N = \{0, 1, 2, \ldots\}$. The mapping

$$f: Z \to Z; \qquad n \mapsto |n| \qquad \text{(where } |n| \text{ is the absolute value of } n)$$

is not surjective. Changing the codomain from Z to N, we obtain a new surjective mapping

$$g: Z \to N; \qquad n \mapsto |n|.$$

We see as follows that the mapping

$$h: N \to N; \qquad n \mapsto n^2$$

is injective. We assume that $h(m) = h(n)$, that is, $m^2 = n^2$. Since neither m nor n is negative, this implies that $m = n$. Thus it follows from Definition 4 that h is injective. However, if the domain is enlarged to Z, then the mapping

$$k: Z \to N; \qquad n \mapsto n^2$$

is not injective, since $-1 \neq 1$ but $k(-1) = 1 = k(1)$.   □

DEFINITION 6   **CHARACTERISTIC FUNCTION**

The *characteristic function* for a subset A of S is the mapping f_A from S to $\{0, 1\}$, with $f_A(s) = 1$ if s is in A and $f_A(s) = 0$ otherwise.

Example 7 The characteristic function for the subset $A = \{b, e\}$ of the set $S = \{a, b, c, d, e\}$ is the mapping f_A from S to $\{0, 1\}$ given by

$$f_A: a \mapsto 0, \quad b \mapsto 1, \quad c \mapsto 0, \quad d \mapsto 0, \quad e \mapsto 1.$$

If $S = \{s_1, s_2, \ldots, s_n\}$ and $\alpha = a_1 a_2 \ldots a_n$ is an n-digit binary string, then the characteristic function for the subset S_α (which was defined in Notation 2 of Section 1.2) is

$$f: s_1 \mapsto a_1, \quad s_2 \mapsto a_2, \quad \ldots, \quad s_n \mapsto a_n.$$

In this example, $A = \{b, e\} = S_{01001}$. □

Example 8 A relation R from A to B is a subset of the cartesian product $A \times B$ and hence its characteristic function is the mapping f_R from $A \times B$ to $\{0, 1\}$, with $f_R(a, b) = 1$ if aRb and $f_R(a, b) = 0$ if $a\bar{R}b$. The matrix table for such a mapping is the relation matrix. □

DEFINITION 7 **PRE-IMAGE, COMPLETE INVERSE IMAGE**

Let $f: X \to Y$. A **pre-image** of a y in Y is an x in X with $f(x) = y$. The set of all pre-images of a given y is the **complete inverse image** of y and is denoted by $f^{-1}(y)$. [If y is not in the image set for f, then $f^{-1}(y)$ is empty.]

In Example 1, $f^{-1}(a) = \{1, 3, 4\}$, $f^{-1}(b)$ is the empty set $\varnothing$, and $f^{-1}(c) = \{2\}$. In Example 2, $f^{-1}(k) = B_{5,k}$ for $k = 0, 1, 2, 3, 4, 5$.

THEOREM 1 **COMPLETE INVERSE IMAGE PARTITION**

For $f: X \to Y$, let Γ be the collection of distinct complete inverse images $f^{-1}(y)$ for all y in Y. Then Γ is a partition of the domain X.

PROOF Each x of X has a unique image $y = f(x)$, and therefore the unique complete inverse image containing x is $f^{-1}(y)$. Hence the complete inverse images are pairwise disjoint and have X as their union. This means that Γ is a partition of X. □

Example 9 Let $X = \{1, 2, 3, 4, 5, 6, 7\}$, $Y = \{a, b, c, d, e\}$, and $f: X \to Y$ be given by the following table:

x	1	2	3	4	5	6	7
$f(x)$	a	c	e	b	a	b	a

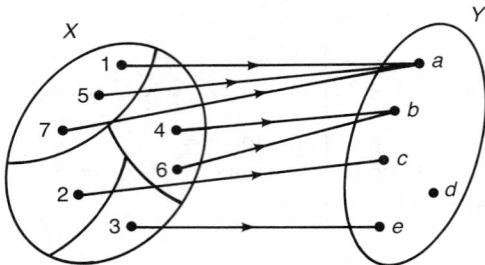

FIGURE 1.8.4

or by Figure 1.8.4. Then the next table gives $f^{-1}(y)$ for each y in Y:

y	a	b	c	d	e
$f^{-1}(y)$	$\{1, 5, 7\}$	$\{4, 6\}$	$\{2\}$	$\varnothing$	$\{3\}$

and $\{\{1, 5, 7\}, \{4, 6\}, \{2\}, \varnothing, \{3\}\}$ is the partition of the domain X discussed in Theorem 1.   □

NOTATION 2   **SET Y^X OF MAPPINGS FROM X TO Y**

The set of all mappings from X to Y is denoted as Y^X.

Thus $f \in Y^X$ has the same meaning as $f: X \to Y$. For example, if $X = \{a, b\}$ and $Y = \{1, 2\}$, then $Y^X = \{f_1, f_2, f_3, f_4\}$, where

$$f_1: a \mapsto 1, \quad b \mapsto 1; \qquad f_2: a \mapsto 1, \quad b \mapsto 2;$$
$$f_3: a \mapsto 2, \quad b \mapsto 1; \qquad f_4: a \mapsto 2, \quad b \mapsto 2.$$

Example 10   Let $X = \{1, 2, \ldots, m\}$ and Y be a nonempty finite set of size n. Then

$$f: 1 \mapsto y_1, \quad 2 \mapsto y_2, \quad \ldots, \quad m \mapsto y_m$$

specifies a mapping f from X to Y whenever the y_i are in Y. Thus there is one and only one mapping f in Y^X for each ordered m-tuple $(y_1, y_2, \ldots, y_m)$ in the cartesian product $Y^m = Y \times Y \times \cdots \times Y$ of m copies of Y. Hence the number of mappings from X to Y is the number of m-tuples $(y_1, y_2, \ldots, y_m)$ in Y^m, that is, $\#(Y^X) = \#(Y^m)$. But $\#(Y^m) = (\# Y)^m$. (See Problem 29 of Section 1.4.) Hence

$$\#(Y^X) = (\# Y)^m = (\# Y)^{\# X}.$$

In particular, if $X = \{1, 2\}$ and $Y = \{a, b, c\}$, then there are $3^2 = 9$ mappings from X to Y.   □

THEOREM 2   **NUMBER OF MAPPINGS FROM X TO Y**

If X and Y are finite sets, the number, $\#(Y^X)$, of mappings from X to Y is $(\#Y)^{\#X}$.

The proof of Theorem 2 is omitted, since it is essentially the discussion in Example 10.

THEOREM 3   **SIZE OF AN IMAGE SET**

Let $\#X = m$, $\#Y = n$, and I be the image set of a mapping f from X to Y. Then:

(i) $\#I \leq \#Y$.
(ii) f is surjective if and only if $\#I = \#Y$.
(iii) $\#I \leq \#X$.
(iv) f is injective if and only if $\#I = \#X$.
(v) if f is surjective, $\#Y \leq \#X$.
(vi) if f is injective, $\#X \leq \#Y$.
(vii) if f is bijective, $\#X = \#Y$.

PROOF   Part (i) follows from the fact that I is a subset of Y. By definition, f is surjective if and only if $I = Y$. Since $I \subseteq Y$, and Y is finite, $I = Y$ if and only if $\#I = \#Y$. These facts prove (ii). Let $X = \{x_1, x_2, \ldots, x_m\}$. If we strike out repetitions in the listing

$$f(x_1), f(x_2), \ldots, f(x_m) \tag{2}$$

of the images of the elements of X, the image set I consists of what remains. Hence $\#I \leq \#X$, and (iii) is proved. The mapping f is injective if and only if there are no repetitions in the listing (2); therefore f is injective if and only if $\#I = \#X$. This proves (iv). If f is surjective, it follows from (ii) and (iii) that $\#Y = \#I \leq \#X$ and hence that $\#Y \leq \#X$. This proves (v). If f is injective, it follows from (iv) and (i) that $\#X = \#I \leq \#Y$ and thus that $\#X \leq \#Y$; this proves (vi). Since a bijection is both a surjection and an injection, (vii) follows from (v) and (vi). □

Example 11   **APPLICATION TO CODES**   Here we apply part of Theorem 3 to a problem that arises in constructing codes. Let $E = \{a, b, \ldots, z\}$ be the English alphabet. We wish to find the smallest positive integer n such that one can represent distinct letters from E by distinct strings in B_n. The representation can be done by a mapping from E into B_n. This mapping has to be injective, since distinct letters must be assigned distinct binary strings. Now, Theorem 3(vi) tells us that we are seeking the smallest n with $26 = \#E \leq \#B_n = 2^n$. Since $2^4 = 16$ and $2^5 = 32$, the desired n is 5. That is, the strings must have length 5 if there are to be enough strings to represent the 26 letters of E.

If we do not insist on representing all the letters of E by strings of the same length, our code could be an injection from E into $B_1 \cup B_2 \cup B_3 \cup B_4$, since there are 2 strings in B_1, 4 other strings in B_2, 8 other strings in B_3, and 16 other strings in B_4; thus there are

$$2 + 4 + 8 + 16 = 30$$

strings of length 4 or less, and this is sufficient for the code.

(See Problem 35 below for an application to the analogous situation for Morse Code, which assigns to each of the 36 symbols in the set

$$\{0, 1, \ldots, 9, a, b, \ldots, z\}$$

a string $a_1 a_2 \ldots a_n$ with each a_i in the set $\{\cdot, -\}$ of size 2.)   □

Example 12   Let $X = \{1, 2, 3\}$ and $Y = \{a, b, c, d, e\}$. An injection f from X to Y is specified by choosing $f(1)$, $f(2)$, and $f(3)$ as distinct elements of Y. Since $\#Y = 5$, there are 5 choices for $f(1)$. After $f(1)$ is chosen, $f(2)$ can be any one of the 4 elements of Y different from $f(1)$. After $f(1)$ and $f(2)$ are selected, $f(3)$ can be any of the remaining 3 elements of Y. Hence there are $5 \cdot 4 \cdot 3 = 60$ injections from X to Y. The following theorem extends this example.   □

THEOREM 4   **NUMBER OF INJECTIONS FROM X TO Y**

Let X and Y be finite sets, $\#X = m$, and $\#Y = n$. If $m \le n$, the number of injections from X to Y is $n(n - 1)(n - 2) \cdots (n - m + 1)$.

PROOF   Let $X = \{x_1, x_2, \ldots, x_m\}$. An injection f from X to Y is specified by choosing

$$f(x_1), f(x_2), \ldots, f(x_m)$$

as distinct elements of Y. Since $\#Y = n$, there are n choices for $f(x_1)$. After $f(x_1)$ is chosen, $f(x_2)$ can be any one of the $n - 1$ remaining elements of Y. After $f(x_1)$ and $f(x_2)$ are selected, $f(x_3)$ can be any of the remaining $n - 2$ elements of Y. Continuing this way one sees that there are $n - m + 1$ choices for $f(x_m)$. Thus the number of injections in Y^X is $n(n - 1)(n - 2) \cdots (n - m + 1)$.   □

Example 13   **APPLICATION TO PROBABILITY**   There are 23 students in a certain class. What is the probability that no two of these students have the same birthday? Assuming that no student in the class was born on February 29th, we reformulate the problem as follows:

Let $S = \{s_1, s_2, \ldots, s_{23}\}$ be the set of students and let $D = \{d_1, d_2, \ldots, d_{365}\}$ be the set of possible birthdays. Let f be the mapping from S to D in which $f(s)$ is the birthday of student s. Then f is injective if and only if no two students have the same birthday. The probability that f is injective is the number of injective mappings from S to D divided by the total number of mappings from S to D. Hence it follows from Theorems 4 and 2 that the desired probability p is

$$p = \frac{365 \cdot 364 \cdots 343}{365^{23}} \approx .494.$$

Most guesses for the number of people required to make $p < .5$ are far greater than 23. ☐

THEOREM 5 **DOMAIN AND CODOMAIN OF THE SAME SIZE**

Let X and Y be finite sets of the same size. Then a mapping f from X to Y is injective if and only if f is surjective.

PROOF Let I be the image set for a mapping f from X to Y. By Theorem 3(iv), f is injective if and only if $\#I = \#X$. Then the hypothesis that $\#X = \#Y$ implies that f is injective if and only if $\#I = \#Y$. But Theorem 3(ii) tells us that f is surjective if and only if $\#I = \#Y$. Hence f is injective if and only if f is surjective, when $\#X = \#Y$. ☐

COROLLARY **BIJECTION**

Let X and Y be finite sets of the same size and f be a mapping from X to Y. If f is injective or f is surjective, it follows that f is bijective.

THEOREM 6 **COUNTING BIJECTIONS**

If $\#X = n = \#Y$, there are $n(n - 1)(n - 2) \cdots 2 \cdot 1$ bijections from X to Y. In particular, if $\#X = n$ there are $n(n - 1)(n - 2) \cdots 2 \cdot 1$ permutations on X.

PROOF With the hypothesis that $\#X = n = \#Y$, it follows from Theorem 5 and its corollary that the bijections from X to Y are the same mappings as the injections from X to Y. The number of these is $n(n - 1)(n - 2) \cdots 2 \cdot 1$ by Theorem 4. This proves the first assertion in the theorem. The second assertion then follows, since a permutation on X is a bijection from X onto itself. ☐

Example 14   Here we use mappings to give formal definitions for a few terms, including some mentioned earlier in this chapter.

Binary String   A binary string $b_1 b_2 \ldots b_n$ in $\boldsymbol{B_n}$ may be thought of as the mapping

$$f: \{1, 2, \ldots, n\} \to \{0, 1\}; \qquad i \mapsto b_i.$$

Listing for a Set   A listing $\{s_1, s_2, \ldots, s_n\}$ for a finite set S is essentially the bijection

$$f: \{1, 2, \ldots, n\} \to S; \qquad i \mapsto s_i.$$

Finite Sequence   A finite sequence $a_1, a_2, \ldots, a_n$ with terms a_i in a set A is essentially the mapping

$$f: \{1, 2, \ldots, n\} \to A; \qquad i \mapsto a_i.$$

Infinite Sequence   An infinite sequence $a_1, a_2, \ldots$ with terms a_i in a set A is essentially the mapping

$$f: \boldsymbol{N} = \{0, 1, \ldots\} \to A; \qquad i \mapsto a_i. \qquad \square$$

PROBLEMS FOR SECTION 1.8

1. Which of the following mappings f are surjective? Which are injective? Which are bijective?
    (a) $f: \boldsymbol{B_4} \to \boldsymbol{B_3}; \quad f(a_1 a_2 a_3 a_4) = a_2 a_3 a_4.$
    (b) $f: \boldsymbol{B_3} \to \boldsymbol{B_4}; \quad f(a_1 a_2 a_3) = 0 a_1 a_2 a_3.$
    (c) $f: \boldsymbol{Z} \to \boldsymbol{Z}; \quad f(n) = n + 1. \quad [\boldsymbol{Z} = \{\ldots, -2, -1, 0, 1, 2, \ldots\}.]$
    (d) $f: \boldsymbol{Z} \to \boldsymbol{Z}; \quad f(n) = n^2.$
    (e) $f: \{1, 2, 3\} \to \{a, b\}; \quad 1 \mapsto a, \quad 2 \mapsto a, \quad 3 \mapsto b.$
    (f) $f: \{1, 2\} \to \{1, 2\}; \quad 1 \mapsto 2, \quad 2 \mapsto 1.$
    (g) $f: \{1, 2\} \to \{a, b, c\}; \quad 1 \mapsto a, \quad 2 \mapsto b.$

2. Answer the questions of Problem 1 for the following functions:
    (a) $f: \boldsymbol{B_n} \to \boldsymbol{B_{n+1}}; \quad f(\alpha)$ is the augmented string 1α.
    (b) $f: \boldsymbol{B_5} \to \boldsymbol{B_4}; \quad f(a_1 a_2 a_3 a_4 a_5) = a_1 a_2 a_3 a_4.$
    (c) $f: \boldsymbol{N} \to \boldsymbol{N}; \quad f(n) = n + 1. \quad [\boldsymbol{N} = \{0, 1, 2, \ldots\}.]$
    (d) $f: \boldsymbol{N} \to \boldsymbol{N}; \quad f(n) = n^2.$
    (e) $f: \{1, 2, 3\} \to \{1, 2, 3\}; \quad 1 \mapsto 2, \quad 2 \mapsto 3, \quad 3 \mapsto 1.$
    (f) $f: P(S) \to P(S); \quad f(A) = \bar{A}.$ [Here S is a nonempty set, $P(S)$ is its power set, and $\bar{A}$ is the complement of A in S.]
    (g) $f: P(S) \to P(S); \quad f(A) = A \cup \{s\}$ where s is a fixed element of S.

3. Let $X = \{1, 2\}$ and $Y = \{a, b, c\}$.
    (i) How many mappings are there from X to Y?
    (ii) In arrow form, show all the injections from X to Y.
    (iii) In arrow form, show the other mappings from X to Y.

4. Let $X = \{1, 2, 3\}$ and $Y = \{a, b\}$.
    (i) How many mappings are there from X to Y?
    (ii) In arrow form, show all surjections from X to Y.
    (iii) In arrow form, show the other mappings from X to Y.

5. Let $X = \{1, 2, 3\}$ and $Y = \{a, b, c\}$.
    (i) How many mappings are there from X to Y?
    (ii) How many injections are there from X to Y?
    (iii) Show all the injections from X to Y in arrow form.
    (iv) Is each mapping of (iii) also a surjection?
    (v) Let f be a surjection from X to Y. Must f be a bijection?

6. Let X be a finite set and f be a mapping from X to itself.
    (a) If f is surjective, must it also be injective and hence bijective? Explain.
    (b) If f is injective, must it be bijective? Explain.

7. Let f be the mapping from $N = \{0, 1, 2, \ldots\}$ to itself, with $f(n) = n/2$ when n is even and $f(n) = (n - 1)/2$ when n is odd. A partial table for f is:

n	0	1	2	3	4	5	6	7	8	...
$f(n)$	0	0	1	1	2	2	3	3	4	...

    (a) What is the complete inverse image $f^{-1}(0)$?
    (b) Describe $f^{-1}(n)$ for n in $Z^+ = \{1, 2, \ldots\}$.
    (c) Is f surjective?   (d) Is f injective?   (e) Is f bijective?

8. Let f be the mapping from N to $Z = \{\ldots, -1, 0, 1, \ldots\}$, with $f(n) = -n/2$ when n is even and $f(n) = (n + 1)/2$ when n is odd. A partial table for f is:

n	0	1	2	3	4	5	6	7	8	...
$f(n)$	0	1	-1	2	-2	3	-3	4	-4	...

    (a) What is the complete inverse image $f^{-1}(3)$?
    (b) Is $f^{-1}(n)$ a singleton for each n in Z?
    (c) Is f surjective? Is f injective? Is f bijective?

9. (i) Describe a surjection f from N to itself such that f is not an injection.
    (ii) Is the answer to Problem 6(a) the same when X is allowed to be infinite?

10. (i) Describe a nonsurjective injection f from N to itself.
    (ii) Is the answer to Problem 6(b) the same when X is infinite?

11. Give the characteristic function for the subset:
    (a) $\{a, d, e\}$ of $T = \{a, b, c, d, e\}$.
    (b) S_{10011} of $S = \{s_1, s_2, s_3, s_4, s_5\}$.

12. Give the characteristic function for the subset:
(a) $\{b, c, e, f\}$ of $T = \{a, b, c, d, e, f\}$.
(b) S_{011011} of $S = \{s_1, s_2, s_3, s_4, s_5, s_6\}$.

13. Let $f: \{1, 2\} \mapsto \{a, b, c\};$ $1 \mapsto a,$ $2 \mapsto b$. Find the following complete inverse images:
(i) $f^{-1}(a);$ (ii) $f^{-1}(b);$ (iii) $f^{-1}(c).$

14. Let $f: \{1, 2, 3\} \to \{a, b\};$ $1 \mapsto a,$ $2 \mapsto a,$ $3 \mapsto b$. Find:
(i) $f^{-1}(a);$ (ii) $f^{-1}(b).$

15. Let f be a mapping from X to Y. If $f^{-1}(y)$ is nonempty for every y in Y, is f surjective? Explain.

16. Let f be a mapping from X to Y. What must be true of each complete inverse image $f^{-1}(y)$ for f to be injective?

17. Let $N = \{0, 1, 2, \ldots\}$. Does the rule $f: (a, b) \mapsto a - b$ make f into a mapping from the cartesian product $N \times N$ to N? Explain.

18. Let $Z = \{\ldots, -2, -1, 0, 1, 2, \ldots\}$. Does the rule $f: (a, b) \mapsto a - b$ make f into a mapping from $Z \times Z$ to Z? Explain.

19. Let $\# A = 4$, $\# B = 5$, and $\# C = 6$.
(a) How many mappings are there from C to $A \times B$?
(b) Of these mappings, how many are injective?

20. Let $\# A = n$, with n in $\{2, 3, 4, \ldots\}$.
(a) How many mappings are there from A to $A \times A$?
(b) Of these mappings, how many are injective?

21. Let $\# A = n$. How many sequences $a_1, a_2, \ldots, a_m$ are there with each of the m terms a_i in A? [*Hint:* There are as many as there are mappings from $X_m = \{1, 2, \ldots, m\}$ to A.]

22. Let $\# A = r$. How many sequences $a_1, a_2, \ldots, a_s$ are there with the a_i as distinct elements of A? Assume that $s \le r$.

23. Let $f: A \to B$ and $g: B \to C$. Let $h(a) = c$ whenever $f(a) = b$ and $g(b) = c$. Does this rule make h into a mapping from A to C? Explain. (One calls h the **composite** of f and g and denotes this composite as $f \circ g$.)

24. Let f and g be mappings from X to itself. Let $h(x) = z$ whenever $f(x) = y$ and $g(y) = z$. Does this rule make h into a mapping from X to itself? Explain.

25. Let f be a bijection from A onto B.
(a) Characterize a bijection g from B onto A such that $g(f(a)) = a$ for each a in A.
(b) Let g be as in Part (a). Does $f(g(b)) = b$ for all b in B?

26. Let β be a permutation on a set S. Is there a permutation α on S such that $\alpha(\beta(s)) = s = \beta(\alpha(s))$ for all s in S? Explain.

27. Let $P = \{p_1, p_2, p_3, p_4, p_5\}$ and $M = \{m_1, m_2, \ldots, m_{12}\}$.

(i) How many injective mappings are there from P to M?

(ii) How many mappings are there from P to M?

(iii) Let P be a set of 5 randomly chosen people. What is the probability that no two people in P were born in the same month? Assume that the 12 months are equally likely as birth months.

28. J. Doe is among the 20 students in a certain class. The instructor selects three of the students at random to do problems at the board—one to do Problem 1, a second to do Problem 2, and a third to do Problem 3. What is the probability that Doe is not among the three selected? [*Hint*: Divide the number of injections from $A = \{1, 2, 3\}$ into $B = \{s_2, s_3, \ldots, s_{20}\}$ by the number of injections from A into $C = \{s_1, s_2, \ldots, s_{20}\}$. We are letting s_1 be J. Doe.]

29. (i) Tabulate the mapping f from B_3 to $N = \{0, 1, \ldots\}$, with

$$f(a_1 a_2 a_3) = 4a_1 + 2a_2 + a_3.$$

(ii) Is f injective?

(iii) What is the image set for f?

30. Repeat Problem 29, but now let f be the mapping from B_4 to N with

$$f(a_1 a_2 a_3 a_4) = 8a_1 + 4a_2 + 2a_3 + a_4.$$

31. Let f be a mapping from X to Y and let R be the relation from X to Y such that $(x, y) \in R$ if and only if $y = f(x)$. By definition of mapping, for each a in X there is one and only one b in Y with $(a, b) \in R$.
(a) What property must R have for f to be injective?
(b) What property must R have for f to be surjective?

32. Let f be a mapping from X to Y. Let T be the binary relation on X for which aTb means that $f(a) = f(b)$. Is T an equivalence relation? If so, what are the equivalence classes of the induced partition of X?

33. How many distinct listings are there for the 3-bit strings of B_3?

34. How many listings are there for the strings of B_4?

35. Find the smallest n for which there is an injection from the set $A = \{0, 1, \ldots, 9, a, b, \ldots, z\}$ of 36 symbols into the union $T = B_1 \cup B_2 \cup \cdots \cup B_n$. (This problem has application in Morse Code. See Example 11 above.)

SUMMARY OF TERMS, CHAPTER 1

Antisymmetric relation R	aRb and bRa together imply $a = b$.	31
aRb [or $(a, b) \in R$]	a is related to b under R.	26
Arrows for mapping	$f: X \to Y$; $\quad x \mapsto f(x)$ indicates that X is the domain, Y is the codomain, and $f(x)$ is the image of x under f.	56
ART	Acronym for antisymmetric, reflexive, and transitive.	36
Associativity for $\cap$ and $\cup$	$A \cap (B \cap C) = (A \cap B) \cap C$, $A \cup (B \cup C) = (A \cup B) \cup C$.	18

Identities S for $\cap$ and $\varnothing$ for $\cup$	$A \cap S = A$, $A \cup \varnothing = A$.	18
Image of x under f	The element $f(x)$ of the codomain assigned to x by the mapping f.	55
Image set for f	Set $\{f(x) : x \in X\}$ of all images under f.	55
Induced:		
equivalence relation from a partition	See Definition 6 of Section 1.7.	49
partition from an equivalence relation E	See Theorem 3 of Section 1.7.	49
Infinite sequence	$a_1, a_2, \ldots$ (with repetitions allowed).	64
Injection (1-to-1 mapping) f	$[f(x) = f(y)]$ implies $x = y$.	57
Integers, set $\mathbf{Z}$ of	$\mathbf{Z} = \{\ldots, -2, -1, 0, 1, 2, \ldots\}$.	46
Integral divisor d of m	For d and m in $\mathbf{Z}$, $d \mid m$ means that $m = cd$ for some c in $\mathbf{Z}$.	48
Integral multiples of d	$d\mathbf{Z} = \{dn : n \in \mathbf{Z}\}$.	48
Intersection of the sets of a collection Γ	The set of all elements that belong to every member of Γ.	13
Inverse image, complete	$f^{-1}(y) = \{x \in X : f(x) = y\}$.	59
Irreflexive binary relation R on S	An R with (s, s) not in R for all s in S, i.e., an R whose matrix has no 1's on the diagonal.	31
Least element a in S under $\preceq$	An a with $a \preceq s$ for all s in S.	38
Length of a binary string β	The number of bits in β.	4
Linearly ordered set	A poset with each pair of elements comparable.	39
Listing of a finite set S	$S = \{s_1, s_2, \ldots, s_n\}$.	2, 64
Loop	An arc from a vertex to itself.	32
Mapping $f: X \to Y$	An assignment to each x in X of a unique element y in Y.	55
Mapping arrows (*see* Arrows for mapping)		56
Matrix table for $\square$	$A \square B$ appears in the spot of the row for A and the column for B. ($\square$ is $\cap$ or $\cup$ here.)	14
Maximal element q in A under $\preceq$	There is no a in A with $q \preceq a$.	39
Member A of a collection Γ	A set A belonging to Γ.	9
Minimal element m in A under $\preceq$	There is no a in A with $a \preceq m$.	39
Minisets M_α	The subsets depicted by the regions of a Venn Diagram.	19
n-ary relation on a set S	Subset of $S^n = S \times S \times \cdots \times S$.	25
n-bit string	$a_1 a_2 \ldots a_n$ with each a_i in $\{0, 1\}$.	2
$\mathbf{N}$, set of natural numbers	$\{0, 1, 2, \ldots\}$.	46
Noncomparable elements a and b under $\preceq$	Neither $a \preceq b$ nor $b \preceq a$.	39
Odd integers	Set $1 + 2\mathbf{Z} = \{\ldots, -3, -1, 1, 3, 5, \ldots\}$.	46
One-to-one (*see* Injection)		57, 58

REVIEW PROBLEMS FOR CHAPTER 1

1. Recall that B_n is the set of n-digit binary strings and that $B_{n,k}$ is the subset of strings of weight k in B_n. For each of the following, tell whether it is true or false and explain your answer.
   (a) $\#B_4 = 2(\#B_2)$.
   (b) $\#B_8 = (\#B_4)^2$.
   (c) If $\alpha \in B_{5,4}$, then wgt $\alpha = 5$.
   (d) If $\alpha \in B_{4,4}$, then wgt $\bar{\alpha} = 1$.
   (e) $B_{5,3} = B_{4,3} \cup B_{4,2}$.
   (f) $\#B_{5,3} = (\#B_{4,3}) + (\#B_{4,2})$.

2. Repeat Problem 1 for the following parts.
   (a) $B_5 = B_4 \cup B_1$.
   (b) $B_5 = \{0\alpha : \alpha \in B_4\} \cup \{1\alpha : \alpha \in B_4\}$.

(c) $\#B_{12} = 4(\#B_{10})$.

(d) $\#B_6 > (\#B_5) + (\#B_4) + (\#B_3) + (\#B_2) + (\#B_1)$.

3. Give a set S such that $\#P(S)$ is:
   (a) 1;   (b) 8;   (c) 256.

4. Is there a set S such that $\#P(S) = 14$? Explain.

5. Given that $\#B_{10,3} = 120$, $\#B_{10,4} = 210$, and $\#B_{10} = 1024$, find:
   (i) $\#B_{11}$;   (ii) $\#B_{11,4}$;   (iii) $\#B_{11,7}$;   (iv) $\binom{11}{4}$;
   (v) $\binom{11}{7}$;   (vi) $\binom{11}{0}$;   (vii) $\binom{11}{11}$.

6. Given that $\#B_{12,4} = 495$, $\#B_{12,5} = 792$, and $\#B_{12} = 4096$, find:
   (i) $\#B_{13}$;   (ii) $\#B_{13,5}$;   (iii) $\#B_{13,8}$;   (iv) $\binom{13}{5}$;
   (v) $\binom{13}{8}$;   (vi) $\binom{13}{0}$;   (vii) $\binom{13}{13}$.

7. Given that $\binom{16}{4} = 1820$ and $\binom{15}{3} = 455$, find $\binom{15}{4}$ and $\binom{15}{11}$.

8. Given that $\binom{20}{5} = 15504$ and $\binom{19}{5} = 11628$, find $\binom{19}{4}$ and $\binom{19}{15}$.

9. Let A, B, and C be sets.
   (a) If $A = B$, must $A \cap C = B \cap C$?
   (b) If $A \cap C = B \cap C$, must $A = B$? Explain.

10. Repeat Problem 9, but with $\cap$ replaced by $\cup$.

11. If $A \subseteq B$ and $B \subseteq C$, must $A \subseteq C$?

12. If $A \subseteq B$, $B \subseteq C$, and $C \subseteq A$, must $A = B = C$?

13. Let A, B, C be subsets of S. Use a case table to show that $\overline{A \cup B \cup C} = \bar{A} \cap \bar{B} \cap \bar{C}$.

14. Let A, B, C be subsets of S. Show with a case table that $\overline{A \cap B \cap C} = \bar{A} \cup \bar{B} \cup \bar{C}$.

15. Let the M_α with α in B_4 be the minisets for A_1, A_2, A_3, A_4. Which of these minisets must be empty when $A_1 \subseteq A_4$?

16. Which of the minisets of Problem 15 must be empty when $A_2 \subseteq A_3$?

17. (a) Does $A \times B = B \times A$ for all sets A and B? Explain.
    (b) Does $A \times \varnothing = A$ for some set A? Explain.

18. (a) Does $A \times \varnothing = \varnothing$ for all sets A? Explain.
    (b) Does $A \times (B \cap C) = (A \times B) \cap (A \times C)$ for all sets A, B, C?

19. Let $\#A = m = \#B$. Give:
    (a) $\#(A \times B)$;   (b) $\#P(A \times B)$.

20. Let $\#A = m = \#B$ and let $\#C = n$. Give:
    (a) $\#(A \times B \times C)$;   (b) $\#P(A \times B \times C)$.

21. Recall that $N = \{0, 1, 2, \ldots\}$. Let

$$R = \{(x, y) : x \text{ and } y \text{ are in } N \text{ and } x + y = 4\}.$$

    (a) Is R reflexive?   (b) Is R symmetric?   (c) Is R transitive?

22. Is the R of Problem 21 antisymmetric? Is it irreflexive?

23. Let $S = \{s_1, s_2, \ldots, s_{10}\}$.
    (i) What is $\#(S \times S)$?
    (ii) How many ordered pairs are there in the complete relation K on S?

24. How many ordered pairs are there in the diagonal relation D on $S = \{1, 2, \ldots, 15\}$?

25. Let $A = \{1, 2, 3, 4\}$.
    (i) Which ordered pairs are in the binary relation R on A in which aRb means $a|b$?
    (ii) Draw the picture for the relation R.
    (iii) Draw the poset diagram for (A, R), that is, $(A, |)$.

26. Let $A = \{1\}$, $B = \{2\}$, $C = \{1, 3\}$, $D = \{2, 3\}$, $E = \{1, 2, 3\}$, and $X = \{A, B, C, D, E\}$.
    (i) Which ordered pairs are in the binary relation $\supset$ on X?
    (ii) Draw the picture for the relation $\supset$ on X.
    (iii) Draw the poset diagram for $(X, \supset)$.

27. Recall that $a + b\mathbf{Z} = \{a + bn : n \in \mathbf{Z}\}$. Which of the following are partitions of $\mathbf{Z}$?
    (a) $\{3\mathbf{Z}, 1 + 6\mathbf{Z}, 2 + 6\mathbf{Z}, 4 + 6\mathbf{Z}, 5 + 6\mathbf{Z}\}$.
    (b) $\{2\mathbf{Z}, 1 + 6\mathbf{Z}, 3 + 6\mathbf{Z}, 5 + 6\mathbf{Z}\}$.
    (c) $\{2\mathbf{Z}, 3\mathbf{Z}, 1 + 6\mathbf{Z}, 5 + 6\mathbf{Z}\}$.

28. Which of the following are partitions of N?
    (a) $\{4N, 1 + 4N, 3 + 4N\}$.
    (b) $\{2N, 1 + 4N, 3 + 4N\}$.
    (c) $\{3N, 1 + 3N, -1 + 3N\}$.

29. Let E be the equivalence relation on $\mathbf{Z}$ induced by the partition of Problem 27(b). Which of the following ordered pairs are in E?
    (a) $(0, 2)$;   (b) $(1, 3)$;   (c) $(1, 5)$;
    (d) $(10, 14)$; (e) $(7, 13)$;   (f) $(11, 23)$.

30. Let E be the equivalence relation on $\mathbf{Z}$ induced by the partition of Problem 27(a). Which of the following are in E?
    (a) $(0, 3)$;   (b) $(1, 4)$;   (c) $(1, 7)$;
    (d) $(3, 9)$;   (e) $(4, 16)$;   (f) $(5, 23)$.

31. Let f and g be the following mappings:

    $$f: \mathbf{B_5} \to \mathbf{B_3}; \quad a_1 a_2 a_3 a_4 a_5 \mapsto a_1 a_3 a_5.$$
    $$g: \mathbf{B_3} \to \mathbf{B_3}; \quad b_1 b_2 b_3 \mapsto 0 b_2 b_3.$$

    (a) Is f surjective?   (b) Is f injective?
    (c) Is g surjective?   (d) Is g injective?

32. Repeat Problem 31 for:

    $$f: \mathbf{B_5} \to \mathbf{B_5}; \quad a_1 a_2 a_3 a_4 a_5 \mapsto a_5 a_4 a_3 a_2 a_1.$$
    $$g: \mathbf{B_3} \to \mathbf{B_5}; \quad b_1 b_2 b_3 \mapsto 0 0 b_1 b_2 b_3.$$

33. Let $S = \{s_1, s_2, s_3, s_4, s_5\}$. The mapping

$$f: \boldsymbol{B_5} \to P(S); \quad \alpha \mapsto S_\alpha$$

is a bijection. Does this mean that $\# P(S) = \# \boldsymbol{B_5} = 2^5$? Explain.

34. Let $S = \{s_1, s_2, \ldots, s_n\}$ and let Q consist of all the subsets A of S with $\# A = k$. The mapping

$$g: \boldsymbol{B_{n,k}} \to Q; \quad \alpha \mapsto S_\alpha$$

is a bijection. Does this mean that $\# Q = \# \boldsymbol{B_{n,k}} = \binom{n}{k}$? Explain.

35. Let $A = \{1, 2, 3\}$, $B = \{a, b, c, d\}$, and $C = \{x_1, x_2, x_3, x_4, x_5\}$.
 (a) How many mappings are there from A to B?
 (b) How many of the mappings from A to B are injective?
 (c) How many of the mappings from A to B are surjective?
 (d) How many mappings are there from B to $A \times C$?

36. (a) How many mappings are there from $\{1, 2, 3, 4, 5\}$ to $\{a, b, c\}$?
 (b) How many of the mappings in (a) are injective?
 (c) Let $\# S = n$. How many mappings are there from $S \times S$ to S?
 (d) If $\# S > 1$, can a mapping from $S \times S$ to S be injective?

37. Let f be the mapping from $N \times N$ to N, with $f(m, n) = 3^m n$.
 (a) Does $f(1, 3) = f(3, 1)$?
 (b) Is f surjective? Explain.
 (c) What is $f^{-1}(18)$? That is, what is the complete inverse image of 18 under f?
 (d) Is f injective? Explain.

38. Repeat Problem 37, but with each N replaced by $\boldsymbol{Z^+}$.

39. Let f be a mapping from X to Y. Match each of the assertions:
 (i) f is surjective,   (ii) f is injective,   (iii) f is bijective,
 with an equivalent assertion chosen from:
 (a) $\# f^{-1}(y) \in \{0, 1\}$ for each y in Y;
 (b) $\# f^{-1}(y) \in \boldsymbol{Z^+} = \{1, 2, \ldots\}$ for each y in Y;
 (c) $\# f^{-1}(y) = 1$ for each y in Y.

40. (i) Which of 10011 and 01110 appears earlier in the standard listing for $\boldsymbol{B_5}$?
 (ii) Which of 1010011 and 1001110 appears earlier in the standard listing for $\boldsymbol{B_7}$?

SUPPLEMENTARY AND CHALLENGING PROBLEMS, CHAPTER 1 _____

1. Let T_n consist of all n-digit *ternary* strings, that is, strings $\alpha = a_1 a_2 \ldots a_n$ with each a_i in $\{0, 1, 2\}$. Let wgt $\alpha = a_1 + a_2 + \cdots + a_n$. For how many α in T_n is wgt α even, that is, in $2N = \{0, 2, 4, \ldots\}$?

2. How many n-digit strings $a_1 a_2 \ldots a_n$ are there with each a_i in $\{0, 1, 2, 3, 4\}$ and $a_1 + a_2 + \cdots + a_n$ in $2N$?

3. Let $\#S = n$ and $P = P(S)$. How many ordered pairs (A, B) are there in $P \times P$ such that $A \subseteq B$?

4. Let $\#S = n$. How many ordered k-tuples $(A_1, A_2, \ldots, A_k)$ are there in $[P(S)]^k$ such that $A_1 \subseteq A_2 \subseteq \cdots \subseteq A_k$?

5. Let $\#S = n$. How many ordered triples (A, B, C) are there in $[P(S)]^3$ such that $A \subseteq C$ and $B \subseteq C$ but neither of A and B is a subset of the other?

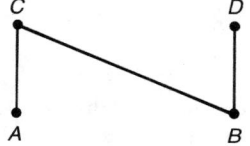

6. Let $\#S = n$. How many ordered quadruples (A, B, C, D) are there in $[P(S)]^4$ such that the poset diagram for $(\{A, B, C, D\}, \subseteq)$ is as shown in the figure?

7. Let m and n be in $\mathbf{Z}^+ = \{1, 2, \ldots\}$ and $(X, \preceq)$ be a poset with $\#X = mn + 1$. Prove that at least one of the following must be true:
(i) There is a subset $A = \{a_1, a_2, \ldots, a_{m+1}\}$ of X with $a_i \prec a_{i+1}$ for $i = 1, 2, \ldots, m$.
(ii) There is a subset $B = \{b_1, b_2, \ldots, b_{n+1}\}$ of X for which $b_i \prec b_j$ is never true with b_i and b_j in B.

8. Let $\#X = m$ and $\#Y = n$. Find the number of surjections from X onto Y when:
(a) $n = 2$ and $m \geq 2$;   (b) $n = 3$ and $m \geq 3$.

2

ALGEBRAIC STRUCTURES

An *algebraic structure* is a set X, called the *carrier* of the structure, with one or more operations on X and possibly with special elements of X such as identities under some of the operations. The type of structure depends on the axioms assumed for the operations.

In the first four sections of this chapter, we study the main algebraic structures that have applications to logic, electrical circuits, and electronic networks. Some of these applications are discussed in Section 2.5. Section 2.6 deals with lattices, which are closely related to the boolean algebras described in Sections 2.3 and 2.4.

2.1

OPERATIONS

When the carrier X is a set of numbers such as $Z = \{\ldots, -1, 0, 1, 2, \ldots\}$ or $N = \{0, 1, \ldots\}$, we are familiar with operations on X, including addition, multiplication, and raising to powers. If X is a power set $P(S)$, we have studied in Chapter 1 such operations on X as forming complements, intersections, and unions. The terms we are about to present, especially Definitions 1 and 4, help us study simultaneously all operations that share some property or properties.

DEFINITION 1   *n*-ARY OPERATION ON *S*

Let S^n be the cartesian product $S \times S \times \cdots \times S$ of n copies of a set S. An *n-ary operation* on S is a mapping f from S^n to S. Usually one replaces 1-ary by *unary*, 2-ary by *binary*, and 3-ary by *ternary*.

NOTATION 1   RESULT OF AN OPERATION

Let f be an *n*-ary operation on S. The *prefix* notation for the image of an *n*-tuple $(s_1, s_2, \ldots, s_n)$ in S^n under f is $f(s_1, s_2, \ldots, s_n)$. With *infix* notation, this image may be written as $s_1 + s_2 + \cdots + s_n$ when f is addition, as $s_1 \cap s_2 \cap \cdots \cap s_n$ when f is the intersection operation, and so on. A miscellaneous or abstract operation may be denoted as $\circ$, $\triangle$, or $\square$.

Example 1 The mapping f from a power set $P(S)$ to itself, in which $f(A)$ is the complement $\bar{A}$ of A in S, is a unary operation on $P(S)$. The mapping g from $P(S) \times P(S)$ to $P(S)$ with $g(A, B) = A \cap B$ is a binary operation on $P(S)$, as is the **symmetric difference** operation $\oplus$ defined by $A \oplus B = (A \cup B) - (A \cap B)$. Also, $h(A, B, C) = A \cup B \cup C$ specifies a ternary operation h on $P(S)$. $\square$

Example 2 Let P be the set of positive real numbers. The mappings f and g with $f(x) = x^3$ and $g(x) = \sqrt[3]{x}$ are unary operations on P. The mappings h and k from P^2 to P with $h(x, y) = x^2 y$ and $k(x, y) = 2x + y$ are binary operations on P. The rule $m(x, y) = x - y$ does not make m into a binary operation on P because there exist (x, y) in P^2 for which $m(x, y)$ is not in P; for example, $1 - 2$ is not in P. The **averaging** operation A with

$$A(x_1, x_2, \ldots, x_n) = \frac{x_1 + x_2 + \cdots + x_n}{n}$$

is an n-ary operation on P. $\square$

DEFINITION 2 **MIN AND MAX OPERATIONS**

Let $(X, \preceq)$ be a linearly ordered set. Then min is the operation on X with $\min(x, y) = x$ if $x \preceq y$ and $\min(x, y) = y$ if $x \succ y$. Also the max operation has $\max(x, y) = x$ if $x \succeq y$ and $\max(x, y) = y$ if $x \prec y$.

Example 3 Let $B_1 = \{0, 1\}$. Then $(B_1, \leq)$ is a linearly ordered set and the min and max operations on B_1 are as shown in Table 2.1.1 or equivalently as shown in Tables 2.1.2(a) and (b).

TABLE 2.1.1

x	y	$\min(x, y)$	$\max(x, y)$
0	0	0	0
0	1	0	1
1	0	0	1
1	1	1	1

TABLE 2.1.2(a)

min	0	1
0	0	0
1	0	1

(b)

max	0	1
0	0	1
1	1	1

$\square$

DEFINITION 3   **CASE TABLE, MATRIX TABLE**

A *case table* for one or more *n*-ary operations on S has a separate row for each ordered *n*-tuple $(s_1, s_2, \ldots, s_n)$ in S^n, a column for each operation, and $f(s_1, \ldots, s_n)$ as the entry on the spot determined by the row labeled with the *n*-tuple $(s_1, \ldots, s_n)$ and the column labeled f. A *matrix table* for a binary operation $\square$ has $a \square b$ as the entry on the place determined by the row labeled a and the column labeled b.

Table 2.1.1 is a case table for the min and max binary operations on B_1; Tables 2.1.2(a) and (b) are matrix tables for these operations.

DEFINITION 4   **PROPERTIES OF SOME BINARY OPERATIONS**

Let $\circ$ be a binary operation on a set X.

Associativity $\circ$ is *associative* if $x \circ (y \circ z) = (x \circ y) \circ z$ for all x, y, z in X.

Commutativity $\circ$ is *commutative* if $x \circ y = y \circ x$ for all x and y in X.

Identity e is an *identity* under $\circ$ if $x \circ e = x = e \circ x$ for all x in X.

Inverse   If there exists an identity e under $\circ$ and if $a \circ h = e = h \circ a$, then h is an *inverse* of a under $\circ$ (with respect to e).

We show in Theorem 1 below ("Uniqueness of the Identity") that a given binary operation has at most one identity; hence we can drop the parenthetical "with respect to e." Then in Theorem 2 ("Uniqueness of the Inverse") we show that if there exists an identity e under a binary operation $\circ$ on X, an element x in X has at most one inverse under $\circ$.

One can see from the case table or the matrix tables of Example 3 that min and max are commutative operations on $B_1 = \{0, 1\}$. In Problems 3 and 4 below, the reader is asked to prove that these operations are associative. The identity for min is 1 and the identity for max is 0 because $\min(x, 1) = x = \min(1, x)$ and $\max(x, 0) = x = \max(0, x)$ for all x in $B_1 = \{0, 1\}$.

Example 4   Let B_n be the set of *n*-bit strings. The complementation mapping $f: \alpha \mapsto \bar{\alpha}$ is a unary operation on B_n. Binary operations $\wedge$ (called "*bitwise and*") and $\vee$ (called "*bitwise or*") are defined as follows. Let $\alpha = a_1 a_2 \ldots a_n$ and $\beta = b_1 b_2 \ldots b_n$ be in B_n. Then $\alpha \wedge \beta$ is the string $c_1 c_2 \ldots c_n$ with $c_i =$

TABLE 2.1.3(a)

∧	00	01	10	11
00	00	00	00	00
01	00	01	00	01
10	00	00	10	10
11	00	01	10	11

(b)

∨	00	01	10	11
00	00	01	10	11
01	01	01	11	11
10	10	11	10	11
11	11	11	11	11

$\min(a_i, b_i)$ for $1 \le i \le n$ and $\alpha \lor \beta$ is the string $d_1 d_2 \ldots d_n$ with $d_i = \max(a_i, b_i)$ for $1 \le i \le n$, with min and max as in Example 3. Tables 2.1.3(a) and (b) are matrix tables for these operations in the case of $n = 2$.

In Problems 3 and 4 below, the reader is asked to show with case tables that each of the min and max operations on $B_1 = \{0, 1\}$ (tabulated in Example 3) is associative. This and the "bitwise" definitions of the operations $\land$ and $\lor$ can be used to show that each of $\land$ and $\lor$ is associative. Using Table 2.1.3(a), one sees that 11 is the identity under $\land$, that 11 is its own inverse under $\land$, and that none of the other elements has an inverse under $\land$. (For example, 01 has no inverse under $\land$ because no entry on its row is the identity 11.) One sees from Table 2.1.3(b) that 00 is the identity under $\lor$, that 00 is its own inverse under $\lor$, and that no other element has an inverse under $\lor$. Since each of these tables is symmetric about its main diagonal, each of $\land$ and $\lor$ is a commutative operation.   □

DEFINITION 5   **LEFT IDENTITY, RIGHT IDENTITY**

A *left identity* under a binary operation ∘ on X is an element f of X such that $f \circ x = x$ for all x in X. A *right identity* under ∘ is an element g such that $x \circ g = x$ for all x in X.

We note that e is an identity under ∘ if and only if e is both a left identity and a right identity. Also f is a left identity under ∘ if and only if the entries on the row for f in the matrix table for ∘ are the same as the column headings. Similarly, g is a right identity if and only if the entries on the column for g are the same as the row labels.

Example 5   Let △ and □ be the binary operations on $X = \{a, b\}$ given by the matrix tables shown below. The table for △ shows that each of a and b is a left identity under △ and that there is no right identity. Similarly, under □, each of a and b is a right identity and there is no left identity.

△	a	b
a	a	b
b	a	b

□	a	b
a	a	a
b	b	b

□

THEOREM 1   **UNIQUENESS OF THE IDENTITY**

If a left identity f and a right identity g exist under a binary operation ∘ on X, then $f = g$.

PROOF   Since f is a left identity, we have $f \circ x = x$ for all x in X. Since g is a right identity, $y \circ g = y$ for all y in X. Substituting g for x and f for y, one has $f \circ g = g$ and $f \circ g = f$; hence $f = g$. □

COROLLARY   There is at most one (2-sided) identity under a binary operation.

THEOREM 2   **UNIQUENESS OF THE INVERSE**

Under an associative binary operation $\circ$ on X, let e be the identity and h be an inverse of a. If either $a \circ k = e$ or $k \circ a = e$, then $h = k$.

PROOF   We prove the case in which $a \circ k = e$ and leave to the reader the proof of the similar case in which $k \circ a = e$. In the case considered here, the hypothesis that h is an inverse of a tells us that $h \circ a = e = a \circ h$. Then, the equations $a \circ h = e$ and $a \circ k = e$ imply that $a \circ h = a \circ k$ and hence that $h \circ (a \circ h) = h \circ (a \circ k)$. By associativity, it follows that $(h \circ a) \circ h = (h \circ a) \circ k$. Since $h \circ a = e$, we have $e \circ h = e \circ k$. Because e is the identity, this implies that $h = k$. □

DEFINITION 6   **CLOSURE OF A SUBSET UNDER AN OPERATION**

Let f be an n-ary operation on X and S be a subset of X. S is **closed** under f if $f(s_1, s_2, \ldots, s_n)$ is in S whenever $s_1, s_2, \ldots, s_n$ are all in S.

Example 6   Subtraction is a binary operation on the set $Z = \{\ldots, -1, 0, 1, 2, \ldots\}$ of integers because $f(m, n) = m - n$ specifies a mapping f from $Z \times Z$ to Z. The subset $N = \{0, 1, 2, \ldots\}$ of Z is not closed under subtraction; for example, 0 and 1 are in N but $0 - 1$ is not in N. Hence the rule $f(m, n) = m - n$ does not make f into a mapping from $N \times N$ to N, and subtraction is not an operation on N. On the other hand, the subset $E = \{\ldots, -2, 0, 2, \ldots\}$ of even integers is closed under subtraction, and so subtraction is an operation on E. □

THEOREM 3   **RESTRICTION OF AN OPERATION TO A SUBSET**

Let $\circ$ be an operation on X and S be a subset of X. Then $\circ$ is an operation on S if and only if S is closed under $\circ$.

The proof of Theorem 3 is similar to the discussion in Example 6.

Example 7 This example has applications in Coding Theory and will be discussed further in Problems 19–24 below and in Section 2.2. The carrier here is the set B_n of n-bit strings. The binary operation $\oplus$ on B_n of "bitwise addition modulo 2" is defined as follows. For $\alpha = a_1 a_2 \ldots a_n$ and $\beta = b_1 b_2 \ldots b_n$ in B_n, $\alpha \oplus \beta$ is the string $c_1 c_2 \ldots c_n$ with (for each i in $\{1, 2, \ldots, n\}$) $c_i = 0$ if $a_i = b_i$ and $c_i = 1$ if $a_i \neq b_i$. In the rest of this example, we consider the special case of $n = 2$.

Table 2.1.4 is the matrix table for $\oplus$ in this case. Since the entries in the row labeled 00 are the same as the column labels and the entries in the column labeled 00 are the same as the row labels, 00 is the identity under $\oplus$. Since each entry on the main diagonal is the identity 00, each string in B_2 is its own inverse under $\oplus$. The symmetry of the table about its main diagonal shows that $\oplus$ is commutative. One can show that $\oplus$ is associative; an easy way to do this for general n is outlined in Problem 21 below. One can see that each of the subsets

$$\{00\}, \quad \{00, 01\}, \quad \{00, 10\}, \quad \{00, 11\}$$

of B_2 is closed under $\oplus$. □

TABLE 2.1.4

$\oplus$	00	01	10	11
00	00	01	10	11
01	01	00	11	10
10	10	11	00	01
11	11	10	01	00

Now we introduce some terms from computer science that will enable us to describe an operation useful in building computer programs.

DEFINITION 7 **ALPHABET *A*, WORD, SET *A** OF ALL WORDS OVER *A***

An *alphabet* is a set of symbols. A *word* of *length* n over an alphabet A is a string $\alpha = a_1 a_2 \ldots a_n$ with each a_i in A. Also, A^* denotes the set of all words over A, including an invented *empty word* ε of length zero.

Example 8 For the alphabet $B = \{0, 1\}$, the set of all words over B is $B^* = \{\varepsilon\} \cup B_1 \cup B_2 \cup \cdots$, where B_n is the set of n-bit strings. For the English lowercase alphabet $E = \{a, b, \ldots, z\}$, E^* includes ordinary English words such as "set" and "monoid" as well as nonsense words such as "qqp" and "jklm." □

DEFINITION 8 **LANGUAGE OVER AN ALPHABET**

A *language* over an alphabet A is a subset of the set A^* of words over A; that is, a language over A is a member of the power set $P(A^*)$.

Definitions 7 and 8 are general enough so that an alphabet A may consist of all the symbols needed to program a given computer and hence any computer program may be considered to be a word. A language over A may consist of all the well-written programs of some system of programming.

DEFINITION 9   **CONCATENATION (OR JUXTAPOSITION)**

The *concatenation* (or *juxtaposition*) of words $\alpha = a_1a_2 \ldots a_m$ and $\beta = b_1b_2 \ldots b_n$ over A is the word $\alpha\beta = a_1a_2 \ldots a_mb_1b_2 \ldots b_n$ over A.

Over the alphabet $B = \{0, 1\}$, the concatenation of $\alpha = 01$ and $\beta = 110$ (in that order) is $\alpha\beta = 01110$; however, the concatenation in the other order is $\beta\alpha = 11001$. The concatenation of the English words $\alpha =$ "over" and $\beta =$ "take" is $\alpha\beta =$ "overtake," whereas $\beta\alpha =$ "takeover," which has a different meaning. Clearly, concatenation is an operation on A^* for every alphabet A. (Only for exceptional A is this operation commutative. See Problem 26 below.)

PROBLEMS FOR SECTION 2.1

1. Let $\cup$ be the binary operation of forming unions on the power set $P(S)$ for a nonempty set S.
    (a) Is $\cup$ associative? Explain.
    (b) Is $\cup$ commutative? Explain.
    (c) What is the identity under $\cup$?
    (d) Does each member A of $P(S)$ have an inverse under $\cup$? Explain.

2. Repeat Problem 1, but with $\cup$ replaced by $\cap$.

3. For x and y in $B_1 = \{0, 1\}$, let $x \triangle y = \min(x, y)$. Give the case table proof that $\triangle$ is associative; that is, show that $x \triangle (y \triangle z) = (x \triangle y) \triangle z$ for all x, y, z in B_1 by appending the other six rows to the following two rows of the case table:

x	y	z	$x \triangle y$	$y \triangle z$	$x \triangle (y \triangle z)$	$(x \triangle y) \triangle z$
0	0	0	0	0	0	0
0	0	1	0	0	0	0

4. Show using a case table with 8 rows that max is an associative operation on $B_1 = \{0, 1\}$.

5. (i) Make the matrix table for the binary operation max on the linearly ordered set $(T, \leq)$ with $T = \{0, 1, 2\}$.
    (ii) Is this operation commutative? Is it associative?

(iii) What is the identity under this operation?

(iv) Does each t of T have an inverse under max?

6. Repeat Problem 5, but with "max" replaced by "min."

7. (i) Give the matrix table for the operation $\vee$ (defined in Example 4) on B_3.

(ii) What is the identity under this operation?

(iii) Is this operation commutative?

(iv) Is this operation associative? Explain.

8. Repeat Problem 7, but with $\vee$ replaced by $\wedge$.

9. Let $\triangle$ be the binary operation on a nonempty set X with $x \triangle y = y$ for all x and y in X.

(a) Which elements of X are left identities under $\triangle$?

(b) Give the condition on $\#X$ for the existence of a right identity.

(c) Give the condition on $\#X$ for $\triangle$ to be commutative.

(d) Prove that $\triangle$ is associative for sets X of all sizes.

10. Repeat Problem 9, but with $\triangle$ replaced by the operation $\square$ such that $x \square y = x$ for all x and y and with "left" and "right" interchanged.

11. Let $\triangle$ be the binary operation on $N = \{0, 1, 2, \ldots\}$ with $m \triangle n = m + n + 1$ for all m and n in N. Prove that:

(a) $\triangle$ is commutative;   (b) $\triangle$ is associative.

12. Let $\square$ be the binary operation on N with $m \square n = 0$ for all m and n in N. Prove that:

(a) $\square$ is commutative;   (b) $\square$ is associative.

13. (i) Is subtraction an operation on $3Z = \{\ldots, -6, -3, 0, 3, 6, \ldots\}$?

(ii) Is the subset $\{0, 3, 6, \ldots\}$ closed under subtraction?

(iii) Is subtraction an operation on $\{0, 3, 6, \ldots\}$?

14. (i) Is subtraction a binary operation on $4Z = \{\ldots, -4, 0, 4, \ldots\}$?

(ii) Is subtraction a binary operation on the subset $\{0, 4, 8, \ldots\}$?

15. Is the binary operation on Z of subtraction of integers commutative? Is it associative? Explain.

16. Let Q^+ be the set of positive rational numbers.

(i) Is $\div$ a binary operation on Q^+?

(ii) Is $\div$ a commutative operation on Q^+? Explain.

(iii) Is $\div$ an associative operation on Q^+? Explain.

17. Let $\oplus$ be the binary operation on a power set $P(S)$ given by $A \oplus B = (A \cup B) - (A \cap B)$; that is, $A \oplus B$ is the complement of $A \cap B$ in $A \cup B$. For the special case in which $S = \{s_1, s_2\}$ and $P(S) = \{S_{00}, S_{01}, S_{10}, S_{11}\}$ do the following parts:

(i) Make the matrix table for $\oplus$.

(ii) Is $\oplus$ commutative? Is $\oplus$ associative?

(iii) Does $A \oplus B$ always equal $(A - B) \cup (B - A)$?

18. Repeat Problem 17, but with $S = \{s_1, s_2, s_3\}$ and

$$P(S) = \{S_{000}, S_{001}, S_{010}, S_{011}, S_{100}, S_{101}, S_{110}, S_{111}\}.$$

19. Let $\oplus$ be the binary operation on $\boldsymbol{B_1} = \{0, 1\}$ for which $0 \oplus 0 = 0 = 1 \oplus 1, 0 \oplus 1 = 1 = 1 \oplus 0$.
    (a) What is the identity under $\oplus$?
    (b) Give the inverse under $\oplus$ of each element of $\boldsymbol{B_1}$.
    (c) Is $\oplus$ commutative?
    (d) Show with a case table that $\oplus$ is associative.

20. Let $\oplus$ be the binary operation on $\boldsymbol{B_n}$ defined as follows: For $\alpha = a_1 a_2 \ldots a_n$ and $\beta = b_1 b_2 \ldots b_n$ in $\boldsymbol{B_n}$, let $\alpha \oplus \beta = c_1 c_2 \ldots c_n$, where $c_i = 0$ if $a_i = b_i$ and $c_i = 1$ if $a_i \neq b_i$.
    (a) Show that the string $O_n = 00 \ldots 0$ of weight 0 in $\boldsymbol{B_n}$ is the identity under $\oplus$.
    (b) Show that each string $\alpha = a_1 a_2 \ldots a_n$ in $\boldsymbol{B_n}$ is its own inverse under $\oplus$.
    (c) Let $S = \{s_1, s_2, \ldots, s_n\}$. How is the operation $\oplus$ on $\boldsymbol{B_n}$ of this problem related to the operation $\oplus$ on $P(S)$ of Problem 17?

21. Use Problem 19(d) to explain why the operation $\oplus$ of Problem 20 is associative for general n.

22. Use Problem 19(c) to explain why the operation $\oplus$ of Problem 20 is commutative.

23. (a) Show with matrix tables that each of the subsets $\{00, 01\}$ and $\{00, 10\}$ is closed under the operation $\oplus$ of Problem 20.
    (b) Show with a counterexample that $\{00, 01, 10\}$ is not closed under $\oplus$.

24. (a) Show that $\{00, 11\}$ is closed under the operation $\oplus$ of Problem 20.
    (b) Show that $\{00, 10, 11\}$ is not closed under $\oplus$.

25. Let A^* be the set of words over the alphabet $A = \{a, b\}$. Show with an example that the operation of concatenation on A^* is not commutative.

26. What must be true of an alphabet A for concatenation to be a commutative operation on the set A^* of words over A?

27. Let $B = \{0, 1\}$ and ε be the invented word of length 0 in the set B^* of all words over the language B.
    (a) Is ε the identity for the concatenation operation on B^*?
    (b) Is concatenation an associative operation on B^*? Explain.

28. Repeat Problem 27, but with B replaced by a general alphabet A.

29. Let the alphabet be $A = \{a, b, c\}$.
    (i) Over A, list the six words of length 2 with no repeated letter.
    (ii) List the three words of length 2 over A not listed in Part (i).

30. Let $A = \{1, 0, \_\}$. List the words xyz of length 3 over A for which:
    (i) just one of x, y, and z is $\_$;
    (ii) exactly two of x, y, and z are $\_$.

31. Let E be the lowercase English alphabet $\{a, b, \ldots, z\}$. Tell how many words there are over E of each of the following lengths:
   (a) 1;   (b) 2;   (c) 3;   (d) m.

32. For each of the following lengths, tell how many words there are over the lowercase English alphabet $\{a, b, c, \ldots, z\}$ in which no letter is repeated:
   (a) 1;   (b) 2;   (c) 3;
   (d) m. (Assume that $m \leq 26$.)

33. (a) Let $A = \{a_1, a_2, \ldots, a_n\}$ and $X = \{1, 2, \ldots, m\}$. Is the number of words $b_1 b_2 \ldots b_m$ of length m over A equal to the number of mappings from X to A? Explain.
   (b) How many words of length m are there over an alphabet of size n?

34. (a) Let $A = \{a_1, a_2, \ldots, a_n\}$ and $X = \{1, 2, \ldots, m\}$. Is the number of words $b_1 b_2 \ldots b_m$ over A with $b_i \neq b_j$ for $i \neq j$ equal to the number of injective mappings from X to A? Explain.
   (b) Over an alphabet A of size n, how many words of length m are there in which no element of A is used more than once in a given word? Assume that $m \leq n$.

2.2

SEMIGROUPS AND MONOIDS

Most of the frequently encountered operations are binary operations and one of the most useful properties a binary operation might have is associativity. Hence there are many important algebraic structures of the types we are about to define. Definitions 1 and 4 below ("Semigroup" and "Monoid, Commutative Monoid") enable us to study simultaneously certain properties of all structures that meet the conditions of the given definition.

DEFINITION 1   SEMIGROUP

A *semigroup* is an ordered pair $(X, \circ)$ with the *carrier* X a nonempty set and $\circ$ an associative binary operation on X. A *commutative semigroup* is one whose operation is commutative.

Example 1   Let $Z^+ = \{1, 2, 3, \ldots\}$. Because addition is an associative binary operation on Z^+, $(Z^+, +)$ is a semigroup. This semigroup is commutative but has no identity since there is no e in Z^+ with $n + e = n = e + n$ for all n in Z^+. In fact, $n + m > n$ for all m and n in Z^+.

The binary operation of subtraction on $Z = \{\ldots, -2, -1, 0, 1, 2, \ldots\}$ is not associative [for example, $(0 - 1) - 2 = -3$ and $0 - (1 - 2) = 1$]; hence the structure $(Z, -)$ is not a semigroup.   □

THEOREM 1   **CLOSED SUBSET**

Let $(X, \circ)$ be a semigroup. In the carrier X, let S be a subset closed under $\circ$. Then $(S, \circ)$ is a semigroup.

PROOF   The hypothesis that S is closed under $\circ$ and Theorem 3 of Section 2.1 ("Restriction of an Operation to a Subset") tell us that $\circ$ is an operation on S. Since $\circ$ is an associative operation on X, $x \circ (y \circ z) = (x \circ y) \circ z$ for all x, y, z in X and therefore for all x, y, z in the subset S of X. Thus the restriction of $\circ$ to S is an associative binary operation on S, and $(S, \circ)$ is a semigroup.   □

DEFINITION 2   **SUBSEMIGROUP**

Let $(X, \circ)$ be a semigroup. Let $S \subseteq X$ and S be closed under $\circ$. Then the semigroup $(S, \circ)$ is a **subsemigroup** in $(X, \circ)$.

Example 2   Since the binary operation of multiplication of positive integers is associative, $(\mathbf{Z}^+, \cdot)$ is a semigroup. This semigroup is commutative and has 1 as its identity. The subset $E = \{2, 4, 6, \ldots\}$ of even positive integers is closed under multiplication; hence $(E, \cdot)$ is a subsemigroup in $(\mathbf{Z}^+, \cdot)$. The subsemigroup $(E, \cdot)$ does not have an identity.   □

DEFINITION 3   **POWERS**

Let $(X, \circ)$ be a semigroup and let x be in X. Then $x^1 = x$, $x^2 = x \circ x$, $x^3 = x^2 \circ x, \ldots, x^{n+1} = x^n \circ x, \ldots$. Also, $\langle x \rangle$ denotes the set $\{x^n : n \in \mathbf{Z}^+\}$ of positive integral **powers** of x.

Example 3   Here we show that $a^3 \circ a^2 = a^5$ in a semigroup. By Definition 3, $a^3 \circ a^2 = a^3 \circ (a \circ a)$. Using the associativity property $x \circ (y \circ z) = (x \circ y) \circ z$ with $x = a^3$, $y = a$, and $z = a$ and the definitions of a^4 and a^5, one has

$$a^3 \circ (a \circ a) = (a^3 \circ a) \circ a = a^4 \circ a = a^5.$$

Hence $a^3 \circ a^2 = a^5$. The following theorem extends these formulas.   □

THEOREM 2   **A LAW OF EXPONENTS**

In a semigroup $(X, \circ)$, $x^m \circ x^n = x^{m+n}$ for all x in X and all m and n in $\mathbf{Z}^+$.

The proof of Theorem 2 is postponed until we take up mathematical induction.

THEOREM 3   SUBSEMIGROUP OF POWERS

Let $(X, \circ)$ be a semigroup and let a be in X. Then $(\langle a \rangle, \circ)$ is a subsemigroup in $(X, \circ)$ (and is called the **subsemigroup generated** by a).

PROOF   In view of Definition 2 ("Subsemigroup"), it suffices to show that $\langle a \rangle$ is closed under $\circ$. Let b and c be in $\langle a \rangle$. Then $b = a^m$ and $c = a^n$ with m and n in $\mathbf{Z}^+$. Now,

$$b \circ c = a^m \circ a^n = a^{m+n}$$

by Theorem 2. Since the sum $m + n$ of positive integers is a positive integer, $b \circ c$ is in $\langle a \rangle$. Thus $\langle a \rangle$ is closed under $\circ$, and the desired result follows.   □

Example 4   Let H be the set of 2-digit decimal numbers $\{00, 01, \ldots, 99\}$. (One usually writes 00 as 0, 01 as 1, ..., 09 as 9.) For x and y in H, let $x \square y$ be the string formed by the two rightmost digits of the ordinary product xy; that is, let $x \square y$ be the remainder when xy is divided by 100. In particular, $05 \square 35 = 75$ since $5 \cdot 35 = 175$, which has 75 as its last two digits. It can be shown that this operation is associative. Hence $(H, \square)$ is a semigroup. It is commutative and has 01 as its identity.

Next we seek the elements of the subsemigroup generated by 06. One finds that

$06^2 = 36,$

$06^3 = 36 \square 06 = 16,$

$06^4 = 16 \square 06 = 96,$

$06^5 = 96 \square 06 = 76,$

$06^6 = 76 \square 06 = 56,$

$06^7 = 56 \square 06 = 36 = 06^2.$

Since $06^7 = 06^2$, one sees that

$$06^8 = 06^7 \square 06 = 06^2 \square 06 = 06^3 = 16.$$

Continuing this way, one can see for any n in $N = \{0, 1, \ldots\}$ that $06^{7+n} = 06^{2+n}$. It follows that

$$\langle 06 \rangle = \{06, 36, 16, 96, 76, 56\}.$$ □

Example 5   Let $\triangle$ be the binary operation on $\mathbf{B}_1 = \{0, 1\}$ with $x \triangle y = y$ for all x and y in $\mathbf{B}_1$. Then $\triangle$ is associative (see Problem 9 of Section 2.1), and so $(\mathbf{B}_1, \triangle)$ is a semigroup. Since $0 \triangle 1 = 1$ and $1 \triangle 0 = 0$, this semigroup is not commutative.   □

NOTATION 1   **ALLOWABLE REMOVAL OF PARENTHESES**

Let $(X, \square)$ be a semigroup and let $a, b, c \in X$. Since $(a \,\square\, b) \,\square\, c = a \,\square\, (b \,\square\, c)$, we can drop the parentheses and write either of these expressions as $a \,\square\, b \,\square\, c$. Similarly, each of the expressions $a \,\square\, (b \,\square\, (c \,\square\, d))$, $a \,\square\, ((b \,\square\, c) \,\square\, d), (a \,\square\, b) \,\square\, (c \,\square\, d), (a \,\square\, (b \,\square\, c)) \,\square\, d, ((a \,\square\, b) \,\square\, c) \,\square\, d$ can be written more simply as $a \,\square\, b \,\square\, c \,\square\, d$. This removal process extends to expressions involving more than three $\square$'s.

DEFINITION 4   **MONOID, COMMUTATIVE MONOID**

A *monoid* is a semigroup $(X, \square)$ that has an identity e under $\square$. We use an ordered triple $[X, \square, e]$ to denote such a monoid. It is *commutative* if its operation is commutative.

The semigroup $(Z^+, +)$ of Example 1 is not a monoid since it lacks an identity. The commutative monoids $[Z^+, \cdot, 1]$ and $[H, \square, 01]$ were dealt with in Examples 2 and 4, respectively. Noncommutative monoids will be encountered in Theorems 4 and 5 below.

Let $\cdot$ be the symbol for the binary operation of concatenation on the set A^* of all words over an alphabet A, and let ε be the word of length 0 in A^*. [See Definitions 7, 8, and 9 of Section 2.1 ("Alphabet," "Language over an Alphabet," and "Concatenation").] The following theorem summarizes, in our present terminology, statements from Problems 26 and 28 of Section 2.1.

THEOREM 4   **MONOID OF WORDS**

$[A^*, \cdot, \varepsilon]$ is a monoid for all alphabets A. Such a monoid is noncommutative if A has at least 2 elements.

The proof of Theorem 4 is illustrated in the solutions to Problems 25 and 27 of Section 2.1 and is essentially the same for a general alphabet A having at least 2 elements.

DEFINITION 5   **SUBMONOID**

Let $M = [X, \circ, e]$ be a monoid. If S is a subset of the carrier X, S is closed under $\circ$, and e is in S, then $[S, \circ, e]$ is a *submonoid* in M.

Example 6 Let Z be the set of integers and $3Z = \{\ldots, -6, -3, 0, 3, 6, \ldots\}$ be the set of integral multiples of 3. Then $[Z, +, 0]$ is a commutative monoid with $[3Z, +, 0]$ as a submonoid. □

Example 7 Let $\oplus$ be the binary operation on B_n defined as follows: For $\alpha = a_1 a_2 \ldots a_n$ and $\beta = b_1 b_2 \ldots b_n$ in B_n, let $\alpha \oplus \beta = \gamma = c_1 c_2 \ldots c_n$, where $c_i = 0$ if $a_i = b_i$ and $c_i = 1$ if $a_i \neq b_i$. Also, let O_n denote the string $00 \ldots 0$ of weight zero in B_n. Then it follows from Problems 20–22 of Section 2.1 that $[B_n, \oplus, O_n]$ is a commutative monoid in which each element is its own inverse. This monoid has applications in Coding Theory. □

We recall that a binary relation R on a set S is a subset of the cartesian product S^2 of S with itself; that is, a binary relation R on S is a member of the power set $P(S^2)$. In the rest of this section, "relation" will mean "binary relation."

DEFINITION 6 **MULTIPLICATION OF RELATIONS ON S**

The *product* $R_1 R_2$ of relations R_1 and R_2 on S is the relation R_3 such that $(a, c) \in R_3$ if and only if there is an element b in S for which both $(a, b) \in R_1$ and $(b, c) \in R_2$; that is, $a R_3 c$ if and only if $a R_1 b$ and $b R_2 c$ for some b in S.

Alternatively,

$R_1 R_2 = \{(a, c) : \text{there is a } b \text{ in } S \text{ with } (a, b) \in R_1 \text{ and } (b, c) \in R_2\}.$

Thus multiplication of relations on S is an operation on $P(S^2)$.

Example 8 Let $S = \{1, 2, 3, 4\}$. Then $U = \{(1, 2), (2, 3), (3, 4), (4, 1)\}$ and $V = \{(1, 3), (2, 4)\}$ are relations on S. Let $W = UV$. By Definition 6, $1U2$ and $2V4$ imply that $1W4$; that is, $(1, 4) \in W$. Also, $4U1$ and $1V3$ imply that $4W3$; that is, $(4, 3) \in W$. Trial shows that these are the only ordered pairs in W, and so $W = UV = \{(1, 4), (4, 3)\}$. Similarly one finds that $VU = \{(1, 4), (2, 1)\}$, and we note that $UV \neq VU$. Also, one can see that $U^2 = UU = \{(1, 3), (2, 4), (3, 1), (4, 2)\}$ and that V^2 is the empty relation $\varnothing$. (Note that here U^2 is not $U \times U$.) □

THEOREM 5 **MONOID OF RELATIONS ON S**

Let $\cdot$ denote multiplication of relations on S and let D be the diagonal relation on S. Then $[P(S^2), \cdot, D]$ is a monoid.

PROOF   Let relations U, V, W be in $P(S^2)$. We wish to show that $U(VW) = (UV)W$, that is, multiplication of relations is associative. Let $a[U(VW)]d$. By definition of multiplication of relations, there is an element b in S with aUb and $b(VW)d$. Similarly, it follows from $b(VW)d$ that there is an element c in S with bVc and cWd. Now, aUb and bVc imply that $a(UV)c$, and then $a(UV)c$ and cWd imply that $a[(UV)W]d$. Thus every (a, d) in $U(VW)$ is also in $(UV)W$; that is, $U(VW) \subseteq (UV)W$. In a similar way, one can show that $(UV)W \subseteq U(VW)$. Since $\subseteq$ is antisymmetric, $(UV)W \subseteq U(VW)$ and $U(VW) \subseteq (UV)W$ imply that $U(VW) = (UV)W$. Hence multiplication of relations is associative, and $(P(S^2), \cdot)$ is a semigroup.

Next we show that the diagonal relation $D = \{(s, s) : s \in S\}$ is the identity in this semigroup. Let R be any relation on S and let (s, t) be any ordered pair in R. By definition of diagonal, (t, t) is in D. Then, $(s, t) \in R$ and $(t, t) \in D$ imply that $(s, t) \in RD$. Thus every ordered pair in R is also in RD, and so $R \subseteq RD$. Conversely, let (x, z) be in RD; that is, let $x(RD)z$. Then xRy and yDz for some y in S. By definition of D, $y = z$. Substituting z for y in xRy, we have xRz. Hence every (x, z) in RD is in R, and so $RD \subseteq R$. This and the previously shown $R \subseteq RD$ give us $RD = R$. We leave it to the reader as Problem 19 below to show similarly that $DR = R$. Thus D is the identity in $(P(S^2), \cdot)$ and $[P(S^2), \cdot, D]$ is a monoid.
$\square$

Problems 21 and 22 below show that the monoid $[P(S), \cdot, D]$ is noncommutative unless S is exceptional.

PROBLEMS FOR SECTION 2.2

1. Let $N = \{0, 1, 2, \ldots\}$.
   (i) Is $(N, +)$ a semigroup?
   (ii) Does $(N, +)$ have an identity? If so, what is it?
   (iii) Is $(N, +)$ commutative?

2. Repeat Problem 1, but with $(N, +)$ replaced by $(N, \cdot)$.

3. Let $Z^+ = \{1, 2, 3, \ldots\}$. Is $(Z^+, +)$ a subsemigroup of $(N, +)$?

4. Is $(Z^+, \cdot)$ a subsemigroup of $(N, \cdot)$?

5. Let $T = \{1, 3, 5, \ldots\}$ be the set of odd positive integers. Is $(T, +)$ a subsemigroup of $(N, +)$? Explain.

6. Let $T = \{1, 3, 5, \ldots\}$. Is $(T, \cdot)$ a subsemigroup of $(N, \cdot)$? Explain.

7. Let $H = \{00, 01, \ldots, 99\}$ and $(H, \square)$ be the semigroup of Example 4.
   (i) Is $[H, \square, 01]$ a monoid? Explain.
   (ii) Does the subsemigroup $(\langle 06 \rangle, \square)$ have an identity? If so, what is it?

(iii) Give an example of elements a, b, c in H with $a \neq b$, $c \neq 01$, but $a \, \square \, c = b \, \square \, c$ and thus show that cancellation is not always valid in a monoid.

8. For the $(H, \square)$ of Problem 7, list the elements of:
(a) $\langle 05 \rangle$;   (b) $\langle 04 \rangle$;   (c) $\langle 02 \rangle$;   (d) $\langle 01 \rangle$.

9. Let $S = \{1, 2, 3, 4, 5\}$. Then $A = \{(1, 2), (2, 3), (3, 4), (4, 2)\}$ and $B = \{(4, 5)\}$ are relations on S. In the monoid of relations on S, find the following:
(a) AB;   (b) BA;   (c) B^2;
(d) the set $\langle B \rangle$ of powers of B.

10. Let S and A be as in Problem 9. Find:
(i) A^2;   (ii) A^3;   (iii) A^4;
(iv) the positive integer r such that $\langle A \rangle = \{A, A^2, \ldots, A^r\}$.

11. Let $P(S)$ be the power set for a nonempty set S.
(a) Is $[P(S), \cap, S]$ a monoid? Explain.
(b) Is $[P(S), \cup, \varnothing]$ a monoid? Explain.

12. Let B_n be the set of n-digit binary strings. Let $\wedge$ and $\vee$ be the binary operations on B_n defined in Example 4 of Section 2.1. Let O_n be the string $00 \ldots 0$ of weight zero and let I_n be the string $11 \ldots 1$ of weight n in B_n.
(a) Is $[B_n, \wedge, I_n]$ a monoid? Explain.
(b) Is $[B_n, \vee, O_n]$ a monoid? Explain.
(*Hint:* See Problems 7 and 8 of Section 2.1.)

13. Make a matrix table for the operation of the monoid $[B_3, \oplus, O_3]$. (This monoid is the case $n = 3$ of the monoids $[B_n, \oplus, O_n]$ described in Example 7 of this section. The table for $n = 2$ is in Example 7 of Section 2.1.)

14. Let $M = [B_3, \oplus, O_3]$ be the monoid of Problem 13.
(a) Show, in a table, the inverse of each string of B_3 under $\oplus$.
(b) Show that the subset $T = \{000, 001, 010, 100\}$ is not closed under $\oplus$.
(c) Let $S = \{000, 001, 010, 011\}$ and show that $[S, \oplus, O_3]$ is a submonoid in M.

15. Let B_1^* be the set of words of all lengths over the alphabet $B_1 = \{0, 1\}$. For each of the following languages (i.e., subsets of B_1^*), tell whether the language is closed under concatenation:
(a) the language $\{\varepsilon, 00, 01, 10, 11, 0000, \ldots\}$ of words of even length. (ε has length 0.)
(b) the language $\{0, 1, 000, 001, 010, 011, 100, \ldots\}$ of words of odd length.
(c) the language $\{0^n : n \in \mathbf{Z}^+\} = \{0, 00, 000, \ldots\}$.

16. For each of the following languages over $B_1 = \{0, 1\}$, tell whether it is closed under concatenation:
(a) the set of all words α over B_1 with the length of α in $3N = \{0, 3, 6, \ldots\}$.

(b) the language of all words α over B_1 in which any 1 appearing in α has a 1 immediately before or immediately after it.

(c) the language $\{1^n : n \in \mathbf{Z}^+\} = \{1, 11, 111, \ldots\}$.

17. In the monoid $[A^*, \cdot, \varepsilon]$ of words over an alphabet A, let an α in A^* have length g and give the lengths of:

(a) α^2,   (b) α^3,   (c) α^n, with n in $\mathbf{Z}^+ = \{1, 2, \ldots\}$.

18. (a) In the monoid $[A^*, \cdot, \varepsilon]$ of words over an alphabet A, what must be the length of a word α such that $\alpha^2 = \alpha$?

(b) In the monoid $[P(S^2), \cdot, D]$ of binary relations on a set S, is there a binary relation E on S such that $ER = E = RE$ for all binary relations R on S? If so, what is E?

19. Let R be a binary relation on S and let D be the diagonal relation on S. Prove that the product $DR = R$. (This is the part of the proof of Theorem 5 left to the reader.)

20. Let U, V, and W be binary relations on S, that is, members of $P(S^2)$. If $U \subseteq V$, must $UW \subseteq VW$? Explain.

21. Let $U = \{(1, 1)\}$ and $V = \{(1, 2)\}$ be relations on $\{1, 2\}$. Does $UV = VU$?

22. What must be true of $\#S$ for $[(P(S^2), \cdot, D]$ to be commutative?

23. Let R be a relation on S. If S is finite, is the set $\langle R \rangle$ of positive integral powers of R also finite? Explain.

24. Let S be finite and let R be a relation on S. Prove that there exist positive integers a and b such that $R^n = R^{n+b}$ for $n = a, a + 1, a + 2, \ldots$ and $\langle R \rangle = \{R, R^2, \ldots, R^{a+b-1}\}$.

25. Let $S = \{1, 2\}$. Also let D and R be the binary relations on S with $D = \{(1, 1), (2, 2)\}$ and $R = \{(1, 1), (1, 2)\}$. Show that there is no binary relation T on S with $TR = D$. (Since D is the identity in $[P(S^2), \cdot, D]$, this shows that R has no inverse in this monoid.)

26. Let $S = \{1, 2\}$ and $R = \{(1, 1), (2, 1)\}$. Show that there is no binary relation T on S such that $RT = D$ and thus show that R does not have an inverse in the monoid $[P(S^2), \cdot, D]$.

27. Find a binary relation R on $S = \{1, 2\}$ such that $(1, 1) \in R$ and R has an inverse in $[P(S^2), \cdot, D]$.

28. Repeat Problem 27, but with $(1, 1) \in R$ replaced by $(1, 2) \in R$.

29. Explain why "inverse of a binary relation R" does not mean the same as "reverse of a binary relation R." (The meaning of "reverse" is given in Definition 5 of Section 1.4.)

30. Let R be the binary relation $\{(n, n + 1) : n \in \mathbf{N}\}$ on $\mathbf{N} = \{0, 1, \ldots\}$ and let V be the reverse $\{(n + 1, n) : n \in \mathbf{N}\}$ of R. Show the following:

(a) $RV = D = \{(0, 0), (1, 1), \ldots\}$.

(b) $VR = \{(1, 1), (2, 2), \ldots\}$, a *proper* subset of D.

31. Let f be a bijection from a set S to itself. Let R be the binary operation on S for which $(a, b) \in R$ if and only if $b = f(a)$. Show that the reverse V of R is the inverse of R in $[P(S^2), \cdot, D]$.

32. Let S be a nonempty set and let R be a binary relation on S with an inverse T in $[P(S^2), \cdot, D]$. Show the following:
    (a) For every a in S there is an element b in S such that (a, b) is in R and (b, a) is in T.
    (b) For every d in S there is an element c in S with (c, d) in R and (d, c) in T.
    (c) If aRb and bTc, then $a = c$.

33. Let $a \in X$ and $\triangle$ be the operation on X with $x \triangle y = a$ for all x and y in X. Is $(X, \triangle)$ a semigroup? Explain.

34. What must be true of the X of Problem 33 for $(X, \triangle)$ to have an identity?

35. For permutations f and g on a nonempty set T, let the **composite** $f \circ g$ be the mapping h from T to itself with $h(x) = z$ when $f(x) = y$ and $g(y) = z$.
    *(a) Prove that the composite $f \circ g$ of permutations f and g on T is also a permutation on T.
    (b) In the special case in which $T = \{1, 2, 3\}$,

    $$e: 1 \mapsto 1, 2 \mapsto 2, 3 \mapsto 3, \quad \text{and} \quad f: 1 \mapsto 2, 2 \mapsto 3, 3 \mapsto 1,$$

    find a permutation g on T such that $f \circ g = e = g \circ f$.
    (c) Find a permutation h on T such that $f \circ h \neq h \circ f$.

36. Let T be a nonempty set and X be the set of all permutations on T. Let $\circ$ be the binary operation on X defined in Problem 35. Prove the following:
    (i) Composition is associative and hence $(X, \circ)$ is a semigroup.
    (ii) There is an identity e in X, and so $[X, \circ, e]$ is a monoid.
    (iii) Each f in X has an inverse f^{-1} in X such that $f \circ f^{-1} = e = f^{-1} \circ f$.

2.3

BOOLEAN ALGEBRAS

The next concept, distributivity, applies to certain structures that have at least two binary operations.

DEFINITION 1 **DISTRIBUTIVITY**

Let $\triangle$ and $\square$ be commutative binary operations on X. Then $\triangle$ is **distributive** over $\square$ if $x \triangle (y \square z) = (x \triangle y) \square (x \triangle z)$ for all x, y, z in X.

Example 1   In the structure $(\mathbf{Z}, \cdot, +)$, each of the operations $\cdot$ and $+$ is commutative, and multiplication is distributive over addition, because $x(y + z) = xy + xz$ for all integers x, y, z. Addition, however, is *not* distributive over multiplication; for example, $3 + (2 \cdot 1) \neq (3 + 2) \cdot (3 + 1)$.   □

Example 2   Let S be a nonempty set. Properties of its power set $P(S)$ listed in Section 1.3 can be rewritten for the structure $[P(S), {}^-, \cap, S, \cup, \varnothing]$ as follows:

1. The structures $[P(S), \cap, S]$ and $[P(S), \cup, \varnothing]$ are commutative monoids.
2. Each of $\cap$ and $\cup$ is distributive over the other.
3. The identities of these monoids are distinct; that is, $\varnothing \neq S$.
4. The unary operation $^-$ of complementation is such that $A \cap \bar{A} = \varnothing$ and $A \cup \bar{A} = S$ for all A in $P(S)$.   □

If the set S is finite and $\#S = n$, then each member of $P(S)$ can be represented as S_α [as defined in Notation 2 ("Subset S_α") of Section 1.2], with α in the set $\mathbf{B}_n$ of n-bit strings. The following example translates the information of Example 2 into the language of binary strings.

Example 3   In $\mathbf{B}_n$, let $O = 00 \ldots 0$ and $I = 11 \ldots 1$ be the strings of weight 0 and n, respectively. For strings $\alpha = a_1 a_2 \ldots a_n$ and $\beta = b_1 b_2 \ldots b_n$ in $\mathbf{B}_n$, we recall that the unary operation $^-$ and the binary operations $\wedge$ and $\vee$ are given by:

$$\bar{\alpha} = h_1 h_2 \ldots h_n, \quad \text{where} \quad h_i = 1 - a_i \quad \text{for } i = 1, 2, \ldots, n;$$
$$\alpha \wedge \beta = d_1 d_2 \ldots d_n, \quad \text{where} \quad d_i = \min(a_i, b_i) \quad \text{for } i = 1, 2, \ldots, n;$$
$$\alpha \vee \beta = c_1 c_2 \ldots c_n, \quad \text{where} \quad c_i = \max(a_i, b_i) \quad \text{for } i = 1, 2, \ldots, n.$$

For each positive integer n, the structure $[\mathbf{B}_n, {}^-, \wedge, I, \vee, O]$ has the following properties:

1. $[\mathbf{B}_n, \wedge, I]$ and $[\mathbf{B}_n, \vee, O]$ are commutative monoids.
2. Each of $\wedge$ and $\vee$ is distributive over the other.
3. $O \neq I$.
4. $\alpha \wedge \bar{\alpha} = O$ and $\alpha \vee \bar{\alpha} = I$ for all α in $\mathbf{B}_n$.   □

Examples 2 and 3 deal with structures that share certain properties. These and other structures possessing the same properties can be studied simultaneously with the help of the following definition. [This is named after the British mathematician George Boole (1815–1864), who used such a structure in his algebraic treatment of logic. A biographical note on George Boole can be found just before the problems for this section.]

The "$\wedge$" symbol in the following definition is called by any one of the names **and**, **conjunction**, or **meet**; the "$\vee$" symbol is called by any one of the names *or*, *disjunction*, or *join*. The symbol ‾ is called *negation* or *complementation*.

DEFINITION 2   **BOOLEAN ALGEBRA**

Let X be a set containing two special elements denoted as 0 and 1. On the carrier X, let ‾ be a unary operation. Also, let $\wedge$ and $\vee$ be binary operations on X. The structure

$$L = [X, ^-, \wedge, 1, \vee, 0]$$

is a *boolean algebra* if it satisfies the following four axioms:

(B1) $[X, \wedge, 1]$ and $[X, \vee, 0]$ are commutative monoids.

(B2)   Each of $\wedge$ and $\vee$ is distributive over the other.

(B3) $0 \neq 1$.

(B4) $x \wedge \bar{x} = 0$ and $x \vee \bar{x} = 1$ for each x in X.

We next present some theorems on boolean algebras.

THEOREM 1   **COMPLEMENTS OF 0 AND 1**

In a boolean algebra, $\bar{0} = 1$ and $\bar{1} = 0$.

PROOF   Since 0 is the identity for $\vee$, one has $0 \vee \bar{0} = \bar{0}$. Letting $x = 0$ in the property $x \vee \bar{x} = 1$ of Axiom (B4), we have $0 \vee \bar{0} = 1$. Hence $\bar{0} = 1$. The remaining part of the proof, that $\bar{1} = 0$, is left to the reader as Problem 2 below.   □

THEOREM 2   **COMPLEMENT OF A COMPLEMENT**

In a boolean algebra, if $\bar{a} = b$ then $\bar{b} = a$; that is, $\bar{\bar{a}} = a$ for all a in the carrier.

PROOF   Let $\bar{a} = b$ and $\bar{b} = c$. We wish to show that $c = a$. Using Axiom (B4), we have

$$a \wedge b = 0 = b \wedge c, \qquad a \vee b = 1 = b \vee c.$$

Since 1 is the identity for $\wedge$, $\wedge$ is distributive over $\vee$, and 0 is the identity for $\vee$, one has

$$a = a \wedge 1 = a \wedge (b \vee c) = (a \wedge b) \vee (a \wedge c) = 0 \vee (a \wedge c) = a \wedge c.$$

Hence $a = a \wedge c$. Similarly,

$$c = c \wedge 1 = c \wedge (a \vee b) = (c \wedge a) \vee (c \wedge b) = (a \wedge c) \vee (b \wedge c)$$
$$= (a \wedge c) \vee 0 = a \wedge c.$$

Thus $c = a$ and $\bar{\bar{a}} = \bar{b} = a$, as desired.   □

THEOREM 3   **COMPLEMENTATION IS A BIJECTION**

The mapping $f: x \mapsto \bar{x}$, from the carrier X of a boolean algebra to itself, is a bijection.

PROOF   To prove that f is injective, we assume that $\bar{a} = \bar{b}$ and seek to show that this implies that $a = b$. Taking complements of both sides of $\bar{a} = \bar{b}$, we have $\bar{\bar{a}} = \bar{\bar{b}}$. By Theorem 2, $\bar{\bar{a}} = a$ and $\bar{\bar{b}} = b$; hence $a = b$ and f is injective.

To show that f is surjective, we let d be any element of the codomain X of the mapping f and seek an element c of the domain X such that $f(c) = d$. Theorem 2 helps us find the desired c; we let $c = \bar{d}$. Then $f(c) = \bar{c} = \bar{\bar{d}} = d$. Thus the image set for f is the entire codomain, and f is surjective. Finally, f is both injective and surjective; hence f is bijective.   □

If one interchanges $\vee$ and $\wedge$ while simultaneously interchanging 0 and 1 in the four axioms for a boolean algebra, each axiom is somewhat re-arranged, although it still retains its meaning. If these same interchanges are made in a statement on general boolean algebras, a new statement, called the **dual** of the original statement, is obtained. The dual of a theorem is also a theorem because the dual can be proved by making the same interchanges in each step and in each justification (that is, reference to an axiom or previous theorem) of the proof of the original statement. We sum this up as Theorem 4.

THEOREM 4   **PRINCIPLE OF DUALITY**

If $\vee$, $\wedge$, 0, and 1 are replaced by $\wedge$, $\vee$, 1, and 0, respectively, in a theorem on boolean algebras, the new statement (that is, the dual statement) is also a theorem.

For example, in Theorem 1 ("Complements of 0 and 1") we proved that $\bar{0} = 1$ and left it to the reader (Problem 2 below) to dualize each step and thus prove the dual result that $\bar{1} = 0$.

Each of Examples 2 and 3 provides, for each n in $\mathbf{Z}^+$, a boolean algebra whose carrier X has 2^n elements. The simplest case, in which $\#X = 2$, is especially valuable in applications to circuits and logic.

DEFINITION 3 **DOUBLETON BOOLEAN ALGEBRA**

The ***doubleton boolean algebra*** is $[\boldsymbol{B}_1, ^-, \wedge, 1, \vee, 0]$, whose carrier is $\boldsymbol{B}_1 = \{0, 1\}$.

TABLE 2.3.1

x	0	1
$\bar{x}$	1	0

TABLE 2.3.2

$\wedge$	0	1
0	0	0
1	0	1

TABLE 2.3.3

$\vee$	0	1
0	0	1
1	1	1

Using Example 3 with $n = 1$, one finds that the basic operations $^-$, $\wedge$, and $\vee$ on the carrier $\boldsymbol{B}_1$ of the doubleton boolean algebra are given by Tables 2.3.1, 2.3.2, and 2.3.3.

Theorems on general boolean algebras have to be proved from Axioms (B1), (B2), (B3), and (B4) of Definition 2, "Boolean Algebra" (and previously proved results on general boolean algebras), as in the proofs of Theorems 1–4 above. Any such theorem applies to any specific boolean algebra such as the doubleton boolean algebra. However, some results in a specific structure may not hold in all boolean algebras.

Since the carrier $\boldsymbol{B}_1 = \{0, 1\}$ of the doubleton boolean algebra has only two elements, identities such as "$x \wedge x = x$ for all x in $\boldsymbol{B}_1$" can be proved by a case table. However, case table proofs should not be attempted for results on general boolean algebras because their carriers may be infinite. Properties of general boolean algebras have to be derived from the axioms of Definition 2 ("Boolean Algebra"). Such a proof of "$x \wedge x = x$ for all x in the carrier X of a boolean algebra" is outlined in Problem 3 below.

We recall that $\boldsymbol{B}_1^n$ consists of all n-tuples $(a_1, a_2, \ldots, a_n)$ with each a_i in $\boldsymbol{B}_1 = \{0, 1\}$ and that an n-ary operation on $\boldsymbol{B}_1$ is a mapping from $\boldsymbol{B}_1^n$ to $\boldsymbol{B}_1$.

DEFINITION 4 ***n*-ARY BOOLEAN OPERATION, BOOLEAN EXPRESSION**

An n-ary ***boolean operation*** is a mapping from $\boldsymbol{B}_1^n$ to $\boldsymbol{B}_1$ with a rule expressible using only operations chosen from $\{^-, \wedge, \vee\}$. Such a rule is called a ***boolean expression***.

Example 4 Let $f(x) = x \wedge \bar{x}$, $g(x, y) = x \vee \bar{y}$, and $h(x, y, z) = (x \wedge y) \vee (x \wedge z)$. Then f, g, and h are boolean operations with f unary, g binary, and h ternary. Using Axiom (B4), one can change the rule for f to $f(x) = 0$. Using distributivity of $\wedge$ over $\vee$, one can change the rule for h to $h(x, y, z) = x \wedge (y \vee z)$. $\square$

Boolean operations have applications in logic and in the design of electrical circuits. The ability to prove that boolean operations f and g are equal, despite having rules with different appearances, can help in designing a simpler (and hence more reliable, more compact, and less expensive) circuit or may help in rewriting a legal document in more understandable form. One way to prove that n-ary boolean operations f

and g are equal is with the 2^n rows of a case table, as shown in the following example. Less tedious methods may also be available, as we see in the next section.

Example 5   Let f and g be the binary boolean operations, that is, mappings from $\boldsymbol{B}_1^2$ to $\boldsymbol{B_1}$, specified by

$$f(x, y) = x \wedge (\bar{x} \vee y), \qquad g(x, y) = x \wedge y.$$

Although these rules may seem different, f and g are equal boolean functions since examination of columns 5 and 6 of the case table (Table 2.3.4) shows that each of the four ordered pairs (x, y) in $\boldsymbol{B}_1^2$ is assigned the same image by f as by g. The $\bar{x}$ column can be made using Table 2.3.1, the $\bar{x} \vee y$ column can come from Table 2.3.3, and the other columns can come from Table 2.3.2. Since $f = g$, the rule for g is a simplified rule for f.

TABLE 2.3.4

x	y	$\bar{x}$	$\bar{x} \vee y$	$f(x, y) = x \wedge (\bar{x} \vee y)$	$g(x, y) = x \wedge y$
0	0	1	1	0	0
0	1	1	1	0	0
1	0	0	0	0	0
1	1	0	1	1	1

$\square$

Example 6   Let f and g be the ternary boolean operations, that is, mappings from $\boldsymbol{B}_1^3$ to $\boldsymbol{B_1}$, with

$$f(x, y, z) = \bar{x} \wedge y \wedge \bar{z} \text{ and } g(x, y, z) = \bar{x} \wedge y \wedge z.$$

Using Tables 2.3.1 and 2.3.2 one finds that

$$f(0, 1, 0) = \bar{0} \wedge 1 \wedge \bar{0} = 1 \wedge 1 \wedge 1 = 1 \wedge 1 = 1,$$
$$g(0, 1, 0) = \bar{0} \wedge 1 \wedge 0 = 1 \wedge 1 \wedge 0 = 1 \wedge 0 = 0.$$

Since at least one ordered triple in $\boldsymbol{B}_1^3$ has different images under f and g, these ternary boolean operations are not equal. Note that we did not have to consider the values of f and g for all eight ordered triples (x, y, z) in $\boldsymbol{B}_1^3$; only one properly selected ordered triple is needed to prove $f \neq g$.

$\square$

TABLE 2.3.5

(x, y)	$f(x, y)$
$(0, 0)$	0
$(0, 1)$	0
$(1, 0)$	0
$(1, 1)$	1

One way to specify an n-ary boolean operation is by giving a table. For example, Table 2.3.5 determines a binary boolean operation f. A more compact way to specify f is to give the complete inverse image of 1 under f. For example, if one knows that $f^{-1}(1)$ is the set $\{(1, 1)\}$, then f is specified completely, since this fact tells us that $f(x, y) = 1$ for (x, y) in this set and that $f(x, y) = 0$ when (x, y) is not in this set. With the help of Table 2.3.2, one can see that a rule for this f is $f(x, y) = x \wedge y$. The ability to determine and to simplify the rule for an n-ary boolean operation f when $f^{-1}(1)$ is given is important for applications. Techniques for accomplishing those tasks are discussed in the next section. Here we prepare for those methods by finding $f^{-1}(1)$ for certain simple boolean operations f.

Example 7 Let f be the binary boolean operation with $f(x, y) = \bar{x} \wedge y$. We seek $f^{-1}(1)$; that is, we try to solve $\bar{x} \wedge y = 1$ for (x, y). Table 2.3.2 shows that $\bar{x} \wedge y = 1$ if and only if $\bar{x} = 1 = y$. Table 2.3.1 shows that $\bar{x} = 1$ if and only if $x = 0$. Hence $f^{-1}(1) = \{(0, 1)\}$. □

Example 8 Let f be the ternary boolean operation with $f(x, y, z) = \bar{x} \wedge y \wedge z$. We seek $f^{-1}(1)$; that is, we solve $\bar{x} \wedge y \wedge z = 1$ for (x, y, z). Since we can think of $\bar{x} \wedge y \wedge z$ as $(\bar{x} \wedge y) \wedge z$, Table 2.3.2 initially implies that $\bar{x} \wedge y = 1$ and $z = 1$ and then that $\bar{x} = 1$ and $y = 1$. Using $\bar{x} = 1$ and Table 2.3.1, we see that $x = 0$. Hence $f^{-1}(1) = \{(0, 1, 1)\}$. □

Example 9 Now we seek a ternary boolean operation h such that $h^{-1}(1)$ is the doubleton $\{(0, 1, 1), (0, 0, 1)\}$. Motivated somewhat by the previous example, we consider the operation k with

$$k(x, y, z) = (\bar{x} \wedge y \wedge z) \vee (\bar{x} \wedge \bar{y} \wedge z).$$

What is $k^{-1}(1)$? That is, what are the solutions (x, y, z) of

$$(\bar{x} \wedge y \wedge z) \vee (\bar{x} \wedge \bar{y} \wedge z) = 1? \tag{1}$$

Let $f(x, y, z) = \bar{x} \wedge y \wedge z$ and $g(x, y, z) = \bar{x} \wedge \bar{y} \wedge z$. Table 2.3.3 tells us that $a \vee b = 1$ if and only if at least one of a and b equals 1. Hence the solutions (x, y, z) of Equation (1) form the union $f^{-1}(1) \cup g^{-1}(1)$. But $f^{-1}(1) = \{(0, 1, 1)\}$, by Example 8, and similarly, $g^{-1}(1) = \{(0, 0, 1)\}$. Thus

$$k^{-1}(1) = f^{-1}(1) \cup g^{-1}(1)$$
$$= \{(0, 1, 1)\} \cup \{(0, 0, 1)\}$$
$$= \{(0, 1, 1), (0, 0, 1)\},$$

and k is the desired ternary boolean operation h. □

We next restate some results from Section 1.3 in the present context.

THEOREM 5 **ABSORPTION LAWS, DE MORGAN'S LAWS**

Let $[\boldsymbol{B_1}, \bar{}, \wedge, 1, \vee, 0]$ be the doubleton boolean algebra. For all x and y in $\boldsymbol{B_1}$,

(a) $x \wedge (x \vee y) = x$, $x \vee (x \wedge y) = x$ (Absorption Laws)
(b) $\overline{x \vee y} = \bar{x} \wedge \bar{y}$, $\overline{x \wedge y} = \bar{x} \vee \bar{y}$ (De Morgan's Laws)

PROOF   Since the doubleton boolean algebra is essentially the power set boolean algebra $[P(S), \bar{\ }, \cap, S, \cup, \varnothing]$ in the special case with $\# S = 1$, these results follow from Problems 5 and 6 and Theorem 1 ("De Morgan's Laws"), all in Section 1.3. $\square$

In the problems for Section 2.6 we will extend Theorem 5 to all boolean algebras.

The set of all n-ary boolean operations is the carrier of a boolean algebra, as we will note after some preliminaries.

NOTATION 1   **SET OF n-ARY BOOLEAN OPERATIONS**

Let P_n denote the set of all n-ary boolean operations.

DEFINITION 5   **NEGATION, "AND" (CONJUNCTION), "OR" (DISJUNCTION)**

Let f and g be in P_n. Then $\bar{f}$, $f \wedge g$, and $f \vee g$ are the following n-ary boolean operations:

Negation $\bar{f}\colon (x_1, x_2, \ldots, x_n) \mapsto \overline{f(x_1, x_2, \ldots, x_n)}$

"And" $f \wedge g\colon (x_1, \ldots, x_n) \mapsto f(x_1, \ldots, x_n) \wedge g(x_1, \ldots, x_n)$

"Or" $f \vee g\colon (x_1, \ldots, x_n) \mapsto f(x_1, \ldots, x_n) \vee g(x_1, \ldots, x_n)$

THEOREM 6   **IDENTITIES UNDER CONJUNCTION AND DISJUNCTION**

Let I_n and O_n be the n-ary boolean operations with $I_n(x_1, \ldots, x_n) = x_1 \vee \bar{x}_1$ and $O_n(x_1, \ldots, x_n) = x_1 \wedge \bar{x}_1$. Then $I_n(x_1, \ldots, x_n) = 1$ and $O_n(x_1, \ldots, x_n) = 0$ for all $(x_1, \ldots, x_n)$ in $\boldsymbol{B_1^n}$. Also, $f \wedge I_n = f = I_n \wedge f$ and $f \vee O_n = f = O_n \vee f$ for all f in P_n.

The proof of Theorem 6 is straightforward and is omitted.

THEOREM 7   **BOOLEAN ALGEBRA OF OPERATIONS**

$[P_n, \bar{\ }, \wedge, I_n, \vee, O_n]$ is a boolean algebra.

The proof of Theorem 7 is left to the interested reader.

In logic, rules for n-ary boolean operations are separated into three categories, as we indicate next.

DEFINITION 6 **TAUTOLOGY, CONTRADICTION, CONTINGENCY**

A rule for an n-ary boolean operation f is a **tautology** if $f = I_n$; the rule is a **contradiction** if $f = O_n$; and the rule is a **contingency** if f does not equal I_n or O_n.

In other words, $f(x_1, x_2, \ldots, x_n)$ is a tautology if $f(\gamma) = 1$ for all n-tuples $\gamma = (x_1, x_2, \ldots, x_n)$ in $\boldsymbol{B_1^n}$ and is a contradiction if $f(\gamma) = 0$ for all γ in $\boldsymbol{B_1^n}$. This rule is a contingency if $f(\gamma_1) = 1$ and $f(\gamma_2) = 0$ for some γ_1 and γ_2 in $\boldsymbol{B_1^n}$. As in Example 10 below, only two properly chosen rows of a case table for f are needed to show that its rule is a contingency, but a case table proof that the rule is a tautology (or is a contradiction) requires all 2^n rows.

Example 10   Let $f(x, y) = \bar{x} \wedge y$. The following two (well-selected) rows of a case table show that f is a contingency:

x	y	$\bar{x}$	$\bar{x} \wedge y$
0	0	1	0
0	1	1	1

Let $g(x, y) = x \vee y \vee (\bar{x} \wedge \bar{y})$ and let $h(x, y) = (x \vee y) \wedge \bar{x} \wedge \bar{y}$. Table 2.3.6, the complete case table, shows that g is a tautology and h is a contradiction.

TABLE 2.3.6

x	y	$\bar{x}$	$\bar{y}$	$x \vee y$	$\bar{x} \wedge \bar{y}$	$g(x, y) =$ $(x \vee y) \vee (\bar{x} \wedge \bar{y})$	$h(x, y) =$ $(x \vee y) \wedge (\bar{x} \wedge \bar{y})$
0	0	1	1	0	1	1	0
0	1	1	0	1	0	1	0
1	0	0	1	1	0	1	0
1	1	0	0	1	0	1	0

$\square$

We now define, in terms of boolean operations, the "implication" sign used in logic and in proofs in other fields.

NOTATION 2   **IMPLICATION**

Let f and g be boolean operations. In logic it is customary to use

$$f(x_1, \ldots, x_n) \Rightarrow g(x_1, \ldots, x_n)$$

to mean the same thing as

$$\overline{f(x_1, \ldots, x_n)} \vee g(x_1, \ldots, x_n).$$

(The *implication* sign $\Rightarrow$ may be read "implies.")

Example 11   Notation 2 tells us that $x \Rightarrow y = \bar{x} \vee y$. We can therefore use Tables 2.3.1 and 2.3.3 to construct Table 2.3.7, the case table for $x \Rightarrow y$.

TABLE 2.3.7

x	y	$\bar{x}$	$\bar{x} \vee y$	$x \Rightarrow y$
0	0	1	1	1
0	1	1	1	1
1	0	0	0	0
1	1	0	1	1

$\square$

Example 12   Let $f(x, y) = x \wedge (x \Rightarrow y)$. We use the following steps to simplify the rule:

$f(x, y) = x \wedge (x \Rightarrow y)$	Given
$= x \wedge (\bar{x} \vee y)$	Notation 2
$= (x \wedge \bar{x}) \vee (x \wedge y)$	Distributivity of $\wedge$ over $\vee$
$= 0 \vee (x \wedge y)$	Axiom (B4)
$= x \wedge y$	0 is the identity for $\vee$

Thus $x \wedge (x \Rightarrow y) = x \wedge y$. This equation is relevant to the discussion of mathematical induction in Chapter 4. If one suspected such an equality, one could use a case table to prove or disprove it. $\square$

George Boole, *born in 1815 into a family of modest means, began his career as an elementary school teacher. Early in his career he became interested in logic and the limitations of the widely held view that mathematics was the study of magnitude and number. In his classic work, Investigations of the Laws of Thought (1854), he introduced an algebra of sets. Bertrand Russell has written that "pure mathematics was discovered by Boole in a work which he called The Laws of Thought." Boole was appointed professor at Queen's College, Cork, Ireland, in 1849 and was elected to the Royal Society. He died in 1864.*

PROBLEMS FOR SECTION 2.3 _____

Here X is always the carrier of a boolean algebra.

1. (a) Explain why $(x \lor y) \land (z \lor w) = (x \land z) \lor (x \land w) \lor (y \land z) \lor (y \land w)$ for all x, y, z, w in X.

(b) Explain why $(x \land y) \lor (z \land w) = (x \lor z) \land (x \lor w) \land (y \lor z) \land (y \lor w)$ for all x, y, z, w in X.

2. Prove that $\bar{1} = 0$ by dualizing the steps of the proof in Theorem 1 ("Complements of 0 and 1") that $\bar{0} = 1$.

3. Let x be in X. Justify the following assertions:

(i) $x = x \land 1 = x \land (x \lor \bar{x}) = (x \land x) \lor (x \land \bar{x})$

(ii) $(x \land x) \lor (x \land \bar{x}) = (x \land x) \lor 0 = x \land x$.

(iii) $x \land x = x$. (This is called the ***idempotent law*** for $\land$.)

4. Dualize the work of Problem 3 and thus prove that $x \lor x = x$ for all x in X. (This is called the ***idempotent law*** for $\lor$.)

5. Prove that $x \lor x \lor x = x$ for all x in X.

6. Prove that $x \land x \land x = x$ for all x in X.

7. Let a be in X.

(i) Show that $a = \bar{a}$ implies that $0 = 1$. [*Hint*: See Problems 3(iii) and 4 as well as Axiom (B4) in Definition 2, "Boolean Algebra."]

(ii) Then deduce that $a \neq \bar{a}$. [See Axiom (B3) in Definition 2.]

(iii) Prove that $\#X \neq 3$.

8. Given that X is finite, prove that $\#X$ is an even integer.

9. Prove that $x \land 0 = 0$ for all x in X by justifying each of the following equalities:

$$x \land 0 = x \land (x \land \bar{x}) = (x \land x) \land \bar{x} = x \land \bar{x} = 0.$$

10. Prove that $x \lor 1 = 1$ for all x in X.

11. In X, let $x \lor y = y$ and $y \lor z = z$. Show that $x \lor z = z$.

12. In X, let $x \land y = x$ and $y \land z = y$. Show that $x \land z = x$.

13. In what sense is Table 2.3.3 the dual of Table 2.3.2?

14. Is Table 2.3.1 its own dual? Explain.

15. (i) Prove that $x \lor (\bar{x} \land y) = x \lor y$ for all x and y in X.

(ii) Explain why this proof cannot be accomplished with a case table.

16. Prove that $x \land (\bar{x} \lor y) = x \land y$ for all x and y in X.

17. Let f and g be the ternary boolean operations with $f(x, y, z) = \bar{x} \land y \land \bar{z}$ and $g(x, y, z) = x \land y \land \bar{z}$. Find one ordered triple (a, b, c) in B_1^3 such that $f(a, b, c) = 1$ and $g(a, b, c) = 0$ and thus show that $f \neq g$.

18. Let f and g be the ternary boolean operations with $f(x, y, z) = x \land \bar{y} \land \bar{z}$ and $g(x, y, z) = \bar{x} \land \bar{y} \land z$. Does $f = g$? Explain.

19. Find a ternary boolean operation f for which $f^{-1}(1) = \{(1, 1, 0)\}$, that is, such that $f(1, 1, 0) = 1$ and $f(a, b, c) = 0$ when (a, b, c) is an ordered triple of $\boldsymbol{B}_1^3$ different from $(1, 1, 0)$.

20. Find a 4-ary boolean operation f with $f^{-1}(1) = \{(1, 0, 0, 1)\}$.

21. Find a ternary boolean operation f with

$$f^{-1}(1) = \{(0, 1, 0), (1, 1, 1)\}.$$

22. Find a 4-ary boolean operation f with

$$f^{-1}(1) = \{(0, 1, 0, 1), (1, 0, 0, 1)\}.$$

23. Find a boolean operation f with

$$f^{-1}(1) = \{(1, 1, 1), (1, 1, 0), (1, 0, 0)\}.$$

24. Find a boolean operation f with

$$f^{-1}(1) = \{(0, 0, 0, 0), (0, 0, 0, 1), (0, 0, 1, 1)\}.$$

25. Let h and k be in the set P_n of n-ary boolean operations. Let $f = h \vee k$ and $g = h \wedge k$. Explain why:
(a) $f^{-1}(1) = h^{-1}(1) \cup k^{-1}(1)$;   (b) $g^{-1}(1) = h^{-1}(1) \cap k^{-1}(1)$.

26. Let $h \in P_n$, $k \in P_n$, $f = h \vee k$, and $g = h \wedge k$. Express each of $f^{-1}(0)$ and $g^{-1}(0)$ in terms of $h^{-1}(0)$ and $k^{-1}(0)$.

27. Let g and h be the 4-ary boolean operations with

$$g(x, y, z, w) = x \wedge \bar{z} \wedge w, \qquad h(x, y, z, w) = \bar{z} \wedge w.$$

(i) Explain why $g^{-1}(1) \subseteq h^{-1}(1)$.   (ii) Find $g^{-1}(1)$.
(iii) List the 4-tuples of $h^{-1}(1)$ that are not in $g^{-1}(1)$.

28. Let h and k be the 4-ary boolean operations with

$$h(x, y, z, w) = \bar{z} \wedge w, \qquad k(x, y, z, w) = \bar{z}.$$

(i) Explain why $\#k^{-1}(1) = 2[\#h^{-1}(1)]$.   (ii) Find $h^{-1}(1)$.
(iii) List the 4-tuples of $k^{-1}(1)$ that are not in $h^{-1}(1)$.

29. Use Table 2.3.7 in Example 11 to give a case table proof that $[x \wedge (x \Rightarrow y)] \Rightarrow y$ is a tautology.

30. Prove each of the following to be a tautology, using a case table:
(a) $x \Rightarrow x$;   (b) $[(x \Rightarrow y) \wedge (y \Rightarrow z)] \Rightarrow (x \Rightarrow z)$;
(c) $[x \wedge (x \Rightarrow y) \wedge (y \Rightarrow z)] \Rightarrow z$.

31. Use a case table to prove that $(x \vee \bar{x}) \Rightarrow (y \wedge \bar{y})$ is a contradiction.

32. Let f and g be n-ary boolean operations with f a tautology and g a contradiction. Is $f \Rightarrow g$ a contradiction? Explain.

33. Use Table 2.3.7 to prove that $(x \Rightarrow y) \Rightarrow (y \Rightarrow x)$ is a contingency.

34. Use two properly selected rows of a case table to prove that $x \vee y \Rightarrow y$ is a contingency.

35. Which of the following are tautologies? Which are the contradictions? Which are contingencies?
    (a) $x \wedge y \Rightarrow x$.
    (b) $x \Rightarrow (x \wedge y)$.
    (c) $\bar{x} \wedge (x \vee y) \wedge (x \vee \bar{y})$.
    (d) $x \vee (y \wedge z)$.
    (e) $[x \wedge (x \Rightarrow y)] \Rightarrow (x \wedge y)$.

36. Repeat Problem 35, but for the following:
    (a) $(x \vee y) \wedge z$.
    (b) $(x \vee y) \Rightarrow x$.
    (c) $x \Rightarrow (x \vee y)$.
    (d) $(x \wedge y) \Rightarrow [x \wedge (x \Rightarrow y)]$.

37. Let f and g be n-ary boolean operations with $f^{-1}(1) \subseteq g^{-1}(1)$. Is

    $$[f(x_1, x_2, \ldots, x_n) \Rightarrow g(x_1, x_2, \ldots, x_n)]$$

    a tautology? Explain.

38. If

    $$f(x_1, x_2, \ldots, x_n) \Rightarrow g(x_1, x_2, \ldots, x_n)$$

    is a tautology, must $f^{-1}(1) \subseteq g^{-1}(1)$? Explain.

39. Let f and g be mappings from a set S to $\{0, 1\}$. If $f^{-1}(0) = g^{-1}(0)$, must $f = g$? Explain.

40. Let f and g be mappings from S to $\{0, 1, 2\}$. If $f^{-1}(0) = g^{-1}(0)$, must $f = g$? Explain.

41. Is the number of mappings from S to $\{0, 1\}$ equal to $\# P(S)$? Explain.

2.4

BOOLEAN FUNCTIONS

TABLE 2.4.1

x	0	1
$\bar{x}$	1	0

TABLE 2.4.2

$\cdot$	0	1
0	0	0
1	0	1

TABLE 2.4.3

$+$	0	1
0	0	1
1	1	1

In Section 2.5, we will describe some applications of boolean operations to switching circuits and to electronic networks. There we will also see that simplifying a rule for a boolean operation can help in designing more efficient and more reliable circuits and networks. This section is devoted mainly to techniques for such simplification.

In engineering courses on applications of boolean algebra, the symbol $\wedge$ is replaced by $\cdot$ and the symbol $\vee$ is replaced by $+$. Also, $\cdot$ is called "multiplication" and $x \cdot y$ is called the "product of x and y"; $+$ is called "addition" and $x + y$ is called the "sum of x and y." In this section, we will use this terminology, and as in ordinary algebra, we adopt the convention that multiplications are to be performed *before* additions, unless otherwise indicated by parentheses. Thus, the $\cdot$ operation is performed first in the expression $x + y \cdot z$, whereas the $+$ operation is performed first in $(x + y) \cdot z$.

With these new notations, the basic operations on the carrier $B_1 = \{0, 1\}$ of a doubleton boolean algebra are as given in Tables 2.4.1, 2.4.2, and 2.4.3. We recall that B_1^n consists of all n-tuples $(a_1, a_2, \ldots, a_n)$ with each a_i in $B_1 = \{0, 1\}$ and that an n-ary operation on B_1 is a mapping from B_1^n to B_1. One way to specify an n-ary boolean operation f is by giving a table. For example, Table 2.4.4 gives a ternary boolean operation f.

TABLE 2.4.4

(x, y, z)	$(0, 0, 0)$	$(0, 0, 1)$	$(0, 1, 0)$	$(0, 1, 1)$	$(1, 0, 0)$	$(1, 0, 1)$	$(1, 1, 0)$	$(1, 1, 1)$
$f(x, y, z)$	0	0	0	1	1	1	1	1

It is convenient to replace the ordered triples (x, y, z) of B_1^3 by the corresponding binary strings xyz of B_3. When this is done, Table 2.4.4 becomes Table 2.4.5. Thus, dropping the commas in a rule $f(x_1, x_2, \ldots, x_n)$ for an n-ary boolean operation—that is, a mapping f from B_1^n to B_1—allows us to think of f as a mapping from the set B_n of n-digit binary strings to B_1; when this is done we call f an *n-ary boolean function*. A direct definition of this term follows.

TABLE 2.4.5

α	000	001	010	011	100	101	110	111
$f(\alpha)$	0	0	0	1	1	1	1	1

DEFINITION 1   *n*-ARY BOOLEAN FUNCTION

An n-ary *boolean function* is a mapping f from B_n to B_1 with a rule expressible using only operations chosen from $\{^-, +, \cdot\}$, that is, with a rule that is a boolean expression.

We see that the mapping f from B_3 to B_1 given in Table 2.4.5 is a boolean function by noting that

$$f^{-1}(1) = \{011, 100, 101, 110, 111\}$$

and then using the technique developed in Section 2.3 to show that

$$f(xyz) = \bar{x} \cdot y \cdot z + x \cdot \bar{y} \cdot \bar{z} + x \cdot \bar{y} \cdot z + x \cdot y \cdot \bar{z} + x \cdot y \cdot z \tag{1}$$

is a rule for f. Since this rule uses only the operations allowed by Definition 1, f is a ternary boolean function. We will see in Example 3 below that the rule for this f can be simplified to

$$f(xyz) = x + y \cdot z.$$

In this section, we formalize the technique for producing a rule such as Equation (1) for a boolean function f when given the complete inverse image of 1 under f and then discuss methods for simplifying some of these rules. It may be helpful to reread the following definition after examining Example 1 below.

DEFINITION 2   *n*-ARY MONOMIAL OF DEGREE *d*

Let $\sigma = s_1 s_2 \ldots s_n$ be a word of length n over the alphabet $\{1, 0, \_\}$. For a fixed *n*-bit string $x_1 x_2 \ldots x_n$ in $\boldsymbol{B_n}$ and each i in $\{1, 2, \ldots, n\}$, let

$$u_i = \begin{cases} x_i & \text{if } s_i = 1 \\ \bar{x}_i & \text{if } s_i = 0 \\ 1 & \text{if } s_i = \_ \end{cases}$$

Then the *n*-ary boolean **monomial** $m[\sigma]$ is the mapping m from $\boldsymbol{B_n}$ to $\boldsymbol{B_1}$ given by

$$m\colon x_1 x_2 \ldots x_n \mapsto u_1 \cdot u_2 \cdots u_n.$$

The **degree** of $m[\sigma]$ is the number of i's for which u_i is x_i or $\bar{x}_i$ (that is, for which s_i is not $\_$).

Using Definitions 1 and 2, one sees that every *n*-ary boolean monomial is an *n*-ary boolean function. Since 1 is the identity for the multiplication (that is, the "and") operation in a boolean algebra, a factor 1 can be dropped from the rule for a monomial when at least one other factor is present. When n is small, we may replace x_1 by x, x_2 by y, x_3 by z, and x_4 by w in these rules.

The only *n*-ary monomial of degree 0 is the m with $m(x_1 x_2 \ldots x_n) = 1 \cdot 1 \cdots 1 = 1$, that is, the *n*-ary identity I_n under multiplication (that is, "and"). The rules for the *n*-ary monomials of degree 1 are

$$x_1, \bar{x}_1, x_2, \bar{x}_2, \ldots, x_n, \bar{x}_n;$$

thus there are $2n$ such monomials.

Example 1   Using Definition 2, one sees that $m[\_01]$ has the monomial rule $\bar{y} \cdot z$. The following table gives the words σ and the monomial rules for $m[\sigma]$ for the twelve ternary monomials of degree 2:

σ	_00	_01	_10	_11	0_0	0_1	1_0	1_1	00_	01_	10_	11_
$m[\sigma]$	$\bar{y} \cdot \bar{z}$	$\bar{y} \cdot z$	$y \cdot \bar{z}$	$y \cdot z$	$\bar{x} \cdot \bar{z}$	$\bar{x} \cdot z$	$x \cdot \bar{z}$	$x \cdot z$	$\bar{x} \cdot \bar{y}$	$\bar{x} \cdot y$	$x \cdot \bar{y}$	$x \cdot y$

The eight ternary monomials of degree 3 are:

σ	000	001	010	011	100	101	110	111
$m[\sigma]$	$\bar{x}\cdot\bar{y}\cdot\bar{z}$	$\bar{x}\cdot\bar{y}\cdot z$	$\bar{x}\cdot y\cdot\bar{z}$	$\bar{x}\cdot y\cdot z$	$x\cdot\bar{y}\cdot\bar{z}$	$x\cdot\bar{y}\cdot z$	$x\cdot y\cdot\bar{z}$	$x\cdot y\cdot z$

□

Example 2   Let $f = m[1001]$, $g = m[1\_01]$, $h = m[\_\_01]$, and $k = m[\_\_0\_]$. That is, let f, g, h, and k be the 4-ary monomials with

$$f(xyzw) = x\cdot\bar{y}\cdot\bar{z}\cdot w, \quad g(xyzw) = x\cdot\bar{z}\cdot w,$$
$$h(xyzw) = \bar{z}\cdot w, \quad k(xyzw) = \bar{z}.$$

We now show that the complete inverse image of 1 under each of these monomials $m[s_1s_2s_3s_4]$ consists of all the strings α of $\boldsymbol{B_4}$ obtainable from the word $s_1s_2s_3s_4$ by replacing each blank among the s_i by either 0 or 1. The equation $f(\alpha) = 1$ (that is, $x\cdot\bar{y}\cdot\bar{z}\cdot w = 1$) gives us $x = \bar{y} = \bar{z} = w = 1$ because a meet (conjunction) of factors chosen from $\{0, 1\}$ equals 1 if and only if each factor is 1. Then $\bar{y} = \bar{z} = 1$ implies that $y = z = 0$. Thus $x\cdot\bar{y}\cdot\bar{z}\cdot w = 1$ has the single solution $xyzw = 1001$, and $f^{-1}(1) = \{1001\}$. In solving the equation $g(\alpha) = 1$ (that is, $x\cdot\bar{z}\cdot w = 1$), we must again have $x = 1$, $z = 0$, and $w = 1$, but now y can be either 0 or 1, since neither y nor $\bar{y}$ is a factor in the rule for g. Thus $g^{-1}(1) = \{1001, 1101\}$. We note that $g = m[1\_01]$ and that $g^{-1}(1)$ consists of the strings of $\boldsymbol{B_4}$ obtained by replacing the blank in 1_01 with 0 and with 1.

The equation $h(\alpha) = 1$ (that is, $\bar{z}\cdot w = 1$) necessitates that $z = 0$ and $w = 1$ but allows x to be 0 or 1 and allows y to be 0 or 1. Thus $h^{-1}(1) = \{0001, 0101, 1001, 1101\}$ consists of the strings of $\boldsymbol{B_4}$ obtainable from $\_\_01$ by replacing each blank independently with either 0 or 1. Finally, $k(\alpha) = 1$ (that is, $\bar{z} = 1$) necessitates that $z = 0$ but allows each of x, y, and w to be 0 or 1. Thus

$$k^{-1}(1) = \{0000, 0001, 0100, 0101, 1000, 1001, 1100, 1101\}$$

consists of the strings obtained by independently replacing each blank of $\_\_0\_$ with 0 or 1. □

Let $\sigma = s_1s_2\ldots s_n$ be a word of length n over the alphabet $\{1, 0, \_\}$ and let m be the monomial $m[\sigma]$. If m has degree n, then each s_i is in $\{1, 0\}$ and so σ is a binary string in $\boldsymbol{B_n}$. The n-ary monomials of degree n are called n-ary **minifunctions**. Minifunctions are analogous to the minisets of Section 1.3, and we next give an independent definition of them.

DEFINITION 3   **MINIFUNCTION FOR A BINARY STRING**

For $\alpha = a_1 a_2 \ldots a_n$ in B_n, the **minifunction** m_α is the n-ary boolean function with

$$m_\alpha(x_1 x_2 \ldots x_n) = v_1 \cdot v_2 \cdots v_n,$$

where $v_i = x_i$ if $a_i = 1$ and $v_i = \bar{x}_i$ if $a_i = 0$.

For example, the f of Example 2, with $f(xyzw) = x \cdot \bar{y} \cdot \bar{z} \cdot w$, is the 4-ary minifunction m_{1001}.

THEOREM 1   **MONOMIAL COMPLETE INVERSE IMAGE OF 1**

Let $\sigma = s_1 s_2 \ldots s_n$ be a word of length n over the alphabet $\{1, 0, \_\}$ and let the monomial $m = m[\sigma]$. Then:

(a) The complete inverse image $m^{-1}(1)$ consists of all the binary strings $\alpha = x_1 x_2 \ldots x_n$ obtained from σ by independently replacing each $\_$ among the s_i with either 0 or 1.
(b) If m has degree n, then σ is in B_n, $m = m_\sigma$, and $m^{-1}(1) = m_\sigma^{-1}(1)$ is the singleton $\{\sigma\}$.
(c) $\# m^{-1}(1) = 2^{n-d}$, where d is the degree of m.

PROOF   (a) By the definition of monomial, $m(x_1 x_2 \ldots x_n) = u_1 \cdot u_2 \cdots u_n$, where $u_i = x_i$ if $s_i = 1$, $u_i = \bar{x}_i$ if $s_i = 0$, and $u_i = 1$ if s_i is $\_$. Let a string $x_1 x_2 \ldots x_n$ of B_n be in $m^{-1}(1)$. Then

$$m(x_1 x_2 \ldots x_n) = u_1 \cdot u_2 \cdots u_n = 1.$$

Since each u_i is in $\{0, 1\}$, we have $u_1 \cdot u_2 \cdots u_n = 1$ if and only if each $u_i = 1$. When $s_i = 1$, this gives $u_i = x_i = 1$; when $s_i = 0$, we have $u_i = \bar{x}_i = 1$ and so $x_i = 0$. Thus $x_i = s_i$ if s_i is either 1 or 0. When s_i is $\_$, the condition $u_i = 1$ is just $1 = 1$, so x_i can be either 0 or 1. These statements imply Part (a).
(b) If the monomial m has degree n, then there are no blanks among the s_i and so the only $x_1 x_2 \ldots x_n$ in $m^{-1}(1)$ is $\sigma = s_1 s_2 \ldots s_n$; that is, $m^{-1}(1) = \{\sigma\}$. This gives us Part (b).
(c) If one thinks of introducing the blanks among the s_i one at a time, as in the sequence of monomials of Example 2,

$$m[1001], \quad m[1\_01], \quad m[\_\_01], \quad m[\_\_0\_],$$

then each added blank doubles the size of $m^{-1}(1)$. If m has degree d, there are $n - d$ blanks in σ and hence $\# m^{-1}(1) = 2^{n-d}$. This gives us Part (c) and completes the proof. $\qquad\qquad\qquad\qquad\qquad\qquad\square$

Problems 19–24 of Section 2.3 illustrate, in the notation and terminology of that section, a technique for producing an n-ary boolean function f when $f^{-1}(1)$ is a given subset of $\boldsymbol{B_n}$. The following result presents this technique for general n and general subsets of $\boldsymbol{B_n}$.

THEOREM 2   **GIVEN INVERSE IMAGE OF 1**

Let f be a mapping from $\boldsymbol{B_n}$ to $\boldsymbol{B_1}$.

(a) If $f^{-1}(1) = \varnothing$, then f is the boolean function O_n, with

$$O_n(x_1 x_2 \ldots x_n) = x_1 \cdot \bar{x}_1 = 0.$$

(b) If $f^{-1}(1) = \{\beta, \gamma, \ldots, \lambda\}$, then f is the boolean function

$$m_\beta + m_\gamma + \cdots + m_\lambda.$$

PROOF   (a) Part (a) is clear because $f^{-1}(1) = \varnothing$ means that $f(\alpha) = 0$ for all α in $\boldsymbol{B_n}$.

(b) We let

$$g = m_\beta + m_\gamma + \cdots + m_\lambda \qquad\qquad\qquad (2)$$

and show in the following that $f = g$. Since a sum (that is, a disjunction) of terms from $\{0, 1\}$ equals 1 if and only if at least one of the terms is 1, it follows from (2) that

$$g^{-1}(1) = m_\beta^{-1}(1) \cup m_\gamma^{-1}(1) \cup \cdots \cup m_\lambda^{-1}(1).$$

Using Part (b) of Theorem 1 ("Monomial Complete Image of 1") this becomes

$$\begin{aligned} g^{-1}(1) &= \{\beta\} \cup \{\gamma\} \cup \cdots \cup \{\lambda\} \\ &= \{\beta, \gamma, \ldots, \lambda\} = f^{-1}(1). \end{aligned}$$

Thus $g(\alpha) = 1 = f(\alpha)$ when α is in the set $\{\beta, \gamma, \ldots, \lambda\}$, and $g(\alpha) = 0 = f(\alpha)$ when α is a string of $\boldsymbol{B_n}$ not in this set. Hence $g = f$, as claimed. Finally, $f = m_\beta + m_\gamma + \cdots + m_\lambda$ is a sum of monomials and so meets the conditions of Definition 1 for being an n-ary boolean function. $\quad\square$

COROLLARY   **BOOLEAN FUNCTION**

Every mapping from $\boldsymbol{B_n}$ to $\boldsymbol{B_1}$ is an n-ary boolean function.

DEFINITION 4   **SUM OF PRODUCTS CANONICAL FORM**

The (*sum of products*) *canonical form* for an n-ary boolean function f with $f^{-1}(1) = \{\beta, \gamma, \ldots, \lambda\}$ is

$$f = m_\beta + m_\gamma + \cdots + m_\lambda.$$

This is also known as the *disjunctive normal form*.

Definition 4 has a dual that defines a "product of sums canonical form," also known as the "conjunctive normal form." We will make little use of this dual.

The next two examples illustrate techniques for simplifying certain sum of products rules. These techniques may seem to require "pulling rabbits out of a hat," but we will try to make them less "magical" in the rest of the section.

Example 3   Let f be the ternary boolean function with

$$f^{-1}(1) = \{011, 100, 101, 110, 111\}. \tag{3}$$

(This f was tabulated in Table 2.4.5 above.) It follows from Display (3) and Theorem 2 that

$$f = m_{011} + m_{100} + m_{101} + m_{110} + m_{111}$$

and hence that a rule for f is

$$f(xyz) = \bar{x} \cdot y \cdot z + x \cdot \bar{y} \cdot \bar{z} + x \cdot \bar{y} \cdot z + x \cdot y \cdot \bar{z} + x \cdot y \cdot z. \tag{4}$$

The following observations enable us to simplify this rule. First we note from Display (3) that

$$f^{-1}(1) = \{100, 101, 110, 111\} \cup \{011\}, \tag{5}$$

where the quadruple in Display (5) has all the strings of B_3 with first digit equal to 1. The proof of Theorem 1 shows that $\{100, 101, 110, 111\} = g^{-1}(1)$, where $g(xyz) = x$, and shows that $\{011\} = h^{-1}(1)$, where $h(xyz) = \bar{x} \cdot y \cdot z$. Then $f^{-1}(1) = g^{-1}(1) \cup h^{-1}(1)$ and hence $f = g + h$, since a sum (that is, a disjunction) of terms from $\{0, 1\}$ is 1 if and only if one of its terms is 1. Thus the rule of Display (4) can be simplified to

$$f(xyz) = x + \bar{x} \cdot y \cdot z.$$

Alternatively, we could let

$$f^{-1}(1) = \{100, 101, 110, 111\} \cup \{111, 011\}$$

play the role of Display (5) and note from the proof of Theorem 1 that $\{111, 011\} = k^{-1}(1)$, where $k(xyz) = y \cdot z$. Then $f^{-1}(1) = g^{-1}(1) \cup k^{-1}(1)$

implies that $f = g + k$ and hence that f has the simple rule

$$f(xyz) = x + y \cdot z. \tag{6}$$

□

Since we are interested in simplifying rules for boolean functions—for example, going from Display (4) to Display (6), it may be helpful to look at the process in reverse, as follows:

$$x + y \cdot z = x \cdot 1 \cdot 1 + 1 \cdot y \cdot z = x \cdot (y + \bar{y}) \cdot (z + \bar{z}) + (x + \bar{x}) \cdot y \cdot z$$
$$= x \cdot (y \cdot z + y \cdot \bar{z} + \bar{y} \cdot z + \bar{y} \cdot \bar{z}) + x \cdot y \cdot z + \bar{x} \cdot y \cdot z$$
$$= x \cdot y \cdot z + x \cdot y \cdot \bar{z} + x \cdot \bar{y} \cdot z + x \cdot \bar{y} \cdot \bar{z} + x \cdot y \cdot z + \bar{x} \cdot y \cdot z.$$

The idempotent law for "or" (see Problem 4 of Section 2.3, with ∨ replaced by +) tells us that $a + a = a$ in a boolean algebra. This, along with $a = x \cdot y \cdot z$, gives us $x \cdot y \cdot z + x \cdot y \cdot z = x \cdot y \cdot z$. Thus we can drop the extra $x \cdot y \cdot z$ and have

$$x + y \cdot z = x \cdot y \cdot \bar{z} + x \cdot \bar{y} \cdot z + x \cdot \bar{y} \cdot \bar{z} + x \cdot y \cdot z + \bar{x} \cdot y \cdot z.$$

We see that the right-hand side of this equation is the right-hand side of Display (4) with the terms rearranged.

Example 4   Let f be the binary boolean function with $f^{-1}(1) = \{00, 10, 11\}$. It follows from Theorem 2 that

$$f = m_{00} + m_{10} + m_{11}.$$

Thus a rule for f is

$$f(xy) = \bar{x} \cdot \bar{y} + x \cdot \bar{y} + x \cdot y. \tag{7}$$

We now simplify this rule as follows: The idempotent law for + tells us that $x \cdot \bar{y} = x \cdot \bar{y} + x \cdot \bar{y}$. This replacement in (7) gives

$$f(xy) = \bar{x} \cdot \bar{y} + x \cdot \bar{y} + x \cdot \bar{y} + x \cdot y$$
$$= (\bar{x} \cdot \bar{y} + x \cdot \bar{y}) + (x \cdot \bar{y} + x \cdot y).$$

Using distributivity of "and" over "or" gives us

$$f(xy) = (\bar{x} + x) \cdot \bar{y} + x \cdot (\bar{y} + y).$$

Since $\bar{a} + a = 1$ and $1 \cdot a = a = a \cdot 1$ in a boolean algebra, we have

$$f(xy) = 1 \cdot \bar{y} + x \cdot 1 = \bar{y} + x.$$

Thus the rule of (7) for f has been simplified to $f(xy) = \bar{y} + x.$ □

We now try to make the simplification techniques of Examples 3 and 4 less magical by introducing **Karnaugh Maps**, which are related to minifunctions somewhat as Venn Diagrams are related to the minisets of Section 1.3. The arrangement of regions in a Karnaugh Map is especially suitable for the purpose of simplifying boolean functions. Also, for $n = 4$, all $2^4 = 16$ minifunctions can be shown in a Karnaugh Map more easily than all 16 minisets can be shown in a Venn Diagram. (There is a biographical note on Maurice Karnaugh at the end of this section.)

We begin with the Karnaugh Map for $n = 2$, shown in Figure 2.4.1. The four regions represent the $2^2 = 4$ minifunctions. Taking the join of the minifunctions of the first row, one has

$$m_{11}(xy) + m_{01}(xy) = x \cdot y + \bar{x} \cdot y = (x + \bar{x}) \cdot y = 1 \cdot y = y,$$

since $x + \bar{x} = 1$ and $1 \cdot y = y$ are axioms for boolean algebras. Thus y is the disjunction $m_{11} + m_{01}$ of the minifunctions of the first row. We use this simple rule y as the label for that row. Similarly, $\bar{y}$ is the disjunction $m_{10} + m_{00}$ of the minifunctions of the second row and is used as the label for that row. Also, $x = m_{11} + m_{10}$ and $\bar{x} = m_{01} + m_{00}$, so we use x and $\bar{x}$ as labels for the first and second columns, respectively.

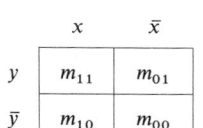

FIGURE 2.4.1

Example 5 Let $f = m_{00} + m_{10} + m_{11}$ be the binary boolean function of Example 4. Since $m_{10} + m_{10} = m_{10}$ by the idempotent law for "or," one can see that f is the sum (that is, the disjunction) of the minifunctions of the second row and of the first column of the Karnaugh Map of Figure 2.4.1. Since $\bar{y}$ is the label for the second row and x is the label for the first column, this indicates quickly that the rule for f can be simplified to $f(xy) = \bar{y} + x$.

□

The following concept will be helpful in labeling the regions of the Karnaugh Maps for $n = 3$ and $n = 4$.

DEFINITION 5   **ADJACENT MONOMIALS**

The n-ary monomials f and g are **adjacent** if their rules (meeting the conditions of Definition 1, "n-ary Boolean Function,") are of the form

$$f(x_1 x_2 \ldots x_n) = u_1 \cdots u_{i-1} \cdot u_i \cdot u_{i+1} \cdots u_n,$$
$$g(x_1 x_2 \ldots x_n) = u_1 \cdots u_{i-1} \cdot \bar{u}_i \cdot u_{i+1} \cdots u_n,$$

with $u_i \neq 1$.

For example, the monomials adjacent to the third-degree 4-ary monomial f with $f(xyzw) = x \cdot \bar{z} \cdot w$ are those whose rules are

$$\bar{x} \cdot \bar{z} \cdot w, \qquad x \cdot z \cdot w, \qquad \text{and} \qquad x \cdot \bar{z} \cdot \bar{w}.$$

We note that a rule for a monomial adjacent to f is obtained by replacing a factor u_i different from 1 in the rule for f with its complement $\bar{u}_i$. Hence, if f and g are adjacent, they must have the same positive degree.

THEOREM 3 **SIMPLIFYING A SUM OF ADJACENT MONOMIALS**

Let f and g be adjacent n-ary monomials of degree d. Then $f + g$ is a monomial of degree $d - 1$.

PROOF   Since f and g are adjacent, they have rules of the form

$$f(x_1 x_2 \ldots x_n) = u_1 \cdots u_{i-1} \cdot u_i \cdot u_{i+1} \cdots u_n,$$
$$g(x_1 x_2 \ldots x_n) = u_1 \cdots u_{i-1} \cdot \bar{u}_i \cdot u_{i+1} \cdots u_n.$$

Hence a rule for $f + g$ is

$$u_1 \cdots u_{i-1} \cdot u_i \cdot u_{i+1} \cdots u_n + u_1 \cdots u_{i-1} \cdot \bar{u}_i \cdot u_{i+1} \cdots u_n.$$

Using distributivity of "and" over "or" gives us

$$u_1 \cdots u_{i-1} \cdot (u_i + \bar{u}_i) \cdot u_{i+1} \cdots u_n.$$

Since $a + \bar{a} = 1$ and $a \cdot 1 = a$ in a boolean algebra, the rule simplifies to the monomial $u_1 \cdots u_{i-1} \cdot 1 \cdot u_{i+1} \cdots u_n$ of degree $d - 1$, as claimed. □

We note from the proof of Theorem 3 that the simplified rule for the disjunction $f + g$ of adjacent monomials can be obtained from the rule for f, or the rule for g, by dropping the only factor that is different in the rules for f and g. For example,

$$x \cdot \bar{z} \cdot w + x \cdot \bar{z} \cdot \bar{w} = x \cdot \bar{z}.$$

Since n-ary minifunctions are n-ary monomials of degree n, Definition 5 can be used to see if n-ary minifunctions m_α and m_β are adjacent. We now define adjacent strings in B_n so that α and β are adjacent if and only if m_α and m_β are adjacent.

DEFINITION 6 **ADJACENT STRINGS**

Strings $\alpha = a_1 a_2 \ldots a_n$ and $\beta = b_1 b_2 \ldots b_n$ in B_n are **adjacent** if $a_i \neq b_i$ for exactly one i in $\{1, 2, \ldots, n\}$.

For example, the strings adjacent to 0110 are 1110, 0010, 0100, and 0111.

A Karnaugh Map for $n = 3$ is shown in Figure 2.4.2. The boxes for the minifunctions are arranged so that a minifunction adjacent (as in Defini-

	$x \cdot y$	$x \cdot \bar{y}$	$\bar{x} \cdot \bar{y}$	$\bar{x} \cdot y$
z	m_{111}	m_{101}	m_{001}	m_{011}
$\bar{z}$	m_{110}	m_{100}	m_{000}	m_{010}

FIGURE 2.4.2

tion 5) to an m_α appears just to the right of m_α, just to the left of m_α, just below m_α, just above m_α, or at the other end of the row when m_α is at one end of a row. For example, the minifunctions adjacent to m_{111} are m_{110} (just below), m_{101} (just to the right), and m_{011} (at the other end of the first row). Using Theorem 3, "Simplifying a Sum of Adjacent Monomials," one sees that each of the column labels is the sum (disjunction) of the minifunctions of its column. One can also show with several applications of Theorem 3 that each row label is the sum of the minifunctions of its row.

We next illustrate the use of the Karnaugh Map in simplifying a rule for a boolean function.

Example 6 Let f be the ternary boolean function with $f(\alpha) = 1$ if and only if wgt $\alpha \geq 2$; that is, let f be the mapping from B_3 to B_1 with

$$f^{-1}(1) = \{011, 101, 110, 111\}. \tag{8}$$

It follows from Display (8) and Theorem 2 ("Given Inverse Image of 1") that

$$f = m_{011} + m_{101} + m_{110} + m_{111}. \tag{9}$$

Thus a rule for f is

$$f(xyz) = \bar{x} \cdot y \cdot z + x \cdot \bar{y} \cdot z + x \cdot y \cdot \bar{z} + x \cdot y \cdot z. \tag{10}$$

Figure 2.4.3 is the Karnaugh Map of Figure 2.4.2, but with each minifunction m_α replaced by its string α and with a check mark in the box of each minifunction of the sum in Display (9). We see from Figure 2.4.3 or Display (9) that f is the sum of m_{111} and its three adjacent minifunctions.

	$x \cdot y$	$x \cdot \bar{y}$	$\bar{x} \cdot \bar{y}$	$\bar{x} \cdot y$
z	111 ✓	101 ✓	001	✓ 011
$\bar{z}$	110 ✓	100	000	010

FIGURE 2.4.3

We therefore use an idempotent law for "or" (see Problem 5 of Section 2.3) to write

$$m_{111} = m_{111} + m_{111} + m_{111},$$

and we substitute this into Display (9) to obtain

$$f = (m_{011} + m_{111}) + (m_{101} + m_{111}) + (m_{110} + m_{111}).$$

Using Theorem 3 ("Simplifying a Sum of Adjacent Monomials"), the rule $\bar{x} \cdot y \cdot z + x \cdot y \cdot z$ for $m_{011} + m_{111}$ is simplified to $y \cdot z$. Similarly, $m_{101} + m_{111}$ has $x \cdot z$ as a simplified rule, and $m_{110} + m_{111}$ has $x \cdot y$ as a simplified rule. Making these replacements, we obtain

$$f(xyz) = y \cdot z + x \cdot z + x \cdot y$$

as a simplified substitute for the rule in Display (10).   □

Now we take up the case of $n = 4$. Figure 2.4.4 shows a Karnaugh Map for $n = 4$ in which we have placed the strings α of $\boldsymbol{B_4}$ in the boxes, rather than the minifunctions m_α. A string $\alpha = a_1 a_2 a_3 a_4$ in $\boldsymbol{B_4}$ has four adjacent strings, obtained by changing just one of the digits a_i from 1 to 0 or from 0 to 1. The sixteen strings of $\boldsymbol{B_4}$ have been placed in these sixteen boxes so that adjacent strings α and β appear in one of the following relationships:

  (i) α and β are at opposite ends of a row; or
 (ii) α and β are at opposite ends of a column; or
(iii) β is just to the right or left of α, or just under or above α.

	$x \cdot y$	$x \cdot \bar{y}$	$\bar{x} \cdot \bar{y}$	$\bar{x} \cdot y$
$z \cdot w$	1111	1011	0011	0111
$z \cdot \bar{w}$	1110	1010	0010	0110
$\bar{z} \cdot \bar{w}$	1100	1000	0000	0100
$\bar{z} \cdot w$	1101	1001	0001	0101

FIGURE 2.4.4

For example, the strings adjacent to 1110 are 1111 (just above), 1010 (just to the right), 1100 (just under), and 0110 (at the opposite end of the row).

It can be shown that each row label in Figure 2.4.4 is the sum (the disjunction) of the minifunctions m_α for the α's in its row and that each column label is the sum of the minifunctions for its column.

Example 7   Let f be the 4-ary boolean function with

$$f^{-1}(1) = \{0011, 1110, 0110, 1100, 0100, 1001, 0001\}. \tag{11}$$

Figure 2.4.5 has the frame of the Karnaugh Map of Figure 2.4.4, but with a string α in its box if and only if α is in $f^{-1}(1)$. Theorem 2 ("Given

	$x \cdot y$	$x \cdot \bar{y}$	$\bar{x} \cdot \bar{y}$	$\bar{x} \cdot y$
$z \cdot w$			0011	
$z \cdot \bar{w}$	1110			0110
$\bar{z} \cdot \bar{w}$	1100			0100
$\bar{z} \cdot w$		1001	0001	

FIGURE 2.4.5

Inverse Image of 1") applied to Display (11) gives

$$f = m_{0011} + m_{1110} + m_{0110} + m_{1100} + m_{0100} + m_{1001} + m_{0001}.$$

As a start in simplifying this sum, we group into pairs of adjacent minifunctions with the help of Figure 2.4.5, as follows:

$$f = (m_{0011} + m_{0001}) + (m_{1110} + m_{1100}) + (m_{0110} + m_{0100}) + m_{1001}.$$
(12)

Using Theorem 3 ("Simplifying a Sum of Adjacent Monomials") on each of the parentheses, we get the simplified rule

$$f(xyzw) = \bar{x} \cdot \bar{y} \cdot w + x \cdot y \cdot \bar{w} + \bar{x} \cdot y \cdot \bar{w} + x \cdot \bar{y} \cdot \bar{z} \cdot w.$$
(13)

Since the middle two terms in Display (13) are adjacent, Theorem 3 tells us that $x \cdot y \cdot \bar{w} + \bar{x} \cdot y \cdot \bar{w} = y \cdot \bar{w}$. Thus Display (13) simplifies to

$$f(xyzw) = \bar{x} \cdot \bar{y} \cdot w + y \cdot \bar{w} + x \cdot \bar{y} \cdot \bar{z} \cdot w.$$
(14)

If m_{0001} were grouped with m_{1001} instead of with m_{0011} as in Display (12), then the rule of Display (14) would be replaced by

$$f(xyzw) = \bar{x} \cdot \bar{y} \cdot z \cdot w + y \cdot \bar{w} + \bar{y} \cdot \bar{z} \cdot w.$$

If m_{0001} were replaced by $m_{0001} + m_{0001}$ and then grouped with both m_{0011} and m_{1001}, one would obtain

$$f(xyzw) = \bar{x} \cdot \bar{y} \cdot w + y \cdot \bar{w} + \bar{y} \cdot \bar{z} \cdot w.$$

The reasoning of the next example can be used to show that f is not representable as a sum of fewer than three monomials. ☐

Example 8 Let f be the 4-ary boolean function with

$$f^{-1}(1) = \{0011, 0111, 1110, 0110, 1000, 0000, 0001, 0101\}.$$

Figure 2.4.6 shows the strings of $f^{-1}(1)$ inside the frame of the Karnaugh Map for $n = 4$. We seek to express $f^{-1}(1)$ as a union

$$f^{-1}(1) = f_1^{-1}(1) \cup f_2^{-1}(1) \cup \cdots \cup f_r^{-1}(1)$$
(15)

	$x \cdot y$	$x \cdot \bar{y}$	$\bar{x} \cdot \bar{y}$	$\bar{x} \cdot y$
$z \cdot w$			0011	0111
$z \cdot \bar{w}$	1110			0110
$\bar{z} \cdot \bar{w}$		1000	0000	
$\bar{z} \cdot w$			0001	0101

FIGURE 2.4.6

with each f_i a 4-ary monomial and r as small as possible, and thus to get f as a sum $f_1 + f_2 + \cdots + f_r$, of monomials.

Let us define a ***batch*** to be a subset S of $f^{-1}(1)$ such that $S = m^{-1}(1)$ for some monomial m. The way the strings of a batch are related to one another is described in Theorem 1, "Monomial Complete Inverse Image of 1." Every singleton subset of $f^{-1}(1)$ is a batch; so is every pair of adjacent strings in $f^{-1}(1)$. If m is a 4-ary monomial with both 1110 and 1000 in $m^{-1}(1)$, then the proof of Theorem 1 implies that m is of the form $m[s_1 -- s_4]$ with s_1 in $\{1, \_\}$ and s_4 in $\{0, \_\}$; this would force 1010 and 1100 to be in $m^{-1}(1)$. Since 1010 is not in $f^{-1}(1)$ (neither is 1100), the strings 1110 and 1000 of $f^{-1}(1)$ are not in the same batch. Similarly, one can see that no two of the three strings 1110, 1000, 0011 of $f^{-1}(1)$ can be in the same batch. Thus r must be at least 3 in Display (15). We can express $f^{-1}(1)$ as the union of three batches as follows:

$$f^{-1}(1) = \{0011, 0111, 0001, 0101\} \cup \{1110, 0110\} \cup \{1000, 0000\}.$$

$$(16)$$

This grouping is indicated in Figure 2.4.6. Theorem 1 and Display (16) imply that

$$f^{-1}(1) = g^{-1}(1) + h^{-1}(1) + k^{-1}(1),$$

where $g(xyzw) = \bar{x} \cdot w$, $h(xyzw) = y \cdot z \cdot \bar{w}$, and $k(xyzw) = \bar{y} \cdot \bar{z} \cdot \bar{w}$. Hence $f = g + h + k$ is the sum of three monomials, and f has the simplified rule

$$f(xyzw) = \bar{x} \cdot w + y \cdot z \cdot \bar{w} + \bar{y} \cdot \bar{z} \cdot \bar{w}.$$

Our discussion above on the impossibility of having $r < 3$ shows that f is not the sum of fewer than three monomials. Problems 41 and 42 below present a 4-ary boolean function that is the sum of four, but not fewer than four, monomials. □

More information on simplification of rules for boolean functions can be found in advanced texts on circuit design under the topics of Karnaugh Maps and the Quine–McCluskey Procedure. Some of these texts are listed in the Bibliography near the back of this book.

Maurice Karnaugh   was born in New York in 1924 and educated in physics at City College of New York and at Yale. From 1952, he worked at Bell Laboratories, and since 1966 he has been on the staff of IBM, currently at Yorktown Heights, New York. His work has largely been on problems of electrical switching.

PROBLEMS FOR SECTION 2.4

1. The formula

$$(x \lor y) \land (z \lor w) = (x \land z) \lor (x \land w) \lor (y \land z) \lor (y \land w)$$

appears in Problem 1 of Section 2.3. Rewrite this formula using $\cdot$ for $\land$ and $+$ for $\lor$. Also, omit unnecessary parentheses.

2. Rewrite De Morgan's Laws $\overline{x \lor y} = \bar{x} \land \bar{y}$ and $\overline{x \land y} = \bar{x} \lor \bar{y}$ using $\cdot$ for $\land$ and $+$ for $\lor$.

3. Let f be the 4-ary boolean function (mapping from B_4 to B_1) with

$$f(xyzw) = (x \cdot y + \bar{x} \cdot \bar{y}) \cdot (z \cdot w + \bar{z} \cdot \bar{w}).$$

   (i) Use distributivity of $\cdot$ over $+$ to expand $f(xyzw)$ into a form requiring no parentheses.
   (ii) Find the complete inverse image $f^{-1}(1)$.

4. Repeat Problem 3, but for $f(xyzw) = (x \cdot y + \bar{x} \cdot y) \cdot (z \cdot w + \bar{z} \cdot w)$.

5. Let $f(xyz) = \bar{x} \cdot y \cdot \bar{z}$ and let $g(xyz) = x \cdot y \cdot \bar{z}$. Find one string α in B_3 for which $f(\alpha) \neq g(\alpha)$, thus showing that $f \neq g$.

6. Let $f(xyz) = x \cdot \bar{y} \cdot \bar{z}$ and let $g(xyz) = \bar{x} \cdot \bar{y} \cdot z$. Does $f = g$? Explain.

7. Give the six rules for ternary monomials of degree 1.

8. Give the eight rules for 4-ary monomials of degree 1.

9. Give the rules for all the 4-ary monomials of degree 2.

10. Give the rules for all the 4-ary monomials of degree 3.

11. For each of the following values of n, tell how many n-ary monomials there are (with the degree unlimited):
    (a) $n = 1$;   (b) $n = 2$;   (c) $n = 3$.

12. How many n-ary monomials are there (with the degree unlimited)?

13. Explain why the number of n-ary monomials of degree d is $2^d \binom{n}{d}$.

14. How many 10-ary monomials of degree 7 are there?

15. Give the rules for the following minifunctions:
    (a) m_1;   (b) m_{00};   (c) m_{101};   (d) m_{1110}.

16. Give the rules for the following minifunctions:
    (a) m_0;   (b) m_{11};   (c) m_{010};   (d) m_{0001}.

17. Find $f^{-1}(1)$ for the 5-ary monomial with $f(x_1x_2x_3x_4x_5) = \bar{x}_2 \cdot x_5$.

18. Find $f^{-1}(1)$ for the 5-ary monomial with $f(x_1x_2x_3x_4x_5) = x_1 \cdot x_4 \cdot \bar{x}_5$.

19. For each of the following sets $f^{-1}(1)$, use Theorem 2 ("Given Inverse Image of 1") to express f as a sum of minifunctions:
    (a) $f^{-1}(1) = \{0000, 1100, 1010, 1001, 0110, 0101, 0011\}$.
    (b) $f^{-1}(1) = \{001, 010, 100, 111\}$.

20. Repeat Problem 19, but for:
(a) $f^{-1}(1) = \{0001, 0100, 0111, 1110, 1101\}$.
(b) $f^{-1}(1) = \{000, 011, 101, 110\}$.

21. Let $f(x_1x_2x_3x_4x_5) = \bar{x}_2 \cdot x_4 \cdot \bar{x}_5$. Use the expansion of

$$\bar{x}_2 \cdot x_4 \cdot \bar{x}_5 = (x_1 + \bar{x}_1) \cdot \bar{x}_2 \cdot (x_3 + \bar{x}_3) \cdot x_4 \cdot \bar{x}_5$$

to express f as a sum of four minifunctions.

22. Let $f(x_1x_2x_3x_4x_5) = x_1 \cdot \bar{x}_4$. Express f as a sum of eight minifunctions.

23. Use Theorem 3, "Simplifying a Sum of Adjacent Monomials," to simplify each of the following:
(a) $\bar{x} \cdot y \cdot z \cdot \bar{w} + \bar{x} \cdot y \cdot \bar{z} \cdot \bar{w}$;
(b) $\bar{x}_1 \cdot \bar{x}_2 \cdot x_3 \cdot \bar{x}_4 \cdot x_5 + \bar{x}_1 \cdot x_2 \cdot x_3 \cdot \bar{x}_4 \cdot x_5$.

24. Rewrite each of the following sums as a single monomial:
(a) $\bar{x} \cdot \bar{y} \cdot z \cdot \bar{w} + \bar{x} \cdot y \cdot z \cdot \bar{w}$;
(b) $x_1 \cdot \bar{x}_2 \cdot x_3 \cdot x_4 \cdot \bar{x}_5 + x_1 \cdot \bar{x}_2 \cdot \bar{x}_3 \cdot x_4 \cdot \bar{x}_5$.

25. For each of the following sets $f^{-1}(1)$, find a monomial f:
(a) $f^{-1}(1) = \{10\}$;   (b) $f^{-1}(1) = \{101, 111\}$;
(c) $f^{-1}(1) = \{1000, 1001, 1100, 1101\}$.

26. Find a monomial f (perhaps with the help of Theorem 1, "Given Inverse Image of 1,") such that:
(a) $f^{-1}(1) = \{00\}$;   (b) $f^{-1}(1) = \{000, 010\}$;
(c) $f^{-1}(1) = \{0010, 0011, 1010, 1011\}$.

27. List all the strings adjacent to 01100.

28. List all the strings adjacent to 101001.

29. If wgt $\alpha = 17$ and wgt $\beta = 19$, can α and β be adjacent? Explain.

30. If α and β are adjacent strings and wgt $\alpha = k$, what are the possibilities for wgt β?

31. Express f as a sum of two monomials, given that

$$f^{-1}(1) = \{111, 110, 101, 011, 010\}.$$

32. Express f as a sum of two monomials, given that

$$f^{-1}(1) = \{110, 101, 100, 001\}.$$

33. Let $m = m[s_1s_2 \ldots s_n]$, with $s_1s_2 \ldots s_n$ a word over $\{0, 1, \_\}$. Let strings $01a_3a_4 \ldots a_n$ and $10a_3a_4 \ldots a_n$ be in $m^{-1}(1)$. Explain why $00a_3a_4 \ldots a_n$ and $11a_3a_4 \ldots a_n$ must be in $m^{-1}(1)$.

34. Let m be an n-ary monomial. Let $00a_3a_4 \ldots a_n$ and $11a_3a_4 \ldots a_n$ be in $m^{-1}(1)$. Explain why $01a_3 \ldots a_n$ and $10a_3 \ldots a_n$ must be in $m^{-1}(1)$.

35. Let m be a 5-ary monomial of degree 2 and let α be in $m^{-1}(1)$. Explain why there must be three strings, each adjacent to α, in $m^{-1}(1)$.

36. Let m be an n-ary monomial, $\alpha \in m^{-1}(1)$, and let $\# m^{-1}(1) = 2^e$, with $e \geq 1$. Explain why $m^{-1}(1)$ must contain e strings adjacent to α.

37. Let f be the ternary boolean function with

$$f^{-1}(1) = \{101, 011, 110, 000\}.$$

Show that f is the sum of four monomials and explain why f cannot be written as the sum of fewer than four monomials.

38. Explain why every ternary boolean function is the sum of four or fewer monomials.

39. Express f as a sum of three monomials, given that

$$f^{-1}(1) = \{1010, 1100, 1000, 0011, 0111, 0001, 0101\}.$$

40. Express f as a sum of three monomials, given that

$$f^{-1}(1) = \{1111, 1011, 1110, 1010, 0010, 1000, 0000, 0101\}.$$

41. Express f as a sum of four monomials, given that

$$f^{-1}(1) = \{0011, 1110, 1010, 0010, 1000, 0000, 0100, 1001\}.$$

42. Explain why the f of Problem 41 cannot be written as the sum of fewer than four monomials.

43. Is every mapping f from $\boldsymbol{B_n}$ to $\boldsymbol{B_1}$ an n-ary boolean function? Explain.

44. (i) Describe a bijection f from the collection $P(\boldsymbol{B_n})$ of subsets S of $\boldsymbol{B_n}$ onto the set F of all n-ary boolean functions f.
(ii) What is $\# F$? That is, how many n-ary boolean functions are there?

45. In Example 3, we proved the equality

$$x + y \cdot z = x + \bar{x} \cdot y \cdot z$$

of rules for boolean functions. Show that this does not imply that $y \cdot z = \bar{x} \cdot y \cdot z$, that is, left cancellation is not always valid.

2.5

APPLICATIONS TO CIRCUITS

In this section we introduce two related applications of boolean functions. The first is the older topic of switches in electrical circuits and the second is the newer one of boolean gates in electronic networks.

Switches are used to turn on or turn off electrical appliances such as lightbulbs, automobile ignitions, and televisions. This "on–off" dichotomy, and the fact that switches can be placed either in series or in parallel, makes it possible to use n-ary boolean functions to model certain electrical circuits.

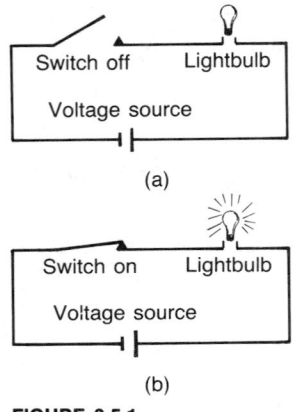

(a)

(b)

FIGURE 2.5.1

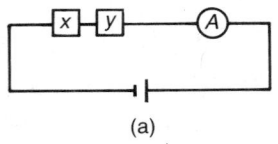

(a)

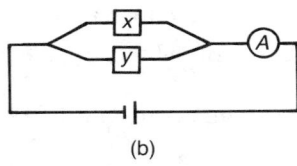

(b)

FIGURE 2.5.2

Figures 2.5.1(a) and 2.5.1(b) depict the two possible states of a switch in an electrical circuit. In Figure 2.5.1(a), the "off" position of the switch breaks the circuit, thus preventing the current from flowing, and so the bulb is unlit. In Figure 2.5.1(b), the "on" position of the switch allows current to flow, thus lighting up the bulb.

Switches x and y can be placed in a circuit either *in series*, as shown in Figure 2.5.2(a), or *in parallel*, as shown in Figure 2.5.2(b). In these figures, A represents an appliance (such as a lightbulb). Frequently, we will drop the part of the circuit containing the appliance and the voltage source because we are interested mainly in the arrangement of the switches. When the switches x and y are in series, as in Figure 2.5.2(a), current can flow if and only if x and y are both in the "on" position. When x and y are in parallel, as in Figure 2.5.2(b), current can flow if either x or y is in the "on" position (assuming there are no defects in the circuit or appliance).

Let 0 for x or y stand for the "off" position and 1 stand for the "on" position. Also, let $f(xy) = 0$ mean that the positions of the switches do not allow current to flow and $f(xy) = 1$ mean that current can flow. Then $f(xy) = x \cdot y$ (that is, $x \wedge y$) is a boolean function that models the circuit of Figure 2.5.2(a), and $g(xy) = x + y$ (that is, $x \vee y$) models the circuit of Figure 2.5.2(b).

In slightly more complicated circuits, a single external switch controls several internal switches by means of relays. If x and w are internal switches controlled by a relay so that they always are either both "on" or both "off," we can replace w by x in a figure or in the boolean function associated with the circuit. If w is "on" when x is "off" and w is "off" when x is "on," then we can replace w by $\bar{x}$. Figure 2.5.3, for Example 1 following, illustrates the control (through a relay) of several internal switches by one external switch.

Example 1   A company keeps important documents and emergency funds in a safe that is opened and closed electronically using three switches. Each of the three top officers controls one of the switches by having the unique key for that switch. The safe is closed if and only if at least two of the three switches are in the closed position. Let 0 represent "open" and 1 represent "closed" for both the safe and each switch. Also, let x, y, and z denote the three switches. Then a ternary function f with $f^{-1}(1) = \{011, 101, 110, 111\}$ models the operation of this safe. Using Theorem 2 of Section 2.4 ("Given Inverse Image of 1"), one obtains the following rule for f:

$$f(xyz) = \bar{x} \cdot y \cdot z + x \cdot \bar{y} \cdot z + x \cdot y \cdot \bar{z} + x \cdot y \cdot z.$$

By using the other techniques of Section 2.4, one can simplify this rule to

$$f(xyz) = x \cdot y + x \cdot z + y \cdot z.$$

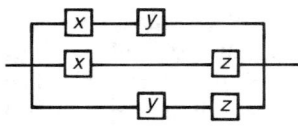

FIGURE 2.5.3

Figure 2.5.3 shows the switching arrangement for this simplified rule; we have dropped the voltage source and appliance from the picture because we assume that they are present in such figures. □

Example 2

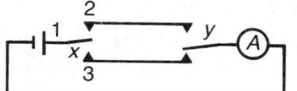

FIGURE 2.5.4

The 2-wire binary boolean switches we have discussed so far are not the only switches in use. If one wants to be able to turn an appliance on or off from either of two locations, 3-wire switches can be used, as shown in Figure 2.5.4. (The three wires for switch x are numbered 1, 2, and 3.) In Problem 17 below, the reader is asked to draw an arrangement of two ordinary 2-wire external switches and four internal switches that works the way this 3-wire circuit does. □

Electronic digital computers store and process data in the form of binary strings, that is, words over the alphabet $\{0, 1\}$. Table 2.5.1 illustrates how a decimal numeral N or a letter L of the English alphabet can be represented by the binary string S below it. Any activity in such a computer has an n-digit binary string $\alpha = x_1 x_2 \ldots x_n$ as initial input and m-digit binary string $\beta = v_1 v_2 \ldots v_m$ as final output. Each output digit v_j is the value $f_j(x_1 x_2 \ldots x_n)$ of a mapping f_j from $\boldsymbol{B}_n$ to $\boldsymbol{B}_1$. Theorem 2 of Section 2.4 tells us that each f_j is either the identity function O_n for $+$ (disjunction) or a sum of monomials. In an n-ary boolean function

$$f: \boldsymbol{B}_n \to \boldsymbol{B}_1, \quad x_1 x_2 \ldots x_n \mapsto f(x_1 x_2 \ldots x_n),$$

each digit x_i can take on only the values in $\boldsymbol{B}_1 = \{0, 1\}$. For present purposes, we call x_i the ith **input**. All the inputs together form the **input string** $x_1 x_2 \ldots x_n$. The image $f(x_1 x_2 \ldots x_n)$ of the input string under the mapping f is called the **output**. The element 1 of $\boldsymbol{B}_1$, when used as an input or an output, can be thought of as representing a relatively high voltage, and 0 represents a low (or zero) voltage.

TABLE 2.5.1

N	0	1	2	3	4	5	6	7
L	a	b	c	d	e	f	g	h
S	00000	00001	00010	00011	00100	00101	00110	00111
N	8	9	10	11	12	13	14	15
L	i	j	k	l	m	n	o	p
S	01000	01001	01010	01011	01100	01101	01110	01111
N	16	17	18	19	20	21	22	23
L	q	r	s	t	u	v	w	x
S	10000	10001	10010	10011	10100	10101	10110	10111
N	24	25	26	27	28	29	30	31
L	y	z						
S	11000	11001	11010	11011	11100	11101	11110	11111

Now we introduce the topic of electronic gates. An n-ary gate is a component of an electronic network associated with a frequently used n-ary boolean function. Table 2.5.2 and Figures 2.5.5(a) through (e) list the most popular gates, along with their rules and pictorial representations. These gates are available to be combined into gate networks that carry out arbitrary mappings from B_n to B_m. In such networks, an output of an early gate may be an input of a following gate. The use of gate networks in electronic computers will be illustrated after we discuss addition of integers in base 2 notation.

TABLE 2.5.2

Name	Arity	Rule	Figure No.
NOT gate (or INVERTER)	Unary	$x \mapsto \bar{x}$	2.5.5(a)
AND gate	n-ary	$x_1 x_2 \ldots x_n \mapsto x_1 \cdot x_2 \cdots x_n$	2.5.5(b)
OR gate	n-ary	$x_1 x_2 \ldots x_n \mapsto x_1 + x_2 + \cdots + x_n$	2.5.5(c)
NAND gate	n-ary	$x_1 x_2 \ldots x_n \mapsto \overline{x_1 \cdot x_2 \cdots x_n}$	2.5.5(d)
NOR gate	n-ary	$x_1 x_2 \ldots x_n \mapsto \overline{x_1 + x_2 + \cdots + x_n}$	2.5.5(e)

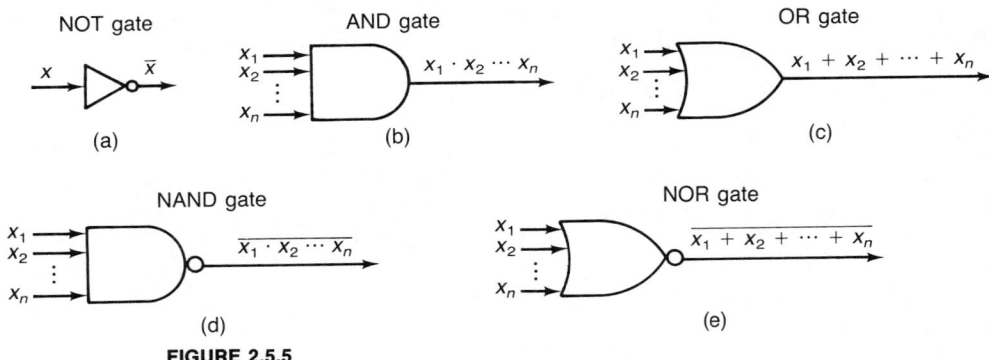

FIGURE 2.5.5

If $\alpha = a_1 a_2 \ldots a_n$ is an n-digit binary string, then $(\alpha)_2$ is called the *base 2* (or binary) ***representation*** for the nonnegative integer

$$(\alpha)_2 = 2^{n-1}a_1 + 2^{n-2}a_2 + \cdots + 2a_{n-1} + a_n.$$

For example, $(111)_2$ is the base 2 representation for $4 \cdot 1 + 2 \cdot 1 + 1 = 7$ and $(1011)_2$ represents $8 \cdot 1 + 4 \cdot 0 + 2 \cdot 1 + 1 = 11$. Such representations were used in making Table 2.5.1. Addition is easy in base 2. For example, the base 2 addition

$$
\begin{array}{r}
1011 \\
111 \\
\hline
10010
\end{array}
$$

shows that $11 + 7 = (1011)_2 + (111)_2 = (10010)_2 = 18$. To perform such an addition, one needs only the following facts about adding single digits:

$$(0)_2 + (0)_2 = (0)_2,$$
$$(0)_2 + (1)_2 = (1)_2 = (1)_2 + (0)_2,$$
$$(1)_2 + (1)_2 = (10)_2,$$
$$(1)_2 + (1)_2 + (1)_2 = (11)_2.$$

Thus in the last (that is, the rightmost) digit place of the base 2 addition of 11 and 7, one has $(1)_2 + (1)_2 = (10)_2$ and puts down 0 and carries 1. Then in the next to last place, one has $(1)_2 + (1)_2 + (1)_2 = (11)_2$ and puts down 1 and carries 1. One proceeds similarly for the other places.

The basic part of addition in base 2 is adding single binary digits. We now set this up so as to be able to picture it in terms of an electronic network.

Let x and y be single binary digits; that is, let x and y be in $\boldsymbol{B_1} = \{0, 1\}$. We write the sum $x + y$ as a 2-digit binary string cw by representing a sum 0 as 00 and a sum 1 as 01. This addition is tabulated in Table 2.5.3, where the binary digit w is the digit to be *written down* and c is the digit to be *carried over* to the next place to the left.

Table 2.5.3 characterizes the digits c and w as binary boolean functions; that is, each of c and w is given by a mapping from $\boldsymbol{B_2}$ to $\boldsymbol{B_1}$. The table shows that the complete inverse images of 1 for these functions are

$$c^{-1}(1) = \{11\}, \qquad w^{-1}(1) = \{01, 10\}.$$

It follows from Theorem 2 of Section 2.4 ("Given Inverse Image of 1") that c and w can be given by the rules

$$c(xy) = x \cdot y, \qquad w(xy) = \bar{x} \cdot y + x \cdot \bar{y}.$$

It can be seen that the network of Figure 2.5.6(a) takes x and y as initial inputs and gives c and w as final outputs. We note that the network begins by splitting the inputs x and y so that each of the inputs appears on different wires. However, it is easy to see that c and w are also produced by

TABLE 2.5.3

x	y	$cw = x + y$
0	0	00
0	1	01
1	0	01
1	1	10

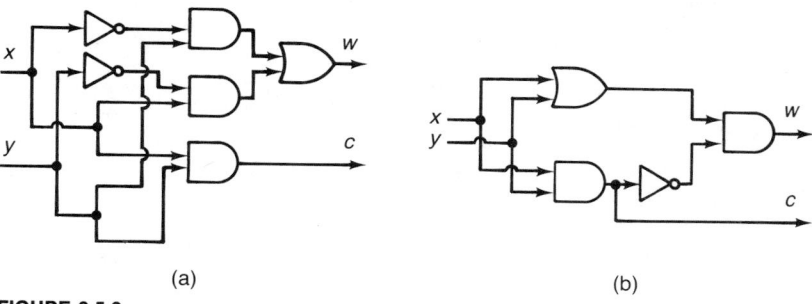

(a)   (b)

FIGURE 2.5.6

the rules

$$c(xy) = x \cdot y, \qquad w(xy) = (x + y) \cdot \overline{x \cdot y}.$$

These rules can be used to obtain the more economical network of Figure 2.5.6(b), which is the one used in practice.

    The device pictured in Figure 2.5.6(b) performs the addition in the last digit place and is called a *half adder*. In other digit places one needs a device that will have as inputs the digits x and y currently being added together with the carry-over digit c from the column to the right; this should have as outputs the digit w to be written down and the digit c' to be carried to the left. Such a device, called an *adder* (or a *full adder*), is shown in Figure 2.5.7. To add 8-digit binaries, one would need a half adder for the last place and a full adder for each of the other places.

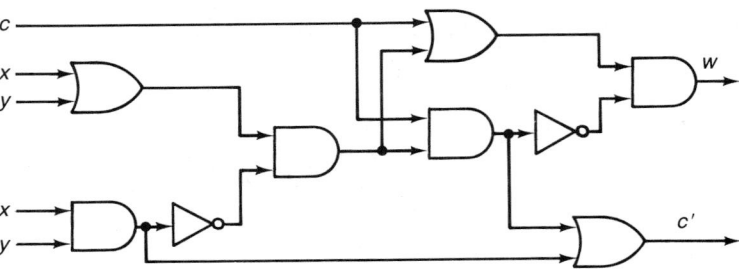

FIGURE 2.5.7

Example 3   Suppose we have a large supply of binary AND gates but no 4-ary AND gate and want to construct a network calling for a 4-ary AND gate. We can use three binary AND gates to do the work of one 4-ary AND gate, as in Figure 2.5.8(a) or as in Figure 2.5.8(b). Which of these is preferable? The network of Figure 2.5.8(a) should perform its function in less time because it involves only two stages, whereas that of Figure 2.5.8(b) has three stages. (The number of *stages* is the maximum number of gates in a path leading directly from an original input to a final output.)

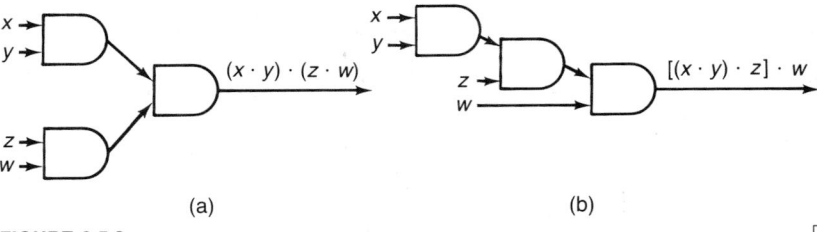

(a)   (b)

FIGURE 2.5.8

If we have an unlimited supply of NOT gates, binary AND gates, and binary OR gates, we can construct a gate network to perform any desired mapping

$$f: B_n \rightarrow B_m, \quad x_1 x_2 \ldots x_n \mapsto v_1 v_2 \ldots v_m \tag{1}$$

because for each j in $\{1, 2, \ldots, m\}$ there is a boolean function f_j with $f_j(x_1 x_2 \ldots x_n) = v_j$ and the rule for each f_j is expressible solely in terms of the unary operation $^-$ and the binary operations $+$ and $\cdot$.

Can one construct a gate network for any desired mapping from B_n to B_m using fewer than three types of gates? We will answer this question after introducing a new term.

DEFINITION 1 **FUNCTIONALLY COMPLETE**

A set of types of gates is **_functionally complete_** if for any mapping $f: B_n \rightarrow B_m$ there is a gate network using only gates of these types that performs the desired mapping.

For example, our above remarks show that the set

$$R = \{\text{NOT gate, binary AND gate, binary OR gate}\} \tag{2}$$

is functionally complete.

LEMMA 1 **TWO TYPES SUFFICE**

The set $S = \{\text{NOT gate, binary AND gate}\}$ of types of gates is functionally complete.

PROOF   Figure 2.5.9 shows a network that can substitute for a binary OR gate and that uses only gates of the types in S. This network performs the desired mapping, since $\bar{x} \cdot \bar{y} = \overline{x + y}$ by one of De Morgan's Laws. Thus we can drop binary OR gates from the functionally complete set R of Display (2) and still have a functionally complete set.

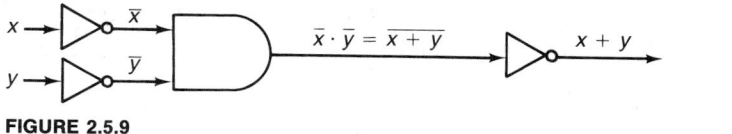

FIGURE 2.5.9   □

THEOREM 1 **ONE TYPE SUFFICES**

The singleton set $T = \{\text{binary NAND gate}\}$ is functionally complete.

PROOF   Figure 2.5.10 shows that a network using only a binary NAND gate performs the function of a NOT gate. This uses the idempotent law $x \cdot x = x$
for "and." Then a binary NAND gate followed by the network of Figure
2.5.10 can substitute for a binary AND gate. These facts and Lemma 1
prove that the singleton set T is functionally complete.   □

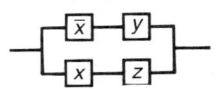

FIGURE 2.5.10

Another functionally complete singleton is presented in Problem 16(ii)
below.

PROBLEMS FOR SECTION 2.5

1.   (a) Give a rule for the boolean function f associated with the switches
         shown in the figure.
     (b) Draw a gate network for the boolean function f of Part (a).

2.   Repeat Problem 1 for the switches shown in the figure below.

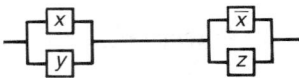

3.   (i) Give the rule for the boolean function f associated with the switching
         arrangement shown in the figure.
     (ii) Simplify this rule.
     (iii) Draw the switching arrangement for the simplified rule.
     (iv) Draw the gate network for the simplified rule.

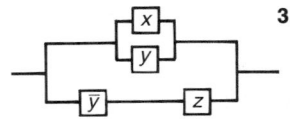

4.   Repeat Problem 3 for the switching arrangement given in the figure.

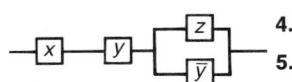

5.   Draw switching arrangements for each of the following boolean functions:
     (a) $f(xyz) = x \cdot y \cdot \bar{z} + x \cdot \bar{y} \cdot z + \bar{x} \cdot y \cdot z + \bar{x} \cdot \bar{y} \cdot \bar{z}$.
     (b) $f(xyzw) = x \cdot y \cdot z \cdot \bar{w} + x \cdot y \cdot \bar{z} \cdot w + x \cdot \bar{y} \cdot z \cdot w + \bar{x} \cdot y \cdot z \cdot w$.

6.   Draw switching arrangements for each of the following boolean functions:
     (a) $f(xyz) = x \cdot \bar{y} \cdot \bar{z} + \bar{x} \cdot y \cdot \bar{z} + \bar{x} \cdot \bar{y} \cdot z$.
     (b) $f(xyzw) = x \cdot y \cdot z \cdot w + x \cdot y \cdot \bar{z} \cdot \bar{w} + x \cdot \bar{y} \cdot \bar{z} \cdot w$.

7.   Draw gate networks for the boolean functions of Problem 5.

8.   Draw gate networks for the boolean functions of Problem 6.

9.   Let f be the 4-ary boolean function with

     $$f^{-1}(1) = \{1111, 1011, 0011, 0110, 1000, 0000, 1001, 0001\}.$$

     (a) Show that f is the sum of four monomials.
     (b) Draw a gate network for this f that uses only four NOT gates, a
         binary AND gate, a ternary AND gate, two 4-ary AND gates, and a
         4-ary OR gate.

10. Let f be the 4-ary boolean function with

$$f^{-1}(1) = \{1110, 1010, 1000, 1001, 0011, 0010, 0000, 0100\}.$$

(a) Show that f is the sum of four monomials.
(b) Draw a gate network for this f that uses just four NOT gates, four ternary AND gates, and one 4-ary OR gate.

11. Does every n-ary boolean function have a gate network using at most n NOT gates, fewer than 2^n AND gates (of various arities), and one OR gate (of some arity)? Explain.

12. Does every 4-ary boolean function have a gate network using at most four NOT gates, at most eight AND gates (of various arities), and one OR gate? Explain.

13. Draw a gate network for the following input-output table:

Input	000	001	010	011	100	101	110	111
Output	00	01	01	10	01	10	10	11

14. Draw a gate network for a computer that would add 2-digit base 2 numbers.

15. Draw a gate network that is equivalent to a binary AND gate and uses only NOT gates and a binary OR gate.

16. Explain why each of the following sets is functionally complete:
(i) {NOT gate, binary OR gate}.   (ii) {binary NOR gate}.

17. Let f be a binary boolean function with $f(11) = 1$ and with

$$f(x\bar{y}) = \overline{f(xy)} = f(\bar{x}y) \quad \text{for all } xy \text{ in } B_2.$$

(This f describes the operation of an appliance that can be turned on or off with either of two switches.)
(i) Tabulate f.   (ii) Find $f^{-1}(1)$.   (iii) Find a rule for f.
(iv) Draw a gate network for f.   (v) Draw a switching circuit for f.

18. How many ternary boolean functions f are there with

$$f(xy\bar{z}) = f(x\bar{y}z) = f(\bar{x}yz) = \overline{f(xyz)} \quad \text{for all } xyz \text{ in } B_3?$$

2.6

LATTICES

In Problems 27 and 29 of this section, two methods are given for using the operations of a boolean algebra $[X, \bar{\ }, \wedge, 1, \vee, 0]$ to introduce a partial order relation $\subseteq$ on X [and thus to make $(X, \subseteq)$ a poset]. Below we convert special posets $(X, \preceq)$ into algebraic structures akin to boolean algebras by using the partial ordering relation $\preceq$ to define binary operations on X similar to the boolean operations $\cdot$ and $+$ (called **meet** and **join**, respectively, in lattice theory).

In this section, $(X, \preceq)$ always denotes a poset; that is, X is a set and $\preceq$ is a reflexive, transitive, and antisymmetric binary relation on X. We recall from Section 1.6 certain notation and terminology concerning a poset $P = (X, \preceq)$. In P, $x \prec y$ means that $x \preceq y$ and $x \neq y$. If S is a subset of X, then a **least element** of S in the poset P is an element m of S such that $m \preceq s$ for all s in S; a **greatest element** of S in P is an element g of S such that $s \preceq g$ for all s in S. In a **poset diagram** for P, the vertices represent the elements of X and there is an upward sloping line or broken line from vertex x to vertex y if and only if $x \prec y$, with as few segments as possible to accomplish this.

Here, X^2 denotes the cartesian product of set X with itself; that is, X^2 is the set of ordered pairs (x, y) with x and y in X.

DEFINITION 1   **LOWER BOUND, GLB, UPPER BOUND, LUB**

Let $P = (X, \preceq)$ be a poset and $x, y \in X$. In P, a **lower bound** for (x, y) is an element m of X such that $m \preceq x$ and $m \preceq y$. If the set of lower bounds for (x, y) is nonempty and has a greatest element g, then this g is the **greatest lower bound** for (x, y) in P and is denoted as $\text{GLB}(x, y)$. An **upper bound** for (x, y) is an element u of X such that $x \preceq u$ and $y \preceq u$. If the set of upper bounds for (x, y) is nonempty and has a least element s, then $s = \text{LUB}(x, y)$ is the **least upper bound** for (x, y) in P.

THEOREM 1   **PROPERTIES OF GLB AND LUB**

Let $\text{GLB}(x, y)$ exist in a poset $(X, \preceq)$. Then

(a) $\text{GLB}(x, y) \preceq x$ and $\text{GLB}(x, y) \preceq y$;
(b) $m \preceq x$ and $m \preceq y$ together imply that $m \preceq \text{GLB}(x, y)$.

Let $\text{LUB}(x, y)$ exist in a poset $(X, \preceq)$. Then

(c) $x \preceq \text{LUB}(x, y)$ and $y \preceq \text{LUB}(x, y)$;
(d) $x \preceq u$ and $y \preceq u$ together imply that $\text{LUB}(x, y) \preceq u$.

PROOF   The parts of this theorem are merely restatements of Definition 1. Part (a) states that $\text{GLB}(x, y)$ is a lower bound for (x, y) with respect to the partial order relation $\preceq$. Part (b) states that $\text{GLB}(x, y)$ is the greatest among such lower bounds. Similarly, Parts (c) and (d) restate the definition of LUB. $\square$

Example 1

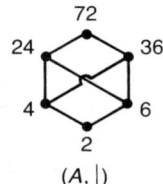

72
24   36
4   6
2
(A, |)

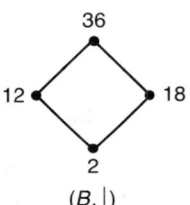

36
12   18
2
(B, |)

FIGURE 2.6.1

As in the case we are about to discuss, the symbol $\preceq$ for the binary relation of a poset may be replaced by symbols such as $|$ or $\subseteq$, which are customary for the particular binary relations of these cases. Let $\mathbf{Z}^+ = \{1, 2, 3, \ldots\}$ and X be a subset of $\mathbf{Z}^+$. We saw in Problem 33 of Section 1.7 that $(X, |)$ is a poset, where $|$ is the binary relation on X in which $d \mid m$ means that d is an integral divisor of m. Let $A = \{2, 4, 6, 24, 36, 72\}$ and $B = \{2, 12, 18, 36\}$. Figure 2.6.1 shows poset diagrams for the posets $(A, |)$ and $(B, |)$.

In $(A, |)$, GLB(24, 36) does not exist, since the set $S = \{2, 4, 6\}$ of lower bounds for (24, 36) has no greatest element with respect to the relation "is divisible by"; that is, there is no g in S such that $2 \mid g$, $4 \mid g$, and $6 \mid g$. Also in $(A, |)$, LUB(4, 6) does not exist, since the set $T = \{24, 36, 72\}$ of upper bounds for (4, 6) has no least element; that is, there is no m in T such that $m \mid 24$, $m \mid 36$, and $m \mid 72$. One sees in the matrix Tables 2.6.1(a) and (b) that GLB(x, y) and LUB(x, y) exist in $(B, |)$ for all (x, y) in B^2.

TABLE 2.6.1(a)

GLB	2	12	18	36
2	2	2	2	2
12	2	12	2	12
18	2	2	18	18
36	2	12	18	36

(b)

LUB	2	12	18	36
2	2	12	18	36
12	12	12	36	36
18	18	36	18	36
36	36	36	36	36

$\square$

THEOREM 2 **DIAGONAL AND SYMMETRY OF GLB AND LUB**

In a poset $(X, \preceq)$, GLB(x, x) $= x =$ LUB(x, x) for all x in X. Also, GLB(x, y) $=$ GLB(y, x) whenever either side exists, and LUB(x, y) $=$ LUB(y, x) if either side exists.

PROOF   Since $\preceq$ is reflexive, one has $x \preceq x$ for all x in X. Hence x is a lower bound for (x, x). If m is a lower bound for (x, x), then $m \preceq x$; this means that x is the greatest lower bound for (x, x). Similarly, $x =$ LUB(x, x). Since x and y have interchangeable roles in Definition 1, one has GLB(x, y) $=$ GLB(y, x) whenever either side exists. For the same reason, LUB(x, y) $=$ LUB(y, x) if either side exists. $\square$

DEFINITION 2 **LATTICE**

A *lattice* is a poset $(X, \preceq)$ in which GLB(x, y) and LUB(x, y) exist for all (x, y) in X^2.

In Example 1, the poset $(A, |)$ is not a lattice because GLB(24, 36) does not exist [or because LUB(4, 6) does not exist]. The poset $(B, |)$ of that example is a lattice because, as Tables 2.6.1(a) and (b) show, GLB(x, y) and LUB(x, y) exist for all (x, y) in B^2.

Definition 2 implies that, in a lattice $(X, \preceq)$, each of GLB and LUB is a binary operation on X; that is, each is a mapping from X^2 to X. Theorem 2 tells us that each of these operations is commutative. In Theorem 5 below ("Lattice Properties"), we will see that GLB and LUB also are associative and that together they satisfy the absorption laws of boolean algebra.

Example 2   Let $P(S)$ be the power set for a set S. Let X be a collection of subsets of S; that is, let $X \subseteq P(S)$. Then $(X, \subseteq)$ is a poset (as we saw in Problem 17 of Section 1.6). Such a poset may or may not be a lattice. The poset $(P(S), \subseteq)$ is a lattice (as we can see from the affirmative answers to all parts of Problems 31 and 32 of Section 1.2); in this lattice, GLB$(A, B) = A \cap B$ and LUB$(A, B) = A \cup B$. The reader is asked in Problem 13 below to show that GLB$(A, B) \subseteq A \cap B$ and $A \cup B \subseteq$ LUB(A, B) in the poset $(X, \subseteq)$ for every $X \subseteq P(S)$.   □

In the expressions GLB(x, y) and LUB(x, y), GLB and LUB are *prefix* notations for the binary operations characterized in Definition 1 because each appears before the ordered pair (x, y). These operations are closely related to the boolean operations of "meet" and "join" and also share some properties with the ordinary algebraic operations of multiplication and addition; hence the following infix notations frequently are substituted for GLB and LUB.

NOTATION 1   **INFIX NOTATIONS**

In a lattice $L = (X, \preceq)$, if one replaces GLB(x, y) by $x \wedge y$ and LUB(x, y) by $x \vee y$, then L may be rewritten as the algebraic structure $[X, \wedge, \vee]$; the operation $\wedge$ is called "meet" and the operation $\vee$ is called "join." Alternatively, if one replaces GLB(x, y) by xy and LUB(x, y) by $x + y$, then L may be rewritten as $[X, \cdot, +]$.

One advantage of the infix notations of $[X, \cdot, +]$ is that they make it easy to use the conventions of ordinary algebra on performing multiplications before additions (unless parentheses indicate otherwise). Although this cuts down on the need for parentheses, it also makes it harder to see "duality." Another disadvantage is the possibility in a lattice of attributing to $\cdot$ and $+$ the properties of ordinary multiplication and addition not possessed by GLB and LUB. For example, as we will see in Problem 17 below, the · operation may not be distributive over + in a lattice. Also, a lattice may not have the complementation unary operation of a boolean algebra.

In the following four displays, the content of Theorem 1, "Properties of GLB and LUB," is rewritten in the infix notations of $[X, \cdot, +]$:

$$xy \leq x \text{ and } xy \leq y; \tag{1}$$

$$m \leq x \text{ and } m \leq y \text{ together imply that } m \leq xy; \tag{2}$$

$$x \leq x + y \text{ and } y \leq x + y; \tag{3}$$

$$x \leq u \text{ and } y \leq u \text{ together imply that } x + y \leq u. \tag{4}$$

Let $(X, \leq)$ be a poset. We saw in Problem 20 of Section 1.6 that the reverse $\geq$ of the partial order relation $\leq$ is also a partial order relation on X; that is, $(X, \geq)$ is also a poset. We can now say something more, and for convenience we will use one of the extra notations for GLB and LUB.

THEOREM 3   **REVERSED LATTICE**

Let $L = (X, \leq) = [X, \wedge, \vee]$ be a lattice. Then $L' = (X, \geq)$ is also a lattice. In L and L', GLB and LUB are interchanged.

PROOF   If m is a lower bound for (x, y) in L, then one has $m \leq x$ and $m \leq y$. These can be rewritten as $x \geq m$ and $y \geq m$; hence m is an upper bound for (x, y) in the "reversed" poset L'. Also, the greatest lower bound $x \wedge y$ for (x, y) in L is easily seen to be LUB(x, y) in L'. Similarly, one can find that $x \vee y$ in L is GLB(x, y) in L'. Hence GLB(x, y) and LUB(x, y) exist in L' for all (x, y) in X^2, and L' is a lattice. $\square$

Theorem 3 enables us to introduce a lattice duality principle related to the duality principle in boolean algebras discussed in Section 2.3.

DEFINITION 3   **DUALITY IN LATTICES**

The *dual* of a statement concerning lattices is the new statement obtained by replacing $\wedge$ with $\vee$, replacing $\vee$ with $\wedge$, and reversing each inequality $x \leq y$ into $x \geq y$ (or its equivalent, $y \leq x$).

THEOREM 4   **LATTICE DUALITY PRINCIPLE**

The dual of a theorem on lattices is also a theorem.

PROOF Consider a theorem applying to all lattices $(X, \preceq) = [X, \wedge, \vee]$. Then its dual is also a theorem, since the dual is the original theorem applied to reversed lattices $(X, \succeq) = [X, \vee, \wedge]$. ☐

The statements "GLB$(x, x) = x$ for all x in X" and "LUB$(x, x) = x$ for all x in X" are duals of each other. Also, the statements "GLB$(x, y) =$ GLB(y, x) if either side exists" and "LUB$(x, y) =$ LUB(y, x) if either side exists" are duals of each other. Thus Theorem 1 ("Properties of GLB and LUB") is self-dual because its dual is merely a rearrangement of the statements in the theorem.

THEOREM 5 LATTICE PROPERTIES

Let $L = (X, \preceq) = [X, \cdot, +]$ be a lattice and let $x, y, z \in X$. Then

(a) $x(yz) = (xy)z$; that is, $\cdot$ is associative;
(b) $x + (y + z) = (x + y) + z$; that is, $+$ is associative;
(c) $x + yz \preceq (x + y)(x + z)$; that is, $+$ is **weakly distributive** over $\cdot$;
(d) $x(y + z) \succeq xy + xz$; that is, $\cdot$ is **reverse weakly distributive** over $+$;
(e) $x + xy = x$ and $x(x + y) = x$. (These are the **absorption laws** for lattices.)

PROOF (a) Let $w = (xy)z$. Then w is a lower bound for (xy, z) and so $w \preceq xy$ and $w \preceq z$. As in Display (1), $xy \preceq x$ and $xy \preceq y$. Using $w \preceq xy$, $xy \preceq y$, and transitivity of the partial ordering $\preceq$, we have $w \preceq y$ and, similarly, $w \preceq x$. From $w \preceq y$, $w \preceq z$, and the result in Display (2), we have $w \preceq yz$. This along with $w \preceq x$ and the result in Display (2) give us $w \preceq x(yz)$. Similarly we can show that $x(yz) \preceq w$. [This is left to the reader as Problem 12(a) below.] These two inequalities and the fact that $\preceq$ is antisymmetric imply that $x(yz) = w$. Thus $x(yz) = (xy)z$, and $\cdot$ is associative.

(b) The proof of the dual result that $+$ is associative is left to the reader as Problem 11 below.

(c) Part (c) is the dual of Part (d) and its independent proof is left to the reader as Problem 12(b) below.

(d) We start by noting from Display (1) that $xy \preceq x$ and $xz \preceq x$. Display (4), with x, y, and u replaced by xy, xz, and x, respectively, gives us $xy + xz \preceq x$. It is clear from Displays (1) and (3) that

$$xy \preceq y \preceq y + z \qquad \text{and} \qquad xz \preceq z \preceq y + z.$$

Since $\preceq$ is transitive, these imply that $xy \preceq y + z$ and $xz \preceq y + z$. Display (4), with x, y, and u replaced by xy, xz, and $y + z$, respectively, gives us $xy + xz \preceq y + z$. Since $xy + xz \preceq x$ and $xy + xz \preceq y + z$, we can replace m, x, and y in Display (2) by $xy + xz$, x, and $y + z$, respectively, and thus get $xy + xz \preceq x(y + z)$. This proves Part (d).

(e) Let $x + xy = u$. Then $x \preceq u$, since u is an upper bound for (x, xy). Also, $x \preceq x$, since $\preceq$ is reflexive, and $xy \preceq x$, since xy is a lower bound for (x, y). Hence x is an upper bound for (x, xy). Since u is the least upper bound for (x, xy), this means that $u \preceq x$. This, the previously shown $x \preceq u$, and the fact that $\preceq$ is antisymmetric imply that $u = x$. Thus $x = x + xy$, and this absorption law is proved. Then the other absorption law in (e) follows because it is the dual result; however, the reader is asked in Problem 12(c) below to give a direct proof. □

In Definition 1, the operations · and + (that is, GLB and LUB) are defined in terms of $\preceq$. The following result, together with Problems 9 and 10 below, shows that in a lattice any two of $x \preceq y$, $xy = x$, and $x + y = y$ are equivalent.

THEOREM 6   EQUIVALENT CONDITIONS IN A LATTICE

Let $L = (X, \preceq) = [X, \cdot, +]$ be a lattice and $x, y \in X$.

(i) If $xy = x$, then $x \preceq y$.
(ii) If $x \preceq y$, then $x + y = y$.
(iii) If $x + y = y$, then $xy = x$.

PROOF   For the proof of Part (i), let $xy = x$. Then x is a lower bound for (x, y) and so $x \preceq y$, as desired.

For Part (ii), let $x \preceq y$. We also have $y \preceq y$, since $\preceq$ is reflexive. Thus y is an upper bound for (x, y). Since $x + y$ is the least upper bound for (x, y), we have $x + y \preceq y$. But by Display (3), $y \preceq x + y$. These inequalities and the antisymmetry of $\preceq$ give us $x + y = y$, as desired.

For the proof of Part (iii), let $x + y = y$. Then $x \preceq y$, since $y = x + y$ is an upper bound for (x, y). Also, $x \preceq x$, since $\preceq$ is reflexive. Hence x is a lower bound for (x, y). Since xy is the greatest lower bound for (x, y), then $x \preceq xy$. But $xy \preceq x$, since xy is a lower bound for (x, y). Finally, $x \preceq xy$, $xy \preceq x$, and the antisymmetry of $\preceq$ imply that $xy = x$, which proves Part (iii). □

Theorem 2, "Diagonal and Symmetry of GLB and LUB," tells us that $xx = x = x + x$ in a lattice. Hence the entries on the (main) diagonal are the same in a matrix table for xy as in a matrix table for $x + y$. Theorem 2 also tells us that each of · and + is a commutative operation; this implies that the entries below the diagonal can be obtained from the entries above the diagonal or vice versa. These facts enable us to pack the information in matrix tables for · and + into one table (using half as much space) by using the spots on or below the diagonal to record xy and the spots on or above the diagonal to record $x + y$.

DEFINITION 4   **MEET-JOIN TABLE**

A *meet-join table* for a lattice $[X, \cdot, +]$ is an economical table for the operations $\cdot$ and $+$ on X of the form described in the previous paragraph.

TABLE 2.6.2

+ ·	2	12	18	36
2	2	12	18	36
12	2	12	36	36
18	2	2	18	36
36	2	12	18	36

As an illustration, the meet-join table replacing Tables 2.6.1(a) and (b) for the lattice $(B, |) = (\{2, 12, 18, 36\}, |)$ of Example 1 is Table 2.6.2.

In texts on Theory of Numbers or on Abstract Algebra, it is shown that the poset $(\mathbf{Z}^+, |)$ has the properties required to make it a lattice. We now introduce the terminology for GLB and LUB in this lattice.

DEFINITION 5   **GREATEST COMMON DIVISOR, LEAST COMMON MULTIPLE**

Let x and y be in $\mathbf{Z}^+ = \{1, 2, 3, \ldots\}$. Then the *greatest common divisor* of x and y, [gcd(x, y), for short] is GLB(x, y) in the lattice $(\mathbf{Z}^+, |)$. The *least common multiple* of x and y (lcm$[x, y]$, for short) is LUB(x, y) in $(\mathbf{Z}^+, |)$.

In the poset $(B, |)$ of Example 1, GLB$(12, 18) = 2$; on the other hand, gcd$(12, 18) = 6$, since GLB$(12, 18) = 6$ in the poset $(\mathbf{Z}^+, |)$. In the poset $(A, |)$ of Example 1, GLB$(24, 36)$ does not exist; however gcd$(24, 36) = 12$, since GLB$(24, 36) = 12$ in $(\mathbf{Z}^+, |)$. We note that gcd(x, y) and lcm$[x, y]$ exist for all positive integers x and y, since $(\mathbf{Z}^+, |)$ is a lattice and hence gcd and lcm are binary operations on $\mathbf{Z}^+$.

Let X be a subset of $\mathbf{Z}^+$. In Problem 14 below, the reader is asked to show that

GLB(x, y)|gcd(x, y) whenever GLB(x, y) exists,

lcm$[x, y]$|LUB(x, y) whenever LUB(x, y) exists,

where GLB and LUB are as defined for the poset $(X, |)$.

PROBLEMS FOR SECTION 2.6

1. Let $A = \{1, 2, 3, 12\}$.
   (a) Construct the matrix tables for GLB(x, y) and LUB(x, y) in $(A, |)$.
   (b) Is $(A, |)$ a lattice? Explain.
   (c) Does LUB$(2, 3) = $ lcm$[2, 3]$?

2. Let $B = \{1, 4, 6, 12\}$.
   (a) Construct matrix tables for GLB and LUB in the poset $(B, |)$.
   (b) Is $(B, |)$ a lattice? Explain.
   (c) Does GLB$(4, 6) = $ gcd$(4, 6)$?

3. For each of the following subsets X of Z^+, draw a poset diagram for $(X, |)$ and explain why the poset is or is not a lattice:
    (a) $X = \{1, 2, 3, 5, 30\}$; (b) $X = \{1, 2, 3, 4, 6\}$;
    (c) $X = \{1, 2, 3, 4, 12\}$; (d) $X = \{2, 3, 4, 12\}$;
    (e) $X = \{1, 3, 6, 30\}$; (f) $X = \{1, 2, 3, 4, 6, 12\}$.

4. Repeat Problem 3, but for each of the following subsets X of Z^+:
    (a) $X = \{2, 5, 15, 30\}$; (b) $X = \{1, 2, 5, 15, 30\}$;
    (c) $X = \{1, 2, 4, 5\}$; (d) $X = \{1, 2, 3, 5, 6, 10, 15, 30\}$;
    (e) $X = \{1, 2, 4\}$; (f) $X = \{1, 2, 4, 8\}$;
    (g) $X = \{1, 2, 3, 4, 6, 8, 12, 24\}$;
    (h) the set X of all positive integral divisors of 72.

5. Let $A = \{1, 2\}$, $B = \{1, 3\}$, $C = \{1, 2, 3\}$, and $X = \{A, B, C\}$.
    (i) Draw a poset diagram for $(X, \subseteq)$.
    (ii) Is $(X, \subseteq)$ a lattice? Explain.
    (iii) Does $\text{GLB}(A, B) = A \cap B$? Explain.

6. Let $A = \{1\}$, $B = \{2\}$, $C = \{1, 2, 3\}$, and $X = \{\varnothing, A, B, C\}$.
    (i) Draw a poset diagram for $(X, \subseteq)$.
    (ii) Is $(X, \subseteq)$ a lattice? Explain.
    (iii) Does $\text{LUB}(A, B) = A \cup B$? Explain.

7. (a) Are Displays (1) and (3) duals of each other?
    (b) Rewrite Displays (1) and (2) in the notations of a lattice $(X, \subseteq) = [X, \wedge, \vee]$.

8. (a) Are Displays (1) and (2) duals of each other?
    (b) Rewrite Displays (3) and (4) in the notations of a lattice $(X, \subseteq) = [X, \wedge, \vee]$.

9. Let $L = (X, \preceq) = [X, \cdot, +]$ be a lattice and $x, y \in X$.
    (a) Given that $xy = x$, prove that $x + y = y$.
    (b) Explain why $xy = x$ if and only if $x + y = y$.

10. Let $L = (X, \preceq) = [X, \cdot, +]$ be a lattice and $x, y \in X$. Prove that:
    (a) $x \preceq y$ if and only if $xy = x$.
    (b) $x \preceq y$ if and only if $x + y = y$.

11. Dualize the steps in the proof of Part (a) of Theorem 5, "Lattice Properties," and thus prove that the binary operation $+$ (that is, LUB) in a lattice is associative.

12. (a) Prove that $x(yz) \preceq (xy)z$ in a lattice $[X, \cdot, +]$. [This is a part of Theorem 5(a), "Lattice Properties," that was left to the reader.]
    (b) Dualize the steps in the proof of Part (d) of Theorem 5 and thus prove Part (c). That is, prove that $x + yz \preceq (x + y)(x + z)$.
    (c) Dualize the steps of the proof of $x + xy = x$ in Theorem 5(e) and thus prove the other absorption law,

    $$x(x + y) = x.$$

13. Let $P(S)$ be the power set for a nonempty set S and let $Y \subseteq P(S)$. Let GLB(A, B) and LUB(A, B) be as defined in the poset $(Y, \subseteq)$. Prove that:
(a) GLB$(A, B) \subseteq A \cap B$ whenever GLB(A, B) exists.
(b) $A \cup B \subseteq$ LUB(A, B) whenever LUB(A, B) exists.

14. Let $X \subseteq \mathbf{Z}^+ = \{1, 2, 3, \ldots\}$. Let GLB$(x, y)$ and LUB(x, y) be as defined in the poset $(X, |)$. Prove the following:
(a) GLB(x, y) is an integral divisor of gcd(x, y) whenever GLB(x, y) exists.
(b) LUB(x, y) is an integral multiple of lcm$[x, y]$ whenever LUB(x, y) exists.
(c) lcm$[x, \gcd(x, y)] = x$ for all x and y in $\mathbf{Z}^+$.
(d) gcd$(x, \text{lcm}[x, y]) = x$ for all x and y in $\mathbf{Z}^+$.

15. Give an example of a lattice $[X, \cdot, +]$ in which $x + (yz) = (x + y)(x + z)$ for all x, y, z in X, that is, in which $+$ is distributive over $\cdot$.

16. Give an example of a lattice $[X, \cdot, +]$ in which $\cdot$ is distributive over $+$.

17. Let $X = \{1, 2, 3, 5, 30\}$.
(i) Use a meet-join table (as described in Definition 4 and the paragraph before it) to show that $(X, |)$ is a lattice.
(ii) Show that $\cdot$ is not distributive over $+$ in this lattice by identifying elements a, b, c in X for which

$$a(b + c) \neq ab + ac.$$

18. Let $A = \{1\}$, $B = \{2\}$, $C = \{3\}$, $D = \{1, 2, 3\}$, and $X = \{\varnothing, A, B, C, D\}$.
(i) Show that $(X, \subseteq)$ is a lattice by tabulating $\cdot$ and $+$ in one meet-join table (see Definition 4).
(ii) Show that $+$ is not distributive over $\cdot$ in this lattice by identifying elements U, V, W in X for which $U + VW$ is a proper subset of $(U + V)(U + W)$.

19. Show that $\cdot$ is not distributive over $+$ in the lattice of Problem 3(c).

20. Show that $+$ is not distributive over $\cdot$ in the lattice of Problem 3(a).

21. Given that $x \leq y$ and $z \leq w$ in a lattice, prove that $xz \leq yw$.

22. Given that $x \leq y$ and $z \leq w$ in a lattice, prove that $x + z \leq y + w$.

23. Let $(X, \leq)$ be a poset and 0 be an element of X such that $0 \leq x$ for all x in X. Find:
(a) $0 \cdot 0$;   (b) $0 + 0$.

24. Let $(X, \leq)$ be a poset and let 1 be an element of X such that $x \leq 1$ for all x in X. Find:
(a) $1 \cdot 1$;   (b) $1 + 1$.

25. In the lattice $(B, |) = [B, \text{GLB}, \text{LUB}]$ of Example 1, is there an identity under the binary operation GLB? If so, what is it?

26. Do as in Problem 25, but with GLB replaced by LUB.

27. Let $[X, ^-, \wedge, 1, \vee, 0]$ be a boolean algebra and let $\subseteq$ be the binary relation on its carrier X in which $x \subseteq y$ means that $x \vee y = y$. Prove that

$(X, \subseteq)$ is a poset by showing that $\subseteq$ is:
(i) reflexive;   (ii) antisymmetric;   (iii) transitive.

28. Prove the following for the relation $\subseteq$ of Problem 27:
    (i) $0 \subseteq x$ for all x in X.
    (ii) $x \subseteq 1$ for all x in X.
    (iii) If $a \subseteq b$, then $(a \vee x) \subseteq (b \vee x)$ for all x in X.
    (iv) If $a \subseteq b$, then $(a \wedge x) \subseteq (b \wedge x)$ for all x in X.
    (v) $x \subseteq (x \vee y)$ and $y \subseteq (x \vee y)$ for all x and y in X. Also, if $x \subseteq z$ and $y \subseteq z$, then $x \vee y \subseteq z$.
    (vi) $(x \wedge y) \subseteq y$ for all x and y in X. [*Hint*: Use Parts (ii) and (iv).]
    (vii) If $a \subseteq b$, then $a \subseteq (a \wedge b)$. [*Hint*: Replace x with a in Part (iv).]
    (viii) If $a \subseteq b$, then $a = a \wedge b$. [*Hint*: Use Parts (vii) and (vi).]

29. Let R be the relation on a set X in which xRy means that $x \wedge y = x$. Prove the following:
    (i) (X, R) is a poset.
    (ii) $0Rx$ and $xR1$ for all x in X.
    (iii) If aRb, then $(x \wedge a)R(x \wedge b)$ and $(x \vee a)R(x \vee b)$ for all x in X.
    (iv) $(x \wedge y)Rx$ and $(x \wedge y)Ry$ for all x and y in X. Also, if zRx and zRy, then $zR(x \wedge y)$.
    (v) $xR(x \vee y)$ for all x and y in X.
    (vi) If aRb, then $a \vee b = b$.

30. Explain why the relation R of Problem 29 is the same as the relation $\subseteq$ of Problems 27 and 28. That is, show that aRb if and only if $a \subseteq b$.

31. In the special case of the boolean algebra $[P(S), ^-, \cap, S, \cup, \varnothing]$, what familiar partial ordering γ on $P(S)$ is such that $A\gamma B$ if and only if $A = A \cap B$?

32. For the boolean algebra of Problem 31, what relation γ on $P(S)$ is such that $A\gamma B$ if and only if $A \cup B = B$?

33. Let $\subseteq$ be the relation of Problems 27, 28, 29, and 30. Let x and y be in X. Explain why:
    (i) $x \subseteq (x \vee y)$ and hence $x = x \wedge x \subseteq x \wedge (x \vee y)$.
    (ii) $x \wedge (x \vee y) \subseteq x$.
    (iii) $x \wedge (x \vee y) = x$ for all x and y in X. (This is one of the *absorption laws* for boolean algebras.)

34. Prove that $x \vee (x \wedge y) = x$ for all x and y in X. (This is the other *absorption law*.)

35. Let $[X, ^-, \wedge, 1, \vee, 0]$ be a boolean algebra and $a, x, y \in X$. Justify the following steps of a proof that $x \wedge a = y \wedge a$ and $x \vee a = y \vee a$ together imply that $x = y$:

    $$x = x \vee (x \wedge a) = x \vee (y \wedge a) = (x \vee y) \wedge (x \vee a)$$
    $$= (x \vee y) \wedge (y \vee a) = (y \vee x) \wedge (y \vee a)$$
    $$= y \vee (x \wedge a) = y \vee (y \wedge a) = y.$$

36. Let a, x, and y be in the carrier of a boolean algebra.
(a) If $x \wedge a = y \wedge a$, must $x = y$? Explain.
(b) If $x \vee a = y \vee a$, must $x = y$? Explain.

37. Let a and b be in X. Given that $a \wedge b = 0$ and $a \vee b = 1$, prove that $b = \bar{a}$.

38. Let a, $b \in X$ and $a \wedge b = 0$. Show that $a \wedge (\bar{a} \vee \bar{b}) = a \wedge \bar{b}$.

39. Let x and y be in X. Let $z = x \vee y$ and $w = \bar{x} \wedge \bar{y}$. Explain why:
(i) $z \vee w = (z \vee \bar{x}) \wedge (z \vee \bar{y}) = (x \vee y \vee \bar{x}) \wedge (x \vee y \vee \bar{y}) = 1 \wedge 1 = 1$.
(ii) $z \wedge w = (x \wedge w) \vee (y \wedge w) = (x \wedge \bar{x} \wedge \bar{y}) \vee (y \wedge \bar{x} \wedge \bar{y}) = 0 \vee 0 = 0$.
(iii) $\overline{x \vee y} = \bar{x} \wedge \bar{y}$. (This is one of *De Morgan's Laws*.)

40. Prove that $\overline{x \wedge y} = \bar{x} \vee \bar{y}$ for all x and y in X. (This is the other of *De Morgan's Laws*.)

SUMMARY OF TERMS, CHAPTER 2

REVIEW PROBLEMS FOR CHAPTER 2

1. Let $\mathbf{Z} = \{\ldots, -1, 0, 1, \ldots\}$. For each of the following, tell whether the given subset of $\mathbf{Z}$ is closed under the given operation on $\mathbf{Z}$:
   (a) the set $1 + 2\mathbf{Z} = \{\ldots, -3, -1, 1, 3, 5, \ldots\}$ of odd integers under addition.
   (b) the set $2\mathbf{Z} = \{\ldots, -2, 0, 2, 4, \ldots\}$ of even integers under subtraction.
   (c) the set $1 + 2\mathbf{Z}$ under multiplication.
   (d) the set $2\mathbf{Z}$ under multiplication.

2. Answer the question of Problem 1 for each of the following:
   (a) the set $S = \{0, 1, 4, 9, \ldots\}$ of squares under addition.
   (b) the set S of Part (a) under multiplication.
   (c) the set $\{\ldots, -8, -1, 0, 1, 8, \ldots\}$ of cubes under multiplication.

3. Let $N = \{0, 1, \ldots\}$. For each of the following parts, tell whether the rule for f specifies a binary operation on N, that is, a mapping from $N \times N$ to N:
   (a) $f(m, n) = mn$.   (b) $f(m, n) = m - n$.
   (c) $f(m, n) = 2^m 3^n$.   (d) $f(m, n) = (m + n)^2$.

4. For each f of Problem 3, if f is an operation on N, tell whether the operation is commutative, whether it is associative, and whether there is an identity under the operation. If there is an identity, name it.

5. (a) Explain why the rule $m \square n = mn + m + n$ specifies $\square$ as a binary operation on $N = \{0, 1, \ldots\}$.
   (b) Is this $\square$ commutative?
   (c) Is this $\square$ associative? Explain.
   (d) Is there an identity e under this $\square$? If so, what is e?

6. (i) For the $\square$ of Problem 5, is $(N, \square)$ a semigroup?
   (ii) For the $\square$ and e of Problem 5, is $[N, \square, e]$ a monoid?

7. Let B_1^* be the set of words of all lengths over the alphabet $B_1 = \{0, 1\}$.
   (a) Complete the concatenation table shown in the margin.
   (b) Is the subset $\{0, 01, 001\}$ of B_1^* closed under concatenation?

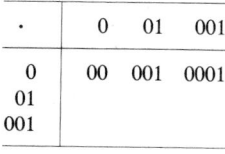

$\cdot$	0	01	001
0	00	001	0001
01			
001			

8. For the B_1^* of Problem 7, is the subset $\{0, 00, 01, 001\}$ closed under concatenation? Explain.

9. Let L be the language over $B_1 = \{0, 1\}$ consisting of the words over B_1 with length in $5N = \{0, 5, 10, \ldots\}$. Is L closed under concatenation? Explain.

10. Let L be the language over $B_1 = \{0, 1\}$ consisting of the words α over B_1 for which each 0 in α has a 1 immediately before it or immediately after it. Is L closed under concatenation?

11. Let $Z^+ = \{1, 2, \ldots\}$, Q^+ be the set of positive rational numbers, and R^+ be the set of positive real numbers. Let $+$, $-$, $\cdot$, and $\div$ denote the usual addition, subtraction, multiplication, and division, respectively.
    (a) Which of the following [(i)–(vi)] are semigroups?
    (b) Which are monoids? If a monoid, give its identity.
        (i) Z^+ under $+$.   (ii) Z^+ under $-$.   (iii) Q^+ under $\cdot$.
        (iv) Q^+ under $\div$.   (v) R^+ under $+$.   (vi) R^+ under $-$.

12. Answer Parts (a) and (b) of Problem 11 for the following:
        (i) Z^+ under $\cdot$.   (ii) Z^+ under $\div$.   (iii) Q^+ under $+$.
        (iv) Q^+ under $-$.   (v) R^+ under $\cdot$.   (vi) R^+ under $\div$.

13. Let $N = \{0, 1, 2, \ldots\}$, $dN = \{0, d, 2d, \ldots\}$, and $M = [N, +, 0]$. Which of the following are submonoids in M? (Note that parentheses are used here instead of brackets so as not to prejudge that the structure is a monoid.)
        (i) $(2N, +, 0)$,   (ii) $(3N, +, 0)$,
        (iii) $(2N \cap 3N, +, 0)$,   (iv) $(2N \cup 3N, +, 0)$.

14. Let $Z^+ = \{1, 2, \ldots\}$ and $r + qZ^+ = \{r + qn : n \in Z^+\}$. Which of the following are carriers of submonoids in $[Z^+, \cdot, 1]$?
        (i) $A = -1 + 2Z^+$,   (ii) $B = -2 + 3Z^+$,
        (iii) $A \cap B$.   (iv) $A \cup B$.

15. Let A be an alphabet and A^* be the set of words of all lengths over A. For a word $\alpha = a_1 a_2 \ldots a_n$ in A^*, let $r(\alpha) = a_n a_{n-1} \ldots a_1$. Also, let $r(\varepsilon) = \varepsilon$, where ε is the word of length 0. Show that $r(\alpha\beta) = r(\beta)r(\alpha)$ for all α and β in A^*, where $\alpha\beta$ is the concatenation of α and β.

16. Using the notation of Problem 15, a **palindrome** is a word α in A^* such that $r(\alpha) = \alpha$. Let P be the language consisting of all the palindromes in A^*. Show that P is not the carrier of a submonoid in $[A^*, \cdot, \varepsilon]$.

17. Let f and g be the ternary boolean operations with $f(x, y, z) = x \wedge \bar{y} \wedge z$ and $g(x, y, z) = \bar{x} \wedge \bar{y} \wedge z$. Find an ordered triple (a, b, c) in B_1^3 such that $f(a, b, c) = 0$ and $g(a, b, c) = 1$ and thus show that $f \neq g$.

18. Let f and g be the ternary boolean operations with $f(x, y, z) = \bar{x} \wedge y \wedge z$ and $g(x, y, z) = \bar{x} \wedge \bar{y} \wedge z$. Show that $f \neq g$.

19. Identify each of the following as a tautology, a contradiction, or a contingency:
    (a) $[x \vee (x \Rightarrow y)] \Rightarrow (x \vee y)$.   (b) $[x \wedge (x \Rightarrow y)] \Rightarrow (x \vee y)$.
    (c) $(x \vee \bar{x}) \Rightarrow (x \wedge \bar{x})$.

20. Identify each of the following as a tautology, a contradiction, or a contingency:
(a) $[x \wedge (y \vee z)] \Rightarrow [x \vee (y \wedge z)]$.   (b) $[x \wedge y \wedge (y \Rightarrow z)] \Rightarrow (x \wedge y \wedge z)$.
(c) $(x \wedge \bar{x}) \Rightarrow (x \vee \bar{x})$.

21. Find $f^{-1}(1)$ for the 5-ary monomial boolean function f of degree 3 with $f(x_1 x_2 x_3 x_4 x_5) = x_2 \cdot \bar{x}_4 \cdot x_5$.

22. Find $g^{-1}(1)$ for the 5-ary monomial g of degree 2 with $g(x_1 x_2 x_3 x_4 x_5) = \bar{x}_1 \cdot x_3$.

23. Express the f of Problem 21 as a sum of minifunctions.

24. Express the g of Problem 22 as a sum of minifunctions.

25. Find a 4-ary monomial f with $f^{-1}(1) = \{0010, 0011, 0110, 0111\}$.

26. Find a 4-ary monomial g with $g^{-1}(1) = \{0100, 0110, 1100, 1110\}$.

27. Express g as a sum of 2 monomials, given that

$$g^{-1}(1) = \{011, 010, 101, 111\}.$$

28. Express f as a sum of 2 monomials given that

$$f^{-1}(1) = \{011, 100, 101, 110, 111\}.$$

	$x \cdot y$	$x \cdot \bar{y}$	$\bar{x} \cdot \bar{y}$	$\bar{x} \cdot y$
z	✓	✓		
$\bar{z}$	✓	✓	✓	✓

29. Use the Karnaugh Map in the margin to express

$$x \cdot y \cdot z + x \cdot \bar{y} \cdot z + x \cdot y \cdot \bar{z} + x \cdot \bar{y} \cdot \bar{z} + \bar{x} \cdot \bar{y} \cdot \bar{z} + \bar{x} \cdot y \cdot \bar{z}$$

as a sum of two monomials.

30. Express $x \cdot y \cdot z + x \cdot y \cdot \bar{z} + x \cdot \bar{y} \cdot \bar{z} + \bar{x} \cdot \bar{y} \cdot \bar{z} + \bar{x} \cdot y \cdot \bar{z} + \bar{x} \cdot y \cdot z$ as a sum of two monomials. (A Karnaugh Map may help.)

31. Give a rule for the boolean function associated with the circuit shown below. (The part of the circuit with the voltage source and appliance has been dropped.)

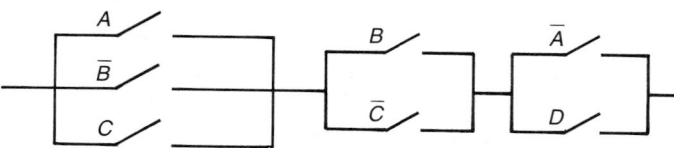

32. Show that the two circuits shown in the margin are associated with equal boolean functions.

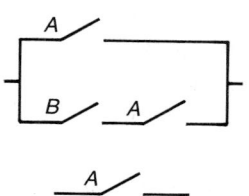

33. (i) Draw a figure for a circuit associated with the boolean expression $\bar{x} \cdot \bar{y} \cdot z + x \cdot \bar{y} \cdot \bar{z} + \bar{x} \cdot y \cdot \bar{z} + x \cdot \bar{y} \cdot z$.

(ii) Simplify the expression in Part (i) and redesign the circuit.

34. Do Problem 33 with circuits replaced by gate networks.

35. The *exclusive* "or" binary operation $\oplus$ on $B_1 = \{0, 1\}$ is defined by $x \oplus y = x \cdot \bar{y} + \bar{x} \cdot y$. Draw a gate network for this operation.

36. Draw a circuit for the $\oplus$ operation of Problem 35.

37. For a and b in Z, recall that $b|c$ means that $ab = c$ for some a in Z. For each of the following sets A, draw the poset diagram for $(A, |)$ and tell whether the poset is a lattice:
(a) $A = \{1, 3, 5, 7, 105\}$. (b) $A = \{1, 2, 3, 4\}$.

38. Do as in Problem 37 for:
(a) $A = \{2, 4, 6, 8\}$. (b) $A = \{4, 8, 16, 32\}$.

39. Let $A = \{1, 3\}$, $B = \{2, 3, 4\}$, $C = \{1, 4\}$, $D = \{1, 3, 4\}$, and $X = \{A, B, C, D\}$. Is $(X, \subseteq)$ a lattice? Explain.

40. Let $A = \{1\}$, $B = \{1, 2\}$, $C = \{1, 3\}$, $D = \{1, 2, 3, 4\}$, and $X = \{A, B, C, D\}$. Use a meet-join table to show that $(X, \subseteq)$ is a lattice $[X, \text{GLB}, \text{LUB}]$.

41. Label each of the following as True or False. If True, give a reference. If False, give a counter-example.
(a) Every lattice is a poset.
(b) Every poset is a lattice.
(c) In a lattice $L = [X, \cdot, +]$, the operations $\cdot$ and $+$ are associative.

42. Let $(X, \preceq) = [X, \cdot, +]$ be a lattice.
(a) Does $(xy)z \preceq x(yz)$ for all x, y, z in X? Explain.
(b) Must $x(y + z) = xy + xz$ for all x, y, z in X?

SUPPLEMENTARY AND CHALLENGING PROBLEMS, CHAPTER 2 _____

1. Let $(A, \circ)$ and $(B, \triangle)$ be semigroups. Let $\square$ be the binary operation on $A \times B$ with $(u, v) \,\square\, (x, y) = (u \circ x, v \triangle y)$. Show that $(A \times B, \square)$ is a semigroup. $(A \times B, \square)$ is called the **direct product** of $(A, \circ)$ and $(B, \triangle)$ (in the order given).

2. Do the analogue of Problem 1 for monoids.

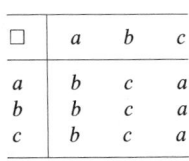

3. Let $\square$ be the binary operation on $X = \{a, b, c\}$ given by the table.
(a) Show that $(x \,\square\, y) \,\square\, z \neq x \,\square\, (y \,\square\, z)$ for all choices of x, y, z in X.
(b) Show that $\square$ has the **left-cancellation** property that whenever $x, y,$ and z are in X and $x \,\square\, y = x \,\square\, z$, then it follows that $y = z$.

4. Develop an analogue of Problem 3 for a set $X = \{a, b, c, d\}$.

5. Let $M = [X, \square, e]$ be a commutative monoid and let I consist of the **idempotents** of M, that is, the x in X with $x^2 = x$. Show that $[I, \square, e]$ is a submonoid in M.

6. Give an example of a monoid $M = [X, \square, e]$ in which the set I of idempotents is not closed under $\square$.

7. Let $(A, \square)$ and $(B, \square)$ be subsemigroups in $(X, \square)$. Prove that $(A \cap B, \square)$ is a subsemigroup in $(X, \square)$.

8. Let $[A, \square, e]$ and $[B, \square, e]$ be submonoids in a monoid $M = [X, \square, e]$ in which each x in A (or in B) has an inverse x^{-1} in A (or in B). Show that $[A \cup B, \square, e]$ is a submonoid in M if and only if A and B are comparable under the binary relation $\subseteq$, that is, either $A \subseteq B$ or $B \subseteq A$.

9. Let R^* denote the reverse of a binary relation R on a set S. In the monoid $[P(S^2), \cdot, D]$ of binary relations on S, show that $(AB)^* = B^*A^*$ for all A and B in $P(S^2)$.

10. Let $(X, \square)$ be a semigroup. Suppose that there is an element f in X such that $f \square x = x$ for all x in X. Also, for each x in X, let there be an element y_x in X such that $y_x \square x = f$. Prove the following:
    (i) If $g \in X$ and $g \square g = g$, then $g = f$.
    (ii) $x \square y_x = f$ for each x in X.
    (iii) $x \square f = x$ for each x in X.

11. Let T_n consist of all words $a_1 a_2 \dots a_n$ of length n over the alphabet $A = \{0, 1, 2\}$. For $k = 0, 1, \dots, 2n$, let $T_{n,k}$ consist of the $a_1 a_2 \dots a_n$ in T_n with $a_1 + a_2 + \cdots + a_n = k$. Prove that:
    (a) $\# T_n = 3^n$ for all n in $\mathbf{Z}^+ = \{1, 2, \dots\}$.
    (b) $\# T_{n,k} = \# T_{n,2n-k}$ for n in $\mathbf{Z}^+$ and $k = 0, 1, \dots, 2n$.
    (c) $\# T_{n,0} = 1 = \# T_{n,2n}$.
    (d) $\# T_{n+1,k+2} = (\# T_{n,k}) + (\# T_{n,k+1}) + (\# T_{n,k+2})$.

12. Given that $\# X = 6$, prove that X cannot be the carrier of a boolean algebra.

13. Find the smallest positive integer m such that every 4-ary boolean function is the sum of m or fewer monomials.

14. Find the smallest positive integers s and t (as functions of n) such that every n-ary boolean function has a gate network using at most s NOT gates, at most t AND gates (of various arities), and one OR gate.

15. Let $(X, \leq) = [X, \cdot, +]$ be a lattice with $\# X = 3$.
    (a) Show that $\leq$ is a well ordering of X.
    (b) Must $\leq$ be a well ordering of X if $\# X = 4$? Explain.

3

LOGIC

For assertions p and q, we will define the negation $\bar{p}$ of p, the conjunction $p \wedge q$ (read as "p and q"), and the disjunction $p \vee q$ (read as "p or q"). This will enable us to apply material on boolean expressions to logic. Frequently we will let 1 stand for "true" and 0 stand for "false" in a fashion similar to our use of 1 for "in" and 0 for "out" in the case tables of Section 1.3 and the use of 1 for "on" and 0 for "off" when describing circuits in Section 2.5.

3.1

PROPOSITIONS AND PREDICATES

DEFINITION 1 **PROPOSITION (ASSERTION), PREDICATE, UNIVERSE, TRUTH SET**

A *proposition* (or *assertion*) is a statement that is either true or false but not both. A *predicate* P on a *universe* X is a mapping from X to a set of propositions; the *truth set* for P is the set $T(P)$ of x in X for which $P(x)$ is true.

Example 1 Let the universe be $N = \{0, 1, 2, \ldots\}$ and let $P(n)$ stand for "n is the square of an integer." Then P is a predicate on N, since $P(n)$ is a proposition for each n in N; the truth set $T(P) = \{0, 1, 4, 9, \ldots, n^2, \ldots\}$. □

Example 2 Let $Z = \{\ldots, -1, 0, 1, \ldots\}$ and let the universe be the cartesian product $C = Z \times Z$. Let $P(m, n)$ denote the equation $m^2 = n^2 + 15$. Then P is a predicate on C, since $P(m, n)$ is a proposition for each ordered pair (m, n) in C. One can show that the truth set $T(P)$ is the finite set

$$\{(8, 7), (8, -7), (-8, 7), (-8, -7), (4, 1), (4, -1), (-4, 1), (-4, -1)\}$$

of solutions in integers m and n of the equation $m^2 = n^2 + 15$. □

Example 3   Let R be a binary relation on a set S. Then one can think of "xRy" or equivalently "$(x, y) \in R$" as a predicate P on the universe $S \times S$ with the set R as the truth set $T(P)$.   □

DEFINITION 2   **BASIC BOOLEAN OPERATIONS ON PROPOSITIONS**

Let p and q be propositions. The **negation** of p is the assertion "p is false" and is denoted as $\bar{p}$ or as $\neg p$. The **conjunction** $p \wedge q$ is the assertion "both p and q are true"; it can be read as "p and q." The **disjunction** $p \vee q$ is the assertion "at least one of p and q is true"; it can be read as "p or q."

The word "or" in the definition of $p \vee q$ is the **logical** "or," also called the **nonexclusive** "or." It has the same meaning as "and/or." When p is a complicated expression, it may be more convenient to use $\neg p$ instead of $\bar{p}$ for the negation of p.

Example 4   Let p stand for "wgt $001 = 2$" and q denote "$001 \in \boldsymbol{B_{3,1}}$." By the definitions of Section 1.1, p is a false proposition and q is a true proposition. The negation $\bar{p}$ of the false statement p is true; $\bar{p}$ can be expressed as "wgt $001 \neq 2$." The negation $\bar{q}$ is false because q is true. The disjunction $p \vee q$ is the true proposition that at least one of p and q is true. The conjunction $p \wedge q$ is the false proposition that p and q are both true.   □

DEFINITION 3   **TRUTH TABLE**

A **truth table** is a case table in which 1 represents "true" and 0 represents "false."

TABLE 3.1.1(a)

p	$\bar{p}$
0	1
1	0

(b)

p	q	$p \wedge q$	$p \vee q$
0	0	0	0
0	1	0	1
1	0	0	1
1	1	1	1

Table 3.1.1(a) is a truth table showing how the truth or falsity of p determines that of $\bar{p}$. Table 3.1.1(b) shows how the truth or falsity of $p \vee q$ and of $p \wedge q$ are determined from the truth or falsity of p and of q.

An n-ary boolean operation f has a rule $f(x_1, x_2, \ldots, x_n)$ that is expressible in terms of the unary operation $^-$ and the binary operations $\wedge$ and $\vee$. Such a rule $f(x_1, \ldots, x_n)$ is called a **boolean expression**. Definition 2 allows us to apply the operations $^-$, $\wedge$, and $\vee$ to propositions. Hence we can replace each x_i in $f(x_1, x_2, \ldots, x_n)$ by a proposition p_i and thus obtain a proposition, denoted as $f(p_1, p_2, \ldots, p_n)$, that is built up from the propositions p_i using Definition 2. The truth or falsity of $f(p_1, p_2, \ldots, p_n)$ can be determined from the truth or falsity of each p_i with the help of Tables 3.1.1(a) and (b).

Example 5   Let $f(x, y, z) = \overline{x \wedge \overline{y}} \vee z = [\neg(x \wedge \overline{y})] \vee z$. If p, q, and r are propositions, then $f(p, q, r) = [\neg(p \wedge \overline{q})] \vee r$ is the proposition asserting that "either (p is true and q is false) is false or r is true." When p, q, and r denote $2 \leq 3$, $2 = 3$, and $2 < 3$, respectively, then p is true, q is false, and r is true. This means that the relevant row of a truth table is the row with 101 as its label:

pqr	$\overline{q}$	$p \wedge \overline{q}$	$\neg(p \wedge \overline{q})$	$[\neg(p \wedge \overline{q})] \vee r$
101	1	1	0	1

The entries of this row can be obtained with the aid of Tables 3.1.1(a) and (b); the last entry shows that $f(p, q, r)$ is true.   □

The procedure used in Example 5 applies to all boolean expressions $f(x_1, x_2, \ldots, x_n)$. We now state it formally.

ALGORITHM 1   **TRUTH OR FALSITY OF A COMPOUND PROPOSITION**

Let $f(x_1, x_2, \ldots, x_n)$ be a boolean expression and let $p_1, p_2, \ldots, p_n$ be propositions. Replace x_i by 1 when p_i is true and by 0 when p_i is false. If these replacements make $f(x_1, x_2, \ldots, x_n) = 1$, then the proposition $f(p_1, p_2, \ldots, p_n)$ is true; otherwise $f(p_1, p_2, \ldots, p_n)$ is false.

THEOREM 1   **PROPOSITIONS FROM TAUTOLOGIES AND CONTRADICTIONS**

If $f(x_1, \ldots, x_n)$ is a tautology, then $f(p_1, \ldots, p_n)$ is true for all propositions $p_1, \ldots, p_n$. If $f(x_1, \ldots, x_n)$ is a contradiction, then $f(p_1, \ldots, p_n)$ is false for all propositions $p_1, \ldots, p_n$.

PROOF   If $f(x_1, \ldots, x_n)$ is a tautology, then it is a rule for the boolean operation I_n with $I_n(a_1, \ldots, a_n) = 1$ for all $(a_1, \ldots, a_n)$ in $\boldsymbol{B_1^n}$. Now, Algorithm 1 tells us that $f(p_1, \ldots, p_n)$ is true for all propositions $p_1, \ldots, p_n$. The other part of the theorem follows similarly from the definition of contradiction.   □

For example, since $x \vee \overline{x}$ is a tautology and $x \wedge \overline{x}$ is a contradiction, $p \vee \overline{p}$ is true and $p \wedge \overline{p}$ is false for every proposition p.

Bearing in mind that a predicate on a universe X is a mapping from X into a set of propositions, we now extend the basic boolean operations of Definition 2 to predicates.

DEFINITION 4   **NEGATION, CONJUNCTION, DISJUNCTION FOR PREDICATES**

Let P and Q be predicates on the same universe X. Then $\bar{P}$, $P \wedge Q$, and $P \vee Q$ are the following predicates on X:

Negation $\bar{P}: x \mapsto \overline{P(x)}$.

Conjunction $P \wedge Q: x \mapsto [P(x) \wedge Q(x)]$.

Disjunction $P \vee Q: x \mapsto [P(x) \vee Q(x)]$.

Example 6   Let $B_{n,k}$ be the set of n-digit binary strings of weight k and let B be the set of binary strings of all lengths. On the universe B, let P and Q be the predicates such that $P(\alpha)$ denotes "α has length 3" and $Q(\alpha)$ denotes "wgt $\alpha = 1$." Then the truth set $T(P)$ is B_3. Also,

$$T(Q) = B_{1,1} \cup B_{2,1} \cup B_{3,1} \cup \cdots,$$
$$T(P \wedge Q) = B_{3,1},$$

and

$$T(P \wedge \bar{Q}) = B_{3,0} \cup B_{3,2} \cup B_{3,3}. \qquad \square$$

THEOREM 2   **TRUTH SETS**

TABLE 3.1.2

pq	$p \Rightarrow q$
00	1
01	1
10	0
11	1

Let P and Q be predicates on X. Then $T(\bar{P}) = \overline{T(P)}$ [that is, the complement of $T(P)$ in X], $T(P \wedge Q) = T(P) \cap T(Q)$, and $T(P \vee Q) = T(P) \cup T(Q)$.

These equalities follow from the parallel nature of the definitions of the operations $^-$, $\cap$, and $\cup$ on the collection of subsets of X and the definitions of the operations $^-$, $\wedge$, and $\vee$ on predicates.

TABLE 3.1.3

pq	$\bar{p}$	$\bar{p} \vee q$
00	1	1
01	1	1
10	0	0
11	0	1

If p and q represent propositions, the notation $p \Rightarrow q$ is used in logic to denote the compound proposition, read as "p implies q," whose truth table is Table 3.1.2. Using Tables 3.1.1(a) and (b), one can make Table 3.1.3, which shows that $p \Rightarrow q$ is true when $\bar{p} \vee q$ is true and that $p \Rightarrow q$ is false when $\bar{p} \vee q$ is false. Thus we can consider $p \Rightarrow q$ to have the same meaning as $\bar{p} \vee q$. This motivates the following definition, in which some related terms are also defined and some other ways of reading $p \Rightarrow q$ are given.

DEFINITION 5   **IMPLICATION, PREMISE, CONCLUSION**

Let p and q be propositions. Then the **implication** $p \Rightarrow q$ has the same meaning as $\bar{p} \vee q$. In $p \Rightarrow q$, p is the **premise** (or **hypothesis**) and q is the *conclusion*. "$p \Rightarrow q$" may be read in any of the following ways:

(i) p implies q.
(ii) If p, then q.
(iii) p only if q.
(iv) p is a sufficient condition for q.
(v) q is a necessary condition for p.

Example 7   Let p be a false proposition such as "$0 = 1$" and let q be any proposition (true or false). Then $\bar{p}$ is true and hence $\bar{p} \vee q$ is true, as one can see from Tables 3.1.1(a) and (b). It then follows from the definition of implication that $p \Rightarrow q$ is true. In other words, a false premise implies any conclusion. For instance, "if $0 = 1$, then we are all fabulously wealthy" is a true proposition, although it would not improve our credit rating with people properly educated in logic.   □

THEOREM 3   **INFERENCES FROM A FALSE IMPLICATION**

Let p and q be propositions. Then the implication $p \Rightarrow q$ is false only when p is true and q is false.

PROOF   This is seen from the following truth table, in which the columns for $\bar{p}$ and $\bar{p} \vee q$ may be obtained using Definition 2 ("Basic Boolean Operations on Propositions") or Tables 3.1.1(a) and (b), and for which Definition 5 tells us that the column for $p \Rightarrow q$ is the same as that for $\bar{p} \vee q$.

p	q	$\bar{p}$	$\bar{p} \vee q$	$p \Rightarrow q$
0	0	1	1	1
0	1	1	1	1
1	0	0	0	0
1	1	0	1	1

□

DEFINITION 6   **IMPLICATION USING PREDICATES**

Let each of P and Q be a predicate on X. Then $P \Rightarrow Q$ is the predicate on X with

$$x \mapsto [P(x) \Rightarrow Q(x)].$$

For predicates P and Q on X, one reads "$P \Rightarrow Q$" in any of the five ways for reading "$p \Rightarrow q$" given in Definition 5. When p and q are propositions, either $p \Rightarrow q$ is true or it is false. For predicates P and Q on X, we see in the next example that $P(x) \Rightarrow Q(x)$ can be true for all x in X, for some but not all x in X, or for no x in X; that is, the truth set $T(P \Rightarrow Q)$ can be all of X, part of X, or the empty set.

Example 8   Let the universe be the set $\boldsymbol{B} = \boldsymbol{B}_1 \cup \boldsymbol{B}_2 \cup \boldsymbol{B}_3 \cup \cdots$ of binary strings of all lengths. Let P, Q, R, and S be the predicates on $\boldsymbol{B}$ for which $P(\alpha)$ denotes "wgt α is less than or equal to the length of α," $Q(\alpha)$ denotes "wgt $\alpha = -1$," $R(\alpha)$ denotes "wgt $\alpha = 5$," and $S(\alpha)$ denotes "the length of α is 7." Then $P(\alpha)$ is true for all α in $\boldsymbol{B}$, $Q(\alpha)$ is false for all α in $\boldsymbol{B}$, $R(\alpha)$ is true if and only if α is in the proper subset $\boldsymbol{B}_{5,5} \cup \boldsymbol{B}_{6,5} \cup \boldsymbol{B}_{7,5} \cup \cdots$ of $\boldsymbol{B}$, and $S(\alpha)$ is true if and only if α is in the proper subset $\boldsymbol{B}_7$ of $\boldsymbol{B}$. It follows that each of $Q(\alpha) \Rightarrow P(\alpha)$, $R(\alpha) \Rightarrow P(\alpha)$, and $S(\alpha) \Rightarrow P(\alpha)$ is true for all α in $\boldsymbol{B}$. Also, $P(\alpha) \Rightarrow Q(\alpha)$ is false for all α in $\boldsymbol{B}$. However, $R(\alpha) \Rightarrow S(\alpha)$ is true for some α's in $\boldsymbol{B}$, such as $\alpha = 1111100$ [since $R(1111100)$ and $S(1111100)$ are both true] and $\alpha = 00$ [since $R(00)$ is false], whereas $R(\alpha) \Rightarrow S(\alpha)$ is false for other α's in $\boldsymbol{B}$, such as $\alpha = 11111$ and $\alpha = 11111000$ [since $R(\alpha)$ is true and $S(\alpha)$ is false for each of these α's]. $\qquad \square$

THEOREM 4   **IMPLICATIONS AND TRUTH SETS**

Let P and Q be predicates on a nonempty universe X. Then $T(P \Rightarrow Q) = \overline{T(P)} \cup T(Q)$. Also, $P(x) \Rightarrow Q(x)$ is true for all x in X if and only if $T(P) \subseteq T(Q)$.

PROOF   Using Definition 5 ("Implication, Premise, Conclusion") and Theorem 2 ("Truth Sets"), we have

$$T(P \Rightarrow Q) = T(\bar{P} \vee Q) = T(\bar{P}) \cup T(Q) = \overline{T(P)} \cup T(Q).$$

Then it follows from Problem 15(iii) of Section 1.3 that $T(P \Rightarrow Q) = X$ if and only if $T(P) \subseteq T(Q)$. $\qquad \square$

Example 9   Let P and Q be the predicates on $\boldsymbol{Z} = \{\ldots, -1, 0, 1, \ldots\}$ for which $P(n)$ denotes "$(n - 5)^2 = 9$" and $Q(n)$ denotes "$n - 5 = 3$." Then $T(P) = \{2, 8\}$ and $T(Q) = \{8\}$. It follows from Theorem 4 that

$$T(P \Rightarrow Q) = \overline{T(P)} \cup T(Q) = (\boldsymbol{Z} - \{2, 8\}) \cup \{8\} = \boldsymbol{Z} - \{2\}, \qquad (1)$$

where $\bar{A}$ and the more explicit notation $\boldsymbol{Z} - A$ each represent the complement of A in $\boldsymbol{Z}$. Checking on Display (1), one sees that $P(n) \Rightarrow Q(n)$ is false for $n = 2$ because $P(2)$ is true and $Q(2)$ is false. The implication is true for $n = 8$ because both $P(8)$ and $Q(8)$ are true. $P(n) \Rightarrow Q(n)$ is true when n is not in $\{2, 8\}$ because $P(n)$ is false for such n's and a false premise implies any assertion. $\qquad \square$

DEFINITION 7 **EQUIVALENCE**

Let P and Q be propositions or predicates on the same universe. Then $P \Leftrightarrow Q$ is an alternate notation for $(P \Rightarrow Q) \wedge (Q \Rightarrow P)$. The *equivalence* $P \Leftrightarrow Q$ may be read in any of the following ways:

(i) P is equivalent to Q.
(ii) P if and only if Q.
(iii) P is a necessary and sufficient condition for Q.
(iv) Q is a necessary and sufficient condition for P.

Example 10 Let S be a nonempty set, $P(S)$ be its power set, and X be the cartesian product $P(S) \times P(S)$. Let f, g, and h be the predicates on X for which $f(A, B)$ denotes "$A \cup B = B$," $g(A, B)$ denotes "$A \subseteq B$," and $h(A, B)$ denotes "$A \cap B = A$." One sees from Problems 25 and 26 of Section 1.2 that $A \cup B = B$ if and only if $A \subseteq B$ and that $A \subseteq B$ if and only if $A \cap B = A$. Hence

$$f(A, B) \Leftrightarrow g(A, B) \qquad \text{and} \qquad g(A, B) \Leftrightarrow h(A, B)$$

for all (A, B) in X. □

Example 11 Let f be a mapping from a set X to itself. Let p denote "f is injective" and q denote "f is surjective." Then $p \Leftrightarrow q$ is true whenever X is a finite set but need not be true when X is infinite. In particular, the mapping f from N to itself, with $f(2n) = n = f(2n + 1)$, is surjective but not injective (see Problem 7 of Section 1.8). For this f, the assertion q is true and the assertion p is false and hence $q \Rightarrow p$ is false. It follows that $p \Leftrightarrow q$ is false for this f, since both $p \Rightarrow q$ and $q \Rightarrow p$ must be true for $p \Leftrightarrow q$ to be true. □

In proving that an equivalence $p \Leftrightarrow q$ is true, one can prove the implications $p \Rightarrow q$ and $q \Rightarrow p$ separately, as in the solution to Problem 11 of Section 1.3, or simultaneously, as in Example 10 above.

NOTATION 1 **REPEATED IMPLICATION OR EQUIVALENCE**

One may abbreviate "$x \Rightarrow y$ and $y \Rightarrow z$" as "$x \Rightarrow y \Rightarrow z$." Also, "$x \Leftrightarrow y \Leftrightarrow z$" denotes "$x \Leftrightarrow y$ and $y \Leftrightarrow z$."

Similarly, one gives meaning to $x_1 \Rightarrow x_2 \Rightarrow \cdots \Rightarrow x_n$ and to $x_1 \Leftrightarrow x_2 \Leftrightarrow \cdots \Leftrightarrow x_n$. Note that

$$(x \Rightarrow y \Rightarrow z) = (\bar{x} \vee y) \wedge (\bar{y} \vee z),$$
$$[x \Rightarrow (y \Rightarrow z)] = [\bar{x} \vee (\bar{y} \vee z)] = \bar{x} \vee \bar{y} \vee z,$$
$$[(x \Rightarrow y) \Rightarrow z] = [\neg(\bar{x} \vee y)] \vee z = [(x \wedge \bar{y}) \vee z].$$

In Problem 31 below we see that these three boolean expressions are rules for three different boolean functions. Hence one should not drop the parentheses in $x \Rightarrow (y \Rightarrow z)$ or in $(x \Rightarrow y) \Rightarrow z$. Thus one sees that the notation $x \Rightarrow y \Rightarrow z$ is *not* analogous to $a + b + c$ but is analogous to the interval notation $a \le x \le b$ and to the set inclusion notation $A \subseteq B \subseteq C$.

DEFINITION 8   **CONVERSE, CONTRAPOSITIVE**

The *converse* of an implication $P \Rightarrow Q$ is the implication $Q \Rightarrow P$. The *contrapositive* of $P \Rightarrow Q$ is the implication $\bar{Q} \Rightarrow \bar{P}$.

Example 12   Let C be the cartesian product $\mathbf{Z} \times \mathbf{Z}$. Let $P(x, y)$ denote "$x = y$," $Q(x, y)$ denote "$x^2 = y^2$," and $R(x, y)$ denote "x is either y or $-y$." Then $P(x, y) \Rightarrow Q(x, y)$ is true for all (x, y) in C; that is, $T(P \Rightarrow Q) = C$. However, the truth set $T(Q \Rightarrow P)$ of the converse is not all of C; for example, $Q(1, -1)$ is true and $P(1, -1)$ is false and hence $Q(1, -1) \Rightarrow P(1, -1)$ is false. The implication $Q(x, y) \Rightarrow R(x, y)$ is true for all (x, y) in C and so is its converse $R(x, y) \Rightarrow Q(x, y)$; hence $T(Q \Rightarrow R) = T(R \Rightarrow Q) = C$.

As just stated, $P(x, y) \Rightarrow Q(x, y)$ is true for all (x, y) in C. So is its contrapositive $\bar{Q}(x, y) \Rightarrow \bar{P}(x, y)$, which can be rewritten as "if $x^2 \ne y^2$, then $x \ne y$." Thus $T(\bar{Q} \Rightarrow \bar{P}) = T(P \Rightarrow Q)$.

We have seen that when p and q are propositions and $p \Rightarrow q$ is true, its converse $q \Rightarrow p$ may or may not be true. However, the contrapositive $\bar{q} \Rightarrow \bar{p}$ of a true implication $p \Rightarrow q$ is always true, as shown in Theorem 5 below. It follows that for predicates A and B on X, $T(B \Rightarrow A)$ may or may not equal $T(A \Rightarrow B)$ but that $T(\bar{B} \Rightarrow \bar{A})$ always equals $T(A \Rightarrow B)$.   □

DEFINITION 9   **REVERSIBLE IMPLICATION**

Let p and q be propositions. A true implication $p \Rightarrow q$ is said to be *reversible* if its converse $q \Rightarrow p$ is also true.

THEOREM 5   **A PROPOSITION IS EQUIVALENT TO ITS CONTRAPOSITIVE**

Let p and q be propositions. Then $p \Rightarrow q$ is true if and only if its contrapositive $\bar{q} \Rightarrow \bar{p}$ is true.

PROOF   By the definition of implication, $p \Rightarrow q$ means $\bar{p} \vee q$ and $\bar{q} \Rightarrow \bar{p}$ means $\bar{\bar{q}} \vee \bar{p}$. Since $\bar{\bar{q}} = q$ and $q \vee \bar{p} = \bar{p} \vee q$, the implication $p \Rightarrow q$ has the same meaning as its contrapositive $\bar{q} \Rightarrow \bar{p}$.   □

COROLLARY Let P and Q be predicates on X. Then

$$T(P \Rightarrow Q) = T(\bar{Q} \Rightarrow \bar{P}).$$

Example 13 By definition, a mapping f from X to Y is injective if

$$[f(x_1) = f(x_2)] \Rightarrow [x_1 = x_2]$$

is true, where x_1 and x_2 denote arbitrary elements of X. Using Theorem 5, one can show that f is injective by proving that the contrapositive

$$[x_1 \neq x_2] \Rightarrow [f(x_1) \neq f(x_2)]$$

is true. □

Example 14 Let P and Q be the predicates on $\mathbf{Z}$ for which $P(n)$ denotes "n^2 is even" and $Q(n)$ denotes "n is even." For all n in $\mathbf{Z}$, one can prove that $P(n) \Rightarrow Q(n)$ is true by showing, as follows, that its contrapositive $\neg Q(n) \Rightarrow \neg P(n)$ is true:

$$\begin{aligned}
\neg Q(n) &\Rightarrow [n \in 1 + 2\mathbf{Z}] \\
&\Rightarrow [n = 2k + 1 \text{ with } k \text{ in } \mathbf{Z}] \\
&\Rightarrow [n^2 = 2(2k^2 + 2k) + 1] \\
&\Rightarrow [n^2 \in 1 + 2\mathbf{Z}] \Rightarrow \neg P(n).
\end{aligned} \qquad (2)$$

This proof uses the fact that the sets $2\mathbf{Z}$ (of even integers) and $1 + 2\mathbf{Z}$ (of odd integers) are disjoint and have $\mathbf{Z}$ as their union; that is, these sets form a partition of $\mathbf{Z}$. It also uses the fact that $\Rightarrow$ is transitive and hence that $\neg Q(n) \Rightarrow \neg P(n)$ follows from the string of true implications in Display (2). □

We note that $\Rightarrow$ and $\Leftrightarrow$ are relations on any set of propositions.

THEOREM 6 **IMPLICATION IS REFLEXIVE AND TRANSITIVE**

The implication $p \Rightarrow p$ is true for all propositions p. Also, if $p \Rightarrow q$ and $q \Rightarrow r$ are both true, so is $p \Rightarrow r$.

PROOF This theorem follows from the facts that

$$x \Rightarrow x$$

and

$$[(x \Rightarrow y) \wedge (y \Rightarrow z)] \Rightarrow (x \Rightarrow z)$$

are tautologies. (See Problem 30 of Section 2.3.) □

THEOREM 7 **EQUIVALENCE IS AN EQUIVALENCE RELATION**

Let S be a set of propositions. Then:

(a) $p \Leftrightarrow p$ is true for all p in S.
(b) If $p \Leftrightarrow q$ is true, so is $q \Leftrightarrow p$.
(c) If $p \Leftrightarrow q$ and $q \Leftrightarrow r$ are true, so is $p \Leftrightarrow r$.

The proof is straightforward and is left to the reader.

Example 15   Here we solve the equation

$$\sqrt{3n + 1} = 8 + \sqrt{n + 1}$$

by writing a sequence of equations (labeled as predicates A, B, C, D, E, F, G, H, I) on $\mathbf{Z} = \{\ldots, -1, 0, 1, \ldots\}$ and noting implications among these predicates.

$A(n)$: $\sqrt{3n + 1} = 8 + \sqrt{n + 1}$

$B(n)$: $(\sqrt{3n + 1})^2 = (8 + \sqrt{n + 1})^2$

$C(n)$: $3n + 1 = 64 + 16\sqrt{n + 1} + n + 1$

$D(n)$: $2n - 64 = 16\sqrt{n + 1}$

$E(n)$: $n - 32 = 8\sqrt{n + 1}$

$F(n)$: $(n - 32)^2 = (8\sqrt{n + 1})^2$

$G(n)$: $n^2 - 64n + 1024 = 64(n + 1)$

$H(n)$: $n^2 - 128n + 960 = 0$

$I(n)$: $(n - 8)(n - 120) = 0$

We note that the truth set $T(I) = \{8, 120\}$. For all n in $\mathbf{Z}$,

$$A(n) \Rightarrow B(n) \Rightarrow C(n) \Rightarrow D(n) \Rightarrow E(n) \Rightarrow F(n) \Rightarrow G(n) \Rightarrow H(n) \Rightarrow I(n).$$

Hence $A(n) \Rightarrow I(n)$ is true for all n in $\mathbf{Z}$. Then it follows from Theorem 4 ("Implications and Truth Sets") that $T(A) \subseteq T(I) = \{8, 120\}$. Substituting each of these candidates 8 and 120 for n in Equation A, one finds that 120 is a solution but 8 is not. Hence the desired set of solutions to Equation A is the proper subset $T(A) = \{120\}$ of $T(I) = \{8, 120\}$. This should not be surprising, since Example 12 warns us that the implications $A(n) \Rightarrow B(n)$ and $E(n) \Rightarrow F(n)$ may not be reversible for some integers n. In particular, the true implication $E(8) \Rightarrow F(8)$ is not reversible because $F(8)$ is true but $E(8)$ is false and hence the converse $F(8) \Rightarrow E(8)$ is false. Thus we have not shown that $I(n)$ implies $A(n)$ for all n in $\mathbf{Z}$ and so we should have been prepared to find that the truth set $T(I)$ is not a subset of $T(A)$. $\square$

PROBLEMS FOR SECTION 3.1

1. Which of the following propositions are true?
   (a) $5 = -5$;   (b) $5^2 = (-5)^2$;   (c) $5^2 = -5^2$;   (d) $5 = 2 + 3$.

2. Which of the following propositions are true?
   (a) $0 \cdot 2 = 0 \cdot 3$;   (b) $2 = 3$;   (c) $2 + 3 = 3 + 2$;   (d) $\dfrac{1+2}{1+3} = \dfrac{2}{3}$.

3. Which of the following implications are true?
   (a) If $5^2 = (-5)^2$, then $5 = -5$.
   (b) If $5^2 = (-5)^2$, then $5 = 3 + 2$.
   (c) If $5 = -5$, then $5 = 3 + 2$.
   (d) If $5 = -5$, then $5 = 4 + 2$.

4. Which of the following implications are true?
   (a) If $2 = 3$, then $2 \cdot 0 = 3 \cdot 0$.   (b) If $2 \cdot 0 = 3 \cdot 0$, then $2 = 3$.
   (c) If $2 \cdot 0 = 3 \cdot 0$, then $2 + 3 = 3 + 2$.
   (d) If $2 = 3$, then $(1 + 2) \div (1 + 3) = 2 \div 3$.

5. Let p denote the assertion "$x > 7$." Which of the following is the negation $\bar{p}$ of p?
   (i) $x < 7$,   (ii) $x \leq 7$.

6. Let p denote "$x \leq 5$." Which of the following is the negation $\bar{p}$ of p?
   (i) $x > 5$,   (ii) $x \geq 5$.

7. Find the truth set for the predicate P on $N \times N$, where $N = \{0, 1, \ldots\}$ and $P(m, n)$ is "$(m - n)(m + n) = 35$."

8. Let $Z = \{\ldots, -1, 0, 1, \ldots\}$ and $P(m, n)$ be "$m^2 - n^2 = 35$." Find the truth set $T(P)$ for the predicate P on $Z \times Z$.

9. On the universe B_5 of five-digit binary strings, let $P(\alpha)$ be "wgt $\alpha \leq 3$" and $Q(\alpha)$ be "wgt $\alpha \geq 2$." Express each of the following truth sets as a $B_{5,k}$ or as a union of sets $B_{5,k}$:
   (a) $T(P)$;   (b) $T(\bar{P})$;   (c) $T(Q)$;   (d) $T(P) \cap T(Q)$;
   (e) $T(P \wedge Q)$;   (f) $T(\bar{P}) \cup T(Q)$;   (g) $T(\bar{P} \vee Q)$;   (h) $T(P \Rightarrow Q)$.

10. On the universe B_6, let $P(\alpha)$ be "wgt $\alpha \leq 3$" and $Q(\alpha)$ be "wgt $\alpha \geq 3$." Express each of the following as a $B_{6,k}$ or as a union of sets $B_{6,k}$:
    (a) $T(P)$;   (b) $T(\bar{P})$;   (c) $T(Q)$;   (d) $T(P) \cap T(Q)$;
    (e) $T(P \wedge Q)$;   (f) $T(\bar{P}) \cup T(Q)$;   (g) $T(\bar{P} \vee Q)$;   (h) $T(P \Rightarrow Q)$.

11. Let M be the set of all mappings f from $N = \{0, 1, 2, \ldots\}$ to itself. On the universe M, let I, S, and B be the predicates for which $I(f)$ is "f is injective," $S(f)$ is "f is surjective," and $B(f)$ is "f is bijective." Which of the following implications are true for all f in M?
    (a) $I(f) \Rightarrow B(f)$;   (b) $B(f) \Rightarrow I(f)$;   (c) $S(f) \Rightarrow B(f)$;
    (d) $B(f) \Rightarrow S(f)$;   (e) $[I(f) \wedge S(f)] \Rightarrow B(f)$.

12.   (i) Which implications of Problem 11 have converses that are true for all mappings f in M?

(ii) Which implications of Problem 11 are reversible for all f in M? That is, which are true and have true converses for all f in M?

13.   Write the converse of each of the following:

(a) If $x^2 = x$, then $x = 0$ or $x = 1$.

(b) $\bar{p} \Rightarrow q$.

(c) You become rich if you work hard or live longer than your rich relatives.

(d) If $[C(a) \cap C(b)] \neq \varnothing$, then $C(a) = C(b)$.

14.   Write the converse of each of the following:

(a) $q \Rightarrow [\neg (q \Rightarrow r)]$.

(b) If n is an integer and n^2 is even, then n is even.

(c) One can make a moon if one has enough green cheese.

15.   Give the contrapositive of each implication in Problem 13.

16.   Give the contrapositive of each implication in Problem 14.

17.   For each of the following, tell whether it is true or false for all assertions p and q; outline a counterexample when it is false.

(a) $(p \Rightarrow q) \Leftrightarrow (p \wedge q)$.   (b) $(\bar{p} \Rightarrow q) \Leftrightarrow (p \vee q)$.   (c) $p \wedge (p \vee q) \Leftrightarrow q$.

18.   Do as in Problem 17 for:

(a) $(p \wedge \bar{q}) \Leftrightarrow (\bar{p} \vee q)$.   (b) $(\bar{p} \wedge q) \Leftrightarrow \neg (p \vee \bar{q})$.   (c) $p \vee (p \wedge q) \Leftrightarrow p$.

19.   Make a truth table for the equivalence $x \Leftrightarrow y$.

20.   Let $f(xy) = (x \Leftrightarrow y)$. Find the complete inverse images $f^{-1}(1)$ and $f^{-1}(0)$. (Here xy ranges over $\{00, 01, 10, 11\}$.)

21.   Use an analysis similar to that in Example 15 to find all solutions in $\mathbf{Z}$ of the equation

$$\sqrt{2n - 1} = 7 + \sqrt{n + 11}.$$

22.   For each of the following equations, find all solutions in $\mathbf{Z}$:

(a) $\sqrt{3n + 1} = 8 - \sqrt{n + 1}$.   (b) $\sqrt{2n - 1} = 7 - \sqrt{n + 11}$.

(c) $\sqrt{n + 80} = 8 + \sqrt{n}$.   (d) $\sqrt{n + 80} = 8 - \sqrt{n}$.

23.   Convert each of the statements (a), (b), (c), and (d) into one of the forms (i), (ii), . . . , (vii) by telling what $P, Q, \ldots$ denote:

(i) $P \Rightarrow Q$;   (ii) $P \Leftrightarrow Q$;   (iii) $(P \wedge Q) \Rightarrow R$;   (iv) $P \Rightarrow (Q \wedge R)$;

(v) $(P \wedge Q \wedge R) \Rightarrow S$;   (vi) $(P \wedge Q) \Rightarrow (R \wedge S)$;   (vii) $P \Rightarrow (Q \wedge R \wedge S)$.

(a) $\# S_\alpha = k$ if and only if wgt $\alpha = k$.

(b) If $C \subseteq A$ and $C \subseteq B$, then $C \subseteq (A \cap B)$.

(c) If e is a left identity and e is a right identity, then e is the identity.

(d) If r, s, and t are in $\mathbf{Z}^+$, $r | s$, and $s | t$, then $r | t$.

24. Do as in Problem 23 for the following parts:
(a) If $n \in 2N$, then $n + 1 \in 1 + 2N$.
(b) If $(X, \preceq)$ is a poset and $A \subseteq X$, then A has no more than one least element and A has no more than one greatest element.
(c) A binary relation R, on a set S, is its own reverse if and only if R is symmetric.
(d) If a quadrilateral is a parallelogram, then opposite sides have equal length, opposite angles have equal measure, and the diagonals bisect each other.

25. Let p and q be assertions such that $p \Rightarrow q$ is true.
(a) If p is true, must q be true? Explain.
(b) If p is false, must q be false? Explain.
(c) If q is false, must p be false? Explain.
(d) If q is true, must p be true? Explain.

26. Let a be an element of the carrier X of a boolean algebra. Let p be the proposition "$a = \bar{a}$" and q be the proposition "$0 = 1$." Axiom (B3) for boolean algebras (Definition 2 of Section 2.3) tells us that q is false. In Problem 7 of Section 2.3, the reader was asked to show that the implication $p \Rightarrow q$ is true and then to infer that p is false. Which part of Problem 25 above justifies that inference?

27. (i) Is $(A \subseteq S) \wedge (B \subseteq S) \Rightarrow (A = B)$ true for all sets A, B, and S? Explain.
(ii) Let $P(x)$, $Q(x)$, and $R(x)$ be the predicates "x is a dog," "x is a cat," and "x is an animal," respectively, on some universe X. Which of the following always (that is, for all sets X) have all of X as the truth set?
(a) $P(x) \Rightarrow R(x)$; (b) $Q(x) \Rightarrow R(x)$;
(c) $[P(x) \Rightarrow R(x)] \wedge [Q(x) \Rightarrow R(x)] \Rightarrow [P(x) = Q(x)]$.

28. (i) Is $[(x \Rightarrow z) \wedge (y \Rightarrow z)] \Rightarrow (x \Rightarrow y)$ a tautology, a contingency, or a contradiction?
(ii) Does it follow from "every dog is an animal" and "every cat is an animal" that "every dog is a cat"?

29. Let $x \Rightarrow y \Rightarrow z \Rightarrow w$ be shorthand for $(x \Rightarrow y) \wedge (y \Rightarrow z) \wedge (z \Rightarrow w)$ and similarly define $x \Leftrightarrow y \Leftrightarrow z$. Prove that

$$(x \Rightarrow y \Rightarrow z \Rightarrow x) \Leftrightarrow (x \Leftrightarrow y \Leftrightarrow z)$$

for all assertions (or predicates) x, y, and z.

30. Prove that $(A \subseteq B \subseteq C \subseteq A) \Leftrightarrow (A = B = C)$ for all sets A, B, and C.

31. Let f, g, and h be the ternary boolean functions with $f(xyz) = (x \Rightarrow y) \Rightarrow z$, $g(xyz) = x \Rightarrow (y \Rightarrow z)$, $h(xyz) = (x \Rightarrow y) \wedge (y \Rightarrow z)$. Find $f^{-1}(1)$, $g^{-1}(1)$, and $h^{-1}(1)$ and thus show that no two of f, g, and h are equal. (The shorthand rule for h is $x \Rightarrow y \Rightarrow z$. This problem shows that $\Rightarrow$ is not associative. It is transitive.)

32. Is the implication $(p \wedge \bar{p}) \Rightarrow q$ true for all propositions p and q? Explain.

3.2

LOGICAL INFERENCE

People frequently try to prove some result by using the incorrect technique of assuming that the result is true and then showing that this assumption implies a result already known to be true.

Example 1   Do the following steps prove that $7 = 11$?

$7 = 11$ Assumption.
$11 = 7$ Symmetry of the "equals" relation.
$18 = 18$ If equals are added to equals, the sums are equal.

No, the assertion has not been proven. Let p denote "$7 = 11$" and q denote "$18 = 18$." Then the implication $p \Rightarrow q$ and the assertion q are both true, yet together they do not imply the assertion p. Replacing these specific assertions p and q by variables x and y, the form of the purported proof becomes

$$[(x \Rightarrow y) \wedge y] \Rightarrow x. \tag{1}$$

The expression in Display (1) is not a tautology, since it equals 0 when $x = 0$ and $y = 1$. Therefore,

$$[(p \Rightarrow q) \wedge q] \Rightarrow p$$

is false when p is false and q is true, as they are in this specific example. The reasoning of this example is fallacious because it treats the contingency given by Display (1) as if it were a tautology. The fallacy involved here is called "Affirming the Consequent." This and a few other fallacies are listed later in this section (Table 3.2.5).   □

Example 2   The prosecution at a trial presents evidence that a murder was committed by either Guest or Butler and then introduces additional evidence indicating that Butler is not the murderer. The prosecutor states that it clearly follows from all the furnished evidence that Guest is guilty. Is this inference correct?

Symbolically the form of the inference is

$$[(G \vee B) \wedge \bar{B}] \Rightarrow G. \tag{2}$$

The boolean function f with $f(xy) =$

$$[(x \vee y) \wedge \bar{y}] \Rightarrow x$$

is easily seen to be a tautology. One way to prove this is by showing with a truth table that $f(xy) = 1$ for each of the four binary strings xy of $\boldsymbol{B_2}$.

Hence Display (2) is a true statement for any assertions B and G; in particular, Display (2) is true when B stands for "Butler is guilty" and G stands for "Guest is guilty."

Think of yourself as a juror. Does this all mean that Guest is really guilty? When we say that Display (2) is true, we mean that if the assertions represented by $B \lor G$ and $\bar{B}$ are true, then so is assertion G. Jurors have to decide on the credibility of the evidence as well as on the validity of the inferences. Let us retreat from the role of being jurors to being just technical advisors on logical inference. □

Suppose that *Mathjournal* receives a paper by Smith that contains a purported proof of a mathematical theorem and that *Mathjournal* asks the well-known mathematicians Jones and Brown to check independently the validity of the proof. Might these referees disagree? The answer is yes. They are more apt to disagree on whether the result is interesting. But they might also disagree on whether the proof is sufficiently complete. In fact, one of them may think the proof is valid while the other shows it to be utterly invalid.

Will mastery of the material of this section eliminate all disagreements about reasoning among jurors and among referees for mathematics journals? No, it will not. The validity of the reasoning cannot always be checked by determining whether or not some boolean function is a tautology. "Reasoning" is a difficult and complicated subject, as one may see by consulting the items under "Logic" in the annotated Bibliography near the end of this book. Our goal here is improvement, not perfection, in reasoning and in proofs.

Example 3 Let O stand for a contradiction such as $y \land \bar{y}$. The following table shows that

$$(\bar{x} \Rightarrow O) \Rightarrow x \tag{3}$$

is a tautology:

x	$\bar{x}$	O	$\bar{x} \Rightarrow O$	$(\bar{x} \Rightarrow O) \Rightarrow x$
0	1	0	0	1
1	0	0	1	1

This means that Display (3) becomes a true statement when x is replaced by any assertion p. Hence one can prove that an assertion p is true by showing that its negation $\bar{p}$ implies a contradiction such as $q \land \bar{q}$, where q is some assertion. Similarly, one can show that $[(x \land \bar{y}) \Rightarrow O] \Rightarrow (x \Rightarrow y)$ is a tautology. (See Problem 25 below.) The tautologies of this example justify the following technique of proof (which will be used for Lemma 3, "Proof by Strong Induction," of Section 4.3).   □

ALGORITHM 1   **PROOF BY CONTRADICTION**

An assertion p can be proved true by showing that the implication $\bar{p} \Rightarrow O$ is true, where O is some contradiction. Also, one can prove an implication $p \Rightarrow q$ true by proving that $(p \wedge \bar{q}) \Rightarrow O$ is true.

We have illustrated, in several examples, the technique of checking the validity of certain reasoning by associating an inference with a boolean function and determining whether or not the function is a tautology. This technique has been used for more than 2000 years, and a number of the tautologies have been named and applied. Table 3.2.1 lists some of the well-known tautologies.

TABLE 3.2.1

	Inference Rule	*Associated Tautology*
(T1)	Contrapositive	$(x \Rightarrow y) \Rightarrow (\bar{y} \Rightarrow \bar{x})$
(T2)	Proof by Contradiction	$(\bar{x} \Rightarrow O) \Rightarrow x$ or $[(x \wedge \bar{y}) \Rightarrow O] \Rightarrow (x \Rightarrow y)$
		(O here denotes some contradiction.)
(T3)	Excluded Middle	$x \vee \bar{x}$
(T4)	Addition	$x \Rightarrow (x \vee y)$
(T5)	Simplification	$(x \wedge y) \Rightarrow x$
(T6)	Modus Ponens	$[x \wedge (x \Rightarrow y)] \Rightarrow y$
(T7)	Modus Tollens	$[\bar{y} \wedge (x \Rightarrow y)] \Rightarrow \bar{x}$
(T8)	Disjunctive Syllogism	$[(x \vee y) \wedge \bar{y}] \Rightarrow x$
(T9)	Hypothetical Syllogism	$[(x \Rightarrow y) \wedge (y \Rightarrow z)] \Rightarrow (x \Rightarrow z)$
(T10)	Constructive Dilemma	$[(x \Rightarrow y) \wedge (z \Rightarrow w) \wedge (x \vee z)] \Rightarrow (y \vee w)$
(T11)	Destructive Dilemma	$[(x \Rightarrow y) \wedge (z \Rightarrow w) \wedge (\bar{y} \vee \bar{w})] \Rightarrow (\bar{x} \vee \bar{z})$

The valid reasoning of Example 2 illustrates "Disjunctive Syllogism," Inference Rule (T8). Each of the boolean functions of Table 3.2.1 can be shown to be a tautology by a truth table. In Problems 5 and 6 below, the reader is asked to give such proofs for Inference Rules (T3), (T4), (T5), and (T7).

We next present some methods for obtaining new tautologies from known tautologies.

THEOREM 1   **CONSTRUCTING NEW TAUTOLOGIES**

(a) If $P(x_1 x_2 \ldots x_n)$ is a rule for a tautology, then some or all of the variables x_i can be replaced by other variables or by rules for boolean functions and one will still have a rule for a tautology.

(b) If P and Q are equal as n-ary boolean functions and P is a tautology, then so is Q.

(c) If P and $P \Rightarrow Q$ are tautologies, then so is Q.

(d) If P and Q are tautologies, then so are $P \wedge Q$ and $P \vee Q$.

PROOF

(a) If P is an n-ary tautology, then $P(x_1 x_2 \ldots x_n) = 1$ for all strings $x_1 x_2 \ldots x_n$ in $\boldsymbol{B_n}$, that is, for all choices of each x_i as either 0 or 1. Since a boolean function A has only 0 and 1 as possible values, replacing an x_i by the rule for A must give a rule for a tautology. This explains why Part (a) holds.

(b) If P and Q are equal n-ary boolean functions and P is a tautology, then $P(x_1 x_2 \ldots x_n) = Q(x_1 x_2 \ldots x_n)$ and $P(x_1 x_2 \ldots x_n) = 1$ for all strings $x_1 x_2 \ldots x_n$ in $\boldsymbol{B_n}$. Hence $Q(x_1 x_2 \ldots x_n) = 1$ for all $x_1 x_2 \ldots x_n$ in $\boldsymbol{B_n}$, and Q is a tautology. This proves Part (b).

(c)–(d) The proofs of Parts (c) and (d) are left to the reader as Problems 21 and 22 below. $\square$

Example 4

The proof in Table 3.2.2, that

$$[(\bar{x} \Rightarrow y) \wedge \bar{y}] \Rightarrow x$$

is a tautology, illustrates a technique for deriving a new tautology from previously established tautologies.

TABLE 3.2.2

Tautology	Justification
$[\bar{y} \wedge (x \Rightarrow y)] \Rightarrow \bar{x}$	"Modus Tollens," that is, Inference Rule (T7).
$[(x \Rightarrow y) \wedge \bar{y}] \Rightarrow \bar{x}$	Commutativity of $\wedge$ [and Theorem 1(b)].
$[(\bar{x} \Rightarrow y) \wedge \bar{y}] \Rightarrow \bar{\bar{x}}$	Replace x with $\bar{x}$ [and use Theorem 1(a)].
$[(\bar{x} \Rightarrow y) \wedge \bar{y}] \Rightarrow x$	$\bar{\bar{x}} = x$ in a boolean algebra.

$\square$

THEOREM 2   **IMPLICATION TAUTOLOGIES**

Let $I = [(P_1 \wedge P_2 \wedge \cdots \wedge P_s) \Rightarrow Q]$, where Q and the P_i are n-ary boolean functions.

(a) If $Q(\alpha) = 1$ whenever α is a string in $\boldsymbol{B_n}$ for which $P_1(\alpha) = P_2(\alpha) = \cdots = P_s(\alpha) = 1$, then I is a tautology.

(b) If I is a tautology and α is a string in $\boldsymbol{B_n}$ for which $P_1(\alpha) = P_2(\alpha) = \cdots = P_s(\alpha) = 1$, then $Q(\alpha) = 1$.

PROOF

(a) We wish to show that $I(\alpha) = 1$ for all α in $\boldsymbol{B_n}$. We consider two cases. For those α with $P_1(\alpha) = P_2(\alpha) = \cdots = P_s(\alpha) = 1$, we are given that $Q(\alpha) = 1$, and so I becomes $1 \wedge 1 \wedge \cdots \wedge 1 \Rightarrow 1$, which equals $1 \Rightarrow 1$

and so equals 1. For the other strings α of B_n, some $P_i(\alpha) = 0$ and hence $P_1(\alpha) \wedge P_2(\alpha) \wedge \cdots \wedge P_s(\alpha) = 0$; then $I(\alpha)$ becomes $0 \Rightarrow Q(\alpha)$, which equals 1. Thus $I(\alpha) = 1$ for all α in B_n and I is a tautology.

(b) Under the hypothesis for Part (b), $I(\alpha)$ becomes $1 \wedge 1 \wedge \cdots \wedge 1 \Rightarrow Q(\alpha)$, or $1 \Rightarrow Q(\alpha)$. Since I is a tautology, $1 \Rightarrow Q(\alpha)$ must equal 1; hence $Q(\alpha) = 1$, as desired. $\square$

Example 5   Here we prove that the ternary boolean function

$$[(x \Rightarrow y) \wedge (y \Rightarrow z) \wedge \bar{z}] \Rightarrow \bar{x}$$

is a tautology. Instead of using the eight lines of a truth table, we use a procedure based on Theorem 2. Theorem 2(a) tells us that we will have a valid proof if we assume that xyz is a string in B_3 for which each of

$$x \Rightarrow y, \qquad y \Rightarrow z, \qquad \text{and} \qquad \bar{z}$$

equals 1 and if we show under this assumption that $\bar{x} = 1$. This is accomplished in Table 3.2.3, where the first column's format

$$\begin{array}{c} \hline P_1 \\ P_2 \\ \vdots \\ P_s \\ \hline Q \\ \hline \end{array}$$

stands for the assertion that

$$\text{“} [P_1(\alpha) \wedge P_2(\alpha) \wedge \cdots \wedge P_s(\alpha)] \Rightarrow Q(\alpha) \text{ is true for all } \alpha \text{ in } B_3 \text{.”} \qquad (4)$$

When dealing with an n-ary boolean function, we replace B_3 in Display (4) with B_n.

TABLE 3.2.3

Boolean Function	Justification
$x \Rightarrow y$	Hypothesis.
$y \Rightarrow z$	Hypothesis.
$x \Rightarrow z$	"Hypothetical Syllogism," Inference Rule (T9) [that is, $(x \Rightarrow y) \wedge (y \Rightarrow z) \Rightarrow (x \Rightarrow z)$] and Theorem 2(b).
$\bar{z}$	Hypothesis.
$\bar{x}$	$(x \Rightarrow z) \wedge \bar{z} \Rightarrow \bar{x}$, which is "Modus Tollens," Inference Rule (T7) (with minor changes allowed by Theorem 1, "Constructing New Tautologies").

$\square$

Example 6 Here we prove that the 4-ary boolean function

$$[(x \Rightarrow y) \wedge (y \Rightarrow z) \wedge (z \Rightarrow w) \wedge \bar{w}] \Rightarrow \bar{x}$$

is a tautology. Instead of using all sixteen lines of a truth table or using the tautology of Example 5, we give the proof in Table 3.2.4, in which the format of Table 3.2.3 is streamlined by omitting reference to Theorem 2(b) and other such amplifications.

TABLE 3.2.4

Boolean Function	Justification
$x \Rightarrow y$	Hypothesis.
$y \Rightarrow z$	Hypothesis.
$x \Rightarrow z$	Inference Rule (T9), "Hypothetical Syllogism."
$z \Rightarrow w$	Hypothesis.
$x \Rightarrow w$	Inference Rule (T9).
$\bar{w}$	Hypothesis.
$\bar{x}$	Inference Rule (T7), "Modus Tollens."

□

Example 7 Let us test the following reasoning: "If a positive integer is an integral multiple of 9, then the sum of its digits is an integral multiple of 9. The sum of the digits of 76,543,210 is 28. The sum of the digits of 28 is 10. The sum of the digits of 10 is 1. The integer 1 is not an integral multiple of 9. Therefore 76,543,210 is not an integral multiple of 9."

To expedite our work, we let M be the predicate on $\mathbf{Z}^+$ for which $M(n)$ asserts that "n is an integral multiple of 9." The theorem stated in the first sentence of the above reasoning plus the facts in the three sentences that follow that theorem tell us that the implications

$$M(76{,}543{,}210) \Rightarrow M(28), \qquad M(28) \Rightarrow M(10), \qquad M(10) \Rightarrow M(1)$$

are all true. We are also told that $M(1)$ is false. The question now is whether these assertions imply that $M(76,543,210)$ is false. Symbolically, the reasoning can be expressed as

$$[(p \Rightarrow q) \wedge (q \Rightarrow r) \wedge (r \Rightarrow t) \wedge \bar{t}] \Rightarrow \bar{p}.$$

This reasoning is valid because, as we saw in Example 6,

$$[(x \Rightarrow y) \wedge (y \Rightarrow z) \wedge (z \Rightarrow w) \wedge \bar{w}] \Rightarrow \bar{x}$$

is a tautology. □

Invalid reasoning has been around so long that some of the fallacies have been named. These are associated with contingencies that some people mistake for tautologies. Some of these are listed in Table 3.2.5.

TABLE 3.2.5

	Fallacy Name	Associated Contingency
(F1)	Affirming the Consequent	$[(x \Rightarrow y) \wedge y] \Rightarrow x$
(F2)	Denying the Antecedent	$[(x \Rightarrow y) \wedge \bar{x}] \Rightarrow \bar{y}$
(F3)	Converse	$(x \Rightarrow y) \Rightarrow (y \Rightarrow x)$
(F4)	Obverse	$(x \Rightarrow y) \Rightarrow (\bar{x} \Rightarrow \bar{y})$

The fallacious reasoning of Example 1 illustrates Fallacy (F1), "Affirming the Consequent." In Problems 7 and 8 below, the reader is asked to show that each of the boolean functions of Table 3.2.5 is *not* a tautology.

PROBLEMS FOR SECTION 3.2

1. Find a tautology in Table 3.2.1 that justifies the following valid reasoning: "Butler is guilty or Guest is guilty. If Guest is guilty, then Guest should be convicted. If Butler is guilty, then Butler should be convicted. Therefore, Butler should be convicted or Guest should be convicted."

2. Find a tautology in Table 3.2.1 that justifies the following valid reasoning: "If I live, I can learn. If I can learn, I can improve my situation. Therefore, if I live, I can improve my situation."

3. What is an easy way to show that $[x \wedge (x \Rightarrow \bar{y})] \Rightarrow \bar{y}$ is a tautology?

4. How can one easily determine that $[(x \Rightarrow \bar{y}) \wedge y] \Rightarrow \bar{x}$ is a tautology?

5. For each of the following boolean functions (selected from Table 3.2.1), use a truth table to prove it a tautology:
(a) $x \vee \bar{x}$;　(b) $(x \wedge y) \Rightarrow x$.

6. For each of the following, use a truth table to prove it a tautology:
(a) $[\bar{y} \wedge (x \Rightarrow y)] \Rightarrow \bar{x}$;　(b) $x \Rightarrow (x \vee y)$.

7. Prove that each of the following is not a tautology:
(a) $[(x \Rightarrow y) \wedge y] \Rightarrow x$.　[This is Fallacy (F1), "Affirming the Consequent."]
(b) $(x \Rightarrow y) \Rightarrow (y \Rightarrow x)$.　[This is Fallacy (F3), "Converse."]

8. Prove that each of the following is not a tautology.
(a) $[(x \Rightarrow y) \wedge \bar{x}] \Rightarrow \bar{y}$.　[This is Fallacy (F2), "Denying the Antecedent."]
(b) $(x \Rightarrow y) \Rightarrow (\bar{x} \Rightarrow \bar{y})$.　[This is Fallacy (F4), "Obverse."]

9. Analyze the following reasoning: "If 5 is in A, then 5^2 is in A. But 5 is not in A. Therefore 5^2 is not in A."

10. Analyze the following reasoning: "If 5 is in A, then 5^2 is in A. Therefore, if 5^2 is in A, then 5 is in A."

11. Let m be an integer. Analyze the following reasoning: "m^2 is odd. Also, if m^2 is odd, then m is odd. Hence m is odd."

12. Let m be an integer. Analyze the following reasoning: "m^2 is not even. If m is even, then m^2 is even. Hence m is not even."

13. Let m be an integer.
    (a) Analyze the following reasoning: "If m is odd, then m^2 is odd. Therefore, if m^2 is odd it follows that m is odd."
    (b) Is the assertion "If m^2 is odd, then m is odd" true for all integers m? Explain.

14. Let m be an integer. Analyze the following reasoning: "The integer m is either even or odd. If m is even, then m^2 is even. Hence, if m^2 is odd, then m must be odd."

15. Prove that $[(x \lor y) \land \bar{y}] \Rightarrow (x \land \bar{y})$ is a tautology using the format of Example 6, that is, a table similar to Table 3.2.4.

16. Do as in Problem 15 for each of the following:
    (a) $[x \land y \land (x \Rightarrow y)] \Rightarrow y$. (b) $(x \land y) \Rightarrow (x \lor y)$.
    (c) $[(\bar{x} \Rightarrow y) \land \bar{y}] \Rightarrow [x \lor (z \land w)]$.

17. Use a procedure similar to that of Example 4 to prove that $x \lor y \lor (\bar{x} \land \bar{y})$ is a tautology.

18. Use a procedure similar to that of Example 4 to prove that $x \lor y \lor z \lor (\bar{x} \land \bar{y} \land \bar{z})$ is a tautology.

19. Let $r = \sqrt{2} + \sqrt{3}$, $A = \{1, -1\}$, and E denote the equation $x^4 - 10x^2 + 1 = 0$. Analyze the following reasoning: "The number r is a root of E. If r is a root of E and r is rational, then r is in A. If r is in A, then r is not a root of E. Hence r is not rational."

20. Let r, A, and E be as in Problem 19. Analyze the following: "The number r is a root of E but is not in A. If r is a root of E and r is rational, then r is in A. Hence r is not rational."

21. Let P and Q be n-ary boolean functions such that both P and $P \Rightarrow Q$ are tautologies. Prove that Q is a tautology. [This is Part (c) of Theorem 1, "Constructing New Tautologies."]

22. Let P and Q be n-ary tautologies. Prove that $P \land Q$ and $P \lor Q$ are tautologies. [This is Part (d) of Theorem 1, "Constructing New Tautologies."]

23. Let q and r be in $\mathbf{Z} = \{\ldots, -2, -1, 0, 1, 2, 3, \ldots\}$. Recall from Section 1.7 that $r + q\mathbf{Z}$ denotes $\{r + qn : n \in \mathbf{Z}\}$. For example, $3\mathbf{Z} = \{\ldots, -3, 0, 3, 6, \ldots\}$, $1 + 3\mathbf{Z} = \{\ldots, -2, 1, 4, 7, \ldots\}$, and $2 + 3\mathbf{Z} = \{\ldots, -1, 2, 5, 8, \ldots\}$. Analyze the following reasoning: "If $n \in 3\mathbf{Z}$, then $n^2 \in 3\mathbf{Z}$. If $n \in 1 + 3\mathbf{Z}$, then $n^2 \in 1 + 3\mathbf{Z}$. Therefore, if n is not in $3\mathbf{Z}$ and n is not in $1 + 3\mathbf{Z}$, it follows that n^2 is not in $3\mathbf{Z}$ and n^2 is not in $1 + 3\mathbf{Z}$."

24. Let $r + q\mathbf{Z}$ be as in Problem 23. Analyze the following: "$(5 - 1) \in 2\mathbf{Z}$ and $5 \neq 1$. If $(5 - 1) \in 2\mathbf{Z}$, then $5 + 2\mathbf{Z} = 1 + 2\mathbf{Z}$. Hence we simultaneously have $5 \neq 1$ and $1 + 2\mathbf{Z} = 5 + 2\mathbf{Z}$."

25. Let O be a contradiction such as $x \wedge \bar{x}$. Prove with a case table that $[(x \wedge \bar{y}) \Rightarrow O] \Rightarrow (x \Rightarrow y)$ is a tautology.

3.3

QUANTIFIERS

Let P be a predicate on a set X. By analogy with Definition 8 of Section 1.2 ("Union of the Sets of a Collection"), one might express the assertion that "$P(x)$ is true for all x in X" in the form

$$\bigwedge_{x \in X} P(x).$$

However, this notation is not used in logic. Instead, the following is the customary usage in logic.

NOTATION 1   **UNIVERSAL QUANTIFIER** $\forall$

The assertion that "$P(x)$ is true for all x in X" may be written as

$\forall x \in X, P(x).$

The symbol $\forall$ is the **universal quantifier**; it may be read as "for all," as "for every," or as "for each."

We recall that an alternative symbolism for the negation $\bar{p}$ of p is $\neg p$, which is the symbol generally used when p is a complicated expression.

Example 1   Let $P(n)$ be "$n^2 \geq 0$" and $\mathbf{Z} = \{\ldots, -1, 0, 1, \ldots\}$. Then $\forall n \in \mathbf{Z}, P(n)$ is the true assertion that "all squares of integers are nonnegative," and hence its negation $\neg[\forall n \in \mathbf{Z}, P(n)]$ is false. If $Q(n)$ denotes "$n^2 > 0$," then $\forall n \in \mathbf{Z}$, $Q(n)$ is false for at least one integer n; specifically, $Q(0)$ is false. Hence the negation $\neg[\forall n \in \mathbf{Z}, Q(n)]$ is true.   □

By analogy with Definition 7 of Section 1.2 ("Intersection of the Sets of a Collection"), one might write "$P(x)$ is true for some x in X" symbolically as

$$\bigvee_{x \in X} P(x).$$

However, the customary notation in logic is as follows.

NOTATION 2   **EXISTENTIAL QUANTIFIER** $\exists$

"$P(x)$ is true for at least one x in X" may be written as

$$\exists x \in X, \, P(x).$$

One can also read this as "There exists an x in X for which $P(x)$ is true." The symbol $\exists$ is the ***existential quantifier***.

Example 2   Let $P(n)$ denote "$n^2 = 16$." Since $P(4)$ is true, as is $P(-4)$, $\exists n \in \mathbf{Z}, \, P(n)$ is the true assertion that "16 is the square of at least one integer." If $Q(n)$ denotes "$n^2 = 15$" then $\exists n \in \mathbf{Z}, \, Q(n)$ is false, since there does not exist an integer whose square is 15. (Neither $\sqrt{15}$ nor $-\sqrt{15}$ is an integer.) Hence the negation $\neg[\exists n \in \mathbf{Z}, \, Q(n)]$ is true. $\square$

Example 3   Let X be a finite set $\{x_1, x_2, \ldots, x_n\}$. Then $\forall x \in X, \, P(x)$ is the same as $P(x_1) \wedge P(x_2) \wedge \cdots \wedge P(x_n)$ and $\exists x \in X, \, P(x)$ is the same as $P(x_1) \vee P(x_2) \vee \cdots \vee P(x_n)$. Using one of De Morgan's Laws (see Problem 40 of Section 2.6 and Problem 24 of Section 4.2), it can be shown that

$$\neg[\forall x \in X, \, P(x)] = \neg[P(x_1) \wedge P(x_2) \wedge \cdots \wedge P(x_n)]$$
$$= [\neg P(x_1)] \vee [\neg P(x_2)] \vee \cdots \vee [\neg P(x_n)].$$

Thus "it is false that $P(x)$ is true for all x in X" is equivalent to "$P(x)$ is false for at least one x in X." That is,

$$\neg[\forall x \in X, \, P(x)] \Leftrightarrow [\exists x \in X, \, \neg P(x)]. \tag{1}$$

Formula (1) is true even when X is an infinite set. We state this and its companion formula, without proof, in the following result. $\square$

THEOREM 1   **DE MORGAN'S LAWS IN LOGIC**

Let P be a predicate on a set X. Then

(a) $\neg[\forall x \in X, \, P(x)] \Leftrightarrow [\exists x \in X, \, \neg P(x)]$.
(b) $\neg[\exists x \in X, \, P(x)] \Leftrightarrow [\forall x \in X, \, \neg P(x)]$.

NOTATION 3   **UNIQUENESS QUANTIFIER** $\exists!$

"$P(x)$ is true for exactly one x in X" may be written as

$$\exists! x \in X, \, P(x).$$

This may also be read as "there is a unique x in X for which $P(x)$ is true" or as "there is one and only one x in X such that $P(x)$ is true."

Example 4   Let $N = \{0, 1, 2, \ldots\}$ and $\mathbf{Z}^+ = \{1, 2, \ldots\}$. Then

$$\exists! n \in N, \, n < 1$$

is the true assertion that "exactly one natural number n is less than 1." Also,

$$\exists! n \in N, \, n^2 = n$$

is false because $n^2 = n$ for both $n = 0$ and $n = 1$. However,

$$\exists! n \in \mathbf{Z}^+, \, n^2 = n$$

is true because the unique positive integer n with $n^2 = n$ is $n = 1$.   □

When P is a predicate on the cartesian product $S_1 \times S_2 \times \cdots \times S_n$ of n sets, up to n quantifiers can be applied to $P(s_1, s_2, \ldots, s_n)$. These quantifiers are to be read from left to right, as illustrated in the following notation.

NOTATION 4   **READING QUANTIFIERS FROM LEFT TO RIGHT**

Let P be a predicate on a cartesian product $S \times T$. Then

$$\exists s \in S, \, \forall t \in T, \, P(s, t)$$

may be read as "there exists an s in S for which $P(s, t)$ is true for all t in T. Also,

$$\forall t \in T, \, \exists s \in S, \, P(s, t) \tag{2}$$

may be read as "for each t in T there exists an s in S for which $P(s, t)$ is true. That is, the choice of s in Display (2) may vary with the choice of t.

Thus we suggest that "$\forall t \in T$" be read as "for all t in T" when it appears after "$\exists s \in S$" and that it be read as "for each t in T" when it appears first.

Example 5   Let $\mathbf{Z} = \{\ldots, -1, 0, 1, \ldots\}$. Then

$$\forall m \in \mathbf{Z}, \, \exists n \in \mathbf{Z}, \, m + n = 0$$

is the true assertion that every integer m has an inverse in $\mathbf{Z}$ under the operation of addition, and

$$\exists n \in \mathbf{Z}, \, \forall m \in \mathbf{Z}, \, m + n = 0$$

is the false assertion that there exists an integer n that is simultaneously the additive inverse of all integers m.   □

Example 5 shows that interchanging $\forall x \in X$ and $\exists y \in Y$ may change the meaning (and the truth value) of a quantified predicate. Our next example shows this pictorially.

Example 6   Let $X = \{\alpha, \beta, \gamma\}$ and $Y = \{d, e, f, g\}$. Let 1 denote "true" and 0 denote "false" and let $P(x, y)$ be the mapping from $X \times Y$ to $\{0, 1\}$ given by the matrix of Table 3.3.1. Then $\exists x \in X, \forall y \in Y, P(x, y) = 1$ is the false assertion that there exists a row having all entries equal to 1; but interchanging $\exists x \in X$ and $\forall y \in Y$ gives us the true assertion

$$\forall y \in Y, \exists x \in X, P(x, y) = 1$$

that each column has a 1 among its entries.   □

TABLE 3.3.1

P	d	e	f	g
α	1	1	0	0
β	0	0	1	0
γ	0	0	0	1

We saw in Examples 5 and 6 that $\exists s \in S, \forall t \in T, P(s, t)$ and $\forall t \in T, \exists s \in S, P(s, t)$ have different meanings. On the other hand, the order of appearance of the quantifications for the variables does not matter when the quantifiers are all $\forall$ or all $\exists$. For example,

$$[\forall s \in S, \forall t \in T, P(s, t)] \Leftrightarrow [\forall t \in T, \forall s \in S, P(s, t)].$$

In fact, each side of this equivalence is also equivalent to

$$\forall (s, t) \in S \times T, P(s, t).$$

It also is true that

$$[\exists s \in S, \exists t \in T, P(s, t)] \Leftrightarrow [\exists t \in T, \exists s \in S, P(s, t)]$$

and that each of these is equivalent to

$$\exists (s, t) \in S \times T, P(s, t).$$

However, order does matter in the use of both $\exists$ and $\exists!$, as we next show.

Example 7   Let $Z = \{\ldots, -1, 0, 1, \ldots\}$. Then

$$\exists m \in Z, \exists! n \in Z, mn = 0$$

is true because there exist integers m (the integer 1 will serve for this purpose) such that $mn = 0$ is true uniquely for $n = 0$. However,

$$\exists! n \in Z, \exists m \in Z, mn = 0$$

is false because now n is not unique. In fact, n can be any integer whatsoever and $\exists m \in Z, mn = 0$ is true because 0 has the property claimed for m.   □

PROBLEMS FOR SECTION 3.3

1. Let $X = \{1, 2, 3\}$. Rewrite $\forall x \in X$, $P(x)$ as a conjunction that uses no quantifiers. (See Example 3.)

2. Let $X = \{1, 2, 3, 4\}$. Rewrite $\exists x \in X$, $P(x)$ as a disjunction.

3. Let $X = \{1, 2, 3\}$. Rewrite $\neg[\forall x \in X, P(x)]$ as a disjunction.

4. Let $X = \{1, 2\}$. Rewrite $\neg[\exists x \in X, P(x)]$ as a conjunction. Negation signs are allowed but quantifiers are not.

5. Let $\mathbf{Z} = \{\ldots, -1, 0, 1, \ldots\}$. Which of the following are true?
   (a) $\exists m \in \mathbf{Z}$, $\forall n \in \mathbf{Z}$, $mn = 0$.   (b) $\forall n \in \mathbf{Z}$, $\exists m \in \mathbf{Z}$, $mn = 0$.
   (c) $\exists! m \in \mathbf{Z}$, $\forall n \in \mathbf{Z}$, $mn = 0$.   (d) $\forall n \in \mathbf{Z}$, $\exists! m \in \mathbf{Z}$, $mn = 0$.

6. Which of the following are true?
   (a) $\exists m \in \mathbf{Z}$, $\forall n \in \mathbf{Z}$, $mn = n$.   (b) $\forall n \in \mathbf{Z}$, $\exists m \in \mathbf{Z}$, $mn = n$.
   (c) $\forall n \in \mathbf{Z}$, $\exists! m \in \mathbf{Z}$, $mn = n$.   (d) $\exists! m \in \mathbf{Z}$, $\forall n \in \mathbf{Z}$, $mn = n$.

7. Let $X = \{0, 1\}$. Which of the following are equivalent to $\exists! x \in X$, $P(x)$?
   (i) $\{P(0) \wedge [\neg P(1)]\} \vee \{P(1) \wedge [\neg P(0)]\}$.
   (ii) $[P(0) \vee P(1)] \wedge \{\neg[P(0) \wedge P(1)]\}$.
   (iii) $P(0) \vee P(1)$.

8. Let $X = \{1, 2, 3\}$. Rewrite $\exists! x \in X$, $P(x)$ in a form analogous to that in Problem 7(i).

9. Let $S = \{a, b\}$ and $T = \{c, d, e\}$. Specify a mapping Q from $S \times T$ to $\{0, 1\}$ by a matrix table similar to the one in Example 6 such that both

   $$[\exists s \in S, \forall t \in T, Q(s, t) = 1]$$

   and

   $$[\forall t \in T, \exists s \in S, Q(s, t) = 1]$$

   are true.

10. Give an example in which both of the following are false:

    $$[\exists s \in S, \forall t \in T, Q(s, t) = 1],$$
    $$[\forall t \in T, \exists s \in S, Q(s, t) = 1].$$

11. Explain why the implication

    $$[\exists s \in S, \forall t \in T, P(s, t)] \Rightarrow [\forall t \in T, \exists s \in S, P(s, t)]$$

    is true for all sets S and T and all predicates P on $S \times T$.

12. Explain why the converse of the implication of Problem 11 is not true for all predicates P on cartesian products $S \times T$.

13. Let R denote a binary relation on a set S and let $S^3 = S \times S \times S$. Then

    $$[R \text{ is transitive}] \Leftrightarrow [\forall(x, y, z) \in S^3, (xRy) \wedge (yRz) \Rightarrow (xRz)]$$

can serve as a definition of transitivity. Give a similar definition of symmetry.

14. Give a definition of reflexivity similar to the definition of transitivity in Problem 13.

15. An operation $\square$ on a set S is commutative if

$$\forall (x, y) \in S \times S, \ x \square y = y \square x.$$

Translate the definition of associativity of $\square$ into similar notation.

16. Translate "$\square$ is distributive over $\triangle$," for commutative binary operations $\square$ and $\triangle$ on S, into notation similar to that of Problem 15.

17. Let A and B be sets. Then

$$(A = B) \Leftrightarrow [(x \in A) \Leftrightarrow (x \in B)].$$

(a) Give a similar equivalence for $A \subseteq B$.
(b) Check your answer for Part (a) in the special case of $A = \varnothing$.

18. Do as in Problem 17(a), but with $\subseteq$ replaced by $\subset$.

19. Let B_n be the set of n-digit binary strings and $B_{n,k}$ be the subset of strings of weight k in B_n. Let $Z^+ = \{1, 2, 3, \ldots\}$ and let $N = \{0, 1, \ldots\}$. Which of the following are true?
(a) $\forall n \in Z^+, \ \forall k \in N, \ [\alpha \in B_{n,k} \Rightarrow \alpha \in B_n]$.
(b) $\forall n \in Z^+, \ (\alpha \in B_n) \Rightarrow [(\alpha \in B_{n,k}) \text{ for some } k \in \{0, 1, \ldots, n\}]$.
(c) $\exists n \in Z^+, \ \{\alpha \in B_n \Rightarrow [(\alpha \in B_1) \vee (\alpha \in B_2)]\}$.
(d) $\exists! n \in Z^+, \ \{\alpha \in B_n \Rightarrow [(\alpha \in B_1) \vee (\alpha \in B_2)]\}$.

20. Let $\alpha\beta$ denote the concatenation (or juxtaposition) of binary strings α and β. Which of the following are true?
(a) $\forall m \in Z^+, \ \forall n \in Z^+, \ [(\alpha \in B_m) \wedge (\beta \in B_n)] \Rightarrow (\alpha\beta \in B_{m+n})$.
(b) $\forall m \in Z^+, \ \forall h \in N, \ \forall n \in Z^+, \ \forall k \in N,$
$[(\alpha \in B_{m,h}) \wedge (\beta \in B_{n,k})] \Rightarrow (\alpha\beta \in B_{m+n,h+k})$.
(c) $\exists n \in Z^+, \ \{(\alpha \in B_n) \Rightarrow [(\alpha \in B_{n,0}) \vee (\alpha \in B_{n,1})]\}$.
(d) $\exists m \in Z^+, \ \forall n \in Z^+, \ (\alpha \in B_m) \wedge (\beta \in B_n) \Rightarrow \text{wgt}(\alpha\beta) \in \{n, n+1, n+2\}$.
(e) $\exists! m \in Z^+, \ \forall n \in Z^+, \ (\alpha \in B_m) \wedge (\beta \in B_n) \Rightarrow \alpha\beta \in \{B_{n+1}, B_{n+2}\}$.

21. Give an example of a universe X and predicates P and Q such that

$$[\forall x \in X, \ P(x)] \Rightarrow [\forall x \in X, \ Q(x)]$$

is true and

$$\forall x \in X, \ [P(x) \Rightarrow Q(x)]$$

is false.

22. Do the following for $X = \{1, 2\}$.
(a) For all predicates P and Q on X, explain why the following implication is true:

$$[\exists x \in X, \ P(x) \wedge Q(x)] \Rightarrow \{[\exists x \in X, \ P(x)] \wedge [\exists x \in X, \ Q(x)]\}.$$

(b) Give an example of predicates P and Q on X for which the converse of the implication in Part (a) is false.

23. Is the implication in Problem 22(a) true for all sets X and all predicates P and Q on X? Explain.

SUMMARY OF TERMS, CHAPTER 3 _____

REVIEW PROBLEMS FOR CHAPTER 3

1. State the premise of each of the following implications and label the premise as true or as false:
   (a) If $3^2 + 4^2 = 5^2$, then $3 + 4 = 5$.
   (b) If $(-2)^3 = 2^3$, then $-2 = 2$.
   (c) If $-6 = 6$, then $(-6)^4 = 6^4$.
   (d) If $3 \mid 72$, then $3 \mid 9$.

2. For each of the implications of Problem 1, state the conclusion and label it as true or as false.

3. Label each of the implications of Problem 1 as reversible (that is, true with a true converse), true but not reversible, false with a true converse, or false with a false converse.

4. State the contrapositive of each implication of Problem 1.

5. If p and q are true propositions, is $(\neg p) \vee (\neg q)$ true or false? Explain.

6. If p and q are false propositions, is $(p \vee q) \wedge [(\neg p) \vee (\neg q)]$ true or false? Explain.

7. Is the implication $[(a \wedge b) \wedge (a \Rightarrow c)] \Rightarrow (b \wedge c)$ true for all propositions a, b, and c? Explain.

8. Is the implication $[(a \vee b) \wedge (a \Rightarrow c)] \Rightarrow (b \vee c)$ true for all a, b, and c? Explain.

9. Use a truth table to show that $[\neg(\neg p)] \Leftrightarrow p$ is true for all propositions p.

10. Find assertions p, q, and r such that $p \wedge (q \vee r) \Leftrightarrow (p \wedge q) \vee r$ is false. [*Hint:* First find x, y, z in $\{0, 1\}$ such that $x \wedge (y \vee z) \neq (x \wedge y) \vee z$ in the doubleton boolean algebra.]

11. Let P and Q be the predicates on the set $\mathbf{Z}$ of integers with $P(n) =$ "$(n - 1)(n - 2)(n - 3) = 0$" and $Q(n) =$ "$(n - 1)(n + 1) = (n - 1)(n + 2)$." Find the following truth sets.
(a) $T(P)$;   (b) $T(Q)$;   (c) $T(P \Rightarrow Q)$;   (d) $T(Q \Rightarrow P)$.

12. For a subset A of $\mathbf{Z}$, let $\bar{A}$ denote the relative complement $\mathbf{Z} - A$ of A in $\mathbf{Z}$. Using the P and Q of Review Problem 11, find:
(a) $T(\neg P)$;   (b) $\overline{T(P)}$;   (c) $T(\neg P) \cup T(Q)$;   (d) $\overline{T(Q)}$;
(e) $\overline{T(Q)} \cup T(P)$.

13. (a) Find all integers satisfying the equation $\sqrt{4x + 5} = \sqrt{x - 2} + 4$.
(b) Does the rational number $\frac{19}{9}$ satisfy the equation?

14. Find all rational numbers x satisfying $\sqrt{5x - 19} = 17 - \sqrt{3x + 4}$.

15. Is the implication $[\forall x \in X, P(x)] \Rightarrow [\exists x \in X, P(x)]$ true for all predicates P on a nonempty set $X = \{x_1, x_2, \ldots\}$? Explain.

16. Give an example of a set X and a predicate P on X for which the converse of the implication in Problem 15 is false.

17. Let $f(x, y, z) = [(x \Rightarrow z) \wedge (y \Rightarrow z)] \Rightarrow [(x \vee y) \Rightarrow z]$. Is $f(x, y, z)$ a tautology? Explain.

18. Let $g(x, y, z) = [(x \wedge y) \Rightarrow z] \Rightarrow [(x \Rightarrow z) \wedge (y \Rightarrow z)]$. Is $g(x, y, z)$ a tautology? Explain.

19. Give an example of predicates P and Q on a set X such that
$$\{\forall x \in X, [P(x) \vee Q(x)]\} \Rightarrow \{[\forall x \in X, P(x)] \vee [\forall x \in X, Q(x)]\} \text{ is false.}$$

20. Is the converse of the implication of Problem 19 true for all predicates P and Q on a set X?

SUPPLEMENTARY AND CHALLENGING PROBLEMS, CHAPTER 3 _____

1. Suppose A, B, and C are identical triplets. When asked a "yes or no" question, A and B always answer truthfully and C always lies. Devise a "yes or no" question such that the answer by any x in $\{A, B, C\}$ will enable you to tell whether x is A.

2. Show that $(\bar{x} \Rightarrow x) \Leftrightarrow x$ is a tautology, and use this tautology to describe a method of proof.

3. Is $(x \Rightarrow \bar{x}) \Leftrightarrow \bar{x}$ a tautology?

4. Let $P(n)$, $Q(n)$, and $R(n)$ be the predicates "$n^2 - 4n = 0$," "$n(2n - 1) = n(n + 3)$," and "$2n - 1 = n + 3$," respectively, on the set $\mathbf{Z}$ of integers.
(a) Are the truth sets $T(P)$ and $T(Q)$ equal?
(b) Explain why $T(R)$ is a proper subset of $T(Q)$.

5.   Which of the following equivalences are true for all predicates P on the cartesian product $N \times N \times N$?

(a) $[\forall x \in N, \forall y \in N, \exists z \in N, P(x, y, z)] \Leftrightarrow$
$[\forall y \in N, \forall x \in N, \exists z \in N, P(x, y, z)]$.

(b) $[\forall x \in N, \exists y \in N, \forall z \in N, P(x, y, z)] \Leftrightarrow$
$[\forall z \in N, \exists y \in N, \forall x \in N, P(x, y, z)]$.

6.   For assertions p and q, let $p \downarrow q$ have the same meaning as $\bar{p} \wedge \bar{q}$. (The symbol $\downarrow$ is called the Peirce arrow or "nor" operator.) Prove that each of the following is a tautology:

(a) $\bar{x} \Leftrightarrow x \downarrow x$;   (b) $x \wedge y \Leftrightarrow [(x \downarrow x) \downarrow (y \downarrow y)]$;

(c) $x \vee y \Leftrightarrow [(x \downarrow x) \downarrow (x \downarrow x)] \downarrow [(y \downarrow y) \downarrow (y \downarrow y)]$.

4

INDUCTION

In this chapter, we introduce a method for defining certain sequences and a technique of proof closely associated with well-ordered sets of integers such as $N = \{0, 1, 2, \ldots\}$ and $Z^+ = \{1, 2, 3, \ldots\}$.

4.1

INDUCTIVE DEFINITION

A sequence $a_1, a_2, a_3, \ldots$ with terms a_i in a set A is essentially the mapping

$$\sigma: Z^+ \to A, \quad n \mapsto a_n$$

from Z^+ to A with $\sigma(n) = a_n$. If the terms of a sequence are written as $a_0, a_1, a_2, \ldots$ with the a_i in A, the sequence may be thought of as a mapping from N to A.

Some sequences are defined directly with a formula for the nth term. Other sequences are **defined inductively** by a two-step procedure that is described in the following algorithm.

ALGORITHM 1   **INDUCTIVELY DEFINED SEQUENCE**

Basis   Give the first term (or the first few terms) explicitly.

Inductive Part   Tell how to obtain any later term from earlier terms.

Now we use this inductive method to define a sequence that occurs frequently in mathematics and its applications.

DEFINITION 1 **FACTORIALS**

For all n in $N = \{0, 1, \ldots\}$, $n!$ is defined by the following two steps:

Basis $0! = 1$.

Inductive Part $(k + 1)! = k!(k + 1)$ for $k \in N$.

(One reads $n!$ as "n factorial.")

Using this definition, one sees that

$1! = (0 + 1)! = 0! \cdot 1 = 1 \cdot 1 = 1,$
$2! = (1 + 1)! = 1! \cdot 2 = 1 \cdot 2 = 2,$
$3! = (2 + 1)! = 2! \cdot 3 = 2 \cdot 3 = 6,$
$4! = (3 + 1)! = 3! \cdot 4 = 6 \cdot 4 = 24,$

and similarly that

$5! = 120,$
$6! = 720,$
$7! = 5040,$
$8! = 40,320,$

and so on. If one had to calculate 200!, one would appreciate the help of a computer. However, it would be rash to program a computer to calculate and print 1,000,000! unless one were prepared for a printout of 5,565,709 digits!

Example 1 The sequence of standard listings $\{0, 1\}$, $\{00, 01, 10, 11\}$, $\{000, 001, 010, 011, 100, 101, 110, 111\}, \ldots$ for the sets B_n of n-digit binary strings was defined inductively in Algorithm 1 of Section 1.1. Formally, the two steps of that definition are:

Basis The standard listing for B_1 is $\{0, 1\}$.

Inductive Part Given the standard listing

$$B_k = \{\alpha_1, \alpha_2, \ldots, \alpha_m\},$$

then the standard listing for B_{k+1} is

$$\{0\alpha_1, 0\alpha_2, \ldots, 0\alpha_m, 1\alpha_1, 1\alpha_2, \ldots, 1\alpha_m\}. \qquad \square$$

A shorthand notation for the sum $a_r + a_{r+1} + \cdots + a_s$ is

$$\sum_{j=r}^{s} a_j.$$

In this notation, the Greek capital letter sigma, $\sum$, is the **summation sign**, j is the **index** of summation, r is the **initial value** of the index, and s is the **final value** of the index. For example,

$$\sum_{i=1}^{3} a_i = a_1 + a_2 + a_3 \qquad \text{and} \qquad \sum_{j=5}^{8} b_j = b_5 + b_6 + b_7 + b_8.$$

The following is an inductive definition of the sigma notation.

DEFINITION 2   **SUMMATION NOTATION**

Let r be any integer and s be an integer of the set $\{r, r + 1, r + 2, \ldots\}$. Then

$$\sum_{j=r}^{s} a_j$$

is defined by the following two statements:

Basis $\quad \sum_{j=r}^{r} a_j = a_r.$

Inductive Part $\quad \sum_{j=r}^{k+1} a_j = \left(\sum_{j=r}^{k} a_j \right) + a_{k+1} \quad \text{for } k \in \{r, r + 1, \ldots\}.$

Example 2   Problem 19 of Section 1.1 involves the formula

$$1 + 2 + 3 + \cdots + 99 = \binom{100}{2}.$$

In the sigma notation, this becomes

$$\sum_{j=1}^{99} j = \binom{100}{2}.$$

Similarly,

$$\binom{2}{2} + \binom{3}{2} + \binom{4}{2} + \cdots + \binom{n}{2} = \binom{n+1}{3}$$

becomes

$$\sum_{j=2}^{n} \binom{j}{2} = \binom{n+1}{3}. \qquad \qquad \square$$

Now we give the analogue for products of the sigma notation for sums. (See Problems 13 and 14 below for inductive definitions.)

NOTATION 1 **PRODUCT SIGN PI, Π**

$$\prod_{j=r}^{s} a_j = a_r a_{r+1} \cdots a_s.$$

The sequence 0, 1, 1, 2, 3, 5, 8, 13, 21, ... of Fibonacci Numbers arises in many contexts. We next define inductively this sequence and its companion sequence 2, 1, 3, 4, 7, 11, 18, ... of Lucas Numbers.

DEFINITION 3 **FIBONACCI NUMBERS AND LUCAS NUMBERS**

For n in $N = \{0, 1, 2, \ldots\}$, the Fibonacci Numbers F_n and Lucas Numbers L_n are determined as follows:

Basis $F_0 = 0$ and $F_1 = 1$; $L_0 = 2$ and $L_1 = 1$.

Inductive Part $F_{k+2} = F_{k+1} + F_k$ and $L_{k+2} = L_{k+1} + L_k$, both for k in N.

Next we inductively define arithmetic and geometric sequences.

DEFINITION 4 **ARITHMETIC PROGRESSION**

A sequence $a_1, a_2, a_3, \ldots$ is an infinite **arithmetic progression** with **initial term** a_1 and **common difference** d if $a_{n+1} = a_n + d$ for all n in $Z^+ = \{1, 2, \ldots\}$. The first n terms $a_1, a_2, \ldots, a_n$ of such a sequence form a finite arithmetic progression.

For example, the arithmetic progression with initial term 2 and common difference 3 is 2, 5, 8, 11, 14, ... ; also, the arithmetic progression with initial term 9 and common difference -4 is 9, 5, 1, -3, -7, -11, ...

DEFINITION 5 **GEOMETRIC PROGRESSION**

A sequence $b_1, b_2, b_3, \ldots$ is an infinite **geometric progression** with **initial term** b_1 and **common ratio** r if $b_{n+1} = r b_n$ for all n in Z^+. The first n terms $b_1, b_2, \ldots, b_n$ of such a sequence form a finite geometric progression.

For example, the geometric progression with initial term 3 and common ratio 2 is 3, 6, 12, 24, ... , and the geometric progression with initial term 1 and common ratio $-\frac{1}{2}$ is 1, $-\frac{1}{2}$, $\frac{1}{4}$, $-\frac{1}{8}$, $\frac{1}{16}$, $-\frac{1}{32}$, ...

Next we illustrate techniques for summing the first n terms of an arithmetic progression and for summing the first n terms of a geometric progression.

Example 3 Let $S = 2 + 5 + 8 + \cdots + 101$ be the sum of a certain number of beginning terms of the arithmetic progression with 2 as the initial term and 3 as the common difference. This is the sequence $a_1, a_2, \ldots$ with $a_1 = 2$, $a_2 = 2 + 3$, $a_3 = 2 + 3 \cdot 2$, $a_4 = 2 + 3 \cdot 3$, $a_5 = 2 + 3 \cdot 4$, and in general

$$a_n = 2 + 3(n - 1) = 3n - 1.$$

Letting $101 = 3n - 1$ and solving for n, we find that $n = (101 + 1)/3 = 34$; hence there are 34 terms in the sum S. Now we write S frontwards and backwards as

$$S = 2 + 5 + 8 + \cdots + 95 + 98 + 101,$$
$$S = 101 + 98 + 95 + \cdots + 8 + 5 + 2.$$

Adding these lines gives us

$$2S = 103 + 103 + 103 + \cdots + 103 + 103 + 103.$$

There are 34 terms in the sum S; so $2S = 34 \cdot 103$ and $S = 17 \cdot 103 = 1751$.
        □

Example 4 Let T_n be the sum of the first n terms of the geometric progression $3, 15, 75, \ldots$. For example,

$$T_5 = 3 + 3 \cdot 5 + 3 \cdot 5^2 + 3 \cdot 5^3 + 3 \cdot 5^4.$$

We find a compact formula for T_n as follows:

$$T_n = 3 + 3 \cdot 5 + 3 \cdot 5^2 + \cdots + 3 \cdot 5^{n-1}$$
$$5T_n = \phantom{3 + {}} 3 \cdot 5 + 3 \cdot 5^2 + \cdots + 3 \cdot 5^{n-1} + 3 \cdot 5^n$$

Subtracting, we see that $5T_n - T_n = 3 \cdot 5^n - 3$, and so $T_n = 3(5^n - 1)/4$.
        □

Example 5 Here we find a simple expression for the sum

$$S = 1 + 2x + 3x^2 + \cdots + nx^{n-1}.$$

The formula we obtain can be applied to problems on searching in binary tree files; for examples, see Problems 21 and 22 of Section 6.2 and Problems 15 and 16 of Section 6.3.

We write S, xS, and their difference in the format

$$S = 1 + 2x + 3x^2 + \cdots + nx^{n-1}$$
$$xS = \phantom{1 + {}} x + 2x^2 + \cdots + (n-1)x^{n-1} + nx^n$$
$$\overline{(1 - x)S = 1 + x + x^2 + \cdots + x^{n-1} - nx^n}$$

We use this method once more, as follows:

$$
\begin{array}{rl}
(1-x)S = & 1 + x + x^2 + \cdots + \quad x^{n-1} - nx^n \\
x(1-x)S = & x + x^2 + \cdots + \quad x^{n-1} + x^n - nx^{n+1} \\
\hline
(1-x)^2 S = & 1 - (n+1)x^n + nx^{n+1}
\end{array}
$$

$$
S = \frac{1 - (n+1)x^n + nx^{n+1}}{(1-x)^2} \qquad \square
$$

An expression such as $x \vee (\bar{y} \wedge z)$ becomes the rule for a boolean operation f if we write $f(x, y, z) = x \vee (\bar{y} \wedge z)$; it becomes the rule for a boolean function f if we drop the commas and write $f(xyz) = x \vee (\bar{y} \wedge z)$. Such an expression is called a "boolean expression." We next define this term inductively.

DEFINITION 6   **BOOLEAN EXPRESSION**

(1) Basis   Each of $x_1, x_2, \ldots, x_n$ is an n-ary boolean expression.

(2) Inductive Part   If p is an n-ary boolean expression, then so is $\bar{p}$. If p and q are n-ary boolean expressions, then so are $p \wedge q$ and $p \vee q$.

(3) Limiting Part   An expression is a ***boolean expression*** if and only if it can be formed using the basis (1) together with a finite number of applications of the procedures of (2).

Giuseppe Peano   *was born in 1858 in Spinetta, Italy, but lived in Turin from the age of 12. He attended schools in Turin, was made professor at the military academy there, and was elected a member of the Academy of Science, Turin. Peano's name is remembered in mathematics for his famous space-filling curve and for his axioms characterizing the positive integers. The technique of "proof by mathematical induction" is based on these axioms. In later years he became involved in the development of Interlingua, an international language combining Latin, German, French, and English. (It never caught on.) Peano's significant contributions remain those in mathematics. He died in 1932.*

PROBLEMS FOR SECTION 4.1

1. Given that $7! = 5040$, find:
   (i) $8!$;   (ii) $9!$;   (iii) $10!$.

2. Given that $11! = 39,916,800$, find:
   (i) $12!$;   (ii) $13!$.

3. Find:
    (i) $3! + 1$;   (ii) $(3 + 1)!$;   (iii) $(2!)(3!)$;   (iv) $(2 \cdot 3)!$.

4. (a) Does $(n + 1)! = n! + 1!$ for all n in N? Explain.
    (b) Does $(m!)(n!) = (mn)!$ for all m and n in N? Explain.

5. (a) Find the a in N such that $a! = 24$.
    (b) Find the b in N such that $3! \cdot 4 \cdot 5 = b!$.
    (c) Find two ordered pairs (c, d) in $N \times N$ such that $9 \cdot 10 \cdot 11 \cdot 12 = c!/d!$.
    (d) Show that $(n + 1)! - n! = n!n$.
    (e) Does $(n - 2)!(n^2 - n) = n!$ for $n = 2, 3, \ldots$? Explain.

6. (a) Find the a in N such that $a! = 120$.
    (b) Find the b in N such that $4! \cdot 210 = b!$
    (c) Find two ordered pairs (c, d) in $N \times N$ such that $c!/d! = 7980$.
    (d) Show that $(n + 2)! = n!(n^2 + 3n + 2)$.
    (e) Show that $n! + (n + 1)! + (n + 2)! = n!(n + 2)^2$.

7. Use a common denominator to write each of the following as a single fraction:

    (a) $\dfrac{1}{3!} + \dfrac{1}{4!}$;   (b) $\dfrac{1}{4!} - \dfrac{29}{6!}$;   (c) $\dfrac{1}{2!4!} + \dfrac{1}{3!3!}$.

8. Use a common denominator to write each of the following as a single fraction:

    (a) $\dfrac{1}{r!} + \dfrac{1}{(r + 1)!}$;   (b) $\dfrac{1}{h!(k + 1)!} + \dfrac{1}{(h + 1)!k!}$.

9. As in Definition 3 of Section 1.1 ("Binomial Coefficient"), let $\binom{n}{r} = \# B_{n,r}$.
    (a) The formula

    $$\binom{n}{2} = \sum_{j=1}^{n-1} j,$$

    motivated by Example 2, tells us that $\binom{2}{2} = 1$, $\binom{3}{2} = 1 + 2 = 3$, $\binom{4}{2} = 1 + 2 + 3 = 6$. Find $\binom{5}{2}$ and $\binom{6}{2}$.
    (b) The formula

    $$\binom{n + 1}{3} = \sum_{j=2}^{n} \binom{j}{2}$$

    of Example 2 tells us that $\binom{3}{3} = \binom{2}{2} = 1$, $\binom{4}{3} = \binom{2}{2} + \binom{3}{2} = 1 + 3 = 4$, and $\binom{5}{3} = \binom{2}{2} + \binom{3}{2} + \binom{4}{2} = 1 + 3 + 6 = 10$. Find $\binom{6}{3}$ and $\binom{7}{3}$.
    (c) Find the a in N such that $\binom{5}{2} \cdot 2! \cdot 3! = a!$.
    (d) Find the b in N such that

    $$\frac{6!}{2!4!} + \frac{6!}{3!3!} = \frac{b!}{3!4!}.$$

10. (a) Find an a in N such that $\binom{6}{3}(3!)(3!) = a!$.

(b) For all r and n in N with $0 \leq r < n$, prove that

$$\frac{n!}{r!(n-r)!} + \frac{n!}{(r+1)!(n-r-1)!} = \frac{(n+1)!}{(r+1)!(n-r)!}.$$

(This result is needed in Problem 10 of Section 4.2.)

11. The sequence $x^1, x^2, x^3, \ldots$ of positive integral powers of x in a semigroup $(X, \circ)$ was defined inductively in Definition 3 ("Powers") of Section 2.2.
(i) Give the basis part of this definition.
(ii) Give the inductive part of this definition.

12. If we assume the standard listings $\boldsymbol{B_{n,0}} = \{00 \ldots 0\}$ and $\boldsymbol{B_{n,n}} = \{11 \ldots 1\}$ to be known, then the standard listings for the sets

$$\boldsymbol{B_{n,1}}, \boldsymbol{B_{n,2}}, \ldots, \boldsymbol{B_{n,n-1}}$$

are defined inductively in Algorithm 2 of Section 1.1. The basis is that $\{01, 10\}$ is the standard listing for $\boldsymbol{B_{2,1}}$. What is the inductive part of this definition?

13. A shorthand notation for the product $a_1 a_2 \cdots a_n$ of n terms, which uses the product sign Π introduced in Notation 1, is

$$\prod_{j=1}^{n} a_j.$$

Define this notation inductively.

14. For integers r and s with $r \leq s$, let

$$\prod_{j=r}^{s} a_j = a_r a_{r+1} \cdots a_s.$$

Define this notation inductively.

15. In the sequence $0, 1, \frac{1}{2}, \frac{3}{4}, \frac{5}{8}, \ldots$, each term (after the first two) is the average of the two preceding terms. Define this sequence $a_1, a_2, \ldots$ inductively.

16. Define a sequence $P_0, P_1, P_2, \ldots$ inductively so that its first ten terms are $0, 1, 2, 5, 12, 29, 70, 169, 408, 985$.

17. Is the following equation true?

$$\sum_{j=1}^{5} \binom{1+j}{2} = \binom{7}{3}.$$

18. Find n such that

$$\sum_{j=3}^{6} \binom{j}{3} = \binom{n}{4}.$$

19. (i) Let $\#X = m$, $\#Y = n$, and $m \leq n$. Show that the number of injective mappings from X to Y is $n!/(n - m)!$

(ii) If $\#X = n = \#Y$, how many injections are there from X to Y?

(iii) If $\#X = n = \#Y$, how many bijections are there from X to Y?

20. Let $\#X = n$.

(i) How many injections are there from X to itself? Write the answer as a factorial.

(ii) How many permutations are there on X? (A permutation on X is a bijection from X to itself.)

21. (a) Find the Fibonacci Number F_{12}.

(b) Make a conjecture concerning the values of n for which the Fibonacci Number F_n is an even integer. (In the next section, we will be able to prove such conjectures.)

(c) Make a conjecture concerning the values of n for which F_n is an integral multiple of 3.

22. Do the analogue of Problem 21 for the Lucas Numbers L_n.

23. Find the terms a_2, a_3, and a_4 for the arithmetic progression $a_1, a_2, \ldots$ with $a_1 = -11$ and common difference 7.

24. Find the terms b_2, b_3, and b_4 for the arithmetic progression $b_1, b_2, \ldots$ with $b_1 = 8$ and common difference -3.

25. Find the next three terms of the arithmetic progression $-3, -7, -11, -15, \ldots$.

26. Find the next three terms of the arithmetic progression $\frac{7}{4}, 1, \frac{1}{4}, -\frac{1}{2}, -\frac{5}{4}, \ldots$.

27. Find the terms b_2, b_3, and b_4 for the geometric progression $b_1, b_2, \ldots$ with $b_1 = 2$ and common ratio 3.

28. Find the terms a_2, a_3, and a_4 for the geometric progression $a_1, a_2, \ldots$ with $a_1 = 5$ and common ratio -1.

29. Find the next three terms of the geometric progression $2, 14, 98, \ldots$.

30. Find the next three terms of the geometric progression $6, -2, \frac{2}{3}, -\frac{2}{9}, \ldots$.

31. Find x and y such that 29, x, y, 5 are four consecutive terms of an arithmetic progression.

32. Find both values of x for which 7, x, 252 are three consecutive terms of a geometric progression.

33. Let $a_1, a_2, \ldots$ be the arithmetic progression $5, 9, 13, 17, \ldots$. Find:

(i) the common difference d;   (ii) the term a_{100};

(iii) the sum $a_1 + a_2 + \cdots + a_{100}$ of the first 100 terms. Use the technique illustrated in Example 3.

34. Do as in Problem 33 for the arithmetic progression $4, 13, 22, 31, \ldots$.

35. Let $b_1, b_2, \ldots$ be the geometric progression $1, \frac{1}{3}, \frac{1}{9}, \frac{1}{27}, \ldots$. Find:
(i) the common ratio r; (ii) the term b_{99};
(iii) the sum $b_1 + b_2 + \cdots + b_{99}$ of the first 99 terms. Use the technique of Example 4.

36. Do as in Problem 35 for the geometric progression $3, \frac{3}{2}, \frac{3}{4}, \ldots$.

37. Use the techniques of Examples 3 and 4 to find simple formulas for:
(a) $a + (a + d) + (a + 2d) + \cdots + (a + nd)$.
(b) $a + ax + ax^2 + \cdots + ax^n$.

38. Find simple formulas for:
(a) $a + [a + d] + [a + 2d] + \cdots + [a + (n - 1)d]$.
(b) $a + ax + ax^2 + \cdots + ax^{n-1}$.

39. Let $S_n = 2 + 2^2 + 2^3 + \cdots + 2^n$.
(i) Show that $S_n = 2^{n+1} - 2$. (ii) Tabulate S_n for $n = 1, 2, 3, 4$.
(iii) Find the smallest n such that $S_n \geq 36$.

40. Find the smallest n such that $\#(B_1 \cup B_2 \cup \cdots \cup B_n) \geq 36$.

41. (i) Use the technique of Example 5 to find a simple formula for

$$S_h = 1 + 2 \cdot 2 + 3 \cdot 2^2 + 4 \cdot 2^3 + \cdots + h \cdot 2^{h-1}.$$

(ii) Check by substituting 2 for x in the formulas of Example 5.

42. Find a simple formula for $T_h = 1 + 2 \cdot 3 + 3 \cdot 3^2 + \cdots + h \cdot 3^{h-1}$.

*43. Differentiate the formula

$$a + ax + ax^2 + \cdots + ax^n = a\frac{1 - x^{n+1}}{1 - x}$$

of Problem 37(b) and thus show that

$$a + 2ax + 3ax^2 + \cdots + nax^{n-1} = a\frac{1 - (n + 1)x^n + nx^{n+1}}{(1 - x)^2}.$$

4.2

PROOF BY MATHEMATICAL INDUCTION

We recall from Section 3.1 that a **proposition** (or **assertion**) is a statement that is either true or false (but not both) and that a **predicate** on a set X is a mapping from X into a set of assertions.

Example 1 Let $F_0, F_1, F_2, \ldots$ be the sequence of Fibonacci Numbers

$$0, 1, 1, 2, 3, 5, 8, 13, 21, 34, 55, 89, \ldots$$

and let P be the predicate on $N = \{0, 1, 2, \ldots\}$ for which $P(n)$ is the assertion that "F_{3n} is even, whereas F_{3n+1} and F_{3n+2} are odd." ☐

If X is a set of the form $\{a, a + 1, a + 2, \ldots\}$, with a an integer, there are many predicates P on X for which one can prove that $P(n)$ is true for all n in X using the following technique.

ALGORITHM 1   **PROOF BY MATHEMATICAL INDUCTION**

Let P be a predicate on $X = \{a, a + 1, a + 2, \ldots\}$. The following two steps constitute a proof by ***mathematical induction on n*** that $P(n)$ is true for all n in X:

Basis   Show that $P(a)$ is true.

Inductive Step   Show that whenever k is an element of X for which $P(k)$ is true, the assertion $P(k + 1)$ is also true.

The implication $x \Rightarrow y$ is the assertion that "if x is true, then y is also true." This implication says nothing about y when x is false. It is conventional in logic that an implication $x \Rightarrow y$ is automatically true when x is false.

The task of the inductive step can be stated as "For all k in X, show that $P(k)$ implies $P(k + 1)$." Using the "implication" arrow $\Rightarrow$, the "and" sign $\wedge$, and the "for all" sign $\forall$, this task can be restated as "Prove that

$$[P(a) \Rightarrow P(a + 1)] \wedge [P(a + 1) \Rightarrow P(a + 2)] \wedge [P(a + 2) \Rightarrow P(a + 3)] \wedge \cdots$$

is true" or as "Prove that $[\forall k \in X, P(k) \Rightarrow P(k + 1)]$ is true." When working on this task, one assumes that k is an integer for which $P(k)$ is true and uses this to show that $P(k + 1)$ is true. In a proof by mathematical induction, the assumption that $P(k)$ is true is called the ***inductive hypothesis***.

The following imaginary situation may help to indicate why Algorithm 1 is a valid technique of proof.

Let an infinite sequence of dominoes be stood on end as in Figure 4.2.1. If one pushes the top of the left-most domino towards its neighbor and if each domino is close enough to its right-hand neighbor, then it seems reasonable to assume that each domino (no matter how far to the right it is located) ultimately will topple. The impetus to the first domino represents $P(1)$, and the effect of the kth domino on the $(k + 1)$th domino represents the fact that $P(k + 1)$ is true whenever $P(k)$ is true. The toppling of all the dominoes represents the conclusion that $P(n)$ is true for all n in X.

In Section 4.3, the well ordering of sets $\{a, a + 1, a + 2, \ldots\}$ under the "less than" relation will be used to justify Algorithm 1 of the present section.

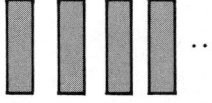

FIGURE 4.2.1

We assume here that proof by mathematical induction is valid and illustrate its use.

Example 2   At one time, 3¢ and 5¢ stamps were in common use. Let $P(n)$ be the assertion that n¢ worth of postage can be made up using only 3¢ and 5¢ stamps. We prove by mathematical induction that $P(n)$ is true for all n in $X = \{8, 9, \ldots\}$.

Basis $P(8)$ is true because $8 = 3 + 5$.

Inductive Step   Let k be an integer in X for which $P(k)$ is true; that is, let us assume that $k \geq 8$ and that k¢ worth of postage can be assembled using only 3¢ and 5¢ stamps. We consider two cases:

A. If the collection of k¢ worth of postage includes a 5¢ stamp, we can replace it with two 3¢ stamps and thus achieve $(k + 1)$¢ worth of postage.

B. If the collection of k¢ worth of postage does not include a 5¢ stamp, then there must be at least three 3¢ stamps in it because $k \geq 8$. Replacing the three 3¢ stamps with two 5¢ stamps, we achieve $(k + 1)$¢ worth of postage.

These two cases show that $[\forall k \in X,\ P(k) \Rightarrow P(k + 1)]$ is true, and our proof is complete.   □

Example 3   Let $f(n) = n^2 - 7n + 12$ and let $P(n)$ be the assertion that "$f(n) > 0$." We use mathematical induction to prove $P(n)$ true for all n in $X = \{5, 6, 7, \ldots\}$.

Basis   When $n = 5$, then $f(n) = f(5) = 5^2 - 7 \cdot 5 + 12 = 2 > 0$; hence $P(5)$ is true.

Inductive Step   Let k be an integer in X for which $P(k)$ is true; that is, let $f(k) = k^2 - 7k + 12 > 0$. Then

$$f(k + 1) - f(k) = [(k + 1)^2 - 7(k + 1) + 12] - [k^2 - 7k + 12]$$
$$= [k^2 + 2k + 1 - 7k - 7 + 12] - [k^2 - 7k + 12]$$
$$= 2k - 6 = 2(k - 3) > 0,$$

since $k \geq 5$. It follows from $f(k + 1) - f(k) > 0$ and the inductive hypothesis $f(k) > 0$ that the sum

$$f(k + 1) = [f(k + 1) - f(k)] + f(k)$$

of two positive numbers is positive. Thus we have shown that if k is an integer in X for which $P(k)$ is true, then $P(k + 1)$ is also true. That is, we have shown that

$$\forall k \in X,\ P(k) \Rightarrow P(k + 1)$$

is true. This completes the inductive step and the proof.   □

Next we prove the assertion in Example 1 concerning the Fibonacci Numbers.

THEOREM 1 **EVEN FIBONACCI NUMBERS**

For all n in $N = \{0, 1, \ldots\}$, F_{3n} is even, whereas F_{3n+1} and F_{3n+2} are odd.

PROOF   We use mathematical induction. Let $P(n)$ be the assertion of this theorem.

Basis   When $n = 0$, $F_{3n} = F_0 = 0$ is even and $F_{3n+1} = F_1 = 1$ is odd, as is $F_{3n+2} = F_2 = 1$. Thus $P(0)$ is true.

Inductive Step   Assume that k is an integer in N for which $P(k)$ is true; that is, assume that F_{3k} is even and that F_{3k+1} and F_{3k+2} are odd. Then

$$F_{3(k+1)} = F_{3k+3} = F_{3k+1} + F_{3k+2} \tag{1}$$

by the recursion relation defining the Fibonacci Numbers. (See Definition 3 of Section 4.1.) Using the inductive hypothesis that F_{3k+1} and F_{3k+2} are odd, Display (1) shows that $F_{3(k+1)}$ is the sum of two odd integers and hence is even. Then

$$F_{3(k+1)+1} = F_{3k+4} = F_{3k+2} + F_{3k+3}$$

is the sum of an odd integer and an even integer and thus is odd. Similarly,

$$F_{3(k+1)+2} = F_{3k+5} = F_{3k+3} + F_{3k+4}$$

is odd. Since $P(k + 1)$ is the assertion that $F_{3(k+1)}$ is even and that $F_{3(k+1)+1}$ and $F_{3(k+1)+2}$ are odd, we have shown that if $P(k)$ is true, then $P(k + 1)$ is also true. That is, $[\forall k \in N, P(k) \Rightarrow P(k + 1)]$ is true. This completes the inductive step, and the theorem is proved.   □

Example 4   Let $S_n = 1 \cdot 1! + 2 \cdot 2! + \cdots + n \cdot n!$ We seek a simple formula for S_n. We let $a_n = n \cdot n!$ and note that $S_{n+1} = S_n + a_{n+1}$. We use this to construct the table below.

n	1	2	3	4	5
$n!$	1	2	6	24	120
$a_n = n \cdot n!$	1	4	18	96	600
S_n	1	5	23	119	719

In filling out the last line of the table, we have used

$S_1 = 1,$

$S_2 = 1 + 4 = 5,$

$S_3 = (1 + 4) + 18 = 5 + 18 = 23,$

$S_4 = (1 + 4 + 18) + 96 = 23 + 96 = 119,$

$S_5 = 119 + 600 = 719.$

The table leads us to conjecture the assertion $P(n)$ that $S_n = (n + 1)! - 1$. We prove this conjecture by induction for all n in $\mathbf{Z}^+ = \{1, 2, \ldots\}$ as follows:

Basis   When $n = 1$, then $S_1 = 1$ and $(n + 1)! - 1 = 2! - 1 = 2 - 1 = 1$. Thus $P(1)$ is true.

Inductive Step   Assume that k is in $\mathbf{Z}^+$ and that $S_k = (k + 1)! - 1$. Then

$S_{k+1} = S_k + (k + 1)[(k + 1)!] = (k + 1)! - 1 + (k + 1)[(k + 1)!]$

$= (1 + k + 1)[(k + 1)!] - 1 = (k + 2)[(k + 1)!] - 1$

$= (k + 2)! - 1$

Since $S_{k+1} = (k + 2)! - 1$ is the assertion $P(k + 1)$, we have shown that $P(k) \Rightarrow P(k + 1)$, and the conjecture has been elevated into a proved result.   □

Example 5   Let $f(n) = n^2 - n + 41$. A partial table for $f(n)$ follows:

n	0	1	2	3	4	5	6	7	8	9
$f(n)$	41	41	43	47	53	61	71	83	97	113

All the values of $f(n)$ shown here are primes. Does this prove that $f(n)$ is a prime for *every* n in $\mathbf{N} = \{0, 1, \ldots\}$? No, for although we have more than enough cases for the basis part of a proof by induction, we do not have the inductive part. Also, the inductive part cannot be provided, because

$f(41) = 41^2 - 41 + 41 = 41^2$

shows that $f(n)$ is not prime when $n = 41$. We can show that $f(n)$ is not prime for an infinite set of n's, including the arithmetic progression 41, 82, 123, ...   □

Example 6   Let $F_0, F_1, \ldots$ be the Fibonacci Sequence and let

$$S_n = \sum_{i=0}^{n} F_i = F_0 + F_1 + \cdots + F_n.$$

Let $P(n)$ be the assertion that $S_n = F_{n+2}$. Then $P(k) \Rightarrow P(k+1)$ for all k in N, since $S_k = F_{k+2}$ implies that

$$S_{k+1} = F_0 + F_1 + \cdots + F_k + F_{k+1}$$
$$= S_k + F_{k+1}$$
$$= F_{k+2} + F_{k+1}$$
$$= F_{k+3},$$

and $S_{k+1} = F_{k+3}$ is the assertion $P(k+1)$. Does this mean that $S_n = F_{n+2}$ for all n in N? No; we have the inductive part of a proof by induction but do not have the basis. In fact, $S_0 = F_0 = 0$ and $F_2 = 1$, so $S_n \neq F_{n+2}$ when $n = 0$. We can see that $S_n \neq F_{n+2}$ for all n in N. The correct formula is

$$F_0 + F_1 + F_2 + \cdots + F_n = F_{n+2} - 1 \quad \text{for all } n \text{ in } N. \qquad \square$$

THEOREM 2   **EXPONENT RULE IN A SEMIGROUP**

In a semigroup $(X, \circ)$, $x^m \circ x^n = x^{m+n}$ for all x in X and all m and n in Z^+.

PROOF   The proof is by induction on n; that is, we think of m as a fixed positive integer and let $P(n)$ be the assertion that $x^m \circ x^n = x^{m+n}$.

Basis $P(1)$ is the assertion that $x^m \circ x^1 = x^{m+1}$. By Definition 3 ("Powers") of Section 2.2, $x^1 = x$ and $x^m \circ x = x^{m+1}$. Hence $x^m \circ x^1 = x^m \circ x = x^{m+1}$, and $P(1)$ is true.

Inductive Step   Let k be in Z^+. The inductive hypothesis is that $P(k)$ is true, that is, $x^m \circ x^k = x^{m+k}$. Now, $x^m \circ x^{k+1} = x^m \circ (x^k \circ x)$ by definition of powers. Using the fact that the operation of a semigroup is associative, this becomes $(x^m \circ x^k) \circ x$, which equals $x^{m+k} \circ x$ by the inductive hypothesis. This is x^{m+k+1} by definition of powers. Thus, for all k in Z^+, $x^m \circ x^k = x^{m+k}$ implies that $x^m \circ x^{k+1} = x^{m+k+1}$. This means that $[\forall k \in Z^+, \; P(k) \Rightarrow P(k+1)]$ is true, and the proof is complete. $\qquad \square$

DEFINITION 1   **BINARY NUMERALS, BASE 2 REPRESENTATION**

For a binary string $\beta = b_1 b_2 \ldots b_n$, let $(\beta)_2$ denote the number $2^{n-1} b_1 + 2^{n-2} b_2 + \cdots + 2 b_{n-1} + b_n$. The string β is the *binary numeral*, or *base 2 representation*, for the number $(\beta)_2$.

Using this definition for the case of $\beta = 110$, one finds that $(110)_2 = 2^2 \cdot 1 + 2 \cdot 1 + 0 = 4 + 2 + 0 = 6$. Similarly, one finds that the numbers

$(\beta)_2$ for all β in $\boldsymbol{B_3}$ are as listed in the following table:

β	000	001	010	011	100	101	110	111
$(\beta)_2$	0	1	2	3	4	5	6	7

We observe that $(\beta_1)_2, (\beta_2)_2, \ldots, (\beta_8)_2$ are the integers $0, 1, \ldots, 7$, respectively, when $\{\beta_1, \beta_2, \ldots, \beta_8\}$ is the standard listing for $\boldsymbol{B_3}$. This is extended to $\boldsymbol{B_n}$, for general n, in the following result.

THEOREM 3   **BASE 2 REPRESENTATION**

Let $n \in \boldsymbol{Z^+}$, $r = 2^n$, and $\{\beta_1, \beta_2, \ldots, \beta_r\}$ be the standard listing for the set $\boldsymbol{B_n}$ of n-digit binary strings. Then $(\beta_1)_2, (\beta_2)_2, (\beta_3)_2, \ldots, (\beta_r)_2$ are the integers $0, 1, 2, \ldots, 2^n - 1$, respectively.

PROOF   Our proof is by mathematical induction. Let $P(n)$ be the assertion that the theorem holds for the positive integer n.

Basis   When $n = 1$, we have $r = 2^n = 2^1 = 2$ and the standard listing for $\boldsymbol{B_1}$ is $\{0, 1\}$. Since $(0)_2 = 1 \cdot 0 = 0$ and $(1)_2 = 1 \cdot 1 = 1$, $P(1)$ is true.

Inductive Step   Let $k \in \boldsymbol{Z^+}$, $s = 2^k$, and $\{\beta_1, \beta_2, \ldots, \beta_s\}$ be the standard listing for $\boldsymbol{B_k}$. From Algorithm 1 of Section 1.1, the standard listing for $\boldsymbol{B_{k+1}}$ is

$$\{0\beta_1, 0\beta_2, \ldots, 0\beta_s, 1\beta_1, 1\beta_2, \ldots, 1\beta_s\}.$$

Let $\beta = b_1 b_2 \ldots b_k$ be in $\boldsymbol{B_k}$. Then $0\beta = c_1 c_2 \ldots c_{k+1}$, where $c_1 = 0$ and $c_{i+1} = b_i$ for $i = 1, 2, \ldots, k$. Hence

$$(0\beta)_2 = 2^k \cdot 0 + 2^{k-1}b_1 + 2^{k-2}b_2 + \cdots + 2b_{k-1} + b_k = (\beta)_2.$$

Thus $(0\beta)_2 = (\beta)_2$, and similarly $(1\beta)_2 = 2^k + (\beta)_2$. The inductive hypothesis is that $(\beta_1)_2, (\beta_2)_2, \ldots, (\beta_s)_2$ are the integers $0, 1, \ldots, 2^k - 1$, respectively. With this assumption and the formulas $(0\beta)_2 = (\beta)_2$ and $(1\beta)_2 = 2^k + (\beta)_2$, one sees that

$$(0\beta_1)_2, (0\beta_2)_2, \ldots, (0\beta_s)_2, (1\beta_1)_2, (1\beta_2)_2, \ldots, (1\beta_s)_2$$

are, respectively, the integers

$$0, 1, \ldots, 2^k - 1, 2^k + 0, 2^k + 1, \ldots, 2^k + 2^k - 1. \tag{2}$$

Since $2^k + 2^k = 2^{k+1}$, the terms of Display (2) are the integers $0, 1, 2, \ldots,$ $2^{k+1} - 1$ in order. Hence, for all k in $\boldsymbol{Z^+}$, $P(k) \Rightarrow P(k+1)$. This proves the theorem.   □

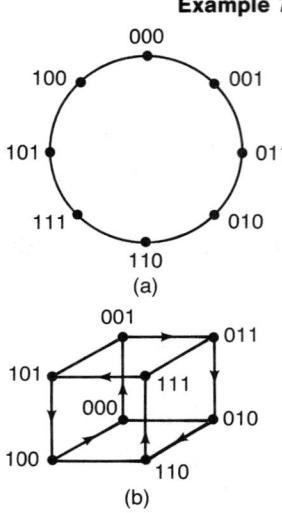

FIGURE 4.2.2

(a)

(b)

Example 7   If a circuit has three switches, a binary string $a_1a_2a_3$ can be used to indicate the state of the switches; this is done by letting a_i be 1 when the ith switch is in the On position and $a_i = 0$ when it is in the Off position. One might want to test the flow of current in all eight states by changing one switch at a time, and in the most efficient manner, that is, without repeating a state. This can be done with any state of the switches as the initial one. One sees this in the cube of Figure 4.2.2(b) by reading the indicators of the states in the order defined by the arrows, or in Figure 4.2.2(a) by circling either clockwise or counter-clockwise. For example, reading clockwise from 101, one obtains the sequence

101, 100, 000, 001, 011, 010, 110, 111

of indicators for the eight states of the switches. We note in this sequence that adjacent strings differ in just one place. In Example 8 we will prove by mathematical induction that for every n in Z^+ the 2^n strings of B_n can be arranged around a circle to provide a similar efficient order for testing all 2^n states of a circuit with n switches.   □

Example 8   Let A be the binary relation on the set B_n of n-digit binary strings for which $\alpha A\beta$ means that $\alpha = a_1a_2 \ldots a_n$ and $\beta = b_1b_2 \ldots b_n$ differ in exactly one position; that is, $a_i \neq b_i$ for exactly one i in $\{1, 2, \ldots, n\}$. (This means that α and β are adjacent, in the sense of Definition 6, "Adjacent Strings," of Section 2.4.) Let $m = 2^n$. A **Gray Code** for B_n is a listing $B_n = \{\alpha_1, \alpha_2, \ldots, \alpha_m\}$ such that $\alpha_i A\alpha_{i+1}$ for $i = 1, 2, \ldots, m - 1$ and $\alpha_m A\alpha_1$. Let P be the predicate on Z^+ for which $P(n)$ is the assertion that a Gray Code exists for B_n. We next prove by mathematical induction that $P(n)$ is true for all n in Z^+.

Basis   When $n = 1$, the listing $B_1 = \{0, 1\}$ has the desired property. Hence $P(1)$ is true.

Inductive Step   Let $k \in Z^+$, $s = 2^k$, and assume that $P(k)$ is true. Then there is a listing $B_k = \{\alpha_1, \alpha_2, \ldots, \alpha_s\}$ such that $\alpha_i A\alpha_{i+1}$ for $i = 1, 2, \ldots, s - 1$ and $\alpha_s A\alpha_1$. Let

$0\alpha_1, 0\alpha_2, \ldots, 0\alpha_s, 1\alpha_s, 1\alpha_{s-1}, \ldots, 1\alpha_1$

be denoted by $\beta_1, \beta_2, \ldots, \beta_{2s}$, respectively. Examination shows that $\{\beta_1, \beta_2, \ldots, \beta_{2s}\}$ is a listing for B_{k+1} such that $\beta_i A\beta_{i+1}$ for $i = 1, 2, \ldots, 2s - 1$ and $\beta_{2s} A\beta_1$. Hence $P(k) \Rightarrow P(k + 1)$ for all k in Z^+. This completes the inductive step, and the result is proved.   □

The following result (Theorem 4) can be skipped by readers unfamiliar with trigonometry or complex numbers.

THEOREM 4   DE MOIVRE'S THEOREM

$$(\cos \theta + i \sin \theta)^n = \cos n\theta + i \sin n\theta \qquad (3)$$

for all n in N.

PROOF   Let $P(n)$ be the assertion in Formula (3). We use the addition formulas

$$\cos(\alpha + \beta) = (\cos \alpha)(\cos \beta) - (\sin \alpha)(\sin \beta) \qquad (4)$$

$$\sin(\alpha + \beta) = (\sin \alpha)(\cos \beta) + (\cos \alpha)(\sin \beta) \qquad (5)$$

and induction on n.

Basis   When $n = 0$, we have $(\cos \theta + i \sin \theta)^n = (\cos \theta + i \sin \theta)^0 = 1$ and $\cos n\theta + i \sin n\theta = \cos 0 + i \sin 0 = 1 + i \cdot 0 = 1$. So $P(0)$ is true.

Inductive Step   Assume that k is in N and that $(\cos \theta + i \sin \theta)^k = \cos k\theta + i \sin k\theta$. Then, using the addition formulas (4) and (5),

$$\begin{aligned}
(\cos \theta + i \sin \theta)^{k+1} &= (\cos \theta + i \sin \theta)^k (\cos \theta + i \sin \theta) \\
&= (\cos k\theta + i \sin k\theta)(\cos \theta + i \sin \theta) \\
&= (\cos k\theta \cos \theta - \sin k\theta \sin \theta) \\
&\quad + i(\sin k\theta \cos \theta + \cos k\theta \sin \theta) \\
&= \cos(k\theta + \theta) + i \sin(k\theta + \theta) \\
&= \cos(k + 1)\theta + i \sin(k + 1)\theta.
\end{aligned}$$

Thus $P(k)$ implies $P(k + 1)$, and we have proved Formula (3) true for all n in N.

Formula (3) also is true when n is a negative integer because

$$\sin(-\alpha) = -\sin \alpha,$$
$$\cos(-\alpha) = \cos \alpha,$$
$$(\cos \alpha + i \sin \alpha)(\cos \alpha - i \sin \alpha) = 1,$$

and

$$\frac{1}{\cos \alpha + i \sin \alpha} = \cos \alpha - i \sin \alpha,$$

and hence

$$\begin{aligned}
(\cos \theta + i \sin \theta)^{-m} &= \frac{1}{(\cos \theta + i \sin \theta)^m} \\
&= \frac{1}{\cos m\theta + i \sin m\theta} \\
&= \cos m\theta - i \sin m\theta \\
&= \cos(-m\theta) + i \sin(-m\theta).
\end{aligned}$$ □

PROBLEMS FOR SECTION 4.2

In each of Problems 1–12, let $P(n)$ be the stated assertion and prove by mathematical induction on n that $P(n)$ is true for all n in the given set.

1. If $x \neq 1$, then for all n in N,

$$1 + x + x^2 + \cdots + x^n = \frac{x^{n+1} - 1}{x - 1}.$$

2. If $x \neq 1$, then for all n in $N = \{0, 1, \ldots\}$,

$$a + ax + ax^2 + \cdots + ax^n = a\frac{x^{n+1} - 1}{x - 1}.$$

3. $F_{n+1}^2 - F_n F_{n+2} = (-1)^n$ for all n in $N = \{0, 1, \ldots\}$. (Here F_0, F_1, $\ldots$ is the Fibonacci Sequence 0, 1, 1, 2, 3, 5, $\ldots$.)

4. Let L_0, L_1, $\ldots$ be the Lucas Numbers 2, 1, 3, 4, 7, 11, $\ldots$. For all n in N,
   (a) L_{3n} is even; also, L_{3n+1} and L_{3n+2} are odd.
   (b) $L_n L_{n+2} - L_{n+1}^2 = 5(-1)^n$.

5. For all n in $X = \{6, 7, 8, \ldots\}$, $n^2 - 9n + 19 > 0$.

6. For all n in $X = \{4, 5, 6, \ldots\}$, one can assemble $n\cent$ worth of postage using only 2¢ stamps and 5¢ stamps.

7. Let $\binom{n}{h}$ denote the binomial coefficient $\#B_{n,h}$. For all h and n in N,

$$\binom{h}{h} + \binom{h+1}{h} + \binom{h+2}{h} + \cdots + \binom{h+n}{h} = \binom{h+n+1}{h+1}.$$

8. For all h and n in N,

$$\binom{h}{0} + \binom{h+1}{1} + \cdots + \binom{h+n}{n} = \binom{h+n+1}{n}.$$

9. For all n in Z^+,

$$(1 + x)^n = \binom{n}{0} + \binom{n}{1}x + \binom{n}{2}x^2 + \cdots + \binom{n}{n}x^n.$$

[Recall that $\binom{k}{r+1} + \binom{k}{r} = \binom{k+1}{r+1}$ for k and r in N with $0 \leq r < k$.]

10. For all n in N and h in $\{0, 1, \ldots, n\}$,

$$\binom{n}{h} = \frac{n!}{(n-h)!h!}.$$

11. $x - y$ is a factor of $x^n - y^n$ for all n in Z^+.

12. $x + y$ is a factor of $x^{2n+1} + y^{2n+1}$ for all n in N.

13. Let

$$S_n = \frac{1}{2!} + \frac{2}{3!} + \cdots + \frac{n}{(n+1)!}.$$

(i) Tabulate S_n for $n = 1, 2, 3, 4, 5$.
(ii) Conjecture a simple form for S_n.
(iii) Prove the conjecture true for all n in $\mathbf{Z}^+$.

14. Using the product notation of Problem 13 of Section 4.1, let

$$p_n = \prod_{j=2}^{n} \left(1 - \frac{1}{j^2}\right).$$

(i) Note that $p_2 = \frac{3}{4}$ and $p_3 = (\frac{3}{4})(\frac{8}{9}) = \frac{2}{3}$. Find p_4, p_5, p_6, p_7, and p_8.
(ii) Conjecture a simple formula for p_n based on the data in Part (i) for p_2, p_4, p_6, and p_8. Is the formula correct for p_{10}? Is it correct for p_3, p_5, and p_7?
(iii) Prove by induction on n that the formula of Part (ii) is true for all n in $\{2, 3, \ldots\}$.

15. Let

$$S_n = \sum_{j=0}^{n} \frac{1}{(2j+1)(2j+3)}.$$

(i) Tabulate S_n for $n = 0, 1, 2, 3, 4, 5$.
(ii) Conjecture a simple formula for S_n.
(iii) Prove that the formula of Part (ii) is true for all n in $\mathbf{N}$.

16. For each of the following parts, let $P(n)$ denote the assertion. In which part is $P(1)$ false? In which part is $[P(k) \Rightarrow P(k+1)]$ false for some k in $\mathbf{Z}^+$? In which part is $P(n)$ true for all n in $\mathbf{Z}^+$?

(i) $\displaystyle\sum_{j=1}^{n} \frac{1}{j(j+1)} = 1 - \frac{1}{n+1}$, (ii) $\displaystyle\sum_{j=1}^{n} j(j+2) = 4n^2 - 4n + 3$;
(iii) $1 + 3 + 5 + \cdots + (2n-1) = n^2 + 1$.

17. Use the formula in Problem 10 to establish the following:

(i) $\dbinom{n}{2} = \dfrac{n(n-1)}{2}$. (ii) $\dbinom{n}{2} + \dbinom{n+1}{2} = n^2$.

(iii) $\dbinom{n}{k+1} = \dfrac{n-k}{k+1}\dbinom{n}{k}$.

18. Use the formula in Problem 10 to establish the following:

(i) $\dbinom{n}{3} = \dfrac{n(n-1)(n-2)}{6}$. (ii) $\dbinom{n}{3} + 4\dbinom{n+1}{3} + \dbinom{n+2}{3} = n^3$.

(iii) $\dbinom{n}{k} = \dfrac{n}{k}\dbinom{n-1}{k-1}$.

19.   Write a listing $B_4 = \{\alpha_1, \alpha_2, \ldots, \alpha_{16}\}$ such that $\alpha_i A\alpha_{i+1}$ for $1 \leq i \leq 15$ and $\alpha_{16}A\alpha_1$, where A is the binary relation of Example 8.

20.   Do as in Problem 19 with B_4 replaced by B_5.

21.   Let $a_1, a_2, \ldots$ be an arithmetic progression with d as the common difference. For all n in $\mathbf{Z}^+$, prove by induction that:
      (i) $a_n = a_1 + (n-1)d$.

      (ii) $\displaystyle\sum_{j=1}^{n} a_j = na_1 + \binom{n}{2}d$, where $\binom{1}{2} = 0$.

22.   Let $b_1, b_2, \ldots$ be a geometric progression with r as the common ratio. For all n in $\mathbf{Z}^+$, prove by induction that:
      (i) $b_n = b_1 r^{n-1}$.

      (ii) $\displaystyle\prod_{j=1}^{n} b_j = b_1^n r^m$, where $m = \binom{n}{2}$ and $\binom{1}{2} = 0$.

      (*Note:* $\displaystyle\prod_{j=1}^{n} b_j = b_1 \cdots b_n$.)

23.   Let $[X, ^-, \wedge, 1, \vee, 0]$ be a boolean algebra. Prove by induction on n that, for all n in $\{2, 3, \ldots\}$,
      $$\overline{x_1 \vee x_2 \vee \cdots \vee x_n} = \bar{x}_1 \wedge \bar{x}_2 \wedge \cdots \wedge \bar{x}_n$$
      for any elements $x_1, x_2, \ldots, x_n$ of the carrier X. (This is a generalized De Morgan's Law.)

24.   Prove the dual of the generalized De Morgan's Law of Problem 23.

25.   Let $(X, \preceq)$ be a poset. A *lower bound* for a subset T of X is an m in X such that $m \preceq t$ for all t in T. Given that $(X, \preceq)$ is a lattice, prove by induction on $\#T$ that, for every nonempty finite subset T of X, the set $\lambda(T)$, of lower bounds for T, has a greatest element g [which can be denoted by GLB(T)].

26.   (i) Define "upper bound for a subset" T of the carrier X of a poset $(X, \preceq)$.
      (ii) Do the dual of Problem 25 with *lower* replaced by *upper*.

27.   Let T be a transitive relation on a set S. Let $a_1, a_2, \ldots$ be a sequence of elements of S such that $a_i T a_{i+1}$ for all i in $\mathbf{Z}^+$. Prove that $a_1 T a_{n+1}$ for all n in $\mathbf{Z}^+$.

28.   Let T be a transitive relation on S. For all n in $\mathbf{Z}^+$, prove that $s_0 T s_n$ whenever there is a directed path $(s_0, s_1, \ldots, s_n)$ of length n from s_0 to s_n in T.

29.   For n in $X = \{2, 3, 4, \ldots\}$, let $f(x_1, x_2, \ldots, x_n)$ be defined inductively by:

      Basis $f(x_1, x_2) = (x_1 \Rightarrow x_2)$.

      Inductive Part $f(x_1, \ldots, x_k, x_{k+1}) = f(x_1, \ldots, x_k) \wedge (x_k \Rightarrow x_{k+1})$.

      Prove by induction on n that

      $$f(x_1, x_2, \ldots, x_n) \Rightarrow (x_1 \Rightarrow x_n) \quad \text{for all } n \text{ in } X.$$

30. For all n in N, conjecture and prove a simple formula for

$$(x + y)(x^2 + y^2)(x^4 + y^4)(x^8 + y^8) \cdots (x^{2^n} + y^{2^n}).$$

4.3

WELL ORDERING AND MATHEMATICAL INDUCTION

We start this section with a presentation of *strong induction*, a variation on the technique of proof by induction presented in the previous section. We illustrate the use of this new algorithm on certain predicates for which ordinary induction is either unfeasible or inconvenient. Then we note that a set $X = \{a, a + 1, \ldots\}$, with a an integer, is well ordered under the "less than" relation; that is, every nonempty subset of X has a least integer. Finally, this property of X is used to prove that both induction algorithms are valid methods of proof.

ALGORITHM 1   **PROOF BY STRONG INDUCTION**

Let P be a predicate on $X = \{a, a + 1, \ldots\}$, with a an integer. The following steps constitute a proof by **strong induction** that $P(n)$ is true for all n in X.

Basis   Show that $P(a)$ is true.

Inductive Step   Assume that h is an integer in $\{a + 1, a + 2, \ldots\}$ for which $P(a)$, $P(a + 1)$, ..., $P(h - 1)$ are true. Show that this **inductive hypothesis** implies that $P(h)$ is true.

Example 1   Let the F_n and L_n be the Fibonacci Numbers and Lucas Numbers of Definition 3, Section 4.1. Let $P(n)$ be the assertion that $F_n + F_{n+2} = L_{n+1}$. We now use strong induction on n to prove that $P(n)$ is true for all n in $N = \{0, 1, \ldots\}$.

Basis $P(0)$ is true because, for $n = 0$, we have

$$F_n + F_{n+2} = F_0 + F_2 = 0 + 1 = 1 \qquad \text{and} \qquad L_{n+1} = L_1 = 1.$$

Inductive Step   For later use, we note that $P(1)$ is true because, for $n = 1$,

$$F_n + F_{n+2} = F_1 + F_3 = 1 + 2 = 3 \qquad \text{and} \qquad L_{n+1} = L_2 = 3. \qquad (1)$$

We assume that h is an integer in $\{1, 2, \ldots\}$ for which

$$P(0), \quad P(1), \quad \ldots, \quad P(h - 1) \quad \text{are all true}, \qquad (2)$$

and we wish to show that this inductive hypothesis implies that $P(h)$ is true. For this process, we can ignore the case in which $h = 1$ because we have already shown in Display (1) that $P(1)$ is true. For the remaining cases, we know that $h \geq 2$, so both $h - 2$ and $h - 1$ are in N. The inductive hypothesis (2) then allows us to assume that both $P(h - 2)$ and $P(h - 1)$ are true; that is,

$$F_{h-2} + F_h = L_{h-1},$$
$$F_{h-1} + F_{h+1} = L_h.$$

Adding gives

$$(F_{h-2} + F_{h-1}) + (F_h + F_{h+1}) = L_{h-1} + L_h.$$

This and the defining recursive properties of the F_n and L_n lead to

$$F_h + F_{h+2} = L_{h+1}.$$

This is the assertion $P(h)$; so the proof that $F_n + F_{n+2} = L_{n+1}$ for all n in N is now complete. □

Example 2   Let $P(n)$ be the assertion that n¢ worth of postage can be assembled using only 5¢ stamps and 17¢ stamps. We use strong induction to prove $P(n)$ true for all n in $X = \{64, 65, \ldots\}$.

It is helpful to consider the first five cases, that is, to see that $P(h)$ is true for $h = 64, 65, 66, 67$, and 68. Table 4.3.1 shows this. For example, the table shows that 64¢ worth of postage can be assembled using six 5¢ stamps and two 17¢ stamps.

TABLE 4.3.1

$h = 5f + 17s$	64	65	66	67	68
f = number of 5¢ stamps	6	13	3	10	0
s = number of 17¢ stamps	2	0	3	1	4

Basis   Since $64 = 5 \cdot 6 + 17 \cdot 2$, we see that P(64) is true.

Inductive Step   Let $h \in \{65, 66, \ldots\}$ and assume that $P(64), P(65), \ldots,$ $P(h - 1)$ are true. We wish to show that these assumptions imply that $P(h)$ is true. As Table 4.3.1 shows, $P(h)$ is true when $64 \leq h \leq 68$; hence we can restrict our attention to the case in which $69 \leq h$. In this case, $64 \leq h - 5 < h$, and the inductive hypothesis allows us to assume that $P(h - 5)$ is true; that is, $(h - 5)$¢ worth of postage can be assembled using only 5¢ stamps and 17¢ stamps. Adding an extra 5¢ stamp gives us

$(h - 5) + 5 = h\cent$ worth of postage. This shows that

$$[P(64) \wedge P(65) \wedge \cdots \wedge P(h - 1)] \Rightarrow P(h)$$

is true for all h in $\{65, 66, \ldots\}$. The proof is complete. $\square$

Let $X = \{2, 3, 4, \ldots\}$, let $P = \{2, 3, 5, 7, 11, \ldots\}$ be the subset of X consisting of the (positive integral) primes, and let $C = \{4, 6, 8, 9, \ldots\}$ be the complement of P in X. An integer c in C is called a **composite**. We recall from Section 1.7 that an integer n in X is a prime if and only if its only positive integral divisors are 1 and n itself. It follows that an integer n in X is composite if and only if n has an integral divisor d that satisfies $1 < d < n$. When this is the case, n/d is an integer e that satisfies $1 < e < n$. Thus an integer c in X is a composite if and only if $c = de$ with d and e in X. For example, 60 is a composite because $60 = 12 \cdot 5$. Since 12 is also a composite, it can be written as the product $3 \cdot 4$, and so $60 = 3 \cdot 4 \cdot 5$. The composite 4 equals $2 \cdot 2$, and hence $60 = 2 \cdot 2 \cdot 3 \cdot 5$. Because each of the numbers 2, 3, and 5 is a prime, we attempt no further breakdown into smaller factors.

This factorization illustrates the following important result in the Theory of Numbers, which goes back at least to Euclid.

THEOREM 1   FACTORIZATION INTO PRIMES

Every n in $X = \{2, 3, 4, \ldots\}$ is expressible as $n = p_1 p_2 \cdots p_r$, with r in $\mathbf{Z}^+ = \{1, 2, \ldots\}$ and each p_i a prime in X. That is, each n in X is either a prime or a product of primes.

PROOF   We use strong induction on n. Let $P(n)$ be the assertion concerning n in this theorem.

Basis   Since 2 is a prime, $P(2)$ is true.

Inductive Step   Assume that h is in $\{3, 4, 5, \ldots\}$ and that $P(2), P(3), \ldots, P(h - 1)$ are true. We wish to show that this assumption implies that $P(h)$ is true. If h is a prime, then $P(h)$ is true; so we need only consider the case in which h is composite. Then $h = de$ with d and e in X, $1 < d < h$, and $1 < e < h$. Since d and e are in $\{2, 3, \ldots, h - 1\}$, the inductive hypothesis includes the assumption that $P(d)$ and $P(e)$ are true. So

$$d = q_1 q_2 \cdots q_s \qquad \text{and} \qquad e = q_1' q_2' \cdots q_t',$$

where s and t are in $\mathbf{Z}^+$ and the q_i and q_j' are primes. Then

$$h = de = q_1 q_2 \cdots q_s q_1' q_2' \cdots q_t'$$

is the desired expression for h as a product of primes. This completes the proof. $\square$

The three following lemmas validate the inductive techniques of proof given in this and the previous section.

LEMMA 1   **CONDITIONS FOR A SUBSET TO BE X**

Let $a \in \mathbf{Z}$, $X = \{a, a + 1, \ldots\}$, and $T \subseteq X$. If $a \in T$ and if $[k \in T] \Rightarrow [(k + 1) \in T]$ is true for all k in X, then $T = X$.

PROOF   Let C be the complement of T in X. Then $C \cap T = \varnothing$ and $C \cup T = X$. Proving that $T = X$ is equivalent to proving that $C = \varnothing$. We assume that $C \neq \varnothing$ and seek a contradiction. With this assumption, the non-empty subset C of X has a least integer c, since X is well ordered under the relation $<$. Then $c \neq a$, since $c \in C$, $a \in T$, and $C \cap T = \varnothing$. But $c \in C$ and $C \subseteq X$ show that $c \in X$. Now, $c \in X$, $c \neq a$, and $X = \{a, a + 1, \ldots\}$ imply that $c - 1$ is in X. Since c is the least integer in C, $c - 1$ is not in C and so must be in the complement T of C in X. The hypothesis $[k \in T] \Rightarrow [(k + 1) \in T]$, with k replaced by $c - 1$, tells us that $(c - 1) + 1 = c$ is in T. This is a contradiction because $c \in C$ and $C \cap T = \varnothing$. Hence the assumption that $C \neq \varnothing$ is false. Thus $C = \varnothing$, $T = X$, and the lemma is proved.   □

We next use Lemma 1 to show that Algorithm 1 of Section 4.2 ("Proof by Mathematical Induction") is a valid technique of proof.

LEMMA 2   **ALGORITHM OF MATHEMATICAL INDUCTION**

Let P be a predicate on $X = \{a, a + 1, \ldots\}$. Then

$$P(a) \wedge [\forall k \in X, P(k) \Rightarrow P(k + 1)] \Rightarrow \forall n \in X, P(n).$$

PROOF   Let T be the truth set for P; that is, let T consist of the t of X for which $P(t)$ is true. We assume that $P(a)$ and $[\forall k \in X, P(k) \Rightarrow P(k + 1)]$ are true. The hypothesis that $P(a)$ is true means that $a \in T$. The hypothesis that $[\forall k \in X, P(k) \Rightarrow P(k + 1)]$ is true means that $[k \in T] \Rightarrow [(k + 1) \in T]$ is true for all k in X. These statements allow us to apply Lemma 1, and it follows that $T = X$, which tells us that $P(n)$ is true for all n in X. This completes the proof of Lemma 2 and justifies the technique of proof by mathematical induction introduced in Section 4.2.   □

Now we present a variation on Lemma 2 in which the inductive hypothesis "$P(k)$ is true" is replaced by the stronger hypothesis "$P(n)$ is true for $n \in \{a, a + 1, \ldots, k\}$." It is convenient to replace k by $h - 1$ in the new version.

LEMMA 3   **PROOF BY STRONG INDUCTION**

Let P be a predicate on $X = \{a, a + 1, \ldots\}$. If $P(a)$ is true and if

$$[P(a) \wedge P(a + 1) \wedge \cdots \wedge P(h - 1)] \Rightarrow P(h) \tag{3}$$

is true for all h in $\{a + 1, a + 2, \ldots\}$, then $P(n)$ is true for all n in X.

PROOF   Let T be the truth set for the predicate P and let $\bar{T}$ be the complement of T in X. Then

$$T \cap \bar{T} = \varnothing \quad \text{and} \quad T \cup \bar{T} = X. \tag{4}$$

We wish to show that $P(n)$ is true for all n in X, that is, to show that $T = X$. This is equivalent to showing that $\bar{T}$ is empty. We assume that $\bar{T} \neq \varnothing$ and seek a contradiction. The assumption that $\bar{T} \neq \varnothing$ and the fact that X is well ordered under $<$ imply that $\bar{T}$ has a least element h. We note that $h \neq a$, since $h \in \bar{T}$, $a \in T$, and $\bar{T} \cap T = \varnothing$. Since h is the least element of $\bar{T}$, the elements $a, a + 1, \ldots, h - 1$ of X are not in $\bar{T}$ and so must be in T. This means that $P(a), P(a + 1), \ldots, P(h - 1)$ are all true. Now, implication (3) in the hypothesis of this lemma tells us that $P(h)$ is true; that is, $h \in T$. Then $h \in T$ and $h \in \bar{T}$ imply that $T \cap \bar{T} \neq \varnothing$. But $T \cap \bar{T} = \varnothing$, as noted in Display (4). Thus we have a contradiction. Since this contradiction follows from the assumption above that $\bar{T} \neq \varnothing$, we must have $\bar{T} = \varnothing$. Hence $T = X$, and $P(n)$ is true for all n in X. This proves the lemma and shows that strong induction is a valid technique of proof. $\square$

We have used the technique of "proof by contradiction," described in Algorithm 1 of Section 3.2 ("Proof by Contradiction"), to prove Lemma 3. Specifically, we showed that $\bar{p} \Rightarrow (q \wedge \bar{q})$ is true, where p is the assertion that "$\bar{T} = \varnothing$" and q is the assertion that "$T \cap \bar{T} = \varnothing$." Since

$$[\bar{x} \Rightarrow (y \wedge \bar{y})] \Rightarrow x \tag{5}$$

is a tautology, we obtain a true statement when x is replaced by p and y is replaced by q in Display (5); that is, the fact that the negation $\bar{p}$ of p implies the contradiction $q \wedge \bar{q}$ shows that p is true.

PROBLEMS FOR SECTION 4.3

1. Let $F_0, F_1, \ldots$ be the Fibonacci Sequence. Let a be in $N = \{0, 1, \ldots\}$. Prove by strong induction on n that

$$F_a F_n + F_{a+1} F_{n+1} = F_{a+n+1} \quad \text{for all } n \text{ in } N.$$

2. With a, F_0, F_1, ... as in Problem 1 and L_0, L_1, ... the Lucas Sequence, prove by strong induction on n that

$$F_n L_a + F_{n+1} L_{a+1} = L_{a+n+1} \quad \text{for all } n \text{ in } N.$$

3. Let a, b, c, r, s, t be fixed integers. Prove that

$$rF_{n+a} = sF_{n+b} + tL_{n+c}$$

holds for all n in N if it holds for $n = 0$ and $n = 1$.

4. Prove that $F_n + L_n = 2F_{n+1}$ for all n in N.

5. Prove that $n\cent$ in postage can be assembled using only 10¢ stamps and 13¢ stamps for all n in $\{108, 109, \ldots\}$.

6. Prove that $n\cent$ in postage can be assembled using only 17¢ stamps and 20¢ stamps for all n in $\{304, 305, \ldots\}$.

7. Use strong induction on n to prove each of the following for all n in $N = \{0, 1, \ldots\}$:
    (a) $F_{n+4} = 3F_{n+2} - F_n$.   (b) $F_{n+6} = 4F_{n+3} + F_n$.
    (c) $F_{n+8} = 7F_{n+4} - F_n$.   (d) $F_{n+10} = 11F_{n+5} + F_n$.

8. Discover and prove formulas similar to those in Problem 7 for the Lucas Numbers.

9. Let $a = (1 + \sqrt{5})/2$ and $b = (1 - \sqrt{5})/2$.
    (i) Show that $a^2 = a + 1$ and $b^2 = b + 1$.
    (ii) Use strong induction on n to prove that

$$F_n = \frac{a^n - b^n}{a - b} \quad \text{for all } n \text{ in } N.$$

    (This is called the **Binet Formula** for F_n.)

10. Let $a = (1 + \sqrt{5})/2$ and $b = (1 - \sqrt{5})/2$. For all n in N:
    (i) Use strong induction on n to prove that $L_n = a^n + b^n$. (This is the **Binet Formula** for L_n.)
    (ii) Use the Binet Formulas to prove that $F_n L_n = F_{2n}$.
    (iii) Show that $ab = -1$; use this and Part (i) to prove that

$$L_{2n} = L_n^2 - 2(-1)^n.$$

11. Prove that $L_n + 2L_{n+1} = L_{n+3}$ for all n in N.

12. Prove that $F_n + 2F_{n+1} = F_{n+3}$ for all n in N.

13. Use (ordinary) mathematical induction on n to prove each of the following properties of the Lucas Numbers for all n in N:

    (a) $\sum_{i=0}^{n} L_i = L_{n+2} - 1$.   (b) $\sum_{i=0}^{n} L_{2i} = L_{2n+1} + 1$.

    (c) $\sum_{i=0}^{n} L_{2i+1} = L_{2n+2} - 2$.   (d) $2\sum_{i=0}^{n} L_{3i} = L_{3n+2} + 1$.

14. Discover and prove Fibonacci analogues of the formulas of Problem 13.

15. Use the formula in Problem 1 to prove that $F_n^2 + F_{n+1}^2 = F_{2n+1}$ for all n in N. (No induction is needed here.)

16. Use the formula $F_{k+1} + F_k = F_{k+2}$ to prove that

$$F_{n+1}^2 - F_n^2 = F_{n-1}F_{n+2} \quad \text{for all } n \text{ in } \{1, 2, \ldots\}.$$

(No induction is required.)

17. A binary string $\alpha = a_1 a_2 \ldots a_n$ in B_n is said to be **unfriendly** if no two adjacent digits are 1's. That is, α is unfriendly if $a_i = 1$ and $1 < i < n$ imply that $a_{i-1} = 0 = a_{i+1}$. Let U_n be the number of unfriendly strings in B_n. Note that $U_1 = 2$ and $U_2 = 3$.
(i) Find U_3, U_4, and U_5.
(ii) Conjecture and prove a simple formula for U_n.

18. Let "unfriendly string" be as defined in Problem 17. Let $V_{n,h}$ be the number of unfriendly strings of weight h in B_n, that is, let $V_{n,h}$ be the number of unfriendly strings in $B_{n,h}$. Conjecture and prove a simple formula for $V_{n,h}$.

19. Let $S_n = L_0^2 + L_1^2 + L_2^2 + \cdots + L_n^2$. Use mathematical induction (ordinary or strong) to prove that

$$S_n = L_{2n+1} + 2 + (-1)^n \quad \text{for all } n \text{ in } N.$$

20. Let $T_n = F_0^2 + F_1^2 + \cdots + F_n^2$.
(i) Tabulate T_n for $n = 0, 1, 2, 3, 4, 5$.
(ii) Conjecture a simple formula for T_n. (This formula is simpler than the one for the analogue in Problem 19.)
(iii) Prove the conjecture true for all n in N.

21. Every rational number r is expressible in an infinite number of ways as a fraction s/t, where s and t are integers and t is positive. For example,

$$-0.75 = \frac{-75}{100} = \frac{-3}{4} = \frac{-6}{8} = \cdots.$$

Justify the assertion that the set of denominators t in these fractions must have a least integer.

22. Let Q be the set of all positive integers t for which there exists a positive integer s with $s^2 = 2t^2$.
*(i) Prove by contradiction that Q does not have a least element.
(ii) Explain why Q must be empty.
(iii) Explain why $\sqrt{2}$ is not a rational number.

SUMMARY OF TERMS, CHAPTER 4

REVIEW PROBLEMS FOR CHAPTER 4

1. Given that $13! = 6{,}227{,}020{,}800$, find $14!$.

2. Find the three smallest positive integers n for which $n! + 1$ is the square of an integer.

3. Find the six smallest positive integers n for which $n \mid [(n-1)! + 1]$.

4. Show that $n! + (n+1)! + (n+2)! = n!(n+2)^2$ for n in N.

5. Let $\#X = 9$ and $\#Y = 15$. Express the number of injective mappings from X to Y as a quotient of factorials.

6. Find the n in N such that
$$\frac{12!}{5! \cdot 7!} + \frac{12!}{6! \cdot 6!} = \frac{n!}{6! \cdot 7!}.$$

7. Give an inductive definition of
$$\sum_{j=1}^n (2j - 1), \quad \text{for } n \text{ in } Z^+.$$

8. Give an inductive definition of

$$\sum_{j=5}^{n} 3^j, \quad \text{for } n \text{ in } \{5, 6, \ldots\}.$$

9. Give an inductive definition of

$$\prod_{j=5}^{n} 3^j = 3^5 \cdot 3^6 \cdots 3^n, \quad \text{for } n \text{ in } \{5, 6, \ldots\}.$$

10. Give an inductive definition of

$$\prod_{j=1}^{n} (2j - 1) = 1 \cdot 3 \cdot 5 \cdots (2n - 1), \quad \text{for } n \text{ in } \mathbf{Z}^+.$$

11. For the arithmetic progression $1001, 1008, 1015, \ldots$, find:
    (i) the 100th term; (ii) the sum of the first 100 terms.

12. For the geometric progression $4^{1000}, 4^{999} \cdot 7, 4^{998} \cdot 7^2, \ldots$, find:
    (i) the 1001st term; (ii) the sum of the first 1001 terms.

13. Find a simple expression for

$$\sum_{j=0}^{n} (-1)^j x^{n-j} y^j.$$

14. Find a simple expression for the sum

$$x^n + x^{n-1}y + x^{n-2}y^2 + \cdots + xy^{n-1} + y^n.$$

15. Prove by mathematical induction that

$$F_0 + F_2 + \cdots + F_{2n} = F_{2n+1} - 1 \quad \text{for } n \text{ in } \mathbf{N} = \{0, 1, \ldots\}.$$

    Here, $F_0, F_1, \ldots$ is the Fibonacci Sequence.

16. Prove that $L_0^2 + L_1^2 + \cdots + L_n^2 = 2 + L_n L_{n+1}$ for n in $\mathbf{N}$. Here $L_0, L_1, \ldots$ is the Lucas Sequence.

17. Prove that $0^2 + 1^2 + 2^2 + \cdots + n^2 = n(n + 1)(2n + 1)/6$ for n in $\mathbf{N}$.

18. Prove that $0^3 + 1^3 + 2^3 + \cdots + n^3 = [n(n + 1)/2]^2$ for n in $\mathbf{N}$.

19. Label each of the following assertions as True or False. If False, give a counterexample. If True, justify the assertion.
    (a) $(m + n)! = m! + n!$ for all m and n in $\mathbf{N}$.
    (b) $(m + n)!/m! \cdot n!$ is an integer for all m and n in $\mathbf{N}$.
    (c) $\binom{2n}{2} = 2n^2 - n$ for all n in $\mathbf{Z}^+ = \{1, 2, \ldots\}$.

20. (a) Show that

$$(2n)! = n! \cdot 2^n \prod_{j=1}^{n} (2j - 1).$$

    (b) Prove by mathematical induction on n that

$$\prod_{j=1}^{n} (2j - 1) = \frac{(2n)!}{n! \cdot 2^n}.$$

21. Let $a_n = n(n + 1)$ and let $b_n = n(n^2 + 5)$.
   (i) Explain why a_n is an even integer for all n in N.
   (ii) Show that $b_{k+1} - b_k = 3a_k + 6$ for all k in N.
   (iii) Explain why $6|(b_{k+1} - b_k)$ for all k in N.
   (iv) Prove by induction on n that $6|b_n$ for all n in N.

22. Let

$$S_n = \frac{1}{1 \cdot 4} + \frac{1}{4 \cdot 7} + \frac{1}{7 \cdot 10} + \cdots + \frac{1}{(3n - 2)(3n + 1)}.$$

   (i) Compute S_n for $n = 1, 2, 3, 4,$ and 5.
   (ii) Conjecture a simple formula for S_n.
   (iii) Prove that the formula of Part (ii) is true for all n in Z^+.

23. Show that $a_1, a_2, \ldots$ is an arithmetic progression if and only if
   $a_{n+2} - 2a_{n+1} + a_n = 0$ for all n in Z^+.

24. Show that $b_1, b_2, \ldots$ is a geometric progression if and only if $b_{n+2}b_n = b_{n+1}^2$ for all n in Z^+.

25. Show that kr^a, kr^b, and kr^c are three consecutive terms of a geometric progression if and only if $a, b,$ and c are three consecutive terms of an arithmetic progression.

26. Prove that $2^n < \binom{2n}{n} < 4^n$ for n in $\{2, 3, \ldots\}$.

27. Let $F_0, F_1, \ldots$ and $L_0, L_1, \ldots$ be the Fibonacci Sequence and the Lucas Sequence, respectively. Prove the following by strong induction.
   (a) $F_n < 2^n$ for n in N.   (b) $L_n < 2^n$ for n in Z^+.

28. Let $a_n = 3^n + 7^n + 6$. Prove that:
   (i) $8|(a_h - a_{h-2})$ for h in $\{2, 3, \ldots\}$.
   (ii) $8|a_n$ for n in N. (Use strong induction.)

29. Explain why $\binom{n}{4} = n(n - 1)(n - 2)(n - 3)/24$ for $n = 4, 5, \ldots$.

30. Explain why $\binom{n}{5} = n(n - 1)(n - 2)(n - 3)(n - 4)/120$ for $n = 5, 6, \ldots$.

SUPPLEMENTARY AND CHALLENGING PROBLEMS, CHAPTER 4

1. (i) Show that

$$\sum_{j=0}^{n} j = \frac{n(n + 1)}{2} \quad \text{for } n \text{ in } N.$$

(ii) Show that

$$\sum_{j=0}^{n} j(n - j) = \frac{n(n^2 - 1)}{6} = \binom{n + 1}{3} \quad \text{for } n \text{ in } \{2, 3, \ldots\}.$$

2. Assume that $3k^2 + 3k + 1 < k^3$ for k in $\{4, 5, 6, \ldots\}$ and prove that $n^3 < 2^n$ for n in $\{10, 11, 12, \ldots\}$.

3. Explain why:

    (i) $\sqrt{n} - \sqrt{n-1} = \dfrac{1}{\sqrt{n} + \sqrt{n-1}} < \dfrac{1}{\sqrt{n}}$ for n in $\{2, 3, \ldots\}$.

    (ii) $\sqrt{n} < \dfrac{1}{\sqrt{1}} + \dfrac{1}{\sqrt{2}} + \dfrac{1}{\sqrt{3}} + \cdots + \dfrac{1}{\sqrt{n}}$ for n in $\{2, 3, \ldots\}$.

4. Let $F_0, F_1, \ldots$ and $L_0, L_1, \ldots$ be the Fibonacci Sequence and the Lucas Sequence, respectively. Prove the following for m and n in N:
    (a) $F_{m+2n} - L_n F_{m+n} + (-1)^n F_m = 0$.
    (b) $\binom{n}{0}F_m + \binom{n}{1}F_{m+1} + \binom{n}{2}F_{m+2} + \cdots + \binom{n}{n}F_{m+n} = F_{m+2n}$.
    (c) $\binom{2n}{0} + \binom{2n-1}{1} + \binom{2n-2}{2} + \cdots + \binom{n}{n} = F_{2n+1}$ and
    $\binom{2n+1}{0} + \binom{2n}{1} + \binom{2n-1}{2} + \cdots + \binom{n+1}{n} = F_{2n+2}$.

5. For n in Z^+ and k in $\{0, 1, \ldots, 2n\}$, let $T_{n,k}$ be the set of all strings $\alpha = a_1 a_2 \ldots a_n$ (of length n) with each digit a_i in $\{0, 1, 2\}$ and with wgt $\alpha = a_1 + a_2 + \cdots + a_n = k$. Let $\# T_{n,k}$ be denoted as $\begin{bmatrix} n \\ k \end{bmatrix}$. Prove the following for all n in Z^+:
    (a) $\begin{bmatrix} n \\ 0 \end{bmatrix} + \begin{bmatrix} n \\ 1 \end{bmatrix}x + \begin{bmatrix} n \\ 2 \end{bmatrix}x^2 + \cdots + \begin{bmatrix} n \\ 2n \end{bmatrix}x^{2n} = (1 + x + x^2)^n$.
    (b) $\begin{bmatrix} n \\ n \end{bmatrix}$ is an odd integer.

6. Let $\begin{bmatrix} n \\ k \end{bmatrix}$ be as in Problem 5. Conjecture and prove a simple formula for $E_n = \begin{bmatrix} n \\ 0 \end{bmatrix} + \begin{bmatrix} n \\ 2 \end{bmatrix} + \begin{bmatrix} n \\ 4 \end{bmatrix} + \cdots + \begin{bmatrix} n \\ 2n \end{bmatrix}$.

5

COMBINATORIAL PRINCIPLES

Computers perform arithmetic operations very rapidly, and more rapid computers are continually being designed. However, for any computer—no matter how speedy—one could write an infinite number of programs each of which would require more than a lifetime to complete. Thus it is important to be able not only to estimate the time needed to execute a given program but also to determine which of several programs for the same project can be carried out in the least amount of time. Such abilities are enhanced by facility with combinatorial principles (that is, advanced counting techniques). For example, in Section 10.2 we will describe two algorithms for solving n first-degree equations in n unknowns. Our combinatorial analyses will show that when $n = 24$, one of these algorithms requires many lifetimes to execute, whereas the other can be carried out in seconds.

The present chapter deals with basic combinatorial principles. Then in Chapter 9 we will show how to obtain explicit formulas for the nth term of a sequence satisfying any of certain types of recursion relations; one principal application of such solving of recursions is to combinatorial problems.

5.1

SUM AND PRODUCT RULES

Let a finite set X be partitioned into k subsets $A_1, A_2, \ldots, A_k$. That is, let the A_i be pairwise disjoint sets whose union is X. We saw in Theorem 1 of Section 1.7 ("Size of a Union of Pairwise Disjoint Finite Sets") that

$$\# X = \# A_1 + \# A_2 + \cdots + \# A_k.$$

Here we restate this in the language of combinatorics (and probability). We start with the case of $k = 2$.

THEOREM 1   SUM RULE

> If an event A can occur in m ways and event B can occur in n disjoint ways, then the event (A or B) can occur in $m + n$ ways.

The word *disjoint* in Theorem 1 is meant to imply that an occurrence of event A is not simultaneously an occurrence of event B. The following two examples help us differentiate between cases in which the sum rule applies and those in which it does not.

Example 1   The intercity transportation to and from Middletown consists of four bus lines and fifteen airlines. Thus the total number of intercity transportation lines serving Middletown is $4 + 15 = 19$. This is a case where the sum rule applies. □

Example 2   Let D be the set $\{1, 2, 3, 4, 5, 6, 7, 8, 9\}$ of digits. Let E be the subset $\{2, 4, 6, 8\}$ of even integers in D and let $P = \{2, 3, 5, 7\}$ be the subset of primes in D. Although $\#E = 4$ and $\#P = 4$, the number of integers in D that are either even or prime is *not* $4 + 4$, since E and P have the integer 2 in common. In the language of Theorem 1, we can let A be the event of choosing an integer from E and B be the event of choosing an integer from P. Then (A or B) is the event of choosing an integer from $E \cup P$. However, this is a case where the sum rule does *not* apply, since these events A and B are not disjoint—that is, $E \cap P$ is not empty. □

Again we let $A_1, A_2, \ldots, A_k$ be pairwise disjoint sets; we now restate the formula

$$\#(A_1 \cup A_2 \cup \cdots \cup A_k) = \#A_1 + \#A_2 + \cdots + \#A_k$$

for general k in the language of combinatorics (and probability).

THEOREM 2   GENERAL SUM RULE

> Let events $A_1, A_2, \ldots, A_m$ be pairwise disjoint. For $i = 1, 2, \ldots, m$, let there be n_i ways in which A_i can occur. Then
>
> $$A_1 \quad \text{or} \quad A_2 \quad \text{or} \quad \ldots \quad \text{or} \quad A_m$$
>
> can occur in $n_1 + n_2 + \cdots + n_m$ ways.

Example 3   **INJECTIONS FOR CODES**   Here we apply the general sum rule to a combinatorial problem involved in creating codes such as the Morse Code. This example is related to Example 11 and Problem 35 of Section 1.8. Let

$A = \{a, b, \ldots, z\}$ be the English alphabet, let $D = \{0, 1, \ldots, 9\}$ be the set of decimal digits, and let $S = A \cup D$. Since A and D are disjoint,

$$\#S = \#(A \cup D) = \#A + \#D = 26 + 10 = 36.$$

The Morse Code assigns a different short string (word) over the alphabet $\{\cdot, -\}$ to each of the thirty-six elements of S. It is convenient to replace the two symbols of the Morse Code with the bits 0 and 1. Thus our code will assign distinct bit strings to distinct elements of S. This is done by an injective mapping from S into

$$C_n = B_1 \cup B_2 \cup \cdots \cup B_n$$

for some well-chosen positive integer n. The mapping must be injective because distinct symbols in S should have distinct representatives. Thus we must have $36 = \#S \le \#C_n$ in order to have enough strings. The sets $B_1, B_2, \ldots$ are pairwise disjoint, so

$$\#C_n = \#(B_1 \cup B_2 \cup \cdots \cup B_n) = \#B_1 + \#B_2 + \cdots + \#B_n.$$

We know that $\#B_k = 2^k$. Hence $\#C_n$ is the sum of the geometric progression $2 + 2^2 + \cdots + 2^n$. Using the technique of Example 4 in Section 4.1 or the formula of Problem 2 of Section 4.2, we find that $\#C_n = 2^{n+1} - 2$. Therefore, we want the smallest n with

$$36 \le 2^{n+1} - 2,$$

that is, with $38 \le 2^{n+1}$. Since $2^5 = 32$ and $2^6 = 64$, we have $n + 1 = 6$, or $n = 5$.   □

Example 4   A store stocks shirts in 7 neck sizes. For each neck size, there are 3 sleeve sizes, as shown in the following table (n is neck size and s is sleeve size):

n	14	$14\frac{1}{2}$	15	$15\frac{1}{2}$	16	$16\frac{1}{2}$	17
s	30, 31, 32	31, 32, 33	31, 32, 33	32, 33, 34	33, 34, 35	34, 35, 36	35, 36, 37

Let C be the set of the ordered pairs $(n, s) = $ (neck size, sleeve size) for shirts in stock. Let C_1 be the subset of (n, s) in C with $n = 14$, C_2 be the subset with $n = 14\frac{1}{2}, \ldots, C_7$ be the subset with $n = 17$. Then $C_1, C_2, \ldots, C_7$ partition C, and so

$$\#C = \#C_1 + \#C_2 + \cdots + \#C_7 = 7 \cdot 3 = 21.$$

That is, there are 21 choices of neck and sleeve sizes in stock.   □

This illustrates the general sum rule, with $m = 7$ and each $n_i = 3$. Theorem 2 for general m but with each n_i equal to n is stated in the language of combinatorics (or probability) in the following theorem.

THEOREM 3 **PRODUCT RULE**

If an event A can occur in m ways and each possibility for A allows exactly n ways for an event B to occur, then the event (A and B) can occur in mn ways.

Example 5 How many two-digit numbers are there for which the sum of the digits is even? We find the answer as follows: The left-hand digit x comes from the set $\{1, 2, \ldots, 9\}$ and so can be chosen in 9 ways. If x is even, the right-hand digit y must be in $\{0, 2, 4, 6, 8\}$. If x is odd, then y must come from $\{1, 3, 5, 7, 9\}$. Each of the 9 possible choices for x permits 5 choices for y, so by the product rule, there are $9 \cdot 5 = 45$ such numbers. □

Next we generalize the product rule by considering any finite number of events.

THEOREM 4 **GENERAL PRODUCT RULE**

Let $A_1, A_2, \ldots, A_k$ be events. Let there be n_1 ways for A_1 to occur. For each way that A_1 can occur let there be n_2 ways for A_2 to occur. For each way that A_1 and A_2 can occur, let there be n_3 ways for A_3 to occur, and so on. Then $(A_1 \wedge A_2 \wedge \cdots \wedge A_k)$ can occur in $n_1 n_2 \cdots n_k$ ways.

Example 6 Here we illustrate the general product rule by assuming that the store of Example 4 has each neck and sleeve size available in 4 colors. By the general product rule, the store has $7 \cdot 3 \cdot 4 = 84$ shirt types in stock. □

Example 7 **TIME REQUIRED TO RUN A COMPUTER PROGRAM** This example will be used in Section 10.2 in a combinatorial analysis of an algorithm for solving n first-degree equations in n unknowns. The present problem is to determine how many years it would take a computer to do 10^{25} multiplications at the rate of 10^9 multiplications per second. First we find the number of seconds in a year. We take a year to have 365 days. Each day has 24 hours, each hour has 60 minutes, and each minute has 60 seconds. Hence it follows from the general product rule that there are

$$365 \cdot 24 \cdot 60 \cdot 60 = 31536000 = 3.1536 \times 10^7$$

seconds in a year. At the rate of 10^9 multiplications per second, the computer would accomplish $(3.1536 \times 10^7) \times 10^9 = 3.1536 \times 10^{16}$ multiplications per year. Thus it would take $10^{25}/(3.1536 \times 10^{16}) = 10^9/3.1536$ years to perform 10^{25} multiplications—that is, more than 300 million years! □

Example 8   **NUMBER OF LICENSE PLATES**   A certain state indicates the year of registration on auto license plates with stickers and so can manufacture plates for an extended period. How many plates can be made if each is identified by three letters followed by three digits? In other words, how many 6-tuples $(L_1, L_2, L_3, d_1, d_2, d_3)$ are there with 26 choices for each letter L_i and 10 choices for each digit d_j? Using the general product rule, one finds that the answer is $26 \cdot 26 \cdot 26 \cdot 10 \cdot 10 \cdot 10 = 17576000$.   □

Example 9   **APPLICATION TO "TRUTH IN ADVERTISING"**   A fast-food emporium advertises that it will prepare a hamburger to your order in any one of over 2500 different ways. What it actually does is give the customer the following choices: (i) seeded or unseeded bun, (ii) toasted or untoasted bun, (iii) any subset of

   {tomato, lettuce, pickle, onion, relish, chili, coleslaw},

and (iv) at most one item from the set

   {mayonnaise, margarine, catsup, mustard}.

We note that there are 2 choices in (i), 2 choices in (ii), $2^7 = 128$ subsets in (iii), and 5 choices in (iv), including the choice "none of these." By the general product rule, the total number of variations is $2 \cdot 2 \cdot 128 \cdot 5 = 2560$. Thus their claim is valid, even if it sounds grander than it is.   □

A permutation on a set X is a bijective mapping from X to itself. (See Definition 5 of Section 1.8, "Bijection, Permutation.") Now we define a related concept that also uses the word *permutation*.

DEFINITION 1   ***k*-PERMUTATION FROM *X***

A ***k-permutation*** from a set X is a sequence $x_1, x_2, \ldots, x_k$ of k distinct elements of X.

If one changes the order of appearance of the terms of a k-permutation from X, one obtains a new k-permutation. We note that the k-permutation $x_1, x_2, \ldots, x_k$ becomes the listing $\{x_1, x_2, \ldots, x_k\}$ of a subset of size k from X if one encloses all the terms in a set of braces.

Example 10   The 3-permutations from $X = \{1, 2, 3, 4\}$ are the following 24 sequences x_1, x_2, x_3:

1, 2, 3;	1, 2, 4;	1, 3, 2;	1, 3, 4;	1, 4, 2;	1, 4, 3;
2, 1, 3;	2, 1, 4;	2, 3, 1;	2, 3, 4;	2, 4, 1;	2, 4, 3;
3, 1, 2;	3, 1, 4;	3, 2, 1;	3, 2, 4;	3, 4, 1;	3, 4, 2;
4, 1, 2;	4, 1, 3;	4, 2, 1;	4, 2, 3;	4, 3, 1;	4, 3, 2.

In a 3-permutation x_1, x_2, x_3 from X, there are 4 choices for x_1. For a fixed x_1 there are 3 choices for x_2, since x_2 must not equal x_1. Having chosen x_1 and x_2, there are then 2 choices for x_3, since $x_3 \neq x_1$ and $x_3 \neq x_2$. Thus, by the general product rule, there are $4 \cdot 3 \cdot 2 = 24$ such sequences, as we have already seen. □

The following example illustrates the relationship of n-permutations from a set X of size n to permutations on X.

Example 11 Let $X = \{1, 2, 3, 4\}$. Then a permutation f on X is a bijective mapping

$$f: X \rightarrow X; \quad 1 \mapsto x_1, \quad 2 \mapsto x_2, \quad 3 \mapsto x_3, \quad 4 \mapsto x_4.$$

This mapping f is characterized completely by the listing of the four elements of X as the sequence x_1, x_2, x_3, x_4; that is, a permutation f on a set X of size 4 is essentially a 4-permutation from X. □

THEOREM 5 **NUMBER OF k-PERMUTATIONS**

Let $\# X = n$ and $k \in \{1, 2, \ldots, n\}$. Then the number of k-permutations from X is

$$n(n - 1)(n - 2) \cdots (n - k + 1).$$

PROOF As in Example 10, for a k-permutation $x_1, x_2, \ldots, x_k$ from X, there are n choices for x_1, then $n - 1$ choices for x_2, $n - 2$ choices for $x_3, \ldots$, $n - k + 1$ choices for x_k. Now the desired formula follows from the general product rule. □

NOTATION 1 **$P(n, k)$**

Let $n \in \mathbf{Z}^+$ and $k \in \{1, 2, \ldots, n\}$. Then $P(n, k)$ denotes the number of k-permutations from a set of size n.

Theorem 5 restated in this notation says that

$$P(n, k) = n(n - 1)(n - 2) \cdots (n - k + 1).$$

For example, the number of 3-permutations from a set of size 15 is $P(15, 3) = 15 \cdot 14 \cdot 13$.

Example 12 How many ways are there to select a president, a secretary, and a treasurer as 3 distinct people from a committee of 15 people? The president can be any one of the 15 people, the secretary can be any one of them except the president, and the treasurer can be anyone different from the 2 selected for the other offices. Thus the answer is $P(15, 3) = 15 \cdot 14 \cdot 13 = 2730$.   □

Example 13   Here we determine the number of arrangements of 3 women and 3 men in a queue (waiting line) in which men and women alternate. Such an arrangement is of one of the following two forms:

$$w_1, m_1, w_2, m_2, w_3, m_3 \quad \text{or} \quad m_1, w_1, m_2, w_2, m_3, w_3.$$

Using the general product rule, we see that there are $3 \cdot 3 \cdot 2 \cdot 2 \cdot 1 \cdot 1 = 36$ arrangements of the first type, since w_1 can be any one of the 3 women, m_1 can be any one of the 3 men, w_2 can be any of the women different from w_1, and so on. Since there also are 36 arrangements of the second type and no arrangement is simultaneously of both types, the sum rule tells us that the total number of arrangements is $36 + 36 = 72$.   □

So far in this section we have discussed linear permutations, that is, arrangements of objects along a straight line. Now we take up arrangements along a circle.

Example 14   In Figure 5.1.1, the elements of $X = \{1, 2, 3, 4, 5\}$ are placed along a circle. This placement determines the mapping $f : X \to X$ in which $f(x)$ is the element of X immediately after x as one traverses the circle counterclockwise. One sees from Figure 5.1.1 that

$$f : 1 \mapsto 3, \quad 2 \mapsto 5, \quad 3 \mapsto 4, \quad 4 \mapsto 2, \quad 5 \mapsto 1,$$

which helps us see that f is a permutation on $X = \{1, 2, 3, 4, 5\}$; that is, f is a bijection from X onto itself.   □

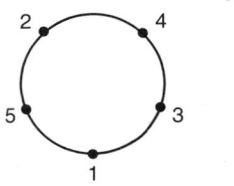

FIGURE 5.1.1

DEFINITION 2   CIRCULAR PERMUTATION

A *circular permutation* on a finite set X is a permutation f with the property that the elements of X can be arranged around a circle so that each x in X is immediately followed by $f(x)$ in counterclockwise traversal of the circle.

We saw in Example 14 that the permutation

$$f : 1 \mapsto 3, \quad 2 \mapsto 5, \quad 3 \mapsto 4, \quad 4 \mapsto 2, \quad 5 \mapsto 1$$

is a circular permutation on $X = \{1, 2, 3, 4, 5\}$. The permutation

$$g : 1 \mapsto 2, \quad 2 \mapsto 3, \quad 3 \mapsto 1, \quad 4 \mapsto 5, \quad 5 \mapsto 4$$

is not a circular permutation on this X because it does not satisfy the condition stated in Definition 2.

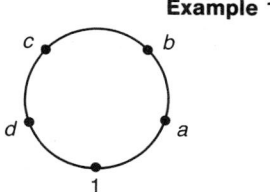

FIGURE 5.1.2

Example 15 How many circular permutations are there on the set $X = \{1, 2, 3, 4, 5\}$? Figure 5.1.2 represents any circular permutation on X where a can be any element of X except 1, b can be any element of X different from 1 and a, and so on. Thus the number of circular permutations on X is $4 \cdot 3 \cdot 2 \cdot 1 = 24$. The generalization to sets X of size n is found in Problem 12 below. ☐

PROBLEMS FOR SECTION 5.1

1. In a World Series, a team from the National League (which currently has 12 teams) competes against a team from the American League (which has 14 teams). No team is in both leagues.
   (a) How many teams have the possibility of winning the World Series?
   (b) At the beginning of the year's competition, how many possibilities are there for the pair of teams that will compete in the next World Series?

2. At a certain point in a primary election campaign there are 3 Democratic and 7 Republican candidates for president.
   (a) Assuming that the president elected will be one of these candidates, how many possibilities are there for the eventual winner of the presidency?
   (b) How many possibilities are there for the pair of candidates who will run against one another in the general election?

3. Let B_n be the set of n-bit strings.
   (i) Are the sets of $B_1, B_2, \ldots$ pairwise disjoint?
   (ii) Let $f_n = \#(B_1 \cup B_2 \cup \cdots \cup B_n)$. Tabulate f_n for $n = 1, 2, 3, 4$.
   (iii) Find the smallest n such that $f_n \geq 50$.
   (iv) Find the smallest n such that $f_n \geq 70$.

4. Let $\#S = 60$. What is the smallest n for which there is an injection from S into the union $B_1 \cup B_2 \cup \cdots \cup B_n$?

5. (a) How many three-digit numbers (that is, integers in $\{100, 101, \ldots, 999\}$) are there with the sum of digits even?
   (b) Do Part (a) with *even* replaced by *odd*.

6. Do Problem 5 for four-digit numbers rather than three-digit numbers.

7. Let $\#A = 10$.
   (i) How many sequences a_1, a_2, a_3 of three terms are there with each a_i in A?
   (ii) Of the sequences for Part (i), how many have the a_i distinct?
   (iii) How many mappings are there from $\{1, 2, 3\}$ into A?
   (iv) Of the mappings for Part (iii), how many are injective?

8. Let A be an alphabet with $\#A = 36$.
   (i) How many words $a_1a_2a_3a_4$ of length 4 are there with each a_i in A?
   (ii) Of the words for Part (i), how many have no repetitions among the a_i?
   (iii) How many mappings are there from $\{1, 2, 3, 4\}$ into A?
   (iv) Of the mappings for Part (iii), how many are injective?
   (v) Which of the previous parts have an answer equal to $P(36, 4)$?

9. In how many ways can one select a president and vice-president from the members of a committee of 9 men and 11 women if one of these officers must be a woman and the other a man?

10. How many 9-permutations are there from $D = \{1, 2, \ldots, 9\}$ in which odd and even integers alternate?

11. How many circular permutations are there on a set of size 10?

12. How many circular permutations are there on a set of size n?

13. Find:
   (a) $P(100, 1)$;   (b) $P(100, 2)$;   (c) $P(100, 3)$.

14. Express as a factorial:
   (a) $P(100, 100)$;   (b) $P(100, 99)$.

15. Express as a ratio of factorials:
   (a) $P(100, 98)$;   (b) $P(100, 3)$.

16. Express as a ratio of factorials:
   (a) $P(100, 97)$;   (b) $P(100, 4)$.

17. Let k and n be integers with $1 \le k \le n$. Express as a ratio of factorials:
   (a) $P(n, n - k)$;   (b) $P(n, k)$.

18. Does $P(n, n) = P(n, n - 1)$ for $n \ge 2$? Explain.

19. Let $\#A = n$. Is the number of n-permutations from A equal to the number of bijections from A to itself? Explain.

20. Is $P(n, k)$ equal to the number of injections from a set of size k into a set of size n? Explain.

21. How many 7-ary boolean functions are there? That is, how many mappings are there from the set B_7 of 7-digit binary strings into $\{0, 1\}$?

22. How many n-ary boolean functions are there?

23. Let X be a set of $2n$ people composed of n couples. Let M_n be the number of circular permutations on X (e.g., seatings at a round dinner table) in which women and men alternate and no person is placed next to his or her spouse. Find M_3.

24. Let M_n be as in Problem 23. Find M_4.

25. Let M_n be as in Problem 23. Prove that M_n is an even integer for $n \ge 3$.

26. A telephone number, including area code, is essentially a 10-digit string $d_1d_2 \ldots d_{10}$ with each d_i in $\{1, 2, \ldots, 9, 0\}$ and with the following restrictions on the digits: (I) None of the digits d_1, d_4, d_5 is 0 or 1; (II) d_2 is either 0 or 1. How many such telephone numbers are there?

27. How many bit strings $a_1 a_2 \ldots a_n$ are there in B_n with $a_1 + a_2 + \cdots + a_n$ an even integer? That is, how many strings α does B_n have with wgt α even?

*28. Let C_n be the set of n-digit **ternary strings** γ, that is, of strings $\gamma = c_1 c_2 \ldots c_n$ with c_i in $\{0, 1, 2\}$. How many of these strings have $c_1 + c_2 + \cdots + c_n$ an even integer?

5.2

BINOMIAL AND MULTINOMIAL EXPANSIONS

Frequently, when all the numbers appearing in an equation are positive integers, those numbers have combinatorial significance; that is, the positive integers are the sizes of certain sets. A good example is the binomial expansion formula

$$(a + b)^n = \binom{n}{0} a^n + \binom{n}{1} a^{n-1}b + \binom{n}{2} a^{n-2}b^2 +$$

$$\cdots + \binom{n}{n-1} ab^{n-1} + \binom{n}{n} b^n$$

(which is proved in upcoming Theorem 1). We recall from Section 1.1 that $\binom{n}{k}$ is the number of subsets of size k from a set of size n. More specifically, $\binom{n}{k}$ is the size of the set $B_{n,k}$ of n-digit binary strings $a_1 a_2 \ldots a_n$ in which $a_i = 1$ for exactly k values of i.

The $\binom{n}{k}$ are called **binomial coefficients** because, for fixed n, they are the coefficients of the terms in the expansion of the nth power of a binomial (that is, two-term expression). One reads $\binom{n}{k}$ as "n choose k" because it is the number of ways of choosing k elements from a set of n elements.

We next give some concrete illustrations of the concepts we will use in proving Theorem 1.

Example 1 Using distributivity of multiplication over addition, we find that

$$(a_1 + b_1)(a_2 + b_2)(a_3 + b_3) = a_1 a_2 a_3 + a_1 a_2 b_3 + a_1 b_2 a_3 + b_1 a_2 a_3 + a_1 b_2 b_3 + b_1 a_2 b_3 + b_1 b_2 a_3 + b_1 b_2 b_3. \quad (1)$$

The right-hand side of Equation (1) is the sum of all triple products $f_1 f_2 f_3$ in which f_i is either a_i or b_i. If we let each $a_i = a$ and each $b_i = b$ in Equation (1), then it becomes

$$(a + b)^3 = a^3 + 3a^2 b + 3ab^2 + b^3. \quad (2)$$

The coefficient of the term $3ab^2$ is 3 because there are $\binom{3}{2} = 3$ ways to choose 2 of the f_i in $f_1 f_2 f_3$ to be b (and the other f_i to be a). Also, the coefficient of the term b^3 is 1 because there is only $\binom{3}{3} = 1$ way to choose each of the three f_i to be b in $f_1 f_2 f_3$. The other coefficients in Equation (2) have similar combinatorial meaning, and thus Equation (2) can be rewritten as

$$(a + b)^3 = \binom{3}{0} a^3 + \binom{3}{1} a^2 b + \binom{3}{2} ab^2 + \binom{3}{3} b^3. \tag{3}$$

The following result generalizes this formula.   □

THEOREM 1   **BINOMIAL EXPANSION**

For n in $\mathbf{Z}^+$,

$$(a + b)^n = \binom{n}{0} a^n + \binom{n}{1} a^{n-1} b + \binom{n}{2} a^{n-2} b^2 +$$

$$\cdots + \binom{n}{n-1} ab^{n-1} + \binom{n}{n} b^n$$

PROOF   As in Example 1, the term $\binom{n}{k} a^{n-k} b^k$ appears in the expansion of $(a + b)^n$ because the expansion of

$$(a_1 + b_1)(a_2 + b_2) \cdots (a_n + b_n)$$

has $\binom{n}{k}$ terms of the form $f_1 f_2 \ldots f_n$ in which $f_i = b_i$ for k values of i (and $f_i = a_i$ for the remaining $n - k$ values of i). That is, the coefficient of $a^{n-k} b^k$ in the expansion of $(a + b)^n$ is the number $\binom{n}{k}$ of subsets of size k from the set $\{1, 2, \ldots, n\}$ of size n.   □

COROLLARY   **SYMMETRY FORMULA FOR $\binom{n}{k}$**

$$\binom{n}{k} = \binom{n}{n-k}.$$

PROOF   This equation follows when a and b in Theorem 1 are interchanged.   □

We give two proofs of the following theorem to illustrate two useful devices.

THEOREM 2   **SUM OF BINOMIAL COEFFICIENTS**

$$\binom{n}{0} + \binom{n}{1} + \binom{n}{2} + \cdots + \binom{n}{n} = 2^n.$$

PROOF **I.** This equation follows immediately by letting $a = b = 1$ in Theorem 1.

II. Another way of looking at this identity is a combinatorial one. Let us calculate the number of subsets of a set S of size n. The null set $\varnothing$ is the unique subset of size 0; that is, there is just $\binom{n}{0} = 1$ subset with 0 elements. There are $\binom{n}{1}$ subsets of size 1, $\binom{n}{2}$ subsets of size 2, and so on. So the total number of subsets is

$$\binom{n}{0} + \binom{n}{1} + \binom{n}{2} + \cdots + \binom{n}{n}. \tag{4}$$

But when forming a subset of S, we can consider each element of S and decide whether or not to include it in the subset. We therefore have 2 choices for each of the n elements. Since the choice for an element is independent of the choice for the other elements, the general product rule (Theorem 4) of Section 5.1 tells us that there are 2^n subsets of S. Thus the sum in Display (4) equals 2^n, and the second proof is complete. $\square$

For each n in $\{0, 1, 2, 3, 4, 5, 6\}$, Table 5.2.1 has a *row* whose entries are the binomial coefficients $\binom{n}{0}$, $\binom{n}{1}$, ..., $\binom{n}{n}$. These entries are arranged so that the numbers $\binom{k}{k}$, $\binom{k+1}{k}$, $\binom{k+2}{k}$, ... for a fixed k appear as a *diagonal* that runs to the left as it goes downward. The unending continuation of this array with a row for each n in $N = \{0, 1, \ldots\}$ is called *Pascal's Triangle*. (See the biographical note on Blaise Pascal at the end of this section.)

TABLE 5.2.1 Pascal's Triangle

n									
0					1				
1				1		1			
2			1		2		1		
3		1		3		3		1	
4	1		4		6		4		1
5	1	5		10		10		5	1
6	1	6	15		20		15	6	1

The table shows that the $\binom{6}{k}$ for $k = 0, 1, \ldots, 6$ are the numbers in the $n = 6$ row

1, 6, 15, 20, 15, 6, 1

and the $\binom{n}{2}$ for $n = 2, 3, 4, 5, 6, \ldots$ are the numbers in the $k = 2$ diagonal

1, 3, 6, 10, 15, ...

These numbers $\binom{2}{2}$, $\binom{3}{2}$, $\binom{4}{2}$, ... are called the *triangular numbers* because they are the numbers of dots in the triangles of Figure 5.2.1.

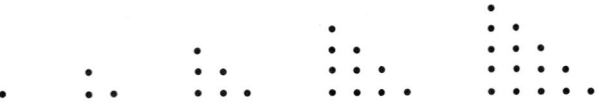

FIGURE 5.2.1

Figure 5.2.1 indicates geometrically that

$$1 + 2 + \cdots + n = \binom{n+1}{2} = \frac{n(n+1)}{2}.$$

Also, if pairs of successive triangles are placed together as in Figure 5.2.2, one sees that $\binom{n+1}{2} + \binom{n}{2} = n^2$.

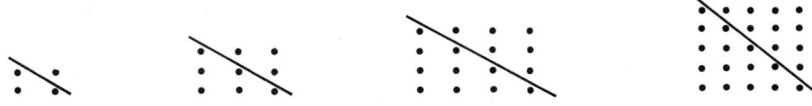

FIGURE 5.2.2

One can add additional rows to Table 5.2.1 by noting that the first and last entries on each row are 1, since $\binom{n}{0} = 1 = \binom{n}{n}$ by Theorem 2(a), "***Borders Formula***," of Section 1.1, and by using the "***Recursion Formula***"

$$\binom{n}{k} = \binom{n-1}{k} + \binom{n-1}{k-1} \quad \text{for integers with } 0 < k < n \tag{5}$$

of Theorem 2(b) of Section 1.1 to obtain additional interior entries. For example, with the help of Table 5.2.1, one sees that

$$\binom{7}{0} = 1,$$

$$\binom{7}{1} = \binom{6}{1} + \binom{6}{0} = 6 + 1 = 7,$$

$$\binom{7}{2} = \binom{6}{2} + \binom{6}{1} = 15 + 6 = 21,$$

$$\binom{7}{3} = \binom{6}{3} + \binom{6}{2} = 20 + 15 = 35.$$

Since each row of Pascal's Triangle reads the same from right to left as from left to right, these facts tell us that the row for $n = 7$ of Pascal's Triangle is

1, 7, 21, 35, 35, 21, 7, 1

and hence

$$(a + b)^7 = a^7 + 7a^6b + 21a^5b^2 + 35a^4b^3 + 35a^3b^4 + 21a^2b^5 + 7ab^6 + b^7.$$

The following result shows the relationship between the number $\binom{n}{k}$ of subsets of size k from a set of size n and the number $P(n, k)$ of k-permutations from a set of size n.

THEOREM 3   **SUBSETS AND PERMUTATIONS**

$P(n, k) = k! \dbinom{n}{k}$ for integers k and n with $1 \le k \le n$.

PROOF   One obtains all the k-permutations $x_1, x_2, \ldots, x_k$ from a set X of size n by first choosing a subset of size k from X in $\binom{n}{k}$ ways and then arranging these k elements on a line in $k!$ ways. Thus the product rule (Theorem 3) of Section 5.1 implies that $P(n, k) = k!\binom{n}{k}$. $\square$

COROLLARY $\dbinom{n}{k} = \dfrac{1}{k!} P(n, k)$ for integers k and n with $1 \le k \le n$.

Next we give a new proof of the formula of Problem 10 in Section 4.2.

THEOREM 4   **FACTORIAL FORMS OF $\binom{n}{k}$**

$$\binom{n}{k} = \frac{n(n-1)(n-2)\cdots(n-k+1)}{1 \cdot 2 \cdot 3 \cdots k} = \frac{n!}{k!(n-k)!}$$

for integers k and n with $0 \le k \le n$.

PROOF   This is true when $k = 0$ because $\binom{n}{0} = 1$ and $n!/(0!n!) = 1$. Hence we assume that $1 \le k$. In Section 5.1, we saw that

$$P(n, k) = n(n-1)(n-2)\cdots(n-k+1) = \frac{n!}{(n-k)!}.$$

Using the corollary to Theorem 3 and these formulas, we have

$$\binom{n}{k} = \frac{1}{k!} P(n, k) = \frac{n(n-1)\cdots(n-k+1)}{1 \cdot 2 \cdots k} = \frac{n!}{k!(n-k)!}.$$ $\square$

Example 2   Let k and n be integers. Here we show that:

(a) $\dbinom{n}{k} = \dfrac{n-k+1}{k} \dbinom{n}{k-1}$ for $0 < k \le n$,   (6)

(b) $\dbinom{n}{k} = \dfrac{n}{k}\dbinom{n-1}{k-1}$ for $0 < k \leq n$. $\hspace{3cm}$ (7)

Formula (a) is equivalent to

$$\frac{\dbinom{n}{k}}{\dbinom{n}{k-1}} = \frac{(n-k+1)}{k}.$$

This follows from Theorem 4, as we now show.

$$\binom{n}{k} \div \binom{n}{k-1} = \frac{n(n-1)\cdots(n-k+1)}{k(k-1)\cdots 2 \cdot 1} \div \frac{n(n-1)\cdots(n-k+2)}{(k-1)(k-2)\cdots 1}$$

$$= \frac{n-k+1}{k}.$$

This formula and the border formula $\binom{n}{0} = 1$ enable us to calculate any row of Pascal's Triangle. For example, we have

$$\binom{10}{0} = 1,$$

$$\binom{10}{1} = \frac{10-1+1}{1}\binom{10}{0} = 10,$$

$$\binom{10}{2} = \frac{10-2+1}{2}\binom{10}{1} = \frac{9}{2}\cdot 10 = 45,$$

and similarly we can find that $\binom{10}{3} = 120$, $\binom{10}{4} = 210$, and $\binom{10}{5} = 252$. Then the symmetry formula $\binom{n}{k} = \binom{n}{n-k}$ gives us

$$\binom{10}{6} = \binom{10}{4} = 210,$$

$$\binom{10}{7} = \binom{10}{3} = 120,$$

$$\binom{10}{8} = 45,$$

$$\binom{10}{9} = 10,$$

$$\binom{10}{10} = 1.$$

Theorem 4 also helps us prove Formula (b), as follows:

$$\binom{n}{k} = \frac{n!}{k!(n-k)!} = \frac{n \cdot (n-1)!}{k \cdot (k-1)!(n-k)!} = \frac{n}{k} \cdot \frac{(n-1)!}{(k-1)!(n-k)!} = \frac{n}{k}\binom{n-1}{k-1}.$$

Now we can rewrite Formula (b) as

$$k\binom{n}{k} = n\binom{n-1}{k-1},$$

which we will apply in Proof III of the following example. ☐

Example 3 **ALTERNATE PROOFS** Let $A_n = \binom{n}{1} + 2\binom{n}{2} + 3\binom{n}{3} + \cdots + n\binom{n}{n}$. We here prove, in four different ways, that $A_n = n \cdot 2^{n-1}$. Although one proof would be sufficient, each of the four techniques is useful in different contexts, and the multiple proofs show that there can be more than one approach to a given problem.

PROOF **I.** Using the binomial coefficient symmetry formula $\binom{n}{n-k} = \binom{n}{k}$ of Theorem 4(d) of Section 1.2, or the corollary to Theorem 1 above ("Binomial Expansion"), we see that

$$A_n = \binom{n}{n-1} + 2\binom{n}{n-2} + 3\binom{n}{n-3} + \cdots + n\binom{n}{0}.$$

Reversing the order of the terms on the right-hand side and also using the original expression for A_n, we have

$$A_n = n\binom{n}{0} + (n-1)\binom{n}{1} + (n-2)\binom{n}{2} + \cdots + \binom{n}{n-1}$$

$$A_n = \binom{n}{1} + 2\binom{n}{2} + \cdots + (n-1)\binom{n}{n-1} + n\binom{n}{n}.$$

Adding these equations gives us

$$2A_n = n\left[\binom{n}{0} + \binom{n}{1} + \binom{n}{2} + \cdots + \binom{n}{n}\right].$$

Then $2A_n = n \cdot 2^n$ by Theorem 2 ("Sum of Binomial Coefficients"), and so $A_n = n \cdot 2^n/2 = n \cdot 2^{n-1}$.

PROOF **II.** This method uses calculus. Letting $a = 1$ and $b = x$ in Theorem 1 ("Binomial Expansion"), we have

$$(1 + x)^n = \binom{n}{0} + \binom{n}{1}x + \binom{n}{2}x^2 + \cdots + \binom{n}{n}x^n.$$

Differentiating with respect to x results in

$$n(1 + x)^{n-1} = \binom{n}{1} + 2\binom{n}{2}x + 3\binom{n}{3}x^2 + \cdots + n\binom{n}{n}x^{n-1}.$$

We let $x = 1$ and get the desired $n \cdot 2^{n-1} = A_n$.

PROOF   **III.**   Using the formula

$$k\binom{n}{k} = n\binom{n-1}{k-1},$$

from Example 2 (with $k = 1, 2, \ldots, n$), we get

$$\binom{n}{1} = n\binom{n-1}{0},$$

$$2\binom{n}{2} = n\binom{n-1}{1},$$

$$3\binom{n}{3} = n\binom{n-1}{2},$$

$$\vdots$$

$$n\binom{n}{n} = n\binom{n-1}{n-1}.$$

Substituting these into the original A_n leads to

$$A_n = n\binom{n-1}{0} + n\binom{n-1}{1} + n\binom{n-1}{2} + \cdots + n\binom{n-1}{n-1}$$

$$= n\left[\binom{n-1}{0} + \binom{n-1}{1} + \cdots + \binom{n-1}{n-1}\right].$$

Theorem 2, "Sum of Binomial Coefficients," with n replaced by $n - 1$, shows that the sum in the brackets equals 2^{n-1}, thus $A_n = n \cdot 2^{n-1}$.

PROOF   **IV.**   Let X be a set of size n, $P(X)$ be its power set, and Q_n be the sum of the sizes of all the members of $P(X)$, that is, of all the subsets of X. We note that X has $\binom{n}{0} = 1$ subset of size 0, $\binom{n}{1}$ subsets of size 1, $\binom{n}{2}$ subsets of size 2, and so on. Therefore the sum Q_n of the sizes of the 2^n subsets of X is

$$\binom{n}{0} \cdot 0 + \binom{n}{1} \cdot 1 + \binom{n}{2} \cdot 2 + \cdots + \binom{n}{n} \cdot n.$$

That is, $Q_n = A_n$. But we can think of $P(X)$ as being partitioned into 2^{n-1} pairs $\{S, \bar{S}\}$, where $\bar{S}$ is the complement of S in X. For each pair, $\#S + \#\bar{S} = n$ because $S \cup \bar{S} = X$ and $S \cap \bar{S} = \emptyset$. As there are 2^{n-1}

such pairs, the sum Q_n (or A_n) of the sizes of all 2^n subsets of X is $2^{n-1} \cdot n$. Thus $A_n = 2^{n-1} \cdot n$. □

Example 4 Here we expand $(x + y + z)^3$. Letting $a = x + y$ and using the binomial expansion, we have

$$(x + y + z)^3 = (a + z)^3 = a^3 + 3a^2z + 3az^2 + z^3$$
$$= (x + y)^3 + 3(x + y)^2z + 3(x + y)z^2 + z^3$$
$$= x^3 + 3x^2y + 3xy^2 + y^3 + 3(x^2 + 2xy + y^2)z + 3xz^2 + 3yz^2 + z^3$$
$$= x^3 + 3x^2y + 3xy^2 + y^3 + 3x^2z + 6xyz + 3y^2z + 3xz^2 + 3yz^2 + z^3$$
$$= x^3 + y^3 + z^3 + 3x^2y + 3x^2z + 3xy^2 + 3xz^2 + 3y^2z + 3yz^2 + 6xyz.$$

□

Example 5 Now we find the coefficient c of the term $cx^3y^5z^4$ in the expansion of $(x + y + z)^{12}$. The technique of Example 4 shows that the desired term can be obtained by letting $n = 12$, $a = x + y$, and $b = z$ in Theorem 1, "Binomial Expansion"; then c is also the coefficient of the term $cx^3y^5z^4$ in the expansion of

$$\binom{12}{4}(x + y)^8 z^4.$$

Using the binomial expansion of $(x + y)^8$ we find that the term we are interested in is $\binom{12}{4}\binom{8}{5}x^3y^5z^4$, and so $c = \binom{12}{4}\binom{8}{5}$.

Alternatively, we can let $a = x$ and $b = y + z$ in Theorem 1 and see that the desired term is the term $cx^3y^5z^4$ in the expansion of $\binom{12}{9}x^3(y + z)^9$. Expanding $(y + z)^9$, we find that this term is $\binom{12}{9}\binom{9}{4}x^3y^5z^4$; hence c can also be written as $\binom{12}{9}\binom{9}{4}$.

With the help of Theorem 4, "Factorial Forms of $\binom{n}{k}$," we see that

$$c = \binom{12}{4}\binom{8}{5} = \frac{12!}{4! \cdot 8!} \cdot \frac{8!}{5! \cdot 3!} = \frac{12!}{3! \cdot 5! \cdot 4!}.$$

□

Example 5 illustrates the following general result.

THEOREM 5 MULTINOMIAL EXPANSION

(i) Let $m = e_1 + e_2 + \cdots + e_n$ with each e_i in $N = \{0, 1, \ldots\}$. Then the coefficient of

$$(x_1)^{e_1}(x_2)^{e_2} \cdots (x_n)^{e_n}$$

in the expansion of $(x_1 + x_2 + \cdots + x_n)^m$ is

$$\frac{m!}{e_1!e_2! \cdots e_n!}$$

(ii) $(x_1 + x_2 + \cdots + x_n)^m = \sum \dfrac{m!}{e_1!e_2!\cdots e_n!}(x_1)^{e_1}(x_2)^{e_2}\cdots(x_n)^{e_n},$

where the sum on the right is over all ordered n-tuples $(e_1, e_2, \ldots, e_n)$ of nonnegative integers e_i with $e_1 + e_2 + \cdots + e_n = m$.

The basis step $n = 2$ of a proof by induction on n is Theorem 1, "Binomial Expansion." The inductive step is left to the reader.

Example 6   Here we find a compact expression for the sum

$$S = \binom{5}{5} + \binom{6}{5} + \binom{7}{5} + \cdots + \binom{94}{5}$$

of the first ninety entries on the $k = 5$ diagonal. Since $\binom{5}{5} = 1 = \binom{6}{6}$,

$$S = \left[\binom{6}{6} + \binom{6}{5}\right] + \binom{7}{5} + \binom{8}{5} + \cdots + \binom{94}{5}.$$

Using the recursion formula $\binom{n}{k} + \binom{n}{k-1} = \binom{n+1}{k}$ we get

$$S = \binom{7}{6} + \binom{7}{5} + \binom{8}{5} + \binom{9}{5} + \cdots + \binom{94}{5}$$

$$= \binom{8}{6} + \binom{8}{5} + \binom{9}{5} + \cdots + \binom{94}{5}.$$

If we continue in this way, the last two steps will be

$$S = \binom{94}{6} + \binom{94}{5} = \binom{95}{6}. \qquad \Box$$

Example 7   Here we give a combinatorial proof of the formula $\binom{5}{5} + \binom{6}{5} + \binom{7}{5} + \cdots + \binom{94}{5} = \binom{95}{6}$ of Example 6. Let $T = \{1, 2, 3, \ldots, 95\}$ and let U be the collection of all the sets A of 6 integers chosen from T. Then $\#U = \binom{95}{6}$. For $r = 6, 7, \ldots, 95$, let V_r consist of the sets A in the collection U such that the largest integer in A is r. Then $\#V_r = \binom{r-1}{5}$, since the other 5 integers of such an A (in addition to r) are to be chosen from $\{1, 2, \ldots, r - 1\}$. The union of the disjoint sets $V_6, V_7, \ldots, V_{95}$ is U, since the largest integer in a set of 6 integers from T must be at least 6. The general sum rule (or Theorem 1, "Size of a Union of Pairwise Disjoint Finite Sets," of Section 1.7) tells us that

$$\#V_6 + \#V_7 + \cdots + \#V_{95} = \#U.$$

Since $\#V_r = \binom{r-1}{5}$ and $\#U = \binom{95}{6}$, we have the desired result:

$$\binom{5}{5} + \binom{6}{5} + \binom{7}{5} + \cdots + \binom{94}{5} = \binom{95}{6}. \qquad \Box$$

Example 8 Now we prove combinatorially that

$$\sum_{h=1}^{n} h(n + 1 - h) = \binom{n + 2}{3};$$

that is, we show combinatorially that

$$1 \cdot n + 2(n - 1) + 3(n - 2) + \cdots + (n - 1) \cdot 2 + n \cdot 1 = \binom{n + 2}{3}.$$

The right-hand side $\binom{n+2}{3}$ is the number of subsets $A = \{g, h, k\}$ of 3 distinct integers chosen from the set

$$T = \{0, 1, 2, \ldots, n, n + 1\}$$

of size $n + 2$. We assume that the elements g, h, and k of the subset A are listed so that $g < h$ and $h < k$. The middle integer h of A can be any integer in $\{1, 2, \ldots, n\}$. Then g can be chosen as any of the h integers in $\{0, 1, \ldots, h - 1\}$ and k can be chosen as any of the $n + 1 - h$ integers in $\{h + 1, h + 2, \ldots, n + 1\}$. Thus for each h in $\{1, 2, \ldots, n\}$ there are $h(n + 1 - h)$ subsets $\{g, h, k\}$ of T with $g < h < k$. Hence the total number of subsets of size 3 from T is

$$\sum_{h=1}^{n} h(n + 1 - h).$$

The number of such subsets also is $\binom{n+2}{3}$, and thus the formula is proved.
□

Example 9 **A PATH PROBLEM** Let each of the small squares in Figure 5.2.3 be a 1 by 1 square. How many paths are there from A to B that consist of 15 segments, each of which is a side of one of these small squares? One such path is shown as the heavy line in the figure. Its five vertical segments are the 2nd, 5th, 7th, 11th, and 13th of the required 15 segments. Thus this particular path can be specified by the subset $\{2, 5, 7, 11, 13\}$ of the set $\{1, 2, \ldots, 15\}$. In a similar way, one sets up a bijection from the set of paths being counted onto the set of subsets of size 5 from the set $\{1, 2, \ldots, 15\}$ of size 15. Hence it follows from Part (vii) of Theorem 3 ("Size of an Image Set") of Section 1.8 that the number of paths of the desired type is

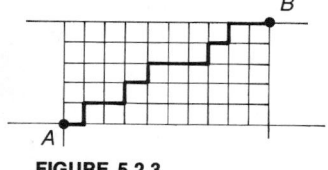

FIGURE 5.2.3

$$\binom{15}{5} = \frac{15 \cdot 14 \cdot 13 \cdot 12 \cdot 11}{5 \cdot 4 \cdot 3 \cdot 2 \cdot 1} = 3003.$$
□

Example 10 **SIGNIFICANCE OF DATA** The data in this example are based on a network TV report. A certain medical procedure involving random elements succeeds approximately 50% of the times it is attempted. The success–failure pattern for a sequence of 33 attempts can be modeled by a 33-bit string $\alpha = a_1 a_2 \ldots a_{33}$, in which $a_i = 1$ if the ith try succeeds and $a_i = 0$ if the

ith try fails. Since each a_i is equally likely to be 1 or 0, each of the 2^{33} strings in B_{33} is equally likely for the success–failure pattern.

A change is made in the procedure, and the new procedure then succeeds in 24 of the first 33 attempts. Does this strongly indicate a significant improvement? The following is one way to answer this question. The number of successes in 33 attempts is

$$\text{wgt } \alpha = a_1 + a_2 + \cdots + a_{33},$$

where $\alpha = a_1 a_2 \ldots a_{33}$ is the success–failure pattern. A high-end portion of the set of possible values of wgt α is the set $\{24, 25, \ldots, 33\}$ of ten integers. The ten integers at the other extreme form the set $\{0, 1, \ldots, 9\}$. Excluding these two extremes, we get a middle range of $\{10, 11, \ldots, 23\}$ for wgt α. With the help of data from Problems 11 and 12 below, we find that approximately 98.65% of the strings α of B_{33} have wgt α in this middle range. Hence a success–failure pattern in the high success set $\{24, \ldots, 33\}$ strongly indicates a significant improvement.   □

Example 11   A student council, C, has 15 members, including the council president, p, and vice-president, v. In how many ways can one select a committee of 5 of these 15 members so that at least one of p and v is on the committee? The total number of subsets of people chosen from C is $\binom{15}{5}$. But $\binom{13}{5}$ of these $\binom{15}{5}$ subsets contain neither p nor v; they are chosen from the other 13 members of C. Hence the answer is $\binom{15}{5} - \binom{13}{5}$.

Alternatively, the answer is found to be $\binom{14}{4} + \binom{13}{4}$, as follows: There are $\binom{14}{4}$ ways to obtain a committee of 5 that consists of p and any 4 of the other 14 members of C. The other committees we want to include in our count are $\binom{13}{4}$ subsets consisting of v and 4 of the 13 members of C different from p and from v. The answers check:

$$\binom{15}{5} - \binom{13}{5} = \left[\binom{14}{5} + \binom{14}{4}\right] - \binom{13}{5}$$

$$= \binom{13}{5} + \binom{13}{4} + \binom{14}{4} - \binom{13}{5} = \binom{13}{4} + \binom{14}{4}.\quad □$$

Blaise Pascal   is one of the most curious individuals in the history of mathematics. Born in 1623 in Clermont-Ferrand, he quickly showed signs of being a mathematical prodigy. His periods of creativity were sporadic, however, due to ill health and a conviction that secular pursuits like mathematics were unworthy. His family had early on converted to an austere brand of Christianity centered at Port Royal outside Paris. Much of his energy went to writing philosophical and theological work supporting the views of the Jansenists in their disputes with the Jesuits. His mathematical contributions are in geometry, combinatorics, probability, and hydrostatics. At the age of 18 he developed a calculating machine, examples of which still survive. This machine gives Pascal a firm position in the history of computing. He died in 1662, at the age of 39.

PROBLEMS FOR SECTION 5.2

1. For each of the following values of k, write all the terms $f_1 f_2 f_3 f_4$ of the expansion of

   $$(a_1 + b_1)(a_2 + b_2)(a_3 + b_3)(a_4 + b_4)$$

   in which $f_i = b_i$ for exactly k values of i and $f_i = a_i$ for the remaining $4 - k$ values of i:
   (a) $k = 2$;   (b) $k = 3$;   (c) $k = 4$.

2. Do as in Problem 1 for:
   (a) $k = 0$;   (b) $k = 1$.

3. Find simple expressions (without summation notation or "...") for each of the following:

   (a) $\binom{7}{0} + \binom{7}{1} + \binom{7}{2} + \binom{7}{3} + \binom{7}{4} + \binom{7}{5} + \binom{7}{6} + \binom{7}{7}$;

   (b) $\binom{7}{1} + 2\binom{7}{2} + 3\binom{7}{3} + 4\binom{7}{4} + 5\binom{7}{5} + 6\binom{7}{6} + 7\binom{7}{7}$;

   (c) $\binom{7}{7} + \binom{8}{7} + \binom{9}{7} + \cdots + \binom{100}{7}$;

   (d) $\binom{7}{0} + \binom{8}{1} + \binom{9}{2} + \cdots + \binom{100}{93}$. $\left[\textit{Hint: Use Part (c) and the sym-} \right.$
   metry formula, that is, $\left. \binom{n}{k} = \binom{n}{n-k}. \right]$

   (e) $\binom{7}{0} + 5\binom{7}{1} + 5^2\binom{7}{2} + 5^3\binom{7}{3} + 5^4\binom{7}{4} + 5^5\binom{7}{5} + 5^6\binom{7}{6} + 5^7\binom{7}{7}$.
   (*Hint:* Use Theorem 1, "Binomial Expansion," with $n = 7$, $a = 1$, and $b = 5$.)

4. Find simple expressions for each of the following:

   (a) $\binom{8}{0} + \binom{8}{1} + \binom{8}{2} + \binom{8}{3} + \binom{8}{4} + \binom{8}{5} + \binom{8}{6} + \binom{8}{7} + \binom{8}{8}$;

   (b) $\binom{8}{1} + 2\binom{8}{2} + 3\binom{8}{3} + \cdots + 8\binom{8}{8}$;

(c) $\binom{8}{8} + \binom{9}{8} + \binom{10}{8} + \cdots + \binom{999}{8}$;

(d) $\binom{8}{0} + \binom{9}{1} + \binom{10}{2} + \cdots + \binom{999}{991}$;

(e) $\binom{8}{0} + 3\binom{8}{1} + 3^2\binom{8}{2} + \cdots + 3^8\binom{8}{8}$;

(f) $4^8\binom{8}{0} + 4^7 \cdot 3\binom{8}{1} + 4^6 \cdot 3^2\binom{8}{2} + 4^5 \cdot 3^3\binom{8}{3} + \cdots + 3^8\binom{8}{8}$.

5. (i) Use Theorem 1, "Binomial Expansion," and Pascal's Triangle (Table 5.2.1) to expand $(a + b)^5$.
    (ii) Use Part (i) with $a = 2x$ and $b = -3y$ to expand $(2x - 3y)^5$.

6. Expand:
    (i) $(a + b)^6$;   (ii) $(3x - 2y)^6$.

7. (i) List the entries $\binom{7}{0}, \binom{7}{1}, \ldots, \binom{7}{7}$ of the $n = 7$ row of Pascal's Triangle.
    (ii) Expand $(a + b)^7$.
    (iii) Expand $(4x - 5y)^7$.

8. (i) List the entries $\binom{8}{k}$ of the $n = 8$ row of Pascal's Triangle.
    (ii) Expand $(a + b)^8$.
    (iii) Expand $(x + 6y)^8$.

9. List the first ten entries $\binom{2}{2}, \binom{3}{2}, \ldots, \binom{11}{2}$ of the $k = 2$ diagonal of Pascal's Triangle. (These are the first ten triangular numbers.)

10. List the first six entries $\binom{3}{3}, \binom{4}{3}, \binom{5}{3}, \binom{6}{3}, \binom{7}{3}, \binom{8}{3}$ of the $k = 3$ diagonal of Pascal's Triangle.

The answers to Problems 11 and 12 are needed in Example 10 above.

11. Use $\binom{33}{0} = 1$ and the formula

$$\binom{n}{k} = \frac{n + 1 - k}{k}\binom{n}{k - 1}$$

to find $\binom{33}{k}$ for $k = 1, 2, \ldots, 9$.

12. Let $L = \binom{33}{0} + \binom{33}{1} + \cdots + \binom{33}{9}$, $M = \binom{33}{10} + \binom{33}{11} + \cdots + \binom{33}{23}$, $H = \binom{33}{24} + \binom{33}{25} + \cdots + \binom{33}{33}$.
    (i) Use Problem 11 to calculate L.
    (ii) Use the symmetry formula $\binom{n}{k} = \binom{n}{n-k}$ to show that $L = H$.
    (iii) Explain why $L + M + H = 2^{33}$ and $M = 2^{33} - 2L$.
    (iv) Show that $M/2^{33}$ is approximately 0.9865 (or 98.65%).

13. (i) Use the special cases $\binom{n}{1} = n$, $\binom{n}{2} = n(n - 1)/2$, $\binom{n}{3} = n(n - 1)(n - 2)/6$ of Theorem 4 to find $\binom{33}{1}, \binom{33}{2}$, and $\binom{33}{3}$.
    (ii) Find $\binom{33}{32}, \binom{33}{31}$, and $\binom{33}{30}$.

14. Calculate $\binom{36}{3}$ and $\binom{36}{4}$ and give the values of $\binom{36}{33}$ and $\binom{36}{32}$.

15. The north–south thoroughfares in a certain section of Salt Lake City are 1st Street, 2nd Street, ..., 13th Street; the east–west thoroughfares are 1st Avenue, 2nd Avenue, ..., 13th Avenue.
  (i) How many 10-block paths are there along these thoroughfares from the intersection of 1st Street and 3rd Avenue to the intersection of 7th Street and 7th Avenue?
  (ii) How many of the paths from Part (i) go through the intersection of 5th Street and 5th Avenue?
  (iii) How many of the paths from Part (i) do *not* go through the intersection of 5th Street and 5th Avenue?
(One can travel at the speed limit along any of these paths and have all traffic lights green.)

16. (i) How many 12-block paths are there along the thoroughfares of Problem 15 from the intersection of 4th Street and 2nd Avenue to the intersection of 9th Street and 9th Avenue?
  (ii) How many of the paths of Part (i) go through the intersection of 7th Street and 5th Avenue?
  (iii) How many of the paths of Part (i) do *not* go through the intersection of 7th Street and 5th Avenue?

17. Use the formula $\binom{n}{k} = n\binom{n-1}{k-1}/k$ of Example 2 and $\binom{80}{2} = 3160$ to find $\binom{81}{3}$. Then find $\binom{80}{78}$ and $\binom{81}{78}$.

18. Use $\binom{80}{3} = 82{,}160$ and $\binom{n}{k} = n\binom{n-1}{k-1}/k$ to find $\binom{81}{4}$. Then find $\binom{81}{77}$.

19. Show that $\binom{n}{2} + \binom{n+1}{2} = n^2$ for $n = 2, 3, \ldots$.

20. Show that $\binom{n}{3} + 4\binom{n+1}{3} + \binom{n+2}{3} = n^3$ for $n = 3, 4, \ldots$.

21. Let X consist of the 20-bit strings $\alpha = a_1 a_2 \ldots a_{20}$ with wgt $\alpha = 10$, that is, with $a_1 + a_2 + \cdots + a_{20} = 10$. How many of the $\binom{20}{10}$ strings α in X have $a_1 + a_2 + \cdots + a_{10}$ in the set $\{0, 1, 2\}$?

22. How many of the 20-bit strings $\alpha = a_1 a_2 \ldots a_{20}$ with wgt $\alpha = 10$ have $a_1 + a_2 + \cdots + a_{10}$ in the set $\{8, 9, 10\}$?

23. A student council has 15 members of whom 8 are women and 7 are men. In how many ways can a committee of 5 council members be selected so that the committee has at least 2 women and at least 2 men?

24. Assume that the U.S. Senate consists of 55 Republicans and 45 Democrats and that the House of Representatives consists of 200 Republicans and 235 Democrats. In how many ways could a conference committee of 10 be selected so that it has 3 Democratic Representatives, 2 Republican Representatives, 3 Republican Senators, and 2 Democratic Senators?

25. Show that:
  (a) $(x + 1)^4 + (x - 1)^4 = 2(x^4 + 6x^2 + 1)$.

(b) $(x + 1)^{100} + (x - 1)^{100}$

$$= 2\left[\binom{100}{0}x^{100} + \binom{100}{2}x^{98} + \binom{100}{4}x^{96} + \cdots + \binom{100}{100}\right].$$

(c) $(x + 1)^{100} - (x - 1)^{100}$

$$= 2\left[\binom{100}{1}x^{99} + \binom{100}{3}x^{97} + \binom{100}{5}x^{95} + \cdots + \binom{100}{99}x\right].$$

(d) $\binom{100}{0} + \binom{100}{2} + \binom{100}{4} + \cdots + \binom{100}{100} = 2^{99}.$

26. Show that:

(a) $(x + 1)^5 + (x - 1)^5 = 2(x^5 + 10x^3 + 5x).$

(b) $(x + 1)^{99} + (x - 1)^{99}$

$$= 2\left[\binom{99}{0}x^{99} + \binom{99}{2}x^{97} + \binom{99}{4}x^{95} + \cdots + \binom{99}{98}x\right].$$

(c) $(x + 1)^{99} - (x - 1)^{99}$

$$= 2\left[\binom{99}{1}x^{98} + \binom{99}{3}x^{96} + \binom{99}{5}x^{94} + \cdots + \binom{99}{99}\right].$$

(d) $\binom{99}{0} + \binom{99}{2} + \binom{99}{4} + \cdots + \binom{99}{98}$

$$= 2^{98} = \binom{99}{1} + \binom{99}{3} + \binom{99}{5} + \cdots + \binom{99}{99}.$$

27. Expand $(x + y + z + w)^2.$

28. Expand $(x + y + z + w)^3.$

29. Explain why $300!/(60! \cdot 70! \cdot 80! \cdot 90!)$ must be an integer.

30. Explain why $(e_1 + e_2 + \cdots + e_k)!/(e_1! \cdot e_2! \cdots e_k!)$ must be an integer whenever $e_1, e_2, \ldots, e_k$ are in $N = \{0, 1, \ldots\}.$

31. (a) Find the coefficient of $x^3 y^4 z^5 w^6$ in the expansion of $(x + y + z + w)^{18}.$
     (b) Find the subset $\{e, f, g, h\}$ of $N = \{0, 1, \ldots\}$ such that $\binom{26}{4}\binom{22}{5}\binom{17}{7}$ is the coefficient of $x^e y^f z^g w^h$ in the expansion of $(x + y + z + w)^{26}.$

32. (a) Find the coefficient of $xy^3 z^3 w^6$ in the expansion of $(x + y + z + w)^{13}.$
     (b) Find the subset $\{e, f, g, h, k\}$ of N such that $\binom{39}{2}\binom{37}{5}\binom{32}{19}\binom{13}{3}$ is the coefficient of $x^e y^f z^g u^h v^k$ in the expansion of $(x + y + z + u + v)^{39}.$

33. Let $a, b,$ and c be in N and let $a + b + c = n.$

(i) Explain why $\dbinom{n}{a}\dbinom{n - a}{b} = \dbinom{n}{c}\dbinom{n - c}{b}.$

(ii) Does $\dbinom{90}{20}\dbinom{70}{30} = \dbinom{90}{40}\dbinom{50}{30}$? Explain.

34. Let $a, b, c,$ and d be in N and let $a + b + c + d = n.$

(i) Explain why $\binom{n}{a}\binom{n-a}{b}\binom{n-a-b}{c} = \binom{n}{d}\binom{n-d}{c}\binom{n-c-d}{b}$.

(ii) Does $\binom{n}{a}\binom{n-a}{b}\binom{n-a-b}{c} = \binom{n}{b}\binom{n-b}{c}\binom{n-b-c}{d}$?

35. Explain why each of the following holds for integers k and n with $2 \le k \le n$:

(a) $\binom{n}{k} + 2\binom{n}{k-1} + \binom{n}{k-2} = \binom{n+2}{k}$.

(b) $\binom{n}{k} - 2\binom{n-1}{k-1} + \binom{n-2}{k-2} = \binom{n-2}{k}$.

36. Explain why the following hold for $3 \le k \le n$:

(a) $\binom{n}{k} + 3\binom{n}{k-1} + 3\binom{n}{k-2} + \binom{n}{k-3} = \binom{n+3}{k}$.

(b) $\binom{n}{k} - 3\binom{n-1}{k-1} + 3\binom{n-2}{k-2} - \binom{n-3}{k-3} = \binom{n-3}{k}$.

37. Find a simple expression for

$$2 \cdot 1 \cdot \binom{n}{2} + 3 \cdot 2 \cdot \binom{n}{3} + 4 \cdot 3 \cdot \binom{n}{4} + \cdots + n(n-1)\binom{n}{n}.$$

38. Find a simple expression for

$$1^2\binom{n}{1} + 2^2\binom{n}{2} + 3^2\binom{n}{3} + \cdots + n^2\binom{n}{n}.$$

39. Explain why

$$\left[\binom{n}{0} + \binom{n}{1} + \cdots + \binom{n}{n}\right]^2 = \binom{2n}{0} + \binom{2n}{1} + \cdots + \binom{2n}{2n}.$$

40. Show that

$$(n+1)\left[\binom{n}{0} + \frac{1}{2}\binom{n}{1} + \frac{1}{3}\binom{n}{2} + \cdots + \frac{1}{n+1}\binom{n}{n}\right] = 2^{n+1} - 1.$$

41. Explain why each of the following is true:

(i) $\left[\binom{60}{0} + \binom{60}{1}x + \cdots + \binom{60}{60}x^{60}\right] \cdot$

$\left[\binom{40}{0} + \binom{40}{1}x + \cdots + \binom{40}{40}x^{40}\right] = (1+x)^{100}$.

(ii) $\binom{60}{0}\binom{40}{33} + \binom{60}{1}\binom{40}{32} + \binom{60}{2}\binom{40}{31} + \cdots + \binom{60}{33}\binom{40}{0} = \binom{100}{33}$.

(iii) $\binom{60}{0}\binom{40}{7} + \binom{60}{1}\binom{40}{8} + \binom{60}{2}\binom{40}{9} + \cdots + \binom{60}{33}\binom{40}{40} = \binom{100}{33}$.

42. Explain why each of the following is true:

(i) $\left[\binom{45}{0} + \binom{45}{1} x + \binom{45}{2} x^2 + \cdots + \binom{45}{45} x^{45} \right]^2 = (1 + x)^{90}.$

(ii) $\binom{45}{0}\binom{45}{45} + \binom{45}{1}\binom{45}{44} + \binom{45}{2}\binom{45}{43} + \cdots + \binom{45}{45}\binom{45}{0} = \binom{90}{45}.$

(iii) $\binom{45}{0}^2 + \binom{45}{1}^2 + \binom{45}{2}^2 + \cdots + \binom{45}{45}^2 = \binom{90}{45}.$

(iv) $\binom{45}{10}\binom{45}{45} + \binom{45}{11}\binom{45}{44} + \binom{45}{12}\binom{45}{43} + \cdots + \binom{45}{45}\binom{45}{10} = \binom{90}{55}.$

(v) $\binom{45}{10}\binom{45}{0} + \binom{45}{11}\binom{45}{1} + \binom{45}{12}\binom{45}{2} + \cdots + \binom{45}{45}\binom{45}{35} = \binom{90}{55}.$

43. Explain why each side of the equation in Problem 41(ii) is the number of ways of choosing a subset of 33 people from a set consisting of 60 women and 40 men.

44. Give an explanation similar to that of Problem 43 but now for the equation

$$\binom{45}{10}\binom{45}{45} + \binom{45}{11}\binom{45}{44} + \binom{45}{12}\binom{45}{43} + \cdots + \binom{45}{45}\binom{45}{10} = \binom{90}{55}.$$

45. Let k, m, and n be integers, with $0 \leq k \leq m \leq n$. Explain why

$$\binom{m}{0}\binom{n}{k} + \binom{m}{1}\binom{n}{k-1} + \binom{m}{2}\binom{n}{k-2} + \cdots + \binom{m}{k}\binom{n}{0}$$
$$= \binom{m+n}{k}.$$

46. Let h, m, and n be integers, with $0 \leq m \leq n$ and $h \leq n - m$. Explain why

$$\binom{m}{0}\binom{n}{m+h} + \binom{m}{1}\binom{n}{m+h-1} + \binom{m}{2}\binom{n}{m+h-2} +$$
$$\cdots + \binom{m}{m}\binom{n}{h} = \binom{m+n}{m+h}.$$

47. Explain why

$$\binom{n}{0}^2 + \binom{n}{1}^2 + \binom{n}{2}^2 + \cdots + \binom{n}{n}^2 = \binom{2n}{n}.$$

48. Find a simple formula for the sum

$$S = \binom{n}{1}^2 + 2\binom{n}{2}^2 + 3\binom{n}{3}^2 + \cdots + n\binom{n}{n}^2.$$

(*Hint*: See Proof I of Example 3 and use Problem 47.)

49. Give a combinatorial proof (as in Example 7) of

$$\binom{7}{7} + \binom{8}{7} + \binom{9}{7} + \cdots + \binom{1000}{7} = \binom{1001}{8}.$$

50. (i) Give a combinatorial proof (as in Example 7) of

$$\binom{11}{11} + \binom{12}{11} + \binom{13}{11} + \cdots + \binom{9999}{11} = \binom{10000}{12}.$$

(ii) Explain why

$$\binom{11}{0} + \binom{12}{1} + \binom{13}{2} + \cdots + \binom{9999}{9988} = \binom{10000}{9988}.$$

51. Use the formula of Problem 47 to show that $2^n < \binom{2n}{n}$ for n in $\{2, 3, \ldots\}$.

52. Show that $2^n \le \binom{2n}{n} < 4^n$ for n in $\mathbf{Z}^+$.

53. Explain why $\binom{2n}{n}$ is even for all n in $\mathbf{Z}^+$.

54. Show that 3 is an integral divisor of $\binom{3n}{n}$ for all n in $\mathbf{Z}^+$.

55. For all n in $\mathbf{Z}^+ = \{1, 2, \ldots\}$, prove by induction on n that

$$(a + b)^n = \binom{n}{0} a^n + \binom{n}{1} a^{n-1}b + \binom{n}{2} a^{n-2}b^2 +$$

$$\cdots + \binom{n}{n-1} ab^{n-1} + \binom{n}{n} b^n.$$

5.3

PIGEONHOLE PRINCIPLE, INCLUSION–EXCLUSION PRINCIPLE

Let us consider the distribution of m distinguishable objects $s_1, s_2, \ldots, s_m$ into n containers $P_1, P_2, \ldots, P_n$. The mathematical model for such a distribution is a mapping f from $S = \{s_1, \ldots, s_m\}$ to $T = \{P_1, \ldots, P_n\}$. What condition on m and n *guarantees* that any such distribution will result in some container having at least two of the objects in it—that is, guarantees that each mapping f from S to T is not injective? Part (vi) of Theorem 3 ("Size of an Image Set") of Section 1.8 tells us that

"f is injective" $\Rightarrow$ "$m \le n$." (1)

Since "$m \le n$" is false if and only if $m > n$, then the contrapositive of Display (1) is "$m > n$" $\Rightarrow$ "f is not injective." So the desired condition on m and n is that there are more objects than containers. This simple result is so useful that we restate it as the following theorem.

THEOREM 1   **PIGEONHOLE PRINCIPLE**

Let m objects be distributed into n containers. If $m > n$, then some container will end up with at least two objects in it.

This principle derives its name from the "pigeonhole" compartments found in old-fashioned desks. It follows from the pigeonhole principle that in any set of 367 or more people there must be two people with the same birthday. (See Example 13 of Section 1.8 for the technique of determining the probability that some pair of people in a smaller set have the same birthday.) The following result is a generalization of Theorem 1.

THEOREM 2   **GENERALIZED PIGEONHOLE PRINCIPLE**

Let m objects be distributed into n containers. If $m > kn$, then some container must end up with more than k objects in it.

PROOF   Let $S = \{s_1, s_2, \ldots, s_m\}$ be the set of objects and let $T = \{P_1, P_2, \ldots, P_n\}$ be the set of containers (that is, pigeonholes). For $j = 1, 2, \ldots, n$, let S_j be the set of all objects from S that end up in P_j. Then $S_1, S_2, \ldots, S_n$ is a partition of S, and hence

$$m = \#S = \#S_1 + \#S_2 + \cdots + \#S_n. \tag{2}$$

If $\#S_j \leq k$ for each j, it would follow from Display (2) that $m \leq kn$. However, this would contradict the hypothesis that $m > kn$, so we see that $\#S_j > k$ for some j, and the theorem is proved.   □

Example 1   It follows from the generalized pigeonhole principle, with $m = 22$, $n = 7$, and $k = 3$, that in any set of 22 people there must be some subset of 4 or more people who were born on the same day of the week.   □

Example 2   John Doe walks into a room containing 5 other people. The generalized pigeonhole principle, with $m = 5$, $n = 2$, and $k = 2$, tells us that either at least 3 of these people were acquaintances of John or at least 3 of them were strangers to John. (This fact will be useful in Problem 15 of this section.)   □

Now we turn to the inclusion–exclusion principle of James Joseph Sylvester. (See the biographical note on Sylvester just before the problems for this section.) The following is the first case of this principle.

THEOREM 3   **THE CASE OF $n = 2$ OF INCLUSION–EXCLUSION**

$$\#(A \cup B) = \#A + \#B - \#(A \cap B) \qquad \text{for finite sets } A \text{ and } B.$$

PROOF   This theorem can be proved quickly by noting that although $\#A + \#B$ counts the elements of $A \cup B$, in the process it also counts each element of $A \cap B$ twice (once for being in A and once for being in B). So $\#(A \cap B)$ has to be subtracted to make the count correct.

Alternatively, one can think of A and B as subsets of a universe X and picture their minisets (as defined in Definition 1 of Section 1.3) in the Venn Diagram of Figure 5.3.1. We note that

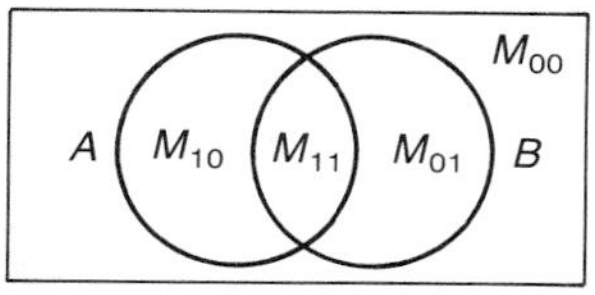

$$A = M_{10} \cup M_{11},$$
$$B = M_{11} \cup M_{01},$$
$$A \cup B = M_{10} \cup M_{11} \cup M_{01},$$
$$A \cap B = M_{11}.$$

FIGURE 5.3.1

Because the minisets are pairwise disjoint, these formulas imply that

$$\begin{aligned}
\#(A \cup B) &= \#M_{10} + \#M_{11} + \#M_{01} \\
&= (\#M_{10} + \#M_{11}) + (\#M_{11} + \#M_{01}) - \#M_{11} \\
&= \#A + \#B - \#(A \cap B). \qquad \square
\end{aligned}$$

Example 3   In a certain set M of 50 mathematics majors, 40 are taking French, 30 are taking German, and 25 are taking both French and German. How many are taking at least one of these languages? Let F be the subset of the members of M taking French and G be the subset of those taking German. Then the number we seek is $\#(F \cup G)$. Theorem 3 implies that this equals

$$\#F + \#G - \#(F \cap G) = 40 + 30 - 25 = 45.$$

The number of mathematics majors in M taking neither French nor German is the size of the complement of $F \cup G$ in M; that is, it is

$$\#M - \#(F \cup G) = 50 - 45 = 5. \qquad \square$$

Example 4   **COUNTING SURJECTIONS**   Let $X = \{1, 2, \ldots, n\}$ and $Y = \{a, b\}$. We show as follows that there are $2^n - 2$ surjections from X onto Y. Theorem 2 ("Number of Mappings from X to Y") of Section 1.8 tells us that there are 2^n mappings f from X into Y. All of these are surjections except for the mapping f_1 and f_2 given by

$$f_1 \colon X \to Y, f_1(x) = a \quad \text{for all } x \text{ in } X;$$
$$f_2 \colon X \to Y, f_2(x) = b \quad \text{for all } x \text{ in } X.$$

Thus there are $2^n - 2$ surjections from X onto Y. In Problems 27 and 28 below, the reader is asked to use the inclusion–exclusion principle to count the number of surjections from X onto $\{a, b, c\}$ and from X onto $\{a, b, c, d\}$. □

Example 5   In how many ways can each of n students be assigned a grade chosen from the set $\Gamma = \{A, B, C, D, F\}$ so that at least one B and at least one C are assigned? (Assume $n \geq 2$.) Let M be the set of all mappings f from the set S of the n students into the set Γ of grades. Let P be the subset of all f in M for which $f(s) \in \{A, C, D, F\}$ for all s in S and let Q consist of the f in M for which $f(s) \in \{A, B, D, F\}$ for all s in S. Then the number we want is the size of the complement of $P \cup Q$ in S, that is,

$$\# M - \#(P \cup Q) = \# M - \# P - \# Q + \#(P \cap Q).$$

In determining a mapping f from S to G, there are 5 choices of a grade for each of the n students. Assuming the choice for a student to be independent of the choices for the other students, it follows from the general product rule (Theorem 1 of Section 5.1) that there are 5^n mappings in M. Similarly, there are 4^n mappings in each of P and Q. Also, there are 3^n mappings f in $P \cap Q$, since the codomain for such an f is $\{A, D, F\}$. Hence the desired number is $5^n - 2 \cdot 4^n + 3^n$. □

THEOREM 4   **THE NEXT CASE OF INCLUSION–EXCLUSION**

For finite sets A, B, and C,

$$\#(A \cup B \cup C) = \# A + \# B + \# C - \#(A \cap B)$$
$$- \#(A \cap C) - \#(B \cap C) + \#(A \cap B \cap C)$$

Two applications of Theorem 3 will yield this result. The details are left to the reader.

Example 6   Let $X = \{1, 2, 3, \ldots, 30\}$. How many of the integers of X are integral multiples of at least one of the integers 2, 3, and 5? How many of the integers of X are not exactly divisible by any of the integers 2, 3, and 5? We answer these questions as follows. Let

$$A = \{2, 4, 6, \ldots, 30\},$$
$$B = \{3, 6, 9, \ldots, 30\},$$
$$C = \{5, 10, 15, \ldots, 30\}$$

be the subsets of X consisting of the multiples of 2, the multiples of 3, and the multiples of 5, respectively. Then

$$A \cap B = \{6, 12, 18, 24, 30\},$$
$$A \cap C = \{10, 20, 30\},$$
$$B \cap C = \{15, 30\},$$
$$A \cap B \cap C = \{30\}$$

and so the answer to the first question is

$$\#(A \cup B \cup C) = \#A + \#B + \#C - \#(A \cap B) - \#(A \cap C)$$
$$- \#(B \cap C) + \#(A \cap B \cap C)$$
$$= 15 + 10 + 6 - 5 - 3 - 2 + 1 = 22.$$

The answer to the second question is

$$\#X - \#(A \cup B \cup C) = 30 - 22 = 8.$$ □

Example 7   Let $X = \{1, 2, 3, \ldots, 6000\}$. How many of the integers in X are integral multiples of at least one of the integers 4, 5, and 6? How many are not exactly divisible by any of the integers 4, 5, and 6? As in Section 1.7, let $d\mathbf{Z}$ denote the set of integral multiples of an integer d. We recall that $\text{lcm}[a, b]$ is the least common multiple of a and b. (See Definition 5 of Section 2.6.) Let

$$A = (4\mathbf{Z}) \cap X, \qquad B = (5\mathbf{Z}) \cap X, \qquad C = (6\mathbf{Z}) \cap X.$$

Since $(a\mathbf{Z}) \cap (b\mathbf{Z}) = m\mathbf{Z}$, where $m = \text{lcm}[a, b]$, then

$$A \cap B = (20\mathbf{Z}) \cap X,$$
$$A \cap C = (12\mathbf{Z}) \cap X,$$
$$B \cap C = (30\mathbf{Z}) \cap X,$$
$$A \cap B \cap C = (60\mathbf{Z}) \cap X.$$

We note that $\#A = \#X/4 = 6000/4 = 1500$, since A has every fourth integer from X. Similarly, $\#B = 6000/5 = 1200$, $\#C = 6000/6 = 1000$, $\#(A \cap B) = 6000/20 = 300$, $\#(A \cap C) = 6000/12 = 500$, $\#(B \cap C) = 6000/30 = 200$, and $\#(A \cap B \cap C) = 6000/60 = 100$. It follows from the inclusion–exclusion principle that the answer $\#(A \cup B \cup C)$ to the first question is

$$1500 + 1200 + 1000 - 300 - 500 - 200 + 100 = 2800.$$

Then the answer to the second question is

$$\#X - \#(A \cup B \cup C) = 6000 - 2800 = 3200.$$ □

We next set up notation for the statement of the inclusion–exclusion principle in general form. Let $A_1, A_2, \ldots, A_n$ be subsets of a universe X. Let σ_1 be the sum of the sizes of the A_i, let σ_2 be the sum of the sizes of the intersections $A_i \cap A_j$ (with $i < j$) of pairs of these subsets, let σ_3 be the sum of the sizes of all intersections of triples $A_i \cap A_j \cap A_k$ (with $i < j < k$), and so on. Let $\bar{A}_i$ be the complement of A_i in X.

THEOREM 5   INCLUSION–EXCLUSION PRINCIPLE

In the notation just given,

(a) $\#(A_1 \cup A_2 \cup \cdots \cup A_n) = \sigma_1 - \sigma_2 + \sigma_3 - \cdots + (-1)^{n+1}\sigma_n.$
(b) $\#(\bar{A}_1 \cap \bar{A}_2 \cap \cdots \cap \bar{A}_n) = \#X - \sigma_1 + \sigma_2 - \cdots + (-1)^n\sigma_n.$

PROOF   By one of De Morgan's Laws, $\bar{A}_1 \cap \bar{A}_2 \cap \cdots \cap \bar{A}_n$ is the complement of $A_1 \cup A_2 \cup \cdots \cup A_n$ in X. Hence Part (b) follows easily from Part (a). We note that the case of $n = 2$ of Part (a) is Theorem 3, and we leave it to the reader to complete a proof of Part (a) for $n \geq 2$ by mathematical induction.   □

James Joseph Sylvester was born in 1814 in London, England, and educated at St. John's College, Cambridge, England. However, he was in the United States for part of his career. In 1841 he became professor of mathematics at the University of Virginia, although he soon returned to England. In 1876 he took a position at the newly founded Johns Hopkins University in Baltimore. During his eight years at Johns Hopkins, Sylvester exerted great influence on the introduction of Ph.D. programs at American universities. During that tenure he also served as the first editor of the American Journal of Mathematics.

In 1884 Sylvester was appointed Savilian Professor of Geometry at Oxford University. Between his stays in the United States, he collaborated with Arthur Cayley on some of the most important research of their era, especially on the theory of invariants. Sylvester died in 1897.

PROBLEMS FOR SECTION 5.3 _____

1.   How many people would be needed to ensure that two of them were born on the same day of the week?

2.   Do Problem 1 with "day of the week" changed to "month of the year."

3. There are m identical blue socks and n identical black socks scrambled in a drawer. If the room is completely dark, how many socks must be taken to be sure of having two differently colored socks?

4. Under the circumstances of Problem 3, how many socks must be taken to be sure of having a matched pair among them? (Because of this problem, the pigeonhole principle is sometimes called the *dresser drawer principle*.)

5. A four-year college has 19,000 students, with more freshmen than either sophomores, juniors, or seniors. What is the minimum number of freshmen the college can have?

6. An elementary school has 141 students in four first-grade classes. Is it living up to its rule of not exceeding 35 students in any one class? Explain.

7. In a certain election for seats on a board, 32 ballots are cast, each for one of 18 candidates. If the 12 candidates with the highest numbers of votes are to be declared winners, how many votes are required to guarantee winning a seat?

8. Given the circumstances of Problem 7, how many votes are required to guarantee at least a tie for a seat on the board? (If necessary, ties will be broken by lot.)

9. Let $S \subseteq \mathbf{Z} \times \mathbf{Z}$ and let $\#S = 5$. Explain why there must exist ordered pairs (a, b) and (c, d) in S such that
$$\left(\frac{a + c}{2}, \frac{b + d}{2} \right) \in \mathbf{Z} \times \mathbf{Z}.$$

10. Let T be a finite subset of $\mathbf{Z} \times \mathbf{Z} \times \mathbf{Z}$. What must be true of $\#T$ to guarantee that there exist ordered triples (a, b, c) and (d, e, f) in T such that
$$\left(\frac{a + d}{2}, \frac{b + e}{2}, \frac{c + f}{2} \right) \in \mathbf{Z} \times \mathbf{Z} \times \mathbf{Z}?$$

11. A, B, and C are subsets of X. Also, $\#X = 60$, $\#A = 30$, $\#B = 28$, $\#C = 14$, $\#(A \cap B) = 11$, $\#(A \cap C) = 4$, $\#(B \cap C) = 3$, and $\#(A \cap B \cap C) = 2$. Use the inclusion–exclusion principle to find $\#(A \cup B \cup C)$.

12. Find the size of each miniset M_α for the subsets A, B, C of X in Problem 11.

13. Let $X = \{1, 2, \ldots, 168\}$. How many of the integers of X are integral multiples of:
    (i) at least one of the integers 6, 7, and 8?
    (ii) none of the integers 6, 7, and 8?

14. Let $X = \{1, 2, 3, \ldots, 600\}$. How many of the integers of X are integral multiples of:
    (i) at least one of the integers 6 and 10?   (ii) neither 6 nor 10?

15. Is it true that for any set S of 6 people there must be a subset of 3 who are mutually acquainted or a subset of 3 who are mutual strangers? Explain.

16. Let S be a set of 6 points in space. Let each of the 15 pairs of points from S be connected by an arc and let each of these 15 arcs be colored red or blue. Must S have a subset of 3 points for which the 3 arcs connecting them have the same color? Explain.

17. Let S be a square whose sides have length 2 units. Show that for any 5 points on or inside S there must be 2 whose distance apart is at most $\sqrt{2}$ units.

18. Let T be an equilateral triangle with sides of length 2 units. If one has 5 points on or inside T, must there be 2 of them that are a unit or less apart? Explain.

19. Let f be a mapping from $X = \{x_1, x_2, \ldots, x_{26}\}$ into $J = \{1, 2, 3\}$. For j in J, let $f^{-1}(j)$ be the complete inverse image of j under f (as in Definition 7 of Section 1.8). Show that at least one of the following must hold:

$$\#f^{-1}(1) \geq 8, \qquad \#f^{-1}(2) \geq 9, \qquad \#f^{-1}(3) \geq 11.$$

20. Let f be a mapping from a finite set X into $J = \{1, 2, 3, \ldots, n\}$. Let $b_1, b_2, \ldots, b_n$ be in $N = \{0, 1, \ldots\}$, and for j in J let $\#f^{-1}(j) < b_j$. Prove that

$$\#X \leq b_1 + b_2 + \cdots + b_n - n.$$

21. For an integer d, let $d\mathbf{Z}$ consist of the integral multiples of d. Let $X = \{1, 2, \ldots, 900\}$, $A = (2\mathbf{Z}) \cap X$, $B = (3\mathbf{Z}) \cap X$, and $C = (5\mathbf{Z}) \cap X$. Let $\bar{A}$, $\bar{B}$, $\bar{C}$ be the complements of A, B, C, respectively, in X. Find:
(a) $\#(A \cup B \cup C)$; (b) $\#(\bar{A} \cap \bar{B} \cap \bar{C})$.

22. Suppose that grades are assigned to each of a set X of n students by a mapping f from X into $\Gamma = \{A, B, C, D, E, F\}$. How many of these mappings f have each of the complete inverse images $f^{-1}(B)$, $f^{-1}(C)$, $f^{-1}(D)$ nonempty?

23. Use the inclusion–exclusion principle to find the number of permutations p on $T = \{1, 2, \ldots, n\}$ such that both $p(1) \neq 1$ and $p(2) \neq 2$. (Assume $n \geq 2$.)

24. How many permutations p on $T = \{1, 2, \ldots, n\}$ simultaneously have $p(1) \neq 1$, $p(2) \neq 2$, and $p(3) \neq 3$? (Assume $n \geq 3$.)

25. Find the answer to Problem 23 without using the inclusion–exclusion principle but using the general product rule and considering two cases:
(i) $p(1) = 2$; (ii) $p(1) \neq 2$.

26. How many of the integers in $\{1, 2, 3, \ldots, 999\}$ have no 5 among their digits?

27. Let $T = \{1, 2, \ldots, n\}$ with $n \geq 3$ and $V = \{a, b, c\}$.
(a) How many mappings f are there from T into V?
(b) How many surjective mappings are there from T onto V?

28. Do Problem 27 with $\{a, b, c\}$ replaced by $\{a, b, c, d\}$ and with $n \geq 4$.

29. A year is a leap year if its A.D. number n satisfies *one* of the following conditions: (I) n is exactly divisible by 4 but not by 100, or (II) $400 \mid n$. How many leap years will there be between 1885 and 4085?

30. (i) Show that calendars repeat in cycles of 400 years.
*(ii) Show that more than $\frac{1}{7}$ of the months, of such a cycle, have the 13th day a Friday.

31. Let $T = \{1, 2, 3, \ldots, 20\}$. How many ordered pairs (A, B) are there with $A \subseteq T$ and $B \subseteq T$ but with neither A nor B a subset of the other? (*Hint*: This is the number of ways of assigning each integer of T to one of the minisets $M_{00}, M_{01}, M_{10}, M_{11}$ of Figure 5.3.1 so that M_{01} and M_{10} are both nonempty.)

32. Do Problem 31 with $\{1, 2, 3, \ldots, 20\}$ replaced by $\{1, 2, \ldots, n\}$.

33. Let $T = \{1, 2, 3, \ldots, 1000000\}$.
(a) How many squares of integers are there in T?
(b) How many cubes of integers are there in T?
(c) How many integers n are there in T such that n is neither a square of an integer nor a cube of an integer?

34. Do Problem 33(c) with *cube* replaced by *fifth power*.

35. What is the one-millionth term of the sequence 2, 3, 5, 6, 7, 10, ... that results when the squares and cubes of integers are removed from the sequence 1, 2, 3, ... of all positive integers?

36. What is the one-millionth term of the sequence that results from the removal of all squares, cubes, and fifth powers of integers from the sequence 1, 2, 3, ... ?

5.4

INTEGER COMPOSITIONS

Here we present a technique for counting the ways of distributing n identical objects into k distinguishable containers $C_1, C_2, \ldots, C_k$. Since the objects cannot be distinguished from one another, a distribution of this type is determined by an ordered k-tuple $(x_1, x_2, \ldots, x_k)$, where x_i specifies the number of objects placed in C_i. Such an ordered k-tuple has each x_i in $N = \{0, 1, \ldots\}$ and has $x_1 + x_2 + \cdots + x_k = n$. This motivates the following definition.

DEFINITION 1   **COMPOSITION OF *n* INTO *k* PARTS**

Let $n \in N$ and $k \in Z^+$. A *composition* of n into k parts is an ordered k-tuple $(x_1, x_2, \ldots, x_k)$ with each x_i in N and $x_1 + x_2 + \cdots + x_k = n$. The x_i are the *parts* of the composition.

Thus $(2, 5, 0, 4)$ is a composition of 11 into 4 parts.

Example 1   How many compositions are there of 11 into 4 parts? A useful technique will enable us to answer this and similar questions easily. Consider 14 dashes on a line

$$- - - - - - - - - - - - - -. \tag{1}$$

There are $\binom{14}{3}$ ways to select a subset of 3 of these dashes for replacement with slashes. One such selection and replacement leads to

$$- / - - - - - / - - / - - -. \tag{2}$$

The 3 slashes in Display (2) split the remaining 11 dashes into 4 batches containing 1, 5, 2, and 3 dashes, respectively. This leads to the composition $(1, 5, 2, 3)$ of 11 into 4 parts. Another selection of 3 of the dashes of Display (1) for replacement with slashes leads to

$$/ - - - - / / - - - - - - -. \tag{3}$$

The composition associated with Display (3) is $(0, 4, 0, 7)$, since the first and third batches of dashes are empty. (The first batch consists of the dashes before the first slash, the second batch consists of the dashes between the first and second slashes, and so on.)

Each selection of 3 of the 14 dashes of Display (1) leads to a composition of 11 into 4 parts in a one-to-one way. Hence there are $\binom{14}{3}$ compositions of 11 into 4 parts. □

Example 2   Let Γ be the set of all compositions C of 4 into 3 parts. Using the technique of Example 1, we show in Table 5.4.1 the bijection between the collection of dash–slash arrangements A with slashes in two of the six positions and

TABLE 5.4.1

A	C	A	C	A	C
$//----$	$(0, 0, 4)$	$-//---$	$(1, 0, 3)$	$--/-/-$	$(2, 1, 1)$
$/-/---$	$(0, 1, 3)$	$-/-/--$	$(1, 1, 2)$	$--/--/$	$(2, 2, 0)$
$/--/--$	$(0, 2, 2)$	$-/--/-$	$(1, 2, 1)$	$---//-$	$(3, 0, 1)$
$/---/-$	$(0, 3, 1)$	$-/---/$	$(1, 3, 0)$	$---/-/$	$(3, 1, 0)$
$/----/$	$(0, 4, 0)$	$--//--$	$(2, 0, 2)$	$----//$	$(4, 0, 0)$

the set Γ of compositions C. The table verifies that $\#\Gamma = \binom{4+3-1}{3-1} = \binom{6}{2} = 6 \cdot 5/2 = 15$. $\qquad\square$

THEOREM 1   **COMPOSITION COUNT**

Let $n \in N$ and $k \in Z^+$. The number of compositions of n into k parts is $\binom{n+k-1}{k-1}$.

PROOF   We use the technique illustrated in Examples 1 and 2. Consider $n + k - 1$ positions on a line. Fill $k - 1$ of these positions with slashes and the remaining n positions with dashes. In each such arrangement, the slashes split the n dashes into k batches. Let x_1 be the number of dashes in the first batch, that is, before the first slash. Let x_2 be the number of dashes in the second batch, that is, between the first and second slashes. Similarly, let $x_3, \ldots, x_k$ be the numbers of dashes in the other batches. Thus each of the $\binom{n+k-1}{k-1}$ ways of selecting $k - 1$ of the $n + k - 1$ positions to be filled by slashes is associated with a composition $(x_1, x_2, \ldots, x_k)$ of n into k parts. This association is one-to-one, so there are $\binom{n+k-1}{k-1}$ such compositions.

$\qquad\square$

MNEMONIC 1 $\binom{n+k-1}{k-1}$

The result in Theorem 1 is easier to remember if one keeps in mind the technique in which $k - 1$ slashes separate the n dashes into k batches.

Now we present techniques for counting compositions satisfying restrictions on one or more of the parts.

THEOREM 2   **COMPOSITIONS WITH POSITIVE PARTS**

For integers k and n, with $1 \le k \le n$, there are $\binom{n-1}{k-1}$ compositions $(x_1, x_2, \ldots, x_k)$ of n into k **positive parts**, that is, parts satisfying $x_i \ge 1$ for all i.

We give two proofs:

PROOF   **I.**   The mapping

$$\beta: (x_1, x_2, \ldots, x_k) \mapsto (x_1 - 1, x_2 - 1, \ldots, x_k - 1)$$

is a bijection from the set A of compositions of n into k positive parts onto the set B of all compositions of $n - k$ into k (nonnegative) parts. Hence it follows from Part (vii) of Theorem 3 ("Size of an Image Set") of Section 1.8 that $\#A = \#B$. But $\#B = \binom{n-k+k-1}{k-1} = \binom{n-1}{k-1}$ by Theorem 1 ("Composition Count") of this section. Thus $\#A = \binom{n-1}{k-1}$, as claimed.

PROOF   **II.**   Let n dashes be placed on a line, with adjacent dashes separated by blank spaces. Thus there will be $n-1$ such blank spaces. Choose $k-1$ of the $n-1$ blank spaces and fill them with $k-1$ slashes; this can be done in $\binom{n-1}{k-1}$ ways. Each of these ways breaks the n dashes into k non-empty batches and thus provides a composition of n into k positive parts. The selection of $k-1$ of the $n-1$ blank spaces to be filled with slashes is associated in a one-to-one manner with the compositions of n into k positive parts, so there are $\binom{n-1}{k-1}$ such compositions.   □

Example 3   We see from Example 2 that the compositions of 4 into 3 positive parts are

$$(1, 1, 2), \qquad (1, 2, 1), \qquad \text{and} \qquad (2, 1, 1). \tag{4}$$

Subtracting 1 from each part, that is, using the bijection of Proof I of Theorem 2, leads to three compositions of 1 into 3 parts:

$$(0, 0, 1), \qquad (0, 1, 0), \qquad \text{and} \qquad (1, 0, 0).$$

To illustrate Proof II of Theorem 2, we place 4 dashes on a line

$$- \ - \ - \ -$$

and insert slashes into 2 of the 3 spaces between adjacent dashes in the $\binom{3}{2} = 3$ possible ways. Each such insertion splits the 4 dashes into 3 non-empty batches and thus associates the dash–slash picture with the indicated composition of 4 into 3 positive parts given below it in Figure 5.4.1.   □

$- / - / - -$

$(1, 1, 2)$

$- / - - / -$

$(1, 2, 1)$

$- - / - / -$

$(2, 1, 1)$

FIGURE 5.4.1

Example 4   Let Γ consist of all the compositions $(x_1, x_2, x_3, x_4, x_5)$ of 100 into 5 parts. By Theorem 1, "Composition Count," we know that $\#\Gamma = \binom{100+5-1}{5-1} = \binom{104}{4}$. For each of the following conditions, we count the compositions in Γ that satisfy the condition:

(a) $10 \le x_1$,
(b) $81 \le x_1$,
(c) $x_1 \le 80$,
(d) $10 \le x_1 \le 80$.

The count for (a) is $\binom{100-10+4}{4} = \binom{94}{4}$, since the mapping

$$(x_1, x_2, x_3, x_4, x_5) \mapsto (x_1 - 10, x_2, x_3, x_4, x_5)$$

is a bijection from the subset of compositions in Γ with $10 \le x_1$ onto the set of all compositions of 90 into 5 parts. Theorem 1 then tells us that there are $\binom{90+4}{4} = \binom{94}{4}$ such compositions. Similarly, the count for (b) is $\binom{100-81+4}{4} = \binom{23}{4}$. Now let A, B, C, and D be the subsets of Γ consisting of the compositions satisfying (a), (b), (c), and (d), respectively. Then C is the complement of B in Γ, and so $\#C = \#\Gamma - \#B = \binom{104}{4} - \binom{23}{4}$. Finally, D is the complement of B in A, so $\#D = \#A - \#B = \binom{94}{4} - \binom{23}{4}$. □

Example 5 Here we find the number of distributions of 100 identical objects into 5 distinguishable containers C_1, C_2, C_3, C_4, C_5 in which at most 40 of the objects go into C_1 and at most 30 go into C_2. Let Γ be the set of all compositions $(x_1, x_2, x_3, x_4, x_5)$ of 100 into 5 parts. Let C be the subset of Γ consisting of the compositions satisfying both $x_1 \leq 40$ and $x_2 \leq 30$. We find $\#C$ as follows: To get the set C, we remove from Γ the subset A of compositions with $41 \leq x_1$ and also the subset B of compositions with $31 \leq x_2$. Hence $\#C = \#\Gamma - \#(A \cup B)$. Using the inclusion–exclusion principle yields

$$\#C = \#\Gamma - \#A - \#B + \#(A \cap B).$$

By Theorem 1 ("Composition Count"), $\#\Gamma = \binom{100+4}{4} = \binom{104}{4}$. Using a technique of Example 4, we see that $\#A = \binom{100-41+4}{4} = \binom{63}{4}$ and $\#B = \binom{100-31+4}{4} = \binom{73}{4}$. The mapping

$$(x_1, x_2, x_3, x_4, x_5) \mapsto (x_1 - 41, x_2 - 31, x_3, x_4, x_5)$$

is a bijection from $A \cap B$ onto the set of all compositions of $100 - 41 - 31 = 28$ into 5 parts, so $\#(A \cap B) = \binom{28+4}{4} = \binom{32}{4}$. Hence

$$\#C = \binom{104}{4} - \binom{63}{4} - \binom{73}{4} + \binom{32}{4}.$$ □

Example 6 Let Γ consist of all compositions $(x_1, x_2, x_3, x_4, x_5)$ of 100 into 5 parts. Let C be the subset of Γ consisting of the compositions with both $x_1 \leq 55$ and $x_2 \leq 65$. We find $\#C$ by using a slight variation of the technique of Example 5. To get the set C, we remove from Γ the subset A of compositions with $56 \leq x_1$ and the subset B of compositions with $66 \leq x_2$. We note that $\#A = \binom{100-56+4}{4} = \binom{48}{4}$ and that $\#B = \binom{100-66+4}{4} = \binom{38}{4}$. Since $A \cap B = \emptyset$, it follows that

$$\#C = \#\Gamma - \#A - \#B = \binom{104}{4} - \binom{48}{4} - \binom{38}{4}.$$ □

Example 7 How many of the integers from 1 to 99999 have 22 as the sum of the digits? Writing 1 as 00001, 2 as 00002, and so on, each of these integers can be represented as $d_1d_2d_3d_4d_5$, with each d_i in $\{0, 1, \ldots, 9\}$. Thus the answer is the number of compositions $(d_1, d_2, d_3, d_4, d_5)$ of 22 into 5 parts d_i, each satisfying $d_i \leq 9$. There are $\binom{26}{4}$ compositions of 22 into 5 parts.

Of these, $\binom{16}{4}$ have $10 \le d_1$ and so have to be deleted from the count. The same holds for each of the conditions $10 \le d_2, \ldots, 10 \le d_5$. If we subtract $5\binom{16}{4}$ from $\binom{26}{4}$, we will be subtracting out twice for each composition with 2 of the d_i being at least 10. Thus we have to correct the count by adding back $\binom{5}{2}\binom{6}{4}$, where $\binom{5}{2}$ is the number of ways of choosing the 2 values of i from $\{1, 2, 3, 4, 5\}$ for which $10 \le d_i$ and $\binom{6}{4}$ is the number of compositions of 22 into 5 parts with 2 chosen parts being at least 10. No further corrections are needed because it is impossible for three of the digits to be at least 10 when their sum is 22. Hence the answer is

$$\binom{26}{4} - \binom{5}{1}\binom{16}{4} + \binom{5}{2}\binom{6}{4} = \binom{26}{4} - 5\binom{16}{4} + 10\binom{6}{4}. \qquad \square$$

PROBLEMS FOR SECTION 5.4

1. (a) List the compositions of 5 into 3 *positive* parts.
   (b) List the remaining compositions of 5 into 3 parts.

2. (a) How many compositions are there of 6 into 3 parts?
   (b) Of these, how many have all the parts positive?

3. For the case of $n = 5$ and $k = 3$, display the bijection

   $$\beta: (x_1, x_2, x_3) \mapsto (x_1 - 1, x_2 - 1, x_3 - 1),$$

   of Proof I of Theorem 2 ("Compositions with Positive Parts"), from the set of compositions of 5 into 3 positive parts onto the set of all compositions of 2 into 3 parts.

4. Do as in Problem 3 for the case of $n = 6$ and $k = 3$.

5. In the following equations, think of $x, y, \ldots$ as the parts $x_1, x_2, \ldots$ of a composition and tell how many solutions each equation has with each unknown in $N = \{0, 1, \ldots\}$.
   (a) $x + y = 27$;   (b) $x + y + z = 40$;
   (c) $x_1 + x_2 + \cdots + x_{20} = 252$; (d) $x_1 + x_2 + \cdots + x_k = 500$.

6. Do as in Problem 5 for the following:
   (a) $x + y = 35$;   (b) $x + y + z = 47$;
   (c) $x_1 + x_2 + \cdots + x_{32} = 647$; (d) $x_1 + x_2 + \cdots + x_k = 901$.

7. For each of the parts of Problem 5, find the number of solutions in positive integers, that is, with each unknown in Z^+.

8. For each of the parts of Problem 6, find the number of solutions in positive integers.

9. (a) In how many ways can one distribute 709 identical objects into 6 boxes $B_1, B_2, \ldots, B_6$?
   (b) In how many of these ways will B_6 be nonempty?

(c) In how many of these ways will each B_i be nonempty?

(d) In how many of these ways will each B_i have at least 5 of the objects?

10. Do as in Problem 9, but with the number of objects now 907 and the number of boxes now 7.

11. Is there a one-to-one correspondence between the terms of $(x + y + z)^{17}$ and the compositions of 17 into 3 parts? Explain.

12. Is there a one-to-one correspondence between the terms of $(x_1 + x_2 + \cdots + x_k)^n$ and the compositions of n into k parts? Explain.

13. Tell how many terms there are in the expansion of each of the following:
(a) $(x + y)^{12}$;   (b) $(x + y + z)^{18}$;   (c) $(x - y + z + 2w)^{81}$.

14. Do as in Problem 13 for:
(a) $(x + y)^{14}$;   (b) $(x + 3y - z)^{23}$;   (c) $(x - 3y + 5z - 7w)^n$.

15. For each part of Problem 13, tell how many of the terms of the expansion have each of the variables appearing to a positive power.

16. For each part of Problem 14, tell how many of the terms of the expansion have each of the variables appearing to a positive power.

17. Suppose that one has an abundant supply of pennies, nickels, dimes, and quarters. (The coins of a particular denomination are identical.)
(a) In how many different ways can one select 7 of these coins?
(b) In how many ways can one select 7 coins with a total value of 49¢?

18. Do Problem 17(a) with a plentiful supply of half-dollars added to the original supply of coins.

19. Let $X = \{1, 2, 3, \ldots, 999999\}$.
(a) How many integers in X have 9 as the sum of the digits?
(b) How many integers in X have 15 as the sum of the digits?
(c) How many integers in X have 23 as the sum of the digits?

20. Let $X = \{1, 2, 3, \ldots, 999999\}$.
(a) How many integers in X have 39 as the sum of the digits?
(b) How many integers in X have 53 as the sum of the digits?

21. Let Γ be the set of all compositions (x_1, x_2, x_3, x_4) of 345 into 4 parts. For each of the following parts, tell how many of the $\binom{348}{3}$ compositions in Γ satisfy the conditions:
(a) $1 \le x_i$ for $i = 1, 2, 3, 4$;   (b) $2 \le x_i$ for $i = 1, 2, 3, 4$;
(c) $5 \le x_4$;   (d) $25 \le x_4$;   (e) $x_4 \le 24$;   (f) $5 \le x_4 \le 24$.

22. Do Problem 21 with 345 replaced by 543 [and $\binom{348}{3}$ by $\binom{546}{3}$].

23. Let Γ be the set of all compositions $(x_1, x_2, x_3, x_4, x_5)$ of 600 into 5 parts.
(a) How many compositions in Γ satisfy $x_1 \le 100$ and $x_2 \le 200$?
(b) How many compositions in Γ satisfy $x_1 \le 300$ and $x_2 \le 400$?

24. Let Γ be the set of all compositions $(x_1, x_2, x_3, x_4, x_5, x_6)$ of 700 into 6 parts.

(a) How many compositions in Γ have $x_1 \leq 100$ and $x_2 \leq 300$?

(b) How many compositions in Γ have $x_1 \leq 300$ and $x_2 \leq 500$?

25. How many integers are products $p_1 p_2 \cdots p_7$ of 7 factors p_i each of which is in $\{2, 3, 5, 7, 11\}$? [The p_i need not (and cannot) be distinct. Also, rearranging the p_i does not change the product.]

26. Do as in Problem 25, but with the p_i now allowed to be in $\{2, 3, 5, 7, 11, 13, 17, 19\}$.

27. How many solutions are there of $x_1 + x_2 + \cdots + x_8 = 15$ in integers x_i chosen from $\{-3, -2, -1, 0, 1, \ldots\}$?

28. How many solutions does $x_1 + x_2 + \cdots + x_{14} = 29$ have in integers x_i each satisfying $-7 \leq x_i$?

29. For n in N, let C_n be the set of compositions (x_1, x_2, x_3) of $3n$ into 3 parts x_i each satisfying $x_i \leq 2n$. Find $\# C_n$.

30. For n in N, let D_n be the set of compositions (x_1, x_2, x_3, x_4) of $2n$ into 4 parts x_i each satisfying $x_i \leq n$. Find $\# D_n$.

5.5

INTEGER PARTITIONS

As noted in Section 5.4, a composition $(x_1, x_2, \ldots, x_k)$ of n into k parts is a mathematical representation for a distribution of n identical objects into k distinguishable containers $C_1, C_2, \ldots, C_k$. In this section we introduce the mathematical model for a distribution of n identical objects into k identical containers.

A composition $(x_1, x_2, \ldots, x_k)$ is an ordered k-tuple. Thus

$$(2, 1, 1), \qquad (1, 2, 1), \qquad (1, 1, 2) \tag{1}$$

are different compositions of 4 into 3 parts. Each represents a distribution of 4 identical objects into 3 distinguishable containers. If we have no reason to distinguish one container from another, the triples of Display (1) would represent the same distribution. For uniqueness of representation, we would use the triple (2, 1, 1), in which the parts are in nonincreasing order. This motivates the following concept.

DEFINITION 1   **PARTITION OF n INTO k PARTS**

A *partition* of n into k parts is a composition $(x_1, x_2, \ldots, x_k)$ of n into k parts x_i satisfying $x_1 \geq x_2 \geq \cdots \geq x_k$.

Example 1 The partitions of 6 into 3 parts are the seven ordered triples $(6, 0, 0)$, $(5, 1, 0)$, $(4, 2, 0)$, $(4, 1, 1)$, $(3, 3, 0)$, $(3, 2, 1)$, $(2, 2, 2)$. Also, the partitions of 9 into 2 parts are the five ordered pairs $(9, 0)$, $(8, 1)$, $(7, 2)$, $(6, 3)$, $(5, 4)$.

□

NOTATION 1 **NUMBER OF PARTITIONS OF n INTO k PARTS**

For $k \in \mathbf{Z}^+ = \{1, 2, \ldots\}$ and $n \in N = \{0, 1, \ldots\}$, $p_k(n)$ denotes the number of partitions of n into k parts.

We see from Example 1 that $p_3(6) = 7$ and $p_2(9) = 5$.

THEOREM 1 **PARTITIONS WITH POSITIVE PARTS**

For $n \geq k$, the number of partitions of n into k positive parts is $p_k(n - k)$.

PROOF The mapping

$$\beta: (x_1, x_2, \ldots, x_k) \mapsto (x_1 - 1, x_2 - 1, \ldots, x_k - 1)$$

is a bijection from the set P of all partitions of n into k positive parts onto the set Q of all partitions of $n - k$ into k parts. Hence $\#P = \#Q = p_k(n - k)$.

□

Example 2 The mapping β of Theorem 1 in the case of $n = 6$ and $k = 3$ is the bijection

$$\beta: (4, 1, 1) \mapsto (3, 0, 0), \quad (3, 2, 1) \mapsto (2, 1, 0), \quad (2, 2, 2) \mapsto (1, 1, 1)$$

from the set P of partitions of 6 into 3 positive parts onto the set Q of all partitions of $6 - 3 = 3$ into 3 parts.

□

We will see in Problems 9 and 10 below that

$$p_1(n) = 1 \quad \text{for all } n \text{ in } N = \{0, 1, \ldots\}; \tag{2}$$

$$p_k(0) = 1 \quad \text{for all } k \text{ in } \mathbf{Z}^+ = \{1, 2, \ldots\}. \tag{3}$$

In other problems of this section, we will see that Displays (2) and (3), together with the recursion relation presented next, enable us readily to compute tables of $p_2(n)$, $p_3(n)$, ...

THEOREM 2 **RECURSION FOR $p_k(n)$**

(a) $p_k(n) = p_n(n)$ for $2 \leq k$ and $0 \leq n \leq k$.
(b) $p_k(n) = p_k(n - k) + p_{k-1}(n)$ for $2 \leq k \leq n$.

PROOF   (a) Let $2 \leq k$, $0 \leq n \leq k$, and $(x_1, \ldots, x_n, x_{n+1}, \ldots, x_k)$ be a partition of n into k parts. Then

$$x_1 + \cdots + x_n + x_{n+1} + \cdots + x_k = n. \tag{4}$$

Since there are no negative parts, it follows from Display (4) that $x_i \geq 1$ for at most n values of i. Since $x_1 \geq x_2 \geq \cdots \geq x_k$ and the parts are in $N = \{0, 1, \ldots\}$, this implies that $0 = x_{n+1} = x_{n+2} = \cdots = x_k$; that is,

$$(x_1, \ldots, x_n, x_{n+1}, \ldots, x_k) = (x_1, \ldots, x_n, 0, \ldots, 0).$$

Then the mapping with

$$(x_1, \ldots, x_n, 0, \ldots, 0) \mapsto (x_1, \ldots, x_n)$$

is a bijection from the set of all partitions of n into k parts onto the set of all partitions of n into n parts. Hence $p_k(n) = p_n(n)$ for $0 \leq n \leq k$.

(b) Now let $2 \leq k \leq n$. Let P be the set of all partitions $(x_1, x_2, \ldots, x_k)$ of n into k parts. Let A consist of the partitions in P with $x_k \geq 1$ (and hence each $x_i \geq 1$) and let B consist of the partitions in P with $x_k = 0$. Since $P = A \cup B$ and $A \cap B = \emptyset$, it follows that $\#P = \#A + \#B$. By Notation 1 ("Number of Partitions of n into k Parts"), $\#P = p_k(n)$. By Theorem 1 ("Partitions with Positive Parts"), $\#A = p_k(n-k)$. The mapping

$$\beta: (x_1, x_2, \ldots, x_{k-1}, 0) \mapsto (x_1, x_2, \ldots, x_{k-1})$$

is a bijection from B onto the set C of all partitions of n into $k-1$ parts. Hence $\#B = \#C = p_{k-1}(n)$ and

$$p_k(n) = \#P = \#A + \#B = p_k(n-k) + p_{k-1}(n). \qquad \square$$

As an illustration of Theorem 2(b), we use $p_3(6) = 7$ and $p_2(9) = 5$ from Example 1 and have $p_3(9) = p_3(6) + p_2(9) = 7 + 5 = 12$.

The following result will be used in Example 9 of Section 9.4 to derive the explicit formula $p_2(n) = [3 + 2n + (-1)^n]/4$ for $n \in N = \{0, 1, \ldots\}$.

LEMMA 1   **RECURSION AND INITIAL CONDITIONS FOR $p_2(n)$**

$$p_2(n) = p_2(n-1) + p_2(n-2) - p_2(n-3) \quad \text{for } n \in \{3, 4, \ldots\}.$$

Also,

$$p_2(0) = 1, \qquad p_2(1) = 1, \qquad \text{and} \qquad p_2(2) = 2.$$

PROOF   Theorem 2(b), with $k = 2$, gives us

$$p_2(n) = p_2(n-2) + p_1(n) \quad \text{for } n \in \{2, 3, \ldots\}. \tag{5}$$

Since the only partition of n into 1 part is the (x_1) with $x_1 = n$, it follows that $p_1(n) = 1$ for all n in $N = \{0, 1, \ldots\}$. Hence Display (5) can be rewritten as

$$p_2(n) = p_2(n-2) + 1 \quad \text{for } n \in \{2, 3, \ldots\},$$

which is equivalent to

$$p_2(n) - p_2(n-2) = 1 \quad \text{for } n \in \{2, 3, \ldots\}. \tag{6}$$

Replacing n by $n-1$ in Display (6) gives us

$$p_2(n-1) - p_2(n-3) = 1 \quad \text{for } n \in \{3, 4, \ldots\}. \tag{7}$$

It follows from Displays (6) and (7) that

$$p_2(n) - p_2(n-2) = p_2(n-1) - p_2(n-3) \quad \text{for } n \in \{3, 4, \ldots\}.$$

Adding $p_2(n-2)$ to both sides gives us the desired formula:

$$p_2(n) = p_2(n-1) + p_2(n-2) - p_2(n-3) \quad \text{for } n \in \{3, 4, \ldots\}.$$

The only partition of 0 into 2 parts is $(0, 0)$; hence $p_2(0) = 1$. Also, $p_2(1) = 1$, since the only partition of 1 into 2 parts is $(1, 0)$, and $p_2(2) = 2$, since the only partitions of 2 into 2 parts are $(2, 0)$ and $(1, 1)$. □

Example 3 Let $P = \{(4), (3, 1), (2, 2), (2, 1, 1), (1, 1, 1, 1)\}$. We see that P is the set of all partitions p of 4 into positive parts (where the number of parts is unrestricted). The mapping β of the following table is a bijection from P onto the set Q of partitions of 4 into 4 parts:

p	(4)	(3, 1)	(2, 2)	(2, 1, 1)	(1, 1, 1, 1)
$\beta(p)$	(4, 0, 0, 0)	(3, 1, 0, 0)	(2, 2, 0, 0)	(2, 1, 1, 0)	(1, 1, 1, 1)

Hence $\#P = \#Q = p_4(4)$. □

NOTATION 2 **UNRESTRICTED NUMBER OF PARTS**

For n in $Z^+ = \{1, 2, \ldots\}$, $p(n)$ denotes the number of partitions of n into positive parts (with the number of parts unrestricted). Also, $p(0) = 1$.

We see from Example 3 that $p(4) = 5$.

THEOREM 3 **FORMULA FOR $p(n)$**

$$p(n) = p_n(n) \quad \text{for all } n \text{ in } Z^+.$$

PROOF   This is established with a bijection, as illustrated in Example 3.   □

A method of depicting a partition with positive parts is due to Norman Macleod Ferrers. (See the biographical note on Ferrers just before the problems for this section.)

DEFINITION 2   FERRERS DIAGRAM

The *Ferrers diagram* for a partition $(x_1, \ldots, x_k)$ with positive parts is an array of dots in left-justified rows with x_i dots in the ith row.

· The term *left-justified* means that the rows are aligned so that the first column holds the first dot of every row. The Ferrers diagrams for the partitions (4, 4, 3, 3, 2) and (5, 5, 4, 2) are shown in Figures 5.5.1(a) and (b), respectively. These two diagrams are related to one another in an interesting way: The number of dots in the ith row of one diagram is the number of dots in the ith column of the other.

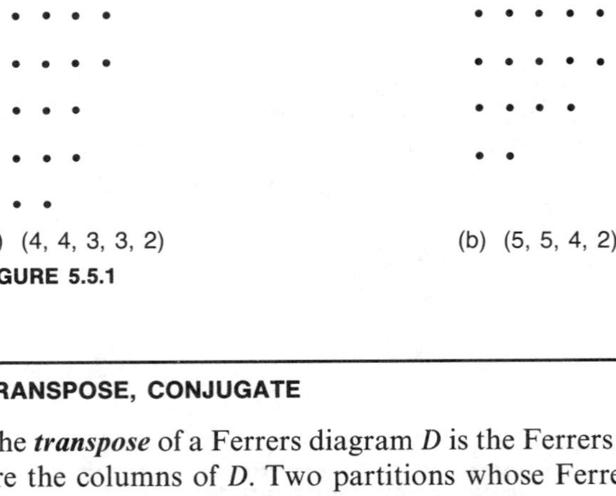

(a) (4, 4, 3, 3, 2)   (b) (5, 5, 4, 2)

FIGURE 5.5.1

DEFINITION 3   TRANSPOSE, CONJUGATE

The *transpose* of a Ferrers diagram D is the Ferrers diagram E whose rows are the columns of D. Two partitions whose Ferrers diagrams are transposes of each other are *conjugate partitions*.

Thus the diagrams of Figures 5.5.1(a) and (b) are transposes of each other; also, the partitions (4, 4, 3, 3, 2) and (5, 5, 4, 2) are conjugates of each other.

Let $\alpha = (x_1, x_2, \ldots, x_k)$ be a partition of n into positive parts and let $\beta = (y_1, y_2, \ldots, y_h)$ be its conjugate. Then β is also a partition of n, since the total number of dots does not change when the rows are made into columns. It is also easily seen that the number k of positive parts in $\alpha = (x_1, x_2, \ldots, x_k)$ is the largest part in its conjugate β. For example, there are 5 positive parts in the $\alpha = (4, 4, 3, 3, 2)$ of Figure 5.5.1(a), and the largest part in its conjugate $\beta = (5, 5, 4, 2)$ is 5. In fact, the mapping f with $f(\alpha)$ the conjugate of α is a bijection from the set of all partitions of n into k positive parts onto the set of positive part partitions of n with the largest part equal to k and an unrestricted number of parts. This bijection proves the following theorem.

THEOREM 4 **PARTITIONS OF _n_ WITH LARGEST PART _k_**

There are as many partitions of n into k positive parts as there are partitions of n into (an unrestricted number of) positive parts of which the largest is k.

Norman Macleod Ferrers, born in 1829 in Prinknash Park, Gloucestershire, England, was head of Gonville and Caius College at Cambridge. Though known during his lifetime largely for his administrative work at Cambridge, he did nevertheless work in a number of areas in pure mathematics. It is for his graphs that Ferrers' name is remembered today, largely due to a citation in James Sylvester's famous 1882 paper on partition theory, given the rather unusual title "A constructive theory of partitions in three acts, an interact and an exodion." Ferrers died in 1903.

PROBLEMS FOR SECTION 5.5

1. (i) List all the partitions of 6 into 2 parts.
    (ii) List all the partitions of 7 into 2 parts.
    (iii) Is the mapping with $(x, y) \mapsto (x + 1, y)$ a bijection from the set of partitions in Part (i) onto the set for Part (ii)?

2. (i) List all the partitions of 8 into 2 parts.
    (ii) Explain why the mapping with $(x, y) \mapsto (x + 1, y)$ is not a surjection (and hence not a bijection) from the set A of partitions of 7 into 2 parts onto the set B of partitions of 8 into 2 parts.

3. (i) List all the partitions of 5 into positive parts (with the number of parts unrestricted).
    (ii) What is $p(5)$?
    (iii) How many of the partitions listed for Part (i) have 3 as the largest part?
    (iv) Does the answer for Part (iii) equal the number of partitions of 5 into 3 positive parts?

4. (i) List all the partitions of 6 into positive parts (with the number of parts unrestricted).
    (ii) What is $p(6)$?
    (iii) How many of the partitions listed for Part (i) have 3 as the largest part?
    (iv) How many partitions are there of 6 into 3 positive parts?

5. (a) Draw the Ferrers diagram for $\alpha = (5, 3, 2, 2)$.
    (b) Use the Ferrers diagram of Part (a) to find the conjugate β of α.

6. (a) Draw the Ferrers diagram for $\alpha = (4, 4, 3)$.
    (b) Find the conjugate β of α.

7. Which of the following partitions is its own conjugate: $(3, 2, 1)$? $(4, 3, 2)$?

8. Which of the following is its own conjugate: $(4, 4, 2)$? $(4, 2, 1, 1)$?

9. Explain why $p_1(n) = 1$ for all n in N.

10. Explain why $p_k(0) = 1$ for all k in Z^+.

11. Explain why $p_k(n) \in N$ for all n in N and k in Z^+.

12. Explain why $p_k(n) = p_{k-1}(n)$ for all $n < k$ and $2 \le k$. [*Hint*: Explain why each side equals $p_n(n)$.]

13. Explain why $p_2(n) = p_2(n - 2) + 1$ for $n \ge 2$.

14. Prove each of the following by induction on m:
    (a) $p_2(2m) = m + 1$ for all m in N.
    (b) $p_2(2m + 1) = m + 1$ for all m in N.

15. (i) Find $p_3(0)$, $p_3(1)$, and $p_3(2)$.
    (ii) Explain why $p_3(2m) = p_3(2m - 3) + m + 1$ for $m \ge 2$.

16. Explain why $p_3(2m + 1) = p_3(2m - 2) + m + 1$ for $m \ge 1$.

17. Use the formulas of Problem 14 to tabulate $p_2(n)$ for $n = 0, 1, \ldots, 11$.

18. Use Theorem 2, "Recursion for $p_k(n)$," and the answer to Problem 17 to tabulate $p_3(n)$ for $n = 0, 1, \ldots, 11$.

19. Tabulate $p_4(n)$ for $n = 0, 1, \ldots, 11$.

20. Tabulate $p_5(n)$ for $n = 0, 1, \ldots, 11$.

21. Use Problems 15(ii) and 16 to show that $p_3(2m) = 2m + p_3(2m - 6)$ for $m \ge 3$.

22. Show that $p_3(2m + 1) = 2m + 1 + p_3(2m - 5)$ for $m \ge 3$.

23. Give references to previous problems to justify the following assertions:
    (a) $p_3(0) = 1$ and $p_3(n) = n$ for $n = 1, 2, 3, 4, 5$.
    (b) $p_3(n) = n + p_3(n - 6)$ for $n \ge 6$.

24. Explain why $p_3(6m) = 6m + (6m - 6) + (6m - 12) + \cdots + 6 + 1$.

25. Show that $p_3(6m) = 3m^2 + 3m + 1$ for all m in $N = \{0, 1, \ldots\}$.

26. Show that $p_3(6m + 1) = 3m^2 + 4m + 1$ for all m in N.

27. Find formulas for:
(a) $p_3(6m + 2)$;   (b) $p_3(6m + 3)$.

28. Find formulas for:
(a) $p_3(6m + 4)$;   (b) $p_3(6m + 5)$.

29. Tabulate $p(n)$ for $n = 0, 1, 2, 3, 4, 5$.

30. Find $p(6)$ and $p(7)$.

31. Let S be the set of all ordered triples (a, b, c) of integers with both $a \geq b \geq c \geq 1$ and $abc = 2^{10}$. Find $\# S$.

32. Let T be the set of all ordered 4-tuples (a, b, c, d) of integers with $a \geq b \geq c \geq d \geq 1$ and $abcd = 3^{20}$. Express $\# T$ in the form $p_k(n)$.

33. For integers $n \geq 10$, explain why there are $p_4(n - 10)$ partitions (x, y, z, w) of n into 4 *distinct positive* parts, that is, integers satisfying $x > y > z > w > 0$.

34. Explain why the number of partitions of n into 3 distinct positive parts is $p_3(n - 6)$.

35. Does $p_6(10) = p_6(4) + p_5(5) + p_4(6) + p_3(7) + p_2(8) + p_1(9)$? Explain.

36. Find k and n such that

$$\sum_{i=1}^{100} p_i(120 - i) = p_k(n).$$

37. Does $p_9(80) = p_8(80) + p_8(71) + p_9(62)$? Explain.

38. Does $p_9(80) = p_8(80) + p_8(71) + p_8(62) + \cdots + p_8(8)$? Explain.

39. Find k and n such that $p_6(0) + p_6(7) + p_6(14) + p_6(21) + p_6(28) = p_k(n)$.

40. Find h and m such that $p_6(1) + p_6(8) + p_6(15) + p_6(22) + p_6(29) = p_h(m)$.

41. Is $p_6(0) + p_6(1) + p_6(2) + \cdots + p_6(33)$ equal to $p_7(28) + p_7(29) + p_7(30) + p_7(31) + p_7(32) + p_7(33)$? Explain.

42. Find two choices for (a, b, h) in terms of k and n such that

$$\sum_{i=0}^{n} p_k(i) = \sum_{j=a}^{b} p_h(j).$$

*43. Write a computer program for the calculation and printing of a table of $p_d(n)$ for $d = 1, 2, 3, 4$ and $n = 1, 2, \ldots, 100$.

5.6

COUNTING DISTRIBUTIONS

In the two preceding sections, we dealt with two cases of counting distributions of n objects into k containers. Here we briefly review these two cases and study two additional cases.

The objects to be distributed may be distinguishable or indistinguishable; the same is true of the containers. This leads to four cases:

I. Indistinguishable objects into distinguishable containers.
II. Indistinguishable objects into indistinguishable containers.
III. Distinguishable objects into indistinguishable containers.
IV. Distinguishable objects into distinguishable containers.

CASE I   INDISTINGUISHABLE OBJECTS INTO DISTINGUISHABLE CONTAINERS

Let the k containers $C_1, C_2, \ldots, C_k$ be distinguishable and the n objects be indistinguishable. Then we consider the distribution of the objects into the containers to be specified by the k-tuple $(x_1, x_2, \ldots, x_k)$, where x_i is the number of these objects placed in C_i. Since each $x_i \in N = \{0, 1, \ldots\}$ and $x_1 + x_2 + \cdots + x_k = n$, such a k-tuple is a composition of n into k (nonnegative integral) parts. We saw in Section 5.4 that the number of compositions of n into k parts is $\binom{n+k-1}{k-1}$. Hence the number of distributions of n indistinguishable objects into k distinguishable containers is $\binom{n+k-1}{k-1}$.

If we are counting the number of such distributions for which each C_i has at least one object placed in it, then the parts x_i of the composition $(x_1, \ldots, x_k)$ must all be positive, and the number of distributions becomes the number $\binom{n-1}{k-1}$ of partitions of n into k positive (integral) parts.

Example 1   Fifty bookstores order a total of 9000 copies of a certain textbook. Each of the 50 orders is for at least 10 copies. The number of ways in which the total of 9000 might be split among these bookstores is the number of compositions $(x_1, x_2, \ldots, x_{50})$ of 9000 into 50 integral parts x_i, with each $x_i \geq 10$. Using a technique from Example 4 of Section 5.4, one finds that the number of such compositions is

$$\binom{9000 - 500 + 49}{49} = \binom{8549}{49}. \qquad \square$$

CASE II   INDISTINGUISHABLE OBJECTS INTO INDISTINGUISHABLE CONTAINERS

Again let the n objects be indistinguishable. In this case, however, the k containers are also indistinguishable. That is, rearranging the containers does not change the distribution. Therefore, after the distribution is made, we arrange the containers in a line and number them as $C_1, C_2, \ldots, C_k$ so that

$$x_1 \geq x_2 \geq \cdots \geq x_k,$$

where x_i is the number of objects placed in container C_i. Then $(x_1, x_2, \ldots, x_k)$ is a partition of n into k (nonnegative integral) parts. This way of assigning a partition of n into k parts to each such distribution is a bijection. Hence the number of distributions of n indistinguishable objects into k indistinguishable containers is the number $p_k(n)$ of partitions of n into k (nonnegative integral) parts. The numbers $p_k(n)$ can be calculated from the following formulas from Section 5.5 [see Example 2 and Theorem 2, "Recursion for $p_k(n)$," of that section]:

$$p_1(n) = 1 \quad \text{for all } n \text{ in } N = \{0, 1, \ldots\},$$
$$p_k(0) = 1 \quad \text{for all } k \text{ in } Z^+ = \{1, 2, \ldots\},$$
$$p_k(n) = p_n(n) \quad \text{for } 2 \leq k \text{ and } 0 \leq n \leq k,$$
$$p_k(n) = p_k(n - k) + p_{k-1}(n) \quad \text{for } 2 \leq k \leq n.$$

If $n \geq k$ and we want to count the number of distributions of n indistinguishable objects into k indistinguishable containers for which each container ends up with at least one object, then the associated partitions $(x_1, \ldots, x_k)$ must have each x_i positive. By Theorem 1 ("Partitions with Positive Parts") of Section 5.5, the number of such distributions is $p_k(n - k)$.

Example 2 An educational TV station announces that its fund drive generated pledges totaling \$24,957 from 1990 people. The number of ways in which the total \$24,957 might be partitioned into 1990 positive integral parts is

$$p_{1990}(24957 - 1990) = p_{1990}(22967). \qquad \square$$

CASE III   DISTINGUISHABLE OBJECTS INTO INDISTINGUISHABLE CONTAINERS

Here we study distributions of a set $X = \{x_1, x_2, \ldots, x_n\}$ of n distinguishable objects into k indistinguishable containers such that each container gets at least one of the objects. The mathematical model for such a distribution is a partition of $T_n = \{1, 2, \ldots, n\}$ into k nonempty subsets— that is, a collection

$$\Gamma = \{A_1, A_2, \ldots, A_k\}$$

of subsets of T_n such that

$$A_i \neq \varnothing \quad \text{for } 1 \leq i \leq k,$$
$$A_i \cap A_j = \varnothing \quad \text{for } i \neq j,$$
$$A_1 \cup A_2 \cup \cdots \cup A_k = T_n.$$

Example 3 A distribution of 4 distinguishable elements x_1, x_2, x_3, x_4 into 2 indistinguishable containers (each of which ends up nonempty) is modeled by the set partitions of $T_4 = \{1, 2, 3, 4\}$ into 2 nonempty subsets. One sees that the following list gives all of the partitions of $\{1, 2, 3, 4\}$ into 2 nonempty subsets:

$$\{\{1\}, \{2, 3, 4\}\}, \qquad \{\{2\}, \{1, 3, 4\}\}, \qquad \{\{3\}, \{1, 2, 4\}\},$$
$$\{\{4\}, \{1, 2, 3\}\}, \qquad \{\{1, 2\}, \{3, 4\}\}, \qquad \{\{1, 3\}, \{2, 4\}\},$$
$$\{\{1, 4\}, \{2, 3\}\}. \qquad\qquad\qquad\qquad\qquad\qquad\qquad\quad \square$$

NOTATION 1   **STIRLING NUMBERS $S(n, k)$ OF THE SECOND KIND**

$S(n, k)$ denotes the number of partitions of a set of size n into k nonempty subsets. Here $k \in \mathbf{Z}^+$ and $n \geq k$.

The $S(n, k)$ are called **Stirling Numbers of the second kind**. (Stirling Numbers of the first kind are discussed in the Supplementary and Challenging Problems of this chapter.) It follows from Example 3 that $S(4, 2) = 7$. In the examples below, we show how to obtain the data of Table 5.6.1, in which the entries for the nth row are $S(n, 1)$, $S(n, 2), \ldots,$ $S(n, n)$.

TABLE 5.6.1 Rows for $n = 1, 2, 3, 4, 5$ of Stirling's Second Triangle

n					
1			1		
2		1	1		
3		1	3	1	
4	1	7	6	1	
5	1	15	25	10	1

Example 4   We want to obtain all the partitions of $\{1, 2, 3, 4\}$ into 3 nonempty subsets. First we note that $\{\{1\}, \{2\}, \{3\}\}$ is the only partition of $\{1, 2, 3\}$ into 3 nonempty subsets. By inserting 4 into one of these subsets in each of the 3 possible ways, we get the partitions

$$\{\{1, 4\}, \{2\}, \{3\}\}, \qquad \{\{1\}, \{2, 4\}, \{3\}\}, \qquad \{\{1\}, \{2\}, \{3, 4\}\}.$$

These are only some of the partitions we are looking for. The others have the singleton $\{4\}$ as one of the subsets and are such that the other two subsets form a partition of $\{1, 2, 3\}$. These other partitions are

$$\{\{4\}, \{1\}, \{2, 3\}\}, \qquad \{\{4\}, \{2\}, \{1, 3\}\}, \qquad \text{and} \qquad \{\{4\}, \{3\}, \{1, 2\}\}.$$

Thus we see that $S(4, 3) = 3S(3, 3) + S(3, 2) = 3 \cdot 1 + 3 = 6$. $\square$

The process illustrated in Example 4 is extended to general positive integers n and k with $1 < k < n$ in Theorem 2 below. As is true of Pascal's

Triangle, additional rows of Stirling's Triangle can be calculated using border formulas and a recursion formula, which the following results state.

THEOREM 1 **BORDER FORMULAS FOR THE $S(n, k)$**

(a) $S(n, 1) = 1$ for $n \in Z^+ = \{1, 2, \ldots\}$.
(b) $S(n, n) = 1$ for $n \in Z^+$.

PROOF (a) The only partition of $T_n = \{1, 2, \ldots, n\}$ into 1 nonempty subset is $\{T_n\}$; hence $S(n, 1) = 1$ for all n in Z^+.
(b) The only partition of T_n into n nonempty subsets is

$$\{\{1\}, \{2\}, \{3\}, \ldots, \{n\}\}.$$

Hence $S(n, n) = 1$ for all n in Z^+. □

For example, $S(100, 1) = 1$ and $S(1000, 1000) = 1$.

THEOREM 2 **RECURSION FORMULA FOR $S(n,k)$**

Let $n \in \{3, 4, \ldots\}$ and $k \in \{2, 3, \ldots, n - 1\}$. Then

$$S(n, k) = kS(n - 1, k) + S(n - 1, k - 1).$$

PROOF Let $\Gamma = \{A_1, A_2, \ldots, A_k\}$ be a partition of $T_n = \{1, 2, \ldots, n\}$ into k nonempty subsets A_i. Since $A_1 \cup A_2 \cup \cdots \cup A_k = T_n$, the number n must be in one of the A_i. We consider two types of such partitions Γ. The first type consists of the Γ's for which the singleton $\{n\}$ is one of the subsets A_i. The Γ's of the first type are of the form

$$\{D_1, D_2, \ldots, D_{k-1}, \{n\}\},$$

where $\{D_1, D_2, \ldots, D_{k-1}\}$ is any partition of $T_{n-1} = \{1, 2, \ldots, n - 1\}$ into $k - 1$ nonempty subsets. Hence there are $S(n - 1, k - 1)$ first-type partitions of T_n. The second-type partitions $\{A_1, \ldots, A_k\}$ of T_n are those in which some A_i contains n and some other numbers of T_n. Such partitions can be constructed by taking $\{C_1, C_2, \ldots, C_k\}$ to be any one of the $S(n - 1, k)$ partitions of T_{n-1} into k nonempty subsets and adjoining n to any one of the k subsets C_i to form a second-type partition

$$\{C_1, \ldots, C_{i-1}, C_i \cup \{n\}, C_{i+1}, \ldots, C_k\}$$

of T_n into k nonempty subsets. By the product rule (Theorem 3) of Section 5.1, the number of second-type partitions of T_n is $kS(n - 1, k)$. Since each partition of T_n into k nonempty subsets is of either the first or second type but not both, it follows from the sum rule (Theorem 1) of Section 5.1 that

$$S(n, k) = kS(n - 1, k) + S(n - 1, k - 1).$$ □

Example 5   It follows from the border formulas of Theorem 1 that $S(3, 1) = 1 = S(2, 2)$. Then the recursion formula of Theorem 2 shows that

$$S(3, 2) = 2S(2, 2) + S(2, 1) = 2 \cdot 1 + 1 = 3.$$

Similarly, the border formulas give us $S(4, 1) = 1 = S(3, 3)$, and the recursion formula then produces

$$S(4, 2) = 2S(3, 2) + S(3, 1) = 2 \cdot 3 + 1 = 7,$$
$$S(4, 3) = 3S(3, 3) + S(3, 2) = 3 \cdot 1 + 3 = 6. \qquad \square$$

THEOREM 3   **SOME SPECIAL CASES OF $S(n, k)$**

(a) $S(n, 2) = 2^{n-1} - 1$ for $n \in \{2, 3, \dots\}$.
(b) $S(n, n - 1) = \binom{n}{2}$ for $n \in \mathbf{Z}^+$.

Ways of establishing these formulas are suggested to the reader in the problems below.

CASE IV   **DISTINGUISHABLE OBJECTS INTO DISTINGUISHABLE CONTAINERS**

Here we count distributions of n distinguishable objects $x_1, x_2, \dots, x_n$ into k distinguishable containers $C_1, C_2, \dots, C_k$ after which each C_j ends up nonempty. Such a distribution can be modeled by a mapping

$$f: X = \{x_1, x_2, \dots, x_n\} \to Y = \{y_1, y_2, \dots, y_k\}$$

if we think of $f(x_i) = y_j$ as indicating that the object x_i is placed by the distribution in container C_j. Since each container C_j should have at least one object placed in it, each complete inverse image $f^{-1}(y_j)$ must be nonempty. This means that the mapping f must be a surjection.

Example 6   **A MAPPING AS A DISTRIBUTION**   Let $X = \{1, 2, \dots, 10\}$ and $Y = \{a, b, c, d\}$. Let f be the mapping from X to Y given by the following table:

x	1	2	3	4	5	6	7	8	9	10
$f(x)$	a	b	c	d	a	b	c	d	a	b

This mapping indicates the distribution of the 10 distinguishable integers from X into 4 distinguishable containers A, B, C, and D in which x is placed in A if $f(x) = a$, x ends up in B if $f(x) = b$, and so on. That is, the set of integers placed in A is the complete inverse image $f^{-1}(a) = \{1, 5, 9\}$, the set of integers placed in B is $f^{-1}(b) = \{2, 6, 10\}$, the set of integers placed in C is $f^{-1}(c) = \{3, 7\}$, and the set of integers placed in D is $f^{-1}(d) = \{4, 8\}$. The mapping f is a surjection, since each element of Y is the image of at least one integer in X; that is, each of the complete inverse images $f^{-1}(a), f^{-1}(b), f^{-1}(c), f^{-1}(d)$ is nonempty. □

Example 7 **A DISTRIBUTION AS A MAPPING** Here we consider the distribution of the 10 integers from $X = \{1, 2, \ldots, 10\}$ into 4 distinguishable containers A, B, C, D in which the integers placed in A form the subset $\{3, 6, 9\}$, those placed in B form the subset $\{1, 4, 7, 10\}$, those placed in C form the subset $\{2, 5\}$, and the subset $\{8\}$ consists of the sole integer placed in D. We note that each container ends up with at least one of the integers. This distribution is modeled by the mapping of X into $Y = \{a, b, c, d\}$ given by the following table, where $g(x) = a$ if x is placed in A, $g(x) = b$ if x is placed in B, and so on.

x	1	2	3	4	5	6	7	8	9	10
$g(x)$	b	c	a	b	c	a	b	d	a	b

Since each of the complete inverse images $g^{-1}(a) = \{3, 6, 9\}$, $g^{-1}(b) = \{1, 4, 7, 10\}$, $g^{-1}(c) = \{2, 5\}$, and $g^{-1}(d) = \{8\}$ is nonempty, the mapping g is a surjection. □

Examples 6 and 7 indicate that we can think of a distribution of the n distinguishable elements of $X = \{x_1, x_2, \ldots, x_n\}$ into k distinguishable containers $C_1, C_2, \ldots, C_k$ as a mapping f from X to a set $\{c_1, c_2, \ldots, c_k\}$ of size k. The distribution will result in each container having at least one object if and only if the mapping f is a surjection. This implies that the number of distributions of any given set of n distinguishable objects into a given set of k distinguishable containers in which the distribution gives at least one of the objects to each container is the number of surjections from a set X of size n onto a set Y of size k.

In the next example we illustrate the technique for counting such surjections; we then prove the formula in general in Theorem 4.

Example 8 Here we count the number of distributions of 4 distinguishable objects into 3 distinguishable containers. This number is also the number of surjections from $X = \{1, 2, 3, 4\}$ onto a set $Y = \{a, b, c\}$ of size 3.

As in Example 4, one of the $S(4, 3)$ partitions of X into 3 nonempty subsets is $\{\{1\}, \{2\}, \{3, 4\}\}$. The 3 subsets in this collection can be permuted in 3! ways to get the 6 listings

$$\{\{1\}, \{2\}, \{3, 4\}\}, \quad \{\{1\}, \{3, 4\}, \{2\}\}, \quad \{\{2\}, \{1\}, \{3, 4\}\},$$
$$\{\{2\}, \{3, 4\}, \{1\}\}, \quad \{\{3, 4\}, \{1\}, \{2\}\}, \quad \{\{3, 4\}, \{2\}, \{1\}\}.$$

Each such listing determines a surjection from X onto Y. The listing $\{\{1\}, \{2\}, \{3, 4\}\}$ determines the surjection f with $f^{-1}(a) = \{1\}$, $f^{-1}(b) = \{2\}$, and $f^{-1}(c) = \{3, 4\}$, that is, the surjection f with the following table:

x	1	2	3	4
$f(x)$	a	b	c	c

The listing $\{\{1\}, \{3, 4\}, \{2\}\}$ determines the surjection g with $g^{-1}(a) = \{1\}$, $g^{-1}(b) = \{3, 4\}$, $g^{-1}(c) = \{2\}$, that is, the g with the following table:

x	1	2	3	4
$g(x)$	a	c	b	b

Each of the $S(4, 3)$ partitions of X into 3 nonempty subsets can be permuted to give us 3! listings of the subsets. This produces $3!S(4, 3)$ listings and the same number of surjections from X onto Y. We see from Table 5.6.1 that $S(4, 3) = 6$. Hence the answer is

$$3!S(4, 3) = 6 \cdot 6 = 36. \qquad \square$$

THEOREM 4   **NUMBER OF SURJECTIONS**

Let $\#X = n$ and $\#Y = k$ with $1 \leq k \leq n$. Then the number of surjections from X onto Y is $k!S(n, k)$.

PROOF   Let $X = \{x_1, x_2, \ldots, x_n\}$, $Y = \{y_1, y_2, \ldots, y_k\}$, and f be a surjection from X onto Y. Since f is a surjection, each y_j in Y is the image of at least one x_i in X and hence the complete inverse image $f^{-1}(y_j)$ is nonempty. By Theorem 1 of Section 1.8, the collection

$$\Gamma = \{f^{-1}(y_1), f^{-1}(y_2), \ldots, f^{-1}(y_k)\} \qquad (1)$$

of all the complete inverse images forms a partition of X. Thus the Γ of Display (1) is a partition of X into k nonempty subsets for every surjection f from X onto Y. Our work in Case III above tells us that there are $S(n, k)$ partitions of a set of size n into k nonempty subsets. However, each partition $\Gamma = \{A_1, A_2, \ldots, A_k\}$ of X into k nonempty subsets can be used to get $k!$ surjections from X onto Y, as follows. Let $\{H_1, H_2, \ldots, H_k\}$ be any one of the $k!$ listings of the collection Γ. Then

$$g^{-1}(y_1) = H_1, \qquad g^{-1}(y_2) = H_2, \qquad \ldots, \qquad g^{-1}(y_k) = H_k$$

determines the surjection g from X onto Y in which $g(x) = y_j$ if x is in H_j. Each surjection from X onto Y is determined in a one-to-one way by such a listing $\{H_1, H_2, \ldots, H_k\}$ of the sets of a collection $\{A_1, A_2, \ldots, A_k\}$ forming a partition of X into k nonempty subsets. There are $S(n, k)$ of these partitions, and each has $k!$ listings. It follows from the product rule that there are $k!S(n, k)$ surjections from X onto Y. $\square$

Theorem 1 above gave the border formulas

$$S(n, 1) = 1 = S(n, n) \quad \text{for } n \in \mathbf{Z}^+;$$

Theorem 2 has the recursion formula

$$S(n, k) = kS(n - 1, k) + S(n - 1, k - 1) \qquad \text{for } 2 \le k < n;$$

and Theorem 3 has the closed forms

$$S(n, 2) = 2^{n-1} - 1 \quad \text{for } n \in \{2, 3, \ldots\},$$

$$S(n, n - 1) = \binom{n}{2} \quad \text{for } n \in \mathbf{Z}^+$$

for the entries of Table 5.6.1 on the diagonals next to the borders. Closed forms can be found for other special cases, but no simple formula is known for $S(n, k)$ for general n and k. The best we can do is the formula involving ellipsis dots or summation notation given in the following result.

THEOREM 5 **FORMULA FOR STIRLING NUMBERS OF THE SECOND KIND**

$$S(n, k) = \frac{1}{k!} \left[k^n - \binom{k}{1}(k - 1)^n + \binom{k}{2}(k - 2)^n - \right.$$

$$\left. \cdots + (-1)^{k-1} \binom{k}{k - 1} \cdot 1^n \right];$$

that is,

$$S(n, k) = \frac{1}{k!} \sum_{i=0}^{k-1} (-1)^i \binom{k}{i} (k - i)^n.$$

PROOF Let $\#X = n$ and $Y = \{y_1, y_2, \ldots, y_k\}$ with $2 \le k \le n$. There are $k!S(n, k)$ surjections from X onto Y. Let us count these surjections in another way. The set of all mappings from X to Y is Y^X, and by Theorem 2 of Section 1.8, the number of such mappings is $(\#Y)^{\#X} = k^n$. We want to count only the mappings f in Y^X with

$$f^{-1}(y_1) \ne \varnothing, \qquad f^{-1}(y_2) \ne \varnothing, \qquad \cdots, \qquad f^{-1}(y_k) \ne \varnothing.$$

For $j = 1, 2, \ldots, k$, let A_j be the subset of mappings f in Y^X with the complete inverse image $f^{-1}(y_j)$ empty. We want to count the mappings in the complement of $A_1 \cup A_2 \cup \cdots \cup A_k$ in the set Y^X. Let σ_1 be the sum of the sizes of the A_j, σ_2 be the sum of the sizes of the intersections $A_i \cap A_j$ of pairs of these subsets, σ_3 be the sum of the sizes of the intersections $A_h \cap A_i \cap A_j$ of triples of these subsets, and so on. Then $\sigma_k = 0$, since there are no mappings f in Y^X with $\varnothing = f^{-1}(y_1) = f^{-1}(y_2) = \cdots = f^{-1}(y_k)$. It then follows from the inclusion–exclusion principle (Theorem 5 of Section 5.3) that the number of surjections in Y^X is

$$k!S(n, k) = \# Y^X - \sigma_1 + \sigma_2 - \sigma_3 + \cdots + (-1)^{k-1}\sigma_{k-1}. \tag{2}$$

We see that $\# A_j = (k - 1)^n$, since A_j consists of the mappings f of Y^X with $f^{-1}(y_j) = \varnothing$, that is, with each image $f(x)$ in the set

$$\{y_1, y_2, \ldots, y_{j-1}, y_{j+1}, \ldots, y_k\}$$

of size $k - 1$. Then

$$\begin{aligned} \sigma_1 &= \# A_1 + \# A_2 + \cdots + \# A_k \\ &= k(k - 1)^n \\ &= \binom{k}{1}(k - 1)^n. \end{aligned}$$

Also, $\#(A_i \cap A_j) = (k - 2)^n$, since $A_i \cap A_j$ consists of the mappings f in Y^X with each image $f(x)$ in a set of size $k - 2$, namely, the complement of $\{y_i, y_j\}$ in Y. There are $\binom{k}{2}$ such pairs $\{A_i, A_j\}$; so $\sigma_2 = \binom{k}{2}(k - 2)^n$. Similarly, $\sigma_3 = \binom{k}{3}(k - 3)^n$ and so on. We make these replacements in Display (2) and have

$$k!S(n, k) = k^n - \binom{k}{1}(k - 1)^n + \binom{k}{2}(k - 2)^n - \cdots + (-1)^{k-1}\binom{k}{k-1} \cdot 1^n.$$

Dividing both sides by $k!$, we get the claimed formula for $S(n, k)$.   □

Example 9   It follows from Theorem 5 that

$$S(n, 3) = \frac{1}{3!}(3^n - 3 \cdot 2^n + 3)$$

and hence that

$$S(6, 3) = \frac{1}{6}(3^6 - 3 \cdot 2^6 + 3) = \frac{1}{6}(729 - 192 + 3) = \frac{540}{6} = 90.   □$$

Table 5.6.2 gives synonyms for some key words in the combinatorial theory of distributions.

TABLE 5.6.2

Word	Synonyms
container	bin, box, batch
distinguishable	different, distinct
indistinguishable	identical, same
distributing	placing, dividing, splitting

PROBLEMS FOR SECTION 5.6

1. (a) In how many ways can 5 identical marbles be distributed into 3 distinguishable boxes?
   (b) In how many of the distributions of Part (a) will each box end up nonempty?

2. (a) In how many ways can one place 8 identical marbles into 5 distinguishable boxes?
   (b) In how many of these distributions will each box end up nonempty?

3. Repeat Problem 1, now with indistinguishable boxes.

4. Repeat Problem 2, now with indistinguishable boxes.

5. In how many ways can one select a set of 7 coins from a plentiful supply of identical pennies, identical nickels, and identical dimes?

6. Repeat Problem 5, but now also add a plentiful supply of identical quarters.

7. Use the border formulas, recursion formula, and the 5th row of Stirling's Second Triangle,

$$S(5, 1) = 1, \quad S(5, 2) = 15, \quad S(5, 3) = 25, \quad S(5, 4) = 10, \quad S(5, 5) = 1,$$

   to find the 6th row.

8. Find the 7th row of Stirling's Second Triangle.

9. Use the following formula to compute $S(7, 3)$:

$$S(n, k) = \frac{1}{k!} \sum_{i=0}^{k-1} (-1)^i \binom{k}{i} (k - i)^n$$

10. Use the formula of Problem 9 to compute $S(8, 4)$.

11. How many subsets $\{a, b, c\}$ are there of the set $\{2, 3, 4, \ldots\}$ such that $abc = 2 \cdot 3 \cdot 5 \cdot 7 \cdot 11 \cdot 13 \cdot 17$?

12. How many subsets $\{a, b, c, d\}$ are there of the set $\{2, 3, 4, \ldots\}$ such that $abcd = 2 \cdot 3 \cdot 5 \cdot 7 \cdot 11 \cdot 13 \cdot 17 \cdot 19 \cdot 23$?

13. Let $S = \{2, 3, 4, \ldots\}$. How many ordered triples (a, b, c) are there in $S \times S \times S$ such that $abc = 2 \cdot 3 \cdot 5 \cdot 7 \cdot 11 \cdot 13 \cdot 17$?

14. Let $S = \{2, 3, 4, \ldots\}$. How many ordered 4-tuples (a, b, c, d) are there in S^4 such that $abcd = 2 \cdot 3 \cdot 5 \cdot 7 \cdot 11 \cdot 13 \cdot 17 \cdot 19 \cdot 23$?

15. Let $\#X = 9$ and $\#Y = 4$.
(a) How many mappings are there from X to Y?
(b) Of these, how many are surjections?

16. Repeat Problem 15, but now with $\#X = 12$ and $\#Y = 5$.

17. In how many ways can one distribute 9 distinguishable objects into 4 distinguishable containers if some containers are allowed to end up empty?

18. Repeat Problem 17 for 12 distinguishable objects and 5 distinguishable containers.

19. Repeat Problem 17, but now do not count distributions in which any container is left empty.

20. In how many ways can 12 distinguishable objects be split into 5 nonempty distinguishable batches?

21. Explain why $S(n, 5) = (5^n - 5 \cdot 4^n + 10 \cdot 3^n - 10 \cdot 2^n + 5)/120$ for $n \in \{5, 6, \ldots\}$.

22. Find a formula for $S(n, 6)$.

23. Prove that $S(n, n - 1) = \binom{n}{2}$. That is, prove Theorem 3(b).

24. Use Theorem 5 ("Formula for Stirling Numbers of the Second Kind") to derive the formula $S(n, 2) = 2^{n-1} - 1$ of Theorem 3(a).

25. How many of the distributions of the integers of $\{1, 2, \ldots, n\}$ into two distinguishable containers C and D are such that 1 is placed in C and D does not end up empty?

26. Does the answer to Problem 25 equal $S(n, 2)$?

27. Explain why $24 | (4^n - 4 \cdot 3^n + 6 \cdot 2^n - 4)$ for $n \in \{4, 5, \ldots\}$.

28. Explain why $120 | (5^n - 5 \cdot 4^n + 10 \cdot 3^n - 10 \cdot 2^n + 5)$ for $n \in \{5, 6, \ldots\}$.

5.7

DISCRETE PROBABILITY

In the seventeenth century, the theory of probability was given impetus toward becoming a branch of mathematics when Blaise Pascal (1623–1662) was asked to calculate odds by a friend who gambled. Probability now helps in making decisions in many situations involving uncertainty and has applications in such varied fields as quality testing, insurance, and predicting election results.

Discrete probability is a branch of probability whose techniques are essentially combinatorial. More advanced branches use a generalization of integral calculus called "measure theory."

The following definition, due to the French mathematician, physicist, and astronomer Pierre Simon Laplace (1749–1827), furnishes us with a combinatorial model for discrete probability. (See the biographical note on Laplace just before the problems for this section.)

DEFINITION 1   **SAMPLE SPACE, FAVORABLE SUBSET, PROBABILITY**

Let S be a finite set, called the **sample space**. Let a subset F of S be designated as the **favorable subset**. The **probability** that a randomly chosen element of S is in F is defined to be $\#F/\#S$.

The word *randomly* is used in this definition to indicate that each element of S has equal probability of being selected.

Example 1   Let the sample space be the set

$$B_3 = \{000, 001, 010, 011, 100, 101, 110, 111\}$$

of binary strings of length 3. What is the probability that a string $\beta = b_1 b_2 b_3$ chosen at random from B_3 has exactly two 1's among its digits b_i, that is, has weight 2? The favorable subset is $B_{3,2} = \{011, 101, 110\}$, and so the desired probability is $\#B_{3,2}/\#B_3 = \frac{3}{8}$. To find the probability that a randomly chosen β in B_3 has wgt $\beta \neq 2$, one would let F be the complement of $B_{3,2}$ in B_3 and get as the answer

$$\frac{\#F}{\#B_3} = \frac{8-3}{8} = 1 - \frac{3}{8} = \frac{5}{8}.$$

The probability that a randomly chosen β in B_3 has weight at least 2 is $\frac{4}{8} = \frac{1}{2}$, since for this case the favorable subset is $B_{3,2} \cup B_{3,3} = \{011, 101, 110, 111\}$.   □

Example 2   Someone is about to shake 8 pennies in a box and toss them onto a table. We assume that each penny will land either heads or tails and that these two outcomes are equally likely. Let p be the probability that exactly 4 of the 8 pennies will land heads. Is $p \geq \frac{1}{2}$? That is, can we reasonably expect exactly 4 heads in at least half of the cases when this experiment is repeated many times? We model this problem by using 1 for heads and 0 for tails, and thus have the set B_8 of eight-digit binary strings $\alpha = a_1 a_2 \ldots a_8$ as the sample space. There are two choices for each a_i, so by the product rule, $\#B_8 = 2^8 = 256$. The favorable subset $B_{8,4}$ consists of the α with $a_i = 1$ for exactly 4 values of i in $\{1, 2, \ldots, 8\}$; hence $\#B_{8,4} = \binom{8}{4}$. Using Theorem 4, "Factorial Forms of $\binom{n}{k}$," of Section 5.2 we have

$$\#B_{8,4} = \binom{8}{4} = \frac{8 \cdot 7 \cdot 6 \cdot 5}{4 \cdot 3 \cdot 2 \cdot 1} = 70.$$

Hence $p = \#B_{8,4}/\#B_8 = \frac{70}{256} = \frac{35}{128}$. Since $p < \frac{1}{2}$, it is not a good "even money" bet.   □

Example 3   What is the probability of throwing a 4 with a pair of dice? A die is a cube whose six faces are numbered 1, 2, 3, 4, 5, 6 in a certain order. We assume that each face is equally likely to be the top face of its die and that the two dice are distinguishable (say one is red and one is blue). We model the problem by taking the set S of ordered pairs (m, n), with each of m and n in $\{1, 2, 3, 4, 5, 6\}$ as the sample space. There are 6 choices for m and 6 choices for n, so by the product rule, $\#S = 6 \cdot 6 = 36$. The favorable subset F consists of the (m, n) of S with $m + n = 4$; that is, $F = \{(1, 3), (2, 2), (3, 1)\}$. Hence the desired probability is $\#F/\#S = \frac{3}{36} = \frac{1}{12}$.   □

Example 4   What is the probability of getting a total of exactly 16 when 5 dice are thrown? We model this problem by taking the sample space S to be the set of all ordered 5-tuples $(x_1, x_2, x_3, x_4, x_5)$ with each x_i in $\{1, 2, 3, 4, 5, 6\}$. By the product rule, $\#S = 6^5 = 7776$. The favorable subset F consists of the compositions of 16 into 5 parts, with each part x_i satisfying $1 \le x_i \le 6$. We find $\#F$ as follows.

Let T consist of all the compositions $(x_1, \ldots, x_5)$ of 16 into 5 positive parts. Let A_i be the subset of the compositions in T with $7 \le x_i$. Then F is the complement of $B = A_1 \cup A_2 \cup A_3 \cup A_4 \cup A_5$ in T. By Theorem 2 ("Compositions with Positive Parts") of Section 5.4, $\#T = \binom{15}{4}$. Using the technique of Example 4 of Section 5.4, we see that $\#A_i = \binom{9}{4}$ for each i. The sets A_i are disjoint; for example, a composition in both A_1 and A_2 would have $7 \le x_1$, $7 \le x_2$, $1 \le x_3$, $1 \le x_4$, and $1 \le x_5$, and these contradict $x_1 + x_2 + x_3 + x_4 + x_5 = 16$. Hence

$$\#B = \#A_1 + \#A_2 + \cdots + \#A_5 = 5\binom{9}{4}.$$

Then $\#F = \#T - \#B = \binom{15}{4} - 5\binom{9}{4}$. Using the binomial coefficient formula from Theorem 4 of Section 5.2 yields

$$\binom{9}{4} = \frac{9 \cdot 8 \cdot 7 \cdot 6}{4 \cdot 3 \cdot 2 \cdot 1} = 3 \cdot 7 \cdot 6 = 126,$$

$$\binom{15}{4} = \frac{15 \cdot 14 \cdot 13 \cdot 12}{4 \cdot 3 \cdot 2 \cdot 1} = 15 \cdot 7 \cdot 13 = 1365.$$

Thus $\#F = 1365 - 5 \cdot 126 = 1365 - 630 = 735$, and the desired probability is $\#F/\#S = \frac{735}{7776} = \frac{245}{2592}$. To four decimal places this fraction is 0.0945.   □

Example 5   What is the probability that a hand in the card game of bridge will contain exactly two aces? For our model, we take a **bridge deck** to be the set

K of all strings xy with x in $\{S, H, D, C\}$ (that is, spades, hearts, diamonds, and clubs) and y in $\{2, 3, \ldots, 9, t, j, q, k, a\}$ (that is, the numbers 2–10 and jack, queen, king, ace). For example, Sa is in K and is known as the ace of spades. A string in K is called a ***card***, and a subset of 13 of the 52 cards of K is called a ***bridge hand***. The sample space B consists of the $\binom{52}{13}$ bridge hands. To be in the favorable subset F, the hand must have 2 cards from the set $\{Sa, Ha, Da, Ca\}$ of the 4 aces, with the remaining 11 cards being chosen from the 48 non-aces. Using the product rule, we get $\#F = \binom{4}{2}\binom{48}{11}$. Since $\binom{4}{2} = 4 \cdot 3/2 = 6$, the desired probability is

$$\frac{\#F}{\#B} = \frac{\binom{4}{2}\binom{48}{11}}{\binom{52}{13}} = \frac{6 \cdot \dfrac{48!}{11! \cdot 37!}}{\dfrac{52!}{13! \cdot 39!}} = \frac{6 \cdot 48! \cdot 13! \cdot 39!}{52! \cdot 11! \cdot 37!} = \frac{6 \cdot 13 \cdot 12 \cdot 39 \cdot 38}{52 \cdot 51 \cdot 50 \cdot 49}$$

$$= \frac{2 \cdot 3 \cdot 13 \cdot 4 \cdot 3 \cdot 39 \cdot 38}{13 \cdot 4 \cdot 17 \cdot 3 \cdot 25 \cdot 2 \cdot 49} = \frac{3 \cdot 39 \cdot 38}{17 \cdot 25 \cdot 49} = \frac{4446}{20825}$$

To five decimal places this is 0.21349. □

Example 6   Let $T = \{t_1, t_2, \ldots, t_{10}\}$. What is the probability that a randomly chosen subset A of T will have an even number of objects in it? We model this by letting the power set $P(T)$ be the sample space S and letting the favorable subset F consist of the members A of $P(T)$ with $\#A$ in $\{0, 2, 4, 6, 8, 10\}$. Using the technique illustrated in Problem 25 of Section 5.2 gives us

$$\#F = \binom{10}{0} + \binom{10}{2} + \binom{10}{4} + \binom{10}{6} + \binom{10}{8} + \binom{10}{10} = 2^9.$$

Hence the desired probability is $\#F/\#S = 2^9/2^{10} = \frac{1}{2}$. □

The following example illustrates some topics that will appear in our analysis of two probabilistic games in Section 5.8.

Example 7   For a listing $\lambda = \{a_1, a_2, a_3\}$ of $\{1, 2, 3\}$, let $f(\lambda)$ be the number of terms a_i that are in their natural positions, that is, the number of a_i with $a_i = i$. Let the set of all 6 listings of $\{1, 2, 3\}$ be $L_3 = \{\lambda_1, \lambda_2, \lambda_3, \lambda_4, \lambda_5, \lambda_6\}$, where

$$\lambda_1 = \{1, 2, 3\}, \qquad \lambda_2 = \{1, 3, 2\}, \qquad \lambda_3 = \{2, 1, 3\},$$
$$\lambda_4 = \{2, 3, 1\}, \qquad \lambda_5 = \{3, 1, 2\}, \qquad \lambda_6 = \{3, 2, 1\}.$$

Now we repeat these listings, with a bar over each term that is in natural position:

$$\lambda_1 = \{\bar{1}, \bar{2}, \bar{3}\}, \qquad \lambda_2 = \{\bar{1}, 3, 2\}, \qquad \lambda_3 = \{2, 1, \bar{3}\},$$
$$\lambda_4 = \{2, 3, 1\}, \qquad \lambda_5 = \{3, 1, 2\}, \qquad \lambda_6 = \{3, \bar{2}, 1\}.$$

By counting the overbars for a given λ_n, we obtain the data for the following table:

n	1	2	3	4	5	6
$f(\lambda_n)$	3	1	1	0	0	1

The set of λ's in L_3 with $f(\lambda) = 0$ is $\{\lambda_4, \lambda_5\}$; hence the probability that $f(\lambda) = 0$ for a randomly chosen λ in L_3 is $\frac{2}{6} = \frac{1}{3}$. The set of λ's in L_3 with $f(\lambda) = 1$ is $\{\lambda_2, \lambda_3, \lambda_6\}$, and so the probability is $\frac{3}{6} = \frac{1}{2}$ that a randomly chosen λ in L_3 has $f(\lambda) = 1$. The probability is 0 that $f(\lambda) = 2$, and the probability is $\frac{1}{6}$ that $f(\lambda) = 3$. We note that the sum of these probabilities is $\frac{1}{3} + \frac{1}{2} + 0 + \frac{1}{6} = \frac{6}{6} = 1$. This should not be surprising because, for a randomly chosen λ in L_3, the probability is 100% that $f(\lambda)$ is in $\{0, 1, 2, 3\}$.   □

*Example 8   This is an illustration of the kind of probability problem that can *not* be solved by combinatorial methods because the sample space is infinite. The specific question is: If x and y are both randomly chosen real numbers in the interval $0 \leq t \leq 3$, what is the probability that the absolute value of their difference is less than 1? The sample space here consists of all ordered pairs (x, y) with x and y in $0 \leq t \leq 3$. An (x, y) in S is favorable if $|x - y| < 1$. Since both S and the subset F of favorable elements are infinite, it is not very constructive to give $\#F/\#S$ as the answer. Instead we note that each (x, y) in S can be associated with the point whose coordinates are (x, y). We picture S as the square in Figure 5.7.1 and F as the shaded region inside the square. Finally, we decide that a reasonable answer to this probability question is the ratio of the area of the shaded region to the area of the square. The unshaded region in the square consists of two triangles, each of area 2. The area of the square is 9. Hence the shaded region has area $9 - 2 \cdot 2 = 5$, and the desired probability (using this interpretation) is $\frac{5}{9}$.   □

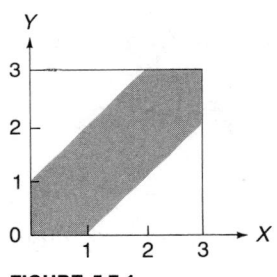

FIGURE 5.7.1

Pierre Simon Laplace   *was born in 1749 in Normandy, the son of a poor farmer. He showed great promise in school and was encouraged to go to military school and eventually to Paris, where he attracted the attention of one of the eminent mathematicians of the day, Jean le Rond D'Alembert. He lived during the dangerous times of the French Revolution, the subsequent Napoleonic period, and the later return of the Bourbons to the throne. Somehow he survived all of these upheavals while others were subject to banishment or the guillotine.*

   Laplace's principal scientific work was in celestial mechanics, mathematical physics, and probability. His most famous work, the

Mécanique Céleste, is a monument in the history of science, though the writing is notoriously lacking in clarity. (His translator into English, the noted American astronomer Nathaniel Bowditch, tried to make it comprehensible with extensive annotations. Many pages of the translation consist of one or two lines of Laplace's original, with the rest of the page devoted entirely to footnotes.)

Though of humble background, Laplace enjoyed favor with the powerful. Napoleon enjoyed his company and is reported to have discussed astronomy with him during battles. Napoleon made him a Count, and later, one of the Bourbon kings made him a Marquis. He held various government positions, but seemed to show little talent for government. Napoleon at one time remarked that Laplace "carried the spirit of the infinitely small into the management of affairs." Laplace died in Paris in 1827.

PROBLEMS FOR SECTION 5.7

1. (a) What is the probability that a randomly chosen string α from $B_2 = \{00, 01, 10, 11\}$ will have exactly one 1 among its digits?
   (b) What is the probability that a randomly chosen α from B_2 will have at least one 1 among its digits?
   (c) What is the probability that a randomly chosen string α from B_7 will have weight 3?
   (d) If α is chosen randomly from B_n, what is the probability that wgt $\alpha = k$?

2. Let $\alpha = a_1 a_2 a_3 a_4$ be a randomly chosen string from B_4. What is the probability that among the digits a_i of α there are:
   (a) no 1's?   (b) exactly one 1?   (c) exactly two 1's?
   (d) at least two 1's?   (e) no more than two 1's?

3. Let $T = \{a, b, c\}$. Let A be a randomly chosen subset of T.
   (i) What is the size $\# P(T)$ of the power set for T?
   (ii) What is the probability that A is a singleton?
   (iii) What is the probability that A is a doubleton?

4. Do as in Problem 3, but with T now a set $\{a, b, c, d\}$ of size 4.

5. Let 8 pennies be tossed (as in Example 2). What is the probability that:
   (a) exactly 5 of the pennies land heads?
   (b) at least 5 of the pennies land heads?

6. Let 8 pennies be tossed (as in Example 2). What is the probability that the number of heads resulting is either 2 or 4?

7. For each of the following values of t, find the probability of throwing a total of t with a pair of dice:
   (a) 2;   (b) 3;   (c) 4;   (d) 12;   (e) 11;   (f) 10.

8. Do as in Problem 7 for the following values of t:
(a) 5;   (b) 6;   (c) 7;   (d) 8;   (e) 9.

9. Let 4 dice be shaken fairly and tossed on a table. What is the probability that the total of their top faces will be:
(a) 4?   (b) 5?   (c) 6?   (d) 22?   (e) 23?   (f) 24?

10. Do as in Problem 9 for the following totals:
(a) 7;   (b) 8;   (c) 20;   (d) 21.

11. Let 10 dice be shaken fairly and tossed on a table. Let $p(t)$ be the probability that the total on the top faces will be t. Explain why $p(t) = p(70 - t)$ for $t = 10, 11, \ldots, 60$.

12. Generalize Problem 11 by letting n dice be tossed.

13. (a) What is the probability that a randomly chosen bridge hand will have exactly k spades, that is, k cards xy with $x = $ S? (The notation is as in Example 5.)
(b) Evaluate the answer to Part (a) when $k = 7$.

14. (a) What is the probability that a randomly chosen bridge hand will have exactly k *red cards*, that is, cards xy with x either H (hearts) or D (diamonds)?
(b) Evaluate the answer to Part (a) when $k = 6$.

15. A *bridge table* is an ordered 4-tuple (A_1, A_2, A_3, A_4) with each A_i a bridge hand and A_1, A_2, A_3, A_4 a partitioning of the bridge deck K. How many bridge tables are there?

16. What is the probability that a randomly obtained bridge table (as defined in Problem 15) will have one ace in each of its hands A_i?

17. Let $\lambda = \{a_1, a_2, a_3, a_4\}$ be a randomly constructed listing of $\{1, 2, 3, 4\}$. As in Example 7, let $f(\lambda)$ be the number of terms a_i in their natural positions; that is, let $f(\lambda)$ be the number of a_i with $a_i = i$. What is the probability that:
(a) $f(\lambda) = 0$?   (b) $f(\lambda) = 1$?   (c) $f(\lambda) = 2$?
(d) $f(\lambda) = 3$?   (e) $f(\lambda) = 4$?

18. Let $\lambda = \{a_1, a_2, \ldots, a_n\}$ be a randomly constructed listing of the set $\{1, 2, \ldots, n\}$. What is the probability that:
(a) $a_1 = 1$?   (b) $a_1 = 1$ and $a_2 = 2$ (simultaneously)?
(c) $a_1 = 1$ or $a_2 = 2$ (or both)?
(The answers can be checked using the cases of $n = 2$ and $n = 3$.)

19. Let n be chosen at random from $S = \{1000, 1001, \ldots, 9999\}$. What is the probability that the 4 digits of n are distinct, that is, different from each other?

20. Let n be chosen at random from $S = \{1000, 1001, \ldots, 9999\}$. What is the probability that:
(a) exactly 1 of the 4 digits of n is odd?
(b) exactly 1 of the 4 digits of n is even?

21. In a random permutation of the 26 letters of the alphabet $\{a, b, \ldots, z\}$, what is the probability that b will appear just after a? That is, for a random permutation

$$a \mapsto L_1, b \mapsto L_2, \ldots, z \mapsto L_{26}$$

on the set $A = \{a, b, \ldots, z\}$, what is the probability that $a = L_i$ and $b = L_{i+1}$ for some i in $\{1, 2, \ldots, 25\}$?

22. In a random permutation of the alphabet $\{a, b, \ldots, z\}$, what is the probability that b will appear just before or just after a?

23. Let X consist of the 20-bit strings $\alpha = a_1 a_2 \ldots a_{20}$ with wgt $\alpha = 10$, that is, with $a_1 + a_2 + \cdots + a_{20} = 10$.
(i) Find $\#X$.
(ii) Find the probability that a randomly chosen α in X has $a_1 + a_2 + \cdots + a_{10}$ in the set $\{0, 1, 2\}$.

24. Let X consist of the 20-bit strings $\alpha = a_1 a_2 \ldots a_{20}$ with wgt $\alpha = 10$. What is the probability that a randomly chosen α in X has $a_1 + a_2 + \cdots + a_{10}$ in the set $\{8, 9, 10\}$?

5.8

DERANGEMENTS, EXPECTED VALUES, AND PROBABILISTIC GAMES

As stated at the beginning of Section 5.7, the probability theory that was originally used to analyze games of chance now helps in many situations in which decisions have to be based on probabilities rather than on certainties. In the twentieth century, the book *Theory of Games and Economic Behavior* by John von Neumann and Oskar Morgenstern (John Wiley & Sons, New York, 1953) gave impetus to a mathematical theory of games and to applications of this theory in economics, political science, and other fields. (See the biographical note on von Neumann just before the problems for this section.)

This section illustrates the application of combinatorial techniques in game theory by developing the basic properties of a particularly interesting sequence of integers and then using these properties to determine the "fairness" of two related games.

We call the first game *Hits*. There is a form of Hits for every integer n in the set $\{2, 3, \ldots\}$. The participants are called *Player* and *Bank*. Each round of the game starts with Player paying Bank a fixed amount, called the *round fee*. Then the participants together produce a random listing $\{a_1, a_2, \ldots, a_n\}$ of the set $\{1, 2, \ldots, n\}$. For example, when $n = 13$, the random listing can be obtained by having each of the participants shuffle the same suit of a bridge deck until both are satisfied that the 13 cards are in random order. The round ends with a *round payoff* from Bank to

Player of $1 for each k such that $a_k = k$ in the listing. That is, the number of dollars in the round payoff is the number of integers k in $\{1, 2, \ldots, n\}$ such that k is in its natural position in the listing $\{a_1, a_2, \ldots, a_n\}$ for the round. If the listing $\{a_1, \ldots, a_{13}\}$ is

$$\{6, 3, 9, 5, 12, 4, 13, 8, 10, 2, 11, 7, 1\},$$

then the k's with $a_k = k$ are 8 and 11, since 8 is the eighth integer in the listing, 11 is the eleventh integer listed, and no other integer is in its natural position. Thus the round payoff for this listing is $2.

The basic mathematical problem of this game is the determination, for each n, of the average of the round payoffs for $n!$ rounds in which each of the $n!$ listings of $\{1, 2, \ldots, n\}$ is used exactly once. This average is called the **expected payoff**. It is reasonable to say that the game is **fair** to both participants when the expected payoff from Bank to Player equals the round fee paid by Player to Bank at the beginning of each round.

Since the number of dollars for a round payoff may be any integer in $\{0, 1, \ldots, n\}$, one might guess that the expected payoff (that is, average payoff) is $n/2$. But as upcoming Theorem 1 ("Expected Payoff in the Game of Hits") will show, this conjecture holds only for $n = 2$. The next two examples contain complete analyses of the cases of $n = 2$ and $n = 3$, which will help us to make a better conjecture.

Example 1   There are only two listings of the set $\{1, 2\}$; these are given in the first column of Table 5.8.1. For a given listing, the second column of the table indicates each integer k that appears in its natural position. Counting these integers k, we obtain the payoff for the given listing. The entries in the Payoff column enable us to see that the expected payoff when $n = 2$ (that is, the average of the payoffs for all possible listings of $\{1, 2\}$) is $(2 + 0)/2 = 1$.

TABLE 5.8.1

Listing	Integers k in Natural Position	Payoff
$\{1, 2\}$	1, 2	2
$\{2, 1\}$	(None)	0

Example 2   Table 5.8.2 indicates the payoff for every listing of $\{1, 2, 3\}$, thus enabling us to find that the expected payoff when $n = 3$ is the average

$$\frac{3 + 1 + 1 + 0 + 0 + 1}{6} = 1.$$

TABLE 5.8.2

Listing	Integers in Natural Position	Payoff
{1, 2, 3}	1, 2, 3	3
{1, 3, 2}	1	1
{2, 1, 3}	3	1
{2, 3, 1}	(None)	0
{3, 1, 2}	(None)	0
{3, 2, 1}	2	1

□

Examples 1 and 2 might lead us to conjecture that the expected payoff is 1 for every n in $\{2, 3, \ldots\}$. After introducing some terminology, we will prove this conjecture correct.

NOTATION 1   **SET L_n OF ALL LISTINGS OF $\{1, 2, \ldots, n\}$**

L_n denotes the set of all $n!$ listings of $\{1, 2, \ldots, n\}$.

For example, $L_2 = \{\{1, 2\}, \{2, 1\}\}$ and L_3 consists of all the listings in the left-most column of Table 5.8.2.

DEFINITION 1   **HIT, $f(\lambda)$**

A **hit** for a listing $\lambda = \{a_1, a_2, \ldots, a_n\}$ is an integer k such that $a_k = k$. The number of hits for a listing λ is denoted as $f(\lambda)$.

For example, Table 5.8.2 shows that 2 is the only hit for the listing $\lambda = \{3, 2, 1\}$ and hence that this $f(\lambda) = 1$. Next we solve the main problem concerning the game of Hits.

THEOREM 1   **EXPECTED PAYOFF IN THE GAME OF HITS**

Let $m = n!$ and $L_n = \{\lambda_1, \lambda_2, \ldots, \lambda_m\}$. Then:

(a) $f(\lambda_1) + f(\lambda_2) + \cdots + f(\lambda_m) = n! = m$;
(b) the expected payoff in the game of Hits is 1 for all n in $\{2, 3, \ldots\}$.

PROOF   (a) One produces a listing $\lambda = \{a_1, a_2, \ldots, a_n\}$ in L_n with 1 as a hit by letting $a_1 = 1$ and taking $\{a_2, a_3, \ldots, a_n\}$ to be any of the $(n-1)!$ listings of the set $\{2, 3, \ldots, n\}$ of size $n - 1$; hence there are $(n-1)!$ listings in L_n with 1 as a hit. Similarly, for each k in $\{1, 2, \ldots, n\}$, there are $(n - 1)!$ listings in L_n with k as a hit, since such a listing

$$\{a_1, \ldots, a_{k-1}, k, a_{k+1}, \ldots, a_n\}$$

is obtained by taking $\{a_1, \ldots, a_{k-1}, a_{k+1}, \ldots, a_n\}$ to be any of the $(n - 1)!$ listings of $\{1, \ldots, k - 1, k + 1, \ldots, n\}$. Thus, for the $n!$ listings in L_n, 1 is a hit $(n - 1)!$ times, 2 is a hit $(n - 1)!$ times, ..., n is a hit $(n - 1)!$ times. This implies that the total number of hits for all the listings in L_n is $(n - 1)!n = n!$ But the total number of hits for all the λ's in L_n is also

$$f(\lambda_1) + f(\lambda_2) + \cdots + f(\lambda_m).$$

Hence this sum equals $n!$, and Part (a) is proved.

(b) The expected payoff in the game of Hits is the average value of $f(\lambda)$ for all λ's in L_n. Using the result we have just proved, this average is

$$\frac{f(\lambda_1) + f(\lambda_2) + \cdots + f(\lambda_m)}{m} = \frac{n!}{n!} = 1.$$

This proves Part (b).   □

Now we introduce a relative of the game Hits called **Nohit**. This new game has the same procedures as the old one except for the determination of the round payoff. In the game of Nohit, the payoff for a listing λ is 1 if $f(\lambda) = 0$, that is, if λ has no hits; the payoff is 0 if $f(\lambda) > 0$, that is, if λ has at least one hit. Again, we would like to know the expected payoff, that is, the average of the payoffs for the $n!$ listings in L_n. This would give us the fair amount to serve as the round fee in Nohit. To help in the analysis of this game, we introduce some additional terminology.

DEFINITION 2   **DERANGEMENT, NUMBER d_n OF DERANGEMENTS IN L_n**

A listing $\lambda = \{a_1, a_2, \ldots, a_n\}$ in L_n is a **derangement** if $a_i \neq i$ for all i. For $n = 2, 3, \ldots$, we use d_n to denote the number of derangements in L_n. Also, we adopt the convention that $d_0 = 1$ and $d_1 = 0$.

In other words, a listing λ in L_n is a derangement if it has no hits, that is, if $f(\lambda) = 0$. As Example 1 shows, the only derangement in L_2 is $\{2, 1\}$; hence $d_2 = 1$. We see from Example 2 that the only derangements in L_3 are $\{2, 3, 1\}$ and $\{3, 1, 2\}$; thus $d_3 = 2$. The listings in L_4 that are derangements are

$$
\begin{array}{lll}
\{2, 1, 4, 3\}, & \{2, 3, 4, 1\}, & \{2, 4, 1, 3\}, \\
\{3, 1, 4, 2\}, & \{3, 4, 1, 2\}, & \{3, 4, 2, 1\}, \\
\{4, 1, 2, 3\}, & \{4, 3, 1, 2\}, & \{4, 3, 2, 1\}.
\end{array}
$$

TABLE 5.8.3

n	0	1	2	3	4
d_n	1	0	1	2	9

This shows that $d_4 = 9$. In Table 5.8.3 we summarize the data we have so far on d_n.

In the game of Nohit, the total of the payoffs for $n!$ rounds in which each listing in L_n is used exactly once is the number d_n of derangements in L_n. Since the size of L_n is $n!$, this implies that the expected (that is, average) payoff in Nohit is $d_n/n!$. This ratio $d_n/n!$ is the number of derangements in L_n divided by the total number of listings in L_n. By Definition 1 ("Sample Space, Favorable Subset, Probability") of Section 5.7, this means that $d_n/n!$ is also the probability that a randomly chosen listing in L_n will be a derangement.

NOTATION 2 **PROBABILITY OF OBTAINING A DERANGEMENT**

The probability $d_n/n!$ that a randomly chosen listing in L_n will be a derangement is denoted as p_n.

For example, $p_4 = d_4/4! = \frac{9}{24} = \frac{3}{8}$. As we have just noted, p_n is also the expected payoff (so is the fair round fee) in the game of Nohit when the listings are obtained from L_n. Table 5.8.4 expands Table 5.8.3 by including a row for $p_n = d_n/n!$. The analysis of the game of Nohit now becomes the study of properties of the sequence $p_1, p_2, \ldots$, which is aided by the study of the sequence $d_1, d_2, \ldots$. The rest of this section is devoted to these intertwined studies. One of the facts we will establish is that p_9, p_{10}, $p_{11}, \ldots$ all agree, to six decimal places.

The next theorem gives the basic formulas for d_n and p_n. Then Theorem 3 gives additional interesting formulas.

TABLE 5.8.4

n	0	1	2	3	4
d_n	1	0	1	2	9
p_n	1	0	$\frac{1}{2}$	$\frac{1}{3}$	$\frac{3}{8}$

THEOREM 2 **FORMULAS FOR d_n AND p_n**

(a) $d_n = n!\left[1 - \dfrac{1}{1!} + \dfrac{1}{2!} - \dfrac{1}{3!} + \cdots + (-1)^n \dfrac{1}{n!}\right]$,

(b) $p_n = 1 - \dfrac{1}{1!} + \dfrac{1}{2!} - \dfrac{1}{3!} + \cdots + (-1)^n \dfrac{1}{n!}$.

PROOF (a) Let $T_n = \{1, 2, \ldots, n\}$. We recall that L_n consists of all listings $\lambda = \{a_1, a_2, \ldots, a_n\}$ of T_n. For k in T_n, let $L_n(k)$ be the subset of L_n consisting of the λ in L_n with $a_k = k$, that is, the λ with k as a hit. For example,

$$L_3(2) = \{\{1, 2, 3\}, \{3, 2, 1\}\}.$$

For distinct integers i and j in T_n, let $L_n(i, j)$ consist of the λ's in L_n with both $a_i = i$ and $a_j = j$, that is, of the λ's having both i and j among their hits. For example,

$$L_4(1, 2) = \{\{1, 2, 3, 4\}, \{1, 2, 4, 3\}\}.$$

In general, for any subset $\{i, j, \ldots, h\}$ of T_n, let $L_n(i, j, \ldots, h)$ consist of the listings λ in L_n satisfying the simultaneous conditions

$$a_i = i, \qquad a_j = j, \qquad \ldots, \qquad a_h = h.$$

That is, let $L_n(i, j, \ldots, h)$ be the subset of the λ's in L_n that have each of $i, j, \ldots, h$ among their hits.

We know that $\# L_n = n!$ and can easily see that $\# L_n(k) = (n - 1)!$ for each k in T_n. In general, if $\{i, j, \ldots, h\}$ is a subset of size s in T_n, then $\# L_n(i, j, \ldots, h) = (n - s)!$ since, in the listings $\{a_1, a_2, \ldots, a_n\}$ that are being counted, the s integers of $\{i, j, \ldots, h\}$ are in their natural positions and the remaining $n - s$ integers of T_n are available to be permuted. It can also be seen that

$$d_n = \#[\overline{L_n(1)} \cap \overline{L_n(2)} \cap \cdots \cap \overline{L_n(n)}],$$

where $\overline{L_n(k)}$ is the complement of $L_n(k)$ in L_n. The number of subsets $\{i, j, \ldots, h\}$ of size s in T_n is $\binom{n}{s}$. It follows from the inclusion–exclusion principle [Theorem 5(b) of Section 5.3] that

$$d_n = n! - (n - 1)!\binom{n}{1} + (n - 2)!\binom{n}{2} - \cdots + (-1)^n 0!\binom{n}{n}.$$

With the aid of the formula $\binom{n}{s} = n!/s!(n - s)!$ of Problem 10 in Section 4.2 this becomes

$$d_n = n! - \frac{(n - 1)!n!}{(n - 1)!1!} + \frac{(n - 2)!n!}{(n - 2)!2!} - \cdots + (-1)^n \frac{0!n!}{0!n!}.$$

By canceling a common factor from the numerator and denominator of each fraction, we get

$$d_n = n! - \frac{n!}{1!} + \frac{n!}{2!} - \frac{n!}{3!} + \cdots + (-1)^n \frac{n!}{n!}. \tag{1}$$

Factoring out $n!$ from each term, we get the formula

$$d_n = n!\left[1 - \frac{1}{1!} + \frac{1}{2!} - \frac{1}{3!} + \cdots + (-1)^n \frac{1}{n!}\right].$$

This proves Formula (a).

(b) Dividing the previous result by $n!$ and using $p_n = d_n/n!$ we get the formula

$$p_n = 1 - \frac{1}{1!} + \frac{1}{2!} - \frac{1}{3!} + \cdots + (-1)^n \frac{1}{n!}.$$

This proves Formula (b). $\square$

Example 3 As an illustration of the use of the formulas of Theorem 2, we calculate d_5 using Display (1), with $n = 5$, as follows:

$$d_5 = 5! - \frac{5!}{1!} + \frac{5!}{2!} - \frac{5!}{3!} + \frac{5!}{4!} - \frac{5!}{5!}$$

$$= 120 - \frac{120}{1} + \frac{120}{2} - \frac{120}{6} + \frac{120}{24} - \frac{120}{120}$$

$$= 120 - 120 + 60 - 20 + 5 - 1 = 44$$

Then $p_5 = d_5/5! = \frac{44}{120} = \frac{11}{30}$. □

We next present some other useful properties of the sequences $d_0, d_1, \ldots$ and $p_0, p_1, \ldots$. The first of these properties makes it easy to calculate p_n when p_{n-1} is known.

THEOREM 3 **ADDITIONAL PROPERTIES OF d_n AND p_n**

(a) $p_n = p_{n-1} + \dfrac{(-1)^n}{n!}$ for n in $\mathbf{Z}^+ = \{1, 2, \ldots\}$.

(b) $p_{2m+1} < p_{2m+3} < p_{2m+2} < p_{2m}$ for m in $\mathbf{N} = \{0, 1, \ldots\}$.

(c) $d_n = nd_{n-1} + (-1)^n$ for n in $\mathbf{Z}^+$.

(d) $d_n = (n-1)(d_{n-1} + d_{n-2})$ for n in $\{2, 3, \ldots\}$.

(e) $\dbinom{n}{0} d_0 + \dbinom{n}{1} d_1 + \dbinom{n}{2} d_2 + \cdots + \dbinom{n}{n} d_n = n!$ for n in $\mathbf{N}$.

(f) $\dbinom{n}{1} d_{n-1} + 2 \dbinom{n}{2} d_{n-2} + 3 \dbinom{n}{3} d_{n-3} + \cdots + n \dbinom{n}{n} d_0 = n!$ for n in $\mathbf{N}$.

PROOF (a) Theorem 2(b) tells us that

$$p_n = 1 - \frac{1}{1!} + \frac{1}{2!} - \frac{1}{3!} + \cdots + (-1)^n \frac{1}{n!}.$$

If we replace n by $n-1$ in this formula, we get

$$p_{n-1} = 1 - \frac{1}{1!} + \frac{1}{2!} - \cdots + (-1)^{n-1} \frac{1}{(n-1)!}.$$

Subtracting corresponding sides of these equations gives us

$$p_n - p_{n-1} = (-1)^n \frac{1}{n!}.$$

This is equivalent to Formula (a).

(b)–(f) The proofs of parts (b)–(f) are left to the reader in the problem set below. □

Example 4   We saw in Example 3 that $d_5 = 44$ and $p_5 = \frac{11}{30}$. These values and Theorem 3(c) and (a), with $n = 6$, give us

$$d_6 = 6 \cdot 44 + (-1)^6 = 264 + 1 = 265,$$

$$p_6 = \frac{11}{30} + (-1)^6 \frac{1}{6!} = \frac{11}{30} + \frac{1}{720} = \frac{264 + 1}{720} = \frac{265}{720} = \frac{53}{144}.$$

Also, it follows from Theorem 3(b), with $m = 1, 2, 3, \ldots$, that

$$p_1 < p_3 < p_5 < p_7 < p_9 < p_{11} < \cdots < p_{10} < p_8 < p_6 < p_4 < p_2. \qquad (2)$$

We note from Theorem 3(a), with $n = 10$, that $p_{10} = p_9 - (1/10!)$. Since $1/10! = 1/3628800 < 0.000001$, this and Display (2) imply that all terms of the sequence $p_9, p_{10}, p_{11}, \ldots$ agree, to six decimal places. With the help of calculus, we could show that the number

$$\frac{1}{e} = 0.36787944117144232 \ldots,$$

where e is the base of natural logarithms, has the property

$$p_{2m+1} < \frac{1}{e} < p_{2m} \quad \text{for all } m \text{ in } \mathbf{Z}^+.$$

Hence $1/e$ is an approximation to p_n, and is an especially good one when n is large. □

John von Neumann   *was born in 1903 in Budapest, where he received his education. While still in his twenties, he solved Hilbert's fifth problem, one of 23 posed by David Hilbert in 1900 and generally viewed as among the most important (and difficult) mathematical problems of the twentieth century. Von Neumann held teaching positions in Berlin (1927 to 1929), in Hamburg (1929 to 1930), and finally at Princeton (1930 to 1933). He then joined the faculty of the newly formed Institute for Advanced Study, from which post he moved increasingly into association with the American government. He participated in the development of the atomic bomb at Los Alamos and in 1954 became a member of the U.S. Atomic Energy Commission. He was influential in the development of some of the earliest high-speed computers and also did important work in mathematical economics. Von Neumann is credited with pioneering work in many branches of mathematics, in particular, the theory of automata. He was renowned for being extraordinarily quick at doing complex computations in his head. Von Neumann died of cancer in 1957, at the age of 54.*

PROBLEMS FOR SECTION 5.8

1. Give the set of hits (integers in their natural positions) for each of the following listings of $\{1, 2, 3, 4, 5\}$:
  (i) $\{2, 3, 4, 5, 1\}$;   (ii) $\{2, 3, 1, 5, 4\}$;
  (iii) $\{2, 3, 5, 4, 1\}$;   (iv) $\{2, 1, 3, 5, 4\}$;
  (v) $\{3, 2, 5, 4, 1\}$;   (vi) $\{5, 4, 3, 2, 1\}$.

2. Give the set of hits for each of the following:
  (i) $\{5, 1, 2, 3, 4\}$;   (ii) $\{2, 3, 4, 1, 5\}$;
  (iii) $\{2, 5, 3, 4, 1\}$;   (iv) $\{3, 1, 2, 5, 4\}$;
  (v) $\{1, 3, 2, 5, 4\}$;   (vi) $\{5, 3, 1, 2, 4\}$.

3. Give $f(\lambda)$ for each λ in Problem 1. That is, give the number of hits for each λ.

4. Give $f(\lambda)$ for each λ in Problem 2.

5. Which of the listings in Problem 1 are derangements?

6. Which of the listings in Problem 2 are derangements?

7. Use $d_6 = 265$ and the formula $d_n = nd_{n-1} + (-1)^n$ to find d_7 and d_8.

8. (i) Use $p_6 = \frac{53}{144}$ and the formula $p_n = p_{n-1} + (-1)^n/n!$ to find p_7 and p_8.
  (ii) Check your answers to Part (i) by using the answers to Problem 7 and $p_n = d_n/n!$.

9. Explain why $p_{2m+1} < p_{2m}$ for all m in $\mathbf{N}$.

10. Explain why $p_{2m-1} < p_{2m}$ for all m in $\mathbf{Z}^+$.

11. Explain why $p_{2m+2} < p_{2m}$ for all m in $\mathbf{N}$.

12. (i) Explain why $p_{2m+1} < p_{2m+3}$ for all m in $\mathbf{N}$.
  (ii) Explain why $p_{2m+1} < p_{2m+3} < p_{2m+2} < p_{2m}$ for all m in $\mathbf{N}$. [That is, prove Formula (b) of Theorem 3, "Additional Properties of d_n and p_n."]
  (iii) Is p_{1000} less than p_3, equal to p_3, or greater than p_3?

13. Explain why $d_n = n!p_n = n!p_{n-1} + (-1)^n = n[(n-1)!p_{n-1}] + (-1)^n$.

14. Prove Formula (c) of Theorem 3, "Additional Properties of d_n and p_n." That is, prove that $d_n = nd_{n-1} + (-1)^n$ for n in $\mathbf{Z}^+$.

15. Explain why $[d_n - nd_{n-1}] + [d_{n-1} - (n-1)d_{n-2}] = 0$ for n in $\{2, 3, \dots\}$.

16. Prove Formula (d) of Theorem 3, "Additional Properties of d_n and p_n." That is, prove that $d_n = (n-1)(d_{n-1} + d_{n-2})$ for n in $\{2, 3, \dots\}$.

17. For which positive integers n is d_n exactly divisible by n? Explain.

18. Is d_n exactly divisible by $n-1$ for all n in $\{2, 3, \dots\}$? Explain.

19. Prove that d_n is an even integer for n in $\{1, 3, 5, \dots\}$.

20. Prove that d_n is odd whenever n is even.

21. How many of the listings $\{a_1, a_2, a_3, a_4, a_5\}$ of $\{1, 2, 3, 4, 5\}$ have:
  (a) 3 as a hit?

    (b) 3 as the only hit?

    (c) 2 and 3 as hits?

    (d) 2 and 3 as the only hits?

22. How many listings of $\{1, 2, 3, 4, 5\}$ have:

    (a) 1 as a hit?

    (b) 1 as the only hit?

    (c) 1 and 2 as hits?

    (d) 1 and 2 as the only hits?

23. Let $i \in \{1, 2, \ldots, n\}$. How many of the listings λ in L_n have:

    (a) i as a hit?   (b) i as the only hit?

24. Let i and j be distinct integers in $\{1, 2, \ldots, n\}$. How many of the listings of $\{1, 2, \ldots, n\}$ have:

    (a) i and j as hits?   (b) i and j as the only hits?

25. For a listing λ in L_n, we recall that $f(\lambda)$ is the number of hits for λ. How many λ in L_n have $f(\lambda) = 1$?

26. How many λ are there in L_n with $f(\lambda) = 2$? (Assume $n > 1$.)

27. How many λ are there in L_n with:

    (a) $f(\lambda) = 3$?   (b) $f(\lambda) = 4$?   (c) $f(\lambda) = 5$?

28. For each of the following values of s, give all the listings λ in L_4 such that $f(\lambda) = s$:

    (a) $s = 0$;   (b) $s = 1$;   (c) $s = 2$;   (d) $s = 3$;   (e) $s = 4$.

29. Explain why the number of λ's in L_n with $f(\lambda) = s$ is $\binom{n}{s} d_{n-s}$ for s in $\{0, 1, \ldots, n\}$.

30. (i) Does $\binom{0}{0} d_0 = 0!$? Explain.

    (ii) For all n in $N = \{0, 1, \ldots\}$, prove that

$$\binom{n}{n} d_0 + \binom{n}{n-1} d_1 + \binom{n}{n-2} d_2 + \cdots + \binom{n}{0} d_n = n!.$$

31. Prove Formula (e) of Theorem 3, "Additional Properties of d_n and p_n." That is, prove that

$$\binom{n}{0} d_0 + \binom{n}{1} d_1 + \binom{n}{2} d_2 + \cdots + \binom{n}{n} d_n = n!.$$

32. Let $L_n = \{\lambda_1, \lambda_2, \ldots, \lambda_m\}$. Use the result in Problem 29 and the formula

$$f(\lambda_1) + f(\lambda_2) + \cdots + f(\lambda_m) = n!$$

of Theorem 1 ("Expected Payoff in the Game of Hits") to prove Formula (f) of Theorem 3, "Additional Properties of d_n and p_n," that is, to show that

$$\binom{n}{1} d_{n-1} + 2\binom{n}{2} d_{n-2} + 3\binom{n}{3} d_{n-3} + \cdots + n\binom{n}{n} d_0 = n!.$$

33. Let $\lambda = \{a_1, a_2, \ldots, a_8\}$ represent an arbitrary listing in L_8.

(a) How many of these λ's have $\{a_1, a_2, a_3\} = \{1, 2, 3\}$, that is, have 1, 2, 3 in some order as the first three a's?

(b) How many of these λ's are derangements with $\{a_1, a_2, a_3\} = \{1, 2, 3\}$?

34. Let $\lambda = \{a_1, a_2, \ldots, a_8\}$ represent an arbitrary listing in L_8.

(a) How many of these λ's have $\{a_1, a_2, a_3\} = \{6, 7, 8\}$?

(b) How many of these λ's are derangements with $\{a_1, a_2, a_3\} = \{6, 7, 8\}$? [*Hint*: Consider the cases of (i) $a_4 = 5$ and (ii) $a_4 \neq 5$.]

35. How many of the listings in L_8 have neither 1 nor 2 as a hit?

36. How many of the listings in L_n have neither 1 nor 2 as a hit?

SUMMARY OF TERMS, CHAPTER 5

REVIEW PROBLEMS FOR CHAPTER 5

1. Let $B_{n,k}$ be the set of n-bit strings of weight k.
   (a) Find $\#(B_{4,2} \cup B_{5,3})$.
   (b) How many strings $a_1a_2 \ldots a_9$ are there such that $a_1a_2a_3a_4$ is in $B_{4,2}$ and $a_5a_6a_7a_8a_9$ is in $B_{5,3}$?

2. Let C_n consist of all the strings $c_1c_2 \ldots c_n$ with each c_i in $\{0, 1, 2\}$.
   (i) Find $\#C_1$, $\#C_2$, and $\#C_3$.
   (ii) Find the smallest k such that $\#(C_1 \cup C_2 \cup \cdots \cup C_k) \ge 200$.

3. Let A be an alphabet with $\#A = 26$.
   (a) How many words $a_1a_2a_3a_4a_5$ (of length 5) are there over A, that is, with each a_i in A?
   (b) How many of these words have no repetitions among the a_i?

4. A local telephone number is a string $d_1d_2 \ldots d_7$ with each d_i in $\{1, 2, \ldots, 9, 0\}$, and with neither d_1 nor d_2 in $\{1, 0\}$. How many such numbers are there?

5. How many circular permutations are there on a set of size 8?

6. In how many ways can 4 women and 4 men be seated at a round table so that women and men alternate? (This is the count for some special circular permutations.)

7. The $n = 8$ row of Pascal's Triangle is 1, 8, 28, 56, 70, 56, 28, 8, 1. Write the $n = 9$ row.

8. Let $\#S = 80$. How many of the subsets of S have:
   (a) an even number of elements?   (b) an odd number of elements?

9. Show that $\binom{90}{50} = \binom{88}{50} + 2\binom{88}{49} + \binom{88}{48}$.

10. Show that $\binom{100}{70} - 2\binom{99}{70} + \binom{98}{70} = \binom{98}{68}$.

11. In Salt Lake City (as described in Problem 15 of Section 5.2), how many 22-block paths are there from the intersection of 1st Street and 1st Avenue to the intersection of 11th Street and 13th Avenue?

12. How many of the paths counted in Problem 11 go through the intersection of 7th Street and 9th Avenue?

13. In terms of factorials, find the coefficient of $x^6 y^7 z^8 w^9$ in the expansion of $(x + y + z + w)^{30}$.

14. Explain why $\binom{80}{20} = \binom{30}{0}\binom{50}{20} + \binom{30}{1}\binom{50}{19} + \binom{30}{2}\binom{50}{18} + \cdots + \binom{30}{20}\binom{50}{0}$.

15. Use the expansion of $(a + b)^5$, with $a = 3$ and $b = 0.01$, to find 3.01^5.

16. Express the sum $\sum_{k=0}^{50} \binom{50}{k} 7^k$ as a power of an integer.

17. Let A be a subset of $\{100, 101, 102, \ldots\}$. How large must $\#A$ be to guarantee that A has two integers x and y such that $x - y$ is an integral multiple of 100?

18. A, B, and C are subsets of X. Also, $\#X = 124$, $\#A = 59$, $\#B = 57$, $\#C = 55$, $\#(A \cap B) = 27$, $\#(A \cap C) = 26$, $\#(B \cap C) = 25$, and $\#(A \cap B \cap C) = 12$. Find $\#(A \cup B \cup C)$ and $\#M_{101}$, where M_{101} is the miniset $A \cap \bar{B} \cap C$.

19. How many compositions $(x_1, x_2, x_3, x_4, x_5)$ of 83 into 5 integral parts have each part $x_i \geq 7$?

20. How many of the compositions of Problem 19 also satisfy both $x_1 \leq 15$ and $x_2 \leq 20$?

21. The number of partitions of n into k parts is denoted as $p_k(n)$. Use the formula $p_k(n) = p_k(n - k) + p_{k-1}(n)$ for $2 \leq k \leq n$ to explain why $p_4(100) = p_4(96) + p_3(97) + p_2(98) + p_1(100)$.

22. Let T be the set of all ordered 5-tuples (a, b, c, d, e) of integers with $a \geq b \geq c \geq d \geq e \geq 1$ and $abcde = 7^{30}$. Express $\#T$ in the form $p_k(n)$.

23. Use $S(5, 2) = 15$ and $S(5, 3) = 25$ to find the Stirling Number $S(6, 3)$.

24. How many collections $\{A, B, C\}$ of pairwise disjoint nonempty sets are there with $A \cup B \cup C = \{1, 2, 3, 4, 5, 6\}$?

25. How many ordered triples (A, B, C) of pairwise disjoint nonempty sets are there with $A \cup B \cup C = \{1, 2, 3, 4, 5, 6\}$?

26. How many surjections are there from $\{1, 2, 3, 4, 5, 6\}$ onto $\{a, b, c\}$?

27. Eight pennies are shaken thoroughly and tossed onto a table. What is the probability that the number of heads will be in the set $\{0, 1, 2\}$?

28. Under the conditions of Problem 27, what is the probability that the number of heads will be in the set $\{3, 4, 5\}$?

29. What is the probability that a bridge hand will contain the ace and king of spades, that is, have $\{Sa, Sk\}$ as a subset?

30. The number of listings $\{a_1, a_2, \ldots, a_n\}$ of $\{1, 2, \ldots, n\}$ with $a_k \neq k$ for all k is denoted as d_n. Use the formula $d_n = (n - 1)(d_{n-1} + d_{n-2})$ for n in $\{2, 3, \ldots\}$ to complete the following table:

n	0	1	2	3	4	5	6	7	8	9
d_n	1	0	1	2	9					

31. How many of the listings $\{a_1, a_2, \ldots, a_{11}\}$ of $\{1, 2, \ldots, 11\}$ have:
    (a) $a_{10} = 10$ and $a_{11} = 11$?
    (b) $a_{10} = 10$, $a_{11} = 11$, and $a_k \neq k$ for k in $\{1, 2, \ldots, 9\}$?
    (c) $a_{11} \neq 11$?
    (d) $a_{10} \neq 10$ and $a_{11} \neq 11$?

SUPPLEMENTARY AND CHALLENGING PROBLEMS, CHAPTER 5

1. Use
$$\binom{2}{2} + \binom{3}{2} + \binom{4}{2} + \cdots + \binom{n}{2} = \binom{n+1}{3} \quad \text{and} \quad k^2 = \binom{k}{2} + \binom{k+1}{2}$$
to find a formula for $1^2 + 2^2 + 3^2 + \cdots + n^2$.

2. Show that
$$1^3 + 2^3 + 3^3 + \cdots + n^3 = \binom{n+1}{4} + 4\binom{n+2}{4} + \binom{n+3}{4} \quad \text{for } n \geq 3.$$

3. Find integers a, b, and c such that
$$0^4 + 1^4 + 2^4 + \cdots + n^4 = \binom{n+4}{5} + a\binom{n+3}{5} + b\binom{n+2}{5} + c\binom{n+1}{5}$$
for n in $\{0, 1, \ldots\}$, where $\binom{m}{5} = 0$ for $m = 0, 1, 2, 3, 4$.

4. Find a relatively simple expression for
$$1^3\binom{n}{1} + 2^3\binom{n}{2} + 3^3\binom{n}{3} + \cdots + n^3\binom{n}{n}.$$

5. Show that $\binom{m+n}{2} - \binom{m}{2} - \binom{n}{2} = mn$ for all m and n in $N = \{0, 1, \ldots\}$, where $\binom{0}{2} = 0 = \binom{1}{2}$.

6. For all r, s, and t in N, show that

$$\binom{r+s+t}{3} - \binom{r+s}{3} - \binom{r+t}{3} - \binom{s+t}{3} + \binom{r}{3} + \binom{s}{3} + \binom{t}{3} = rst,$$

where $\binom{0}{3} = \binom{1}{3} = \binom{2}{3} = 0$.

7. For every subset $\{x_1, x_2, \ldots, x_{10}\}$ of $\{1, 2, \ldots, 100\}$, explain why there must be an x_i and an x_j such that $0 < \sqrt{x_i} - \sqrt{x_j} \le 1$.

8. For integers k and n with $1 \le k \le n$, let $s_k(n)$ be the coefficient of x^k in the expansion of $x(x + 1)(x + 2) \cdots (x + n - 1)$. For example, $x(x + 1)(x + 2) = x^3 + 3x^2 + 2x$, and thus

$$s_3(3) = 1, \qquad s_2(3) = 3, \qquad \text{and} \qquad s_1(3) = 2.$$

Show that $s_n(n) = 1$, $s_1(n) = (n - 1)!$, and $s_k(n + 1) = ns_k(n) + s_{k-1}(n)$ for $1 < k \le n$. [The $s_k(n)$ are the **Stirling Numbers of the first kind.**]

9. For the Stirling Numbers $s_k(n)$ of the first kind, show that $s_{n-1}(n) = \binom{n}{2}$ and $s_1(n) + s_2(n) + \cdots + s_n(n) = n!$.

10. Let the $S(n, k)$ be the Stirling Numbers of the second kind. Explain why the number of ways of distributing n distinguishable objects into k indistinguishable containers is $S(n, 1) + S(n, 2) + \cdots + S(n, k)$.

11. Explain why $S(n, n - 2) = \binom{n}{3} + 3\binom{n}{4}$, and find a similar formula for $S(n, n - 3)$.

12. For n in $Z^+ = \{1, 2, \ldots\}$, let $x^{(n)} = x(x - 1)(x - 2) \cdots (x - n + 1)$. For example, $x^{(1)} = x$, $x^{(2)} = x^2 - x$, and $x^{(3)} = x^3 - 3x^2 + 2x$. Show that:
    (a) $x^n = s_n(n)x^n - s_{n-1}(n)x^{n-1} + s_{n-2}(n)x^{n-2} - \cdots - (-1)^n s_1(n)x$.
    (b) $x^n = S(n, 1)x^{(1)} + S(n, 2)x^{(2)} + \cdots + S(n, n)x^{(n)}$.

13. Explain why $\sum_{j=0}^{n} (-1)^j \binom{n}{j}(n - j)^n = n!$.

14. For all real numbers x and all n in Z^+, prove that $\sum_{j=0}^{n} (-1)^j \binom{n}{j}(x - j)^n = n!$.

15. As usual, $\boldsymbol{B_{2n+1,n}}$ consists of the $(2n + 1)$-bit strings $\alpha = a_1 a_2 \ldots a_{2n+1}$ of weight n. Such an α is a **Singmaster String** if $2(a_1 + a_2 + \cdots + a_k) < k$ whenever $a_k = 1$. For example, the only Singmaster Strings in $\boldsymbol{B_{5,2}}$ are 00011 and 00101. For every $\beta = b_1 b_2 \ldots b_{2n+1}$ in $\boldsymbol{B_{2n+1,n}}$, prove that $b_j b_{j+1} \ldots b_{2n+1} b_1 b_2 \ldots b_{j-1}$ is a Singmaster String for one and only one j in $\{0, 1, \ldots, 2n + 1\}$.

16. Let c_n be the number of Singmaster Strings in $\boldsymbol{B_{2n+1,n}}$. Prove that

$$c_n = \frac{1}{2n+1}\binom{2n+1}{n} = \frac{1}{n+1}\binom{2n}{n} = \binom{2n}{n} - \binom{2n}{n-1}.$$

(David Singmaster is currently a professor of mathematics at the Polytechnic of the South Bank, London, England.)

6

DIGRAPHS AND GRAPHS

Digraphs and graphs have a number of applications, including:

(a) The flowchart analysis of computer programs.
(b) The design of transmission networks, such as telephone lines, so as to minimize construction costs and minimize vulnerability to accidental disruption.
(c) The determination of travel routes that will minimize travel costs.
(d) The design of the layers of circuits in a computer chip.

In Section 1.5, Definition 2, we saw that a binary relation on a finite set can be characterized by a picture. In the first four sections of this chapter, we use geometrical language suggested by such pictures to help in the study and application of such relations. As part of this process, we call the elements of the finite set "vertices," and use V to designate the set. Also, we call an ordered pair (v, w) in the binary relation on V an "edge," and use E to designate the binary relation on V consisting of such edges.

6.1

DIRECTED PATHS, CIRCUITS, AND CYCLES

DEFINITION 1   DIGRAPH, VERTEX, EDGE

A *digraph* (short for "directed graph") is an ordered pair $D = \langle V, E \rangle$ in which E is a binary relation on the finite set V. An element of V is a *vertex* of D (or in V), and an ordered pair (v, w) with vEw is an *edge* of D (or in E) *from v to w.*

As we shall see in the examples that follow, the binary relation E of a digraph $D = \langle V, E \rangle$ can be specified in any one of several ways. In a particular case, E may be given as a subset of ordered pairs in $V \times V$, by a relation matrix, or by a picture. When E is given by one of these methods, it may also be helpful to look at one or more of the other representations.

Since the relation matrix for E also shows the vertices of V, we can call it the (digraph) **matrix** for D. Similarly, a picture (or figure) for E can be called a **picture** (or figure) for D.

Example 1   Let $V = \{1, 2, 3, 4\}$ and $E = \{(1, 1), (1, 2), (1, 3), (1, 4), (2, 3), (3, 1), (3, 4)\}$. This specifies a digraph $D = \langle V, E \rangle$, which is given alternatively by the matrix of Table 6.1.1 or by the picture of Figure 6.1.1.

TABLE 6.1.1

E	1	2	3	4
1	1	1	1	1
2	0	0	1	0
3	1	0	0	1
4	0	0	0	0

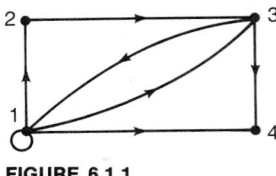

FIGURE 6.1.1

DEFINITION 2   **INDEGREE, OUTDEGREE**

The **indegree** of a vertex v of a digraph $\langle V, E \rangle$ is the number of vertices u such that uEv; we use indg(v) to denote this number. The **outdegree** of v is the number of vertices w such that vEw; it is denoted as outdg(v).

In other words, indg$(v) = \#\{u : uEv\}$ and outdg$(v) = \#\{w : vEw\}$. In a digraph matrix, the sum of the entries in the row for a vertex v is outdg(v) and the sum of the entries in the column for v is indg(v). Thus Table 6.1.1 shows that

$$\text{outdg}(1) = 1 + 1 + 1 + 1 = 4, \qquad \text{indg}(1) = 1 + 0 + 1 + 0 = 2.$$

Example 2   Let $V = \{a, b, c, d, e\}$ and $E = \{(a, b), (a, e), (b, c), (b, d), (c, d), (d, a), (d, e), (e, b)\}$. Figure 6.1.2 is a picture for the digraph $\langle V, E \rangle$. One sees that indg$(a) = 1$, since (d, a) is the only edge to a, and that outdg$(a) = 2$, since (a, b) and (a, e) are the only edges from a.

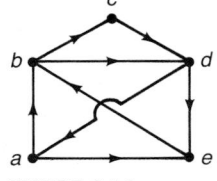

FIGURE 6.1.2

DEFINITION 3   **PATH IN A DIGRAPH**

A **path** of **length** s from v to w in a digraph $D = \langle V, E \rangle$ is an ordered $(s + 1)$-tuple $(v_0, v_1, \ldots, v_s)$ with $v_0 = v$, $v_s = w$, and $(v_{i-1}, v_i) \in E$ for $i = 1, 2, \ldots, s$. This path has v_0 as its **initial vertex** and v_s as its **final vertex**.

We interpret this to include (v) as a path of length 0 from v to itself for every vertex v. If $s \geq 1$, each of $(v_0, v_1), (v_1, v_2), \ldots, (v_{s-1}, v_s)$ is an **edge** of the path $(v_0, v_1, \ldots, v_s)$; also, each of $v_0, v_1, \ldots, v_s$ is a **vertex** of this path. For example, in Figure 6.1.2 the path (a, b, d, a, b, d, e, b) of length 7 from a to b has $(a, b), (b, d), (d, a), (d, e)$, and (e, b) as its 5 (distinct) edges and a, b, d, e as its 4 vertices.

| NOTATION 1 | **ALTERNATE NOTATION FOR A PATH** |

A path $(v_0, v_1, \ldots, v_s)$ of positive length s will sometimes be denoted as $[e_1, e_2, \ldots, e_s]$, where e_i is the edge (v_{i-1}, v_i) for $i = 1, 2, \ldots, s$.

| Example 3 | **ALL THE EDGES WITHOUT REPETITION** |

Let $D = \langle V, E \rangle$ be a digraph in which V is a set of lodging places and E is a set of scenic trips, each from one of these places to another. A tourist might be interested in a path that contains all of these scenic trips with no trip repeated. Using the next definition, we call such a path an *eulerian path*. □

| DEFINITION 4 | **ELEMENTARY, HAMILTONIAN, SIMPLE, EULERIAN** |

A path $(v_0, v_1, \ldots, v_s)$ of length s in a digraph $D = \langle V, E \rangle$ is **elementary** if $v_0, v_1, \ldots, v_s$ are $s + 1$ distinct vertices. A path is **hamiltonian** if it is elementary and its vertices are all the vertices in V. A path $[e_1, e_2, \ldots, e_s]$ is **simple** if $e_1, e_2, \ldots, e_s$ are s distinct edges. A path is **eulerian** if it is simple and its edges are all the edges in E.

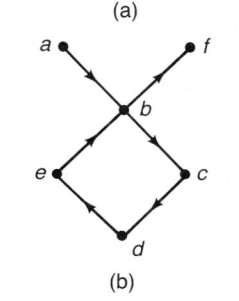

(a)

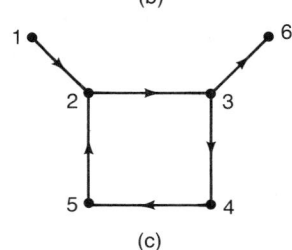

(b)

In Figure 6.1.3(a), the path $(1, 2, 3, 4, 5, 6, 7, 8)$, of length seven from 1 to 8, is elementary because no vertex is repeated and is simple because no edge occurs more than once in it. This same path is also hamiltonian because its vertices are all the vertices of the digraph; but the path is not eulerian because its edges are only seven of the twelve edges of the digraph.

In Figure 6.1.3(b), the path $P = (a, b, c, d, e, b, f)$, of length 6 from a to f, is not elementary, and hence not hamiltonian, because the vertex b appears more than once in this ordered 7-tuple. The path P is simple because $(a, b), (b, c), (c, d), (d, e), (e, b), (b, f)$ are 6 distinct edges. Also, P is eulerian because its 6 edges are all the edges of the digraph. Because the vertex b is repeated in P, this nonelementary path of length 6 can be shortened to the path (a, b, f), of length 2 from a to f.

In Figure 6.1.3(c), the path $Q = (1, 2, 3, 4, 5, 2, 3, 6)$, of length seven from 1 to 6, is not simple because the edge $(2, 3)$ occurs more than once in it. This guarantees that the vertices 2 and 3 are repeated in the 8-tuple Q; hence Q is not elementary. Since the edge $(2, 3)$ occurs twice in Q, this nonsimple path of length seven can be shortened to the path $(1, 2, 3, 6)$, of length three from 1 to 6.

We next prove that every elementary path is simple and that the shortest path from v to w in a digraph must be elementary and hence also simple.

(c)

FIGURE 6.1.3

| THEOREM 1 | **ELEMENTARY $\Rightarrow$ SIMPLE** |

If $P = (v_0, v_1, \ldots, v_s)$ is an elementary path, it is also a simple path.

PROOF   If P were not simple, an edge (v_{i-1}, v_i) would be repeated as an edge (v_{j-1}, v_j), with $i \neq j$. This would imply that the vertex v_i is repeated, and so P would not be elementary. Thus we have proved the desired implication by proving its contrapositive

(not simple) $\Rightarrow$ (not elementary).   □

THEOREM 2   **SHORTEST PATHS ARE ELEMENTARY**

If there exists a path from v to w in a digraph D, there exists an elementary path from v to w in D.

PROOF   Let $P = (v_0, v_1, \ldots, v_s)$ be some path of length s from v to w. If P is not elementary, a vertex v_i is repeated as a vertex v_j, with $1 \leq i < j \leq s$, and so $(v_0, \ldots, v_{i-1}, v_j, \ldots, v_s)$ is a shorter path from v to w. The set S of lengths of paths from v to w is a nonempty subset of $N = \{0, 1, 2, \ldots\}$ since $s \in S$. As N is well ordered, it follows that S has a least element. That is, there is a path from v to w with a least possible length. Such a shortest path must be elementary because, as we just showed, a nonelementary path can be shortened.   □

DEFINITION 5   **CIRCUIT, SIMPLE CIRCUIT, EULERIAN CIRCUIT**

A *circuit* in a digraph $D = \langle V, E \rangle$ is a path $C = (v_0, v_1, \ldots, v_s)$ of positive length in which the initial vertex v_0 is the same as the final vertex v_s. C is a *simple circuit* if its edges (v_{i-1}, v_i) are distinct. An *eulerian circuit* is a simple circuit whose edges are all the edges in E.

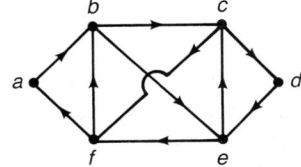

FIGURE 6.1.4

In Figure 6.1.4, (a, b, c, d, e, f, a) is a simple circuit of length 6 because its 6 edges are distinct; it is not eulerian because it does not have all 10 of the edges of the digraph. However, the circuit $(a, b, c, d, e, f, b, e, c, f, a)$ of length 10 is simple and eulerian.

DEFINITION 6   **CYCLE, HAMILTONIAN CYCLE**

A *cycle* in a digraph $\langle V, E \rangle$ is a circuit $(v_0, v_1, \ldots, v_s)$ in which the only repetition of vertices is $v_0 = v_s$. A cycle is *hamiltonian* if its vertices are all the vertices in V.

For example, (b, c, d, e, f, b) is a cycle of length 5 in Figure 6.1.4 because the final vertex is the same as the initial vertex and there are no other repetitions of vertices. This cycle is not hamiltonian because its vertices do not include a. The cycle (a, b, c, d, e, f, a), of length 6, is hamiltonian.

Example 4   **PROVIDING SERVICES TO A SET OF LOCATIONS**   Let $D = \langle V, E \rangle$ be a digraph in which V consists of a traveling salesperson's home city and a number of other cities to be visited and E is a set of airplane flights, each from one such city to another. The salesperson would be interested in paths in D that start and end at the home city and go through all the cities of V without repetition. Such a path is a hamiltonian cycle.   □

Example 5   **FLOWCHART FOR THE DIVISION ALGORITHM**   In Algorithm 1 of Section 1.7, we described the "Division Algorithm." One case of this process has an ordered pair (a, b) of positive integers as its input and produces as its output an ordered pair (q, r) of integers such that

$$a = qb + r \qquad \text{and} \qquad r \in \{0, 1, \ldots, b - 1\}.$$

Figure 6.1.5 is a flowchart for this case of the algorithm. In this figure, the circled B denotes the instruction to begin the process, the punched card outlining the ordered pair (a, b) denotes the input, the diamonds represent tests, the rectangles represent operations, the printout-tearsheets represent

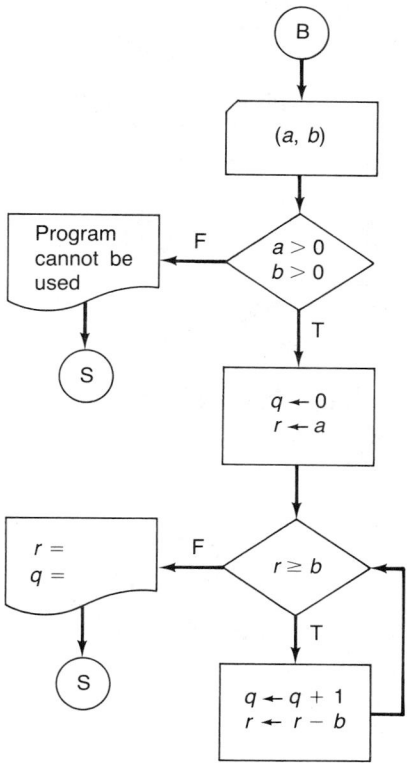

FIGURE 6.1.5

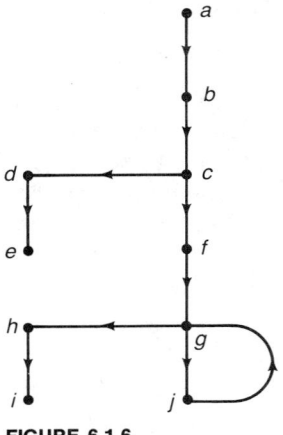

FIGURE 6.1.6

outputs, and the circled S is an order to stop. The diamond containing "$a > 0$, $b > 0$" tests for whether or not the algorithm applies. When this test fails, the next step is to print "Program cannot be used" and then to stop. This is indicated by the F arrow from the diamond. When the test is passed, the T arrow indicates that the process continues with the operation that places 0 in the q position and a in the r position. Then it tests whether $r \geq b$. If not, the r and q are given as output and the process is stopped. If $r \geq b$, the next step adds 1 in the q position and subtracts b in the r position; then the program goes back to the "$r \geq b$" test.

Figure 6.1.6 shows the digraph obtained from the flowchart of Figure 6.1.5 by replacing the circles, punched card, diamonds, rectangles, and tearsheets with vertices.

When writing a computer program, one must be careful to ensure that it will stop after a finite number of steps. The flowchart of Figure 6.1.5 is an outline of a program for the Division Algorithm. The possibility for an unending sequence of steps in the program shows up as an infinite path in the digraph of Figure 6.1.6. Such an infinite path would have to use the infinite sequence $g, j, g, j, g, j, \ldots$. This possibility arises because the digraph has the cycle (g, j, g). However, this part of the program will only be used a finite number of times because the numbers in the r position will be the sequence $a, a - b, a - 2b, a - 3b, \ldots$. Since b is positive, sooner or later one will obtain a term less than b in the sequence. Then the test at vertex g will fail, the desired (q, r) will be printed as the output, and the process will stop. $\qquad\square$

PROBLEMS FOR SECTION 6.1 _____

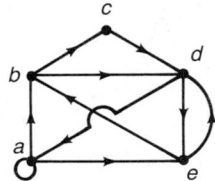

In Problems 1 through 4, the answers should be for the digraph $D = \langle V, E \rangle$ shown in the margin.

1. Complete the following table of indegrees.

vertex v	a	b	c	d	e
indg(v)	2				

2. Complete the following table of outdegrees.

v	a	b	c	d	e
outdg(v)	3				

3. (i) How many edges are there? That is, what is $\#E$?
(ii) What is the sum of the indegrees of the vertices?
(iii) What is the sum of the outdegrees of the vertices?

4. Do the three parts of Problem 3 have equal answers? Will this also hold when the digraph is changed to any other digraph? Explain.

For Problems 5 through 12, use the new figure in the margin.

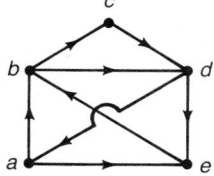

5. (i) Find all the paths of length 2 with a as the initial vertex.
(ii) Are all these paths simple? Are they all elementary? Is any one of them eulerian? Is any one hamiltonian?

6. (i) Find a path of length 3 from e to a.
(ii) Is the path of Part (i) simple? Is it elementary? Is it eulerian? Is it hamiltonian?

7. (i) Find an elementary path of length 4 from a to d.
(ii) Is the path of Part (i) hamiltonian? Explain.

8. (i) Find an elementary path of length 4 from e to a.
(ii) Is every elementary path of length 4 in this digraph hamiltonian? Explain.

9. (i) Find a simple circuit of length 5 with b as the initial and final vertex.
(ii) Is the circuit of Part (i) eulerian? Explain.
(iii) Is the circuit of Part (i) a cycle? Explain.

10. Repeat Problem 9, but with vertex b replaced by vertex c.

11. (i) Find a simple path of length 8 from vertex a to some vertex.
(ii) Is the path of Part (i) eulerian? Explain.

12. (i) Find a simple path of length 8 from some vertex to vertex e.
(ii) Must every simple path of length 8 be eulerian? Explain.

In Problems 13 through 18, take $D = \langle V, E \rangle$ to be a general digraph.

13. Let P be a path of shortest length from v to w in D. Is P simple? Explain.

14. If a path from v to w exists in D, must there be a simple path from v to w in D? Explain.

15. If $\#V = n$, what are the possibilities for the length of a hamiltonian path in D? Explain.

16. If $\#E = m$, what are the possibilities for the length of an eulerian path in D? Explain.

17. Let $(v_0, v_1, \ldots, v_s)$ be an eulerian path in D, with $v_0 \neq v_s$. Justify each of the following assertions.
(a) $\text{outdg}(v_0) = 1 + \text{indg}(v_0)$.   (b) $\text{indg}(v_s) = 1 + \text{outdg}(v_s)$.
(c) $\text{indg}(v_i) = \text{outdg}(v_i)$ for $i = 1, 2, \ldots, s - 1$.

18. Let $(v_0, v_1, \ldots, v_s)$ be an eulerian circuit in D. Must $indg(v) = outdg(v)$ for every v in V? Explain.

19. (a) What are the possibilities for the length of an elementary path in the figure for Problems 5–12?
   (b) In that same figure, what are the possibilities for the length of a simple path?

20. Must every eulerian path in the figure for Problems 5–12 have length 8, a as the initial vertex, and e as the terminal vertex? Explain.

21. Let $V = \{r, a, b, c, d, e, f\}$. In a figure, show all the digraphs $\langle V, E \rangle$ such that $(a, b), (a, c), (r, a)$, and (r, e) are among the edges in E and the indegrees and outdegrees are given by the following table.

vertex v	r	a	b	c	d	e	f
indg(v)	0	1	1	1	1	1	1
outdg(v)	2	2	1	0	0	1	0

22. Let $V = \{r, a, b, c\}$. Show in a figure all digraphs $\langle V, E \rangle$ with no loops and having the indegrees and outdegrees shown in the following table. [A *loop* is an edge (v, v).]

vertex v	r	a	b	c
indg(v)	0	1	1	1
outdg(v)	1	1	1	0

23. Let $D = \langle V, E \rangle$ be a digraph in which $indg(v) \leq 1$ for all v in V. Let $(v_0, v_1, \ldots, v_s)$ be a path in D. Let $v_k = v_s$ with $0 \leq k < s$. Prove that $v_{k-i} = v_{s-i}$ for $i = 0, 1, \ldots, k$.

24. Let $D = \langle V, E \rangle$ be a digraph with $indg(v) \leq 1$ for all v in V. Let $(v_0, v_1, \ldots, v_s)$ and $(w_0, w_1, \ldots, w_t)$ be paths in D with $v_s = w_t$ and $s \leq t$. Prove that $v_{s-i} = w_{t-i}$ for $i = 0, 1, \ldots, s$.

25. Let $(v_0, v_1, \ldots, v_s)$ be a cycle in a digraph. Is $(v_{s-1}, v_0, v_1, \ldots, v_{s-1})$ also a cycle? Explain.

26. Let $(v_0, v_1, \ldots, v_s)$ be a cycle in a digraph. Is $(v_1, v_2, \ldots, v_s, v_1)$ also a cycle? Explain.

27. Let $\langle V, E \rangle$ be a digraph with $\#V = n$. Explain why $\#E \leq n^2$.

28. Let $\langle V, E \rangle$ be a digraph with no loops, that is, a digraph such that $(v, w) \in E$ implies that $v \neq w$. Also, let $\# V = n$. Explain why $\# E \leq n^2 - n$.

29. Let $D = \langle V, E \rangle$ be a digraph. Let P be the binary relation on V for which vPw means that there is a path from v to w in D. Prove that P is reflexive and transitive.

30. Show with an example that the binary relation P of Problem 29 may not be symmetric.

31. Let F be the reverse (as characterized in Definition 5 of Section 1.4) of a binary relation E on a set V. How are indegree and outdegree in the digraph $\langle V, F \rangle$ expressed in terms of indegree and outdegree in $\langle V, E \rangle$?

32. Let $\langle V, E \rangle$ and $\langle V, F \rangle$ be as in Problem 31. How could one convert a picture for $\langle V, E \rangle$ into a picture for $\langle V, F \rangle$?

33. Let $D = \langle V, E \rangle$ be a digraph in which $\# V \geq 1$ and $\text{outdg}(v) \geq 1$ for each v in V. Prove that a circuit exists in D.

34. Let D be as in Problem 33. Must D have a cycle? Explain.

35. Let E be an irreflexive binary relation on V such that exactly one of the ordered pairs (v, w) and (w, v) is in E for every pair $\{v, w\}$ of elements of V. Let $\# V = n$.
(a) What is $\# E$?
*(b) Prove that there is a hamiltonian path in the digraph $\langle V, E \rangle$.

*36. Let $D = \langle V, E \rangle$ be a digraph with a vertex r such that there is a path from r to v for each v in V. Let $\# V = n$. Prove that $\# E \geq n - 1$.

6.2

ROOTED TREES

Here we deal with a type of digraph whose applications include methods of storing data and of searching files for desired data. These applications are discussed in the next section.

DEFINITION 1   **ROOTED TREE, ROOT**

$T = [V, E, r]$ is a *rooted tree* with r as its *root* if:

(a) $\langle V, E \rangle$ is a digraph,
(b) r is a vertex in V with indegree 0,
(c) every other vertex has indegree 1, and
(d) there is a path in $\langle V, E \rangle$ from r to each vertex in V.

Whenever we consider a rooted tree $[V, E, r]$ to be a digraph, we mean the digraph $\langle V, E \rangle$. In a figure for a rooted tree the root r will always be the topmost vertex. As we will see, it is always possible to draw the figure so that v is higher than w whenever vEw, that is, so that all edges are directed downward. This enables us to omit arrowheads in diagrams for rooted trees. Figure 6.2.1 depicts four rooted trees.

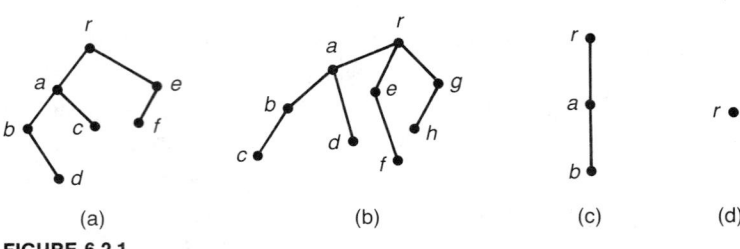

(a)   (b)   (c)   (d)

FIGURE 6.2.1

Let v be a vertex different from the root r in a rooted tree $T = [V, E, r]$. It follows from Definition 1(c) that $\text{indg}(v) = 1$ and hence that there is a unique vertex u in V such that uEv.

DEFINITION 2   PARENT, CHILD, LEAF

Let $T = [V, E, r]$ be a rooted tree, $v \in V$, and $v \neq r$. The unique u in V with uEv is called *the parent* of v, and v is said to be *a child* of u. A *leaf* of T is a vertex with no children.

For example, in Figure 6.2.1(b), the vertices a, e, and g are the children of the root r; a is the parent of b and d; also b, e, and g each have one child; and c, d, f, and h are leaves.

DEFINITION 3   *n*-ARY TREE, BINARY TREE

An *n-ary tree* is a rooted tree in which no vertex has more than n children and some vertex has n children. A *binary tree* is a 2-ary tree in which each child is specified as the left child or the right child of its parent (and no vertex has two left children or two right children).

The specification of "left" or "right" is usually given by a diagram. For example, Figure 6.2.1(a) shows a binary tree in which the root r has a as its left child and e as its right child, e has f as its left child and has no right child, and b has d as its right child and has no left child. The graphs depicted in Figures 6.2.1(b), (c), and (d) are a 3-ary tree, a 1-ary tree, and a 0-ary tree, respectively.

The following example can be used to illustrate the results on paths in a rooted tree that are stated and proved for general rooted trees in the four lemmas of this section.

Example 1   Let $T = [V, E, r]$ be the rooted tree of Figure 6.2.2. In the matrix of Table 6.2.1, the entry on the location of the row for a vertex v and the column for a vertex w is the sole path from v to w, if such a path exists; the entry is a dash if no such path exists from v to w.

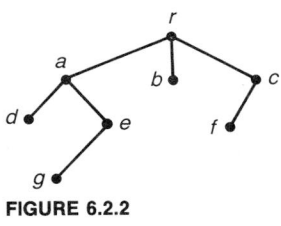

FIGURE 6.2.2

TABLE 6.2.1

	r	a	b	c	d	e	f	g
r	(r)	(r, a)	(r, b)	(r, c)	(r, a, d)	(r, a, e)	(r, c, f)	(r, a, e, g)
a	—	(a)	—	—	(a, d)	(a, e)	—	(a, e, g)
b	—	—	(b)	—	—	—	—	—
c	—	—	—	(c)	—	—	(c, f)	—
d	—	—	—	—	(d)	—	—	—
e	—	—	—	—	—	(e)	—	(e, g)
f	—	—	—	—	—	—	(f)	—
g	—	—	—	—	—	—	—	(g)

$\square$

LEMMA 1   PATHS IN ROOTED TREES

Let $P = (v_0, v_1, \ldots, v_n)$ be a path in a rooted tree $[V, E, r]$. Then:

(a) The only vertex v_i that can be r is v_0.
(b) The path P is determined uniquely by its length n and its final vertex v_n.

PROOF   (a) The root r has no parent. Since each v_i for $1 \le i \le n$ has v_{i-1} as its parent, r cannot be one of $v_1, v_2, \ldots, v_n$. This proves Part (a).

(b) Now let n and v_n be given. If $n > 0$, it follows from $v_{n-1} E v_n$ that v_{n-1} is the unique parent of v_n. Similarly, if $n > 1$, then v_{n-2} is the unique parent of v_{n-1}. Continuing this way, one sees that the entire path P is determined uniquely by n and v_n. (A formal proof can be given using induction on the length n of the path.) $\square$

LEMMA 2   **HOW PATHS IN ROOTED TREES CAN INTERSECT**

Let $(v_0, v_1, \ldots, v_m)$ and $(w_0, w_1, \ldots, w_n)$ be paths in a rooted tree. If $v_h = w_k$ for some fixed h and k with $0 \le h \le k \le n$, then $v_{h-i} = w_{k-i}$ for $i = 0, 1, \ldots, h$.

PROOF   We note that

$$(v_0, v_1, \ldots, v_h) \qquad \text{and} \qquad (w_{k-h}, w_{k-h+1}, \ldots, w_k) \qquad (1)$$

are paths with the same length h and the same final vertex (since $v_h = w_k$). Hence, by Lemma 1(b), the paths of Display (1) are identical, which is the content of this lemma.   □

LEMMA 3   **UNIQUE PATH FROM r TO A GIVEN VERTEX**

There is exactly one path from the root r to a given vertex x of a rooted tree.

PROOF   Let each of $(v_0, v_1, \ldots, v_m)$ and $(w_0, w_1, \ldots, w_n)$ be a path from r to x. Then $v_0 = r = w_0$ and $v_m = x = w_n$. In the case of $m \le n$, it follows from Lemma 2 that

$$v_{m-i} = w_{n-i} \quad \text{for } i = 0, 1, \ldots, m. \qquad (2)$$

In particular, $r = v_0 = v_{m-m} = w_{n-m}$. Now, $r = w_{n-m}$ and Lemma 1(a) tell us that $w_{n-m} = w_0$; that is, $n = m$. This and Display (2) imply that the paths are identical. The case of $m \ge n$ is similar. Definition 1(d) tells us that there is at least one path from r to x, and we have proved here that there cannot be more than one such path.   □

LEMMA 4   **UNIQUENESS OF PATHS**

Let x and y be vertices in a rooted tree. Then there is at most one path from x to y.

PROOF   Let each of $(v_0, v_1, \ldots, v_m)$ and $(w_0, w_1, \ldots, w_n)$ be a path from x to y; that is, let these paths have $v_0 = x = w_0$ and $v_m = y = w_n$. By Definition 1(d) there is a path $(u_0, u_1, \ldots, u_h)$ with $r = u_0$ and $x = u_h$. Then

$$(u_0, u_1, \ldots, u_h, v_1, \ldots, v_m) \qquad \text{and} \qquad (u_0, u_1, \ldots, u_h, w_1, \ldots, w_n)$$

are paths from r to y. Since these must be identical by Lemma 3, the paths from x to y must also be identical.   □

DEFINITION 4   LEVEL, HEIGHT

The *level* of vertex x in a rooted tree is the length of the unique path from the root to x. The *height* of a tree is the maximum of the levels of its vertices.

Example 2

The level $\lambda(v)$ of each vertex v for the rooted tree $T = [V, E, r]$ of Figure 6.2.3 is given in the following table:

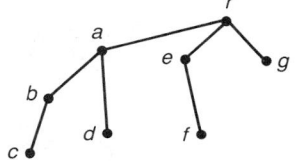

FIGURE 6.2.3

v	r	a	b	c	d	e	f	g
$\lambda(v)$	0	1	2	3	2	1	2	1

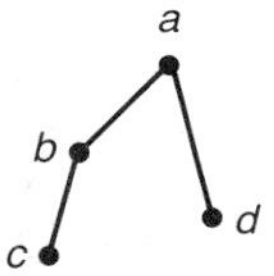

The maximum 3 of these levels is the height of T. For this tree T, let V_a consist of all the vertices w of T for which there is a path in T from a to w; one sees easily that $V_a = \{a, b, c, d\}$. Also, let E_a consist of the edges (v, w) of T for which both v and w are in the subset V_a; then $E_a = \{(a, b), (a, d), (b, c)\}$, and $[V_a, E_a, a]$ is the rooted tree of Figure 6.2.4. This process for obtaining smaller rooted trees within a given rooted tree has certain applications which will be discussed in the next section. The following theorem extends our observation that this $[V_a, E_a, a]$ is a rooted tree to a more general context.   □

FIGURE 6.2.4

THEOREM 1   ROOTED TREE STARTING FROM VERTEX x

Let $T = [V, E, r]$ be a rooted tree and $x \in V$. Let V_x consist of all vertices y for which there is a path in T from x to y. Let E_x consist of the edges (v, w) in E with both v and w in V_x. Then $T_x = \langle V_x, E_x \rangle$ is a rooted tree $[V_x, E_x, x]$ (with x as its root).

PROOF

If $x = r$, then $T_x = T$ and we are done. So let $x \neq r$ and let p be the unique parent of x. By definition of V_x, if p were in V_x, there would be a path $(x, v_1, \ldots, v_{n-1}, p)$ from x to p; then (p) and $(p, x, v_1, \ldots, v_{n-1}, p)$ would be distinct paths from p to p, contradicting Lemma 4. Hence p is not in V_x, and so the indegree of x in T_x is 0. Thus x can serve as the root. Now, let y be in V_x and $y \neq x$. By definition of V_x, there is a path $P = (w_0, w_1, \ldots, w_m)$ in T with $x = w_0$, $y = w_m$, and $m \geq 1$. For $0 \leq i \leq m$, $(w_0, w_1, \ldots, w_i)$ is a path in T from x to w_i and hence w_i is in V_x. This means that P is a path in T_x from x to y. The indegree of y in T_x is 1, since (w_{m-1}, w_m) is the one and only edge in E_x with y as final point. Thus the digraph $\langle V_x, E_x \rangle$ is a rooted tree $[V_x, E_x, x]$.   □

DEFINITION 5 **SUBTREE WITH x AS ROOT**

Let the rooted trees T and T_x be as in Theorem 1. Then T_x is called the *subtree of T with x as its root*.

For the rooted tree $T = [V, E, r]$ of Figure 6.2.3, one sees that a, e, and g are the children of the root r. The sets of vertices for the subtrees for these children are

$$V_a = \{a, b, c, d\}, \qquad V_e = \{e, f\}, \qquad V_g = \{g\},$$

and the collection $\{\{r\}, V_a, V_e, V_g\}$ forms a partition of the set V of vertices of the original tree T. The statement and proof of such a result for a general rooted tree follow.

THEOREM 2 **PARTITIONING A ROOTED TREE**

Let $c_1, c_2, \ldots, c_s$ be a listing of the children of the root r of a rooted tree $T = [V, E, r]$. For $i = 1, 2, \ldots, s$, let $T_i = [V_i, E_i, c_i]$ be the subtree of T with c_i as its root. Then

$$\{r\}, V_1, V_2, \ldots, V_s \tag{3}$$

is a partition of V.

PROOF Let x be in V. If x has level 0, x must be r. If x has positive level, the vertex w_1 in the unique path $(r, w_1, \ldots, w_{n-1}, x)$ from r to x must be a child c_i of r, and so x is in this V_i. Hence each x of V is in exactly one of the sets of Display (3). $\square$

DEFINITION 6 **LEFT SUBTREE, RIGHT SUBTREE**

Suppose that in a binary tree $T = [V, E, r]$, the root r has both a left child f and a right child g. Then the subtree T_f with f as root is the *left subtree* of T and the subtree T_g with g as root is the *right subtree* of T.

If r has no left child (or has no right child), then the left subtree (or the right subtree) is defined to be the *null rooted tree* with no vertices and hence no edges.

Example 3 Figure 6.2.5 depicts the binary tree $T = [V, E, \varepsilon]$ in which the root is the empty word ε, $V = \{\varepsilon\} \cup \boldsymbol{B_1} \cup \boldsymbol{B_2} \cup \boldsymbol{B_3}$, the leaves are the strings of $\boldsymbol{B_3}$, and a nonleaf α has the string $\alpha 0$ (with 0 postfixed) as its left child and has $\alpha 1$ as its right child. For $n = 1, 2$, and 3, the strings of $\boldsymbol{B_n}$ are the vertices with level n. Also, at each level the strings appear in the order of the standard listing for $\boldsymbol{B_n}$.

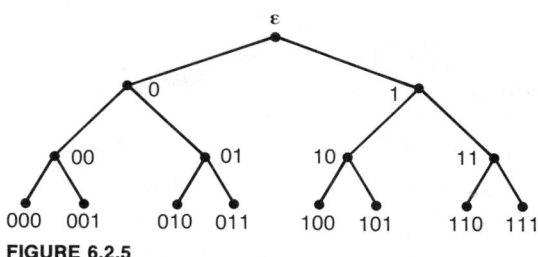

FIGURE 6.2.5

PROBLEMS FOR SECTION 6.2

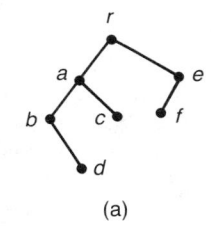

(a)

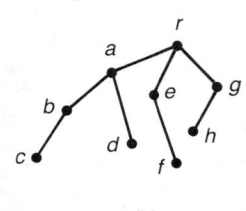

(b)

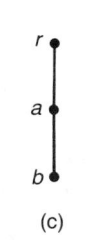

(c)

r •

(d)

FIGURE 6.2.1

1. (a) Can a rooted tree have two vertices each of which has no parent? Explain.
    (b) What is the sum of the indegrees of the vertices of a rooted tree with n vertices?

2. Let $T = [V, E, r]$ be a rooted tree with $\# V = n$.
    (a) What is the outdegree of a leaf in T?
    (b) What is the sum of the outdegrees of the vertices of T?
    (c) What is $\# E$?

3. Give the level of each vertex in the rooted tree of Figure 6.2.1(a), repeated here in the margin.

4. Give the level of each vertex in the rooted tree of Figure 6.2.1(b).

5. What is the height of the rooted tree of Figure 6.2.1(b)?

6. Give the heights of the rooted trees of:
    (a) Figure 6.2.1(c),   (b) Figure 6.2.1(d).

7. For the binary tree of Figure 6.2.1(a), draw figures for:
    (a) the left subtree,   (b) the right subtree.

8. For the 3-ary tree of Figure 6.2.1(b), draw figures for the subtrees with a, e, and g as their respective roots.

9. Explain why the left and right subtrees in a binary tree are n-ary trees with $n = 0$, 1, or 2.

10. (a) Let x be a vertex in an n-ary tree T. Explain why the subtree T_x with x as its root is an m-ary tree with $m \le n$.
    (b) Show by an example that the T_x of Part (a) may be an m-ary tree with $m < n$.

11. Let T_f be the left subtree and T_g be the right subtree of a binary tree T of height $h \ge 1$. Explain why:
    (a) The height of T_f is at most $h - 1$ and the same is true for T_g.
    (b) The height of at least one of T_f and T_g is $h - 1$.

12. Let $c_1, \ldots, c_m$ be the children of the root r of an n-ary tree T of height h. Justify the following assertions.
(a) For $i = 1, \ldots, m$, the height of the subtree with c_i as root is at most $h - 1$.
(b) At least one of the subtrees of Part (a) has height $h - 1$.

13. Find the maximum number of vertices in a binary tree of height:
(i) 0;   (ii) 1;   (iii) 2;   (iv) 3;   (v) 4;   (vi) h.

14. Repeat Problem 13, but with "binary" replaced by:
(a) 3-ary,   (b) n-ary.

15. In a binary tree $T = [V, E, r]$, let $[V_f, E_f, f]$ be the left subtree and $[V_g, E_g, g]$ be the right subtree. Explain why the three subsets $\{(r, f), (r, g)\}$, E_f, E_g partition E.

16. Let $c_1, c_2, \ldots, c_m$ be the children of r in an n-ary tree $T = [V, E, r]$. Let $[V_i, E_i, c_i]$ be the subtree with c_i as root. Explain why

$$\{(r, c_1), (r, c_2), \ldots, (r, c_m)\}, E_1, E_2, \ldots, E_m$$

is a partition of E.

17. Prove that there are no circuits in a rooted tree.

18. Let $[V, E, r]$ be a rooted tree. Prove the following.
(a) The binary relation E is irreflexive; that is, no vertex is its own child.
(b) $vEw \Rightarrow w\bar{E}v$; that is, no vertex is its own grandchild.
(c) E is antisymmetric.

19. A binary tree of height h is **maximal** if every leaf has level h and every nonleaf has outdegree 2. Let $[V, E, r]$ be a maximal binary tree of height 3.
(i) Explain why $\#V = 15$.
(ii) Find the sum of the levels of these 15 vertices.
(iii) Find the average (that is, arithmetic mean) of these 15 levels.

20. Let $[V, E, r]$ be a maximal binary tree of height 4. (See Problem 19 for the definition of *maximal*.)
(i) Explain why $\#V = 31$.
(ii) Find the average of the levels of the vertices.

21. Find the average of the levels of the vertices in a maximal binary tree of height h.

22. An n-ary tree of height h is **maximal** if every leaf has level h and every nonleaf has outdegree n. Find the average of the levels of the vertices in such a tree.

23. Let $[V, E, r]$ be a rooted tree with $V = \{v_1, v_2, \ldots, v_n\}$. Explain why:
(i) $\text{indg}(v_1) + \text{indg}(v_2) + \cdots + \text{indg}(v_n) = n - 1$.
(ii) $\#E = n - 1 = \#V - 1$.

6.3

TRAVERSING BINARY TREES

Here we discuss three algorithms for listing the vertices of a binary tree. Two of these algorithms lead to efficient parenthesis-free methods for writing algebraic expressions, and the third corresponds to the method of ordinary algebra.

Let $T = [V, E, r]$ be a binary tree with $T_f = [V_f, E_f, f]$ as its left subtree and $T_g = [V_g, E_g, g]$ as its right subtree. Then each of T_f and T_g has smaller height than T. [See Problem 11(a) of Section 6.2.]

The three methods are called **preorder**, **inorder**, and **postorder**. If T has height 0, then $V = \{r\}$ and hence each algorithm must give the only possible listing $\{r\}$. If T has height 1 (as in Figure 6.3.1), the listings are:

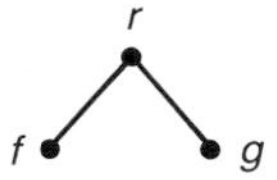

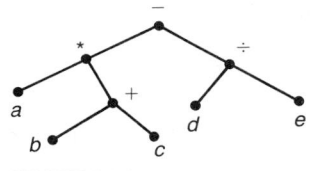

FIGURE 6.3.1

Preorder:	$\{r, f, g\}$;
Inorder:	$\{f, r, g\}$;
Postorder:	$\{f, g, r\}$.

Thus left always comes before right and the root is first for preorder, the root is between left and right for inorder, and the root is last for postorder.

We now give formal inductive definitions of inorder listing and postorder listing, and leave the formal definition of preorder listing to the reader as Problems 1 and 2 below.

DEFINITION 1 **INORDER LISTING**

Basis If T has height 0, the inorder listing for V is $\{r\}$.

Inductive Part If $\{x_1, x_2, \ldots, x_s\}$ and $\{y_1, y_2, \ldots, y_t\}$ are the inorder listings for the left and right subtrees of T, respectively, the inorder listing for V is $\{x_1, x_2, \ldots, x_s, r, y_1, y_2, \ldots, y_t\}$.

Example 1 Let $T = [V, E, -]$ be the rooted tree of Figure 6.3.2. For each vertex x in V let $T_x = [V(x), E_x, x]$ be the subtree of T with x as root. Note that here $V(x)$ replaces the notation V_x of Section 6.2. We now use Definition 1 to find the inorder listing for V. The basis part tells us that the inorder listing for $V(+)$ is $\{b, +, c\}$. Clearly, $\{a\}$ is the only listing for the singleton $V(a)$. Hence the inductive part of Definition 1 implies that $\{a, *, b, +, c\}$ is the inorder listing for $V(*)$. Since $\{d, \div, e\}$ is the inorder listing for $V(\div)$, it follows from the inductive part that the inorder listing for all the vertices of T is

FIGURE 6.3.2

$$V = \{a, *, b, +, c, -, d, \div, e\}. \tag{1}$$

$\square$

DEFINITION 2   **POSTORDER LISTING**

Basis   If T has height 0, the postorder listing for V is $\{r\}$.

Inductive Part   If $\{x_1, x_2, \ldots, x_s\}$ and $\{y_1, y_2, \ldots, y_t\}$ are the postorder listings for V_f and V_g, respectively, the postorder listing for V is $\{x_1, x_2, \ldots, x_s, y_1, y_2, \ldots, y_t, r\}$.

Example 2   Now we use Definition 2 to find the postorder listing for the vertices of the tree $T = [V, E, -]$ of Figure 6.3.2. As in Example 1, we use $V(x)$ to denote V_x. The only listing for the singleton $V(a)$ is $\{a\}$. The basis part of Definition 2 tells us that $V(+) = \{b, c, +\}$ and $V(\div) = \{d, e, \div\}$ are the postorder listings. Then it follows from the inductive part of Definition 2 that $V(*) = \{a, b, c, +, *\}$ is the postorder listing for the vertices of the left subtree of T and that

$$V = \{a, b, c, +, *, d, e, \div, -\} \tag{2}$$

is the postorder listing for all the vertices of T.   □

In the rest of this section, we will assume that B is a set $\{+, -, *, \div, \ldots\}$ of binary operations on a set $X = \{a, b, c, d, e, \ldots\}$, $A = X \cup B$, and $A' = A \cup \{(,)\}$ is the alphabet A augmented with a pair of parentheses.

We note that an ordinary algebraic expression such as

$$(a * (b + c)) - (d \div e) \tag{3}$$

is a word over the alphabet A'. In Example 3, we will represent this expression by a binary tree. The process for doing this is inductive, and hence we start with the simplest form of an algebraic expression, namely, an expression $x \,\square\, y$ with x and y standing for elements of X and $\square$ for an element of the set B of operations. This expression $x \,\square\, y$ is represented by the rooted tree of Figure 6.3.3 in which x and y are the leaves and $\square$ is the only nonleaf. Next we illustrate the algorithm for representing a more complicated expression, in particular Display (3), by a rooted tree.

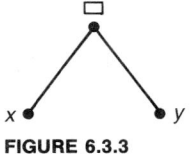

FIGURE 6.3.3

Example 3   Using Display (3) as a specific case, we now illustrate the method for representing an algebraic expression by a rooted tree. If we let $x = (a * (b + c))$ and $y = (d \div e)$, then Display (3) becomes $x - y$, which is represented by Figure 6.3.4(a). The rooted tree for the expression $a * z$ is Figure 6.3.3 with x, $\square$, and y replaced by a, $*$, and z, respectively. If this tree for $a * z$ is superimposed on Figure 6.3.4(a) so that $*$ takes the place of x, we obtain Figure 6.3.4(b). We use Figure 6.3.4(b) to represent the expression $(a * z) - y$ that results from $x - y$ by replacing x with $(a * z)$. In the expression $(a * z) - y$, if we replace z with $(b + c)$ and y with $(d \div e)$, we obtain the expression $(a * (b + c)) - (d \div e)$ of Display (3). Using the method that

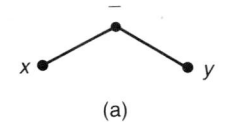

(a)

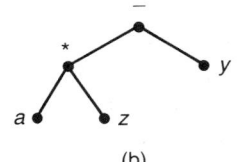

(b)

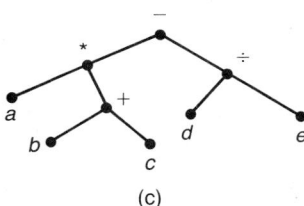

(c)

FIGURE 6.3.4

produced Figure 6.3.4(b) from Figure 6.3.4(a), we superimpose on Figure 6.3.4(b) the rooted tree for $b + c$ so that $+$ takes the place of z and superimpose the rooted tree for $d \div e$ so that $\div$ takes the place of y. This produces Figure 6.3.4(c), which we use to represent the expression of Display (3), now repeated:

$$(a * (b + c)) - (d \div e). \tag{3}$$

Since Figure 6.3.4(c) is the same as Figure 6.3.2, we have shown in Examples 1 and 2 that

$$\{a, *, b, +, c, -, d, \div, e\} \tag{4}$$

is the inorder listing for the set V of vertices for the rooted tree of Figure 6.3.4(c) and that

$$\{a, b, c, +, *, d, e, \div, -\} \tag{5}$$

is the postorder listing for V.

The inorder listing of Display (4) for the set V of vertices of the rooted tree T of Figure 6.3.4(c) is not sufficient by itself to determine T or to determine the algebraic expression (3) that T represents. We can see this by noting that Display (4) results from Display (3) by removing the parentheses to get $a * b + c - d \div e$ and then listing these nine symbols, in this order, as a set. Hence the same inorder listing of Display (4) would result if we had started with the expression

$$(((a * b) + c) - d) \div e \tag{6}$$

instead of Display (3). But the expressions of Displays (3) and (6) are not equal, as we see in the counterexample in which $*$ represents multiplication and in which $a = 5$, $b = 4$, $c = 3$, $d = 2$, and $e = 1$; then

$$(5 * (4 + 3)) - (2 \div 1) = (5 * 7) - 2 = 35 - 2 = 33,$$
$$(((5 * 4) + 3) - 2) \div 1 = ((20 + 3) - 2) \div 1 = (23 - 2) \div 1 = 21.$$

Although the inorder listing (4) does not enable us to determine uniquely the original algebraic expression (3), the postorder listing (5) does determine the expression (3) uniquely by using Algorithm 1 below.   □

NOTATION 1   REVERSE POLISH NOTATION

Reverse Polish notation for an algebraic expression is the postorder listing for the vertices of the binary tree representing the expression, with the braces and commas omitted. (This notation is due to the Polish logician Jan Lukasiewicz; see the biographical sketch appearing just before the problems for this section.)

For example, the reverse Polish notation for the expression $(a * (b + c)) - (d \div e)$ of Display (3) is

$$abc + *de \div -, \tag{7}$$

which is obtained from the postorder listing (5) by omitting braces and commas.

We see that the reverse Polish notation for an algebraic expression involving elements from X and binary operations from B is a word over the alphabet $A = X \cup B$. The word of length 9 in Display (7) substitutes for the word of length 15 in Display (3) over the augmented alphabet $A' = A \cup \{(,)\}$ because we can obtain Display (3) from Display (7) by using Algorithm 1 below. Such shortening makes reverse Polish notation a valuable tool for storage in computer memories.

We next characterize the words, over the alphabet $A = X \cup B$, that are reverse Polish notation for meaningful algebraic expressions.

DEFINITION 3   **MEANINGFUL REVERSE POLISH EXPRESSION (MRPE)**

A word $W = u_1 u_2 \ldots u_n$ over $X \cup B = \{a, b, c, \ldots\} \cup \{+, -, *, \div, \ldots\}$ is a *meaningful reverse Polish expression* (MRPE) if it satisfies the following two conditions:

(a) The length n of the word $W = u_1 u_2 \ldots u_n$ must be an odd integer $2h + 1$. Also, $h + 1$ of the symbols u_i must be from X and the remaining h symbols must be from B.

(b) For each i such that u_i is in B, the subword $u_1 u_2 \ldots u_i$ must have more symbols from X than from B.

Condition (a) of Definition 3 tells us that the length of an MRPE is an odd integer. Clearly, an MRPE of length 1 is of the form x with x in X, and an MRPE of length 3 has the form $xy\square$ with x and y in X and $\square$ in B. The words

$$ab + -, \qquad a + b - c, \qquad ab + - *, \qquad \text{and} \qquad abc + - * d$$

over $X \cup B = \{a, b, c, d, \ldots\} \cup \{+, -, *, \div, \ldots\}$ are not MRPE's. The words $ab + -$ and $ab + - *$ fail to be MRPE's because they do not satisfy Condition (a) of Definition 3. The word $a + b - c$ fails Condition (b) when i is 2, since the subword $a+$ has an element of B as its rightmost symbol and does not have more symbols from X than from B. The word $abc + - * d$ fails Condition (b) when i is 6, since the subword $abc + - *$ ends with an element of B and does not have more symbols from X than from B.

Example 4 Let $X = \{a, b, c, d, e, \ldots\}$ and $B = \{+, -, *, \div, \ldots\}$. The word $W = abcd \div e - + *$ over $X \cup B$ is an MRPE because it satisfies the conditions of Definition 3. We now illustrate an algorithm for converting W into an ordinary algebraic expression S. In the process, we will see why W determines a unique expression S and hence the unique rooted tree T that represents S. The leaves of T will be the symbols a, b, c, d, e from X, and the nonleaves will be the operation symbols $\div$, $-$, $+$, $*$ from B.

The leftmost operation symbol in $W = abcd \div e - + *$ is $\div$. There are four symbols from X to the left of $\div$ in W; we are guaranteed at least two such symbols by Condition (b) of Definition 3, since the subword $abcd \div$, which ends with $\div$, must have more symbols from X than from B. The two elements of X immediately preceding $\div$ are c and d. These must be the leaves of the subtree with $\div$ as its root. The ordinary algebraic expression for this subtree is $c \div d$. Therefore the first step of the procedure is to let $x = c \div d$ and to replace the string $cd \div$ in W by x thus getting $W' = abxe - + *$. The number of operation symbols in W' is one less than the number in W; the same is true of the number of elements of X. This decrease occurs in such a way that W' satisfies the conditions of Definition 3 for being an MRPE. The second step of the procedure is to treat W' as we have just treated W. In W', the leftmost operation symbol is $-$ and the two elements of X immediately preceding $-$ are x and e. So we let $y = x - e$ and replace the string $xe-$ in W' by y, thus obtaining $W'' = aby + *$. Repeating this process, we let $z = b + y$ and $W''' = az*$. Finally we have $w = a * z$. Substituting back, we obtain

$$w = a * z = a * (b + y) = a * (b + (x - e)) = a * (b + ((c \div d) - e)).$$

It is left to the reader as Problem 6 below to make a binary tree for $w = a * (b + ((c \div d) - e))$ and then to use postorder listing of the vertices of this tree to show that W is the reverse Polish notation for w. $\square$

The formal description of the algorithm used in Example 1 follows.

ALGORITHM 1 **CONVERTING AN MRPE**

Let $W = u_1 u_2 \ldots u_n$ be an MRPE.

(a) If $n = 3$, then W is of the form $xy\square$, with x and y in X and $\square$ in B; such a W is converted to $x \square y$.

(b) If $n > 3$, let u_i be the leftmost operation symbol in W (which symbol we denote as $\square$). Replace the string $u_{i-2}u_{i-1}u_i$ in W by a new letter x thus getting a shorter word W', which is also an MRPE. When W' is converted into an ordinary algebraic expression, substitute back $x = u_{i-2} \square u_{i-1}$.

(c) Continue the process until you have an MRPE of length 3, and then do as in Part (a).

Example 5　We want to replace the symbols labeling the nine vertices of the binary tree $T = [V, E, r]$ of Figure 6.3.5 with the numbers $1, 2, \ldots, 9$ so that the inorder listing of the vertices will have these new labels appearing in their natural order. Using Definition 1, we find that the inorder listing is

$$V = \{c, a, g, d, h, r, e, b, f\}.$$

Replacing c by 1, a by 2, and so on gives the desired labeling. (See Figure 6.3.6 in Example 6 below for the new labeling.)　□

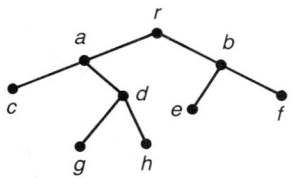

FIGURE 6.3.5

Computer storage of data is an application of n-ary trees. The word **_record_** is used to denote a packet of data. A finite collection of records is called a **_file_**. In a given file, each record is given a **key** chosen from a linearly ordered set. In our examples and problems, we will use keys from $N = \{0, 1, 2, \ldots\}$. The keys for the records of a given file are used as labels for the vertices of a binary tree $T = [V, E, r]$ in such a way that the inorder listing $V = \{k_1, k_2, \ldots, k_n\}$ of these keys has $k_1 < k_2 < \cdots < k_n$. (Example 5 illustrates the technique for such a labeling.) Let $T_f = [V_f, E_f, f]$ be the left subtree of T and $T_g = [V_g, E_g, g]$ be the right subtree of T. The inductive description of the method of searching for the record having a given k as its key (that is, searching for the vertex labeled k) is given in the following algorithm.

ALGORITHM 2　**SEARCHING IN A BINARY TREE FILE**

Basis　If the height of T is 0, then V consists of just the root r and its key k_r is examined to see if it is the desired k.

Inductive Part　If k equals the key k_r of the root, the desired vertex has been found. If $k < k_r$, the rest of the search is conducted in the left subtree of T. If $k > k_r$, the rest of the search is done in the right subtree of T.

Example 6　Figure 6.3.6 is Figure 6.3.5 with its vertices relabeled so that the inorder listing of its vertices is $\{1, 2, 3, \ldots, 9\}$. Table 6.3.1 gives the level of each vertex and the number of comparisons needed to find the vertex using Algorithm 2.

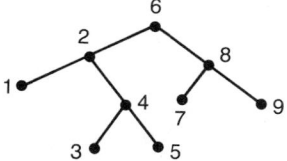

FIGURE 6.3.6

TABLE 6.3.1

vertex	6	2	8	1	4	7	9	3	5
level	0	1	1	2	2	2	2	3	3
number of comparisons	1	2	2	3	3	3	3	4	4

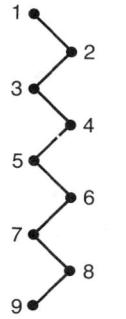

FIGURE 6.3.7

Clearly, the number of comparisons needed to find a vertex v using Algorithm 2 is one more than the level of v. The sum of the levels is

$$S = 0 + 1 + 1 + 2 + 2 + 2 + 2 + 3 + 3 = 2 \cdot 1 + 4 \cdot 2 + 2 \cdot 3 = 16,$$

and so the average level of the nine vertices is $A = \frac{16}{9}$. Hence the average number of comparisons needed is $1 + A = \frac{25}{9}$.

If the nine records were arranged in a 1-ary file, as in Figure 6.3.7, the levels of the nine vertices would be $0, 1, 2, \ldots, 8$. Then the average of the levels would be 4 and the average number of comparisons would be 5, which is greater than $\frac{25}{9}$. $\qquad\square$

We next illustrate another application of n-ary trees. (The classical version of this problem deals with pennies, but we have introduced coins of greater value.)

Example 7 Suppose that we have nine seemingly identical coins, that eight of them are gold coins identical in all respects (including weight), and that the remaining coin is of much cheaper material and of lower weight. We wish to find the bad coin using weighings on a two-pan balance scale. Let us number the coins $1, 2, \ldots, 9$ and use these numbers as symbols to represent the coins. In the *decision tree* of Figure 6.3.8, each nonleaf has the label "S vs. T," indicating that we are placing the subset S of the coins on one pan of the scale and T on the other pan. The edges have labels such as $S < T$, $S = T$, or $S > T$, indicating the possible results of a given weighing. ($S < T$ gives the case in which the coins of S have smaller total weight than those of T.) Each possible outcome of the weighings leads to a leaf, which is labeled with the number of the coin found to be the bad one in that case. The decision tree of Figure 6.3.8 gives a strategy for finding the bad coin using just two weighings.

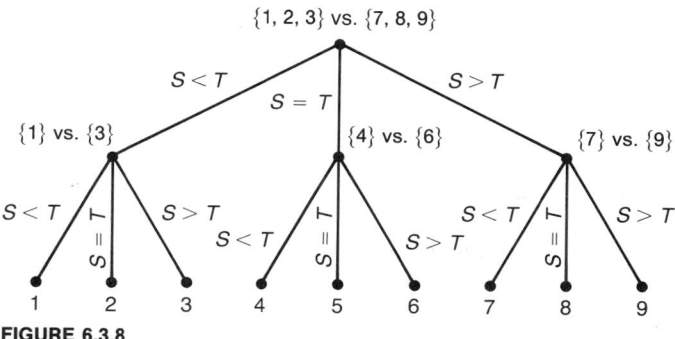

FIGURE 6.3.8 $\qquad\square$

Jan Lukasiewicz, *an eminent Polish logician, was born in Lwow, Poland, in 1878. He studied at the University of Lwow, where he later became docent before moving on to professorships in Warsaw and, after World War II, at the Royal Irish Academy in Dublin. In 1921 he published a paper in which he described a three-valued logic, though this was soon superseded by a paper of E. L. Post that described an m valued logic for m > 2. Lukasiewicz continued his work in many-valued logic and other branches of the subject. Among mathematicians not working in logic, he is known primarily for his parenthesis-free notation. He died in 1956.*

PROBLEMS FOR SECTION 6.3

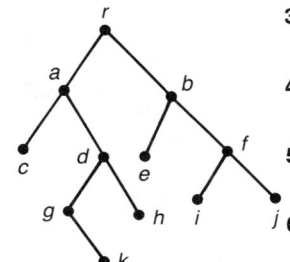

1. Give the basis part of the algorithm for preorder listing.

2. Give the inductive part of the algorithm for preorder listing.

3. Give the inorder listing for the vertices of the binary tree shown in the figure.

4. Give the preorder listing for the vertices of the binary tree shown in Problem 3.

5. (i) Make a binary tree that represents $((a - (b \div c)) + d) * e$.
(ii) Give the reverse Polish notation for the expression in Part (i).

6. (i) Make a binary tree for $w = a * (b + ((c \div d) - e))$.
(ii) Give the reverse Polish notation for the expression in Part (i).

7. Which of the following words over $\{a, b, c, d, e, \ldots\} \cup \{+, -, *, \div, \ldots\}$ are meaningful reverse Polish expressions (MRPE's)?
(a) $abcd+$,   (b) $a+bcd-$,   (c) $abcd+-*$,   (d) $ab+cd-*$.

8. Which of the following are MRPE's?
(a) $ab+-*$,   (b) $abc+-d*$,   (c) $abc+-*d$,   (d) $ab+c-d*$.

9. Let $B = \{\triangle, \square\}$ and $X = \{x, y, z\}$. Write the 2 MRPE's of length 5 over $X \cup B$ in which $\triangle$ appears to the left of $\square$, x appears to the left of y, and y appears to the left of z.

10. Let $B = \{\circ, \triangle, \square\}$ and $X = \{a, b, c, d\}$. Write the MRPE's of length 7 over $X \cup B$ in which $\circ$ appears to the left of $\triangle$, $\triangle$ appears to the left of $\square$, and the four elements of X appear in alphabetical order from left to right.

11. Let C_n be the number of MRPE's of length $2n + 1$ over $X \cup B$ in which all n operation symbols appear from left to right in the order of the listing $B = \{b_1, b_2, \ldots, b_n\}$ and all $n + 1$ elements of X appear in the order of the listing $\{x_1, x_2, \ldots, x_{n+1}\}$ (for example, $C_0 = 1 = C_1$, $C_2 = 2$, and $C_3 = 5$). Find the 5 MRPE's of this type for $n = 3$.

12. Let C_n be as in Problem 11. Find C_4.

13. Let $X = \{x_1, x_2, \ldots, x_{n+1}\}$ and $B = \{\square\}$. Let Q_n be the number of MRPE's of length $2n + 1$ over $X \cup B$ in which all $n + 1$ elements x_i of X appear from left to right in numerical order of their subscripts i. (Each of these MRPE's will have $\square$ appearing n times.) Find:
(a) Q_1;   (b) Q_2;   (c) Q_3.

14. Let Q_n be as in Problem 13. Find Q_4.

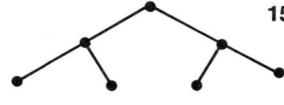

15. Label the vertices of the figure so that $\{1, 2, 3, 4, 5, 6, 7\}$ is the inorder listing of its vertices. Then use a table like Table 6.3.1 in Example 6 to find the average number of comparisons in using Algorithm 2, "Searching in a Binary Tree File."

16. Do the analogue of Problem 15 for a maximal binary tree of height 3. (See Problem 19 of Section 6.2 for the meaning of "maximal.")

17. Let $\{1, 2, 3, 4\}$ be labels for four coins. Assume that coin 4 and two of the other coins are identical genuine coins but that one of $\{1, 2, 3\}$ is fake and either too light or too heavy. Show with a decision tree that the bad coin can be found and classified as light or heavy with two tests on a balance scale.

18. Let $\{1, 2, \ldots, 27\}$ designate a set of coins. Twenty-six of the coins are identical, and the remaining coin is too light. Use a decision tree to show that the bad coin can be found with three tests on a balance scale.

19. Let $\{1, 2, \ldots, 12\}$ designate a set of coins. Eleven of them are identical, and the other coin is either too light or too heavy. Show with a decision tree that the different coin can be found and classified as too light or too heavy with three tests on a balance scale.

20. Let D_n be the number of binary trees for which the postorder listing of the vertices is $\{1, 2, 3, \ldots, 2n + 1\}$ and there are $n + 1$ leaves. Find:
(a) D_0;   (b) D_1;   (c) D_2;   (d) D_3.

21. Let D_n be as in Problem 20. Find:
(a) D_4;   *(b) D_5.

*22. Let C_n be as in Problem 11. Explain why

$$C_{n+1} = \sum_{k=0}^{n} C_k C_{n-k} \quad \text{for all } n \text{ in } N = \{0, 1, \ldots\}.$$

*23. Let D_n be as in Problem 20. Explain why

$$D_{n+1} = \sum_{k=0}^{n} D_k D_{n-k} \quad \text{for all } n \text{ in } N.$$

24. Let C_n, Q_n, and D_n be as in Problems 11, 13, and 20, respectively. Does $C_n = Q_n = D_n$ for all n in N? Explain. (The C_n are called the **Catalan Numbers**. This problem asks whether the Q_n and the D_n are also the Catalan Numbers. See the biographical sketch below.)

Eugène Charles Catalan was born in 1814 in Liège, Belgium. He worked in various branches of mathematics—differential equations, mathematical physics, and algebra. Jacobians, as used in calculus today, are due to Catalan. But his name is mainly associated with the sequence of Catalan Numbers that arises in so many contexts. Catalan died in 1894.

6.4

SUBDIGRAPHS, ISOMORPHISMS, MAPPING DIGRAPHS

One of the concepts we are about to introduce is that of "subdigraph of a digraph." This is the analogue for digraphs of "subsemigroup of a semigroup" and "submonoid of a monoid," which were studied in Section 2.2. We will also discuss "digraph isomorphism," which will help us determine whether digraphs $\langle V, E \rangle$ and $\langle V', E' \rangle$ differ merely in the symbols for their vertices. The topic of "mapping digraph" helps in the geometrical analysis of a mapping f from a finite set to itself, as we will see in our study of permutations in Chapter 7.

DEFINITION 1   **SUBDIGRAPH, SPANNING SUBDIGRAPH**

A **subdigraph** of a digraph $D = \langle V, E \rangle$ is a digraph $D_1 = \langle V_1, E_1 \rangle$ such that $V_1 \subseteq V$ and $E_1 \subseteq E$. This D_1 is a **spanning subdigraph** if $V_1 = V$ (and $E_1 \subseteq E$).

Example 1   In Figure 6.4.1, the digraphs D_1, D_2, and D_3 are some of the subdigraphs of D. Of these, only D_1 is a spanning subdigraph of D, since neither D_2 nor D_3 has all the vertices of D.

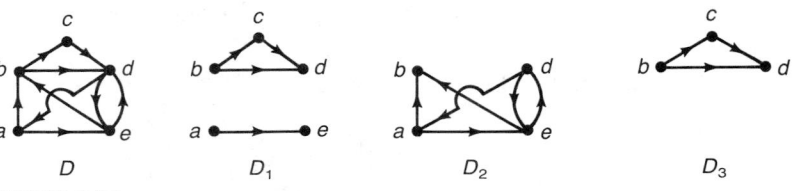

D D_1 D_2 D_3

FIGURE 6.4.1   □

DEFINITION 2   **SUBDIGRAPH INDUCED BY A SUBSET OF VERTICES**

Let $D = \langle V, E \rangle$ be a digraph and let $U \subseteq V$. Then the ***subdigraph of D induced by*** U is the digraph $\langle U, K \rangle$, in which K consists of all the edges (v, w) in E for which v and w are in U.

DEFINITION 3   **SUBDIGRAPH EVOKED BY A SUBSET OF EDGES**

Let $D = \langle V, E \rangle$ be a digraph and let $F \subseteq E$. Then the subdigraph of D ***evoked by F*** is the digraph $\langle W, F \rangle$ in which W consists of all vertices v that are endpoints of edges in F.

Example 2   In Figure 6.4.1, D_3 is the subdigraph of D induced by the subset $\{b, c, d\}$ of vertices. Also, D_3 is the subdigraph of D evoked by the subset $\{(b, c), (b, d), (c, d)\}$ of edges.   □

DEFINITION 4   **COMPLEMENTARY SUBDIGRAPHS**

Let $D = \langle V, E \rangle$ be a digraph. Let E_1 and E_2 form a partition of the set E of edges. Let $D_1 = \langle W_1, E_1 \rangle$ and $D_2 = \langle W_2, E_2 \rangle$ be the subdigraphs of D evoked by E_1 and E_2, respectively. Then D_1 and D_2 are ***complementary subdigraphs*** in D, and D_2 is the complement of D_1 in D.

Example 3   In Figure 6.4.1, D_2 and D_3 are complementary subdigraphs in D.   □

DEFINITION 5   **PARTITION OF A DIGRAPH**

Digraphs $\langle V_1, E_1 \rangle$, $\langle V_2, E_2 \rangle$, ..., $\langle V_n, E_n \rangle$ form a (***digraph***) ***partition*** of $\langle V, E \rangle$ if $V_1, V_2, \ldots, V_n$ form a (set) partition of V and $E_1, E_2, \ldots, E_n$ form a partition of E.

Example 4   Let D_1 be as in Figure 6.4.1, $V_4 = \{b, c, d\}$, $E_4 = \{(b, c), (b, d), (c, d)\}$, $V_5 = \{a, e\}$, and $E_5 = \{(a, e)\}$. Then the digraphs $\langle V_4, E_4 \rangle$ and $\langle V_5, E_5 \rangle$ form a partition of D_1.   □

DEFINITION 6   **ISOMORPHIC DIGRAPHS**

Digraphs $D = \langle V, E \rangle$ and $D' = \langle V', E' \rangle$ are ***isomorphic*** if there exists at least one bijection β from V onto V' such that vEw if and only if $\beta(v)E'\beta(w)$. Such a bijection β is an ***isomorphism*** from D onto D'.

In other words, D and D' are isomorphic when there is a one-to-one correspondence between V and V' such that there is an edge from a vertex v to a vertex w in D if and only if there is an edge from the corresponding vertex v' to the corresponding vertex w' in D'. Digraphs D and D' are isomorphic when they differ only in the names (that is, symbols) for their vertices. One can prove that $D = \langle V, E \rangle$ and $D' = \langle V', E' \rangle$ are isomorphic by establishing a bijection β from V onto V' such that the relation matrix for E' is obtained from the relation matrix for E by replacing each row and column label v with its image $\beta(v)$. This method is used in the following example.

Example 5 Let $D = \langle V, E \rangle$ and $D' = \langle V', E' \rangle$ be the digraphs of Figure 6.4.2(a) and (b). Relation matrices for the binary relations E and E' are the following:

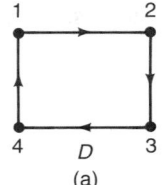

(a)

E	1	2	3	4
1	0	1	0	0
2	0	0	1	0
3	0	0	0	1
4	1	0	0	0

E'	a	c	b	d
a	0	1	0	0
c	0	0	1	0
b	0	0	0	1
d	1	0	0	0

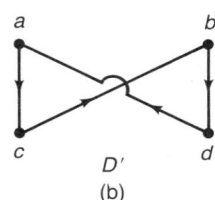

(b)

Clearly, the bijection β from V onto V' with

$$\beta: 1 \mapsto a, \quad 2 \mapsto c, \quad 3 \mapsto b, \quad 4 \mapsto d$$

is such that one obtains the relation matrix for E' from the relation matrix for E by replacing each row and column label v with its image $\beta(v)$ under the bijection β. This shows that the digraphs D and D' are isomorphic and that β is one of the isomorphisms from D onto D'. Problems 15 and 16 below deal with other isomorphisms from D onto D'.

One can see geometrically that D and D' are isomorphic by changing Figure 6.4.2(b) for D' into Figure 6.4.2(c) and then noting that Figures 6.4.2(a) and (c) differ only in the labels for their vertices. □

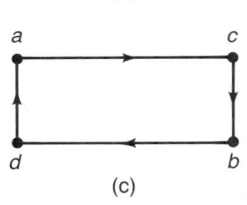

(c)

FIGURE 6.4.2

Example 6 Let D and D' be the digraphs of Figure 6.4.3. Let us try to determine whether D and D' are isomorphic. Our strategy is to assume that there is an isomorphism β from D onto D' and to try to either find such a β or prove that no such β exists by obtaining a contradiction. We start by noting that $\text{outdg}(1) = 0$; that is, there is no edge of the form $(1, v)$ in E. With Definition 6 (and the assumption that β is an isomorphism), this fact implies that there is no edge of the form $(\beta(1), \beta(v))$ in E'; that is,

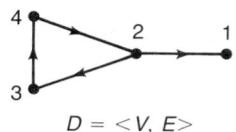

$$D = \langle V, E \rangle$$

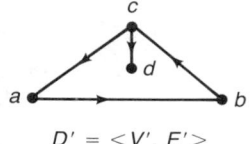

$$D' = \langle V', E' \rangle$$

FIGURE 6.4.3

outdg($\beta(1)$) = 0 in D'. Hence $\beta(1)$ must be d. Since (2, 1) is an edge in E, Definition 6 tells us that $(\beta(2), \beta(1)) = (\beta(2), d)$ is an edge in E'. As (c, d) is the only edge to d in E', this forces $\beta(2)$ to be c. Similarly, one finds that $\beta(3)$ must be a and $\beta(4)$ must be b. Thus the only possibility for an isomorphism from D onto D' is

$$\beta: 1 \mapsto d, \quad 2 \mapsto c, \quad 3 \mapsto a, \quad 4 \mapsto b.$$

The reader can confirm that β is in fact an isomorphism by performing the following three steps:

1. Make the relation matrix for E.
2. For each v in V, replace the row label v and the column label v in this matrix with $\beta(v)$ and thus obtain a new matrix.
3. Check that the new matrix is the relation matrix for E'. ☐

Example 7, which follows, deals with a case in which the two digraphs are found to be nonisomorphic.

Example 7

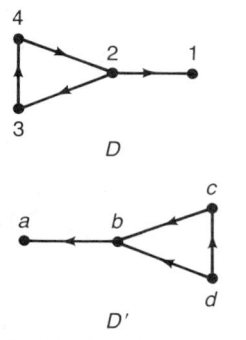

$$D$$

$$D'$$

FIGURE 6.4.4

Let $D = \langle V, E \rangle$ and $D' = \langle V', E' \rangle$ be the digraphs of Figure 6.4.4. Let us see whether D and D' are isomorphic. We tentatively consider β to be a digraph isomorphism from D onto D'. Since outdg(1) = 0 in D and a is the only vertex of D' with outdegree equal to 0, $\beta(1)$ would have to be a. Since (2, 1) is an edge of D, it follows that $(\beta(2), \beta(1)) = (\beta(2), a)$ would have to be an edge of D'. As (b, a) is the only edge to a in D', this would imply that $\beta(2) = b$. Since (2, 3) is an edge of D, $(\beta(2), \beta(3)) = (b, \beta(3))$ must be an edge of D'. As (b, a) is the only edge from b in D', this would force $\beta(3)$ to be a. But $\beta(1) = a = \beta(3)$ (with $1 \neq 3$) shows that β is not injective and hence is not bijective. This contradiction proves that there is no digraph isomorphism from D onto D'; that is, D and D' are not isomorphic. ☐

DEFINITION 7 | **MAPPING RELATION AND DIGRAPH FOR A MAPPING**

Let f be a mapping from a set V into itself. The **relation for f** is the binary relation R_f consisting of the ordered pairs $(v, f(v))$ for all v in V. The **mapping digraph for f** is the digraph $D_f = \langle V, R_f \rangle$.

Example 8 | Let f be the mapping from $V = \{a, b, c, d\}$ to itself given by

$$f: a \mapsto a, \quad b \mapsto c, \quad c \mapsto a, \quad d \mapsto a.$$

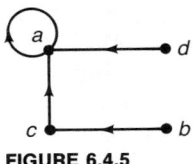

FIGURE 6.4.5

Figure 6.4.5 is a picture of the digraph D_f for this mapping. The following table gives the outdegree and indegree of each vertex in V:

v	a	b	c	d
outdg(v)	1	1	1	1
indg(v)	3	0	1	0

Example 9   Let $V = \{1, 2, 3, 4, 5, 6, 7, 8, 9, 10\}$ and let β be the permutation on V, that is, the bijective mapping from V onto itself, given by

$$\beta: 1 \mapsto 2, \quad 2 \mapsto 3, \quad 3 \mapsto 4, \quad 4 \mapsto 1, \quad 5 \mapsto 6, \quad 6 \mapsto 7, \quad 7 \mapsto 5, \quad 8 \mapsto 9,$$
$$9 \mapsto 8, \quad 10, \mapsto 10.$$

Figure 6.4.6 is a picture of the digraph D_β for this permutation. Clearly, indg(v) = 1 = outdg(v) for all vertices v of this digraph. We note that D_β is partitioned into four subdigraphs; the last of these is a loop and each of the other three parts is the subdigraph determined by the edges of a cycle.

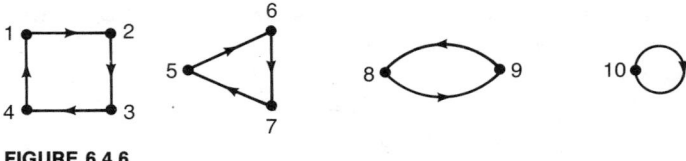

FIGURE 6.4.6

PROBLEMS FOR SECTION 6.4

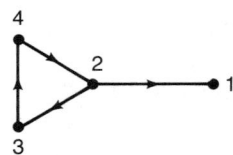

1.   Let $D = \langle V, E \rangle$ be the digraph shown in the margin. Let $E_1 = \{(3, 4), (2, 1)\}$ and $D_1 = \langle V, E_1 \rangle$.
(a) Is D_1 a subdigraph of D? Explain.
(b) Is D_1 a spanning subdigraph of D? Explain.
(c) Is D_1 the subdigraph of D evoked by E_1? Explain.

2.   Let $D = \langle V, E \rangle$ be as in the figure of Problem 1. Let $V_3 = \{2, 3, 4\}$, $E_3 = \{(3, 4), (4, 2)\}$, and $D_3 = \langle V_3, E_3 \rangle$.
(a) Is D_3 a subdigraph of D? Explain.
(b) Is D_3 a spanning digraph of D? Explain.
(c) Is D_3 the subdigraph of D induced by V_3? Explain.
(d) Is D_3 the subdigraph of D evoked by E_3? Explain.

3.   Let D and D_1 be as in Problem 1. What is the complement of D_1 in D?

4.   Let D and D_3 be as in Problem 2. Give the complement of D_3 in D.

5.   Let D be as in the figure of Problem 1 and let $V_1 = \{2, 3, 4\}$.
(i) Find E_1 so that $\langle V_1, E_1 \rangle$ is the subdigraph of D induced by V_1.
(ii) Give the complement of $\langle V_1, E_1 \rangle$ in D.

6.   Let D be as in the figure of Problem 1 and let $E_2 = \{(2, 3), (2, 1)\}$.
(i) Find V_2 so that $\langle V_2, E_2 \rangle$ is the subdigraph of D evoked by E_2.
(ii) Give the complement of $\langle V_2, E_2 \rangle$ in D.

7.   Let $\langle V_1, E_1 \rangle$ be a spanning subdigraph of $\langle V, E \rangle$. If $\#V = n$, what is $\#V_1$? Explain.

8.   Let $D = \langle V, E \rangle$ be a digraph.
(a) What is the subdigraph of D induced by V? Explain.
(b) What is the subdigraph of D evoked by E? Explain.

9.   Find V' and E' such that the mapping

$$\beta: 1 \mapsto a, \quad 2 \mapsto b, \quad 3 \mapsto c, \quad 4 \mapsto d$$

is a digraph isomorphism from the D of the figure of Problem 1 onto $D' = \langle V', E' \rangle$.

10. Let D and D' be as in Problem 9. Is the subdigraph D_1 of D induced by $\{1, 2, 3\}$ isomorphic with the subdigraph D_1' of D' induced by $\{a, b, c\}$?

11. Let $D = \langle V, E \rangle$ be the digraph shown in Problem 1. Give the relation matrix for the binary relation E on V.

12. Let $D' = \langle V', E' \rangle$ be the digraph of Problem 9. Give the relation matrix for E'.

13. Let $(v_0, v_1, \ldots, v_s)$ be a hamiltonian path in a digraph $D = \langle V, E \rangle$. Let

$$E_1 = \{(v_0, v_1), (v_1, v_2), \ldots, (v_{s-1}, v_s)\}.$$

Is the digraph D_1 evoked by E_1 a spanning subdigraph of D? Explain.

14. Let $D = \langle V, E \rangle$ be a digraph with $\#E = m$. How many spanning subdigraphs of D are there? Explain.

15. Let $D = \langle V, E \rangle$ and $D' = \langle V', E' \rangle$ be as in Figure 6.4.2 of Example 5.
(a) Give an isomorphism α from D onto D' with $\alpha(1) = b$.
(b) Give an isomorphism γ from D onto itself with $\gamma(1) = 4$.
(c) How many bijections are there from V onto itself?
(d) How many isomorphisms are there from D onto itself? Explain.

16. Let $D = \langle V, E \rangle$ and $D' = \langle V', E' \rangle$ be as in Figure 6.4.2 of Example 5.
(a) Give an isomorphism α from D onto D' with $\alpha(1) = c$.
(b) Give an isomorphism γ from D onto itself with $\gamma(1) = 2$.
(c) How many bijections are there from V onto V'?
(d) How many isomorphisms are there from D onto D'?

17. Let β be a digraph isomorphism from $D = \langle V, E \rangle$ onto $D' = \langle V', E' \rangle$.
    (a) Must $\text{indg}(v) = \text{indg}(\beta(v))$ for each v in V? Explain.
    (b) If there is a path from v to w in D, must there be a path from $\beta(v)$ to $\beta(w)$ in D'? Explain.

18. Repeat Problem 17(a), but with "indegree" replaced with "outdegree."

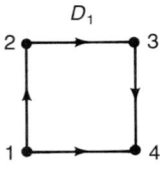

19. Let D_1 and D_2 be the digraphs shown in the top two figures in the margin. Are D_1 and D_2 isomorphic? Explain.

20. Let D_2 and D_3 be as shown in the margin. Are D_2 and D_3 isomorphic? Explain.

21. Let $V = \{1, 2, 3, 4, 5\}$ and β be the permutation on V given by

    $$\beta: 1 \mapsto 3, \quad 2 \mapsto 4, \quad 3 \mapsto 5, \quad 4 \mapsto 2, \quad 5 \mapsto 1.$$

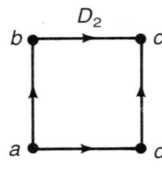

    (i) Give the ordered pairs of the relation R_β for β.
    (ii) Draw a picture of the digraph D_β for β.
    (iii) Give the values of $\text{indg}(v)$ and $\text{outdg}(v)$ for each v in V.

22. Let $V = \{1, 2, 3, 4, 5\}$ and f be the mapping from V to V given by

    $$f: 1 \mapsto 1, \quad 2 \mapsto 1, \quad 3 \mapsto 4, \quad 4 \mapsto 5, \quad 5 \mapsto 4.$$

    (i) Give the ordered pairs of the relation R_f for f.
    (ii) Draw a picture of the digraph D_f for f.
    (iii) Tabulate the indegrees and outdegrees of the vertices of V.

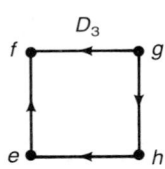

In Problems 23 through 26, assume that V is a finite set and $D_f = \langle V, E \rangle$ is the digraph for a mapping f from V to itself.

23. Does $\text{outdg}(v) = 1$ for each vertex of D_f? Explain.

24. Does $\text{indg}(v)$ equal the size of the complete inverse image $f^{-1}(v)$ for each vertex v? Explain.

25. Is $[\forall v \in V, \text{indg}(v) \geq 1] \Leftrightarrow [f \text{ is surjective}]$ true? Explain.

26. (i) State and explain the equivalence analogous to that in Problem 25 in which "surjective" is replaced with "injective."
    (ii) Do as in Part (i), but with "injective" replaced with "bijective."

27. Let $D = \langle V, E \rangle$ be a digraph with $\text{outdg}(v) = 1$ for each v in V. Does there exist a mapping f from V to itself such that D is the digraph D_f for f? Explain.

28. Let α be a permutation on a finite set X. Let A be the binary relation R_α on X for the mapping α. Let B be the reverse of the binary relation A (as defined in Definition 5 of Section 1.4). Does there exist a permutation β on X such that $R_\beta = B$? If so, how does one obtain the digraph D_β from D_α?

29. Let f be a permutation on a finite set V. Let $v \in V$ and $v_0, v_1, \ldots$ be the sequence defined inductively by $v_0 = v$ and $v_{k+1} = f(v_k)$ for $k = 0, 1, 2, \ldots$. Given that $v_s = v_t$, with $0 \leq s < t$, prove that $v_0 = v_{t-s}$.

6.5 _____

UNDIRECTED GRAPHS

In a digraph (that is, directed graph) $D = \langle V, E \rangle$, the set E of edges consists of ordered pairs (v, w) with v and w in V. Changing the edges from ordered pairs to pairs, we obtain the following concept.

DEFINITION 1   **GRAPH**

A *graph* G is an ordered pair (V, E) in which E is a collection of pairs $\{v, w\}$ with v and w in V.

As noted in Section 1.1, a pair $\{v, w\}$ must have $v \neq w$. Also, $\{v, w\} = \{w, v\}$. Let (V, E) be a graph and R be the binary relation on V in which vRw if and only if $\{v, w\} \in E$. Then R is irreflexive, since $v\bar{R}v$ for all v in V, and R is symmetric, since $vRw \Leftrightarrow wRv$. Conversely, if R is an irreflexive symmetric binary relation on a set V and E consists of the pairs $\{v, w\}$ such that vRw, then (V, E) is a graph.

DEFINITION 2   **ADJACENCY MATRIX FOR A GRAPH**

The *adjacency matrix* for a graph (V, E) is the relation matrix for the irreflexive symmetric binary relation R on V with vRw if and only if $\{v, w\} \in E$.

Example 1   Let $V = \{a, b, c\}$ and $E = \{\{a, b\}, \{b, c\}\}$. Then Table 6.5.1 is the adjacency matrix for the graph (V, E). Since we know that Table 6.5.1 is the relation matrix for an irreflexive symmetric binary relation R on V, one could construct it from that part given in Table 6.5.2 by placing 0's down the main diagonal of Table 6.5.2 and using symmetry to obtain the entries below the main diagonal.

TABLE 6.5.1

R	a	b	c
a	0	1	0
b	1	0	1
c	0	1	0

TABLE 6.5.2

	b	c
a	1	0
b		1

□

The following definitions are not numbered and are not displayed separately because they are analogous to the definitions of Sections 6.1–6.4 for directed graphs.

Let $G = (V, E)$ be a graph. An element v in V is a **vertex** of G (or in V). A pair $\{v, w\}$ in E is an **edge** of G (or in E) **joining** the vertices v and w; the vertices v and w are the **endpoints** of this edge. In a **picture** (or **figure**) for the graph G, each vertex is represented by a dot, and an edge $\{v, w\}$ is represented by one arc (or segment) joining the dots for v and w. Since the edges are pairs instead of ordered pairs, there are neither arrowheads nor loops in a picture for a graph.

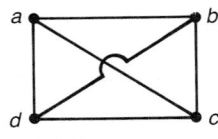

FIGURE 6.5.1

Either Figure 6.5.1 or Figure 6.5.2 is a picture for the graph $G = (V, E)$, with $V = \{a, b, c, d\}$ and

$$E = \{\{a, b\}, \{a, c\}, \{a, d\}, \{b, c\}, \{b, d\}, \{c, d\}\}.$$

Figure 6.5.3 is not a picture of a graph because there is more than one arc joining the vertices a and b.

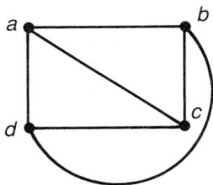

FIGURE 6.5.2

The **degree** of a vertex v is the number $\mathrm{dg}(v)$ of vertices w such that $\{v, w\}$ is an edge in E. In Figure 6.5.1, each vertex has degree 3, that is, $\mathrm{dg}(v) = 3$ for each v in V.

A **path** of **length** s between vertices v_0 and v_s is an ordered $(s + 1)$-tuple $P = (v_0, v_1, \ldots, v_s)$ such that $\{v_{i-1}, v_i\}$ is an edge in E for $i = 1$, $2, \ldots, s$. This path P is **elementary** if $v_i \neq v_j$ for $i \neq j$. P is **hamiltonian** if it is elementary and its vertices v_i are all the vertices in V. The path P is **simple** if

$$\{v_0, v_1\}, \{v_1, v_2\}, \ldots, \{v_{s-1}, v_s\}$$

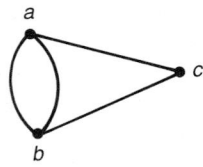

FIGURE 6.5.3

are s distinct edges. P is **eulerian** if it is simple and its edges $\{v_{i-1}, v_i\}$ are all the edges in E.

A **circuit** in a graph $G = (V, E)$ is a path $C = (v_0, v_1, \ldots, v_s)$ of positive length in which $v_0 = v_s$. C is a **simple circuit** if its edges $\{v_{i-1}, v_i\}$ are distinct pairs. An **eulerian circuit** is a simple circuit whose edges are all the edges in E. A **cycle** in G is a circuit $(v_0, v_1, \ldots, v_s)$, with $s \geq 3$, in which the only repetition of vertices is that given by $v_0 = v_s$. A cycle is **hamiltonian** if its vertices are all the vertices in V.

Example 2 Let $V = \{a, b, c, d\}$ and

$$E = \{\{a, b\}, \{a, c\}, \{b, c\}, \{b, d\}, \{c, d\}\}.$$

Then Figure 6.5.4 represents the graph $G = (V, E)$. We note that $\mathrm{dg}(a) = 2 = \mathrm{dg}(d)$ and $\mathrm{dg}(b) = 3 = \mathrm{dg}(c)$. Also, (a, b, c, d, b, a, c) is a path of length 6 between a and c. It is not simple because the edge $\{a, b\}$ is repeated in the path; it is not elementary because the vertices a, b, and c are repeated. The path (a, b, c, d) is hamiltonian and so is elementary and simple. The path (c, b, a, c, d, b) is eulerian (and hence simple) but is not elementary since vertex c (or vertex b) is repeated. □

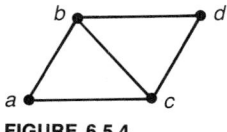

FIGURE 6.5.4

Now we continue the definitions for graphs that are analogous to those for digraphs.

A graph $G_1 = (V_1, E_1)$ is a **subgraph** of $G = (V, E)$ if $V_1 \subseteq V$ and $E_1 \subseteq E$; this G_1 is a **spanning subgraph** of G if $V_1 = V$ and $E_1 \subseteq E$. The subgraph of G **induced** by a subset U of V is the graph (U, K) such that

$$[\{v, w\} \in K] \Leftrightarrow [(v \in U) \wedge (w \in U) \wedge (\{v, w\} \in E)].$$

The subgraph of G **evoked** by a subset F of E is the graph (W, F) in which W consists of the endpoints of all the edges in F. Graphs (V_1, E_1), $(V_2, E_2), \ldots, (V_m, E_m)$ form a **partition** of a graph (V, E) if $V_1, V_2, \ldots, V_m$ form a partition of V and $E_1, E_2, \ldots, E_m$ form a partition of E. Graphs $G = (V, E)$ and $G' = (V', E')$ are **isomorphic** if there exists a bijection β from V onto V' such that $\{v, w\}$ is in E if and only if $\{\beta(v), \beta(w)\}$ is in E'; such a bijection β is an **isomorphism** from G onto G'.

Example 3

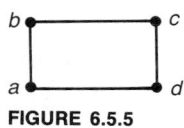

FIGURE 6.5.5

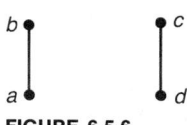

FIGURE 6.5.6

Let $G = (V, E)$ be the graph of Figure 6.5.5. We can think of V as representing a set of four cities and E as the set of roads connecting pairs of these cities. It is easy to see that there is a path between any two vertices in V; this means that one can get from any one of the four cities to any other city in the set via these roads. This is true even when any one of the edges in E is removed. (Such a removal could represent the destruction of a bridge on the given road.) However, if the edges $\{b, c\}$ and $\{a, d\}$ are removed, as in Figure 6.5.6, then there no longer is a path joining a (or b) to d (or c). Such matters also are considered by utility companies, including electric companies and telephone companies, when they construct their transmission lines. □

We now introduce terminology for situations like that described in Example 3.

DEFINITION 3   CONNECTED GRAPH

A graph $G = (V, E)$ is **connected** if there is a path between any two vertices in V.

The statements in Example 3 tell us that the graph of Figure 6.5.5 is connected whereas that of Figure 6.5.6 is not.

Example 4

Let $G = (V, E)$ be a graph in which V is a set of airports and $\{v, w\}$ is in E if and only if there exist scheduled flights between v and w. Then G is connected if and only if it is possible to get from any airport v in V to any other airport w in V by a sequence of scheduled flights. Especially when G is not connected, we might be interested in the subset of airports that can be reached in this way from a given v; the following definition and theorem deal with such subsets of vertices.   □

DEFINITION 4   **COMPONENT OF A GRAPH**

A connected subgraph $G_1 = (V_1, E_1)$ of a graph $G = (V, E)$ is a ***component*** of G if whenever $G_2 = (V_2, E_2)$ is a connected subgraph of G with $V_1 \subseteq V_2$ and $E_1 \subseteq E_2$ one must have $V_1 = V_2$ and $E_1 = E_2$.

In other words, a connected subgraph $G_1 = (V_1, E_1)$ of a graph $G = (V, E)$ is a component of G if and only if any graph G_2 produced by adjoining additional vertices of G to V_1 and/or adjoining additional edges of G to E_1 is a nonconnected graph.

The only component of the connected graph of Figure 6.5.5 is the graph itself. The disconnected (that is, not connected) graph $G = (V, E)$ with

$$V = \{a, b, c, d\} \qquad \text{and} \qquad E = \{\{a, b\}, \{c, d\}\}$$

of Figure 6.5.6 has as its two components the subgraphs (V_1, E_1) and (V_2, E_2) with

$$V_1 = \{a, b\}, \qquad E_1 = \{\{a, b\}\},$$
$$V_2 = \{c, d\}, \qquad E_2 = \{\{c, d\}\}.$$

Example 5   The components of the graph G shown in Figure 6.5.7 are the subgraphs of G shown in Figures 6.5.8 and 6.5.9.

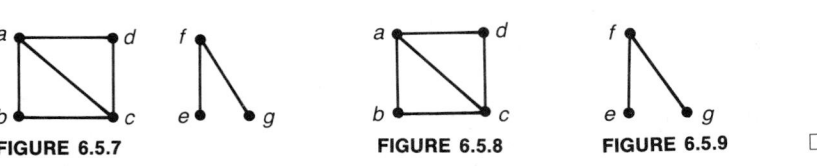

FIGURE 6.5.7   FIGURE 6.5.8   FIGURE 6.5.9   □

THEOREM 1   **COMPONENT CONTAINING A GIVEN VERTEX**

Let u be a vertex of a graph $G = (V, E)$. Let U be the subset of V consisting of u and all the vertices v such that there is a path between u and v in G. Let $G_1 = (U, K)$ be the subgraph of G induced by U. Then G_1 is a component of G (and is called ***the component of G containing U***).

PROOF   Let x and y be any vertices in U. By definition of U, there are paths $(v_0, v_1, \ldots, v_s)$ and $(w_0, w_1, \ldots, w_t)$ in G with $v_0 = u = w_0$, $v_s = x$, and $w_t = y$.

The definition of U clearly implies that each v_i and each w_j is in U. Hence

$$(v_s, v_{s-1}, \ldots, v_1, w_0, w_1, \ldots, w_t)$$

is a path between x and y in G_1, and so G_1 is connected.

Now let $G_2 = (V_2, E_2)$ be a connected subgraph of G with $U \subseteq V_2$ and $K \subseteq E_2$. Let $v \in V_2$ and $v \neq u$. Since G_2 is connected, there is a path between u and v in G_2 and hence in G. By definition of U, one has $v \in U$. This means that $V_2 \subseteq U$. Since we also have $U \subseteq V_2$, it follows that $V_2 = U$. Also, the definition of G_1 implies that $E_2 \subseteq K$. This and $K \subseteq E_2$ imply that $E_2 = K$. Finally, $V_2 = U$, $E_2 = K$, and Definition 4 together imply that G_1 is a component of G. $\qquad\square$

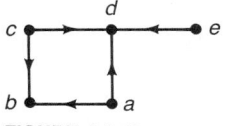

FIGURE 6.5.10

Now we consider the question: When does a picture for a digraph $D = \langle V, R \rangle$ become a picture for a graph $G = \langle V, E \rangle$ by just removing all arrowheads from arcs? Since a picture for a graph has no loops, the picture for the digraph should not have loops; that is, the binary relation R on V should be irreflexive. Also, since a picture for a graph has at most one arc joining a given pair of vertices, one should not have both (v, w) and (w, v) in the binary relation R for distinct vertices v and w; that is, R should be antisymmetric. For example, each of Figures 6.5.10, 6.5.11, and 6.5.12 is the picture of a digraph, but only that of Figure 6.5.10 becomes the picture of a graph when all arrowheads are removed. The picture of Figure 6.5.11 does not because it has a loop; the picture of Figure 6.5.12 does not because it has more than one arc joining a and b. When the binary relation R, of a digraph $D = \langle V, R \rangle$, is both irreflexive and antisymmetric, then its picture becomes a picture for a graph $G = (V, E)$ if one removes all arrowheads. We name this graph G in the following definition.

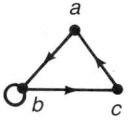

FIGURE 6.5.11

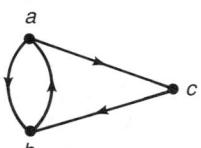

FIGURE 6.5.12

DEFINITION 5 | **UNDERLYING GRAPH**

Let $D = \langle V, R \rangle$ be a digraph in which the binary relation R is irreflexive and antisymmetric. Let E consist of all pairs $\{v, w\}$ such that vRw. Then $G = (V, E)$ is called the **underlying graph** for the digraph D.

In a rooted tree $T = [V, R, r]$, the binary relation R is irreflexive and antisymmetric (as stated in Problem 18 of Section 6.2); hence T has an underlying graph $G = (V, E)$.

DEFINITION 6 | **(UNDIRECTED) TREE**

A **tree** is a graph underlying a rooted tree.

In Theorems 2 and 3 below, we give two other characterizations of trees.

THEOREM 2   **CHARACTERIZATION OF TREES**

A graph (V, E) is a tree if and only if it is connected and $\#V = 1 + \#E$.

PROOF   First we let $T = (V, E)$ be a tree and seek to prove that T is connected and that $\#V = 1 + \#E$. By the definition of tree, there is a rooted tree $T^* = [V, E^*, r]$ such that T is the underlying graph for T^*. Let $V = \{v_1, v_2, \ldots, v_n\}$. By the definition of rooted tree, $\text{indg}(r) = 0$ and $\text{indg}(v) = 1$ for $v \neq r$. Hence, in T^*,

$$\text{indg}(v_1) + \text{indg}(v_2) + \cdots + \text{indg}(v_n) = n - 1. \tag{1}$$

Since each edge in E^* contributes 1 to the sum of the indegrees, it follows from Display (1) that $\#E^* = n - 1$. By the definition of underlying graph, we also have $\#E = n - 1$. Hence $\#V = n = 1 + \#E$.

Now let v and w be distinct vertices in V. Since T^* is a rooted tree, there are paths $(r, x_1, x_2, \ldots, x_s)$ and $(r, y_1, y_2, \ldots, y_t)$ in T^* with $x_s = v$ and $y_t = w$. Let

$$(x_s, x_{s-1}, \ldots, x_1, r, y_1, y_2, \ldots, y_t)$$

be denoted as $P = (z_0, z_1, \ldots, z_{s+t})$. For $i = 1, 2, \ldots, s + t$, $\{z_{i-1}, z_i\}$ is an edge in E because either (z_{i-1}, z_i) or (z_i, z_{i-1}) is an edge in E^*. Hence P is a path in T between v and w. This means that T is connected.

Conversely, we now let $G = (V, E)$ be a connected graph with $\#V = n$ and $\#E = n - 1$; we prove that G is a tree by induction on n. Clearly, G is a tree if $n = 1$, and hence the basis of the induction holds. Let k be a positive integer and assume inductively that the desired result is true when $n = k$. Let $H = (W, F)$ be a connected graph with $\#W = k + 1$ and $\#F = (k + 1) - 1 = k$. Let $W = \{w_0, w_1, \ldots, w_k\}$. Since each edge in F contributes 2 to the sum of the degrees of the vertices in W, it follows that

$$\text{dg}(w_0) + \text{dg}(w_1) + \cdots + \text{dg}(w_k) = 2(\#F) = 2k.$$

This implies that $\text{dg}(w_i) \leq 1$ for some i; for otherwise we would have the contradiction

$$\text{dg}(w_0) + \cdots + \text{dg}(w_k) \geq 2(k + 1).$$

Let us use g to denote some vertex in W with $\text{dg}(g) \leq 1$. Since (W, F) is connected and $\#W \geq 2$, there is a path in (W, F) between g and some vertex; thus $\text{dg}(g) \geq 1$. This and $\text{dg}(g) \leq 1$ imply that $\text{dg}(g) = 1$. Let $\{g, h\}$ be the sole edge in F involving g.

Let V result by deleting g from the set W and let E result by deleting $\{g, h\}$ from F. Then (V, E) is the subgraph of (W, F) induced by the subset V of W. Also, $\#V = \#W - 1 = (k + 1) - 1 = k$ and $\#E = k - 1$.

Let a and b be distinct vertices in V. Since (W, F) is connected, this graph has a path connecting a and b. Of all such paths, let $P = (x_0, x_1, \ldots, x_m)$ be one with shortest possible length. Then $x_{i-1} \neq x_{i+1}$ for $1 \leq i < m$, since otherwise $(x_0, x_1, \ldots, x_{i-1}, x_{i+2}, \ldots, x_m)$ would be a shorter path connecting a and b. The fact that $x_{i-1} \neq x_{i+1}$ tells us that $\{x_{i-1}, x_i\}$ and $\{x_i, x_{i+1}\}$ are distinct edges in F and hence that $\mathrm{dg}(x_i) \geq 2$ for $1 \leq i < m$. Since $\mathrm{dg}(g) = 1$, this means that no x_i is g. Thus P is a path in (V, E). Since this argument applies to all a and b in V, it follows that (V, E) is connected. Since $\#V = 1 + \#E$, the inductive hypothesis allows us to assume that (V, E) is a tree T. By the definition of tree, there is a rooted tree $T^* = [V, E^*, r]$ such that T underlies T^*. Let F^* be the result of adjoining (g, h) to E^*. We can easily see that $T' = [W, F^*, r]$ is a rooted tree such that (W, F) underlies T'. By the definition of tree, this means that (W, F) is a tree. This completes the proof. □

THEOREM 3   ANOTHER CHARACTERIZATION OF TREES

A graph is a tree if and only if it is connected and has no cycles.

The proof is left to the reader as Problems 19 and 20 below.

DEFINITION 7   FOREST

A *forest* is a graph with each component a tree.

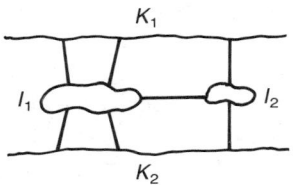

FIGURE 6.5.13

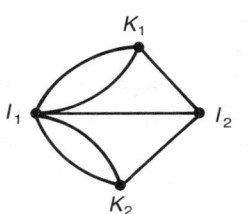

FIGURE 6.5.14

Graph theory probably began when the great Swiss mathematician Leonhard Euler (1707–1783) solved the following puzzle: The Pregel River has two islands where it passes through the then Prussian city of Königsberg. There were seven bridges connecting the islands and riverbanks, as indicated in Figure 6.5.13. The problem was to design a walking tour that would take a person over each of the seven bridges exactly once. This problem is equivalent to that of tracing Figure 6.5.14 without lifting the pencil and without going over an arc already traced. In 1736, Euler proved that each of these tasks is impossible to perform. Figure 6.5.14 depicts a *multigraph* rather than a graph, since certain pairs of vertices are joined by more than one arc; however, the reader easily will be able to apply the material in Sections 6.1 and 6.5 on eulerian paths in digraphs and graphs to the more general situation of multigraphs and thus to obtain Euler's disposition of this puzzle.

Leonhard Euler   *was born in 1707 in Basel, Switzerland, the son of a Calvinist minister. He initially studied theology and Hebrew before moving to mathematics. In mathematics he established himself as a major figure in Europe, moving in 1727 to St. Petersburg, the city of Peter the Great, where he worked for Catherine the Great in the St. Petersburg Academy. In 1740 he moved to the Berlin Academy (where he worked for Frederick the Great), but in 1766 he returned to St. Petersburg, where he died in 1783.*

Euler was one of the most prolific mathematicians in history, producing major results in a wide variety of areas, from analysis to number theory to ship design to the theory of music. Many well-known formulas and theorems are named for Euler, and the origins of several branches of mathematics can be traced to his work: partitions in the theory of numbers, topology, and—relevant to the present context—graph theory. During his first stay in Russia he lost the sight in one eye, and on his return from Berlin he became totally blind. His creativity was not diminished however, and he continued to publish mathematics, dictating his theorems and calculations to assistants. New volumes in the set of his collected works are still appearing, over 200 years after his death, with more to come.

Sir William Rowan Hamilton,   *born in Dublin in 1805, early on demonstrated prodigious abilities in mathematics and languages. He entered Trinity College, Dublin, at the age of 18, and in 1827 was appointed Astronomer Royal of Ireland. He lived and worked at Dunsink Observatory outside Dublin until his death in 1865. His principal contributions were in physics and algebra. With the discovery of quaternions in 1843, he freed algebra of the constraints of ordinary arithmetic. Multiplication of quaternions is noncommutative. The appropriate method of multiplication came to him on a walk along a canal in Dublin; he was so taken with his discovery that he carved the formulas in the stone of a bridge across the canal. A plaque marks the spot today. Hamilton's contribution to algebra is somewhat analogous to Bolyai's and Lobachevsky's non-Euclidean geometry in that it broke completely from the widely accepted, conventional views of the subject.*

It was in the study of a noncommutative algebra that Hamilton came up with his "Icosian calculus" that can be interpreted in terms of paths on the graph of the regular dodecahedron. This became the idea for a puzzle marketed in nineteenth-century England. These investigations assure Hamilton a place in the history of graph theory.

PROBLEMS FOR SECTION 6.5 _____

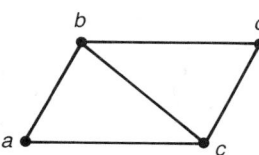

1. Let $G = (V, E)$ be a graph. How are E and the power set $P(V)$ related?

2. Let $G = (V, E)$ be a graph and $\#V = n$. Explain why $\#E \leq \binom{n}{2}$.

3. How many edges are there in the accompanying graph?

4. How is the answer to Problem 3 related to the sum of the degrees of the vertices?

5. In the graph shown in Problem 3, find a simple path of length 5 connecting vertex b to some vertex.

6. In the graph shown in Problem 3, find an elementary path of length 3 connecting c to some vertex.

7. In the graph shown in Problem 3, find an elementary circuit of length 4 connecting d to itself.

8. In the graph shown in Problem 3, find a simple circuit of length 4 connecting a to itself.

9. Let $U = \{a, b, c\}$. Find K so that (U, K) is the subgraph induced by U in the graph shown in Problem 3.

10. Repeat Problem 9, but with $\{a, b, c\}$ replaced by $\{b, c, d\}$.

11. Let $V = \{a, b, c, d\}$, $E = \{\{a, b\}, \{b, c\}, \{b, d\}\}$, and $H = (V, E)$. Let G be the graph shown in Problem 3.
(a) Is H a subgraph of G?   (b) Is H a spanning subgraph of G?
(c) Is H a tree?

12. Repeat Problem 11, but with E now $\{\{a, b\}, \{b, c\}, \{c, d\}\}$.

13. Let the graph $G = (V, E)$ underlie a digraph $D = \langle V, R \rangle$.
(a) Can both (v, w) and (w, v) be in R for some v and w in V? Explain.
(b) Must $\#E = \#R$? Explain.

14. Let $G = (V, E)$ be a graph with $\#E = m$.
(a) How many digraphs D are there such that G underlies D? Explain.
(b) How can one make a picture for G into a picture for a digraph D with G as its underlying graph?

15. Let (V, E) be a graph with $V = \{v_1, v_2, \ldots, v_n\}$. Explain why

$$\text{dg}(v_1) + \text{dg}(v_2) + \cdots + \text{dg}(v_n) = 2(\#E).$$

16. Explain why in a graph there must be an even number of vertices whose degree is odd.

17. Let $[V, E, r]$ be a rooted tree with $V = \{v_1, v_2, \ldots, v_n\}$. Explain why:
(i) $\text{indg}(v_1) + \text{indg}(v_2) + \cdots + \text{indg}(v_n) = n - 1$.
(ii) $\text{outdg}(v_1) + \text{outdg}(v_2) + \cdots + \text{outdg}(v_n) = n - 1$.
(iii) $\#E = n - 1$.

18. Let (V, E) be a tree with $V = \{v_1, v_2, \ldots, v_n\}$. Explain why:
   (a) $\#E = n - 1$;   (b) $\mathrm{dg}(v_1) + \mathrm{dg}(v_2) + \cdots + \mathrm{dg}(v_n) = 2(n - 1)$.

19. Prove that every tree $T = (V, E)$ is connected.

*20. Prove Theorem 3, that is, prove that a graph is a tree if and only if it is connected and has no cycles.

21. In each of the following parts, use the given vertex as the root r and draw a picture for a rooted tree $T = [V, R, r]$ such that the tree $H = (V, E)$ of Problem 11 underlies T.
   (a) $r = a$;   (b) $r = b$;   (c) $r = c$;   (d) $r = d$.

22. Repeat Problem 21, but with H replaced by the tree of Problem 12.

23. Let $(v_0, v_1, \ldots, v_n)$ be an eulerian path in a graph. Justify the following.
   (a) If $v_0 \neq v_n$, then $\mathrm{dg}(v_0)$ and $\mathrm{dg}(v_n)$ are odd integers.
   (b) $\mathrm{dg}(v_i)$ is an even integer if $v_i \neq v_0$ and $v_i \neq v_n$.

24. Let $(v_0, v_1, \ldots, v_n)$ be an eulerian circuit in a graph (V, E). Must $\mathrm{dg}(v)$ be an even integer for every v in V? Explain.

25. Must every eulerian path in the graph shown in Problem 3 be a path between b and c? Explain.

26. Let G be the graph shown in Problem 3.
   (a) Does G have an elementary path of length 4? Explain.
   (b) What must be the length of a hamiltonian cycle in G? Explain.

27. Let $G = (V, E)$ be the graph with $V = \{a, b, c, d, e, f\}$ and

$$E = \{\{a, b\}, \{a, c\}, \{b, c\}, \{d, e\}\}.$$

   (a) Give the component $G_1 = (V_1, E_1)$ of G containing a.
   (b) Give the component $G_2 = (V_2, E_2)$ of G containing d.
   (c) Give the component $G_3 = (V_3, E_3)$ of G containing f.
   (d) Is V_1, V_2, V_3 a partition of V?
   (e) Is E_1, E_2, E_3 a partition of E?

28. Let $G = (V, E)$, where $V = \{1, 2, 3, 4, 5, 6, 7, 8, 9, 10\}$ and

$$E = \{\{1, 2\}, \{2, 3\}, \{3, 4\}, \{4, 1\}, \{5, 6\}, \{6, 7\}, \{7, 5\}, \{8, 9\}\}.$$

   Give all the components of G.

29. (i) Give the adjacency matrix for the graph G_1 of Problem 27(a).
   (ii) For the graph of Problem 28, give the adjacency matrix for the component H containing the vertex 5.
   (iii) Are the G_1 and H of Parts (i) and (ii) isomorphic? Explain.

30. (i) Give the adjacency matrix for the graph G_2 of Problem 27(b).
   (ii) Is some component of the graph of Problem 28 isomorphic with the G_2 of Part (i)? Explain.

31. Let $G_1 = (V_1, E_1)$ and $G_2 = (V_2, E_2)$ be graphs. Let $V = V_1 \cup V_2$ and $E = E_1 \cup E_2$. Prove that (V, E) is a graph (which may be denoted as $G_1 \cup G_2$).

32. Repeat Problem 31, but with unions replaced by intersections.

33. Let $G = (V, E)$ be a graph in which $\mathrm{dg}(v) \geq 2$ for every v in V. Prove that a cycle exists in G. Assume that $\#V \geq 1$.

*34. Let $G = (V, E)$ be a connected graph. Prove that $1 + \#E \geq \#V$.

*35. Let $T = (V, E)$ be a tree. Prove that each vertex x in V is the root of a rooted tree $T_x = [V, R, x]$ with T as its underlying tree.

*36. Prove that the rooted tree T_x in Problem 35 is uniquely determined by the tree T and the vertex x.

6.6

COMPLETE, BIPARTITE, AND PLANAR GRAPHS

The complete binary relation on a set S was defined in Section 1.5 to be the cartesian product $S^2 = S \times S$. Thus it is natural to call $\langle S, S^2 \rangle$ the *complete digraph* on S. We now define the analogue for (undirected) graphs of this digraph.

DEFINITION 1   COMPLETE GRAPH

A graph (V, E) is *complete* if there is an edge $\{v, w\}$ in E whenever v and w are distinct vertices in V.

In other words, a graph (V, E) is complete if and only if

$$[(v \in V) \wedge (w \in V) \wedge (v \neq w)] \Rightarrow [\{v, w\} \in E].$$

Since there are $\binom{n}{2} = n(n-1)/2$ pairs that can be chosen from a set V of size n, a graph (V, E) with $\#V = n$ is complete if and only if $\#E = \binom{n}{2}$.

THEOREM 1   ISOMORPHIC COMPLETE GRAPHS

Let $G = (V, E)$ and $G' = (V', E')$ be complete graphs. Then G and G' are isomorphic if and only if $\#V = \#V'$.

The proof is straightforward and is left to the reader.
In view of Theorem 1, the following notation is appropriate.

NOTATION 1   **COMPLETE GRAPH K_n**

K_n denotes a complete graph with n vertices.

Figure 6.6.1 has pictures of complete graphs with 1, 2, 3, 4, and 5 vertices, respectively. K_5 is also called the ***star graph***.

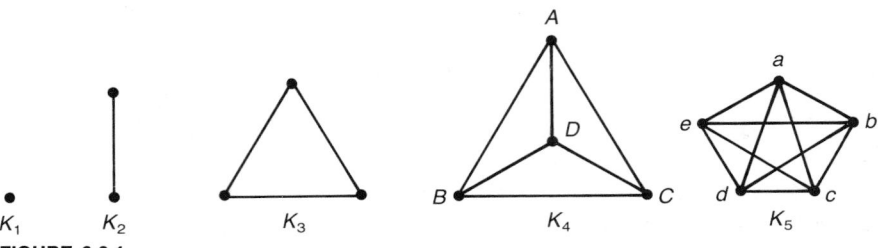

FIGURE 6.6.1

Example 1   **WEIGHTED GRAPH, TRAVELING SALESPERSON PROBLEM**   Figure 6.6.2 shows a complete graph $G = (V, E)$ in which $V = \{D, L, R, S\}$ represents the set {Denver, Los Angeles, Reno, Seattle} of four cities and each edge is labeled with the distance between the cities it joins. (A graph whose edges are labeled with nonnegative real numbers is called a ***weighted graph***.) A salesperson who lives in Denver and wants to visit each of the other three cities seeks in this graph a hamiltonian cycle beginning and ending at D such that the sum of the distances is a minimum. There are $3! = 6$ such cycles $(v_1, v_2, v_3, v_4, v_5)$; since each of v_1 and v_5 must be D, there are 3 choices for v_2, there are 2 choices for v_3 (as it cannot be v_1 or v_2), and 1 choice for v_4. Because the sum of distances is the same for a cycle $(v_1, v_2, \dots, v_5)$ as for the reversed cycle $(v_5, v_4, \dots, v_1)$, we only have to consider half of these cycles, as has been done in Table 6.6.1. The table entries show that the minimum occurs for the cycle (D, L, R, S, D) [or its reversed cycle (D, S, R, L, D)].

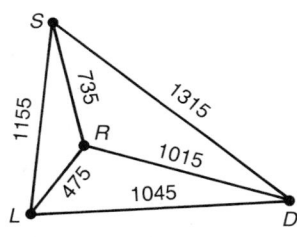

FIGURE 6.6.2

TABLE 6.6.1

cycle	(D, L, R, S, D)	(D, L, S, R, D)	(D, R, L, S, D)
mileage sum	3570	3950	3960

The general problem in which each edge in the complete graph K_n is given a positive real number as its weight (representing distance, cost, or something else) and one seeks a hamiltonian cycle such that the sum of the weights is minimal is called the ***traveling salesperson problem***. The technique we have just used for $n = 4$ would involve $(n - 1)!/2$ cycles. When $n = 11$ this number is 1814400, and when $n = 21$ it is more than $1.2 \times 10^{18} = 1200000000000000000$. Because the numbers $(n - 1)!/2$ grow so rapidly as n increases, the simpleminded technique we have described has been replaced by better algorithms, but there still is no really practical method for exact solution when n is large. Some people are happy with a practical algorithm for finding near-optimal cycles. [For a good survey of the general problem, see M. Bellmore and G. Nemhauser, "The traveling salesman problem," *Operations Research* 16 (1968), 538–558.] □

In some applications it is convenient to partition the set V of vertices into two subsets A and B, as we see in the next example.

Example 2

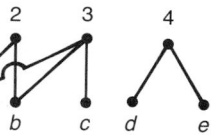

FIGURE 6.6.3

TASK ASSIGNMENT GRAPH   Let $A = \{1, 2, 3, 4\}$ represent a set of four tasks and $B = \{a, b, c, d, e\}$ stand for a set of five people. In the graph $G = (V, E)$ of Figure 6.6.3, $V = A \cup B$ and there is an edge $\{n, x\}$ in E if and only if task n can be performed adequately by person x. The injective mapping f from A to B with

$$f: 1 \mapsto a, \quad 2 \mapsto b, \quad 3 \mapsto c, \quad 4 \mapsto d$$

provides an assignment of people for tasks such that each task can be performed and no person has more than one of these tasks. In Problem 1 below, the reader is asked to give the only other injection from A to B with these properties. The following concept generalizes on this example. □

DEFINITION 2   **BIPARTITE GRAPH**

A graph $G = (V, E)$ is ***bipartite*** with ***parts*** A and B if the sets A and B partition V and every edge in E joins a vertex in A with a vertex in B.

In this definition, $A = \{a_1, a_2, \ldots, a_m\}$ and $B = \{b_1, b_2, \ldots, b_n\}$ are disjoint sets, $V = \{a_1, \ldots, a_m, b_1, \ldots, b_n\}$, and each edge in E is of the form $\{a_i, b_j\}$. It follows that there are at most mn edges; that is, $\#E \le (\#A)(\#B)$. The case in which $\#E = (\#A)(\#B)$ is defined next.

DEFINITION 3   **COMPLETE BIPARTITE GRAPH**

$G = (V, E)$ is a ***complete bipartite graph*** with parts A and B if $V = A \cup B$, $A \cap B = \varnothing$, and E consists of all pairs $\{a, b\}$ with a in A and b in B.

NOTATION 2   **COMPLETE BIPARTITE GRAPH $K_{m,n}$**

$K_{m,n}$ denotes a complete bipartite graph with parts A and B such that $\#A = m$ and $\#B = n$. Customarily, $m \leq n$ in this notation. (Any two such graphs are isomorphic.)

Example 3   Figure 6.6.4 shows three bipartite graphs. The first two of these are the complete bipartite graphs $K_{2,2}$ and $K_{2,3}$. The third graph, G, has parts $A = \{a_1, a_2\}$ and $B = \{b_1, b_2\}$; this graph is not complete because $\{a_2, b_1\}$ is not an edge.

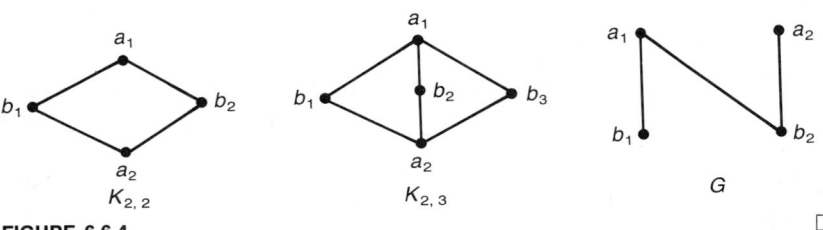

FIGURE 6.6.4

Example 4   **THE UTILITIES GRAPH $K_{3,3}$**   Let the parts for a complete bipartite graph $K_{3,3}$ be a set $A = \{1, 2, 3\}$ representing three homes and a set $B = \{e, g, w\}$ representing three utilities (electricity, gas, and water, for example). The nine edges in a picture for $K_{3,3}$ then stand for the utility lines connecting each of these homes to each of these utilities. Is it possible to draw such a picture in a plane so that no two of these lines intersect at a nonvertex? We now prove that the answer is negative by assuming that the picture can be drawn this way and showing that this assumption leads to a contradiction.

Since the graph is bipartite with $\{1, 2, 3\}$ and $\{e, g, w\}$ as its parts, it follows that $(1, e, 2, g, 1)$ is a path. Clearly, this path is a cycle C. On the basis of the nonintersection assumption, the edge $\{3, w\}$ must be completely inside or completely outside of this cycle. In the case in which $\{3, w\}$ is inside C, the region inside C is cut up into the region inside cycle $(1, e, 3, g, 1)$ and the region inside cycle $(2, e, 3, g, 2)$. In Figure 6.6.5, we show the subcase in which w is inside $(2, e, 3, g, 2)$. In this subcase, there is no way to connect 1 and w without crossing another edge or introducing an edge $\{1, 3\}$ that does not belong in $K_{3,3}$. Each case (and each subcase) leads to a similar contradiction. Thus the answer to our question is "no." This example motivates the following concept.

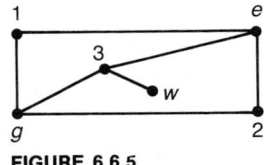

FIGURE 6.6.5

PLANAR GRAPH

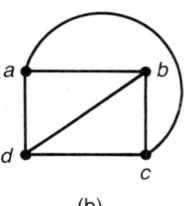

(a)

(b)

FIGURE 6.6.6

A graph $G = (V, E)$ is **planar** if it has a picture in a plane such that no two edges intersect at a nonvertex. Such a picture is a **planar picture** (for G).

The graph in Figure 6.6.6(a) is planar because it can be redrawn as in Figure 6.6.6(b).

One of the applications of planar graphs is to printed circuits in which each layer is represented by a planar graph. Figure 6.6.1 shows that K_n is planar for $n \leq 4$. In Theorem 6 below, it is proved that K_n is not planar when $n \geq 5$. Figure 6.6.4 in Example 3 shows that the complete bipartite graphs $K_{2,2}$ and $K_{2,3}$ are planar. One can easily generalize from these pictures for $K_{2,2}$ and $K_{2,3}$ to see that $K_{2,n}$ is planar for $n \geq 2$. The discussion in Example 4 shows that $K_{3,3}$ is not planar. It is left to the reader in Problems 23, 24, 25, and 26 below to show that $K_{m,n}$ is not planar when $3 \leq m \leq n$.

Example 4 illustrates the usefulness of the following concept.

DEFINITION 5   **FACE IN A PLANAR GRAPH**

Let P be a planar picture for a planar graph G. A **region** in P is a set ρ of points of the plane such that any two points of ρ can be connected by a curve that does not meet any of the vertices or edges drawn in P. A **face** in P is a region ρ for P such that ρ is not a proper part of any other region for P.

For example, the four faces in the picture for the complete graph K_4 in Figure 6.6.1 are the insides of $\triangle ABD$, $\triangle ACD$, and $\triangle BCD$ and the outside of $\triangle ABC$. In the picture for the bipartite graph $K_{2,3}$ in Figure 6.6.4, the three faces are the insides of cycles $(a_1, b_1, a_2, b_2, a_1)$ and $(a_1, b_2, a_2, b_3, a_1)$ and the outside of cycle $(a_1, b_1, a_2, b_3, a_1)$.

DEFINITION 6   **DEGREE OF A FACE**

The **degree** of a face f in a planar picture P is the number $\deg(f)$ of edges in P bounding f.

For example, in the picture for K_4 in Figure 6.6.1, each face has degree 3 because each face is bounded by a triangle. In the picture for $K_{2,3}$ in Figure 6.6.4, each face has degree 4 because each face is bounded by 4 edges.

Example 5

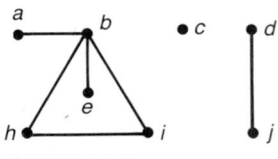

FIGURE 6.6.7

Let $G = (V, E)$ be the planar graph depicted in Figure 6.6.7. This picture has two faces, f_1 and f_2; the face f_1 is the inside of $\triangle bhi$ with edge $\{b, e\}$ removed. Face f_2 is the outside of $\triangle bhi$ with edges $\{a, b\}$ and $\{d, j\}$ and vertex c removed. We see that $\deg(f_1) = 4$, since f_1 is bounded by the 4 edges $\{b, e\}$, $\{b, h\}$, $\{h, i\}$, and $\{i, b\}$. Also, $\deg(f_2) = 5$, since f_2 is bounded by the 5 edges $\{a, b\}$, $\{b, h\}$, $\{h, i\}$ $\{i, b\}$, and $\{d, j\}$. We note that the edges $\{a, b\}$ and $\{d, j\}$ are only in the boundary of face f_2, that $\{b, e\}$ is only in the boundary of f_1, and that each other edge in E is part of the boundary of both faces. $\qquad\square$

THEOREM 2   **EULER'S FORMULA FOR CONNECTED PLANAR GRAPHS**

Let F be the set of faces in a planar picture for a connected graph $G = (V, E)$. Then $\#V - \#E + \#F = 2$ if $\#V > 0$.

PROOF

We give an informal proof that is somewhat inductive. Let us draw a planar picture for G in stages. We start by putting down a dot to represent a vertex v in V. At this stage, the picture has one vertex, no edges, and one face; so Euler's Formula holds. When we introduce a new vertex w, we simultaneously add an edge connecting w to a vertex previously put into the picture. This is possible because G is connected. These additions can be done so that both $\#V$ and $\#E$ increase by one and thus do not change $\#V - \#E + \#F$. When we add an edge $\{x, y\}$ joining two vertices already present in the previous stage, we break a face into two new faces; this increases each of $\#E$ and $\#F$ by one and so does not change $\#V - \#E + \#F$. Using such procedures, we draw a planar picture for G in stages and see that $\#V - \#E + \#F = 2$ in all stages, including the final stage. $\qquad\square$

In the planar picture of Figure 6.6.7, $\#V - \#E + \#F = 8 - 6 + 2 = 4$. This does not contradict Theorem 2 because the graph shown in this picture is not connected.

We now state a generalization of Euler's Formula applying to nonconnected and connected graphs.

THEOREM 3   **GENERALIZED EULER FORMULA FOR PLANAR GRAPHS**

Let a planar graph $G = (V, E)$ have m components and let F be the set of faces in a planar picture for G. Then $\#V - \#E + \#F = 1 + m$.

The proof is left to the reader.

We next obtain inequalities that are helpful in showing that certain graphs are not planar.

THEOREM 4   **INEQUALITIES FOR PLANAR GRAPHS**

Let $G = (V, E)$ be a planar graph with $\#E \geq 2$. Let F be the set of faces in a picture for G. Then

$$\frac{3}{2}(\#F) \leq \#E \leq 3(\#V) - 6. \tag{1}$$

PROOF   Let s be the sum of the degrees of all the faces in F. Each edge in E is in the boundary of at most 2 faces; hence each edge contributes at most 2 to the sum s. Thus

$$s \leq 2(\#E). \tag{2}$$

Now we consider the case in which $\#F > 1$. Then each face f in F must have a cycle in its boundary (to separate f from the other faces). Since a cycle in a graph has length at least 3, it follows that $\deg(f) \geq 3$ for each f in F. This implies that

$$3(\#F) \leq s. \tag{3}$$

Displays (2) and (3) give us the first inequality in Display (1) in the case in which $\#F > 1$. But this inequality obviously also holds when $\#F = 1$, since $\#E \geq 2$. The inequality just proved can be rewritten as

$$\#F \leq \frac{2}{3}(\#E). \tag{4}$$

The Generalized Euler Formula (Theorem 3) implies that

$$2 \leq \#V - \#E + \#F. \tag{5}$$

Displays (4) and (5) give us

$$2 \leq \#V - \#E + \frac{2}{3}(\#E) = \#V - \frac{1}{3}(\#E).$$

Thus $6 \leq 3(\#V) - \#E$, and the second inequality in Display (1) follows.

□

THEOREM 5   **VERTEX WITH LIMITED DEGREE**

In a planar graph $G = (V, E)$, $\mathrm{dg}(v) \leq 5$ for at least one vertex v.

PROOF   We assume that $\mathrm{dg}(v) \geq 6$ for all v in V and seek a contradiction. This assumption implies that the sum t of the degrees of all the vertices in V is at least $6(\#V)$. But $t = 2(\#E)$, since each edge in E contributes 2 to the sum t. These statements imply that $6(\#V) \leq 2(\#E)$, or equivalently, that $3(\#V) \le \#E$. In the case in which $\#E \ge 2$, Theorem 4 then gives us $3(\#V) \le \#E \le 3(\#V) - 6$. The contradiction $3(\#V) \le 3(\#V) - 6$ shows that $\mathrm{dg}(v) \le 5$ for some v in V, in the case in which $\#E \ge 2$. When $\#E \le 1$, we have the stronger result that $\mathrm{dg}(v) \le 1$ for all v in V. ☐

Figure 6.6.1 shows that the complete graphs K_1, K_2, K_3, and K_4 are planar. We are now able to show that a complete graph K_n with $n \ge 5$ is not planar.

THEOREM 6   **NONPLANAR COMPLETE GRAPHS**

K_n is not planar for $n \ge 5$.

PROOF   Let $K_n = (V, E)$. Then $\#V = n$ and $\#E = \binom{n}{2} = n(n-1)/2$. For $n \ge 5$, we have $\#E \ge 2$ and can use Theorem 4. The second inequality in Display (1) of Theorem 4 tells us that K_n, for $n \ge 5$, could only be planar if

$$\frac{n(n-1)}{2} \le 3n - 6.$$

This would imply that $n^2 - n \le 6n - 12$, and so $n^2 - 7n + 12 \le 0$. But the graph of the parabola $y = x^2 - 7x + 12$ shows that $n^2 - 7n + 12 > 0$ for $n \ge 5$. Hence, for each $n \ge 5$, K_n is not planar. ☐

Next we present without proof an interesting result on planar graphs.

THEOREM 7   **FARY'S THEOREM**

A planar graph has a picture in which each edge is represented by a straight-line segment.

This was proved by I. Fary in his paper "On straight-line-representations of planar graphs," *Acta Sci. Math. Szeged*, 11 (1948): 229–233.

PROBLEMS FOR SECTION 6.6

1.   In Example 2, find the injective mapping g from A to B such that $g \ne f$ and $\{n, g(n)\}$ is an edge in Figure 6.6.3 for all tasks n in A.

2.   (a) What are the parts A and B for the bipartite graph of Figure 6.6.3?
     (b) Is the graph of Figure 6.6.3 a complete bipartite graph? Explain.

3. Solve the traveling salesperson problem for the weighted complete graph shown in the figure below. (Start and end at a.)

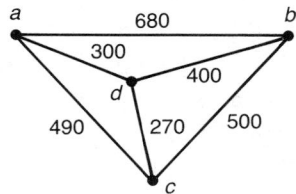

4. Solve the traveling salesperson problem for the graph shown in the figure in the margin. (Start at a).

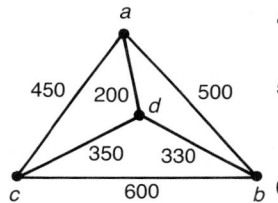

5. (a) How many edges are there in the complete graph K_6?
   (b) How many edges are there in the complete bipartite graph $K_{4,5}$?
   (c) Explain why K_n is connected for each n in Z^+.

6. (a) How many edges are there in K_7?
   (b) How many edges are there in $K_{3,6}$?
   (c) Let v and w be vertices of $K_{m,n}$. Explain why v and w are joined by a path of length at most 2 and hence $K_{m,n}$ is connected for all m and n in Z^+.

7. Let $T = (V, E)$ be a tree with $\#V = n$.
   (i) What is $\#E$?
   (ii) How many faces are there in a planar picture for T?
   (iii) Verify Euler's Formula for T.

8. A *forest* is a graph in which each component is a tree. Does Theorem 3 ("Generalized Euler Formula for Planar Graphs") apply to a forest? Explain.

9. Let $K_3 = (V, E)$ be a complete graph with $V = \{a, b, c\}$. Give all the mappings $f: V \to V$ that are isomorphisms from K_3 onto itself.

10. How many isomorphisms are there from K_4 onto itself?

11. Let $K_{2,2} = (V, E)$ be a complete bipartite graph with parts $A = \{h, k\}$ and $B = \{v, w\}$. Give all the isomorphisms from $K_{2,2}$ onto itself.

12. How many isomorphisms are there from the complete bipartite graph $K_{m,n}$ onto itself? Consider the following two cases:
    (i) $m < n$;   (ii) $m = n$.

13. How many faces are there in a planar picture for a planar connected graph (V, E) with $\#V = 10$ and $\#E = 20$?

14. How many edges are there in a planar picture for a planar connected graph (V, E) with 7 vertices and 7 faces?

15. How many faces are there in a planar picture for a planar graph with 3 components and having $\#V = 17$ and $\#E = 27$?

16. How many vertices are there in a planar picture for a planar graph with 2 components and having 18 faces and 32 edges?

17. Let (V, E) be a connected planar graph. Does there exist a planar graph (V', E') with $\#V' = 3(\#V)$ and $\#E' = 3(\#E)$? Explain.

18. Let (V_1, E_1) and (V_2, E_2) be planar graphs. Does there exist a planar graph (V, E) with $\#V = \#V_1 + \#V_2$ and $\#E = \#E_1 + \#E_2$? Explain.

19. Let F be the set of faces in a picture for a planar graph $G = (V, E)$. Let s be the sum of the degrees of the faces of F. If $\deg(f) \geq 4$ for some f in F, is $3(\#F) < s$? Explain.

20. Let (V, E) and s be as in Problem 19. If some edge in E is part of the boundary of only one face, is $s < 2(\#E)$? Explain.

21. Explain why the length of a cycle in a bipartite graph must be an even integer.

22. Let $G = (V, E)$, F, and s be as in Problem 19. Explain why $4(\#F) \leq s$ if G is bipartite.

23. Explain why a subgraph of a planar graph is also planar.

24. Let G_1 be a subgraph of G. If G_1 is not planar, can G be planar? Explain.

25. Is $K_{3,4}$ planar? Explain.

26. Let $3 \leq m \leq n$. Is $K_{m,n}$ planar? Explain.

27. Let $G = (V, E)$ be a planar graph with $\#E = 24$.
(a) Can a planar picture for G have 17 faces? Explain.
(b) Can $\#V = 9$? Explain.

28. Let $G = (V, E)$ be a planar graph with $\#V = 15$.
(a) Can $\#E = 40$? Explain.
(b) Can a planar picture for G have 12 faces? Explain.

29. Let F be the set of faces in a picture for a planar graph $G = (V, E)$. Show that $\#F \leq 2(\#V) - 4$.

30. Let $T = [V, E, r]$ be a rooted tree and $G = (V, E^*)$ be the graph underlying T. Let A consist of the vertices v in V such that the level of v in T is an even integer and let B be the complement of A in V. Show that G is a bipartite graph with A and B as parts.

SUMMARY OF TERMS, CHAPTER 6 _____

Adjacency matrix for (V, E)	The matrix for the binary relation R on V in which vRw if and only if $\{v, w\} \in E$.	325
Binary tree	A 2-ary rooted tree in which each child is specified as the left child or right child.	302

Bipartite graph with parts A and B	A graph $G = (V, E)$ in which $\{A, B\}$ is a partition of V and each edge joins some a in A to some b in B.	337
Catalan Numbers	See Problem 24 of Section 6.3.	318
Characterizations of trees	See Definition 6, Theorem 2, and Theorem 3 of Section 6.5.	329–331
Child c of p	A vertex c in a rooted tree $[V, E, r]$ such that pEc.	302
Circuit	A path $(v_0, v_1, \ldots, v_s)$ with $v_0 = v_s$ and $s > 0$.	296, 326
Complementary subdigraphs	Two subdigraphs evoked by sets partitioning the edges.	319
Complete bipartite graph $K_{m,n}$	Bipartite graph with parts A and B, $\#A = m$, $\#B = n$, and an edge $\{a, b\}$ for every a in A and b in B.	337
Complete graph K_n	Graph (V, E) with $\#V = n$ and an edge $\{v, w\}$ for each v and w in V.	335
Component containing a given vertex u	The subgraph induced by the set U of vertices v having a path from u.	328
Component of a graph	See Definition 4 of Section 6.5.	328
Connected graph	A graph in which there is a path between any two vertices.	327
Converting an MRPE	See Algorithm 1 of Section 6.3.	313
Cycle	A path $(v_0, v_1, \ldots, v_s)$ with $v_0 = v_s$ as the only repetition and $s \geq 3$.	296, 326
Decision tree	See Example 7 of Section 6.3.	315
Degree $dg(v)$ of a vertex v in (V, E)	The number of vertices w such that $\{v, w\}$ is in E.	326
Degree of a face F	The number of edges bounding F.	339
Digraph	$\langle V, E \rangle$, with E a binary relation on V.	293
Directed path	A path in a digraph.	294
Division Algorithm	See Example 5 of Section 6.1.	297
Edge of a digraph $\langle V, E \rangle$	An ordered pair (v, w) in E.	293
Edge of a graph (V, E)	A pair $\{v, w\}$ in E.	326
Elementary path	A path with no vertex repeated.	295, 326
Endpoints	The vertices of an edge.	326
Eulerian circuit	A circuit using each edge once.	296, 326
Eulerian path	A path using each edge once.	295, 326
Euler's Formulas	See Theorems 2 and 3 of Section 6.6.	340
Evoked subdigraph	See Definition 3 of Section 6.4.	319
Evoked subgraph	See the analogues in Section 6.5 for graphs of definitions previously given for digraphs.	327
Face	See Definition 5 of Section 6.6.	339
Fary's Theorem	Each edge of a planar picture can be straight.	342
File	A finite collection of records.	314
Final vertex	The v_s of a path $(v_0, v_1, \ldots, v_s)$ in a digraph.	294
Flowchart	See Example 5 of Section 6.1.	297
Forest	A graph whose components are trees.	331, 343
Generalized Euler Formula	See Theorem 3 of Section 6.6.	340

REVIEW PROBLEMS FOR CHAPTER 6 _____

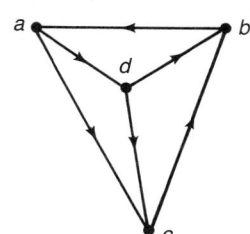

1. Do the following for the digraph depicted in the margin.
   (a) Show the indegree and outdegree for each vertex (in a table).
   (b) Give the digraph matrix.

2. Do the following for the digraph shown in Problem 1.
   (a) Find a hamiltonian path of length 3 from d to a.
   (b) Find a simple path of length 5 from d to b.

3. Does the digraph shown in Problem 1 have a hamiltonian cycle?

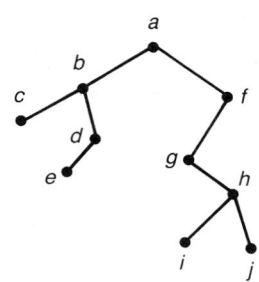

4. Does the digraph shown in Problem 1 have an eulerian circuit?

5. For the binary tree shown in the margin, give the following listings of the vertices:
(a) preorder,　　(b) inorder,　　(c) postorder.

6. Do the following for the rooted tree shown in Problem 5.
(a) Show the level of each vertex (in a table).
(b) What is the height of this tree?
(c) Which vertices are leaves?

7. (a) Draw a picture for a binary tree having eleven vertices of which five have level 3.
(b) What is the maximum number of vertices having level n in a binary tree?

8. (a) What is the maximum number of vertices of an n-ary tree of height h?
(b) What is the sum of the levels of all the vertices of the tree of Part (a)?

9. Let $[V, E, r]$ be a rooted tree with $V = \{v_1, v_2, \ldots, v_{100}\}$. Find:
(a) $\text{indg}(v_1) + \text{indg}(v_2) + \cdots + \text{indg}(v_{100})$.
(b) $\text{outdg}(v_1) + \text{outdg}(v_2) + \cdots + \text{outdg}(v_{100})$.

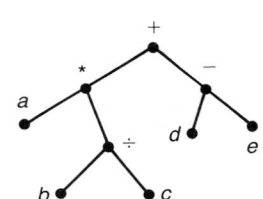

10. Write the algebraic expression represented by the accompanying figure.

11. Make a binary tree that represents the expression $((a + b) - c) \div (d * e)$.

12. Give the reverse Polish notation for the expression in Problem 11.

13. Let $X = \{a, b, c, d, \ldots\}$ and $B = \{+, -, *, \div, \ldots\}$.
(a) Is $ab + *cd\div$ an MRPE over $X \cup B$? Explain.
(b) Is $abc + d - *$ an MRPE over $X \cup B$? Explain.

14. Evaluate the MRPE $abcd \div e - + +$ for $a = 2, b = 3, c = 4, d = 5, e = 6$.

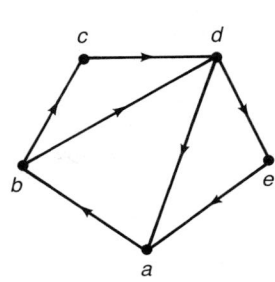

15. Do the following for the digraph D shown in the margin.
(a) Give the E_1 for the subdigraph $\langle V_1, E_1 \rangle$ induced by $V_1 = \{a, b, d, e\}$.
(b) Give the V_2 for the subdigraph $\langle V_2, E_2 \rangle$ evoked by $E_2 = \{(b, c), (b, d), (d, a), (e, a)\}$.
(c) Find a spanning subdigraph $\langle V_3, E_3 \rangle$ in which $\#E_3 = 4$ and (a, b, c, d, e) is a path.

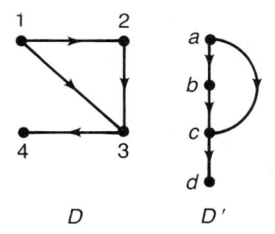

16. (i) Give the relation matrices for the digraphs D and D' shown here.
(ii) Are these digraphs isomorphic? Explain.

17. Let $V = \{a, b, c, d, e\}$ and let β be the permutation on V given by

$$\beta: a \mapsto d, \quad b \mapsto a, \quad c \mapsto e, \quad d \mapsto b, \quad e \mapsto c.$$

(i) Give the ordered pairs of the relation R_β for β.
(ii) Draw a picture of the digraph D_β for β.

18. Draw nonisomorphic graphs G and G', each having 4 vertices and 2 components.

19. Draw graphs G, G', and G'' such that no two are isomorphic and each has 5 vertices and 3 components.

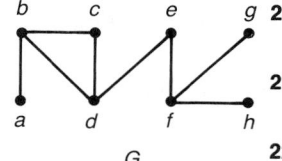

G

20. For the accompanying graph G, give a set of three edges such that the removal of any one of these edges from G results in a connected graph.

21. A *spanning tree* of a graph G is a spanning subgraph T of G such that T is a tree. Describe three spanning trees for the graph G shown in Problem 20.

22. Consider the rooted tree shown in Problem 5 to be a picture for a tree $T = (V, E)$. Draw a picture for a rooted tree $T^* = [V, E^*, g]$ with g as its root and such that T is the underlying graph for T^*.

23. How many isomorphisms are there from:
    (a) the complete graph K_7 to itself?
    (b) the complete bipartite graph $K_{8,9}$ to itself?
    (c) the complete bipartite graph $K_{10,10}$ to itself?

24. Let $G = (V, E)$ be a graph and let R denote the binary relation on V in which vRw means that there is a path between v and w.
    (i) Show that R is an equivalence relation. [Note that (v) is a path between v and itself.]
    (ii) What are the equivalence classes for R, that is, the sets $C(x) = \{y : xRy\}$?

25. Let G and G' be isomorphic graphs.
    (a) If G is connected, must G' be connected?
    (b) Must G and G' have the same number of components?

26. Can a planar graph have 10 vertices and 25 edges? Explain.

27. Can a planar picture for a graph have 30 vertices and 17 faces? Explain.

28. For each of the following assertions, tell whether it is true (T) or false (F):
    (a) If a path is hamiltonian, it is elementary.
    (b) If a path is elementary, it is simple.
    (c) A path in $\langle V, E \rangle$ is eulerian whenever it contains all the edges in E.
    (d) Every circuit is a cycle.
    (e) Every cycle is a circuit.
    (f) Every hamiltonian cycle is simple.
    (g) If a graph is connected, it has exactly one component.
    (h) Every tree is connected.
    (i) Every connected graph is a tree.
    (j) If H is a component of a graph G, then H is connected.
    (k) The complete graph K_n is connected for every n in $\mathbf{Z}^+$.
    (l) The complete bipartite graph $K_{m,n}$ is connected for all m and n in $\mathbf{Z}^+$.
    (m) Every connected bipartite graph is a complete graph.

SUPPLEMENTARY AND CHALLENGING PROBLEMS, CHAPTER 6 _____

1.   Prove that a connected digraph has an eulerian path if it has exactly one vertex x with $\text{outdg}(x) = 1 + \text{indg}(x)$ and has exactly one vertex y with $\text{indg}(y) = 1 + \text{outdg}(y)$.

2.   Prove that a digraph does not have an eulerian path if any one of the following is true:
     (a) There are two or more vertices x with $\text{outdg}(x) = 1 + \text{indg}(x)$.
     (b) There is a vertex x with $\text{outdg}(x) > 1 + \text{indg}(x)$.
     (c) There are two or more vertices y with $\text{indg}(y) = 1 + \text{outdg}(y)$
     (d) There is a vertex y with $\text{indg}(y) > 1 + \text{outdg}(y)$.

3.   The "rotating drum" relation R_n on the set B_n of n-bit strings is the binary relation R in which $a_1 a_2 \ldots a_n R b_1 b_2 \ldots b_n$ means that $a_2 a_3 \ldots a_n = b_1 b_2 \ldots b_{n-1}$.
     (a) Find a hamiltonian circuit in the digraph $\langle B_3, R_3 \rangle$.
     (b) Prove that $\langle B_n, R_n \rangle$ has a hamiltonian circuit for $n \geq 2$.

4.   Let $(x_0, x_1, \ldots, x_s)$ be a path in a rooted tree. Prove that $x_i \neq x_j$ for $i \neq j$.

5.   Let $T = [V, E, r]$ be a rooted tree with $\#V = n > 1$. Explain why the following are true.
     (i) There is a vertex f in V whose level is at least as large as the level of every other vertex in V.
     (ii) The f of Part (i) is a leaf.
     (iii) Let pEf, V' be V with f deleted, and E' be E with (p, f) deleted. Then $T' = [V', E', r]$ is a rooted tree with $\#V' = n - 1$ and $\#E' = \#E - 1$.

6.   Prove that for each vertex v in a tree $T = (V, E)$ there is a rooted tree $T^* = [V, E^*, v]$ with v as its root and with T underlying T^*.

7.   Prove that every connected graph G has a spanning subgraph that is a tree.

8.   Prove that a finite graph G is a tree if and only if it is connected and has no cycles.

9.   Prove that a connected graph has an eulerian path if and only if the number of vertices with odd degree is 0 or 2.

10. Prove that a connected graph has an eulerian circuit if and only if each vertex has even degree.

7

GROUPS

In Sections 2.1 and 2.2, we studied semigroups, a type of algebraic structure that arises frequently in computer-related fields. Special attention was given to monoids, that is, semigroups having identities. Here we specialize further by considering monoids in which each element of the carrier has an inverse; such a monoid is called a *group*.

Groups are involved in the study of systems of numbers, vectors, matrices, and so on. Among the disciplines in which group theory is applied are coding, combinatorics, mathematical physics, chemistry, and, not least, the art of M. C. Escher.

7.1

BASIC PROPERTIES OF GROUPS AND SUBGROUPS

We recall from Section 2.2 that a monoid is an algebraic structure $[X, \Box, e]$ in which $\Box$ is an associative binary operation on the carrier X and e is the identity under $\Box$. Let $Z = \{\ldots, -2, -1, 0, 1, 2, \ldots\}$ and Q^+ be the set of positive rational numbers. Then each of $[Z, +, 0]$ and $[Q^+, \cdot, 1]$ is a monoid with the additional property that each element of the carrier has an inverse under the respective operation. The same is true of the "bitwise modulo 2 addition" monoids $[B_n, \oplus, 0_n]$, which will be applied to coding theory in Chapter 11. The following definition helps us study simultaneously all the structures that have these properties.

DEFINITION 1 **GROUP**

A *group* is a monoid $G = [X, \Box, e]$ in which each element of the carrier has an inverse under $\Box$; that is, for every x in X there is an x^{-1} in X such that $x \Box x^{-1} = e = x^{-1} \Box x$. We use the notation $G = \langle X, \Box, e \rangle$ to indicate that this G is a group.

Thus $\langle \mathbf{Z}, +, 0 \rangle$ and $\langle \mathbf{Q}^+, \cdot, 1 \rangle$ are groups. The monoid $[\mathbf{Z}^+, +, 0]$ is not a group; for example, the element 1 of $\mathbf{Z}^+$ does not have an inverse under $+$ in $\mathbf{Z}^+$. Similarly, the monoid $[\mathbf{Z}^+, \cdot, 1]$ is not a group because the number 2 in $\mathbf{Z}^+$ does not have an inverse under multiplication in $\mathbf{Z}^+$.

Since a group is a special kind of monoid, any property that is possessed by all monoids is automatically possessed by all groups. For example, it follows from Theorem 1 of Section 2.1 that the identity in a group is unique. Other examples are contained in the following result.

THEOREM 1   **UNIQUE INVERSE, INVERSE OF THE INVERSE**

Let $G = \langle X, \square, e \rangle$ be a group. Let a and h be in X.

(a) If either $a \,\square\, h = e$ or $h \,\square\, a = e$, then $h = a^{-1}$.
(b) Also, $(x^{-1})^{-1} = x$ for all x in X.

PROOF   (a) By definition of inverse,

$$a \,\square\, a^{-1} = e = a^{-1} \,\square\, a. \tag{1}$$

With the help of Theorem 2 of Section 2.1 ("Uniqueness of the Inverse") concerning monoids and Display (1), one sees that either $a \,\square\, h = e$ or $h \,\square\, a = e$ implies that $h = a^{-1}$. This proves Part (a).

(b) One of the things we have just noted is that

$$[a \,\square\, h = e] \qquad \text{implies} \qquad [h = a^{-1}].$$

Replacing a by x^{-1} and h by x, this becomes

$$[x^{-1} \,\square\, x = e] \qquad \text{implies} \qquad [x = (x^{-1})^{-1}].$$

Since $x^{-1} \,\square\, x = e$ for all x in X, it follows that $x = (x^{-1})^{-1}$ for all x in X. This proves Part (b). $\square$

The following is a definition of group that does not refer back to the definition of monoid.

DEFINITION 1′   **ALTERNATE DEFINITION OF GROUP**

A *group* is an ordered triple $G = \langle X, \square, e \rangle$ in which $\square$ is a binary operation on X and G has the following three properties:

Associativity $x \,\square\, (y \,\square\, z) = (x \,\square\, y) \,\square\, z$ for all x, y, z in X.

Identity $e \in X$ and $e \,\square\, x = x = x \,\square\, e$ for all x in X.

Inverses   For each x in X there is an x^{-1} in X such that $x \,\square\, x^{-1} = e = x^{-1} \,\square\, x$.

Example 1 Let $U_4 = \{1, \mathbf{i}, -1, -\mathbf{i}\}$, where $\mathbf{i}$ and $-\mathbf{i}$ are the complex roots of the equation $z^2 = -1$. Table 7.1.1 shows that U_4 is closed under multiplication and hence that $\cdot$ is a binary operation on U_4. Since the first row is the same as the column labels and the first column is the same as the row labels in this table, we see that 1 is the identity under multiplication. Table 7.1.2, which can be obtained using Table 7.1.1, shows that each number z in U_4 has a multiplicative inverse z^{-1} in U_4. We assume it to be known that multiplication of complex numbers is associative and commutative. Thus $\langle U_4, \cdot, 1 \rangle$ is a group whose operation is commutative. We can easily see that U_4 consists of the four fourth roots of unity, that is, of the four roots of the equation $z^4 = 1$, which is equivalent to $z^4 - 1 = 0$ or to $(z^2 - 1)(z^2 + 1) = 0$.

TABLE 7.1.1

$\cdot$	1	$\mathbf{i}$	-1	$-\mathbf{i}$
1	1	$\mathbf{i}$	-1	$-\mathbf{i}$
$\mathbf{i}$	$\mathbf{i}$	-1	$-\mathbf{i}$	1
-1	-1	$-\mathbf{i}$	1	$\mathbf{i}$
$-\mathbf{i}$	$-\mathbf{i}$	1	$\mathbf{i}$	-1

TABLE 7.1.2

z	1	$\mathbf{i}$	-1	$-\mathbf{i}$
z^{-1}	1	$-\mathbf{i}$	-1	$\mathbf{i}$

$\square$

DEFINITION 2 **ABELIAN (OR COMMUTATIVE) GROUP**

A group $G = \langle X, \square, e \rangle$ is *abelian* (or *commutative*) if the operation $\square$ is commutative, that is, if $x \square y = y \square x$ for all x and y in X.

The group $\langle U_4, \cdot, 1 \rangle$ in Example 1 is an abelian group with a finite carrier. The groups $\langle \mathbf{Z}, +, 0 \rangle$ and $\langle \mathbf{Q}^+, \cdot, 1 \rangle$ are abelian groups with infinite carriers. An infinite sequence of nonabelian groups will be introduced in Section 7.2. One such group is presented in Example 6 of this section. In mathematics, the $+$ symbol is used for the operation of a group only when the group is abelian; also, in such a group the identity is usually denoted by 0 and the inverse of x under $+$ is written as $-x$ and is called the *negative* of x or the *additive inverse* of x.

NOTATION 1 **ADDITIVE GROUP**

An *additive group* is an abelian group $\langle X, +, 0 \rangle$ in which $+$ denotes the operation, 0 is the identity under $+$, and $-x$ is the inverse of x under $+$.

Thus $\langle \mathbf{Z}, +, 0 \rangle$ is an additive group.

Example 2

Let $\oplus$ be the binary operation of "bitwise addition modulo 2" on the set B_n of n-bit strings; that is, for $\alpha = a_1a_2\ldots a_n$ and $\beta = b_1b_2\ldots b_n$ in B_n let $\alpha \oplus \beta = c_1c_2\ldots c_n$, where $c_i = 0$ if $a_i = b_i$ and $c_i = 1$ if $a_i \neq b_i$. Also let 0_n be the string $00\ldots 0$ of weight zero in B_n. We saw in Example 7 of Section 2.2 that $[B_n, \oplus, 0_n]$ is a commutative monoid such that each string α in B_n is its own inverse under $\oplus$. It follows that $\langle B_n, \oplus, 0_n \rangle$ is an abelian (that is, commutative) group in which $\alpha \oplus \alpha = 0_n$ for each α in B_n. In the case of $n = 2$, the operation table for $\langle B_2, \oplus, 0_2 \rangle$ is Table 7.1.3. □

TABLE 7.1.3   Operation Table for $\langle B_2, \oplus, 0_2 \rangle$

$\oplus$	00	01	10	11
00	00	01	10	11
01	01	00	11	10
10	10	11	00	01
11	11	10	01	00

In Example 1, the carrier U_4 of the group has four elements and z^4 is the identity for each z in U_4. We will generalize on this when we see in Section 7.5 below that $x^m = e$ for all x in X when $\langle X, \square, e \rangle$ is a group with $\#X = m$. Thus the number of elements in the carrier can provide information concerning the group.

DEFINITION 3   **ORDER OF A GROUP**

Let $G = \langle X, \square, e \rangle$ be a group. If X is finite, G is a **finite group** and the **order** of G is $\#X$ and is denoted ord G. If X is infinite, G is an **infinite group** or a group of **infinite order**.

For example, the group $\langle U_4, \cdot, 1 \rangle$ of Example 1 has order 4 since $\#U_4 = 4$; the group $\langle B_n, \oplus, 0_n \rangle$ of Example 2 has order $\#B_n = 2^n$; and the group $\langle Z, +, 0 \rangle$ has infinite order.

THEOREM 2   **SUBSETS OF THE CARRIER**

Let $G = \langle X, \square, e \rangle$ be a group. In the carrier X, let Y be a subset closed under $\square$. Let $e \in Y$. Also, let $y^{-1} \in Y$ for each y in Y. Then $\langle Y, \square, e \rangle$ is a group.

PROOF

By Theorem 1 of Section 2.2, $(Y, \square)$ is a semigroup. Since $x \square e = x = e \square x$ for all x in X and $Y \subseteq X$, one has $y \square e = y = e \square y$ for all y in Y. As $e \in Y$, this means that e is the identity for this semigroup, and so $[Y, \square, e]$ is a monoid. This monoid is a group $\langle Y, \square, e \rangle$ because $y^{-1} \in Y$ for each $y \in Y$; that is, the inverse y^{-1} in X serves as an inverse in Y. □

We now introduce terminology for the relationship between the groups $\langle Y, \square, e \rangle$ and $\langle X, \square, e \rangle$ of Theorem 2.

DEFINITION 4 SUBGROUP IN A GROUP

Let $G = \langle X, \square, e \rangle$ be a group. Let $Y \subseteq X$, Y be closed under $\square$, $e \in Y$, and $y^{-1} \in Y$ for each $y \in Y$. Then the group $H = \langle Y, \square, e \rangle$ is a *subgroup* in G. If Y is a proper subset of X, H is said to be a *proper subgroup* in G.

Example 3 Here we find all the subgroups $H = \langle Y, \cdot, 1 \rangle$ in the group $G = \langle U_4, \cdot, 1 \rangle$ of Example 1. To do this, we find the subsets Y of the carrier $U_4 = \{1, \mathbf{i}, -1, -\mathbf{i}\}$ such that simultaneously $1 \in Y$, Y is closed under multiplication, and $y^{-1} \in Y$ whenever $y \in Y$. First we note that if $\mathbf{i}$ is in such a subset Y, then Y must be U_4, since

$$\mathbf{i} \cdot \mathbf{i} = -1, \qquad -1 \cdot \mathbf{i} = -\mathbf{i}, \qquad \text{and} \qquad \mathbf{i}^4 = \mathbf{i}^2 \cdot \mathbf{i}^2 = (-1)^2 = 1$$

have to be in Y by closure under the operation. Similarly, we see that the only such subset Y with $-\mathbf{i} \in Y$ is $Y = U_4$. Now we can conclude that the only possibilities for Y are U_4 itself and the subsets $\{1\}$ and $\{1, -1\}$ of U_4 that include 1 but do not include $\mathbf{i}$ or $-\mathbf{i}$. Let

$$\Gamma = \{\{1\}, \{1, -1\}, \{1, \mathbf{i}, -1, -\mathbf{i}\}\}.$$

Using Table 7.1.1 in Example 1, one can see that each Y in Γ is closed under multiplication. Also, the identity 1 is in each Y. Finally, one finds that $y^{-1} \in Y$ whenever $y \in Y$ for each Y in Γ by noting that each of 1 and -1 is its own inverse whereas $\mathbf{i}$ and $-\mathbf{i}$ are inverses of each other. Thus we have shown that $\langle Y, \cdot, 1 \rangle$ is a subgroup in G if and only if Y is a member of Γ. $\square$

THEOREM 3 TRIVIAL SUBGROUP, IMPROPER SUBGROUP

Let $G = \langle X, \square, e \rangle$ be a group. Then $E = \langle \{e\}, \square, e \rangle$ and G itself are subgroups in G. (One calls E the *trivial subgroup* and G the *improper subgroup* in G.)

PROOF Each of the subsets $\{e\}$ and X of X has all the properties required of Y in Definition 4 for $\langle Y, \square, e \rangle$ to be a subgroup in G. $\square$

Of the three subgroups of $G = \langle U_4, \cdot, 1 \rangle$ found in Example 3, one is the trivial subgroup $\langle \{1\}, \cdot, 1 \rangle$, the second is a proper subgroup $\langle \{1, -1\}, \cdot, 1 \rangle$, and the third is the improper subgroup G itself.

If X is any set, the inclusion relation $\subseteq$ is a partial ordering on its power set $P(X)$; that is, $(P(X), \subseteq)$ is a poset. In fact, if Γ is any subcollection of $P(X)$, that is, any collection of subsets of X, then $(\Gamma, \subseteq)$ is a poset. (See Problem 11 of Section 1.6.)

DEFINITION 5   **SUBGROUP POSET FOR A GROUP**

Let $G = \langle X, \square, e \rangle$ be a group and Γ be the collection of the carriers of all the subgroups in G. Then $(\Gamma, \subseteq)$ is called the **subgroup poset** for G. Also, a poset diagram for $(\Gamma, \subseteq)$ is a **subgroup poset diagram** for G.

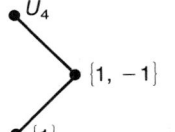

U_4

$\{1, -1\}$

$\{1\}$

FIGURE 7.1.1

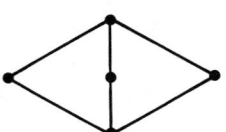

FIGURE 7.1.2

It follows from the work in Example 3 that the subgroup poset for $G = \langle U_4, \cdot, 1 \rangle$ is $(\Gamma, \subseteq)$, where

$$\Gamma = \{\{1\}, \{1, -1\}, \{1, \mathbf{i}, -1, -\mathbf{i}\}\}.$$

Figure 7.1.1 is a subgroup poset diagram for this G. The figure shows that this poset is linearly ordered; that is, here $(\Gamma, \subseteq)$ is a chain.

In Problem 18 below, the reader is asked to show that the subgroup poset diagram for $\langle B_2, \oplus, 0_2 \rangle$ is Figure 7.1.2.

A group $G = \langle X, \square, e \rangle$ is a special kind of semigroup; therefore powers a^n are defined for each a in X and each n in $\mathbf{Z}^+ = \{1, 2, \ldots\}$ as in Definition 3 of Section 2.2. That is, $a^1 = a$, $a^2 = a \square a$, $a^3 = a^2 \square a = a \square a \square a$, and so on. For each a in the carrier X of a group, we next define a^n when the exponent n is 0 or a negative integer. We also give the notation for the set of all integral powers of a and terminology for the number of distinct integral powers of a.

DEFINITION 6   **SET $[a]$ OF ALL INTEGRAL POWERS OF a, ORDER OF a**

Let $\langle X, \square, e \rangle$ be a group and $a \in X$. Then $a^0 = e$ and $a^{-n} = (a^n)^{-1}$ for n in $\mathbf{Z}^+$. Also, $[a]$ is a notation for the set $\{a^n : n \in \mathbf{Z}\}$ of all integral powers of a. The **order** of a is the number of distinct integral powers of a, that is, the order of a is $\#[a]$.

Note that the order of a equals the order of the cyclic subgroup $\langle [a], \square, e \rangle$ generated by a. For example, in the group $\langle Q^+, \cdot, 1 \rangle$, in which Q^+ is the set of positive rational numbers, one has

$$[2] = \{\ldots, 2^{-2}, 2^{-1}, 2^0, 2^1, 2^2, \ldots\} = \{\ldots, \tfrac{1}{4}, \tfrac{1}{2}, 1, 2, 4, \ldots\},$$

$$[\tfrac{1}{3}] = \{\ldots, (\tfrac{1}{3})^{-2}, (\tfrac{1}{3})^{-1}, (\tfrac{1}{3})^0, (\tfrac{1}{3})^1, (\tfrac{1}{3})^2, \ldots\}$$

$$= \{\ldots, 9, 3, 1, \tfrac{1}{3}, \tfrac{1}{9}, \ldots\}.$$

Thus we see that each of the numbers 2 and $\tfrac{1}{3}$ has infinite order in $\langle Q^+, \cdot, 1 \rangle$. In this group, $[-1] = \{1, -1\}$ since $(-1)^n = 1$ for even integers n and $(-1)^n = -1$ for odd n; hence the order of -1 is $\#[-1] = 2$.

In all groups $\langle X, \square, e \rangle$, we have $e^n = e$ for all integers n and hence $[e]$ is the singleton $\{e\}$. Since $\#[e] = 1$, the order of the identity is always 1.

NOTATION 2   **POWERS IN AN ADDITIVE GROUP**

In an additive group $\langle X, +, 0 \rangle$, the notation x^n for an integral power is customarily replaced by $n \cdot x$; however, the set $\{n \cdot x : n \in \mathbf{Z}\}$ of all (additively written) integral powers of x is still denoted as $[x]$.

Thus, in an additive group $\langle X, +, 0 \rangle$, the set $[x]$ consists of the distinct elements among the (additive) integral powers

$$\dots, (-2) \cdot x, (-1) \cdot x, 0 \cdot x, 1 \cdot x, 2 \cdot x, 3 \cdot x, \dots,$$

where $0 \cdot x = 0$, $1 \cdot x = x$, $2 \cdot x = x + x$, $3 \cdot x = x + x + x$, and so on. Also, $(-1)x$ is the additive inverse $-x$ of x, $(-2) \cdot x = -(2 \cdot x) = -(x + x)$, and so on.

In the additive group $\langle \mathbf{Z}, +, 0 \rangle$, this notation is consistent with the notation $n \cdot x = nx$ for integral multiples of x because, when $n > 0$, the sum $x + x + \cdots + x$ of n terms each equal to x is n times x. In this group $\langle \mathbf{Z}, +, 0 \rangle$,

$$[3] = \{n \cdot 3 : n \in \mathbf{Z}\} = \{\dots, (-1) \cdot 3, 0 \cdot 3, 1 \cdot 3, 2 \cdot 3, \dots\}$$
$$= \{\dots, -3, 0, 3, 6, \dots\}.$$

Also, $[-3] = [3]$ because

$$[-3] = \{n \cdot (-3) : n \in \mathbf{Z}\}$$
$$= \{\dots, (-2) \cdot (-3), (-1) \cdot (-3), 0 \cdot (-3), 1 \cdot (-3), 2 \cdot (-3), \dots\}$$
$$= \{\dots, 6, 3, 0, -3, -6, \dots\}.$$

Hence each of 3 and -3 has infinite order in $\langle \mathbf{Z}, +, 0 \rangle$.

We can consider the abelian groups $\langle \mathbf{B}_n, \oplus, 0_n \rangle$ of Example 2 to be additive groups since $\oplus$ and 0_n are modifications of $+$ and 0. Then in $\langle \mathbf{B}_2, \oplus, 0_2 \rangle$, one has

$$0 \cdot 01 = 0_2 = 00,$$
$$1 \cdot 01 = 01,$$
$$2 \cdot 01 = 01 \oplus 01 = 00,$$
$$3 \cdot 01 = 2 \cdot 01 \oplus 01 = 00 \oplus 01 = 01,$$
$$(-1) \cdot 01 = -01 = 01.$$

These cases suggest that $n \cdot 01 = 00$ when n is an even integer and $n \cdot 01 = 01$ when n is odd. This is easily proved by mathematical induction. Hence the set $[01]$ of all integral powers of 01 is $\{00, 01\}$ and the string 01 has order 2.

THEOREM 4   **[a] ⊆ X FOR EACH a ∈ X**

Let $\langle X, \Box, e \rangle$ be a group and let $a \in X$. Then $[a]$ is a subset of X.

PROOF   The positive integral powers $a^1 = a$, $a^2 = a \,\Box\, a$, $a^3 = a^2 \,\Box\, a, \ldots$ are in X by the hypothesis that $a \in X$ and the fact that the carrier X is closed under $\Box$. Also, $a^0 = e$ is in X and the negative powers $a^{-n} = (a^n)^{-1}$ are in X, since X contains the inverses of all of its elements.   □

We next show that $[a]$ is the carrier of a subgroup for each a in X.

THEOREM 5   **SUBGROUP OF INTEGRAL POWERS**

Let $G = \langle X, \Box, e \rangle$ be a group and let $a \in X$. Then $\langle [a], \Box, e \rangle$ is a subgroup in G.

PROOF $[a]$ consists of the distinct elements among the integral powers

$$\ldots, a^{-2}, a^{-1}, e, a, a^2, a^3, \ldots.$$

We show that $[a]$ is closed under $\Box$ as follows: If x and y are in $[a]$, then $x = a^r$ and $y = a^s$, with r and s integers. Thus $x \,\Box\, y = a^r \,\Box\, a^s = a^{r+s}$, with $r + s$ an integer, and $[a]$ is closed under $\Box$. Also, $e = a^0$ is in $[a]$. Finally, if $y = a^s$ is in $[a]$, then $y^{-1} = (a^s)^{-1} = a^{-s}$, with $-s$ an integer. Hence y^{-1} is in $[a]$ for every y in $[a]$. Now Theorem 2 tells us that $\langle [a], \Box, e \rangle$ is a group and Definition 4 tells us that $\langle [a], \Box, e \rangle$ is a subgroup in G.   □

DEFINITION 7   **CYCLIC SUBGROUP GENERATED BY a, CYCLIC GROUP**

Let $G = \langle X, \Box, e \rangle$ be a group and let $a \in X$. The subgroup $\langle [a], \Box, e \rangle$ described in Theorem 5 is called the **(cyclic) subgroup generated** by a. If there exists an element g of X such that $[g] = X$, then G is a **cyclic group** and g is a **generator** of G.

Example 4   As in Examples 1 and 3, let $G = \langle U_4, \cdot, 1 \rangle$ with $U_4 = \{1, \mathbf{i}, -1, -\mathbf{i}\}$. We note that

$$\mathbf{i}^1 = \mathbf{i}, \quad \mathbf{i}^2 = -1, \quad \mathbf{i}^3 = \mathbf{i}^2 \mathbf{i} = -\mathbf{i}, \quad \text{and} \quad \mathbf{i}^4 = \mathbf{i}^2 \mathbf{i}^2 = (-1)(-1) = 1,$$

and thus see that $U_4 = \{1, \mathbf{i}, -1, -\mathbf{i}\} \subseteq [\mathbf{i}]$. But $[\mathbf{i}] \subseteq U_4$ by Theorem 4. Hence $[\mathbf{i}] = U_4$, $\#[\mathbf{i}] = 4$, and $\mathbf{i}$ has order 4. Since $[\mathbf{i}]$ is the entire carrier U_4, the group G is cyclic with $\mathbf{i}$ as a generator. Similarly we find that $[-\mathbf{i}] = U_4$; thus $-\mathbf{i}$ also is a generator of G.

Clearly, $[1]$ is the singleton $\{1\}$. Hence 1 has order 1 and the (cyclic) subgroup generated by 1 is the trivial subgroup $\langle\{1\}, \cdot, 1\rangle$. Also, $[-1] = \{1, -1\}$ and so the subgroup generated by -1 is the proper subgroup $\langle\{1, -1\}, \cdot, 1\rangle$. Since $[1] = \{1\}$ and $[-1] = \{1, -1\}$ are proper subsets of the carrier U_4, neither 1 nor -1 is a generator of G. $\quad\square$

The infinite abelian group $\langle Q^+, \cdot, 1\rangle$, with Q^+ the set of positive rational numbers, is not cyclic, because $[a]$ is a proper subset of Q^+ for every a in Q^+. The finite abelian group $\langle B_2, \oplus, 0_2\rangle$ of Example 2 is not cyclic, as we will see in Problem 18 below. In Example 6, we will present a finite nonabelian group that is not cyclic.

The following theorem gives a method, different from that of Definition 6, for determining $[a]$ and the order of a.

THEOREM 6   **A METHOD FOR FINDING $[a]$ AND $\#[a]$**

Let $G = \langle X, \square, e \rangle$ be a group and let $a \in X$.

(a) If $a^n \neq e$ for all positive integers n, then the integral powers of a are all distinct; that is,

$$[a] = \{\ldots, a^{-2}, a^{-1}, e, a, a^2, a^3, \ldots\}$$

and a has infinite order.
(b) If s is the smallest positive integer with $a^s = e$, then $[a] = \{e, a, a^2, \ldots, a^{s-1}\}$ and a has order s.

PROOF   (a) Given that $a^n \neq e$ for all n in Z^+, we prove that the integral powers of a are distinct by proving the contrapositive. That is, we assume that $a^i = a^j$ with $i \neq j$ and seek to contradict the hypothesis. Since $i \neq j$, we have either $i < j$ or $i > j$. The two cases are similar, so we assume that $i < j$. Now $a^i = a^j$ helps us see that

$$a^{j-i} = a^j \square a^{-i} = a^i \square a^{-i} = a^0 = e.$$

Since $i < j$, we have $j - i > 0$; thus $a^{j-i} = e$ contradicts the hypothesis that $a^n \neq e$ for all positive integers n. This proves Part (a).
(b) Let s be the smallest positive integer with $a^s = e$. The "Division Algorithm" (Algorithm 1 of Section 1.7) expresses any integer n as $n = qs + r$, with q an integer and r in $\{0, 1, \ldots, s-1\}$. Then

$$a^n = a^{qs+r} = (a^s)^q \square a^r = e^q \square a^r = e \square a^r = a^r.$$

Thus each integral power a^n equals one of the powers $a^0, a^1, \ldots, a^{s-1}$. These powers are distinct because, as in the proof of Part (a), $a^i = a^j$ with $0 \leq i < j < s$ implies that $a^{j-i} = e$ with $0 < j - i < s$. But this would contradict the hypothesis that s is the smallest positive integer with $a^s = e$. Hence $[a] = \{e, a, \ldots, a^{s-1}\}$ and a has order s. $\quad\square$

The following result does not hold in all monoids, but the fact that in a group $\langle X, \Box, e \rangle$ one has an inverse x^{-1} in X for each x in X enables us to establish this property for groups.

THEOREM 7 **LEFT OR RIGHT CANCELLATION**

In a group $G = \langle X, \Box, e \rangle$, either $c \Box a = c \Box b$ or $a \Box c = b \Box c$ implies that $a = b$.

PROOF Let the hypothesis be that $c \Box a = c \Box b$. (The other case is left to the reader as Problem 26 below.) Since G is a group, the element c of X has an inverse c^{-1} in X. Substituting $c \Box b$ for its equal $c \Box a$, we have $c^{-1} \Box (c \Box a) = c^{-1} \Box (c \Box b)$. This and associativity of $\Box$ give us $(c^{-1} \Box c) \Box a = (c^{-1} \Box c) \Box b$. By the definition of inverse, $c^{-1} \Box c = e$. Hence $e \Box a = e \Box b$. Since e is the identity under $\Box$, this implies that $a = b$, as desired. $\qquad \Box$

One sees from Theorem 7, as follows, that an element of X does not appear more than once in any row (or in any column) of the operation table for a group $\langle X, \Box, e \rangle$. If there were repetition on the row for an element c, one would have $c \Box a = c \Box b$ with $a \neq b$. But the left cancellation part of Theorem 7 tells us that $c \Box a = c \Box b$ implies that $a = b$. Similarly, it follows from right cancellation that no element appears more than once in any column.

Example 5 Let $G = \langle X, \Box, e \rangle$ be a group with $\#X = 4$ and let $x^2 = x \Box x = e$ for each x in X. Here we show that there is only one possibility for the table of the binary operation $\Box$ on X. Since $\#X = 4$, we can list X in the form $X = \{e, b, c, d\}$. Since e is the identity, we can fill in the first row and first column as shown in Table 7.1.4. Also, the fact that $x^2 = e$ for each x in X means that e is the entry for each spot on the main diagonal. Since b and e already appear in the row for b and no element of X can appear more than once in a given row, $b \Box c$ cannot be b or e. Since c already appears in the column for c and no element appears more than once in a given column, $b \Box c \neq c$. As X is closed under $\Box$, these facts imply that $b \Box c = d$. Similarly one finds the other entries missing from Table 7.1.4. Thus Table 7.1.5 is the only possibility for the operation $\Box$ on $X = \{e, b, c, d\}$ when $\langle X, \Box, e \rangle$ is a group with $x^2 = e$ for all x in X. $\qquad \Box$

TABLE 7.1.4

$\Box$	e	b	c	d
e	e	b	c	d
b	b	e		
c	c		e	
d	d			e

TABLE 7.1.5

$\Box$	e	b	c	d
e	e	b	c	d
b	b	e	d	c
c	c	d	e	b
d	d	c	b	e

Let $G = \langle X, \Box, e \rangle$ be a group. Each of the following two theorems sometimes provides an easier way of showing that certain subsets Y of X are carriers of subgroups in G, that is, easier than demonstrating all the properties asked for in Definition 4 ("Subgroup in a Group").

THEOREM 8   **NONEMPTY SUBSET CLOSED UNDER DIVISION**

Let $G = \langle X, \square, e \rangle$ be a group. Let $\div$ be the binary operation on X given by $x \div y = x \;\square\; y^{-1}$. If Y is a nonempty subset of X and Y is closed under $\div$, then e is in Y and $\langle Y, \square, e \rangle$ is a subgroup in G.

PROOF   Since $Y \neq \varnothing$, there is some a in Y. Now $a \div a = a \;\square\; a^{-1} = e$. Hence it follows from the closure of Y under $\div$ that $e \in Y$. Similarly, for every y in Y, $e \div y = e \;\square\; y^{-1} = y^{-1}$ is in Y. Then for any x and y in Y, one sees that $x \;\square\; y = x \;\square\; (y^{-1})^{-1} = x \div y^{-1}$. Thus closure of Y under $\div$ implies closure of Y under $\square$. Now we conclude that $\langle Y, \square, e \rangle$ is a subgroup in G since it meets all the conditions of Definition 4, "Subgroup in a Group." □

With the help of Theorem 8 one could shorten the proof of Theorem 5 that $\langle [a], \square, e \rangle$ is a subgroup in a group $G = \langle X, \square, e \rangle$ for each a in X by showing merely that $[a]$ is nonempty and is closed under the binary operation $\div$ given by $x \div y = x \;\square\; y^{-1}$.

THEOREM 9   **FINITE SUBSET CLOSED UNDER GROUP OPERATION**

Let $G = \langle X, \square, e \rangle$ be a group, Y be a nonempty finite subset of X, and Y be closed under $\square$. Then $\langle Y, \square, e \rangle$ is a subgroup in G.

PROOF   Since Y is closed under $\square$, the positive integral powers $y, y^2, y^3, \ldots$ of an element y of Y are all in Y. The finiteness of Y implies that these powers are not distinct. Hence $y^i = y^j$ for some integers i and j with $0 < i < j$. As in the proof of Theorem 6, it follows that $y^s = e$ where $s = j - i$. This implies that the identity e is in Y. It also tells us that $y^{s-1} \;\square\; y = e$, which implies that y^{s-1} is the inverse of y. Therefore the inverse of y is in Y. All together, we have shown that $\langle Y, \square, e \rangle$ satisfies the conditions of Definition 4 to be a subgroup in $\langle X, \square, e \rangle$. □

Example 6   Let S consist of all the rational numbers except 0 and 1. Let $X = \{f_1, f_2, f_3, f_4, f_5, f_6\}$, where the f_i are the mappings from S to itself given by the following rules:

$$f_1(s) = s,$$

$$f_2(s) = \frac{1}{1 - s},$$

$$f_3(s) = \frac{s - 1}{s},$$

$$f_4(s) = 1 - s,$$

$$f_5(s) = \frac{1}{s},$$

$$f_6(s) = \frac{s}{s-1}.$$

If f and g are in X, let their **composite**, denoted as $f \circ g$, be the mapping h with $h(s) = g(f(s))$ for each s in S. That is, $h(s) = u$ whenever $f(s) = t$ and $g(t) = u$. As an illustration of this definition of composite, we note that

$$f_4(f_2(s)) = 1 - f_2(s) = 1 - \frac{1}{1-s} = \frac{1-s-1}{1-s} = \frac{s}{s-1} = f_6(s),$$

and hence $f_2 \circ f_4 = f_6$. In a similar fashion one finds all the entries shown in Table 7.1.6. This table shows that X is closed under $\circ$ and hence that $\circ$ is a binary operation on X. The fact that the first row is the same as the column labels and the first column is the same as the row labels shows that f_1 is the identity under $\circ$. Using the table, one sees that each of f_1, f_4, f_5, f_6 is its own inverse and that f_2 and f_3 are inverses of each other. In Theorem 1 of Section 7.2 we will prove that the operation $\circ$ on X is associative. All of these facts together establish that $\langle X, \circ, f_1 \rangle$ is a group. This group is nonabelian; for example, $f_4 \circ f_2 = f_5$ and $f_2 \circ f_4 = f_6$, and so $f_4 \circ f_2 \neq f_2 \circ f_4$.

TABLE 7.1.6

$\circ$	f_1	f_2	f_3	f_4	f_5	f_6
f_1	f_1	f_2	f_3	f_4	f_5	f_6
f_2	f_2	f_3	f_1	f_6	f_4	f_5
f_3	f_3	f_1	f_2	f_5	f_6	f_4
f_4	f_4	f_5	f_6	f_1	f_2	f_3
f_5	f_5	f_6	f_4	f_3	f_1	f_2
f_6	f_6	f_4	f_5	f_2	f_3	f_1

Using Table 7.1.6, we find that $f_2^2 = f_2 \circ f_2 = f_3$ and $f_2^3 = f_2^2 \circ f_2 = f_3 \circ f_2 = f_1$. Since f_1 is the identity, the smallest positive integer s with f_2^s equal to the identity is $s = 3$. It now follows from Part (b) of Theorem 6 ("A Method for Finding $[a]$ and $\#[a]$") that

$$[f_2] = \{f_2^0, f_2^1, f_2^2\} = \{f_1, f_2, f_3\}.$$

This shows that the order of f_2 is 3 and that $[f_2]$ is a proper subset of X. We leave it to the reader in Problem 27 below to show that $[x]$ is a proper subset of X for each x in X and hence that this group is not cyclic.

□

PROBLEMS FOR SECTION 7.1

1. Describe an infinite set X of numbers such that $\langle X, +, 0 \rangle$ is a group.

2. Describe an infinite set X of numbers such that $\langle X, \cdot, 1 \rangle$ is a group.

3. Is the monoid $[N, +, 0]$ a group? Explain. ($N = \{0, 1, \ldots\}$.)

4. Is the monoid $[Z^+, \cdot, 1]$ a group? Explain. ($Z^+ = \{1, 2, \ldots\}$.)

5. What is the order of the group $\langle B_2, \oplus, 00 \rangle$?

6. Can a group of order n have a subgroup with order greater than n? Explain.

7. Let $\langle X, \square, e \rangle$ be a group. Does $x^m \square x^n = x^n \square x^m$ for each x in X and all integers m and n? Explain.

8. Explain why every cyclic group $\langle [g], \square, e \rangle$ is abelian.

9. Let v be the complex number $(1 + \sqrt{3}i)/2$ and let $U_6 = \{1, v, v^2, v^3, v^4, v^5\}$.
　(i) Show that $v^2 = (-1 + \sqrt{3}i)/2$, $v^3 = -1$, and $v^6 = 1$.
　(ii) Construct the multiplication table for U_6.
　(iii) Tabulate x^{-1} for each x in U_6.
　(iv) Explain why $G = \langle U_6, \cdot, 1 \rangle$ is a group.
　(v) For each x in U_6, list the elements of the carrier $[x]$ of the cyclic subgroup $\langle [x], \cdot, 1 \rangle$ and give the order of x.
　(vi) Is G cyclic? If so, name each generator of G.
　(vii) Is G abelian?
　(viii) Is each x in U_6 a sixth root of 1?
　(ix) Assume as given that every subgroup in G is a cyclic subgroup. Give the subgroup poset diagram for G.

10. Let u be the complex number $(1 + i)/\sqrt{2}$ and let $U_8 = \{1, u, u^2, \ldots, u^7\}$.
　(i) Show that $u^2 = i$, $u^4 = -1$, $u^8 = 1$.
　(ii) Complete the following table:

n	0	1	2	3	4	5	6	7
u^n	1	$\dfrac{1+i}{\sqrt{2}}$	i	$\dfrac{-1+i}{\sqrt{2}}$	-1			

　(iii) Make the multiplication table for U_8.
　(iv) Use $1 = 1 \cdot 1 = uu^7 = u^2 u^6 = u^3 u^5 = u^4 u^4$ to tabulate x^{-1} for each x in U_8.
　(v) Explain why $G = \langle U_8, \cdot, 1 \rangle$ is a group.
　(vi) For each x in U_8, give $[x]$ and the order of x.
　(vii) Is G cyclic? If so, which elements are generators of G?
　(viii) Is G abelian?
　(ix) Is each number in U_8 an eighth root of 1?

(x) Assume as given that every subgroup in G is one of the cyclic subgroups $\langle [x], \cdot, 1 \rangle$ and give the subgroup poset diagram for G.

11. For each of the following subsets Y of the set $\boldsymbol{B_3}$, of 3-bit strings, determine whether Y is closed under the binary operation $\oplus$ of "bitwise addition modulo 2" defined in Example 2. If Y is not closed under $\oplus$, name strings α and β in Y such that $\alpha \oplus \beta$ is not in Y.
    (a) $Y = \{001\}$.   (b) $Y = \{000, 001\}$.   (c) $Y = \{000, 001, 010\}$.
    (d) $Y = \{000, 001, 010, 011\}$.

12. Do as in Problem 11 for the following subsets of $\boldsymbol{B_3}$.
    (a) $Y = \{000\}$.   (b) $Y = \{100\}$.   (c) $Y = \{000, 100, 010\}$.
    (d) $Y = \{000, 010, 100, 110\}$.   (e) $Y = \{000, 001, 010, 100\}$.

13. For which subsets Y in Problem 11 is $(Y, \oplus, 0_3)$ a subgroup in $\langle \boldsymbol{B_3}, \oplus, 0_3 \rangle$?

14. For which subsets Y in Problem 12 is $(Y, \oplus, 0_3)$ a subgroup in $\langle \boldsymbol{B_3}, \oplus, 0_3 \rangle$?

15. Let a and b be in the carrier X of a group $\langle X, \square, e \rangle$.
    (a) Solve the equation $a \,\square\, x = b$ for x (in terms of a and b).
    (b) Show that $(a \,\square\, b)^{-1} = b^{-1} \,\square\, a^{-1}$.
    (c) Name a group in which $(a \,\square\, b)^{-1} \neq a^{-1} \,\square\, b^{-1}$ for some a and b.

16. Let $\langle X, \square, e \rangle$ be a group with a, b, and c in X.
    (a) Solve $x \,\square\, a = b$ for x (in terms of a and b).
    (b) Express $(a \,\square\, b \,\square\, c)^{-1}$ in terms of a^{-1}, b^{-1}, and c^{-1}.

17. Let $\langle Y, \oplus, 0_2 \rangle$ be a subgroup in $\langle \boldsymbol{B_2}, \oplus, 0_2 \rangle$. Use the fact that $01 \oplus 10 = 11$ to explain why the subset Y cannot contain two of the three strings 01, 10, 11 without containing the third string.

18. Let $G = \langle \boldsymbol{B_2}, \oplus, 0_2 \rangle$.
    (i) For each string α in $\boldsymbol{B_2}$, list the elements of the carrier $[\alpha]$ of the cyclic subgroup $\langle [\alpha], \oplus, 0_2 \rangle$ and give the order of α.
    (ii) Is G cyclic? Explain.
    (iii) Is G abelian?
    (iv) Use Problem 17 to show that the only noncyclic subgroup in G is the improper subgroup G itself.
    (v) Give the subgroup poset diagram for G.

19. Let $X = \{e, b, c\}$ and assume that $G = \langle X, \square, e \rangle$ is a group.
    (i) Use the facts that e is the identity and that no element appears more than once in a row or column to make the operation table for G.
    (ii) Find the set $[b]$ of integral powers of b and the order of b.
    (iii) Find $[c]$ and the order of c.
    (iv) Is G cyclic?
    (v) Is every group of order 3 cyclic and abelian? Explain.

20. Let $X = \{e, f, g, h\}$ and assume that $G = \langle X, \square, e \rangle$ is a group (of order 4) with $f^2 = g$.

(i) Use the facts that e is the identity, that $f^2 = g$, and that no element appears more than once in a row or column to make the operation table for G.

(ii) Show that G is cyclic and name its generators.

(iii) Can e, f, g, h be four complex numbers and $\Box$ be multiplication of complex numbers? Explain.

(iv) Is every group of order 4 cyclic? (*Hint*: Consider $\langle B_2, \oplus, 0_2 \rangle$.)

21. Let $G = \langle [g], \Box, e \rangle$ be a cyclic group of order 15. Show that G has a subgroup of order 5.

22. Show that the group G of Problem 21 has a subgroup of order 3.

23. Let $G = \langle [g], \Box, e \rangle$ be a cyclic group of order 16. List the carriers of subgroups H in G with the following orders for H:
(i) 1,   (ii) 2,   (iii) 4,   (iv) 8,   (v) 16.

24. Let $G = \langle X, \Box, e \rangle$ be a group of finite order n. Explain why G is cyclic if and only if there is an x of order n in X.

25. Let $G = \langle X, \Box, e \rangle$ be a group. Explain why:
(a) $(a \Box b)^2 = a \Box b \Box a \Box b$ for all a and b in X.
(b) $(a \Box b)^2 = a^2 \Box b^2$ when G is abelian.

26. Prove the right cancellation part of Theorem 7 that was left to the reader. That is, show that $a \Box c = b \Box c$ implies $a = b$ in a group $\langle X, \Box, e \rangle$.

27. Let $G = \langle X, \circ, f_1 \rangle$ with $X = \{f_1, f_2, f_3, f_4, f_5, f_6\}$ be the group of Example 6.
(i) Use Table 7.1.6 in Example 6 to find $[x]$ for each x in X.
(ii) Explain why G is not cyclic.
(iii) Assume that the only noncyclic subgroup in G is the improper subgroup G itself and draw the subgroup poset diagram for G.

28. As in Example 6, let $f_1, f_2, f_3, f_4, f_5, f_6$ be the mappings with $f_1(s) = s$, $f_2(s) = 1/(1 - s)$, $f_3(s) = (s - 1)/s$, $f_4(s) = 1 - s$, $f_5(s) = 1/s$, $f_6(s) = s/(s - 1)$.
(a) Show directly (that is, without using Table 7.1.6) that $f_5(f_4(s)) = 1/(1 - s)$, that is, $f_4 \circ f_5 = f_2$.
(b) Show that $(f_4 \circ f_5)^2 \neq f_4^2 \circ f_5^2$.
(c) Find an f_i such that $f_i \circ f_2 = f_2 \circ f_4$ with $f_i \neq f_4$ and thus show that "*mixed cancellation*" is not always valid in a nonabelian group.

29. Describe a subset Y of $Z = \{\ldots, -2, -1, 0, 1, 2, \ldots\}$ such that Y is closed under addition and $0 \in Y$ but $(Y, +, 0)$ is not a group (and hence is not a subgroup in $\langle Z, +, 0 \rangle$).

30. Describe a subset Y of the set Q^+ of positive rational numbers such that Y is closed under multiplication and $1 \in Y$ but $(Y, \cdot, 1)$ is not a subgroup in $\langle Q^+, \cdot, 1 \rangle$.

31. Let Y be the subset $\{5^n : n \in N\} = \{1, 5, 25, \ldots\}$ of Q^+.
   (i) Is Y closed under multiplication?
   (ii) Is Y the carrier of a subgroup in $\langle Q^+, \cdot, 1\rangle$? Explain.
   (iii) Does Theorem 9 ("Finite Groups Closed under Group Operation") still hold when the word *finite* is deleted? Explain.

32. For d in Z^+, let dZ be the set $\{\ldots, -2d, -d, 0, d, 2d, \ldots\}$. Is dZ the carrier of a subgroup in $\langle Z, +, 0\rangle$ for each d in Z^+? If so, is this subgroup cyclic? If it is cyclic, name all generators of $\langle dZ, +, 0\rangle$.

33. Let $G = \langle X, \square, e\rangle$ be a group. For a fixed element c in X, let f be the mapping from X to itself with $f(x) = c \square x$. Explain why:
   (i) f is injective;   (ii) f is surjective;
   (iii) f is a permutation on X.

34. Do as in Problem 33 with now $f(x) = x \square c$.

35. Let $\langle X, \square, e\rangle$ be a group and $a \in X$. Prove that the set $[a] = \{a^n : n \in Z\}$ is closed under division.

36. Use Problem 35 and Theorem 8 ("Nonempty Subset Closed under Division") to prove that $\langle [a], \square, e\rangle$ is a subgroup in $\langle X, \square, e\rangle$ for every a in X. Do *not* use Theorem 5 ("Subgroup of Integral Powers") or Definition 7 ("Cyclic Subgroup Generated by a Cyclic Group").

37. Let $\langle X, \square, e\rangle$ be a group with a and b in X. Show that $(a \square b)^{-1} = a^{-1} \square b^{-1}$ if and only if $a \square b = b \square a$.

38. Let $G = \langle X, \square, e\rangle$ be a group with a and b in X.
   (i) Show that $(a \square b)^2 = a^2 \square b^2$ if and only if $a \square b = b \square a$.
  *(ii) If $x^2 = e$ for every x in X, show that G is abelian.

39. Let $F = \langle A, \square, e\rangle$ and $G = \langle B, \triangle, e'\rangle$ be groups. Let $*$ be the binary operation on the cartesian product $A \times B$ with $(a_1, b_1) * (a_2, b_2) = (a_1 \square a_2, b_1 \triangle b_2)$. Show that $\langle A \times B, *, (e, e')\rangle$ is a group. (This is called the **direct product** of F and G and is denoted $F \times G$.)

40. Show that the direct product $F \times G$ (as defined in Problem 39) is abelian if and only if both F and G are abelian.

41. In a group $\langle X, \square, e\rangle$, does $(a \square c \neq b \square c) \Rightarrow (a \neq b)$? Explain.

42. In a group $\langle X, \square, e\rangle$, is $(a \square c = b \square c) \Leftrightarrow (a = b)$? Explain.

43. Let $G = \langle X, \square, e\rangle$ be a group, let Γ be a collection of carriers of subgroups in G, and let I be the intersection of the members of Γ. Prove that $\langle I, \square, e\rangle$ is a subgroup in G.

44. Give an example of subgroups $\langle A, \square, e\rangle$ and $\langle B, \square, e\rangle$ in a group $G = \langle X, \square, e\rangle$ such that $\langle A \cup B, \square, e\rangle$ is not a group.

*45. Let Γ be the collection of the carriers of all the subgroups in G. Prove that $(\Gamma, \subseteq)$ is a lattice in which $\text{GLB}(A, B) = A \cap B$ and $\text{LUB}(A, B)$ is the intersection of all the upper bounds for (A, B).

7.2

PERMUTATION GROUPS, GROUP HOMOMORPHISMS

Group theory as a formal subject began with the work of Lagrange and Galois on permutation groups, one of the topics of this section. One of the reasons for the importance of permutation groups is that they exhibit all of the phenomena possible in groups.

In Example 6 of Section 7.1, we met a nonabelian group in which the operation is composition of mappings. In this section, an infinite sequence of such groups is introduced. First we define composition in its most general setting.

DEFINITION 1   **COMPOSITION OF MAPPINGS**

Let f be a mapping from A to B and g be a mapping from B to C. Then the **composite** $f \circ g$ of f and g is the mapping h from A to C for which $f(a) = b$ and $g(b) = c$ imply that $h(a) = c$. In this section, the composite $f \circ g$ is usually written as fg.

Example 1   Let $A = \{a, b, c\}$, $B_2 = \{00, 01, 10, 11\}$, and $N = \{0, 1, 2, \ldots\}$. Let $f\colon A \to B_2$ and $g\colon B_2 \to N$ be the mappings given by

$$f\colon a \mapsto 00, \quad b \mapsto 00, \quad c \mapsto 01;$$
$$g\colon 00 \mapsto 0, \quad 01 \mapsto 1, \quad 10 \mapsto 1, \quad 11 \mapsto 2.$$

Let h be the composite fg of these mappings. Writing

$$[f(x) = y] \wedge [g(y) = z] \Rightarrow [h(x) = z]$$

in the form

$$x \overset{f}{\mapsto} y \overset{g}{\mapsto} z \Rightarrow x \overset{h}{\mapsto} z,$$

one finds that

$$a \overset{f}{\mapsto} 00 \overset{g}{\mapsto} 0 \Rightarrow a \overset{h}{\mapsto} 0,$$
$$b \overset{f}{\mapsto} 00 \overset{g}{\mapsto} 0 \Rightarrow b \overset{h}{\mapsto} 0,$$
$$c \overset{f}{\mapsto} 01 \overset{g}{\mapsto} 1 \Rightarrow c \overset{h}{\mapsto} 1.$$

Thus the composite $h = fg$ is the mapping

$$fg\colon a \mapsto 0, \quad b \mapsto 0, \quad c \mapsto 1. \qquad \square$$

In Example 6 of Section 7.1, we promised to prove that composition of mappings is associative; now we present the proof.

THEOREM 1   **COMPOSITION OF MAPPINGS IS ASSOCIATIVE**

Let f, g, and h be mappings whose domains and codomains are as follows:

$$f: S \to T; \qquad g: T \to U; \qquad h: U \to V.$$

Then $(fg)h = f(gh)$.

PROOF   Let s be a general element of S, $f(s) = t$, $g(t) = u$, and $h(u) = v$. Then

$$s \xmapsto{f} t \xmapsto{g} u \Rightarrow s \xmapsto{fg} u, \tag{1}$$

$$s \xmapsto{fg} u \xmapsto{h} v \Rightarrow s \xmapsto{(fg)h} v, \tag{2}$$

$$t \xmapsto{g} u \xmapsto{h} v \Rightarrow t \xmapsto{gh} v, \tag{3}$$

$$s \xmapsto{f} t \xmapsto{gh} v \Rightarrow s \xmapsto{f(gh)} v. \tag{4}$$

Displays (2) and (4) show that $(fg)h = f(gh)$, as desired.   □

We recall from Section 1.8 that a permutation on a set T is a bijective mapping from T to itself. The next example deals with composites of such mappings.

Example 2   Let $T_3 = \{1, 2, 3\}$. Let f and g be the permutations on T_3 given by

$$f: 1 \mapsto 2, \quad 2 \mapsto 3, \quad 3 \mapsto 1 \qquad \text{and} \qquad g: 1 \mapsto 2, \quad 2 \mapsto 1, \quad 3 \mapsto 3.$$

Let h be the composite fg of these mappings. Writing

$$[f(x) = y] \wedge [g(y) = z] \Rightarrow [h(x) = z]$$

in the form

$$x \xmapsto{f} y \xmapsto{g} z \Rightarrow x \xmapsto{h} z$$

one finds that

$$1 \xmapsto{f} 2 \xmapsto{g} 1 \Rightarrow 1 \xmapsto{h} 1,$$

$$2 \xmapsto{f} 3 \xmapsto{g} 3 \Rightarrow 2 \xmapsto{h} 3,$$

$$3 \xmapsto{f} 1 \xmapsto{g} 2 \Rightarrow 3 \xmapsto{h} 2.$$

Thus the composite $h = fg$ is the permutation

$$h = fg: 1 \mapsto 1, \quad 2 \mapsto 3, \quad 3 \mapsto 2.$$

Similarly one finds that the composite $k = gf$ in the other order is

$$k = gf: 1 \mapsto 3, \quad 2 \mapsto 2, \quad 3 \mapsto 1.$$

Hence $fg \neq gf$ in this example. Using Definition 7 of Section 6.4 ("Mapping Relation and Digraph for a Mapping"), one finds that the digraphs D_f, D_g, D_h, and D_k for the mappings f, g, h, and k, respectively, are as shown in Figure 7.2.1.

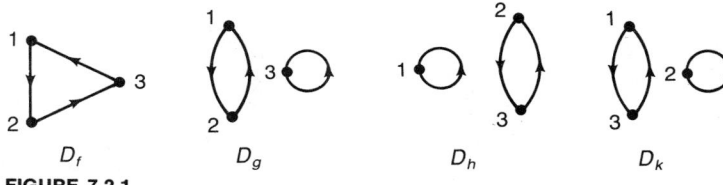

$$D_f \qquad D_g \qquad D_h \qquad D_k$$

FIGURE 7.2.1

We prove in Theorem 3 below that composition of permutations is a binary operation on the set X of all permutations on a nonempty set T and that this operation makes X into a group. The following notation is convenient for parts of that proof.

NOTATION 1   **MATRIX FORM OF A PERMUTATION**

Let

$$f: a_1 \mapsto b_1, \quad a_2 \mapsto b_2, \quad \dots, \quad a_n \mapsto b_n$$

be a permutation on $T = \{a_1, a_2, \dots, a_n\}$. Then the **matrix form** for f is

$$f = \begin{pmatrix} a_1 & a_2 & \dots & a_n \\ b_1 & b_2 & \dots & b_n \end{pmatrix}.$$

For example, if

$$f: 1 \mapsto 2, \quad 2 \mapsto 3, \quad 3 \mapsto 1,$$

then its matrix form is

$$f = \begin{pmatrix} 1 & 2 & 3 \\ 2 & 3 & 1 \end{pmatrix}.$$

Interchanging the columns in the matrix form does not change the permutation. Thus f could also be written as

$$\begin{pmatrix} 2 & 1 & 3 \\ 3 & 2 & 1 \end{pmatrix}.$$

The noteworthy characteristic of a matrix representation of a permutation f is that $f(t)$ appears directly below t for each t in T.

THEOREM 2   **COMPOSITE USING MATRIX FORM**

Let

$$f = \begin{pmatrix} a_1 & a_2 & \cdots & a_n \\ b_1 & b_2 & \cdots & b_n \end{pmatrix} \quad \text{and} \quad g = \begin{pmatrix} b_1 & b_2 & \cdots & b_n \\ c_1 & c_2 & \cdots & c_n \end{pmatrix}$$

be permutations on $T = \{a_1, a_2, \ldots, a_n\}$. Then the composite fg is

$$fg = \begin{pmatrix} a_1 & a_2 & \cdots & a_n \\ c_1 & c_2 & \cdots & c_n \end{pmatrix}.$$

PROOF   Let $fg = h$. Then $f(a_i) = b_i$ and $g(b_i) = c_i$ implies that $h(a_i) = c_i$ for $i = 1, 2, \ldots, n$. Hence the composite fg is given by the matrix

$$\begin{pmatrix} a_1 & a_2 & \cdots & a_n \\ c_1 & c_2 & \cdots & c_n \end{pmatrix}. \qquad \square$$

ALGORITHM 1   **COMPOSITE OF PERMUTATIONS**

To find the composite fg of permutations on $T = \{a_1, a_2, \ldots, a_n\}$, express f as

$$\begin{pmatrix} a_1 & a_2 & \cdots & a_n \\ b_1 & b_2 & \cdots & b_n \end{pmatrix}$$

and reorder the columns of the matrix form for g so that the top row of g is the bottom row of f, that is, so that

$$g = \begin{pmatrix} b_1 & b_2 & \cdots & b_n \\ c_1 & c_2 & \cdots & c_n \end{pmatrix}.$$

Then

$$fg = \begin{pmatrix} a_1 & a_2 & \cdots & a_n \\ c_1 & c_2 & \cdots & c_n \end{pmatrix}.$$

For example, using Algorithm 1, the composites of the permutations

$$f: 1 \mapsto 2, \quad 2 \mapsto 3, \quad 3 \mapsto 1 \qquad \text{and} \qquad g: 1 \mapsto 2, \quad 2 \mapsto 1, \quad 3 \mapsto 3$$

of Example 2 are obtained as follows:

$$fg = \begin{pmatrix} 1 & 2 & 3 \\ 2 & 3 & 1 \end{pmatrix} \begin{pmatrix} 2 & 3 & 1 \\ 1 & 3 & 2 \end{pmatrix} = \begin{pmatrix} 1 & 2 & 3 \\ 1 & 3 & 2 \end{pmatrix},$$

$$gf = \begin{pmatrix} 1 & 2 & 3 \\ 2 & 1 & 3 \end{pmatrix} \begin{pmatrix} 2 & 1 & 3 \\ 3 & 2 & 1 \end{pmatrix} = \begin{pmatrix} 1 & 2 & 3 \\ 3 & 2 & 1 \end{pmatrix}.$$

THEOREM 3 **GROUP OF PERMUTATIONS ON A FINITE SET**

Let $T = \{a_1, a_2, \ldots, a_n\}$, X consist of all permutations on T, and e be the permutation with $e(t) = t$ for each t in T. Then $\langle X, \circ, e \rangle$ is a group, where $\circ$ is composition of mappings.

PROOF   We have to show that X is closed under $\circ$ and hence that $\circ$ is a binary operation on X. Then we can use Theorem 1 to see that $\circ$ is associative. Next we have to produce an identity e for X under $\circ$ and finally have to show that each x in X has an inverse under $\circ$.

Let $f, g \in X$. Using Notation 1, we write f in the form

$$f = \begin{pmatrix} a_1 & a_2 & \cdots & a_n \\ b_1 & b_2 & \cdots & b_n \end{pmatrix}. \tag{5}$$

Since f is a bijection from T onto T, it follows that $\{b_1, b_2, \ldots, b_n\}$ is also the set T. This allows us to write g in the form

$$g = \begin{pmatrix} b_1 & b_2 & \cdots & b_n \\ c_1 & c_2 & \cdots & c_n \end{pmatrix},$$

where $\{c_1, c_2, \ldots, c_n\} = T$. Then

$$fg = \begin{pmatrix} a_1 & a_2 & \cdots & a_n \\ c_1 & c_2 & \cdots & c_n \end{pmatrix}$$

is in X (that is, fg is a permutation on T). Thus X is closed under composition and hence composition is a binary operation on X. Theorem 1 tells us that this operation is associative. Let e be the permutation on T with $e(t) = t$ for each t in T. Then

$$a_i \xoverset{f}\mapsto b_i \xoverset{e}\mapsto b_i \Rightarrow a_i \xoverset{fe}\mapsto b_i,$$

$$a_i \xoverset{e}\mapsto a_i \xoverset{f}\mapsto b_i \Rightarrow a_i \xoverset{ef}\mapsto b_i.$$

These show that $fe = f = ef$; that is, e is the identity for the semigroup $(X, \circ)$. Thus $[X, \circ, e]$ is a monoid. Finally we see that

$$\begin{pmatrix} a_1 & a_2 & \cdots & a_n \\ b_1 & b_2 & \cdots & b_n \end{pmatrix}\begin{pmatrix} b_1 & b_2 & \cdots & b_n \\ a_1 & a_2 & \cdots & a_n \end{pmatrix} = \begin{pmatrix} a_1 & a_2 & \cdots & a_n \\ a_1 & a_2 & \cdots & a_n \end{pmatrix} = e,$$

$$\begin{pmatrix} b_1 & b_2 & \cdots & b_n \\ a_1 & a_2 & \cdots & a_n \end{pmatrix}\begin{pmatrix} a_1 & a_2 & \cdots & a_n \\ b_1 & b_2 & \cdots & b_n \end{pmatrix} = \begin{pmatrix} b_1 & b_2 & \cdots & b_n \\ b_1 & b_2 & \cdots & b_n \end{pmatrix} = e.$$

These show that the inverse of the permutation f of Display (5) is the permutation

$$f^{-1} = \begin{pmatrix} b_1 & b_2 & \cdots & b_n \\ a_1 & a_2 & \cdots & a_n \end{pmatrix}$$

obtained by interchanging the rows of f in Display (5). Since this f^{-1} is in X, we see that $\langle X, \circ, e \rangle$ meets the conditions of Definition 1 of Section 7.1 to be a group. □

When we consider group isomorphisms later in this section, we will see that the structure of the group $\langle X, \circ, e \rangle$ of Theorem 3 is not affected by the nature of the elements of T that are being permuted but depends only on the size of T. Therefore we can take T to be the specific set $T_n = \{1, 2, \ldots, n\}$ when studying permutations on a set of size n.

NOTATION 2 **SYMMETRIC GROUP $S_n = \langle X_n, \circ, e \rangle$ OF PERMUTATIONS**

Let $T_n = \{1, 2, \ldots, n\}$ and X_n consist of all permutations on T_n. Let e be the permutation in X_n with $e(t) = t$ for all t in T_n. Then $S_n = \langle X_n, \circ, e \rangle$ is called the *symmetric group*. In the rest of this chapter, the symbols T_n, X_n, and S_n will have this fixed meaning when printed in boldface type.

Example 3 The only permutations on $T_2 = \{1, 2\}$ are

$$e: 1 \mapsto 1, \quad 2 \mapsto 2 \quad \text{and} \quad f: 1 \mapsto 2, \quad 2 \mapsto 1.$$

We note that e is the identity of the symmetric group $S_2 = \langle X_2, \circ, e \rangle$ and that $X_2 = \{e, f\}$. Since e is the identity, we know that $ee = e$, $ef = f$, and $fe = f$. We find ff as follows:

$$(1 \overset{f}{\mapsto} 2 \overset{f}{\mapsto} 1) \Rightarrow 1 \overset{ff}{\longmapsto} 1, \quad (2 \overset{f}{\mapsto} 1 \overset{f}{\mapsto} 2) \Rightarrow 2 \overset{ff}{\longmapsto} 2.$$

This shows that $f^2 = ff = e$. Now we have all the data needed for the operation table for S_2 (Table 7.2.1). □

TABLE 7.2.1

$\circ$	e	f
e	e	f
f	f	e

THEOREM 4 **ORDER OF S_n**

The order of the symmetric group S_n is $n!$.

PROOF   The order of $S_n = \langle X_n, \circ, e \rangle$ is the size of the set X_n of all permutations on $T_n = \{1, 2, \ldots, n\}$. Since T_n is finite, the permutations on T_n are the same as the injections from T_n to itself. Hence Theorem 4 ("Number of Injections from X to Y") of Section 1.8 tells us that the order of S_n is $n(n - 1)(n - 2) \cdots 2 \cdot 1 = n!$. $\square$

Example 4   **THE SYMMETRIC GROUP S_3**   For $S_3 = \langle X_3, \circ, e \rangle$, the elements of X_3 are the permutations

$$e\colon 1 \mapsto 1, \quad 2 \mapsto 2, \quad 3 \mapsto 3; \qquad g\colon 1 \mapsto 2, \quad 2 \mapsto 3, \quad 3 \mapsto 1;$$
$$h\colon 1 \mapsto 3, \quad 2 \mapsto 1, \quad 3 \mapsto 2; \qquad i\colon 1 \mapsto 1, \quad 2 \mapsto 3, \quad 3 \mapsto 2;$$
$$j\colon 1 \mapsto 3, \quad 2 \mapsto 2, \quad 3 \mapsto 1; \qquad k\colon 1 \mapsto 2, \quad 2 \mapsto 1, \quad 3 \mapsto 3.$$

One can see that

$$gi = \begin{pmatrix} 1 & 2 & 3 \\ 2 & 3 & 1 \end{pmatrix}\begin{pmatrix} 2 & 3 & 1 \\ 3 & 2 & 1 \end{pmatrix} = \begin{pmatrix} 1 & 2 & 3 \\ 3 & 2 & 1 \end{pmatrix} = j,$$

$$ig = \begin{pmatrix} 1 & 2 & 3 \\ 1 & 3 & 2 \end{pmatrix}\begin{pmatrix} 1 & 3 & 2 \\ 2 & 1 & 3 \end{pmatrix} = \begin{pmatrix} 1 & 2 & 3 \\ 2 & 1 & 3 \end{pmatrix} = k.$$

Hence $gi \neq ig$ and S_3 is nonabelian. Table 7.2.2 is the operation table for S_3; its entries can be found by the technique used to find the products gi and ig.

TABLE 7.2.2

$\circ$	e	g	h	i	j	k
e	e	g	h	i	j	k
g	g	h	e	j	k	i
h	h	e	g	k	i	j
i	i	k	j	e	h	g
j	j	i	k	g	e	h
k	k	j	i	h	g	e

$\square$

The following concepts deal with situations in which equations can be transferred from one group to another.

DEFINITION 2   **GROUP HOMOMORPHISM, GROUP ISOMORPHISM**

Let $G = \langle X, \square, e \rangle$ and $G' = \langle X', \triangle, e' \rangle$ be groups. A ***homomorphism*** from G to G' is a mapping α from X to X' such that

$$\alpha(x \square y) = \alpha(x) \triangle \alpha(y) \qquad \text{for all } x \text{ and } y \text{ in } X. \tag{6}$$

If this homomorphism α is a bijection from X onto X', one says that α is an ***isomorphism*** from G onto G' and that G and G' are ***isomorphic groups***.

The defining property of a homomorphism α shown in Display (6) can be rephrased as follows:

$$[x \,\square\, y = z \text{ in } G] \Rightarrow [\alpha(x) \,\triangle\, \alpha(y) = \alpha(z) \text{ in } G']. \tag{7}$$

This property is called **preservation of the operations**. If one thinks of each operation as "multiplication," this property states that "the image of a product is the product of the images."

Let G and G' be as in Definition 2. To prove that a mapping α from X to X' is not a group homomorphism (and hence is not a group isomorphism), one just has to find specific elements a and b in X such that $\alpha(a \,\square\, b) \neq \alpha(a) \,\triangle\, \alpha(b)$. To prove that α is a group homomorphism, one has to show that $\alpha(x \,\square\, y) = \alpha(x) \,\triangle\, \alpha(y)$ for all x and y in X.

Example 5 **A NONHOMOMORPHISM** Here we give a mapping $f: B_3 \to B_2$ and strings α, β and γ in B_3 such that

$$\alpha \oplus \beta = \gamma \qquad \text{but} \qquad f(\alpha) \oplus f(\beta) \neq f(\gamma).$$

TABLE 7.2.3

α	$f(\alpha)$
000	00
001	01
010	10
011	00
100	00
101	01
110	10
111	11

Such a mapping is not a homomorphism. The mapping f is that of Table 7.2.3. In the group $\langle B_3, \oplus, 000 \rangle$, we have the equality

$$001 \oplus 010 = 011.$$

When each string in this equation is replaced by its image under f, the result is not an equality in $\langle B_2, \oplus, 00 \rangle$, since the left-hand side becomes

$$f(001) \oplus f(010) = 01 \oplus 10 = 11$$

and the right-hand side becomes $f(011) = 00$. Hence this f is not a homomorphism from $\langle B_3, \oplus, 000 \rangle$ to $\langle B_2, \oplus, 00 \rangle$. $\square$

Example 6 **A NONINJECTIVE HOMOMORPHISM** Here we show that the mapping $f: B_3 \to B_2$ given by Table 7.2.4 is a homomorphism from $G = \langle B_3, \oplus, 000 \rangle$ to $G' = \langle B_2, \oplus, 00 \rangle$. This mapping can also be specified by the rule $f(a_1 a_2 a_3) = a_2 a_3$. Since the operation $\oplus$ is bitwise addition modulo 2, an equation

$$a_1 a_2 a_3 \oplus b_1 b_2 b_3 = c_1 c_2 c_3 \tag{8}$$

TABLE 7.2.4

α	$f(\alpha)$
000	00
001	01
010	10
011	11
100	00
101	01
110	10
111	11

in G means that

$$a_1 \oplus b_1 = c_1, \qquad a_2 \oplus b_2 = c_2, \qquad a_3 \oplus b_3 = c_3.$$

Hence, when each string α in Display (8) is replaced by its image $f(\alpha)$, one gets a valid equation

$$a_2 a_3 \oplus b_2 b_3 = c_2 c_3$$

in G'. That is, $f(\alpha \oplus \beta) = f(\alpha) \oplus f(\beta)$ for all α and β in B_3, and f is a homomorphism from G to G'. Since $f(000) = f(100)$, f is not injective. Therefore f is not a bijection and is not an isomorphism. $\square$

TABLE 7.2.5

α	$f(\alpha)$
00	000
01	001
10	010
11	011

Example 7 **A NONSURJECTIVE HOMOMORPHISM** Now let us consider the mapping $f\colon B_2 \to B_3$ given in Table 7.2.5. This can also be specified by the rule $f(a_1 a_2) = 0 a_1 a_2$. As in Example 6, the "bitwise" nature of $\oplus$ enables us to see that $f(\alpha \oplus \beta) = f(\alpha) \oplus f(\beta)$ for all α and β in B_2. Hence f is a homomorphism from $\langle B_2, \oplus, 00 \rangle$ to $\langle B_3, \oplus, 000 \rangle$. Since the image set is a proper subset of B_3, f is not a surjection. Hence f is not a bijection and is not an isomorphism. □

Example 8 **AN ISOMORPHISM** Let R^+ be the subset of positive real numbers in the set R of all real numbers. Then $G = \langle R, +, 0 \rangle$ is an additive group and $G' = \langle R^+, \cdot, 1 \rangle$ is a multiplicative group. Let

$$f\colon R \to R^+; \quad x \mapsto 2^x.$$

Then $f(x + y) = 2^{x+y} = 2^x \cdot 2^y = f(x) \cdot f(y)$ for all x and y in R. Hence f is a group homomorphism from G to G'. In calculus courses, one shows that $f(x)$ is an increasing function with R^+ as its image set (called *range* in calculus). This implies that f is a bijection from R onto R^+, and so G and G' are isomorphic. □

Example 9 Let $G = \langle R, +, 0 \rangle$ be as in Example 8. Let $X = R - \{0\}$; that is, let X consist of all real numbers except 0. Then $V = \langle X, \cdot, 1 \rangle$ is a group. Let

$$h\colon X \to R; \quad x \mapsto \ln |x|,$$

where $\ln |x|$ is the natural logarithm of the absolute value of x. The mapping h is a group homomorphism from V to G because $h(xy) = \ln |xy| = \ln |x| + \ln |y| = h(x) + h(y)$ for all x and y in X. This h is not a group isomorphism because $h(1) = \ln 1 = 0 = \ln |-1| = h(-1)$ shows that h is not injective (and so is not bijective). □

THEOREM 5 **PROPERTIES OF GROUP HOMOMORPHISMS**

Let h be a homomorphism from $G = \langle X, \square, e \rangle$ to $G' = \langle X', \triangle, e' \rangle$. Then

(a) $h(e) = e'$.
(b) $h(x^{-1}) = [h(x)]^{-1}$ for each x in X.
(c) $h(x^n) = [h(x)]^n$ for each x in X and each n in Z.

PROOF (a) Using preservation of the operations and properties of the identities, we have

$$h(e) \triangle h(e) = h(e \square e) = h(e) = e' \triangle h(e).$$

The equality $h(e) \triangle h(e) = e' \triangle h(e)$ and right cancellation give us $h(e) = e'$. This proves Part (a).

(b) For each x in X, we have $x \square x^{-1} = e$. This and preservation of the operations give us $h(x) \triangle h(x^{-1}) = h(e)$. Since $h(e) = e'$ by Part (a), we have $h(x) \triangle h(x^{-1}) = e'$. This and "Unique Inverse" [Theorem 1(a) of Section 7.1] imply that $h(x^{-1}) = [h(x)]^{-1}$; this proves Part (b).

(c) The formula in Part (c) can be proved for n in $N = \{0, 1, \dots\}$ by induction on n and then be shown for negative integers n using Part (b). ◻

One can see from Definition 2 here ("Group Homomorphism, Group Isomorphism"), Definition 3 of Section 7.1 ("Order of a Group"), and Part (vii) of Theorem 3 of Section 1.8 ("Size of an Image Set") that isomorphic groups must have the same order. The converse is not true; that is, groups G and G' can have the same order without being isomorphic, as we shall see in Example 11 below.

We saw in Chapter 6 that digraphs $\langle V, E \rangle$ and $\langle V', E' \rangle$ are isomorphic if and only if they differ merely in the labels for their vertices. The same is true of graphs (V, E) and (V', E'). Similarly, if $G = \langle X, \square, e \rangle$ and $G' = \langle X', \triangle, e' \rangle$ are groups of the same finite order n and β is a bijection from X onto X', then β is an isomorphism from G onto G' if and only if one can change from G to G' merely by replacing each x of X by its image $\beta(x)$ in X' and replacing $\square$ by $\triangle$. When the common order n is fairly small, this provides the following technique for checking whether a given bijection β from X onto X' is an isomorphism from G onto G'.

ALGORITHM 2   **PROVING A GROUP ISOMORPHISM**

Let $G = \langle X, \square, e \rangle$ and $G' = \langle X', \triangle, e' \rangle$ be finite groups. Let β be a bijection from X onto X'. Use a table for the operation $\square$ on X to construct a second table as follows: For each x in X replace the row label x, the column label x, and each entry x within the table by $\beta(x)$. Then β is a group isomorphism from G onto G' if and only if the new table is a table for the operation $\triangle$ on X'.

Example 10

TABLE 7.2.6

$\square$	e	b	c	d
e	e	b	c	d
b	b	e	d	c
c	c	d	e	b
d	d	c	b	e

Let $X = \{e, b, c, d\}$ and let $G = \langle X, \square, e \rangle$ be the group of Example 5 in Section 7.1 whose operation was given in Table 7.1.5, which we repeat here as Table 7.2.6. Let $Y = \{e, b\}$ and $W = \{e, c\}$. We see from the table that each of Y and W is closed under $\square$ and that

$$H = \langle Y, \square, e \rangle \qquad \text{and} \qquad K = \langle W, \square, e \rangle$$

are subgroups in G whose tables are Table 7.2.7(a) and (b), respectively. Let β be the bijection from Y onto W given by

$$\beta: e \mapsto e, \quad b \mapsto c.$$

We use Table 7.2.7(a) to make a new table as follows: For each y in Y, we replace the row label y, the column label y, and each entry y inside the

TABLE 7.2.7(a)   **(b)**

□	e	b
e	e	b
b	b	e

□	e	c
e	e	c
c	c	e

table by $\beta(y)$. Since this converts Table 7.2.7(a) into Table 7.2.7(b), β is an isomorphism from H onto K, and so these groups of order 2 are isomorphic.   □

The following result may be helpful in setting up an isomorphism β from a group G onto a group G' or in proving that no such isomorphism exists.

THEOREM 6   **ISOMORPHISMS PRESERVE ORDER**

Let $\beta: X \to X'$ be an isomorphism from $G = \langle X, \square, e \rangle$ onto $G' = \langle X', \triangle, e' \rangle$. For each x in X, the order of x in G equals the order of $\beta(x)$ in G'.

The proof is left to the reader as Problem 29 below.

Example 11   **NONISOMORPHIC GROUPS OF ORDER 4**   Let $U_4 = \{1, \mathbf{i}, -1, -\mathbf{i}\}$, $G = \langle U_4, \cdot, 1 \rangle$, and $G' = \langle B_2, \oplus, 00 \rangle$. Then each of G and G' has order 4. However, these groups are not isomorphic, since $\mathbf{i}$ has order 4 but there is no string of order 4 in B_2 to act as the image of $\mathbf{i}$ under an isomorphism. (The string 00 has order 1 and every other string in B_2 has order 2 because $\alpha \oplus \alpha = 00$ for each α in B_2.)   □

PROBLEMS FOR SECTION 7.2

1. (a) Draw a figure for the digraph D_f (as defined in Definition 7 of Section 6.2), where f is the permutation

$$f = \begin{pmatrix} 1 & 2 & 3 & 4 & 5 & 6 & 7 & 8 \\ 5 & 4 & 3 & 8 & 6 & 1 & 2 & 7 \end{pmatrix}.$$

   (b) Find all paths of length 2 in D_f.
   (c) Give the matrix form of f^2.

2. (a) Draw a figure for the digraph D_g, where

$$g = \begin{pmatrix} 1 & 2 & 3 & 4 & 5 & 6 & 7 & 8 & 9 \\ 1 & 5 & 8 & 7 & 2 & 3 & 9 & 6 & 4 \end{pmatrix}.$$

(b) Find all paths of length 3 in D_g.

(c) Give the matrix form of g^3.

3.   Let f and g be the permutations on $T_4 = \{1, 2, 3, 4\}$ with

$$f: 1 \mapsto 2, \quad 2 \mapsto 1, \quad 3 \mapsto 4, \quad 4 \mapsto 3$$

and

$$g: 1 \mapsto 2, \quad 2 \mapsto 3, \quad 3 \mapsto 4, \quad 4 \mapsto 1.$$

(i) In S_4, find $h = fg$ (that is, $f \circ g$) using

$$x \overset{f}{\mapsto} y \overset{g}{\mapsto} z \Rightarrow x \overset{h}{\mapsto} z.$$

(ii) Check using the matrix forms for f and g and Algorithm 1, "Composite of Permutations."

4.   Let f and g be as in Problem 3.

(i) Find $k = gf$ and check (as in Problem 3).

(ii) Is S_4 abelian? Explain.

5.   (i) Draw a picture of the digraph D_g (as defined in Definition 7 of Section 6.4) for the g of Problem 3.

(ii) How does one get a picture of the digraph for g^{-1}?

6.   Do as in Problem 5 with g replaced by the f of Problem 3.

7.   For the f of Problem 3, find in S_4 the powers:

(i) $f^2 = f \circ f$;   (ii) $f^3 = f^2 \circ f$;   (iii) f^4;   (iv) f^{99};   (v) f^{100}.

8.   For the g of Problem 3, find in S_4:

(i) g^2;   (ii) g^3;   (iii) g^4;   (iv) g^5;   (v) g^{99};   (vi) g^{100}.

9.   Let f be the permutation on $T_6 = \{1, 2, 3, 4, 5, 6\}$ with

$$f: 1 \mapsto 2, \quad 2 \mapsto 3, \quad 3 \mapsto 4, \quad 4 \mapsto 5, \quad 5 \mapsto 6, \quad 6 \mapsto 1.$$

For each of the following values of m, draw a picture of the digraph for the power f^m in $S_6 = \langle X_6, \circ, e \rangle$.

(i) $m = 1$.   (ii) $m = 2$.   (iii) $m = 3$.   (iv) $m = 4$.   (v) $m = 5$.

(vi) $m = 6$.   (vii) $m = 7$.   (viii) $m = 100$.

10.   Do as in Problem 9, but with S_6 replaced by S_5 and f replaced by

$$g: 1 \mapsto 2, \quad 2 \mapsto 3, \quad 3 \mapsto 4, \quad 4 \mapsto 5, \quad 5 \mapsto 1.$$

11.   Assume that h is a homomorphism from $\langle B_3, \oplus, 000 \rangle$ to $\langle B_2, \oplus, 00 \rangle$ with $h(001) = 11$ and $h(010) = 01$. Find:

(a) $h(000)$.   (b) $h(011)$.

12.   Let h be a homomorphism from $\langle B_2, \oplus, 00 \rangle$ to $\langle B_3, \oplus, 000 \rangle$ with $h(01) = 110$ and $h(10) = 011$. Find:

(a) $h(00)$.   (b) $h(11)$.

13. Does there exist a homomorphism h from $\langle B_2, \oplus, 00 \rangle$ to $\langle B_3, \oplus, 000 \rangle$ with $h(01) = 100$, $h(10) = 010$, and $h(11) = 111$? Explain.

14. Does there exist a homomorphism h from $\langle B_3, \oplus, 000 \rangle$ to $\langle B_2, \oplus, 00 \rangle$ with $h(011) = 01$, $h(101) = 10$, and $h(110) = 00$? Explain.

15. For each of the following mappings, prove or disprove that it is a homomorphism from $\langle Z, +, 0 \rangle$ to itself:
(a) $f: Z \to Z$; $n \mapsto 2n$.   (b) $g: Z \to Z$; $n \mapsto n^2$.

16. For each of the following mappings, prove or disprove that it is a homomorphism from $\langle Q^+, \cdot, 1 \rangle$ to itself. (Q^+ is the set of positive rational numbers.)
(a) $f: Q^+ \to Q^+$; $x \mapsto 2x$.   (b) $g: Q^+ \to Q^+$; $x \mapsto x^2$.

17. Let e, r, and f be the permutations on $T_3 = \{1, 2, 3\}$ with

$e: 1 \mapsto 1$, $2 \mapsto 2$, $3 \mapsto 3$; $r: 1 \mapsto 2$, $2 \mapsto 3$, $3 \mapsto 1$;
$f: 1 \mapsto 1$, $2 \mapsto 3$, $3 \mapsto 2$.

(i) In the symmetric group $S_3 = \langle X_3, \circ, e \rangle$, find r^2, rf, and r^2f in arrow form.
(ii) Is $\{e, r, r^2, f, rf, r^2f\}$ the set X_3 of all permutations on T_3?
(iii) Show that $fr = r^2f$ and then make the operation table for S_3 using the notation of Part (ii) for the permutations in X_3.
(iv) Using the table of Part (iii), find the sets of integral powers $[e]$, $[r^2]$, and $[rf]$, where $[x]$ is as in Definition 6 of Section 7.1.

18. (a) Using the notation of Problem 17, find $[r]$, $[f]$, and $[r^2f]$.
(b) Use the table of Problem 17(iii) and Algorithm 2 ("Proving a Group Isomorphism") to show that there is an isomorphism β from S_3 to the group of Example 6 in Section 7.1 with $\beta(r) = f_2$ and $\beta(f) = f_4$.
(c) Find permutations α, β, and γ on $\{1, 2, 3\}$ such that $\gamma\alpha = \beta\gamma$ but $\alpha \neq \beta$ and thus show that "mixed cancellation" need not be valid in a nonabelian group.

19. Let

$f: T_4 \to T_4$; $1 \mapsto 2$, $2 \mapsto 3$, $3 \mapsto 4$, $4 \mapsto 1$.

Find the subset Y of smallest size in X_4 such that $f \in Y$, and $\langle Y, \circ, e \rangle$ is a subgroup in the symmetric group $S_4 = \langle X_4, \circ, e \rangle$.

20. Do as in Problem 19, but with f now given by

$f: 1 \mapsto 3$, $2 \mapsto 4$, $3 \mapsto 1$, $4 \mapsto 2$.

21. Let $U_4 = \{1, i, -1, -i\}$ and $G = \langle U_4, \cdot, 1 \rangle$ be the group of Example 1 in Section 7.1. Let $G' = \langle Y, \circ, e \rangle$ be the group of Problem 19.
(a) Explain why

$\alpha: 1 \mapsto e$, $i \mapsto f$, $-1 \mapsto f^2$, $-i \mapsto f^3$

is a group isomorphism from G onto G'.

(b) Show that

$$\beta: 1 \mapsto e, \quad \mathbf{i} \mapsto f^2, \quad -1 \mapsto f^3, \quad -\mathbf{i} \mapsto f$$

is not a group isomorphism from G onto G'.

22. Let $U_2 = \{1, -1\}$ and G be the multiplicative group $\langle U_2, \cdot, 1 \rangle$. Let S_2 be the symmetric group of Example 3.
(a) Show that

$$\alpha: 1 \mapsto e, \quad -1 \mapsto f$$

is a group isomorphism from G onto S_2.
(b) Show that

$$\beta: 1 \mapsto f, \quad -1 \mapsto e$$

is not a group isomorphism from G onto S_2.

23. Let $G = \langle X, \square, e \rangle$ and $G' = \langle X', \triangle, e' \rangle$ be groups of order 2 with $X = \{e, a\}$ and $X' = \{e', b\}$.
  (i) Explain why $e \,\square\, a = a$ and $a \,\square\, a = e$.
  (ii) Make the operation tables for G and G'.
  (iii) Explain why G and G' are isomorphic.

24. Prove that any two groups G and G' of order 3 are isomorphic.

25. Let f be a permutation on $T_n = \{1, 2, \ldots, n\}$. Let $a_1 \in T_n$, $a_2 = f(a_1)$, $a_3 = f(a_2)$, and so on. Explain why:
  (i) $a_i = a_j$ for some i and j with $1 \le i < j$.
  (ii) If j is the smallest positive integer such that $a_i = a_j$ for some i with $1 \le i < j$, then this i must be 1.

26. Let f be a permutation on $T_n = \{1, 2, \ldots, n\}$. Let $a_1, b_1 \in T_n$ and let sequences $a_1, a_2, \ldots$ and $b_1, b_2, \ldots$ be defined inductively by $a_{k+1} = f(a_k)$ and $b_{k+1} = f(b_k)$ for all k in Z^+. Prove that either (i) no term a_i equals a term b_j or (ii) each term a_i equals a term b_j and each b_j equals an a_i.

27. Find 6 subsets A_i of the set $X_3 = \{e, r, r^2, f, rf, r^2f\}$ of Problem 17 such that $\langle A_i, \circ, e \rangle$ is a subgroup in S_3 for $1 \le i \le 6$.

28. For the A_i of Problem 27, let $\Gamma = \{A_1, A_2, A_3, A_4, A_5, A_6\}$. Draw the poset diagram for $(\Gamma, \subseteq)$. (It happens to be the subgroup poset diagram for S_3.) What are the minimal and maximal elements of the poset $(\Gamma, \subseteq)$?

29. Let $\beta: X \to X'$ be an isomorphism from $G = \langle X, \square, e \rangle$ onto $G' = \langle X', \triangle, e' \rangle$. Prove that each x in X has the same order in G as its image $\beta(x)$ has in G'. (This is the proof of Theorem 6 that was left to the reader.)

30. Let $U_8 = \{1, u, u^2, \ldots, u^7\}$ be the set of all eight 8th roots of 1. (This implies that 8 is the smallest positive integer n with $u^n = 1$.) Prove that the groups $G = \langle U_8, \cdot, 1 \rangle$ and $G' = \langle B_3, \oplus, 000 \rangle$ are not isomorphic.

31. Let $G = \langle [a], \square, e \rangle$ and $G' = \langle [b], \triangle, e' \rangle$ be cyclic groups of order 5. Prove that G and G' are isomorphic.

32. Prove that cyclic groups $G = \langle [a], \square, e \rangle$ and $G' = \langle [b], \triangle, e' \rangle$ are isomorphic if and only if they have the same order.

33. Let $G = \langle [a], \square, e \rangle$ and $G' = \langle Y, \triangle, e' \rangle$ be isomorphic groups with G cyclic. Prove that G' is cyclic.

7.3

CYCLE NOTATION

The notations for permutations used in the previous section are standard notations for mappings. A permutation is a special kind of mapping in that its codomain is the same as its domain and it is bijective. These special properties make possible a notation, given in Definition 3 below, that is less cumbersome and is especially suited for certain applications. But first we need the following notation for some special permutations.

DEFINITION 1 **CYCLE, TRANSPOSITION**

Let $\{a_1, a_2, \ldots, a_s\}$ be a listing for a subset A of $T_n = \{1, 2, \ldots, n\}$. Then

$$g = (a_1 \quad a_2 \quad \ldots \quad a_s)$$

denotes the permutation g on T_n with

$$g(a_i) = a_{i+1} \quad \text{for } 1 \leq i < s,$$
$$g(a_s) = a_1,$$

and

$$g(t) = t \quad \text{for } t \text{ not in } A.$$

Such a permutation is an **s-cycle** (or a **cycle** of **length** s). A 2-cycle is also called a **transposition**.

Example 1 Let

$$f = \begin{pmatrix} 1 & 2 & 3 & 4 & 5 \\ 4 & 2 & 1 & 3 & 5 \end{pmatrix}.$$

Since $f(1) = 4$, $f(4) = 3$, $f(3) = 1$, and $f(t) = t$ when t is not in the set $\{1, 4, 3\}$, it follows from Definition 1 that f can be represented by any one of the 3-cycles

$$(1 \quad 4 \quad 3), \quad (4 \quad 3 \quad 1), \quad \text{or} \quad (3 \quad 1 \quad 4).$$

Each of these cycle representations indicates that f is in some X_n with $n \geq 4$ but does not give the n any more specifically. $\square$

Example 2   **THE SYMMETRIC GROUP $S_2 = \langle X_2, \circ, (1) \rangle$**   The set of permutations on $\{1, 2\}$ is $X_2 = \{e, f\}$, where

$$e: 1 \mapsto 1, \quad 2 \mapsto 2 \quad \text{and} \quad f: 1 \mapsto 2, \quad 2 \mapsto 1.$$

It follows from Definition 1 that e can be written as the 1-cycle (1) or as the 1-cycle (2). It also follows that f is the transposition (1   2).   □

Example 3   **THE SYMMETRIC GROUP $S_3 = \langle X_3, \circ, (1) \rangle$**   Using the notation of Problem 17(ii) of Section 7.2, the set of permutations on $\{1, 2, 3\}$ is $X_3 = \{e, r, r^2, f, rf, r^2f\}$, where the previous notation and the new cycle notation for e, r, and f are as follows:

Old Notation	Cycle Notation
$e: 1 \mapsto 1, \quad 2 \mapsto 2, \quad 3 \mapsto 3$	(1) or (2) or (3)
$r: 1 \mapsto 2, \quad 2 \mapsto 3, \quad 3 \mapsto 1$	(1 2 3)
$f: 1 \mapsto 1, \quad 2 \mapsto 3, \quad 3 \mapsto 2$	(2 3)

One sees from

$$1 \overset{r}{\mapsto} 2 \overset{r}{\mapsto} 3, \quad 2 \overset{r}{\mapsto} 3 \overset{r}{\mapsto} 1, \quad 3 \overset{r}{\mapsto} 1 \overset{r}{\mapsto} 2$$

that

$$r^2: 1 \mapsto 3, \quad 2 \mapsto 1, \quad 3 \mapsto 2.$$

This shows that r^2 is the 3-cycle (1   3   2). Also,

$$1 \overset{r}{\mapsto} 2 \overset{f}{\mapsto} 3, \quad 2 \overset{r}{\mapsto} 3 \overset{f}{\mapsto} 2, \quad 3 \overset{r}{\mapsto} 1 \overset{f}{\mapsto} 1$$

shows that

$$rf: 1 \mapsto 3, \quad 2 \mapsto 2, \quad 3 \mapsto 1.$$

Hence, in cycle notation, one has $rf = (1 \quad 3)$. Similarly, one can show that $r^2f = (1 \quad 2)$.

     Problem 17(iii) of Section 7.2 asked for the operation table for S_3. In Table 7.3.1, we give that table in cycle notation.

TABLE 7.3.1   **Operation Table for the Symmetric Group S_3**

$\circ$	(1)	(1 2 3)	(1 3 2)	(2 3)	(1 3)	(1 2)
$e = (1)$	(1)	(1 2 3)	(1 3 2)	(2 3)	(1 3)	(1 2)
$r = (1 \ 2 \ 3)$	(1 2 3)	(1 3 2)	(1)	(1 3)	(1 2)	(2 3)
$r^2 = (1 \ 3 \ 2)$	(1 3 2)	(1)	(1 2 3)	(1 2)	(2 3)	(1 3)
$f = (2 \ 3)$	(2 3)	(1 2)	(1 3)	(1)	(1 3 2)	(1 2 3)
$rf = (1 \ 3)$	(1 3)	(2 3)	(1 2)	(1 2 3)	(1)	(1 3 2)
$r^2f = (1 \ 2)$	(1 2)	(1 3)	(2 3)	(1 3 2)	(1 2 3)	(1)

□

DEFINITION 2   **DISJOINT CYCLES**

In a symmetric group $S_n = \langle X_n, \circ, e \rangle$, let $f = (a_1 \quad a_2 \quad \ldots \quad a_r)$, $g = (b_1 \quad b_2 \quad \ldots \quad b_s), \ldots$, and $h = (c_1 \quad c_2 \quad \ldots \quad c_t)$ be cycles such that $\{a_1, \ldots, a_r\}$, $\{b_1, \ldots, b_s\}, \ldots$, and $\{c_1, \ldots, c_t\}$ are disjoint sets. Then $f, g, \ldots, h$ are said to be ***disjoint cycles***.

Example 4   In the symmetric group $S_4 = \langle X_4, \circ, (1) \rangle$, let

$$f: 1 \mapsto 2, \quad 2 \mapsto 1, \quad 3 \mapsto 3, \quad 4 \mapsto 4,$$
$$g: 1 \mapsto 1, \quad 2 \mapsto 2, \quad 3 \mapsto 4, \quad 4 \mapsto 3.$$

In cycle notation, $f = (1 \quad 2)$ and $g = (3 \quad 4)$. Using

$$1 \overset{f}{\mapsto} 2 \overset{g}{\mapsto} 2, \quad 2 \overset{f}{\mapsto} 1 \overset{g}{\mapsto} 1, \quad 3 \overset{f}{\mapsto} 3 \overset{g}{\mapsto} 4, \quad 4 \overset{f}{\mapsto} 4 \overset{g}{\mapsto} 3,$$

one sees that

$$fg: 1 \mapsto 2, \quad 2 \mapsto 1, \quad 3 \mapsto 4, \quad 4 \mapsto 3.$$

This permutation fg is not a cycle because it is not one of the special permutations described in Definition 1. However, $fg = (1 \quad 2)(3 \quad 4)$ is a product of disjoint cycles. Using the results in Problems 25 and 26 of Section 7.2, one can show that every permutation on $\{1, 2, \ldots, n\}$ is either a cycle or a product of disjoint cycles. The algorithm for getting such a cycle representation is illustrated in Example 5 below.   □

THEOREM 1   **DISJOINT CYCLES COMMUTE**

Let $f = (a_1 \quad a_2 \quad \ldots \quad a_r)$ and $g = (b_1 \quad b_2 \quad \ldots \quad b_s)$ be a pair of disjoint cycles in X_n. Then $fg = gf$.

PROOF   Let $h = fg$ and $k = gf$. No a_i is a b_j. Thus

$$a_i \overset{f}{\mapsto} a_{i+1} \overset{g}{\mapsto} a_{i+1} \Rightarrow a_i \overset{h}{\mapsto} a_{i+1},$$
$$a_i \overset{g}{\mapsto} a_i \overset{f}{\mapsto} a_{i+1} \Rightarrow a_i \overset{k}{\mapsto} a_{i+1}$$

shows that $h(a_i) = k(a_i)$ for $i = 1, 2, \ldots, r - 1$. Similarly one can see that $h(t) = k(t)$ for all t in T_n; that is, $fg = gf$. (See Problems 19 and 20 below for parts of the remaining details.)   □

For example, it follows from Theorem 1 that

$$(1 \quad 4 \quad 3)(2 \quad 5) = (2 \quad 5)(1 \quad 4 \quad 3).$$

THEOREM 2 **POWERS OF AN s-CYCLE**

Let $c = (a_1 \quad a_2 \quad \ldots \quad a_s)$ be an s-cycle. Then c^s equals the identity (1) and, for each integer n, $c^n = c^r$ where r is the remainder in the division of n by s.

PROOF   For a 1-cycle $c = (a_1)$, Definition 1 tells us that $c(a_1) = a_1$ and that $c(t) = t$ for $t \neq a_1$. Thus $c(t) = t$ for all t in T_n; this means that (a_1) is the identity (1). Now let c be a transposition $(a_1 \quad a_2)$ and let $c^2 = d$. Then $d(a_1) = c(c(a_1)) = c(a_2) = a_1$, $d(a_2) = c(c(a_2)) = c(a_1) = a_2$, and $d(t) = c(c(t)) = c(t) = t$ for all t not in $\{a_1, a_2\}$. Hence $d(t) = t$ for all t in T_n, and so $d = c^2 = (1)$ when c is a transposition.

In the general case in which c is an s-cycle, one sees similarly that $c^s = (1)$. Now let $n \in Z$. The "Division Algorithm" (Algorithm 1 of Section 1.7) expresses n as $n = qs + r$, where q and r are integers and $r \in \{0, 1, \ldots, s - 1\}$. Then

$$c^n = c^{qs+r} = (c^s)^q c^r = (1)^q c^r = (1)c^r = c^r.$$

Thus $c^n = c^r$, where r is the remainder in the division of n by s.   □

COROLLARY **SET [c] OF INTEGRAL POWERS OF AN s-CYCLE c**

If c is an s-cycle, then

$$[c] = \{c^n : n \in Z\} = \{(1), c, c^2, \ldots, c^{s-1}\}.$$

Example 5   In S_{10}, let

$$f = \begin{pmatrix} 1 & 2 & 3 & 4 & 5 & 6 & 7 & 8 & 9 & 10 \\ 7 & 5 & 3 & 1 & 10 & 8 & 9 & 6 & 4 & 2 \end{pmatrix}.$$

The following algorithm expresses f as a product of disjoint cycles. First we inductively define a sequence $a_1, a_2, \ldots$ by

$$a_1 = 1, \quad a_{k+1} = f(a_k) \quad \text{for all } k \text{ in } Z^+ = \{1, 2, 3, \ldots\}.$$

Using the matrix form of f, we see that this sequence is

1, 7, 9, 4, 1, 7, 9, 4, 1, 7, 9, 4, ...

This indicates that $(1 \quad 7 \quad 9 \quad 4)$ is the first of the cycles we are seeking. Since 2 is the smallest integer of T_{10} not in $A = \{1, 7, 9, 4\}$, we use it to start a new sequence as follows:

$$b_1 = 2, \quad b_{k+1} = f(b_k) \quad \text{for all } k \text{ in } Z^+.$$

The matrix form of f shows that this new sequence is

2, 5, 10, 2, 5, 10, ...

Thus our second cycle is (2 5 10). Let $B = \{2, 5, 10\}$. Since 3 is the smallest integer of T_{10} not in $A \cup B$, we use it to find the next cycle, which turns out to be just the cycle (3). Similarly we find that the remaining cycle is (6 8). The reader can easily verify that the product

$$(1 \quad 7 \quad 9 \quad 4)(2 \quad 5 \quad 10)(3)(6 \quad 8) \tag{1}$$

of disjoint cycles is the f given above. Figure 7.3.1 is a picture of the digraph D_f for this permutation.

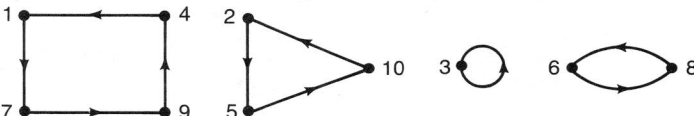

FIGURE 7.3.1

The picture clearly shows $f(t)$ for every t in T_{10}, and Display (1) compactly contains the relevant information of the figure. □

Using the results in Problems 25 and 26 of Section 7.2 and the technique illustrated in Example 5, one can show that any permutation on $T_n = \{1, 2, \ldots, n\}$ is a cycle or a product of disjoint cycles. Since

$$(a_1 \quad a_2 \quad \ldots \quad a_r) = (a_2 \quad a_3 \quad \ldots \quad a_r \quad a_1)$$
$$= (a_3 \quad a_4 \quad \ldots \quad a_r \quad a_1 \quad a_2)$$

and so on, and since disjoint cycles commute, there can be a number of ways of expressing a given permutation in such form. It is helpful to restrict the expression to the following unique form.

DEFINITION 3 **CANONICAL FORM FOR A PERMUTATION**

Let a permutation f on T_n be a product

$$(a_1 \quad a_2 \quad \ldots \quad a_r)(b_1 \quad b_2 \quad \ldots \quad b_s) \cdots (c_1 \quad c_2 \quad \ldots \quad c_t) \tag{2}$$

of disjoint cycles. Then Display (2) is the **canonical form** of f if f is not the identity; $a_1 < a_i$ for $2 \leq i \leq r$; $b_1 < b_j$ for $2 \leq j \leq s, \ldots$; $c_1 < c_k$ for $2 \leq k \leq t$; $a_1 < b_1 < \cdots < c_1$; and there are no 1-cycles in Display (2). The canonical form of the identity permutation is (1).

Example 6 Let $f = (5 \quad 2 \quad 7)(4 \quad 1)$. Since $(5 \quad 2 \quad 7) = (2 \quad 7 \quad 5)$, $(4 \quad 1) = (1 \quad 4)$, and disjoint cycles commute, it follows that $f = (1 \quad 4)(2 \quad 7 \quad 5)$. This is the canonical form of f because

$$f \neq e, \qquad 1 < 4, \qquad 2 < 7, \qquad 2 < 5, \qquad \text{and} \qquad 1 < 2;$$

that is, this representation satisfies the conditions of Definition 3. Now let $g = (2 \quad 4 \quad 7)(5 \quad 6 \quad 7)(1 \quad 3)$. Since these cycles are not disjoint (7 appears in two of them), we let $b = (2 \quad 4 \quad 7)$, $c = (5 \quad 6 \quad 7)$, and use the technique of Example 5 to find the canonical form of $d = bc$, as follows:

$$2 \overset{b}{\mapsto} 4 \overset{c}{\mapsto} 4 \Rightarrow 2 \overset{d}{\mapsto} 4; \qquad 4 \overset{b}{\mapsto} 7 \overset{c}{\mapsto} 5 \Rightarrow 4 \overset{d}{\mapsto} 5;$$

$$5 \overset{b}{\mapsto} 5 \overset{c}{\mapsto} 6 \Rightarrow 5 \overset{d}{\mapsto} 6; \qquad 6 \overset{b}{\mapsto} 6 \overset{c}{\mapsto} 7 \Rightarrow 6 \overset{d}{\mapsto} 7;$$

$$7 \overset{b}{\mapsto} 2 \overset{c}{\mapsto} 2 \Rightarrow 7 \overset{d}{\mapsto} 2.$$

Hence

$$d = bc = (2 \quad 4 \quad 7)(5 \quad 6 \quad 7) = (2 \quad 4 \quad 5 \quad 6 \quad 7),$$

and so $g = (2 \quad 4 \quad 5 \quad 6 \quad 7)(1 \quad 3)$. The canonical form of g is $(1 \quad 3)(2 \quad 4 \quad 5 \quad 6 \quad 7)$. $\qquad\square$

Example 7   We wish to show that the special products

$$(1 \quad 2)(1 \quad 3) \qquad \text{and} \qquad (1 \quad 2)(1 \quad 3)(1 \quad 4)$$

of transpositions can be rewritten as cycles. Let $a = (1 \quad 2)$, $b = (1 \quad 3)$, $c = (1 \quad 4)$, $d = ab$, and $f = dc$. Then

$$(1 \overset{a}{\mapsto} 2 \overset{b}{\mapsto} 2) \Rightarrow (1 \overset{d}{\mapsto} 2), \qquad (2 \overset{a}{\mapsto} 1 \overset{b}{\mapsto} 3) \Rightarrow (2 \overset{d}{\mapsto} 3),$$

$$(3 \overset{a}{\mapsto} 3 \overset{b}{\mapsto} 1) \Rightarrow (3 \overset{d}{\mapsto} 1).$$

This helps us see that $(1 \quad 2)(1 \quad 3) = (1 \quad 2 \quad 3)$. Similarly, we find that $abc = dc = f = (1 \quad 2 \quad 3 \quad 4)$; that is,

$$(1 \quad 2)(1 \quad 3)(1 \quad 4) = (1 \quad 2 \quad 3)(1 \quad 4) = (1 \quad 2 \quad 3 \quad 4). \qquad\square$$

Example 8   Let c be the 6-cycle $(1 \quad 2 \quad 3 \quad 4 \quad 5 \quad 6)$ in some S_n with $n \geq 6$. Let $G = \langle [c], \circ, (1) \rangle$ be the subgroup generated by c in S_n. The corollary to Theorem 2 ("Set $[c]$ of Integral Powers of an s-Cycle c") tells us that

$$[c] = \{c^n : n \in \mathbf{Z}\} = \{(1), c, c^2, c^3, c^4, c^5\}.$$

Let $d = c^2$. Then

$$[d] = \{d^n : n \in \mathbf{Z}\} = \{c^{2n} : n \in \mathbf{Z}\} = \{(1), c^2, c^4\}$$

since $d^0 = (1)$, $d = c^2$, $d^2 = c^4$, $d^3 = c^6 = (1)$, $d^4 = c^8 = c^2$, $d^{-1} = c^{-2} = c^4$, $d^{-2} = c^{-4} = c^2$, and so on. Similarly, one can show that

$$[c^3] = \{(1), c^3\}, \qquad [c^4] = [c^2], \qquad \text{and} \qquad [c^5] = [c]. \qquad\square$$

Example 9 In S_9 let $f = (1 \quad 3 \quad 5 \quad 7)(2 \quad 4 \quad 6)$, $g = (1 \quad 2 \quad 3 \quad 4 \quad 5)$, and $h = fg$. We seek the order of this product h. It seems helpful to express h as a cycle or product of disjoint cycles. To do this, we let $c = (1 \quad 3 \quad 5 \quad 7)$ and $d = (2 \quad 4 \quad 6)$. Then $f = cd$ and $h = cdg$. Now

$$1 \xmapsto{c} 3 \xmapsto{d} 3 \xmapsto{g} 4 \Rightarrow 1 \xmapsto{h} 4; \qquad 4 \xmapsto{c} 4 \xmapsto{d} 6 \xmapsto{g} 6 \Rightarrow 4 \xmapsto{h} 6;$$

$$6 \xmapsto{c} 6 \xmapsto{d} 2 \xmapsto{g} 3 \Rightarrow 6 \xmapsto{h} 3; \qquad 3 \xmapsto{c} 5 \xmapsto{d} 5 \xmapsto{g} 1 \Rightarrow 3 \xmapsto{h} 1.$$

Thus $(1 \quad 4 \quad 6 \quad 3)$ is the first of the disjoint cycles for h. Similarly we find that $h(2) = 5$, $h(5) = 7$, and $h(7) = 2$. Hence the desired product of disjoint cycles is $h = uv$, where $u = (1 \quad 4 \quad 6 \quad 3)$ and $v = (2 \quad 5 \quad 7)$. Since u and v are disjoint, they commute, and hence

$$h^2 = (uv)^2 = uvuv = u^2v^2 = (1 \quad 6)(4 \quad 3)(2 \quad 7 \quad 5),$$
$$h^3 = u^3v^3 = (1 \quad 3 \quad 6 \quad 4),$$
$$h^4 = u^4v^4 = (2 \quad 5 \quad 7),$$
$$h^5 = (1 \quad 4 \quad 6 \quad 3)(2 \quad 7 \quad 5),$$
$$h^6 = (1 \quad 6)(4 \quad 3).$$

These cases illustrate the fact that, for every n in $\mathbf{Z}$, $h^n = u^r v^s$ where r and s are the remainders in the division of n by 4 and by 3, respectively. Hence $h^n = (1)$ if and only if both $4 | n$ and $3 | n$, that is, if and only if $12 | n$. Then Theorem 6 of Section 7.1 tells us that

$$\{h^n : n \in \mathbf{Z}\} = \{(1), h, h^2, \ldots, h^{11}\}$$

and hence that h has order 12. $\square$

An important procedure in computer science is the sorting of data. A key result on algorithms for sorting is that any rearrangement of the terms of a sequence $a_1, a_2, \ldots, a_n$ can be performed just by some finite number of interchanges of pairs of terms. The formal statement of this in terms of permutations is Part (b) of the following theorem.

THEOREM 3 **PRODUCT OF TRANSPOSITIONS**

(a) Every s-cycle $(a_1 \quad a_2 \quad \ldots \quad a_s)$ is the product

$$(a_1 \quad a_2)(a_1 \quad a_3)(a_1 \quad a_4) \cdots (a_1 \quad a_s)$$

of $s - 1$ transpositions. Here $s \geq 3$.

(b) If $n \geq 2$, every permutation on $\{1, 2, \ldots, n\}$ is a transposition or a product of transpositions.

PROOF   (a) We prove this by mathematical induction on s.

Basis   For $s = 3$ we have to prove that

$$(a_1 \quad a_2 \quad a_3) = (a_1 \quad a_2)(a_1 \quad a_3).$$

This is similar to part of Example 7 and is left to the reader.

Inductive Step   Let $k \in \{3, 4, \ldots\}$ and assume that

$$(a_1 \quad a_2)(a_1 \quad a_3) \cdots (a_1 \quad a_k) = (a_1 \quad a_2 \quad a_3 \quad \ldots \quad a_k).$$

Then

$$(a_1 \quad a_2)(a_1 \quad a_3) \cdots (a_1 \quad a_{k+1}) = (a_1 \quad a_2 \quad \ldots \quad a_k)(a_1 \quad a_{k+1}).$$

Let $f = (a_1 \quad a_2 \quad \ldots \quad a_k)$, $g = (a_1 \quad a_{k+1})$, and $h = fg$. Then

$$(a_1 \overset{f}{\mapsto} a_2 \overset{g}{\mapsto} a_2) \Rightarrow (a_1 \overset{h}{\mapsto} a_2),$$

and similarly $a_i \overset{h}{\mapsto} a_{i+1}$ for $i = 2, 3, \ldots, k - 1$. Also,

$$(a_k \overset{f}{\mapsto} a_1 \overset{g}{\mapsto} a_{k+1}) \Rightarrow (a_k \overset{h}{\mapsto} a_{k+1}),$$

$$(a_{k+1} \overset{f}{\mapsto} a_{k+1} \overset{g}{\mapsto} a_1) \Rightarrow (a_{k+1} \overset{h}{\mapsto} a_1).$$

All together, these help us see that

$$h = (a_1 \quad a_2 \quad \ldots \quad a_{k+1}).$$

This completes the induction.

(b) Let f be a permutation on $\{1, 2, \ldots, n\}$. The canonical form for f is a product $g_1 g_2 \cdots g_r$ of cycles. Using the result in Part (a), we can replace each cycle g_i of length greater than 2 by a product of transpositions. If f is not the identity (1), this rewrites f as a transposition or product of transpositions. If f is the identity (1) and $n \geq 2$, we write f as the product $(1 \quad 2)(1 \quad 2)$ of transpositions.   □

Let us agree that for $r = 1$ a product of r transpositions is just a transposition. Then Theorem 3(b) asserts that every permutation on $\{1, 2, \ldots, n\}$ is a product of transpositions when $n \geq 2$. The transpositions in such a product are not necessarily disjoint. Also, there are many such products for a given permutation. For example,

$$(1 \quad 2 \quad 3) = (1 \quad 2)(1 \quad 3) = (1 \quad 3)(2 \quad 3).$$

Since $(1 \quad 2)(1 \quad 2)$ is the identity (1), we can also write

$$(1 \quad 2 \quad 3) = (1 \quad 2)(1 \quad 2)(1 \quad 2)(1 \quad 3)$$
$$= (1 \quad 3)(2 \quad 3)(1 \quad 2)(1 \quad 2).$$

In this way we can obtain an infinite number of expressions for the given permutation (1 2 3) as a product of transpositions. One thing that we can prove about any possible expression for (1 2 3) as a product $g_1 g_2 \cdots g_u$ of transpositions is that the number u of transpositions must be even. This is done in Theorem 5 below which also implies that whenever (1 2 3 4) = (1 2)(1 3)(1 4) is expressed as a product $h_1 h_2 \cdots h_v$ of transpositions, the number v of transpositions is odd.

THEOREM 4   **(1) AS A PRODUCT OF TRANSPOSITIONS**

Let $(1) = t_1 t_2 \cdots t_m$, where each t_i is a transposition. Then the number m of transpositions must be even.

PROOF   Let $T = \{1, 2, \ldots, n\}$. Also, assume that $n \geq 2$, since there are no transpositions in X_n when $n = 1$. In the expression $(1) = t_1 t_2 \cdots t_m$ for the identity as a product of transpositions, let k be some integer of T that appears in at least one of these transpositions. [That is, one of the transpositions has the form $(j \quad k)$ or the form $(k \quad j)$.] Let t_i be the first of the transpositions in which k appears. If t_i were t_m, the integer k would be mapped to itself by each of $t_1, t_2, \ldots, t_{m-1}$ and then sent to some other integer by t_m. This is not possible because $t_1 t_2 \cdots t_m = (1)$ and the identity (1) sends k to itself. Therefore $i < m$. Now let us consider $t_i t_{i+1}$. Either k appears in both t_i and t_{i+1} or it appears only in t_i, and we can express $t_i t_{i+1}$ in one of four ways:

$(k \quad a)(k \quad a) = (1)$

or

$(k \quad a)(k \quad b) = (a \quad b)(a \quad k)$

or

$(k \quad a)(a \quad b) = (a \quad b)(b \quad k)$

or

$(k \quad a)(b \quad c) = (b \quad c)(a \quad k), \qquad a, b, c \in T.$

If we then substitute the appropriate expression on the right for the pair of transpositions on the left in $(1) = t_1 t_2 \cdots t_m$, we will succeed in pushing the first appearance of k one transposition to the right or eliminating it altogether. If k is not eliminated by applying the first of the above substitutions, we continue until we do succeed in eliminating k completely. It cannot appear in t_m only, as we have already seen, so sooner or later, for any k, we have to substitute the cycle (1) for $t_i t_{i+1}$. We do this for all the values of k and end up with $(1) = (1)(1) \cdots (1)$. But since the number of transpositions remains the same or is reduced by two at each step, we must have had an even number of transpositions in the beginning.   □

THEOREM 5   **PRESERVATION OF PARITY**

Let p be a permutation on $\{1, 2, \ldots, n\}$ and let $p = g_1 g_2 \cdots g_u = h_1 h_2 \cdots h_v$, where each g_i and each h_j is a transposition. Then u and v are both even or are both odd.

PROOF   Using the hypothesis, one has

$$(1) = pp^{-1} = (g_1 g_2 \cdots g_u)(h_1 h_2 \cdots h_v)^{-1}.$$

Since $(h_1 h_2 \cdots h_v)^{-1} = h_v^{-1} h_{v-1}^{-1} \cdots h_1^{-1}$ and each transposition is its own inverse, this becomes

$$(1) = g_1 g_2 \cdots g_u h_v h_{v-1} \cdots h_1.$$

It follows from Theorem 4 that the number $u + v$ of transpositions in this representation for the identity is even. Since $u + v$ is even, both u and v are even or both are odd.   □

DEFINITION 4   **EVEN PERMUTATION, ODD PERMUTATION**

In a symmetric group $S_n = \langle X_n, \circ, (1) \rangle$, a permutation f is **even** if f is expressible as the product of an even number of transpositions and f is **odd** if it is expressible as the product of an odd number of transpositions. In S_1, the only permutation (1) is said to be even.

Thus (1 2 3) is an even permutation, since it is the product (1 2)(1 3) of an even number of transpositions, and (1 2 3)(3 4) = (1 2)(1 3)(3 4) is an odd permutation, since it is the product of an odd number of transpositions.

In Problem 32 below, the reader is asked to show that the subset E_n of all even permutations in X_n is nonempty and is closed under division. Given that this is so, it follows from Theorem 8 of Section 7.1 ("Nonempty Subset Closed under Division") that $\langle E_n, \circ, (1) \rangle$ is a subgroup in the symmetric group S_n.

NOTATION 1   **SET E_n OF EVEN PERMUTATIONS, ALTERNATING SUBGROUP A_n**

E_n denotes the set of all even permutations in X_n. The subgroup $\langle E_n, \circ, (1) \rangle$ in S_n is denoted A_n and is called the **alternating subgroup in S_n**.

PROBLEMS FOR SECTION 7.3

1. Express

    $$f: 1 \mapsto 9, \quad 2 \mapsto 8, \quad 3 \mapsto 5, \quad 4 \mapsto 4, \quad 5 \mapsto 1,$$
    $$6 \mapsto 6, \quad 7 \mapsto 3, \quad 8 \mapsto 2, \quad 9 \mapsto 7$$

    as a product of disjoint cycles.

2. Express each of the following as a cycle or product of disjoint cycles:
    (a) $f: 1 \mapsto 6, \quad 2 \mapsto 5, \quad 3 \mapsto 4, \quad 4 \mapsto 1, \quad 5 \mapsto 3, \quad 6 \mapsto 7, \quad 7 \mapsto 2.$
    (b) $g: 1 \mapsto 3, \quad 2 \mapsto 6, \quad 3 \mapsto 1, \quad 4 \mapsto 5, \quad 5 \mapsto 2, \quad 6 \mapsto 4.$

3. In S_4, let $r = (1 \quad 2 \quad 3 \quad 4)$, and $f = (2 \quad 4)$. Express each of the following as a cycle or product of disjoint cycles:
    (i) r^2; (ii) r^3; (iii) r^4; (iv) rf; (v) $r^2 f$.

4. In S_4, let $r = (1 \quad 2 \quad 3 \quad 4)$ and $f = (2 \quad 4)$. Show that $r^{-1} = r^3$ and that $fr = r^3 f$.

5. In S_4, let $b = (1 \quad 2)(3 \quad 4)$, $c = (1 \quad 3)(2 \quad 4)$, $d = bc$, and $g = (1 \quad 2 \quad 3)$. Express each of the following as a cycle or product of disjoint cycles:
    (i) d; (ii) gb; (iii) gc; (iv) gd;
    (v) g^2; (vi) $g^2 b$; (vii) $g^2 c$; (viii) $g^2 d$.

6. Let b, c, and d be as in Problem 5. Show that:
    (a) $b^2 = c^2 = d^2 = (1)$.
    (b) $cb = d$, $bd = c = db$, and $cd = b = dc$.

7. Let b, c, and d be as in Problem 5 and let $Y = \{(1), b, c, d\}$. Show that $G = \langle Y, \circ, (1) \rangle$ is a subgroup in S_4 and make its table.

8. Let r and f be as in Problems 3 and 4. Let $W = \{(1), r, r^2, r^3, f, rf, r^2 f, r^3 f\}$. After making its table, show that $\langle W, \circ, (1) \rangle$ is a subgroup in S_4.

9. In S_8, let $h = (1 \quad 2 \quad 3 \quad 4 \quad 5 \quad 6 \quad 7 \quad 8)$. Express each of the following as a cycle or product of disjoint cycles:
    (i) h^2; (ii) h^3; (iii) h^4; (iv) h^5.

10. Let h be as in Problem 9. Do as in Problem 9 for:
    (i) h^6; (ii) h^7; (iii) h^8.

11. Let h be as in Problem 9.
    (a) Explain why $[h^2] = \{(1), h^2, h^4, h^6\}$.
    (b) Express $[h^4]$ similarly.

12. Let h be as in Problem 9.
    (a) For which m in $\{0, 1, 3, 4, 5, 6, 7\}$ does $[h^m] = [h^2]$?
    (b) For which m's in $\{0, 1, \ldots, 7\}$ is h^m a generator of $\langle [h], \circ, (1) \rangle$?

13. Express each of the following as a cycle:
    (i) $(1 \quad 2)(1 \quad 3)$. (ii) $(1 \quad 2)(1 \quad 3)(1 \quad 4)$.
    (iii) $(1 \quad 2)(1 \quad 3)(1 \quad 4)(1 \quad 5)$.

14. Express each of the following as a cycle:
(i) $(1 \quad 3)(2 \quad 3)$.   (ii) $(1 \quad 4)(2 \quad 4)(3 \quad 4)$.
(iii) $(1 \quad 5)(2 \quad 5)(3 \quad 5)(4 \quad 5)$.

15. Express $(1 \quad 2 \quad 3 \quad 4 \quad 5 \quad 6)$ as a product of five transpositions. (They will not be disjoint.)

16. Express $(1 \quad 2 \quad 3 \quad 4 \quad 5 \quad 6 \quad 7)$ as a product of six transpositions.

17. Let f, g, and h be three disjoint cycles in S_n. Does $fgh = ghf$? Explain.

18. Prove that S_n is nonabelian for $n \geq 3$.

19. Let $f = (a_1 \quad a_2 \quad \ldots \quad a_r)$ and $g = (b_1 \quad b_2 \quad \ldots \quad b_s)$ be disjoint cycles in X_n. Let $h = fg$ and $k = gf$. Without using Theorem 1, explain why:
(i) $f(b_j) = b_j$ for $j = 1, 2, \ldots, s$.
(ii) $h(b_j) = k(b_j)$ for $j = 1, 2, \ldots, s$.

20. Let f, g, h, and k be as in Problem 19. Without using Theorem 1, explain why $h(t) = k(t)$ for all integers t that are in $\{1, 2, \ldots, n\}$ but not in $\{a_1, a_2, \ldots, a_r\} \cup \{b_1, b_2, \ldots, b_s\}$.

21. Let $u = (1 \quad 2 \quad 3)$ and $v = (1 \quad 2)$. Show that $(uv)^2 \neq u^2 v^2$.

22. Let $u = (1 \quad 2 \quad 3)$ and $v = (1 \quad 2)$. Find the order of the cyclic group $\langle [uv], \circ, (1) \rangle$.

23. Let c be an r-cycle and d be an s-cycle. If c and d are disjoint, what is the order of the cyclic group $\langle [cd], \circ, (1) \rangle$?

24. Show with an example that the answer in Problem 23 may change when c and d are not disjoint.

25. (a) Give the canonical forms of all the permutations on $T_2 = \{1, 2\}$.
(b) Give the 3 canonical forms of the type $(a_1 \quad a_2)$ for permutations on T_3.
(c) Give the 2 canonical forms of the type $(a_1 \quad a_2 \quad a_3)$ for permutations on T_3.

26. Let $S_4 = \langle X_4, \circ, e \rangle$, as usual. In X_4, give:
(a) the 6 canonical forms of the type $(a_1 \quad a_2)$.
(b) the 8 canonical forms of the type $(a_1 \quad a_2 \quad a_3)$.
(c) the 6 canonical forms of the type $(a_1 \quad a_2 \quad a_3 \quad a_4)$.
(d) the 3 canonical forms of the type $(a_1 \quad a_2)(a_3 \quad a_4)$.
(e) the canonical form for the permutation in X_4 not listed in Parts (a), (b), (c), or (d).

27. Give all the types for permutations in X_5, that is, permutations on $\{1, 2, 3, 4, 5\}$.

28. How many permutations with canonical forms of the type $(a_1 \quad a_2 \quad a_3 \quad a_4 \quad a_5)$ are there in:
(a) S_5?   (b) S_6?   (c) S_7?

29. Let $G = \langle [a], \square, e \rangle$ be a cyclic group of order 10. Make a table showing the order of each element a^k in $[a]$.

30. Do as in Problem 29 but with G now cyclic of order 12.

31. In $S_n = \langle X_n, \circ, (1) \rangle$, let $p = t_1 t_2 \cdots t_{2h}$ and $q = u_1 u_2 \cdots u_{2k}$, where each t_i and u_j is a transposition. Explain why:
  (i) p and q are even permutations.
  (ii) pq^{-1} is an even permutation.

32. Let E_n be the set of even permutations in $S_n = \langle X_n, \circ, (1) \rangle$. For $n \geq 2$, show that E_n is nonempty and is closed under division and thus prove that $\langle E_n, \circ, (1) \rangle$ is a subgroup in S_n. (This is the proof of the result stated before Notation 1.)

33. Let G be the group $\langle U_4, \cdot, 1 \rangle$ of Example 4 in Section 7.1 and let G' be the group $\langle Y, \circ, (1) \rangle$ of Problem 7. Show that G and G' are not isomorphic.

7.4

GEOMETRIC SYMMETRIES AND THE SYMMETRIC GROUP

Let X_n be the set of all permutations on $T_n = \{1, 2, \ldots, n\}$. Since the elements of X_2 are (1) (the identity) and $(1 \quad 2)$, we see that one permutation is even and the other odd. In S_3, we see that (1), $r = (1 \quad 2 \quad 3)$, and $r^2 = (1 \quad 3 \quad 2)$ are even and $f = (1 \quad 2)$, $g = (2 \quad 3)$, and $h = (1 \quad 3)$ are odd.

Before listing the permutations in X_4, it is convenient to give all the partitions of 4 as a sum of positive integers:

$$4 = 4$$
$$= 3 + 1$$
$$= 2 + 2$$
$$= 2 + 1 + 1$$
$$= 1 + 1 + 1 + 1$$

and to note that each partition corresponds to a different kind of product of disjoint cycles. We can write down typical canonical forms corresponding to these partitions:

$(a \quad b \quad c \quad d)$
$(a \quad b \quad c)(d)$
$(a \quad b)(c \quad d)$
$(a \quad b)(c)(d)$
$(a)(b)(c)(d)$

These are usually written simply as $(a \quad b \quad c \quad d), (a \quad b \quad c), (a \quad b)(c \quad d),$ $(a \quad b)$, and (1), respectively.

There are $\binom{4}{4}3! = 6$ permutations with canonical forms of the type $(a \quad b \quad c \quad d)$, since a must be 1, and then $\{b, c, d\}$ can be any listing of $\{2, 3, 4\}$. There are $\binom{4}{3}2! = 8$ elements of the form $(a \quad b \quad c)$ by a similar argument. We have $\binom{4}{2}\binom{2}{2}$ choices for $(a \quad b)(c \quad d)$. But disjoint transpositions $(a \quad b)$ and $(c \quad d)$ commute and thus we have counted each product twice. So we divide by 2 to get $\binom{4}{2}\binom{2}{2}/2 = 3$. There are $\binom{4}{2} = 6$ transpositions and 1 identity. Since permutations of the forms $(a \quad b \quad c)$ and $(a \quad b)(c \quad d)$ and the identity are even, we see that there are $8 + 3 + 1 = 12$ even permutations. The other 12 permutations are odd.

These data strongly suggest the following theorem.

THEOREM 1   **EQUAL NUMBER OF EVEN AND ODD PERMUTATIONS**

Let $n \geq 2$. In S_n, the number of even permutations equals the number of odd permutations.

PROOF   Let E_n be the set of even permutations and let D_n be the set of odd permutations in S_n. Choose a fixed transposition—say, $t = (1 \quad 2)$. If a is in E_n, then the product ta is in D_n because a can be expressed as the product of an even number of transpositions and hence ta is the product of an odd number of transpositions. Thus $f: a \mapsto ta$ is a mapping from E_n to D_n. Since $ta = tb$ implies that $a = b$ (by left cancellation), f is injective. An odd permutation c in D_n has tc in E_n, and then $f(tc) = t(tc) = c$, since the transposition t is its own inverse. Now $f(tc) = c$ shows that f is surjective. Hence f is bijective. It then follows from Part (vii) of Theorem 3 of Section 1.8 ("Size of an Image Set") that $\#E_n = \#D_n$. □

Example 1   **THE ALTERNATING SUBGROUP A_3**   The alternating subgroup in S_3 is $A_3 = \langle E_3, \circ, (1) \rangle$ where $E_3 = \{(1), (1 \quad 2 \quad 3), (1 \quad 3 \quad 2)\}$. Table 7.4.1 shows its operation.

TABLE 7.4.1

A_3	(1)	$(1 \ 2 \ 3)$	$(1 \ 3 \ 2)$
(1)	(1)	$(1 \ 2 \ 3)$	$(1 \ 3 \ 2)$
$(1 \ 2 \ 3)$	$(1 \ 2 \ 3)$	$(1 \ 3 \ 2)$	(1)
$(1 \ 3 \ 2)$	$(1 \ 3 \ 2)$	(1)	$(1 \ 2 \ 3)$

□

Example 2 THE ALTERNATING SUBGROUP A_4 Since the order of S_4 is $4! = 24$, Theorem 1 tells us that A_4 has order $\frac{24}{2} = 12$. We let the 12 even permutations in A_4 be $a_1, a_2, \ldots, a_{12}$, where the a_i are as given in the leftmost column of Table 7.4.2. In this table, we have placed the integer k in the position of the row for a_i and the column for a_j to denote that $a_i a_j = a_k$; that is, in the main body of the table, k stands for a_k.

TABLE 7.4.2

A_4		a_1	a_2	a_3	a_4	a_5	a_6	a_7	a_8	a_9	a_{10}	a_{11}	a_{12}
	$(1) = a_1$	1	2	3	4	5	6	7	8	9	10	11	12
$(1\ 2)(3\ 4) = a_2$		2	1	4	3	8	7	6	5	11	12	9	10
$(1\ 3)(2\ 4) = a_3$		3	4	1	2	6	5	8	7	12	11	10	9
$(1\ 4)(2\ 3) = a_4$		4	3	2	1	7	8	5	6	10	9	12	11
$(1\ 2\ 3) = a_5$		5	6	7	8	9	10	11	12	1	2	3	4
$(2\ 4\ 3) = a_6$		6	5	8	7	12	11	10	9	3	4	1	2
$(1\ 4\ 2) = a_7$		7	8	5	6	10	9	12	11	4	3	2	1
$(1\ 3\ 4) = a_8$		8	7	6	5	11	12	9	10	2	1	4	3
$(1\ 3\ 2) = a_9$		9	10	11	12	1	2	3	4	5	6	7	8
$(1\ 4\ 3) = a_{10}$		10	9	12	11	4	3	2	1	7	8	5	6
$(2\ 3\ 4) = a_{11}$		11	12	9	10	2	1	4	3	8	7	6	5
$(1\ 2\ 4) = a_{12}$		12	11	10	9	3	4	1	2	6	5	8	7

☐

Now let us check to see what the groups S_n and A_n tell us about symmetries of geometric figures.

Example 3 Let us consider an equilateral triangle with vertices labeled 1, 2, and 3, as in Figure 7.4.1(a). We are interested in transformations of this triangle that leave it in exactly the same position but, possibly, where the vertices have been permuted. For example, if we take the triangle and rotate it counterclockwise 120° about its centroid, the position of vertices will have changed but the triangle will cover the same region in the plane, as shown in Figure 7.4.1(b). (The original vertex labels are on the inside, the new ones on the outside.) This gives us the permutation

$$r: 1 \mapsto 2, \quad 2 \mapsto 3, \quad 3 \mapsto 1,$$

where $i \mapsto j$ indicates that the vertex with old label i has j as its new label. We could also rotate it through 240° or through 360° (which is equivalent to no rotation at all) or we could flip the triangle about any of its medians. These transformations are summarized in Figure 7.4.2.

The rotations about the centroid are the even permutations of A_3; all six of the symmetries of the equilateral triangle are the elements of S_3.

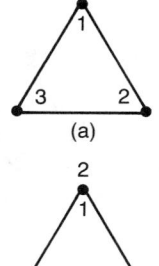

FIGURE 7.4.1

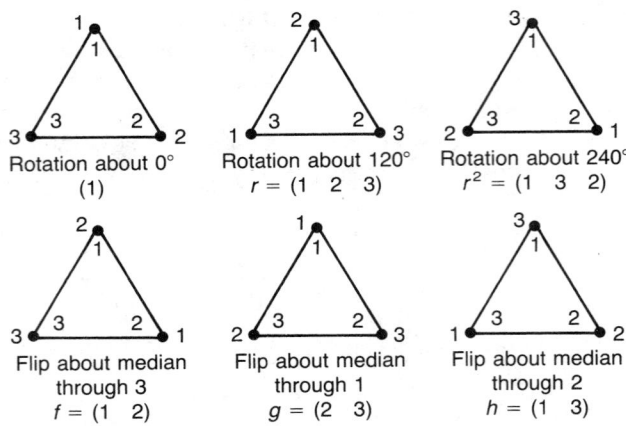

Rotation about 0°
(1)

Rotation about 120°
$r = (1 \quad 2 \quad 3)$

Rotation about 240°
$r^2 = (1 \quad 3 \quad 2)$

Flip about median
through 3
$f = (1 \quad 2)$

Flip about median
through 1
$g = (2 \quad 3)$

Flip about median
through 2
$h = (1 \quad 3)$

FIGURE 7.4.2

Example 4   **SYMMETRIES OF A REGULAR TETRAHEDRON**   Let us look at the regular tetrahedron shown in Figure 7.4.3. There are rotations of 120° and 240° about the four altitudes, as shown in Figure 7.4.4, and rotations through 180° about lines connecting midpoints of opposite edges, as in Figure 7.4.5. We see that the group of symmetries of the regular tetrahedron is A_4.

FIGURE 7.4.3

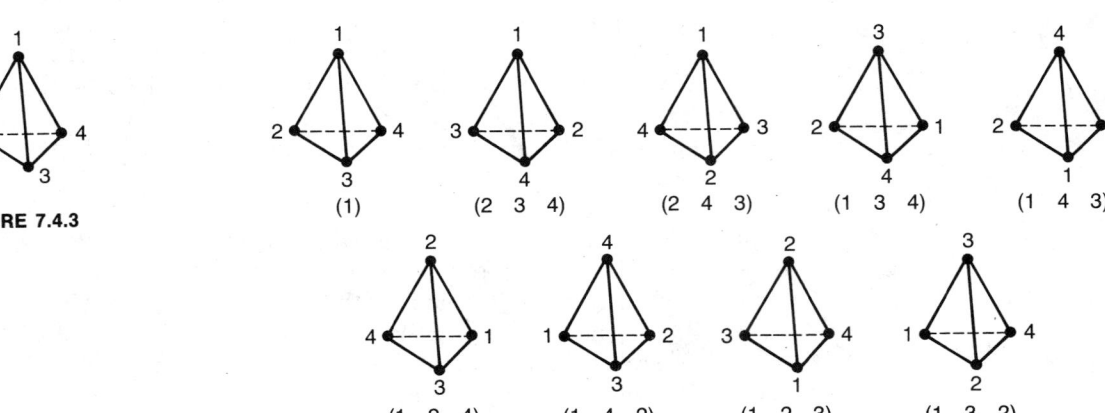

(1)   (2 3 4)   (2 4 3)   (1 3 4)   (1 4 3)

(1 2 4)   (1 4 2)   (1 2 3)   (1 3 2)

FIGURE 7.4.4

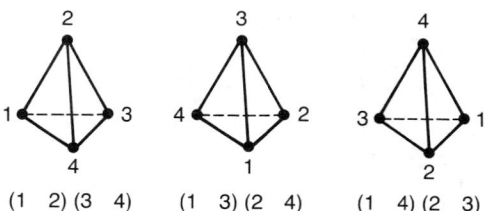

FIGURE 7.4.5   (1   2) (3   4)   (1   3) (2   4)   (1   4) (2   3)

PROBLEMS FOR SECTION 7.4

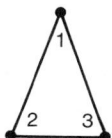

1. List the permutations of the group of symmetries of the isosceles triangle shown in the figure.

2. List the permutations of the group of symmetries of a regular pentagon (whose vertices in cyclic order are labeled 1, 2, 3, 4, 5).

3. List the permutations of the group of symmetries of a square (with vertices 1, 2, 3, 4 in cyclic order). This group of symmetries is a subgroup of order 8 in S_4 and is called *the octic group*.

4. Let $r = (1 \quad 2 \quad 3 \quad 4)$. Is $\langle [r], \circ, (1) \rangle$ a cyclic subgroup of order 4 in the octic group of Problem 3? Explain.

5. Let $r = (1 \quad 2 \quad 3 \quad 4)$ and $f = (2 \quad 4)$. Is $\{(1), r, r^2, r^3, f, rf, r^2f, r^3f\}$ the carrier of the octic group of Problem 3?

6. Let $r = (1 \quad 2 \quad 3 \quad 4)$ and $f = (2 \quad 4)$. Show that $fr = r^3f$.

7. Use the notation for the eight symmetries of a square given in Problem 5 and the formula $fr = r^3f$ of Problem 6 to construct the multiplication table for the octic group.

8. (a) Tabulate the orders of the permutations in the octic group.
    (b) Find the carriers of two noncyclic subgroups of order 4 in the octic group.
    (c) Find the carriers of three subgroups of order 2 in the octic group.

9. Some of the types of canonical forms for permutations in S_5 are $(a \quad b \quad c \quad d \quad e), (a \quad b \quad c \quad d)$, and $(a \quad b \quad c)(d \quad e)$. Give *all* the types of canonical forms for S_5.

10. Which of the types listed in the answer to Problem 9 represent even permutations?

11. For each type of canonical form for even permutations in S_5, give the number of permutations of that type. [For example, $(a \quad b \quad c \quad d \quad e)$ is a type for even permutations and there are 24 permutations of this type in S_5.] The sum of the answers should be $5!/2 = 120/2 = 60$.

12. Do as in Problem 11, but now for the odd permutations.

13. Using the notation of Table 7.4.2, let $E_4 = \{a_1, a_2, \ldots, a_{12}\}$ and $Y = \{a_1, a_2\}$.
    (i) Is Y closed under multiplication?

(ii) Is $\langle Y, \circ, a_1 \rangle$ a subgroup in A_4? Explain.

(iii) For each x in E_4, let xY denote the set $\{xa_1, xa_2\}$ and let Yx denote $\{a_1x, a_2x\}$. Does $xY = Yx$ for each x in E_4?

14. Using the notation of Table 7.4.2, let $E_4 = \{a_1, a_2, \ldots, a_{12}\}$ and $W = \{a_1, a_2, a_3, a_4\}$.

(i) Is W closed under multiplication?

(ii) Is $\langle W, \circ, a_1 \rangle$ a subgroup in A_4? Explain.

(iii) For each x in E_4 let $xW = \{xa_1, xa_2, xa_3, xa_4\}$ and $Wx = \{a_1x, a_2x, a_3x, a_4x\}$. For which permutations x in E_4 does $xW = Wx$?

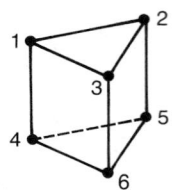

*15. What is the order of the group of symmetries of a cube? (This is a subgroup in S_8. See the figure in the margin.)

16. List the elements of the group of symmetries of the triangular prism with an equilateral triangle as its base shown in the figure below.

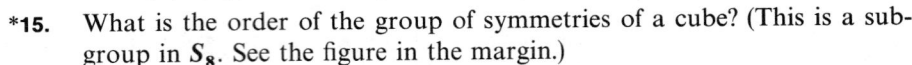

7.5

COSETS OF A SUBGROUP IN A GROUP, LAGRANGE'S THEOREM

Using the notation $r = (1 \quad 2 \quad 3)$ and $f = (2 \quad 3)$, the set of all permutations on $T_3 = \{1, 2, 3\}$ is

$$X_3 = \{(1), r, r^2, f, rf, r^2f\},$$

and the table for the symmetric group $S_3 = \langle X_3, \circ, (1) \rangle$ is Table 7.5.1.

The set of even permutations in X_3 is $E_3 = \{(1), r, r^2\}$ and the set of odd permutations in X_3 is $D_3 = \{f, rf, r^2f\}$. The nine entries in the upper

TABLE 7.5.1

	(1)	r	r^2	f	rf	r^2f
(1)	(1)	r	r^2	f	rf	r^2f
$(1 \quad 2 \quad 3) = r$	r	r^2	(1)	rf	r^2f	f
$(1 \quad 3 \quad 2) = r^2$	r^2	(1)	r	r^2f	f	rf
$(2 \quad 3) = f$	f	r^2f	rf	(1)	r^2	r
$(1 \quad 3) = rf$	rf	f	r^2f	r	(1)	r^2
$(1 \quad 2) = r^2f$	r^2f	rf	f	r^2	r	(1)

TABLE 7.5.2

	E	D
E	E	D
D	D	E

left quarter of Table 7.5.1 are all even permutations because a product pq of even permutations is even. The nine entries in the lower right quarter of the table also are all even because a product of two odd permutations is even. All the other entries are odd. These statements are summarized in Table 7.5.2, which is an operation table for a group $\langle \{E, D\}, \Box, E \rangle$ of order 2.

At this point some words of caution are in order. We will see below that any proper subgroup H in a group G enables one to obtain a partition $\Gamma = \{A_1, A_2, \ldots, A_q\}$ of the carrier of G, but this partitioning does not always produce a new group whose carrier is Γ.

DEFINITION 1   **SUBGROUP COSETS**

Let $H = \langle Y, \Box, e \rangle$ be a subgroup in $G = \langle X, \Box, e \rangle$. For each a in X, the set $\{a \Box y : y \in Y\}$ is called the **left coset for a of Y in G** and is denoted as $a \Box Y$. Similarly, $Y \Box a = \{y \Box a : y \in Y\}$ is the **right coset for a of Y in G**.

If Y is a finite set $\{y_1, y_2, \ldots, y_m\}$, then $a \Box Y = \{a \Box y_1, a \Box y_2, \ldots, a \Box y_m\}$ and $Y \Box a = \{y_1 \Box a, y_2 \Box a, \ldots, y_m \Box a\}$.

Example 1   The group $S_3 = \langle X_3, \circ, (1) \rangle$ has

$$X_3 = \{(1), r, r^2, f, rf, r^2f\}$$

as its carrier, where $r = (1 \quad 2 \quad 3)$ and $f = (2 \quad 3)$. Let $E = \{(1), r, r^2\}$. Then $A = \langle E, \circ, (1) \rangle$ is a subgroup in S_3. For this subgroup we have $xE = Ex$ for each x in X_3, since

$$\{(1), r, r^2\} = (1)E = E(1) = rE = Er = r^2E = Er^2,$$
$$\{f, rf, r^2f\} = fE = Ef = (rf)E = E(rf) = (r^2f)E = E(r^2f).$$

Thus in this example each left coset xE is identical with the right coset Ex. This is not true in the next example. We also note that the cosets $\{(1), r, r^2\}$ and $\{f, rf, r^2f\}$ form a partition of X_3.   □

Example 2   Let $r = (1 \quad 2 \quad 3)$ and $f = (2 \quad 3)$, as in Example 1, and let $Y = \{(1), f\}$. For some x's in X_3 one has $xY = Yx$, as one can see from

$$(1)Y = \{(1)(1), (1)f\} = \{(1), f\}, \qquad Y(1) = \{(1)(1), f(1)\} = \{(1), f\},$$
$$fY = \{f(1), ff\} = \{f, (1)\}, \qquad Yf = \{(1)f, ff\} = \{f, (1)\}.$$

However, for other x's one has $xY \neq Yx$. For example,

$$rY = \{r(1), rf\} = \{r, rf\}, \qquad Yr = \{(1)r, fr\} = \{r, r^2f\}.$$

The left cosets xY for the six x's of X_3 turn out to be only three distinct sets, since

$$(1)Y = fY, \qquad rY = (rf)Y, \qquad r^2Y = (r^2f)Y.$$

The three distinct left cosets form the partition $\{\{(1), f\}, \{r, rf\}, \{r^2, r^2f\}\}$ of the carrier X_3 of S_3. Similarly, there are only three distinct right cosets, since

$$Y(1) = Yf, \qquad Yr = Y(r^2f), \qquad Yr^2 = Y(rf).$$

The three distinct right cosets form another partition of X_3, namely, the collection $\{\{(1), f\}, \{r, r^2f\}, \{r^2, rf\}\}$. □

THEOREM 1   NUMBER OF ELEMENTS IN A COSET

The number of elements in a left coset $a \square Y$ is the same as the order $\# Y$ of the subgroup $H = \langle Y, \square, e \rangle$.

PROOF   Let $Y = \{y_1, y_2, \ldots, y_r\}$, where it is assumed that the y_1 are distinct elements and $\# Y = r$. Since $a \square Y = \{a \square y_1, \ldots, a \square y_r\}$, the number of elements in $a \square Y$ will be r if all of the elements in $a \square Y$ are distinct. What if $a \square y_i = a \square y_j$? Then by left cancellation, $y_i = y_j$, which contradicts the assumption that the elements listed in Y are distinct. Hence $\#(a \square Y) = \# Y$. □

THEOREM 2   DISTINCT LEFT COSETS ARE DISJOINT

Let $H = \langle Y, \square, e \rangle$ be a subgroup in $G = \langle X, \square, e \rangle$. For a and b in X, the left cosets $a \square Y$ and $b \square Y$ are either identical or they are disjoint. That is, either $a \square Y = b \square Y$ or $(a \square Y) \cap (b \square Y) = \varnothing$.

PROOF   Either $a \square Y$ and $b \square Y$ are disjoint or they have some element in common. Let x be a common element; that is, let $x \in a \square Y$ and $x \in b \square Y$. Then there exist elements y_1 and y_2 in Y such that $x = a \square y_1 = b \square y_2$. By definition of a subgroup, y_1^{-1} is in Y. So $(a \square y_1) \square y_1^{-1} = (b \square y_2) \square y_1^{-1}$ and thus $a = b \square (y_2 \square y_1^{-1})$. Since y_2 and y_1^{-1} are in Y and Y is closed under $\square$, it follows that $y_2 \square y_1^{-1}$ is some y_3 in Y and $a = b \square y_3$. Now, each $a \square y$ in $a \square Y$ is of the form $a \square y = (b \square y_3) \square y = b \square (y_3 \square y)$, with $y_3 \square y$ some element y_4 in Y. Thus $a \square y = b \square y_4$, and we see that every $a \square y$ in $a \square Y$ is also in $b \square Y$. This means that $a \square Y \subseteq b \square Y$. Similarly we can show that $b \square Y \subseteq a \square Y$. Hence $a \square Y = b \square Y$, and we have shown that left cosets that have some element in common must be identical. □

The statements in Theorem 2 are illustrated in Examples 1 and 2 above, as is the analogue of Theorem 2 for right cosets. The proof of the analogue is left to the reader.

THEOREM 3   **LEFT COSET PARTITION**

Let $H = \langle Y, \square, e \rangle$ be a subgroup in $G = \langle X, \square, e \rangle$. Then the collection $\Gamma = \{x \square Y : x \in X\}$ of the distinct left cosets of Y in G is a partition of X.

PROOF   Theorem 2 tells us that distinct left cosets $a \square Y$ and $b \square Y$ are disjoint; hence we merely have to show that the union of all the left cosets is X. We see this by noting that the identity e is in Y and hence that $x = x \square e$ is in $x \square Y$ for each x in X. Also, each left coset $x \square Y$ is a subset of X. Therefore the union of all these left cosets is X, and the theorem is proved. $\square$

The statement in Theorem 3 was also illustrated in Examples 1 and 2. The analogue of Theorem 3 for right cosets is left to the reader.

THEOREM 4   **LAGRANGE'S THEOREM**

Let $H = \langle Y, \square, e \rangle$ be a subgroup in a finite group $G = \langle X, \square, e \rangle$. Let $\#X = n$ and $\#Y = s$. Then $n = st$, where t is the number of left cosets of Y in G.

PROOF   Since X is finite, there are a finite number of left cosets. Therefore, let there be t distinct left cosets, denoted $C_1, C_2, \ldots, C_t$. By Theorem 3, $\{C_1, C_2, \ldots, C_t\}$ is a partition of X. Hence

$$\#X = (\#C_1) + (\#C_2) + \cdots + (\#C_t).$$

By Theorem 1, $\#C_i = \#Y = s$ for $i = 1, 2, \ldots, t$. Thus $n = \#X = st$, as claimed. $\square$

COROLLARY 1   **POSSIBLE ORDERS FOR SUBGROUPS**

Let $H = \langle Y, \square, e \rangle$ be a subgroup in a finite group $G = \langle X, \square, e \rangle$. Then the order of H is an integral divisor of the order of G.

COROLLARY 2   **POSSIBLE ORDERS FOR ELEMENTS**

Let $G = \langle X, \square, e \rangle$ have order m and let an x in X have order q. Then q is an integral divisor of m and $x^m = e$.

Corollary 2 follows from Corollary 1 because the order q of an element x is the order of the cyclic subgroup $\langle [x], \Box, e \rangle$ that it generates. Hence $m = qd$ with $d \in \mathbf{Z}^+$ and $x^m = (x^q)^d = e^d = e$.

For example, in the alternating subgroup $A_4 = \langle E_4, \circ, (1) \rangle$ of order 12 tabulated in Example 2 of Section 7.4, the permutation (1) has order 1, (1 2)(3 4) has order 2, and (1 2 3) has order 3. Each of these orders 1, 2, and 3 is an integral divisor of the order 12 of A_4. The other possibilities for orders of elements in a group of order 12 are 4, 6, and 12 (the other positive integral divisors of 12), however, A_4 has no elements of order 4, 6, or 12. Also, it can be shown (not easily) that the set of orders of subgroups in A_4 is $\{1, 2, 3, 4, 12\}$.

DEFINITION 2 **INDEX OF A SUBGROUP H IN A GROUP G**

Let $H = \langle Y, \Box, e \rangle$ be a subgroup in $G = \langle X, \Box, e \rangle$. The ***index*** of H in G is the number of distinct left cosets of Y in G.

In other words, the index of H in G is $\#\{x \Box Y : x \in X\}$. If X is finite, it follows from the proof of Lagrange's Theorem that

(index of H in G) = (order of G) ÷ (order of H).

For example, the index of the alternating subgroup $A_n = \langle E_n, \circ, (1) \rangle$ in the symmetric group $S_n = \langle X_n, \circ, (1) \rangle$ is $n! \div (n!/2) = 2$.

DEFINITION 3 **NORMAL SUBGROUP IN A GROUP**

A subgroup $N = \langle Y, \Box, e \rangle$ in a group $G = \langle X, \Box, e \rangle$ is said to be ***normal*** in G if $x \Box N = N \Box x$ for each x in X.

We saw in Example 1 that $xA = Ax$ for each x in X_3; hence the alternating subgroup $A_3 = \langle E_3, \circ, (1) \rangle$ is a normal subgroup in S_3. In Example 2 we saw that $rY \neq Yr$. Thus some left coset xY is not identical with the right coset Yx, and the subgroup $\langle Y, \circ, (1) \rangle$ with $Y = \{(1), f\}$ is not normal in S_3.

Joseph-Louis Lagrange, though French, was born in Turin, in 1736. Usually viewed as the only rival to Euler for the position of most important mathematician of the eighteenth century, Lagrange's view of mathematics was much different from Euler's. Euler's approach was algorithmic, often concerned with formulas and techniques. Lagrange was interested in clarity, precision, and rigor. He worked extensively in analysis (specifically, differential equations and calculus of variations), in the theory of equations, and in number theory. He replaced Euler at the Berlin Academy when Euler returned to St. Petersburg in 1766, wooed by Frederick's argument that the greatest of Europe's geometers should live close to the greatest of kings. Lagrange left for Paris in 1787, where he worked in several governmental positions and taught at the École Normale. He died in 1813.

PROBLEMS FOR SECTION 7.5

1. In $S_4 = \langle X_4, \circ, (1) \rangle$, let Y consist of the permutations f with $f(4) = 4$.
   (i) List the six permutations in Y.
   (ii) Is Y closed under multiplication (that is, composition of mappings)?
   (iii) Is $\langle Y, \circ, (1) \rangle$ a subgroup in S_4?
   (iv) Is $\langle Y, \circ, (1) \rangle$ isomorphic to S_3?
   (v) Let $t = (1 \quad 4)$. Show that $tY \neq Yt$.
   (vi) Is $\langle Y, \circ, (1) \rangle$ a normal subgroup in S_4?

2. Consider $Y = \{(1), (1 \quad 2)\}$ to be a subset of the carrier X_3 of the symmetric group S_3.
   (i) Is $H = \langle Y, \circ, (1) \rangle$ a subgroup in S_3?
   (ii) Is H a normal subgroup in S_3?
   (iii) Is H isomorphic to S_2?

3. In the set B_5 of 5-bit strings, let $\alpha = 10010$, $\beta = 01011$, and $\gamma = 00101$. Let G be the "bitwise addition modulo 2" group $\langle B_5, \oplus, 0_5 \rangle$ given in Example 2 of Section 7.1 and let $Y = \{0_5, \alpha, \beta, \gamma, \alpha \oplus \beta, \alpha \oplus \gamma, \beta \oplus \gamma, \alpha \oplus \beta \oplus \gamma\}$.
   (i) Show that Y is closed under $\oplus$.
   (ii) Explain why $H = \langle Y, \oplus, 0_5 \rangle$ is a subgroup in G.
   (iii) Show that the collection of cosets $\Gamma = \{00000 \oplus Y, 10000 \oplus Y, 01000 \oplus Y, 00100 \oplus Y\}$ is a partition of B_5.
   (iv) What is the index of H in G?

4. Let $G = \langle B_5, \oplus, 0_5 \rangle$ and $H = \langle Y, \oplus, 0_5 \rangle$ be as in Problem 3.
   (i) Does $\sigma \oplus Y = Y \oplus \sigma$ for each σ in B_5? Explain.
   (ii) Is H a normal subgroup in G?

5. Let $G = \langle X, \square, e \rangle$ be abelian. Explain why every subgroup $H = \langle Y, \square, e \rangle$ is normal in G.

6. Find an abelian subgroup H in the symmetric group $S_3 = \langle X_3, \circ, (1) \rangle$ such that H is not normal in S_3.

7. Prove the analogue of Theorem 1 ("Number of Elements in a Coset") for right cosets.

8.   (a) Prove the analogue of Theorem 2 ("Distinct Left Cosets Are Disjoint")
      for right cosets.
      (b) Prove the analogue of Theorem 3 ("Left Coset Partition") for right
      cosets.

9.   Let $H = \langle Y, \square, e \rangle$ be a subgroup in $G = \langle X, \square, e \rangle$.
      (i) Show that $e \square Y = Y$.
      (ii) Show that x is in $x \square Y$ for each x in X.
      (iii) Show that $y \square Y = Y$ for each y in Y.
      (iv) Show that $x \square Y \neq Y$ if x is in X but is not in Y.
      (v) Show that $x \square Y = w \square Y$ if x is in $w \square Y$.

10. Do the analogue of Problem 9 for right cosets.

11. Let $H = \langle Y, \square, e \rangle$ be a subgroup in $G = \langle X, \square, e \rangle$ with Y a doubleton
      $\{e, y\}$. Let x be in X. Explain why $x \square Y = Y \square x$ if and only if $x \square y = y \square x$.

12. Let $r = (1 \quad 2 \quad 3)$, $E_3 = \{(1), r, r^2\}$, and $A_3 = \langle E_3, \circ, (1) \rangle$ be the alter-
      nating subgroup in $S_3 = \langle X_3, \circ, (1) \rangle$.
      (i) Find an f in X_3 such that $fr \neq rf$.
      (ii) Show that $fE_3 = E_3 f$ despite the fact that $fr \neq rf$.
      (iii) Show that A_3 is a normal subgroup in S_3.

13. Let $H = \langle Y, \square, e \rangle$ be a subgroup of index 2 in a finite group $G = \langle X, \square, e \rangle$. Explain why H must be a normal subgroup in G.

14. In the alternating group $A_4 = \langle E_4, \circ, (1) \rangle$, let $H = \langle Y, \circ, (1) \rangle$ be the sub-
      group of index 3 with

$$Y = \{(1), (1 \quad 2)(3 \quad 4), (1 \quad 3)(2 \quad 4), (1 \quad 4)(2 \quad 3)\}.$$

      Show that H is a normal subgroup in A_4.

15. For a and b in Z, let $a + bZ = \{a + bn : n \in Z\}$. For example,

$$2 + 3Z = \{2 + 3n : n \in Z\} = \{\ldots, -4, -1, 2, 5, \ldots\}.$$

      (i) Does $-4 + 3Z = -1 + 3Z = 2 + 3Z = 5 + 3Z$?
      (ii) Explain why $H = \langle 3Z, +, 0 \rangle$ is a normal subgroup in $G = \langle Z, +, 0 \rangle$.
      (iii) Find the index q of H in G.
      (iv) List q distinct cosets of H in G.

16. (i) Does $-3 + 4Z = 1 + 4Z = 5 + 4Z$?
      (ii) Find the index q of $K = \langle 4Z, +, 0 \rangle$ in $G = \langle Z, +, 0 \rangle$.
      (iii) List q distinct cosets of K in G.

17. Let $G = \langle X, \square, e \rangle$ be a group of order 5. Justify the following:
      (i) Each element x of X has order 1 or 5.
      (ii) Only the identity e has order 1.
      (iii) If $x \neq e$, then x has order 5.
      (iv) G is cyclic.

18. Let $G = \langle X, \square, e \rangle$ be a group of order 7. Explain why G is cyclic and $[x] = X$ if $x \in X$ and $x \neq e$.

19. What integers can be orders of subgroups in a group of order 24?

20. What integers can be orders of subgroups in a group of order 54?

7.6

RINGS AND FIELDS

A boolean algebra $L = [X, ^-, \wedge, 1, \vee, 0]$ is an algebraic structure with a unary operation of complementation and two binary operations $\wedge$ and $\vee$ related by the distributive laws

$$x \wedge (y \vee z) = (x \wedge y) \vee (x \wedge z),$$
$$x \vee (y \wedge z) = (x \vee y) \wedge (x \vee z),$$

which state that each of $\wedge$ and $\vee$ is distributive over the other. Our familiar number systems give us examples of algebraic structures with addition and multiplication as two binary operations related by the left and right distributive laws

$$x(y + z) = xy + xz, \qquad (y + z)x = yx + zx,$$

which tell us that multiplication is distributive over addition. We now formally define such structures.

DEFINITION 1   **RING**

A *ring* is an algebraic structure $R = (X, +, 0, \cdot)$ in which $+$ and $\cdot$ are associative binary operations on X such that $\langle X, +, 0 \rangle$ is an abelian group and R has the distributive properties

$$x(y + z) = xy + xz, \qquad (y + z)x = yx + zx$$

for all x, y, z in X. The ring is *commutative* if multiplication is a commutative operation on X.

For example, $(Z, +, 0, \cdot)$, $(Q, +, 0, \cdot)$, $(R, +, 0, \cdot)$, and $(C, +, 0, \cdot)$ are infinite commutative rings whose carriers are the integers Z, the rational numbers Q, the real numbers R, and the complex numbers C, respectively. The structure $(N, +, 0, \cdot)$ is not a ring because $(N, +, 0)$ is not a group. (The integer 1 in N does not have an additive inverse in N.)

It follows from Definition 1 here and Definition 1 "Semigroup" in Section 2.2 that a ring $(X, +, 0, \cdot)$ is an abelian group $\langle X, +, 0 \rangle$ when multiplication is ignored and is a semigroup $(X, \cdot)$ when addition is ignored. In each of the number systems mentioned above, the semigroup $(X, \cdot)$ is a monoid $[X, \cdot, 1]$, since each has 1 as a multiplicative identity. However, this is not true of the ring $(2Z, +, 0, \cdot)$ with $2Z = \{\ldots, -4, -2, 0, 2, 4, \ldots\}$, which has no multiplicative identity.

DEFINITION 2   **RING WITH UNITY, FIELD**

A *ring with unity* is a ring $U = (X, +, 0, \cdot)$ in which there is a multiplicative identity 1 in X. Such a ring may be written as $U = [X, +, 0, \cdot, 1]$. A *field* is a ring U with unity such that $\langle X - \{0\}, \cdot, 1\rangle$ is an abelian group. A field may be written as $\langle X, +, 0, \cdot, 1\rangle$.

Example 1   Let $+$ and $\cdot$ be the binary operations on $X = \{0, 1, c\}$ given by Tables 7.6.1 and 7.6.2. These operations make $F = \langle X, +, 0, \cdot, 1\rangle$ into a *finite field*, that is, a field with a finite carrier. The details for showing that F is a field are easy but tedious and are omitted.

TABLE 7.6.1

+	0	1	c
0	0	1	c
1	1	c	0
c	c	0	1

TABLE 7.6.2

·	0	1	c
0	0	0	0
1	0	1	c
c	0	c	1

□

Example 2   Let $G = \langle X, +, 0\rangle$ be an additive (abelian) group. If we define $\cdot$ to be the binary operation on X for which $x \cdot y = 0$ for all x and y in X, then $(X, +, 0, \cdot)$ is a commutative ring. If $\#X > 1$, that is, if $X \neq \{0\}$, then this ring has no unity 1, since there is an x in X with $x \neq 0$ and $x \cdot 1 = 0 \neq x$ for such an x.   □

Example 3   Let M consist of all 2×2 matrices

$$\begin{bmatrix} x & y \\ z & w \end{bmatrix},$$

with x, y, z, w in Z. Then $[M, +, O, \cdot, I]$ is a noncommutative ring with unity if addition and multiplication of these matrices are defined by

$$\begin{bmatrix} a & b \\ c & d \end{bmatrix} + \begin{bmatrix} g & h \\ i & j \end{bmatrix} = \begin{bmatrix} a+g & b+h \\ c+i & d+j \end{bmatrix},$$

$$\begin{bmatrix} a & b \\ c & d \end{bmatrix} \cdot \begin{bmatrix} g & h \\ i & j \end{bmatrix} = \begin{bmatrix} ag+bi & ah+bj \\ cg+di & ch+dj \end{bmatrix},$$

and the zero and unity matrices are

$$O = \begin{bmatrix} 0 & 0 \\ 0 & 0 \end{bmatrix}, \quad I = \begin{bmatrix} 1 & 0 \\ 0 & 1 \end{bmatrix}.$$

Let

$$A = \begin{bmatrix} 0 & 1 \\ 0 & 1 \end{bmatrix}, \quad B = \begin{bmatrix} 1 & 1 \\ 0 & 0 \end{bmatrix}.$$

Then

$$A \cdot B = \begin{bmatrix} 0 & 0 \\ 0 & 0 \end{bmatrix} = O, \quad B \cdot A = \begin{bmatrix} 1 & 1 \\ 0 & 0 \end{bmatrix} \cdot \begin{bmatrix} 0 & 1 \\ 0 & 1 \end{bmatrix} = \begin{bmatrix} 0 & 2 \\ 0 & 0 \end{bmatrix}.$$

Since $A \cdot B \neq B \cdot A$, this ring of matrices is noncommutative. □

In our familiar number systems, a product ab equals zero if and only if at least one of the factors a and b is zero. In Example 3, neither of the matrices A and B is the zero matrix but the product $A \cdot B$ is the zero matrix. So there exist rings in which a product can be zero despite the fact that the factors are nonzero. However, in all rings it is sufficient to have one zero factor to make a product zero, as we see in the following theorem.

THEOREM 1 **ZERO FACTOR IMPLIES ZERO PRODUCT**

Let $R = (X, +, 0, \cdot)$ be a ring. For all x in X, $x \cdot 0 = 0 = 0 \cdot x$.

PROOF Since 0 is the identity in the group $\langle X, +, 0 \rangle$, it follows that $0 + 0 = 0$, and so $(0 + 0)x = 0 \cdot x$. Using right distributivity, one gets

$$0 \cdot x + 0 \cdot x = 0 \cdot x. \tag{1}$$

By uniqueness of the identity (that is, Theorem 1 of Section 7.1) in the additive group $\langle X, +, 0 \rangle$, Display (1) implies that $0 \cdot x = 0$. It is left to the reader to prove the analogous fact that $x \cdot 0 = 0$ for all x in X. □

PROBLEMS FOR SECTION 7.6

1. Let $3\mathbf{Z} = \{\ldots, -6, -3, 0, 3, 6, \ldots\}$. Is $(3\mathbf{Z}, +, 0, \cdot)$ a ring? Is it a ring with unity?

2. Let $4\mathbf{Z} = \{\ldots, -8, -4, 0, 4, 8, \ldots\}$. Is $(4\mathbf{Z}, +, 0, \cdot)$ a ring? Is it a ring with unity?

3. Let $2N = \{0, 2, 4, 6, \ldots\}$. Is $(2N, +, 0, \cdot)$ a ring?

4. Let $3N = \{0, 3, 6, 9, \ldots\}$. Is $(3N, +, 0, \cdot)$ a ring?

5. Let $X = \{0, 1, g, h, k\}$ and $R = \langle X, +, 0, \cdot, 1\rangle$ be a field in which $1 + 1 = g$, $g + 1 = h$, and $h + 1 = k$. Explain why the following are true.
    (i) $k + 1 = 0$.   (ii) $g + g = k$.
    (iii) $gg = (1 + 1)g = 1 \cdot g + 1 \cdot g = g + g = k$.
    (iv) $gh = g(g + 1) = gg + g = k + g = 1$.

6. Make the addition and multiplication tables for the field $R = \langle X, +, 0, \cdot, 1\rangle$ of Problem 5.

7. Let $F = \langle X, +, 0, \cdot, 1\rangle$ be a field with $\#X = 5$. It follows from Problem 17 of Section 7.5 that $\langle X, +, 0\rangle$ is a cyclic group with 1 as a generator; that is, $X = [1] = \{0, 1, 2 \cdot 1, 3 \cdot 1, 4 \cdot 1\}$, where $2 \cdot 1 = 1 + 1$, $3 \cdot 1 = 1 + 1 + 1$, $4 \cdot 1 = 1 + 1 + 1 + 1$, and $5 \cdot 1 = 0$.
    (i) Explain why $(2 \cdot 1)(2 \cdot 1) = (1 + 1)(2 \cdot 1) = 2 \cdot 1 + 2 \cdot 1 = 4 \cdot 1$.
    (ii) Make the addition and multiplication tables for F using the notation $\bar{n}$ for $n \cdot 1$.

8. Let $F = \langle X, +, 0, \cdot, 1\rangle$ be a field with $\#X = 7$.
    (i) Explain why $X = [1] = \{0, 1, 2 \cdot 1, 3 \cdot 1, 4 \cdot 1, 5 \cdot 1, 6 \cdot 1\}$.
    (ii) Using the notation $\bar{n}$ for $n \cdot 1$, make the addition and multiplication tables for F.

9. Let X consist of all the 2×2 matrices

    $$\begin{bmatrix} x & y \\ 0 & w \end{bmatrix} \quad \text{with } x, y, \text{ and } w \text{ integers.}$$

    Show that $[X, +, O, \cdot, I]$ is a ring with unity.

10. Let Y consist of all the matrices

    $$\begin{bmatrix} x & 0 \\ z & w \end{bmatrix} \quad \text{with } x, z, \text{ and } w \text{ integers.}$$

    Show that $[Y, +, O, \cdot, I]$ is a ring with unity.

---

*7.7

POLYA'S ENUMERATION FORMULA

A number of combinatorial problems involve the labeling of points or arcs or regions in geometric figures. Labelings that at first glance appear to be different can sometimes be considered to be the same labeling viewed from different vantage points; this complicates the problem of counting essentially different labelings. A powerful tool for dealing with this problem was brought to the attention of the mathematical community in a theorem proved in 1937 by G. Polya. In recent years, it has been discovered that it was proved in another context by J. Redfield in 1927.

In our discussions, we assume that the labeling of the geometric objects is accomplished by coloring them, using several colors. Therefore we shall refer consistently to "colorings" rather than "labelings." Since the technique is by no means transparent, let us look at an example before outlining the general method.

Example 1

2-COLORINGS OF THE SIDES OF A SQUARE Let us consider a square with each of its 4 sides colored either red or blue. Since there are 2 choices of color for each of the 4 sides, the general product rule of Section 5.1 tells us that there are $2^4 = 16$ possible colorings. If we use a solid line for red and a dotted line for blue, these 16 colorings would be as shown in Figures 7.7.1 through 7.7.6. Clearly, Figure 7.7.1 gives the only coloring with all sides red. The four colorings with exactly one side blue are given in Figure 7.7.2; these four colorings may be considered to be the same coloring viewed from above, from the right, from below, and from the left. Instead of moving our vantage point, we could transform any one of these four colorings into any other in this set by a rigid motion of the square. Thus, there is essentially only one coloring with three red sides (and the remaining side blue). However, there are two essentially different types of colorings in which two of the sides are red (and two are blue). The colorings with the two red sides meeting at a vertex are shown in Figure 7.7.3; the colorings having the sides of the same color opposite each other are shown in Figure 7.7.4. No square from Figure 7.7.3 can be transformed into a square from Figure 7.7.4 by a rigid motion of the square.

Each of Figures 7.7.1–7.7.6 shows a set of colorings. Any coloring shown can be changed into any other of the same set by a rigid motion of the square. However, no coloring from one set can be transformed into a coloring from a different set by such a motion. Thus there are 6 essentially different colorings of the sides of a square using 2 colors. □

FIGURE 7.7.1

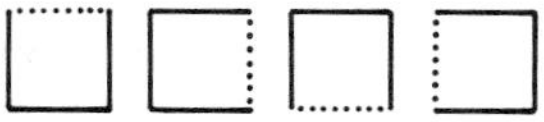

FIGURE 7.7.2

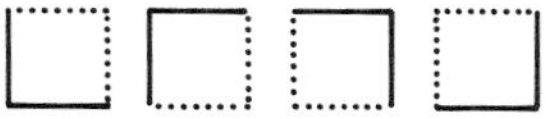

FIGURE 7.7.3

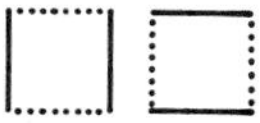

FIGURE 7.7.4

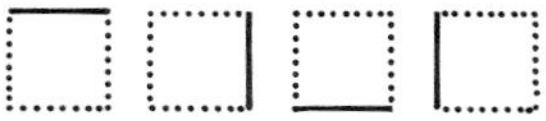

FIGURE 7.7.5

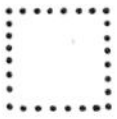

FIGURE 7.7.6

We will illustrate the concepts and techniques introduced in this section by seeing how they apply to the problem discussed in Example 1. We now expand the discussion, in that example, of rigid motions of a square and the permutations associated with these motions.

Let r be the 4-cycle (1 2 3 4) and f be the 2-cycle (2 4). Then Problems 3–7 of Section 7.4 tell us that the octic group of symmetries of a square is $\langle X, \circ, e \rangle$, where

$$X = \{e, r, r^2, r^3, f, rf, r^2f, r^3f\}.$$

In Section 7.4, we thought of an element g of X as a permutation of the vertices of a square; now we consider g to be a permutation of the sides.

TABLE 7.7.1

g	Cycle Representation	Rigid Motion
e	$(1)(2)(3)(4)$	The identity
r	$(1\ \ 2\ \ 3\ \ 4)$	A 90° rotation (about the center)
r^2	$(1\ \ 3)(2\ \ 4)$	A 180° rotation
r^3	$(1\ \ 4\ \ 3\ \ 2)$	A 270° rotation
f	$(1)(2\ \ 4)(3)$	A flip about the vertical line connecting the midpoints of sides 1 and 3
rf	$(1\ \ 4)(2\ \ 3)$	A flip about diagonal d_2
r^2f	$(1\ \ 3)(2)(4)$	A flip about a horizontal line
r^3f	$(1\ \ 2)(3\ \ 4)$	A flip about diagonal d_1

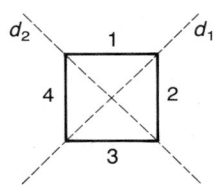

FIGURE 7.7.7

Table 7.7.1 gives each permutation g in the octic group of symmetries of a square, the cycle representation of g, and a description of g as a rigid motion of the square. We include all 1-cycles for reasons that will become apparent later. Figure 7.7.7 shows how the sides of the square are represented by the integers of the set $T = \{1, 2, 3, 4\}$ and also shows the diagonals mentioned in Table 7.7.1.

The general problem involves a finite set T of vertices, edges, faces, or other objects and a group $G = \langle X, \circ, e \rangle$ of permutations on T. Let C be a set of s colors. Then an *s-coloring* of T is an assignment to each t in T of one of the s colors in C, that is, a mapping

$$c: T \to C; \quad t \mapsto c(t).$$

Let g be a permutation in X, that is, a bijective mapping

$$g: T \to T; \quad t \mapsto g(t).$$

Then the permutation g **transforms** the coloring c into a new coloring, denoted as $g(c)$, given by

$$g(c): T \to C; \quad t \mapsto c(g(t)). \tag{1}$$

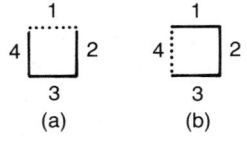

FIGURE 7.7.8

For example, let $T = \{1, 2, 3, 4\}$ with the elements of T representing the sides of a square. Figure 7.7.8(a) shows the coloring

$$c: 1 \mapsto \text{blue}, \quad 2 \mapsto \text{red}, \quad 3 \mapsto \text{red}, \quad 4 \mapsto \text{red}.$$

Let g be the permutation $(1\ \ 2\ \ 3\ \ 4)$ on T, that is, the mapping

$$g: 1 \mapsto 2, \quad 2 \mapsto 3, \quad 3 \mapsto 4, \quad 4 \mapsto 1.$$

Then the permutation g transforms the coloring c into the new coloring $c' = g(c)$ with

$$c'(1) = c(g(1)) = c(2) = \text{red}, \qquad c'(2) = c(g(2)) = c(3) = \text{red},$$
$$c'(3) = c(g(3)) = c(4) = \text{red}, \qquad c'(4) = c(g(4)) = c(1) = \text{blue}.$$

That is, the new coloring is

$$c': 1 \mapsto \text{red}, \quad 2 \mapsto \text{red}, \quad 3 \mapsto \text{red}, \quad 4 \mapsto \text{blue}.$$

This coloring is shown in Figure 7.7.8(b). If the square of Figure 7.7.8(b) is rotated $90°$ clockwise around its center, it turns into the square of Figure 7.7.8(a).

Since the set T is finite, it can be listed as $T = \{t_1, t_2, \ldots, t_n\}$. Frequently we find it convenient to use the subscript i as a representation of t_i, that is, to think of T as being the set $\{1, 2, \ldots, n\}$. Let C be a set of s colors. Using Notation 2 of Section 1.8, the set of all mappings from T into C is denoted as C^T, that is, the set of all s-colorings of T is C^T. With respect to a group $G = \langle X, \circ, e \rangle$ of permutations on T, we now introduce a binary relation $\sim$ on C^T. Let c and c' be s-colorings of T, that is, mappings in C^T. If c is transformed into c' by some permutation g in X, we say that c is *equivalent* to c' (with respect to the group G) and write $c \sim c'$. It is left to the reader as Problem 12 below to show that $\sim$ is an equivalence relation. As in Theorem 3 of Section 1.7, this equivalence relation induces a partition of C^T into equivalence classes.

When we said that colorings c_1 and c_2 are essentially different, we meant that c_1 and c_2 are not equivalent with respect to the group G of allowable permutations of the set T being colored. Thus the number of essentially different colorings is the number of equivalence classes in the partition of C^T induced by $\sim$.

In the situation discussed in Example 1, there are 6 essentially different colorings. Each of the 6 equivalence classes is shown in one of the sets of squares given in Figures 7.7.1 through 7.7.6.

When T and C are larger sets, it may not be practical to count the essentially different colorings as we did in Example 1. Therefore, we now introduce some additional aids for this combinatorial problem.

Let g be a permutation on $T = \{1, 2, \ldots, n\}$ and c be an s-coloring of T. If c is transformed into itself by g, we say that c is *fixed under* g. It follows from the definition of the transform $g(c)$ given in Display (1) that each of the following assertions is equivalent to each of the other two assertions:

(a) The coloring c is fixed under the permutation g.
(b) The transform $g(c)$ equals c.
(c) $c(t) = c(g(t))$, that is, t and $g(t)$ have the same color, for each t in T.

NOTATION 1   **SET $F(g)$ OF COLORINGS FIXED UNDER g**

For each fixed permutation g on T, the set $\{c : c \in C^T, g(c) = c\}$ of colorings fixed under g is denoted by $F(g)$.

In the specific example in which $T = \{1, 2, 3, 4\}$ and $C = \{$red, blue$\}$, what colorings of T are fixed under the permutation $g = (1 \quad 3)(2)(4)$? For this permutation,

$$g(1) = 3, \qquad g(3) = 1, \qquad g(2) = 2, \qquad \text{and} \qquad g(4) = 4.$$

Thus a coloring c of T is fixed under this g if and only if $c(1) = c(3)$, that is, if and only if elements 1 and 3 have the same color. To get such a coloring, we can let each of $c(1)$, $c(2)$, and $c(4)$ be either red or blue and then take $c(3)$ to be the same as $c(1)$. It now follows from the general product rule of Section 5.1 that there are $2^3 = 8$ fixed colorings under $(1 \quad 3)(2)(4)$. Table 7.7.2 gives each permutation g of the octic group of symmetries of a square, the set $F(g)$ of 2-colorings fixed under g, and the number of such colorings. (One should consider the sides of each square in the table to be numbered as in Figure 7.7.7, repeated here.)

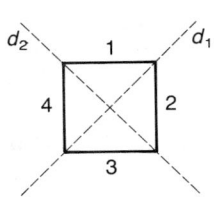

FIGURE 7.7.7

TABLE 7.7.2

g	Set $F(g)$ of 2-Colorings Fixed under g	$\# F(g)$
$(1)(2)(3)(4)$	All of the 2-colorings	$2^4 = 16$
$(1 \ 2 \ 3 \ 4)$		2
$(1 \ 3)(2 \ 4)$		$2^2 = 4$
$(1 \ 4 \ 3 \ 2)$	Same as for $(1 \ 2 \ 3 \ 4)$	2
$(1)(2 \ 4)(3)$		$2^3 = 8$
$(1 \ 4)(2 \ 3)$		$2^2 = 4$
$(1 \ 3)(2)(4)$		$2^3 = 8$
$(1 \ 2)(3 \ 4)$		$2^2 = 4$

In general, a permutation g on $T = \{1, 2, \ldots, n\}$ can be written as a product

$$g = (a_1 \quad a_2 \quad \cdots \quad a_u)(b_1 \quad b_2 \quad \cdots \quad b_v) \cdots (k_1 \quad k_2 \quad \cdots \quad k_w) \qquad (2)$$

of disjoint cycles such that each t in T is present in exactly one of these cycles, that is, such that

$$T = \{a_1, a_2, \ldots, a_u, b_1, b_2, \ldots, b_v, \ldots, k_1, k_2, \ldots, k_w\}. \tag{3}$$

For this g, we have $g(a_1) = a_2, g(a_2) = a_3, \ldots, g(a_u) = a_1$ and similarly for the other cycles in g. Hence an s-coloring c of T is fixed under this product of disjoint cycles if and only if each of the elements of T in a given cycle has the same color. It then follows from the general product rule of Section 5.1 that the number of s-colorings fixed under g is s^r, where r is the number of cycles in Display (2).

We have seen that $\# F(g)$ is s^r, where r is the number of cycles in the representation of Display (2) for g as a product of disjoint cycles. This formula and the following powerful (and hard to prove) theorem enable us to calculate the number of essentially different s-colorings of T, that is, the number of equivalence classes in the partition of C^T induced by the equivalence relation $\sim$.

THEOREM 1   **BURNSIDE'S LEMMA**

With respect to a group $G = \langle X, \circ, e \rangle$ with $X = \{g_1, g_2, \ldots, g_m\}$, the number of essentially different colorings is

$$\frac{1}{\# X} \left[\# F(g_1) + \# F(g_2) + \cdots + \# F(g_m) \right].$$

For a proof, see Alan Tucker's *Applied Combinatorics*, 2nd ed. (New York: John Wiley and Sons, 1984).

Burnside's Lemma tells us that to count the number of equivalence classes, we need only look at each permutation, count the number of colorings it leaves fixed, sum these numbers, and divide the sum by the number of permutations. For the 2-colorings of the edges of a square, Table 7.7.2 helps us see that this procedure gives

$$\frac{1}{8}(16 + 2 + 4 + 2 + 8 + 4 + 8 + 4) = \frac{48}{8} = 6$$

as the number of equivalence classes, that is, the number of essentially different 2-colorings.

Let $G = \langle X, \circ, e \rangle$ be a group of permutations on $T = \{1, 2, \ldots, n\}$. Let a permutation g in X be the product of disjoint cycles given in Display (2). Let each integer in T be present in exactly one of these cycles, as is implied by Display (3). We now assign a monomial to each such permutation g and a polynomial to the group G.

DEFINITION 1   **MONOMIAL FOR g, CYCLE INDEX FOR G**

In Display (2), let the number of i-cycles be a, the number of j-cycles be $b, \ldots,$ the number of k-cycles be c. Then the monomial for g is $x_i^a x_j^b \cdots x_k^c$. The **cycle index** for the group G is $\sigma/\#X$, where σ is the sum of the monomials for all permutations g in X.

TABLE 7.7.3

g	Monomial
(1)(2)(3)(4)	x_1^4
(1 2 3 4)	x_4^1
(1 3)(2 4)	x_2^2
(1 4 3 2)	x_4^1
(1)(2 4)(3)	$x_1^2 x_2^1$
(1 4)(2 3)	x_2^2
(1 3)(2)(4)	$x_1^2 x_2^1$
(1 2)(3 4)	x_2^2

Table 7.7.3 gives the monomials for all the permutations of the octic group. This table shows that the cycle index for the octic subgroup G in S_4 is

$$\frac{1}{8}(x_1^4 + 2x_4^1 + 3x_2^2 + 2x_1^2 x_2^1).$$

Inside the parentheses of the cycle index, we have the sum of the 8 monomials with like terms combined. Hence the sum

$$1 + 2 + 3 + 2$$

of the coefficients of these terms should be 8, as it is. We also note that, in each monomial $x_i^a x_j^b \cdots x_k^c$, the sum of products $ai + bj + \cdots + ck$ must equal $\#T$. In this example, each such sum of products is 4.

Now we examine the set $F(g)$ of 8 colorings left fixed under the specific permutation $g = (1 \ \ 3)(2)(4)$. This set is shown in Table 7.7.2 and consists of the colorings in which sides 1 and 3 are both red or are both blue, side 2 is red or blue, and side 4 is red or blue. Using r for "red," b for "blue," $+$ for "or," and $\cdot$ for "and," we translate this description of $F(g)$ into the algebraic expression

$$(r \cdot r + b \cdot b) \cdot (r + b) \cdot (r + b) = (r + b)^2(r^2 + b^2).$$

Let us note the relationship between the monomial $x_1^2 x_2^1$ for this g and the expression $(r + b)^2(r^2 + b^2)$. One gets the algebraic expression by replacing each factor x_i^a in the monomial with $(r^i + b^i)^a$. The permutation $(1)(2 \ \ 4)(3)$ has the same monomial as $(1 \ \ 3)(2)(4)$ and hence its set of fixed colorings is also described by $(r + b)^2(r^2 + b^2)$. Each of the permutations $(1 \ \ 2 \ \ 3 \ \ 4)$ and $(1 \ \ 4 \ \ 3 \ \ 2)$ has x_4^1 as its monomial and has its set of fixed colorings described by $r^4 + b^4$. If h is $(1 \ \ 2)(3 \ \ 4)$ or $(1 \ \ 3)(2 \ \ 4)$ or $(1 \ \ 4)(2 \ \ 3)$, the monomial for h is x_2^2 and $F(h)$ is described by $(r^2 + b^2)^2$.

If we substitute these expressions for the monomials in the cycle index

$$P = \frac{1}{8}(x_1^4 + 2x_4^1 + 3x_2^2 + 2x_1^2 x_2^1)$$

for the octic group G, we get the following polynomial P^*, called the **pattern inventory** for G:

$$P^* = \frac{1}{8}\left[(r + b)^4 + 2(r^4 + b^4) + 3(r^2 + b^2)^2 + 2(r + b)^2(r^2 + b^2)\right].$$

Expanding and collecting like terms, this becomes

$$
\begin{aligned}
P^* = \frac{1}{8}[\ & r^4 + 4r^3b + 6r^2b^2 + 4rb^3 + b^4 \\
& + 2r^4 \qquad\qquad\qquad\qquad\ + 2b^4 \\
& + 3r^4 \qquad\quad + 6r^2b^2 \qquad\ + 3b^4 \\
& + 2r^4 + 4r^3b + 4r^2b^2 + 4rb^3 + 2b^4]
\end{aligned}
$$

$$P^* = \frac{1}{8}\left[8r^4 + 8r^3b + 16r^2b^2 + 8rb^3 + 8b^4\right]$$

$$P^* = r^4 + r^3b + 2r^2b^2 + rb^3 + b^4.$$

Here, miraculously, the coefficients give the important information that there is one way of coloring all the sides red, one way of coloring three red and one blue, two essentially different ways of coloring two sides red and two sides blue, and so on.

In the example just discussed, there were only sixteen colorings possible, so it was easy to examine them to decide how many are essentially different. One may ask, therefore, why it was necessary to use all the machinery from the symmetry group, the cycle index, and so on. It should also be emphasized that we have presented no proof to indicate that the machinery will always work. Let us look at another case, one where an examination of all the colorings would not be so easy.

What if we could color the sides of our square with the colors red, white, or blue? Then there would be $3^4 = 81$ possible colorings. Again, we are interested in knowing how many of the colorings are really different, that is, not the same as another coloring when viewed from a different vantage point.

Following in a natural way what we did in the earlier case, we substitute $(r^i + w^i + b^i)^a$ for each factor x_i^a in the cycle index. This yields the following pattern inventory:

$$
\begin{aligned}
P^* = \frac{1}{8}[&(r + w + b)^4 + 2(r^4 + w^4 + b^4) + 3(r^2 + w^2 + b^2)^2 \\
& + 2(r + w + b)^2(r^2 + w^2 + b^2)].
\end{aligned}
$$

Expanding and collecting like terms, we get

$$
\begin{aligned}
P^* = {}& r^4 + w^4 + b^4 + r^3w + wr^3 + r^3b + rb^3 + w^3b + wb^3 \\
& + 2r^2w^2 + 2r^2b^2 + 2w^2b^2 + 2r^2wb + 2rw^2b + 2rwb^2.
\end{aligned}
$$

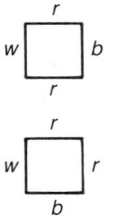

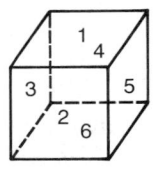

FIGURE 7.7.9

If our generalization is correct, this tells us, for example, that there are two essentially different ways to color two sides of a square red and two sides blue; but we already knew that. And it is not surprising that this should also be true for two white and two blue sides or for two white and two red sides. The new information in this pattern inventory concerns the actual use of three colors. The term $2r^2wb$ tells us that there are two essentially different ways of using red for two of the sides and each of white and blue for one of the sides. Figure 7.7.9 shows these two colorings. The terms $2rw^2b$ and $2rwb^2$ give similar information.

Let us now look at other examples.

Example 2   **2-COLORINGS OF A CUBE**   Here we count the essentially different 2-colorings of the faces of a cube and find the pattern inventory as well. We use red and blue as the colors.

Assigning the numbers 1, 2, 3, 4, 5, 6 to the cube faces so that 1 is the top face, 2 the front face, 3 the left, 4 the back, 5 the right, and 6 the bottom (Figure 7.7.10), we see that the group of symmetries is $G = \langle X, \circ, (1) \rangle$, where the permutations in X are listed after their monomials in Table 7.7.4.

FIGURE 7.7.10

TABLE 7.7.4

Monomial	Symmetries of a Cube
x_1^6	(1)(2)(3)(4)(5)(6).
$x_1^2x_4^1$	(1)(2 3 4 5)(6), (1)(2 5 4 3)(6), (1 2 6 4)(3)(5),
	(1 4 6 2)(3)(5), (1 3 6 5)(2)(4), (1 5 6 3)(2)(4).
$x_1^2x_2^2$	(1)(2 4)(3 5)(6), (1 6)(2 4)(3)(5), (1 6)(3 5)(2)(4).
x_3^2	(1 2 5)(3 6 4), (1 5 2)(3 4 6), (1 5 4)(2 6 3),
	(1 4 5)(2 3 6), (1 3 4)(2 6 5), (1 4 3)(2 5 6),
	(1 2 3)(4 5 6), (1 3 2)(4 6 5).
x_2^3	(1 2)(3 5)(4 6), (1 5)(2 4)(3 6), (1 4)(2 6)(3 5),
	(1 3)(2 4)(5 6), (1 6)(2 5)(3 4), (1 6)(2 3)(4 5).

Table 7.7.4 helps us see that the cycle index for this group is

$$P = \frac{1}{24}(x_1^6 + 6x_1^2x_4^1 + 3x_1^2x_2^2 + 8x_3^2 + 6x_2^3).$$

As in Example 2, we obtain the pattern inventory P^* from the cycle index

$$P = \frac{1}{24}(x_1^6 + 6x_1^2x_4^1 + 3x_1^2x_2^2 + 8x_3^2 + 6x_2^3)$$

by substituting $(r^i + b^i)^a$ for each x_i^a. This gives us

$$P^* = \frac{1}{24} \left[(r + b)^6 + 6(r + b)^2(r^4 + b^4) + 3(r + b)^2(r^2 + b^2)^2 \right.$$
$$\left. + 8(r^3 + b^3)^2 + 6(r^2 + b^2)^3 \right].$$

A short calculation yields

$$P^* = r^6 + r^5 b + 2r^4 b^2 + 2r^3 b^3 + 2r^2 b^4 + rb^5 + b^6.$$

The terms of P^* furnish an inventory of the essentially different 2-colorings of the faces of a cube. For example, the term $2r^4 b^2$ tells us that 2 of these colorings involve 4 red faces and 2 blue faces. All of the terms together inform us that there are 10 essentially different colorings, that is, 10 equivalence classes induced by the binary relation $\sim$ on the set of all 64 colorings. In Table 7.7.5, each of the 10 columns headed by $c_1, c_2, \ldots, c_{10}$ gives a representative chosen from a different equivalence class.

TABLE 7.7.5

Side	c_1	c_2	c_3	c_4	c_5	c_6	c_7	c_8	c_9	c_{10}
1	r	b	b	b	b	b	r	r	r	b
2	r	r	b	r	b	b	b	r	b	b
3	r	r	r	r	b	r	b	b	b	b
4	r	r	r	r	r	r	b	b	b	b
5	r	r	r	r	r	r	b	b	b	b
6	r	r	r	b	r	b	r	b	b	b

Alternatively, we can find the number of essentially different colorings using the cycle index P and Burnside's Lemma. For a permutation g with $x_i^a x_j^b \cdots x_k^c$ as its monomial, the number of 2-colorings fixed under g is 2^r, where r is the number of cycles in the representation of Table 7.7.4 for g. Hence r is $a + b + \cdots + c$. This fact and Burnside's Lemma together imply that the number of essentially different 2-colorings of the cube is obtained from the cycle index by replacing each x_i with 2. Hence this number is

$$\frac{1}{24} (2^6 + 6 \cdot 2^3 + 3 \cdot 2^4 + 8 \cdot 2^2 + 6 \cdot 2^3)$$

$$= \frac{1}{24} (64 + 48 + 48 + 32 + 48) = 10. \qquad \square$$

Example 3 **COUNTING NONISOMORPHIC GRAPHS** Here we find the maximum number of nonisomorphic graphs (V, E) with $\# V = 3$. If we let $V = \{u, v, w\}$, then the only possibilities for edges are the pairs $\{u, v\}$, $\{u, w\}$, and $\{v, w\}$.

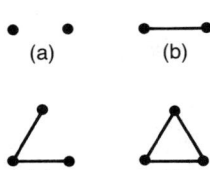

(a)   (b)

(c)   (d)

FIGURE 7.7.11

We can think of a selection of some or all of these pairs as a coloring of each of these possible edges with two colors, say p (for present) and n (for not present). Every graph with 3 vertices is isomorphic to one of the graphs in Figure 7.7.11. Can we obtain these possibilities from a cycle index? We number the possible edges as 1, 2, and 3 and consider the symmetric group $S_3 = \langle X_3, \circ, e \rangle$ whose carrier is the set

$$X_3 = \{(1)(2)(3), (1\ \ 2\ \ 3), (1\ \ 3\ \ 2), (1\ \ 2)(3), (1\ \ 3)(2), (1)(2\ \ 3)\}$$

of all permutations on $\{1, 2, 3\}$. The cycle index for this group is

$$P = \frac{1}{6}(x_1^3 + 2x_3^1 + 3x_1^1x_2^1).$$

Replacing each x_i by 2, we find that the maximum number of nonisomorphic graphs with 3 vertices is

$$\frac{1}{6}(2^3 + 2 \cdot 2 + 3 \cdot 2 \cdot 2) = \frac{1}{6}(8 + 4 + 12) = 4. \qquad \square$$

Example 4   **3-COLORINGS OF A TETRAHEDRON**   Here we find the number of essentially different 3-colorings of the vertices of the regular tetrahedron shown in Figure 7.7.12. We saw in Example 4 of Section 7.4 that the group of symmetries of a regular tetrahedron is the alternating group $A_4 = \langle E_4, \circ, e \rangle$ of even permutations on $T_4 = \{1, 2, 3, 4\}$. Table 7.4.2 in Example 2 of Section 7.2 can be used to see that the cycle index for A_4 is

$$P = \frac{1}{12}(x_1^4 + 8x_1^1x_3^1 + 3x_2^2).$$

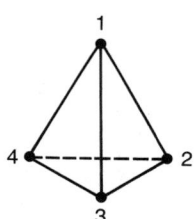

FIGURE 7.7.12

Since we are interested in 3-colorings, we replace each x_i by 3 and thus find the number of essentially different colorings is

$$\frac{1}{12}(3^4 + 8 \cdot 3 \cdot 3 + 3 \cdot 3^2) = \frac{1}{12}(81 + 72 + 27) = 15. \qquad \square$$

The Polya technique outlines an algorithm for finding the number of essentially different colorings of the elements of a set T, that is, the number of equivalence classes of colorings induced by the binary relation $\sim$ on the colorings. If we find the pattern inventory P^*, a term $mr^dw^e \cdots b^f$ in P^* tells us that there are m classes in which d of the elements of T are colored red, e of the elements are colored white, ..., and f of the elements are colored blue.

If one wants just the total number of equivalence classes induced by the binary relation $\sim$ on C^T (with respect to a group G) in a case with $\#C = s$, then this can be found by substituting s for each x_i in the cycle index for G.

George Polya   *was born in 1887 in Budapest. After studying there
and in Göttingen, he became professor at the Swiss Federal Institute of
Technology in Zurich. In 1942 he was made professor at Stanford
University. Known widely for his writings on problem solving as well as
for major contributions to a wide range of mathematical fields, Polya
made his principal contribution to combinatorics, his enumeration
technique, when studying chemical compounds. The original motivation
came from a study of alternate models proposed for the benzene molecule.
Polya died in 1985.*

PROBLEMS FOR SECTION 7.7

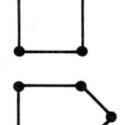

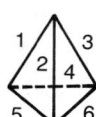

1.   Find the number of 2-colorings of the vertices of a regular tetrahedron.

2.   Find the number of 4-colorings of the vertices of a regular tetrahedron.

*3.   Find the maximum number of nonisomorphic spanning subgraphs of the graph in the accompanying figure.

*4.   Find the maximum number of nonisomorphic spanning subgraphs of the graph in the figure in the margin.

5.   In how many ways can we 2-color the faces of a pyramid with square base?

6.   In how many ways can we 2-color the edges of a pyramid with square base?

7.   Find the number of 3-colorings of the vertices of a regular hexagon if only rotations about the center are allowed in the group of symmetries.

8.   Find the number of 3-colorings of the vertices of a regular hexagon if rotations and flips about lines are allowed in the group.

9.   Find the pattern inventory for the 2-colorings of the edges of the regular tetrahedron shown in the figure, where the two colors are red (r) and blue (b).

10.   Find the pattern inventory for the 2-colorings of the vertices of a regular octahedron, where the two colors are red (r) and white (w).

11.   For a regular p-gon, with p a prime and $p > 2$, find the number of m-colorings if:
(a) rotations about the center are the only symmetries allowed.
(b) rotations about the center and flips about lines are allowed.

12.   Show that the binary relation $\sim$ on C^T is an equivalence relation.

SUMMARY OF TERMS, CHAPTER 7 _____

Abelian group	$\langle X, \square, e \rangle$ with $x \square y = y \square x$ for all x, y.	353
Additive group	$\langle X, +, 0 \rangle$ with $x + y = y + x$ for all x, y.	353
Additive inverse of x	The element $-x$ such that $x + (-x) = 0$.	353
Additive powers of x	$n \cdot x$ written for x^n.	357
Alternate definition of group	See Definition 1' of Section 7.1.	352
Alternating subgroup:		
A_n in S_n	$\langle E_n, \circ, (1) \rangle$ with E_n the set of even permutations on $\{1, \ldots, n\}$.	390
A_3	See Table 7.4.1 in Section 7.4.	394
A_4	See Table 7.4.2 in Section 7.4.	395
Associativity of composition	See Theorem 1 of Section 7.2.	368
Bitwise addition modulo 2	See Example 2 of Section 7.1.	354
Burnside's Lemma	See Theorem 1 of Section 7.7.	413
Cancellation:		
Left	$(c \square a = c \square b) \Rightarrow (a = b)$ in a group.	360
Mixed	$c \square a = b \square c$ does NOT necessarily imply $a = b$.	365
Right	$(a \square c = b \square c) \Rightarrow (a = b)$ in a group.	360
Canonical form	See Definition 3 of Section 7.3.	385
Closed subsets	See Theorem 2 of Section 7.1.	354
Colorings	See Section 7.7.	409
Commutative group	*See* Abelian group.	353
Commutative ring	$(X, +, 0, \cdot)$ with $xy = yx$ for all x, y.	405
Composite of mappings	See Definition 1 and Theorem 1 of Section 7.2.	367
Composite of permutations	See Theorem 2 and Algorithm 1 of Section 7.2.	370
Coset for a of Y in G	See Definition 1 of Section 7.5.	399
Counting labelings	See Section 7.7.	408
Cycle index	See Section 7.7.	414
Cycles, product of disjoint	See Definition 3 of Section 7.3.	385
Cyclic group	See Definition 7 of Section 7.1.	358
Cyclic subgroup generated by a	See Definition 7 of Section 7.1.	358
Direct product of groups	See Problem 39 of Section 7.1.	366
Disjoint cycles	See Definition 2 and Theorem 1 of Section 7.3.	383
Disjoint left (right) cosets	See Theorem 2 of Section 7.5.	400
D_n	Set of odd permutations on $\{1, 2, \ldots, n\}$.	394
E_n	Set of even permutations on $\{1, 2, \ldots, n\}$.	390
Equal size of E_n and D_n	See Theorem 1 of Section 7.4.	394
Equivalent colorings	See Section 7.7.	411
Even permutation	Product of an even number of transpositions.	390
Field $\langle X, +, 0, \cdot, 1 \rangle$	See Definition 2 of Section 7.6.	406
Finite closed subset	See Theorem 9 of Section 7.1.	361
Finite field	Field with a finite carrier.	406
Finite group	Group with a finite carrier.	354

REVIEW PROBLEMS FOR CHAPTER 7

1. Which of the following are subgroups in $\langle Z, +, 0 \rangle$?

(a) $\langle 2Z, +, 0 \rangle$;   (b) $\langle 3Z, +, 0 \rangle$;

(c) $\langle (2Z) \cup (3Z), +, 0 \rangle$;   (d) $\langle (2Z) \cap (3Z), +, 0 \rangle$.

2. Which of the following sets Y are carriers of subgroups in the multiplicative group $\langle Q^+, \cdot, 1 \rangle$ of the positive rational numbers?
    (a) $Y = \{3^n : n \in N\} = \{1, 3, 9, \ldots\}$.
    (b) $Y = \{3^n : n \in Z^+\} = \{3, 9, 27, \ldots\}$.
    (c) $Y = \{3^n : n \in Z\} = \{\ldots, \frac{1}{9}, \frac{1}{3}, 1, 3, 9, \ldots\}$.
    (d) $Y = \{3n : n \in Z\} = \{\ldots, -6, -3, 0, 3, 6, \ldots\}$.

3. Which of the following sets Y are carriers of subgroups in the bitwise addition modulo 2 group $\langle B_4, \oplus, 0_4 \rangle$?
    (a) $Y = \{0000, 1111\}$;   (b) $Y = \{0000, 0011, 1100, 1111\}$;
    (c) $Y = \{0011, 1100, 1111\}$;   (d) $Y = \{0001, 0010, 0100, 1000\}$.

4. (a) For which n's in Z^+ is $\langle B_n, \oplus, 0_2 \rangle$ abelian?
    (b) For which n's in Z^+ is $\langle B_n, \oplus, 0_2 \rangle$ cyclic?

5. Let $G = \langle [g], \square, e \rangle$ be a cyclic group of order 12. Give the order of g^n for $n = 0, 1, \ldots, 11$.

6. Let $G = \langle [g], \square, e \rangle$ be a cyclic group of order 28. List the elements of the carrier of a subgroup:
    (a) of order 4.   (b) of index 4.

7. Let $G = \langle [g], \square, e \rangle$ be a cyclic group of order n and let d be a positive integral divisor of n. Must G have a subgroup of order d? Explain.

8. (i) Is every monoid a group?   (ii) Is every group a monoid?
    (iii) If a property is possessed by all monoids, must it be possessed by all groups?

9. Let $U_2 = \{1, -1\}$, $U_4 = \{1, \mathbf{i}, -1, -\mathbf{i}\}$, $G = \langle U_4, \cdot, 1 \rangle$, $G' = \langle U_2, \cdot, 1 \rangle$.
    (a) Tabulate a homomorphism α from G to G' with $\alpha(\mathbf{i}) = -1$.
    (b) Tabulate an isomorphism β from G to a cyclic group $\langle [g], \square, e \rangle$ of order 4 in which $\beta(-\mathbf{i}) = g$.

10. Let R and R^+ be the sets of the real numbers and of the positive real numbers, respectively. Is
    $$f: R \to R^+; \quad x \mapsto 10^x$$
    an isomorphism from $\langle R, +, 0 \rangle$ onto $\langle R^+, \cdot, 1 \rangle$? Explain.

11. Let $\alpha: X_3 \to E_3 = \{(1), (1\ \ 2\ \ 3), (1\ \ 3\ \ 2)\}$ be given by the following table:

p	(1)	(1 2 3)	(1 3 2)	(2 3)	(1 3)	(1 2)
$\alpha(p)$	(1)	(1 3 2)	(1 2 3)	(1 2 3)	(1 3 2)	(1 2 3)

    Is α a homomorphism from S_3 to $A_3 = \langle [(1\ \ 2\ \ 3)], \circ, (1) \rangle$? Explain.

12. If h is a homomorphism from $G = \langle X, \square, e \rangle$ to $G' = \langle X', \square, e' \rangle$, then $h(e) = e'$ and $h(x^n) = [h(x)]^n$ for each x in X and each n in Z. Is this still true when h is an isomorphism? Explain.

13. Let

$$p = \begin{pmatrix} 1 & 2 & 3 & 4 & 5 & 6 & 7 & 8 & 9 \\ 1 & 3 & 4 & 2 & 6 & 7 & 8 & 9 & 5 \end{pmatrix}.$$

(i) Find the canonical form for p.   (ii) Find the order of p in S_9.

14. Let $p = (1 \quad 2 \quad 3 \quad 4 \quad 5)(4 \quad 5 \quad 6 \quad 7)$.
(i) Find the canonical form for p.   (ii) Find the order of p.

15. Make the operation tables for the groups $G = \langle X, \circ, (1) \rangle$ and $G' = \langle X', \circ, (1) \rangle$ with $X = \{(1), (1 \quad 2)(3 \quad 4), (1 \quad 3)(2 \quad 4), (1 \quad 4)(2 \quad 3)\}$ and $X' = \{(1), (1 \quad 2 \quad 3 \quad 4), (1 \quad 3)(2 \quad 4), (1 \quad 4 \quad 3 \quad 2)\}$.

16. Are the groups of Problem 15 isomorphic? Explain.

17. Let p and q be permutations on $\{1, 2, \ldots, n\}$.
(i) If p is even, must p^{-1} be even? Explain.
(ii) If p is odd, must p^{-1} be odd? Explain.
(iii) Explain why $q^{-1}(1 \quad 2)q$ is odd and $q^{-1}(1 \quad 2 \quad 3)q$ is even.

18. (a) If $g = t_1 t_2 \cdots t_m$ with each t_i a transposition, does $g^2 = (1)$?
(b) Let g be a permutation on $\{1, 2, \ldots, n\}$. If $g^2 = (1)$, must g be a product of transpositions?

19. The types of canonical forms for permutations in S_5 are: (1), $(a \quad b)$, $(a \quad b \quad c)$, $(a \quad b \quad c \quad d)$, $(a \quad b \quad c \quad d \quad e)$, $(a \quad b)(c \quad d)$, $(a \quad b \quad c)(d \quad e)$, $(a \quad b)(c \quad d \quad e)$.
(a) Give all the types of canonical forms for even permutations in S_6. For each type give the number of such permutations in S_6.
(b) Do Part (a) with *even* replaced by *odd*.

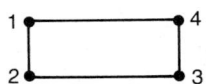

20. List the symmetries of the (nonsquare) rectangle shown in the margin.

21. Let $r = (1 \quad 2 \quad 3 \quad 4)$ and $f = (2 \quad 4)$.
(i) Does $fr = r^3 f$?

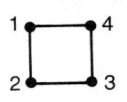

(ii) Is $\{(1), r, r^2, r^3, f, rf, r^2 f, r^3 f\}$ the set of symmetries of the square shown in the margin?

22. (i) Show that the subset $Y = \{00000, 11000, 00110, 11110\}$ of B_5 is closed under bitwise addition modulo 2.
(ii) Find eight distinct left cosets of $\langle Y, \oplus, 0_5 \rangle$ in $\langle B_5, \oplus, 0_5 \rangle$.
(iii) Is each left coset $\alpha \oplus Y$ in (ii) equal to $Y \oplus \alpha$? Explain.

23. Let K be a subgroup in H and H be a subgroup in G. Let the orders of K and G be 5 and 60, respectively. What are the possibilities for the order of H?

24. Explain why every group of prime order is cyclic.

25. Let $\langle X, +, 0, \cdot, 1 \rangle$ be a field with $\#X = 11$. Let X^* be the complement $X - \{0\}$ of $\{0\}$ in X. Explain why:
(i) $M = \langle X^*, \cdot, 1 \rangle$ is a group of order 10.
(ii) the order of each x in X^* is in the set $\{1, 2, 5, 10\}$.

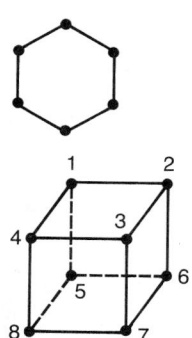

(iii) $x^{10} = 1$ for each x in X^*.

(iv) $x^{11} = x$ for each x in X.

26. What is the largest number of subgraphs of the graph of the figure in the margin that we can have without having two isomorphic subgraphs? (Sketch each subgraph of such a collection.)

27. (a) Find the cycle index for the labelings (colorings) of the vertices of the cube shown here.

(b) Find the number of 2-colorings of the vertices.

(c) Find the corresponding pattern inventory for colors black (*b*) and white (*w*).

SUPPLEMENTARY PROBLEMS, CHAPTER 7

1. Let $\langle C, +, 0, \cdot, 1 \rangle$ be the field of complex numbers. Describe all the finite subgroups of the multiplicative group $\langle C - \{0\}, \cdot, 1 \rangle$.

2. Let "direct product" of groups be as described in Problem 39 of Section 7.1. Prove that the direct product $\langle B_2, \oplus, 0_2 \rangle \times \langle B_3, \oplus, 0_3 \rangle$ is isomorphic to $\langle B_5, \oplus, 0_5 \rangle$.

3. Let $G = \langle [g], \square, e \rangle$ be a cyclic group.

(a) Show that every subgroup in G is cyclic.

(b) Show that G is isomorphic to a proper subgroup in G if and only if $[g]$ is infinite.

4. Let $\langle H, \square, e \rangle$ and $\langle N, \square, e \rangle$ be normal subgroups in $G = \langle X, \square, e \rangle$. Prove that $\langle H \cap N, \square, e \rangle$ is a normal subgroup in G.

5. Prove that there is no field $\langle X, +, 0, \cdot, 1 \rangle$ with $\# X = 6$.

6. Let $G = \langle X, \square, e \rangle$ be a group. The *center* in G is the set C of elements c such that $c \square x = x \square c$ for all x in X. The *centralizer for a* in G is the set C_a of all y in X such that $a \square y = y \square a$. Prove that:

(a) $\langle C, \square, e \rangle$ is a subgroup in G.

(b) $\langle C_a, \square, e \rangle$ is a subgroup in G for each a in X.

(c) $\langle C, \square, e \rangle$ is a subgroup in $\langle C_a, \square, e \rangle$ for each a in X.

7. Find the center in the symmetric group S_n.

8. Find the center in the octic group of symmetries of a square.

9. Let $G = \langle X, \square, e \rangle$ be a group and $a \in X$. Prove that

$$\beta: X \to X; \quad x \mapsto a^{-1}xa$$

is an isomorphism from G onto itself. (Such a mapping is called an ***inner automorphism***.)

8
POLYNOMIALS, PARTIAL FRACTIONS

Polynomial functions are the most frequently used functions because they arise naturally and because they can provide helpful approximations to other functions. In the next chapter, we will need techniques for solving polynomial equations, for factoring polynomials, and for expressing quotients of polynomials in terms of partial fractions. The purpose of this chapter is to develop these aids for solving recursions.

8.1
POLYNOMIALS

This section contains a brief review of solving first and second degree polynomial equations. Then, for polynomials of all degrees, we present the "Synthetic Division" algorithm for finding values of polynomial functions, methods for finding rational roots and for using roots as an aid in factoring, and a discussion of multiple, or repeated, roots.

A *polynomial* in x of *degree* d with complex *coefficients* a_i is of the form

$$a_0 x^d + a_1 x^{d-1} + \cdots + a_{d-1} x + a_d, \tag{1}$$

with the a_i complex numbers and with $a_0 \neq 0$. (Of course, the coefficients a_i may be real numbers, rational numbers, or integers, since these are special cases of complex numbers.) A nonzero constant c is a polynomial of degree 0; the constant zero is also a polynomial but it is not assigned a degree. A *first degree polynomial* has the form $ax + b$, with $a \neq 0$, and a *second degree polynomial* is of the form $ax^2 + bx + c$, with $a \neq 0$.

Let C be the set of complex numbers and D be a subset of C (such as the real numbers, the rational numbers, or the integers). A *polynomial function* on D is a mapping

$$p: D \to C, \quad x \mapsto p(x) = a_0 x^d + a_1 x^{d-1} + \cdots + a_d$$

whose rule $p(x)$ is a polynomial.

A *polynomial equation* has the form $p(x) = 0$, with $p(x)$ a polynomial. For $p(x) = a_0 x^d + \cdots + a_d$, a *root* of $p(x) = 0$ is a number h such that $p(h) = 0$, that is, such that

$$a_0 h^d + a_1 h^{d-1} + \cdots + a_{d-1} h + a_d = 0.$$

FIRST DEGREE EQUATIONS

The only root of a first degree equation $ax + b = 0$, with $a \neq 0$, is $x = -b/a$. For example, the sole root of $12x - 8 = 0$ is $x = \frac{8}{12} = \frac{2}{3}$.

SECOND DEGREE EQUATIONS

A second degree polynomial equation has the form

$$ax^2 + bx + c = 0, \qquad a \neq 0.$$

If the polynomial can be factored so that the equation becomes

$$a(x - r)(x - s) = 0, \qquad a \neq 0,$$

then the roots r and s are found by setting the factors $x - r$ and $x - s$ equal to zero and solving for x.

Example 1   We solve the equation $3x^2 - 6x - 45 = 0$ as follows:

$$3x^2 - 6x - 45 = 0$$
$$3(x^2 - 2x - 15) = 0$$
$$3(x - 5)(x + 3) = 0$$
$$x - 5 = 0 \qquad \text{or} \qquad x + 3 = 0$$
$$x = 5 \qquad \text{or} \qquad x = -3.$$

Thus the roots are 5 and -3.   □

Example 2   Here we solve $x^2 + 12x + 36 = 0$. Factoring, we have

$$(x + 6)(x + 6) = 0.$$

We equate each factor to zero and solve for x. This shows that -6 is the only root.   □

Example 3   Now we solve the equation $3x^2 - 7 = 0$. Adding 7 to both sides and dividing by 3 gives us

$$3x^2 = 7$$
$$x^2 = \tfrac{7}{3}.$$

Taking square roots results in $x = \pm\sqrt{\frac{7}{3}}$. Hence the two roots are $\sqrt{\frac{7}{3}}$ and $-\sqrt{\frac{7}{3}}$.

Alternatively, we can use the "difference of squares factorization"

$$A^2 - B^2 = (A - B)(A + B)$$

to rewrite $3x^2 - 7 = 0$ as

$$(\sqrt{3}x - \sqrt{7})(\sqrt{3}x + \sqrt{7}) = 0$$

and thus find that the roots are $\sqrt{7}/\sqrt{3} = \sqrt{\frac{7}{3}}$ and $-\sqrt{7}/\sqrt{3} = -\sqrt{\frac{7}{3}}$. □

Next we present a formula for factoring a general quadratic polynomial and for solving a general quadratic equation.

THEOREM 1   **THE QUADRATIC FORMULA**

(a) Let $a \neq 0$. Then $ax^2 + bx + c = a(x - r)(x - s)$, where r and s are the numbers $(-b \pm \sqrt{b^2 - 4ac})/2a$. If $b^2 - 4ac = 0$, then $r = s = -b/2a$.

(b) The roots of $ax^2 + bx + c = 0$, with $a \neq 0$, are

$$\frac{-b \pm \sqrt{b^2 - 4ac}}{2a}.$$

PROOF   (a) We use completing squares and the difference of squares factorization $y^2 - d = (y - \sqrt{d})(y + \sqrt{d})$. Let $Q = ax^2 + bx + c$. Then

$$4aQ = 4a^2x^2 + 4abx + 4ac$$
$$= 4a^2x^2 + 4abx + b^2 - b^2 + 4ac$$
$$= (2ax + b)^2 - (b^2 - 4ac)$$
$$= (2ax + b - \sqrt{b^2 - 4ac})(2ax + b + \sqrt{b^2 - 4ac})$$
$$4a^2Q = a(2ax + b - \sqrt{b^2 - 4ac})(2ax + b + \sqrt{b^2 - 4ac})$$
$$Q = a\left(\frac{2ax + b - \sqrt{b^2 - 4ac}}{2a}\right)\left(\frac{2ax + b + \sqrt{b^2 - 4ac}}{2a}\right)$$
$$Q = a\left(x + \frac{b - \sqrt{b^2 - 4ac}}{2a}\right)\left(x + \frac{b + \sqrt{b^2 - 4ac}}{2a}\right)$$
$$Q = a\left(x - \frac{-b + \sqrt{b^2 - 4ac}}{2a}\right)\left(x - \frac{-b - \sqrt{b^2 - 4ac}}{2a}\right)$$

This proves Part (a).

(b) One obtains r and s by solving each of $x - r = 0$ and $x - s = 0$ for x. □

Example 4   We solve the quadratic equation $7x^2 - 8x - 9 = 0$ by setting $a = 7$, $b = -8$, and $c = -9$ in the quadratic formula and thus finding that the roots are

$$\frac{-b \pm \sqrt{b^2 - 4ac}}{2a} = \frac{8 \pm \sqrt{64 - 4 \cdot 7(-9)}}{2 \cdot 7} = \frac{8 \pm \sqrt{64 + 252}}{14}$$

$$= \frac{8 \pm \sqrt{316}}{14} = \frac{8 \pm \sqrt{4 \cdot 79}}{14} = \frac{8 \pm 2\sqrt{79}}{14} = \frac{4 \pm \sqrt{79}}{7}.$$

$\square$

In the next chapter, we will need the following variation on the factorization formula of Theorem 1.

THEOREM 2   **ALTERNATE FACTORING FORM**

$1 + bx + cx^2 = (1 - rx)(1 - sx)$, where r and s are the numbers $(-b \pm \sqrt{b^2 - 4c})/2$. If $b^2 - 4c = 0$, then $r = s = -b/2$.

PROOF   We use Theorem 1(a) with $a = 1$ and x replaced by y; this gives

$$y^2 + by + c = (y - r)(y - s).$$

where r and s are the numbers $(-b \pm \sqrt{b^2 - 4c})/2$. We replace y by $1/x$ and get

$$\frac{1}{x^2} + \frac{b}{x} + c = \left(\frac{1}{x} - r\right)\left(\frac{1}{x} - s\right).$$

Then we multiply each side by x^2 and have the desired factorization

$$1 + bx + cx^2 = (1 - rx)(1 - sx).$$

$\square$

Example 5   The factored form of Theorem 2 for $1 - 3x - 10x^2$ is $(1 - 5x)(1 + 2x)$. This can be seen by inspection or by letting $b = -3$ and $c = -10$ in the formula of Theorem 2. Similarly, this type of factorization for $1 - 8x + 16x^2$ is $(1 - 4x)(1 - 4x)$.

$\square$

There are formulas for solving third and fourth degree polynomial equations. These formulas are very complicated and are rarely used; hence they are not presented here. For a discussion of exact solution of all third and fourth degree polynomial equations, see A. P. Hillman and G. L. Alexanderson, *A First Undergraduate Course in Abstract Algebra*, 3rd ed. (Belmont, Calif.: Wadsworth Publishing Co., 1983).

Here we present some easier methods that apply in special cases and in the next section give algorithms for refining, to any desired accuracy, an approximation to a real root of a polynomial equation with real coefficients. First we introduce the efficient "Synthetic Division" algorithm for evaluating polynomials.

Example 6   Let $p(x) = 5x^3 - 13x^2 + 7x + 8$. How should we find $p(2)$? It may seem natural to do this in the form

$$p(2) = 5 \cdot 2^3 - 13 \cdot 2^2 + 7 \cdot 2 + 8$$
$$= 5 \cdot 8 - 13 \cdot 4 + 7 \cdot 2 + 8$$
$$= 40 - 52 + 14 + 8 = 10.$$

Alternatively, we can rewrite $p(x)$ as $p(x) = [(5x - 13)x + 7]x + 8$ and thus find that

$$p(2) = [(10 - 13)2 + 7]2 + 8$$
$$= [(-3)2 + 7]2 + 8$$
$$= [-6 + 7]2 + 8 = 1 \cdot 2 + 8 = 10. \qquad \square$$

When the degree d of $p(x)$ is large, the second method in Example 6 is recommended, since it involves only d multiplications whereas the first requires $2d - 1$ multiplications. The number of additions and subtractions is the same for both methods.

Next we generalize the second method of Example 6 so that it applies to general polynomials.

ALGORITHM 1   EVALUATING A POLYNOMIAL BY SYNTHETIC DIVISION

Let $p(x) = a_0 x^d + a_1 x^{d-1} + \cdots + a_d$. To find $p(h)$ one finds numbers $b_0, c_0, b_1, c_1, \ldots, b_d, c_d$ using $b_0 = 0$, $b_i = hc_{i-1}$ for $1 \le i \le d$, and $c_i = a_i + b_i$ for $0 \le i \le d$. Then $c_d = p(h)$.

The calculations using Algorithm 1 are arranged as follows:

h	a_0	a_1	a_2	$\cdots$	a_{d-1}	a_d
	b_0	b_1	b_2	$\cdots$	b_{d-1}	b_d
	c_0	c_1	c_2	$\cdots$	c_{d-1}	c_d

Example 7   As in Example 6, let $p(x) = 5x^3 - 13x^2 + 7x + 8$. The following application of Algorithm 1 gives us $p(2) = 10$:

2	5	-13	7	8
	0	10	-6	2
	5	-3	1	10

In this array, the coefficients of $p(x)$ appear on the first row, the top two numbers in each column are added to get the number below the line in that column, each of these sums except the last is multiplied by h (2 in this example), and the products $c_{i-1}h$ are placed as indicated by the arrows on the row of the b_i. $\square$

Example 8 As in Example 6, let $p(x) = 5x^3 - 13x^2 + 7x + 8$. Now we perform long division of $p(x)$ by $x - 2$, as follows:

$$
\begin{array}{r}
5x^2 - 3x + 1 \\
x-2\ \overline{\smash{\big)}\ 5x^3 - 13x^2 + 7x + 8} \\
\underline{5x^3 - 10x^2} \\
-3x^2 + 7x \\
\underline{-3x^2 + 6x} \\
x + 8 \\
\underline{x - 2} \\
10
\end{array}
$$

This shows that the quotient is $5x^2 - 3x + 1$ and the remainder is 10; that is,

$$5x^3 - 13x^2 + 7x + 8 = (x - 2)(5x^2 - 3x + 1) + 10. \quad \square$$

If we examine Examples 7 and 8, it can be noted that the quotient $5x^2 - 3x + 1$ is $c_0 x^2 + c_1 x + c_2$ and the remainder 10 is c_3, where c_0, c_1, c_2, and c_3 are the numbers on the last line of the array for finding $p(2)$ using Algorithm 1. Let us see if this is true for all polynomials $p(x)$ and all numbers h.

If $p(x) = a_0 x^d + a_1 x^{d-1} + \cdots + a_d$ is divided by $x - h$, one gets a quotient $q(x)$ with degree one less than that of $p(x)$ and a constant remainder r. We can write the quotient as $q(x) = c_0 x^{d-1} + c_1 x^{d-2} + \cdots + c_{d-1}$ and the remainder r as c_d. Then $p(x) = (x - h)q(x) + r$ or

$$
\begin{aligned}
a_0 x^d + a_1 x^{d-1} + \cdots + a_d &= (x - h)(c_0 x^{d-1} + c_1 x^{d-2} + \cdots + c_{d-1}) + c_d \\
&= c_0 x^d + (c_1 - hc_0)x^{d-1} + (c_2 - hc_1)x^{d-2} \\
&\quad + \cdots + (c_{d-1} - hc_{d-2})x + (c_d - hc_{d-1}).
\end{aligned}
$$

Equating coefficients of like powers on both sides of this equation, we get

$$c_0 = a_0 \quad \text{and} \quad c_i - hc_{i-1} = a_i \quad \text{for } i = 1, 2, \ldots, d.$$

It follows that $c_i = a_i + hc_{i-1}$ for $i = 1, 2, \ldots, d$. Letting $hc_{i-1} = b_i$, we get the formula $c_i = a_i + b_i$ of Algorithm 1. Thus the coefficients $c_0, c_1, \ldots, c_{d-1}$ of the quotient $q(x)$ and the remainder $r = c_d$ in the division of $p(x)$ by $x - h$ are produced as in Algorithm 1. We now state this formally.

ALGORITHM 2   **SYNTHETIC DIVISION**

Let $p(x) = a_0 x^d + a_1 x^{d-1} + \cdots + a_d$. To divide $p(x)$ by $x - h$, one produces $c_0, c_1, \ldots, c_d$ as in Algorithm 1, lets $q(x) = c_0 x^{d-1} + c_1 x^{d-2} + \cdots + c_{d-1}$ and $r = c_d$, and has

$$p(x) = (x - h)q(x) + r.$$

Since each of $p(h)$ and the remainder r in the division of $p(x)$ by $x - h$ equals the c_d of Algorithm 1, we have the following result.

THEOREM 3   **REMAINDER THEOREM**

Let $p(x) = (x - h)q(x) + r$, with r a number. Then the remainder $r = p(h)$.

PROOF   Although we have given a long indirect proof above, a short direct proof is available; we give it now. Substituting h for x in the given equality, one gets

$$p(h) = (h - h)q(h) + r = 0 \cdot q(h) + r = 0 + r = r.$$

Thus $p(h) = r$, as claimed.   □

Example 9   Let $p(x) = 2x^4 + 15x - 4$. We use synthetic division, as follows, to find the quotient $q(x)$ and the remainder r in the division of $p(x)$ by $x + 3$.

$$
\begin{array}{r|rrrrr}
-3 & 2 & 0 & 0 & 15 & -4 \\
   &   & 0 & -6 & 18 & -54 & 117 \\
\hline
   & 2 & -6 & 18 & -39 & \boxed{113}
\end{array}
$$

Thus $2x^4 + 15x - 4 = (x + 3)(2x^3 - 6x^2 + 18x - 39) + 113$, with $2x^3 - 6x^2 + 18x - 39$ as the quotient and 113 as the remainder.

Note: One of the errors frequently made in using synthetic division is to omit the 0's for coefficients of missing terms on the top line. In this $p(x)$, no x^3 or x^2 is present. This means that the coefficients of x^3 and x^2 in $p(x)$ are each 0. These 0 coefficients must be placed in their required positions in order to perform the division accurately.   □

The following result helps us find first degree factors of a polynomial.

THEOREM 4   **FACTOR THEOREM**

Let $p(x)$ be a polynomial of degree $d \geq 1$. Then h is a root of $p(x) = 0$ if and only if $p(x) = (x - h)q(x)$, with $q(x)$ a polynomial of degree $d - 1$.

PROOF Using synthetic (or long) division, one can obtain $p(x) = (x - h)q(x) + r$, with $q(x)$ a polynomial of degree $d - 1$ and $r = p(h)$. Clearly, h is a root of $p(x) = 0$ if and only if $p(h) = 0$, and $r = p(h) = 0$ if and only if $p(x)$ is of the form $(x - h)q(x)$. $\square$

When the coefficients a_i of a polynomial $p(x)$ are integers, there is only a limited number of possibilities for rational roots (and hence for integer roots) of $p(x) = 0$. We state this, without proof, as the following theorem.

THEOREM 5 **RATIONAL ROOT THEOREM**

Let $p(x) = a_0 x^d + a_1 x^{d-1} + \cdots + a_d$, with the a_i integers and with $a_0 \neq 0$. If $h = s/t$ is a root of $p(x) = 0$ with s and t integers having 1 as their greatest common integral divisor, then $s \mid a_d$ and $t \mid a_0$. We can take t to be positive.

The notation $u \mid v$ is as in Notation 3 of Section 1.7 and means that u is an exact divisor of v.

Example 10 Let us try to solve $p(x) = 0$ where $p(x) = x^4 - 2x^3 + 2x^2 - 2x + 1$. Since the coefficients of $p(x)$ are integers, the Rational Root Theorem is applicable. The "leading" coefficient a_0 is 1. The degree d of $p(x)$ is 4 and the "caboose" coefficient is $a_d = a_4 = 1$. The only possibilities for rational roots of $p(x) = 0$ are fractions s/t, with $s \mid 1$, $t \mid 1$, and $t > 0$. For such s/t, one must have s in $\{1, -1\}$ and $t = 1$. Thus 1 and -1 are the only possibilities for rational roots. We try $x = 1$ by synthetic division as follows.

$$
\begin{array}{r|rrrrr}
1 & 1 & -2 & 2 & -2 & 1 \\
  & 0 & 1 & -1 & 1 & -1 \\
\hline
  & 1 & -1 & 1 & -1 & 0
\end{array}
$$

This shows that 1 is a root and that $p(x) = (x - 1)q(x)$, where $q(x) = x^3 - x^2 + x - 1$. To find the other roots of $p(x) = 0$, we solve $q(x) = 0$. Applying the Rational Root Theorem once more, we see that 1 and -1 are the only possible rational roots. Trying $x = 1$ by synthetic division, we find that it is a root and that $q(x) = (x - 1)(x^2 + 1)$. Hence $p(x) = (x - 1)(x - 1)(x^2 + 1) = (x - 1)(x - 1)(x - \mathbf{i})(x + \mathbf{i})$. Setting these factors equal to zero, one finds that the roots of $p(x) = 0$ are

$$1, 1, \mathbf{i}, \text{ and } -\mathbf{i}. \tag{2}$$

$\square$

We repeated the root 1 in Display (2) because $x - 1$ appeared twice in the factorization of $p(x)$. This phenomenon is generalized in the following definition.

DEFINITION 1   **MULTIPLE ROOT, MULTIPLICITY OF A ROOT**

If $p(x) = (x - h)^m q(x)$, with m a positive integer and $q(h) \neq 0$, we say that h is a root of $p(x) = 0$ with **multiplicity** m. If $m \geq 2$, then h is a **multiple root**, or **repeated root**.

In Example 10, the root 1 is a multiple root with multiplicity 2, whereas the roots $\mathbf{i}$ and $-\mathbf{i}$ are **simple roots** (that is, they have multiplicity 1). Note that $p(x)$ must have degree at least 2 to have a multiple root.

Example 11   Here we solve $p(x) = 0$ with $p(x) = 3x^3 + 2x^2 + 12x + 8$. Since the co-efficients are integers, the Rational Root Theorem is applicable. The possibilities for rational roots are the s/t, with $s|8$, $t|3$, and $t > 0$. Thus we can restrict ourselves to s in $\{1, -1, 2, -2, 4, -4, 8, -8\}$ and t in $\{1, 3\}$. If $h > 0$, then $p(h)$ is a sum of positive numbers and so is not zero. Hence a set of possibilities for rational roots is

$$\{-1, -2, -4, -8, -\tfrac{1}{3}, -\tfrac{2}{3}, -\tfrac{4}{3}, -\tfrac{8}{3}\}.$$

We try these in order; the first that turns out to be a root is $-\tfrac{2}{3}$. Its test by synthetic division is:

$$
\begin{array}{r|rrrr}
-\tfrac{2}{3} & 3 & 2 & 12 & 8 \\
 & 0 & -2 & 0 & -8 \\
\hline
 & 3 & 0 & 12 & \;0 \\
\end{array}
$$

This shows that

$$p(x) = (x + \tfrac{2}{3})(3x^2 + 12) = (3x + 2)(x^2 + 4).$$

The roots of $p(x) = 0$ besides $-\tfrac{2}{3}$ are the roots of $x^2 + 4 = 0$. These satisfy $x^2 = -4$ and hence are $\pm\sqrt{-4}$, or $\pm 2\mathbf{i}$. Thus the roots of $p(x) = 0$ are $-\tfrac{2}{3}$, $2\mathbf{i}$, and $-2\mathbf{i}$.   □

Example 12   How might we prove that $\sqrt{2} + \sqrt{3}$ is irrational? One way is to show that it is a root of an equation $p(x) = 0$, where $p(x)$ is a polynomial with in-teger coefficients and no rational roots. We start by letting $u = \sqrt{2} + \sqrt{3}$. Then

$$u - \sqrt{2} = \sqrt{3}$$
$$(u - \sqrt{2})^2 = 3$$
$$u^2 - 2\sqrt{2}u + 2 = 3$$
$$u^2 - 1 = 2\sqrt{2}u$$
$$u^4 - 2u^2 + 1 = 8u^2$$
$$u^4 - 10u^2 + 1 = 0.$$

Thus u is a root of $x^4 - 10x^2 + 1 = 0$. The only possibilities for rational roots of this equation are 1 and -1. Testing, one finds that neither possibility is a root. (It is also clear that neither 1 nor -1 is $\sqrt{2} + \sqrt{3}$ because $\sqrt{2} + \sqrt{3} > 1 + 1$.) But if u were rational, it would be 1 or -1. Hence $u = \sqrt{2} + \sqrt{3}$ is not rational. $\qquad\square$

Table 8.1.1 contains a number of additional examples.

TABLE 8.1.1

Polynomial $p(x)$	Degree of $p(x)$	Roots of $p(x) = 0$	Multiple Roots
0	Not defined	Every number	
5	0	No roots	
$x + 8$	1	-8	
$3x - 5i$	1	$\frac{5}{3}i$	
$x^2 + 9$	2	$3i, -3i$	
$x^2 - 7$	2	$\sqrt{7}, -\sqrt{7}$	
$x^2 - 8x + 15$	2	$3, 5$	
$x^3 - 6x^2 + 12x - 8$	3	$2, 2, 2$	2 is a root of multiplicity 3.
$x^4 + 6x^3 + 9x^2$	4	$0, 0, -3, -3$	Each of 0 and -3 is a root of multiplicity 2.
$(x - 1)^3(x + 2)^2$	5	$1, 1, 1, -2, -2$	1 is a root of multiplicity 3; -2 has multiplicity 2.

PROBLEMS FOR SECTION 8.1

1. Solve each of the following equations for x:
   (a) $7x + 4 = 0$.
   (b) $(2x + 5)(9x - 8) = 0$.
   (c) $(x + 6)^2 = 0$.
   (d) $5x^2 = 8$.

2. Solve for x:
   (a) $4x - 7 = 0$.
   (b) $(x + 2)(3x - 4) = 0$.
   (c) $4x^2 = 9$.
   (d) $(x - 10)^2 = 0$.

3. Use the quadratic formula to solve $4x^2 + 5x - 3 = 0$ for x.

4. Use the quadratic formula to solve $2x^2 - 3x - 4 = 0$ for x.

5. Use Theorem 2 ("Alternate Factoring Form") to find r and s such that $1 - 6x - 5x^2 = (1 - rx)(1 - sx)$.

6. Find r and s such that $1 + 2x - 3x^2 = (1 - rx)(1 - sx)$.

7. Use the factorization $x^2 - 30x + 144 = (x - 6)(x - 24)$ to factor $1 - 30x + 144x^2$ in the form $(1 - rx)(1 - sx)$.

8. Use the factorization $x^2 + 30x + 216 = (x + 12)(x + 18)$ to factor $1 + 30x + 216x^2$ in the form $(1 - rx)(1 - sx)$.

9. Let $p(x) = x^4 - 5x^3 + 10x - 12$.

   (i) Find a polynomial $q(x)$ and a number r such that $p(x) = (x - 2)q(x) + r$.

   (ii) What is $p(2)$?

10. Express $f(x) = 5x^5 + x^4 - x^3 + x^2 - x + 2$ in the form $(x + 1)g(x) + f(-1)$, with $g(x)$ a polynomial.

11. (i) Find a positive integral root of $x^3 - 3x^2 + 2 = 0$.

   (ii) Find the other roots of this equation.

12. (i) Find a negative integral root of $x^3 - 6x - 4 = 0$.

   (ii) Find all the roots of this equation.

13. (i) Find all the roots of $x^3 - x^2 - x + 1 = 0$.

   (ii) Express $x^3 - x^2 - x + 1$ as the product of three first degree factors.

14. (i) Show that $(x^3 - 1)(x^3 - x^2 - x + 1) = x^6 - x^5 - x^4 + x^2 + x - 1$.

   (ii) Find all the roots of $x^6 - x^5 - x^4 + x^2 + x - 1 = 0$.

   (iii) Factor $x^6 - x^5 - x^4 + x^2 + x - 1$ as a product of four first degree polynomials and one second degree polynomial.

15. Find b, given that 4 is a root of $5x^6 + 7x^5 - 11x + b = 0$.

16. Find b, given that -3 is a root of $x^7 - 10x^5 + 8x^3 - 4x^2 + 3x - b = 0$.

17. Let $f(x) = x^4 + 2x^3 - x^2 + 4x - 6$.

   (i) Find integers a and b and a second degree polynomial $g(x)$ such that $f(x) = (x - a)(x - b)g(x)$.

   (ii) Find the roots of $f(x) = 0$.

18. Let $p(x) = x^5 + 8x^4 + 15x^3 - 8x^2 - 64x - 120$.

   (i) Find integers a, b, and c and a second degree polynomial $q(x)$ such that $p(x) = (x - a)(x - b)(x - c)q(x)$.

   (ii) Find all the roots of $p(x) = 0$.

19. Let $p(x) = (x - c)^3 - x^3 + c^3$.

   (i) Find $p(0)$ and $p(c)$.   (ii) Factor $p(x)$.

20. Let $f(x) = (x - d)^5 - x^5 + d^5$.

   (i) Find $f(0)$ and $f(d)$.   (ii) Find the roots of $f(x) = 0$.

21. (i) Find a rational root of $3x^3 - 4x^2 - 21x - 10 = 0$.

   (ii) Find all the roots of this equation.

22. (i) Find two rational roots for $81x^4 + 54x^3 - 3x - 2 = 0$.

   (ii) Find all the roots of this equation.

   (iii) Find all the roots of $81x^5 + 54x^4 - 3x^2 - 2x = 0$.

23. (i) Find all the roots of $12x^3 + 11x^2 - 13x - 10 = 0$.

   (ii) Find all the roots of $12x^4 + 11x^3 - 13x^2 - 10x = 0$.

24. (i) Find all the roots of $8x^4 - 4x^3 - 6x^2 + 5x - 1 = 0$.

   (ii) Find all the roots of $8x^5 - 4x^4 - 6x^3 + 5x^2 - x = 0$.

25. Let a and b be integers.

   (a) What are the possibilities for integral roots of $7x^3 + ax^2 + bx - 15 = 0$?

   (b) What are the possibilities for rational roots of this equation?

26. Let a, b, and c be integers and $f(x) = 14x^4 + ax^3 + bx^2 + cx + 3$.
    (a) What are the possibilities for integral roots of $f(x) = 0$?
    (b) What are the possibilities for rational roots of $f(x) = 0$?

27. Given that a and b are integers, can $\frac{65}{39}$ be a root of $9x^3 + ax^2 + bx - 10 = 0$? Explain.

28. Let a, b, and c be integers and let $\frac{48}{21}$ be a root of $14x^3 + ax^2 + bx + c = 0$. Explain why $16|c$ but it is not necessarily true that $48|c$.

29. Let $p(x) = x^d + a_1 x^{d-1} + a_2 x^{d-2} + \cdots + a_{d-1}x + a_d$, with $a_1, a_2, \ldots, a_d$ integers. Let h be a rational root of $p(x) = 0$. Explain why h must be an integer.

30. Let $f(x) = a_0 x^d + a_1 x^{d-1} + \cdots + a_{d-1}x$. (Note that $a_d = 0$.)
    (i) Explain why the roots of $f(x) = 0$ are 0 and the roots of $a_0 x^{d-1} + a_1 x^{d-2} + \cdots + a_{d-1} = 0$.
    (ii) If n is an integral root of $f(x) = 0$ and $n \neq 0$, must $n|a_{d-1}$?
    (iii) If s/t is a rational root of $f(x) = 0$, with s and t having no common integral divisor greater than 1 and $s \neq 0$, what conditions must s and t satisfy?

31. Let b be an integer and $p(x) = x^5 + x^4 + 20bx - 3$. Explain why:
    (i) $n^5 + n^4$ is an even integer for every n in $\mathbf{Z}$.
    (ii) $p(n)$ is an odd integer for every n in $\mathbf{Z}$.
    (iii) $p(x) = 0$ has no integral roots.

32. Let b and $p(x)$ be as in Problem 31. Can $p(x) = 0$ have a rational root? Explain.

33. (i) Explain why $x^5 - 3 = 0$ has no rational roots.
    (ii) Explain why $\sqrt[5]{3}$ is irrational.

34. Explain why $\sqrt[7]{11}$ is not rational.

35. Prove that $\sqrt{7} - \sqrt{2}$ is irrational.

36. Prove that $\sqrt{5} - \sqrt{3}$ is irrational.

37. For the equation $(x - 2)^3(x + 1)^8(x^2 - 5x + 6) = 0$, list each root with its multiplicity.

38. Give each root of $x^2(x^2 - 25)^3(x^2 - 2x - 15)^4 = 0$ with its multiplicity.

39. Give each root, with its multiplicity, for

$$(x - 1)^6(x + 2)^7(x - 3)^8 + (x - 1)^6(x + 2)^6(x - 3)^9 = 0.$$

40. Give each root, with its multiplicity, for

$$2(x + 3)^2(x + 2)^5(x + 5)^4 + (x + 3)(x + 2)^6(x + 5)^5 = 0.$$

41. Find the multiplicity of the root $\mathbf{i}$ of the equation $x^6 + 3x^4 + 3x^2 + 1 = 0$.

42. Find the multiplicity of the root 1 of the equation $5x^6 - 6x^5 + 1 = 0$.

43. Express $(n + 4)! \div n!$ as a polynomial in n.

44. Express $(n + 5)! \div (n + 1)!$ as a polynomial in n.

45. Let $1 + bx + cx^2 = (1 - rx)(1 - sx)$, where b, c, r, and s are numbers with $r \geq s$. Show that $r - s = \sqrt{b^2 - 4c}$.

46. Let b, c, r, and s be as in Problem 45. Show that $r + s = -b$.

8.2

ALGORITHMS FOR IMPROVING APPROXIMATIONS TO ROOTS

In Section 8.1, we showed how to solve any first or second degree polynomial equation and how to solve certain higher degree polynomial equations that have some rational roots. Although that material enables one to solve in exact form all the polynomial equations found in many elementary textbooks, unfortunately it is insufficient for certain real-life applications. Here we present two methods for isolating, in narrower and narrower intervals, real roots of polynomial equations $p(x) = 0$ with real coefficients. These methods enable one to improve an approximation for a real root to any desired accuracy. In calculus textbooks, it is shown that each of these methods applies to a wider class of functions than dealt with here.

First we note that there are polynomial equations, with real coefficients, that have no real roots. For example, the equation $x^2 + 1 = 0$ has no real roots because it is equivalent to $x^2 = -1$ and the square roots $\pm i$ of -1 are not real numbers.

Next we present, without proof, a result that enables us to find intervals containing a root of an equation $p(x) = 0$ for certain polynomials p.

THEOREM 1   **CHANGE OF SIGN IMPLIES ROOT IN INTERVAL**

Let p be a polynomial of positive degree with real coefficients. Let u and v be real numbers, with $u < v$. If $p(u)$ and $p(v)$ have opposite signs, then there exists a real number r with $u < r < v$ and $p(r) = 0$.

This is proved in most advanced calculus textbooks.

Example 1   We seek a real root of the polynomial equation $x^5 - 4x^3 - 2 = 0$. There is no formula for the roots of a general fifth degree equation, but we can try to find rational roots. It follows from the Rational Root Theorem (Theorem 5 of Section 8.1) that the possibilities for rational roots are the numbers ± 1 and ± 2. Let $p(x) = x^5 - 4x^3 - 2$. As an aid in the following calculations, we observe that

$$p(x) = x^3(x^2 - 4) - 2. \tag{1}$$

We now test our possibilities for rational roots:

$$p(-2) = -8(4-4) - 2 = 0 - 2 = -2,$$
$$p(-1) = -(1-4) - 2 = 3 - 2 = 1,$$
$$p(1) = 1(1-4) - 2 = -3 - 2 = -5,$$
$$p(2) = 8(4-4) - 2 = 0 - 2 = -2.$$

These calculations show that none of the possibilities -2, -1, 1, 2 is actually a root of $p(x) = 0$. But, with the help of Theorem 1, we have found two intervals each of which contains a root. Specifically, since $p(-1)$ is positive and $p(1)$ is negative, there is a root between -1 and 1, that is, in the interval $-1 < x < 1$. Similarly, $p(-2)$ and $p(-1)$ have opposite signs, and so there is another root in the interval $-2 < x < -1$. We can also calculate

$$p(3) = 27(9-4) - 2 = 135 - 2 = 133,$$

and then we note that $p(2) < 0$ and $p(3) > 0$. This change of sign tells us that there is a third root in the interval $2 < x < 3$.

Let us call these three real roots r, s, and t. The Factor Theorem (Theorem 4 of Section 8.1) can then be used to show that

$$p(x) = (x - r)(x - s)(x - t)q(x),$$

where $q(x)$ is a second degree polynomial. If one finds r, s, and t accurately enough, one can show that the quadratic equation $q(x) = 0$ has no real roots. Hence $p(x) = 0$ has three real roots and two complex roots. □

In several following examples, we illustrate techniques for approximating one of the real roots to any desired accuracy.

TECHNIQUE I   EDUCATED GUESSING

Example 2   As in Example 1, let

$$p(x) = x^5 - 4x^3 - 2 = x^3(x^2 - 4) - 2.$$

We saw that $p(2) = -2$ and $p(3) = 133$ and hence that there is a root in the interval $2 < x < 3$. Since -2 is much closer to 0 than is 133, we might be tempted to calculate $p(2.1)$ and see if we get a sign change between $x = 2$ and $x = 2.1$. This try succeeds, since

$$p(2.1) = (2.1)^3[(2.1)^2 - 4] - 2$$
$$= 9.261(4.41 - 4) - 2$$
$$= 3.79701 - 2 = 1.79701.$$

Now, $p(2) = -2$ and $p(2.1) \approx 1.8$ show that there is a root in the interval $2 < x < 2.1$. (The $\approx$ sign can be read "is approximately.") To localize the root in a smaller interval, we calculate

$$p(2.05) = 8.615125(4.2025 - 4) - 2$$
$$\approx 1.7445628 - 2 \approx -0.2554372.$$

Since $p(2.05)$ is negative and $p(2.10)$ is positive, there is a root in the interval $2.05 < x < 2.10$. Since the distance from -0.3 to 0 is $\frac{1}{6}$ the distance from 1.8 to 0, we guess that there is a root in the interval $2.05 < x < 2.06$ and confirm this guess with the calculation

$$p(2.06) = 8.741816(4.2436 - 4) - 2$$
$$\approx 2.1295064 - 2 \approx 0.1295064.$$

Thus $p(2.05)$ and $p(2.06)$ have opposite signs and, as guessed, there is a root in the interval $2.05 < x < 2.06$.

What would the situation be if $p(2.06)$ had turned out to be negative? Then, instead of knowing that there is a root in the interval $2.05 < x < 2.06$, we would have found that there is a root in the wider interval $2.06 < x < 2.10$.

If one continues in this way, the root can be found to any desired number of decimal places. Similarly, one can narrow the intervals containing each of the other two real roots.   □

TECHNIQUE II   BISECTION

Here we modify slightly the previous method. We remove the "guessing" and thus make it easier to program the algorithm. This change also enables us to predict the number of steps needed to achieve a specific accuracy. The advantage of the first method is that it is quicker when used by an expert guesser.

Example 3   As in Examples 1 and 2, let

$$p(x) = x^5 - 4x^3 - 2 = x^3(x^2 - 4) - 2.$$

We saw in Example 2 that $p(2.05) < 0$ and $p(2.06) > 0$. Hence $p(x) = 0$ has a root r in the interval $2.05 < x < 2.06$. Instead of making an educated guess as to whether r is closer to 2.05 than to 2.06 and trying to predict how close r might be to the closer endpoint of the interval, here we just cut the interval in half by noting that 2.055 is the midpoint of the interval and calculating

$$p(2.055) = (2.055)^3[(2.055)^2 - 4] - 2$$
$$= (8.6783164)(0.223025) - 2 \approx -0.0645185.$$

Since $p(2.055) < 0$ and $p(2.06) > 0$, we now know that there is a root in the interval $2.055 < x < 2.06$. As before, we cut this interval in half. First we note that the midpoint of the interval is $(2.055 + 2.06)/2 = 2.0575$. Then we calculate

$$p(2.0575) = (2.0575)^3[(2.0575)^2 - 4] - 2$$
$$= (8.7100275)(0.23330625) - 2 \approx 0.0321038.$$

Since $p(2.055) < 0$ and $p(2.0575) > 0$, there is a root in the interval $2.055 < x < 2.0575$. This bisection technique can be continued until the root is known to the desired accuracy. Once an interval containing a root has been found, this technique for narrowing the size of the interval, though slow, is sure and is easy to program.

We have isolated the root in an interval of size $2.0575 - 2.055 = 0.0025$. With n more bisections, the size of the interval would be cut down to $0.0025/2^n$. If we want the root to six decimal places, the number of additional bisections is the smallest integer n such that

$$\frac{0.0025}{2^n} < 0.000001.$$

This n is the smallest integer n that satisfies

$$2^n > \frac{0.0025}{0.000001} = 2500.$$

Calculating $2, 2^2, 2^3, \ldots$, we find that $2^{11} = 2048$ and $2^{12} = 4096$. Hence 12 more bisections are needed to get the root to six decimal places. □

ALGORITHM 1   BISECTION

Now we describe the bisection technique for a general polynomial equation $p(x) = 0$, where p is a polynomial with real coefficients. Let u and v be real numbers such that $p(u)$ and $p(v)$ have opposite signs. If $p(u) < 0$ and $p(v) > 0$, we say that the interval $u < x < v$ is a $(-, +)$ interval for the polynomial p. If $p(u) > 0$ and $p(v) < 0$, we change the signs of all coefficients in the equation $p(x) = 0$ and thus replace the old polynomial p with a new polynomial p having $u < x < v$ as a $(-, +)$ interval.

We define a sequence of $(-, +)$ intervals $u_n < x < v_n$ for p inductively. We let $u_0 = u$ and $v_0 = v$; that is, for $n = 0$ the interval is the original $u < x < v$. Assuming that the $(-, +)$ interval $u_k < x < v_k$ has been found, we obtain a $(-, +)$ interval $u_{k+1} < x < v_{k+1}$ as follows: Let m_k be the midpoint $(u_k + v_k)/2$ of the interval $u_k < x < v_k$. Calculate $p(m_k)$ by synthetic division, that is, Algorithm 1 of Section 8.1. The next $(-, +)$ interval $u_{k+1} < x < v_{k+1}$ is the interval $u_k < x < m_k$ when $p(m_k) > 0$ and is $m_k < x < v_k$ when $p(m_k) < 0$. If $p(m_k)$ is 0 to the number of decimal places being used, then m_k is the desired root of $p(x) = 0$ and the process should be stopped. Otherwise, one continues until one obtains the first interval

$u_n < x < v_n$ with

$$\frac{v - u}{2^n} < \frac{1}{10^q},$$

where q is the number of decimal places to which one wants the root. This implies that the number of bisections should be the smallest integer n with $2^n > 10^q(v - u)$.

Example 4   As in the previous examples, let $p(x) = x^5 - 4x^3 - 2$. We saw in Example 1 that $p(x) = 0$ has a root in the interval $-1 < x < 1$ of length 2. If we use the "Bisection Algorithm" to get this root to six decimal places, the number n of bisections has to be the smallest integer n with

$$2^n > 10^q(v - u) = 10^6[1 - (-1)] = 2000000.$$

Calculating $2, 2^2, 2^3, \ldots$, we find that

$$2^{20} = 1048576 \qquad \text{and} \qquad 2^{21} = 2097152.$$

Hence 21 bisections would be required to isolate the root in an interval whose length is less than 0.000001.   □

TECHNIQUE III   **NEWTON'S METHOD**

We are about to describe another algorithm for improving an approximation to a root of a polynomial equation $p(x) = 0$. The advantage of this method is that it generally is considerably faster; the disadvantage is that it sometimes does not work. One way to find out if it works in a given situation is to try it. Justification for the algorithm and a discussion of when it fails can be found in calculus textbooks. We need a definition before we can describe the algorithm.

DEFINITION 1   **DERIVATIVE $p'(x)$ OF A POLYNOMIAL $p(x)$**

Let $p(x) = a_0x^d + a_1x^{d-1} + \cdots + a_{d-1}x + a_d$, where the a_i are real numbers. The (first) *derivative* of $p(x)$ is

$$p'(x) = da_0x^{d-1} + (d-1)a_1x^{d-2} + (d-2)a_2x^{d-3} + \cdots + a_{d-1}.$$

[One reads $p'(x)$ as "p prime of x."]

For example, if

$$p(x) = x^5 - 4x^3 - 2 = x^5 + 0 \cdot x^4 - 4x^3 + 0 \cdot x^2 + 0 \cdot x - 2$$

then

$$p'(x) = 5x^4 - 12x^2 = 5x^4 + 4 \cdot 0x^3 - 3 \cdot 4x^2 + 2 \cdot 0x + 1 \cdot 0.$$

ALGORITHM 2 **NEWTON'S METHOD FOR REFINING APPROXIMATIONS**

(a) Let a be an approximation to a root of a polynomial equation $p(x) = 0$. Let the sequence $x_0, x_1, \ldots$ be determined inductively, as follows:

$$x_0 = a, \qquad x_{k+1} = x_k - \frac{p(x_k)}{p'(x_k)} \qquad \text{for } k \in \mathbf{Z}^+.$$

(b) If the terms of $x_0, x_1, \ldots$ agree to increasing numbers of decimal places, continue obtaining the terms until x_k and x_{k+1} agree to the desired number of places. Then x_{k+1} is the sought approximation.

One cannot continue with Algorithm 2 if at some stage $p'(x_k) = 0$, since then the formula for x_{k+1} involves division by 0 and so is meaningless. Even if $p'(x_k) \neq 0$ for all k, the terms of the sequence $x_1, x_2, \ldots$ will not necessarily agree to more and more places. If either of these difficulties arises, Algorithm 2 will not work for the given $p(x)$ and approximation a. It might work for the given $p(x)$ and some other approximation a. Generally, neither difficulty arises if the approximation is fairly good. If trouble occurs, one can switch to Algorithm 1.

Example 5 We continue with the polynomial

$$p(x) = x^5 - 4x^3 - 2 = x^3(x^2 - 4) - 2$$

of the previous examples. Here we use Newton's Method starting with the approximation $x_0 = 2$ to the root of $p(x) = 0$ known to be in the interval $2 < x < 3$. First we note that

$$p'(x) = 5x^4 - 12x^2 = x^2(5x^2 - 12).$$

The basis step of the inductive definition of $x_0, x_1, \ldots$ is $x_0 = 2$. The inductive step tells us that

$$x_1 = x_0 - \frac{p(x_0)}{p'(x_0)}.$$

We calculate

$$p(x_0) = p(2) = 8(4 - 4) - 2 = 8 \cdot 0 - 2 = -2,$$
$$p'(x_0) = p'(2) = 4(5 \cdot 4 - 12) = 4 \cdot 8 = 32.$$

Hence $x_1 = x_0 - p(x_0)/p'(x_0) = 2 - (-\frac{2}{32}) = 2 + (\frac{1}{16}) = 2.0625.$

For the second round, we use $x_1 = 2.0625$ as the approximation to be improved. We get

$$p(x_1) = p(2.0625) = (2.0625)^3[(2.0625)^2 - 4] - 2$$
$$= (8.7736816)(0.25390625) - 2 \approx 0.2276926,$$

$$p'(x_1) = p'(2.0625) = (2.0625)^2[5(2.0625)^2 - 12]$$
$$= (4.25390625)(21.26953125 - 12) \approx 39.431716,$$

$$x_2 = x_1 - \frac{p(x_1)}{p'(x_1)} \approx 2.0625 - \frac{0.2276926}{39.431716}$$

$$\approx 2.0625 - 0.0057744 \approx 2.0567256.$$

For the third round, we get

$$p(x_2) = p(2.0567256) = (2.0567256)^3[(2.0567256)^2 - 4] - 2$$
$$\approx (8.7001963)(0.2301201) - 2 \approx 0.002091,$$

$$p'(x_2) = p'(2.0567256) = (2.0567256)^2[5(2.0567256)^2 - 12]$$
$$\approx (4.2301201)(21.1506005 - 12) \approx 38.70814,$$

$$x_3 = x_2 - \frac{p(x_2)}{p'(x_2)} \approx 2.0567256 - \frac{0.002091}{38.70814}$$

$$x_3 \approx 2.0567256 - 0.0000540 \approx 2.0566716.$$

TABLE 8.2.1

n	x_n	$x_n - x_4$
0	2.0000000	−0.0566716
1	2.0625000	0.0058284
2	2.0569505	0.0002789
3	2.0566716	0.0000000

Similarly, one can calculate x_4 and find that it agrees with x_3 to seven decimal places. Therefore we stop the process with x_4 (or x_3) as the desired approximation. Table 8.2.1 shows the closeness of the terms x_0, x_1, x_2, x_3 to the end result x_4. □

PROBLEMS FOR SECTION 8.2

1. Let $p(x) = x^2 - x - 1$.
   (i) Complete the table:

x	−2	−1	0	1	2
$p(x)$			−1	−1	

   (ii) Find two integers a such that $p(a)$ and $p(a + 1)$ have opposite signs.
2. Let $p(x) = x^2 - 5$. Find two integers a such that $p(a)$ and $p(a + 1)$ have opposite signs.
3. Let $p(x) = x^3 + 3x - 2$.

    (i) What are the possibilities for rational roots of $p(x) = 0$?

    (ii) Are any of the possibilities in Part (i) actually roots? Justify your answer.

    (iii) Find an integer a such that $p(a) < 0$ and $p(a + 1) > 0$.

4. Do as in Problem 3 for $p(x) = x^3 + x - 3$.

5. There is a root of $x^2 - x - 1 = 0$ in the interval $1 < x < 2$. Use 3 rounds of Algorithm 1 ("Bisection") to find a positive rational number r such that there is a root in the interval $r < x < r + \frac{1}{8}$.

6. Let $q(x) = x^2 - x - 1$. We see easily that $q(-1) > 0$ and $q(0) < 0$. So we let $p(x) = -q(x) = -x^2 + x + 1$ and have $p(-1) < 0$ and $p(0) > 0$. Now use 3 rounds of the "Bisection Algorithm" (Algorithm 1) to find a negative rational number s such that $p(x) = 0$ [or $q(x) = 0$] has a root in the interval $s < x < s + \frac{1}{8}$.

7. Use Newton's Method (Algorithm 2), with $x_0 = -1$, to find approximations x_1, x_2, and x_3 to the negative root of $x^2 - x - 1 = 0$.

8. Use Newton's Method (Algorithm 2), with $x_0 = 1$, to find approximations x_1, x_2, and x_3 to the positive root of $x^2 - x - 1 = 0$.

9. Let $q(x) = 3 - x - x^3$. One sees easily that $q(1) = 1$ and $q(2) = -7$. Then if $p(x) = -q(x)$, one has $p(1) < 0$ and $p(2) > 0$.

    (i) Use the "Bisection Algorithm" (Algorithm 1) to find a number r such that $p(x) = 0$ has a root in the interval $r < x < r + \frac{1}{4}$.

    (ii) Use Newton's Method (Algorithm 2), with x_0 the r of Part (i), to find approximations x_1 and x_2.

10. Let $p(x) = x^3 + 3x - 2$. One sees easily that $p(0) = -2$ and $p(1) = 2$. Thus there is a root of $p(x) = 0$ in the interval $0 < x < 1$.

    (i) Use the "Bisection Algorithm" (Algorithm 1) to find a fraction r such that $p(x) = 0$ has a root in the interval $r < x < r + \frac{1}{4}$.

    (ii) Use Newton's Method (Algorithm 2), with x_0 the r of Part (i), to find approximations x_1 and x_2.

11. Let $p(x) = x^4 - 2x^3 - 9x^2 + 14x + 14$.

    (i) Find $p(2)$ and $p(3)$.

    (ii) Can one be sure that there is no root of $p(x) = 0$ in the interval $2 < x < 3$?

    (iii) Find $p(2.7)$.

    (iv) Are there at least two roots of $p(x) = 0$ in the interval $2 < x < 3$? Explain.

12. Let $p(x)$ be as in Problem 11. Show that $p(x) = 0$ has a root in the interval $2.6 < x < 2.7$ and another root in the interval $2.7 < x < 2.8$.

13. Let x_0, x_1, ... be the sequence obtained by using Newton's Method (Algorithm 2), with $x_0 = 1$, to approximate the positive root of $x^2 - 3 = 0$, that is, to approximate $\sqrt{3}$. Show that

$$x_{n+1} = \frac{1}{2}\left(x_n + \frac{3}{x_n}\right) \qquad \text{for } n \in N = \{0, 1, \ldots\}.$$

14. Find the terms x_1, x_2, x_3, and x_4 for the sequence $x_0, x_1, \ldots$ of Problem 13.

15. Let c be a positive real number and $x_0, x_1, \ldots$ be the sequence obtained by Newton's Method (Algorithm 2), with $x_0 = 1$, for approximating the positive root of $x^2 - c = 0$, that is, to approximate $\sqrt{c}$. Derive a formula for x_{n+1} in terms of x_n. (This should become the formula of Problem 13 when c is replaced by 3.)

16. Approximate $\sqrt{2}$ to six decimal places.

17. Let p be a polynomial with real coefficients. Also, let $p(5) < 0$ and $p(8) > 0$. How many bisections are needed to reduce the size of the interval containing the root to less than 10^{-8}?

18. How many bisections are needed to replace the interval $8 < x < 13$ containing a root with an interval whose size is less than 10^{-10}?

19. Let $p(x) = a_0x^d + a_1x^{d-1} + \cdots + a_{d-1}x + a_d$, with no a_i negative and at least one a_i positive. Explain why $p(x) = 0$ cannot have a positive root.

20. Let $q(x) = a_d - a_{d-1}x + a_{d-2}x^2 - \cdots + (-1)^d a_0 x^d$ and let $p(x)$ be as in Problem 19. Show that:
(i) $q(-x) = p(x)$.   (ii) $q(x) = 0$ cannot have a negative root.

21. (i) Explain why $x^6 + x + 1 = 0$ has no positive roots.
(ii) Explain why $x^6 - x + 1 = 0$ has no negative roots.

22. (i) Explain why $x^5 + x + 1 = 0$ has no positive roots.
(ii) Explain why $1 - x - x^5 = 0$ has no negative roots.

23. Let $p(x) = a_0x^d + a_1x^{d-1} + \cdots + a_{d-1}x + a_d$, with each a_i a real number and $a_0 \neq 0$. Let the calculations of Algorithm 1 of Section 8.1 for evaluating $p(h)$ by "Synthetic Division" be arranged as follows:

h	a_0	a_1	a_2	$\cdots$	a_{d-1}	a_d
	b_0	b_1	b_2	$\cdots$	b_{d-1}	b_d
	c_0	c_1	c_2	$\cdots$	c_{d-1}	c_d

If none of $c_0, c_1, \ldots, c_d$ is negative and at least one c_i is positive, explain why $p(k) > 0$ for $k > h$.

24. Let $p(x) = x^4 - x^3 + x^2 - x + 1$.
(i) Use "Synthetic Division" (Algorithm 1 of Section 8.1) to find $p(1)$.
(ii) Use Part (i) and Problem 23 to show that $p(k) > 0$ for $k \geq 1$.
(iii) Use the result in Problem 20 to show that $p(x) = 0$ has no negative roots.

(iv) In what interval would a real root have to be, if there were a real root?

25. What happens if one uses Newton's Method with $x_0 = 1$, for the equation $x^5 - 3x + 2 = 0$?

26. What happens if one uses Newton's Method with $x_0 = -2$, for the equation $x^4 - 5x^3 - 56 = 0$?

27. Suppose that Newton's Method is attempted for the equation $x^2 - x - 1 = 0$.

(a) Explain why the method fails if $x_0 = 0.5$.

(b) Show that if $x_0 = 0.4$, then x_1 is farther from the roots than is x_0 but fairly soon the terms $x_1, x_2, \ldots$ get close to the negative root $(1 - \sqrt{5})/2 \approx -0.618034$.

28. (i) Show that the equation $x^3 - 3x - 1 = 0$ has three real roots, r, s, and t such that $-2 < r < -1$, $-1 < s < 0$, and $1 < t < 2$.

(ii) What happens if Newton's Method is used with $x_0 = -1$ or $x_0 = 1$?

(iii) When Newton's Method is used with $x_0 = 1.1$, show that ultimately the terms of $x_1, x_2, \ldots$ get close to t.

(iv) What happens if Newton's Method is used with $x_0 = 0.9$?

(v) Find r to four decimal places using Newton's Method with $x_0 = -2$.

(vi) Find s to four decimal places using Newton's Method with $x_0 = 0$.

(vii) Find t to four decimal places using Newton's Method with $x_0 = 2$.

8.3

PARTIAL FRACTIONS

Partial fractions will be applied in the next chapter to the solution of recursions.

The sum, difference, or product of polynomials is also a polynomial. For example, if $F = x^2 - 1$ and $G = x - 1$, then

$F + G = x^2 + x - 2,$

$F - G = x^2 - x,$

$FG = (x^2 - 1)(x - 1) = x^3 - x^2 - x + 1.$

We will discuss quotients of polynomials after introducing some terminology.

DEFINITION 1 **x-FRACTION, EQUALITY, PROPER x-FRACTION**

If A and B are polynomials in x, with B not the zero polynomial, then A/B is an **x-fraction**. If A/B and C/D are x-fractions with $AD = BC$, then $A/B = C/D$. An x-fraction A/B is **proper** if the **numerator** A has lower degree than the **denominator** B.

Any polynomial A can be thought of as the x-fraction $A/1$. Let $G = x^2 - 1$, $H = x - 1$, and $K = x + 1$. Since $HK = G$, it follows from Definition 1 that

$$\frac{G}{H} = \frac{x^2 - 1}{x - 1} = x + 1 = K, \qquad \frac{H}{G} = \frac{x - 1}{x^2 - 1} = \frac{1}{x + 1} = \frac{1}{K}.$$

Clearly, if A and B are polynomials with $B \neq 0$, then A/B is an x-fraction that may in special cases equal a polynomial. The sum, difference, product, and quotient of x-fractions A/B and C/D are given by the following formulas:

$$\frac{A}{B} \pm \frac{C}{D} = \frac{AD \pm BC}{BD},$$

$$\frac{A}{B} \cdot \frac{C}{D} = \frac{AC}{BD},$$

$$\frac{A}{B} \div \frac{C}{D} = \frac{AD}{BC} \qquad \text{if } C \neq 0.$$

Next we define a close relative of an x-fraction. Let

$$A(x) = a_0 x^d + a_1 x^{d-1} + \cdots + a_d$$

and

$$B(x) = b_0 x^e + b_1 x^{e-1} + \cdots + b_e$$

be rules for polynomial functions and let $b_0 \neq 0$. Let S be a set of complex numbers that does not contain any roots of $B(x) = 0$. The mapping from S into the set of complex numbers with the rule

$$x \mapsto \frac{A(x)}{B(x)} = \frac{a_0 x^d + \cdots + a_d}{b_0 x^e + \cdots + b_e}$$

is a **rational function** on S. Rational functions R and T are **equal** if they have the same domain and $R(x) = T(x)$ for every x in that domain. For example, the rational functions R and T with the rules

$$R(x) = \frac{x^2 - 1}{x - 1}, \qquad T(x) = x + 1$$

are equal if the domain of each is the set of all real numbers except 1; but they are not equal if 1 is in the domain of T, since the rule for R is meaningless when $x = 1$. As we have seen above, $(x^2 - 1)/(x - 1)$ and $x + 1$ are equal as x-fractions.

Most textbooks use the term *rational function* for the related concept we call *x-fraction*. Since it is desirable to have distinct language for distinct concepts, we have coined a new term and shown the difference between these concepts.

In Chapter 9, we will apply x-fractions to recursively defined sequences and generating functions. For those purposes, it is helpful to be able to express a given x-fraction as a sum of x-fractions of the following special form.

DEFINITION 2 **SPECIAL x-FRACTION**

A *special x-fraction* is of the form $c/(1 - rx)^d$, with c and r nonzero numbers and d in $\mathbf{Z}^+ = \{1, 2, \ldots\}$.

Example 1 Let $A = 12x^2 - 4x + 6$, $B = (1 - 2x)^3$, and $F = A/B$. We express the proper x-fraction F as a sum of special x-fractions in the following manner: Let $y = 1 - 2x$. Then $x = (1 - y)/2$. Substituting this into A gives us

$$A = 12 \cdot \frac{(1 - y)^2}{4} - 4 \cdot \frac{1 - y}{2} + 6 = 3(1 - y)^2 - 2(1 - y) + 6$$

$$= 3(1 - 2y + y^2) - 2 + 2y + 6 = 3y^2 - 4y + 7.$$

Since $B = y^3$,

$$F = \frac{A}{B} = \frac{3y^2 - 4y + 7}{y^3} = \frac{3}{y} + \frac{-4}{y^2} + \frac{7}{y^3}.$$

Substituting back $y = 1 - 2x$, we get the sum of special x-fractions

$$F = \frac{3}{1 - 2x} + \frac{-4}{(1 - 2x)^2} + \frac{7}{(1 - 2x)^3},$$

which can also be written as

$$F = \frac{3}{1 - 2x} - \frac{4}{(1 - 2x)^2} + \frac{7}{(1 - 2x)^3}. \qquad \square$$

LEMMA 1 **DENOMINATOR A POWER OF $1 - rx$**

Let r be a nonzero complex number and d be in $\mathbf{Z}^+$. Let F be a proper x-fraction $A/(1 - rx)^d$ (with A a polynomial whose degree is less than d). Then F is a sum of special x-fractions

$$F = \frac{k_1}{1 - rx} + \frac{k_2}{(1 - rx)^2} + \cdots + \frac{k_d}{(1 - rx)^d}.$$

PROOF   Expressing F as such a sum of special x-fractions is accomplished as in Example 1.   □

In the next two lemmas and their accompanying examples, we show how to express a proper x-fraction

$$\frac{e + fx}{1 + bx + cx^2},$$

where e, f, b, and c are given numbers with $c \neq 0$, as a sum of special x-fractions. We factor the denominator in the form

$$1 + bx + cx^2 = (1 - rx)(1 - sx),$$

where r and s are the numbers $(-b \pm \sqrt{b^2 - 4c})/2$ (as stated in Theorem 2, "Alternate Factoring Form," of Section 8.1) and consider two cases.

CASE I $r \neq s$

LEMMA 2   **DISTINCT FACTORS**

Let e, f, r, and s be numbers, with $r \neq s$. Then

$$\frac{e + fx}{(1 - rx)(1 - sx)} = \frac{h}{1 - rx} + \frac{k}{1 - sx}, \tag{1}$$

where

$$h = \frac{er + f}{r - s} \quad \text{and} \quad k = \frac{es + f}{s - r}. \tag{2}$$

PROOF   Clearing fractions, one finds that the equality in Display (1) is equivalent to each of the following:

$$e + fx = h(1 - sx) + k(1 - rx),$$
$$e + fx = (h + k) - (hs + kr)x. \tag{3}$$

Equation (3) is equivalent to the system

$$\begin{cases} h + k = e & (4) \\ hs + kr = -f. & (5) \end{cases}$$

Equation (4) implies that $k = e - h$. We substitute $e - h$ for k in Equation (5) and get

$$hs + (e - h)r = -f.$$

This gives us

$$hs + er - hr = -f,$$
$$er + f = hr - hs = h(r - s).$$

Since $r \neq s$, we have $r - s \neq 0$ and can divide by $r - s$. This leads to $h = (er + f)/(r - s)$. Then

$$k = e - h = e - \frac{er + f}{r - s} = \frac{er - es - er - f}{r - s}$$

$$= \frac{-es - f}{r - s} = \frac{es + f}{s - r}.$$

This completes the proof.   □

Example 2   Let $F = (5 - 4x)/(1 - x - 6x^2)$. We use a modification of the method of Lemma 2 to express F as a sum of special x-fractions and then check using the formulas of Lemma 2.

The denominator of F factors as follows:

$$1 - x - 6x^2 = (1 - 3x)(1 + 2x).$$

This has the form $(1 - rx)(1 - sx)$ with $r = 3$ and $s = -2$. Since $r \neq s$, it follows from Lemma 2 that F is expressible in the form

$$\frac{5 - 4x}{(1 - 3x)(1 + 2x)} = \frac{h}{1 - 3x} + \frac{k}{1 + 2x},$$

where h and k are numbers to be determined. Clearing fractions, we have

$$5 - 4x = h(1 + 2x) + k(1 - 3x). \tag{6}$$

We know from Lemma 2 that there exist constants h and k that make Equation (6) a true statement. The easiest way to find k is to let $x = -\frac{1}{2}$ in Equation (6) and get

$$5 - 4\left(-\frac{1}{2}\right) = h\left[1 + 2\left(-\frac{1}{2}\right)\right] + k\left[1 - 3\left(-\frac{1}{2}\right)\right],$$

$$5 + 2 = h \cdot 0 + k \cdot \frac{5}{2},$$

$$7 = \frac{5}{2}k.$$

Thus $k = \frac{14}{5}$. Similarly, one can let $x = \frac{1}{3}$ in Equation (6), and find that $h = \frac{11}{5}$. Hence the desired expression for F as a sum of special x-fractions is

$$F = \frac{\frac{11}{5}}{1 - 3x} + \frac{\frac{14}{5}}{1 + 2x}.$$

For the check, we use $e = 5$, $f = -4$, $r = 3$, and $s = -2$ in the formula of Lemma 2 and obtain

$$h = \frac{er + f}{r - s} = \frac{5 \cdot 3 - 4}{3 - (-2)} = \frac{11}{5},$$

$$k = \frac{es + f}{s - r} = \frac{5(-2) - 4}{-2 - 3} = \frac{-14}{-5} = \frac{14}{5}.$$

These agree with the values for h and k found above. $\qquad\qquad\square$

CASE II $r = s$

Let

$$F = \frac{e + fx}{1 + bx + cx^2} \qquad \text{and} \qquad 1 + bx + cx^2 = (1 - rx)(1 - sx).$$

When $r = s$ (that is, when $b^2 - 4c = 0$), we have

$$F = \frac{e + fx}{(1 - rx)^2}.$$

Then it follows from Lemma 1 that there exist constants k_1 and k_2 such that

$$\frac{e + fx}{(1 - rx)^2} = \frac{k_1}{1 - rx} + \frac{k_2}{(1 - rx)^2}.$$

In the following result, we give an independent proof of this and also derive explicit formulas for k_1 and k_2 in terms of e, f, and r.

LEMMA 3   **SQUARE DENOMINATOR**

Let

$$F = \frac{e + fx}{(1 - rx)^2},$$

where e, f, and r are numbers and $r \neq 0$. Then

$$F = \frac{k_1}{1 - rx} + \frac{k_2}{(1 - rx)^2},$$

where $k_1 = -f/r$ and $k_2 = e + (f/r)$.

PROOF $$F = \frac{e + fx}{(1 - rx)^2} = \frac{(-f/r)(1 - rx) + e + (f/r)}{(1 - rx)^2}$$

$$= \frac{(-f/r)(1 - rx)}{(1 - rx)^2} + \frac{e + (f/r)}{(1 - rx)^2}$$

$$= \frac{-f/r}{1 - rx} + \frac{e + (f/r)}{(1 - rx)^2},$$

as claimed. □

Example 3 Here we express $F = (5 - 6x)/(1 - 4x + 4x^2)$ as a sum of special x-fractions. The denominator factors as $1 - 4x + 4x^2 = (1 - 2x)(1 - 2x)$. Then

$$F = \frac{5 - 6x}{(1 - 2x)^2} = \frac{2 + 3 - 6x}{(1 - 2x)^2} = \frac{2 + 3(1 - 2x)}{(1 - 2x)^2}$$

$$= \frac{2}{(1 - 2x)^2} + \frac{3(1 - 2x)}{(1 - 2x)^2} = \frac{2}{(1 - 2x)^2} + \frac{3}{1 - 2x}.$$

Thus the desired expression for F as a sum of special x-fractions is

$$F = \frac{3}{1 - 2x} + \frac{2}{(1 - 2x)^2}.$$

This result can also be found with the method of Example 1 or the formulas of Lemma 3. We use these formulas as a check: In the notation of Lemma 3 we have $e = 5$, $f = -6$, and $r = 2$. Then $k_1 = -f/r = 6/2 = 3$ and $k_2 = e + (f/r) = 5 + (-6/2) = 5 - 3 = 2$. These values check with the numerators of the special x-fractions found above. □

We can now state procedures for expressing a proper x-fraction A/B, with B of second degree, as a sum of special x-fractions.

ALGORITHM 1 **PROPER x-FRACTION WITH QUADRATIC DENOMINATOR**

Let

$$F = \frac{e + fx}{1 + bx + cx^2},$$

where b, c, e, and f are numbers and $c \neq 0$. The following steps express F as a sum of special x-fractions.

(I) Factor $1 + bx + cx^2$ as $(1 - rx)(1 - sx)$, where r and s are $(-b \pm \sqrt{b^2 - 4c})/2$. Then rewrite F as

$$\frac{e + fx}{(1 - rx)(1 - sx)}.$$

(II) If $b^2 - 4c \neq 0$, then $r \neq s$ and

$$F = \frac{h}{1 - rx} + \frac{k}{1 - sx},$$

where $h = (re + f)/(r - s)$ and $k = (se + f)/(s - r)$.

(III) If $b^2 - 4c = 0$, then $r = s = -b/2$ and we can write $F = (e + fx)/(1 - rx)^2$. This is expressible as the sum

$$F = \frac{k_1}{1 - rx} + \frac{k_2}{(1 - rx)^2}$$

of special x-fractions, with $k_1 = -f/r = 2f/b$ and $k_2 = e + (f/r) = e - (2f/b)$.

The factorization in Step (I) is as in Theorem 2 ("Alternate Factoring Form") of Section 8.1. Then the formula in Step (II) follows from Lemma 2 ("Distinct Factors"), and the formula in Step (III) follows from Lemma 3 ("Square Denominator").

Next we state, without proof, a theorem that helps us extend Algorithm 1 to x-fractions A/B with B having arbitrary degree.

THEOREM 1   **PARTIAL-FRACTIONS DECOMPOSITION**

Let $B = (1 - r_1 x)^{d_1}(1 - r_2 x)^{d_2} \cdots (1 - r_m x)^{d_m}$, with the r_i distinct complex numbers and the d_i in $\mathbf{Z}^+$. Let A be a polynomial in x with degree less than the degree $d_1 + d_2 + \cdots + d_m$ of B. Then the x-fraction $F = A/B$ is a sum of special x-fractions of the form $c/(1 - r_i x)^e$, with r_i in $\{r_1, r_2, \ldots, r_m\}$ and $e \leq d_i$. This sum is called the ***partial-fractions decomposition*** for A/B.

The proof of Theorem 1 is too advanced for this text. A proof is given in A. P. Hillman and G. L. Alexanderson, *A First Undergraduate Course in Abstract Algebra*, 3rd ed. (Belmont, Calif.: Wadsworth Publishing Co., 1983). However, below we give Algorithm 2 for obtaining the sum promised by Theorem 1. First we present a specific illustration.

Example 4   Let $A = 57x^2 - 20x + 7$, $B = (1 + 2x)(1 - 3x)^2$, and $F = A/B$. Then Theorem 1 tells us that

$$F = \frac{A}{B} = \frac{57x^2 - 20x + 7}{(1 + 2x)(1 - 3x)^2} = \frac{a}{1 + 2x} + \frac{b}{1 - 3x} + \frac{c}{(1 - 3x)^2}, \qquad (7)$$

with a, b, and c numbers. To solve for these numbers, we first clear denominators by multiplying both sides of the last equation of Display (7) by B, yielding

$$57x^2 - 20x + 7 = a(1 - 3x)^2 + b(1 + 2x)(1 - 3x) + c(1 + 2x). \qquad (8)$$

Letting $x = \frac{1}{3}$ in Equation (8), the first two terms on the right-hand side become 0 and we have

$$57 \cdot \frac{1}{9} - 20 \cdot \frac{1}{3} + 7 = c\left(1 + \frac{2}{3}\right),$$

$$\frac{19}{3} - \frac{20}{3} + 7 = \frac{5}{3}c.$$

This gives $20/3 = 5c/3$, $20 = 5c$, and so $c = 4$. Similarly, letting $x = -\frac{1}{2}$ makes the last two terms of the right-hand side of Equation (8) zero and we get

$$\frac{57}{4} + 10 + 7 = a\left(1 + \frac{3}{2}\right)^2,$$

$$\frac{125}{4} = \frac{25a}{4},$$

$$a = 5.$$

Equation (8) with $a = 5$ and $c = 4$ becomes

$$57x^2 - 20x + 7 = 5(1 - 3x)^2 + b(1 + 2x)(1 - 3x) + 4(1 + 2x).$$

We can find b by replacing x with any number not in $\{-\frac{1}{2}, \frac{1}{3}\}$. It is convenient to let $x = 0$. Then we get $7 = 5 + b + 4$, which shows that $b = -2$. Hence the desired sum of special x-fractions for F is

$$\frac{57x^2 - 20x + 7}{(1 + 2x)(1 - 3x)^2} = \frac{5}{1 + 2x} - \frac{2}{1 - 3x} + \frac{4}{(1 - 3x)^2}. \qquad \square$$

Example 5   In Example 4, we wanted numbers a, b, and c such that

$$57x^2 - 20x + 7 = a(1 - 3x)^2 + b(1 + 2x)(1 - 3x) + c(1 + 2x). \qquad (9)$$

Alternatively, we can find these numbers starting by expanding the right-hand side of Equation (9) and collecting like terms, as follows:

$$57x^2 - 20x + 7 = a(1 - 6x + 9x^2) + b(1 - x - 6x^2) + c(1 + 2x)$$
$$= (9a - 6b)x^2 - (6a + b - 2c)x + (a + b + c).$$

Then equating coefficients of like powers gives us the following system of simultaneous equations:

$$\begin{cases} 9a - 6b & = 57 \\ 6a + b - 2c = 20 \\ a + b + c = 7. \end{cases}$$

This system can be solved by elimination, as in elementary algebra. $\square$

Example 6   Here we show how to find the constants a, b, and c of Examples 4 and 5 using a variation of the method of Example 2. Since there are three constants to be found, we get a system of three equations in these unknowns by substituting three different numbers for x in Equation (9). Small integers usually are convenient, so we replace x with -1, then with 0, and finally with 1. Thus we obtain the system

$$\begin{cases} 84 = 16a - 4b - c \\ 7 = a + b + c \\ 44 = 4a - 6b + 3c. \end{cases}$$

This system can then be solved by elimination.   □

In any specific problem, one can get enough equations to solve for the constants using one or more of the techniques illustrated in Examples 4, 5, and 6.

In the following example, we show the nature of the terms of the partial-fractions forms for some proper x-fractions but leave the constants undetermined.

Example 7   Let $B = (1 - 4x)^5(1 + 5x)^3$ and let A be a polynomial in x of degree at most 7. Then Theorem 1 tells us that the partial-fractions decomposition for the x-fraction A/B is of the following type:

$$\frac{A}{B} = \frac{a}{1 - 4x} + \frac{b}{(1 - 4x)^2} + \frac{c}{(1 - 4x)^3} + \frac{d}{(1 - 4x)^4} + \frac{e}{(1 - 4x)^5}$$

$$+ \frac{f}{1 + 5x} + \frac{g}{(1 + 5x)^2} + \frac{h}{(1 + 5x)^3},$$

where $a, b, \ldots, h$ are constants to be determined. If $D = (1 + 7x)(1 - 8x)(1 - 4x)$ and C is a polynomial in x of degree at most 2, then C/D has a partial-fractions form

$$\frac{C}{D} = \frac{a}{1 + 7x} + \frac{b}{1 - 8x} + \frac{c}{1 - 4x},$$

with a, b, and c constants to be found.   □

ALGORITHM 2   **DETERMINING THE CONSTANTS**

Let $F = A/B$ be as in Theorem 1 ("Partial-Fractions Decomposition"). One finds the partial-fractions form for F as follows: Express F as a sum of special x-fractions, of the type described in Theorem 1, using constants to be determined. Clear denominators by multiplying through by B. Obtain enough equations to solve for the constants by the techniques of Examples 4, 5, and 6. Solve the system of equations for the constants and use the determined constants in the sum of special x-fractions.

Example 8   Let $F = 120/(x - 5)(x + 3)(x + 4)$. We convert F into the form to which Theorem 1 applies as follows:

$$\frac{120}{(x - 5)(x + 3)(x + 4)} = \frac{5 \cdot 3 \cdot 4 \cdot 2}{5(\frac{1}{5}x - 1) \cdot 3(\frac{1}{3}x + 1) \cdot 4(\frac{1}{4}x + 1)}$$

$$= \frac{2}{(\frac{1}{5}x - 1)(\frac{1}{3}x + 1)(\frac{1}{4}x + 1)}$$

$$= \frac{-2}{(1 - \frac{1}{5}x)(1 + \frac{1}{3}x)(1 + \frac{1}{4}x)}. \qquad \square$$

PROBLEMS FOR SECTION 8.3

1.   Which of the following x-fractions are proper?

   (i) $\dfrac{x^3}{(x - 1)(x - 2)}$,   (ii) $\dfrac{x^2 + x + 1}{x^3 + x^2 + x + 1}$,

   (iii) $\dfrac{1}{x^4 - 1}$,   (iv) $\dfrac{2 + x^2}{x + 3}$.

2.   Which of the following x-fractions are proper?

   (i) $\dfrac{x^3 + x}{x^6 + x^3 + 1}$,   (ii) $\dfrac{5}{(x + 2)(x - 3)}$,

   (iii) $\dfrac{x^5}{(x + 2)(x - 3)}$,   (iv) $\dfrac{1 + x^3}{x^2 - x - 6}$.

3.   (i) Use the method of Example 2 to find the partial-fractions decomposition for $F = (3 + 23x)/(1 - x - 12x^2)$. That is, express F in the form

$$\frac{3 + 23x}{1 - x - 12x^2} = \frac{h}{1 - rx} + \frac{k}{1 - sx}.$$

   (ii) Check using the formulas in Lemma 2, "Distinct Factors."

4.   (i) Use the method of Example 2 to find the partial-fractions decomposition for $F = (8 - 17x)/(1 - 5x + 4x^2)$.
   (ii) Check using the formulas in Lemma 2, "Distinct Factors."

5.   Use the method of Example 3 to find and check the partial-fractions decomposition for $F = (3 + 35x)/(1 + 10x + 25x^2)$.

6.   Use the method of Example 3 to find and check the partial-fractions decomposition for $F = (5 + 12x)/(1 - 8x + 16x^2)$, that is, to express F in the form

$$\frac{5 + 12x}{1 - 8x + 16x^2} = \frac{k_1}{1 - rx} + \frac{k_2}{(1 - rx)^2}.$$

7. Use the substitution $y = 1 + 3x$ [with its companion $x = (y - 1)/3$] to find numbers a, b, and c such that

$$9 + 21x + 54x^2 = a + b(1 + 3x) + c(1 + 3x)^2.$$

8. Find the a, b, and c of Problem 7 by the method of Example 5.

9. Find the a, b, and c of Problem 7 by replacing x with $-\frac{1}{3}$ to find a, equating coefficients of x^2 to find c, and then using the found values of a and c with $x = 0$ to find b.

10. Use the answer to Problem 7 (or Problem 8) to express $(9 + 21x + 54x^2)/(1 + 3x)^3$ as a sum of special x-fractions, that is, to find the partial-fractions form for this proper x-fraction.

11. Let $A = 5x^4 - 6x^3 - 3x^2 + 8x + 2$ and $B = (1 - \frac{1}{2}x)^5$. Take as given that

$$A = 5(x - 2)^4 + 34(x - 2)^3 + 81(x - 2)^2 + 84(x - 2) + 38.$$

Let $y = 1 - \frac{1}{2}x$.
(i) Express $x - 2$ in terms of y.   (ii) Express A/B in terms of y.
(iii) Use Part (ii) to find the partial-fractions form for A/B.

12. Let $A = 5x^4 + 6x^3 - 3x^2 - 8x + 2$ and $B = (1 + \frac{1}{2}x)^5$. Take as given that

$$A = 5(x + 2)^4 - 34(x + 2)^3 + 81(x + 2)^2 - 84(x + 2) + 38.$$

Use this to find the partial-fractions decomposition for A/B.

13. Let $B = (1 + x)^4(1 - 2x)^5(1 + 3x)^2$ and let A/B be a proper x-fraction.
(i) What is the largest that the degree of A can be?
(ii) Write the partial-fractions form for A/B in terms of undetermined constants. (*Hint:* See Example 7.)

14. Repeat Problem 13, but with B now $(1 - 5x)^3(1 + 6x)^6(1 - 7x)$.

15. Find the partial-fractions form for each of the following:

(a) $\dfrac{x^2 - 7}{(1 - x)^4}.$
(b) $\dfrac{2x + 1}{(1 - x)(1 - 2x)}.$

(c) $\dfrac{8x^2 + 4x + 5}{(1 + x)^2(1 - 2x)}.$
(d) $\dfrac{2}{(1 - x)(1 - \frac{1}{2}x)(1 - \frac{1}{3}x)}.$

16. Find the partial-fractions form for each of the following:

(a) $\dfrac{x^4 - 3x}{(1 + x)^5}.$
(b) $\dfrac{11x + 1}{(1 - 4x)(1 + x)}.$

(c) $\dfrac{18x^2 - 22x - 1}{(1 - 2x)^2(1 + 3x)}.$
(d) $\dfrac{60}{(1 + 3x)(1 - 4x)(1 - 5x)}.$

17. Let **i** be the complex number with $\mathbf{i}^2 = -1$. Find the partial-fractions form for

$$\frac{1}{(1 + 4x)(1 - \mathbf{i}x)(1 + \mathbf{i}x)}.$$

18. Find the partial-fractions form for

$$\frac{1}{(1 + x)(1 - x)(1 + \mathbf{i}x)(1 - \mathbf{i}x)}.$$

19. Convert $12(x^3 - 4x^2 - 3x + 1)/(x - 1)^2(x + 2)(x - 3)$ into the form to which Theorem 1 ("Partial-Fractions Decomposition") applies.

20. Repeat Problem 19 for $80/(x + 4)^2(x - 5)$.

21. (i) Use the "Rational Root Theorem" (Theorem 5) of Section 8.1 to factor $x^3 - x^2 - 8x + 12$ into first degree factors, that is, in the form $(x - a)(x - b)(x - c)$.

(ii) Let a, b, c be the constants found in Part (i). Show that

$$1 - x - 8x^2 + 12x^3 = (1 - ax)(1 - bx)(1 - cx).$$

(iii) Find the partial-fractions form for

$$\frac{18x^2 - 22x - 1}{1 - x - 8x^2 + 12x^3}.$$

22. (i) Find the partial-fractions form for

$$\frac{1}{(1 - x)(1 - \frac{1}{2}x)(1 - \frac{1}{3}x)}.$$

(ii) Use Part (i) to find the partial-fractions form for

$$\frac{6}{(1 - x)(2 - x)(3 - x)}.$$

(iii) Use Part (ii) to find the partial-fractions form for

$$\frac{-6}{(x - 1)(x - 2)(x - 3)}.$$

23. Find the partial-fractions form for

$$\frac{24}{x^3 - 6x^2 + 12x - 8}.$$

24. Find the partial-fractions form for

$$\frac{54}{x^3 + 7x^2 + 15x + 9}.$$

25. Let $A(x)$ be a polynomial of degree 0, 1, or 2. Let r, s, and t be three distinct numbers. Prove that

$$\frac{A(x)}{(x-r)(x-s)(x-t)} = \frac{A(r)}{(r-s)(r-t)} \cdot \frac{1}{x-r} + \frac{A(s)}{(s-r)(s-t)} \cdot \frac{1}{x-s}$$

$$+ \frac{A(t)}{(t-r)(t-s)} \cdot \frac{1}{x-t}.$$

26. Let $A(x)$ be a polynomial of degree 0, 1, 2, or 3. Let r, s, t, and u be four distinct numbers, let $B = (x-r)(x-s)(x-t)(x-u)$, and let

$$a = \frac{A(r)}{(r-s)(r-t)(r-u)}, \qquad b = \frac{A(s)}{(s-r)(s-t)(s-u)},$$

$$c = \frac{A(t)}{(t-r)(t-s)(t-u)}, \qquad d = \frac{A(u)}{(u-r)(u-s)(u-t)}.$$

Prove that

$$\frac{A}{B} = \frac{a}{x-r} + \frac{b}{x-s} + \frac{c}{x-t} + \frac{d}{x-u}.$$

27. Use the formula of Problem 25 with $\{r, s, t\} = \{1, 2, 3\}$ to solve Problem 15(d).

28. Use Problem 25 with $\{r, s, t\} = \{-\frac{1}{3}, \frac{1}{4}, \frac{1}{5}\}$ to solve Problem 16(d).

29. State and prove the analogue of Problems 25 and 26 for a proper x-fraction $A(x)/(x-r)(x-s)$.

30. Use Problem 29 to solve Problem 16(b).

31. Use long division to express each improper (that is, not proper) x-fraction of Problem 1 as a polynomial plus a proper x-fraction.

32. Express each improper x-fraction of Problem 2 as a polynomial plus a proper x-fraction.

33. What happens in the formula of Problem 25 when $r = s$?

34. What happens in the formula of Problem 26 when the numbers r, s, t, u are not distinct?

35. In Theorem 1 ("Partial-Fractions Decomposition"), let some $d_i = 1$. Show that the constant c in the term $c/(1 - r_i x)$ of the partial-fractions form for A/B is $A(1/r_i)/h$, where

$$h = \left(1 - \frac{r_1}{r_i}\right)^{d_1} \cdots \left(1 - \frac{r_{i-1}}{r_i}\right)^{d_{i-1}} \left(1 - \frac{r_{i+1}}{r_i}\right)^{d_{i+1}} \cdots \left(1 - \frac{r_m}{r_i}\right)^{d_m}.$$

SUMMARY OF TERMS, CHAPTER 8 _____

Alternate factoring	$1 + bx + cx^2 = (1 - rx)(1 - sx)$, where r and s are $(-b \pm \sqrt{b^2 - 4c})/2$.	429
Bisection Algorithm	Successively bisecting intervals containing a root.	440
Change of sign	Sufficient condition for a root of $p(x) = 0$.	438
Coefficients	The a_i of $a_0 x^d + a_1 x^{d-1} + \cdots + a_d$.	426
Degree of $p(x)$	The d of $p(x) = a_0 x^d + \cdots + a_d$, where $a_0 \neq 0$.	426
Denominator	The B of a fraction A/B.	447
Derivative of $p(x)$	If $p(x) = a_0 x^d + a_1 x^{d-1} + \cdots + a_{d-1} x + a_d$, its derivative is $p'(x) = da_0 x^{d-1} + (d-1)a_1 x^{d-2} + \cdots + a_{d-1}$.	442
Educated guessing	A technique for refining an approximation to a root of $p(x) = 0$.	439
Factor Theorem	$x - h$ is a factor of $p(x)$ if and only if h is a root of $p(x) = 0$.	432
First degree equation	$ax + b = 0$, with $a \neq 0$.	427
First degree polynomial	$ax + b$, with $a \neq 0$.	426
Multiple root of $p(x) = 0$	An r such that $(x - r)^2$ is a factor of $p(x)$.	434
Multiplicity of a root r of $p(x) = 0$	The largest m such that $(x - r)^m$ is a factor of $p(x)$.	434
Newton's Method	A technique for refining an approximation to a root of $p(x) = 0$.	442
Numerator	The A of a fraction A/B.	447
Partial-fractions decomposition	Expression for a proper x-fraction as a sum of terms $c/(1 - rx)^m$.	454
Polynomial in x	$a_0 x^d + a_1 x^{d-1} + \cdots + a_d$.	426
Polynomial equation	$p(x) = 0$ with $p(x)$ a polynomial in x.	427
Polynomial function	A mapping $x \mapsto a_0 x^d + a_1 x^{d-1} + \cdots + a_0$.	426
Proper x-fraction	Quotient $p(x)/q(x)$ of polynomials, with $p(x)$ of lower degree than $q(x)$.	447
Quadratic equation	*See* Second degree equation.	427
Quadratic formula	The roots of $ax^2 + bx + c = 0$, with $a \neq 0$, are $(-b \pm \sqrt{b^2 - 4ac})/2a$.	428
Quadratic polynomial	*See* Second degree polynomial.	426
Rational function	A mapping $x \mapsto p(x)/q(x)$, with $p(x)$ and $q(x)$ polynomials in x.	448
Rational Root Theorem	See Theorem 5 of Section 8.1.	433
Remainder Theorem	If $p(x) = (x - h)q(x) + r$, then $r = p(h)$.	432
Repeated root of $p(x) = 0$	*See* Multiple root of $p(x) = 0$.	434
Root of $p(x) = 0$	A number h such that $p(h) = 0$.	427
Second degree equation	$ax^2 + bx + c = 0$, with $a \neq 0$.	427
Second degree polynomial	$ax^2 + bx + c$, with $a \neq 0$.	426
Simple root	A root of multiplicity 1.	434
Special x-fraction	$c/(1 - rx)^m$, with $m \in \mathbf{Z}^+$.	449

REVIEW PROBLEMS FOR CHAPTER 8

1. Find the root of $5x + 10 = 0$.

2. Find the root of $10x - 5 = 0$.

3. Express each of the following polynomials $p(x)$ as a product of first degree polynomials:
    (a) $x^2 + 4x - 21$;   (b) $1 + 4x - 21x^2$;
    (c) $x^2 - 14x + 49$;   (d) $1 - 14x + 49x^2$.

4. Express each of the following polynomials $p(x)$ as a product of first degree polynomials:
    (a) $x^2 - 4x - 21$;   (b) $1 - 4x - 21x^2$;
    (c) $x^2 + 14x + 49$;   (d) $1 + 14x + 49x^2$.

5. Find the roots of $p(x) = 0$ for each $p(x)$ of Problem 3.

6. Find the roots of $p(x) = 0$ for each $p(x)$ of Problem 4.

7. (i) Find the rational roots of $x^3 + 8x^2 + 17x + 10 = 0$.
    (ii) Find numbers r, s, and t such that
    $$x^3 + 8x^2 + 17x + 10 = (x - r)(x - s)(x - t).$$
    (iii) Find numbers r, s, and t such that
    $$1 + 8x + 17x^2 + 10x^3 = (1 - rx)(1 - sx)(1 - tx).$$

8. (i) Find the rational roots of $x^3 - 8x^2 + 17x - 10 = 0$.
    (ii) Find numbers r, s, and t such that
    $$x^3 - 8x^2 + 17x - 10 = (x - r)(x - s)(x - t).$$
    (iii) Find numbers r, s, and t such that
    $$1 - 8x + 17x^2 - 10x^3 = (1 - rx)(1 - sx)(1 - tx).$$

9. Let $p(x) = x^3 - x^2 + 4x - 4$.
    (i) Find a rational root of $p(x) = 0$.
    (ii) Find all the roots of $p(x) = 0$.
    (iii) Express $p(x)$ as a product of first degree factors.

10. Repeat Problem 9 for $p(x) = x^3 + x^2 + 9x + 9$.

11. List each root, with its multiplicity, for the equation
    $$(x - 3)^2(x + 2)^3(x^2 - 5x + 6)(x - 0.5)(x + 3.6) = 0.$$

12. Find all roots and their multiplicities for the equation
    $$x^5 - x^4 - 9x^3 + 5x^2 + 16x - 12 = 0.$$

13. Let $p(x) = 3x^4 + ax^3 + bx + 15$, where a and b are integers. What are the possibilities for rational roots of $p(x) = 0$?

14. Let $p(x) = 15x^5 + ax^4 + bx^3 - 14x^2 - 3$, where a and b are integers. What are the possibilities for rational roots of $p(x) = 0$?

15. Let $p(x) = x^2 - 10$. Find two integers a such that $p(a)$ and $p(a + 1)$ have opposite signs.

16. Let $p(x) = x^3 - x^2 - 2$. Find an integer a such that $p(a)$ and $p(a + 1)$ have opposite signs.

17. Let $p(x) = x^4 - x - 3$.
(i) Show that there is a root of $p(x) = 0$ in the interval $1 < x < 2$.
(ii) Use the "Bisection Algorithm" (Algorithm 1 of Section 8.2) to isolate the root in an interval $a < x < a + 0.25$.

18. Let $p(x) = x^3 + 2x^2 - 30$.
(i) Show that there is a root of $p(x) = 0$ in the interval $2 < x < 3$.
(ii) Use the "Bisection Algorithm" (Algorithm 1 of Section 8.2) to isolate the root in an interval $a < x < a + 0.25$.

19. Given that $p(x) = 0$ has a root in the interval $-6 < x < -5$, how many bisections may be needed to find the root to seven decimal places?

20. Given that $p(x) = 0$ has a root in the interval $8 < x < 12$, how many bisections may be needed to find the root to six decimal places?

21. Let $p(x) = x^4 + x - 3$.
(i) Show that $p(x) = 0$ has a root in the interval $1 < x < 2$.
(ii) Use Newton's Method (Algorithm 2 of Section 8.2) with $x_0 = 1$ and compute $x_1, x_2, \ldots$ until terms x_k and x_{k+1} differ by less than 0.00001.

22. Repeat Problem 21(ii), but now use $x_0 = 2$.

23. Find the partial-fractions decompositions for:
(a) $\dfrac{1}{1 - 8x + 12x^2}$;   (b) $\dfrac{1 + 2x}{1 - 8x + 16x^2}$.

24. Find the partial-fractions decompositions for:
(a) $\dfrac{3 - x}{1 + 14x + 49x^2}$;   (b) $\dfrac{x}{4 - x^2}$.

25. Find the partial-fractions decomposition for $(2 - x^3)/(1 + x)^4$.

26. Find the partial-fractions decomposition for $(4 - 9x + 2x^2)/(1 - 2x)^3$.

27. Find the partial-fractions decompositions for:
(a) $\dfrac{2 - 36x + 14x^2}{(1 - 2x)(1 + 3x)(1 - 4x)}$;   (b) $\dfrac{3 - 2x + 27x^2}{(1 + x)(1 - 3x)^2}$.

28. Find the partial-fractions decompositions for:
(a) $\dfrac{4 - 12x + 20x^2}{1 - x - 4x^2 + 4x^3}$;   (b) $\dfrac{21 + 10x + x^2}{1 + x - x^2 - x^3}$.

SUPPLEMENTARY AND CHALLENGING PROBLEMS, CHAPTER 8 _____

1. Use synthetic division to find the polynomial $q(x)$ such that
$$x^4 + 4x^3 + 8x^2 + 11x + 6 = (x^2 + 3x + 2)q(x).$$

2. Let $p(x) = x^4 + 2bx^2 - 207x - 1575$, where b is an integer. Explain why:
   (i) An integer r that satisfies $p(x) = 0$ would have to be odd.
   (ii) An integer r that satisfies $p(x) = 0$ could not be odd.
   (iii) The equation $p(x) = 0$ has no rational roots.

3. Prove that $\sqrt[3]{2} + \sqrt[3]{4}$ is not a rational number.

4. Choose x_0 as any number in the interval $0 < x < 2$. Then let the sequence $x_0, x_1, \ldots$ be defined inductively by
$$x_{k+1} = \begin{cases} 2x_k & \text{if } 0 < x_k \le 1 \\ 4 - 2x_k & \text{if } 1 < x_k < 2. \end{cases}$$
   For which numbers x_0 will $x_n = x_{n+1}$ for some n in N?

5. Let the sequence $x_0, x_1, \ldots$ be defined inductively by $x_0 = 1$ and
$$x_{k+1} = \frac{1}{2}\left(x_k + \frac{2}{x_k}\right) \quad \text{for } k \in N = \{0, 1, \ldots\}.$$
   Prove that $\sqrt{2} < x_{n+1} < x_n$ for $n \in N$.

6. Let $x_0, x_1, \ldots$ be defined inductively by $x_0 = 1$ and
$$x_{k+1} = \frac{x_k^2 + 1}{2x_k - 1} \quad \text{for } k \in N.$$
   (i) For $n \in N$ and $m = 2^n$, prove that x_n is the quotient F_{m+1}/F_m of Fibonacci Numbers.
   (ii) How is this problem related to Problem 8 of Section 8.2?

7. Let $x_0, x_1, \ldots$ be defined inductively by $x_0 = -1$ and
$$x_{k+1} = \frac{x_k^2 + 1}{2x_k - 1} \quad \text{for } k \in N.$$
   For $n \in N$ and $m = 2^n$, prove that $x_n = -F_{2m-1}/F_{2m}$.

8. Let Newton's Method for approximating a root be used for the equation $x^2 - 2x - 1 = 0$. Let x_0 be the starting value for the sequence $x_0, x_1, \ldots$ of that method. Show that:
   (i) If $x_0 = 1$, the method fails.
   (ii) If $x_0 > 1$, the terms ultimately will agree to more and more decimal places with $1 + \sqrt{2} \approx 2.414$.
   (iii) If $x_0 < 1$, the terms ultimately will agree to more and more places with $1 - \sqrt{2} \approx -0.414$.

9. Find integers $a, b, c,$ and d such that $x^4 + 324 = (x^2 + ax + b)(x^2 + cx + d)$.

9

GENERATING FUNCTIONS AND RECURSIONS

A sequence satisfies a recursion relation if there is a rule for determining each term, except for a few at the beginning of the sequence, from previous terms. Such sequences occur in many applications, including estimation of the time or memory space required for carrying out various computer algorithms. One such application is given in Section 10.1, where we discuss a "divide-and-conquer" algorithm for sorting and show that a measure of its efficiency involves the sequence $v_1, v_2, \ldots$ having $v_1 = 1$ and

$$v_n = 2v_{n-1} + 2^n - 1 \qquad \text{for } n \in \{2, 3, \ldots\}. \tag{1}$$

If we want the term v_{20} of this sequence, we can use the recursion 19 times as follows:

$$v_2 = 2v_1 + 2^2 - 1 = 2 \cdot 1 + 4 - 1 = 5,$$
$$v_3 = 2v_2 + 2^3 - 1 = 2 \cdot 5 + 8 - 1 = 17,$$
$$\vdots$$
$$v_{20} = 2v_{19} + 2^{20} - 1.$$

This method for finding v_n can be tedious, especially when n is large. In this chapter, we will learn how to find an explicit formula for the term v_n of a sequence satisfying certain types of recursions. In particular, we will show that the sequence satisfying the recursion in Display (1) and having the initial term $v_1 = 1$ is given by the explicit formula

$$v_n = 2^n(n - 1) + 1.$$

Then one can find directly that

$$v_{20} = 2^{20}(20 - 1) + 1 = 1048576 \cdot 19 + 1 = 19922945.$$

Several of the sequences considered in earlier chapters satisfy recursions. The sequence $0!, 1!, 2!, \ldots$ of factorials is the sequence $u_0, u_1, u_2, \ldots$ with the initial condition $u_0 = 1$ and satisfying the recursion

$$u_n = nu_{n-1} \qquad \text{for } n \in \mathbf{Z}^+ = \{1, 2, \ldots\}.$$

Both the Fibonacci Sequence $0, 1, 1, 2, 3, 5, \ldots$ and the Lucas Sequence $2, 1, 3, 4, 7, 11, \ldots$ satisfy the recursion

$$u_n = u_{n-1} + u_{n-2} \qquad \text{for } n \in \{2, 3, \ldots\}.$$

The Fibonacci Sequence is the specific solution to this recursion with the initial conditions $u_0 = 0$ and $u_1 = 1$, whereas the Lucas Sequence is the specific solution with $u_0 = 2$ and $u_1 = 1$. A method in Section 9.2 will enable us to derive the explicit formulas

$$F_n = \frac{1}{\sqrt{5}}\left[\left(\frac{1+\sqrt{5}}{2}\right)^n - \left(\frac{1-\sqrt{5}}{2}\right)^n\right], \quad L_n = \left(\frac{1+\sqrt{5}}{2}\right)^n + \left(\frac{1-\sqrt{5}}{2}\right)^n$$

for the Fibonacci Numbers F_n and the Lucas Numbers L_n. These are called the **Binet Formulas** for F_n and L_n.

An arithmetic progression $a_0, a_1, \ldots$ with constant difference d satisfies the recursion $a_n = a_{n-1} + d$. Using this formula several times, we get

$$a_1 = a_0 + d,$$
$$a_2 = a_1 + d = (a_0 + d) + d = a_0 + 2d,$$
$$a_3 = a_2 + d = (a_0 + 2d) + d = a_0 + 3d.$$

This suggests the formula $a_n = a_0 + nd$ for $n \in \mathbf{Z}^+$; this explicit formula is easily proved by mathematical induction.

Similarly, a geometric progression $g_0, g_1, \ldots$ with constant ratio r satisfies the recursion $g_n = rg_{n-1}$, and one can show that $g_n = r^n g_0$ for n in $\mathbf{N} = \{0, 1, \ldots\}$.

Also, as we saw in Section 5.8, the number d_n of derangements of $\{1, 2, \ldots, n\}$ satisfies each of the recursions

$$d_n = nd_{n-1} + (-1)^n \qquad \text{for } n \in \{1, 2, \ldots\},$$
$$d_n = (n-1)(d_{n-1} + d_{n-2}) \qquad \text{for } n \in \{2, 3, \ldots\}.$$

A recursion is "solved" when one obtains a formula for the nth term as a function of n. This chapter contains methods for solving certain categories of recursion relations. Section 9.1 develops a tool for this effort, called "generating series." Then Sections 9.2 through 9.5 present characteristic root techniques. The chapter concludes in Section 9.6 with some miscellaneous techniques.

9.1

GENERATING SERIES

The following concept is a powerful tool for the study of sequences, especially those satisfying recursions.

DEFINITION 1   **GENERATING SERIES, COEFFICIENT SEQUENCE**

The *generating series* for an infinite sequence

$$a_0, a_1, a_2, \ldots \tag{1}$$

is the unending power series

$$a_0 + a_1 x + a_2 x^2 + \cdots + a_n x^n + \cdots. \tag{2}$$

Also, (1) is the *coefficient sequence* for Series (2).

The series in Display (2) is sometimes denoted by $\sum_{n=0}^{\infty} a_n x^n$. Readers who have studied infinite series in calculus may note that we are making no assumptions concerning convergence of any series dealt with here.

The main role of the powers x^0, x, x^2, x^3, ... in Definition 1 is to indicate the positions of the terms $a_0, a_1, a_2, a_3, \ldots$ of the sequence. Hence x may be replaced by another letter when this is convenient.

The generating series for the sequence 0!, 1!, 2!, ... of factorials (Definition 1, "Factorials," of Section 4.1) is

$$0! + 1!x + 2!x^2 + 3!x^3 + 4!x^4 + \cdots + n!x^n + \cdots$$
$$= 1 + x + 2x^2 + 6x^3 + 24x^4 + \cdots + n!x^n + \cdots.$$

The generating series for the Lucas Sequence $L_0, L_1, \ldots$ defined inductively in Definition 3 of Section 4.1 is

$$L_0 + L_1 x + L_2 x^2 + L_3 x^3 + L_4 x^4 + \cdots + L_n x^n + \cdots$$
$$= 2 + x + 3x^2 + 4x^3 + 7x^4 + \cdots + L_n x^n + \cdots,$$

and the generating series for the Fibonacci Sequence 0, 1, 1, 2, 3, ... is

$$F_0 + F_1 x + F_2 x^2 + F_3 x^3 + F_4 x^4 + \cdots + F_n x^n + \cdots$$
$$= x + x^2 + 2x^3 + 3x^4 + \cdots + F_n x^n + \cdots.$$

DEFINITION 2   **EQUALITY OF GENERATING SERIES**

$$a_0 + a_1 x + a_2 x^2 + \cdots = b_0 + b_1 x + b_2 x^2 + \cdots$$

if and only if $a_n = b_n$ for each n in $N = \{0, 1, 2, \ldots\}$.

DEFINITION 3   **ADDITION OF GENERATING SERIES**

Let

$$A = a_0 + a_1x + a_2x^2 + \cdots + a_nx^n + \cdots$$

and

$$B = b_0 + b_1x + b_2x^2 + \cdots + b_nx^n + \cdots.$$

Then

$$A + B = (a_0 + b_0) + (a_1 + b_1)x + \cdots + (a_n + b_n)x^n + \cdots.$$

Example 1   Let

$$A = 2 + x + 3x^2 + 4x^3 + 7x^4 + \cdots + L_nx^n + \cdots,$$
$$B = x + x^2 + 2x^3 + 3x^4 + \cdots + F_nx^n + \cdots.$$

Then

$$A + B = 2 + 2x + 4x^2 + 6x^3 + 10x^4 + \cdots + (L_n + F_n)x^n + \cdots.$$

The coefficient sequence $2, 2, 4, 6, \ldots, L_n + F_n, \ldots$ seems to be the sequence $2F_1, 2F_2, 2F_3, 2F_4, \ldots, 2F_{n+1}, \ldots$. These two sequences are equal since one can use mathematical induction to prove that $L_n + F_n = 2F_{n+1}$ for all n in $N = \{0, 1, \ldots\}$.   □

LEMMA 1   **GENERATING SERIES FOR A SUM OF SEQUENCES**

Let A and B be the generating series for the sequences $a_0, a_1, \ldots$ and $b_0, b_1, \ldots$, respectively. Then $A + B$ is the generating series for the sequence $a_0 + b_0, a_1 + b_1, \ldots$.

PROOF   This follows directly from Definition 3.   □

DEFINITION 4   **MULTIPLICATION OF GENERATING SERIES**

Let

$$A = \sum_{n=0}^{\infty} a_nx^n = a_0 + a_1x + \cdots + a_nx^n + \cdots$$

and

$$B = \sum_{n=0}^{\infty} b_nx^n = b_0 + b_1x + \cdots + b_nx^n + \cdots.$$

Then their product

$$AB = a_0b_0 + (a_0b_1 + a_1b_0)x + (a_0b_2 + a_1b_1 + a_2b_0)x^2 + \cdots.$$

That is,

$$AB = \sum_{n=0}^{\infty} c_n x^n, \quad \text{where } c_n = \sum_{k=0}^{n} a_k b_{n-k}.$$

Example 2   Let

$$A = 1 + 2x + 3x^2 + 4x^3 + \cdots + (n+1)x^n + \cdots,$$

$$B = 1 + 3x + 6x^2 + 10x^3 + \cdots + \binom{n+2}{2}x^n + \cdots.$$

Then their product is

$$AB = 1 \cdot 1 + (1 \cdot 3 + 2 \cdot 1)x + (1 \cdot 6 + 2 \cdot 3 + 3 \cdot 1)x^2 + (1 \cdot 10 + 2 \cdot 6 + 3 \cdot 3 + 4 \cdot 1)x^3 + \cdots$$
$$= 1 + 5x + 15x^2 + 35x^3 + \cdots + c_n x^n + \cdots,$$

where

$$c_n = \binom{n+2}{2} + 2\binom{n+1}{2} + 3\binom{n}{2} + \cdots + (n+1)\binom{2}{2}$$

$$= \sum_{k=0}^{n} (k+1)\binom{n+2-k}{2}.$$

It is left to the reader as Problem 36 below to show that $c_n = \binom{n+4}{4}$.   □

The following notation enables us to consider a polynomial to be a generating series.

NOTATION 1   **POLYNOMIAL AS A SERIES**

The polynomial $a_0 + a_1 x + \cdots + a_d x^d$ is the generating series for the sequence $a_0, a_1, a_2, \ldots$ in which $a_n = 0$ for $n > d$.

For example, $1 - x - x^2$ is the generating series for the sequence 1, -1, -1, 0, 0, ... in which all terms not shown explicitly are zeros.

The following result will enable us to show a nice relationship between generating series such as the G and H given by

$$G = 1 + 2x + 3x^2 + \cdots + (n+1)x^n + \cdots,$$
$$H = 1 + x + x^2 + \cdots + x^n + \cdots.$$

THEOREM 1   **DIFFERENCING**

Let $G = g_0 + g_1 x + \cdots + g_n x^n + \cdots$. Then $(1 - x)G$ is the series $H = h_0 + h_1 x + \cdots + h_n x^n + \cdots$ in which $h_0 = g_0$ and $h_n = g_n - g_{n-1}$ for $n \in \{1, 2, \ldots\}$.

PROOF   Let $A = 1 - x$. Since A is a polynomial, we find it convenient to perform the multiplication AG with the following format:

$$G = g_0 + g_1 x + g_2 x^2 + \cdots + \quad g_n x^n + \cdots$$
$$-xG = \quad -g_0 x - g_1 x^2 - \cdots - g_{n-1} x^n - \cdots.$$

We add these equations and let $(1 - x)G = H = h_0 + h_1 x + \cdots$; this gives us

$$h_0 + h_1 x + h_2 x^2 + \cdots + h_n x^n + \cdots$$
$$= g_0 + (g_1 - g_0)x + (g_2 - g_1)x^2 + \cdots + (g_n - g_{n-1})x^n + \cdots.$$

Equating coefficients of like powers of x, we get

$$h_0 = g_0 \quad \text{and} \quad h_n = g_n - g_{n-1} \quad \text{for } n \in \{1, 2, \ldots\}. \qquad \square$$

Example 3   Using Theorem 1, one obtains

$$(1 - x)(1 + x + x^2 + \cdots) = 1 + (1 - 1)x + (1 - 1)x^2 + \cdots.$$

That is,

$$(1 - x)(1 + x + x^2 + x^3 + \cdots) = 1. \qquad (3)$$

This formula tempts us to write

$$1 + x + x^2 + \cdots = \frac{1}{1 - x} = (1 - x)^{-1}$$

and thus motivates the following notation. $\qquad \square$

NOTATION 2   **QUOTIENT OF POLYNOMIALS, GENERATING FUNCTION**

Let $G = g_0 + g_1 x + g_2 x^2 + \cdots$. If there exist polynomials A and B, with $B \neq 0$, such that $BG = A$, we can write $G = A/B$, or $G = AB^{-1}$. The quotient A/B then is called the **generating function** for the sequence $g_0, g_1, g_2, \ldots$.

Example 4   Let $G = 1 + 2x + 3x^2 + \cdots + (n + 1)x^n + \cdots$. Using Theorem 1 ("Differencing") or Definition 4 ("Multiplication of Generating Series"), one has

$$(1 - x)G = 1 + (2 - 1)x + (3 - 2)x^2 + \cdots$$
$$(1 - x)G = 1 + x + x^2 + \cdots + x^n + \cdots.$$

Multiplying each side of this equation by $1 - x$ and using Display (3) in Example 3, gives one

$$(1 - x)^2 G = (1 - x)(1 + x + x^2 + \cdots) = 1.$$

Hence $G = 1/(1 - x)^2 = (1 - x)^{-2}$ is the generating function for the sequence 1, 2, 3, ... □

Example 5 **GENERATING FUNCTION FOR AN ARITHMETIC PROGRESSION** Let us now find the generating function C for the arithmetic progression 2, 5, 8, 11, ..., $3n + 2$, ... The generating series for the sequence is

$$\begin{aligned} C &= 2 + 5x + 8x^2 + \cdots + (3n + 2)x^n + \cdots \\ &= 2 + (3 + 2)x + (3 \cdot 2 + 2)x^2 + \cdots + (3n + 2)x^n + \cdots \\ &= (2 + 2x + 2x^2 + \cdots + 2x^n + \cdots) + (3x + 3 \cdot 2x^2 + 3 \cdot 3x^3 + \cdots) \\ &= 2(1 + x + x^2 + \cdots) + 3x(1 + 2x + 3x^2 + \cdots). \end{aligned}$$

Using the results of Examples 3 and 4, this becomes

$$C = \frac{2}{1 - x} + \frac{3x}{(1 - x)^2} = \frac{2(1 - x) + 3x}{(1 - x)^2} = \frac{2 + x}{(1 - x)^2}.$$

Hence the desired generating function is $C = (2 + x)/(1 - x)^2$.

This formula can also be obtained using Theorem 1 ("Differencing"), as we now show:

$$\begin{aligned} C &= 2 + 5x + 8x^2 + \cdots + (3n + 2)x^n + \cdots \\ (1 - x)C &= 2 + (5 - 2)x + (8 - 5)x^2 + \cdots \\ &\quad + [(3n + 2) - (3n - 1)]x^n + \cdots \\ (1 - x)C &= 2 + 3x + 3x^2 + \cdots + 3x^n + \cdots \\ (1 - x)(1 - x)C &= 2 + (3 - 2)x + (3 - 3)x^2 + \cdots + (3 - 3)x^n + \cdots \\ (1 - x)^2 C &= 2 + x \\ C &= \frac{(2 + x)}{(1 - x)^2}. \end{aligned}$$

□

Example 6 Here we find the generating function G for the geometric progression 3, 6, 12, 24, ..., $3 \cdot 2^n$, ... We have

$$\begin{aligned} G &= 3 + 6x + 12x^2 + \cdots + 3 \cdot 2^n x^n + \cdots \\ -2xG &= - 6x - 12x^2 - \cdots - 3 \cdot 2^n x^n - \cdots \\ \hline (1 - 2x)G &= 3. \end{aligned}$$

Hence $G = 3/(1 - 2x)$.

□

THEOREM 2   **GENERATING FUNCTIONS RELATED TO GEOMETRIC PROGRESSIONS**

(a) $a/(1 - rx)$ is the generating function for the geometric progression a, $ar, ar^2, \ldots, ar^n, \ldots$.

(b) $a/(1 - rx)^2$ is the generating function for the sequence $u_0, u_1, \ldots$ with $u_n = a(n + 1)r^n$.

PROOF   (a) Let $G = a + arx + ar^2x^2 + \cdots$ be the generating series for the geometric progression $a, ar, ar^2, \ldots$. Then we find $(1 - rx)G$ as follows:

$$G = a + arx + ar^2x^2 + \cdots + ar^nx^n + \cdots$$
$$-rxG = \quad - arx - ar^2x^2 - \cdots - ar^nx^n - \cdots$$
$$\overline{G - rxG = a \qquad\qquad\qquad \cdots \qquad\qquad ..}$$

Hence $(1 - rx)G = a$ and $G = a/(1 - rx)$.

(b) Let $H = a + 2arx + 3ar^2x^2 + \cdots + (n + 1)ar^nx^n + \cdots$. We find $(1 - rx)H$ as follows:

$$H = a + 2arx + 3ar^2x^2 + \cdots + (n + 1)ar^nx^n + \cdots$$
$$-rxH = \quad - arx - 2ar^2x^2 - \cdots - \quad nar^nx^n - \cdots$$
$$\overline{(1 - rx)H = a + \quad arx + \quad ar^2x^2 + \cdots + \qquad ar^nx^n + \cdots.}$$

This shows that $(1 - rx)H$ is the G of Part (a). Thus $(1 - rx)H = a/(1 - rx)$ and hence $H = a/(1 - rx)^2$. □

Example 7   It follows from Theorem 2(b), with $r = 1$ and $a = 1$, that $(1 - x)^{-2} = 1/(1 - x)^2$ is the generating function for the sequence $u_0, u_1, \ldots$ with $u_n = n + 1$, that is, for the sequence

$1, 2, 3, \ldots, (n + 1), \ldots$.

Also, the generating function for the sequence $u_0, u_1, \ldots$ with $u_n = 5(n + 1)3^n$ is $5/(1 - 3x)^2$, and the generating function for the sequence $w_0, w_1, \ldots$ with $w_n = 4(n + 1)(-7)^n$ is $4/(1 + 7x)^2$. □

Let G and H be generating series related (as in Theorem 1, "Differencing") by the equation $(1 - x)G = H$. Then one might be motivated to write $G = (1 - x)^{-1}H$. This and the formula

$(1 - x)^{-1} = 1 + x + x^2 + \cdots + x^n + \cdots$

from Example 3 would lead to

$G = (1 + x + x^2 + \cdots + x^n + \cdots)H.$ (4)

In the following theorem, we show directly how to get G from H when these generating series are related as in Display (4).

THEOREM 3   **GENERATING SERIES FOR PARTIAL SUMS**

Let $G = BH$, where

$$B = 1 + x + x^2 + \cdots + x^n + \cdots$$
$$G = g_0 + g_1 x + g_2 x^2 + \cdots + g_n x^n + \cdots$$
$$H = h_0 + h_1 x + h_2 x^2 + \cdots + h_n x^n + \cdots$$

Then:

(a) $g_0 = h_0,$

$\quad g_1 = h_0 + h_1,$

$\quad g_2 = h_0 + h_1 + h_2,$

$\quad \vdots$

$\quad g_n = \displaystyle\sum_{k=0}^{n} h_k = h_0 + h_1 + \cdots + h_n.$

(b) $H = (1 - x)G.$

PROOF   (a) This follows immediately from Definition 4, "Multiplication of Generating Series."

(b) Theorem 1 ("Differencing") tells us that

$$(1 - x)G = g_0 + (g_1 - g_0)x + (g_2 - g_1)x^2$$
$$+ \cdots + (g_n - g_{n-1})x^n + \cdots. \qquad (5)$$

Using Part (a), we see that

$$g_0 = h_0,$$
$$g_1 - g_0 = (h_0 + h_1) - h_0 = h_1,$$
$$\vdots$$
$$g_n - g_{n-1} = (h_0 + h_1 + \cdots + h_{n-1} + h_n) - (h_0 + h_1 + \cdots + h_{n-1})$$
$$= h_n.$$

We make these substitutions in Display (5) and get the claimed

$$(1 - x)G = h_0 + h_1 x + h_2 x^2 + \cdots = H. \qquad \square$$

Example 8   Let $G = g_0 + g_1 x + g_2 x^2 + \cdots + g_n x^n + \cdots$ be the generating series for the sequence

$$g_0, g_1, g_2, \ldots, g_n, \ldots.$$

Then what sequence has xG as its generating series? Since

$$xG = 0 + g_0 x + g_1 x^2 + g_2 x^3 + \cdots + g_{n-1} x^n + \cdots,$$

TABLE 9.1.1

Operation	Sequence	Generating Function	Generating Series
	$a_0, a_1, a_2, a_3, \ldots, a_n, \ldots$	A	$a_0 + a_1 x + a_2 x^2 + a_3 x^3 + \cdots + a_n x^n + \cdots$
	$b_0, b_1, b_2, b_3, \ldots, b_n, \ldots$	B	$b_0 + b_1 x + b_2 x^2 + b_3 x^3 + \cdots + b_n x^n + \cdots$
Addition	$a_0 + b_0, a_1 + b_1, a_2 + b_2, \ldots$	$A + B$	$(a_0 + b_0) + (a_1 + b_1)x + (a_2 + b_2)x^2 + \cdots + (a_n + b_n)x^n + \cdots$
Differencing	$a_0, a_1 - a_0, a_2 - a_1, a_3 - a_2, \ldots$	$(1 - x)A$	$a_0 + (a_1 - a_0)x + (a_2 - a_1)x^2 + (a_3 - a_2)x^3 + \cdots + (a_n - a_{n-1})x^n + \cdots$
Summing	$a_0, a_0 + a_1, a_0 + a_1 + a_2, \ldots$	$\dfrac{A}{1 - x}$	$a_0 + (a_0 + a_1)x + (a_0 + a_1 + a_2)x^2 + \cdots + \left(\sum_{k=0}^{n} a_k\right)x^n + \cdots$
Shifting	$0, a_0, a_1, a_2, \ldots$	xA	$a_0 x + a_1 x^2 + a_2 x^3 + \cdots + a_{n-1}x^n + \cdots$
Multiplication	$a_0 b_0, a_0 b_1 + a_1 b_0, \ldots$	AB	$a_0 b_0 + (a_0 b_1 + a_1 b_0)x + (a_0 b_2 + a_1 b_1 + a_2 b_0)x^2 + \cdots + \left(\sum_{i=0}^{n} a_i b_{n-i}\right)x^n + \cdots$

the answer is that xG is the generating series for the sequence

$$0, g_0, g_1, \ldots, g_{n-1}, \ldots.$$

That is, xG is the generating series for the sequence $k_0, k_1, \ldots$ with $k_0 = 0$ and $k_n = g_{n-1}$ for $n \in \{1, 2, \ldots\}$. □

Example 9 Here we obtain the generating function for the sequence $2, 1, 3, 4, 7, \ldots$ of Lucas Numbers $L_0, L_1, L_2, \ldots$. Let

$$G = 2 + x + 3x^2 + 4x^3 + 7x^4 + \cdots + L_n x^n + \cdots.$$

By Definition 3 ("Fibonacci Numbers and Lucas Numbers") of Section 4.1,

$$L_{n+2} = L_{n+1} + L_n \quad \text{for all } n \text{ in } N = \{0, 1, 2, \ldots\}.$$

This recursion relation can be rewritten as $L_n - L_{n-1} - L_{n-2} = 0$ for $n = 2, 3, \ldots$. We see, as follows, that this equation causes all but the beginning terms to be zero in the product $(1 - x - x^2)G$:

$$
\begin{array}{llllll}
G = & 2 + & x + & 3x^2 + & 4x^3 + \cdots + & L_n x^n + \cdots \\
-xG = & & -2x - & x^2 - & 3x^3 - \cdots - & L_{n-1}x^n - \cdots \\
-x^2 G = & & & -2x^2 - & x^3 - \cdots - & L_{n-2}x^n - \cdots \\
\hline
(1 - x - x^2)G = & 2 - & x + & 0 \cdot x^2 + & 0 \cdot x^3 + \cdots + & 0 \cdot x^n + \cdots = 2 - x
\end{array}
$$

and so $G = (2 - x)/(1 - x - x^2)$. □

Table 9.1.1 summarizes some of the definitions and theorems of this section.

PROBLEMS FOR SECTION 9.1

1. Give the generating series for each of the following sequences.
   (i) $0, 1, 4, \ldots, n^2, \ldots$.   (ii) $1, 4, 9, \ldots, (n+1)^2, \ldots$.

2. Give the generating series for each of the following sequences.
   (i) $0, 1, 8, 27, \ldots, n^3, \ldots$.   (ii) $1, 8, 27, \ldots, (n+1)^3, \ldots$.

3. Give the generating series for $\binom{3}{3}, \binom{4}{3}, \ldots, \binom{n+3}{3}, \ldots$.

4. Give the generating series for $\binom{4}{4}, \binom{5}{4}, \ldots, \binom{n+4}{4}, \ldots$.

5. Let A and C be the series of Problems 1(ii) and 3. Find:
   (a) $A + C$;   (b) AC.

6. Let B and D be the series of Problems 2(ii) and 4. Find:
   (a) $B + D$;   (b) BD.

7. (i) Use the technique in Example 6 to find the generating function for the geometric progression $2, 10, 50, \ldots, 2 \cdot 5^n, \ldots$, that is, for the sequence $u_0, u_1, \ldots$ with $u_n = 2 \cdot 5^n$.
   (ii) Check using Theorem 2(a).

8. (i) Use the technique in Example 6 to find the generating function for the geometric progression $u_0, u_1, \ldots$ with $u_n = 6(-7)^n$.

(ii) Check using Theorem 2(a).

9. Use the technique in Example 6 or in the proof of Theorem 2 to find the generating function for each of the following geometric progressions:

(a) $1, \dfrac{1}{2}, \ldots, \dfrac{1}{2^n}, \ldots;$ (b) $2, 6, \ldots, 2 \cdot 3^n, \ldots;$

(c) $3, 3, \ldots, 3, \ldots;$ (d) $5, -5, \ldots, 5(-1)^n, \ldots.$

10. Do as in Problem 9 for each of the following:

(a) $1, -2, 4, \ldots, (-2)^n, \ldots;$ (b) $-8, -8, \ldots, -8, \ldots;$

(c) $4, \dfrac{4}{5}, \dfrac{4}{25}, \ldots, \dfrac{4}{5^n}, \ldots;$ (d) $1, -1, 1, \ldots, (-1)^n, \ldots.$

11. Let $a_n = 3(-4)^n$, $b_n = 5 \cdot 3^n$, and $c_n = a_n + b_n$. Find the generating functions for the following sequences.

(i) $a_0, a_1, a_2, \ldots.$ [*Hint:* Use Part (a) of Theorem 2, "Generating Functions Related to Geometric Progressions."]

(ii) $b_0, b_1, b_2, \ldots.$

(iii) $c_0, c_1, c_2, \ldots.$ (*Hint:* Use Lemma 1, "Generating Series for a Sum of Sequences.")

12. Repeat Problem 11, but with $a_n = 2 \cdot 8^n$, $b_n = 9(-5)^n$, and $c_n = a_n + b_n$.

13. Which geometric progression has $5/(1 + 2x)$ as its generating function?

14. Which geometric progression has $7/(1 - 3x)$ as its generating function?

15. For each of the following x-fractions G, give the formula for the term u_n of the sequence $u_0, u_1, \ldots$ having G as its generating function.

(i) $G = \dfrac{-4}{1 + 6x}$.   [*Hint:* Use Part (a) of Theorem 2, "Generating Functions Related to Geometric Progressions."]

(ii) $G = \dfrac{7}{1 - 9x}$.

(iii) $G = \dfrac{-4}{1 + 6x} + \dfrac{7}{1 - 9x} = \dfrac{3 + 78x}{(1 + 6x)(1 - 9x)}$.   [*Hint:* Use Parts (i) and (ii) together with Lemma 1, "Generating Series for a Sum of Sequences."

16. Repeat Problem 15, but for the following:

(i) $G = \dfrac{1}{1 - 8x}$,   (ii) $G = \dfrac{2}{1 + 7x}$,

(iii) $G = \dfrac{1}{1 - 8x} + \dfrac{2}{1 + 7x}$,   (iv) $G = \dfrac{3 - 9x}{1 - x - 56x^2}$

17. What sequence has $5/(1 - 2x) + 4/(1 + 3x)$ as its generating function?

18. What sequence has $3/(1 + 4x) - 2/(1 - 5x)$ as its generating function?

19. Let $F_0, F_1, \ldots$ be the Fibonacci Sequence 0, 1, 1, 2, 3, 5, $\ldots$ and $V = F_0 + F_1 x + F_2 x^2 + \cdots + F_n x^n + \cdots$.
  (i) Show that $(1 - x - x^2)V$ is a polynomial.
  (ii) Express V as a quotient of polynomials; that is, give the generating function for the Fibonacci Sequence.

20. Let F_n be the nth Fibonacci Number and let $G_n = F_{2n}$. Let

$$W = G_0 + G_1 x + G_2 x^2 + \cdots = F_0 + F_2 x + F_4 x^2 + \cdots.$$

  Accept as given that $G_n - 3G_{n-1} + G_{n-2} = 0$ for $n = 2, 3, \ldots$.
  (i) Show that $(1 - 3x + x^2)W$ is a polynomial.
  (ii) Find the generating function for the sequence $G_0, G_1, \ldots$.

21. Find the generating function for the arithmetic progression $a_0, a_1, \ldots$ with $a_n = 4n + 1$, that is, for 1, 5, 9, 13, $\ldots$, $4n + 1, \ldots$.

22. Find the generating function for the arithmetic progression 3, 10, 17, 24, $\ldots$, $7n + 3, \ldots$.

23. Let $G = a + (a + d)x + (a + 2d)x^2 + \cdots + (a + nd)x^n + \cdots$. Show that:
  (i) $(1 - x)G = a + dx + dx^2 + \cdots + dx^n + \cdots$.

  (ii) $(1 - x)^2 G = a + (d - a)x$.   (iii) $G = \dfrac{a + (d - a)x}{(1 - x)^2}$.

24. In each of the following parts, find the arithmetic progression that has the given x-fraction as its generating function.

  (a) $\dfrac{1 + 5x}{(1 - x)^2}$.   [*Hint*: Use Problem 23(iii).]

  (b) $\dfrac{3 - 4x}{(1 - x)^2}$.

25. Let G be the generating series for a sequence $g_0, g_1, \ldots, g_n, \ldots$. What sequence has $x^2 G$ as its generating series?

26. Do Problem 25 with $x^2 G$ replaced by $x^3 G$.

27. Let $G = 1 + 2x^2 + 3x^4 + 4x^6 + \cdots + (n + 1)x^{2n} + \cdots$. Find the following series.
  (i) $(1 - x^2)G$.   (ii) $(1 - x^2)^2 G$.

28. What is the generating function for the sequence 1, 0, 2, 0, 3, 0, 4, 0, $\ldots$?

29. Let $A = 1 - x^3$ and $B = 1 + x^3 + x^6 + \cdots + x^{3n} + \cdots$.
  (i) Find AB.
  (ii) Find the generating function for the sequence 1, 0, 0, 1, 0, 0, 1, 0, 0, $\ldots$.

30. Find the generating function for each of the following sequences.
  (i) 1, 0, 1, 0, 1, 0, $\ldots$;   (ii) 0, -1, 0, -1, 0, -1, $\ldots$;
  (iii) 1, -1, 1, -1, 1, -1, $\ldots$.

31. Let $u_n = (n + 1)^2$ and $U = \sum_{n=0}^{\infty} u_n x^n = 1 + 4x + \cdots + (n + 1)^2 x^n + \cdots$.
(i) Show that $u_n - 3u_{n-1} + 3u_{n-2} - u_{n-3} = 0$.
(ii) Show that $(1 - 3x + 3x^2 - x^3)U$ is a polynomial.
(iii) Find the generating function for the sequence $u_0, u_1, \ldots$.

32. Let $u_n = (n + 1)^3$ and $U = u_0 + u_1 x + u_2 x^2 + \cdots = 1 + 8x + 27x^2 + \cdots + (n + 1)^3 x^n + \cdots$.
(i) Show that $(1 - x)^4 U$ is a polynomial A, and find A.
(ii) Find the generating function for $u_0, u_1, u_2, \ldots$.

33. Let $C = 1 + 3x + 6x^2 + 10x^3 + \cdots + \binom{n+2}{2}x^n + \cdots$ be the generating series for the sequence $\binom{2}{2}, \binom{3}{2}, \binom{4}{2}, \ldots$ of binomial coefficients. Use Theorem 1 ("Differencing") to show the following.
(i) $(1 - x)C = 1 + 2x + 3x^2 + 4x^3 + \cdots + (n + 1)x^n + \cdots$.
(ii) $(1 - x)^2 C = 1 + x + x^2 + \cdots + x^n + \cdots$.
(iii) $(1 - x)^3 C = 1$ and so $C = 1/(1 - x)^3 = (1 - x)^{-3}$.

34. Let $D = 1 + 4x + 10x^2 + 20x^3 + \cdots + \binom{n+3}{3}x^n + \cdots$ be the generating series for the sequence $\binom{3}{3}, \binom{4}{3}, \binom{5}{3}, \ldots$.
(i) Show that $(1 - x)D = C$, where C is as in Problem 33.
(ii) Express D as a quotient of polynomials.

35. Find the generating function (that is, quotient of polynomials) for each of the following sequences.
(i) $\binom{4}{4}, \binom{5}{4}, \binom{6}{4}, \ldots, \binom{n+4}{4}, \ldots$
(ii) $\binom{5}{5}, \binom{6}{5}, \binom{7}{5}, \ldots, \binom{n+5}{5}, \ldots$
(iii) $\binom{6}{6}, \binom{7}{6}, \binom{8}{6}, \ldots, \binom{n+6}{6}, \ldots$

36. Example 4 and Problem 33 tell us that
$$(1 - x)^{-2} = 1 + 2x + 3x^2 + \cdots + (n + 1)x^n + \cdots,$$
$$(1 - x)^{-3} = 1 + 3x + 6x^2 + \cdots + \binom{n + 2}{2}x^n + \cdots.$$
Use these and Problem 35(i) to show (as promised in Example 2) that
$$\binom{n + 2}{2} + 2\binom{n + 1}{2} + 3\binom{n}{2} + \cdots + (n + 1)\binom{2}{2} = \binom{n + 4}{4}.$$

37. Let $b_n = \sum_{k=1}^{n+1} k^2$. Note that $b_0 = 1, b_1 = 1 + 4 = 5$, and $b_2 = 1 + 4 + 9 = 14$. Use Theorem 3 ("Generating Series for Partial Sums") and the formula
$$\frac{1 + x}{(1 - x)^3} = 1 + 4x + 9x^2 + \cdots + (n + 1)^2 x^n + \cdots$$
resulting from Problem 31 to find the generating function for the sequence $b_0, b_1, \ldots$.

38. Let $a_n = \sum_{k=1}^{n+1} k^3$. Use Theorem 3 ("Generating Series for Partial Sums") and the formula

$$\frac{1 + 4x + x^2}{(1-x)^4} = 1 + 8x + 27x^2 + \cdots + (n+1)^3 x^n + \cdots$$

resulting from Problem 32 to find the generating function for a_0, a_1, $a_2, \ldots$.

39. Let $x/(1 - 2x - x^2)$ be the generating function for a sequence p_0, p_1, $p_2, \ldots$; that is, let

$$(1 - 2x - x^2)(p_0 + p_1 x + p_2 x^2 + \cdots) = x.$$

(i) Find p_0 and p_1. (*Hint*: Multiply out and equate coefficients of like powers.)

(ii) Find integers c and d such that $p_n - cp_{n-1} - dp_{n-2} = 0$, that is, such that $p_n = cp_{n-1} + dp_{n-2}$ for $n = 2, 3, \ldots$.

(iii) Find p_2, p_3, p_4, and p_5.

40. Let $1/(1 - x + x^2)$ be the generating function for q_0, $q_1, \ldots$; that is, let

$$(1 - x + x^2)(q_0 + q_1 x + q_2 x^2 + \cdots) = 1.$$

(i) Find q_0 and q_1.

(ii) Find a and b such that $q_n - aq_{n-1} - bq_{n-2} = 0$ for $n = 2, 3, \ldots$.

(iii) Use Part (ii) to find q_2, q_3, q_4, q_5, q_6, and q_7.

41. Prove by mathematical induction on m that $(1 - x)^{-m-1}$ is the generating function for the sequence

$$\binom{m}{m}, \binom{m+1}{m}, \binom{m+2}{m}, \ldots, \binom{m+n}{m}, \ldots.$$

42. Find real numbers a, b, r, and s such that $a/(1 - rx) + b/(1 - sx)$ is the generating function for the Fibonacci Sequence $0, 1, 1, \ldots, F_n, \ldots$.

43. Let $A = 1 + 2x + 3x^2 + \cdots + (n+1)x^n + \cdots$. Explain why:

(i) $A^2 = (1 - x)^{-4} = \sum_{n=0}^{\infty} \binom{n+3}{3} x^n$.

(ii) $A^2 = b_0 + b_1 x + b_2 x^2 + \cdots + b_n x^n + \cdots$ with

$$b_n = 1 \cdot (n+1) + 2n + 3(n-1) + 4(n-2) + \cdots + (n+1) \cdot 1$$

$$= \sum_{k=0}^{n} (k+1)(n+1-k).$$

(iii) $b_n = \binom{n+3}{3}$ for all n in $N = \{0, 1, \ldots\}$.

44.   Show that:

(a) $\displaystyle\sum_{k=0}^{n} \binom{k+2}{2}\binom{n+2-k}{2} = \binom{n+5}{5}$ for all n in N.

(b) $\displaystyle\sum_{k=0}^{n} \binom{k+2}{2}\binom{n+3-k}{3} = \binom{n+6}{6}$ for all n in N.

9.2

SOME FIRST AND SECOND ORDER HOMOGENEOUS LINEAR RECURSIONS

A ***dth order recursion*** for a sequence $u_0, u_1, \ldots$ is a rule $u_n = f(u_{n-1}, u_{n-2}, \ldots, u_{n-d})$ for finding u_n when the d terms preceding it are known.

Example 1   If a sequence $u_0, u_1, \ldots$ satisfies the first order recursion

$u_n = 5u_{n-1}$ for $n \in Z^+ = \{1, 2, \ldots\}$,

then

$u_1 = 5u_0,$
$u_2 = 5u_1 = 5(5u_0) = 5^2 u_0,$
$u_3 = 5u_2 = 5(5^2 u_0) = 5^3 u_0,$

and one can easily prove by mathematical induction that $u_n = 5^n u_0$. Clearly, this recursion for $u_0, u_1, \ldots$ states that the sequence is the geometric progression with u_0 as initial term and with 5 as the constant ratio. A sequence satisfying this first order recursion can have any number as its initial term u_0 and then all other terms are determined uniquely by the recursion.   □

Example 2   If a sequence $u_0, u_1, \ldots$ satisfies the first order recursion $u_n = nu_{n-1}$, then

$u_1 = 1 \cdot u_0 = u_0,$
$u_2 = 2u_1 = 2u_0,$
$u_3 = 3u_2 = 3 \cdot 2u_0 = 6u_0,$

and it follows from the inductive definition of the factorials (Definition 1) in Section 4.1 that $u_n = n!u_0$. We note that the initial term u_0 of a sequence satisfying this first order recursion can be any number and then all the other terms are determined uniquely by the recursion. The sequence with $u_0 = 1$ that satisfies this recursion is the sequence $0!, 1!, 2!, \ldots, n!, \ldots$ of factorials.   □

Example 3   If a sequence $u_0, u_1, \ldots$ satisfies the second order recursion $u_n = u_{n-1} + u_{n-2}$, then

$$u_2 = u_1 + u_0,$$
$$u_3 = u_2 + u_1 = (u_1 + u_0) + u_1 = 2u_1 + u_0,$$
$$u_4 = u_3 + u_2 = (2u_1 + u_0) + (u_1 + u_0) = 3u_1 + 2u_0,$$
$$u_5 = u_4 + u_3 = (3u_1 + 2u_0) + (2u_1 + u_0) = 5u_1 + 3u_0,$$

and one can prove by mathematical induction that

$$u_n = F_n u_1 + F_{n-1} u_0 \qquad \text{for } n \in \{2, 3, \ldots\},$$

where $F_0, F_1, \ldots$ is the Fibonacci Sequence. We note that the two initial terms u_0 and u_1 of a sequence satisfying this second order recursion can be any numbers and then all the other terms are determined uniquely by the recursion. The specific solution to this recursion with $u_0 = 0$ and $u_1 = 1$ is $u_n = F_n$—that is, the Fibonacci Sequence 0, 1, 1, 2, 3, 5, . . . ; and the specific solution with $u_0 = 2$ and $u_1 = 1$ is the Lucas Sequence 2, 1, 3, 4, 7, 11, ...   □

Example 4   Here, let $u_0, u_1, \ldots$ satisfy the first order recursion

$$u_n = u_{n-1}(u_{n-1} - 1) + 1 \qquad \text{for } n \in \mathbf{Z}^+ = \{1, 2, \ldots\}$$

and the initial condition $u_0 = 2$. Then

$$u_1 = u_0(u_0 - 1) + 1 = 2(2 - 1) + 1 = 3,$$
$$u_2 = u_1(u_1 - 1) + 1 = 3(3 - 1) + 1 = 7,$$
$$u_3 = u_2(u_2 - 1) + 1 = 7(7 - 1) + 1 = 43.$$

The number of terms we can calculate in this manner is limited only by our willingness and ability to expend the necessary effort. No simple formula is known that gives u_n directly as a function of n. This sequence has some interesting properties, such as the fact that, of all the sums of reciprocals of $n + 1$ distinct positive integers, the sum

$$\frac{1}{u_0} + \frac{1}{u_1} + \cdots + \frac{1}{u_n}$$

comes closest to 1 without equaling 1. For example,

$$\frac{1}{2} + \frac{1}{3} + \frac{1}{7} + \frac{1}{43} = \frac{1805}{1806}$$

is closer to 1 than any other sum of reciprocals of four distinct positive integers.   □

In the remainder of this chapter, we will show how to *solve* certain types of recursions, that is, how to get an explicit formula for the general term u_n as a function of n. When the recursion is of the dth order, the explicit formula will involve d arbitrary constants. We will also show how these constants can be determined specifically when the initial terms $u_0, u_1, \ldots, u_{d-1}$ are given.

First we consider recursions of the type

$$u_n - ru_{n-1} = 0 \qquad \text{for } n \in \mathbf{Z}^+ = \{1, 2, \ldots\}, \tag{1}$$

where r is a nonzero constant. Such a relationship is called a ***first order homogeneous linear recursion with constant coefficients***. (This is abbreviated as first order H.L.R.W.C.C.)

Of the recursions in Examples 1, 2, 3, and 4, only that of Example 1 is a first order H.L.R.W.C.C.; it is the special case of Display (1) with $r = 5$. The first order recursion $u_n = nu_{n-1}$ of Example 2 is not of this type, since the coefficient n of u_{n-1} is not a constant. The first order recursion $u_n = u_{n-1}(u_{n-1} - 1) + 1$ of Example 4 also is not an H.L.R.W.C.C., since $u_{n-1}(u_{n-1} - 1) + 1$ is not a constant times u_{n-1}.

TYPE I   **FIRST ORDER H.L.R.W.C.C.**

Here we solve the first order homogeneous linear recursion with constant coefficient

$$u_n - ru_{n-1} = 0 \qquad \text{for } n \in \mathbf{Z}^+, r \text{ constant.}$$

We rewrite this as $u_n = ru_{n-1}$ and replace n with 1, 2, 3, respectively. Then we have:

$$u_1 = ru_0,$$
$$u_2 = ru_1 = r(ru_0) = r^2u_0,$$
$$u_3 = ru_2 = r(r^2u_0) = r^3u_0.$$

These suggest that the term u_n of this geometric progression is given by $u_n = r^nu_0$. This is easily proved by mathematical induction. (Problem 22 of Section 4.2 requested a proof of this result in different notation.)

DEFINITION 1   **CLOSED-FORM SOLUTIONS OF FIRST ORDER H.L.R.W.C.C.**

For the recursion $u_n - ru_{n-1} = 0$ with r constant, the formula $u_n = r^nu_0$ is called the ***closed-form*** (or ***explicit***) ***solution***. When u_0 is considered as an arbitrary constant k, the formula $u_n = r^nk$ is also called the ***general solution*** to the recursion. If u_0 is given, then $u_n = r^nu_0$ is the ***specific solution*** to the recursion for the given initial condition.

We next apply the closed-form solution for a first order H.L.R.W.C.C. to a compound-interest problem.

Example 5 Let $10000 be deposited in a savings account that has an annual interest rate of 10.8%, with the interest compounded and credited monthly. Let P_0 be the $10000 deposit and P_n be the balance in the account after the nth month's interest is credited. We assume that no withdrawals are made from the account and seek the closed form for P_n.

The monthly interest rate is $\frac{1}{12}$ of the annual rate; that is, the monthly interest rate is

$$\frac{10.8\%}{12} = \frac{.108}{12} = .009.$$

The interest for the nth month is .009 times the previous balance P_{n-1}, that is, $.009P_{n-1}$. This has to be added to the previous balance to get the new balance. Hence $P_n = P_{n-1} + .009P_{n-1} = 1.009P_{n-1}$. The recursion

$$P_n = 1.009P_{n-1} \qquad \text{for } n \in \{1, 2, \ldots\}$$

is a first order H.L.R.W.C.C. The closed-form solution is

$$P_n = 1.009^n P_0 \qquad \text{for } n \in N = \{0, 1, \ldots\},$$

and the specific solution with $P_0 = 10000$ is

$$P_n = 10000(1.009^n) \qquad \text{for } n \in N.$$

In the next section, we will show how to solve variations of this problem in which the depositor withdraws a fixed amount after the crediting of interest for each period. $\qquad\square$

Example 6 How much does one have to deposit in a savings account paying an annual rate of 12% compounded quarterly in order to have a balance of $15000 after 5 years? The quarterly interest rate is $12\%/4 = .12/4 = .03$. The balance P_n after n quarters therefore is $1.03^n P_0$. Since 5 years is 20 quarters, we let $n = 20$ in the formula $P_n = 1.03^n P_0$ and seek the amount P_0 such that

$$\$15000 = P_{20} = 1.03^{20} P_0.$$

With the help of a calculator or a compound interest table, we find that

$$P_0 = \frac{\$15000}{1.03^{20}} = \frac{\$15000}{1.806111} = \$8305.14. \qquad\square$$

TYPE II **SECOND ORDER H.L.R.W.C.C.**

Next we show how to solve recursions of the form

$$u_n + bu_{n-1} + cu_{n-2} = 0 \qquad \text{for } n \in \{2, 3, \ldots\}, \tag{2}$$

with b and c constants and $c \neq 0$. Such a recursion is called a *second order homogeneous linear recursion with constant coefficients*. (This is abbreviated as second order H.L.R.W.C.C.) If the restriction $c \neq 0$ is not met, these recursions become first order recursions $u_n + bu_{n-1} = 0$ (provided that $b \neq 0$).

The Fibonacci recursion $u_n = u_{n-1} + u_{n-2}$ can be rewritten as $u_n - u_{n-1} - u_{n-2} = 0$; it then is the special case of the recursion in Display (2) with $b = -1 = c$.

We find it helpful in solving a recursion of the type in Display (2) to introduce the generating series

$$G = u_0 + u_1 x + u_2 x^2 + \cdots + u_n x^n + \cdots$$

for the sequence $u_0, u_1, \ldots$. Then we use the recursion to express G as an x-fraction, that is, a quotient of polynomials, as follows: We multiply G by the polynomial $B = 1 + bx + cx^2$ whose coefficients 1, b, and c are the coefficients in the recursion. The format for this multiplication is that used in Example 9 of Section 9.1.

$$
\begin{array}{llll}
G = u_0 + & u_1 x + & u_2 x^2 + \cdots + & u_n x^n + \cdots \\
bxG = & bu_0 x + & bu_1 x^2 + \cdots + & bu_{n-1} x^n + \cdots \\
cx^2 G = & & cu_0 x^2 + \cdots + & cu_{n-2} x^n + \cdots \\
\hline
\end{array}
$$

$$(1 + bx + cx^2)G = u_0 + (u_1 + bu_0)x + (u_2 + bu_1 + cu_0)x^2 + \cdots + (u_n + bu_{n-1} + cu_{n-2})x^n + \cdots \quad (3)$$

Since the sequence $u_0, u_1, \ldots$ satisfies the recursion $u_n + bu_{n-1} + cu_{n-2} = 0$, the coefficients of $x^2, x^3, \ldots, x^n, \ldots$ in Display (3) are all 0. Thus

$$(1 + bx + cx^2)G = u_0 + (u_1 + bu_0)x$$

and hence the generating function is the x-fraction

$$G = \frac{u_0 + (u_1 + bu_0)x}{1 + bx + cx^2}. \quad (4)$$

The denominator of this x-fraction and a related quadratic polynomial play important roles in the algorithm for finding u_n as an explicit function of n. To aid in this process, we introduce some terminology.

DEFINITION 2   **RECURSION POLYNOMIAL, CHARACTERISTIC POLYNOMIAL**

The *recursion polynomial* for the second order H.L.R.W.C.C. $u_n + bu_{n-1} + cu_{n-2} = 0$ is $B(x) = 1 + bx + cx^2$. The *characteristic polynomial* for this recursion is $K(x) = x^2 + bx + c$. The roots

$$\frac{-b \pm \sqrt{b^2 - 4c}}{2}$$

of the *characteristic equation* $K(x) = 0$ are the *characteristic roots* r and s for the recursion.

We note that the characteristic roots r and s can be found by factoring the characteristic polynomial in the form

$$x^2 + bx + c = (x - r)(x - s)$$

or by factoring the recursion polynomial in the form

$$1 + bx + cx^2 = (1 - rx)(1 - sx).$$

We now break up the type II recursions

$$u_n + bu_{n-1} + cu_{n-2} = 0$$

into two subcases. Case IIA deals with such recursions having distinct characteristic roots r and s, that is, the case with $b^2 - 4c \neq 0$. Case IIB treats the second order H.L.R.W.C.C. having a multiple characteristic root $r = -b/2$, that is, the case with $b^2 - 4c = 0$.

CASE IIA   **DISTINCT CHARACTERISTIC ROOTS**

Because of the importance of the technique we are about to present, we will illustrate the entire theoretical process in Example 7, then state and prove the solution formula for second order H.L.R.W.C.C. having distinct characteristic roots in Theorem 1, and after that show in Example 8 how this theorem can be used to solve such a recursion.

Example 7   Let $u_0, u_1, \ldots$ satisfy the recursion

$$u_n - u_{n-1} - 12u_{n-2} = 0 \qquad \text{for } n \in \{2, 3, \ldots\} \tag{5}$$

and the initial conditions $u_0 = 3$ and $u_1 = 26$. We seek an explicit formula for u_n. The recursion polynomial here is

$$B = 1 - x - 12x^2 = (1 - 4x)(1 + 3x)$$

and the characteristic polynomial is

$$K = x^2 - x - 12 = (x - 4)(x + 3).$$

Thus the recursion has distinct characteristic roots $r = 4$ and $s = -3$. Let

$$G = \sum_{n=0}^{\infty} u_n x^n = 3 + 26x + u_2 x^2 + u_3 x^3 + \cdots + u_n x^n + \cdots$$

be the generating series for the sequence $u_0, u_1, \ldots$. Then

$$
\begin{aligned}
BG = (1 - x - 12x^2)G &= (1 - x - 12x^2)(3 + 26x + u_2 x^2 + \cdots) \\
&= 3 + (26 - 3)x + (u_2 - u_1 - 12u_0)x^2 + \cdots \\
&\quad + (u_n - u_{n-1} - 12u_{n-2})x^n + \cdots.
\end{aligned}
$$

The recursion in Display (5) implies that the coefficients of $x^2, x^3, \ldots$ are all 0. Hence

$$BG = 3 + 23x.$$

Thus

$$G = \frac{3 + 23x}{B} = \frac{3 + 23x}{1 - x - 12x^2} = \frac{3 + 23x}{(1 - 4x)(1 + 3x)}.$$

Since the characteristic roots $r = 4$ and $s = -3$ are unequal, Lemma 2 ("Distinct Factors") of Section 8.3 tells us that there is a partial-fractions decomposition

$$G = \frac{3 + 23x}{(1 - 4x)(1 + 3x)} = \frac{h}{1 - 4x} + \frac{k}{1 + 3x}, \tag{6}$$

where h and k are constants. Clearing fractions, we have

$$3 + 23x = h(1 + 3x) + k(1 - 4x). \tag{7}$$

In this, we let $x = \frac{1}{4}$ and get

$$3 + \frac{23}{4} = h\left(1 + \frac{3}{4}\right) + k\left(1 - \frac{4}{4}\right) = \frac{7}{4}h + 0 \cdot k.$$

Hence $7h/4 = 35/4$, $7h = 35$, and $h = 5$. Similarly, we let $x = -\frac{1}{3}$ in (7) and have

$$3 - \frac{23}{3} = h\left(1 - \frac{3}{3}\right) + k\left(1 + \frac{4}{3}\right) = 0 \cdot h + \frac{7}{3}k.$$

Thus $7k/3 = (9 - 23)/3$, $7k = -14$, and $k = -2$. Now we substitute $h = 5$ and $k = -2$ in Display (6) and see that

$$G = \frac{5}{1 - 4x} - \frac{2}{1 + 3x}. \tag{8}$$

By Theorem 2(a) ("Generating Functions Related to Geometric Progressions") of Section 9.1, we have

$$\frac{5}{1 - 4x} = 5 + 5 \cdot 4x + 5 \cdot 4^2 x^2 + \cdots + 5 \cdot 4^n x^n + \cdots$$

$$\frac{-2}{1 + 3x} = -2 - 2(-3)x - 2(-3)^2 x^2 - \cdots - 2(-3)^n x^n - \cdots.$$

We add corresponding sides of these equations and use the formula of Display (8); this gives us

$$G = \sum_{n=0}^{\infty} u_n x^n = 3 + 26x + \cdots + [5 \cdot 4^n - 2(-3)^n]x^n + \cdots.$$

By equating coefficients of x^n on both sides, we get the specific solution

$$u_n = 5 \cdot 4^n - 2(-3)^n$$

for the given recursion and initial conditions. $\square$

Example 7 illustrates the following result.

THEOREM 1

DISTINCT CHARACTERISTIC ROOTS

Let $u_0, u_1, \ldots$ satisfy $u_n + bu_{n-1} + cu_{n-2} = 0$ for $n \in \{2, 3, \ldots\}$, with b and c constants and $c \neq 0$. Let $1 + bx + cx^2 = (1 - rx)(1 - sx)$, with $r \neq s$. Then for each n in $N = \{0, 1, \ldots\}$,

$$u_n = hr^n + ks^n, \qquad \text{with } h \text{ and } k \text{ constants.} \tag{9}$$

If the initial terms u_0 and u_1 are known, then

$$u_n = \frac{u_1 - u_0 s}{r - s} r^n + \frac{u_1 - u_0 r}{s - r} s^n. \tag{10}$$

PROOF

Let G be the generating series for $u_0, u_1, \ldots$. Also, let $e = u_0$ and $f = u_1 + bu_0$. We have seen in Display (4) above that

$$G = \frac{u_0 + (u_1 + bu_0)x}{1 + bx + cx^2} = \frac{e + fx}{(1 - rx)(1 - sx)}.$$

Then Lemma 2 ("Distinct Factors") of Section 8.3 tells us that G has a partial-fractions decomposition

$$G = \frac{h}{1 - rx} + \frac{k}{1 - sx}. \tag{11}$$

We replace each term of this equation by its generating series [with the help of Theorem 2(a), "Generating Functions Related to Geometric Progressions," of Section 9.1] and get

$$u_0 + u_1 x + \cdots + u_n x^n + \cdots = (h + hrx + \cdots + hr^n x^n + \cdots)$$
$$+ (k + ksx + \cdots + ks^n x^n + \cdots).$$

Equating coefficients of x^n gives us the formula

$$u_n = hr^n + ks^n.$$

If u_0 and u_1 are known, we let $n = 0$ in this formula and get

$$u_0 = h + k.$$

Hence $k = u_0 - h$. Making this substitution and letting $n = 1$ in the formula, we have

$$u_1 = hr + (u_0 - h)s = h(r - s) + u_0 s.$$

This implies that $h(r - s) = u_1 - u_0 s$, and so $h = (u_1 - u_0 s)/(r - s)$. Then

$$k = u_0 - h = u_0 - \frac{u_1 - u_0 s}{r - s} = \frac{u_0 r - u_0 s - u_1 + u_0 s}{r - s}$$

$$= \frac{u_0 r - u_1}{r - s} = \frac{u_1 - u_0 r}{s - r}.$$

Substituting $h = (u_1 - u_0 s)/(r - s)$ and $k = (u_1 - u_0 r)/(s - r)$ in Display (11) gives us the specific solution stated in Display (10). □

DEFINITION 3   **CLOSED-FORM SOLUTIONS WHEN $r \neq s$**

For the recursion $u_n + b u_{n-1} + c u_{n-2} = 0$ with b and c constant, $c \neq 0$, and having distinct characteristic roots r and s, the formula $u_n = hr^n + ks^n$ is the **closed-form solution.** When h and k are considered to be arbitrary constants, the closed-form solution is also called the **general solution.** When the initial terms u_0 and u_1 are given, then

$$u_n = \frac{u_1 - u_0 s}{r - s} r^n + \frac{u_1 - u_0 r}{s - r} s^n$$

is the **specific solution** to the recursion for the given initial conditions.

Example 8   Let us consider sequences $u_0, u_1, \ldots$ that satisfy the second order H.L.R.W.C.C.

$$u_n - 2u_{n-1} - 15u_{n-2} = 0 \quad \text{for } n \in \{2, 3, \ldots\}.$$

The characteristic polynomial for this recursion (with $b = -2$ and $c = -15$) is

$$x^2 - 2x - 15 = (x - 5)(x + 3).$$

Thus the characteristic roots are $r = 5$ and $s = -3$. Since $5 \neq -3$, the general solution is

$$u_n = 5^n h + (-3)^n k,$$

where h and k are arbitrary constants. There are infinitely many sequences satisfying this recursion since we can replace h and k by any numbers. However, when we are given the values of the initial terms u_0 and u_1, then we can determine h and k specifically and thus get a unique solution to the problem. To illustrate this, we find the specific solution satisfying the initial conditions

$$u_0 = 10 \quad \text{and} \quad u_1 = 2.$$

As above, we have the closed form

$$u_n = 5^n h + (-3)^n k. \tag{12}$$

Here h and k are not arbitrary constants but instead are constants to be determined from the initial conditions, as follows: We replace n first by 0 and then by 1 in Equation (12) and get

$$10 = h + k,$$
$$2 = 5h - 3k.$$

Multiplying the first of these equations through by 3 and adding to the second equation, we get $32 = 8h$, or $h = 4$. Then $k = 10 - h = 10 - 4 = 6$. Thus the specific solution for the given initial conditions is

$$u_n = 4 \cdot 5^n + 6(-3)^n.$$

As a check, we calculate u_2 both from the closed form and from the recursion, as follows:

$$u_2 = 4 \cdot 5^2 + 6(-3)^2 = 4 \cdot 25 + 6 \cdot 9 = 154,$$
$$u_2 = 2u_1 + 15u_0 = 2 \cdot 2 + 15 \cdot 10 = 154. \qquad \square$$

CASE IIB   **REPEATED CHARACTERISTIC ROOT**

As in Case IIA, let the sequence satisfy

$$u_n + bu_{n-1} + cu_{n-2} = 0 \qquad \text{for } n \in \{2, 3, \ldots\} \tag{13}$$

for some constants b and c with $c \neq 0$. Again the generating series $G = u_0 + u_1x + u_2x^2 + \cdots$ is expressible as the x-fraction

$$G = \frac{e + fx}{(1 - rx)(1 - sx)},$$

where r and s are the characteristic roots for Recursion (13). But in this case let $b^2 - 4c = 0$. Then the characteristic equation $x^2 + bx + c = 0$ has only one root; that is, $r = s = -b/2$. Hence

$$G = \frac{e + fx}{(1 - rx)^2}.$$

Then from Lemma 3 ("Square Denominator") of Section 8.3, we have

$$G = \frac{k_1}{1 - rx} + \frac{k_2}{(1 - rx)^2},$$

where k_1 and k_2 are constants. Theorem 2 ("Generating Functions Related to Geometric Progressions") of Section 9.1 tells us that $k_1/(1 - rx)$ and $k_2/(1 - rx)^2$ are the generating functions for the sequences

$$k_1, k_1r, k_1r^2, \ldots, k_1r^n, \ldots,$$
$$k_2, 2k_2r, 3k_2r^2, \ldots, (n + 1)k_2r^n, \ldots.$$

Then it follows from Lemma 1 ("Generating Series for a Sum of Sequences") of Section 9.1 that the sum G of these special x-fractions is the generating function for the sum of the sequences. This means that

$$u_n = k_1 r^n + (n + 1)k_2 r^n.$$

Letting $h_1 = k_1 + k_2$ and $h_2 = k_2$, we can rewrite this as

$$u_n = (h_1 + h_2 n)r^n. \tag{14}$$

Any replacement of h_1 and h_2 by numbers in Display (14) will give us a solution to Recursion (13). When the initial terms u_0 and u_1 are known, we find the specific solution for these initial conditions by letting $n = 0$ and $n = 1$ in Display (14) as follows:

$$u_0 = (h_1 + h_2 \cdot 0)r^0 = h_1,$$
$$u_1 = (h_1 + h_2 \cdot 1)r = (u_0 + h_2)r = u_0 r + h_2 r.$$

Then $h_2 r = u_1 - u_0 r$, and so $h_2 = (u_1/r) - u_0$. This gives us the specific solution

$$u_n = \left[u_0 + \left(\frac{u_1}{r} - u_0\right)n\right]r^n. \tag{15}$$

The formula in Display (15) is meaningless when $r = 0$ because one cannot divide by 0. However, the characteristic roots of a second order H.L.R.W.C.C. are nonzero, since

$$1 + bx + cx^2 = (1 - rx)(1 - sx) = 1 - (r + s)x + rsx^2$$

implies that $c = rs$ and we have assumed that $c \neq 0$. (When $c = 0$, the recursion is not second order.) We can now give the analogue of Definition 3 for the case in which $r = s = -b/2$.

DEFINITION 4   **CLOSED FORMS, REPEATED ROOT CASE**

The *closed-form solution* to the second order H.L.R.W.C.C. with r as a multiple characteristic root is

$$u_n = (h_1 + h_2 n)r^n.$$

When h_1 and h_2 are considered to be arbitrary constants, this is also called the *general solution*. If the initial terms u_0 and u_1 are given, then

$$u_n = \left[u_0 + \left(\frac{u_1}{r} - u_0\right)n\right]r^n$$

is the *specific solution* to the recursion for the given initial conditions.

Example 9   Here we solve the second order H.L.R.W.C.C.

$$u_n + 8u_{n-1} + 16u_{n-2} = 0 \qquad \text{for } n \in \{2, 3, \ldots\}.$$

The characteristic polynomial is

$$x^2 + 8x + 16 = (x + 4)^2.$$

Thus this is a case of equal characteristic roots $r = -4 = s$. (One can check that $r = s$ by noting that $b^2 - 4c = 8^2 - 4 \cdot 16 = 0$.) Hence the general solution is

$$u_n = (h_1 + h_2 n)(-4)^n \qquad \text{for } n \in N = \{0, 1, \ldots\}, \tag{16}$$

where h_1 and h_2 are arbitrary constants.

However, if we are given the initial conditions

$$u_0 = -3, \qquad u_1 = 4,$$

then we determine h_1 and h_2 specifically by letting $n = 0$ and $n = 1$ in Display (16), thus getting the simultaneous equations

$$-3 = h_1,$$
$$4 = (h_1 + h_2)(-4).$$

We replace h_1 by -3 in the second equation and solve for h_2:

$$4 = (-3 + h_2)(-4),$$
$$-1 = -3 + h_2,$$
$$h_2 = -1 + 3 = 2.$$

Replacing h_1 by -3 and h_2 by 2 in Display (16) gives us the specific solution

$$u_n = (-3 + 2n)(-4)^n$$

to the recursion for the given initial conditions. We check by getting u_2 both from this closed form and from the recursion, as follows:

$$u_2 = (-3 + 2 \cdot 2)(-4)^2 = 16,$$
$$u_2 = -8u_1 - 16u_0 = -8 \cdot 4 - 16(-3) = -32 + 48 = 16. \qquad \square$$

We now summarize the procedures for solving a second order homogeneous linear recursion

$$u_n + bu_{n-1} + cu_{n-2} = 0 \qquad \text{for } n \in \{2, 3, \ldots\}$$

with constant coefficients b and c and $c \neq 0$.

ALGORITHM 1   **CLOSED-FORM SOLUTION FOR SECOND ORDER H.L.R.W.C.C.**

(a) Solve the characteristic equation $x^2 + bx + c = 0$ for the characteristic roots r and s [or find r and s from the factorization $1 + bx + cx^2 = (1 - rx)(1 - sx)$].

(b) If $r \neq s$, the general solution is $u_n = hr^n + ks^n$, with h and k arbitrary constants. When u_0 and u_1 are given, use this formula with $n = 0$ and $n = 1$ to get

$$\begin{cases} h + k = u_0 \\ hr + ks = u_1. \end{cases}$$

Solve this system for h and k and use these values to write the specific solution to the recursion for the given initial conditions.

(c) If $r = s$, the general solution is $u_n = (h_1 + h_2 n)r^n$, with h_1 and h_2 arbitrary constants. When u_0 and u_1 are given, one determines the h_1 and h_2 for the specific solution to the recursion for the given initial conditions by letting n equal 0 and 1 and solving

$$\begin{cases} h_1 = u_0 \\ (h_1 + h_2)r = u_1. \end{cases}$$

PROBLEMS FOR SECTION 9.2

1.   (i) Write the closed-form general solution of the recursion $u_n + 1.03u_{n-1} = 0$.
(ii) Use $u_0 = 1000$ and the recursion to find u_1 and u_2.
(iii) Make the closed form of Part (i) specific using $u_0 = 1000$.
(iv) Check Part (ii) using the specific closed form of Part (iii).

2.   (i) Write the closed-form general solution of the recursion $u_n - 5u_{n-1} = 0$.
(ii) Use $u_0 = 2$ and the recursion to find u_1 and u_2.
(iii) Make the closed form of Part (i) specific using $u_0 = 2$.
(iv) Check Part (ii) using the specific closed form of Part (iii).

3.   Suppose that $5000 is deposited in a savings account crediting interest at an annual rate of 10% compounded each quarter (of a year). Find the closed form for the balance P_n after n quarters. (Assume that there are no withdrawals.)

4.   Repeat Problem 3, but with the annual interest rate now 12%.

5.   A savings account gives interest at an annual rate of 10.8% credited and compounded monthly. Find the amount of the opening deposit, given that the first month's interest is $72.

6. Assume that in Problem 5 the depositor withdraws \$72 immediately after *each month's* interest is credited. What is the balance P_n in the account just after the withdrawal for the nth month?

7. (i) Find the general solution of the recursion

$$u_n - \frac{3}{2} u_{n-1} = 0 \qquad \text{for } n \in \mathbf{Z}^+ = \{1, 2, \ldots\}.$$

(ii) Find the general solution of $2u_n - 3u_{n-1} = 0$ for $n \in \mathbf{Z}^+$.

8. Find the general solution of $5u_n + 4u_{n-1} = 0$ for $n \in \mathbf{Z}^+$.

9. Give the recursion polynomial $B(x)$ and the characteristic polynomial $K(x)$ for each of the following second order recursions $u_n + bu_{n-1} + cu_{n-2} = 0$.
(a) $u_n - 6u_{n-1} + 8u_{n-2} = 0.$ (b) $u_n + 14u_{n-1} + 49u_{n-2} = 0.$
(c) $u_n - 9u_{n-2} = 0.$ (Note that $b = 0$ and $c = -9$ here.)

10. Give the recursion polynomial $B(x)$ and characteristic polynomial $K(x)$ for each of the following.
(a) $u_n - 6u_{n-1} - 7u_{n-2} = 0.$ (b) $u_n - 12u_{n-1} + 36u_{n-2} = 0.$
(c) $u_n - 25u_{n-2} = 0.$

11. For each recursion in Problem 9, find the characteristic roots r and s and tell whether $r = s$ or $r \neq s$.

12. For each recursion in Problem 10, find the characteristic roots r and s and tell whether $r = s$ or $r \neq s$.

13. For each recursion in Problem 9, find the general solution. [That is, write u_n as $hr^n + ks^n$ when $r \neq s$ or as $(h_1 + h_2 n)r^n$ when $r = s$.]

14. Find the general solution for each recursion in Problem 10.

15. For the recursion $u_n - u_{n-1} - u_{n-2} = 0$, find the closed forms of:
(i) the general solution;
(ii) the specific solution with $u_0 = 0$ and $u_1 = 1$;
(iii) the specific solution with $u_0 = 2$ and $u_1 = 1$.
[The answers to (ii) and (iii) are called the **Binet Formulas** for the Fibonacci Numbers and Lucas Numbers, respectively.]

16. For the recursion $u_n - 2u_{n-1} - u_{n-2} = 0$, find the closed forms of:
(i) the general solution;
(ii) the specific solution with $u_0 = 0$ and $u_1 = 1$;
(iii) the specific solution with $u_0 = 2 = u_1$.

17. Let $u_n = h \cdot 5^n + k(-4)^n$ for $n \in \mathbf{N}$, with h and k constants.
(a) Given that $u_0 = 5$ and $u_1 = -2$, find h and k.
(b) Find the recursion $u_n + bu_{n-1} + cu_{n-2} = 0$ satisfied by the sequence $u_0, u_1, \ldots$.

18. Let $u_n = h \cdot 3^n + k(-1)^n$ for $n \in \mathbf{N}$, with h and k constants.
(a) Given that $u_0 = 1$ and $u_1 = 15$, find h and k.
(b) Find the second order H.L.R.W.C.C. satisfied by $u_0, u_1, \ldots$.

19. Let $u_n = (h_1 + h_2 n)(-3)^n$ for $n \in N$, with h_1 and h_2 constants.
(a) Given that $u_0 = 4$ and $u_1 = 6$, find h_1 and h_2.
(b) Find the second order H.L.R.W.C.C. satisfied by $u_0, u_1, \ldots$.

20. Let $u_n = (h_1 + h_2 n)4^n$ for $n \in N$, with h_1 and h_2 constants.
(a) Given that $u_0 = 5$ and $u_1 = 8$, find h_1 and h_2.
(b) Find the second order H.L.R.W.C.C. satisfied by $u_0, u_1, \ldots$.

21. Solve each recursion with initial conditions:
(a) $u_0 = 3$, $u_1 = 3$, $u_n - u_{n-1} - 20u_{n-2} = 0$ for $n \in \{2, 3, \ldots\}$.
(b) $u_0 = 5$, $u_1 = 8$, $u_n - 8u_{n-1} + 16u_{n-2} = 0$ for $n \in \{2, 3, \ldots\}$.

22. Solve each recursion with initial conditions:
(a) $u_0 = 4$, $u_1 = 6$, $u_n + 6u_{n-1} + 9u_{n-2} = 0$ for $n \in \{2, 3, \ldots\}$.
(b) $u_0 = 5$, $u_1 = -2$, $u_n + u_{n-1} - 20u_{n-2} = 0$ for $n \in \{2, 3, \ldots\}$.

23. Of the following recursions, which are satisfied by $u_n = \binom{n+2}{2}$?
(a) $u_n - u_{n-1} = n + 1$ for $n \in \{1, 2, \ldots\}$.
(b) $u_n - 2u_{n-1} + u_{n-2} = 1$ for $n \in \{2, 3, \ldots\}$.
(c) $u_n - 3u_{n-1} + 3u_{n-2} - u_{n-3} = 0$ for $n \in \{3, 4, \ldots\}$.
(d) $u_n = \dfrac{n+2}{n} u_{n-1}$ for $n \in \{1, 2, \ldots\}$.

24. Of the following recursions, which are satisfied by $u_n = \binom{n+3}{3}$?
(a) $u_n - u_{n-1} = \begin{pmatrix} n+2 \\ 2 \end{pmatrix}$ for $n \in \{1, 2, \ldots\}$.
(b) $u_n - 2u_{n-1} + u_{n-2} = n + 1$ for $n \in \{2, 3, \ldots\}$.
(c) $u_n - 3u_{n-1} + 3u_{n-2} - u_{n-3} = 1$ for $n \in \{3, 4, \ldots\}$.
(d) $u_n = \dfrac{n+3}{n} u_{n-1}$ for $n \in \{1, 2, \ldots\}$.

25. Let $u_0, u_1, \ldots$ satisfy $u_n - u_{n-1} + u_{n-2} = 0$ for $n \in \{2, 3, \ldots\}$. Show that:
(i) $u_n = \left(\dfrac{1 + \sqrt{3}i}{2}\right)^n h + \left(\dfrac{1 - \sqrt{3}i}{2}\right)^n k,$ with h and k constants.

(ii) If $u_0 = 0$ and $u_1 = 1$, then

$$u_n = \frac{1}{\sqrt{3}i}\left[\left(\frac{1 + \sqrt{3}i}{2}\right)^n - \left(\frac{1 - \sqrt{3}i}{2}\right)^n\right].$$

26. Let $u_0, u_1, \ldots$ satisfy $u_n - u_{n-1} + u_{n-2} = 0$ for $n \in \{2, 3, \ldots\}$.
(i) Show that $u_n = -u_{n-3}$ for $n \in \{3, 4, \ldots\}$.
(ii) Given that $u_0 = 0$ and $u_1 = 1$, tabulate u_n for $n = 2, 3, \ldots, 10$.

27. Let \$10 be deposited in an account giving interest at an annual rate of 10.95% compounded daily, that is, an interest rate of .03% ($=.0003$) per day.
(i) Find the interest for the first day. Round to the nearest cent.

(ii) How much interest will be credited for 90 days if *each day* interest is calculated, rounded to the nearest cent, and credited to the account?

(iii) Explain why the closed form for 90 days interest is $\$10(1.0003^{90} - 1)$.

(iv) Should the depositor prefer that the rounding be done only once, that is, only after 90 days? [Use the closed form of Part (iii) and the approximation $1.0003^{90} \approx 1.0273636$.]

28. As in Problem 27, let $\$10$ be deposited in an account giving interest at .03% per day. Explain why:

(i) the interest after 2 days is $\$10(1.0003^2 - 1) = \$10(1.00060009 - 1) = \$0.0060009$.

(ii) the depositor should prefer that rounding of the interest to the nearest cent take place every 2 days rather than every day.

29. Let $x_0, x_1, \ldots$ and $y_0, y_1, \ldots$ each satisfy the recursion

$$u_n + b(n)u_{n-1} + c(n)u_{n-2} = 0 \qquad \text{for } n \in \{2, 3, \ldots\}, \tag{R}$$

where $b(0), b(1), \ldots$ and $c(0), c(1), \ldots$ are known sequences. Show that the sequence $z_0, z_1, \ldots$ with $z_n = x_n + y_n$ for n in $N = \{0, 1, \ldots\}$ also satisfies the Recursion (R).

30. Repeat Problem 29, but here let $z_n = ex_n + fy_n$, where e and f are constants.

31. Let $u_0, u_1, \ldots$ satisfy the recursion

$$u_n - 3u_{n-1} + 3u_{n-2} - u_{n-3} = 0 \qquad \text{for } n \in \{3, 4, \ldots\}$$

and let

$$G = u_0 + u_1 x + u_2 x^2 + \cdots + u_n x^n + \cdots.$$

Explain why:

(i) $(1 - 3x + 3x^2 - x^3)G = u_0 + (u_1 - 3u_0)x + (u_2 - 3u_1 + 3u_0)x^2$.

(ii) $G = \dfrac{u_0 + (u_1 - 3u_0)x + (u_2 - 3u_1 + 3u_0)x^2}{(1 - x)^3}$.

(iii) there exist constants a, b, and c such that

$$G = \frac{a}{1 - x} + \frac{b}{(1 - x)^2} + \frac{c}{(1 - x)^3}.$$

(iv) $u_n = a + b(n + 1) + c\binom{n+2}{2}$, where a, b, c are as in Part (iii).

32. Let $u_0, u_1, \ldots$ satisfy $u_n - 2u_{n-1} + u_{n-2} = 5$ for $n \in \{2, 3, \ldots\}$.

(i) Show that the sequence also satisfies

$$u_n - 3u_{n-1} + 3u_{n-2} - u_{n-3} = 0 \qquad \text{for } n \in \{3, 4, \ldots\}.$$

(ii) Use Problem 31 to explain why there exist constants a, b, c such that $u_n = a + b(n + 1) + c\binom{n+2}{2}$.

*(iii) Show that $c = 5$ in Part (ii).

9.3

FIRST AND SECOND ORDER NONHOMOGENEOUS RECURSIONS

We next apply recursions to a variation of the compound-interest problems of Section 9.2. This will help us learn how to use the general solutions of the recursions studied in Section 9.2 as aids in solving associated recursions that are slightly more complicated.

Example 1   As in Example 5 of Section 9.2, let \$10000 be deposited in a savings account having an annual interest rate of 10.8% compounded monthly. But here let \$72 be withdrawn from the account each month immediately after the interest is credited. We let P_0 be the \$10000 opening deposit and let P_n be the balance in the account after both the crediting of the interest for the nth month and the withdrawal of the nth \$72. We seek an explicit formula for P_n.

The monthly interest rate is $\frac{1}{12}$ of the annual interest rate, that is, $10.8\%/12 = .108/12 = .009$. Hence the interest for the nth month is $.009P_{n-1}$. The balance after adding this interest to the old balance P_{n-1} and subtracting \$72 is

$$P_n = P_{n-1} + .009P_{n-1} - \$72 = 1.009P_{n-1} - \$72.$$

We drop the dollar sign and also rewrite this as the recursion

$$P_n - 1.009P_{n-1} = -72. \tag{1}$$

The initial term $P_0 = 10000$ and the recursion in Display (1) completely determine our desired sequence $P_0, P_1, \ldots$ since the recursion implies that

$$P_1 = 1.009P_0 - 72, \qquad P_2 = 1.009P_1 - 72 = 1.009(1.009P_0 - 72) - 72,$$

and so on. Our technique for finding an explicit formula for P_n involves thinking of the 10000 opening deposit as having been split into amounts A and B, which are used to open two accounts. Let A be the amount required to have 72 as the first month's interest. That is, A is found from the equation $.009A = 72$ to be $72/.009 = 8000$. Then $B = 10000 - 8000 = 2000$. If the withdrawal of 72 per month is made from the first account (the one with opening deposit of 8000), the balance A_n after the withdrawal of 72 for the nth month will be the constant 8000. There are no withdrawals from the other account; hence its balance B_n after n months satisfies the recursion $B_n = 1.009B_{n-1}$, which is equivalent to the first order homogeneous linear recursion

$$B_n - 1.009B_n = 0 \qquad \text{for } n \in \mathbf{Z}^+. \tag{2}$$

Hence, as in Example 5 of Section 9.2, we have the closed-form solution

$$B_n = B_0 \cdot 1.009^n = 2000(1.009^n).$$

A little reflection convinces us that $P_n = A_n + B_n$. Thus we have the desired explicit formula

$$P_n = 8000 + 2000(1.009^n). \qquad \square$$

We now embark on a study of sequences satisfying a pair of recursions related to each other as the recursions in Displays (1) and (2) are related. First we present some terminology.

FIRST ORDER LINEAR RECURSIONS

A *first order linear recursion* for a sequence $v_0, v_1, \ldots$ has the form

$$v_n + b(n)v_{n-1} = g(n) \qquad \text{for } n \in \mathbf{Z}^+, \tag{3}$$

where $b(1), b(2), \ldots$ and $g(1), g(2), \ldots$ are known sequences with $b(n) \neq 0$ for at least one n. If $g(n) = 0$ for all n in $\mathbf{Z}^+$, this recursion is *homogeneous*; otherwise it is *nonhomogeneous*. When the recursion in Display (3) is non-homogeneous, its *associated homogeneous recursion* is

$$u_n + b(n)u_{n-1} = 0 \qquad \text{for } n \in \mathbf{Z}^+. \tag{4}$$

LEMMA 1 **DIFFERENCE OF SOLUTIONS OF A NONHOMOGENEOUS LINEAR RECURSION**

Let each of the sequences $x_0, x_1, \ldots$ and $y_0, y_1, \ldots$ satisfy

$$v_n + b(n)v_{n-1} = g(n) \qquad \text{for } n \in \mathbf{Z}^+ \tag{5}$$

and let $z_n = x_n - y_n$ for $n \in \mathbf{N} = \{0, 1, \ldots\}$. Then $z_0, z_1, \ldots$ satisfies the associated homogeneous recursion

$$u_n + b(n)u_{n-1} = 0 \qquad \text{for } n \in \mathbf{Z}^+. \tag{6}$$

PROOF   For n in $\mathbf{Z}^+$, we are given that

$$x_n + b(n)x_{n-1} = g(n),$$
$$y_n + b(n)y_{n-1} = g(n).$$

We subtract and get

$$(x_n - y_n) + b(n)(x_{n-1} - y_{n-1}) = 0.$$

Since $x_n - y_n = z_n$ and $x_{n-1} - y_{n-1} = z_{n-1}$, this is the claimed $z_n + b(n)z_{n-1} = 0.$ $\square$

Example 2   Let us take another look at Example 1, this time having Lemma 1 available. The nonhomogeneous recursion we dealt with there was

$$v_n - 1.009v_{n-1} = -72; \tag{7}$$

and its associated homogeneous recursion is

$$u_n - 1.009u_{n-1} = 0. \tag{8}$$

We know all of the solutions of the first order H.L.R.W.C.C. in Display (8); they are of the form $u_n = 1.009^n k$, with k any constant. One solution to Recursion (7) is easy to find; it is the one with v_n constant. We find this solution by replacing each of v_n and v_{n-1} by a constant h in (7), thus getting

$$h - 1.009h = -72.$$

This leads to $-.009h = -72$, $h = 72/.009 = 8000$. Thus the sequence x_0, $x_1, \ldots$ with each $x_n = 8000$ satisfies Recursion (7). What we really want is the sequence $P_0, P_1, \ldots$ satisfying Recursion (7) and also having the initial condition $P_0 = 10000$. Lemma 1 tells us that the term-by-term difference

$$P_0 - 8000, P_1 - 8000, \ldots, P_n - 8000, \ldots$$

of solutions of Recursion (7) satisfies the associated homogeneous Recursion (8). Since $u_n = 1.009^n k$, with k some constant, for every solution to Recursion (8), this means that

$$P_n - 8000 = 1.009^n k.$$

Adding 8000 to both sides, we get

$$P_n = 8000 + 1.009^n k. \tag{9}$$

To determine the constant k, we use the initial condition $P_0 = 10000$. That is, we let $n = 0$ in Display (9) and have

$$P_0 = 10000 = 8000 + k.$$

This gives us $k = 10000 - 8000 = 2000$. Substituting $k = 2000$ in Display (9), we see again that the specific solution to our compound-interest problem with monthly withdrawals of 72 has the closed form $P_n = 8000 + 1.009^n \cdot 2000$. $\quad\square$

A first order nonhomogeneous linear recursion has the form

$$v_n + b(n)v_{n-1} = g(n) \qquad \text{for } n \in \mathbf{Z}^+, \tag{10}$$

where $b(1), b(2), \ldots$ and $g(1), g(2), \ldots$ are given sequences. In this section, we show how to solve some special cases of such recursions. In all of these cases, $b(n)$ will be a constant $-r$; that is, the recursion has the form

$$v_n - rv_{n-1} = g(n) \qquad \text{for } n \in \mathbf{Z}^+. \tag{11}$$

The main reason why recursions of the type in Display (11) are easier to solve than those of the more general type in Display (10) is that we know that the associated homogeneous recursion

$$u_n - ru_{n-1} = 0 \qquad \text{for } n \in \mathbf{Z}^+$$

for Display (11) has $u_n = r^n k$, with k an arbitrary constant, as its general solution. Having this fact and Lemma 1, we merely need some *particular solution* $x_0, x_1, \ldots$ to the nonhomogeneous Recursion (11) and then have every solution to Recursion (11) expressible as

$$v_n = x_n + r^n k \qquad \text{for } n \in N = \{0, 1, \ldots\}.$$

This was the procedure used in Example 2; we prove it to be valid in the following result.

THEOREM 1   **COMPLETE SOLUTION FOR A FIRST ORDER NONHOMOGENEOUS LINEAR RECURSION**

If $x_0, x_1, \ldots$ is a particular solution to the first order nonhomogeneous linear recursion

$$v_n - rv_{n-1} = g(n) \qquad \text{for } n \in \mathbf{Z}^+, \tag{12}$$

with r constant, then every solution has the form

$$v_n = x_n + r^n k,$$

where k is an arbitrary constant.

PROOF   Let us think of $x_0, x_1, \ldots$ as a known solution to Recursion (12) and $v_0, v_1, \ldots$ as a sought solution, satisfying some given initial condition, to Recursion (12). Lemma 1 tells us that the term-by-term differences $u_0 = v_0 - x_0$, $u_1 = v_1 - x_1, \ldots$ satisfy the associated homogeneous recursion

$$u_n - ru_{n-1} = 0. \tag{13}$$

But we know that every solution to the first order H.L.R.W.C.C. in Display (13) has the form

$$u_n = r^n k, \qquad \text{with } k \text{ constant.}$$

This means that $v_n - x_n = r^n k$. Adding x_n to both sides gives us the claimed

$$v_n = x_n + r^n k, \qquad \text{with } k \text{ constant.} \qquad \square$$

COROLLARY   **SPECIFIC SOLUTION**

The specific solution to Recursion (12) with a given initial term v_0 is $v_n = x_n + (v_0 - x_0)r^n$.

The proof of the corollary is left to the reader as Problem 13 below.

DEFINITION 1   **GENERAL SOLUTION, SPECIFIC SOLUTION**

The *general solution* to the nonhomogeneous recursion

$$v_n - rv_{n-1} = g(n) \qquad \text{for } n \in \mathbf{Z}^+$$

is the solution $v_n = x_n + r^n k$, with $x_0, x_1, \ldots$ any particular solution and k an arbitrary constant, given in Theorem 1. The *specific solution* to this recursion with a given v_0 is $v_n = x_n + (v_0 - x_0)r^n$.

We next apply Theorem 1 for several special types of right-hand sides $g(n)$ of the recursion

$$v_n - rv_{n-1} = g(n).$$

CASE I   **CONSTANT RIGHT-HAND SIDE**

Here we show how to solve recursions

$$v_n - rv_{n-1} = g \qquad \text{for } n \in \mathbf{Z}^+,$$

in which r and g are constants. There are two subcases: the first is the one with $r = 1$ and the other has $r \neq 1$. The following lemmas take care of these subcases.

LEMMA 2   **CASE OF $r = 1$**

The solution to the recursion

$$v_n - v_{n-1} = g \qquad \text{for } n \in \mathbf{Z}^+ = \{1, 2, \ldots\},$$

with g constant, is $v_n = v_0 + ng$.

PROOF   We use mathematical induction on n. Clearly $v_0 = v_0 + 0 \cdot g$. This furnishes the basis step. Now we assume that $v_k = v_0 + kg$. Then the recursion helps us get

$$v_{k+1} = v_k + g = (v_0 + kg) + g = v_0 + (k+1)g.$$

Since $v_{k+1} = v_0 + (k+1)g$ is the claimed formula when $n = k + 1$, the inductive step is finished and the lemma is proved.   □

The formula in Lemma 2 applies to the problem of determining the amount v_n in a safe deposit box that originally contained v_0 dollars and to which g dollars are added each month for n months. (No interest is paid on funds in a safe deposit box. In fact, an annual fee usually is charged for rental of the box.)

LEMMA 3   **CASE OF $r \neq 1$**

The general solution to the recursion

$$v_n - rv_{n-1} = g \qquad \text{for } n \in \mathbf{Z}^+, \tag{14}$$

with r and g constants and $r \neq 1$, is

$$v_n = \frac{g}{1-r} + r^n k, \qquad \text{with } k \text{ an arbitrary constant.} \tag{15}$$

The particular solution for a given v_0 is

$$v_n = \frac{g}{1-r} + \left(v_0 - \frac{g}{1-r}\right)r^n.$$

PROOF   One particular solution to Recursion (14) is easy to find; it is the solution with v_n a constant h. We find h by replacing each of v_n and v_{n-1} by h in Recursion (14), thus getting

$$h - rh = g$$
$$h(1-r) = g.$$

Since $r \neq 1$, we have $1 - r \neq 0$ and can solve for h. Thus we get the particular solution $v_n = g/(1-r)$. Using this particular solution and Theorem 1, we obtain the general solution claimed in Display (15).

If v_0 is given, we let $n = 0$ in Display (15) and solve for k. This gives us

$$v_0 = \frac{g}{1-r} + k,$$

$$k = v_0 - \frac{g}{1-r}.$$

Substituting this formula for k into Display (15), we get the specific solution stated in this lemma.   □

Example 3   Here we solve the recursion

$$v_n - 2v_{n-1} = 3,$$

that is, the specific illustration of the recursion $v_n - rv_{n-1} = g$ in which $r = 2$ and $g = 3$. Replacing each of v_n and v_{n-1} by h, we get

$$h = 2h + 3,$$
$$-h = 3,$$
$$h = -3.$$

Hence the particular solution is $v_n = -3$ and, using Theorem 1, the general solution is

$$v_n = -3 + 2^n k, \qquad \text{with } k \text{ an arbitrary constant.}$$

If we are given that $v_0 = 5$, we let $n = 0$ in the general solution and have

$$5 = -3 + k,$$
$$k = 5 + 3 = 8.$$

Replacing k by 8 in the general solution, we get the specific solution

$$v_n = -3 + 8 \cdot 2^n \qquad \text{for } n \in N$$

to the recursion with given initial condition. We check this by calculating v_1 both from this formula and from the recursion, as follows:

$$v_1 = -3 + 8 \cdot 2 = -3 + 16 = 13,$$
$$v_1 = 2v_0 + 3 = 2 \cdot 5 + 3 = 13. \qquad \square$$

CASE II   **RECURSION $v_n - rv_{n-1} = fs^n$**

Here we show how to solve a first order nonhomogeneous linear recursion

$$v_n - rv_{n-1} = fs^n \qquad \text{for } n \in Z^+, \tag{16}$$

where f, r, and s are fixed numbers. We replace n by $n - 1$ in Recursion (16) and see that

$$v_{n-1} - rv_{n-2} = fs^{n-1}.$$

We multiply each side by s and have

$$sv_{n-1} - srv_{n-2} = fs^n.$$

Subtracting corresponding sides of this from the sides of Recursion (16) leads to

$$v_n - (r + s)v_{n-1} + srv_{n-2} = 0. \tag{17}$$

Thus we have shown that every solution to the first order nonhomogeneous Recursion (16) also is a solution of the second order homogeneous Recursion (17). The steps used to show this are not reversible; that is, the equality in Recursion (17) does not imply the equality in Recursion (16).

It will turn out that Recursion (17) has more solutions than Recursion (16) has. In other words, Recursion (17) has all the desired solutions to Recursion (16) together with *extraneous* solutions, that is, sequences not satisfying Recursion (16). But the important thing is that we need just one particular solution to the first order nonhomogeneous Recursion (16) and it can be found among the solutions, which are given by Algorithm 1 of Section 9.2, to the second order H.L.R.W.C.C.

The characteristic polynomial for the second order H.L.R.W.C.C. in Display (17) is

$$x^2 - (r + s)x + rs = (x - r)(x - s),$$

and hence the characteristic roots are r and s. Using Algorithm 1 ("Closed-Form Solution for Second Order H.L.R.W.C.C.") of Section 9.2, we find that every solution of Recursion (17) with $r \neq s$ has the form

$$v_n = r^n h + s^n k, \qquad \text{with } h \text{ and } k \text{ constants.}$$

If $r = s$, every solution of Recursion (17) is of the form

$$v_n = (h_1 + h_2 n)r^n, \qquad \text{with } h_1 \text{ and } h_2 \text{ constants.}$$

We now consider these two subcases.

CASE IIA $r \neq s$

Let us assume that $r \neq s$ in the recursion

$$v_n - rv_{n-1} = fs^n. \tag{18}$$

We have just noted that every solution of Recursion (18) is of the form

$$v_n = hr^n + ks^n, \qquad \text{with } h \text{ and } k \text{ constants.} \tag{19}$$

As we will see, h is an arbitrary constant but k is a constant to be determined specifically so as to eliminate the sequences of Display (19) that are not solutions of Recursion (18). Theorem 1 above tells us that every solution of Recursion (18) is of the form

$$v_n = hr^n + x_n, \tag{20}$$

where h is a constant and $x_0, x_1, \ldots$ is a particular solution of Recursion (18). Comparing Recursions (19) and (20), we see that the particular solution should be sought in the form

$$x_n = ks^n. \tag{21}$$

Substituting this and $x_{n-1} = ks^{n-1}$ for v_n and v_{n-1} in Recursion (18), we get

$$ks^n - rks^{n-1} = fs^n.$$

We divide by s^{n-1} and have

$$ks - rk = fs,$$
$$k(s - r) = fs,$$
$$k = \frac{fs}{s - r}.$$

Substituting this value of k in Display (21), we have

$$x_n = \left(\frac{fs}{s - r}\right)s^n \tag{22}$$

as a particular solution of Recursion (18). Then all solutions of Recursion (18) are of the form

$$v_n = hr^n + \left(\frac{fs}{s - r}\right)s^n, \qquad \text{with } h \text{ constant.} \tag{23}$$

When v_0 is known, we let $n = 0$ in Display (23) and have

$$v_0 = h + \frac{fs}{s - r},$$

$$h = v_0 - \frac{fs}{s - r}.$$

We substitute this h in Display (23) and thus get the solution

$$v_n = \left(v_0 - \frac{fs}{s - r}\right)r^n + \left(\frac{fs}{s - r}\right)s^n \tag{24}$$

to Recursion (18) for the given initial value v_0.

DEFINITION 2   **CLOSED-FORM SOLUTIONS**

The formula of Display (23) is the ***closed-form solution*** to the first order nonhomogeneous recursion

$$v_n - rv_{n-1} = fs^n, \qquad r \neq s.$$

When h is an arbitrary constant, Display (23) is also called the ***general solution***. When v_0 is known, Formula (24) is the ***specific solution*** to this recursion for the given initial value v_0.

Example 4   Here we solve the first order nonhomogeneous recursion

$$v_n + 4v_{n-1} = 3 \cdot 5^n \qquad \text{for } n \in \mathbf{Z}^+. \tag{25}$$

Since $r \neq s$, we seek a particular solution of the form

$$v_n = 5^n k.$$

We substitute this and $v_{n-1} = 5^{n-1}k$ in the recursion and get

$$5^n k + 4 \cdot 5^{n-1}k = 3 \cdot 5^n.$$

We divide by 5^{n-1} and have

$$5k + 4k = 3 \cdot 5,$$
$$9k = 15,$$
$$k = \tfrac{5}{3}.$$

Thus $v_n = (\tfrac{5}{3})5^n$ is a particular solution. Now we use Theorem 1 and see that

$$v_n = (\tfrac{5}{3})5^n + (-4)^n h, \tag{26}$$

with h an arbitrary constant, is the general solution of Recursion (25).

If we are given that $v_0 = 7$, then we let $n = 0$ in Display (26) and determine h as follows:

$$7 = \tfrac{5}{3} + h,$$
$$h = 7 - \tfrac{5}{3} = \tfrac{16}{3}.$$

Replacing h with $\tfrac{16}{3}$ in Display (26), we obtain

$$v_n = (\tfrac{5}{3})5^n + (\tfrac{16}{3})(-4)^n$$

as the specific solution to Recursion (25) for the given initial condition $v_0 = 7$. We check by calculating the next term v_1 both from this formula and from the recursion, as follows:

$$v_1 = \frac{5}{3} \cdot 5 + \frac{16}{3}(-4) = \frac{25 - 64}{3} = \frac{-39}{3} = -13,$$

$$v_1 = -4v_0 + 3 \cdot 5 = -4 \cdot 7 + 15 = -28 + 15 = -13. \qquad \square$$

CASE IIB $r = s$

Now we solve the first order nonhomogeneous recursion

$$v_n - r v_{n-1} = fr^n, \tag{27}$$

with r and f known constants. Theorem 1 ("Complete Solution for a First Order Nonhomogeneous Linear Recursion") tells us that all solutions have the form

$$v_n = r^n h + x_n, \tag{28}$$

with h constant and $x_0, x_1, \ldots$ any particular solution to Recursion (27). We saw just before the start of Case IIA that all solutions are also of the form

$$v_n = (h + kn)r^n. \tag{29}$$

We compare Displays (28) and (29) and thus see that we should seek a particular solution of the form

$$x_n = knr^n.$$

Substituting $v_n = knr^n$ and $v_{n-1} = k(n-1)r^{n-1}$ into Recursion (27) gives us

$$knr^n - k(n-1)r^n = fr^n.$$

We divide by r^n and get

$$kn - k(n-1) = f,$$
$$kn - kn + k = f,$$
$$k = f.$$

Thus the particular solution to Recursion (27) is

$$x_n = fnr^n, \tag{30}$$

and the general solution to Recursion (27) is

$$v_n = (h + fn)r^n, \qquad \text{with } h \text{ constant.} \tag{31}$$

When v_0 is given, we let $n = 0$ in this and solve for h, as follows:

$$v_0 = (h + f \cdot 0)r^0 = h.$$

Hence the specific solution to Recursion (27) with given initial term v_0 is

$$v_n = (v_0 + fn)r^n. \tag{32}$$

Example 5   Here we solve the first order nonhomogeneous recursion

$$v_n + 5v_{n-1} = 6(-5)^n.$$

This is of the type given in Display (27) with $r = -5$ and $f = 6$. Using the formula of Display (31), we see that the general solution is

$$v_n = (h + 6n)(-5)^n.$$

To find the specific solution with $v_0 = 9$, we let $n = 0$ in this formula and get

$$9 = v_0 = h(-5)^0 = h.$$

Replacing h by 9 in the general solution, we get

$$v_n = (9 + 6n)(-5)^n$$

as the specific solution with the initial condition $v_0 = 9$. We check this by calculating v_1 both from this closed form and from the recursion, as follows:

$$v_1 = (9 + 6 \cdot 1)(-5) = 15(-5) = -75,$$
$$v_1 = -5v_0 + 6(-5) = -5 \cdot 9 - 30 = -45 - 30 = -75. \qquad \square$$

CASE III   COMPOUND RIGHT-HAND SIDE

The next result makes it possible to solve a recursion whose left-hand side is of a type we have studied and whose right-hand side is a sum of terms $g(n)$ of the forms we have considered.

THEOREM 2   NONHOMOGENEOUS RECURSIONS WITH SAME HOMOGENEOUS PART

Let $x_0, x_1, \ldots$ satisfy

$$v_n + b(n)v_{n-1} = f(n)$$

and $y_0, y_1, \ldots$ satisfy

$$v_n + b(n)v_{n-1} = g(n),$$

where $b(1), b(2), \ldots$; $f(1), f(2), \ldots$; and $g(1), g(2), \ldots$ are given sequences. Then the sequence $z_0, z_1, \ldots$ with $z_n = x_n + y_n$ satisfies

$$v_n + b(n)v_{n-1} = f(n) + g(n).$$

PROOF   We are given, for $n \in \mathbf{Z}^+$, that

$$x_n + b(n)x_{n-1} = f(n),$$
$$y_n + b(n)y_{n-1} = g(n).$$

Adding these leads to

$$(x_n + y_n) + b(n)(x_{n-1} + y_{n-1}) = f(n) + g(n).$$

Substituting $x_n + y_n = z_n$ and $x_{n-1} + y_{n-1} = z_{n-1}$, we get

$$z_n + b(n)z_{n-1} = f(n) + g(n),$$

as claimed. $\qquad \square$

Example 6   Here we solve the recursion

$$v_n - 2v_{n-1} = 3 + 6(-2)^n - 4 \cdot 2^n. \qquad (33)$$

We intend to use Theorem 2 and therefore consider the following three related recursions:

$$x_n - 2x_{n-1} = 3, \tag{34}$$
$$y_n - 2y_{n-1} = 6(-2)^n, \tag{35}$$
$$z_n - 2z_{n-1} = -4 \cdot 2^n. \tag{36}$$

We find with the method of Case I above that a particular solution to Recursion (34) is the constant solution

$$x_n = -3.$$

Recursion (35) is a Case IIA recursion with $r = 2$ and $s = -2$; the method of Case IIA or the formula of Display (22) gives us the particular solutions

$$y_n = \left(\frac{fs}{s-r}\right)s^n = \frac{6(-2)}{-2-2}(-2)^n = 3(-2)^n.$$

Display (36) is a Case IIB recursion with $r = 2$ and $f = -4$. The method of Case IIB or the formula of Display (30) tells us that a particular solution to Recursion (36) is

$$z_n = fnr^n = -4n \cdot 2^n.$$

Using Theorem 2 and the particular solution $x_n = -3$ to Recursion (34) together with the particular solution $y_n = 3(-2)^n$ to Recursion (35), we find that

$$w_n = x_n + y_n = -3 + 3(-2)^n$$

is a particular solution to

$$w_n - 2w_{n-1} = 3 + 6(-2)^n.$$

This and the fact that $z_n = -4n \cdot 2^n$ is a particular solution to Recursion (36) can be used with Theorem 2 to find that

$$v_n = w_n + z_n = -3 + 3(-2)^n - 4n \cdot 2^n$$

is a particular solution to our original recursion

$$v_n - 2v_{n-1} = 3 + 6(-2)^n - 4 \cdot 2^n. \tag{37}$$

Then Theorem 1 ("Complete Solution for a First Order Nonhomogeneous Linear Recursion") tells us that the general solution to Recursion (37) is

$$v_n = -3 + 3(-2)^n - 4n \cdot 2^n + 2^n h, \qquad \text{with } h \text{ an arbitrary constant.}$$

If we are given v_0, we can determine h using $n = 0$ in this formula. For example, if $v_0 = 6$, then

$$6 = -3 + 3 + h,$$
$$h = 6.$$

Hence the specific solution to Display (37) with given initial term $v_0 = 6$ is

$$v_n = -3 + 3(-2)^n - 4n \cdot 2^n + 6 \cdot 2^n = -3 + 3(-2)^n + (6 - 4n)2^n.$$

We check by calculating v_1 from this and from the recursion, as follows:

$$v_1 = -3 + 3(-2) + (6 - 4)2 = -3 - 6 + 4 = -5,$$
$$v_1 = 2v_0 + 3 + 6(-2) - 4 \cdot 2 = 12 + 3 - 12 - 8 = -5. \qquad \square$$

PROBLEMS FOR SECTION 9.3

1. Do the following for the nonhomogeneous L.R.W.C.C.

   $$v_n - 1.025v_{n-1} = -200. \qquad (R)$$

   (i) Find the constant solution.
   (ii) Use Part (i) and the general solution $u_n = 1.025^n k$ to the associated homogeneous recursion $u_n - 1.025u_{n-1} = 0$ to write the general solution to the nonhomogeneous Recursion (R).
   (iii) Write the specific solution to Recursion (R) for the initial condition $v_0 = 10000$.

2. Do the following for the nonhomogeneous L.R.W.C.C.

   $$v_n - 1.03v_{n-1} = -200.$$

   (i) Find the constant solution.   (ii) Write the general solution.
   (iii) Write the specific solution having $v_0 = 10000$.

3. Suppose that \$10000 is deposited in an account with an annual interest rate of 10% compounded quarterly. Each quarter, there is a withdrawal of \$200 immediately after interest is credited.
   (i) Find the closed form for the balance P_n after the nth such withdrawal.
   (ii) Tell how the answer to Part (i) is related to the answer to Problem 1(iii).

4. Repeat Problem 3(i), but with the annual interest rate changed from 10% to 12%.

5. (i) Find the general solution to $v_n + 3v_{n-1} = 7$.
   (ii) Find the specific solution (to this recursion) with initial condition $v_0 = 1$.
   (iii) Check the answer in Part (ii) by finding v_1 in two ways.

6. (i) Find the general solution to $v_n - 4v_{n-1} = 3$.
   (ii) Find the specific solution (to this recursion) with $v_0 = 2$.
   (iii) Check the answer in Part (ii) by finding v_1 in two ways.

7. (i) Find the general solution to $v_n - 3v_{n-1} = 6(-5)^n$.
   (ii) Find the specific solution with $v_0 = -4$.

8. (i) Find the general solution to $v_n + 2v_{n-1} = 5 \cdot 4^n$.
   (ii) Find the specific solution with $v_0 = 9$.

9. (i) Find the general solution to $v_n + 7v_{n-1} = 6(-7)^n$.
    (ii) Find the specific solution with $v_0 = 11$.

10. (i) Find the general solution to $v_n - 8v_{n-1} = 7 \cdot 8^n$.
    (ii) Find the specific solution with $v_0 = -3$.

11. (i) Find a particular solution to $x_n + 2x_{n-1} = 6$.
    (ii) Find a particular solution to $y_n + 2y_{n-1} = -5 \cdot 3^n$.
    (iii) Find a particular solution to $z_n + 2z_{n-1} = 4(-2)^n$.
    (iv) Write a particular solution to $w_n + 2w_{n-1} = 6 - 5 \cdot 3^n$.
    (v) Write a particular solution to $v_n + 2v_{n-1} = 6 - 5 \cdot 3^n + 4(-2)^n$.
    (vi) Write the general solution to the recursion in Part (v).
    (vii) Find the specific solution to the recursion in Part (v) with $v_0 = 18$.

12. (i) Find a particular solution to $x_n - 3x_{n-1} = 2$.
    (ii) Find a particular solution to $y_n - 3y_{n-1} = -3 \cdot 4^n$.
    (iii) Find a particular solution to $z_n - 3z_{n-1} = 5 \cdot 3^n$.
    (iv) Write a particular solution to $v_n - 3v_{n-1} = 2 - 3 \cdot 4^n + 5 \cdot 3^n$.
    (v) Write the general solution to the recursion in Part (iv).
    (vi) Find the specific solution to the recursion in Part (iv) with $v_0 = 6$.

13. Let $x_0, x_1, \ldots$ be a particular solution to the nonhomogeneous recursion $v_n - rv_{n-1} = g(n)$, with r some constant. Prove that the specific solution with a given initial term v_0 is $v_n = x_n + (v_0 - x_0)r^n$. [This is the proof of the Corollary ("Specific Solution") to Theorem 1, which was left to the reader.]

14. Let $y_0, y_1, \ldots$ satisfy $y_n + b(n)y_{n-1} = g(n)$ for $n \in \mathbf{Z}^+$ and $z_0, z_1, \ldots$ satisfy $z_n + b(n)z_{n-1} = 0$ for $n \in \mathbf{Z}^+$. Also, let $x_n = y_n + z_n$ for $n \in \mathbf{N}$. Show that $x_n + b(n)x_{n-1} = g(n)$ for $n \in \mathbf{Z}^+$.

9.4

HOMOGENEOUS LINEAR RECURSIONS OF ALL ORDERS

In this section, we extend the results in Section 9.2 to homogeneous linear recursions of all orders.

A sequence $u_0, u_1, \ldots$ is defined *inductively* (or *recursively*) if the beginning terms are given together with a rule for obtaining each of the remaining terms u_n from previous terms. A rule for expressing u_n as a function of the terms $u_{n-1}, u_{n-2}, \ldots, u_{n-d}$ is called a *recursion of order d*, or *dth order recursion*. A dth order *linear recursion* is a rule of the form

$$u_n = b_0(n) - b_1(n)u_{n-1} - b_2(n)u_{n-2} - \cdots - b_d(n)u_{n-d}$$
$$\text{for } n \in \{d, d+1, \ldots\} \quad (1)$$

or, equivalently, of the form

$$u_n + b_1(n)u_{n-1} + b_2(n)u_{n-2} + \cdots + b_d(n)u_{n-d} = b_0(n)$$
$$\text{for } n \in \{d, d+1, \ldots\}, \quad (2)$$

where $b_i(d)$, $b_i(d+1)$, ... is a given sequence for each i in $\{0, 1, \ldots, d\}$ and $b_d(n) \neq 0$ for some n in $\{d, d+1, \ldots\}$. If $b_d(d)$, $b_d(d+1)$, ... is the sequence $0, 0, \ldots$ with all terms equal to 0, then the linear recursion in Display (1) or Display (2) has order less than d.

Now let us consider the case in which $b_0(n) = 0$ for all n in $\{d, d+1, \ldots\}$. Then the rule

$$u_n + b_1(n)u_{n-1} + b_2(n)u_{n-2} + \cdots + b_d(n)u_{n-d} = 0$$
$$\text{for } n \in \{d, d+1, \ldots\} \quad (3)$$

is a ***homogeneous*** linear recursion of order d if $b_d(n) \neq 0$ for at least one n. Next we replace each $b_i(n)$ by a constant b_i. Then the rule

$$u_n + b_1 u_{n-1} + b_2 u_{n-2} + \cdots + b_d u_{n-d} = 0 \quad \text{for } n \in \{d, d+1, \ldots\}, \quad (4)$$

in which the coefficients $b_1, b_2, \ldots, b_d$ are known constants with $b_d \neq 0$, is a dth order homogeneous linear recursion with ***constant coefficients***. (This is abbreviated as dth order H.L.R.W.C.C.) Most of this section deals with such H.L.R.W.C.C.

In all of the phrases defined above, the word *recursion* may be replaced by ***difference equation***.

Example 1　　The first order linear recursion

$$u_n = nu_{n-1} + (-1)^n \qquad \text{for } n \in \mathbf{Z}^+ = \{1, 2, \ldots\} \quad (5)$$

is the special case of Display (1) with $d = 1$, $b_0(n) = (-1)^n$, and $b_1(n) = -n$; it does not have constant coefficients. The first order H.L.R.W.C.C.

$$u_n - 3u_{n-1} = 0 \qquad \text{for } n \in \mathbf{Z}^+ \quad (6)$$

is the case of Display (4) with $d = 1$ and $b_1 = -3$. The second order H.L.R.W.C.C.

$$u_n - u_{n-1} - u_{n-2} = 0 \qquad \text{for } n \in \{2, 3, \ldots\} \quad (7)$$

is the case of Display (4) with $d = 2$ and $b_1 = -1 = b_2$. The second order recursion $u_n = u_{n-1}^2 / u_{n-2}$ or its equivalent

$$u_n = u_{n-1}^2 u_{n-2}^{-1} \qquad \text{for } n \in \{2, 3, \ldots\} \quad (8)$$

is not linear, since u_{n-1} does not appear only with degree 1. (The same is true of u_{n-2}.) The second order H.L.R.W.C.C.

$$u_n - 2u_{n-1} + u_{n-2} = 0 \qquad \text{for } n \in \{2, 3, \ldots\} \quad (9)$$

is the case of Display (4) with $d = 2$, $b_1 = -2$, and $b_2 = 1$. The third order H.L.R.W.C.C.

$$u_n - 6u_{n-1} + 12u_{n-2} - 8u_{n-3} = 0 \qquad \text{for } n \in \{3, 4, \ldots\} \quad (10)$$

is the case of Display (4) with $d = 3$, $b_1 = -6$, $b_2 = 12$, and $b_3 = -8$.　□

We will see in Theorem 3 below that there is an explicit formula for the general term u_n of a sequence $u_0, u_1, \ldots$ satisfying an H.L.R.W.C.C. of any order. In Examples 3, 4, 5, 6, 7 and 9 below, we illustrate the techniques for finding explicit solutions to an H.L.R.W.C.C.

Example 2　One of the solutions of the second order linear homogeneous recursion with constant coefficients

$$u_n - 4u_{n-1} - 5u_{n-2} = 0$$

is the sequence $u_0, u_1, \ldots$ with $u_n = 2 \cdot 5^n - 4(-1)^n$, as we see from the following direct substitution:

$$
\begin{aligned}
u_n - 4u_{n-1} - 5u_{n-2} &= [2 \cdot 5^n - 4(-1)^n] - 4[2 \cdot 5^{n-1} - 4(-1)^{n-1}] - 5[2 \cdot 5^{n-2} - 4(-1)^{n-2}] \\
&= (2 \cdot 5^n - 8 \cdot 5^{n-1} - 10 \cdot 5^{n-2}) + [-4(-1)^n + 16(-1)^{n-1} + 20(-1)^{n-2}] \\
&= 5^{n-2}(50 - 40 - 10) + (-1)^{n-2}(-4 - 16 + 20) \\
&= 5^{n-2} \cdot 0 + (-1)^{n-2} \cdot 0 = 0 + 0 = 0. \qquad \square
\end{aligned}
$$

THEOREM 1　**GENERATING FUNCTION FOR H.L.R.W.C.C. SOLUTIONS**

Let $u_0, u_1, \ldots$ satisfy the dth order H.L.R.W.C.C.

$$u_n + b_1 u_{n-1} + b_2 u_{n-2} + \cdots + b_d u_{n-d} = 0 \quad \text{for } n \in \{d, d+1, \ldots\}. \quad (11)$$

Then the generating function $G = u_0 + u_1 x + u_2 x^2 + \cdots$ is expressible as the proper x-fraction A/B with

$$
\begin{aligned}
A = u_0 &+ (u_1 + b_1 u_0)x + (u_2 + b_1 u_1 + b_2 u_0)x^2 \\
&+ \cdots + (u_{d-1} + b_1 u_{d-2} + \cdots + b_{d-1} u_0)x^{d-1}
\end{aligned}
$$

and

$$B = 1 + b_1 x + b_2 x^2 + \cdots + b_d x^d.$$

ILLUSTRATION OF PROOF　We deal with the case of $d = 3$ in which

$$A = u_0 + (u_1 + b_1 u_0)x + (u_2 + b_1 u_1 + b_2 u_0)x^2$$

and

$$B = 1 + b_1 x + b_2 x^2 + b_3 x^3.$$

The proof for general d is entirely analogous.

We see that

$$
\begin{array}{llllll}
G = u_0 + & u_1 x + & u_2 x^2 + & u_3 x^3 + \cdots + & u_n x^n + \cdots \\
b_1 x G = & b_1 u_0 x + & b_1 u_1 x^2 + & b_1 u_2 x^3 + \cdots + b_1 u_{n-1} x^n + \cdots \\
b_2 x^2 G = & & b_2 u_0 x^2 + & b_2 u_1 x^3 + \cdots + b_2 u_{n-2} x^n + \cdots \\
b_3 x^3 G = & & & b_3 u_0 x^3 + \cdots + b_3 u_{n-3} x^n + \cdots
\end{array}
$$

Adding these equations gives us

$$BG = [u_0 + (u_1 + b_1 u_0)x + (u_2 + b_1 u_1 + b_2 u_0)x^2] + (u_3 + b_1 u_2 + b_2 u_1 + b_3 u_0)x^3 + \cdots$$
$$BG = A + (u_3 + b_1 u_2 + b_2 u_1 + b_3 u_0)x^3 + \cdots + (u_n + b_1 u_{n-1} + b_2 u_{n-2} + b_3 u_{n-3})x^n + \cdots.$$

The right-hand side of this last equation is just A if and only if the sequence $u_0, u_1, \ldots$ satisfies Recursion (11) (with d replaced by 3). When it does, $G = A/B$. ☐

Example 3 Let $u_0, u_1, \ldots$ be the sequence given by the initial conditions

$$u_0 = 1, \qquad u_1 = 8$$

and the linear homogeneous recursion with constant coefficients

$$u_n = u_{n-1} + 2u_{n-2} \qquad \text{for } n \text{ in } \{2, 3, \ldots\}.$$

We rewrite this recursion in the form of Theorem 1 as

$$u_n - u_{n-1} - 2u_{n-2} = 0.$$

Then Theorem 1 tells us that the generating function for $u_0, u_1, \ldots$ is $G = A/B$, where

$$B = 1 + b_1 x + b_2 x^2 = 1 - x - 2x^2 = (1 + x)(1 - 2x),$$
$$A = u_0 + (u_1 + b_1 u_0)x = 1 + 7x.$$

That is, $G = (1 + 7x)/[(1 + x)(1 - 2x)]$. Using the technique of Section 8.3, the partial-fractions form of G is found to be

$$G = \frac{3}{1 - 2x} - \frac{2}{1 + x}.$$

Theorem 2(a) ("Generating Functions Related to Geometric Progressions") of Section 9.1, tells us that

$$\frac{3}{1 - 2x} = 3 + 6x + 12x^2 + \cdots + 3 \cdot 2^n x^n + \cdots$$

$$\frac{-2}{1 + x} = -2 + 2x - 2x^2 + \cdots - 2(-1)^n x^n + \cdots.$$

Adding these two equations gives us

$$G = 1 + 8x + 10x^2 + \cdots + [3 \cdot 2^n - 2(-1)^n]x^n + \cdots.$$

But

$$G = u_0 + u_1 x + u_2 x^2 + \cdots + u_n x^n + \cdots.$$

Equating coefficients of x^n leads to the explicit formula

$$u_n = 3 \cdot 2^n - 2(-1)^n.$$

☐

Theorem 1 of this section tells us that a sequence satisfying an H.L.R.W.C.C. has a proper x-fraction as its generating function. Theorem 1 ("Partial-Fractions Decomposition") of Section 8.3 states that every proper x-fraction G is a finite sum of special x-fractions of the form $c/(1 - rx)^d$, with c, r, and d constants and d in $Z^+ = \{1, 2, \ldots\}$. In Lemma 1 below, we give the explicit sequence having such a special x-fraction as its generating function. Together, these results will enable us to find an explicit formula for the general term u_n of a sequence $u_0, u_1, \ldots$ satisfying an H.L.R.W.C.C.

It follows from Theorem 2 of Section 9.1 that

$$\frac{c}{1 - rx} = c + crx + cr^2x^2 + \cdots + cr^nx^n + \cdots,$$

$$\frac{c}{(1 - rx)^2} = c + 2crx + 3cr^2x^2 + \cdots + (n + 1)cr^nx^n + \cdots.$$

The special cases of these with $c = 1 = r$ are

$$(1 - x)^{-1} = 1 + x + x^2 + \cdots + x^n + \cdots,$$
$$(1 - x)^{-2} = 1 + 2x + 3x^2 + \cdots + (n + 1)x^n + \cdots.$$

These were obtained in Examples 3 and 4 of Section 9.1. The following result extends these formulas to arbitrary special x-fractions $c/(1 - rx)^d$.

LEMMA 1   **GENERATING FUNCTION FOR** $c\binom{h + n}{h}r^n$

Let h be in $N = \{0, 1, \ldots\}$. Then:

(a) $(1 - x)^{-h-1} = \binom{h}{h} + \binom{h + 1}{h}x + \cdots + \binom{h + n}{h}x^n + \cdots.$

(b) $(1 - rx)^{-h-1} = \binom{h}{h} + \binom{h + 1}{h}rx + \cdots + \binom{h + n}{h}r^nx^n + \cdots.$

(c) $c(1 - rx)^{-h-1} = c\binom{h}{h} + c\binom{h + 1}{h}rx + \cdots + c\binom{h + n}{h}r^nx^n + \cdots.$

PROOF   We prove Part (a) by mathematical induction on h. Then Part (b) follows if we replace x by rx. Part (c) is obtained by multiplying both sides of the equation in Part (b) by the constant c.

Basis of the Induction   When $h = 0$, the left-hand side of Part (a) is $(1 - x)^{-1}$ and the right-hand side is $1 + x + \cdots + x^n + \cdots$, since $\binom{n}{0} = 1$ for all n in N. The two sides are equal by Theorem 2(a) ("Generating Functions Related to Geometric Progressions") of Section 9.1, with $a = 1 = r$. This establishes the basis.

Inductive Part We assume that k is in N and that

$$(1 - x)^{-k-1} = \binom{k}{k} + \binom{k+1}{k}x + \cdots + \binom{k+n}{k}x^n + \cdots.$$

Then it follows from Theorem 3 ("Generating Series for Partial Sums") of Section 9.1 and $(1 - x)^{-1}(1 - x)^{-k-1} = (1 - x)^{-(k+1)-1}$ that

$$(1 - x)^{-(k+1)-1} = c_0 + c_1 x + \cdots + c_n x^n + \cdots,$$

where

$$c_n = \binom{k}{k} + \binom{k+1}{k} + \binom{k+2}{k} + \cdots + \binom{k+n}{k}.$$

But this sum, of binomial coefficients along diagonal k of the Pascal Triangle, equals $\binom{k+n+1}{k+1}$ by Problem 7 of Section 4.2. Hence

$$(1 - x)^{-(k+1)-1} = \binom{k+1}{k+1} + \binom{k+2}{k+1}x + \cdots + \binom{k+1+n}{k+1}x^n + \cdots.$$

Since this is Part (a) with h replaced by $k + 1$, the lemma is proved. $\square$

Example 4 Here we find an explicit formula for the term u_n of the sequence $u_0, u_1, \ldots$ satisfying the homogeneous linear recursion of order 3

$$u_n - 6u_{n-1} + 12u_{n-2} - 8u_{n-3} = 0 \qquad \text{for } n = 3, 4, \ldots$$

and the initial conditions

$$u_0 = 1, \qquad u_1 = 6, \qquad u_2 = 24.$$

Let G be the generating series $u_0 + u_1 x + u_2 x^2 + \cdots$. It can be seen from Theorem 1 ("Generating Function for H.L.R.W.C.C. Solutions") that

$$G = \frac{1}{1 - 6x + 12x^2 - 8x^3} = \frac{1}{(1 - 2x)^3} = (1 - 2x)^{-3}.$$

But Lemma 1(b), with $r = 2$ and $h = 2$, tells us that

$$(1 - 2x)^{-3} = \binom{2}{2} + 2\binom{3}{2}x + 4\binom{4}{2}x^2 + \cdots + 2^n\binom{2+n}{2}x^n + \cdots.$$

Since u_n is the coefficient of x^n in the series G, we have the desired explicit formulas

$$u_n = 2^n\binom{2+n}{2} = \frac{2^n(n+2)(n+1)}{2} = 2^{n-1}(n+2)(n+1). \qquad \square$$

LEMMA 2   **ROOTS AND FACTORS**

Let $K(x) = x^d + b_1 x^{d-1} + b_2 x^{d-2} + \cdots + b_d$ and $B(x) = 1 + b_1 x + \cdots + b_d x^d$, with the b_i complex numbers. Then:

(a) $K(x) = 0$ has a complex root.

(b) $K(x) = (x - r_1)^{d_1}(x - r_2)^{d_2} \cdots (x - r_s)^{d_s}$, where the r_i are the distinct roots of $K(x) = 0$ and d_i is the multiplicity of r_i.

(c) $B(x) = x^d K\left(\dfrac{1}{x}\right)$.

(d) $B(x) = (1 - r_1 x)^{d_1}(1 - r_2 x)^{d_2} \cdots (1 - r_s x)^{d_s}$.

DISCUSSION
OF PROOF

(a) Part (a), called the ***Fundamental Theorem of Algebra***, is due to Carl Friedrich Gauss (1777–1855). The proof is too difficult for a text of this level.

(b) Part (b) can be proved by mathematical induction on the degree of $K(x)$, with the help of Part (a) and the Factor Theorem of Section 8.1.

PROOF

(c) $B(x) = 1 + b_1 x + b_2 x^2 + \cdots + b_d x^d$

$$= x^d \left[\left(\frac{1}{x}\right)^d + b_1 \left(\frac{1}{x}\right)^{d-1} + \cdots + b_d \right]$$

$$= x^d K\left(\frac{1}{x}\right).$$

(d) Using the results in Parts (b) and (c), we get

$$B(x) = x^d \left[\left(\frac{1}{x} - r_1\right)^{d_1} \left(\frac{1}{x} - r_2\right)^{d_2} \cdots \left(\frac{1}{x} - r_s\right)^{d_s} \right]$$

$$= x^{d_1} x^{d_2} \cdots x^{d_s} \left(\frac{1}{x} - r_1\right)^{d_1} \left(\frac{1}{x} - r_2\right)^{d_2} \cdots \left(\frac{1}{x} - r_s\right)^{d_s}$$

$$= \left[x^{d_1} \left(\frac{1}{x} - r_1\right)^{d_1} \right] \left[x^{d_2} \left(\frac{1}{x} - r_2\right)^{d_2} \right] \cdots \left[x^{d_s} \left(\frac{1}{x} - r_s\right)^{d_s} \right]$$

$$= (1 - r_1 x)^{d_1}(1 - r_2 x)^{d_2} \cdots (1 - r_s x)^{d_s}. \qquad \square$$

Let us once again consider a linear homogeneous recursion

$$u_n + b_1 u_{n-1} + b_2 u_{n-2} + \cdots + b_d u_{n-d} = 0 \tag{12}$$

with constant coefficients b_i. Theorem 1 ("Generating Function for H.L.R.W.C.C. Solutions") tells us that a solution $u_0, u_1, \ldots$ to this recursion has a generating function $G = A/B$, where

$$B(x) = 1 + b_1 x + b_2 x^2 + \cdots + b_d x^d. \tag{13}$$

We now give names to this B and its associated polynomial K of Lemma 2.

DEFINITION 1

RECURSION POLYNOMIAL, CHARACTERISTIC POLYNOMIAL

The polynomial $B(x)$ of Display (13) is the *recursion polynomial* for Recursion (12). The *characteristic polynomial* for Recursion (12) is $K(x) = x^d + b_1 x^{d-1} + b_2 x^{d-2} + \cdots + b_d$. The equation $K(x) = 0$ is the *characteristic equation*; its roots are the *characteristic roots* for Recursion (12).

THEOREM 2

EXPLICIT SOLUTION OF AN H.L.R.W.C.C.

A sequence $u_0, u_1, \ldots$ satisfies the H.L.R.W.C.C.

$$u_n + b_1 u_{n-1} + b_2 u_{n-2} + \cdots + b_d u_{n-d} = 0 \quad \text{for } n \in \{d, d+1, \ldots\} \quad (14)$$

if and only if u_n is a finite sum of expressions

$$c\binom{h+n}{h} r^n$$

in each of which c is a constant, r is a characteristic root for the recursion, and h is an integer in $\{0, 1, \ldots\}$ that is less than the multiplicity of the root r of the characteristic equation $K(x) = 0$.

PROOF

Let the characteristic roots for Recursion (14) be $r_1, r_2, \ldots, r_s$ and let their multiplicities as roots of $K(x) = 0$ be $d_1, d_2, \ldots, d_s$, respectively. By Theorem 1, the sequence $u_0, u_1, \ldots$ satisfies Recursion (14) if and only if it has a proper x-fraction $G = A/B$ as its generating function, with B the recursion polynomial for Recursion (14). Lemma 2(c) implies that

$$B = (1 - r_1 x)^{d_1}(1 - r_2 x)^{d_2} \cdots (1 - r_s x)^{d_s}. \quad (15)$$

When G is a proper x-fraction A/B, with B as in Display (15), then Theorem 1 ("Partial-Fractions Decomposition") of Section 8.3 states that G is a sum of special x-fractions $c/(1 - r_i x)^g$, with c constant and g in $\{1, 2, \ldots, d_i\}$. We let $g = h + 1$ and use Lemma 1(c); this gives us

$$\frac{c}{(1 - r_i x)^g} = c(1 - r_i x)^{-h-1}$$

$$= c\binom{h}{h} + c\binom{h+1}{h} r_i x + \cdots + c\binom{h+n}{h} r_i^n x^n + \cdots, \quad (16)$$

where h is in $\{0, 1, \ldots, d_i - 1\}$. Now G is a sum of such special x-fractions if and only if the coefficient u_n of x^n in the series for G is a sum of the coefficients $c\binom{h+n}{h}r_i^n$ of x^n in series such as the right-most side of Display (16). This proves the theorem.   □

Example 5   Here we use the specific recursion

$$u_n + u_{n-1} - 11u_{n-2} - 13u_{n-3} + 26u_{n-4} + 20u_{n-5} - 24u_{n-6} = 0 \quad (17)$$

to illustrate Theorem 2. The characteristic polynomial is

$$K(x) = x^6 + x^5 - 11x^4 - 13x^3 + 26x^2 + 20x - 24.$$

Since we are lucky enough for this to have only integer roots, the techniques of Section 8.1 can be used to factor it as

$$K(x) = (x - 1)^2(x - 3)(x + 2)^3.$$

Now the recursion polynomial is

$$B = (1 - x)^2(1 - 3x)(1 + 2x)^3$$

and Theorem 2 states that $u_0, u_1, \ldots$ satisfies Recursion (17) if and only if

$$u_n = a\binom{n}{0} \cdot 1^n + b\binom{1+n}{1} \cdot 1^n + c\binom{n}{0} \cdot 3^n + d\binom{n}{0}(-2)^n$$

$$+ e\binom{1+n}{1}(-2)^n + f\binom{2+n}{2}(-2)^n \quad (18)$$

with a, b, c, d, e, and f constants. Display (18) can be simplified to

$$u_n = a + b(1 + n) + c \cdot 3^n + d(-2)^n + e(1 + n)(-2)^n$$

$$+ f\left[\frac{(2 + n)(1 + n)}{2}\right](-2)^n.$$

Letting $h = a + b$, $r = d + e + f$, $s = e + (\frac{3}{2})f$, and $t = f/2$, we have

$$u_n = h + bn + c \cdot 3^n + (r + sn + tn^2)(-2)^n. \quad (19)$$

The constants, in any of these forms, can be found explicitly if we know enough terms of the sequence $u_0, u_1, \ldots$. For example, if we are given the initial conditions

$$u_0 = 7, \quad u_1 = 4, \quad u_2 = 37, \quad u_3 = 32, \quad u_4 = 163, \quad u_5 = 646, \quad (20)$$

then it can be shown that

$$u_n = 5 - n + 2 \cdot 3^n + (4n - n^2)(-2)^n. \quad (21)$$

One way to do this is to find the A of the generating function $G = A/B$ using Theorem 1 ("Generating Function for H.L.R.W.C.C. Solutions"), then find the partial fractions form of G, next expand each special x-fraction (that is, partial fraction) using Lemma 2(b) ("Roots and Factors"), and finally equate coefficients of x^n.

Alternatively, one can substitute the values 0, 1, 2, 3, 4, 5 for n in Display (19); use the initial conditions in Display (20); solve the resulting system of equations

$$
\begin{cases}
7 = a & + & c + & g \\
4 = a + & b + & 3c - & 2g - & 2h - & 2k \\
37 = a + & 2b + & 9c + & 4g + & 8h + & 16k \\
32 = a + & 3b + & 27c - & 8g - & 24h - & 72k \\
163 = a + & 4b + & 81c + & 16g + & 64h + & 256k \\
646 = a + & 5b + & 243c - & 32g - & 160h - & 800k
\end{cases}
$$

for the constants a, b, c, g, h, and k; and finally substitute the found values of these constants in Display (19) and so end up with Display (21). $\square$

The change from Display (18) to Display (19) in Example 5 suggests the following alternate form of Theorem 2.

THEOREM 3   **EXPLICIT SOLUTION WITH POLYNOMIAL COEFFICIENTS**

Let $r, s, \ldots, t$ be the distinct characteristic roots for the linear homogeneous recursion with constant coefficients

$$u_n + b_1 u_{n-1} + b_2 u_{n-2} + \cdots + b_d u_{n-d} = 0 \quad \text{for } n = d, d+1, \ldots \quad (22)$$

and let $e, f, \ldots, g$ be the multiplicities for the roots $r, s, \ldots, t$, respectively. Then $u_0, u_1, \ldots$ satisfies Recursion (22) if and only if

$$
\begin{aligned}
u_n = {}&(a_0 + a_1 n + \cdots + a_{e-1} n^{e-1})r^n + (b_0 + b_1 n + \cdots + b_{f-1} n^{f-1})s^n \\
&+ \cdots + (c_0 + c_1 n + \cdots + c_{g-1} n^{g-1})t^n,
\end{aligned}
\quad (23)
$$

where the $a_i, b_j, \ldots, c_k$ are constants.

DISCUSSION   This theorem is obtained from Theorem 2 in the same way that we went
OF PROOF   from Display (18) to Display (19) in Example 5. $\square$

COROLLARY   **CASE OF SIMPLE ROOTS**

In Theorem 3, let each of the roots $r, s, \ldots, t$ have multiplicity 1; that is, let $e = f = \cdots = g = 1$. Then $u_0, u_1, \ldots$ satisfies the recursion if and only if

$$u_n = ar^n + bs^n + \cdots + ct^n,$$

where $a, b, \ldots, c$ are constants.

DEFINITION 2   **GENERAL SOLUTION, PARTICULAR SOLUTION, TO AN H.L.R.W.C.C.**

One calls Display (23) the **general solution** to Recursion (22). To **solve** Recursion (22) is to find the general solution given in Display (23). The u_n of Display (23) with given constants $a_i, b_j, \ldots, c_k$ is a **particular solution**. A **specific solution** is one with these constants determined from initial conditions.

Thus the general solution to an H.L.R.W.C.C. of order d involves d arbitrary constants. Each replacement of all d of these arbitrary constants by specific numbers leads to a particular solution.

Example 6   First we find the general solution of the recursion

$$u_n - 9u_{n-1} + 26u_{n-2} - 24u_{n-3} = 0 \qquad \text{for } n \in \{3, 4, \ldots\},$$

and then we find the specific solution for the initial conditions

$$u_0 = 6, \qquad u_1 = 17, \qquad u_2 = 53.$$

The characteristic polynomial for this recursion is

$$K(x) = x^3 - 9x^2 + 26x - 24.$$

The possibilities for rational roots are $\pm 1, \pm 2, \pm 3, \pm 4, \pm 6, \pm 8, \pm 12, \pm 24$. Testing some of these using synthetic division, we find that 2 is a root:

$$
\begin{array}{r|rrrr}
2 & 1 & -9 & 26 & -24 \\
  & 0 & 2 & -14 & 24 \\
\hline
  & 1 & -7 & 12 & \boxed{0}
\end{array}
$$

This also shows that $K(x) = (x - 2)(x^2 - 7x + 12)$. By inspection we factor the quadratic and have

$$K(x) = (x - 2)(x - 3)(x - 4).$$

The roots of $K(x) = 0$ are 2, 3, and 4. Since each root has multiplicity 1, it follows from the corollary to Theorem 3 that the general solution is

$$u_n = 2^n a + 3^n b + 4^n c; \qquad a, b, \text{ and } c \text{ arbitrary constants.}$$

We determine these constants specifically so as to satisfy the initial conditions by letting $n = 0, 1,$ and 2 in the general solution. This gives us the system of equations

$$\begin{cases} 6 = a + b + c \\ 17 = 2a + 3b + 4c \\ 53 = 4a + 9b + 16c. \end{cases}$$

Using elimination (or determinants) we find that

$$a = 3, \qquad b = 1, \qquad \text{and} \qquad c = 2.$$

Hence the specific solution is $u_n = 3 \cdot 2^n + 3^n + 2 \cdot 4^n$. $\square$

Example 7 Now we solve the problem of Example 6 by a somewhat different method. Let $G = u_0 + u_1 x + u_2 x^2 + \cdots$ be the generating series for $u_0, u_1, \ldots$. Using Theorem 1 ("Generating Function for H.L.R.W.C.C. Solutions"), we obtain $G = A/B$, where $B = 1 - 9x + 26x^2 - 24x^3$ and

$$\begin{aligned}
A &= u_0 + (u_1 + b_1 u_0)x + (u_2 + b_1 u_1 + b_2 u_0)x^2 \\
&= 6 + (17 - 9 \cdot 6)x + (53 - 9 \cdot 17 + 26 \cdot 6)x^2,
\end{aligned}$$

that is, $A(x) = 6 - 37x + 56x^2$. The factorization of $K(x)$ in Example 6 shows that $B = (1 - 2x)(1 - 3x)(1 - 4x)$. Theorem 1 ("Partial-Fractions Decomposition") of Section 8.3 tells us that $G = A/B$ is of the form

$$\frac{6 - 37x + 56x^2}{(1 - 2x)(1 - 3x)(1 - 4x)} = \frac{a}{1 - 2x} + \frac{b}{1 - 3x} + \frac{c}{1 - 4x},$$

with a, b, and c constants. Using the formula of Problem 31 of Section 8.3, we find that

$$a = \frac{A(\frac{1}{2})}{[1 - (\frac{3}{2})][1 - (\frac{4}{2})]} = \frac{6 - (\frac{37}{2}) + 14}{\frac{1}{2}} = \frac{\frac{3}{2}}{\frac{1}{2}} = 3,$$

$$b = \frac{A(\frac{1}{3})}{[1 - (\frac{2}{3})][1 - (\frac{4}{3})]} = \frac{6 - (\frac{37}{3}) + (\frac{56}{9})}{-\frac{1}{9}} = \frac{54 - 111 + 56}{-1} = \frac{-1}{-1} = 1,$$

$$c = \frac{A(\frac{1}{4})}{[1 - (\frac{2}{4})][1 - (\frac{3}{4})]} = \frac{6 - (\frac{37}{4}) + (\frac{56}{16})}{\frac{1}{8}} = 48 - 74 + 28 = 2.$$

Using these values and the fact that $1/(1 - rx) = 1 + rx + r^2 x^2 + \cdots$, we have $u_n = 3 \cdot 2^n + 3^n + 2 \cdot 4^n$. This agrees with Example 6. $\square$

Examples 6 and 7 apply the "only if" part of Theorem 3. Next we apply the "if" part.

Example 8 Given that $u_n = (5 + n^2)4^n + (-3)^n$, let us express the generating series $G = u_0 + u_1 x + \cdots$ as a proper x-fraction. It follows from Theorem 3 that u_n satisfies the H.L.R.W.C.C. whose characteristic polynomial and recursion polynomial are:

$$\begin{aligned}
K &= (x - 4)^3(x + 3) = (x^3 - 12x^2 + 48x - 64)(x + 3) \\
&= x^4 - 9x^3 + 12x^2 + 80x - 192,
\end{aligned}$$

$$B = 1 - 9x + 12x^2 + 80x^3 - 192x^4.$$

Now, Theorem 1 tells us that $G = A/B$, where A is a polynomial with degree at most 3, that is,

$$A = a_0 + a_1 x + a_2 x^2 + a_3 x^3, \tag{24}$$

with the a_i constants given in terms of u_0, u_1, u_2, and u_3 by formulas of Theorem 1. We tabulate u_n for the first four n's as follows:

n	$5 + n^2$	4^n	$(5 + n^2)4^n$	$(-3)^n$	u_n
0	5	1	5	1	6
1	6	4	24	-3	21
2	9	16	144	9	153
3	14	64	896	-27	869

Thus, $G = 6 + 21x + 153x^2 + 869x^3 + \cdots$, and so

$$A = BG = (1 - 9x + 12x^2 + 80x^3 - 192x^4)(6 + 21x + 153x^2 + 869x^3 + \cdots).$$

Since A has degree at most 3,

$$A = 1 \cdot 6 + (1 \cdot 21 - 9 \cdot 6)x + (1 \cdot 153 - 9 \cdot 21 + 12 \cdot 6)x^2 + (1 \cdot 869 - 9 \cdot 153 + 12 \cdot 21 + 80 \cdot 6)x^3$$
$$= 6 + (21 - 54)x + (153 - 189 + 72)x^2 + (869 - 1377 + 252 + 480)x^3$$
$$= 6 - 33x + 36x^2 + 224x^3.$$

The work here is as in the formula of Theorem 1 for A. Thus

$$G = \frac{A}{B} = \frac{6 - 33x + 36x^2 + 224x^3}{1 - 9x + 12x^2 + 80x^3 - 192x^4}. \qquad \square$$

Example 9   Here we find an explicit formula for the number $p_2(n)$ of partitions of an n in N into two parts. Let $u_n = p_2(n)$. Then Lemma 1 of Section 5.5 implies that $u_0, u_1, \ldots$ satisfies the initial conditions $u_0 = 1 = u_1$, $u_2 = 2$ and the third order H.L.R.W.C.C.

$$u_n - u_{n-1} - u_{n-2} + u_{n-3} = 0 \qquad \text{for } n \in \{3, 4, \ldots\}.$$

The characteristic polynomial for this recursion is

$$x^3 - x^2 - x + 1 = (x - 1)^2(x + 1).$$

Thus the characteristic roots are 1, a root of multiplicity two, and -1, a simple root. It now follows from Theorem 3 ("Explicit Solution with Polynomial Coefficients") that

$$u_n = a + bn + (-1)^n c$$

for some constants a, b, and c. Letting $n = 0, 1, 2$ and using the initial conditions, we get the system of equations

$$\begin{cases} 1 = a \quad\quad + c \\ 1 = a + \ b - c \\ 2 = a + 2b + c. \end{cases}$$

The solution of this system is $a = \frac{3}{4}$, $b = \frac{1}{2}$, $c = \frac{1}{4}$. Hence we have the explicit formula

$$u_n = p_2(n) = \frac{3}{4} + \frac{n}{2} + \frac{1}{4}(-1)^n. \qquad\qquad \square$$

We close this section with Table 9.4.1, which shows the nature of the general solution of a third order H.L.R.W.C.C.

$$u_n + b_1 u_{n-1} + b_2 u_{n-2} + b_3 u_{n-3} = 0 \qquad \text{for } n = \{3, 4, \ldots\} \qquad (25)$$

for all possible cases of equality or distinctness among the characteristic roots r, s, and t of the recursion. Let

$$1 + b_1 x + b_2 x^2 + b_3 x^3 = (1 - rx)(1 - sx)(1 - tx).$$

In the table, a, b, and c are arbitrary constants.

TABLE 9.4.1

Case	General Solution of Recursion (25)
$r \neq s, r \neq t$, and $s \neq t$	$u_n = ar^n + bs^n + ct^n$
$r = s$ and $r \neq t$	$u_n = (a + bn)r^n + ct^n$
$r = s = t$	$u_n = (a + bn + cn^2)r^n$

PROBLEMS FOR SECTION 9.4

1. For each of the following recursion formulas, give its order and tell whether it is linear. If it is linear, tell whether it is homogeneous and whether its coefficients are constants (that is, independent of n).
   (a) $u_n - (n - 1)u_{n-1} - (n - 1)u_{n-2} = 0$.
   (b) $u_n - 3u_{n-1} + 3u_{n-2} - u_{n-3} = 0$.
   (c) $u_n - u_{n-1}(u_{n-1} - 1) - 1 = 0$.
   (d) $u_n - u_{n-1} - u_{n-2} - 1 = 0$.

2. Do as in Problem 1 for the following recursions.
   (a) $u_n - 3u_{n-1} + 1 = 0$.   (b) $u_n - 5u_{n-1} + 6u_{n-2} = 0$.
   (c) $u_n - u_{n-1}^3 - u_{n-2}^2 - u_{n-3} = 0$.   (d) $u_n = nu_{n-1}$.
   (e) $u_n = 3u_{n-1} - 2u_{n-3}$.

3. Find u_3, u_4, and u_5 for the solution to the recursion of Problem 1(b) with $u_0 = 0$, $u_1 = 1$, and $u_2 = 4$. [*Hint:* First rewrite the recursion as $u_n = 3(u_{n-1} - u_{n-2}) + u_{n-3}$.]

4. Find u_1, u_2, and u_3 for the solution to the recursion of Problem 1(c) with $u_0 = 2$.

5. Let F_0, $F_1, \ldots$ be the Fibonacci Sequence 0, 1, 1, ... Prove by direct substitution that $u_n = F_{n+2} - 1$ satisfies the recursion of Problem 1(d).

6. Prove by direct substitution that $u_n = (3^n + 1)/2$ satisfies the recursion $u_n - 3u_{n-1} + 1 = 0$ for all n in $\mathbf{Z}^+$.

7. Let $G = u_0 + u_1 x + u_2 x^2 + \cdots$. Find u_n explicitly, given that:

(a) $G = \dfrac{1}{1 - 2x}$,   (b) $G = \dfrac{5}{(1 - 3x)^2}$,   (c) $G = \dfrac{5}{(1 + 2x)^3}$,

(d) $G = \dfrac{4}{(1 - 3x)^7}$,   (e) $G = \dfrac{4}{(1 - 3x)^7} - \dfrac{5}{(1 + 2x)^3}$.

8. Let $G = u_0 + u_1 x + \cdots$. Find u_n explicitly, given that:

(a) $G = \dfrac{1}{1 + 5x}$,   (b) $G = \dfrac{8}{(1 + 5x)^2}$,   (c) $G = \dfrac{5}{(1 - 7x)^6}$,

(d) $G = \dfrac{5}{(1 - 7x)^6} + \dfrac{8}{(1 + 5x)^2}$.

9. For the Fibonacci recursion $u_n - u_{n-1} - u_{n-2} = 0$, find:
(i) the recursion polynomial B and characteristic polynomial K;
(ii) each characteristic root, with its multiplicity.

10. Do as in Problem 9 for $u_n - 3u_{n-1} + 3u_{n-2} - u_{n-3} = 0$.

11. Let $K = (x + 4)(x - 5)^3$ be the characteristic polynomial for a homogeneous linear recursion of order 4.
(i) Give the recursion polynomial B.
(ii) Write out the recursion.
(iii) Write the general solution of the recursion.

12. Do as in Problem 11 for $K(x) = (x - 6)^3(x + 7)^2$.

13. Find the homogeneous linear recursion of order 4 with -3, -4, 2, and 5 as its characteristic roots.

14. Find constants b_1 and b_2 for the recursion $u_n + b_1 u_{n-1} + b_2 u_{n-2} = 0$ whose characteristic roots are $1 + \mathbf{i}$ and $1 - \mathbf{i}$. (Here, $\mathbf{i}^2 = -1$.)

15. Find b_1 and b_2 so that $u_n = c(-4)^n + k \cdot 9^n$ satisfies $u_n = -b_1 u_{n-1} - b_2 u_{n-2}$ for all constants c and k.

16. Do as in Problem 15 for $u_n = c \cdot 4^n + k(-9)^n$.

17. Find the general solution of the recursion

$$u_n - 5u_{n-1} - 14u_{n-2} = 0 \qquad \text{for } n \in \{2, 3, \ldots\}.$$

Then find the specific solution for each of the following sets of initial conditions:

(i) $u_0 = 1, u_1 = 7.$ (ii) $u_0 = 1, u_1 = -2.$
(iii) $u_0 = 2, u_1 = 5.$ [$Hint$: $1 + 1 = 2$ and $7 + (-2) = 5.$]
(iv) $u_0 = 0, u_1 = 9.$ (v) $u_0 = 3, u_1 = 3.$

18. Find the general solution of the recursion

$$u_n - 4u_{n-1} + 3u_{n-2} = 0 \qquad \text{for } n \in \{2, 3, \ldots\}.$$

Then find the specific solution for each set of initial conditions:

(i) $u_0 = 1, u_1 = 1.$ (ii) $u_0 = 1, u_1 = 3.$
(iii) $u_0 = 2, u_1 = 4.$ [See hint for Problem 17(iii).]
(iv) $u_0 = 0, u_1 = 2.$ (v) $u_0 = 1, u_1 = 2.$

19. Let the characteristic polynomial for a homogeneous linear recursion of order 4 be $K(x) = (x + 4)(x - 5)^3$. Let $u_0, u_1, \ldots$ satisfy the recursion. For each of the following sets of initial conditions, find u_n explicitly.
(i) $u_0 = 1, u_1 = 5, u_2 = 25, u_3 = 125.$
(ii) $u_0 = 2, u_1 = 10, u_2 = 50, u_3 = 250.$

20. Do as in Problem 19 for each of the following.
(i) $u_0 = 0, u_1 = 5, u_2 = 50, u_3 = 375.$
(ii) $u_0 = 0, u_1 = 10, u_2 = 100, u_3 = 750.$

21. Do as in Problem 19 for:
(i) $u_0 = 1, u_1 = -4, u_2 = 16, u_3 = -64.$
(ii) $u_0 = 3, u_1 = -12, u_2 = 48, u_3 = -192.$

22. Do as in Problem 19 for the initial conditions $u_0 = 1 + 1 = 2$, $u_1 = 5 - 4 = 1$, $u_2 = 25 + 16 = 41$, and $u_3 = 125 - 64 = 61$.

23. Which of the following sequences $u_0, u_1, \ldots$ satisfy

$$u_n = u_{n-1} + 5u_{n-2} \qquad \text{for } n = 2, 3, \text{ and } 4?$$

(a) $0, 1, 1, 6, 11, \ldots$ (b) $1, 0, 5, 5, 30, \ldots$
(c) $1, 1, 6, 11, 41, \ldots$ (d) $1, -1, 4, -1, 19, \ldots$
(e) $2, 3, 7, 8, 27, \ldots$

24. For each of the following sets of initial conditions, find u_2, u_3, and u_4 for the sequence satisfying the recursion

$$u_n = 3u_{n-1} - 2u_{n-2} \qquad \text{for } n \geq 2.$$

(a) $u_0 = 0, u_1 = 1;$ (b) $u_0 = 1, u_1 = 0;$
(c) $u_0 = 1, u_1 = 1;$ (d) $u_0 = 1, u_1 = -1;$
(e) $u_0 = c, u_1 = k$ (with c and k constants).

25. For each of the following recursions for $n \in \{2, 3, \ldots\}$, with accompanying initial conditions, find u_n specifically.
(a) $u_0 = 1, u_1 = 0,$ and $u_n = 5u_{n-1} - 6u_{n-2}.$
(b) $u_0 = 5, u_1 = -2,$ and $u_n + 4u_{n-1} + 4u_{n-2} = 0.$

(c) $u_0 = 1$, $u_1 = 3$, and $u_n = 6u_{n-1} - 13u_{n-2}$.

(d) $u_0 = 0$, $u_1 = 1$, and $u_n = 2u_{n-1} + u_{n-2}$.

26. Do as in Problem 25 for:

(a) $u_0 = 5$, $u_1 = 0$, and $u_n = u_{n-1} + 6u_{n-2}$.

(b) $u_0 = 2$, $u_1 = 15$, and $u_n - 10u_{n-1} + 25u_{n-2} = 0$.

(c) $u_0 = 0$, $u_1 = 1$, and $u_n = 3u_{n-1} - u_{n-2}$.

(d) $u_0 = 2$, $u_1 = 8$, and $u_n - 8u_{n-1} + 17u_{n-2} = 0$.

27. Find u_n specifically, given that $u_0 = 6$, $u_1 = 2$, $u_2 = 34$, and

$$u_n - 3u_{n-1} - 4u_{n-2} + 12u_{n-3} = 0 \qquad \text{for } n = 3, 4, \dots.$$

28. Find u_n specifically, given that $u_0 = 0$, $u_1 = 6$, $u_2 = 24$, and

$$u_n + u_{n-1} - 9u_{n-2} - 9u_{n-3} = 0 \qquad \text{for } n = 3, 4, \dots.$$

29. Express $G = u_0 + u_1 x + u_2 x^2 + \cdots$ as a proper x-fraction, given that:

(a) $u_n = 2$.   (b) $u_n = 7(-1)^n$.   (c) $u_n = n$.

(d) $u_n = 4 \cdot 3^n$.   (e) $u_n = 4 \cdot 3^n + 7(-1)^n$.   (f) $u_n = 2^n n$.

(g) $u_n = 2^n n - 4 \cdot 3^n$.

30. Do as in Problem 29 for:

(a) $u_n = -6$.   (b) $u_n = 4(-1)^n$.

(c) $u_n = (-4)^n$.   (d) $u_n = (7 - 6n)4^n$.

(e) $u_n = 1 + n^2$. (*Hint: r = 1.*)   (f) $u_n = 8 + (-4)^n$.

(g) $u_n = 3 \cdot 2^n - 2(-3)^n$.

31. Let $K(x) = (x - 1)(x + 1)(x - 2)(x + 2)$ be the characteristic polynomial for an H.L.R.W.C.C. of order 4 for $u_0, u_1, \dots$.

(i) Write the recursion.

(ii) Find u_4 given that $u_0 = 2$ and $u_2 = 1$. Then find u_6.

(iii) Find u_5 and u_7 given that $u_1 = -1$ and $u_3 = 3$.

(iv) Find a formula for u_n given that $u_0 = 2$, $u_1 = -1$, $u_2 = 1$, and $u_3 = 3$.

32. Let $K(x) = (x - 3)(x + 1)(x + 2)$ be the characteristic polynomial for an H.L.R.W.C.C. of order 3 for $u_0, u_1, \dots$.

(i) Write the recursion.

(ii) Find u_3 and u_4 given that $u_0 = 2$, $u_1 = 0$, $u_2 = 16$.

(iii) Find a formula for u_n for the initial conditions of Part (ii).

33. Let $G = u_0 + u_1 x + u_2 x^2 + \cdots$ with $u_1 = (5 - 4n + n^2)(-7)^n + 4^n$. Express G as a proper x-fraction.

34. Do as in Problem 33 for $u_n = 3 \cdot 2^n - 2(-3)^n + (7 - 6n)4^n$.

35. Let $(6 - 13x)/(1 - 2x + 9x^2)$ be the generating function for $u_0, u_1, \dots$. Use Theorem 3 ("Generating Series for Partial Sums") of Section 9.1 to find the generating function for $v_0, v_1, \dots$ where

$$v_0 = u_0, \qquad v_1 = u_0 + u_1, \qquad \dots, \qquad v_n = u_0 + u_1 + \cdots + u_n, \qquad \dots.$$

36. Let $(4 - 3x)/[(1 - x)(1 + x - x^3)]$ be the generating function for u_0, $u_1, \ldots$ and let

$$w_0 = u_0, \qquad w_1 = u_1 - u_0, \qquad \ldots, \qquad w_n = u_n - u_{n-1}, \qquad \ldots.$$

Use Theorem 1 ("Differencing") of Section 9.1 to find the generating function for $w_0, w_1, \ldots$.

37. Let $G = u_0 + u_1 x + u_2 x^2 + \cdots$, where $u_0 = 1$ and

$$u_n = u_0 u_{n-1} + u_1 u_{n-2} + u_2 u_{n-3} + \cdots + u_{n-1} u_0 \qquad \text{for } n \text{ in } \mathbf{Z}^+.$$

(i) Explain why this recursion does not have an order.
(ii) Note that the recursion implies that $u_1 = u_0^2$, $u_2 = u_0 u_1 + u_1 u_0$, and $u_3 = u_0 u_2 + u_1 u_1 + u_2 u_0$. Find similar formulas for u_4 and u_5.
(iii) Show that $1 + xG^2 = G$.

38. Let $V = x + x^2 + 2x^3 + \cdots + F_n x^n + \cdots$ and $W = 2 + x + 3x^2 + \cdots + L_n x^n + \cdots$, where F_n and L_n denote, respectively, Fibonacci Numbers and Lucas Numbers. Let $u_0 = F_0 L_0$, $u_1 = F_0 L_1 + F_1 L_0, \ldots, u_n = F_0 L_n + F_1 L_{n-1} + F_2 L_{n-2} + \cdots + F_n L_0, \ldots$. Express each of the following as a proper x-fraction.

(i) V. (See Problem 19 of Section 9.1.)
(ii) W.
(iii) $M = VW = u_0 + u_1 x + \cdots + u_n x^n + \cdots$.

39. Let $v_0, v_1, \ldots$ and $w_0, w_1, \ldots$ be sequences such that each of $u_n = v_n$ and $u_n = w_n$ satisfies the homogeneous linear recursion

$$u_n + b_1 u_{n-1} + b_2 u_{n-2} + \cdots + b_d u_{n-d} = 0 \qquad \text{for } n = d, d + 1, \ldots.$$

Show that $u_n = v_n + w_n$ also satisfies this recursion.

40. Let $u_n = v_n$ satisfy the recursion of Problem 39. Prove that $u_n = cv_n$ also satisfies the recursion for all constants c.

41. Let $v_0, v_1, \ldots$ and $w_0, w_1, \ldots$ be sequences such that each of $u_n = v_n$ and $u_n = w_n$ satisfies the recursion

$$u_n + b_1 u_{n-1} + b_2 u_{n-2} + \cdots + b_d u_{n-d} = 0 \qquad \text{for } n = d, d + 1, \ldots.$$

Show that $u_n = c_1 v_n + c_2 w_n$ satisfies this recursion for all constants c_1 and c_2.

42. State and prove the analogue of Problem 41 for a linear combination $c_1 v_n + c_2 w_n + c_3 z_n$.

43. Let $r = 3 + 4i$ and $s = 3 - 4i$ (where $i^2 = -1$). Show that:
(i) the recursion $u_n - 6u_{n-1} + 25u_{n-2} = 0$ has $K = (x - r)(x - s)$ as its characteristic polynomial.
(ii) every solution $u_0, u_1, \ldots$ of the recursion has $u_n = cr^n + ks^n$ for some constants c and k.

44. Let $r = 3 + 4i$, $s = 3 - 4i$, α be the acute angle with $\cos \alpha = \frac{3}{5}$ (and $\sin \alpha = \frac{4}{5}$), and $e = 2.71828\ldots$ be the base of natural logarithms. Also, assume that $e^{\beta i} = \cos \beta + i \sin \beta$ for all real numbers β. Show that:

(i) $r = 5e^{\alpha i}$ and $s = 5e^{-\alpha i}$.

(ii) every solution $u_0, u_1, \ldots$ of the recursion of Problem 43(i) has $u_n = c_1 \cdot 5^n \cos(n\alpha) + c_2 \cdot 5^n \sin(n\alpha)$ for some constants c_1 and c_2. [*Hint*: Use Problem 43(ii) and Theorem 4 (De Moivre's Theorem) of Section 4.2.]

45. Generalize the result in Problem 41 by replacing each b_i with a function $b_i(n)$.

46. Generalize the result in Problem 42 by replacing each b_i with a function $b_i(n)$.

9.5

NONHOMOGENEOUS LINEAR RECURSIONS OF ALL ORDERS

In this section, we show how to solve dth order linear recursions

$$v_n + b_1 v_{n-1} + b_2 v_{n-2} + \cdots + b_d v_{n-d} = g_n; \qquad n \in \{d, d+1, \ldots\}, \qquad (1)$$

where the b_i are known constants, $b_d \neq 0$, and

$$g_n = A(n)r^n + B(n)s^n + \cdots + C(n)t^n \qquad (2)$$

for known constants $r, s, \ldots, t$ and known polynomials $A(n), B(n), \ldots, C(n)$. We recall from Theorem 3, "Explicit Solution with Polynomial Coefficients," of Section 9.4 that a sequence $g_d, g_{d+1}, \ldots$ has a rule of the form shown in Display (2) if and only if it satisfies an H.L.R.W.C.C. (that is, a homogeneous linear recursion with constant coefficients).

The recursion

$$v_n - 3v_{n-1} + 2v_{n-2} = \frac{1}{n}; \qquad n \in \{2, 3, \ldots\}$$

is not of the type shown in Displays (1) and (2), since $g_n = 1/n$ is not of the form given in Display (2). On the other hand, the recursion

$$v_n - 3v_{n-1} + 2v_{n-2} = (7 - 6n)2^n + (5 + 4n - 3n^2)(-5)^n;$$

$$n \in \{2, 3, \ldots\}$$

is of the type shown in Displays (1) and (2) and can be solved by the methods of this section.

It usually helps in solving a recursion of the type shown in Display (1) to consider the H.L.R.W.C.C.

$$u_n + b_1 u_{n-1} + b_2 u_{n-2} + \cdots + b_d u_{n-d} = 0; \qquad n \in \{d, d+1, \ldots\}, \qquad (3)$$

which we can solve by the methods of Section 9.4.

DEFINITION 1   **ASSOCIATED HOMOGENEOUS RECURSION**

The *associated homogeneous recursion* for Recursion (1) is Recursion (3). The *characteristic polynomial and roots* for Recursion (1) are the same as those for Recursion (3).

The following two results enable us to use the solution of the associated homogeneous Recursion (3) as an aid in solving a nonhomogeneous Recursion (1). One indication of the importance of the next lemma is seen when one thinks of $v_0, v_1, \ldots$ as a sought solution to Recursion (1) (for example, a solution satisfying given initial conditions); of $w_0, w_1, \ldots$ as a particular solution to Recursion (1) that one can find more easily; and of $u_0, u_1, \ldots$ as a solution to the H.L.R.W.C.C. (3) that can be obtained by the methods of Section 9.4.

LEMMA 1   **DIFFERENCE OF SOLUTIONS**

Let $v_0, v_1, \ldots$ and $w_0, w_1, \ldots$ be sequences each satisfying the nonhomogeneous Recursion (1). Then the sequence $u_0, u_1, \ldots$ with $u_n = v_n - w_n$ satisfies the associated homogeneous Recursion (3).

PROOF   For $n \in \{d, d + 1, \ldots\}$, the hypothesis is that

$$v_n + b_1 v_{n-1} + b_2 v_{n-2} + \cdots + b_d v_{n-d} = g_n,$$
$$w_n + b_1 w_{n-1} + b_2 w_{n-2} + \cdots + b_d w_{n-d} = g_n.$$

We subtract and let each $v_k - w_k = u_k$. This gives us the claimed homogeneous recursion

$$u_n + b_1 u_{n-1} + b_2 u_{n-2} + \cdots + b_d u_{n-d} = 0. \qquad \square$$

For example, the difference $v_0 - w_0, v_1 - w_1, \ldots$ of solutions $v_0, v_1, \ldots$ and $w_0, w_1, \ldots$ of the nonhomogeneous recursion

$$v_n - v_{n-1} - 6v_{n-2} = 5 \cdot 4^n; \qquad n \in \{2, 3, \ldots\}$$

satisfies the associated homogeneous recursion

$$u_n - u_{n-1} - 6u_{n-2} = 0; \qquad n \in \{2, 3, \ldots\}.$$

The following result is a reinterpretation of Lemma 1.

THEOREM 1   **GENERAL SOLUTION FROM A PARTICULAR SOLUTION**

Every solution $v_0, v_1, \ldots$ of a nonhomogeneous Recursion (1) is expressible as $w_0 + u_0, w_1 + u_1, \ldots$, where $w_0, w_1, \ldots$ is one particular solution to the nonhomogeneous Recursion (1) and $u_0, u_1, \ldots$ is a solution to the associated homogeneous Recursion (3).

PROOF   This follows by rewriting the formula $u_n = v_n - w_n$ of Lemma 1 as $v_n = w_n + u_n$ and thinking of the sequence $w_0, w_1, \ldots$ as a fixed solution to Recursion (1).   □

Example 1   Here we solve the recursion

$$v_n - v_{n-1} - 6v_{n-2} = 5 \cdot 4^n; \qquad n \in \{2, 3, \ldots\}. \tag{4}$$

This is the special case of the recursion in Display (1) with $d = 2$, $b_1 = -1$, $b_2 = -6$, and $g_n = 5 \cdot 4^n$. We will soon see that a particular solution to Recursion (4) exists in the form $w_n = 4^n c$, with c a constant to be determined by substituting

$$v_n = 4^n c, \qquad v_{n-1} = 4^{n-1} c, \qquad v_{n-2} = 4^{n-2} c$$

into Recursion (4). These substitutions give us

$$4^n c - 4^{n-1} c - 6 \cdot 4^{n-2} c = 5 \cdot 4^n.$$

We divide by 4^{n-2} and get

$$16c - 4c - 6c = 5 \cdot 16.$$

Then $6c = 80$ and $c = \frac{40}{3}$. Hence we have found by actual substitution that

$$w_n = \frac{40}{3} \cdot 4^n$$

is a particular solution to Recursion (4). The associated homogeneous recursion

$$u_n - u_{n-1} - 6u_{n-2} = 0; \qquad n \in \{2, 3, \ldots\}, \tag{5}$$

for Recursion (4) has $x^2 - x - 6 = (x - 3)(x + 2)$ as its characteristic polynomial. Thus the characteristic roots are 3 and -2, each with multiplicity one, and it follows from the corollary ("Case of Simple Roots") to Theorem 3 of Section 9.4 that

$$u_n = 3^n a + (-2)^n b, \qquad a \text{ and } b \text{ arbitrary constants,}$$

is its general solution. Now Theorem 1 above implies that every solution of Recursion (4) has a rule of the form

$$v_n = \frac{40}{3} \cdot 4^n + 3^n a + (-2)^n b, \qquad a \text{ and } b \text{ constants.}$$

We summarize by noting that all solutions $v_0, v_1, \ldots$ to Recursion (4) are given by $v_n = w_n + u_n$, where $w_0, w_1, \ldots$ is any particular solution to Recursion (4) and u_n stands for the general solution of the associated homogeneous Recursion (5).

If we want the specific solution that satisfies the initial conditions

$$v_0 = -2, \qquad v_1 = 3,$$

then we determine the constants a and b as follows: We rewrite the above solution as

$$3^n a + (-2)^n b = v_n - \frac{40}{3} \cdot 4^n.$$

We substitute $n = 0$ and $n = 1$ in this to get the system of equations

$$\begin{cases} a + b = -2 - \dfrac{40}{3} = -\dfrac{46}{3} \\[2mm] 3a - 2b = 3 - \dfrac{160}{3} = -\dfrac{151}{3}. \end{cases}$$

Multiplying the first of these equations by 2 and adding to the second gives us

$$5a = -\frac{92}{3} - \frac{151}{3} = -\frac{243}{3} = -81.$$

Hence $a = -\frac{81}{5}$. Then

$$b = -\frac{46}{3} - a = -\frac{46}{3} + \frac{81}{5} = \frac{-230 + 243}{15} = \frac{13}{15}.$$

Thus the desired specific solutions for the given initial conditions is

$$v_n = \frac{40}{3} \cdot 4^n - \frac{81}{5} \cdot 3^n + \frac{13}{15}(-2)^n.$$

We check this by obtaining v_2 both from this closed form and from the recursion, as follows:

$$v_2 = \frac{40}{3} \cdot 16 - \frac{81}{5} \cdot 9 + \frac{13}{15} \cdot 4 = \frac{3200 - 2187 + 52}{15} = \frac{1065}{15} = 71,$$

$$v_2 = v_1 + 6v_0 + 5 \cdot 16 = 3 - 12 + 80 = 71. \qquad \qquad \square$$

It follows from Theorem 1 that if $w_0, w_1, \ldots$ is a particular solution to a dth order nonhomogeneous recursion

$$v_n + b_1 v_{n-1} + b_2 v_{n-2} + \cdots + b_d v_{n-d} = g_n; \qquad n \in \{d, d+1, \ldots\}, \qquad (6)$$

then every solution $v_0, v_1, \ldots$ to Recursion (6) is given by

$$v_n = w_n + u_n,$$

where u_n is the general solution, involving d arbitrary constants, to the associated homogeneous recursion

$$u_n + b_1 u_{n-1} + b_2 u_{n-2} + \cdots + b_d u_{n-d} = 0; \qquad n \in \{d, d+1, \ldots\}. \qquad (7)$$

DEFINITION 2   **GENERAL SOLUTION, SPECIFIC SOLUTION**

The **general solution** to Recursion (6) is $v_n = w_n + u_n$, with $w_0, w_1, \ldots$ a particular solution to Recursion (6) and u_n the general solution (involving d arbitrary constants) to the associated homogeneous Recursion (7). When these d constants are determined specifically from conditions such as given values of $v_0, v_1, \ldots, v_{d-1}$, then $v_0, v_1, \ldots$ is the **specific solution** for these given conditions.

Example 2   Here we solve the nonhomogeneous linear recursion

$$v_n - v_{n-1} - 6v_{n-2} = 3^n \qquad \text{for } n \in \{2, 3, \ldots\}. \qquad (8)$$

This recursion and Recursion (4) have the same associated homogeneous recursion

$$u_n - u_{n-1} - 6u_{n-2} = 0 \qquad \text{for } n \in \{2, 3, \ldots\}. \qquad (9)$$

We noted in Example 1 that the characteristic polynomial for Recursion (4) is

$$H(x) = x^2 - x - 6 = (x - 3)(x + 2) \qquad (10)$$

and that the general solution of Recursion (9) is

$$u_n = 3^n a + (-2)^n b, \qquad \text{with } a \text{ and } b \text{ arbitrary constants.}$$

It now follows from Theorem 1 that the general solution of Recursion (8) can be written as

$$v_n = w_n + 3^n a + (-2)^n b, \qquad \text{with } a \text{ and } b \text{ constants,} \qquad (11)$$

if one can find a particular solution w_n to Recursion (8). If we try for w_n in the form $3^n c$, with c a constant, we will not succeed, since $u_n = 3^n c$ satisfies the associated homogeneous Recursion (9) and hence the substitution $v_n = 3^n c$ in Recursion (8) will lead to the contradiction $0 = 3^n$. Thus the method of Example 1 has to be modified, as follows.

We replace n by $n - 1$ in Recursion (8) and multiply by -3; this gives us

$$-3v_{n-1} + 3v_{n-2} + 18v_{n-3} = -3 \cdot 3^{n-1} = -3^n.$$

This and Recursion (8) can be arranged as the following system of equations:

$$\begin{cases} v_n - v_{n-1} - 6v_{n-2} &= 3^n, \qquad\qquad (12) \\ -3v_{n-1} + 3v_{n-2} + 18v_{n-3} = -3^n. \qquad (13) \end{cases}$$

We add these equations and get the third order H.L.R.W.C.C.

$$v_n - 4v_{n-1} - 3v_{n-2} + 18v_{n-3} = 0. \qquad (14)$$

We can see from the way that Recursion (14) is obtained from Equations (12) and (13) that the characteristic polynomial $K(x)$ for Recursion (14) is

$$K(x) = (x - 3)H(x) = (x - 3)^2(x + 2), \qquad (15)$$

where $H(x)$ is the characteristic polynomial for Recursion (8) given in Display (10). Thus the characteristic roots for Recursion (14) are 3 and -2, with 3 a root of multiplicity two. These facts and Theorem 3 ("Explicit Solution with Polynomial Coefficients") of Section 9.4 tell us that the general solution of Recursion (14) is

$$v_n = (a + cn)3^n + (-2)^n b, \qquad \text{with } a, b, \text{ and } c \text{ constants.}$$

We compare this with Display (10) and thus see that the desired particular solution to Recursion (8) should be sought in the form

$$w_n = 3^n nc, \qquad \text{with } c \text{ a constant.}$$

So we substitute $3^n nc$ for v_n in Recursion (8). This means that we must also replace v_{n-1} by $3^{n-1}(n - 1)c$ and v_{n-2} by $3^{n-2}(n - 2)c$. Then we get

$$3^n nc - 3^{n-1}(n - 1)c - 6 \cdot 3^{n-2}(n - 2)c = 3^n.$$

We divide by 3^{n-2} and factor out c on the left-hand side. This gives us

$$[9n - 3(n - 1) - 6(n - 2)]c = 9,$$
$$[(9 - 3 - 6)n + (3 + 12)]c = 9,$$
$$15c = 9.$$

Thus $c = \frac{9}{15} = \frac{3}{5}$, and so

$$w_n = \left(\frac{3}{5}\right)3^n n$$

is a particular solution to our original nonhomogeneous Recursion (8). Hence the general solution to Recursion (8) is

$$v_n = \frac{3}{5}3^n n + 3^n a + (-2)^n b, \qquad a \text{ and } b \text{ arbitrary constants.} \qquad (16)$$

Now let us seek the specific solution for the initial conditions

$$v_0 = 1 \quad \text{and} \quad v_1 = 2.$$

We substitute $n = 0$ and $n = 1$ in the general solution in Display (16) and get the system of equations

$$\begin{cases} 1 = a + b \\ 2 = \dfrac{9}{5} + 3a - 2b. \end{cases}$$

The first of these equations gives us $b = 1 - a$. Substituting this in the second equation leads to

$$2 = \frac{9}{5} + 3a - 2(1 - a) = 5a - \frac{1}{5}.$$

Then

$$5a = 2 + \frac{1}{5} = \frac{10 + 1}{5} = \frac{11}{5}$$

and so $a = \frac{11}{25}$ and $b = 1 - a = \frac{14}{25}$. Hence the specific solution for the given initial conditions is

$$v_n = \frac{3}{5} \cdot 3^n n + \frac{11}{25} \cdot 3^n + \frac{14}{25}(-2)^n. \tag{17}$$

$\square$

Generalizing on Examples 1 and 2, we now give the form of a particular solution to a nonhomogeneous linear recursion with constant coefficients for certain right-hand sides g_n.

THEOREM 2 **FORM OF A PARTICULAR SOLUTION**

Let r be a complex number and $P(n)$ be a polynomial in n of degree p. Let $K(x)$ be the characteristic polynomial for the nonhomogeneous linear recursion with constant coefficients

$$v_n + b_1 v_{n-1} + b_2 v_{n-2} + \cdots + b_d v_{n-d} = r^n P(n). \tag{18}$$

If r is a root of $K(x) = 0$, let m be its multiplicity; otherwise let $m = 0$. Then a particular solution to Recursion (18) has the form

$$w_n = r^n(c_0 n^m + c_1 n^{m+1} + \cdots + c_p n^{m+p}), \tag{19}$$

where the c_i are constants to be determined by substitution in Recursion (18).

The proof is illustrated in Example 2 and is omitted.

Example 3   Here we solve the nonhomogeneous recursion

$$v_n + 3v_{n-1} - 10v_{n-2} = (-7)^n n. \tag{20}$$

The associated homogeneous recursion is

$$u_n + 3u_{n-1} - 10u_{n-2} = 0. \tag{21}$$

The characteristic polynomial for Recursion (20), or for Recursion (21), is

$$K(x) = x^2 + 3x - 10 = (x + 5)(x - 2).$$

We are dealing with a special case of Recursion (18) with $r = -7$ and $p = 1$. Since -7 is not a root of $K(x) = 0$, the m of (19) equals 0. Hence the w_n of Display (19) for our desired particular solution to Recursion (20) should be of the form

$$w_n = (-7)^n(c_0 + c_1 n), \qquad c_0 \text{ and } c_1 \text{ to be found.}$$

Substituting this in Recursion (20), we get

$$(-7)^n[c_0 + c_1 n] + 3(-7)^{n-1}[c_0 + c_1(n-1)] - 10(-7)^{n-2}[c_0 + c_1(n-2)] = (-7)^n n.$$

Dividing by $(-7)^{n-2}$ gives us

$$49[c_0 + c_1 n] - 21[c_0 + c_1(n-1)] - 10[c_0 + c_1(n-2)] = 49n.$$

Writing the left-hand side in the form $An + B$, this becomes

$$(49c_1 - 21c_1 - 10c_1)n + (49c_0 - 21c_0 + 21c_1 - 10c_0 + 20c_1) = 49n,$$

which simplifies to

$$18c_1 n + (18c_0 + 41c_1) = 49n.$$

This is satisfied for all n if

$$18c_1 = 49 \qquad \text{and} \qquad 18c_0 + 41c_1 = 0.$$

Hence we let $c_1 = \frac{49}{18}$ and solve

$$18c_0 + 41\left(\frac{49}{18}\right) = 0$$

to find that $c_0 = -41 \cdot 49/(18)^2 = -2009/324$. Thus a particular solution to Recursion (20) is

$$w_n = (-7)^n\left[\frac{-2009}{324} + \left(\frac{49}{18}\right)n\right].$$

Since every solution of the associated homogeneous Recursion (21) is of the form

$$u_n = (-5)^n a + 2^n b, \qquad \text{with } a \text{ and } b \text{ arbitrary constants,}$$

every solution of Recursion (20) has the form

$$v_n = (-7)^n\left[\frac{-2009}{324} + \left(\frac{49}{18}\right)n\right] + (-5)^n a + 2^n b. \qquad \square$$

Example 4   Here we solve the nonhomogeneous recursion

$$v_n + 3v_{n-1} - 10v_{n-2} = 2^n(5 + n). \tag{22}$$

The associated homogeneous recursion is the same as in Example 3, and its characteristic polynomial is

$$K(x) = x^2 + 3x - 10 = (x + 5)(x - 2).$$

Recursion (22) is a special case of Recursion (18) with $r = 2$ and $p = 1$. Since 2 is a root of $K(x) = 0$ with multiplicity 1, the m of Display (19) is 1. Thus we look for a particular solution to Recursion (22) of the form

$$w_n = 2^n(c_0 n + c_1 n^2), \qquad c_0 \text{ and } c_1 \text{ to be determined.}$$

Substituting this into Recursion (22) gives us

$$2^n(c_0 n + c_1 n^2) + 3 \cdot 2^{n-1}[c_0(n - 1) + c_1(n - 1)^2] - 10 \cdot 2^{n-2}[c_0(n - 2) + c_1(n - 2)^2] = 2^n(5 + n).$$

Dividing by 2^{n-2} results in

$$4(c_0 n + c_1 n^2) + 6[c_0(n - 1) + c_1(n - 1)^2] - 10[c_0(n - 2) + c_1(n - 2)^2] = 20 + 4n. \tag{23}$$

Since we want this to be true for $n = 2, 3, \ldots$, we substitute $n = 2$ and $n = 3$ in Equation (23) and obtain

$$4(2c_0 + 4c_1) + 6(c_0 + c_1) = 28,$$
$$4(3c_0 + 9c_1) + 6(2c_0 + 4c_1) - 10(c_0 + c_1) = 32.$$

These equations simplify to

$$14c_0 + 22c_1 = 28,$$
$$14c_0 + 50c_1 = 32.$$

Subtracting the first of these equations from the second gives $28c_1 = 4$, or $c_1 = \frac{1}{7}$. Substituting this into one of the equations leads to $c_0 = \frac{87}{49}$. It can be shown that these values make Equation (23) true for all n in $\{2, 3, \ldots\}$. Hence a particular solution to Recursion (22) is

$$w_n = 2^n\left(\frac{87}{49} n + \frac{1}{7} n^2\right).$$

Using the solution to the associated homogeneous recursion found in Example 3, we see that every solution of Recursion (22) has the form

$$v_n = 2^n\left(\frac{87}{49} n + \frac{1}{7} n^2\right) + (-5)^n a + 2^n b,$$

with a and b arbitrary constants. $\square$

Example 5   Here we solve the recursion

$$v_n - 3v_{n-1} + 2v_{n-2} = 6n^2 \qquad \text{for } n \text{ in } \{2, 3, \ldots\} \tag{24}$$

together with the initial conditions

$$v_0 = 6, \qquad v_1 = 7. \tag{25}$$

The characteristic polynomial is

$$K(x) = x^2 - 3x + 2 = (x - 1)(x - 2).$$

In the notation of Theorem 2, $g_n = 6n^2$ has $r = 1$, $p = 2$, and $m = 1$. Also, Recursion (24) shows that the order $d = 2$. Hence a particular solution to Recursion (24) exists in the form

$$w_n = an + bn^2 + cn^3, \qquad \text{with } a, b, \text{ and } c \text{ to be found.}$$

Substituting this into Recursion (24), we have for $n \in \{2, 3, \ldots\}$,

$$(an + bn^2 + cn^3) - 3[a(n-1) + b(n-1)^2 + c(n-1)^3] + 2[a(n-2) + b(n-2)^2 + c(n-2)^3] = 6n^2.$$

Letting $n = d$, $d + 1$, and $d + 2$, that is, letting $n = 2$, 3, and 4 in this, gives the system

$$\begin{cases} (2a + 4b + 8c) - 3(a + b + c) & = 24 \\ (3a + 9b + 27c) - 3(2a + 4b + 8c) + 2(a + b + c) & = 54 \\ (4a + 16b + 64c) - 3(3a + 9b + 27c) + 2(2a + 4b + 8c) & = 96. \end{cases}$$

These equations can be simplified to

$$\begin{cases} -a + b + 5c = 24 \\ -a - b + 5c = 54 \\ -a - 3b - c = 96. \end{cases}$$

Subtracting the second of these equations from the first, we get $2b = -30$, and so $b = -15$. Subtracting the third from the first gives us $4b + 6c = -72$. This and $b = -15$ lead to

$$-60 + 6c = -72,$$
$$6c = -12,$$
$$c = -2.$$

Then, using the first equation, we get

$$a = b + 5c - 24 = -15 - 10 - 24 = -49.$$

Hence a particular solution to Recursion (24) is

$$w_n = -49n - 15n^2 - 2n^3.$$

Since the complete solution to the associated homogeneous recursion for Recursion (24) is

$$u_n = d + 2^n e, \qquad \text{with } d \text{ and } e \text{ arbitrary constants,}$$

every solution of Recursion (24) is of the form

$$v_n = -49n - 15n^2 - 2n^3 + d + 2^n e.$$

Letting $n = 0$ and 1 and using the initial conditions in Display (25) gives us

$$6 = d + e$$
$$7 = -49 - 15 - 2 + d + 2e.$$

These simplify to

$$d + e = 6$$
$$d + 2e = 73.$$

Subtracting the first equation from the second gives us $e = 67$. Then $d + 67 = 6$ leads to $d = -61$. Hence the specific solution to the recursion with initial conditions given in Displays (24) and (25) is

$$v_n = -61 + 67 \cdot 2^n - 49n - 15n^2 - 2n^3. \qquad \square$$

The following result sometimes simplifies the algebra of obtaining a particular solution to a nonhomogeneous linear recursion when the right-hand side is a sum of several terms.

THEOREM 3   **SAME ASSOCIATED HOMOGENEOUS RECURSION**

Let $y_0, y_1, \ldots$ be a particular solution to

$$v_n + b_1 v_{n-1} + b_2 v_{n-2} + \cdots + b_d v_{n-d} = f_n$$

and $z_0, z_1, \ldots$ be a particular solution to

$$v_n + b_1 v_{n-1} + b_2 v_{n-2} + \cdots + b_d v_{n-d} = g_n.$$

Let h and k be constants. Then $w_n = hy_n + kz_n$ is a particular solution to

$$v_n + b_1 v_{n-1} + \cdots + b_d v_{n-d} = hf_n + kg_n.$$

PROOF   The hypotheses tell us that

$$y_n + b_1 y_{n-1} + b_2 y_{n-2} + \cdots + b_d y_{n-d} = f_n,$$
$$z_n + b_1 z_{n-1} + b_2 z_{n-2} + \cdots + b_d z_{n-d} = g_n.$$

Multiplying the first of these by h and the second by k and then adding, we find that $w_n = hy_n + kz_n$ satisfies

$$w_n + b_1 w_{n-1} + b_2 w_{n-2} + \cdots + b_d w_{n-d} = hf_n + kg_n,$$

as claimed. $\square$

Example 6   Here we solve

$$v_n - v_{n-1} - 6v_{n-2} = 10 \cdot 4^n - 7 \cdot 3^n, \qquad n \in \{2, 3, \ldots\}. \tag{26}$$

We note that the nonhomogeneous Recursions (4), (8), and (26) of Examples 1, 2, and 6, respectively, all have the same associated homogeneous recursion

$$u_n - u_{n-1} - 6u_{n-2} = 0. \tag{27}$$

Let $f_n = 5 \cdot 4^n$ be the right-hand side of Recursion (4) and $g_n = 3^n$ be the right-hand side of Recursion (8). Then the right-hand side of Recursion (26) is $2f_n - 7g_n$. It follows from Theorem 3 that a particular solution to Recursion (26) is

$$w_n = 2\left(\frac{40}{3}\right)4^n - 7\left(\frac{3}{5}\right)3^n n = 2y_n - 7z_n,$$

where $y_n = (\frac{40}{3})4^n$ and $z_n = (\frac{3}{5})3^n n$ are the particular solutions to Recursions (4) and (8), respectively, found in Examples 1 and 2. Since the general solution of the associated homogeneous Recursion (27) is

$$u_n = (-2)^n a + 3^n b, \qquad \text{with } a \text{ and } b \text{ arbitrary constants,}$$

it follows from Theorem 1 ("General Solution from a Particular Solution") that the general solution of Recursion (26) is

$$v_n = \frac{80}{3} \cdot 4^n - \frac{21}{5} \cdot 3^n n + (-2)^n a + 3^n b. \tag{28}$$

If one wants the specific solution of Recursion (26) that satisfies the initial conditions

$$v_0 = 27, \qquad v_1 = \frac{1426}{15}, \tag{29}$$

one substitutes $n = 0$ and $n = 1$ in Equation (28) and solves for a and b. This can be shown to result in $a = 0$ and $b = \frac{1}{3}$. Then the specific solution for the initial conditions in Display (29) is

$$v_n = \frac{80}{3} \cdot 4^n - \frac{21}{5} \cdot 3^n n + \frac{1}{3} \cdot 3^n = \frac{80}{3} \cdot 4^n + \left(\frac{1}{3} - \frac{21}{5}n\right)3^n. \qquad \square$$

PROBLEMS FOR SECTION 9.5

1. Solve $v_n - 4v_{n-1} = 5^n$; that is, find the general solution.

2. Solve $v_n + 6v_{n-1} = 5 \cdot 3^n$.

3. Solve $v_n - 4v_{n-1} = 4^n$.

4.   Solve $v_n + 6v_{n-1} = 4(-6)^n$.

5.   Use the answers to Problems 1 and 3 and Theorem 3 to solve

$$v_n - 4v_{n-1} = 2 \cdot 5^n - 3 \cdot 4^n.$$

6.   Do as in Problem 5 for $v_n - 4v_{n-1} = 7 \cdot 4^n - 6 \cdot 5^n$.

7.   Solve $v_n + 6v_{n-1} = (-6)^n(2n - 3n^2)$.

8.   Solve $v_n - 4v_{n-1} = 4^n(n - n^2)$.

9.   Solve each of the following.
(a) $v_n - v_{n-1} = 2^n$.
(b) $v_n - v_{n-1} = 3$.   [Here the r of Display (19) equals 1.]
(c) $v_n - v_{n-1} = 4n^3 - 6n^2 + 4n - 1$.

10.   Solve each of the following.
(a) $v_n - v_{n-1} = 3^n$.   (b) $v_n - v_{n-1} = 2$.   (c) $v_n - v_{n-1} = 6n^2$.

11.   For each of the following nonhomogeneous linear recursions, find the characteristic roots; their multiplicities; and the r, p, and m of Theorem 2, "Form of a Particular Solution."
(a) $v_n - 7v_{n-1} + 10v_{n-2} = 3^n(2 - n^2)$.
(b) $v_n - 7v_{n-1} + 10v_{n-2} = 2^n(n + n^3)$.

12.   Do as in Problem 11 for:
(a) $v_n + 5v_{n-1} + 4v_{n-2} = 2^n(3 - 4n)$.
(b) $v_n + 5v_{n-1} + 4v_{n-2} = (-1)^n(2n - 3n^2)$.

13.   For the recursion of Problem 11(a), express a particular solution in terms of constants to be determined.

14.   Do as in Problem 13 for the recursion of Problem 11(b).

15.   Solve the following recursions; that is, find their general solutions.
(i) $v_n - 7v_{n-1} + 12v_{n-2} = 2^n$.   (ii) $v_n - 7v_{n-1} + 12v_{n-2} = 3^n$.
(iii) $v_n - 7v_{n-1} + 12v_{n-2} = 5 \cdot 2^n - 4 \cdot 3^n$.

16.   Solve the recursion $v_n + 2v_{n-1} - 8v_{n-2} = g_n$ for:
(i) $g_n = 7 \cdot 3^n$,   (ii) $g_n = 3(-4)^n$,   (iii) $g_n = 3(-4)^n - 14 \cdot 3^n$.

17.   Solve the recursion $v_n - 2v_{n-1} = g_n$ for:
(i) $g_n = 1$,   (ii) $g_n = 2^n$,   (iii) $g_n = 2^n - 1$.

18.   (a) Find the specific solution to Problem 17(iii) that has $v_0 = 0$.
(b) As a check, calculate v_1, v_2, and v_3 two ways:
     (i) using $v_0 = 0$ and the recursion,   (ii) using the answer to Part (a).

19.   Solve the recursion $v_n - 3v_{n-1} - 4v_{n-2} = 2^n$, with initial conditions $v_0 = 0$ and $v_1 = -1$, using the following steps:
(i) Find the characteristic polynomial $K(x)$ (for the associated homogeneous recursion) and the roots s and t of $K(x) = 0$.
(ii) What are the r, m and p of Display (19) for the present recursion?
(iii) Find the c_i of Display (19) by substituting the w_n of Display (19) into Display (18). Thus find w_n.

(iv) Write the solution of the present nonhomogeneous recursion in the form $v_n = w_n + a \cdot s^n + b \cdot t^n$.

(v) Determine a and b using the initial conditions.

20. Using the outline of Problem 19, solve the recursion $v_n - 3v_{n-1} - 10v_{n-2} = 3 \cdot 4^n$ with initial conditions $v_0 = -5$ and $v_1 = -24$.

21. For each of the following nonhomogeneous recursions, find the specific solution that satisfies the given initial condition:

(a) $v_n - 3v_{n-1} = -2$; $v_0 = 2$.   (b) $v_n - 2v_{n-1} = n - 1$; $v_0 = 1$.
(c) $v_n - v_{n-1} = 3n - 3$; $v_0 = 0$.

22. Do as in Problem 21 for the following.

(a) $v_n - 3v_{n-1} = 4n$; $v_0 = 5$.   (b) $v_n - 3v_{n-1} = 6(n^2 - 3)$; $v_0 = 12$.
(c) $v_n - v_{n-1} = 3(n^2 + n + 1)$; $v_0 = 3$.

23. Do as in Problem 21 for:

(a) $v_n - 5v_{n-1} + 6v_{n-2} = 2$; $v_0 = 1$, $v_1 = 0$.
(b) $v_n - 6v_{n-1} + 9v_{n-2} = 3^n$; $v_0 = 1$, $v_1 = 2$.

24. Do as in Problem 21 for:

(a) $v_n - 3v_{n-1} + 2v_{n-2} = 4$; $v_0 = 1 = v_1$.
(b) $v_n - 7v_{n-1} + 16v_{n-2} - 12v_{n-3} = 2^n + 3^n$; $v_0 = 1$, $v_1 = 0$, $v_2 = 1$.

25. Let $v_0, v_1, \ldots$ satisfy the nonhomogeneous recursion

$$v_n + b_1 v_{n-1} + b_2 v_{n-2} + b_3 v_{n-3} + b_4 v_{n-4} = g_n$$

for which the associated homogeneous recursion has

$$H(x) = (x - 2)(x - 3)(x - 4)^2$$

as its characteristic polynomial. Let g_n satisfy a 5th order H.L.R.W.C.C. whose characteristic polynomial is

$$L(x) = (x - 2)^2(x - 3)(x - 5)^2.$$

Express v_n as $w_n + u_n$, with u_n involving arbitrary constants and the particular solution w_n involving constants to be determined.

26. Do as in Problem 25, but now with $H(x) = (x + 2)(x - 3)^3$ and $L(x) = (x + 2)(x - 1)(x - 2)^2(x - 3)$.

27. State an analogue of Theorem 3 ("Same Associated Homogeneous Recursion") involving three nonhomogeneous linear recursions with the same associated linear recursion.

28. Solve the recursion $v_n - 2v_{n-1} = g_n$ for each of the following right-hand sides g_n.

(i) $g_n = 2^n$;   (ii) $g_n = 3^n$;   (iii) $g_n = 4^n$;
(iv) $g_n = 2^n + 3^n + 4^n$.

29. Use the substitution $v_n = \log_2(y_n)$ to solve the recursion $y_n = 8y_{n-1}^2$ with the initial condition $y_0 = 1$.

30. Use the substitution $v_n = \log_2(y_n)$ to solve $y_n = 4y_{n-1}^3$ with $y_0 = 1$.

31. Let F_0, F_1, ... be the Fibonacci Sequence $0, 1, 1, \ldots$. Show that $y_n = 2^{F_n}$ satisfies $y_n = y_{n-1}y_{n-2}$ for $n \in \{2, 3, \ldots\}$.

32. Let L_0, L_1, ... be the Lucas Sequence. Show that $y_n = 2^{L_n}$ satisfies $y_n = y_{n-1}y_{n-2}$ for $n \in \{2, 3, \ldots\}$.

33. Use the substitution $v_n = \log_2(y_n)$ to find all solutions to the recursion $y_n = y_{n-1}^3 y_{n-2}^{10}$ for $n \in \{2, 3, \ldots\}$.

34. Use the substitution $v_n = \log_2(y_n)$ to find all solutions to the recursion $y_n = y_{n-1}y_{n-2}$ for $n \in \{2, 3, \ldots\}$.

35. Solve the recursion $y_n = y_{n-1}^2 y_{n-2}^3$ with the initial conditions $y_0 = 1$ and $y_1 = 2$.

36. Solve the recursion $y_n = y_{n-1}^7 / y_{n-2}^{12}$ with $y_0 = 1$ and $y_1 = 2$.

9.6

MISCELLANEOUS TECHNIQUES FOR SOLVING RECURSIONS

We saw in Theorem 3 of Section 9.4 that a linear homogeneous recursion with constant coefficients can be solved explicitly in terms of the characteristic roots. In Section 9.5 this was extended to nonhomogeneous recursions

$$v_n + b_1 v_{n-1} + b_2 v_{n-2} + \cdots + b_d v_{n-d} = g_n, \qquad b_i \text{ constant,}$$

for certain right-hand sides g_n. Here we present, through examples, some other techniques that sometimes apply to these types of recursions and to other types, including some nonlinear recursions and some linear recursions with nonconstant coefficients. Techniques for solving recursions also are shown to apply to the finding of explicit formulas for sums

$$S_n = a_1 + a_2 + \cdots + a_n.$$

TECHNIQUE I   INSPECTION

Example 1   Let us look at three related problems of recursion with initial conditions (in which F_0, F_1, ... is the Fibonacci Sequence):

(a) $v_n - v_{n-1} = F_{n+2} - F_{n+1}$ for n in $\mathbf{Z}^+$, $v_0 = 1$.
(b) $v_n - v_{n-1} = F_{n+2} - F_{n+1}$ for n in $\mathbf{Z}^+$, $v_0 = 4$.
(c) $v_n - v_{n-1} = F_n$ for n in $\mathbf{Z}^+$, $v_0 = 4$.

One sees easily that $v_n = F_{n+2}$ satisfies both the recursion and initial condition of (a) and similarly that $v_n = 3 + F_n$ satisfies (b). Since $F_{n+2} - F_{n+1} = F_n$, the solution to (c) is the same as the solution to (b).   □

TECHNIQUE II   **INDUCTION**

Example 2   Here we solve

$$v_n = v_{n-1} + n!n \qquad \text{for } n \in \mathbf{Z}^+, v_0 = 0.$$

First we present some data:

n	0	1	2	3	4
$n!$	1	1	2	6	24
$n!n$	0	1	4	18	96
v_n	0	1	5	23	119

The last line of the table is obtained from left to right using the initial condition $v_0 = 0$ and the recursion in the form

$$v_1 = v_0 + 1! \cdot 1 = 0 + 1 = 1,$$
$$v_2 = v_1 + 2! \cdot 2 = 1 + 4 = 5,$$
$$v_3 = 5 + 18 = 23,$$
$$v_4 = 23 + 96 = 119.$$

The data suggest the conjecture that

$$v_n = (n + 1)! - 1. \qquad (1)$$

This conjecture can be proved by mathematical induction to be true for all n in $\mathbf{N}$. The basis step is the verification

$$(0 + 1)! - 1 = 1! - 1 = 1 - 1 = 0$$

of the initial condition. The algebra of the inductive step is equivalent to verifying that the v_n of Display (1) satisfies the recursion, that is, showing that

$$(n + 1)! - 1 = (n! - 1) + n!n.$$

This holds because

$$n! - 1 + n!n = n!(1 + n) - 1 = (n + 1)! - 1.$$

Thus the explicit formula of Display (1) satisfies the given recursion and initial condition.   □

As one sees in this example, a proof by mathematical induction that a sequence satisfies a recursion with given initial conditions is equivalent to a proof by direct substitution.

Example 3   Here we seek an explicit formula for

$$S_n = 1! \cdot 1 + 2! \cdot 2 + 3! \cdot 3 + \cdots + n!n. \tag{2}$$

Replacing n by $n - 1$ in Display (2) gives us

$$S_{n-1} = 1! \cdot 1 + 2! \cdot 2 + 3! \cdot 3 + \cdots + (n - 1)!(n - 1). \tag{3}$$

Subtracting Display (3) from Display (2) leads to the recursion

$$S_n - S_{n-1} = n!n.$$

We also obtain the initial condition $S_1 = 1$ by replacing n by 1 in Display (2). It follows that the sequence $S_1, S_2, \ldots$ is the sequence $v_0, v_1, v_2, \ldots$ of Example 2, but with the term v_0 deleted. Hence $S_n = (n + 1)! - 1$ for all n in $\mathbf{Z}^+$.   □

TECHNIQUE III   **COLLAPSING SUMS**

Example 4   Here $F_0, F_1, \ldots$ is the Fibonacci Sequence and we solve the recursion with initial condition:

$$v_n - v_{n-1} = F_{n+2} - F_n \quad \text{for } n \text{ in } \mathbf{Z}^+, v_0 = 6. \tag{4}$$

Recursion (4) for $n, n - 1, n - 2, \ldots, 2, 1$ gives us the system

$$\begin{cases} v_n \quad\;\; - v_{n-1} = F_{n+2} - F_n \\ v_{n-1} - v_{n-2} = F_{n+1} - F_{n-1} \\ v_{n-2} - v_{n-3} = F_n \quad\;\; - F_{n-2} \\ \vdots \qquad\qquad \vdots \\ v_2 \quad\; - v_1 \;\;= F_4 \quad - F_2 \\ v_1 \quad\; - v_0 \;\;= F_3 \quad - F_1 \end{cases}$$

Adding these equations, and noting the cancellations, we have

$$v_n - v_0 = F_{n+2} + F_{n+1} - F_2 - F_1.$$

Since $v_0 = 6$, $F_{n+2} + F_{n+1} = F_{n+3}$, $F_2 = 1$, and $F_1 = 1$, this becomes

$$v_n = F_{n+3} + 4. \qquad\qquad □$$

Example 5   Here we find an explicit formula for

$$S_n = \frac{1}{1 \cdot 3} + \frac{1}{2 \cdot 4} + \frac{1}{3 \cdot 5} + \cdots + \frac{1}{n(n + 2)}. \tag{5}$$

Using the partial-fractions technique of Section 8.3, we find that

$$\frac{1}{x(x + 2)} = \frac{\frac{1}{2}}{x} - \frac{\frac{1}{2}}{x + 2}. \tag{6}$$

Replacing x by $1, 2, \ldots, n$ in Display (6) and substituting in Display (5), we get

$$S_n = \frac{1}{2}\left(\frac{1}{1} - \frac{1}{3}\right) + \frac{1}{2}\left(\frac{1}{2} - \frac{1}{4}\right) + \frac{1}{2}\left(\frac{1}{3} - \frac{1}{5}\right) + \cdots + \frac{1}{2}\left(\frac{1}{n-1} - \frac{1}{n+1}\right) + \frac{1}{2}\left(\frac{1}{n} - \frac{1}{n+2}\right)$$

$$S_n = \frac{1}{2}\left(\frac{1}{1} - \frac{1}{3} + \frac{1}{2} - \frac{1}{4} + \frac{1}{3} - \frac{1}{5} + \cdots + \frac{1}{n-1} - \frac{1}{n+1} + \frac{1}{n} - \frac{1}{n+2}\right)$$

$$S_n = \frac{1}{2}\left(\frac{1}{1} + \frac{1}{2} - \frac{1}{3} + \frac{1}{3} - \frac{1}{4} + \frac{1}{4} - \cdots - \frac{1}{n} + \frac{1}{n} - \frac{1}{n+1} - \frac{1}{n+2}\right)$$

$$S_n = \frac{1}{2}\left(\frac{1}{1} + \frac{1}{2} - \frac{1}{n+1} - \frac{1}{n+2}\right) = \frac{1}{2}\left[\frac{3}{2} - \frac{2n+3}{(n+1)(n+2)}\right]. \qquad \square$$

TECHNIQUE IV   ITERATION

Example 6   Here we solve

$$v_n = 2v_{n-1} + 2^n - 1, \qquad v_0 = 0. \tag{7}$$

Replacing n by $n - 1$ in Recursion (7) gives us

$$v_{n-1} = 2v_{n-2} + 2^{n-1} - 1.$$

Substituting this back into Recursion (7) leads to

$$v_n = 2(2v_{n-2} + 2^{n-1} - 1) + 2^n - 1 = 2^2 v_{n-2} + 2^n - 2 + 2^n - 1$$

$$v_n = 2^2 v_{n-2} + 2 \cdot 2^n - (2 + 1). \tag{8}$$

Replacing n by $n - 2$ in Recursion (7), we have

$$v_{n-2} = 2v_{n-3} + 2^{n-2} - 1.$$

Substituting this into Display (8), we get

$$v_n = 2^2(2v_{n-3} + 2^{n-2} - 1) + 2 \cdot 2^n - (2 + 1)$$
$$= 2^3 v_{n-3} + 2^n - 2^2 + 2 \cdot 2^n - (2 + 1)$$
$$v_n = 2^3 v_{n-3} + 3 \cdot 2^n - (2^2 + 2 + 1).$$

Continuing this process, we obtain

$$v_n = 2^n v_0 + n \cdot 2^n - (2^{n-1} + 2^{n-2} + \cdots + 2 + 1).$$

Since $v_0 = 0$ and $2^{n-1} + 2^{n-2} + \cdots + 2 + 1 = 2^n - 1$ by the technique for summing a geometric progression in Example 4 of Section 4.1, this becomes the explicit formula

$$v_n = n \cdot 2^n - (2^n - 1) = (n - 1)2^n + 1. \qquad \square$$

TECHNIQUE V   SUBSTITUTIONS

Example 7   The first order recursion

$$y_n - \frac{1}{n} y_{n-1} = \frac{1}{n!}$$

is of the form $y_n + b_1 y_{n-1} = g_n$, with b_1 not constant. The substitution $y_n = v_n/n!$ leads to

$$\frac{v_n}{n!} - \frac{1}{n} \cdot \frac{v_{n-1}}{(n-1)!} = \frac{1}{n!}$$

Multiplying through by $n!$ gives

$$v_n - v_{n-1} = 1.$$

Solving this by induction, or iteration, or telescoping, or the techniques of Section 9.3 or Section 9.5, one obtains the explicit formula

$$v_n = n + v_0.$$

Substituting back $v_n = n! y_n$ and $v_0 = 0! y_0 = y_0$, one has

$$n! y_n = n + y_0,$$

$$y_n = \frac{n + y_0}{n!}.$$ □

TECHNIQUE VI   GENERATING FUNCTIONS

Example 8   Here we solve

$$v_n - 3v_{n-1} - 10v_{n-2} - 28 \cdot 5^n = 0; \qquad v_0 = 25, \, v_1 = 120.$$

Let G be the generating series

$$G = v_0 + v_1 x + v_2 x^2 + \cdots + v_n x^n + \cdots.$$

Multiplying this by 1, by $-3x$, and by $-10x^2$ and using the series for $28/(1 - 5x)$ from Theorem 2 ("Nonhomogeneous Recursions with Same Homogeneous Part") of Section 9.3, we have

$$G = \quad v_0 + \quad v_1 x + \quad v_2 x^2 + \cdots + \quad v_n x^n + \cdots,$$

$$-3xG = \qquad - \quad 3v_0 x - \quad 3v_1 x^2 - \cdots - \quad 3v_{n-1} x^n - \cdots,$$

$$-10x^2 G = \qquad\qquad - \quad 10v_0 x^2 - \cdots - \quad 10v_{n-2} x^n - \cdots,$$

$$\frac{-28}{1 - 5x} = -28 - 28 \cdot 5x - 28 \cdot 5^2 x^2 - \cdots - 28 \cdot 5^n x^n - \cdots.$$

Adding, and using the recursion, we have

$$(1 - 3x - 10x^2)G - \frac{28}{1 - 5x} = (v_0 - 28) + (v_1 - 3v_0 - 140)x.$$

Using the initial conditions $v_0 = 25$ and $v_1 = 120$ and transposing gives us

$$(1 - 3x - 10x^2)G = \frac{28}{1 - 5x} - 3 - 95x$$

$$= \frac{28 + (1 - 5x)(-3 - 95x)}{1 - 5x}$$

$$= \frac{25 - 80x + 475x^2}{1 - 5x}.$$

Dividing by $1 - 3x - 10x^2 = (1 + 2x)(1 - 5x)$ yields

$$G = \frac{25 - 80x + 475x^2}{(1 + 2x)(1 - 5x)^2}.$$

The partial-fractions technique of Section 8.3 enables us to express G in the form

$$G = \frac{15}{1 + 2x} - \frac{10}{1 - 5x} + \frac{20}{(1 - 5x)^2}.$$

Using the definition of G and Lemma 1(b) of Section 9.4, we have

$$\sum_{n=0}^{\infty} v_n x^n = 15 \sum_{n=0}^{\infty} (-2)^n x^n - 10 \sum_{n=0}^{\infty} 5^n x^n + 20 \sum_{n=0}^{\infty} (n + 1)5^n x^n.$$

Equating coefficients of x^n, we get the explicit formula

$$v_n = 15(-2)^n - 10 \cdot 5^n + 20(n + 1)5^n = 15(-2)^n + 5^n(10 + 20n). \qquad \square$$

PROBLEMS FOR SECTION 9.6

1. Solve each of the following by inspection.

   (i) $v_n - v_{n-1} = \log(2 + n) - \log(1 + n)$, $v_0 = \log 2$.

   (ii) $v_n - v_{n-1} = \log(2 + n) - \log(1 + n)$, $v_0 = 3 + \log 2$.

   (iii) $v_n - v_{n-1} = \log[(2 + n)/(1 + n)]$, $v_0 = 3 + \log 2$.

2. Solve each of the following by inspection.

   (i) $v_n - v_{n-1} = n^2 - (n - 1)^2$, $v_0 = 0$.

   (ii) $v_n - v_{n-1} = n^2 - (n - 1)^2$, $v_0 = 5$.

   (iii) $v_n - v_{n-1} = 2n - 1$, $v_0 = 5$.

3. Solve the recursion (with initial condition)

$$v_n - v_{n-1} = \frac{n}{(n+1)!} \qquad \text{for } n \text{ in } \mathbf{Z}^+ = \{1, 2, \ldots\}, v_0 = 0,$$

by doing the following:
(i) Find v_n for $n = 1, 2, 3, 4,$ and 5.
(ii) Conjecture a formula for v_n.
(iii) Show that the v_n of Part (ii) satisfies the initial condition and the recursion.

4. Do as in Problem 3 for

$$v_n = \frac{n}{n+1} v_{n-1} \qquad \text{for } n \text{ in } \mathbf{Z}^+, v_0 = 1.$$

5. Show that $y_n = \binom{2n}{n}$ satisfies the recursion

$$y_n = \left[\frac{2(2n-1)}{n} \right] y_{n-1} \qquad \text{for all } n \text{ in } \mathbf{Z}^+.$$

6. Given that $y_0 = 1$ and $y_n = n y_{n-1}$ for all n in $\mathbf{Z}^+$, what is y_n? (Use a notation of Section 4.1.)

7. Use collapsing sums to solve

$$v_n - v_{n-1} = \frac{1}{2^n} \qquad \text{for } n \text{ in } \mathbf{Z}^+, v_0 = 7.$$

8. Use collapsing sums to solve

$$v_n - v_{n-1} = \frac{1}{3^n} \qquad \text{for } n \text{ in } \mathbf{Z}^+, v_0 = 5.$$

9. Let $L_0, L_1, \ldots$ be the Lucas Sequence. Solve

$$v_n - v_{n-1} = L_{n+2} - L_n \qquad \text{for } n \text{ in } \mathbf{Z}^+, v_0 = 0.$$

10. Let $F_0, F_1, \ldots$ be the Fibonacci Sequence. Solve

$$v_n - v_{n-1} = F_{n+2} F_{n-1} \qquad \text{for } n \text{ in } \mathbf{Z}^+, v_0 = 10.$$

[*Hint:* $F_{n+2} F_{n-1} = (F_{n+1} + F_n)(F_{n+1} - F_n) = F_{n+1}^2 - F_n^2.$]

11. Given that $v_0 = 0$ and $v_n = v_{n-1} + \binom{n+2}{3}$ for n in $\mathbf{Z}^+$, find an explicit formula for v_n.

12. Given that $v_0 = 0$ and $v_n - v_{n-1} = \binom{n+3}{4}$ for n in $\mathbf{Z}^+$, find an explicit formula for v_n.

13. Use iteration to solve

$$v_n = 3v_{n-1} + 3^n - 1 \qquad \text{for } n \text{ in } \mathbf{Z}^+, v_0 = 0.$$

14. Use iteration to solve

$$v_n = 4v_{n-1} + 4^n \quad \text{for } n \text{ in } \mathbf{Z}^+, v_0 = 0.$$

15. Use the substitution $y_n = v_n^2$ to solve

$$y_n = (2\sqrt{y_{n-1}} + 3\sqrt{y_{n-2}})^2 \quad \text{for } n \text{ in } \mathbf{Z}^+; y_0 = 1, y_1 = 4.$$

16. Use a substitution to solve

$$y_n = (5\sqrt{y_{n-1}} + 6\sqrt{y_{n-2}})^2 \quad \text{for } n \text{ in } \mathbf{Z}^+; y_0 = 1, y_1 = 4.$$

17. Use $y_n = n!v_n$ to solve

$$y_n = 2ny_{n-1} + 7n! \quad \text{for } n \text{ in } \mathbf{Z}^+, y_0 = 1.$$

18. Use $y_n = v_n/n$ to solve

$$y_n = \frac{n-1}{n} y_{n-1} + \frac{1}{n} \quad \text{for } n \text{ in } \mathbf{Z}^+, y_0 = 5.$$

19. Use a substitution to solve

$$y_n = 4n(n-1)y_{n-2} + \frac{5}{9} n! \cdot 3^n \quad \text{for } n \text{ in } \{2, 3, \ldots\}; y_0 = 1, y_1 = -1.$$

20. Solve

$$y_n = 9n(n-1)y_{n-2} + 14n! \cdot 2^n \quad \text{for } n \in \{2, 3, \ldots\}; y_0 = 42, y_1 = 28.$$

21. (i) Solve $v_n - v_{n-1} = 3, v_0 = 0.$
(ii) Use the substitution $w_n = 2^n v_n$ and Part (i) to solve

$$w_n - 2w_{n-1} = 3 \cdot 2^n, \quad w_0 = 0.$$

22. Use the substitution $w_n = 3^n v_n$ to solve

$$w_n - 3w_{n-1} = 5 \cdot 3^n, \quad w_0 = 0.$$

23. Let $P(x)$ be a polynomial in x of degree d and let

$$S_n = P(0) + P(1) + P(2) + \cdots + P(n).$$

Explain why there exists a polynomial $Q(x)$ of degree $d + 1$ such that $S_n = Q(n)$ for all n in $\mathbf{N} = \{0, 1, \ldots\}$.

24. Let $S_n = 0^3 + 1^3 + 2^3 + \cdots + n^3$.
(i) Does there exist a fourth degree polynomial $Q(x)$ such that $S_n = Q(n)$ for all n in $\mathbf{N}$? Explain.
(ii) Find S_n for $n = 0, 1, 2, 3$, and 4.
(iii) Assume that the $Q(x)$ of Part (i) is of the form

$$Q(x) = a + bx + cx(x - 1) + dx(x - 1)(x - 2)$$
$$+ ex(x - 1)(x - 2)(x - 3),$$

with a, b, c, d, e constants. Then use Part (ii) to find these constants and so obtain S_n as a polynomial in n.

(iv) Check by obtaining S_5 in two ways.

25. Use the technique of Problem 24 to get a polynomial formula for $S_n = 0^4 + 1^4 + 2^4 + \cdots + n^4$.

26. Find a polynomial formula for $S_n = 0^5 + 1^5 + 2^5 + \cdots + n^5$.

SUMMARY OF TERMS, CHAPTER 9

REVIEW PROBLEMS FOR CHAPTER 9

1. Find the generating function for:
   (a) the arithmetic progression $3, 7, \ldots, 3 + 4n, \ldots$;
   (b) the geometric progression $4, 12, \ldots, 4 \cdot 3^n, \ldots$.

2. Find the generating function for the sequence $5, 4, \ldots$ that satisfies the recursion $u_n - 3u_{n-1} - u_{n-2} = 0$ for $n \geq 2$.

3. Find the generating function for the sequence $u_0, u_1, \ldots$ with $u_n = 3 \cdot 4^n - 5 \cdot 3^n$ for n in $N = \{0, 1, \ldots\}$.

4. For each of the following functions G, give the formula for the term u_n of the sequence $u_0, u_1, \ldots$ having G as its generating function.

   (a) $G = \dfrac{2}{1-6x} - \dfrac{4}{1+3x}$.   (b) $G = \dfrac{7+24x}{1-3x-18x^2}$.

   (c) $G = \dfrac{7}{(1-5x)^2}$.

5. If G is the generating series for $a_0, a_1, \ldots$, what sequence has $(1 - x)^2 G$ as its generating series?

6. Find the generating function for the sequence $\binom{3}{3}, 0, \binom{4}{3}, 0, \binom{5}{3}, 0, \ldots$.

7. Find the general solution of the recursion $u_n = 1.1u_{n-1}$ for $n \in \mathbf{Z}^+$.

8. Find the specific solution of $u_n = 1.1u_{n-1}$ with $u_0 = 3000$.

9. For the recursion $u_n - u_{n-1} - 42u_{n-2} = 0$, find:
    (i) the characteristic polynomial $K(x)$.
    (ii) the characteristic roots.
    (iii) the general solution of the recursion.
    (iv) the specific solution with $u_0 = 13$ and $u_1 = 1$.

10. Find the specific solution to $u_n - 8u_{n-1} + 16u_{n-2} = 0$ for the initial conditions $u_0 = 8$, $u_1 = 12$.

11. Find the second order H.L.R.W.C.C. satisfied by the sequence $u_0, u_1, \ldots$ with:
    (a) $u_n = (1 + n)(-3)^n$;   (b) $u_n = 3(-2)^n - 7 \cdot 5^n$.

12. Find the general solution of the second order recursion $u_n - 16u_{n-2} = 0$.

13. For each of the following recursions with an initial condition find:
    (i) a particular solution of the recursion,
    (ii) the general solution of the recursion,
    (iii) the specific solution for the given initial condition.
    (a) $v_n - 3v_{n-1} = 4$, $v_0 = 2$.   (b) $v_n - 6v_{n-1} = 2 \cdot 5^n$, $v_0 = 2$.
    (c) $v_n - 6v_{n-1} = 5 \cdot 6^n$, $v_0 = 4$.   (d) $v_n - 6v_{n-1} = 2 \cdot 5^n + 5 \cdot 6^n$, $v_0 = 6$.

14. Find the generating function for the series

$$\binom{5}{5} - \binom{6}{5}(3x) + \binom{7}{5}(3x)^2 - \cdots + \binom{n+5}{5}(-3x)^n + \cdots.$$

15. For the recursion $u_n + 3u_{n-1} - 4u_{n-2} - 12u_{n-3} = 0$, find:
    (i) the characteristic roots and their multiplicities;
    (ii) the general solution;
    (iii) the specific solution with $u_0 = 1$, $u_1 = 0$, $u_2 = 2$.

16. Find the general solutions of:
    (a) $u_n + 6u_{n-1} + 12u_{n-2} + 8u_{n-3} = 0$.
    (b) $u_n - 9u_{n-1} + 27u_{n-2} - 27u_{n-3} = 0$.

17. Let $G = u_0 + u_1 x + \cdots + u_n x^n + \cdots$. Find u_n when:

    (a) $G = \dfrac{4}{(1 + 3x)^2}$;   (b) $G = \dfrac{5 + 6x}{(1 + 3x)^2}$;

    (c) $G = \dfrac{4}{(1 - 5x)^4} - \dfrac{7}{(1 + 2x)^6}$.

18. For the recursion $v_n - 7v_{n-1} + 16v_{n-2} - 12v_{n-3} = 3$, find:
(i) a particular solution; (ii) the general solution;
(iii) the specific solution with $v_0 = 0$, $v_1 = 4$, $v_2 = 15$.

19. Find the general solution of the recursion

$$v_n - 7v_{n-1} + 16v_{n-2} - 12v_{n-3} = g(n)$$

for each of the following functions $g(n)$.
(a) $g(n) = 5^n$, (b) $g(n) = 3^n$, (c) $g(n) = 2^n$,
(d) $g(n) = 6 + 4 \cdot 3^n - 5 \cdot 2^n$.

20. Find the solution with $v_0 = 2$ of the recursion

$$v_n - 3v_{n-1} = \sqrt[5]{n + 32} - 3\sqrt[5]{n + 31}.$$

21. Find the solution with $u_0 = 4$ and $u_1 = 25$ of

$$\sqrt{u_n} - 5\sqrt{u_{n-1}} + 6\sqrt{u_{n-2}} = 0.$$

SUPPLEMENTARY AND CHALLENGING PROBLEMS, CHAPTER 9 ⎯⎯⎯⎯⎯⎯

1. Let $v_0, v_1, \ldots$ satisfy the second order recursion

$$v_n + b_1 v_{n-1} + b_2 v_{n-2} = 5r^n,$$

with b_1, b_2, and r constants. Prove that the sequence also satisfies the third order H.L.R.W.C.C. having $(x^2 + b_1 x + b_2)(x - r)$ as its characteristic polynomial.

2. Let $x_0, x_1, \ldots$ satisfy $x_n - x_{n-1} - x_{n-2} = 0$ and $y_0, y_1, \ldots$ satisfy $y_n - 2y_{n-1} - y_{n-2} = 0$. Find a fourth order H.L.R.W.C.C. satisfied by the sequence $u_0, u_1, \ldots$ with $u_n = x_n + y_n$.

3. Repeat Problem 2, but now with $u_n = x_n y_n$.

4. Let $x_0, x_1, \ldots$ and $y_0, y_1, \ldots$ both satisfy $u_n + b_1 u_{n-1} + b_2 u_{n-2} = 0$, where b_1 and b_2 are constants.
(a) Show that $x_0 y_0, x_1 y_1, x_2 y_2, \ldots$ satisfies a third order H.L.R.W.C.C.
(b) Show that $x_0, x_2, x_4, \ldots$ satisfies a second order H.L.R.W.C.C.

5. Let $F_0, F_1, \ldots$ be the Fibonacci Sequence.
(a) Find constants a, b, c, d such that, for all n in N,

$$F_{3n} = aF_n F_{n+1} F_{n+2} + bF_{n+1} F_{n+2} F_{n+3} + cF_{n+2} F_{n+3} F_{n+4}$$
$$+ dF_{n+3} F_{n+4} F_{n+5}.$$

(b) For all r, s, and t in N, prove that

$$F_{r+s+t+3} = F_{r+2}(F_{s+2} F_{t+1} + F_{s+1} F_t) + F_{r+1}(F_{s+1} F_{t+1} + F_s F_t).$$

6. If a, b, and r are positive real numbers, it can be shown using calculus that there exists a positive integer m such that

$$(a + bn)r^n < n! \qquad \text{for } n \text{ in } \{m, m + 1, m + 2, \ldots\}.$$

Use this to prove that there does not exist any second order H.L.R.W.C.C. satisfied by the sequence $u_0, u_1, \ldots$ with $u_n = n!$. (Actually, there is no H.L.R.W.C.C. of any order satisfied by the sequence of factorials.)

10

COMBINATORIAL
ANALYSIS
OF ALGORITHMS

In this chapter, we apply some of the topics of previous chapters to obtain indicators of the time required to execute certain algorithms.

10.1

ALGORITHMS FOR SORTING

Suppose that we have n cards, with a positive integer a_i on the ith card. To *sort* the cards is to arrange them so that

$$a_1 \leq a_2 \leq a_3 \leq \cdots \leq a_n.$$

For example, if $n = 6$ and $a_1, \ldots, a_6$ are

13, 4, 14, 4, 19, 14,

the cards are not sorted but become sorted when rearranged so that $a_1, \ldots, a_6$ are

4, 4, 13, 14, 14, 19.

We will describe two algorithms for sorting. The first has programming and machine storage advantages; the other requires less computer time when n is relatively large. Since these techniques also apply to sorting numbers in a computer, we will deal with this problem as if it involved rearranging the entries a_i of an ordered n-tuple $(a_1, a_2, \ldots, a_n)$. Here it is helpful to use the synonym *n-vector* for "ordered n-tuple" (which was defined in Section 1.4), since "ordered" may convey the mistaken impression that the a_i are already in numerical order.

Each of the sorting algorithms is aided by a preliminary algorithm. For the first, we also need some terminology.

NOTATION 1   **MIN OF THE ENTRIES OF AN n-VECTOR**

$\min(a_1, a_2, \ldots, a_n)$ is an entry a_h such that $a_h \leq a_i$ for $i = 1, 2, \ldots, n$.

For example, if $(a_1, a_2, \ldots, a_6) = (13, 4, 14, 4, 19, 14)$, then either a_2 or a_4 is $\min(a_1, \ldots, a_6) = 4$.

ALGORITHM 1   **FINDING THE MIN**

We give an inductive description:

Basis   When $n = 1$, $\min(a_1) = a_1$.

Inductive Part   Let $(a_1, a_2, \ldots, a_n)$ be an n-vector with $n \geq 2$. Let $m = \min(a_2, a_3, \ldots, a_n)$. Then

$$\min(a_1, a_2, \ldots, a_n) = \begin{cases} a_1 & \text{if } a_1 \leq m, \\ m & \text{if } a_1 > m. \end{cases}$$

We note that this algorithm is based on comparing integers a and b and doing one thing when $a \leq b$ and another when $a > b$. A good indicator of the time required to execute the algorithm is the number of comparisons required.

NOTATION 2   **NUMBER $A(n)$ OF COMPARISONS FOR MIN**

Let $A(n)$ be the number of comparisons made in using Algorithm 1 to find the min of an n-vector.

THEOREM 1   **FORMULA FOR $A(n)$**

$A(n) = n - 1$.

PROOF   The basis part of Algorithm 1 shows that $A(1) = 0$ and the inductive part shows that $A(n) = 1 + A(n - 1)$. An easy proof by mathematical induction establishes that $A(n) = n - 1$. $\square$

We are now ready to give an inductive technique for arranging the entries a_i of an n-vector $(a_1, \ldots, a_n)$ as a sorted n-vector $(s_1, \ldots, s_n)$.

ALGORITHM 2 **BUBBLE SORTING**

Basis   Every 1-vector (a_1) is already sorted.

Inductive Part   Let $n \geq 2$ and $a_h = \min(a_1, \ldots, a_n)$. Let $(b_1, \ldots, b_{n-1})$ be the $(n-1)$-vector resulting when the entry a_h is deleted from $(a_1, \ldots, a_n)$; that is, $b_i = a_i$ if $i < h$, and $b_i = a_{i+1}$ if $i \geq h$. Let $(s_2, \ldots, s_n)$ be the sorted $(n-1)$-vector for $(b_1, \ldots, b_{n-1})$. Then the sorted n-vector for $(a_1, \ldots, a_n)$ is

$$(a_h, s_2, s_3, \ldots, s_n).$$

Bubble sorting has a dual that we call "sinker sorting" in which $s_n = \max(a_1, \ldots, a_n)$. This is dealt with in Problems 1 and 2 below.

NOTATION 3 **NUMBER $B(n)$ OF COMPARISONS IN BUBBLE SORTING**

Let $B(n)$ be the number of comparisons performed in using Algorithm 2 to sort an n-vector.

THEOREM 2 **FORMULA FOR $B(n)$**

$$B(n) = \frac{n(n-1)}{2} = \binom{n}{2}.$$

PROOF   The basis part of Algorithm 2 shows that $B(1) = 0$, and the inductive part shows that $B(n) = A(n) + B(n-1)$ for $n \geq 2$. Using Theorem 1, we see that this becomes

$$B(n) = n - 1 + B(n-1).$$

Using this repeatedly, we have

$$B(n) = (n-1) + [(n-2) + B(n-2)]$$
$$= (n-1) + (n-2) + (n-3) + B(n-3)$$
$$\vdots$$
$$= (n-1) + (n-2) + \cdots + 2 + 1 + 0.$$

Summing the arithmetic progression, we have the claimed

$$B(n) = \binom{n}{2} = \frac{n(n-1)}{2}. \qquad \square$$

The other algorithm for sorting that we will discuss involves the concept of ***merging*** a sorted m-vector $(a_1, \ldots, a_m)$ and a sorted n-vector $(b_1, \ldots, b_n)$

to produce a sorted $(m + n)$-vector $(s_1, \ldots, s_{m+n})$ whose entries are the a_i and b_j. For example, the merged vector for the sorted 6-vector (4, 4, 13, 14, 14, 19) and the sorted 5-vector (5, 8, 14, 16, 20) is the sorted 11-vector (4, 4, 5, 8, 13, 14, 14, 14, 16, 19, 20). The following is an inductive description of a technique for merging.

ALGORITHM 3   **MERGING SORTED VECTORS**

Let $(a_1, \ldots, a_m)$ and $(b_1, \ldots, b_n)$ be sorted vectors.

Basis   If $m = 1 = n$, compare a_1 and b_1. Then the merged vector (s_1, s_2) for the 1-vectors (a_1) and (b_1) is (a_1, b_1) if $a_1 \leq b_1$ and is (b_1, a_1) if $a_1 > b_1$.

Inductive Part   If $m + n \geq 3$, compare a_1 and b_1. If $a_1 \leq b_1$, let the merged vector $(s_1, \ldots, s_{m+n})$ have $s_1 = a_1$ and $(s_2, \ldots, s_{m+n})$ as the merged vector for $(a_2, \ldots, a_m)$ and $(b_1, \ldots, b_n)$. [If $m = 1$, then $(s_2, \ldots, s_{1+n}) = (b_1, \ldots, b_n)$.] If $a_1 > b_1$, let $s_1 = b_1$ and $(s_2, \ldots, s_{m+n})$ be the merged vector for $(a_1, \ldots, a_m)$ and $(b_2, \ldots, b_n)$.

NOTATION 4   **NUMBER $C(m, n)$ OF COMPARISONS FOR MERGING**

Let $C(m, n)$ denote the maximum number of comparisons that might be needed in using Algorithm 3 to merge a sorted m-vector and a sorted n-vector.

THEOREM 3   **FORMULA FOR $C(m, n)$**

$C(m, n) = m + n - 1.$

PROOF   Let $h = m + n$. We prove this formula for $h = 2, 3, \ldots$ by mathematical induction on h.

Basis   When $h = 2$, we must have $m = 1 = n$, and the desired formula $C(1, 1) = 1$ follows from the basis part of Algorithm 3.

Inductive Step   Let $h \geq 3$. Then either m or n is at least 2. Let us consider the case in which $m \geq 2$ and $a_1 \leq b_1$. Then the number of comparisons needed to merge $(a_1, \ldots, a_m)$ and $(b_1, \ldots, b_n)$ is at most $1 + C(m - 1, n)$, as we see from the inductive part of Algorithm 3. The inductive hypothesis of this proof allows us to assume that $C(m - 1, n) = m + n - 2$. Thus the number of comparisons that might be needed in this case is at most

$1 + (m + n - 2) = m + n - 1.$

One can easily see that no more than this number of comparisons is needed in any other case. In the problems below, we will indicate how one can produce an m-vector and an n-vector whose merger actually requires $m + n - 1$ comparisons. [When $n = m + q$, $(q + 2, q + 4, \ldots, q + 2m)$ and $(1, 2, \ldots, q, q + 1, q + 3, q + 5, \ldots, q + 2m - 1)$ are such vectors.] This shows that $m + n - 1$ is the maximum, as claimed. □

The following example and algorithm give an inductive description of a "divide-and-conquer" algorithm for sorting an n-vector.

Example 1 We start by noting again that every 1-vector (a_1) is sorted. To sort a 2-vector (a_1, a_2), we compare a_1 and a_2. If $a_1 \leq a_2$, then the vector is already sorted; if $a_1 > a_2$, then we interchange a_1 and a_2 to get the sorted 2-vector (s_1, s_2).

When $n = 3$, we make (a_1, a_2, a_3) into a sorted 3-vector (s_1, s_2, s_3) as follows:

(a) Split (a_1, a_2, a_3) into a 1-vector (a_1) and a 2-vector (a_2, a_3).
(b) Make (a_2, a_3) into a sorted 2-vector (b_1, b_2) using the procedure of this example for $n = 2$.
(c) Merge (a_1) and (b_1, b_2) using Algorithm 3. □

ALGORITHM 4 **DIVIDE-AND-CONQUER SORTING**

Basis The algorithm for $n = 1$, 2, and 3 is described in Example 1.

Inductive Part When $n \geq 4$, let $k = n/2$ if n is even and $k = (n - 1)/2$ if n is odd. Then use the following steps:

(a) Sort each of $(a_1, \ldots, a_k)$ and $(a_{k+1}, \ldots, a_n)$ using this algorithm with shorter vector lengths.
(b) Merge the sorted parts using Algorithm 3.

NOTATION 5 **NUMBER $D(n)$ FOR DIVIDE-AND-CONQUER**

Let $D(n)$ denote the maximum number of comparisons that might be needed to sort an n-vector using Algorithm 4.

THEOREM 4 **RECURSION FOR $D(n)$**

For all m in $\mathbf{Z}^+ = \{1, 2, \ldots\}$:

(a) $D(2m) = 2D(m) + 2m - 1$,
(b) $D(2m + 1) = D(m + 1) + D(m) + 2m$.

PROOF   We use strong mathematical induction on m.

Basis   Counting the numbers of comparisons that might be needed in Example 1, we see that $D(1) = 0$, $D(2) = 1$, and $D(3) = 3$. These show that the claimed formulas hold for $m = 1$.

Inductive Step   Let $h \in \{2, 3, \ldots\}$ and assume that the stated formulas hold for $m = 1, 2, \ldots, h - 1$. We deal with Part (a) and leave the similar Part (b) to the reader. To sort $(a_1, \ldots, a_{2h})$ using Algorithm 4, one sorts $(a_1, \ldots, a_h)$ into $(r_1, \ldots, r_h)$, sorts $(a_{h+1}, a_{h+2}, \ldots, a_{2h})$ into $(t_1, \ldots, t_h)$, and then merges the sorted h-vectors. Sorting the pieces of the original vector requires at most $D(h) + D(h)$ comparisons, and Theorem 3, "Formula for $C(m, n)$," tells us that merging the sorted parts requires at most $C(h, h) = 2h - 1$ comparisons. Hence the total number of comparisons needed to sort $(a_1, \ldots, a_{2h})$ is at most $2D(h) + 2h - 1$. We will see in the problems below that certain $2h$-vectors require this number of comparisons for the complete sorting. This will prove Part (a). The proof of Part (b) is very similar.   □

Example 2   We have seen that

$$D(1) = 0, \qquad D(2) = 1, \qquad \text{and} \qquad D(3) = 3.$$

We now use Theorem 4 to find $D(n)$ for additional values of n. Letting $m = 2$ in Theorem 4 gives us

$$D(4) = 2D(2) + 3 = 2 \cdot 1 + 3 = 5,$$
$$D(5) = D(2) + D(3) + 4 = 1 + 3 + 4 = 8.$$

Theorem 4 with $m = 3$ leads to

$$D(6) = 2D(3) + 5 = 2 \cdot 3 + 5 = 11,$$
$$D(7) = D(4) + D(3) + 6 = 5 + 3 + 6 = 14.$$

Similarly, we find that $D(8) = 17$ and $D(9) = 21$. Do we need to find $D(10)$, $D(11), \ldots, D(15)$ in order to find $D(16)$? No; Theorem 4(a) shows that

$$D(16) = 2D(8) + 15 = 2 \cdot 17 + 15 = 49.$$

Similarly, $D(32) = 2D(16) + 31 = 2 \cdot 49 + 31 = 129.$ □

Example 3   Replacing m by 2^{n-1} in the formula $D(2m) = 2D(m) + 2m - 1$ of Theorem 4, gives us

$$D(2^n) = 2D(2^{n-1}) + 2^n - 1.$$

Letting $v_n = D(2^n)$, we see that this goes into $v_n = 2v_{n-1} + 2^n - 1$, or $v_n - 2v_{n-1} = 2^n - 1$. We also have $v_0 = D(2^0) = D(1) = 0$. The solution of this nonhomogeneous linear recursion with this initial condition can be shown, as in Problem 17(iii) of Section 9.5, to be

$$v_n = 2^n(n - 1) + 1.$$

Substituting back, we have

$$D(2^n) = 2^n(n-1) + 1. \tag{1}$$

This formula will enable us to see the advantage of divide-and-conquer sorting over bubble sorting when n is large. □

There are analogues of Algorithm 4, "Divide-and-Conquer Sorting," in which the n-vector to be sorted is split into more than two parts. Let $T(n)$ be the maximum number of comparisons needed for the algorithm in which the n-vector is split into three parts. Then it can be shown that

$$T(0) = 0 = T(1),$$
$$T(2) = 1,$$
$$T(3m) = 3T(m) + 5m - 2,$$
$$T(3m + 1) = 2T(m) + T(m + 1) + 5m - 1,$$
$$T(3m + 2) = T(m) + 2T(m + 1) + 5m + 1.$$

In Problems 21 and 22 below, the reader is asked to use these formulas to find $T(n)$ for $n = 1, 2, \ldots, 27$ and to compare $T(n)$ with $D(n)$ for these n's. Problems 23 and 24 deal with $T(3^m)$ for m in N.

PROBLEMS FOR SECTION 10.1

1. Define $\max(a_1, a_2, \ldots, a_n)$ inductively.

2. Inductively define the **sinker sorting** algorithm for converting $(a_1, a_2, \ldots, a_n)$ into a sorted n-vector $(s_1, s_2, \ldots, s_n)$ in which $s_n = \max(a_1, a_2, \ldots, a_n)$, where max is as in Problem 1.

3. Tabulate $B(n)$ and $D(n)$ for $n = 1, 2, \ldots, 12$.

4. Find:
   (a) $B(13)$ and $D(13)$;   (b) $B(14)$ and $D(14)$.

5. Find $B(1024)$ and $D(1024)$. (*Hint:* $1024 = 2^{10}$.)

6. Find $B(2^{20})$ and $D(2^{20})$.

7. Give an example of sorted vectors (a_1) and $(b_1, \ldots, b_n)$ whose merging by Algorithm 3 ("Merging Sorted Vectors") requires:
   (i) n comparisons;   (ii) only 1 comparison.

8. Give an example of sorted vectors (a_1, a_2) and $(b_1, \ldots, b_n)$ whose merging by Algorithm 3 ("Merging Sorted Vectors") requires only 2 comparisons.

9. Give an example of sorted vectors (a_1, a_2) and $(b_1, \ldots, b_n)$ whose merging by Algorithm 3 ("Merging Sorted Vectors") requires $n + 1$ comparisons.

10. Give an example of sorted vectors (a_1, a_2, a_3) and $(b_1, \ldots, b_n)$ whose merging by Algorithm 3 ("Merging Sorted Vectors") requires $n + 2$ comparisons.

11. How many comparisons are needed to use Algorithm 3 to merge the following?
    (i) (1, 2) and (3, 4);   (ii) (1, 3) and (2, 4);
    (iii) (1, 3, 5, 7) and (2, 4, 6, 8).

12. How many comparisons are needed for Algorithm 3 to merge the following?
    (i) (1, 3) and (5, 7);   (ii) (1, 5) and (3, 7);
    (iii) (1, 2, 3, 4) and (5, 6, 7, 8).

13. How many comparisons are needed to use Algorithm 4 ("Divide-and-Conquer Sorting") to sort the following?
    (i) (3, 1, 4, 2);   (ii) (1, 2, 3, 4).

14. How many comparisons are needed to use Algorithm 4 ("Divide-and-Conquer Sorting") to sort the following?
    (i) (5, 1, 7, 3);   (ii) (6, 2, 8, 4).

15. How many comparisons are needed to use Algorithm 4 to sort the following?
    (i) (5, 1, 7, 3, 6, 2, 8, 4);   (ii) (1, 2, 3, 4, 5, 6, 7, 8).

16. Make a 16-vector for which sorting by Algorithm 4 requires $D(16)$ comparisons.

17. Explain why merging sorted vectors (a_1) and $(b_1, \ldots, b_n)$ using Algorithm 3 ("Merging Sorted Vectors") requires n comparisons when $a_1 > b_{n-1}$. (We are assuming that $n \geq 2$.)

18. Let $m \geq 2$ and $n \geq 2$. Explain why merging sorted vectors $(a_1, \ldots, a_m)$ and $(b_1, \ldots, b_n)$ using Algorithm 3 requires $m + n - 1$ comparisons when both $a_m > b_{n-1}$ and $b_n > a_{m-1}$.

19. Explain why the number of comparisons made in using Algorithm 3 to merge sorted vectors $(a_1, \ldots, a_m)$ and $(b_1, \ldots, b_n)$ is $m + k$ when $b_k < a_m \leq b_{k+1}$.

20. How many comparisons are needed to merge sorted vectors $(a_1, \ldots, a_m)$ and $(b_1, \ldots, b_n)$ using Algorithm 3 when $a_m \leq b_1$?

21. Use $T(0) = 0 = T(1)$ and $T(2) = 1$ with the recursion formulas

$$T(3m) = 3T(m) + 5m - 2,$$
$$T(3m + 1) = 2T(m) + T(m + 1) + 5m - 1,$$
$$T(3m + 2) = T(m) + 2T(m + 1) + 5m + 1,$$

to tabulate $T(n)$ for n in $\{0, 1, \ldots, 27\}$.

22. (i) Extend the table of $D(n)$ in Problem 3 to include $n = 13, 14, \ldots, 27$.
    (ii) For which n's in $\{1, 2, \ldots, 27\}$ is $D(n) < T(n)$? [$T(n)$ is as in Problem 21.]
    (iii) Are there n's in $\{1, 2, \ldots, 27\}$ for which $D(n) > T(n)$?

23. Use $T(1) = 0$ and $T(3m) = 3T(m) + 5m - 2$ to find $T(n)$ for:
(i) $n = 3$;   (ii) $n = 9$;   (iii) $n = 27$;   (iv) $n = 81$;   (v) $n = 243$.

24. (i) Solve the recursion $v_n - 3v_{n-1} = (\frac{5}{3})3^n - 2$, with initial condition $v_0 = 0$.
(ii) Use Part (i) and the substitution $v_n = T(3^n)$ to solve $T(3^n) - 3T(3^{n-1}) = 5 \cdot 3^{n-1} - 2$, $T(1) = T(3^0) = 0$.

10.2

SOLVING SYSTEMS OF SIMULTANEOUS LINEAR EQUATIONS

In this section, we describe and compare two algorithms for solving a system of n simultaneous linear equations in n unknowns. For each of these algorithms, the time required for an electronic computer to carry out the algorithm is essentially proportional to the number of multiplications performed. Let f_n be the number of multiplications needed for the first algorithm and let g_n be the number needed for the other algorithm. Our work below shows that for small values of n, f_n and g_n are as shown in Table 10.2.1. When n is large, the second method is feasible for computer calculation, whereas the first method ceases to be practical even for moderately large n. For example, $g_{24} = 5176$ and

$$f_{24} > 150000000000000000000000000 = 1.5 \times 10^{25}.$$

We deal with the easiest cases and then discuss the algorithms for general n.

TABLE 10.2.1

n	1	2	3	4
f_n	1	8	39	204
g_n	1	6	17	36

THE CASE OF $n = 1$

One linear equation in one unknown x has the form

$$ax = b,$$

where a and b are considered to be known. If $a \neq 0$ the solution to this equation is $x = b/a$.

THE CASE OF $n = 2$

A system of two simultaneous linear equations in unknowns x_1 and x_2 has the form

$$(S) \quad \begin{cases} a_{11}x_1 + a_{12}x_2 = b_1 & \text{(1)} \\ a_{21}x_1 + a_{22}x_2 = b_2, & \text{(2)} \end{cases}$$

where the a_{ij} and b_i are considered to be known numbers. The first method of solving the system (S) for x_1 and x_2 is as follows: Multiply each term in Display (1) by a_{22} and multiply each term in Display (2) by a_{12}; this produces the system

$$(S_1) \quad \begin{cases} a_{11}a_{22}x_1 + a_{12}a_{22}x_2 = b_1a_{22} \\ a_{21}a_{12}x_1 + a_{12}a_{22}x_2 = b_2a_{12}. \end{cases}$$

We subtract the second of these equations from the first and get

$$(a_{11}a_{22} - a_{21}a_{12})x_1 = b_1a_{22} - b_2a_{12}. \tag{3}$$

By multiplying Equation (2) by a_{11} and Equation (1) by a_{21} and subtracting, we get

$$(a_{11}a_{22} - a_{21}a_{12})x_2 = a_{11}b_2 - a_{21}b_1. \tag{4}$$

If $a_{11}a_{22} - a_{21}a_{12} \neq 0$, it follows from Equations (3) and (4) that the solution to the system of equations (S) is

$$x_1 = \frac{b_1a_{22} - b_2a_{12}}{a_{11}a_{22} - a_{21}a_{12}}, \qquad x_2 = \frac{a_{11}b_2 - a_{21}b_1}{a_{11}a_{22} - a_{21}a_{12}}. \tag{5}$$

The following observations will help us to remember the formulas in Display (5) and to generalize to systems of n linear equations in n unknowns.

An m by n **matrix** of numbers is a rectangular arrangement of mn numbers in m rows and n columns. If $m = n$, the matrix is **square**. The coefficients of the unknowns x_1 and x_2 in the system (S) can be written as the 2 by 2 matrix

$$M = \begin{bmatrix} a_{11} & a_{12} \\ a_{21} & a_{22} \end{bmatrix}. \tag{6}$$

M is called the **matrix of the system** of these simultaneous equations. The **determinant** of the square matrix M in Display (6) is defined to be

$$\det M = a_{11}a_{22} - a_{21}a_{12}. \tag{7}$$

We now note that in the solution of the system (S) given in Display (5), each of x_1 and x_2 is a quotient of determinants. Specifically, if we let M_1 and M_2 be the matrices

$$M_1 = \begin{bmatrix} b_1 & a_{12} \\ b_2 & a_{22} \end{bmatrix}, \qquad M_2 = \begin{bmatrix} a_{11} & b_1 \\ a_{21} & b_2 \end{bmatrix},$$

then the solution of (S) can be written

$$x_1 = \frac{\det M_1}{\det M}, \qquad x_2 = \frac{\det M_2}{\det M}, \qquad \text{if } \det M \neq 0. \tag{8}$$

The solution to (S) given in Display (8) is called **Cramer's Rule** for $n = 2$.

Example 1   **CRAMER'S RULE WITH $n = 2$**   Here we solve the system of simultaneous equations

$$(T) \quad \begin{cases} 2x_1 + 3x_2 = 5 \\ 4x_1 + 5x_2 = 7. \end{cases}$$

For this system,

$$M = \begin{bmatrix} 2 & 3 \\ 4 & 5 \end{bmatrix}, \qquad M_1 = \begin{bmatrix} 5 & 3 \\ 7 & 5 \end{bmatrix}, \qquad M_2 = \begin{bmatrix} 2 & 5 \\ 4 & 7 \end{bmatrix}.$$

By the definition of determinant given in Display (7),

$$\det M = 2 \cdot 5 - 4 \cdot 3 = 10 - 12 = -2,$$
$$\det M_1 = 5 \cdot 5 - 7 \cdot 3 = 4,$$
$$\det M_2 = 2 \cdot 7 - 4 \cdot 5 = -6.$$

Since $\det M = -2 \neq 0$, Cramer's Rule gives us the solution

$$x_1 = \frac{\det M_1}{\det M} = \frac{4}{-2} = -2, \qquad x_2 = \frac{\det M_2}{\det M} = \frac{-6}{-2} = 3.$$

It is easy to substitute these values into the original equations and thus to check that $(x_1, x_2) = (-2, 3)$ does satisfy the system.   □

Now we repeat our original system of two simultaneous linear equations

$$(S) \quad \begin{cases} a_{11}x_1 + a_{12}x_2 = b_1 \\ a_{21}x_1 + a_{22}x_2 = b_2 \end{cases}$$

and describe another algorithm for solving the system. If each of the coefficients a_{ij} in this system is 0, the system is of the form

$$\begin{cases} 0 = b_1 \\ 0 = b_2 \end{cases}$$

and one cannot solve for x_1 and x_2. So we assume that some coefficient a_{ij} is not 0. Renumbering the unknowns and/or the equations if necessary, we can get a system with $a_{11} \neq 0$. Assuming that $a_{11} \neq 0$ in (S), we multiply each term in the first equation of (S) by the reciprocal a_{11}^{-1} of a_{11} and get

$$x_1 + a_{11}^{-1}a_{12}x_2 = a_{11}^{-1}b_1.$$

We multiply this equation by a_{21} and subtract from the second equation in (S); this gives us

$$(a_{22} - a_{21}a_{11}^{-1}a_{12})x_2 = b_2 - a_{21}a_{11}^{-1}b_1.$$

Thus the system (S) has been converted to the form

$$(S_2) \quad \begin{cases} x_1 + cx_2 = d \\ \phantom{x_1 + {}} ex_2 = f, \end{cases}$$

where $c = a_{11}^{-1}a_{12}$, $d = a_{11}^{-1}b_1$, $e = a_{22} - a_{11}^{-1}a_{21}a_{12}$, and $f = b_2 - a_{11}^{-1}a_{21}b_1$. In (S_2), if $e \neq 0$, we get $x_2 = e^{-1}f$ and then

$$x_1 = d - cx_2 = d - ce^{-1}f.$$

This algorithm is called **Gaussian Elimination** for $n = 2$.

Example 2   **GAUSSIAN ELIMINATION WITH $n = 2$**   Now we use the new algorithm to solve the same system considered in Example 1:

$$(T) \qquad \begin{cases} 2x_1 + 3x_2 = 5 \\ 4x_1 + 5x_2 = 7. \end{cases}$$

We multiply each term in the first equation by $\frac{1}{2}$ and get

$$x_1 + \frac{3}{2}x_2 = \frac{5}{2}.$$

We subtract 4 times this from the second equation and get

$$\left(5 - 4 \cdot \frac{3}{2}\right)x_2 = 7 - 4 \cdot \frac{5}{2}.$$

Thus the system (T) has been converted into the system

$$(T_1) \qquad \begin{cases} x_1 + \frac{3}{2}x_2 = \frac{5}{2} \\ \qquad\quad -x_2 = -3. \end{cases} \tag{9}$$

The second of these equations gives us $x_2 = 3$. Substituting $x_2 = 3$ into Equation (9), we have

$$x_1 = \frac{5}{2} - \frac{3}{2}x_2 = \frac{5}{2} - \frac{3}{2} \cdot 3 = \frac{5 - 9}{2} = \frac{-4}{2} = -2.$$

Hence we have $(x_1, x_2) = (-2, 3)$, which checks with the solution found in Example 1.   □

THE CASE OF $n = 3$

A 3 by 3 matrix has the form

$$M = \begin{bmatrix} a_{11} & a_{12} & a_{13} \\ a_{21} & a_{22} & a_{23} \\ a_{31} & a_{32} & a_{33} \end{bmatrix}. \tag{10}$$

As an aid in defining the determinant of this square matrix M, we introduce some associated 2 by 2 matrices, which are called minors of M. The **minor**

P_{ij} of M is the matrix obtained by deleting the ith row and jth column of M. Thus

$$P_{11} = \begin{bmatrix} a_{22} & a_{23} \\ a_{32} & a_{33} \end{bmatrix}, \qquad P_{21} = \begin{bmatrix} a_{12} & a_{13} \\ a_{32} & a_{33} \end{bmatrix}, \qquad P_{31} = \begin{bmatrix} a_{12} & a_{13} \\ a_{22} & a_{23} \end{bmatrix}. \tag{11}$$

Of the many formulas for det M, we choose

$$\det M = a_{11} \det P_{11} - a_{21} \det P_{21} + a_{31} \det P_{31} \tag{12}$$

as a definition of the determinant of the 3 by 3 matrix M.

Now we consider a system of 3 simultaneous linear equations in unknowns x_1, x_2, and x_3:

$$(U) \quad \begin{cases} a_{11}x_1 + a_{12}x_2 + a_{13}x_3 = b_1 \\ a_{21}x_1 + a_{22}x_2 + a_{23}x_3 = b_2 \\ a_{31}x_1 + a_{32}x_2 + a_{33}x_3 = b_3. \end{cases}$$

The **matrix of the system** is the M of Equation (10). If we replace the columns of M, one at a time, by the column of b's, we get the three matrices

$$M_1 = \begin{bmatrix} b_1 & a_{12} & a_{13} \\ b_2 & a_{22} & a_{23} \\ b_3 & a_{32} & a_{33} \end{bmatrix}, \qquad M_2 = \begin{bmatrix} a_{11} & b_1 & a_{13} \\ a_{21} & b_2 & a_{23} \\ a_{31} & b_3 & a_{33} \end{bmatrix}, \qquad M_3 = \begin{bmatrix} a_{11} & a_{12} & b_1 \\ a_{21} & a_{22} & b_2 \\ a_{31} & a_{32} & b_3 \end{bmatrix}.$$

It can be shown that if det $M \neq 0$, then the system (U) of 3 simultaneous linear equations has a unique solution given by

$$x_1 = \frac{\det M_1}{\det M}, \qquad x_2 = \frac{\det M_2}{\det M}, \qquad x_3 = \frac{\det M_3}{\det M}. \tag{13}$$

The formulas of Display (13) are **Cramer's Rule** for solving 3 linear equations in 3 unknowns. If det $M = 0$ and one of det M_1, det M_2, and det M_3 is not zero, then the system (U) has no solution. If

$$0 = \det M = \det M_1 = \det M_2 = \det M_3,$$

then the system (U) either has no solution or has an infinite number of solutions. We are interested here in counting the number of uses of some operation (such as multiplication) in an algorithm for finding the solution when the solution is unique, that is, the case of det $M \neq 0$.

Example 3   **CRAMER'S RULE WITH $n = 3$**   Here we use Cramer's Rule to solve the system

$$(V) \quad \begin{cases} 2x_1 + 6x_2 - 5x_3 = 1 \\ 3x_1 - 4x_2 = -17 \\ x_1 + 7x_2 - x_3 = 10. \end{cases}$$

The matrix of this system is

$$M = \begin{bmatrix} 2 & 6 & -5 \\ 3 & -4 & 0 \\ 1 & 7 & -1 \end{bmatrix}.$$

The minors of this matrix that are needed for the formula of Display (12) are

$$P_{11} = \begin{bmatrix} -4 & 0 \\ 7 & -1 \end{bmatrix}, \quad P_{21} = \begin{bmatrix} 6 & -5 \\ 7 & -1 \end{bmatrix}, \quad P_{31} = \begin{bmatrix} 6 & -5 \\ -4 & 0 \end{bmatrix}.$$

Using the formula of Display (7), we find that

$$\det P_{11} = 4, \qquad \det P_{21} = 29, \qquad \det P_{31} = -20.$$

Now it follows from the formula of Display (12) that

$$\det M = 2 \cdot 4 - 3 \cdot 29 + 1(-20) = 8 - 87 - 20 = -99.$$

Since $\det M = -99 \neq 0$, we continue with Cramer's Rule. The matrices M_1, M_2, and M_3 for the system (V) are

$$M_1 = \begin{bmatrix} 1 & 6 & -5 \\ -17 & -4 & 0 \\ 10 & 7 & -1 \end{bmatrix}, \quad M_2 = \begin{bmatrix} 2 & 1 & -5 \\ 3 & -17 & 0 \\ 1 & 10 & -1 \end{bmatrix}, \quad M_3 = \begin{bmatrix} 2 & 6 & 1 \\ 3 & -4 & -17 \\ 1 & 7 & 10 \end{bmatrix}.$$

We can use the formulas of Displays (11) and (12) to evaluate the determinants of these matrices; thus we find that

$$\det M_1 = 297, \qquad \det M_2 = -198, \qquad \det M_3 = -99.$$

Hence it follows from Display (13) that the unique solution to the system (V) is given by

$$x_1 = \frac{\det M_1}{\det M} = \frac{297}{-99} = -3, \quad x_2 = \frac{-198}{-99} = 2, \quad x_3 = \frac{-99}{-99} = 1. \quad \square$$

Example 4   **GAUSSIAN ELIMINATION WITH $n = 3$**   Now we solve the system of Example 3,

$$(V) \quad \begin{cases} 2x_1 + 6x_2 - 5x_3 = 1 \\ 3x_1 - 4x_2 \qquad = -17 \\ x_1 + 7x_2 - x_3 = 10, \end{cases}$$

using another algorithm. We convert the coefficient of x_1 in the first equation into 1 by multiplying each term of this equation by $\frac{1}{2}$; thus we get

$$x_1 + 3x_2 - \frac{5}{2}x_3 = \frac{1}{2}. \tag{14}$$

We eliminate x_1 from the second and third equations in the system (V) by subtracting 3 times Equation (14) from the second equation and subtracting Equation (14) from the third equation in (V). All of these steps replace the system (V) by

$$(V_1) \quad \begin{cases} x_1 + 3x_2 - \dfrac{5}{2}x_3 = \dfrac{1}{2} \\ \quad\quad bx_2 + cx_3 = d \\ \quad\quad ex_2 + fx_3 = g, \end{cases}$$

where

$$b = -4 - 3 \cdot 3 = -13, \qquad c = 0 - 3 \cdot \frac{5}{2} = -\frac{15}{2},$$

$$d = -17 - 3 \cdot \frac{1}{2} = -\frac{37}{2}, \qquad e = 7 - 3 = 4,$$

$$f = -1 - \frac{5}{2} = -\frac{7}{2}, \qquad g = 10 - \frac{1}{2} = \frac{19}{2}.$$

The next steps are to solve the last two equations of (V_1) simultaneously for x_2 and x_3, using the Gaussian Elimination algorithm illustrated in Example 2. Then one finds x_1 after substituting the found values of x_2 and x_3 in the first equation of (V_1). These steps should produce the solution $(x_1, x_2, x_3) = (-3, 2, 1)$ found in Example 3. ☐

THE GENERAL CASE

A system of n linear equations in n unknowns has the form

$$(L) \quad \begin{cases} a_{11}x_1 + a_{12}x_2 + \cdots + a_{1n}x_n = b_1 \\ a_{21}x_1 + a_{22}x_2 + \cdots + a_{2n}x_n = b_2 \\ \quad\vdots \quad\quad\quad \vdots \quad\quad\quad\quad \vdots \quad\quad \vdots \\ a_{n1}x_1 + a_{n2}x_2 + \cdots + a_{nn}x_n = b_n. \end{cases}$$

The *matrix of the system* (L) is

$$M = \begin{bmatrix} a_{11} & a_{12} & \cdots & a_{1n} \\ a_{21} & a_{22} & \cdots & a_{2n} \\ \vdots & \vdots & & \vdots \\ a_{n1} & a_{n2} & \cdots & a_{nn} \end{bmatrix}.$$

The minor P_{ij} of M is the $(n-1)$ by $(n-1)$ matrix obtained by deleting the ith row and the jth column of M. We give an inductive definition of the **determinant**, det M, of the square matrix M. The basis of this definition is the case of $n = 2$ given in Display (7). The inductive part is

$$\det M = a_{11} \det P_{11} - a_{21} \det P_{21} + \cdots + (-1)^{n+1} a_{n1} \det P_{n1}. \qquad (15)$$

For $j = 1, 2, \ldots, n$, let M_j be the n by n matrix resulting when the jth column of M is replaced by the column of b's, which appear after the equal signs in (L). It can be proved that if $\det M \neq 0$, then the system (L) has a unique solution, given by

$$x_1 = \frac{\det M_1}{\det M}, \quad x_2 = \frac{\det M_2}{\det M}, \quad \ldots, \quad x_n = \frac{\det M_n}{\det M}.$$

These formulas are called **Cramer's Rule**. We rewrite these formulas as

$$x_1 = (\det M)^{-1}(\det M_1), \quad x_2 = (\det M)^{-1}(\det M_2), \quad \ldots, \quad x_n = (\det M)^{-1}(\det M_n). \qquad (16)$$

Let us count the number of multiplications required in using Cramer's Rule to solve n linear equations in n unknowns, with the assumption that the determinants will be evaluated by the inductive definition given in Display (15). Let h_n be the number of multiplications in such an evaluation of an n by n determinant. Display (7) shows that $h_2 = 2$. Using the formula of Display (15), it takes h_{n-1} multiplications to evaluate a single det P_{i1}, and so it takes $1 + h_{n-1}$ multiplications to get $a_{i1} \cdot \det P_{i1}$. Since there are n terms in Display (15), we see that

$$h_n = n(1 + h_{n-1}). \qquad (17)$$

Hence $h_3 = 3(1 + h_2) = 3(1 + 2) = 9$, $h_4 = 4(1 + h_3) = 4(1 + 9) = 40$. It is left as Problem 8 below to prove by mathematical induction that

$$h_n = n! \left[\frac{1}{1!} + \frac{1}{2!} + \frac{1}{3!} + \cdots + \frac{1}{(n-1)!} \right] \qquad \text{for } n \text{ in } \{2, 3, \ldots\}. \qquad (18)$$

This implies that $h_n > n!$. Since there are $n + 1$ determinants, each n by n, and n multiplications by $(\det M)^{-1}$ in Display (16), the number f_n of multiplications required by these formulas for Cramer's Rule is given by

$$f_n = (n + 1)h_n + n. \qquad (19)$$

Since $h_n > n!$, it follows that $f_n > (n + 1)!$.

Now we give an inductive discussion of **Gaussian Elimination**. For this algorithm we have to make the coefficient a_{11} in (L) nonzero. This may involve relabeling the equations or unknowns in the system. Then we calculate a_{11}^{-1} and replace the first equation of (L) with

$$x_1 + a_{11}^{-1} a_{12} x_2 + a_{11}^{-1} a_{13} x_3 + \cdots + a_{11}^{-1} a_{1n} x_n = a_{11}^{-1} b_1.$$

For $i = 2, 3, \ldots, n$, we subtract a_{i1} times this equation from the ith equation in (L). These steps replace the system (L) with a system having the form

$$(L_1) \quad \begin{cases} x_1 + c_{12}x_2 + c_{13}x_3 + \cdots + c_{1n}x_n = d_1 \\ \quad\;\; c_{22}x_2 + c_{23}x_3 + \cdots + c_{2n}x_n = d_2 \\ \quad\;\; c_{32}x_2 + c_{33}x_3 + \cdots + c_{3n}x_n = d_3 \\ \qquad \vdots \qquad\; \vdots \qquad\qquad\; \vdots \qquad\; \vdots \\ \quad\;\; c_{n2}x_2 + c_{n3}x_3 + \cdots + c_{nn}x_n = d_n. \end{cases}$$

The basis for this inductive algorithm is the solution $x = a^{-1}b$ of the equation $ax = b$ in the case of $n = 1$. The inductive part uses the fact that the last $n - 1$ equations in the system (L_1) form a system of $n - 1$ linear equations in $n - 1$ unknowns. We solve this system for $x_2, x_3, \ldots, x_n$ using Gaussian Elimination for $n - 1$ equations in $n - 1$ unknowns. Then we substitute these values into the first equation of (L_1) and solve for x_1.

Let g_n be the number of multiplications needed to solve a system (L) by Gaussian Elimination. To go from (L) to (L_1) requires n^2 multiplications. Solving the system of the last $n - 1$ equations in (L_1) for $x_2, x_3, \ldots,$ x_n requires g_{n-1} multiplications. Then one needs $n - 1$ multiplications to use the first equation in (L_1) to solve for x_1. Thus

$$g_n = n^2 + n - 1 + g_{n-1}. \tag{20}$$

The case of $n = 1$ above shows that $g_1 = 1$. Then $g_1, g_2, \ldots$ is the solution of the recursion with initial condition

$$g_n - g_{n-1} = n^2 + n - 1, \qquad g_1 = 1.$$

Using the methods of Chapter 9, one can show that

$$g_n = \frac{1}{3} n^3 + n^2 - \frac{1}{3} n \qquad \text{for } n \text{ in } \mathbf{Z}^+.$$

Since $g_{24} = 5176$, Gaussian Elimination is certainly feasible when $n = 24$; Problem 7 below helps us judge whether Cramer's Rule is practical when $n \geq 24$.

PROBLEMS FOR SECTION 10.2

1. Use Cramer's Rule to solve the system
$$\begin{cases} 5x_1 + 3x_2 = -4 \\ 8x_1 + 5x_2 = 11. \end{cases}$$

2. Use Cramer's Rule to solve the system
$$\begin{cases} 7x_1 - 8x_2 = 6 \\ 2x_1 + 3x_2 = 7. \end{cases}$$

3. Evaluate the determinant of the 3 by 3 matrix

$$M = \begin{bmatrix} 2 & 3 & 4 \\ 5 & -6 & 7 \\ 8 & -9 & -10 \end{bmatrix}.$$

4. Evaluate the determinant of the 3 by 3 matrix

$$M = \begin{bmatrix} 5 & -11 & 8 \\ 0 & -6 & 3 \\ 0 & 3 & -2 \end{bmatrix}.$$

5. Use Gaussian Elimination to solve the system

$$\begin{cases} 2x_1 + 4x_2 - 10x_3 = 6 \\ 3x_1 + 5x_2 + 11x_3 = -14 \\ -4x_1 - 3x_2 + 8x_3 = -15. \end{cases}$$

6. Use Gaussian Elimination to solve the system

$$\begin{cases} 3x_1 - 9x_2 + 15x_3 = -15 \\ 4x_1 - 13x_2 - 6x_3 = 33 \\ 6x_1 + 7x_2 + 2x_3 = 9. \end{cases}$$

7. Assume that a particular computer does one billion multiplications per second. How many years will it take this computer to do 1.5×10^{25} multiplications? (This helps us decide whether Cramer's Rule is practical for $n \geq 24$, since $f_{24} > 1.5 \times 10^{25}$.)

8. Let $h_1, h_2, \ldots$ be the infinite sequence with $h_1 = 0$ and $h_n = n(1 + h_{n-1})$ for n in $\{2, 3, \ldots\}$. Prove by mathematical induction on n that

$$h_n = n! \left[\frac{1}{1!} + \frac{1}{2!} + \cdots + \frac{1}{(n-1)!} \right] \quad \text{for } n \text{ in } \{2, 3, \ldots\}$$

9. Show that $\det M = aehj$ when

$$M = \begin{bmatrix} a & b & c & d \\ 0 & e & f & g \\ 0 & 0 & h & i \\ 0 & 0 & 0 & j \end{bmatrix}.$$

10. For the n by n matrix

$$M = \begin{bmatrix} a_{11} & a_{12} & a_{13} & \cdots & a_{1,n-1} & a_{1n} \\ 0 & a_{22} & a_{23} & \cdots & a_{2,n-1} & a_{2n} \\ \vdots & \vdots & \vdots & & \vdots & \vdots \\ 0 & 0 & 0 & \cdots & 0 & a_{nn} \end{bmatrix}$$

with each entry below the main diagonal equal to 0, prove by induction on n that $\det M = a_{11}a_{22}\cdots a_{nn}$.

11. Find $\det M$ explicitly for

$$M = \begin{bmatrix} a_{11} & a_{12} & a_{13} \\ a_{21} & a_{22} & a_{23} \\ a_{31} & a_{32} & a_{33} \end{bmatrix}.$$

12. Use the answer to Problem 11 to find $\det M$ for

$$M = \begin{bmatrix} a & 0 & 0 \\ b & c & 0 \\ d & e & f \end{bmatrix}.$$

13. Use the answer to Problem 11 to show that $\det M = \det T$, where

$$M = \begin{bmatrix} a_{11} & a_{12} & a_{13} \\ a_{21} & a_{22} & a_{23} \\ a_{31} & a_{32} & a_{33} \end{bmatrix}, \qquad T = \begin{bmatrix} a_{11} & a_{21} & a_{31} \\ a_{12} & a_{22} & a_{32} \\ a_{13} & a_{23} & a_{33} \end{bmatrix}.$$

14. Use $h_n = n(1 + h_{n-1})$ and $f_n = (n+1)h_n + n$ to show that $f_n = (n+1)f_{n-1} + 2n + 1$.

15. Use $f_4 = 204$ and $f_n = (n+1)f_{n-1} + 2n + 1$ to calculate f_5, f_6, and f_7.

16. Use $g_4 = 36$ and $g_n = n^2 + n - 1 + g_{n-1}$ to calculate g_5, g_6, and g_7.

17. Let

$$A = \begin{bmatrix} 3 & 4 \\ s & 2 \end{bmatrix}.$$

Find s, given that $\det A = 0$.

18. Let

$$B = \begin{bmatrix} 0 & 1 & 4 \\ t & 2 & 1 \\ -3 & -1 & 3 \end{bmatrix}.$$

Find t, given that $\det B = 0$.

19. Find a number s for which there is no solution to the system

$$\begin{cases} 3x + 4y = -10 \\ sx - 2y = 6. \end{cases}$$

20. Find a number t for which there are infinitely many solutions to the system

$$\begin{cases} 5x - 6y = 7 \\ 10x - 12y = t. \end{cases}$$

21. Let M be a 2 by 2 matrix and let M' be the matrix obtained by interchanging the rows of M. What is the relationship between det M and det M'?

22. Repeat Problem 21, but with "rows" replaced by "columns."

23. Let

$$M = \begin{bmatrix} a & b \\ c & d \end{bmatrix} \quad \text{and} \quad K = \begin{bmatrix} ka & b \\ kc & d \end{bmatrix}.$$

What is the relationship between det M and det K?

24. Repeat Problem 23, but with K now

$$\begin{bmatrix} a & b \\ kc & kd \end{bmatrix}.$$

25. Let $g_n = (n^3 + 3n^2 - n)/3$. Find the largest positive integer n for which a computer that performs 10^9 multiplications per second could do g_n multiplications within one hour.

26. Repeat Problem 25 with "one hour" replaced by "one day."

10.3

ASYMPTOTIC BEHAVIOR OF COMPLEXITY FUNCTIONS

This section is a brief introduction to some concepts that help in answering the three following types of questions:

(I) Can a given algorithm perform a desired task in the available time or within the available budget?

(II) Which of several algorithms would perform a desired task in the least time or with the least cost?

(III) If one has a feasible algorithm, should one try to find a better one?

If a positive integer n specifies the extent of a task in some way, we call n a *parameter* for the task. For example, the number n of entries in an n-vector $(a_1, a_2, \ldots, a_n)$ is the most appropriate parameter for the task of sorting n-vectors by a given algorithm. Also, the number n of equations (or unknowns) in a system of n linear equations in n unknowns is usually the parameter for the task of solving such a system using a given algorithm. In the traveling salesperson problem of Example 1 in Section 6.6, the natural parameter is the number n of vertices of the weighted graph.

Let Z^+ and R^+ denote the sets of positive integers and of positive real numbers, respectively.

DEFINITION 1   **COMPLEXITY FUNCTION FOR AN ALGORITHM**

Let n be a parameter for some task and let f be a mapping from Z^+ to R^+ such that $f(n)$ is a measure of the time or cost of performing the task for given n using a given algorithm A. Then f is called a *complexity function* for A (with respect to the parameter n).

In Section 10.1, we used $B(n)$ to denote the maximum number of comparisons that might be needed in the bubble sorting algorithm for sorting an n-vector and used $D(n)$ as the analogous function for the divide-and-conquer sorting algorithm. Each of the mappings

$$B: n \mapsto B(n), \qquad D: n \mapsto D(n)$$

is a complexity function for its own algorithm.

Similarly, in Section 10.2, we used f_n to denote the number of multiplications in the Cramer's Rule algorithm for solving n linear equations in n unknowns and used g_n for the number of multiplications in the Gaussian Elimination algorithm for the same task. Each of the mappings

$$f: n \mapsto f_n, \qquad g: n \mapsto g_n$$

is a complexity function for its respective algorithm.

Let us consider a computer that can perform 10^9 multiplications per second. Such a computer can do g_n multiplications in less than one hour if $n \le 22091$. However, it can accomplish f_n multiplications within an hour only if $n \le 14$. In fact, we saw in Problem 7 of Section 10.2 that it would take more than $4.7 \times 10^8 = 470000000$ years to do f_{24} multiplications. These facts show that Cramer's Rule is a practical algorithm only for fairly small values of the parameter n and that Gaussian Elimination is feasible for a much larger range of values of n.

Example 1

TABLE 10.3.1

n	$F(n) = 2^n$	$G(n) = n^3$
1	2	1
2	4	8
3	8	27
4	16	64
5	32	125
6	64	216
7	128	343
8	256	512
9	512	729
10	1024	1000

Let us assume that $F(n) = 2^n$ and $G(n) = n^3$ specify complexity functions F and G for two different algorithms for a given task. Table 10.3.1 shows that $F(n) < G(n)$ for $2 \le n \le 9$. However, it can be shown that $G(n) < F(n)$ for $n \ge 10$. We note that

$$F(20) = 1048576 \quad \text{and} \quad G(20) = 8000.$$

The ratio $F(n)/G(n)$ grows very rapidly, and hence the ratio $G(n)/F(n)$ becomes very small, as the parameter n increases. For example, $G(n) <$ .001 $F(n)$ for $n \ge 24$ and $G(n) < .00001 F(n)$ for $n \ge 32$. Since $2^{10} = 1024$, we easily see that $F(100) = 2^{100} = (2^{10})^{10} > (10^3)^{10} = 10^{30}$. Hence

$$\frac{F(100)}{G(100)} > \frac{10^{30}}{(10^2)^3} = \frac{10^{30}}{10^6} = 10^{24}.$$

The ratio $F(n)/G(n)$ increases without bound as n increases. In the notation of calculus, one can write

$$\lim_{n \to \infty} \frac{F(n)}{G(n)} = \infty.$$

Which algorithm should one consider in programming the given task for a computer? The decision might be made on the basis of ease of programming when the parameter n is small; but when n is large, the algorithm with G as its complexity function would take much less time (or money). Moreover, the values of $G(100)$ and $F(100)$ show that the G algorithm may be feasible when the F algorithm is completely impractical.   □

Notations 1 and 2, which follow, introduce relations "is big Oh of" and "is little oh of" that may apply to complexity functions.

NOTATION 1   **IS BIG OH OF**

Let g and f be mappings from Z^+ to R^+. Then "$g(n)$ is $O[f(n)]$" means that there exist positive real numbers c and n_0 such that $g(n) \leq cf(n)$ for $n \geq n_0$.

For the $G(n) = n^3$ and $F(n) = 2^n$ of Example 1, *any one* of the statements

$G(n) \leq F(n)$ for $n \geq 10$,

$G(n) \leq .001\, F(n)$ for $n \geq 24$,

$G(n) \leq .00001\, F(n)$ for $n \geq 32$

is sufficient to establish that $G(n)$ is $O[F(n)]$. If $K(n) = 1000G(n) = 1000n^3$ and $H(n) = F(n)/100 = 2^n/100$, then $G(n) \leq F(n)$ for $n \geq 10$ implies that

$K(n) = 1000G(n) \leq 1000F(n) = 100000H(n)$ for $n \geq 10$.

Then $K(n) \leq 10^5\, H(n)$ for $n \geq 10$ and Notation 1 with $c = 10^5$ and $n_0 = 10$ tell us that $K(n)$ is $O[H(n)]$.

The statements that "$G(n)$ is $O[F(n)]$" and "$K(n)$ is $O[H(n)]$" can be strengthened so as to contain more of the observations made in Example 1; the following notation is an aid for such stronger statements.

NOTATION 2   **IS LITTLE OH OF**

Let g and f be mappings from Z^+ to R^+. Then "$g(n)$ is $o[f(n)]$" means that for every positive real number s there exists a positive integer n_0 such that $g(n) \leq sf(n)$ for $n \geq n_0$.

Let $G(n) = n^3$ and $F(n) = 2^n$. Statements in Example 1 tell us that with the s of Notation 2 taken to be 1, we have

$$n^3 \leq 2^n \qquad \text{for } n \geq 10$$

and with $s = .00001$ we have

$$n^3 \leq .00001 \cdot 2^n \qquad \text{for } n \geq 32.$$

It can be proved that for every positive real number s, no matter how small, there exists a positive integer n_0 such that $n^3 \leq s \cdot 2^n$ for $n \geq n_0$. This means that n^3 is $o[2^n]$. Thus the statement that "$G(n)$ is $O[F(n)]$" can be strengthened to "$G(n)$ is $o[F(n)]$" for these complexity functions. We will see in Example 2 that such strengthening is not always possible.

Examination of Notations 1 and 2 shows that the essential difference between "big oh" and "little oh" is the fact that "big oh" involves "some positive number c," whereas "little oh" requires the same type of statement for "every positive number s (no matter how small)."

Let there be two algorithms A and B for some task and let their complexity functions be $g(n)$ and $f(n)$, respectively. By building a faster computer, one extends the range of values of the parameter n for which each algorithm is practical. If $g(n)$ is $o[f(n)]$, such extension makes the advantage of the A algorithm more dramatic. For example, let $g(n) = n^3$ and $f(n) = 2^n$ and let each of these complexity functions give the time needed to complete its program. Then for the range $\{10, 11, \ldots, 31\}$ of values of the parameter n, one can say that the A algorithm requires less time. On the other hand, for a range of values of n in the set $\{32, 33, \ldots\}$, the A algorithm takes less than $\frac{1}{100000}$ of the time that B requires. Thus the advantage of the A algorithm over the B algorithm grows dramatically as the parameter n increases; this is a consequence of the fact that $g(n)$ is $o[f(n)]$.

Example 2   The complexity function for the Gaussian Elimination algorithm described in Section 10.2 is the mapping

$$g: n \mapsto g_n = \frac{1}{3} n^3 + n^2 - \frac{1}{3} n.$$

Here we show that g_n is $O[n^3]$ and that n^3 is $O[g_n]$. We use the facts that $n^2 \leq n^3$ and $n \leq n^2$ for all n in $\mathbf{Z}^+$. The inequality $n^2 \leq n^3$ helps us see that

$$g_n = \frac{1}{3} n^3 + n^2 - \frac{1}{3} n \leq \frac{1}{3} n^3 + n^3 - \frac{1}{3} n \leq \frac{1}{3} n^3 + n^3 = \frac{4}{3} n^3 \qquad \text{for } n \geq 1.$$

This and Notation 1 with $c = \frac{4}{3}$ and $n_0 = 1$ show us that g_n is $O[n^3]$. For n in $\mathbf{Z}^+$, the inequality $n \leq n^2$ implies that $n \leq 3n^2$. Hence $3n^2 - n \geq 0$

and

$$n^3 \leq n^3 + 3n^2 - n = 3g_n \qquad \text{for } n \geq 1.$$

This and Notation 1 with $c = 3$ and $n_0 = 1$ imply that n^3 is $O[g_n]$.

The statement that "g_n is $O[n^3]$" *cannot* be replaced by the stronger statement that "g_n is $o[n^3]$." We see this by noting that for $s = \frac{1}{4}$, there is no positive integer n_0 such that $g_n \leq n^3/4$ for $n \geq n_0$, since such inequalities would imply that

$$\frac{1}{3} n^3 \leq \frac{1}{3} n^3 + \left(n^2 - \frac{1}{3} n\right) = g_n \leq \frac{1}{4} n^3 \qquad \text{for } n \geq n_0$$

and thus would give the contradiction $\frac{1}{3} < \frac{1}{4}$. $\square$

NOTATION 3   **EQUIVALENT COMPLEXITY FUNCTIONS**

Complexity functions f and g are said to be ***equivalent***, and we write $f(n) \sim g(n)$, if $f(n)$ is $O[g(n)]$ and $g(n)$ is $O[f(n)]$.

For example, if $g(n) = n^3$ and $f(n) = (n^3 + 3n^2 - n)/3$, then statements in Example 2 imply that $g(n)$ is $O[f(n)]$ and that $f(n)$ is $O[g(n)]$. Hence $f(n) \sim g(n)$; that is, f and g are equivalent.

Let A and B be algorithms for some task with f and g, respectively, as complexity functions. If $f(n) \sim g(n)$, then the algorithms are roughly equivalent; that is, one algorithm may be better than the other by some factor, but the advantage of the better algorithm does not grow dramatically as n increases. For the specific f and g with $f(n) = (n^3 + 3n^2 - n)/3$ and $g(n) = n^3$, the ratio $g(n)/f(n)$ is close to 3 for almost all positive integers n.

THEOREM 1   **A POLYNOMIAL IS EQUIVALENT TO ITS DOMINANT TERM**

Let p be a polynomial function from $\mathbf{Z}^+$ to $\mathbf{R}^+$ given by

$$p(n) = a_0 n^d + a_1 n^{d-1} + \cdots + a_n,$$

with the a_i constants and $a_0 > 0$. Then $p(n) \sim n^d$.

PARTIAL PROOF   If $i < j$, one has $n^i \leq n^j$ for all n in $\mathbf{Z}^+$. Hence

$$p(n) = a_0 n^d + a_1 n^{d-1} + \cdots + a_n \leq |a_0| n^d + |a_1| n^d + \cdots + |a_n| n^d,$$

where $|x|$ denotes the absolute value of x. This inequality and

$$c = |a_0| + |a_1| + \cdots + |a_n|$$

give us $p(n) \leq cn^d$ for $n \geq 1$. Hence $p(n)$ is $O[n^d]$. The proof that n^d is $O[p(n)]$ is omitted. Together these statements give $p(n) \sim n^d$.   □

Logarithms are involved in complexity functions for certain algorithms. We now define $\log_b x$ for a **base** b greater than 1 and for any positive real number x.

DEFINITION 2   **LOGARITHM OF x TO THE BASE b**

Let b and x be real numbers, with $b > 1$ and $x > 0$. Then **$\log_b x$** is the unique real number t such that $b^t = x$. Also, $\log x$ means $\log_2 x$; that is, when the **base** b is omitted, we assume the base to be 2.

For example, $\log_3 81 = 4$ because $3^4 = 81$. Also, it follows from $1000 = 10^3$ that $\log_{10} 1000 = 3$, and it follows from $8^{1/3} = \sqrt[3]{8} = 2$ that $\log_8 2 = \frac{1}{3}$. These statements can be rewritten as

$$\log_3 3^4 = 4, \qquad \log_{10} 10^3 = 3, \qquad \log_8 8^{1/3} = \frac{1}{3}. \tag{1}$$

The equalities in Display (1) are all special cases of $\log_b b^t = t$, which is a restatement of Definition 2.

Since $\log x = \log_2 x$, it follows from $64 = 2^6$ that $\log 64 = 6$ and from $\sqrt{2} = 2^{1/2}$ that $\log \sqrt{2} = \frac{1}{2}$. In general, $\log 2^t = t$ for all real numbers t.

DEFINITION 3   **ORDERING OF COMPLEXITY FUNCTIONS**

A statement such as "$g(n)$ is $O[f(n)]$" or "$g(n)$ is $o[f(n)]$" is called an **ordering** of the complexity functions $g(n)$ and $f(n)$.

We next state, without proof, some orderings of specific complexity functions.

THEOREM 2   **ORDERINGS OF SOME COMPLEXITY FUNCTIONS**

(a) $\log n$ is $o[n]$.
(b) If $0 < d < e$, then n^d is $o[n^e]$.
(c) If d is in N and $b > 1$, then n^d is $o[b^n]$.
(d) If $b > 1$, then b^n is $o[n!]$.
(e) $n!$ is $o[n^n]$.

For example, it follows from Part (b) of Theorem 2 that $\sqrt{n} = n^{1/2}$ is $o[n]$. If follows from Part (c) that n^{100} is $o[1.1^n]$, and it follows from Part (d) that 1000^n is $o(n!)$.

The following general result, also presented without proof, allows us to get new specific orderings from other orderings.

THEOREM 3   **TRANSITIVITY OF ORDERINGS**

Let f, g, and h be complexity functions.

(a) If $f(n)$ is $O[g(n)]$ and $g(n)$ is $O[h(n)]$, then $f(n)$ is $O[h(n)]$.
(b) If $f(n)$ is $o[g(n)]$ and $g(n)$ is $o[h(n)]$, then $f(n)$ is $o[h(n)]$.
(c) If $f(n)$ is $O[g(n)]$ and $g(n)$ is $o[h(n)]$, then $f(n)$ is $o[h(n)]$.
(d) If $f(n)$ is $o[g(n)]$ and $g(n)$ is $O[h(n)]$, then $f(n)$ is $o[h(n)]$.

For example, it follows from Theorem 2 that $\log n$ is $o(n)$ and that n is $o[n^3]$; these facts and Theorem 3(b) tell us that $\log n$ is $o[n^3]$. Also, we know from Example 2 that $\frac{1}{3}n^3 + n^2 - \frac{1}{3}n$ is $O[n^3]$ and from Theorem 2(c) that n^3 is $o[1.01^n]$; hence it follows from Theorem 3(c) that $\frac{1}{3}n^3 + n^2 - \frac{1}{3}n$ is $o[1.01^n]$.

Another useful result follows.

THEOREM 4   **MULTIPLYING AN ORDERING**

(a) Let f, g, and h be complexity functions. If $g(n)$ is $O[f(n)]$, then $h(n)g(n)$ is $O[h(n)f(n)]$.
(b) Part (a) remains true when each "big oh" is replaced by a "little oh."

PROOF   (a) The hypothesis that $g(n)$ is $O[f(n)]$ means that there exist positive numbers c and n_0 such that

$$g(n) \le cf(n) \qquad \text{for } n \ge n_0. \tag{2}$$

Since h is a complexity function, that is, a mapping from $\mathbf{Z}^+$ to the set $\mathbf{R}^+$ of positive real numbers, we have $h(n) > 0$ for all n in $\mathbf{Z}^+$. Therefore we can multiply the inequality in Display (2) by $h(n)$ and get

$$h(n)g(n) \le ch(n)f(n) \qquad \text{for } n \ge n_0.$$

This means that $h(n)g(n)$ is $O[h(n)f(n)]$.
(b) The proof of Part (b) is very similar and is left to the reader.   □

Example 3   Here we show that, as n increases, the advantage of an algorithm with $n \log n$ as its complexity function increases vastly over an algorithm with

n^2 as its complexity function. We see from Theorem 2(a) that $\log n$ is $o[n]$. Then Theorem 4(b) allows us to multiply by n and thus see that $n \log n$ is $o[n^2]$. This means that for any positive real numbers s, no matter how small, there is a range $n \geq n_0$ of values of the parameter n for which $n \log n$ is less than sn^2. $\qquad \square$

Next we present, without proof, another general result on orderings of complexity functions.

THEOREM 5　**LINEAR COMBINATIONS**

(a) Let $f, g_1, g_2, \ldots, g_r$ be complexity functions such that $g_i(n)$ is $o[f(n)]$ for $i = 1, 2, \ldots, r$. Then $a_1 g_1(n) + a_2 g_2(n) + \cdots + a_r g_r(n)$ is $o[f(n)]$ for any constants $a_1, a_2, \ldots, a_r$.

(b) Part (a) remains true when each "little oh" is replaced by a "big oh."

For example, it follows from Theorem 2(c) that n^3 is $o[1.001^n]$ and that n^4 is $o[1.001^n]$; hence it follows from Theorem 5(a) that $(100n^4 + 1000n^3)$ is $o[1.001^n]$.

Example 4　In Example 3 of Section 10.1, we showed that the complexity function $D: n \mapsto D(n)$ for the divide-and-conquer sorting algorithm satisfies

$$D(2^n) = 2^n(n-1) + 1 \qquad \text{for all } n \text{ in } \mathbf{Z}^+. \tag{3}$$

Let $m = 2^n$. Then $n = \log m$ and Display (3) can be rewritten as

$$D(m) = m(\log m - 1) + 1 \qquad \text{for } m \text{ in } \{2, 4, 8, \ldots\}. \tag{4}$$

Since $D(n)$ does not decrease when n increases, it can be shown that the statement in Display (4) implies that $D(n)$ is $O[n \log n]$. In fact $D(n) \sim n \log n$.

We note that the bubble sorting algorithm (Algorithm 2) of Section 10.1 has $B(n) = (n^2 - n)/2$ as its complexity function. It follows from Theorem 1 that $B(n) \sim n^2$. Hence n^2 is $O[B(n)]$. We see from Theorem 2(a) that $\log n$ is $o[n]$. This and Theorem 4(b) tell us that $n \log n$ is $o[n^2]$. Now, the statements that $D(n)$ is $O[n \log n]$, $n \log n$ is $o[n^2]$, and n^2 is $O[B(n)]$, together with the transitivity results of Theorem 3, imply that $D(n)$ is $o[B(n)]$. Hence the advantage of divide-and-conquer sorting over bubble sorting increases with increasing n and thus increases for faster computers.

Using the "decision tree" concept illustrated in the "bad coin" examples and problems of Section 6.3, it can be shown that the best algorithm for sorting that one might discover would share with the divide-and-conquer algorithm the property that its complexity function is equivalent to $n \log n$. This means that any advantage such an optimal algorithm might have over "divide and conquer" would not grow much greater with increasing n.   □

PROBLEMS FOR SECTION 10.3

1. Tabulate $g(n) = 2^n$ and $f(n) = n!$ for $n = 1, 2, \ldots, 10$.

2. Tabulate $k(n) = 4^n$ and $f(n) = n!$ for $n = 8, 9, 10, 11, 12$.

3. Let $g(n) = 2^n$ and $f(n) = n!$. Find the smallest positive integers r, s, and t such that:
(a) $g(n) \leq f(n)$ *for* $n \geq r$.   (b) $g(n) \leq .1f(n)$ for $n \geq s$.
(c) $g(n) \leq .01f(n)$ for $n \geq t$.

4. Find the smallest positive integer n_0 such that $2^n \leq .001(n!)$ for $n \geq n_0$.

5. A computer does 10^9 multiplications per second.
(i) Find the largest positive integer n such that the computer can do 2^n multiplications within one hour.
(ii) Find the largest n such that the computer can do $n!$ multiplications within one hour.

6. (a) Repeat the parts of Problem 5 with "one hour" replaced with "one year."
(b) Repeat the parts of Problem 5, but for a computer that could do 10^{12} multiplications per second.

7. Given that r is a positive real number and that $g(n)$ is $O[f(n)]$, prove that $g(n)$ is $O[rf(n)]$.

8. Given that r is a positive real number and that $g(n)$ is $o[f(n)]$, prove that $g(n)$ is $o[rf(n)]$.

9. Justify the assertion that 1000^n is $o[.01(n!)]$. (It is irrelevant that $1000^n > .01(n!)$ at least for $n = 1, 2, \ldots, 1000$.)

10. Justify the assertion that n^{100000} is $o[.001 \cdot 1.0001^n]$.

11. Label the following functions as $g_1(n), g_2(n), \ldots, g_6(n)$ so that $g_i(n)$ is $o[g_{i+1}(n)]$ for $n = 1, 2, 3, 4, 5$.
(a) $.00001(n^n)$,   (b) $.0001(n!)$,   (c) $.001(100^n)$,   (d) $.01(2^n)$,
(e) $.1(n^{99})$,   (f) $n^{98} \log n$.

12. Repeat Problem 11 for the following functions:
(a) $3 \cdot 7^n$,   (b) n^n,   (c) $4 \cdot 2^n$,   (d) $5n^8$,   (e) $n^8 \log n$,
(f) $2n!$. [Note that $2n! = 2(n!)$, which is different from $(2n)!$.]

13. Show that $2n! \sim n!$.

*14. Show that $(2n)!$ and $n!$ are not equivalent and that $n!$ is $o[(2n)!]$.

SUMMARY OF TERMS, CHAPTER 10 _____

$A(n)$	Number of comparisons in using Algorithm 1 of Section 10.1 to find the min of an n-vector.	556
Base of a logarithm	The b of $(b^t = x) \Leftrightarrow (\log_b x = t)$.	579
Big oh	$g(n)$ is $O[f(n)]$ if there are positive c and n_0 such that $g(n) \leq cf(n)$ for $n \geq n_0$.	576
$B(n)$	Number of comparisons in using "Bubble Sorting," (Algorithm 2 of Section 10.1) to sort an n-vector.	557
Bubble sorting	See Algorithm 2 of Section 10.1.	557
$C(m, n)$	Maximum number of comparisons needed to merge a sorted m-vector and a sorted n-vector.	558
Complexity function	A mapping $n \mapsto f(n)$, where n is a parameter and $f(n)$ is a measure of the time or cost of an algorithm for a given n.	575
Cramer's Rule	An algorithm for solving systems of linear equations using determinants.	564, 570
Determinant	See Section 10.2.	564, 570
Divide-and-conquer sorting	See Algorithm 4 of Section 10.1.	559
$D(n)$	The maximum number of comparisons in sorting an n-vector by Algorithm 4 ("Divide-and-Conquer Sorting") of Section 10.1.	559
Dominant term	See Theorem 1 of Section 10.3.	578
Equivalent complexity functions	$f(n) \sim g(n)$ if $f(n)$ is $O[g(n)]$ and $g(n)$ is $O[f(n)]$.	578
Gaussian Elimination	An efficient algorithm for solving systems of n linear equations in n unknowns.	566, 570
Linear combinations	See Theorem 5 of Section 10.3.	581
Little oh	$g(n)$ is $o[f(n)]$ if for every positive s there is an n_0 such that $g(n) \leq sf(n)$ for $n \geq n_0$.	576
Logarithm to base b	$(\log_b x = t) \Leftrightarrow (b^t = x)$.	579
Matrix	An array of numbers in rows and columns.	564, 569
Merging	Making a sorted $(m + n)$-vector out of a sorted m-vector and a sorted n-vector.	557–558
Min	$\min(a_1, \ldots, a_n)$ is the smallest a_i.	556
Minor M_{ij}	Matrix obtained by striking out the ith row and the jth column of a square matrix M.	566
Multiplying an ordering	See Theorem 4 of Section 10.3.	580
n-vector	An ordered n-tuple $(a_1, a_2, \ldots, a_n)$.	555
Ordering of complexity functions	See Definition 3 of Section 10.3.	579
Parameter	A measure of the extent of an algorithm.	574
Recursion for $D(n)$	$D(2m) = 2D(m) + 2m - 1$, $D(2m + 1) = D(m) + D(m + 1) + 2m$.	559
Sinker sorting	See Problem 2 of Section 10.1.	561
Sort	To arrange in numerical order.	555

REVIEW PROBLEMS FOR CHAPTER 10

1. Consider the following algorithm for finding $m = \min(a_1, a_2, \ldots, a_{2m})$:
Use Algorithm 1 ("Finding the Min") of Section 10.1 to find

$$m' = \min(a_1, a_2, \ldots, a_m), \qquad m'' = \min(a_{m+1}, a_{m+2}, \ldots, a_{2m}),$$

and then $m = \min(m', m'')$.
(i) What is the number of comparisons needed for this new algorithm?
(ii) Is the answer to Part (i) less than, equal to, or greater than the number $A(2m)$ for Algorithm 1 of Section 10.1?

2. How many comparisons are needed to use Algorithm 3 ("Merging Sorted Vectors") of Section 10.1 to merge the sorted vectors $A = (1, 2, 3, 4)$ and $B = (5, 6, 7, 8)$?

3. Let $A = (a_1, a_2, a_3, 7)$ and $B = (b_1, b_2, b_3, 8)$ be sorted vectors with $\{a_1, a_2, a_3, b_1, b_2, b_3\} = \{1, 2, 3, 4, 5, 6\}$. How many comparisons are needed when using Algorithm 3 ("Merging Sorted Vectors") of Section 10.1 to merge A and B?

4. Give an example of sorted vectors (a_1, a_2, a_3) and (b_1, b_2, b_3, b_4) whose merging, using Algorithm 3 ("Merging Sorted Vectors") of Section 10.1, requires 3 comparisons.

5. Give an example of sorted vectors (a_1, a_2, a_3) and (b_1, b_2, b_3, b_4) whose merging, using Algorithm 3 ("Merging Sorted Vectors") of Section 10.1, requires 6 comparisons.

6. (i) Use $D(11) = 29$, $D(12) = 33$, and $D(2m + 1) = D(m + 1) + D(m) + 2m$ to find $D(23)$.
(ii) Use $B(n) = \binom{n}{2}$ to find $B(23)$.

7. (i) Use $D(12) = 33$ and $D(2m) = 2D(m) + 2m - 1$ to find $D(24)$.
(ii) Use $B(n) = \binom{n}{2}$ to find $B(24)$.

8. Evaluate det M where

$$M = \begin{bmatrix} 1 & -2 & 1 \\ 2 & 1 & -3 \\ 3 & -1 & -2 \end{bmatrix}.$$

9. (a) Use Cramer's Rule to solve the system

$$\begin{cases} x - 2y + z = 4 \\ 2x + y - 3z = 5 \\ 3x - y + 2z = 10. \end{cases}$$

(b) Check using Gaussian Elimination.

10. Find the value of s for which there is no solution to the system

$$\begin{cases} 3x + 4y = -10 \\ sx - 2y = 6. \end{cases}$$

11. Find the value of t for which there are infinitely many solutions to the system

$$\begin{cases} 3x - 12y = 7 \\ 2x - 8y = t. \end{cases}$$

12. Given that $f_2 = 8$ and $f_n = (n + 1)f_{n-1} + 2n + 1$ for $n \geq 3$, show that

$$f_n = n + (n + 1)! \left[\frac{1}{1!} + \frac{1}{2!} + \cdots + \frac{1}{(n-1)!} \right].$$

13. Use the formula in Problem 12 to find the number f_5 of multiplications in using Cramer's Rule to solve 5 linear equations in 5 unknowns.

14. Use $g_n = (n^3 + 3n^2 - n)/3$ to find the number g_{22091} of multiplications in the Gaussian Elimination algorithm for solving 22091 linear equations in 22091 unknowns.

15. Does there exist a positive integer n_0 such that

$$n^{100} \leq .000001(1.001^n) \qquad \text{for } n \geq n_0?$$

Justify your answer.

16. Is there a largest positive integer m_0 such that

$$n^{100} \geq .000001(1.001^n) \qquad \text{for } n \leq m_0?$$

Justify your answer.

17. Let $g(n) = 3^n$ and $f(n) = n!$. Find the smallest positive integers r, s, and t such that $g(n) \leq f(n)$ for $n \geq r$, $g(n) \leq .1f(n)$ for $n \geq s$, and $g(n) \leq .01f(n)$ for $n \geq t$.

18. Label the following functions as $g_i(n)$, with $i = 1, 2, 3, 4$, so that $g_i(n)$ is $o[g_{i+1}(n)]$ for $i = 1, 2, 3$.
(a) $10(1.1^n)$;   (b) $(2n)!$;   (c) $8n^3 \log n$;   (d) $n^4 - n^3 + 5$.

19. Find the number d such that $(1 + 2 + 3 + \cdots + n) \sim n^d$, where $g(n) \sim f(n)$ means that $g(n)$ is $O[f(n)]$ and $f(n)$ is $O[g(n)]$.

20. Find e (in terms of d) so that

$$\left[\binom{d}{d} + \binom{d+1}{d} + \binom{d+2}{d} + \cdots + \binom{d+n}{d}\right] \sim n^e.$$

21. Let

$$g(n) = \binom{2n}{0} + \binom{2n}{1} + \binom{2n}{2} + \cdots + \binom{2n}{2n}.$$

Find b so that $g(n) \sim b^n$.

SUPPLEMENTARY AND CHALLENGING PROBLEMS, CHAPTER 10

1. Use $D(1) = 0$ and the formulas $D(2m - 1) = D(m - 1) + D(m) + 2m - 2$ and $D(2^n) = 2^n(n - 1) + 1$ to find a formula for $D(2^n - 1)$.

2. Find a formula for $D(2^n + 1)$.

3. Let M be an n by n matrix. Prove by induction on n that if each entry on a fixed row is multiplied by a constant k, then M goes into a matrix M' with det $M' = k$ det M.

4. Repeat Problem 3, but with "row" replaced with "column."

5. Let M be an n by n matrix and let M' result from the interchange of two rows of M. Prove that det $M' = -$det M.

6. Repeat Problem 5, but with "rows" replaced with "columns."

7. Let p be a complexity function given by

$$p(n) = a_0 n^d + a_1 n^{d-1} + \cdots + a_n,$$

with fixed numbers a_i. Prove that n^d is $O[p(n)]$. [This is the part of Theorem 1 ("A Polynomial Is Equivalent to Its Dominant Term") of Section 10.3 that was left to the reader.]

8. Prove that $n!$ is $o[n^n]$. [This is Theorem 2(e) of Section 10.3, whose proof was omitted.]

11

INTRODUCTION TO CODING

In everyday language, a code implies a "secret code," a means of sending a message in a form that only the intended receiver of the message can read. This idea of a code is, of course, still useful and is the subject of cryptography. Such codes are an area of active research, and interesting developments have occurred in this area even in recent years. These codes are frequently encountered in spy thrillers.

The subject of this chapter, however, is not such "secret codes" but a code far less sinister and only somewhat less romantic. Our concern here is the problem of putting a message in a form that can be transmitted accurately to an intended recipient. This could be a picture of Saturn sent back by a space probe, or a signal sent from a television studio to a satellite or from the satellite to a dish antenna atop someone's house. It could be a message sent from one computer to another, or a message sent over telephone lines. It could be data stored in computer memory and later retrieved.

Messages can be sent in many forms, but these days, messages tend to be sent in digital form because of the ubiquity of computers in modern life. For this reason we shall here concern ourselves with messages in the form of binary strings.

If, say, we wish to transmit a message in the English language, we need 26 letters, along with some punctuation. So we need binary strings of length adequate to distinguish among these 26 letters and some punctuation marks. The fifth power of two, 32 (strings of length 5), would be adequate for a few punctuation marks; but since we wish to convey some numbers and other symbols as well, let us instead use binary strings of length 6. Then 000000 can represent A, 000001 can represent B, and so on down to 011001 to represent Z. If we wanted to send the message SOS, for example, we would send 010010001110010010. This is easier to see if we write it 010010/001110/010010.

In the best of all possible worlds, that would be the end of the problem. To send the message SOS we would just put into our transmitting machine, in whatever form it takes, that string of 0's and 1's, and the person on the other end, knowing the code we are using, would translate it back to "SOS." In this world, unfortunately, machines have faulty components;

there are other powerful machines working in the area that can cause interference; there may be great distances involved so that atmospheric conditions can cause trouble with radio transmissions; and so on and on. Thus, the message received, though a string of 0's and 1's, may not be exactly the string of 0's and 1's sent. And when the recipient translates the string back into a string of letters from the English alphabet (if lucky), the message may make no sense. And it may not even correspond to a string of letters, because a string of six digits may look something like 101111, which does not correspond to a letter at all and may not even correspond to any punctuation according to the scheme determined. Then the message will be read as the wrong letters or as no letters at all. We must therefore devise a scheme for detecting errors in received messages and, even better, correcting them.

The science of devising error-detecting and error-correcting codes began, roughly, in 1950. One of the pioneers was Richard W. Hamming of Bell Laboratories. (See the biographical note just before the problems for Section 11.1.) Since that time the field has grown into a large and active branch of applied mathematics, moving into areas far too sophisticated for this short introduction. The subject does provide, however, a beautiful example of the application of abstract algebra to practical questions.

11.1

ERROR DETECTING AND ERROR CORRECTING

Let us begin by introducing a few words and phrases that will make the discussion easier. The interference in the transmitting system that we referred to earlier, in this context we shall call *noise*. Figure 11.1.1 indicates the various stages of the message. The messages will be made up of binary strings from B_n (see Section 1.1). We shall assume that the probability of sending a 0 and receiving a 1 is the same as that of sending a 1 and receiving a 0. Because of this symmetry, we call this a *binary symmetric channel*. If we let p be the probability that one digit is sent and the other digit of the two is received, then naturally, since p is a probability, $0 \le p \le 1$. If $p = 0$, then the transmission is perfect and the problem is of no real interest. Furthermore, if p were greater than $\frac{1}{2}$, then it would only make sense to read a 0 as a 1 and a 1 as a 0. So we shall consider only the case of $0 < p \le \frac{1}{2}$.

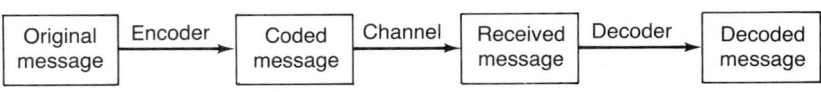

FIGURE 11.1.1

In order to be able to detect errors and then to correct them, it is necessary to build into the message additional information. This could take the form of redundancy. For example, one could repeat a string several times and then read the digit in a particular position to be the digit that appears most often in that position. We shall examine this possibility in more detail later. Or one could add to each string some additional digits that relate to the earlier digits. In extremely simple cases this might not be necessary. For example, if one has only two possible messages, say 000000 and 111111, and one receives 001000, then one could safely interpret this as 000000. Similarly, one would interpret 001001 as 000000, but without the same degree of confidence. But then what would one do with 000111, for example? One could as easily interpret this as 000000 or as 111111. This system leaves certain strings with two equally acceptable interpretations. So in general it is better to move on to a more sophisticated method. One slightly better method would be to add to the string a digit that would be 0 if the sum of the digits in the message string is even and 1 if the sum of the digits in the message string is odd. In other words, if the weight of the string is even we attach a 0 at the end, and if it is odd we attach a 1. When the message is received, if the last digit is 1 and the sum of the digits in the message string is even, one knows there is an error, and similarly for a final 0 on a message string of odd weight. This method, called a *parity code*, can detect some errors, but it neither locates them precisely nor corrects them.

For a fixed n, let $\boldsymbol{B_n}$ be the set of binary strings of length n. A string from this set we can call a *word*; a message, then, is made up of a set of words. Another set, $\boldsymbol{B_c}$, is the set of binary strings of length c, where we take c to be greater than n. An element of $\boldsymbol{B_c}$ is called a *codeword*. The first n digits of this codeword make up the *information digits* of the codeword; the remaining $c - n$ digits make up the *check digits*.

Since distinct words should be represented by distinct codewords, this means that the *encoding* is really an injective mapping $E: \boldsymbol{B_n} \to \boldsymbol{B_c}$. The set of images $E(\boldsymbol{B_n})$ is a subset of the codomain made up of all possible codewords. *Decoding* is done by a mapping D, where the domain is $\boldsymbol{B_c}$ and the codomain is either $\boldsymbol{B_n}$ or $\boldsymbol{B_n} \cup \{\text{error}\}$. The decoding mapping D must be such that $D(\beta) = \alpha$ whenever $E(\alpha) = \beta$. But if β is not a codeword, then $D(\beta)$ must be $D(\beta')$, where β' is closest to β in some sense, that sense to be determined by the system one devises. If there is no way to determine such a "closest β'," then $D(\beta)$ should be "error."

DEFINITION 1   **BLOCK CODE**

An ordered pair $[E, D]$, where E and D are as described in the preceding paragraph, is called an (n, c) *block code*.

Example 1   If in a parity code (as described earlier) we consider two words, say 011100 and 101000, then the corresponding codewords would be 0111001 (we add a 1 at the end of the word because the weight of the word is odd) and 1010000 (in this case we add a 0 at the end of the word because the weight is even). If the words received from these two transmissions are 1111001 and 1011010, then we know that in the first case there has been an error because now the weight is even and the last digit is a 1. In the second case there are indeed two errors in the transmission, but we will not detect this because the weight is even and the last digit is a 0. This example shows two words and corresponding codewords from a $(6, 7)$ block code. In general, with a parity code transmitting words taken from B_n, the parity code will be an $(n, n + 1)$ block code. $\square$

Example 2   If we transmit a word of length n using a **triple repetition code**, we just form the codeword made up by repeating the original word three times. Therefore $E: B_n \rightarrow B_{3n}$ takes the word $a_1 a_2 \ldots a_n$ to $a_1 a_2 \ldots a_n a_1 a_2 \ldots a_n a_1 a_2 \ldots a_n$, and the decoding mapping $D: B_{3n} \rightarrow B_n$ takes $b_1 b_2 \ldots b_{3n}$ to $c_1 c_2 \ldots c_n$, where c_i is the digit that appears at least twice in the ordered triple (b_i, b_{i+n}, b_{i+2n}). $\square$

Since, as mentioned above, in decoding one has to decide, given a received string, what codeword is "closest" to it, we need a concept of distance between words.

DEFINITION 2   **HAMMING DISTANCE**

Given two strings in B_n, $\alpha = a_1 a_2 \ldots a_n$ and $\beta = b_1 b_2 \ldots b_n$, the **Hamming distance** between them is the number of values of i, $i = 1, 2, 3, \ldots, n$, for which $a_i \neq b_i$. It is denoted $d(\alpha, \beta)$.

It should be noted here that the weight wgt α of a string α, defined in Definition 2 ("Length and Weight") of Section 1.1, is—in the context of coding—often called the **Hamming weight**.

DEFINITION 3   **SUM OF STRINGS**

The sum $\alpha \oplus \beta$ of two binary strings $\alpha = a_1 a_2 \ldots a_n$ and $\beta = b_1 b_2 \ldots b_n$ is $c_1 c_2 \ldots c_n$, where $c_i = 0$ if $a_i = b_i$ and $c_i = 1$ if $a_i \neq b_i$.

Definition 3 says that in each position we add the bits modulo 2; that is, $0 \oplus 0 = 1 \oplus 1 = 0$ and $1 \oplus 0 = 0 \oplus 1 = 1$. Definition 3 is actually that of Example 2 of Section 7.1.

THEOREM 1 **DISTANCE GIVEN AS WEIGHT**

If α and β are strings in $\boldsymbol{B_n}$, then $d(\alpha, \beta) = \text{wgt}(\alpha \oplus \beta)$.

PROOF In $\alpha \oplus \beta$, a 1 will appear only when the corresponding elements in α and β differ, so the wgt of $\alpha \oplus \beta$ is just the number of times corresponding elements differ. But this is exactly the definition of Hamming distance. □

One remarkable aspect of the Hamming distance is that it behaves much like the distance we are used to dealing with. For example, it satisfies the *triangle inequality*,

$$d(\alpha, \gamma) \leq d(\alpha, \beta) + d(\beta, \gamma),$$

as we will note in Problem 5 below.

DEFINITION 4 **MINIMUM DISTANCE OF A CODE**

The smallest distance between any two codewords in a code is called the *minimum distance* of the code.

Example 3 Let us consider a very simple code, one with only four words: 10000, 01100, 00111, 11011. The distance between the first and second words is 3, between the first and third is 4, and so on. If we check out all the pairs, we will find that the minimum distance for this code is 3. Let us see what that implies. There are only four codewords in our code, but we are receiving five-digit binary strings and there are 32 of those. So whereas we can receive any one of these 32 strings, we have to decide which of the four codewords was really sent. As we noted before, if we were to receive the word 00000, we would almost certainly assume that 10000 was sent. In fact, we can devise a table where any string in a column is assumed to be the codeword at the head of the column, as in Table 11.1.1.

TABLE 11.1.1

	10000	01100	00111	11011
Received words	00000	11100	10111	01011
with 1 error	11000	00100	01111	10011
	10100	01000	00011	11111
	10010	01110	00101	11001
	10001	01101	00110	11010
Received words	00010	01010	10110	11101
with 2 errors	00001	01001	10101	11110

With this assumption, Table 11.1.1 corrects errors in just 1 digit and detects errors in 1 or 2 digits. For example, the 1-digit error in the received word $\alpha = 00000$ is corrected since $\beta = 10000$ is the only codeword with $d(\alpha, \beta) = 1$. The received word $\alpha = 00010$ could be the result of a 2-digit error in either the codeword $\beta = 10000$ or the codeword $\gamma = 00111$. This decoding scheme detects either error since α is not a codeword but does not correct the error when γ is the intended codeword. More generally, we can say that a code with minimum distance $k + 1$ will detect k or fewer errors. Furthermore, if the minimum distance of a code is $2k + 1$, no received word can be a distance k from more than one codeword (it would violate the triangle inequality); so in this case any word resulting from k or fewer errors can be corrected.   □

Richard W. Hamming, born in Chicago in 1915, studied at the University of Chicago, at the University of Nebraska, and at the University of Illinois. He served on the staff of the Manhattan Project at Los Alamos in 1945–1946. For many years he was at Bell Laboratories. He became a professor at the Naval Postgraduate School in Monterey, California in 1977. His mathematical contributions have been largely in numerical methods and coding theory.

PROBLEMS FOR SECTION 11.1

1.   If $\alpha = 001110$ and $\beta = 010011$, find:
     (a) wgt α;   (b) wgt β;   (c) $d(\alpha, \beta)$;   (d) $\alpha \oplus \beta$;   (e) wgt$(\alpha \oplus \beta)$.

2.   Repeat Problem 1 with the following values of α and β: $\alpha = 000011101$, $\beta = 101011011$.

3.   What is the minimum distance of a code consisting of the following codewords: 001010, 011100, 010111, 011110, 101001?

4.   What is the minimum distance of a code consisting of the following codewords: 00110010, 01111001, 11100110, 11000111?

5.   Show that Hamming distance satisfies the triangle inequality; that is, show that $d(\alpha, \beta) + d(\beta, \gamma) \geq d(\alpha, \gamma)$ for all α, β, γ in B_n.

6.   What is the largest number of wrong digits in a word that can be corrected by a code with minimum distance 5?

7.   For a (2, 6) triple repetition code, find:
     (a) $E(10)$;   (b) $D(001010)$;   (c) $D(101010)$.

8. For a (3, 9) triple repetition code, find:
   (a) $E(100)$;   (b) $E(011)$;   (c) $D(100100110)$;   (d) $D(110110000)$.

9. In the (6, 7) block parity code, which of the following errors will be detected?

	Codeword Sent	Codeword Received
(a)	0110101	0110001
(b)	0111111	0011011
(c)	0111100	0111001
(d)	1111101	1111100

10. In Problem 7, which of the errors will be corrected?

11.2

GROUP CODES AND COSET DECODING

Here we use some ideas from group theory to assist in the decoding process.

NOTATION 1   **THE BITWISE ADDITION MODULO 2 GROUP G_n**

We use G_n to denote the group $\langle B_n, \oplus, 0_n \rangle$.

We recall that 0_n is the string $00 \ldots 0$ of weight zero in the set B_n of n-bit strings and that $\oplus$ is the bitwise addition modulo 2 binary operation on B_n with

$$a_1 a_2 \ldots a_n \oplus b_1 b_2 \ldots b_n = c_1 c_2 \ldots c_n,$$

where $c_i = 0$ if $a_i = b_i$ and $c_i = 1$ if $a_i \neq b_i$. In G_n, each string α is its own inverse; that is, $-\alpha = \alpha$.

As in the previous section, encoding of messages is accomplished by an injective mapping

$$E: B_n \to B_c,$$

where $n \leq c$. Let C be the set of images under this mapping. That is, let

$$C = \{E(\alpha) : \alpha \in B_n\}.$$

Since E is injective, it follows from Theorem 3(iv) ("Size of an Image Set") of Section 1.8 that $\#C = \#B_n = 2^n$. Normally C is not all of B_c. It is helpful to have C be the carrier of a group; hence we assume that the encoding mapping E has the property that $\langle C, \oplus, 0_c \rangle$ is a subgroup H in G_c.

Since G_c is abelian, each left coset $\alpha \oplus C$ equals the corresponding right coset $C \oplus \alpha$. The index of the subgroup H in G_c is the number of distinct cosets $\alpha \oplus C$ (see Definition 2, "Index of a Subgroup H in a Group G," of Section 7.5). It follows from Lagrange's Theorem (Theorem 4 of Section 7.5) that the index of H in G_c is $\#B_c / \#C = 2^c/2^n = 2^{c-n}$; we use h to denote this index 2^{c-n}. Let

$$\gamma_1 \oplus C, \gamma_2 \oplus C, \ldots, \gamma_h \oplus C \tag{1}$$

be the h distinct cosets of C in G_c. We recall from Problem 9(v) of Section 7.5, that in writing a coset as $\gamma \oplus C$ we can let γ be any element of the particular coset. We shall choose, in a special way, the "coset representatives" $\gamma_1, \gamma_2, \ldots, \gamma_h$ for the h cosets listed in Display (1) after introducing some additional terms.

DEFINITION 1   ERROR PATTERN

If $\alpha = a_1 a_2 \ldots a_n$ is a codeword transmitted and $\beta = b_1 b_2 \ldots b_n$ is the string received, the ***error pattern*** is the string (of equal length) $\varepsilon = e_1 e_2 \ldots e_n$, where $e_i = 0$ if $a_i = b_i$ and $e_i = 1$ if $a_i \neq b_i$.

THEOREM 1   NUMBER OF ERRORS

If α, β, and ε are, respectively, the codeword transmitted, the string received, and the error pattern, then $\varepsilon = \alpha \oplus \beta$ and the number of errors is wgt ε or $d(\alpha, \beta)$.

The proof is left as an exercise (Problem 17 below).

DEFINITION 2   COSET LEADER

Let strings $\gamma_1, \gamma_2, \ldots, \gamma_h$ be in B_c and let the cosets $\gamma_1 \oplus C, \gamma_2 \oplus C, \ldots, \gamma_h \oplus C$ partition B_c, where $\langle C, \oplus, 0_c \rangle$ is a subgroup in G_c. If for each coset, γ_i has minimal weight of all the elements in that coset, then γ_i is called the ***coset leader*** for any string in its coset.

In the present context, we cannot use the codewords of Example 3 of Section 11.1, since these do not form a group. In the following example, the codewords do, in fact, form a group under $\oplus$ and we can then use the concept of coset leaders to outline a method of decoding.

Example 1   **GROUP CODE WITH COSET DECODING**   Let $E: B_3 \to B_5$ be a (3, 5)-block code in which

$$C = \{00000, 00101, 01011, 01110, 10010, 10111, 11001, 11100\}$$

is the set of codewords, that is, the set $\{E(\sigma) : \sigma \in B_3\}$ of images of the 8 strings of B_3 under the encoding mapping E. An operation table would show that C is closed under bitwise addition modulo 2. Since C is finite, it follows from Theorem 9 ("Finite Subset Closed under Group Operation") of Section 7.1 that $H = \langle C, \oplus, 0_5 \rangle$ is a subgroup in G_5. Since H has order 8 and G_5 has order $2^5 = 32$, there are 4 distinct cosets of C in G_5. One of these cosets is C itself. The string of least weight in C is $0_5 = 00000$; hence we take 00000 as the coset leader for this coset. Since 00000 is the only string of weight zero in B_5 and the string 10000 of weight one is not in C, 10000 must be a string of minimal weight in its coset and hence we can take 10000 to be the coset leader for the coset $10000 \oplus C$. Similarly, one can show that 01000 is neither in C nor in $10000 \oplus C$; thus 01000 can be used as the coset leader for a third coset $01000 \oplus C$. Of the eight remaining strings that are not in any of these three cosets, a string with minimal weight is 00100, and we let it be the coset leader for the fourth (and final) coset $00100 \oplus C$.

The 32 strings of B_5 are placed in the main body of Table 11.2.1 in the following fashion: Each coset has its own row. The row label (in the leftmost column) is the coset leader. The entries in the first row are the strings $\alpha_1, \alpha_2, \ldots, \alpha_8$ of C in some order. The entries of the row having a string γ as the coset leader are

$$\gamma \oplus \alpha_1, \gamma \oplus \alpha_2, \ldots, \gamma \oplus \alpha_8,$$

in this order.

TABLE 11.2.1

00000	00000	00101	01011	01110	10010	10111	11001	11100
10000	10000	10101	11011	11110	00010	00111	01001	01100
01000	01000	01101	00011	00110	11010	11111	10001	10100
00100	00100	00001	01111	01010	10110	10011	11101	11000

The decoding process proceeds as follows: If we receive a certain string β, we look for it in the table. If β appears in the first row, that is, if β is one of the codewords α_i in C, we assume that no error was made in transmission and decode β as the string σ in B_3 with $E(\sigma) = \beta$. If the received string β is not a codeword, that is, if it is not an entry on the first row, we assume that the error pattern in the transmission is the coset leader γ for that row. With this assumption, the intended codeword α is such that $\beta = \gamma \oplus \alpha$. Then

$$\gamma \oplus \beta = \gamma \oplus \gamma \oplus \alpha = \alpha$$

since $\gamma \oplus \gamma = 0_5$ for every string γ in $\boldsymbol{B_5}$. It follows that the intended codeword α is the string in the first row for the column containing β.

Whether or not the received string β is a codeword, the decoding process assumes that the intended codeword is the string α in C that appears in the first row of the table and in the column containing β. The received string is decoded as the string σ in $\boldsymbol{B_3}$ such that $E(\sigma) = \alpha$.

As an illustration, if the string 10111 is received, we note that it is in the set C of codewords, that is, the entries on the first row. Hence we assume that no error was made in transmission and decode it as the σ in $\boldsymbol{B_3}$ with $E(\sigma) = 10111$.

However, if $\beta = 10101$ is the string received, we find it on the second row in the coset $10000 \oplus C$ with $\gamma = 10000$ as coset leader. We assume that 10000 is the error pattern. Then the intended codeword is the string $\alpha = 00101$ at the top of the column containing 10101 and we decode the erroneous string 10101 as the σ in $\boldsymbol{B_3}$ with $E(\sigma) = 00101$. □

DEFINITION 3   **(SLEPIAN) STANDARD ARRAY**

Let $H = \langle C, \oplus, 0_c \rangle$ be a subgroup of index h in $G_c = \langle \boldsymbol{B_c}, \oplus, 0_c \rangle$. A table for the h cosets $\gamma_1 \oplus C, \gamma_2 \oplus C, \dots, \gamma_h \oplus C$, of C in G_c, having the properties described in Example 1 is called a *Slepian standard array* or *standard array*.

When constructing a standard array, one may find that there is more than one string of minimal weight in some coset. Should this happen, one can choose arbitrarily any one of these minimal-weight strings to be the coset leader.

PROBLEMS FOR SECTION 11.2

1. Using the standard array of Example 1, identify the intended codeword that we would associate with each of the following received strings:
   (a) 00110;   (b) 11101;   (c) 10100;   (d) 01001.

2. Using the standard array of Example 1, identify the intended codeword that we would associate with each of the following received strings:
   (a) 11110;   (b) 11111;   (c) 00000;   (d) 01000.

3. If 010110 is sent and 011110 is received, what is the error pattern?

4. If 11110010 is sent and 10111011 is received, what is the error pattern?

5. For the coset decoding scheme of Example 1, what is the error pattern for each of the following?
   (a) 11010;   (b) 11000.

6. For the coset decoding scheme of Example 1, what is the error pattern for each of the following?
   (a) 01010;   (b) 00011.

7. (a) Construct the last row of the standard array of Example 1 if 00001 were chosen as the coset leader instead of 00100.
   (b) With the new table of Part (a), which codeword would be identified with 01111?
   (c) Is this the same codeword as that identified with this string in the original standard array?

8. Is there a choice for coset leader of the last row of Example 1 other than 00100 and 00001?

9. Verify that the set of strings {000000, 001110, 010011, 011101, 100101, 101011, 110110, 111000} is the carrier of a subgroup in G_6.

10. What is the index in G_6 of the subgroup of Problem 9?

11. The table below gives the first seven rows of the Slepian standard array using the subgroup of Problem 9 as the subgroup of codewords in the group G_6. Construct the eighth row using 001001 as coset leader.

000000	000000	001110	010011	011101	100101	101011	110110	111000
100000	100000	101110	110011	111101	000101	001011	010110	011000
010000	010000	011110	000011	001101	110101	111011	100110	101000
001000	001000	000110	011011	010101	101101	100011	111110	110000
000100	000100	001010	010111	011001	100001	101111	110010	111100
000010	000010	001100	010001	011111	100111	101001	110100	111010
000001	000001	001111	010010	011100	100100	101010	110111	111001

12. Construct the eighth row of the standard array of Problem 11 using 010100 as coset leader.

13. Are there any other possibilities for coset leader for the eighth row of the standard array of Problem 11? If so, construct the corresponding eighth row.

14. Would 110001 be a suitable coset leader for the eighth row of the standard array of Problem 11? Give reasons.

15. Which codewords correspond to the following in the standard array of Problem 11?
    (a) 010101;   (b) 110011.

16. Which codewords correspond to the following in the standard array of Problem 11?
    (a) 110100;   (b) 111010.

17. Prove Theorem 1 ("Number of Errors") of this section.

18. Prove that the set of codewords in Example 1 is the carrier of a subgroup in G_n.

SUMMARY OF TERMS, CHAPTER 11

Binary symmetric channel	A channel for the transmission of binary strings where it is equiprobable that a digit received be the opposite of the digit sent.	588
Block code	Encoding and decoding mappings that allow for error detection and/or correction.	589
Check digits	The added part of a codeword allowing for error detection and/or correction.	589
Codeword	A binary string carrying information beyond the message itself.	589
Coset decoding	A method of decoding making use of cosets and quotient groups.	595
Coset leader	A representative of least weight in a coset of strings in B_c.	594
Decoder	The mapping that transforms a coded message back into the original message.	588
Encoder	The mapping that transforms a message into code.	588
Error pattern	The binary string with 1's in the positions where the received string differs from the transmitted codeword.	594
Group code	A code that makes use of a group structure for decoding.	593–597
Hamming distance	The number of places where two codewords of equal length differ.	590
Hamming weight	The number of 1's in a binary string.	590
Information digits	That part of a codeword containing the original message.	589
Minimum distance	The smallest (Hamming) distance between any two codewords in a code.	591
Noise	Interference in the transmission of a coded message.	588
Number of errors	The weight of the error pattern.	594
Parity code	A code that adds to a message word a digit telling whether the weight of the message is even or odd.	589
Slepian standard array	The array of elements of B_c displaying the coset elements on rows of the array.	596
Triple repetition code	A code that repeats each message three times.	590
Word	A binary string.	589

REVIEW PROBLEMS FOR CHAPTER 11

1. For the (3, 9) triple repetition code, find:
   (a) $E(001)$;   (b) $E(101)$;   (c) $D(100000100)$;   (d) $D(010010110)$.

2. For the (4, 12) triple repetition code, find:
   (a) $E(1001)$;   (b) $E(0000)$;   (c) $D(000010001000)$;   (d) $D(101010101000)$.

3. What are the advantages and disadvantages of a double repetition code, that is, one where each encoded message word consists of the original message word repeated once?

4. What are the advantages and disadvantages of a quintuple repetition code, that is, one where each encoded message word consists of the original message word given five times?

5. What minimum distance between codewords is required to be able to detect all error patterns of weight 5 or less?

6. What minimum distance between codewords is required to be able to correct all error patterns of weight 5 or less?

7. If the minimum distance between codewords is 4, for what weights of error patterns would errors be detected?

8. If the minimum distance between codewords is 7, for what weights of error patterns would errors be corrected?

9. Can one construct a code with three codewords of length 3 such that the minimum distance is 2? If so, find three such codewords.

10. Can one construct a code with three codewords of length 4 such that the minimum distance is 3? If so, find three such codewords.

SUPPLEMENTARY AND CHALLENGING PROBLEMS, CHAPTER 11 _____

1. Let $\alpha = a_1 a_2 \ldots a_n$ and $\beta = b_1 b_2 \ldots b_n$. We define the product $\alpha\beta = c_1 c_2 \ldots c_n$ to be the string with $c_i = 1$ when $a_i = b_i = 1$ and with $c_i = 0$ when either a_i or $b_i = 0$. Show that

$$\text{wgt}(\alpha \oplus \beta) = \text{wgt }\alpha + \text{wgt }\beta - 2 \cdot \text{wgt}(\alpha\beta).$$

2. Construct a Slepian standard array for the subgroup $\langle C, \oplus, 0_5 \rangle$ of $\boldsymbol{B_5}$ with $C = \{00000, 00110, 01011, 01101, 10001, 10111, 11010, 11100\}$.

12

FINITE STATE MACHINES AND LANGUAGES

The types of languages considered in Sections 2.1 and 2.2 and those to be defined in Section 12.1 are meant to encompass the languages humans use to communicate with one another or with machines, as well as the languages machines use to communicate among themselves.

The finite state machines discussed in Section 12.2 are mathematical models of machines such as toasters, clothes washers, microwave ovens, remote control televisions, automated bank tellers, and computers of various degrees of sophistication.

12.1

FORMAL LANGUAGES AND GRAMMARS

Here we repeat some definitions from Section 2.1 and develop these topics further.

We recall that an *alphabet* is a finite nonempty set A whose elements are called *symbols* or *letters*. A *word* of *length* n over an alphabet A is a string $\alpha = a_1 a_2 \ldots a_n$ with each a_i in A. The set of all words, of all lengths, over an alphabet A is called the *closure* of A and is denoted as A^*; we note that A^* includes the empty word ε of length zero. We also add to the definition of an alphabet A the requirement that no letter x in A is a word over the complement $A - \{x\}$ of $\{x\}$ in A. Thus $\{a, b, c\}$ is an alphabet but $\{a, b, ab\}$ is not.

A *language* over an alphabet A is a set of words over A; that is, a language L over A is a subset of the closure A^*. Thus a language L over A is a member of the power set $P(A^*)$.

Example 1   We can define the finite English language E over the alphabet $A = \{a, b, \ldots, z\}$ to be the set of all the words in the alphabetical listing of some given dictionary. Then E should contain the words a, i, act, cat, and dog but probably would not contain any of the words tt, wzev, or nwg of the closure A^* of A.   □

Example 2   If the alphabet is $B_1 = \{0, 1\}$, then the closure B_1^* is the set $\{\varepsilon\} \cup B_1 \cup B_2 \cup B_3 \cup \cdots$ consisting of the binary strings of all possible lengths. A string $\alpha = a_1 a_2 \ldots a_n$ in B_1^* is **unfriendly** if consecutive digits a_i and a_{i+1} are never both 1. The infinite language U consisting of all the unfriendly strings in B_1^* has ε, 0, 1, 00, 01, 10, and 101 among its words but does not contain 11, 110, 011, or 111.   □

Example 3   Let $C = B_{6,0} \cup B_{6,2} \cup B_{6,4} \cup B_{6,6}$ be the set of 6-bit strings of even weight. As we recall from Example 1 of Section 11.1, C is the set of codewords in the (5, 6)-block parity check code. This C is a finite language over the alphabet $\{0, 1\}$.   □

An alphabet A is nonempty; hence it contains some letter x and its closure A^* contains the infinite sequence

$$x, xx, xxx, \ldots.$$

It follows that A^* is infinite for every alphabet A and that a language over A may be finite or infinite. For example, if $x \in A$ then $\{x, xx, xxx\}$ is a finite language and $\{x, xx, xxx, \ldots\}$ is an infinite language over A. The languages used in computer science are generally infinite but have logical structures that make it possible for each such language to be generated using some algorithm, as we will see in Definition 4 below and the examples that follow it.

We also recall from Section 2.1 that the **concatenation** of words $\alpha = a_1 a_2 \ldots a_m$ and $\beta = b_1 b_2 \ldots b_n$ (in this order) over an alphabet A is the word

$$\alpha\beta = a_1 a_2 \ldots a_m b_1 b_2 \ldots b_n$$

over A. For every alphabet A, concatenation is an associative binary operation on the closure A^*, and the empty word ε is the identity under this operation. Using $\cdot$ as the symbol for concatenation, $[A^*, \cdot, \varepsilon]$ is thus a monoid for every alphabet A. This monoid is noncommutative unless A is a singleton $\{a\}$.

Since languages over A are members of the power set $P(A^*)$, the unary operation of complementation and the binary operations of intersection and union can be performed on languages over a fixed alphabet. One can also extend the binary operation of concatenation on the carrier A^* so that it is a binary operation on $P(A^*)$.

DEFINITION 1   **CONCATENATION OF LANGUAGES OVER A**

Let L_1 and L_2 be languages over an alphabet A. The **concatenation** of L_1 and L_2 (in this order) is the set

$$L_1L_2 = \{\alpha\beta : \alpha \in L_1, \beta \in L_2\}.$$

Example 4

Let the alphabet be $A = \{a, b, c\}$. Then $L_1 = \{\varepsilon, a, ab, abc\}$ and $L_2 = \{\varepsilon, b, bc\}$ are languages over A. We see that $L_1 \cap L_2 = \{\varepsilon\}$ and $L_1 \cup L_2 = \{\varepsilon, a, b, ab, bc, abc\}$. As an aid in finding the concatenations L_1L_2 and L_2L_1, we construct some tables. In Table 12.1.1, the row labels come from L_1 and the column labels from L_2. The entry in this table in the position of the row for α and the column for β is the concatenation $\alpha\beta$. Interchanging the roles of L_1 and L_2 in Table 12.1.1 yields the analogous Table 12.1.2. The entries of Table 12.1.1 show that

$$L_1L_2 = \{\varepsilon, a, b, ab, bc, abb, abc, abbc, abcb, abcbc\}$$

and the entries of Table 12.1.2 show that

$$L_2L_1 = \{\varepsilon, a, b, ab, ba, bc, abc, bab, bca, babc, bcab, bcabc\}.$$

We note that L_1L_2 and L_2L_1 are not equal. In fact, they do not even have the same size, since $\#(L_1L_2) = 10$ and $\#(L_2L_1) = 12$. The discrepancy in sizes is explained by the fact that each of ab and abc appears twice as an entry in Table 12.1.1; therefore $\#(L_1L_2) = (\#L_1)(\#L_2) - 2 = 4 \cdot 3 - 2 = 10$. On the other hand, there are no repetitions of entries in Table 12.1.2, and hence $\#(L_2L_1) = (\#L_2)(\#L_1) = 3 \cdot 4 = 12$.   □

TABLE 12.1.1

$\cdot$	ε	b	bc
ε	ε	b	bc
a	a	ab	abc
ab	ab	abb	abbc
abc	abc	abcb	abcbc

TABLE 12.1.2

$\cdot$	ε	a	ab	abc
ε	ε	a	ab	abc
b	b	ba	bab	babc
bc	bc	bca	bcab	bcabc

THEOREM 1   **PROPERTIES OF CONCATENATION OF LANGUAGES**

Let E, F, and G be languages over an alphabet A. Then:

(a) $G\{\varepsilon\} = \{\varepsilon\}G = G$.
(b) If $E \subseteq F$, then $EG \subseteq FG$ and $GE \subseteq GF$.

The proof is left to the reader.

The operation of concatenation of languages over A enables us to define nonnegative integral powers of a language L.

DEFINITION 2   **POWERS L^n OF A LANGUAGE L**

Let L be a language over A. **Powers L^n** are defined inductively for all n in $N = \{0, 1, \ldots\}$ by $L^0 = \{\varepsilon\}$, $L^1 = L$, and $L^{k+1} = L^kL$ for k in N.

This definition tells us that L^2 is the concatenation of L and itself, L^3 is the concatenation of L^2 and L, and so on. We next use all of the non-negative integral powers L^n of L.

DEFINITION 3

KLEENE CLOSURE L^* OF A LANGUAGE L

Let L be a language over an alphabet A. Then the infinite union

$$L^* = \{\varepsilon\} \cup L \cup L^2 \cup L^3 \cup \cdots$$

is called the ***Kleene closure*** of L.

This concept is named after the American logician and mathematician Stephen Kleene, born in 1909.

An alphabet A is also a language over itself; A is the language consisting of all the words of length 1 over A. Thinking of A as a language over itself, the Kleene closure of A turns out to be the language of all words of all possible lengths (including the empty word ε of length zero). Hence the new notation L^*, when L is A, has the same meaning as the A^* given in Definition 7 of Section 2.1 and recalled in the second paragraph of this section. Thus we do not have to worry about whether a set S is an alphabet or a language when using the notation S^*.

Example 5 Let the alphabet be $B_1 = \{0, 1\}$. Then $B_2 = \{00, 01, 10, 11\}$ is a language over B_1. It can be shown that $B_2^n = B_{2n}$ for every n in $Z^+ = \{1, 2, \ldots\}$. Hence the Kleene closure of the language B_2 is the set

$$B_2^* = \{\varepsilon\} \cup B_2 \cup B_2^2 \cup B_2^3 \cup \cdots = \{\varepsilon\} \cup B_2 \cup B_4 \cup B_6 \cup \cdots,$$

which consists of all the binary strings of even length. □

THEOREM 2

PROPERTIES OF KLEENE CLOSURES

Let L and M be languages over the alphabet A.

(a) If $L \subset M$, then $L^* \subseteq M^*$.
(b) $(L^*)^* = L^* = L^* L^*$.
(c) $L^* \cup M^* \subseteq (L \cup M)^* = (L^* \cup M^*)^*$.

The proof is left to the reader.

The concept introduced next enables us to generate certain languages algorithmicly.

DEFINITION 4   PHRASE-STRUCTURE GRAMMAR

A *phrase-structure grammar* is an ordered 4-tuple $G = (A, S, T, P)$ with the following properties:

(a) A is an alphabet.

(b) S is a singleton subset $\{s\}$ of A. This s is called the *start symbol*.

(c) T is a subset of A such that s is not in T. Each t in T is called a *terminal symbol*.

(d) P is a finite binary relation on the closure A^* of A (that is, a finite subset of $A^* \times A^*$) such that no word of T^* is the α of an ordered pair (α, β) in P. The ordered pairs (α, β) of P are called *productions* and are written as $\alpha \rightarrow \beta$.

If $\alpha \rightarrow \beta$ is a production, it follows from Condition (d) of Definition 4 that some letter of the word α is not a terminal symbol. We will see in Definitions 5 and 6 below that the productions $\alpha \rightarrow \beta$ are substitution rules for generating new words in A^* from old words. One of the applications is that we can generate infinite languages from finite languages.

NOTATION 1   SUCCESSIVE PRODUCTIONS

We use $\alpha \rightarrow \beta \rightarrow \gamma$ to mean that $\alpha \rightarrow \beta$ and $\beta \rightarrow \gamma$ are both productions. We write $\alpha \rightarrow \beta \rightarrow \gamma \rightarrow \delta$ to indicate that $\alpha \rightarrow \beta$, $\beta \rightarrow \gamma$, and $\gamma \rightarrow \delta$ are all productions. Similarly, one defines larger *successions* $\alpha \rightarrow \beta \rightarrow \gamma \rightarrow \cdots \rightarrow \sigma$.

Example 6   Let $A = \{s, 0, 1\}$, $S = \{s\}$, $T = \{0, 1\}$, and $P = \{s \rightarrow 1, s \rightarrow 0s, s \rightarrow 10s, s \rightarrow \varepsilon\}$. We note that S and T are subsets of A, that S is a singleton, that the start letter s is not in T, and that $\rightarrow$ is a finite binary relation on the closure A^* with the property that $\alpha \rightarrow \beta$ implies that α is not in T^*. In fact, $\alpha \rightarrow \beta$ implies that $\alpha = s$. Hence the ordered 4-tuple $G = (A, S, T, P)$ is a phrase-structure grammar. In Example 7 below, we will see how this grammar generates the infinite language U of Example 2 from the finite language $\{s\}$. $\square$

Let $G = (A, S, T, P)$ be a phrase-structure grammar. Next we use the finite binary relation $\rightarrow$ on A^* to define an infinite binary relation $\Rightarrow$ on A^*.

DEFINITION 5 **DIRECTLY GENERATED WORDS**

Let $G = (A, S, T, P)$ be a phrase-structure grammar. If α, β, γ, and δ are words in A^* and $\alpha \to \beta$ is a production in P, then $\gamma\alpha\delta$ *directly generates* $\gamma\beta\delta$ and we write $\gamma\alpha\delta \Rightarrow \gamma\beta\delta$.

THEOREM 3 **WORDS GENERATED BY A PRODUCTION**

Let $G = (A, S, T, P)$ be a phrase-structure grammar. Let α, β, γ, and δ be words in A^* and $\alpha \to \beta$ be a production in P. Then:

(a) $\alpha \Rightarrow \beta$,   (b) $\gamma\alpha \Rightarrow \gamma\beta$,
(c) $\alpha\delta \Rightarrow \beta\delta$,   (d) $\gamma\alpha\delta \Rightarrow \gamma\beta\delta$.

PROOF   (a) Definition 5 with $\gamma = \varepsilon = \delta$ tells us that $\varepsilon\alpha\varepsilon \Rightarrow \varepsilon\beta\varepsilon$. Since ε is the empty word (that is, identity in the monoid $[A^*, \cdot, \varepsilon]$), this gives us $\alpha \Rightarrow \beta$.
(b) Here we let $\delta = \varepsilon$ in Definition 5.
(c) Here we let $\gamma = \varepsilon$ in Definition 5.
(d) This follows immediately from Definition 5.   □

Next we give the analogue of Notation 1, "Successive Productions," for the relation $\Rightarrow$.

NOTATION 2 **SUCCESSIVE GENERATIONS**

$\alpha \Rightarrow \beta \Rightarrow \gamma$ means that both $\alpha \Rightarrow \beta$ and $\beta \Rightarrow \gamma$. In general, $\alpha \Rightarrow \beta \Rightarrow \gamma \Rightarrow \cdots \Rightarrow \rho \Rightarrow \sigma$ means that $\alpha \Rightarrow \beta$, $\beta \Rightarrow \gamma, \ldots, \rho \Rightarrow \sigma$.

Notation 2 is useful in the following definition of the transitive closure $\overset{*}{\Rightarrow}$ of the binary relation $\Rightarrow$. (Transitive closure was introduced in Problem 31 of Section 1.5.)

DEFINITION 6 **INDIRECTLY GENERATED WORDS**

Let $G = (A, S, T, P)$ be a phrase-structure grammar. We say that w_1 (indirectly) generates w_n and we write $w_1 \overset{*}{\Rightarrow} w_n$ if there exist words w_i in A^* such that

$$w_1 \Rightarrow w_2 \Rightarrow w_3 \Rightarrow \cdots \Rightarrow w_n.$$

We also agree that $w \overset{*}{\Rightarrow} w$ for each word w in A^*.

Example 7

As in Example 6, let $G = (A, S, T, P)$ be the phrase-structure grammar with $A = \{s, 0, 1\}$, $S = \{s\}$, $T = \{0, 1\}$ and $P = \{s \rightarrow 1, s \rightarrow 0s, s \rightarrow 10s, s \rightarrow \varepsilon\}$. We are interested in characterizing the set L of all words β in T^* such that $s \stackrel{*}{\Rightarrow} \beta$, that is, the set of all words (directly or indirectly) generated by the start symbol s. It can be shown that this set L is the language U, of unfriendly binary strings, described in Example 2. Let us find some of the strings in L.

Since $s \rightarrow 1$ is in P, it follows from Theorem 3(a) that $s \Rightarrow 1$. Then Definition 6 with $n = 2$ tells us that $s \stackrel{*}{\Rightarrow} 1$; so 1 is in L. Using the production $s \rightarrow 0s$ and Theorem 3(a), we get $s \Rightarrow 0s$. From the production $s \rightarrow \varepsilon$ and Theorem 3(b) with $\gamma = 0$, we obtain $0s \Rightarrow 0\varepsilon = 0$. Now, $s \Rightarrow 0s \Rightarrow 0$ and Definition 6 with $n = 3$ give us $s \stackrel{*}{\Rightarrow} 0$. Thus 0 is also in L, and L has both of the strings of length 1. Similarly, we can show that

$$s \rightarrow 0s \Rightarrow 00s \Rightarrow 00 = 00.$$

Hence $s \stackrel{*}{\Rightarrow} 00$, and 00 is in L. Also, $s \rightarrow 0s \Rightarrow 01$ shows that 01 is in L. Thus L contains all the unfriendly strings 00, 01, and 10 of length 2; the string 11 is friendly and is not in L.

Let β be in L; that is, let β be a string in T^* such that $s \stackrel{*}{\Rightarrow} \beta$. Using Theorem 3(b), we can show that $0s \stackrel{*}{\Rightarrow} 0\beta$ and $10s \stackrel{*}{\Rightarrow} 10\beta$. Then $s \rightarrow 0s \stackrel{*}{\Rightarrow} 0\beta$ implies that $s \stackrel{*}{\Rightarrow} 0\beta$. Similarly, $s \rightarrow 10s \stackrel{*}{\Rightarrow} 10\beta$ implies that $s \stackrel{*}{\Rightarrow} 10\beta$. Hence the concatenations 0β and 10β are in L whenever β is in L. We have noted above that the strings β in the first column of Table 12.1.3 are all in L; it then follows that the strings in the columns headed 0β and 10β are also in L. This gives us more strings that could be placed in the first column and thus produces more of the strings of L, as shown in Table 12.1.4. Continuing in this way, one could obtain longer unfriendly strings.

The grammar used in this example is helpful in establishing the recursion formula $u_n = u_{n-1} + u_{n-2}$ for the number u_n of unfriendly binary strings of length n. In Example 9 below, we generate the same language using a different grammar, which is of the type suitable for machine recognition of the words of the language.   □

TABLE 12.1.3

β	0β	10β
0	00	100
1	01	101
00	000	1000
01	001	1001
10	010	1010

TABLE 12.1.4

β	0β	10β
000	0000	10000
001	0001	10001
010	0010	10010
100	0100	10100
101	0101	10101

DEFINITION 7

LANGUAGE GENERATED BY A PHRASE-STRUCTURE GRAMMAR

Let $G = (A, S, T, P)$ be a phrase-structure grammar with $S = \{s\}$. Then the set of all words β in T^* such that $s \stackrel{*}{\Rightarrow} \beta$ is called the ***language generated by*** G and is denoted as $L(G)$.

We emphasize that a word $\beta = b_1 b_2 \dots b_n$ in $L(G)$ must have only terminal symbols among its letters b_i. As an illustration, we consider the grammar G of Example 7 and the word 00s. Material in Example 7 implies that $s \stackrel{*}{\Rightarrow} 00s$. Thus 00s is (indirectly) generated by s. But 00s is not in the language $L(G)$ generated by the grammar G, since one of its letters—

namely, s—is not a terminal symbol. All the words of this language $L(G)$ are bit strings—in fact, unfriendly bit strings.

DEFINITION 8 | **FORMAL LANGUAGE**

A *formal language* over an alphabet T is a language $L(G)$ generated by a phrase-structure grammar $G = (A, S, T, P)$.

Example 8 Let $F = \{4, 34, 334, 3334, \ldots\}$ and let Q consist of the squares of the integers in F. It can be shown that

$$Q = \{16, 1156, 111556, 11115556, \ldots\}.$$

We can think of Q as the language $\{w_0, w_1, \ldots\}$ over the alphabet $T = \{1, 5, 6\}$ in which $w_n = 1^{n+1}5^n6$, where 1^{n+1} denotes a string of $n + 1$ ones and 5^n represents a string of n fives. We now construct a phrase-structure grammar $G = (A, S, T, P)$ such that $Q = L(G)$ and thus show that L is a formal language. We let $S = \{s\}$, $A = \{s, a, 1, 5, 6\}$, and $P = \{s \to 1a6, a \to 1a5, a \to \varepsilon\}$. Then $a \to 1a5$ and Theorem 3(d) with $\gamma = 1$ and $\delta = 6$ gives us $1a6 \Rightarrow 11a56$. Now $s \to 1a6 \Rightarrow 11a56$ implies that $s \overset{*}{\Rightarrow} 11a56$. Similarly, we can prove by induction on n that $s \overset{*}{\Rightarrow} 1^{n+1}a5^n6$ for each n in $N = \{0, 1, \ldots\}$. Then the production $a \to \varepsilon$ enables us to get $s \overset{*}{\Rightarrow} 1^{n+1}\varepsilon 5^n6 = 1^{n+1}5^n6$. Thus $1^{n+1}5^n6$ is in $L(G)$ for every n in N. We omit the proof that $L(G)$ has no other strings. □

In the next section, we will discuss finite state machines. One of the interesting questions about such machines is the following: If L is a language over an alphabet T, is there a finite state machine that can decide whether any word α in T^* is in L? The answer is given in advanced texts such as J. E. Hopcroft and J. D. Ullman, *Introduction to Automata Theory, Languages, and Computation* (Reading, Mass.: Addison-Wesley, 1979). Our very limited answer in Section 12.2 uses the following concept.

DEFINITION 9 | **REGULAR GRAMMAR, REGULAR LANGUAGE**

A *regular grammar* is a phrase-structure grammar $G = (A, S, T, P)$ for which $S = \{s\}$ and each production is one of the following three forms:

(a) $s \to \varepsilon$.
(b) $x \to t$, where x is (a single letter) in the complement $A - T$ of T in A and t is (a single letter) in T.
(c) $x \to ty$, where t is in T, x and y are in $A - T$, and $y \neq s$.

A *regular language* is a language $L(G)$ generated by a regular grammar G.

The grammar in Example 8 is not regular; for example, the production s → 1a6 satisfies none of the conditions given in Definition 9. In the next example, we give a regular grammar that generates the language U of Examples 6 and 7.

Example 9 Let $G = (A, S, T, P)$ with $A = \{s, a, b, 0, 1\}$, $S = \{s\}$, $T = \{0, 1\}$, and $P = \{s → ε, s → 0, s → 1, s → 0a, s → 1b, a → 0, a → 1, a → 0a, a → 1b, b → 0, b → 0a\}$. G is a phrase-structure grammar because it meets the conditions of Definition 4. G is a regular grammar because each of the productions in P satisfies one of the conditions given in Definition 9. Using the productions

$$s → 1b, b → 0a, a → 0a, a → 1b, b → 0 \tag{1}$$

in order, we get

$$s → 1b ⇒ 10a ⇒ 100a ⇒ 1001b ⇒ 10010. \tag{2}$$

Display (2) shows that $s \overset{*}{⇒} 10010$. Each symbol of 10010 is in T. These two facts imply that 10010 is in the regular language $L(G)$ generated by the regular grammar G. It can be shown that $L(G)$ is the language U, of unfriendly strings, described in Example 2. ☐

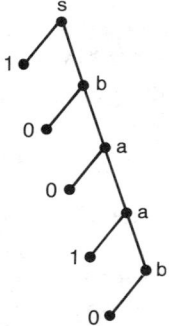

FIGURE 12.1.1

The use of the productions of Display (1), starting with s and getting the word 10010 as generated in Display (2), is represented in Figure 12.1.1. This figure differs from a (rooted) binary tree only by allowing more than one node to have a given label. The root is the start symbol s. The first production s → 1b is represented by giving s a left child labeled 1 and a right child labeled b. In turn, each production of the form $x → ty$ is indicated by giving a left child t and a right child y to the lowest node thus far obtained with x as its label. The production b → 0 is represented by giving the last b node a left child 0. We note that the symbols of the word 10010 generated by these productions appear, in descending order, as the labels of the leaves of the diagram.

DEFINITION 10   **PARSE TREE**

Let w be a word in a regular language. A *parse tree* for w is a diagram, as described in Example 9, that shows how to generate w from the start symbol s using productions.

PROBLEMS FOR SECTION 12.1

1. Is an alphabet A also a language over A? Explain.

2. If A is an alphabet, is A^* a language over A? Explain.

3. Which of the following are alphabets?
    (a) $A = \{0, 1, 2, 12\}$;   (b) $B = \{a, b, c, 0, 1\}$;   (c) $C = \{a, b, sh, th\}$.

4. Which of the following are alphabets?
   (a) $A = \{0, 1, \ldots, 9, a, b, \ldots, z\}$;   (b) $B = \{a, b, c, bc\}$;
   (c) $C = \{a, bc, d, ef\}$.

5. For the languages $L = \{a, b, c\}$ and $L' = \{ba, cb, ac\}$ over the alphabet $A = \{a, b, c, d\}$, construct a matrix table showing xy for each x in L and each y in L'. (This should be similar to Table 12.1.1.)

6. Let L and L' be as in Problem 5. Construct the matrix table showing xy for each x in L' and each y in L. (This should be related to the table for Problem 5 as Table 12.1.2 is related to Table 12.1.1.)

7. Find the concatenation LL' for the L and L' of Problem 5.

8. (i) Find the concatenation $L'L$ for the L and L' of Problem 5.
   (ii) Does $LL' = L'L$?

9. Let $A = \{a, b\}$, $L = \{a, b, ab\}$, and $L' = \{a, b, ab, ba\}$.
   (i) Are L and L' languages over A?   (ii) Is L a proper subset of L'?
   (iii) Does $A^* = L^* = (L')^*$?

10. Let $A = \{a, b, c, d\}$, $L = \{ab, ac, bc\}$, and $L' = \{ab, ba, ac, ca, bc, cb\}$.
    (i) Are L and L' languages over A?   (ii) Is L a proper subset of L'?
    (iii) Is L^* a proper subset of $(L')^*$? Explain.

11. For each of the following, tell whether or not (A, S, T, P) is a phrase-structure grammar. If not, give a reason for your answer.
    (a) $A = \{s, a, t\}$, $S = \{s\}$, $T = \{t\}$, and $P = \{s \to \varepsilon, s \to a, a \to t, t \to s\}$.
    (b) $A = \{s, t\}$, $S = \{s\}$, $T = \{t\}$, and $P = \{s \to \varepsilon, s \to t, st \to tt\}$.

12. Repeat Problem 11 for the following parts:
    (a) $A = \{s, 0, 1\}$, $S = \{s\}$, $T = \{0, 1\}$, $P = \{s \to 0, s \to 01s, s \to \varepsilon\}$.
    (b) $A = \{s, 0, 1\}$, $S = \{s\}$, $T = \{0, 1\}$, $P = \{s \to 0, s \to \varepsilon, 0 \to \varepsilon\}$.

13. Let $A = \{s, a, b, 0, 1\}$, $S = \{s\}$, $T = \{0, 1\}$. For each of the following finite binary relations P on A^*, tell whether the phrase-structure grammar $G = (A, S, T, P)$ is regular. If not, give a production in P that does not meet the conditions of Definition 9, "Regular Grammar, Regular Language."
    (a) $P = \{s \to \varepsilon, s \to 0s, s \to 0, s \to 1\}$.
    (b) $P = \{s \to \varepsilon, s \to 0, s \to 1, s \to 0a, a \to b\}$.
    (c) $P = \{s \to \varepsilon, s \to 0a, s \to 1b, a \to 1, b \to 0\}$.

14. Do as in Problem 13 for the following parts:
    (a) $P = \{s \to \varepsilon, s \to 0a, a \to 1b, b \to 0\}$.
    (b) $P = \{s \to \varepsilon, s \to 0a, a \to b, b \to 1\}$.
    (c) $P = \{s \to \varepsilon, s \to 1s, s \to 0a, a \to 1\}$.

15. Let G be the regular grammar (A, S, T, P) with $A = \{s, a, b, 0, 1\}$, $S = \{s\}$, $T = \{0, 1\}$, and $P = \{s \to \varepsilon, s \to 0, s \to 1, s \to 0a, s \to 1b, a \to 0, a \to 1, a \to 0a, a \to 1b, b \to 0, b \to 0a\}$. Give a succession of productions that generates the word 101001 in $L(G)$ from s.

16. Repeat Problem 15 with the word 101001 replaced by 100101.

17. Let G be as in Problem 15. Is 110001 in $L(G)$? Explain. [*Hint*: G is the grammar of Example 9 and $L(G)$ consists of the unfriendly strings.]

18. Let G be as in Problem 15. Which of the following are in $L(G)$?
(a) 10001,   (b) 001100,   (c) 0010100,   (d) 11011011.

19. For the G of Problem 15, draw the parse tree for the unfriendly string 101001.

20. For the G of Problem 15, draw the parse tree for 0010001.

21. Let $G = (A, S, T, P)$ with $A = \{s, a, b, c\}$, $S = \{s\}$, $T = \{a, b, c\}$, and $P = \{s \rightarrow as, s \rightarrow b, s \rightarrow \varepsilon\}$. Find all the words in $L(G)$ that are words of length 3 (over the alphabet T).

22. For the G of Problem 21, find all the words of length 4 in $L(G)$.

23. Prove Theorem 1. That is, for languages E, F, and G over A, prove that:
(a) $G\{\varepsilon\} = \{\varepsilon\}G = G$.   (b) If $E \subseteq F$, then $EG \subseteq FG$ and $GE \subseteq GF$.

24. Prove Theorem 2. That is, for languages L and M over A, prove that:
(a) If $L \subset M$, then $L^* \subseteq M^*$.   (b) $(L^*)^* = L^* = L^*L^*$.
(c) $L^* \cup M^* \subseteq (L \cup M)^* = (L^* \cup M^*)^*$.

25. Find a phrase-structure grammar G such that $L(G)$ is the language $\{1089, 110889, 11108889, \ldots, 1^n08^n9, \ldots\}$ over the alphabet $\{0, 1, 8, 9\}$. Note that 1^n denotes a string of n 1's and 8^n a string of n 8's.

12.2

FINITE STATE MACHINES

We illustrate the major concept of this section by considering a coin-operated food dispenser that accepts just 25¢ and 50¢ coins and, at a cost of 75¢ apiece, produces two apples, a box of chocolates, a granola bar, or a container of popcorn. We ignore certain aspects of the machine, such as the storing of multiples of 75¢ in the till, the periodic stocking of the machine with merchandise, and the periodic emptying of the till.

We use x_0 to denote the normal state of the machine when a customer approaches, x_1 to indicate that 25¢ has been accepted, x_2 to indicate that 50¢ has been inserted, and x_3 to represent the state in which 75¢ has been placed in the slots. An input for this machine is the depositing of a 25¢ coin or a 50¢ coin or the pushing of one of four buttons, labeled A, C, G, and P (for apples, chocolates, granola bar, and popcorn, respectively). For each ordered pair (x, i) with x a state and i an input, the output of the machine may be nothing (represented by $\varnothing$), or one of the items of merchandise, or such an item plus 25¢ when two 50¢ coins had been accepted. Table 12.2.1 records the states, inputs, and outputs for the case in which the machine starts in the state x_0, then 25¢ is deposited at time

TABLE 12.2.1 Food Dispenser

State	Time	Input	Next State	Output
x_0	t_1	25¢	x_1	$\varnothing$
x_1	t_2	50¢	x_3	$\varnothing$
x_3	t_3	G	x_0	Granola bar
x_0				

t_1, 50¢ is deposited at time t_2, and finally the G button is pressed at time t_3.

We lose no information by deleting the time column because its entry on the kth row is always t_k. Also, the next state column can be omitted because each entry is indicated as the state (in the first column) on the next line. Table 12.2.2, embodying these changes, describes the case in which two 50¢ coins are deposited and then the C button is pressed.

TABLE 12.2.2

State	Input	Output
x_0	50¢	$\varnothing$
x_2	50¢	25¢ change
x_3	C	Chocolates
x_0		

We next introduce a mathematical model for the type of machine we are considering here.

DEFINITION 1   **FINITE STATE MACHINE (FSM)**

A *finite state machine* (FSM) is an ordered 5-tuple $M = (X, I, F, G, U)$ in which X, I, and U are finite sets and

$$F: X \times I \to X, \quad G: X \times I \to U$$

are mappings. The set I is the **input alphabet**, U is the **output alphabet**, X is the set of **states**, F is the **next state function**, and G is the **output function**. An **input symbol** is an element of I, an **input word** is a word over I, and similarly for **output symbols** and **output words**. One of the states in X is designated as the **initial state** x_0.

Example 1   **BINARY ADDER** We describe an FSM that adds nonnegative integers given in base 2. Since addition is performed from right to left, we reverse the usual indexing for binary strings and use $\alpha = a_n a_{n-1} \ldots a_1$ as a typical n-bit string. Then

$$(\alpha)_2 = a_1 + 2a_2 + 2^2 a_3 + \cdots + 2^{n-1} a_n$$

is the integer in $N = \{0, 1, \ldots\}$ represented in base 2 by this α. Given n-bit strings $\alpha = a_n a_{n-1} \ldots a_1$ and $\beta = b_n b_{n-1} \ldots b_1$, we want the FSM to find the $(n+1)$-bit string $\gamma = c_{n+1} c_n \ldots c_1$ such that $(\gamma)_2 = (\alpha)_2 + (\beta)_2$. This operation was previously discussed near Table 2.5.3 in Section 2.5.

We consider the input to be the strings α and β merged to form the $2n$-bit string $a_1 b_1 a_2 b_2 a_3 b_3 \ldots a_n b_n$. More specifically, we let the input at time t_j be the 2-bit string $a_j b_j$. Therefore, we take the input alphabet to be the set $I = \{00, 01, 10, 11\}$ of 2-bit strings. We use $U = \{0, 1\}$ as the output alphabet, since each output word is a bit string. The set X of states is also $\{0, 1\}$, with 0 indicating no carryover from the previous digit position and 1 representing a carryover. The next state function $F(x, i)$ and the output function $G(x, i)$ are given by Table 12.2.3.

TABLE 12.2.3

State x	Input ab	Next State $F(x, ab)$	Output $G(x, ab)$
0	00	0	0
0	01	0	1
0	10	0	1
0	11	1	0
1	00	0	1
1	01	1	0
1	10	1	0
1	11	1	1

Then Table 12.2.4 illustrates the action of the FSM in the case of $\alpha = 1011$ and $\beta = 111$, that is, the adding of $11 = (1011)_2$ and $7 = (111)_2$ to get $18 = (10010)_2$. Since γ has 5 bits, we make α and β into 5-bit strings by prefixing zeros; that is, we let $\alpha = a_5a_4a_3a_2a_1 = 01011$ and $\beta = b_5b_4b_3b_2b_1 = 00111$. Note that the prefixing of zeros does not change the integers $(\alpha)_2$ and $(\beta)_2$ represented in base 2 by α and β. The input at time t_j is a_jb_j; for example, the first input is $a_1b_1 = 11$. The entries in the output column, from bottom to top, give us the bits from left to right of the sum string γ. The state on the first line is 0, to indicate that the carryover memory position was cleared before the operation began. Similarly, the bottom entry in the next state column is 0 because the addition is not complete if a carryover remains to be made. Each entry in the next state column appears on the next line in the state column. Hence the next state column can be omitted without loss of information. The time column can also be omitted. These deletions have been made in Table 12.2.5, which records the addition of $9 = (01001)_2$ and $13 = (01101)_2$, to get $22 = (10110)_2$.

TABLE 12.2.4

State	Time	Input	Next State	Output
0	t_1	11	1	0
1	t_2	11	1	1
1	t_3	01	1	0
1	t_4	10	1	0
1	t_5	00	0	1
0	t_6			

TABLE 12.2.5

State	Input	Output
0	11	0
1	00	1
0	01	1
0	11	0
1	00	1
0		

□

The next state function $F(x, i)$ and the output function $G(x, i)$ of an FSM can also be given by matrix tables in which the states are the row labels and the input symbols are the column labels. The matrix substitutes for Table 12.2.3 are Tables 12.2.6 and 12.2.7.

TABLE 12.2.6 Next State Function $F(x, i)$

x \ i	00	01	10	11
0	0	0	0	1
1	0	1	1	1

TABLE 12.2.7 Output Function $G(x, i)$

x \ i	00	01	10	11
0	0	1	1	0
1	1	0	0	1

[00, 0]
[01, 1]
[10, 1]

[11, 0]   [00, 1]

[01, 0]
[10, 0]
[11, 1]

FIGURE 12.2.1

An FSM (X, I, F, G, U) can also be represented by a *labeled digraph*, which is somewhat similar to the "weighted graphs" introduced in Example 1 of Section 6.6. In a labeled digraph for an FSM, the states are represented as vertices. If x and x' are states and $F(x, i) = x'$ for at least one input symbol i, there is a directed arc from x to x' labeled with all the ordered pairs $[i, G(x, i)]$ for which $F(x, i) = x'$. The diagram of this type for the binary adder of Example 1 is Figure 12.2.1.

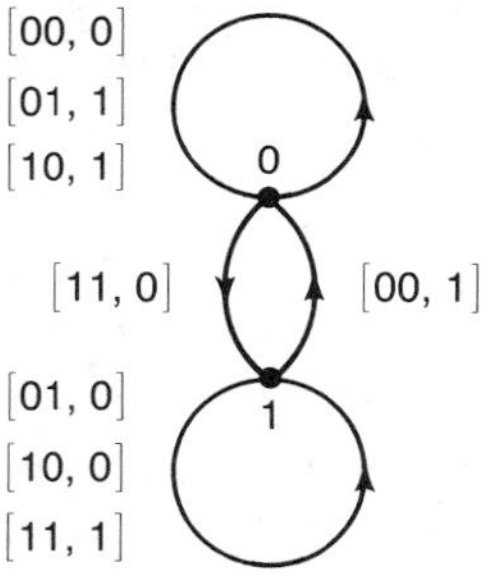

The next example describes an FSM that detects certain transmission errors for one of the codes considered in Section 11.1.

Example 2 **PARITY CHECK MACHINE** In the parity check code of Example 1 in Section 11.1, a valid codeword is a binary string α of even weight, that is, a bit string α with wgt α in $2N = \{0, 2, 4, \ldots\}$. Thus a machine that classifies binary strings as having even or odd weight is helpful in the detection of some transmission errors. Here we describe an FSM that serves this purpose.

An input string is an n-bit string $\alpha = a_1 a_2 \ldots a_n$, with the bit a_j as the input symbol considered by the machine at time t_j. We want the state x_j at time t_j to be 0 if the partial string $a_1 \ldots a_{j-1}$ has even weight and x_j to be 1 if $a_1 \ldots a_{j-1}$ has odd weight. The next state function $F(x, i)$ given by Table 12.2.8 achieves this purpose because $F(x, 0) = x$ and $F(x, 1)$ is the symbol in $\{0, 1\}$ different from x. Here we can, and do, choose the output function $G(x, i)$ to be the same as the next state function $F(x, i)$.

Table 12.2.9 illustrates the operation of this FSM for the case of $\alpha = a_1 a_2 a_3 a_4 a_5 = 11001$. The bits of α, from left to right, are the input symbol entries, from top to bottom. On the first row, the state is the initial state 0 (indicating that the empty binary string ε has 0 weight) and the input symbol is $a_1 = 1$. On this row, the next state entry is $F(0, 1) = 1$, found from Table 12.2.8, and the output symbol is also 1, since $G(x, i) = F(x, i)$. The next state entry 1 on the first row becomes the state entry x on the second row. On the second row, $x = 1$ and the input $a_2 = 1$ give us the

TABLE 12.2.8

State	Input	Next State
0	0	0
0	1	1
1	0	1
1	1	0

TABLE 12.2.9

State	Input	Next State	Output
0	1	1	1
1	1	0	0
0	0	0	0
0	0	0	0
0	1	1	1

next state entry $F(1, 1)$, which is found to be 0 using Table 12.2.8. The output on this row is $G(1, 1) = F(1, 1) = 0$. We similarly find the other rows of Table 12.2.9. The machine is designed so that input strings α of even weight cause the output on the last row to be 0 and the inputs α of odd weight cause the last output to be 1. In the case shown in Table 12.2.9, the last output symbol is 1; hence we know that α has odd weight and so is not a valid codeword. This tells us that at least one error, actually an odd number of errors, occurred in transmission. □

Let E consist of all the binary strings α of even weight and with the length any integer in $N = \{0, 1, \dots\}$. The FSM of Example 2 "recognizes" this language E over $\{0, 1\}$ in the sense that the final output symbol is 0 if and only if the input word α has even weight. (We interpret the operation of the machine to be such that the output symbol is the initial state 0 when the input word is the empty word ε.)

DEFINITION 2   **RECOGNITION OF A LANGUAGE BY AN FSM**

Let $M = (X, I, F, G, U)$ be an FSM and let L be a language over the input alphabet I. We say that M *recognizes* L if, for some u_0 in U, an input word α produces u_0 as the final output symbol if and only if α is in L.

The next example illustrates how a finite state machine M that recognizes a language L can be used to devise a regular grammar G such that L is generated by G. In the example after that, we start with a regular grammar G having a special property (that of being "deterministic," which is defined there) and use G to devise a finite state machine that recognizes the language L generated by G.

Example 3   Let $M = (X, I, F, G, U)$ be the parity check FSM of Example 2 that recognizes the language E consisting of all binary strings of even weight. Here we build a regular grammar $G = (A, S, T, P)$ that generates E. We use the input alphabet I for M as the set T of terminal symbols for G and let $S = \{s\}$. Essentially we want the alphabet A for G to be the union of S, I, and the set X of states for M. But first we must replace the symbols for the states with symbols that are not words over I. Since $I = \{0, 1\}$ and $X = \{0, 1\}$, we replace the state 0 by b and the state 1 by c. This gives us a new set $X = \{b, c\}$ of states and we let the alphabet G be

$$A = \{s\} \cup I \cup X = \{s, b, c, 0, 1\}.$$

Let $F(x, i)$ now denote the next state function for M in terms of the new symbols for the states. Table 12.2.10 gives both $F(x, i)$ and the output function $G(x, i)$. We use this table to obtain the set P of productions for G.

TABLE 12.2.10

State	Input	$F(x, i)$	$G(x, i)$
b	0	b	0
b	1	c	1
c	0	c	1
c	1	b	0

For the machine M and the language E it recognizes, an input word α is in E if and only if the last output $G(x_n, i_n)$ is 0. Therefore, we let the ordered pairs (x, i) such that $G(x, i) = 0$ produce "terminal type" productions of the form $x \to i$ as well as "continuing type" productions $x \to iy$. Let x be a state in X and let i be an input in I. Also let $F(x, i) = y$. If $G(x, i) = 0$, we let both $x \to i$ and $x \to iy$ be productions in P. If $G(x, i) \neq 0$, then only $x \to iy$ is added to the set P of productions. Using these rules, $G(b, 0) = 0$ and $F(b, 0) = b$ give us both $b \to 0$ and $b \to 0b$. Also, $G(c, 1) = 0$ and $F(c, 1) = b$ give us both $c \to 1$ and $c \to 1b$. On the other hand, $G(b, 1) = 1$ and $F(b, 1) = c$ give us only $b \to 1c$, and similarly, $G(c, 0) = 1$ and $F(c, 0) = c$ give us only $c \to 0c$. Together, these rules lead to the productions

$$b \to 0, \ b \to 0b, \ b \to 1c, \ c \to 1, \ c \to 1b, \ c \to 0c.$$

The symbol b represents the state in which the partial input string $a_1 \ldots a_j$ has even weight. Before the machine starts, the input is the empty word ε, which has even weight. The start symbol s can be thought of as the special case of the symbol b used only at this initial state. To allow this interpretation, we must also introduce the three productions

$$s \to 0, \ s \to 0b, \ s \to 1c$$

obtained from productions of the form $b \to i$ and $b \to iy$ by replacing b with s. So the complete set of productions is

$$P = \{s \to 0, s \to 0b, s \to 1c, b \to 0, b \to 0b, b \to 1c, c \to 1, c \to 1b, c \to 0c\},$$

and $G = (A, S, T, P)$ is the regular grammar that generates E.   □

Next we use a grammar G to devise an FSM that recognizes $L(G)$.

Example 4   Here let L be the language of unfriendly strings and let G be the regular grammar that generates L. We recall from Example 9 of Section 12.1 that $G = (A, S, T, P)$ with $A = \{s, a, b, 0, 1\}$, $S = \{s\}$, $T = \{0, 1\}$, and $P = \{s \to \varepsilon, s \to 0, s \to 1, s \to 0a, s \to 1b, a \to 0, a \to 1, a \to 0a, a \to 1b, b \to 0, b \to 0a\}$. The set P of productions has the property that $x \to ty$ and $x \to tz$, with t in T and x and y in $A - T$, imply that $y = z$. Such a regular grammar is called a ***deterministic grammar***. This property of P enables us to devise a finite state machine $M = (X, I, F, G, U)$ that recognizes L. We recall that L consists of the binary strings $\alpha = a_1 a_2 \ldots a_n$ (of all lengths) such that two consecutive bits $a_{j-1} a_j$ are never 11. For this language, there are strings, such as 011, that cannot be extended into words of L. That is, $011a_4 a_5 \ldots a_n$ is not in L no matter what $a_4, a_5, \ldots, a_n$ equal. If an input word $\alpha = a_1 a_2 \ldots . a_n$ has 11 appearing as adjacent bits in the partial string $a_1 \ldots a_{j-1}$, we will use r (for "reject") as the symbol for the state x_j during which the input symbol a_j is being read.

We take the complete set of states to be $X = \{s, a, b, r\}$. We let $I = T = \{0, 1\}$. Here we need only two output symbols, so we also let $U = \{0, 1\}$. Now we have to define the next state function $F(x, i)$ and the output function $G(x, i)$. Let x be in X and i be in I. If there exists a state y in X such that $x \rightarrow iy$ is a production in P, we let $F(x, i) = y$. There is no ambiguity about the value of $F(x, i)$ because the grammar is deterministic. If $x \rightarrow iy$ and $x \rightarrow i$ are both productions, we let $G(x, i) = 0$; otherwise we let $G(x, i) = 1$. What is the value of $F(x, i)$ when there is no state y such that $x \rightarrow iy$ is a production? In such cases we let $F(x, i) = r$. We also let $F(r, i) = r$ and $G(r, i) = 1$ for all inputs i. The matrix table for F is given in Table 12.2.11. It can be seen that $G(r, i) = 1$ when $F(x, i) = r$ and that $G(r, i) = 0$ otherwise. The machine $M = (X, I, F, G, U)$ recognizes L by having the last output $G(x_n, i_n) = 0$ if and only if the input word α is in L. Since the entries on the rows with s and a as labels are identical, the machine would also recognize L if s were deleted from the set of states and we agreed that the initial state, before any input bits are read, is a. $\square$

TABLE 12.2.11
Next State Function

x \ i	0	1
s	a	b
a	a	b
b	a	r
r	r	r

PROBLEMS FOR SECTION 12.2

1. Using the binary adder of Example 1, construct a table showing the states, inputs, and outputs for the addition of $9 = (1001)_2$ and $12 = (1100)_2$. (The table should be similar to Table 12.2.5.) Then give the γ such that $(\gamma)_2 = (1001)_2 + (1100)_2$.

2. Repeat Problem 1, but with $9 + 12$ replaced by $11 + 10$.

3. For each of the following input strings α, construct a table showing how the parity check machine of Example 2 determines whether α has even or odd weight.
   (a) $\alpha = 1011$,   (b) $\alpha = 0110$.

4. Do as in Problem 3 for the following parts.
   (a) $\alpha = 01110$,   (b) $\alpha = 11101$.

5. Give the matrix table for the next state function $F(x, i)$ of the parity check machine of Example 2.

6. Give the matrix table for the output function G of the parity check machine of Example 2.

7. Give the labeled digraph for the parity check machine of Example 2.

8. Let $M = (X, I, F, G, U)$ with $X = \{a, b, r\}$, $I = U = \{0, 1\}$, and F and G given by the two tables in the margin.
   (a) Draw the labeled digraph for M.
   (b) Does M recognize the language of unfriendly strings? Explain.

9. Let L consist of all binary strings $\alpha = a_1 a_2 \ldots a_n$ (of all lengths) such that $a_{j-1} a_j$ is never 00. Devise an FSM (X, I, F, G, U) that recognizes L.

Next State Function F

x \ i	0	1
a	a	b
b	a	r
r	r	r

Output Function G

x \ i	0	1
a	0	0
b	0	1
r	1	1

$a_{j-2}a_{j-1}$	x_j
$\varepsilon\varepsilon$	s
$\varepsilon 0$	b
$\varepsilon 1$	c
00	d
01	e
10	f
11	g

10. Construct a regular grammar G that generates the L of Problem 9.

11. Let L consist of all binary strings $\alpha = a_1 a_2 \ldots a_n$ (of all lengths) such that $a_{j-2}a_{j-1}a_j$ is never 101. Let $I = U = \{0, 1\}$ and $X = \{s, b, c, d, e, f, g, r\}$. Give the matrix table for a next state function F of a finite state machine $M = (X, I, F, G, U)$ that recognizes L. (*Hint*: If 101 has already appeared in the partial input word $a_1 \ldots a_{j-1}$, let the state x_j at the time of reading a_j be r. Otherwise, let x_j be determined from $a_{j-2}a_{j-1}$ using the table in the margin.)

12. Give the matrix table for the output function G of the FSM of Problem 11, using $G(x, i) = 0$ when $F(x, i) \neq r$ and $G(x, i) = 1$ when $F(x, i) = r$.

*13. Draw a labeled digraph for the FSM of Problem 11.

SUMMARY OF TERMS, CHAPTER 12

REVIEW PROBLEMS FOR CHAPTER 12 _____

1. For the languages $L = \{01, 12, 20\}$ and $L' = \{012, 120, 201\}$ over the alphabet $A = \{0, 1, 2\}$, construct a matrix table showing $\alpha\beta$ for each α in L and β in L'.

2. Let L and L' be as in Problem 1. Does $LL' = L'L$? Explain.

3. Let $A = \{s, b, 0, 1, 2\}$, $S = \{s\}$, and $T = \{0, 1, 2\}$. For which of the following sets P is (A, S, T, P) a phrase-structure grammar?
   (a) $P = \{s \rightarrow \varepsilon, s \rightarrow 0, s \rightarrow 0s, 0s \rightarrow 12, 12 \rightarrow 0\}$.
   (b) $P = \{s \rightarrow \varepsilon, s \rightarrow 0b, b \rightarrow 1b, b \rightarrow 0\}$.
   (c) $P = \{s \rightarrow \varepsilon, s \rightarrow 0s, s \rightarrow 1b, b \rightarrow 0\}$.

4. For the part of Problem 3 that does not give a phrase-structure grammar, tell which alleged production $\alpha \rightarrow \beta$ causes it to fail.

5. Which one of the parts of Problem 3 gives a regular grammar?

6. For the phrase-structure grammar of Problem 3 that is not a regular grammar, tell which $\alpha \rightarrow \beta$ causes it to fail.

7. Let L be the language generated by the grammar G of Problem 3(b). (Recall that L is a language over the set $T = \{0, 1, 2\}$ of terminal symbols.) Which of the following words are in L?
    (a) ε,   (b) 00,   (c) 01,   (d) 010,   (e) 011.

8. Give the sequence of productions that generates 01110 as a word in the language L of Problem 7.

Next State Function *F*

x \ i	0	1	2
s	s	b	c
b	b	c	s
c	c	s	b

Output Function *G*

x \ i	0	1	2
s	0	1	2
b	1	2	0
c	2	0	1

9. Let $M = (X, I, F, G, U)$ be an FSM with $X = \{s, b, c\}$, $I = \{0, 1, 2\} = U$, and F and G given by the two tables in the margin. The state before any input symbols are read is the initial state s. Find the final output symbol for each of the following input words.
    (a) 2021,   (b) 00012,   (c) 111100.

10. Let L be the language of all words $a_1 a_2 \ldots a_n$ (of all lengths) over $\{0, 1, 2\}$ such that $a_1 + a_2 + \cdots + a_n$ is an integral multiple of 3, that is, such that $a_1 + a_2 + \cdots + a_n$ is in $3N = \{0, 3, 6, \ldots\}$. Does the machine M of Problem 9 recognize L?

11. Draw the labeled digraph for the M of Problem 9.

12. Give a regular grammar G that generates the language L of Problem 10.

13. A *palindrome* over $A = \{0, 1\}$ is a word $\alpha = a_1 a_2 \ldots a_n$ in A^* such that $a_n \ldots a_2 a_1 = a_1 a_2 \ldots a_n$. Also, the empty word ε is a palindrome. Construct a phrase-structure grammar G that generates the language L of palindromes over A.

14. Construct a phrase-structure grammar G that generates the language L of palindromes of even length (over $\{0, 1\}$).

SUPPLEMENTARY AND CHALLENGING PROBLEMS, CHAPTER 12

1. Let $L = \{16, 1156, 111556, \ldots, 1^{n+1}5^n 6, \ldots\}$, where 5^n denotes a string of n 5's and 1^{n+1} denotes a string $11 \ldots 1$ of length $n + 1$. Prove that the decimal representations of $\{4^2, 34^2, 334^2, 3334^2, \ldots\}$ form the language L.

2. Is there a regular grammar G that generates the language L of Problem 1?

3. Is there an FSM that recognizes the language $\{\varepsilon\} \cup L$, where L is as in Problem 1?

4. A *palindrome* over $A = \{0, 1\}$ is a word $\alpha = a_1 a_2 \ldots a_n$ in A^* such that $a_1 a_2 \ldots a_n = a_n \ldots a_2 a_1$. Also, let ε be a palindrome. Is the language L of palindromes over A a regular language?

5. Is the union $L \cup L'$ of two regular languages also regular?

6. Is the concatenation LL' of two regular languages also a regular language?

7. Let L be a regular language. Must the Kleene closure L^* also be a regular language?

ANNOTATED BIBLIOGRAPHY

GENERAL

Campbell, Douglas M., and John C. Higgins. *Mathematics: People, Problems, Results.* Belmont, CA: Wadsworth, 1984.
> A collection of essays on various aspects of mathematics and computer science. Entertaining reading.

Knuth, Donald E. *The Art of Computer Programming.* Volume I. "Fundamental Algorithms." Reading, MA: Addison-Wesley, 1973.
> Applications of algebra, combinatorics, number theory, graph theory to computer science. Good historical notes. The first of a series of books on computer science by one of the foremost computer scientists of the day.

Knuth, Donald E. *The Art of Computer Programming.* Volume II. "Seminumerical Algorithms." Reading, MA: Addison-Wesley, 1969.
> Topics from the theory of numbers and algebra looked at from the point of view of someone interested in computation.

Knuth, Donald E. *The Art of Computer Programming.* Volume III. "Sorting and Searching." Reading, MA: Addison-Wesley, 1973.
> Binary tree searching and many other topics of interest to computer scientists.

Pollack, S. V., ed. *Studies in Computer Science.* Washington, D.C.: Mathematical Association of America, 1982.
> A series of essays on history and varied topics in computer science.

SETS AND LOGIC

Arnold, B. H. *Logic and Boolean Algebra.* Englewood Cliffs, N.J.: Prentice-Hall, 1962.
> A rather old book but still an easy introduction to the subject.

Dodge, Clayton W. *Sets, Logic, Numbers.* Boston: Prindle, Weber, & Schmidt, 1969.
> A readable, well-written account of logic, set theory, boolean algebra, and

number systems. Contains many of the interesting "extras" of mathematics like synthetic division, infinity, fundamental theorem of algebra, modular arithmetic, induction, Peano postulates, switching circuits, among others.

Halmos, Paul R. *Naive Set Theory*. New York: Van Nostrand, 1960.
A classic text, a standard against which others are measured.

Quine, Willard Van Orman. *Set Theory and Its Logic*. Cambridge, MA: Belknap, 1969.
A sophisticated but readable coverage of many useful topics in logic.

Stoll, Robert R. *Set Theory and Logic*. San Francisco: Freeman, 1963.
A text that includes boolean algebras and algebraic theories in addition to the standard treatment of sets and logic.

Suppes, Patrick. *Axiomatic Set Theory*. New York: Van Nostrand, 1960.
A well-written, rigorous treatment of set theory; again a classic in the field.

Suppes, Patrick. *Introduction to Logic*. Princeton: Van Nostrand, 1957.
This remains the classic in the field.

ALGEBRAIC STRUCTURES

Birkhoff, Garrett. *Lattice Theory*, Third Edition. Providence: American Mathematical Society, 1967.
This is the classic, definitive treatment of lattice theory, for experienced readers.

Birkhoff, Garrett, and T. C. Bartee. *Modern Applied Algebra*. New York: McGraw-Hill, 1970.
An early, pace-setting treatment of applications of algebra to a variety of physical and engineering problems.

Davis, Philip J. *The Mathematics of Matrices*. Waltham, MA: Blaisdell, 1965.
Beginning level discourse on elementary theory of matrices.

Dornhoff, Larry L., and Franz E. Hohn. *Applied Modern Algebra*. New York: Macmillan, 1978.
A readable account of applications of boolean algebra and classical abstract algebra to a wide variety of applications, including coding theory. Some topics in graph theory and combinatorics are included.

Fraleigh, John B. *A First Course in Abstract Algebra*, Second Edition. Reading, MA: Addison-Wesley, 1976.
A very clearly written junior–senior level text with beautiful problems and relationships to other parts of mathematics.

Gill, Arthur. *Applied Algebra for the Computer Sciences*. Englewood Cliffs, N.J.: Prentice-Hall, 1976.
Boolean algebra and switching theory, coding, networks, finite state machines, automata, with appropriate algebraic ideas.

Herstein, I. N. *Topics in Algebra*, Second Edition. Lexington, MA: Xerox, 1975.
A classic text, at the junior–senior level.

Hillman, A. P., and G. L. Alexanderson. *A First Undergraduate Course in Abstract Algebra*, Third Edition. Belmont, CA: Wadsworth, 1983.
A sophomore–junior level text in abstract algebra distinguished by its concrete examples, its problems, and its historical notes.

Hohn, Franz E. *Applied Boolean Algebra*, Second Edition. New York: Macmillan, 1966.
An introduction to the subject for the beginner.

Kohavi, Zvi. *Switching and Finite Automata Theory*, Second Edition. New York: McGraw-Hill, 1978.
Boolean algebra and lattices with application to switching, coding, and various more advanced topics.

MacKiw, George. *Applications of Abstract Algebra.* New York: Wiley, 1985.
This paperback is an exceptionally well-written text on a variety of applications in algebra with a concentration on group codes.

MacWilliams, F. J., and N. J. A. Sloane. *The Theory of Error-Correcting Codes.* Amsterdam: North-Holland, 1978.
An extensive survey of error-correcting codes.

Marcus, Mitchell P. *Switching Circuits for Engineers*, Second Edition. Englewood Cliffs, N.J.: Prentice-Hall, 1967.
Boolean algebra, switching theory, and codes from an engineer's viewpoint.

Stone, Harold S. *Discrete Mathematical Structures.* Chicago: Science Research Associates, 1973.
An advanced treatment of groups, theory of enumeration, group codes, finite state machines, rings and fields, boolean algebra, among others.

Whitesitt, J. Eldon. *Boolean Algebra and Its Applications.* Reading, MA: Addison-Wesley, 1961.
Covers in a readable fashion symbolic logic, truth sets, valid arguments, set algebra, switching algebra, circuits, binary number systems.

Williams, Gerald E. *Boolean Algebra with Computer Applications.* New York: McGraw-Hill, 1970.
A very clear but detailed account of truth tables, boolean algebra, simplification of boolean functions. Freshman–sophomore level, no proofs.

COMBINATORICS, GENERATING FUNCTIONS, AND RECURSION

Beckenbach, Edwin F. *Applied Combinatorial Mathematics.* New York: Wiley, 1964.
A set of essays on a variety of combinatorial topics, some more accessible than others.

Berge, Claude. *Principles of Combinatorics*. New York: Academic Press, 1971.
A rather sophisticated treatment of combinatorics that uses some ideas from abstract algebra.

Even, Shimon. *Algorithmic Combinatorics*. New York: Macmillan, 1973.
Major ideas from combinatorics and graph theory with emphasis on computing.

Goldberg, Samuel. *Introduction to Difference Equations*. New York: Wiley, 1958.
An attractive presentation of applications of difference equations.

Hu, T. C. *Combinatorial Algorithms*. Reading, MA: Addison-Wesley, 1982.
A graduate–undergraduate treatment of a number of combinatorial techniques used in computer science, many not readily available elsewhere.

Levy, Hyman, and F. Lessman. *Finite Difference Equations*. New York: Macmillan, 1961.
A survey of difference equation methods.

Liu, C. L. *Introduction to Combinatorial Mathematics*. New York: McGraw-Hill, 1968.
An advanced undergraduate level text, written by a well-known expert in the field. Extensive problem sets.

Riordan, John. *An Introduction to Combinatorial Analysis*. New York: Wiley, 1958.
General survey of combinatorics at the senior–graduate level.

Rota, Gian-Carlo, ed. *Studies in Combinatorics*. Washington, D.C.: Mathematical Association of America, 1978.
A set of essays on various combinatorial topics, for those with some experience with the subject.

DIGRAPHS AND GRAPHS

Behzad, Mehdi, Gary Chartrand, and Linda Lezniak-Foster. *Graphs and Digraphs*. Belmont, CA: Wadsworth, 1979.
An accessible, extensive treatment of graphs and digraphs.

Bellmore, M., and G. L. Nemhauser. "The Travelling Salesman Problem," *Operations Research* 16 (1968), 538–558.
A good survey of a famous old problem.

Berge, Claude. *Graphs and Hypergraphs*. Amsterdam: North-Holland, 1973.
A high level treatment of a wide range of topics; a good reference.

Biggs, Norman L., E. Keith Lloyd, and Robin J. Wilson. *Graph Theory, 1736–1936*. Oxford: Oxford University Press, 1976.
A beautiful historical account of graph theory from Euler's examination of the Königsberg bridge problem to the early twentieth century.

Chartrand, Gary. *Graphs as Mathematical Models*. Boston: Prindle, Weber & Schmidt, 1977.

A pleasant, easy-to-read account of important topics in graph theory. Most chapters end with interesting applications.

Grossman, Israel, and Wilhelm Magnus. *Groups and Their Graphs.* Washington, D.C.: Mathematical Association of America, 1964.
   Readable by a student with little mathematical background. The abstraction of group theory is softened by "picturing" the structures of groups.

Harary, Frank. *Graph Theory.* Reading, MA: Addison-Wesley, 1969.
   An excellent, comprehensive reference on graph theory.

Marshall, Clifford W. *Applied Graph Theory.* New York: Wiley-Interscience, 1971.
   Readable by undergraduate and graduate students, though some knowledge of probability and linear algebra is necessary. Applications are in operations research, physics, psychology, and other social sciences.

Ore, Øystein. *Graphs and Their Uses.* Washington, D.C.: Mathematical Association of America, 1963.
   A survey of elementary ideas in graph theory for beginners.

Trudeau, Richard J. *Dots and Lines.* Kent, OH: Kent State University Press, 1976.
   A light, gentle introduction to the ideas of graph theory, far from comprehensive.

DATA STRUCTURES, ALGORITHMS, SEARCHING

Aho, Alfred V., John E. Hopcroft, and Jeffrey D. Ullman. *Data Structures and Algorithms.* Reading, MA: Addison-Wesley, 1983.
   A good computer science book dealing with searching, sorting, and graph algorithms.

Aho, Alfred V., John E. Hopcroft, and Jeffrey D. Ullman. *The Design and Analysis of Computer Algorithms.* Reading, MA: Addison-Wesley, 1974.
   This text on the analysis of algorithms gives a careful treatment of the following procedures: merge sort, quick-sort, bubble sort, and heapsort.

Hopcroft, J. E, and J. D. Ullman. *Introduction to Automata Theory, Languages and Computation.* Reading, MA: Addison-Wesley, 1979.
   Concentrates on the use of language-theory concepts and the application of language-theory ideas such as regular expressions and context-free grammars. This is a senior-level text in finite automata theory. Good reference text on computational complexity.

Lucas, Éduard. *Recréations Mathématiques.* Paris: Gauthier-Villars, 1891.
   Early account of searching methods.

Ullman, Jeffrey D. *Principles of Database Systems.* Potomac, MD: Computer Science Press, 1980.
   Excellent in-depth work on accessing the data stored in a relational database.

HISTORY

Ashurst, F. Gareth. *Pioneers of Computing*. London: Frederick Muller, 1983.
Short biographical sketches of giants in the history of computing from Napier, Pascal, Leibniz, and Babbage down to more recent figures like Turing and von Neumann.

Boyer, Carl. *A History of Mathematics*. New York: Wiley, 1967.
A broad history of mathematics that covers some twentieth century developments.

Kline, Morris. *Mathematical Thought from Ancient to Modern Times*. New York: Oxford University Press, 1972.
A detailed history of mathematics covering a broad range of topics, some twentieth century, but favoring slightly analysis and applied mathematics.

Metropolis, N., J. Howlett, and G.-C. Rota. *A History of Computing in the Twentieth Century*. New York: Academic Press, 1980.
A collection of essays on the history of various aspects of computing by people who were, in many cases, part of that history: Richard W. Hamming, Donald E. Knuth, D. H. Lehmer, Edsger W. Dijkstra, among many others.

ANSWERS FOR ODD-NUMBERED PROBLEMS

1. $\{0000, 0001, 0010, 0011, 0100, 0101, 0110, 0111, 1000, 1001, 1010, 1011, 1100, 1101, 1110, 1111\}$.

3. (a) 2; (b) 4; (c) 3; (d) 4.

5. (i) $\{001, 010, 100\}$; (ii) $\{0001, 0010, 0100, 1000\}$; (iii) $\binom{2}{1} = 2, \binom{2}{0} = 1, \binom{3}{1} = 3, \binom{3}{0} = 1, \binom{4}{1} = 4$.

7. (i) $\{0011, 0101, 0110, 1001, 1010, 1100\}$; (ii) $\binom{3}{2} = 3, \binom{3}{1} = 3, \binom{4}{2} = 6$.

9. $\binom{8}{3} = \binom{7}{3} + \binom{7}{2} = 35 + 21 = 56$. 11. (a) 1; (b) 1. 13. The only string in $\boldsymbol{B}_{n,0}$ is $00 \ldots 0$.

15. Yes; $a_1 a_2 \ldots a_n$ is in $\boldsymbol{B}_{n,1}$ if just one of the a_i is 1. There are n possible positions in which to place the single 1.

17. This follows from the formula $\binom{n}{k} = \binom{n-1}{k} + \binom{n-1}{k-1}$ of Theorem 2(b) and the formula $\binom{n}{1} = n$ of Problem 15.

19. This is the end result of the techniques of Problem 17 and the symmetry formula of Theorem 2(c).

1. (i) $\{4, 8\}$; (ii) yes; (iii) 00110; (iv) 5. 3. Yes.

5.

A	$\varnothing$	$\{s_3\}$	$\{s_2\}$	$\{s_2, s_3\}$	$\{s_1\}$	$\{s_1, s_3\}$	$\{s_1, s_2\}$	S
$\bar{A}$	S	$\{s_1, s_2\}$	$\{s_1, s_3\}$	$\{s_1\}$	$\{s_2, s_3\}$	$\{s_2\}$	$\{s_3\}$	$\varnothing$

7. (i) $\{1, 2, 3, 5, 7, 9\}$; (ii) $\{3, 5, 7\}$; (iii) yes.

9.

$\cap$	$\varnothing$	$\{s_2\}$	$\{s_1\}$	S
$\varnothing$	$\varnothing$	$\varnothing$	$\varnothing$	$\varnothing$
$\{s_2\}$	$\varnothing$	$\{s_2\}$	$\varnothing$	$\{s_2\}$
$\{s_1\}$	$\varnothing$	$\varnothing$	$\{s_1\}$	$\{s_1\}$
S	$\varnothing$	$\{s_2\}$	$\{s_1\}$	S

11. (i)

$\cap$	$\varnothing$	$\{s_3\}$	$\{s_2\}$	$\{s_2, s_3\}$	$\{s_1\}$	$\{s_1, s_3\}$	$\{s_1, s_2\}$	S
$\varnothing$	$\varnothing$	$\varnothing$	$\varnothing$	$\varnothing$	$\varnothing$	$\varnothing$	$\varnothing$	$\varnothing$
$\{s_3\}$	$\varnothing$	$\{s_3\}$	$\varnothing$	$\{s_3\}$	$\varnothing$	$\{s_3\}$	$\varnothing$	$\{s_3\}$
$\{s_2\}$	$\varnothing$	$\varnothing$	$\{s_2\}$	$\{s_2\}$	$\varnothing$	$\varnothing$	$\{s_2\}$	$\{s_2\}$
$\{s_2, s_3\}$	$\varnothing$	$\{s_3\}$	$\{s_2\}$	$\{s_2, s_3\}$	$\varnothing$	$\{s_3\}$	$\{s_2\}$	$\{s_2, s_3\}$
$\{s_1\}$	$\varnothing$	$\varnothing$	$\varnothing$	$\varnothing$	$\{s_1\}$	$\{s_1\}$	$\{s_1\}$	$\{s_1\}$
$\{s_1, s_3\}$	$\varnothing$	$\{s_3\}$	$\varnothing$	$\{s_3\}$	$\{s_1\}$	$\{s_1, s_3\}$	$\{s_1\}$	$\{s_1, s_3\}$
$\{s_1, s_2\}$	$\varnothing$	$\varnothing$	$\{s_2\}$	$\{s_2\}$	$\{s_1\}$	$\{s_1\}$	$\{s_1, s_2\}$	$\{s_1, s_2\}$
S	$\varnothing$	$\{s_3\}$	$\{s_2\}$	$\{s_2, s_3\}$	$\{s_1\}$	$\{s_1, s_3\}$	$\{s_1, s_2\}$	S

(ii) Yes; $E = S$.

13. (i)

$\cap$	000	001	010	011	100	101	110	111
000	000	000	000	000	000	000	000	000
001	000	001	000	001	000	001	000	001
010	000	000	010	010	000	000	010	010
011	000	001	010	011	000	001	010	011
100	000	000	000	000	100	100	100	100
101	000	001	000	001	100	101	100	101
110	000	000	010	010	100	100	110	110
111	000	001	010	011	100	101	110	111

(ii) $\sigma = 111$.

15. $S_{00101} \cap S_{01100} = \{s_3, s_5\} \cap \{s_2, s_3\} = \{s_3\} = S_{00100}; \alpha = 00100.$
$S_{00101} \cup S_{01100} = \{s_3, s_5\} \cup \{s_2, s_3\} = \{s_2, s_3, s_5\} = S_{01101}; \beta = 01101.$
$\overline{S_{00101}} = \overline{\{s_3, s_5\}} = \{s_1, s_2, s_4\} = S_{11010}; \gamma = 11010.$

17. $c_i = 0$ if $a_i = 0 = b_i$; otherwise, $c_i = 1$.
$d_i = 1$ if $a_i = 1 = b_i$; otherwise, $d_i = 0$.

19. (i) $\#A + \#B$ counts the number of elements in $A \cup B$, except that it counts the elements of $A \cap B$ twice.
One has to subtract $\#(A \cap B)$ to correct this overcount.
(ii) Using Part (i), one sees that $\#(A \cup B) = \#A + \#B$ if and only if $\#(A \cap B) = 0$. But $\#(A \cap B) = 0$
if and only if $A \cap B = \varnothing$, that is, if and only if A and B are disjoint.
(iii) This follows from Part (i) and the fact that $\#(A \cap B) \geq 0$.

21, 23, 25, & 27. "Yes" for each part.   **29.** $\#S = 1$.   **31.** (a) Yes.   (b) Yes.

33. (i) $a + b - u$, using Problem 19(i).
(ii) 2^{a+b-u}; C must be a subset of $A \cap B$, by Problem 31(b), and the number of subsets of $A \cap B$ is 2^{a+b-u},
by Theorem 2.

SECTION 1.3

1. $\varnothing \cup \varnothing = \varnothing.$ **3.**

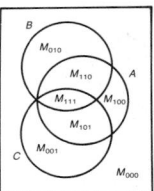

5.

A	B	$A \cup B$	$A \cap (A \cup B)$
0	0	0	0
0	1	1	0
1	0	1	1
1	1	1	1

7.

A	B	$A \cap B$	$\bar{A}$	$\bar{B}$	$\overline{A \cap B}$	$\bar{A} \cup \bar{B}$
0	0	0	1	1	1	1
0	1	0	1	0	1	1
1	0	0	0	1	1	1
1	1	1	0	0	0	0

9. (a) $M_{010} \cup M_{011} \cup M_{110} \cup M_{111};$ (b) $M_{010} \cup M_{011};$
(c) $M_{001} \cup M_{010} \cup M_{011} \cup M_{101} \cup M_{110} \cup M_{111}.$

11. (i) If $M_{100} = \varnothing = M_{101}$, then $A = M_{110} \cup M_{111} \subseteq M_{010} \cup M_{011} \cup M_{110} \cup M_{111} = B$, i.e., $A \subseteq B$.
(ii) $A \subseteq B$ means that $M_{100} \cup M_{101} \cup M_{110} \cup M_{111} \subseteq M_{010} \cup M_{011} \cup M_{110} \cup M_{111}$. Since the minisets are disjoint, this implies that $M_{100} = \varnothing = M_{101}$. (See the Venn Diagram of Figure 1.3.2.)

13. (a) Property (8);   (b) Property (6).   **15.** All true.

17. No. Since $A \neq \varnothing$, there is some a in A. Since $A \cap B = \varnothing$, a is not in B. Hence $A \neq B$.

19. One example is $A = \{1, 2\}$, $B = \{1\} = C$.

SECTION 1.4

1. (a) Pair.   (b) Ordered triple.   (c) Ordered pair.   (d) Triple.   **3.** (a) Yes.   (b) No.

5. (i) $\{(1, 1), (1, 2), (1, 3), (2, 1), (2, 2), (2, 3)\}.$ (ii) $\{(1, 1), (2, 1), (3, 1), (1, 2), (2, 2), (3, 2)\}.$
(iii) $(1, 1), (1, 2), (2, 1), (2, 2).$ (iv) Yes, $(1, 3)$ and $(2, 3)$.   (v) No.

7. (a) $\bar{R} = \{(1, 1), (1, 3), (2, 1), (2, 2), (3, 2), (3, 3)\}.$ (b) $V = \{(2, 1), (3, 2), (1, 3)\}.$

(c)

R	1	2	3	$\bar{R}$	1	2	3	V	1	2	3
1	0	1	0	1	1	0	1	1	0	0	1
2	0	0	1	2	1	1	0	2	1	0	0
3	1	0	0	3	0	1	1	3	0	1	0

9. (a) $00\bar{R}01, 00\bar{R}10, 01\bar{R}00, 01\bar{R}01, 01\bar{R}10, 01\bar{R}11, 10\bar{R}00, 10\bar{R}01, 10\bar{R}10, 10\bar{R}11, 11\bar{R}01, 11\bar{R}10.$
(b) $V = \{(00, 00), (11, 00), (00, 11), (11, 11)\} = R.$

11. (i) Interchange 0's and 1's. [See answer to Problem 7(c).]
(ii) No. The matrix changes when 0's and 1's are interchanged.

13. (a) <;   (b) ≥.   **15.** ⊂.

17. $(0, 0, 0)$, $(1, 0, 1)$, $(1, 1, 0)$, $(2, 1, 1)$, $(3, 0, 3)$, $(3, 3, 0)$, $(4, 1, 3)$, $(4, 3, 1)$, $(6, 3, 3)$.

19. $(3, 4, 5)$, $(4, 3, 5)$, $(6, 8, 10)$, $(8, 6, 10)$, $(5, 12, 13)$, $(12, 5, 13)$, $(9, 12, 15)$, $(12, 9, 15)$, $(8, 15, 17)$, $(15, 8, 17)$, $(12, 16, 20)$, $(16, 12, 20)$.

21. (i) $\{(0, a), (0, b), (0, c), (1, a), (1, b), (1, c)\}$.   (ii) $\{(0, d), (0, e), (1, d), (1, e)\}$.
(iii) $\{(0, a), (0, b), (0, c), (0, d), (0, e), (1, a), (1, b), (1, c), (1, d), (1, e)\}$.   (iv) $\{a, b, c, d, e\}$.
(v) Same as answer to Part (iii).

23. (i) 5;   (ii) 5;   (iii) $5 + 5 + 5 = 3 \cdot 5 = 15$;   (iv) 2^{15}.

25. (i) $4 \cdot 8 = 32$;   (ii) 32;   (iii) 32;   (iv) $3 \cdot 32 = 96$;   (v) 2^{96}.

27. Yes. Let $\# S = s$ and $\# T = t$. Then $\#(S \times T) = st = ts = \#(T \times S)$.

29. $r_1 \cdot r_2 \cdots r_n$.   **31.** $13 \cdot 5 \cdot 7 = 455$.

SECTION 1.5

1. (a) (S_{00}, S_{01}), (S_{00}, S_{10}), (S_{00}, S_{11}), (S_{01}, S_{11}), (S_{10}, S_{11}).
(b) See table in Example 6 of Section 1.4.
(c)   (d) Add a loop at each vertex.

3. (a) $(1, 1, 1, 1)$, $(1, 1, 1, 2)$, $(1, 1, 2, 3)$, $(1, 2, 3, 3)$, $(1, 2, 3, 4)$.
(b) $(1, 1, 1, 1)$, $(4, 1, 1, 1)$, $(3, 4, 1, 1)$, $(3, 3, 4, 1)$, $(2, 3, 4, 1)$.   (c) $(2, 3, 3, 4)$.

5. R is not reflexive, since $2\bar{R}2$. R is not symmetric, since $1R2$ but $2\bar{R}1$. R is not transitive, since $1R2$ and $2R3$ but $1\bar{R}3$.

7. (a)   (b) Yes. No. Yes. Yes. Yes.

9. $\leq$ is reflexive, antisymmetric, and transitive but neither irreflexive nor symmetric.

11. (a) If there is an arc from vertex v to vertex w, then there must also be an arc from w to v.
(b) If $v \neq w$, then there cannot be arcs both from v to w and from w to v.

13. (a) R is reflexive if all the entries on the main diagonal are 1's.
(b) R is irreflexive if all the entries on the main diagonal are 0's.

15. (a) No. If R is reflexive, then (s, s) is in R for all s in S. If R is irreflexive, then there is no (s, s) in R.
(b) Yes. See Example 1 of this section.

17. Reverse all arrowheads.   **19.** D is its own reverse.   **21.** $V = R$.

23. $R \cap D = \varnothing$.   **25.** Yes, since $V = R$ by Problem 21.

27. Yes. If aRb and bRc, then (a, b, c) is a path in R. Also, we are given that such a path implies that aRc. Hence R is transitive.

29. (a)   (b) A is symmetric but neither reflexive nor transitive.

31. (a) $\{(1, 2), (2, 3), (1, 3)\}$.   (b) S^2.   (c) $T = R = \{(1, 2)\}$.

33. (a) $\{(1, 2), (2, 1), (2, 3), (3, 2)\}$.   (b) $\{(1, 2), (2, 1), (2, 3), (3, 2), (3, 1), (1, 3)\}$.   (c) $\{(1, 2), (2, 1)\}$.

35. $2^{(n^2)}$.   **37.** They are the same.

SECTION 1.6

1. (i) 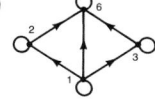   (ii) Yes.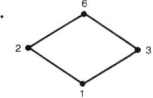

(iii) No, 2 and 3 are noncomparable.   (iv) No, since it is not linearly ordered.

3. Yes, since $P(S) = \{\varnothing, S\}$ and the following table shows that every nonempty subcollection of $P(S)$ has a least element under $\subseteq$.

subcollection X	$\{\varnothing\}$	$\{S\}$	$\{\varnothing, S\}$
least element of X	$\varnothing$	S	$\varnothing$

5. Yes, because $\leq$ represents a partial ordering and so is reflexive.
7. (i) $\Gamma = \{\varnothing, A, B, C, E\}$.   (ii) $\Delta = \{\varnothing, B, C, D, F\}$.   (iii) $\Gamma \cap \Delta = \{\varnothing, B, C\}$.   (iv) No.
(v) B and C.   (vi) No, since A and B (for example) are not comparable. No, since it is not a linear ordering.
9. Yes. $A \cap B$ is the greatest member of Γ.
13. (i) $V = (1, 1), (2, 1), (3, 1), (6, 1), (2, 2), (6, 2), (3, 3), (6, 3), (6, 6)$.
(ii) Yes. The diagram is that of Problem 1(ii) turned upside down.
15. Yes. $\subseteq$ is a reflexive, antisymmetric, and transitive binary relation on any $X \subseteq P(S)$.
17. (i) Yes. $\leq$ is a reflexive, antisymmetric, and transitive binary relation on N.
(ii) Yes. $\geq$ is reflexive, antisymmetric, and transitive.   (iii) Yes, 0.   No.   (iv) No.   (v) Yes, 0.
19. (i) Yes.   (ii) $\varnothing$ is the least and S is the greatest.   (iii) S is the least and $\varnothing$ is the greatest.
21. g is the least and m is the greatest.
23. No. The subset N of N has no least with respect to $\geq$.
25. Let W be the binary relation on E for which aWb means that either $a = b$ or a appears to the left of b in the listing $E = \{0, 2, -2, 4, -4, 6, -6, \dots\}$.
27. A greatest element g of S would have $m \leq g$ and $m' \leq g$. Since m and m' are maximal, we cannot have $m \prec g$ nor $m' \prec g$. Hence we would have $m = g = m'$. This would give us $m = m'$ and contradict the hypothesis that m and m' are distinct. So, no such g exists.
29. 6. The ordered quadruples are columns of the following table:

A	$\{1\}$	$\{2\}$	$\{1\}$	$\{3\}$	$\{2\}$	$\{3\}$
B	$\{2\}$	$\{1\}$	$\{3\}$	$\{1\}$	$\{3\}$	$\{2\}$
C	$\{1, 2\}$	$\{1, 2\}$	$\{1, 3\}$	$\{1, 3\}$	$\{2, 3\}$	$\{2, 3\}$
D	$\{2, 3\}$	$\{1, 3\}$	$\{2, 3\}$	$\{1, 2\}$	$\{1, 3\}$	$\{1, 2\}$

SECTION 1.7

1. (a) Not a partition, since the element 6 of X is not in $A \cup B \cup C$.
(b) Not a partition, since $B \cap C = \{5\} \neq \varnothing$.
(c) A partition, since $A \cap B = A \cap C = B \cap C = \varnothing$ and $A \cup B \cup C = X$.

3. (a) It is reflexive, symmetric, and transitive (RST) and so is an equivalence relation.
   (b) It is not transitive and so is not an equivalence relation.
   (c) It is not reflexive and so is not an equivalence relation.
   (d) It is not symmetric and so is not an equivalence relation.

5. (i) Yes.   (ii) $B_1, B_2, B_3, \ldots$ (iii) The rank is infinite.

7. (i) Eight; they are 7, 13, 19, 31, 37, 43, 61, and 67.   (ii) One, only the prime 2.
   (iii) One, only the prime 3.   (iv) Ten; they are 5, 11, 17, 23, 29, 41, 47, 53, 59, and 71.
   (v) No.   (vi) $8 + 1 + 1 + 10 + 0 = 20$.

9. (i) Yes.   (ii) Yes.   (iii) Yes.

11. Yes, σ is reflexive, symmetric, and transitive.

13. No. This relation is not reflexive (and is not transitive).

15. (a) No, $3Z$ is not a subset of $2Z$ or of $1 + 2Z$.
   (b) Yes. Each member of Γ' is a subset of some member of Γ.

17. (i) Yes; $0 = n \cdot 0 \in nZ$.   (ii) Yes.   (iii) Yes; $0 = 0 \cdot n$.   (iv) $0Z = \{0\}$.   (v) 0.
   (vi) Yes; $n = n \cdot 1$.   (vii) Yes; $n = 1 \cdot n$.   (viii) No, 2 is in $2Z$ but not in $6Z$.

19. (a) $1, -1, 7, -7$.   (b) $1, -1, 5, -5, 25, -25$.   (c) $1, -1, 5, -5, 7, -7, 35, -35$.
   (d) Same as in Part (c).   (e) 1, 2, 5, 7, 10, 14, 35, 70.

21. (i) $\{-3, 3\}, \{-2, 2\}, \{-1, 1\}, \{0\}$.   (ii) $2 + 2 + 2 + 1 = 7$.   (iii) 4.

23. (1, 1), (1, 2), (2, 1), (2, 2), (3, 3), (3, 4), (4, 3), (4, 4), (5, 5).   **25.** $n_1^2 + n_2^2 + n_3^2 + n_4^2$.

27. (i) If $n \in 3Z$, then $n = 3k$, with $k \in Z$, and $n^2 = 3(3k^2) \in 3Z$.
   (ii) If $n \in 1 + 3Z$, then $n = 1 + 3k$, with $k \in Z$, and $n^2 = 1 + 3(2k + 3k^2) \in 1 + 3Z$.
      If $n \in 2 + 3Z$, then $n = 2 + 3k$, with $k \in Z$, and $n^2 = 1 + 3(1 + 4k + 3k^2) \in 1 + 3Z$.
   (iii) This follows from (i) and (ii), since n^2 is in $3Z$ or $1 + 3Z$.

29. (i) Since E is reflexive, xEx and hence $x \in C(x)$ for all x in X.
   (ii) Let $c \in C(a)$ and $c \in C(b)$. Then aEc and bEc by definition of $C(a)$ and $C(b)$. Since E is symmetric, we have cEb. Since aEc, cEb, and E is transitive, then aEb, and so $b \in C(a)$.
   (iii) Let $b \in C(a)$ and $x \in C(b)$. Then aEb and bEx by definition of the equivalence classes. Since E is transitive, these imply that aEx, and so $x \in C(a)$.
   (iv) Let $C(a) \cap C(b) \neq \varnothing$; i.e., let $c \in C(a) \cap C(b)$ for some c in X. Then $c \in C(a)$ and $c \in C(b)$. Now it follows from Part (ii) that $b \in C(a)$. This and Part (iii) tell us that for every $x \in C(b)$ we have $x \in C(a)$. Hence $C(b) \subseteq C(a)$. Similarly, $C(a) \subseteq C(b)$. Since $\subseteq$ is antisymmetric, these imply that $C(a) = C(b)$.
   (v) It follows from Part (iv) that distinct classes $C(a)$ and $C(b)$ are disjoint and from Part (i) that X is the union of all the equivalence classes. This means that the collection of the distinct classes $C(a)$ is a partition of X.

31. (a) Yes. Let $d \mid m$. Then $m = cd$, with c in Z. Thus $-m = (-c)d$, with $-c$ in Z, and so $d \mid (-m)$.
   (b) Yes.   (c) $bZ \subseteq aZ$.

33. The relation $\mid$ on P is reflexive by Problem 17(vii), it is transitive by Problem 18(vi), and it is antisymmetric by Problem 32(b).

35. (a)   (b)   (c)

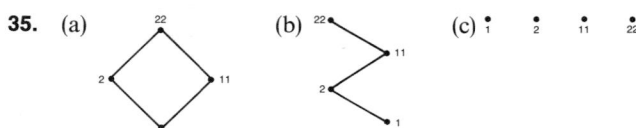

37. (a)   (b)

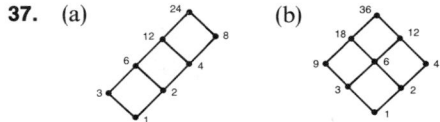

39. (i) $A = \{4, 24, 36, 72\}$.　　(ii) $B = \{6, 24, 36, 72\}$.　　(iii) $I = \{24, 36, 72\}$.　　(iv) 24 and 36.　　(v) No.

41. (i) $\{2, 4, 6, 24\}$.　　(ii) $\{2, 4, 6, 36\}$.　　(iii) $\{2, 4, 6\}$.　　(iv) $\{4, 6\}$.　　(v) No.

43. (i)

(ii) $A = \{1, 2, 5, 10\}$, $B = \{1, 3, 5, 15\}$, $I = \{1, 5\}$.　　(iii) Yes; $g = 5$.

(iv) Just the number 5.

45. (i) $D = \{1, 2, 11, 22\}$.　　(ii) Yes; $g = 22$.　　(iii) Yes; 22.

47. Yes. One obtains Γ' by splitting some or all of the S_i into several subsets. Thus Γ' has more members than Γ has.

SECTION 1.8

1. Surjective: (a), (c), (e), (f). Injective: (b), (c), (f), (g). Bijective: (c), (f).

3. (i) $3^2 = 9$.

(ii) $1 \mapsto a, 2 \mapsto b$;　　$1 \mapsto a, 2 \mapsto c$;　　$1 \mapsto b, 2 \mapsto a$;　　$1 \mapsto b, 2 \mapsto c$;　　$1 \mapsto c, 2 \mapsto a$;　　$1 \mapsto c, 2 \mapsto b$.

(iii) $1 \mapsto a, 2 \mapsto a$;　　$1 \mapsto b, 2 \mapsto b$;　　$1 \mapsto c, 2 \mapsto c$.

5. (i) $3^3 = 27$.　　(ii) $3 \cdot 2 \cdot 1 = 6$.

(iii) $1 \mapsto a, 2 \mapsto b, 3 \mapsto c$;　　$1 \mapsto a, 2 \mapsto c, 3 \mapsto b$;　　$1 \mapsto c, 2 \mapsto b, 3 \mapsto a$;　　$1 \mapsto b, 2 \mapsto a, 3 \mapsto c$;

$1 \mapsto b, 2 \mapsto c, 3 \mapsto a$;　　$1 \mapsto c, 2 \mapsto a, 3 \mapsto b$.

(iv) Yes.　　(v) Yes.

7. (a) $\{0, 1\}$.　　(b) $\{2n, 2n + 1\}$.　　(c) Yes.　　(d) No.　　(e) No.

9. (i) The f of Problem 7.　　(ii) No, as one sees in Problem 7.

11. (a) $a \mapsto 1, b \mapsto 0, c \mapsto 0, d \mapsto 1, e \mapsto 1$.　　(b) $s_1 \mapsto 1, s_2 \mapsto 0, s_3 \mapsto 0, s_4 \mapsto 1, s_5 \mapsto 1$.

13. (i) $\{1\}$.　　(ii) $\{2\}$.　　(iii) $\varnothing$.

15. Yes. If $f^{-1}(y)$ has at least one element x for each y in Y, then $f(x) = y$ shows that each y in Y is an image under f. Thus f is surjective.

17. No, since $(0, 1)$ is in N^2 but $f(0, 1) = 0 - 1 = -1$ is not in N.

19. (a) 20^6.　　(b) $20 \cdot 19 \cdot 18 \cdot 17 \cdot 16 \cdot 15$.　　**21.** n^m.

23. Yes. This rule assigns to each element a in A a unique element c in C.

25. (a) For each b in B, let $g(b)$ be the unique element a of A such that $f(a) = b$. Then $g(f(a)) = g(b) = a$ for all a in A.

(b) Yes.

27. (i) $12 \cdot 11 \cdot 10 \cdot 9 \cdot 8$.　　(ii) 12^5.　　(iii) $\dfrac{12 \cdot 11 \cdot 10 \cdot 9 \cdot 8}{12^5} = \dfrac{55}{144}$.

29. (i)

α	000	001	010	011	100	101	110	111
$f(\alpha)$	0	1	2	3	4	5	6	7

(ii) Yes.

(iii) $\{0, 1, 2, 3, 4, 5, 6, 7\}$.

31. (a) Whenever (a, b) and (c, b) are in R, one must have $a = c$.

(b) For every b in Y there must be at least one a in X with $(a, b) \in R$.

33. Since $\# B_3 = 8$ and a listing for B_3 is characterized by a bijection from $\{1, 2, \ldots, 8\}$ onto B_3, it follows from Theorem 6 that B_3 has $8 \cdot 7 \cdot 6 \cdot 5 \cdot 4 \cdot 3 \cdot 2 \cdot 1 = 5040$ listings.

35. $n = 5$, since $\# B_1 + \# B_2 + \# B_3 + \# B_4 = 2 + 4 + 8 + 16 = 30$ and

$\# B_1 + \# B_2 + \# B_3 + \# B_4 + \# B_5 = 2 + 4 + 8 + 16 + 32 = 62$.

REVIEW PROBLEMS FOR CHAPTER 1

1. (a) False; $\# B_4 = 16 \neq 8 = 2 \cdot 4 = 2(\# B_2)$.   (b) True; $\# B_8 = 2^8 = (2^4)^2 = (\# B_4)^2$.
   (c) False; if $\alpha \in B_{5,4}$ then wgt $\alpha = 4$.   (d) False; if $\alpha \in B_{4,4}$ then wgt $\bar{\alpha} = 4 - 4 = 0$.
   (e) False; $B_{5,3}$ has 5-digit strings, whereas $B_{4,3}$ and $B_{4,2}$ have 4-digit strings.
   (f) True; this follows from Theorem 2(b) of Section 1.1.

3. (a) $\varnothing$;   (b) $\{1, 2, 3\}$;   (c) $\{1, 2, 3, 4, 5, 6, 7, 8\}$.

5. (i) 2048;   (ii) 330;   (iii) 330;   (iv) 330;   (v) 330;   (vi) 1;   (vii) 1.

7. $\binom{15}{4} = 1820 - 455 = 1365 = \binom{15}{11}$.

9. (a) Yes.   (b) No. A counterexample is $A = \{1\}$, $B = \{2\}$, and $C = \{3\}$.

11. Yes.

13.

ABC	$\bar{A}$	$\bar{B}$	$\bar{C}$	$A \cup B \cup C$	$\overline{A \cup B} \cup C$	$\bar{A} \cap \bar{B} \cap \bar{C}$
000	1	1	1	0	1	1
001	1	1	0	1	0	0
010	1	0	1	1	0	0
011	1	0	0	1	0	0
100	0	1	1	1	0	0
101	0	1	0	1	0	0
110	0	0	1	1	0	0
111	0	0	0	1	0	0

15. M_{1000}, M_{1010}, M_{1100}, and M_{1110}.

17. (a) No. For a counterexample, let $A = \{1\}$ and $B = \{2\}$. Then $A \times B = \{(1, 2)\} \neq \{(2, 1)\} = B \times A$.
   (b) Yes. $A \times \varnothing = A$ if $A = \varnothing$.

19. (a) m^2;   (b) 2^{m^2}.   **21.** $R = \{(0, 4), (1, 3), (2, 2), (3, 1), (4, 0)\}$.   (a) No.   (b) Yes.   (c) No.

23. (i) 100.   (ii) 100.

25. (i) $(1, 1)$, $(1, 2)$, $(1, 3)$, $(1, 4)$, $(2, 2)$, $(2, 4)$, $(3, 3)$, $(4, 4)$.   (ii) 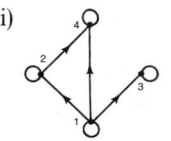   (iii)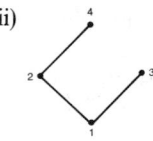

27. (a) and (b) are partitions; (c) is not, since $2\mathbf{Z}$ and $3\mathbf{Z}$ are not disjoint.

29. (a), (d), (e), and (f).   **31.** (a) Yes.   (b) No.   (c) No.   (d) No.

33. Yes; see Theorem 3(vii) of Section 1.8 and Theorem 1 of Section 1.1.

35. $4^3 = 64$.   (b) $4 \cdot 3 \cdot 2 = 24$.   (c) None.   (d) 15^4.

37. (a) No; $3^1 \cdot 3 = 9 \neq 27 = 3^3 \cdot 1$.   (b) Yes; for every n in $\mathbf{N}$, $f(0, n) = 3^0 n = n$.
   (c) $\{(0, 18), (1, 6), (2, 2)\}$.   (d) No; see (c).

39. (i) $\leftrightarrow$ (b),   (ii) $\leftrightarrow$ (a),   (iii) $\leftrightarrow$ (c).

SECTION 2.1

1. (a) Yes. See Property (6) in Section 1.3.   (b) Yes. See Property (5) in Section 1.3.
   (c) $\varnothing$.   (d) No. Only $\varnothing$ has an inverse (itself) under $\cup$.

3.

x	y	z	$x \triangle y$	$y \triangle z$	$x \triangle (y \triangle z)$	$(x \triangle y) \triangle z$
0	1	0	0	0	0	0
0	1	1	0	1	0	0
1	0	0	0	0	0	0
1	0	1	0	0	0	0
1	1	0	1	0	0	0
1	1	1	1	1	1	1

5. (i)

max	0	1	2
0	0	1	2
1	1	1	2
2	2	2	2

(ii) Yes. Yes.   (iii) 0.
(iv) No. For example, 1 has no inverse because $\max(1, t) \neq 0$ for all t in T.

7. (i)

$\vee$	000	001	010	011	100	101	110	111
000	000	001	010	011	100	101	110	111
001	001	001	011	011	101	101	111	111
010	010	011	010	011	110	111	110	111
011	011	011	011	011	111	111	111	111
100	100	101	110	111	100	101	110	111
101	101	101	111	111	101	101	111	111
110	110	111	110	111	110	111	110	111
111	111	111	111	111	111	111	111	111

(ii) 000.   (iii) Yes.
(iv) Yes. This follows from Problem 4 and the definition of $\vee$ in terms of max.

9. (a) All elements of X.   (b) $\# X = 1$.   (c) $\# X = 1$.
(d) $(x \triangle y) \triangle z = y \triangle z = z$ and $x \triangle (y \triangle z) = x \triangle z = z$, and so $(x \triangle y) \triangle z = x \triangle (y \triangle z)$ for all x, y, z in X.

11. (a) $x \triangle y = x + y + 1 = y + x + 1 = y \triangle x$ for all x and y in N because $+$ is a commutative operation on N.
(b) $(x \triangle y) \triangle z = (x + y + 1) \triangle z = x + y + 1 + z + 1 = x + y + z + 2$ and
$x \triangle (y \triangle z) = x \triangle (y + z + 1) = x + y + z + 1 + 1 = x + y + z + 2$.
Thus $(x \triangle y) \triangle z = x \triangle (y \triangle z)$ for all x, y, z in N.

13. (i) Yes.   (ii) No, $0 - 3$ is not in the subset.   (iii) No.
15. No; $0 - 1 \neq 1 - 0$.   No; $-3 = (0 - 1) - 2 \neq 0 - (1 - 2) = 1$.

17. (i)

$\oplus$	S_{00}	S_{01}	S_{10}	S_{11}
S_{00}	S_{00}	S_{01}	S_{10}	S_{11}
S_{01}	S_{01}	S_{00}	S_{11}	S_{10}
S_{10}	S_{10}	S_{11}	S_{00}	S_{01}
S_{11}	S_{11}	S_{10}	S_{01}	S_{00}

(ii) Yes. Yes.
(iii) Yes, as one might see from a Venn Diagram or as one can prove with a case table.

19. (a) 0.   (b) Each of 0 and 1 is its own inverse under $\oplus$.   (c) Yes.

(d) xyz	$x \oplus y$	$y \oplus z$	$(x \oplus y) \oplus z$	$x \oplus (y \oplus z)$
000	0	0	0	0
001	0	1	1	1
010	1	1	1	1
011	1	0	0	0
100	1	0	1	1
101	1	1	0	0
110	0	1	0	0
111	0	0	1	1

$\oplus$ is associative, since the last two columns are the same.

21. Let α, β, and γ be in B_n. Then the ith bit of $(\alpha \oplus \beta) \oplus \gamma$ is the same as the ith bit of $\alpha \oplus (\beta \oplus \gamma)$ since $\oplus$ is defined "bitwise" and Problem 19(d) shows that $\oplus$ is associative for single-bit strings.

23. (a)

$\oplus$	00	01
00	00	01
01	01	00

$\oplus$	00	10
00	00	10
10	10	00

(b) 01 and 10 are in this set, but $01 \oplus 10 = 11$ is not.

25. The concatenation of a and b (in this order) is ab, whereas the concatenation of b and a is ba. Since $a \neq b$, ab and ba are unequal words.

27. (a) Yes.
    (b) Yes. If $\alpha = a_1 a_2 \ldots a_r$, $\beta = b_1 b_2 \ldots b_s$, and $\gamma = c_1 c_2 \ldots c_t$, then each $(\alpha\beta)\gamma$ and $\alpha(\beta\gamma)$ is the word $a_1 a_2 \ldots a_r b_1 b_2 \ldots b_s c_1 c_2 \ldots c_t$.

29. (i) ab, ac, ba, bc, ca, cb.   (ii) aa, bb, cc.

31. (a) 26;   (b) $(26)^2$;   (c) $(26)^3$;   (d) $(26)^m$.

33. (a) Yes. For each word $w = b_1 b_2 \ldots b_m$ let f_w be the mapping
    $f_w: X \to A$; $1 \mapsto b_1$, $2 \mapsto b_2$, $\ldots$, $m \mapsto b_m$. Then $w \leftrightarrow f_w$ is a bijection from
    the set of words of length m over A onto the set A^X of mappings from X to A.
    (b) n^m.

SECTION 2.2

1. (i) Yes.   (ii) Yes, 0 is the identity.   (iii) Yes.   **3.** Yes.

5. No. T is not closed under $+$; for example, $1 + 1$ is not in T.

7. (i) Yes, since 01 is the identity under $\square$.
    (ii) No. The closest thing to an identity is 76, but $76 \square 06 \neq 06$.
    (iii) One example is $a = 56$, $b = 06 = c$.

9. (a) $\{(3, 5)\}$;   (b) $\varnothing$;   (c) $\varnothing$;   (d) $\{\varnothing, B\}$.

11. (a) Yes; $\cap$ is an associative operation with S as the identity.
    (b) Yes; $\cup$ is an associative operation with $\varnothing$ as the identity.

13.

$\oplus$	000	001	010	011	100	101	110	111
000	000	001	010	011	100	101	110	111
001	001	000	011	010	101	100	111	110
010	010	011	000	001	110	111	100	101
011	011	010	001	000	111	110	101	100
100	100	101	110	111	000	001	010	011
101	101	100	111	110	001	000	011	010
110	110	111	100	101	010	011	000	001
111	111	110	101	100	011	010	001	000

15. (a) Yes. (b) No. (c) Yes. **17.** (a) $2g$. (b) $3g$. (c) ng.

19. Let $(s, t) \in R$. Then $(s, s) \in D$. Now, sDs, sRt, and the definition of multiplication of relations give us $s(DR)t$. Hence (s, t) is in DR whenever (s, t) is in R and $R \subseteq DR$. Conversely, let (x, z) be in DR. By definition of multiplication, there is some y in S with xDy and yRz. By definition of D, $x = y$, and so xRz. Hence $DR \subseteq R$. This, $R \subseteq DR$, and antisymmetry of $\subseteq$ imply that $DR = R$.

21. No. $UV = \{(1, 2)\}$ and $VU = \varnothing$.

23. Yes. If S is finite, so is $P(S^2)$, and thus each power of R is one of the relations in the finite set $P(S^2)$.

25. Assume that there is such a T. Then $1D1$ and $D = TR$ would imply $1(TR)1$. This would imply that $1Tx$ and $xR1$ for some x in S. But $x = 1$ is the only x in S with $xR1$. Thus we would have $1T1$. This and $1R2$ would give $1(TR)2$, and so $1D2$. But $(1, 2)$ is not in the diagonal D. This contradiction shows that no such T exists.

27. $R = \{(1, 1), (2, 2)\}$. This R is its own inverse.

29. Every binary relation has a reverse, but there are binary relations, such as the R of Problem 25, that have no inverses.

31. For every a in S, $aRf(a)$ and $f(a)Va$, so $a(RV)a$; i.e., $(a, a) \in RV$. This implies that $D \subseteq RV$. Also, if $cRVe$, then there exists an element d of S with cRd and dVe. Then the rules for R and V tell us that $d = f(c)$ and $d = f(e)$. Since f is injective, $c = e$. Thus $(c, e) = (c, c)$, and so $RV \subseteq D$. This and $D \subseteq RV$ imply that $RV = D$. Similarly, one can use the fact that f is a surjection to show that $VR = D$. Thus V is the inverse of R.

33. Yes. The operation $\triangle$ is associative, because $(x \triangle y) \triangle z = a \triangle z = a$ and $x \triangle (y \triangle z) = x \triangle a = a$.

35. (b) $g: 1 \mapsto 3, \quad 2 \mapsto 1, \quad 3 \mapsto 2.$
(c) $h_1: 1 \mapsto 1, \quad 2 \mapsto 3, \quad 3 \mapsto 2$ or $h_2: 1 \mapsto 3, \quad 2 \mapsto 2, \quad 3 \mapsto 1$ or $h_3: 1 \mapsto 2, \quad 2 \mapsto 1, \quad 3 \mapsto 3.$

SECTION 2.3

1. (a) Let $A = (x \vee y) \wedge (z \vee w)$. Then $A = [x \wedge (z \vee w)] \vee [y \wedge (z \vee w)]$ by distributivity of $\wedge$ over $\vee$. Using this distributivity twice more, $A = (x \wedge z) \vee (x \wedge w) \vee (y \wedge z) \vee (y \wedge w)$.
(b) This follows because it is the dual of Part (a) (or it is shown using the distributivity of $\vee$ over $\wedge$).

3. (i) $x = x \wedge 1$ because Axiom (B1) in Definition 2 tells us that 1 is the identity under $\wedge$. By Axiom (B4), $1 = x \vee \bar{x}$. Then $x \wedge 1 = x \wedge (x \vee \bar{x}) = (x \wedge x) \vee (x \wedge \bar{x})$ by the distributivity of $\wedge$ over $\vee$ in Axiom (B2).
(ii) $x \wedge \bar{x} = 0$ by Axiom (B4), and $(x \wedge x) \vee 0 = x \wedge x$ because 0 is the identity under $\vee$, as one sees in Axiom (B1).
(iii) This follows from (i), (ii), and the transitivity of equality.

5. $x \vee x \vee x = (x \vee x) \vee x$ Associativity for $\vee$
     $= x \vee x$ Idempotent law (Problem 4)
     $= x$ Idempotent law for $\vee$

7.   (i) $a = \bar{a}$ and Problem 3(iii) give us $a = a \wedge \bar{a}$. This implies that $a = 0$, using Axiom (B4). Also, $a = \bar{a}$ and Problem 4 give us $a = a \vee \bar{a}$, which with Axiom (B4) leads to $a = 1$. Hence $a = \bar{a}$ implies $0 = 1$.

(ii) Since $a = \bar{a}$ implies the contradiction to Axiom (B3), $0 = 1$, one has $a \neq \bar{a}$ for all a in X.

(iii) Since the mapping $f: x \mapsto \bar{x}$ is a bijection from X to X by Theorem 3, if $X = \{0, 1, c\}$ one would have $f: 0 \mapsto 1$, $1 \mapsto 0$, $c \mapsto c$, thus contradicting Part (ii).

9. $x \wedge 0 = x \wedge (x \wedge \bar{x})$ by part of Axiom (B4). Also, $x \wedge (x \wedge \bar{x}) = (x \wedge x) \wedge \bar{x}$ by the associativity of $\wedge$. By Problem 3(iii), $x \wedge x = x$. Then by Axiom (B4), $x \wedge \bar{x} = 0$.

11. $x \vee z = x \vee (y \vee z) = (x \vee y) \vee z = y \vee z = z$.

13.   Essentially, Table 2.3.3 results when $\wedge$, 0, 1 in Table 2.3.2 are replaced by $\vee$, 1, 0, respectively.

15.   (i) $x \vee (\bar{x} \wedge y) = (x \vee \bar{x}) \wedge (x \vee y)$ Distributivity of $\vee$ over $\wedge$

$\qquad\qquad\quad\; = 1 \wedge (x \vee y)$ Axiom (B4)

$\qquad\qquad\quad\; = x \vee y$ 1 is the identity for $\wedge$

(ii) We are not given a listing for the carrier X; in fact, X may be infinite. A case table proof could be used in Example 5 because the carrier there was the known $B_1 = \{0, 1\}$.

17. $(a, b, c) = (0, 1, 0)$.   **19.** $f(x, y, z) = x \wedge y \wedge \bar{z}$.

21. $f(x, y, z) = (\bar{x} \wedge y \wedge \bar{z}) \vee (x \wedge y \wedge z)$.   **23.** $f(x, y, z) = (x \wedge y \wedge z) \vee (x \wedge y \wedge \bar{z}) \vee (x \wedge \bar{y} \wedge \bar{z})$.

25.   (a) An n-tuple $(x_1, \ldots, x_n)$ of B_1^n is in $f^{-1}(1)$ if and only if $f(x_1, \ldots, x_n) = h(x_1, \ldots, x_n) \vee k(x_1, \ldots, x_n) = 1$. Since $h(x_1, \ldots, x_n)$ and $k(x_1, \ldots, x_n)$ are in $\{0, 1\}$, one can use Table 2.3.3 to confirm that $f = h \vee k = 1$ if and only if at least one of h and k is 1. Thus $f^{-1}(1) = h^{-1}(1) \cup k^{-1}(1)$.

(b) Similarly, one can use Table 2.3.2 to confirm that $g^{-1}(1) = h^{-1}(1) \cap k^{-1}(1)$.

27.   (i) Let $k(x, y, z, w) = x$. Then $g = k \wedge h = h \wedge k$ and Problem 25(b) tell us that $g^{-1}(1) = h^{-1}(1) \cap k^{-1}(1)$. Hence $g^{-1}(1) \subseteq h^{-1}(1)$.

(ii) $\{(1, 1, 0, 1), (1, 0, 0, 1)\}$.   (iii) $(0, 1, 0, 1)$, $(0, 0, 0, 1)$.

29.

x	y	$x \Rightarrow y$	$x \wedge (x \Rightarrow y)$	$[x \wedge (x \Rightarrow y)] \Rightarrow y$
0	0	1	0	1
0	1	1	0	1
1	0	0	0	1
1	1	1	1	1

31.

x	y	$\bar{x}$	$\bar{y}$	$x \vee \bar{x}$	$y \wedge \bar{y}$	$(x \vee \bar{x}) \Rightarrow (y \wedge \bar{y})$
0	0	1	1	1	0	0
0	1	1	0	1	0	0
1	0	0	1	1	0	0
1	1	0	0	1	0	0

33.   The following two lines of a case table suffice:

x	y	$x \Rightarrow y$	$y \Rightarrow x$	$(x \Rightarrow y) \Rightarrow (y \Rightarrow x)$
0	0	1	1	1
0	1	1	0	0

35.   (a) and (e) are tautologies, (c) is a contradiction, and (b) and (d) are contingencies.

37. Yes; $f(x_1, \ldots, x_n) \Rightarrow g(x_1, \ldots, x_n)$ is a tautology if there is no n-tuple $(a_1, \ldots, a_n)$ in $\mathbf{B}_1^n$ with $f(a_1, \ldots, a_n) = 1$ and $g(a_1, \ldots, a_n) = 0$. There is no such n-tuple, since $f^{-1}(1) \subseteq g^{-1}(1)$.

39. Yes. Let $f^{-1}(0) = A = g^{-1}(0)$. Then $f(s) = 0 = g(s)$ for s in A, and $f(s) = 1 = g(s)$ for an element s of S not in A. Hence f and g are equal mappings. (This uses the fact that the codomain $\{0, 1\}$ has two elements.)

41. Yes; each is $2^{\#S}$.

SECTION 2.4

1. $(x + y) \cdot (z + w) = x \cdot z + x \cdot w + y \cdot z + y \cdot w$.

3. (i) $x \cdot y \cdot z \cdot w + x \cdot y \cdot \bar{z} \cdot \bar{w} + \bar{x} \cdot \bar{y} \cdot z \cdot w + \bar{x} \cdot \bar{y} \cdot \bar{z} \cdot \bar{w}$.   (ii) $\{1111, 1100, 0011, 0000\}$.

5. 110 (or 010).   **7.** $x_1, \bar{x}_1, x_2, \bar{x}_2, x_3, \bar{x}_3$ (or $x, \bar{x}, y, \bar{y}, z, \bar{z}$).

9. $x \cdot y, x \cdot \bar{y}, \bar{x} \cdot y, \bar{x} \cdot \bar{y}, x \cdot z, x \cdot \bar{z}, \bar{x} \cdot z, \bar{x} \cdot \bar{z}, x \cdot w, x \cdot \bar{w}, \bar{x} \cdot w, \bar{x} \cdot \bar{w}, y \cdot z, y \cdot \bar{z}, \bar{y} \cdot z, \bar{y} \cdot \bar{z}, y \cdot w, y \cdot \bar{w}, \bar{y} \cdot w,$
$\bar{y} \cdot \bar{w}, z \cdot w, z \cdot \bar{w}, \bar{z} \cdot w, \bar{z} \cdot \bar{w}$.

11. (a) 3;   (b) $3^2 = 9$;   (c) $3^3 = 27$.

13. One can choose the d variables x_i, for which either x_i or $\bar{x}_i$ appears, in $\binom{n}{d}$ ways, and for each of these x_i one has two choices (x_i or $\bar{x}_i$).

15. (a) x;   (b) $\bar{x} \cdot \bar{y}$;   (c) $x \cdot \bar{y} \cdot z$;   (d) $x \cdot y \cdot z \cdot \bar{w}$.

17. $\{00001, 00011, 00101, 00111, 10001, 10011, 10101, 10111\}$.

19. (a) $m_{0000} + m_{1100} + m_{1010} + m_{1001} + m_{0110} + m_{0101} + m_{0011}$.   (b) $m_{001} + m_{010} + m_{100} + m_{111}$.

21. $m_{10110} + m_{10010} + m_{00110} + m_{00010}$.   **23.** (a) $\bar{x} \cdot y \cdot \bar{w}$;   (b) $\bar{x}_1 \cdot x_3 \cdot \bar{x}_4 \cdot x_5$.

25. (a) $x \cdot \bar{y}$;   (b) $x \cdot z$;   (c) $x \cdot \bar{z}$.   **27.** 11100, 00100, 01000, 01110, 01101.

29. No; the weights of adjacent strings differ by exactly 1.   **31.** $y + x \cdot z$.

33. Since $01a_3 \ldots a_n$ and $10a_3 \ldots a_n$ are in $m^{-1}(1)$, s_1 and s_2 are blanks. Thus when a string α is in $m^{-1}(1)$, one gets a new string in $m^{-1}(1)$ when either (or both) of the first two digits of α is changed.

35. This m is of the form $m[s_1 s_2 s_3 s_4 s_5]$ with three blanks among the s_i. Changing just one of the digits of α in a place for which s_i is a blank gives a string adjacent to α and in $m^{-1}(1)$.

37. $f(xyz) = x \cdot \bar{y} \cdot z + \bar{x} \cdot y \cdot z + x \cdot y \cdot \bar{z} + \bar{x} \cdot \bar{y} \cdot \bar{z}$; f is not a sum of fewer than four monomials, because Problems 33 and 34 (and analogous results for other digit places) can be used to show that no two of the strings of $f^{-1}(1)$ are in the same "batch," that is, in an $m^{-1}(1)$ for a monomial m with $m^{-1}(1) \subseteq f^{-1}(1)$.

39. With the help of $f^{-1}(1)$ written as the union of three batches:

$$f^{-1}(1) = \{1010\} \cup \{1100, 1000\} \cup \{0011, 0111, 0001, 0101\},$$

one sees that $f(xyzw) = x \cdot \bar{y} \cdot z \cdot \bar{w} + x \cdot \bar{z} \cdot \bar{w} + \bar{x} \cdot w$.

41. We rewrite $f^{-1}(1)$ as $\{0011, 0010\} \cup \{1110, 1010\} \cup \{1000, 1001\} \cup \{0000, 0100\}$.
Then $f(xyzw) = \bar{x} \cdot \bar{y} \cdot z + x \cdot z \cdot \bar{w} + x \cdot \bar{y} \cdot \bar{z} + \bar{x} \cdot \bar{z} \cdot \bar{w}$.

43. Yes; this follows from Theorem 2.

45. When $x = y = z = 1$, we have $y \cdot z = 1$ and $\bar{x} \cdot y \cdot z = 0$. Thus they are not equal as rules for boolean functions.

SECTION 2.5

1. (a) $\bar{x} \cdot y + x \cdot z$ (b)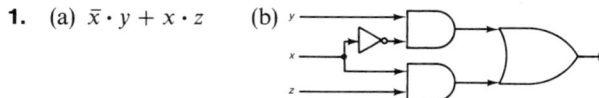

3. (i) $x + y + \bar{y} \cdot z$.   (ii) $x + y + z$.   (iii) 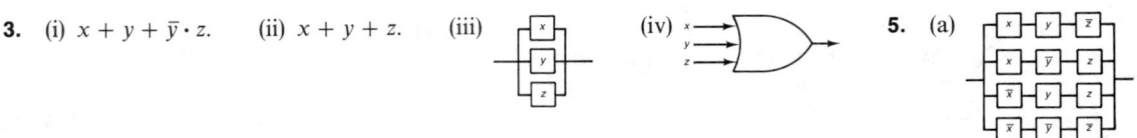 (iv)   **5.** (a)

7. (a) 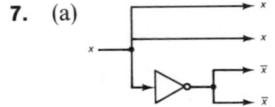   The figure to the left shows how one produces the needed x's and $\bar{x}$'s using splitting of pulses and one NOT gate. Similarly one produces the y's, $\bar{y}$'s, z's, and $\bar{z}$'s needed for the rest of the network, which is shown in the figure below.

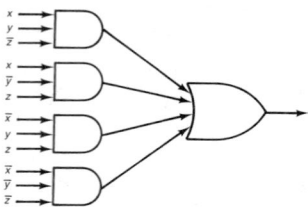

9. (a) $f(xyzw) = \bar{y} \cdot w + \bar{y} \cdot \bar{z} \cdot \bar{w} + x \cdot y \cdot z \cdot w + \bar{x} \cdot y \cdot z \cdot \bar{w}$ because $f^{-1}(1) = \{1011, 0011, 1001, 0001\} \cup \{1000, 0000\} \cup \{1111\} \cup \{0110\}$. (There is more than one way to do this problem.)

     (b) Using splitting of pulses and four NOT gates one produces enough x's, $\bar{x}$'s, y's, $\bar{y}$'s, z's, $\bar{z}$'s, w's, and $\bar{w}$'s in a manner similar to the figure in solution 7(a). The figure below shows the rest of the network.

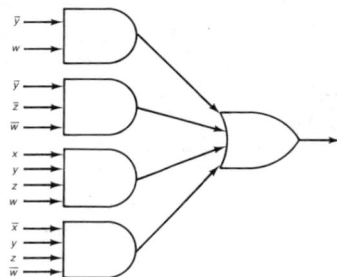

11. Yes. If the function f is O_n, this is easily done from the rule $x \cdot \bar{x}$. If $f \neq O_n$, then f is the sum of at most 2^n minifunctions, by Theorem 2 of Section 2.4. If all 2^n minifunctions are present, then some of them must be adjacent and Theorem 3 of Section 2.4 helps us see that f is the sum of fewer than 2^n monomials. With at most n NOT gates (and splitting of pulses) one produces enough x_1's, $\bar{x}_1$'s, ..., x_n's, $\bar{x}_n$'s, as in the figure in solution 7(a). Then one needs an AND gate for each monomial and one OR gate to sum them.

13. This is the full adder of Figure 2.5.7, with cxy as the input and $c'w$ as the output.

15.

17. (i)

α	00	01	10	11
$f(\alpha)$	1	0	0	1

   (ii) $\{00, 11\}$.   (iii) $x \cdot y + \bar{x} \cdot \bar{y}$

(iv)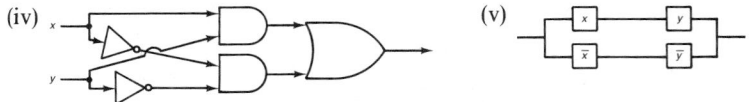

(v)

SECTION 2.6

1. (a)

GLB	1	2	3	12
1	1	1	1	1
2	1	2	1	2
3	1	1	3	3
12	1	2	3	12

LUB	1	2	3	12
1	1	2	3	12
2	2	2	12	12
3	3	12	3	12
12	12	12	12	12

(b) Yes, since GLB(x, y) and LUB(x, y) exist for all (x, y) in A^2.

(c) No. LUB$(2, 3) = 12$ and lcm$[2, 3] = 6$.

3. (a) 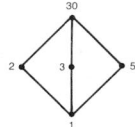 (b) 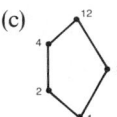 (c) (d) 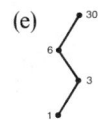 (e) 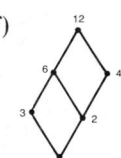 (f)

(a), (c), (e), (f) are lattices since GLB and LUB exist for all (x, y) in X^2; (b) is not a lattice since LUB$(4, 6)$ does not exist; (d) is not a lattice since GLB$(2, 3)$ does not exist.

5. (i) (ii) No, GLB(A, B) does not exist.

(iii) No, GLB(A, B) does not exist, but $A \cap B = \{1\}$.

7. (a) Yes.

(b) $x \wedge y \subseteq x$ and $x \wedge y \subseteq y$; $m \subseteq x$ and $m \subseteq y$ together imply that $m \subseteq x \wedge y$.

9. (a) If $xy = x$, then $x \preceq y$ by Part (i) of Theorem 6 ("Equivalent Conditions in a Lattice"), and hence $x + y = y$ by Theorem 6(ii).

(b) The "if" part is Theorem 6(iii); the "only if" part is Part (a).

11. Let $w = (x + y) + z$. Then w is an upper bound for $(x + y, z)$ and so $x + y \preceq w$ and $z \preceq w$. Similarly, $x \preceq x + y$ and $y \preceq x + y$. Using $y \preceq x + y$, $x + y \preceq w$, and transitivity of $\preceq$, one has $y \preceq w$ and similarly $x \preceq w$. From $y \preceq w$, $z \preceq w$, and Display (4), one has $y + z \preceq w$. This, with $x \preceq w$ and Display (4), gives us $x + (y + z) \preceq w$. Similarly one can show that $w \preceq x + (y + z)$. These two inequalities and the antisymmetry of $\preceq$ imply that $x + (y + z) = w = (x + y) + z$, and so $+$ is associative.

13. (a) GLB$(A, B) \subseteq A$ and GLB$(A, B) \subseteq B$ by definition of GLB in $(Y, \subseteq)$. Since GLB(A, B), A, and B are all in $P(S)$ and since $A \cap B$ is the greatest lower bound for (A, B) in $(P(S), \subseteq)$, one has GLB$(A, B) \subseteq A \cap B$ by Part (b) of Theorem 1, "Properties of GLB and LUB" [with GLB(x, y) replaced by $A \cap B$].

(b) This is essentially the dual of Part (a).

15. $[P(S), \cap, \cup]$, where S is a nonempty set.

17. (i)

$\cdot$ \ $+$	1	2	3	5	30
1	1	2	3	5	30
2	1	2	30	30	30
3	1	1	3	30	30
5	1	1	1	5	30
30	1	2	3	5	30

(ii) Let $a = 2, b = 3, c = 5$. Then $b + c = 30$, $a(b + c) = 2$, $ab = 1$, $ac = 1$, and $ab + ac = 1$. Hence $a(b + c) \neq ab + ac$.

19. Let $a = 4, b = 3$, and $c = 2$. Then $a(b + c) = 4 \cdot 12 = 4$ and $ab + ac = 4 \cdot 3 + 4 \cdot 2 = 1 + 2 = 2$.

21. By definition of GLB, $xz \preceq x$. This, $x \preceq y$, and transitivity of $\preceq$ give us $xz \preceq y$. Similarly, $xz \preceq w$. Now, $xz \preceq y$, $xz \preceq w$, and Theorem 1(b) give us $xz \preceq yw$.

23. (a) 0;   (b) 0.   **25.**   Yes, 36 is the identity under GLB.

27.
(i) Since $x \vee x = x$ by the idempotent law for $\vee$, one has $x \subseteq x$ by the definition of $\subseteq$, and so $\subseteq$ is reflexive.

(ii) $x \subseteq y$ and $y \subseteq x$ mean that $x \vee y = y$ and $y \vee x = x$. Since $x \vee y = y \vee x$, this gives us $x = y$, and so $\subseteq$ is antisymmetric.

(iii) By definition of $\subseteq$ and the hypotheses, $x \vee y = y$ and $y \vee z = z$. Then $x \vee z = x \vee (y \vee z) = (x \vee y) \vee z = y \vee z = z$, and so $x \subseteq z$. Hence $\subseteq$ is transitive.

29.
(i) $x \wedge x = x$ by an idempotent law; so xRx for all x in X, and R is reflexive. Since xRy and yRx imply that $x = x \wedge y = y \wedge x = y$, then R is antisymmetric. Since xRy and yRz imply that $x = x \wedge y = x \wedge (y \wedge z) = (x \wedge y) \wedge z = x \wedge z$ and hence imply that $x = x \wedge z$ and that xRz, then R is transitive. Thus R is a partial ordering and (X, R) is a poset.

(ii) $0Rx$, since $0 \wedge x = x \wedge 0 = 0$ by Problem 9 of Section 2.3. $xR1$, since $x \wedge 1 = x$ by the fact that 1 is the identity under $\wedge$.

(iii) If aRb, then $a = a \wedge b$. Also, $(x \wedge a) \wedge (x \wedge b) = (a \wedge b) \wedge (x \wedge x)$ by associativity and commutativity of $\wedge$. Since $x \wedge x = x$ (idempotent law), we have $(x \wedge a) \wedge (x \wedge b) = (a \wedge b) \wedge (x \wedge x) = a \wedge x$, and so $(x \wedge a)R(x \wedge b)$. Finally, $(x \vee a) \wedge (x \vee b) = (a \wedge b) \vee x$ by distributivity of $\vee$ over $\wedge$. Since aRb implies that $a \wedge b = a$ and $(x \vee a) \wedge (x \vee b) = (a \wedge b) \vee x = a \vee x$, we have $(x \vee a)R(x \vee b)$.

(iv) $(x \wedge y) \wedge x = (x \wedge x) \wedge y$ by associativity and commutativity of $\wedge$. As stated in Part (i), $x \wedge x = x$, and so $(x \wedge y) \wedge x = x \wedge y$. Thus $(x \wedge y)Rx$. Similarly, $(x \wedge y)Ry$. If zRx and zRy, then $z \wedge x = z = z \wedge y$. Now, $z \wedge (x \wedge y) = (z \wedge x) \wedge y = z \wedge y = z$. Finally, $z \wedge (x \wedge y) = z$ implies that $zR(x \wedge y)$.

(v) By Part (ii), $0Ry$. This and the second conclusion in Part (iii) give us $(x \vee 0)R(x \vee y)$. Since 0 is the identity under $\vee$, one has $x \vee 0 = x$, and so $xR(x \vee y)$.

(vi) If aRb, then $a = a \wedge b$. Then $a \vee b = (a \wedge b) \vee b = (a \vee b) \wedge (b \vee b) = (a \vee b) \wedge b$. Now, $a \vee b = (a \vee b) \wedge b$ means that $(a \vee b)Rb$. But $bR(a \vee b)$ by Part (v). Since R is antisymmetric, $a \vee b = b$.

31. γ is $\subseteq$.

33.
(i) Let R be the relation of Problem 29. Then $xR(x \vee y)$ by Problem 29(v). Using the answer to Problem 30, this gives us $x \subseteq (x \vee y)$. Also, $x \wedge x \subseteq x \wedge (x \vee y)$ by the first conclusion of Problem 29(iii), and so $x = x \wedge x \subseteq x \wedge (x \vee y)$.

(ii) $x \vee y \subseteq 1$ by Problem 28(ii). Hence $x \wedge (x \vee y) \subseteq x \wedge 1 = x$ by the first conclusion of Problem 29(iii). Thus $x \wedge (x \vee y) \subseteq x$.

(iii) This follows from Parts (i) and (ii) and the fact that $\subseteq$ is antisymmetric [that is, Problem 27(ii)].

35.
$$\begin{aligned}
x &= x \vee (x \wedge a) & &\text{Absorption law (Problem 34)}\\
&= x \vee (y \wedge a) & &\text{Hypothesis } x \wedge a = y \wedge a\\
&= (x \vee y) \wedge (x \vee a) & &\text{Distributivity of } \vee \text{ over } \wedge\\
&= (x \vee y) \wedge (y \vee a) & &\text{Hypothesis } x \vee a = y \vee a\\
&= (y \vee x) \wedge (y \vee a) & &\text{Commutativity of } \vee\\
&= y \vee (x \wedge a) & &\text{Distributivity of } \vee \text{ over } \wedge\\
&= y \vee (y \wedge a) & &\text{Hypothesis } x \wedge a = y \wedge a\\
&= y & &\text{Absorption law (Problem 34).}
\end{aligned}$$

37. $a \wedge \bar{a} = 0$ and $a \vee \bar{a} = 1$ by Axiom (B4). These and the hypotheses that $a \wedge b = 0$ and $a \vee b = 1$ together with Problem 35 imply that $b = \bar{a}$.

39. (i)
$$\begin{aligned}
z \vee w &= z \vee (\bar{x} \wedge \bar{y}) & &\text{Since } w = \bar{x} \wedge \bar{y}\\
&= (z \vee \bar{x}) \wedge (z \vee \bar{y}) & &\text{By distributivity of } \vee \text{ over } \wedge\\
&= (x \vee y \vee \bar{x}) \wedge (x \vee y \vee \bar{y}) & &\text{Since } z = x \vee y\\
&= (y \vee 1) \wedge (x \vee 1) & &\text{Since } t \vee \bar{t} = 1\\
&= 1 \wedge 1 & &\text{By Problem 10 of Section 2.3}\\
&= 1 & &\text{Since the identity under } \wedge \text{ is 1.}
\end{aligned}$$

(ii) This is essentially the dual of Part (i).

(iii) Since $z \vee w = 1$ and $z \wedge w = 0$ by Parts (i) and (ii), it follows from Problem 37 that $\bar{z} = w$; that is, $\overline{x \vee y} = \bar{x} \wedge \bar{y}$.

REVIEW PROBLEMS FOR CHAPTER 2

1. (a) No.   (b) Yes.   (c) Yes.   (d) Yes.   **3.** (a) Yes.   (b) No.   (c) Yes.   (d) Yes.

5. (a) $mn + m + n$ is in N for every (m, n) in $N \times N$.   (b) Yes.   (c) Yes.   (d) Yes, 0.

7. (a)

	0	01	001
01	010	0101	01001
001	0010	00101	001001

(b) No. The concatenation of 01 and 0 is not in the subset.

9. Yes. If α has length h and β has length k with h and k in $5N$, $\alpha\beta$ has length $h + k$, which is also in $5N$.

11. (a) The semigroups are (i), (iii), and (v).   (b) Only (iii) is a monoid; its identity is 1.

13. The submonoids are (i), (ii), and (iii). $X = 2N \cup 3N$ is not closed under $+$ because 2 and 3 are in X but their sum is not.

15. Let $\alpha = a_1 a_2 \ldots a_m$ and $\beta = b_1 b_2 \ldots b_n$. Then $\alpha\beta = a_1 \ldots a_m b_1 \ldots b_n$, $r(\alpha) = a_m \ldots a_1$, $r(\beta) = b_n \ldots b_1$, and $r(\alpha\beta) = b_n \ldots b_1 a_m \ldots a_1 = r(\beta)r(\alpha)$.

17. $(0, 0, 1)$.   **19.** (a) Contingency.   (b) Tautology.   (c) Contradiction.

21. $\{01001, 01101, 11001, 11101\}$.   **23.** $m_{01001} + m_{01101} + m_{11001} + m_{11101}$.   **25.** $\bar{x} \cdot z$.

27. $g(xyz) = \bar{x} \cdot y + x \cdot z$ or $g = m[01\_] + m[1\_1]$.   **29.** $m[1\_\_] + m[0\_0]$ or $x + \bar{x} \cdot \bar{z}$.

31. $(A \vee \bar{B} \vee C) \wedge (B \vee \bar{C}) \wedge (\bar{A} \vee D)$ or $(A + \bar{B} + C) \cdot (B + \bar{C}) \cdot (\bar{A} + D)$.

33. (i)

(ii) $\bar{y} \cdot z + (x \cdot \bar{y} + \bar{x} \cdot y) \cdot \bar{z}$

35.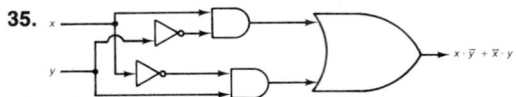

37. (a) A lattice.   (b) Not a lattice. LUB(2, 3) does not exist in A.

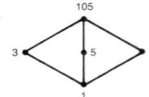   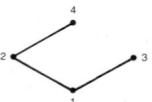

39. No. GLB(A, C) does not exist in X.

41. (a) True. See Definition 2 ("Lattice") of Section 2.6.
(b) False. See the poset $(A, |)$ of Example 1 in Section 2.6 or Problem 39 or Problem 37(b) of this set.
(c) True. See Parts (a) and (b) of Theorem 5 ("Lattice Properties") in Section 2.6.

SECTION 3.1

1. (b) and (d) are true.   **3.** (b), (c), and (d) are true.   **5.** (ii).   **7.** (6, 1), (18, 17).

9. (a) $B_{5,0} \cup B_{5,1} \cup B_{5,2} \cup B_{5,3}$;   (b) $B_{5,4} \cup B_{5,5}$;   (c), (f), (g), (h) $B_{5,2} \cup B_{5,3} \cup B_{5,4} \cup B_{5,5}$;
(d), (e) $B_{5,2} \cup B_{5,3}$.

11. (b), (d), and (e).

13. (a) If $x = 0$ or $x = 1$, then $x^2 = x$.   (b) $q \Rightarrow \bar{p}$.
(c) You work hard or live longer than your rich relatives if you become rich.
(d) If $C(a) = C(b)$, then $[C(a) \cap C(b)] \neq \emptyset$.

15. (a) If x is neither 0 nor 1, then $x^2 \neq x$.   (b) $\bar{q} \Rightarrow p$ or $\bar{q} \Rightarrow \bar{p}$.
(c) You do not work hard or live longer than your rich relatives if you do not become rich.
(d) If $C(a) \neq C(b)$, then $[C(a) \cap C(b)] = \emptyset$.

17. (a) False (when p is false).
(b) True; let $P = \bar{p}$ and $Q = q$ in Definition 5 ("Implication, Premise, Conclusion").
(c) False, for example, when p is true and q is false.

19.

x	y	$x \Leftrightarrow y$
0	0	1
0	1	0
1	0	0
1	1	1

21. $n = 313$.

23. (a) Form (ii), where P denotes "$\#S_\alpha = k$" and Q denotes "wgt $\alpha = k$."
(b) Form (iii), where P = "$C \subseteq A$," Q = "$C \subseteq B$," and R = "$C \subseteq A \cap B$."
(c) Form (iii), where P = "e is a left identity," Q = "e is a right identity," and R = "e is the identity."
(d) Form (v), where P = "r, s, and t are in $\mathbf{Z}^+$," Q = "$r|s$," R = "$s|t$," and S = "$r|t$."

25. One sees from Table 3.1.2 (the truth table for $p \Rightarrow q$) that the answers to the parts of the problem are as follows: (a) Yes.   (b) No, $p \Rightarrow q$ is true when p is false and q is true.   (c) Yes.   (d) Same as (b).

27. (i) No. It is false—for example, when $A = \emptyset$, $B = \{1\}$, and $S = \{1, 2\}$.   (ii) (a) and (b).

29. Let $A = (x \Rightarrow y \Rightarrow z \Rightarrow x)$ and $B = (x \Leftrightarrow y \Leftrightarrow z)$. The following truth table shows that $A \Leftrightarrow B$ is a tautology and hence that the desired equivalence holds for all assertions or predicates.

xyz	$x \Rightarrow y$	$y \Rightarrow z$	$z \Rightarrow x$	A	$x \Leftrightarrow y$	$y \Leftrightarrow z$	B
000	1	1	1	1	1	1	1
001	1	1	0	0	1	0	0
010	1	0	1	0	0	0	0
011	1	1	0	0	0	1	0
100	0	1	1	0	0	1	0
101	0	1	1	0	0	0	0
110	1	0	1	0	1	0	0
111	1	1	1	1	1	1	1

31. $f^{-1}(1) = \{001, 011, 100, 101, 111\}, g^{-1}(1) = \{000, 001, 010, 011, 100, 101, 111\}, h^{-1}(1) = \{000, 001, 011, 111\}.$

SECTION 3.2

1. Inference Rule (T10), "Constructive Dilemma," modified slightly.
3. Replace y by $\bar{y}$ in Inference Rule (T6), "Modus Ponens."

5. (a)

x	$\bar{x}$	$x \vee \bar{x}$
0	1	1
1	0	1

(b)

x	y	$x \wedge y$	$x \wedge y \Rightarrow x$
0	0	0	1
0	1	0	1
1	0	0	1
1	1	1	1

7. (a) This equals 0 when $xy = 01$.   (b) Same as (a).
9. Invalid reasoning; an example of Fallacy (F2) or Fallacy (F4).
11. Valid reasoning; an example of Inference Rule (T6), "Modus Ponens."
13. (a) Invalid reasoning; an example of Fallacy (F3), "Converse."
    (b) Yes. This can be deduced from "If $m \in 2\mathbf{Z}$, then $m^2 \in 2\mathbf{Z}$," which is easily proved by the technique of Example 10 of Section 1.7. (A true statement may arise from faulty reasoning.)

15.

Boolean Function	Justification
(a) $(x \vee y) \wedge \bar{y}$	Hypothesis.
(b) x	Inference Rule (T8), "Disjunctive Syllogism," applied to Step (a).
(c) $\bar{y}$	Hypothesis.
(d) $x \wedge \bar{y}$	Definition of $\wedge$ as applied to Steps (b) and (c).

17.

Tautology	Justification
(a) $x \vee \bar{x}$	Inference Rule (T3), "Excluded Middle."
(b) $(x \vee y) \vee \overline{(x \vee y)}$	Step (a) with x replaced by $x \vee y$.
(c) $(x \vee y) \vee (\bar{x} \wedge \bar{y})$	De Morgan's Law, $\overline{x \vee y} = \bar{x} \wedge \bar{y}$.

19. Valid reasoning; an example of the tautology $\{x \wedge [(x \wedge y) \Rightarrow z] \wedge (z \Rightarrow \bar{x})\} \Rightarrow \bar{y}$, which can be established with a truth table.

21. Since P is a tautology, we have $P(\alpha) = 1$ for all α in B_n. Since $P \Rightarrow Q$ is a tautology, we have $P(\alpha) \Rightarrow Q(\alpha)$ equals 1 for all α in B_n. Thus $1 \Rightarrow Q(\alpha)$ equals 1 for all α in B_n. It follows that $Q(\alpha) = 1$ for all α in B_n, and so Q is a tautology.

23. Invalid reasoning; $[(x \Rightarrow y) \wedge (z \Rightarrow w) \wedge \bar{x} \wedge \bar{z}] \Rightarrow (\bar{y} \wedge \bar{w})$ is false when x and z are false and y or w is true.

25.

xy	$\bar{y}$	$x \wedge \bar{y}$	0	$(x \wedge \bar{y}) \Rightarrow 0$	$x \Rightarrow y$	$[(x \wedge \bar{y}) \Rightarrow 0] \Rightarrow (x \Rightarrow y)$
00	1	0	0	1	1	1
01	0	0	0	1	1	1
10	1	1	0	0	0	1
11	0	0	0	1	1	1

SECTION 3.3

1. $P(1) \wedge P(2) \wedge P(3)$.   **3.** $[\neg P(1)] \vee [\neg P(2)] \vee [\neg P(3)]$.   **5.** (a), (b), and (c) are true.
7. (i) and (ii).   **9.** Any 2×3 table with all entries equal to 1 on some row.
11. The implication is true whenever the premise is false. Also, when the premise is true, there is an a in S such that $P(a, t)$ is true for all t in T; this a will do as the s that is claimed to exist in the conclusion. Thus the conclusion is true when the premise is true. Hence the implication is always true.
13. $[R \text{ is symmetric}] \Leftrightarrow [\forall (x, y) \in S^2, (xRy) \Rightarrow (yRx)]$.   **15.** $\forall (x, y, z) \in S^3, (x \ \Box \ y) \ \Box \ z = x \ \Box \ (y \ \Box \ z)$.
17. (a) $(A \subseteq B) \Leftrightarrow [(x \in A) \Rightarrow (x \in B)]$.
(b) For all sets B, $\varnothing \subseteq B$ is true, since $(x \in \varnothing)$ is false and hence $[(x \in \varnothing) \Rightarrow (x \in B)]$ is true for all objects x.
19. (a), (b), and (c) are true.
21. Let X be $\{0, 1\}$, $P(x)$ be "$x^2 = 1$," and $Q(x)$ be "$x^2 = 0$." Then $P(0)$ and $Q(1)$ are false, and $P(1)$ and $Q(0)$ are true. Thus $[\forall x \in X, P(x)]$ is false and hence the implication $[\forall x \in X, P(x)] \Rightarrow [\forall x \in X, Q(x)]$ is true. The other implication is false because $[P(1) \Rightarrow Q(1)]$ is false.
23. Yes. If $[\exists x \in X, P(x) \wedge Q(x)]$ is true, then $P(a)$ and $Q(a)$ are both true for some a in X, and hence both $[\exists x \in X, P(x)]$ and $[\exists x \in X, Q(x)]$ are true.

REVIEW PROBLEMS FOR CHAPTER 3

1. (a) $3^2 + 4^2 = 5^2$, true.   (b) $(-2)^3 = 2^3$, false.   (c) $-6 = 6$, false.   (d) $3 | 72$, true.
3. (a) False with a true converse.
(b) Reversible, i.e., true with a true converse.
(c) True with a false converse.
(d) Reversible, i.e., true with a true converse.
5. False. In the doubleton boolean algebra, if $x = 1$ and $y = 1$, then $(\neg x) \vee (\neg y) = 0 \vee 0 = 0$.
7. Yes. One can show that $[(x \wedge y) \wedge (x \Rightarrow z)] \Rightarrow (y \wedge z)$ is a tautology, using all eight rows of a truth table.

9.

p	$\neg p$	$\neg(\neg p)$
0	1	0
1	0	1

11. (a) $\{1, 2, 3\}$;   (b) $\{1\}$;   (c) $Z - \{2, 3\}$;   (d) Z.

13. (a) $x = 11$.   (b) No.

15. Yes. Let $H = [\forall x \in X, P(x)]$, $C = [\exists x \in X, P(x)]$, and $I = (H \Rightarrow C)$. The only way the implication I can be false is for the hypothesis H to be true with the conclusion C false. But if H is true, then $P(x_1)$ is true, and so x_1 is the claimed x whose existence makes C true. Thus $\neg I$ implies the contradiction $C \wedge (\neg C)$. Now Algorithm 1 of Section 3.2 ("Proof by Contradiction") tells us that I is true.

17. Yes. This can be shown using all eight lines of a case table.

19. Let $X = \{0, 1\}$, $P(x)$ be "$x = 0$." and $Q(x)$ be "$x = 1$." Then the premise is true and the conclusion is false, and so the implication is false.

SECTION 4.1

1. (i) 40320;   (ii) 362880;   (iii) 3628800.   **3.** (i) 7;   (ii) 24;   (iii) 12;   (iv) 720.

5. (a) 4.   (b) 5.   (c) (12, 8) and (11880, 11879).   (d) $(n + 1)! - n! = n![(n + 1) - 1] = n!n$.

     (e) Yes; $(n - 2)!(n^2 - n) = (n - 2)!(n - 1)n = n!$ for $n \geq 2$.

7. (a) $5/4!$;   (b) $1/6!$;   (c) $7/(3!4!)$.

9. (a) $\binom{5}{2} = 10$, $\binom{6}{2} = 15$;   (b) $\binom{6}{3} = 20$, $\binom{7}{3} = 35$;   (c) 5;   (d) 7.

11. (i) $x^1 = x$.   (ii) For all k in $\mathbf{Z}^+$, $x^{k+1} = x^k \cdot x$.

13. **Basis** $\prod_{j=1}^{1} a_j = a_1$.   **Inductive Part** $\prod_{j=1}^{k+1} a_j = \left(\prod_{j=1}^{k} a_j\right) a_{k+1}$.

15. **Basis** $a_1 = 0$ and $a_2 = 1$.   **Inductive Part** For all k in $\mathbf{Z}^+$, $a_{k+2} = (a_k + a_{k+1})/2$.   **17.** Yes.

19. (ii) $n!$.   (iii) $n!$.   **21.** (a) $F_{12} = 144$.   (b) $2 | F_n$ if and only if $3 | n$.   (c) $3 | F_n$ if and only if $4 | n$.

23. $-4, 3, 10$.   **25.** $-19, -23, -27$.   **27.** 6, 18, 54.   **29.** 686, 4802, 33614.   **31.** 21, 13.

33. (i) 4;   (ii) $a_{100} = 5 + 99 \cdot 4 = 401$;   (iii) $100 \cdot \dfrac{5 + 401}{2} = 20300$.

35. (i) $\frac{1}{3}$;   (ii) $(\frac{1}{3})^{98}$;   (iii) $\dfrac{1 - (\frac{1}{3})^{99}}{1 - (\frac{1}{3})} = (\frac{3}{2})[1 - (\frac{1}{3})^{99}]$.

37. (a) $(2a + nd)(n + 1)/2$.   (b) $a(1 - x^{n+1})/(1 - x)$.

39. (ii) $S_1 = 2$, $S_2 = 6$, $S_3 = 14$, $S_4 = 30$.   (iii) 5.   **41.** (i) $(h - 1)2^h + 1$.   (ii) Same as for Part (i).

SECTION 4.2

1. **Basis** $P(0)$ is true because it asserts that $1 = (x - 1)/(x - 1)$.

    Inductive Step Assume that $1 + x + \cdots + x^k = (x^{k+1} - 1)/(x - 1)$. Then

$$(1 + x + \cdots + x^k) + x^{k+1} = \frac{x^{k+1} - 1}{x - 1} + x^{k+1} = \frac{x^{k+1} - 1 + x^{k+2} - x^{k+1}}{x - 1} = \frac{x^{k+2} - 1}{x - 1}.$$

    Thus $P(k) \Rightarrow P(k + 1)$ for all k in $\mathbf{N}$.

3. **Basis** For $n = 0$, the left side is $F_1^2 - F_0 F_2 = 1^2 - 0 \cdot 1 = 1$ and the right side is $(-1)^0 = 1$; so the result holds for $n = 0$.

    Inductive Step Assume the desired result for $n = k$; that is, let $F_{k+1}^2 - F_k F_{k+2} = (-1)^k$. Since $F_{k+3} = F_{k+2} + F_{k+1}$ and $F_{k+2} = F_{k+1} + F_k$, we have $F_{k+2}^2 - F_{k+1} F_{k+3} = F_{k+2}(F_{k+1} + F_k) - F_{k+1}(F_{k+2} + F_{k+1}) = F_{k+2} F_k - F_{k+1}^2 = -(F_{k+1}^2 - F_k F_{k+2}) = -(-1)^k = (-1)^{k+1}$. This is the desired result for $n = k + 1$, and the proof is done.

5. *Hint*: This is similar to Example 3.

7. **Basis** For $n = 0$, the left side is $\binom{h}{h} = 1$ and the right side is $\binom{h+1}{h+1} = 1$. So the assertion is true for $n = 0$.

Inductive Step   Assume the desired result for $n = k$; that is, assume that $\binom{h}{h} + \binom{h+1}{h} + \cdots + \binom{h+k}{h} =$

$\binom{h+k+1}{h+1}$. Adding $\binom{h+k+1}{h}$ to each side gives $\binom{h}{h} + \binom{h+1}{h} + \cdots + \binom{h+k+1}{h} = \binom{h+k+1}{h+1} +$

$\binom{h+k+1}{h} = \binom{h+k+2}{h+1}$. Since this is the desired result for $n = k + 1$, the theorem is proved.

9. **Basis**   When $n = 1$, the left side is $1 + x$ and the right side is $\binom{1}{0} + \binom{1}{1}x = 1 + x$; so the assertion is true for $n = 1$.

   Inductive Step   Let the result hold for $n = k$; that is, let $(1 + x)^k = \binom{k}{0} + \binom{k}{1}x + \cdots + \binom{k}{k}x^k$. Multiplying

   each side by $1 + x$ gives $(1 + x)^{k+1} = \left[\binom{k}{0} + \binom{k}{1}x + \cdots + \binom{k}{k}x^k\right](1 + x) = \binom{k}{0} + \left[\binom{k}{1} + \binom{k}{0}\right]x +$

   $\left[\binom{k}{2} + \binom{k}{1}\right]x^2 + \cdots + \left[\binom{k}{k} + \binom{k}{k-1}\right]x^k + \binom{k}{k}x^{k+1}$. Since $\binom{k}{0} = 1 = \binom{k+1}{0}$, $\binom{k}{k} = 1 = \binom{k+1}{k+1}$,

   and $\binom{k}{i} + \binom{k}{i-1} = \binom{k+1}{i}$ for $1 \le i \le k$, one has $(1 + x)^{k+1} = \binom{k+1}{0} + \binom{k+1}{1}x + \cdots + \binom{k+1}{k+1}x^{k+1}$.

   This is the desired result for $n = k + 1$, and the theorem is proved.

11. **Basis** $P(1)$ is true because $x - y$ is a factor of $x - y$.
   Inductive Step   Assume that $x - y$ is a factor of $x^k - y^k$; that is, assume that $x^k - y^k = (x - y)Q$. Then $x^{k+1} - y^{k+1} = x^{k+1} - xy^k + xy^k - y^{k+1} = x(x^k - y^k) + y^k(x - y) = x(x - y)Q + y^k(x - y) = (x - y)(xQ + y^k)$, which shows that $x - y$ is a factor of $x^{k+1} - y^{k+1}$. Thus $P(k) \Rightarrow P(k + 1)$.

13. (i) $S_1 = \frac{1}{2}$, $S_2 = \frac{1}{2} + \frac{2}{6} = \frac{5}{6}$, $S_3 = \frac{5}{6} + \frac{3}{24} = \frac{23}{24}$, $S_4 = \frac{23}{24} + \frac{4}{120} = \frac{119}{120}$, $S_5 = \frac{119}{120} + \frac{5}{720} = \frac{719}{720}$.
   (ii) We conjecture that $S_n = [(n + 1)! - 1]/(n + 1)!$.
   (iii) **Basis** $P(1)$ is true because $S_1 = 1/2 = (2! - 1)/2!$.
      Inductive Step   Assume that $S_k = [(k + 1)! - 1]/(k + 1)!$. Then

$$S_{k+1} = \frac{(k+1)! - 1}{(k+1)!} + \frac{k+1}{(k+2)!} = \frac{(k+2)[(k+1)! - 1]}{(k+2)!} + \frac{k+1}{(k+2)!}$$

$$= \frac{(k+2)! - (k+2) + (k+1)}{(k+2)!} = \frac{(k+2)! - 1}{(k+2)!}.$$

   Since $P(k + 1)$ is the assertion that $S_{k+1} = [(k + 2)! - 1]/(k + 2)!$, $P(k)$ implies $P(k + 1)$ for all n in $\mathbf{Z}^+$ and we are done.

15. (i) $S_0 = 1/(1 \cdot 3) = 1/3$, $S_1 = 1/3 + 1/(3 \cdot 5) = 6/(3 \cdot 5) = 2/5$, $S_2 = 2/5 + 1/(5 \cdot 7) = 15/(5 \cdot 7) = 3/7$, $S_3 = 4/9$, $S_4 = 5/11$, $S_5 = 6/13$.
   (ii) $S_n = (n + 1)/(2n + 3)$.
   (iii) **Basis** $P(0)$ is true because $S_0 = 1/3 = (0 + 1)/(2 \cdot 0 + 3)$.
      Inductive Step   Assume that $S_k = (k + 1)/(2k + 3)$. Then

$$S_{k+1} = S_k + \frac{1}{[2(k+1)+1][2(k+1)+3]} = \frac{k+1}{2k+3} + \frac{1}{(2k+3)(2k+5)}$$

$$= \frac{(k+1)(2k+5) + 1}{(2k+3)(2k+5)} = \frac{2k^2 + 7k + 6}{(2k+3)(2k+5)} = \frac{(2k+3)(k+2)}{(2k+3)(2k+5)} = \frac{k+2}{2k+5}.$$

   Since $S_{k+1} = (k + 2)/(2k + 5)$ is $P(k + 1)$, then $P(k) \Rightarrow P(k + 1)$ for all k in N, and the proof by mathematical induction is done.

17. (i) $\binom{n}{2} = \dfrac{n!}{(n-2)!2!} = \dfrac{n!}{2!(n-2)!} = \dfrac{n(n-1)(n-2)(n-3)\cdots 1}{2\cdot(n-2)(n-3)\cdots 1} = \dfrac{n(n-1)}{2}.$

(ii) $\binom{n}{2} + \binom{n+1}{2} = \dfrac{n(n-1)}{2} + \dfrac{(n+1)n}{2} = \dfrac{n^2-n+n^2+n}{2} = \dfrac{2n^2}{2} = n^2.$

19. One such listing is

$B_4 = \{0000,\ 0001,\ 0011,\ 0010,\ 0110,\ 0111,\ 0101,\ 0100,\ 1100,\ 1101,\ 1111,\ 1110,\ 1010,\ 1011,\ 1001,\ 1000\}.$

21. (i) **Basis** Since $a_1 = a_1 + (1-1)d$, $P(1)$ is true.

Inductive Step Assume that $a_k = a_1 + (k-1)d$. Then $a_{k+1} = a_k + d = a_1 + (k-1)d + d = a_1 + kd$. Since $P(k+1)$ asserts that $a_{k+1} = a_1 + kd$, one has $P(k) \Rightarrow P(k+1)$ for all k in $\mathbf{Z}^+$, and the induction is done.

(ii) **Basis** Since $\displaystyle\sum_{j=1}^{1} a_j = a_1$ and $1\cdot a_1 + \binom{1}{2}d = a_1$, $P(1)$ is true.

Inductive Step Assume that $P(k)$ is true; that is, assume that $\displaystyle\sum_{j=1}^{k} a_j = ka_1 + \binom{k}{2}d$. Since $k = \binom{k}{1}$,

$$\sum_{j=1}^{k+1} a_j = \left(\sum_{j=1}^{k} a_j\right) + a_{k+1} = ka_1 + \binom{k}{2}d + a_1 + kd$$

$$= (k+1)a_1 + \left[\binom{k}{2} + \binom{k}{1}\right]d = (k+1)a_1 + \binom{k+1}{2}d.$$

Because $\displaystyle\sum_{j=1}^{k+1} a_j = (k+1)a_1 + \binom{k+1}{2}d$ is $P(k+1)$, we have shown that $P(k) \Rightarrow P(k+1)$. The induction is complete.

SECTION 4.3

1. Let $P(n)$ be the assertion to be proved.

Basis When $n = 0$, we have $F_a F_n + F_{a+1}F_{n+1} = F_a F_0 + F_{a+1}F_1 = F_a\cdot 0 + F_{a+1}\cdot 1 = F_{a+1}$ and $F_{a+n+1} = F_{a+1}$. Thus $P(0)$ is true. **Inductive Step** $P(1)$ is true because $F_a F_1 + F_{a+1}F_2 = F_a + F_{a+1} = F_{a+2}$. Let h be in $\{1, 2, \ldots\}$ and let $P(0), P(1), \ldots, P(h-1)$ be true. We wish to use this inductive hypothesis to show that $P(h)$ is true. Since $P(1)$ is true, we let $h \geq 2$. Then the inductive hypothesis tells us that $P(h-2)$ and $P(h-1)$ are true. That is,

$$F_a F_{h-2} + F_{a+1}F_{h-1} = F_{a+h-1}$$
$$F_a F_{h-1} + F_{a+1}F_h = F_{a+h}.$$

Adding these, we have $F_a(F_{h-2} + F_{h-1}) + F_{a+1}(F_{h-1} + F_h) = F_{a+h-1} + F_{a+h}$. Then the recursive property of the F_n gives us $F_a F_h + F_{a+1}F_{h+1} = F_{a+h+1}$. Since this is $P(h)$, the proof is complete.

3. Let $P(n)$ denote the assertion to be proved.

Basis We are given that $P(0)$ is true. **Inductive Step** Let $P(0), P(1), \ldots, P(h-1)$ all be true. We wish to use this hypothesis to show that $P(h)$ is true. Since $P(0)$ and $P(1)$ are true, we can let $h \geq 2$. Then the inductive hypothesis includes the assumption that $P(h-2)$ and $P(h-1)$ are true; namely,

$$rF_{h-2+a} = sF_{h-2+b} + tL_{h-2+c}$$
$$rF_{h-1+a} = sF_{h-1+b} + tL_{h-1+c}.$$

Adding, and using the recursion formulas for the F_n and L_n, yields $rF_{h+a} = sF_{h+b} + tL_{h+c}$. Since this is $P(h)$, the proof is complete.

5. *Hint*: See Example 2 and use the following table, in which a is the number of 10¢ stamps, b is the number of 13¢ stamps, and $n = 10a + 13b$.

n	108	109	110	111	112	113	114	115	116	117
a	3	7	11	2	6	10	1	5	9	0
b	6	3	0	7	4	1	8	5	2	9

7. *Hint*: These proofs are similar to those of Problems 1 and 3.

9. (i) $a^2 = (1 + \sqrt{5})^2/4 = (1 + 2\sqrt{5} + 5)/4 = (6 + 2\sqrt{5})/4 = (3 + \sqrt{5})/2 = a + 1$. Similarly, $b^2 = b + 1$.
   (ii) Let $P(n)$ be the assertion to be proved.
   Basis Since $F_0 = 0$ and $(a^0 - b^0)/(a - b) = (1 - 1)/\sqrt{5} = 0$, $P(0)$ is true. **Inductive Step** $P(1)$ is true because $F_1 = 1$ and $(a^1 - b^1)/(a - b) = 1$. Let $h \geq 2$ and let $P(0), P(1), \ldots, P(h - 1)$ be true. Then $P(h - 2)$ and $P(h - 1)$ are true; that is, $F_{h-2} = (a^{h-2} - b^{h-2})/(a - b)$ and $F_{h-1} = (a^{h-1} - b^{h-1})/(a - b)$. Adding, we get

$$F_{h-2} + F_{h-1} = \frac{a^{h-2} + a^{h-1} - b^{h-2} - b^{h-1}}{a - b} = \frac{a^{h-2}(1 + a) - b^{h-2}(1 + b)}{a - b}.$$

   Using Part (i) gives

$$F_{h-2} + F_{h-1} = \frac{a^{h-2}a^2 - b^{h-2}b^2}{a - b} = \frac{a^h - b^h}{a - b}.$$

   Since $F_{h-2} + F_{h-1} = F_h$, we have $P(h)$—the proof is complete.

11. Using the recursion formula for the Lucas Numbers gives
   $L_{n+3} = L_{n+2} + L_{n+1} = (L_{n+1} + L_n) + L_{n+1} = 2L_{n+1} + L_n$.

13. (d) Let $S_n = L_0 + L_3 + \cdots + L_{3n}$ and let $P(n)$ assert that $2S_n = L_{3n+2} + 1$.
   Basis $2S_0 = 2L_0 = 2 \cdot 2 = 4$ and $L_{3 \cdot 0 + 2} + 1 = L_2 + 1 = 3 + 1 = 4$. So $P(0)$ is true.
   Inductive Step Assume that $2S_k = L_{3k+2} + 1$. Then $2S_{k+1} = 2S_k + 2L_{3(k+1)} = 2L_{3k+3} + L_{3k+2} + 1$. Using Problem 11, this becomes $2S_{k+1} = L_{3k+5} + 1 = L_{3(k+1)+2} + 1$. Since this is $P(k + 1)$, the proof is complete.

15. Replace a by n in the formula of Problem 1.

17. (i) $U_3 = 5$, $U_4 = 8$, and $U_5 = 13$.
   (ii) Let $P(n)$ be the assertion that $U_n = F_{n+2}$. Our conjecture is that $P(n)$ is true for all n in $\mathbf{Z}^+$. The proof by strong induction follows.
   Basis $U_1 = 2$ and $F_{1+2} = F_3 = 2$, so $P(1)$ is true. **Inductive Step** We assume that $h \in \{2, 3, \ldots\}$ and that $P(1), P(2), \ldots, P(h - 1)$ are true, and we wish to show that $P(h)$ is true. By Part (i), $P(2)$ is true, so we deal now with the case of $h \geq 3$. Then $P(h - 2)$ and $P(h - 1)$ are true, that is, $U_{h-2} = F_h$ and $U_{h-1} = F_{h+1}$. Let $\alpha = a_1 a_2 \ldots a_h$ be an unfriendly string in $\mathbf{B}_h$. If $a_1 = 1$, then a_2 must be 0 and $a_3 \ldots a_h$ is an unfriendly string in $\mathbf{B}_{h-2}$. If $a_1 = 0$, then $a_2 \ldots a_h$ is an unfriendly string in $\mathbf{B}_{h-1}$. Conversely, if β is an unfriendly string in $\mathbf{B}_{h-2}$ and we prefix the digits 10 to it, we obtain an unfriendly string 10β in $\mathbf{B}_h$, with leftmost digit 1. Also if γ is an unfriendly string in $\mathbf{B}_{h-1}$ and we prefix 0 to it, then 0γ is an unfriendly string in $\mathbf{B}_h$ starting with 0. Since the strings of these types 10β and 0γ are all the unfriendly strings of $\mathbf{B}_h$ with no overlap, we have $U_h = U_{h-2} + U_{h-1} = F_h + F_{h+1} = F_{h+2}$. This is $P(h)$, so the proof is complete.

19. **Basis** $S_0 = L_0^2 = 2^2 = 4$ and $L_1 + 2 + (-1)^0 = 1 + 2 + 1 = 4$, so $P(0)$ is true. **Inductive Step** Assume that $S_k = L_{2k+1} + 2 + (-1)^k$. Then $S_{k+1} = S_k + L_{k+1}^2$. It follows from Problem 10(iii) that $L_{k+1}^2 = L_{2k+2} + 2(-1)^{k+1}$. Hence $S_{k+1} = [L_{2k+1} + 2 + (-1)^k] + L_{2k+2} + 2(-1)^{k+1} = L_{2k+3} + 2 - (-1)^{k+1} + 2(-1)^{k+1} = L_{2(k+1)+1} + 2 + (-1)^{k+1}$. Since this is the desired result for $n = k + 1$, the formula is proved by (ordinary) induction.

21. Since r is rational, the set A of denominators t is nonempty (and a subset of $\mathbf{Z}^+$). Since $\mathbf{Z}^+$ is well ordered, A must have a least element.

REVIEW PROBLEMS FOR CHAPTER 4

1. 87178291200. **3.** 1, 2, 3, 5, 7, 11. **5.** 15!/6!.

7. Let $S_n = \sum\limits_{j=1}^{n} (2j - 1)$. Then S_n is defined inductively as follows:

   Basis $S_1 = 1$. **Inductive Part** $S_{k+1} = S_k + [2(k + 1) - 1] = S_k + 2k + 1$.

9. Let $P_n = \prod\limits_{j=5}^{n} 3^j$. Then P_n is defined for n in $A = \{5, 6, \dots\}$ by:

   Basis $P_5 = 3^5$. **Inductive Part** $P_{k+1} = 3^{k+1}P_k$ for k in A.

11. (i) 1694; (ii) 134750. **13.** $[x^{n+1} - (-y)^{n+1}]/(x + y)$.

15. Let $S_n = F_0 + F_2 + \cdots + F_{2n}$. **Basis** When $n = 0$, we have $S_n = S_0 = 0$ and $F_{2n+1} - 1 = F_1 - 1 = 1 - 1 = 0$. So the formula holds for $n = 0$. **Inductive Part** Assume that $S_k = F_{2k+1} - 1$. Then $S_{k+1} = S_k + F_{2(k+1)} = F_{2k+1} - 1 + F_{2k+2} = F_{2k+3} - 1 = F_{2(k+1)+1} - 1$. This is the desired formula for $n = k + 1$, and the proof is accomplished.

17. Let $S_n = 0^2 + 1^2 + \cdots + n^2$. **Basis** When $n = 0$, we have $S_n = S_0 = 0$ and $n(n + 1)(2n + 1)/6 = 0 \cdot 1 \cdot 1/6 = 0$. So the formula holds for $n = 0$. **Inductive Part** Assume that $S_k = k(k + 1)(2k + 1)/6$. Then

$$S_{k+1} = S_k + (k + 1)^2 = \frac{1}{6} k(k + 1)(2k + 1) + (k + 1)^2$$

$$= (k + 1)\left[\frac{1}{6} k(2k + 1) + k + 1\right] = \frac{k + 1}{6}[2k^2 + k + 6k + 6] = \frac{k + 1}{6}[2k^2 + 7k + 6]$$

$$= \frac{(k + 1)(k + 2)(2k + 3)}{6} = \frac{(k + 1)[(k + 1) + 1][2(k + 1) + 1]}{6}.$$

   Since this is the claimed formula for $n = k + 1$, the proof is complete.

19. (a) False. Let $m = 2$ and $n = 1$. Then $(2 + 1)! = 3! = 6$, $2! + 1! = 2 + 1 = 3$, and $6 \neq 3$.

   (b) True. This equals $\binom{m + n}{m}$, which is $\#B_{m+n,m}$ and so is an integer.

   (c) True. $\binom{2n}{2} = \frac{2n(2n - 1)}{2} = n(2n - 1) = 2n^2 - n.$

21. (i) For all n in N, either n or $n + 1$ is even, and a product of integers is even if at least one factor is even.

   (ii) $b_{k+1} - b_k = (k + 1)[(k + 1)^2 + 5] - k(k^2 + 5) = (k + 1)(k^2 + 2k + 6) - k(k^2 + 5)$
   $= k^3 + 3k^2 + 8k + 6 - k^3 - 5k = 3k^2 + 3k + 6 = 3(k^2 + k) + 6 = 3a_k + 6.$

   (iii) Since $a_k = 2m$ with m in Z by Part (i), we have $b_{k+1} - b_k = 3(2m) + 6 = 6(m + 1)$ by Part (ii).

   (iv) **Basis** Since $b_0 = 0$ and $6|0$, the result holds for $n = 0$. **Inductive Part** Assume that $6|b_k$, that is, $b_k = 6c$ with c in Z. Also, $b_{k+1} - b_k = 6d$ with d in Z by Part (iii). Thus $b_{k+1} = b_k + 6d = 6c + 6d = 6(c + d)$, and so $6|b_{k+1}$. This is the claimed result for $n = k + 1$ and completes the proof.

23. $a_1, a_2, \dots$ is an arithmetic progression if and only if the difference of consecutive terms is constant, that is, if and only if $a_{n+2} - a_{n+1} = a_{n+1} - a_n$. This is equivalent to $a_{n+2} - 2a_{n+1} + a_n = 0$.

25. kr^a, kr^b, and kr^c are consecutive terms of a geometric progression if and only if $kr^c \div kr^b = kr^b \div kr^a$. This is true if and only if $r^{c-b} = r^{b-a}$, which holds if and only if $c - b = b - a$. Finally, $c - b = b - a$ if and only if a, b, and c are consecutive terms of an arithmetic progression.

27. (a) **Basis** The inequality holds for $n = 0$ and $n = 1$ because $F_0 = 0 < 1 = 2^0$ and $F_1 = 1 < 2 = 2^1$. **Inductive Part** Assume that h is in $\{2, 3, \dots\}$ and that $F_n < 2^n$ for n in $\{0, 1, \dots, h - 1\}$. Then $F_{h-2} < 2^{h-2}$ and $F_{h-1} < 2^{h-1}$. Hence $F_h = F_{h-2} + F_{h-1} < 2^{h-2} + 2^{h-1} = 2^{h-2}(1 + 2) < 4 \cdot 2^{h-2} = 2^h$. Since $F_h < 2^h$ is the claimed result for $n = h$, the proof is complete.

   (b) The proof of Part (b) is very similar to that of Part (a).

29. Using the formula of Problem 10 of Section 4.2 gives

$$\binom{n}{4} = \frac{n!}{4!(n-4)!} = \frac{n(n-1)(n-2)(n-3)(n-4)\cdots 2\cdot 1}{24(n-4)\cdots 2\cdot 1} = \frac{n(n-1)(n-2)(n-3)}{24}.$$

SECTION 5.1

1. (a) $12 + 14 = 26$; (b) $12\cdot 14 = 168$.
3. (i) Yes; (ii) $f_1 = 2$, $f_2 = 6$, $f_3 = 14$, $f_4 = 30$; (iii) $n = 5$; (iv) $n = 6$.
5. (a) $9\cdot 10\cdot 5 = 450$; (b) $9\cdot 10\cdot 5 = 450$.
7. (i) $10^3 = 1000$; (ii) $10\cdot 9\cdot 8 = 720$; (iii) $10^3 = 1000$; (iv) $10\cdot 9\cdot 8 = 720$.
9. $9\cdot 11 + 11\cdot 9 = 198$. **11.** $9! = 362880$. **13.** (a) 100; (b) 9900; (c) $100\cdot 99\cdot 98 = 970200$.
15. (a) $100!/2!$; (b) $100!/97!$. **17.** (a) $n!/k!$; (b) $n!/(n-k)!$.
19. Yes; the reasoning is the same as in Example 11.
21. $2^{2^7} = 2^{128}$. **23.** $M_3 = 2$; see the figure, in which (w_i, h_i) is the ith couple.

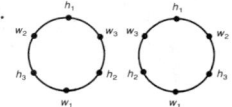

25. The appropriate circular permutations come in pairs of "mirror images," as in the figure for the solution to Problem 23.
27. 2^{n-1}. We can take $a_1 a_2 \ldots a_{n-1}$ to be any of the 2^{n-1} strings in $\mathbf{B}_{n-1}$. Then a_n must be 0 if $a_1 + a_2 + \cdots + a_{n-1}$ is even, and $a_n = 1$ otherwise.

SECTION 5.2

1. (a) $a_1 a_2 b_3 b_4$, $a_1 b_2 a_3 b_4$, $a_1 b_2 b_3 a_4$, $b_1 a_2 a_3 b_4$, $b_1 a_2 b_3 a_4$, $b_1 b_2 a_3 a_4$;
  (b) $a_1 b_2 b_3 b_4$, $b_1 a_2 b_3 b_4$, $b_1 b_2 a_3 b_4$, $b_1 b_2 b_3 a_4$; (c) $b_1 b_2 b_3 b_4$.

3. (a) 2^7; (b) $7\cdot 2^6$; (c) $\binom{101}{8}$; (d) $\binom{101}{8}$; (e) 6^7.

5. (i) $a^5 + 5a^4 b + 10a^3 b^2 + 10a^2 b^3 + 5ab^4 + b^5$.
  (ii) $(2x)^5 + 5(2x)^4(-3y) + 10(2x)^3(-3y)^2 + 10(2x)^2(-3y)^3 + 5(2x)(-3y)^4 + (-3y)^5$
    $= 32x^5 - 240x^4 y + 720x^3 y^2 - 1080x^2 y^3 + 810xy^4 - 243y^5$.

7. (i) $1, 7, 21, 35, 35, 21, 7, 1$;
  (ii) $a^7 + 7a^6 b + 21a^5 b^2 + 35a^4 b^3 + 35a^3 b^4 + 21a^2 b^5 + 7ab^6 + b^7$;
  (iii) Replace a by $4x$ and b by $-5y$ in Part (ii).

9. $1, 3, 6, 10, 15, 21, 28, 36, 45, 55$.

11.

k	1	2	3	4	5	6	7	8	9
$\binom{33}{k}$	33	528	5456	40920	237336	1107568	4272048	13884156	38567100

13. $\binom{33}{1} = 33 = \binom{33}{32}$, $\binom{33}{2} = 528 = \binom{33}{31}$, $\binom{33}{3} = 5456 = \binom{33}{30}$.

15. (i) $\binom{10}{4}$; (ii) $\binom{6}{2}\binom{4}{2}$; (iii) $\binom{10}{4} - \binom{6}{2}\binom{4}{2}$. **17.** $\binom{81}{3} = 85320 = \binom{81}{78}$, $\binom{80}{78} = 3160$.

19. Using Theorem 4, $\binom{n}{2} + \binom{n+1}{2} = \dfrac{n(n-1)}{2} + \dfrac{(n+1)n}{2} = \binom{n}{2}(n-1+n+1) = \binom{n}{2}(2n) = n^2$. This can also be seen geometrically by placing together two adjacent triangles from Figure 5.2.1 to form a square array of dots, as in Figure 5.2.2.

21. $\binom{10}{0}\binom{10}{10} + \binom{10}{1}\binom{10}{9} + \binom{10}{2}\binom{10}{8}$. **23.** $\binom{8}{3}\binom{7}{2} + \binom{8}{2}\binom{7}{3}$.

25. (a), (b), and (c): Expand and collect terms. (d) Let $x = 1$ in Part (b) and divide by 2.

27. $x^2 + y^2 + z^2 + w^2 + 2xy + 2xz + 2xw + 2yz + 2yw + 2zw$.

29. It is the product $\binom{300}{60}\binom{240}{70}\binom{170}{80}$ of integers. **31.** (a) $18!/(3! \cdot 4! \cdot 5! \cdot 6!)$; (b) $\{4, 5, 7, 10\}$.

33. (i) Each is the coefficient of $x^a y^b z^c$ in the expansion of $(x + y + z)^n$.
(ii) Yes. Each is the coefficient of $x^{20} y^{30} z^{40}$ in the expansion of $(x + y + z)^{90}$.

35. (a) Using Display (5), Recursion Formula:

$$\binom{n}{k} + 2\binom{n}{k-1} + \binom{n}{k-2} = \left[\binom{n}{k} + \binom{n}{k-1}\right] + \left[\binom{n}{k-1} + \binom{n}{k-2}\right]$$

$$= \binom{n+1}{k} + \binom{n+1}{k-1} = \binom{n+2}{k}.$$

(b) It follows from Display (5) that $\binom{n}{k} - \binom{n-1}{k-1} = \binom{n-1}{k}$. Then

$$\binom{n}{k} - 2\binom{n-1}{k-1} + \binom{n-2}{k-2} = \left[\binom{n}{k} - \binom{n-1}{k-1}\right] - \left[\binom{n-1}{k-1} - \binom{n-2}{k-2}\right]$$

$$= \binom{n-1}{k} - \binom{n-2}{k-1} = \binom{n-2}{k}.$$

37. Using the formula $k\binom{n}{k} = n\binom{n-1}{k-1}$ of Display (7) in Example 2 and Theorem 2 with n replaced by $n-2$, the present sum becomes

$$n\left[\binom{n-1}{1} + 2\binom{n-1}{2} + 3\binom{n-1}{3} + \cdots + (n-1)\binom{n-1}{n-1}\right]$$

$$= n(n-1)\left[\binom{n-2}{0} + \binom{n-2}{1} + \binom{n-2}{2} + \cdots + \binom{n-2}{n-2}\right] = n(n-1)2^{n-2}.$$

39. By Theorem 2, the left-hand side is $(2^n)^2 = 2^{2n}$ and the right side is 2^{2n}.

41. (i) The left-hand side equals $(1 + x)^{60}(1 + x)^{40} = (1 + x)^{100}$.
(ii) Equate coefficients of x^{33} in the equation of Part (i).
(iii) Use Part (ii) and the symmetry formula $\binom{40}{k} = \binom{40}{40-k}$.

43. Let T be a set of 100 people of whom 60 are women and 40 are men. For $k = 0, 1, \ldots, 33$, let V_k be the collection of subsets A of T with $\#A = 33$ and with k women in A. Also, let $V_0 \cup V_1 \cup \cdots \cup V_{33} = U$. Since the V_i are pairwise disjoint, it follows from the general sum rule that $\#V_0 + \#V_1 + \cdots + \#V_{33} = \#U = \binom{100}{33}$. Let T_k be the number of ways of choosing k of the 60 women and independently choosing

33 − k of the 40 men. By the product rule, $\# T_k = \binom{60}{k}\binom{40}{33-k}$. Hence $\binom{60}{0}\binom{40}{33} + \binom{60}{1}\binom{40}{32} + \cdots + \binom{60}{33}\binom{40}{0} = \binom{100}{33}$.

45. Each side is the number of ways of choosing a subset of k people from a set of m men and n women.

47. Let each of m and k be replaced by n in the formula of Problem 45 and then use the symmetry formula $\binom{n}{n-h} = \binom{n}{h}$.

49. $\binom{1001}{8}$ is the number of ways of choosing a set A of 8 integers from $\{1, 2, \ldots, 1001\}$. For $r = 8, 9, \ldots,$ 1001, $\binom{r-1}{7}$ is the number of ways of choosing such an A with r as the largest integer in A (and the remaining 7 integers of A in $\{1, 2, \ldots, r-1\}$).

51. $2^n = \sum_{k=0}^{n} \binom{n}{k} < \sum_{k=0}^{n} \binom{n}{k}^2 = \binom{2n}{n}$ for n in $\{2, 3, \ldots\}$.

53. Using the formula $\binom{n}{k} = n\binom{n-1}{k-1}\Big/ k$ from Example 2, $\binom{2n}{n} = 2n\binom{2n-1}{n-1}\Big/ n = 2\binom{2n-1}{n-1}$ is double an integer.

SECTION 5.3

1. 8.   3. $1 + \max(m, n)$, where max is as in Definition 2 of Section 2.1.   5. 4751.   7. 3.

9. Let A, B, C, D consist of the (s, t) in S for which, respectively, s and t are even, s is even and t is odd, s is odd and t is even, and both s and t are odd. These sets partition S. It follows from the generalized pigeonhole principle that one of the subsets A, B, C, D has at least two ordered pairs in it. Two ordered pairs in the same subset will do as the (a, b) and (c, d) because $(a + c)/2$ and $(b + d)/2$ will be integers.

11. 56.   13. (i) $28 + 24 + 21 - 4 - 7 - 3 + 1 = 60$.   (ii) $168 - 60 = 108$.

15. Yes. Let A be one of the 6 people. As in Example 2, either at least 3 of the others are acquaintances of A or at least 3 of the others are not acquainted with A. In the first case, let B, C, and D be acquaintances of A. If there is a subset $\{X, Y\}$ of $\{B, C, D\}$ such that X and Y are acquainted, then $\{A, X, Y\}$ is a set of 3 mutually acquainted people in S. If there is no such pair $\{X, Y\}$, then $\{B, C, D\}$ is a set of 3 mutual strangers in S. The other case, in which S has at least 3 people not acquainted with A, is similar.

17. One of the regions A, B, C, D in the figure must have at least 2 of the 5 points in it, and 2 points in the same region are at most $\sqrt{2}$ units apart.

19. If not, one has the contradiction $26 = \#X = \#f^{-1}(1) + \#f^{-1}(2) + \#f^{-1}(3) \le 7 + 8 + 10 = 25$.

21. (a) $450 + 300 + 180 - 150 - 90 - 60 + 30 = 660$;   (b) $900 - 660 = 240$.

23. $n! - 2[(n-1)!] + (n-2)! = (n^2 - 3n + 3)[(n-2)!]$.

25. $(n-1)! + (n-2)^2[(n-2)!] = (n^2 - 3n + 3)[(n-2)!]$.   27. (a) 3^n.   (b) $3^n - 3 \cdot 2^n + 3$.

29. $550 - 22 + 6 = 534$.   **31.** $4^{20} - 2 \cdot 3^{20} + 2^{20}$.

33. (a) 1000.   (b) 100.   (c) $1000000 - 1000 - 100 + 10 = 998910$. (Ten of these are the sixth powers.)

35. 1001090, using Problem 33 and the fact that there are neither squares nor cubes between 1000000 and 1001090.

SECTION 5.4

1. (a) (3, 1, 1), (1, 3, 1), (1, 1, 3), (2, 2, 1), (2, 1, 2), (1, 2, 2).

(b) (5, 0, 0), (0, 5, 0), (0, 0, 5), (4, 1, 0), (4, 0, 1), (1, 4, 0), (1, 0, 4), (0, 4, 1), (0, 1, 4), (3, 2, 0), (3, 0, 2), (2, 3, 0), (2, 0, 3), (0, 3, 2), (0, 2, 3).

3. β: (3, 1, 1) $\mapsto$ (2, 0, 0),   (1, 3, 1) $\mapsto$ (0, 2, 0),   (1, 1, 3) $\mapsto$ (0, 0, 2),   (2, 2, 1) $\mapsto$ (1, 1, 0),   (2, 1, 2) $\mapsto$ (1, 0, 1), (1, 2, 2) $\mapsto$ (0, 1, 1).

5. (a) $\binom{28}{1} = 28$;   (b) $\binom{42}{2} = 861$;   (c) $\binom{271}{19}$;   (d) $\binom{500 + k - 1}{k - 1} = \binom{499 + k}{k - 1}$.

7. (a) $\binom{26}{1} = 26$;   (b) $\binom{39}{2} = 741$;   (c) $\binom{251}{19}$;   (d) $\binom{499}{k - 1}$.

9. (a) $\binom{714}{5}$;   (b) $\binom{713}{5}$;   (c) $\binom{708}{5}$;   (d) $\binom{684}{5}$.

11. Yes. See Theorem 5 ("Multinomial Expansion") of Section 5.2.

13. (a) $\binom{13}{1} = 13$;   (b) $\binom{20}{2} = 190$;   (c) $\binom{84}{3}$.

15. (a) $\binom{11}{1} = 11$;   (b) $\binom{17}{2} = 136$;   (c) $\binom{80}{3}$.

17. (a) $\binom{10}{3} = 120$;   (b) 1 way: 4 pennies, 2 dimes, and 1 quarter.

19. (a) $\binom{14}{5}$;

(b) $\binom{20}{5} - 6\binom{10}{5}$, that is, the number of compositions of 15 into 6 parts no one of which is 10 or more.

(c) $\binom{28}{5} - \binom{6}{1}\binom{18}{5} + \binom{6}{2}\binom{8}{5}$, that is, the number of compositions of 23 into 6 parts no one of which is 10 or more.

21. (a) $\binom{344}{3}$;   (b) $\binom{340}{3}$;   (c) $\binom{343}{3}$;   (d) $\binom{323}{3}$;   (e) $\binom{348}{3} - \binom{323}{3}$;   (f) $\binom{343}{3} - \binom{323}{3}$.

23. (a) $\binom{604}{4} - \binom{503}{4} - \binom{403}{4} + \binom{302}{4}$;   (b) $\binom{604}{4} - \binom{303}{4} - \binom{203}{4}$.

25. $\binom{7 + 5 - 1}{5 - 1} = \binom{11}{4}$. This is found as follows: Let x_1 be the number of 2's, x_2 be the number of 3's, $\ldots$, x_5 be the number of 11's; then the answer is the number of compositions of 7 into 5 parts.

27. $\binom{15 + 24 + 7}{7} = \binom{46}{7}$; this is found using the bijection $(x_1, x_2, \ldots, x_8) \mapsto (x_1 + 3, x_2 + 3, \ldots, x_8 + 3)$ from the set of solutions onto the set of compositions of $15 + 8 \cdot 3 = 39$ into 8 parts.

29. $\binom{3n + 2}{2} - 3\binom{n + 1}{2}$.

SECTION 5.5

1. (i) (6, 0), (5, 1), (4, 2), (3, 3).   (ii) (7, 0), (6, 1), (5, 2), (4, 3).   (iii) Yes.

3. (i) (5), (4, 1), (3, 2), (3, 1, 1), (2, 2, 1), (2, 1, 1, 1), (1, 1, 1, 1, 1).   (ii) 7.   (iii) 2.   (iv) Yes.

5. (a) $\begin{smallmatrix} \bullet & \bullet & \bullet & \bullet & \bullet \\ \bullet & \bullet & \bullet \\ \bullet & \bullet \\ \bullet & \bullet \end{smallmatrix}$ (b) $\beta = (4, 4, 2, 1, 1)$.   **7.** (3, 2, 1).

9. The only partition of n into 1 part is the 1-tuple (n).

11. $p_k(n)$ is in N because it is the size of a finite set of k-tuples.

13. $p_2(n) = p_2(n - 2) + p_1(n)$ by Theorem 2, "Recursion for $p_k(n)$," and $p_1(n) = 1$ by Problem 9, so $p_2(n) = p_2(n - 2) + 1$ for $n \geq 2$.

15. (i) $p_3(0) = 1 = p_3(1)$, $p_3(2) = 2$.
(ii) $p_3(2m) = p_3(2m - 3) + p_2(2m)$ by Theorem 2, "Recursion for $p_k(n)$," and $p_2(2m) = m + 1$ by Problem 14(a).

17.

n	0	1	2	3	4	5	6	7	8	9	10	11
$p_2(n)$	1	1	2	2	3	3	4	4	5	5	6	6

19.

n	0	1	2	3	4	5	6	7	8	9	10	11
$p_4(n)$	1	1	2	3	5	6	9	11	15	18	23	27

21. $p_3(2m) = m + 1 + p_3(2m - 3) = (m + 1) + [(m - 1) + p_3(2m - 6)]$.

23. (a) This follows from the table for Problem 18.
(b) Since each n in N is of the form $2m$ or the form $2m + 1$ with m in N, this follows from Problems 21 and 22.

25. By Problem 24, $p_3(6m) = 6[m + (m - 1) + (m - 2) + \cdots + 2 + 1] + 1$. The sum of the arithmetic progression in the brackets is found to be $m(m + 1)/2$ by the technique of Example 3 of Section 4.1. Hence $p_3(6m) = 6[m(m + 1)/2] + 1 = 3m(m + 1) + 1 = 3m^2 + 3m + 1$.

27. (a) $3m^2 + 5m + 2$;   (b) $3m^2 + 6m + 3$.   **29.**

n	0	1	2	3	4	5
$p(n)$	1	1	2	3	5	7

31. The hypotheses imply that $a = 2^x$, $b = 2^y$, $c = 2^z$, with (x, y, z) a partition of 10 into 3 parts. Hence $\#S = p_3(10) = 14$.

33. This follows because the mapping with $(x, y, z, w) \mapsto (x - 4, y - 3, z - 2, w - 1)$ is a bijection from the set A of partitions of n into 4 distinct positive parts onto the set B of partitions of $n - 10$ into 4 parts.

35. Yes. Theorem 2, "Recursion with $p_k(n)$," with $n = 10$, is $p_k(10) = p_k(10 - k) + p_{k-1}(10)$. Use this with $k = 6, 5, 4, 3, 2$ and also use $p_1(10) = 1 = p_1(9)$.

37. Yes; $p_9(80) = p_8(80) + p_9(80 - 9) = p_8(80) + p_9(71) = p_8(80) + p_8(71) + p_9(71 - 9) = p_8(80) + p_8(71) + p_9(62)$.

39. $k = 7$ and $n = 28$.

41. Yes. This follows from the formulas in Problems 39 and 40 and four similar formulas.

SECTION 5.6

1. (a) $\binom{5 + 2}{2} = \binom{7}{2} = 21$. (b) $\binom{7 - 3}{2} = \binom{4}{2} = 6$. **3.** (a) $p_3(5) = 5$. (b) $p_3(5 - 3) = p_3(2) = 2$.

5. $\binom{9}{2} = 36$. **7.**

k	1	2	3	4	5	6
$S(6, k)$	1	31	90	65	15	1

9. $(3^7 - 3 \cdot 2^7 + 3)/6 = (2187 - 384 + 3)/6 = 1806/6 = 301$. **11.** $S(7, 3) = 301$.

13. $3! S(7, 3) = 6 \cdot 301 = 1806$. **15.** (a) 4^9. (b) $4! S(9, 4) = 4^9 - 4 \cdot 3^9 + 6 \cdot 2^9 - 4$.

17. 4^9, as in Problem 15(a). **19.** $4! S(9, 4) = 4^9 - 4 \cdot 3^9 + 6 \cdot 2^9 - 4$, as in Problem 15(b).

21. This is the special case of $k = 5$ of Theorem 5, "Stirling Numbers of the Second Kind."

23. In a partition $\{A_1, A_2, \ldots, A_k\}$ of $T = \{1, 2, \ldots, n\}$ into k nonempty parts, one of the A_i is a pair $\{a, b\}$ that can be chosen in $\binom{n}{2}$ ways from T; the rest of the A_i are uniquely determined as singletons from the complement of $\{a, b\}$ in T.

25. We can assign each of the $n - 1$ integers in $\{2, 3, \ldots, n\}$ to C or D in 2^{n-1} ways. But we do not want to count the one distribution in which D ends up empty, so the answer is $2^{n-1} - 1$.

27. $(4^n - 4 \cdot 3^n + 6 \cdot 2^n - 4)/24$ is an integer because it is the number of partitions of $\{1, 2, \ldots, n\}$ into 4 nonempty subsets.

SECTION 5.7

1. (a) $\frac{1}{2}$. (b) $\frac{3}{4}$. (c) $\binom{7}{3}\Big/2^7$. (d) $\binom{n}{k}\Big/2^n$. **3.** (i) 8. (ii) $\frac{3}{8}$. (iii) $\frac{3}{8}$.

5. (a) $\binom{8}{5}\Big/2^8 = \frac{56}{256} = \frac{7}{32}$. (b) $\left[\binom{8}{5} + \binom{8}{6} + \binom{8}{7} + \binom{8}{8}\right]\Big/2^8 = [56 + 28 + 8 + 1]/256 = 93/256$.

7. (a) $\frac{1}{36}$. (b) $\frac{1}{18}$. (c) $\frac{1}{12}$. (d) $\frac{1}{36}$. (e) $\frac{1}{18}$. (f) $\frac{1}{12}$.

9. (a) and (f): $1/6^4 = 1/1296$. (b) and (e): $4/6^4 = 1/324$.

(c) and (d): $\left[\binom{4}{2} + \binom{4}{1}\right]\Big/6^4 = \frac{10}{1296} = \frac{5}{648}$.

11. The mapping $\beta \colon (a_1, a_2, \ldots, a_{10}) \mapsto (7 - a_1, 7 - a_2, \ldots, 7 - a_{10})$ is a bijection from the set of 10-tuples of dice readings totaling t to the set of 10-tuples of dice readings totaling $70 - t$. (See Problems 7 through 10.)

13. (a) $\binom{13}{k}\binom{39}{13 - k}\Big/\binom{52}{13}$. (b) $\binom{13}{7}\binom{39}{6}\Big/\binom{52}{13}$. **15.** $\binom{52}{13}\binom{39}{13}\binom{26}{13}$.

17. (a) $\frac{9}{24} = \frac{3}{8}$. (b) $\frac{8}{24} = \frac{1}{3}$. (c) $\frac{6}{24} = \frac{1}{4}$. (d) 0. (e) $\frac{1}{24}$. **19.** $9 \cdot 9 \cdot 8 \cdot 7/9000 = 63/125$.

21. $25!/26! = 1/26$. **23.** (i) $\binom{20}{10}$. (ii) $\left[\binom{10}{0}\binom{10}{10} + \binom{10}{1}\binom{10}{9} + \binom{10}{2}\binom{10}{8}\right]\Big/\binom{20}{10}$.

SECTION 5.8

1. (i) $\emptyset$;   (ii) $\emptyset$;   (iii) $\{4\}$;   (iv) $\{3\}$;   (v) $\{2, 4\}$;   (vi) $\{3\}$.

3. (i) 0;   (ii) 0;   (iii) 1;   (iv) 1;   (v) 2;   (vi) 1.   **5.** (i) and (ii).

7. $d_7 = 7 \cdot 265 - 1 = 1854$, $d_8 = 8 \cdot 1854 + 1 = 14833$.

9. By Theorem 3(a), with $n = 2m + 1$,

$$p_{2m+1} = p_{2m} + \frac{(-1)^{2m+1}}{(2m+1)!} = p_{2m} - \frac{1}{(2m+1)!} < p_{2m}.$$

11. Using Theorem 3(a), with n equal to $2m + 2$ and $2m + 1$, one has

$$p_{2m+2} = p_{2m+1} + \frac{1}{(2m+2)!} = p_{2m} - \frac{1}{(2m+1)!} + \frac{1}{(2m+2)!}$$

$$= p_{2m} - \frac{2m+2-1}{(2m+2)!} = p_{2m} - \frac{2m+1}{(2m+2)!} < p_{2m}.$$

13. This uses Notation 2 ("Probability of Obtaining a Derangement"), Formula (a) of Theorem 3 ("Additional Properties of d_n and p_n"), and Definition 1 ("Factorials") of Section 4.1.

15. Using Problem 14, we see that $[d_n - nd_{n-1}] + [d_{n-1} - (n-1)d_{n-2}] = (-1)^n + (-1)^{n-1} = (-1)^n - (-1)^n = 0$.

17. Only for $n = 1$, as one sees from $d_n = nd_{n-1} + (-1)^n$.

19. $d_1 = 0$ is even. Also, for $n = 3, 5, 7, \ldots$, the integer $n - 1$ is even, and hence $d_n = (n-1)(d_{n-1} + d_{n-2})$ is even.

21. (a) $4! = 24$.   (b) $d_4 = 9$.   (c) $3! = 6$.   (d) $d_3 = 2$.   **23.** (a) $(n-1)!$.   (b) d_{n-1}.

25. There are nd_{n-1} listings λ in L_n with $f(\lambda) = 1$, since—for each of the n values of i in $\{1, 2, \ldots, n\}$—there are d_{n-1} listings with i as the only hit.

27. (a) There are $\binom{n}{3} d_{n-3}$ listings in L_n with $f(\lambda) = 3$ because we can choose the 3 hits in $\binom{n}{3}$ ways and then "derange" the other $n - 3$ integers of $\{1, 2, \ldots, n\}$ in d_{n-3} ways.

(b) $\binom{n}{4} d_{n-4}$.   (c) $\binom{n}{5} d_{n-5}$.

29. There are $\binom{n}{s} d_{n-s}$ listings λ in L_n with $f(\lambda) = s$, since we can choose the s hits in $\binom{n}{s}$ ways and then derange the other $n - s$ integers of $\{1, 2, \ldots, n\}$ in d_{n-s} ways.

31. This follows from the formula of Problem 30(ii) and the symmetry formula $\binom{n}{n-k} = \binom{n}{k}$ for the binomial coefficients.

33. (a) $3! \cdot 5! = 6 \cdot 120 = 720$.   (b) $d_3 d_5 = 2 \cdot 44 = 88$.

35. Using the inclusion–exclusion principle, one can see that the number of listings in L_8 with neither 1 nor 2 as a hit is $8! - 7! - 7! + 6! = (56 - 7 - 7 + 1)6! = 43 \cdot 720 = 30960$.

REVIEW PROBLEMS FOR CHAPTER 5

1. (a) $\binom{4}{2} + \binom{5}{3} = 6 + 10 = 16$.   (b) $\binom{4}{2}\binom{5}{3} = 6 \cdot 10 = 60$.

2. (i) $\#C_1 = 3$, $\#C_2 = 9$, $\#C_3 = 27$.   (ii) 5.   **3.** (a) 26^5.   (b) $26 \cdot 25 \cdot 24 \cdot 23 \cdot 22$.

4. $8^2 \cdot 10^5 = 6400000$.   **5.** $7! = 5040$.   **6.** $3! \cdot 4! = 6 \cdot 24 = 144$.

7. 1, 9, 36, 84, 126, 126, 84, 36, 9, 1. **8.** (a) 2^{79}; (b) 2^{79}.

9. $\binom{90}{50} = \binom{89}{50} + \binom{89}{49} = \left[\binom{88}{50} + \binom{88}{49}\right] + \left[\binom{88}{49} + \binom{88}{48}\right] = \binom{88}{50} + 2\binom{88}{49} + \binom{88}{48}.$

10. The formula $\binom{n}{k} = \binom{n-1}{k} + \binom{n-1}{k-1}$ can be rewritten as $\binom{n-1}{k-1} = \binom{n}{k} - \binom{n-1}{k}$. This gives us

$\binom{98}{68} = \binom{99}{69} - \binom{98}{69} = \left[\binom{100}{70} - \binom{99}{70}\right] - \left[\binom{99}{70} - \binom{98}{70}\right] = \binom{100}{70} - 2\binom{99}{70} + \binom{98}{70}.$

11. $\binom{22}{10}.$ **12.** $\binom{14}{6}\binom{8}{4}.$ **13.** $\dfrac{30!}{6!7!8!9!}.$

14. Each side is the number of ways of choosing 20 people from a set of 30 men and 50 women.

15. 247.0770901501. **16.** $8^{50}.$ **17.** $\#A$ must be at least 101.

18. $\#(A \cup B \cup C) = 105, \#M_{101} = 14.$

19. $\binom{83 - 35 + 4}{4} = \binom{52}{4}.$ **20.** $\binom{52}{4} - \binom{43}{4} - \binom{38}{4} + \binom{29}{4}.$

21. $p_4(100) = p_4(96) + p_3(100) = p_4(96) + [p_3(97) + p_2(100)] = p_4(96) + p_3(97) + [p_2(98) + p_1(100)].$

22. $p_5(30).$ **23.** $S(6, 3) = 3S(5, 3) + S(5, 2) = 3 \cdot 25 + 15 = 90.$ **24.** $S(6, 3) = 90.$

25. $3!S(6, 3) = 6 \cdot 90 = 540.$ **26.** $3!S(6, 3) = 540.$ **27.** $\dfrac{\binom{8}{0} + \binom{8}{1} + \binom{8}{2}}{2^8} = \dfrac{1 + 8 + 28}{256} = \dfrac{37}{256}.$

28. $\dfrac{\binom{8}{3} + \binom{8}{4} + \binom{8}{5}}{2^8} = \dfrac{56 + 70 + 56}{256} = \dfrac{182}{256} = \dfrac{91}{128}.$ **29.** $\dfrac{\binom{50}{11}}{\binom{52}{13}} = \dfrac{13 \cdot 12}{52 \cdot 51} = \dfrac{1}{17}.$

30.

n	5	6	7	8	9
d_n	44	265	1854	14833	133496

31. (a) 9!. (b) $d_9 = 133496.$ (c) $10 \cdot 10!$ or $11! - 10!.$ (d) $11! - 2 \cdot 10! + 9!.$

SECTION 6.1

1.

v	a	b	c	d	e
indg(v)	2	2	1	3	2

3. (i) 10. (ii) 10. (iii) 10.

5. (i) $(a, b, c), (a, b, d), (a, e, b).$ (ii) Each is simple and elementary. No one is eulerian or hamiltonian.

7. (i) $(a, e, b, c, d).$ (ii) Yes. Its vertices are all the vertices in V.

9. (i) $(b, c, d, a, e, b).$ (ii) No. Its edges are only 5 of the 8 edges of E.

(iii) Yes. The only repetition of vertices is that the initial one is also the final one.

11. (i) $(a, b, c, d, e, b, d, a, e).$ (ii) Yes. Its edges are all the edges in E.

13. Yes. See the proof of Theorem 2, "Shortest Paths Are Elementary."

15. The length must be $n - 1$ because a hamiltonian path must have all n vertices with no repetitions.

17. (a) The edge (v_0, v_1) contributes 1 to $\text{outdg}(v_0)$. For every i with $0 < i < s$ such that $v_i = v_0$, (v_{i-1}, v_i) contributes 1 to $\text{outdg}(v_0)$ and (v_i, v_{i+1}) contributes 1 to $\text{indg}(v_0)$.

(b) and (c) are similar.

19. (a) 0, 1, 2, 3, 4   (b) 0, 1, 2, 3, 4, 5, 6, 7, or 8.   **21.**

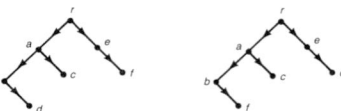

23. $v_{k-1} = v_{s-1}$, since each is a vertex x with (x, v_s) an edge and we have $\text{indg}(v_s) \le 1$. Similarly, $v_{k-2} = v_{s-2}$, and so on. (A formal proof would use induction on k.)

25. Yes. The only repetition of vertices is that of the initial one being the final one.

27. For an edge (v, w) to be in E, there are n choices for v and n choices for w and so at most n^2 edges.

29. For every v in V, (v) is a path (of length 0) from v to v. Hence vPv for all v in V, and P is reflexive. If aPb and bPc, there is a path $(x_0, x_1, \ldots, x_s)$ from a to b and a path $(y_0, y_1, \ldots, y_t)$ from b to c; then $(x_0, \ldots, x_s, y_1, \ldots, y_t)$ is a path from a to c. Hence $(aPb) \wedge (bPc) \Rightarrow (aPc)$, and P is transitive.

31. $\text{indg}(v)$ in $\langle V, E \rangle$ equals $\text{outdg}(v)$ in $\langle V, F \rangle$, and $\text{outdg}(v)$ in $\langle V, E \rangle$ equals $\text{indg}(v)$ in $\langle V, F \rangle$, for each v in V.

33. Since $\#V \ge 1$, there is a vertex v_0 in V. Since $\text{outdg}(v_0) \ge 1$, there is a vertex v_1 such that $v_0 E v_1$. Similarly, there is a vertex v_2 with $v_1 E v_2$. Continuing this way (that is, using an inductive definition) one obtains a sequence $v_0, v_1, v_2, \ldots$ such that $v_{i-1} E v_i$ for each i in $\mathbf{Z}^+$. Since V is finite there must be repetitions in this sequence; that is, $v_j = v_k$ with $j < k$. Then $(v_j, v_{j+1}, \ldots, v_k)$ is a circuit in D.

35. (a) $\dbinom{n}{2} = \dfrac{n(n-1)}{2}$.

SECTION 6.2

1. (a) No. See Part (c) of Definition 1 ("Rooted Tree, Root").   (b) $n - 1$.

3.

v	r	a	b	c	d	e	f
level of v	0	1	2	2	3	1	2

5. 3.   **7.** (a)   (b)

9. Each vertex in a binary tree has 0, 1, or 2 children. Hence the maximum number of children for a vertex in the left, or right, subtree is 0, 1, or 2.

11. (a) The level of each vertex is one less in T_f, or in T_g, than in T. Hence in T_f or in T_g no vertex has level more than $h - 1$.

(b) There is a vertex v with level h in T. This v is in T_f or in T_g and has level $h - 1$ in the subtree, thus giving the subtree a height of $h - 1$.

13. (i) 1;   (ii) 3;   (iii) 7;   (iv) 15;   (v) 31;   (vi) $2^{h+1} - 1$.

15. Each edge in E is in one and only one of the subsets.

17. A circuit is a path $P = (v_0, v_1, \ldots, v_s)$ with $s \ge 1$ and $v_0 = v_s$. If such a circuit existed in a tree, (v_0) and P would be distinct paths from v_0 to v_0. Since this would contradict Lemma 4 ("Uniqueness of Paths"), a tree has no circuits.

19. (i) There is one vertex of level 0, two vertices of level 1, four vertices of level 2, and eight vertices of level 3.

(ii) $1 \cdot 0 + 2 \cdot 1 + 4 \cdot 2 + 8 \cdot 3 = 2 + 8 + 24 = 34$.   (iii) $\frac{34}{15}$.

21. $(2 \cdot 1 + 4 \cdot 2 + 8 \cdot 3 + \cdots + 2^h \cdot h)/(2^{h+1} - 1)$.

23.   (i) By definition of rooted tree, $\text{indg}(r) = 0$ and $\text{indg}(v) = 1$ for $v \neq r$.
     (ii) Each edge in E contributes 1 to the sum of the indegrees in Part (i).

SECTION 6.3

1.   **Basis**   If T has height 0, the preorder listing for V is $\{r\}$.   **3.** $\{c, a, g, k, d, h, r, e, b, i, f, j\}$.
5.   (i) 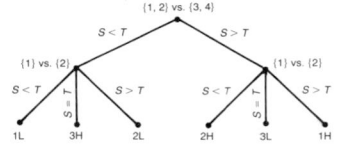   (ii) $abc \div -d + e*$.   **7.**   (c) and (d) are MRPE's.   **9.** $xyz \triangle \square, xy \triangle z \square$.

11. $x_1 x_2 x_3 x_4 b_1 b_2 b_3, x_1 x_2 x_3 b_1 x_4 b_2 b_3, x_1 x_2 x_3 b_1 b_2 x_4 b_3, x_1 x_2 b_1 x_3 x_4 b_2 b_3, x_1 x_2 b_1 x_3 b_2 x_4 b_3$.
13.   (a) $Q_1 = 1$;   (b) $Q_2 = 2$;   (c) $Q_3 = 5$.

15.

vertex	4	2	6	1	3	5	7
level	0	1	1	2	2	2	2
number of comparisons	1	2	2	3	3	3	3

Average number of comparisons is $\frac{17}{7}$.

17.   ("1L" means that 1 is the bad coin and is too light, "3H" means that 3 is the bad coin and is too heavy, and so on.)

19.

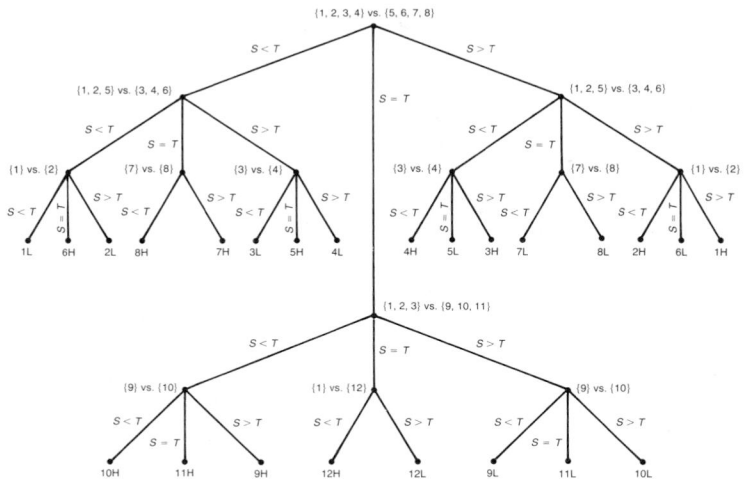

("1L" means that 1 is too light, "6H" means that 6 is too heavy, and so on.)
21.   (a) 14;   (b) 42.

SECTION 6.4

1. (a) Yes, since $V \subseteq V$ and $E_1 \subseteq E$.   (b) Yes, since D_1 has all the vertices of D.
(c) Yes, since each vertex in V is involved in some edge in E_1.

3. $\langle V_2, E_2 \rangle$, where $E_2 = \{(2, 3), (4, 2)\}$ and $V_2 = \{2, 3, 4\}$.

5. (i) $\{(2, 3), (3, 4), (4, 2)\}$.   (ii) $\langle V_2, E_2 \rangle$, where $E_2 = \{(2, 1)\}$ and $V_2 = \{1, 2\}$.

7. $\# V_1 = n$ because $V_1 = V$. (See Definition 1.)   **9.** $V' = \{a, b, c, d\}$ and $E' = \{(b, a), (b, c), (c, d), (d, b)\}$.

11.

E	1	2	3	4
1	0	0	0	0
2	1	0	1	0
3	0	0	0	1
4	0	1	0	0

13. Yes. Since $(v_0, v_1, \ldots, v_s)$ is a path, it follows that $E_1 \subseteq E$; also, the vertices of D_1 are all the vertices of D because the path is hamiltonian.

15. (a) $\alpha: 1 \mapsto b, \quad 2 \mapsto d, \quad 3 \mapsto a, \quad 4 \mapsto c$.   (b) $\gamma: 1 \mapsto 4, \quad 2 \mapsto 1, \quad 3 \mapsto 2, \quad 4 \mapsto 3$.   (c) $4! = 24$.
(d) Four. There are four choices for the image of 1 and each such choice determines a unique isomorphism.

17. (a) Yes. Let $\text{indg}(v) = s$ and $\text{indg}(\beta(v)) = t$. Let $x_1, x_2, \ldots, x_s$ be the s vertices u such that uEv, and let $y_1, y_2, \ldots, y_t$ be the t vertices w such that $wE'\beta(v)$. By Definition 6 ("Isomorphic Digraphs"), $\beta(x_i)E'\beta(v)$ for $i = 1, \ldots, s$; and these $\beta(x_i)$ are distinct because β is injective. Hence the s $\beta(x_i)$ are among the y_j, and so $s \leq t$. Since β is surjective, there exist t vertices z_j in V such that $\beta(z_j) = y_j$ for $j = 1, \ldots, t$. Then $\beta(z_j)E'\beta(v)$ implies z_jEv. Hence the z_j are among the x_i, and $t \leq s$. This and $s \leq t$ give us $s = t$, as desired.
(b) Yes. If $(x_0, x_1, \ldots, x_s)$ is a path from v to w in D, then $(\beta(x_0), \beta(x_1), \ldots, \beta(x_s))$ is a path from $\beta(v)$ to $\beta(w)$ in D'.

19. No. Using Problems 17(a) and 18, together with the two tables below, one sees that an isomorphism β from D_1 onto D_2 would have $\beta(1) = a$ and $\beta(4) = c$. Since $(1, 4)$ is an edge of D_1 but (a, c) is not an edge of D_2, such a β is not an isomorphism.

v	1	2	3	4
indg(v)	0	1	1	2
outdg(v)	2	1	1	0

v	a	b	c	d
indg(v)	0	1	2	1
outdg(v)	2	1	0	1

21. (i) $\{(1, 3), (2, 4), (3, 5), (4, 2), (5, 1)\}$.   (ii)

(iii) $\text{indg}(v) = 1 = \text{outdg}(v)$ for each vertex v.

23. Yes; each v has a unique image $f(v)$.

25. Yes; $\text{indg}(v) \geq 1$ means that there exists at least one u in V with $f(u) = v$; this being true for all v in V is equivalent to f being surjective.

27. Yes. Let f be the mapping from V to V for which $f(v)$ is the unique w in V with vEw.

29. This follows when the result in Problem 23 of Section 6.1 is applied to the digraph D_f [since $\text{indg}(v) = 1$ for all v in V in this digraph].

SECTION 6.5

1. E is a set of pairs each of which is in $P(V)$. That is, $E \subseteq P(V)$.   **3.**   5.

5. (b, a, c, d, b, c) or (b, a, c, b, d, c) or (b, c, a, b, d, c) or (b, c, d, b, a, c) or (b, d, c, a, b, c) or (b, d, c, b, a, c).

7. (d, b, a, c, d) or (d, c, a, b, d).   **9.** $\{\{a, b\}, \{a, c\}, \{b, c\}\}$.   **11.**   (a) Yes.   (b) Yes.   (c) Yes.

13. (a) No. In Definition 5, R must be irreflexive and antisymmetric. Antisymmetry, vRw, and wRv imply that $v = w$, which contradicts irreflexivity.
(b) Yes. See Definition 5.

15. Each edge $\{v, w\}$ in E contributes 2 [1 to dg(v) and 1 to dg(w)] to the sum of the degrees.

17. (i) indg(r) = 0 and indg(v) = 1 for each vertex $v \neq r$.
(ii) The sum of the outdegrees equals the sum of the indegrees.
(iii) $\#E$ equals the sum of the indegrees (or of the outdegrees).

19. See Theorem 2, "Characterization of Trees."

21. (a)   (b)   (c)   (d)

23. (a) The edge $\{v_0, v_1\}$ contributes 1 to dg(v_0), and each v_i that equals v_0, with $0 < i < n$, contributes 2 to dg(v_0) (1 from $\{v_{i-1}, v_i\}$ and 1 from $\{v_i, v_{i+1}\}$). This shows that dg(v_0) is odd. Similarly for dg(v_n).
(b) For each j such that $v_j = v_i$, there is a contribution of 2 to dg(v_i) (1 from $\{v_{j-1}, v_j\}$ and 1 from $\{v_j, v_{j+1}\}$).

25. Yes. The only vertices with odd degree are b and c. Problem 23 tells us that these must be the initial and final vertices.

27. (a) $V_1 = \{a, b, c\}$, $E_1 = \{\{a, b\}, \{a, c\}, \{b, c\}\}$.   (b) $V_2 = \{d, e\}$, $E_2 = \{\{d, e\}\}$.   (c) $V_3 = \{f\}$, $E_3 = \varnothing$.
(d) Yes.   (e) Yes.

29. (i)

E_1	a	b	c
a	0	1	1
b	1	0	1
c	1	1	0

(ii)

	5	6	7
5	0	1	1
6	1	0	1
7	1	1	0

(iii) Yes. The bijection $\beta: a \mapsto 5$, $b \mapsto 6$, $c \mapsto 7$ converts the table of Part (i) into the table of Part (ii). Hence β is an isomorphism between G_1 and H.

31. For each pair $\{v, w\}$ in $E_1 \cup E_2$, both v and w are in V_1 or in V_2 and so both are in $V_1 \cup V_2$.

33. Let $v_0 \in V$. Since dg(v_0) ≥ 1, there is a vertex v_1 in V such that $\{v_0, v_1\} \in E$. Since dg(v_1) ≥ 2, there is a vertex v_2 with $v_2 \neq v_0$ and $\{v_1, v_2\} \in E$. Similarly there is a v_3 with $v_3 \neq v_1$ and $\{v_2, v_3\} \in E$. Continuing this way, we obtain a sequence $v_0, v_1, v_2, \ldots$. Since V is finite, this sequence must have repetitions. Let j be the smallest integer with $v_j = v_i$ and $i < j$. Then $(v_i, v_{i+1}, \ldots, v_j)$ is a cycle in G.

SECTION 6.6

1. $g: 1 \mapsto a, \ 2 \mapsto b, \ 3 \mapsto c, \ 4 \mapsto e$.   **3.**   The cycle (a, d, b, c, a) gives 1690 as the minimal sum.

5. (a) $\binom{6}{2} = \dfrac{6 \cdot 5}{2} = 15$.   (b) $5 \cdot 4 = 20$.
(c) Let $K_n = (V, E)$. If $v, w \in V$ and $v \neq w$, then $\{v, w\} \in E$, and so (v, w) is a path joining v and w. If $v = w$, then (v) is such a path.

7. (i) $n - 1$.   (ii) 1.   (iii) $\#V - \#E + \#F = n - (n - 1) + 1 = 2$.

9. $f_1: a \mapsto a, \;\; b \mapsto b, \;\; c \mapsto c;$ $f_2: a \mapsto b, \;\; b \mapsto c, \;\; c \mapsto a;$ $f_3: a \mapsto c, \;\; b \mapsto a, \;\; c \mapsto b;$ $f_4: a \mapsto a, \;\; b \mapsto c, \;\; c \mapsto b;$ $f_5: a \mapsto c, \;\; b \mapsto b, \;\; c \mapsto a;$ $f_6: a \mapsto b, \;\; b \mapsto a, \;\; c \mapsto c$.

11.

x	$f_1(x)$	$f_2(x)$	$f_3(x)$	$f_4(x)$	$f_5(x)$	$f_6(x)$	$f_7(x)$	$f_8(x)$
h	h	h	k	k	v	v	w	w
k	k	k	h	h	w	w	v	v
v	v	w	v	w	h	k	h	k
w	w	v	w	v	k	h	k	h

13. $\#F = 12$.   **15.** $\#F = 14$.   **17.** Yes, a graph with three components, each isomorphic to (V, E).

19. Yes. To show this, one can rewrite the proof of Theorem 4 up to Display (3) and use $\deg(f) \geq 4$ for some f to change Display (3) to $3(\#F) < s$.

21. If the cycle starts at a vertex in A, it has the form $(a_1, b_1, a_2, b_2, \ldots, a_h, b_h, a_1)$, with the a_i in A and the b_j in B; thus it has length $2h$. If the cycle starts at a vertex in B, the reasoning is similar.

23. Removing some vertices and some edges from a planar picture does not introduce any intersections at nonvertices.

25. No. This follows from Problem 23 and the fact that $K_{3,3}$ can be considered to be a nonplanar subgraph of $K_{3,4}$.

27. (a) No; $\#E = 24$ and $\#F = 17$ would contradict the inequality $3(\#F)/2 \leq \#E$ of Theorem 4, "Inequalities for a Planar Graph."

(b) No; this would contradict the inequality $\#E \leq 3(\#V) - 6$ of Theorem 4.

29. By Theorem 2, $\#F = \#E - \#V + 2$. Using the inequality $\#E \leq 3(\#V) - 6$ of Theorem 4, this becomes $\#F \leq 3(\#V) - 6 - \#V + 2 = 2(\#V) - 4$.

REVIEW PROBLEMS FOR CHAPTER 6

1. (a)

v	a	b	c	d
indg(v)	1	2	2	1
outdg(v)	2	1	1	2

(b)

	a	b	c	d
a	0	0	1	1
b	1	0	0	0
c	0	1	0	0
d	0	1	1	0

2. (a) (d, c, b, a).   (b) (d, c, b, a, d, b).   **3.** Yes: (a, d, c, b, a), for example.   **4.** No.

5. (a) $\{a, b, c, d, e, f, g, h, i, j\}$.   (b) $\{c, b, e, d, a, g, i, h, j, f\}$.   (c) $\{c, e, d, b, i, j, h, g, f, a\}$.

6. (a)

vertex	a	b	c	d	e	f	g	h	i	j
level	0	1	2	2	3	1	2	3	4	4

(b) 4.   (c) c, e, i, and j.

7. (a) 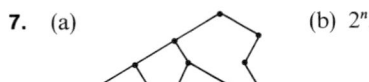   (b) 2^n.

8. (a) $1 + n + n^2 + \cdots + n^h = (n^{h+1} - 1)/(n - 1)$. (b) $n + 2n^2 + 3n^3 + \cdots + hn^h$.

9. (a) 99. (b) 99. **10.** $[a * (b \div c)] + (d - e)$. **11.** 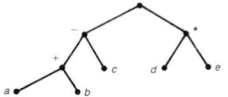 **12.** $ab + c - de* \div$.

13. (a) No; the subword $ab + *$ does not have more symbols from X than from B.

    (b) Yes; it meets the conditions of the definition of an MRPE (Definition 3 of Section 6.3).

14. $-\frac{1}{5}$.

15. (a) $\{(a, b), (b, d), (d, a), (d, e), (e, a)\}$. (b) $\{a, b, c, d, e,\}$.

    (c) $V_3 = \{a, b, c, d, e\}$, $E_3 = \{(a, b), (b, c), (c, d), (d, e)\}$.

16. (i)

D	1	2	3	4
1	0	1	1	0
2	0	0	1	0
3	0	0	0	1
4	0	0	0	0

D'	a	b	c	d
a	0	1	1	0
b	0	0	1	0
c	0	0	0	1
d	0	0	0	0

    (ii) Yes. The replacements of the bijection β: $1 \mapsto a$, $2 \mapsto b$, $3 \mapsto c$, $4 \mapsto d$ convert the table for D into the table for D'.

17. (i) $\{(a, d), (b, a), (c, e), (d, b), (e, c)\}$. (ii)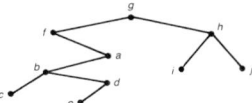

18.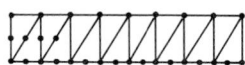

19.

20. $\{\{b, c\}, \{b, d\}, \{c, d\}\}$.

21. The graph of Problem 20 with just one of the arcs $\{b, c\}$, $\{b, d\}$, or $\{c, d\}$ removed.

22.

23. (a) $7! = 5040$. (b) $8! \cdot 9!$. (c) $(10!)^2 \cdot 2$.

24. (i) vRv for all v in V since (v) is a path. vRw implies wRv, since a path between v and w in a graph reverses into a path between w and v. Also, uRv and vRw imply uRw, since a path $(u, \ldots, v)$ and a path $(v, \ldots, w)$ can be placed together to get a path $(u, \ldots, v, \ldots, w)$.

    (ii) $C(x)$ is the set of vertices of the component containing x.

25. (a) Yes. (b) Yes.

26. No; this fails the inequality $\#E \leq 3(\#V) - 6$ of Theorem 4, Section 6.6 ("Inequalities for a Planar Graph").

27. Yes, as the figure shows.

28. (a) T. (b) T. (c) F. (d) F. (e) T. (f) T. (g) T. (h) T. (i) F. (j) T.

    (k) T. (l) T. (m) F.

SECTION 7.1

1. The set Z of all the integers, or the set Q of all the rational numbers, or the set R of all the real numbers, or the set C of all the complex numbers.

3. No; the integer 1, for example, has no inverse under $+$ in N.　　**5.** $\#B_2 = 2^2 = 4.$

7. Yes; $x^m \square x^n = x^{m+n} = x^{n+m} = x^n \square x^m$ because addition of integers is commutative.

9. (ii)

·	1	v	v^2	v^3	v^4	v^5
1	1	v	v^2	v^3	v^4	v^5
v	v	v^2	v^3	v^4	v^5	1
v^2	v^2	v^3	v^4	v^5	1	v
v^3	v^3	v^4	v^5	1	v	v^2
v^4	v^4	v^5	1	v	v^2	v^3
v^5	v^5	1	v	v^2	v^3	v^4

(iii)

x	1	v	v^2	v^3	v^4	v^5
x^{-1}	1	v^5	v^4	v^3	v^2	v

(iv) The table of Part (ii) shows that $\cdot$ is an operation on U_6. The operation of complex-number multiplication is associative. The table in Part (ii) shows that 1 is the identity. The table in Part (iii) shows that each number in U_6 has an inverse under $\cdot$ in U_6. Thus $\langle U_6, \cdot, 1 \rangle$ satisfies the axioms for groups.

(v) $[1] = \{1\}, [v] = U_6 = [v^5], [v^2] = \{1, v^2, v^4\} = [v^4], [v^3] = \{1, v^3\}.$

x	1	v	v^2	v^3	v^4	v^5
Order of x	1	6	3	2	3	6

(vi) Yes; each of v and v^5 is a generator.

(vii) Yes; see Problem 8.　　(viii) Yes.　　(ix)

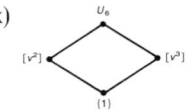

11. (a) No; $001 \oplus 001 = 000$ is not in Y.　　(b) Yes.　　(c) No; $001 \oplus 010 = 011$ is not in Y.　　(d) Yes.

13. (b) and (d).

15. (a) $x = a^{-1} \square b.$

(b) $(a \square b) \square (b^{-1} \square a^{-1}) = a \square (b \square b^{-1}) \square a^{-1} = a \square e \square a^{-1} = a \square a^{-1} = e.$ Then Theorem 1(a) ("Unique Inverse") and $(a \square b) \square (b^{-1} \square a^{-1}) = e$ imply that $(a \square b)^{-1} = b^{-1} \square a^{-1}.$

(c) The group of Example 6. Let $a = f_4$ and $b = f_5.$

17. Since $01 \oplus 10 = 11$, if 01 and 10 are in a Y closed under $\oplus$, so is 11. Since $10 \oplus 11 = 01$, 01 must be in Y when 10 and 11 are in Y. Similarly, 10 is in Y when 01 and 11 are in Y.

19. (i)

$\square$	e	b	c
e	e	b	c
b	b	c	e
c	c	e	b

(ii) $[b] = \{e, b, c\}$; b has order 3.　　(iii) $[c] = [b]$; c has order 3.

(iv) Yes.　　(v) Yes; this follows from the table in Part (i).

21. Since $[g^3] = \{e, g^3, g^6, g^9, g^{12}\}$, it follows that $\langle [g^3], \square, e \rangle$ is a subgroup of order 5 in G.

23. (i) $[e] = \{e\}$, (ii) $[g^8] = \{e, g^8\}$, (iii) $[g^4] = \{e, g^4, g^8, g^{12}\}$,
(iv) $[g^2] = \{e, g^2, g^4, g^6, g^8, g^{10}, g^{12}, g^{14}\}$, (v) $[g]$.

25. (a) $(a \,\square\, b)^2 = (a \,\square\, b) \,\square\, (a \,\square\, b) = a \,\square\, b \,\square\, a \,\square\, b$, by associativity.
(b) $(a \,\square\, b)^2 = a \,\square\, b \,\square\, a \,\square\, b = a \,\square\, a \,\square\, b \,\square\, b = a^2 \,\square\, b^2$ when G is abelian.

27. (i) $[f_1] = \{f_1\}$, $[f_2] = \{f_1, f_2, f_3\} = [f_3]$, $[f_4] = \{f_1, f_4\}$, $[f_5] = \{f_1, f_5\}$, $[f_6] = \{f_1, f_6\}$.

(ii) There is no x with $[x] = X$. (iii)

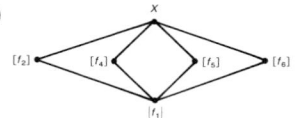

29. One example is $Y = \{0, 2, 4, \ldots\}$.

31. (i) Yes. (ii) No; 5 has no inverse in Y. (iii) No, as one sees in Part (ii).

33. (i) If $c \,\square\, x = c \,\square\, y$, then $x = y$, by left cancellation.
(ii) For every y in X, $f(c^{-1} \,\square\, y) = c \,\square\, c^{-1} \,\square\, y = y$ shows that y is an image under f.
(iii) The mapping f is a bijective mapping from X onto itself.

35. $a^r \div a^s = a^{r-s}$ is in $[a]$ for all r and s in $\mathbf{Z}$, since $\mathbf{Z}$ is closed under subtraction.

37. If $a \,\square\, b = b \,\square\, a$, then $(a \,\square\, b)^{-1} = (b \,\square\, a)^{-1} = a^{-1} \,\square\, b^{-1}$, by Problem 15(b). If $(a \,\square\, b)^{-1} = a^{-1} \,\square\, b^{-1}$,
then $b^{-1} \,\square\, a^{-1} = a^{-1} \,\square\, b^{-1}$, by Problem 15(b). Then

$$(b^{-1} \,\square\, a^{-1})^{-1} = (a^{-1} \,\square\, b^{-1})^{-1},$$
$$(a^{-1})^{-1} \,\square\, (b^{-1})^{-1} = (b^{-1})^{-1} \,\square\, (a^{-1})^{-1},$$
$$a \,\square\, b = b \,\square\, a.$$

39. One can show that Definition 1, "Group," (or 1', "Alternate Definition of Group") is satisfied.

41. Yes; we prove the contrapositive easily as follows: $(a = b) \Rightarrow (a \,\square\, c = b \,\square\, c)$.

43. One can show that $\langle I, \square, e \rangle$ satisfies Definition 4, "Subgroup in a Group."

SECTION 7.2

1. (a)

(b) $(1, 5, 6), (2, 4, 8), (3, 3, 3), (4, 8, 7), (5, 6, 1), (6, 1, 5), (7, 2, 4), (8, 7, 2)$.

(c) $f^2 = \begin{pmatrix} 1 & 2 & 3 & 4 & 5 & 6 & 7 & 8 \\ 6 & 8 & 3 & 7 & 1 & 5 & 4 & 2 \end{pmatrix}$.

3. (i) $1 \overset{f}{\mapsto} 2 \overset{g}{\mapsto} 3$, $2 \overset{f}{\mapsto} 1 \overset{g}{\mapsto} 2$, $3 \overset{f}{\mapsto} 4 \overset{g}{\mapsto} 1$, $4 \overset{f}{\mapsto} 3 \overset{g}{\mapsto} 4$, so fg is
$h: 1 \mapsto 3$, $2 \mapsto 2$, $3 \mapsto 1$, $4 \mapsto 4$.

(ii) $\begin{pmatrix} 1 & 2 & 3 & 4 \\ 2 & 1 & 4 & 3 \end{pmatrix} \begin{pmatrix} 2 & 1 & 4 & 3 \\ 3 & 2 & 1 & 4 \end{pmatrix} = \begin{pmatrix} 1 & 2 & 3 & 4 \\ 3 & 2 & 1 & 4 \end{pmatrix}$.

5. (i) (ii) Reverse all arrowheads.

7. (i) $f^2: 1 \mapsto 1$, $2 \mapsto 2$, $3 \mapsto 3$, $4 \mapsto 4$; (ii) $f^3 = f$; (iii) $f^4 = f^2$; (iv) $f^{99} = f$; (v) $f^{100} = f^2$.

9.   (i)   (ii)   (iii)   (iv)

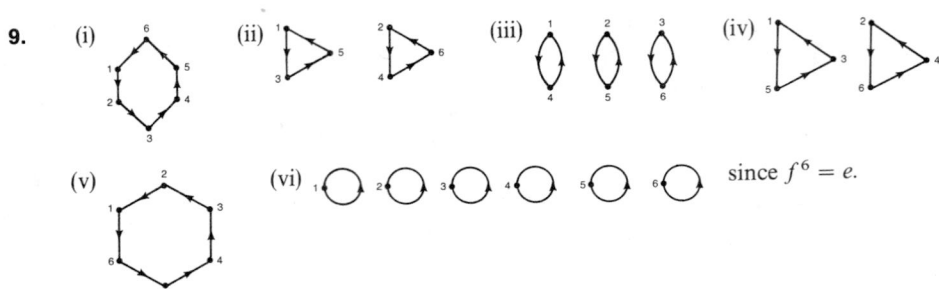

(v)   (vi)   since $f^6 = e$.

(vii) Same as Part (i), since $f^7 = f^6 f = ef = f$.

(viii) Same as Part (iv), since $f^{100} = (f^6)^{16} f^4 = e^{16} f^4 = f^4$.

11.   (a) $h(000) = h(001 \oplus 001) = h(001) \oplus h(001) = 11 \cdot \oplus 11 = 00$.

(b) $h(011) = h(001 \oplus 010) = h(001) \oplus h(010) = 11 \oplus 01 = 10$.

13.   No; if h is a homomorphism with $h(01) = 100$ and $h(10) = 010$, then $h(11) = h(01 \oplus 10) = h(01) \oplus h(10) = 100 \oplus 010 = 110$.

15.   (a) f is a homomorphism because $f(m + n) = 2(m + n) = 2m + 2n = f(m) + f(n)$.

(b) g is not a homomorphism; for example, $g(1) = 1$, $g(2) = 4$, and $g(3) = 9$ and hence $g(1 + 2) \neq g(1) + g(2)$.

17.   (i) $r^2: 1 \mapsto 3, \quad 2 \mapsto 1, \quad 3 \mapsto 2; \qquad rf: 1 \mapsto 3, \quad 2 \mapsto 2, \quad 3 \mapsto 1; \qquad r^2 f: 1 \mapsto 2, \quad 2 \mapsto 1, \quad 3 \mapsto 3$.

(ii) Yes.   (iii)

$\circ$	e	r	r^2	f	rf	$r^2 f$
e	e	r	r^2	f	rf	$r^2 f$
r	r	r^2	e	rf	$r^2 f$	f
r^2	r^2	e	r	$r^2 f$	f	rf
f	f	$r^2 f$	rf	e	r^2	r
rf	rf	f	$r^2 f$	r	e	r^2
$r^2 f$	$r^2 f$	rf	f	r^2	r	e

(iv) $[e] = \{e\}$, $[r^2] = \{e, r, r^2\}$, $[rf] = \{e, rf\}$.

19. $Y = \{e, f, f^2, f^3\}$. One can use $f^4 = e$ to see that $\langle Y, \circ, e \rangle$ is a subgroup in S_4.

21.   (a) The permutation α is bijective and the substitutions described in Algorithm 2 convert the table for G into the table for G'.

(b) $\mathbf{i} \cdot \mathbf{i} = -1$, but $\beta(\mathbf{i})\beta(\mathbf{i}) \neq \beta(-1)$ because $\beta(\mathbf{i})\beta(\mathbf{i}) = f^2 f^2 = e$ and $\beta(-1) = f^3$. Thus β is not a homomorphism and so is not an isomorphism.

23.   (i) $e \,\square\, a = a$ because e is the identity. Then $e \neq a$ implies that $e \,\square\, a \neq a \,\square\, a$, using the contrapositive of Theorem 7 of Section 7.1 ("Left or Right Cancellation"). Thus $a \,\square\, a \neq a$, and so $a \,\square\, a$ is the only other element e of X.

(ii)

$\square$	e	a
e	e	a
a	a	e

$\triangle$	e'	b
e'	e'	b
b	b	e'

(iii) This follows from Algorithm 2 ("Proving a Group Isomorphism") and the tables of Part (ii).

25.   (i) There are only a finite number of elements in T_n.

(ii) If $a_i = a_j$ with $1 < i < j$, then $f(a_{i-1}) = a_i = a_j = f(a_{j-1})$. This and the fact that f is injective imply that $a_{i-1} = a_{j-1}$. This contradicts the minimal nature of j. To avoid the contradiction, one must have $i = 1$.

27. $A_1 = \{e\}$, $A_2 = \{e, r, r^2\}$, $A_3 = \{e, f\}$, $A_4 = \{e, rf\}$, $A_5 = \{e, r^2f\}$, $A_6 = \{e, r, r^2, f, rf, r^2f\}$.

29. Let x have order r in G and $\beta(x)$ have order s in G'. Then $x^r = e$, $x^n \neq e$ for $0 < n < r$, $[\beta(x)]^s = e'$, and $[\beta(x)]^n \neq e'$ for $0 < n < s$. Theorem 5 ("Properties of Group Isomorphisms") tells us that $\beta(e) = e'$ and $\beta(x^n) = [\beta(x)]^n$ for all n in **Z**. Hence $\beta(x^s) = [\beta(x)]^s = e'$. Now, $\beta(x^s) = e'$ and $\beta(e) = e'$ [given by Theorem 5(a)] and the fact that β is a bijection imply that $x^s = e$. Since $x^n \neq e$ for $0 < n < r$, this implies that $r \leq s$. Also, $e' = \beta(e) = \beta(x^r) = [\beta(x)]^r$ implies that $s \leq r$. Then $r \leq s$ and $s \leq r$ force r and s to be equal.

31. The mapping

$$\beta: [a] \to [b]; \quad a^i \mapsto b^i \qquad \text{for } i = 0, 1, 2, 3, 4$$

is an isomorphism because it is a bijection and $\beta(a^i \square a^j) = \beta(a^{i+j}) = b^{i+j} = b^i \triangle b^j = \beta(a^i) \triangle \beta(a^j)$.

33. Let $\beta: [a] \to Y$ be an isomorphism from G onto G'. Then each element of the carrier $[a]$ of G is of the form a^n with n in **Z**. The images $\beta(a^n)$ make up all of Y, since β is surjective. But $\beta(a^n) = (\beta(a))^n$ by Part (c) of Theorem 5 ("Properties of Group Isomorphisms"). Hence Y consists of the integral powers of $\beta(a)$, and so $G' = \langle [\beta(a)], \triangle, e' \rangle$ is cyclic.

SECTION 7.3

1. $(1\ 9\ 7\ 3\ 5)(2\ 8)(4)(6)$ or $(1\ 9\ 7\ 3\ 5)(2\ 8)$.

3. (i) $(1\ 3)(2\ 4)$; (ii) $(1\ 4\ 3\ 2)$; (iii) (1); (iv) $(1\ 4)(2\ 3)$; (v) $(1\ 3)$.

5. (i) $(1\ 4)(2\ 3)$; (ii) $(2\ 4\ 3)$; (iii) $(1\ 4\ 2)$; (iv) $(1\ 3\ 4)$; (v) $(1\ 3\ 2)$; (vi) $(1\ 4\ 3)$; (vii) $(2\ 3\ 4)$; (viii) $(1\ 2\ 4)$.

7. Problem 6(a) shows that $y^{-1} = y \in Y$ for each y in Y. The table shows that Y is closed under $\circ$. So $\langle Y, \circ, (1) \rangle$ is a subgroup in S_4, by Definition 4 of Section 7.1.

$\circ$	(1)	b	c	d
(1)	(1)	b	c	d
b	b	(1)	d	c
c	c	d	(1)	b
d	d	c	b	(1)

9. (i) $(1\ 3\ 5\ 7)(2\ 4\ 6\ 8)$; (ii) $(1\ 4\ 7\ 2\ 5\ 8\ 3\ 6)$; (iii) $(1\ 5)(2\ 6)(3\ 7)(4\ 8)$; (iv) $(1\ 6\ 3\ 8\ 5\ 2\ 7\ 4)$.

11. (a) The smallest m in $\mathbf{Z}^+$ with $(h^2)^m = (1)$ is $m = 4$. Hence the cyclic subgroup generated by h^2 in S_8 has $\{(1), h^2, (h^2)^2, (h^2)^3\}$ as its carrier.
(b) $[h^4] = \{(1), h^4\}$. **13.** (i) $(1\ 2\ 3)$. (ii) $(1\ 2\ 3\ 4)$. (iii) $(1\ 2\ 3\ 4\ 5)$.

15. $(1\ 6)(2\ 6)(3\ 6)(4\ 6)(5\ 6)$. **17.** Yes. Using Theorem 1 ("Disjoint Cycles Commute"), $f(gh) = (gh)f$.

19. (i) Since f and g are disjoint cycles, no b_j is an a_i, and so $f(b_j) = b_j$ by the definition of a cycle.

(ii) $b_j \overset{f}{\mapsto} b_j \overset{g}{\mapsto} b_{j+1} \Rightarrow b_j \overset{h}{\mapsto} b_{j+1}$ for $j = 1, 2, \ldots, s-1$;

$b_j \overset{g}{\mapsto} b_{j+1} \overset{f}{\mapsto} b_{j+1} \Rightarrow b_j \overset{k}{\mapsto} b_{j+1}$ for $1 \leq j < s$;

$b_s \overset{f}{\mapsto} b_s \overset{g}{\mapsto} b_1 \Rightarrow b_s \overset{h}{\mapsto} b_1$;

$b_s \overset{g}{\mapsto} b_1 \overset{f}{\mapsto} b_1 \Rightarrow b_s \overset{k}{\mapsto} b_1$.

21. $uv = (2\ 3)$, $(uv)^2 = (1)$, $u^2 = (1\ 3\ 2)$, $v^2 = (1)$, $u^2v^2 = (1\ 3\ 2)$. Hence $(uv)^2 \neq u^2v^2$.

23. The least common multiple of r and s.

25. (a) (1), $(1\ 2)$. (b) $(1\ 2)$, $(1\ 3)$, $(2\ 3)$. (c) $(1\ 2\ 3)$, $(1\ 3\ 2)$.

27. (1), $(a\ b)$, $(a\ b\ c)$, $(a\ b\ c\ d)$, $(a\ b)(c\ d)$, $(a\ b\ c\ d\ e)$, $(a\ b\ c)(d\ e)$, $(a\ b)(c\ d\ e)$.

29.

g	e	a	a^2	a^3	a^4	a^5	a^6	a^7	a^8	a^9
Order of g	1	10	5	10	5	2	5	10	5	10

31. (i) The permutations p and q are even because each is a product of an even number of transpositions.
(ii) $pq^{-1} = (t_1 t_2 \cdots t_{2h})(u_1 u_2 \cdots u_{2k})^{-1} = t_1 t_2 \cdots t_{2h} u_{2k}^{-1} \cdots u_2^{-1} u_1^{-1} = t_1 t_2 \cdots t_{2h} u_{2k} \cdots u_2 u_1$ because a transposition is its own inverse. Thus pq^{-1} is the product of $2(h+k)$ transpositions and so is an even permutation.

33. Example 4 of Section 7.1 shows that **i** has order 4 in G. For each y in Y, the table for Problem 7 shows that $y^2 = (1)$; hence y has order 1 or 2. Theorem 6 of Section 7.2 implies that there is no isomorphism f from G onto G', since **i** has order 4 and no y in Y can serve as $f(\mathbf{i})$.

SECTION 7.4

1. (1) and (2 3).

3. (1 2 3 4), (1 3)(2 4), (1 4 3 2), (2 4), (1 4)(2 3), (1 3), (1 2)(3 4).

5. Yes.

7.

$\circ$	(1)	r	r^2	r^3	f	rf	r^2f	r^3f
(1)	(1)	r	r^2	r^3	f	rf	r^2f	r^3f
r	r	r^2	r^3	(1)	rf	r^2f	r^3f	f
r^2	r^2	r^3	(1)	r	r^2f	r^3f	f	rf
r^3	r^3	(1)	r	r^2	r^3f	f	rf	r^2f
f	f	r^3f	r^2f	rf	(1)	r^3	r^2	r
rf	rf	f	r^3f	r^2f	r	(1)	r^3	r^2
r^2f	r^2f	rf	f	r^3f	r^2	r	(1)	r^3
r^3f	r^3f	r^2f	rf	f	r^3	r^2	r	(1)

9. $(a\ b\ c\ d\ e), (a\ b\ c\ d), (a\ b\ c), (a\ b), (1), (a\ b\ c)(d\ e), (a\ b)(c\ d), (a\ b)(c\ d\ e)$.

11.

Type	(1)	$(a\ b\ c\ d\ e)$	$(a\ b\ c)$	$(a\ b)(c\ d)$
Number	1	$4! = 24$	$\binom{5}{3} 2! = 20$	$\binom{5}{1} 3 = 15$

13. (i) Yes. (ii) Yes, see Theorem 9 of Section 7.1 ("Finite Subset Closed under Group Operation").
(iii) No; for example $a_5 Y = \{a_5, a_6\}$ and $Y a_5 = \{a_5, a_8\}$.

15. 24.

SECTION 7.5

1. (i) (1), (1 2 3), (1 3 2), (2 3), (1 3), (1 2). (ii) Yes. (iii) Yes. (iv) Yes.
(v) $tY = \{(1\ 4), (1\ 4\ 2\ 3), (1\ 4\ 3\ 2), (1\ 4)(2\ 3), (1\ 4\ 3), (1\ 4\ 2)\}$. Then $Yt \neq tY$, since $(1\ 2\ 3)(1\ 4) = (1\ 2\ 3\ 4)$ is in Yt but not in tY.
(vi) No. This follows from Part (v).

3. $\quad$ (ii) Y is nonempty, finite, and closed under $\oplus$.

$\quad$ (iii) $00000 \oplus Y = Y$; $10000 \oplus Y = \{10000, 00010, 11011, 10101, 01001, 00111, 11110, 01100\}$;
$\quad$ $01000 \oplus Y = \{01000, 11010, 00011, 01101, 10001, 11111, 00110, 10100\}$;
$\quad$ $00100 \oplus Y = \{00100, 10110, 01111, 00001, 11101, 10011, 01010, 11000\}$; and thus the union of these four cosets is $\boldsymbol{B_5}$.

$\quad$ (iv) 4.

5. $\quad$ Since G is abelian, for each x in X, $x \,\square\, Y = \{x \,\square\, y : y \in Y\} = \{y \,\square\, x : y \in Y\} = Y \,\square\, x$.

9. $\quad$ (i) $e \,\square\, Y = \{e \,\square\, y : y \in Y\} = \{y : y \in Y\} = Y$.

$\quad$ (ii) Since the identity e is in the carrier Y of every subgroup H, it follows that $x = x \,\square\, e$ is in $x \,\square\, Y = \{x \,\square\, y : y \in Y\}$.

$\quad$ (iii) For $y \in Y$, $y \in e \,\square\, Y$ by Part (i). Also, $y \in y \,\square\, Y$ by Part (ii). Since $(y \,\square\, Y) \cap (e \,\square\, Y) \neq \varnothing$, it follows that $y \,\square\, Y = e \,\square\, Y = Y$ by Theorem 2 ("Distinct Left Cosets Are Disjoint").

$\quad$ (iv) By Part (ii), $x \in x \,\square\, Y$. Hence $x \,\square\, Y \neq Y$ if x is not in Y.

$\quad$ (v) By Part (ii), x is in $x \,\square\, Y$. If x is also in $w \,\square\, Y$, then by Theorem 2 we have $x \,\square\, Y = w \,\square\, Y$.

11. $\quad$ $x \,\square\, Y = \{x \,\square\, e, x \,\square\, y\} = \{x, x \,\square\, y\}$ and $Y \,\square\, x = \{e \,\square\, x, y \,\square\, x\} = \{x, y \,\square\, x\}$.
$\quad$ Then $\{x, x \,\square\, y\} = \{x, y \,\square\, x\}$ if and only if $x \,\square\, y = y \,\square\, x$.

13. $\quad$ Since the index of H in G is 2, Y has 2 left cosets in G. One of these cosets is Y itself, by Problem 9(i). Let the other left coset be L. Let $\#Y = m$. Then $\#L = m$ by Theorem 1 ("Number of Elements in a Coset") and $\#X = 2m$ because $\{Y, L\}$ is a partition of X. By the analogues for right cosets, Y is the right coset Ye. Since only m of the $2m$ elements of X are in Y, there must be another right coset R with $\#R = m$ and with $\{Y, R\}$ a partition of X. Since each of L and R has the m elements of X that are not in Y, it follows that $L = R$. By Problem 9(iii) and (iv), for x in X one has $x \,\square\, Y = Y$ if $x \in Y$ and $x \,\square\, Y \neq Y$ for x not in Y. Hence $x \,\square\, Y = Y$ if x is in Y and $x \,\square\, Y = L$ if x is not in Y. By the analogues for right cosets, $Y \,\square\, x = Y$ if x is in Y and $Y \,\square\, x = R = L$ if x is not in Y. Thus $x \,\square\, Y = Y \,\square\, x$ for each x in X, and H is a normal subgroup in G.

15. $\quad$ (i) Yes.

$\quad$ (ii) H is a subgroup in G because $3\mathbf{Z}$ is nonempty and closed under subtraction. ($a \,\square\, b^{-1} = a - b$ when $\square$ is addition.) H is normal in G because G is abelian.

$\quad$ (iii) $q = 3$. $\quad$ (iv) $3\mathbf{Z}, 1 + 3\mathbf{Z}, 2 + 3\mathbf{Z}$.

17. $\quad$ (i) This follows from Corollary 2 ("Possible Orders for Elements") of Lagrange's Theorem.

$\quad$ (ii) x has order 1 only if $x^1 = e$. $\quad$ (iii) This follows from Parts (i) and (ii).

$\quad$ (iv) Let x be one of the 4 elements of X different from e. Then $\#[x] = 5$ and so $[x] = X$. Hence $G = \langle [x], \square, e \rangle$ is cyclic.

19. $\quad$ 1, 2, 3, 4, 6, 8, 12, 24.

SECTION 7.6

1. $\quad$ $(3\mathbf{Z}, +, 0, \cdot)$ is a ring but has no unity. $\quad$ **3.** $\quad$ No; 2 has no additive inverse in $2\mathbf{N}$.

5. $\quad$ (i) $g = 2 \cdot 1$, $h = 3 \cdot 1$, $k = 4 \cdot 1$, and $k + 1 = 5 \cdot 1 = 0$ by Corollary 2 ("Possible Orders for Elements") of Lagrange's Theorem because $\#X = 5$.

$\quad$ (ii) $g + g = 2 \cdot 1 + 2 \cdot 1 = 4 \cdot 1 = k$.

$\quad$ (iii) This follows by using distributivity and the fact that 1 is a multiplicative identity.

$\quad$ (iv) $g(g + 1) = gg + g$ by distributivity, $gg = k$ by Part (iii), $k + g = 4 \cdot 1 + 2 \cdot 1 = 6 \cdot 1 = 1 \cdot 1 = 1$ because $5 \cdot 1 = 0$.

7. $\quad$ (i) This uses distributivity and the fact that 1 is a multiplicative identity.

(ii)

+	$\bar{0}$	$\bar{1}$	$\bar{2}$	$\bar{3}$	$\bar{4}$
$\bar{0}$	$\bar{0}$	$\bar{1}$	$\bar{2}$	$\bar{3}$	$\bar{4}$
$\bar{1}$	$\bar{1}$	$\bar{2}$	$\bar{3}$	$\bar{4}$	$\bar{0}$
$\bar{2}$	$\bar{2}$	$\bar{3}$	$\bar{4}$	$\bar{0}$	$\bar{1}$
$\bar{3}$	$\bar{3}$	$\bar{4}$	$\bar{0}$	$\bar{1}$	$\bar{2}$
$\bar{4}$	$\bar{4}$	$\bar{0}$	$\bar{1}$	$\bar{2}$	$\bar{3}$

$\cdot$	$\bar{0}$	$\bar{1}$	$\bar{2}$	$\bar{3}$	$\bar{4}$
$\bar{0}$	$\bar{0}$	$\bar{0}$	$\bar{0}$	$\bar{0}$	$\bar{0}$
$\bar{1}$	$\bar{0}$	$\bar{1}$	$\bar{2}$	$\bar{3}$	$\bar{4}$
$\bar{2}$	$\bar{0}$	$\bar{2}$	$\bar{4}$	$\bar{1}$	$\bar{3}$
$\bar{3}$	$\bar{0}$	$\bar{3}$	$\bar{1}$	$\bar{4}$	$\bar{2}$
$\bar{4}$	$\bar{0}$	$\bar{4}$	$\bar{3}$	$\bar{2}$	$\bar{1}$

9. X is closed under the commutative operation of addition of matrices, the additive identity O and the multiplicative identity I are in X, and the additive inverse of

$$\begin{bmatrix} x & y \\ 0 & w \end{bmatrix} \quad \text{is} \quad \begin{bmatrix} -x & -y \\ 0 & -w \end{bmatrix}.$$

Closure under multiplication is seen from

$$\begin{bmatrix} a & b \\ 0 & d \end{bmatrix} \cdot \begin{bmatrix} g & h \\ 0 & j \end{bmatrix} = \begin{bmatrix} ag & ah + bj \\ 0 & dj \end{bmatrix}.$$

The associative and distributive properties are inherited from the set of all 2×2 matrices.

SECTION 7.7

1. $P(x_1, x_2, x_3) = (x_1^4 + 8x_1^1 x_3^1 + 3x_2^2)/12$, so $P(2, 2, 2) = 5$.

3. $P(x_1, x_2, x_3, x_4) = (x_1^4 + 2x_4^1 + 2x_1^2 x_2^1 + 3x_2^2)/8$, so $P(2, 2, 2, 2) = 6$.

5. $P(x_1, x_2, x_3, x_4) = (x_1^5 + 2x_4^1 x_1^1 + x_2^2 x_1^1)/4$, so $P(2, 2, 2, 2) = 12$.

7. $P(x_1, x_2, x_3, x_4, x_5, x_6) = (x_1^6 + x_2^3 + 2x_3^2 + 2x_6^1)/6$, so $P(3, 3, 3, 3, 3, 3) = 130$.

9. $P^* = r^6 + r^5 b + 2r^4 b^2 + 4r^3 b^3 + 2r^2 b^4 + rb^5 + b^6$.

11. (a) $P(x_1, x_2, \ldots, x_p) = [x_1^p + (p-1)x_p^1]/p$, so $P(m, m, \ldots, m) = [m^p + (p-1)m]/p$.

(b) $P(x_1, x_2, \ldots, x_p) = [x_1^p + (p-1)x_p^1 + px_1^1 x_2^{(p-1)/2}]/2p$,

so $P(m, m, \ldots, m) = [m^p + (p-1)m + pm^{(p+1)/2}]/2p$.

REVIEW PROBLEMS FOR CHAPTER 7

1. (a), (b), and (d) but not (c).   **2.** Only (c).   **3.** (a) and (b).

4. (a) All n's in Z^+.   (b) Only for $n = 1$.

5.

n	0	1	2	3	4	5	6	7	8	9	10	11
Order of g^n	1	12	6	4	3	12	2	12	3	4	6	12

6. (a) $\{e, g^7, g^{14}, g^{21}\}$.   (b) $\{e, g^4, g^8, g^{12}, g^{16}, g^{20}, g^{24}\}$.

7. Yes. If $n = cd$, then $\langle [g^c], \square, e \rangle$ is such a subgroup.   **8.** (i) No.   (ii) Yes.   (iii) Yes.

9. (a)

x	1	i	-1	$-i$
$\alpha(x)$	1	-1	1	-1

(b)

x	1	i	-1	$-i$
$\beta(x)$	e	g^3	g^2	g

10. Yes. It is a bijection with $f(x + y) = 10^{x+y} = 10^x 10^y = f(x)f(y)$.

11. No; $\alpha[(1 \quad 3)(1 \quad 2)] = \alpha[(1 \quad 3 \quad 2)] = (1 \quad 2 \quad 3)$, which does *not* equal
$\alpha[(1 \quad 3)]\alpha[(1 \quad 2)] = (1 \quad 3 \quad 2)(1 \quad 2 \quad 3) = (1)$.

12. Yes. Every isomorphism is a homomorphism.   **13.** (i) $(2 \quad 3 \quad 4)(5 \quad 6 \quad 7 \quad 8 \quad 9)$.   (ii) 15.

14. (i) $(1 \quad 2 \quad 3 \quad 5)(4 \quad 6 \quad 7)$.   (ii) 12.

15.

G	e	b	c	d
$e = (1)$	e	b	c	d
$b = (1 \quad 2)(3 \quad 4)$	b	e	d	c
$c = (1 \quad 3)(2 \quad 4)$	c	d	e	b
$d = (1 \quad 4)(2 \quad 3)$	d	c	b	e

G'	e	r	r^2	r^3
$e = (1)$	e	r	r^2	r^3
$r = (1 \quad 2 \quad 3 \quad 4)$	r	r^2	r^3	e
$r^2 = (1 \quad 3)(2 \quad 4)$	r^2	r^3	e	r
$r^3 = (1 \quad 4 \quad 3 \quad 2)$	r^3	e	r	r^2

16. No. The element r of G' has order 4. The group G has no element of order 4 and so has no element to map onto r under an isomorphism.

17. (i) Yes. If $p = t_1 t_2 \cdots t_{2h}$ with the t_i transpositions, then $p^{-1} = t_{2h} \cdots t_2 t_1$ is also a product of an even number of transpositions.

(ii) Yes. This is similar to Part (i).

(iii) The permutation q is a product $t_1 t_2 \cdots t_h$ of transpositions.
Then $q^{-1}(1 \quad 2)q = t_h \cdots t_2 t_1 (1 \quad 2)t_1 t_2 \cdots t_h$ is a product of an odd number,
$2h + 1$, of transpositions, and $q^{-1}(1 \quad 2 \quad 3)q = t_h \cdots t_2 t_1 (1 \quad 3)(2 \quad 3)t_1 t_2 \cdots t_h$
is a product of an even number, $2h + 2$, of transpositions.

18. (a) Yes.   (b) Yes.

19. (a)

Type	(1)	$(a \quad b \quad c)$	$(a \quad b \quad c \quad d \quad e)$	$(a \quad b)(c \quad d)$
#	1	40	144	45

Type	$(a \quad b)(c \quad d \quad e \quad f)$	$(a \quad b \quad c \quad d)(e \quad f)$	$(a \quad b \quad c)(d \quad e \quad f)$
#	30	60	40

(b)

Type	$(a \quad b)$	$(a \quad b \quad c \quad d)$	$(a \quad b \quad c \quad d \quad e \quad f)$	$(a \quad b)(c \quad d \quad e)$
#	15	90	120	48

Type	$(a \quad b \quad c)(d \quad e)$	$(a \quad b)(c \quad d)(e \quad f)$
#	72	15

20. $(1), (1 \quad 2)(3 \quad 4), (1 \quad 4)(2 \quad 3), (1 \quad 3)(2 \quad 4)$.   **21.** (i) Yes.   (ii) Yes.

22. (ii) $\quad\quad Y = \{00000, 11000, 00110, 11110\}$,   (iii) Yes. The group $\langle B_5, \oplus, 0_5 \rangle$ is abelian.
$00001 \oplus Y = \{00001, 11001, 00111, 11111\}$,
$00010 \oplus Y = \{00010, 11010, 00100, 11100\}$,
$00011 \oplus Y = \{00011, 11011, 00101, 11101\}$,
$01000 \oplus Y = \{01000, 10000, 01110, 10110\}$,
$01100 \oplus Y = \{01100, 10100, 01010, 10010\}$,
$01101 \oplus Y = \{01101, 10101, 01011, 10011\}$,
$01111 \oplus Y = \{01111, 10111, 01001, 10001\}$.

23. Let q be the order of H. Then $5|q$ and $q|60$; hence q must be in the set $\{5, 10, 15, 20, 30, 60\}$.

24. Let $G = \langle X, \square, e \rangle$ have prime order p. By Corollary 2 of Lagrange's Theorem, every x in X has order 1 or p. But only e has order 1. Hence $X = [g]$ for any g in X with $g \neq e$, and $G = \langle [g], \square, e \rangle$ is cyclic.

25. (i) This follows from the definition of a field.

(ii) and (iii) These follow from Corollary 2 of Lagrange's Theorem.

(iv) If $x \neq 0$, then $x^{10} = 1$ by Part (iii), and thus $x^{11} = x^{10}x = 1 \cdot x = x$. If $x = 0$, then $x^{11} = 0^{11} = 0 = x$.

26. 13.

27. (a) $P(x_1, x_2, x_3, x_4) = (x_1^8 + 8x_1^2 x_3^2 + 9x_2^4 + 6x_4^2)/24$.　　(b) 23.

(c) $P^* = b^8 + b^7 w + 3b^6 w^2 + 3b^5 w^3 + 7b^4 w^4 + 3b^3 w^5 + 3b^2 w^6 + bw^7 + w^8$.

SECTION 8.1

1. (a) $x = -\frac{4}{7}$.　　(b) $x \in \{-\frac{5}{2}, \frac{8}{9}\}$.　　(c) $x = -6$, a root of multiplicity 2.　　(d) $x = \pm\sqrt{\frac{8}{5}} = \pm 2\sqrt{10}/5$.

3. $x = (-5 \pm \sqrt{73})/8$.　　**5.** r and s are $3 + \sqrt{14}$ and $3 - \sqrt{14}$.

7. $1 - 30x + 144x^2 = (1 - 6x)(1 - 24x)$.　　**9.** (i) $q(x) = x^3 - 3x^2 - 6x - 2, r = -16$.　　(ii) -16.

11. (i) 1.　　(ii) $1 + \sqrt{3}$ and $1 - \sqrt{3}$.　　**13.** (i) $1, 1, -1$.　　(ii) $(x - 1)(x - 1)(x + 1)$.

15. $b = -27604$.　　**17.** (i) $\{a, b\} = \{1, -3\}$ and $g(x) = x^2 + 2$.　　(ii) $1, -3, \sqrt{2}\mathbf{i}, -\sqrt{2}\mathbf{i}$.

19. (i) $p(0) = 0 = p(c)$.　　(ii) $p(x) = -3cx(x - c)$.　　**21.** (i) $-\frac{5}{3}$.　　(ii) $-\frac{5}{3}, (3 + \sqrt{17})/2, (3 - \sqrt{17})/2$.

23. (i) $1, -\frac{2}{3}, -\frac{5}{4}$.　　(ii) $0, 1, -\frac{2}{3}, -\frac{5}{4}$.

25. (a) $1, -1, 3, -3, 5, -5, 15, -15$.　　(b) $\pm 1, \pm 3, \pm 5, \pm 15, \pm\frac{1}{7}, \pm\frac{3}{7}, \pm\frac{5}{7}, \pm\frac{15}{7}$.

27. Yes; $\frac{65}{39} = \frac{5}{3}$ with $5|10$ and $3|9$. But the best evidence is that $(3x - 5)(3x^2 + 2) = 0$ is such an equation with $\frac{5}{3}$ as a root.

29. Let $h = s/t$, with s and t integers having no common integral divisor greater than 1. Since the a_i are integers, we can use Theorem 5 ("Rational Root Theorem") which tells us that $t|a_0$, that is, $t|1$. Since $t > 0$, this means that $t = 1$, and so $h = s/1 = s$ is an integer.

31. (i) If n is even, so are n^5, n^4, and their sum $n^5 + n^4$. If n is odd, so are n^5 and n^4, but their sum $n^5 + n^4$ again is even.

(ii) $p(n)$ is the sum of the even integers $n^5 + n^4$ and $20bn$ and the odd integer -3; thus $p(n)$ is odd.

(iii) If n is an integer, then $p(n)$ is not zero because it is odd.

33. (i) The possibilities for rational roots are $1, -1, 3$, and -3, but no one of these numbers satisfies the equation.

(ii) $\sqrt[5]{3}$ is a root of the equation $x^5 - 3 = 0$, but the equation has no rational roots.

35. It can be shown that $\sqrt{7} - \sqrt{2}$ is a root of $x^4 - 18x^2 + 25 = 0$ and that this equation has no rational roots.

37. Rewriting the polynomial as $(x - 2)^4(x + 1)^8(x - 3)$, one sees that the roots h and their multiplicities m_h are as in the table below.

h	2	-1	3
m_h	4	8	1

39. Rewriting the polynomial as $(x - 1)^6(x + 2)^6(x - 3)^8(2x - 1)$, one sees that the roots h and their multiplicities m_h are as in the table below.

h	1	-2	3	$\frac{1}{2}$
m_h	6	6	8	1

41. Since $x^6 + 3x^4 + 3x^2 + 1 = (x^2 + 1)^3 = (x - \mathbf{i})^3(x + \mathbf{i})^3$, the root $\mathbf{i}$ has multiplicity 3. This multiplicity can also be found with repeated synthetic division by $x - \mathbf{i}$.

43. $(n + 1)(n + 2)(n + 3)(n + 4) = n^4 + 10n^3 + 35n^2 + 50n + 24$.

45. $r = (-b + \sqrt{b^2 - 4c})/2$ and $s = (-b - \sqrt{b^2 - 4c})/2$. Hence $r - s = 2\sqrt{b^2 - 4c}/2 = \sqrt{b^2 - 4c}$.

SECTION 8.2

1. (i)

x	-2	-1	0	1	2
$p(x)$	5	1	-1	-1	1

(ii) -1 and 1.

3. (i) $-2, -1, 1, 2$.   (ii) No, since $p(-2) = -16$, $p(-1) = -6$, $p(1) = 2$, and $p(2) = 12$.   (iii) $a = 0$.

5. $r = \frac{3}{2}$.

7. $x_1 = -2/3 = -F_3/F_4$, $x_2 = -13/21 = -F_7/F_8$, $x_3 = -610/987 = -F_{15}/F_{16}$. (Here the F_n are the Fibonacci Numbers.)

9. (i) $r = 1$.   (ii) $x_1 = \frac{5}{4}$, $x_2 = \frac{221}{182} \approx 1.214286$.

11. (i) $p(2) = 6$, $p(3) = 2$.   (ii) No; see answer to Part (iv).   (iii) $p(2.7) = -0.0319$.
(iv) Yes; Theorem 1 ("Change of Sign Implies Root in Interval") tells us that there is a root in the interval $2 < x < 2.7$ and a root in the interval $2.7 < x < 3$.

13. $x_{n+1} = x_n - \dfrac{p(x_n)}{p'(x_n)} = x_n - \dfrac{x_n^2 - 3}{2x_n} = \dfrac{1}{2}\left(x_n + \dfrac{3}{x_n}\right)$.   **15.** $x_{n+1} = x_n - \dfrac{x_n^2 - c}{2x_n} = \dfrac{1}{2}\left(x_n + \dfrac{c}{x_n}\right)$.

17. 29, since $2^{28} < 3 \cdot 10^8 < 2^{29}$.   **19.** For $x > 0$, each $a_i x^{d-i} \geq 0$ and their sum is positive.

21. (i) This follows from the result in Problem 19.   (ii) This follows from Part (i) and Problem 20.

23. Let $c_0', c_1', \ldots, c_d'$ be the new c's when h is replaced by a number k with $k > h$. With the given hypotheses, one has $c_i' > c_i$ for $i = 1, 2, \ldots, d$, and so $p(k) = c_d' > c_d \geq 0$. This implies that $p(k) > 0$ for $k > h$.

25. One finds quickly that $x = 1$ is a root.

27. (a) Let $p(x) = x^2 - x - 1$. Then $p'(x) = 2x - 1$ and $p'(0.5) = 0$. The method fails because it involves division by 0.
(b) $x_1 = -5.8$, $x_2 \approx -2.7$, $x_3 \approx -1.3$, $x_4 \approx -0.747$, $x_5 \approx -0.625$, $x_6 \approx -0.61806$, $x_7 \approx -0.618034$, $x_8 \approx x_7 \approx -0.618034$.

SECTION 8.3

1. (ii) and (iii).   **3.** $F = \dfrac{5}{1 - 4x} - \dfrac{2}{1 + 3x}$.

5. $\dfrac{3 + 35x}{1 + 10x + 25x^2} = \dfrac{-4 + 7 + 35x}{(1 + 5x)^2} = \dfrac{-4}{(1 + 5x)^2} + \dfrac{7(1 + 5x)}{(1 + 5x)^2} = \dfrac{-4}{(1 + 5x)^2} + \dfrac{7}{1 + 5x}$.

7. $a = 8$, $b = -5$, $c = 6$.   **9.** $a = 8$, $b = -5$, $c = 6$.

11. (i) $x - 2 = -2y$.   (ii) $\dfrac{A}{B} = \dfrac{80}{y} - \dfrac{272}{y^2} + \dfrac{324}{y^3} - \dfrac{168}{y^4} + \dfrac{38}{y^5}$.   (iii) Replace y by $1 - \frac{1}{2}x$ in Part (ii).

13. (i) 10.
(ii) Let $H = 1/(1 + x)$, $K = 1/(1 - 2x)$, and $L = 1/(1 + 3x)$.
Then $A/B = aH + bH^2 + cH^3 + dH^4 + eK + fK^2 + gK^3 + hK^4 + iK^5 + jL + kL^2$.

15. (a) $\dfrac{1}{(1-x)^2} - \dfrac{2}{(1-x)^3} - \dfrac{6}{(1-x)^4}$. (b) $\dfrac{-3}{1-x} + \dfrac{4}{1-2x}$. (c) $\dfrac{-2}{1+x} + \dfrac{3}{(1+x)^2} + \dfrac{4}{1-2x}$.

(d) $\dfrac{6}{1-x} - \dfrac{6}{1-\frac{1}{2}x} + \dfrac{2}{1-\frac{1}{3}x}$.

17. $\dfrac{a}{1+4x} + \dfrac{b}{1-ix} + \dfrac{c}{1+ix}$, where $a = \frac{16}{17}$, $b = \dfrac{1}{2-8i} = \frac{1}{34} + \frac{2}{17}i$, and $c = \frac{1}{34} - \frac{2}{17}i$.

19. $\dfrac{-2x^3 + 8x^2 + 6x - 2}{(1-x)^2(1+\frac{1}{2}x)(1-\frac{1}{3}x)}$.

21. (i) $(x-2)(x-2)(x+3) = (x-2)^2(x+3)$.

(ii) Replacing x with $1/x$ and then multiplying by x^3, one has

$$\frac{1}{x^3} - \frac{1}{x^2} - \frac{8}{x} + 12 = \left(\frac{1}{x} - 2\right)^2 \left(\frac{1}{x} + 3\right), \quad 1 - x - 2x^2 + 12x^3 = (1-2x)^2(1+3x).$$

(iii) $\dfrac{3}{1+3x} - \dfrac{1}{1-2x} - \dfrac{3}{(1-2x)^2}$.

23. $\dfrac{-3}{(1-\frac{1}{2}x)^3}$.

25. *Hint*: Multiply by $(x-r)(x-s)(x-t)$ and then set x equal to r, to s, and finally to t.

27. See answer to Problem 15(d).

29. Let A be a polynomial of degree 0 or 1 and let $r \neq s$. Then

$$\frac{A(x)}{(x-r)(x-s)} = \frac{A(r)}{r-s} \cdot \frac{1}{x-r} + \frac{A(s)}{s-r} \cdot \frac{1}{x-s}.$$

31. (i) $x + 3 + \dfrac{7x-6}{x^2 - 3x + 2}$. (iv) $x - 3 + \dfrac{11}{x+3}$.

33. It becomes meaningless because it involves division by 0.

REVIEW PROBLEMS FOR CHAPTER 8

1. $x = -2$.

3. (a) $(x+7)(x-3)$; (b) $(1+7x)(1-3x)$; (c) $(x-7)(x-7) = (x-7)^2$; (d) $(1-7x)^2$.

5. (a) $-7, 3$; (b) $-\frac{1}{7}, \frac{1}{3}$; (c) 7, a root of multiplicity 2; (d) $\frac{1}{7}$, a root of multiplicity 2.

7. (i) $-1, -2, -5$. (ii) and (iii) r, s, and t are -1, -2, and -5.

9. (i) 1. (ii) 1, $2i$, and $-2i$. (iii) $(x-1)(x-2i)(x+2i)$.

11.

Root	-3.6	-2	0.5	2	3
Multiplicity	1	3	1	1	3

13. $\pm 1, \pm 3, \pm 5, \pm 15, \pm\frac{1}{3}, \pm\frac{5}{3}$. **15.** -4 and 3.

17. (i) Since $p(1) = -3$ and $p(2) = 11$, there is a root in the interval $1 < x < 2$ by the "Change of Sign Theorem" (Theorem 1 of Section 8.2).

(ii) Since $p(1.5) = 0.5625$, there is a root in the interval $1 < x < 1.5$. Then $p(1.25) \approx -1.8$ shows that there is a root in the interval $1.25 < x < 1.5$.

19. Since $2^{23} < 10^7 < 2^{24}$, it requires 24 bisections.

21. (i) $p(1) = -1$ and $p(2) = 15$ have opposite signs. (ii) $x_1 = 1.2$, $x_2 \approx 1.16542$, $x_3 \approx 1.16404 \approx x_4$.

23. (a) $\dfrac{-\frac{1}{2}}{1-2x}+\dfrac{\frac{3}{2}}{1-6x}$.   (b) $\dfrac{-\frac{1}{2}}{1-4x}+\dfrac{\frac{3}{2}}{(1-4x)^2}$.   **25.** $\dfrac{-1}{1+x}+\dfrac{3}{(1+x)^2}-\dfrac{3}{(1+x)^3}+\dfrac{3}{(1+x)^4}$.

27. (a) $\dfrac{5}{1-2x}+\dfrac{4}{1+3x}-\dfrac{7}{1-4x}$.   (b) $\dfrac{2}{1+x}-\dfrac{3}{1-3x}+\dfrac{4}{(1-3x)^2}$.

SECTION 9.1

1. (i) $x+4x^2+\cdots+n^2x^n+\cdots$.   (ii) $1+4x+9x^2+\cdots+(n+1)^2x^n+\cdots$.

3. $\dbinom{3}{3}+\dbinom{4}{3}x+\dbinom{5}{3}x^2+\cdots+\dbinom{n+3}{3}x^n+\cdots$ or $1+4x+10x^2+\cdots+\dbinom{n+3}{3}x^n+\cdots$.

5. (a) $2+8+19x^2+\cdots+\left[(n+1)^2+\dbinom{n+3}{3}\right]x^n+\cdots$.

(b) $1+8x+35x^2+\cdots+e_nx^n+\cdots$, where $e_n=\dbinom{n+3}{3}+4\dbinom{n+2}{3}+9\dbinom{n+1}{3}+\cdots+(n+1)^2\dbinom{3}{3}$.

7. (i) and (ii) $2/(1-5x)$.   **9.** (a) $1/(1-0.5x)$;   (b) $2/(1-3x)$;   (c) $3/(1-x)$;   (d) $5/(1+x)$.

11. (i) $3/(1+4x)$;   (ii) $5/(1-3x)$;   (iii) $[3/(1+4x)]+[5/(1-3x)]=(8+11x)/(1+x-12x^2)$.

13. $5,-10,20,-40,\ldots,5(-2)^n,\ldots$ **15.** (i) $-4(-6)^n$;   (ii) $7\cdot9^n$;   (iii) $-4(-6)^n+7\cdot9^n$.

17. $u_0,u_1,\ldots$ with $u_n=5\cdot2^n+4(-3)^n$.   **19.** (i) $(1-x-x^2)V=x$;   (ii) $V=x/(1-x-x^2)$.

21. $(1+3x)/(1-x)^2$.   **25.** $0,0,g_0,g_1,\ldots,g_{n-2},\ldots$.

27. (i) $1+x^2+x^4+\cdots+x^{2n}+\cdots$;   (ii) 1.   **29.** (i) $AB=1$;   (ii) $1/(1-x^3)$.

31. (i) $u_n-3u_{n-1}+3u_{n-2}-u_{n-3}=(n+1)^2-3n^2+3(n-1)^2-(n-2)^2$
$$=(n^2+2n+1)-3n^2+3(n^2-2n+1)-(n^2-4n+4)=0.$$

(iii) $(1+x)/(1-3x+3x^2-x^3)$.

33. (i) Let $(1-x)C=e_0+e_1x+e_2x^2+\cdots$. Then $e_n=\dbinom{n+2}{2}-\dbinom{n+1}{2}=\dbinom{n+1}{1}=n+1$ using Theo-

rem 2(b) of Section 1.1 and Problem 15 of Section 1.1.

(ii) See Example 4.   (iii) See Example 3.

35. (i) $1/(1-x)^5=(1-x)^{-5}$;   (ii) $(1-x)^{-6}$;   (iii) $(1-x)^{-7}$.   **37.** $(1+x)/(1-x)^4$.

39. (i) $p_0=0,p_1=1$;   (ii) $c=2,d=1$;   (iii) $p_2=2,p_3=5,p_4=12,p_5=29$.

43. (i) $A^2=[(1-x)^{-2}]^2=(1-x)^{-4}=\displaystyle\sum_{n=0}^{\infty}\dbinom{n+3}{3}x^n$ by Example 4 and Problem 34.

(ii) This uses Definition 4 ("Multiplication of Generating Series").

(iii) Equate coefficients of x^n in the equations of Parts (i) and (ii).

SECTION 9.2

1. (i) $u_n=(-1.03)^nu_0$.   (ii) $u_1=-1030,u_2=1060.9$.   (iii) $u_n=1000(-1.03)^n$.

3. $P_n=\$5000(1.025^n)$.   **5.** $P_0=\$72/0.009=\$8000$.   **7.** (i) and (ii) $u_n=(\frac{3}{2})^nu_0$.

9. (a) $B(x)=1-6x+8x^2$, $K(x)=x^2-6x+8$.   (b) $B(x)=1+14x+49x^2$, $K(x)=x^2+14x+49$.

(c) $B(x)=1-9x^2$, $K(x)=x^2-9$.

11. (a) $\{r,s\}=\{2,4\},r\neq s$.   (b) $r=s=-7$.   (c) $\{r,s\}=\{-3,3\},r\neq s$.

13. (a) $u_n=2^nh+4^nk$ (with h and k arbitrary constants).   (b) $u_n=(h_1+h_2n)(-7)^n$.

(c) $u_n=(-3)^nh+3^nk$.

15.   (i) $u_n = [(1 + \sqrt{5})/2]^n h + [(1 - \sqrt{5})/2]^n k.$ (ii) $u_n = \dfrac{1}{\sqrt{5}}\left[\left(\dfrac{1 + \sqrt{5}}{2}\right)^n - \left(\dfrac{1 - \sqrt{5}}{2}\right)^n\right].$

     (iii) $u_n = \left(\dfrac{1 + \sqrt{5}}{2}\right)^n + \left(\dfrac{1 - \sqrt{5}}{2}\right)^n.$

17.   (a) $h = 2, k = 3.$ (b) $u_n - u_{n-1} - 20u_{n-2} = 0.$

19.   (a) $h_1 = 4, h_2 = -6.$ (b) $u_n + 6u_{n-1} + 9u_{n-2} = 0.$

21.   (a) $u_n = (\tfrac{5}{3})5^n + (\tfrac{4}{3})(-4)^n.$ (b) $u_n = (5 - 3n)4^n.$

23.   All of these recursions are satisfied by $u_n = \dbinom{n + 2}{2}.$

25.   The characteristic polynomial is $K(x) = x^2 - x + 1.$ The characteristic roots are $(1 \pm i\sqrt{3})/2.$ Then the formulas in Parts (i) and (ii) follow.

27.   (i) \$0.003 rounded to the nearest cent is zero cents.   (ii) Zero cents.

     (iii) The interest for 90 days is the balance $\$10(1.0003^{90})$ after 90 days minus the original \$10 deposit.

     (iv) Yes; the depositor would receive 27 cents interest instead of zero cents.

29.   We are given that

$$x_n + b(n)x_{n-1} + c(n)x_{n-2} = 0,$$

$$y_n + b(n)y_{n-1} + c(n)y_{n-2} = 0.$$

     Adding these gives us $z_n + b(n)z_{n-1} + c(n)z_{n-2} = 0.$

31.   (i) When G is multiplied by $1 - 3x + 3x^2 - x^3$, the coefficient of x^n in the product is $u_n - 3u_{n-1} + 3u_{n-2} - u_{n-3}$ for $n \geq 3$, and this coefficient equals zero by the given recursion. The coefficients of x^n for $n = 0, 1,$ and 2 turn out to be as stated.

     (ii) This follows by solving for G in Part (i) and using $1 - 3x + 3x^2 - x^3 = (1 - x)^3.$

     (iii) This follows from Part (ii) and Lemma 1 ("Denominator a Power of $1 - rx$") of Section 8.3.

     (iv) Using Example 3, Example 4, and Problem 33 of Section 9.1, one gets

$$\frac{a}{1 - x} = a + ax + ax^2 + \cdots + ax^n + \cdots,$$

$$\frac{b}{(1 - x)^2} = b + 2bx + 3bx^2 + \cdots + (n + 1)bx^n + \cdots,$$

$$\frac{c}{(1 - x)^3} = c + 3cx + 6cx^2 + \cdots + \binom{n + 2}{2}cx^n + \cdots.$$

     Using Part (iii), one sees that the sum of the left-hand sides of these three equations is $G = u_0 + u_1 x + \cdots + u_n x^n + \cdots.$ Hence u_n equals the sum $a + (n + 1)b + \dbinom{n + 2}{2}c$ of the coefficients of x^n on the right-hand sides of these equations.

SECTION 9.3

1.   (i) $v_n = 8000.$ (ii) $v_n = 8000 + 1.025^n k.$ (iii) $v_n = 8000 + 2000(1.025^n).$

3.   (i) $P_n = 8000 + 2000(1.025^n).$ (ii) The P_n of Part (i) equals the v_n of Problem 1(iii).

5.   (i) $v_n = 1.75 + (-3)^n k.$ (ii) $v_n = 1.75 - 0.75(-3)^n;$ (iii) $v_1 = 4.$

7.   (i) $v_n = 3^n h + 3.75(-5)^n.$ (ii) $v_n = -7.75(3^n) + 3.75(-5)^n.$

9.   (i) $v_n = (h + 6n)(-7)^n.$ (ii) $v_n = (11 + 6n)(-7)^n.$

11. (i) $x_n = 2$. (ii) $y_n = -3(3^n)$. (iii) $z_n = 4n(-2)^n$. (iv) $w_n = 2 - 3(3^n)$.
(v) $v_n = 2 - 3(3^n) + 4n(-2)^n$. (vi) $v_n = 2 - 3(3^n) + 4n(-2)^n + (-2)^n h$.
(vii) $v_n = 2 - 3(3^n) + 4n(-2)^n + 19(-2)^n$.

13. The general solution is $v_n = x_n + r^n k$. We let $n = 0$ and get $v_0 = x_0 + k$. Then $k = v_0 - x_0$. Making this substitution in the general solution, we get $v_n = x_n + (v_0 - x_0)r^n$ as the specific solution for the given initial term v_0.

SECTION 9.4

1. (a) Order is 2, linear homogeneous, coefficients are not constants.
(b) Order is 3, linear homogeneous, constant coefficients. (c) Order is 1, nonlinear.
(d) Order is 2, linear but not homogeneous, constant coefficients.

3. $u_3 = 9$, $u_4 = 16$, $u_5 = 25$.

5. $u_n - u_{n-1} - u_{n-2} - 1 = (F_{n+2} - 1) - (F_{n+1} - 1) - (F_n - 1) - 1$
$$= (F_{n+2} - F_{n+1} - F_n) + (-1 + 1 + 1 - 1) = 0 + 0 = 0.$$

7. (a) $u_n = 2^n$, using Lemma 1(b) with $r = 2$ and $h = 0$.
(b) $u_n = 5(n + 1)3^n$, multiplying the equation of Lemma 1(b), with $r = 3$ and $h = 1$, on both sides by 5.
(c) $5\binom{2+n}{2}(-2)^n$. (d) $4\binom{6+n}{6}3^n$. (e) $4\binom{6+n}{6}3^n - 5\binom{2+n}{2}(-2)^n$.

9. (i) $B = 1 - x - x^2$, $K = x^2 - x - 1$;
(ii) $(1 + \sqrt{5})/2$ and $(1 - \sqrt{5})/2$ are the characteristic roots; each has multiplicity 1.

11. (i) $B = (1 + 4x)(1 - 5x)^3 = 1 - 11x + 15x^2 + 175x^3 - 500x^4$.
(ii) $u_n - 11u_{n-1} + 15u_{n-2} + 175u_{n-3} - 500u_{n-4} = 0$. (iii) $u_n = a(-4)^n + (b + cn + dn^2)5^n$.

13. $u_n - 27u_{n-2} - 14u_{n-3} + 120u_{n-4} = 0$. **15.** $b_1 = -5$, $b_2 = -36$.

17. The general solution is $7^n a + (-2)^n b$, with a and b arbitrary constants. (i) $u_n = 7^n$,
(ii) $u_n = (-2)^n$, (iii) $u_n = 7^n + (-2)^n$, (iv) $u_n = 7^n - (-2)^n$, (v) $u_n = 7^n + 2(-2)^n$.

19. (i) $u_n = 5^n$. (ii) $u_n = 2 \cdot 5^n$. **21.** (i) $u_n = (-4)^n$. (ii) $u_n = 3(-4)^n$. **23.** All but sequence (e).

25. (a) $u_n = 3 \cdot 2^n - 2 \cdot 3^n$, (b) $u_n = (5 - 4n)(-2)^n$,
(c) $K = x^2 - 6x + 13 = (x - r)(x - s)$ with $r = 3 + 2i$ and $s = 3 - 2i$. Then $u_n = cr^n + ks^n$ with $n = 0$ and $n = 1$ gives

$$1 = c + k,$$
$$3 = c(3 + 2i) + k(3 - 2i).$$

From the first equation, we see that $k = 1 - c$. Substituting this in the second equation gives

$$3 = c(3 + 2i) + (1 - c)(3 - 2i) = c(3 + 2i - 3 + 2i) + (3 - 2i) = 4ic + (3 - 2i).$$

Hence $4ic = 3 - 3 + 2i = 2i$, and so $c = \frac{1}{2}$ and $k = 1 - \frac{1}{2} = \frac{1}{2}$. Thus $u_n = [(3 + 2i)^n/2] + [(3 - 2i)^n/2]$.
(d) $[(1 + \sqrt{2})^n/2\sqrt{2}] - [(1 - \sqrt{2})^n/2\sqrt{2}]$.

27. $u_n = 2^n + 3(-2)^n + 2 \cdot 3^n$.

29. (a) $2/(1 - x)$; (b) $7/(1 + x)$; (c) $x/(1 - x)^2$; (d) $4/(1 - 3x)$;
(e) $[4/(1 - 3x)] + [7/(1 + x)] = (11 - 17x)/(1 - 2x - 3x^2)$; (f) $2x/(1 - 4x + 4x^2)$;
(g) $(-4 + 18x - 22x^2)/(1 - 7x + 16x^2 - 12x^3)$.

31. (i) $u_n - 5u_{n-2} + 4u_{n-4} = 0$; (ii) $u_4 = -3$, $u_6 = -19$; (iii) $u_5 = 19$, $u_7 = 83$;
(iv) $[14(-1)^n + 2^n - 3(-2)^n]/6$.

33. $G = (6 + 92x + 273x^2 - 1617x^3)/(1 + 17x + 63x^2 - 245x^3 - 1372x^4)$.

35. $(6 - 13x)/[(1 - x)(1 - 2x + 9x^2)] = (6 - 13x)/(1 - 3x + 11x^2 - 9x^3)$.

37. (i) The formula for u_n does not involve a fixed number of previous terms, as required in Display (2).

(ii) $u_4 = u_0 u_3 + u_1 u_2 + u_2 u_1 + u_3 u_0$, $u_5 = u_0 u_4 + u_1 u_3 + u_2 u_2 + u_3 u_1 + u_4 u_0$.

(iii)
$$G^2 = (u_0 + u_1 x + u_2 x^2 + \cdots)^2$$
$$= u_0^2 + (u_0 u_1 + u_1 u_0)x + (u_0 u_2 + u_1 u_1 + u_2 u_0)x^2 + \cdots$$
$$= u_1 + u_2 x + u_3 x^2 + \cdots,$$
$$xG^2 = u_1 x + u_2 x^2 + \cdots,$$
$$1 + xG^2 = u_0 + u_1 x + u_2 x^2 + \cdots = G.$$

39. We are given that
$$v_n + b_1 v_{n-1} + b_2 v_{n-2} + \cdots + b_d v_{n-d} = 0,$$
$$w_n + b_1 w_{n-1} + b_2 w_{n-2} + \cdots + b_d w_{n-d} = 0.$$

Adding term by term, we have the desired result:
$$(v_n + w_n) + b_1(v_{n-1} + w_{n-1}) + \cdots + b_d(v_{n-d} + w_{n-d}) = 0.$$

41. Substituting $u_n = cv_n + kw_n$ into the recursion gives
$$(cv_n + kw_n) + b_1(cv_{n-1} + kw_{n-1}) + \cdots + b_d(cv_{n-d} + kw_{n-d})$$
$$= c(v_n + b_1 v_{n-1} + \cdots + b_d v_{n-d}) + k(w_n + b_1 w_{n-1} + \cdots + b_d w_{n-d}).$$

Using the hypotheses, this becomes $c \cdot 0 + k \cdot 0 = 0$, as desired.

43. (i) The characteristic polynomial is $K(x) = x^2 - 6x + 25$, and the roots of $K(x) = 0$ are $3 \pm 4\mathbf{i}$, that is, r and s.

(ii) This follows from Part (i) and the corollary to Theorem 3.

SECTION 9.5

1. $v_n = 5 \cdot 5^n + 4^n a$, with a an arbitrary constant.   **3.** $v_n = 4^n(a + n)$, with a an arbitrary constant.

5. $v_n = 10 \cdot 5^n - 3 \cdot 4^n n + 4^n a$, with a an arbitrary constant.   **7.** $v_n = (-6)^n[a + (\frac{1}{2})n - (\frac{1}{2})n^2 - n^3]$.

9. (a) $v_n = 2 \cdot 2^n + a$.   (b) $v_n = 3n + a$.   (c) $v_n = n^4 + a$.

11. The characteristic roots are 2 and 5, each of multiplicity 1.   (a) $r = 3$, $p = 2$, $m = 0$.

(b) $r = 2$, $p = 3$, $m = 1$.

13. $w_n = 3^n(c_0 + c_1 n + c_2 n^2)$.

15. (i) $v_n = 2 \cdot 2^n + 3^n a + 4^n b$.   (ii) $v_n = 3^n(a - 3n) + 4^n b$.   (iii) $v_n = 10 \cdot 2^n + 12 \cdot 3^n n + 3^n a + 4^n b$.

17. (i) $v_n = -1 + 2^n a$.   (ii) $v_n = 2^n(n + a)$.   (iii) $v_n = 1 + 2^n(n + a)$.

19. (i) $K(x) = x^2 - 3x - 4$, $s = 4$, $t = -1$.   (ii) $r = 2$, $m = 0$, $p = 0$.

(iii) $c_0 = -\frac{2}{3}$; $w_n = (-\frac{2}{3})2^n$.   (iv) $v_n = -(\frac{2}{3})2^n + a \cdot 4^n + b(-1)^n$.

(v) $a = \frac{1}{5}$, $b = \frac{7}{15}$, and so $v_n = -(\frac{2}{3})2^n + (\frac{1}{5})4^n + (\frac{7}{15})(-1)^n$.

21. (a) $v_n = 1 + 3^n$;   (b) $v_n = 2 \cdot 2^n - (n + 1)$;   (c) $v_n = (\frac{3}{2})n^2 - (\frac{3}{2})n$.

23. (a) $v_n = 1 + 2^n - 3^n$;   (b) $v_n = 3^n[1 - (\frac{5}{6})n + (\frac{1}{2})n^2]$.

25. $v_n = w_n + u_n$, $u_n = 2^n a_1 + 3^n a_2 + 4^n(a_3 + a_4 n)$, and $w_n = 2^n(c_1 n + c_2 n^2) + 3^n(c_3 n) + 5^n(c_4 + c_5 n)$, where the a_i are arbitrary and the c_i are to be determined.

27. Let L_n denote $v_n + b_1 v_{n-1} + \cdots + b_d v_{n-d}$. Let $y_0, y_1, \ldots$ be a solution to $L_n = g_n$; let $z_0, z_1, \ldots$ be a solution to $L_n = h_n$; and let $w_0, w_1, \ldots$ be a solution to $L_n = k_n$. Let r, s, and t be constants and let $f_n = ry_n + sz_n + tw_n$. Then $f_0, f_1, \ldots$ is a solution to $L_n = rg_n + sh_n + tk_n$.

29. $y_n = 2^{v_n}$, where $v_n = 3 \cdot 2^n - 3$.   **31.** $y_{n-1} y_{n-2} = 2^{F_{n-1}} \cdot 2^{F_{n-2}} = 2^{F_{n-1} + F_{n-2}} = 2^{F_n} = y_n$.

33. $y_n = 2^{v_n}$, where $v_n = 5^n a + (-2)^n b$, with a and b arbitrary constants.

35. $y_n = 2^{v_n}$, where $v_n = [3^n - (-1)^n]/4$.

SECTION 9.6

1. (i) $v_n = \log(2 + n)$; (ii) $v_n = 3 + \log(2 + n)$; (iii) Same as Part (ii).

3. (i)

n	0	1	2	3	4	5
v_n	0	$\frac{1}{2}$	$\frac{5}{6}$	$\frac{23}{24}$	$\frac{119}{120}$	$\frac{719}{720}$

(ii) $v_n = 1 - [1/(n + 1)!]$.

(iii) $1 - \dfrac{1}{(0 + 1)!} = 1 - 1 = 0,$ $\left[1 - \dfrac{1}{(n + 1)!}\right] - \left[1 - \dfrac{1}{n!}\right] = \dfrac{1}{n!} - \dfrac{1}{(n + 1)!} = \dfrac{n + 1 - 1}{(n + 1)!} = \dfrac{n}{(n + 1)!}$.

5. $\dbinom{2n}{n} = \dfrac{(2n)!}{n!n!} = \dfrac{2n(2n - 1)[(2n - 2)!]}{n[(n - 1)!]n[(n - 1)!]} = \dfrac{2(2n - 1)}{n} \cdot \dfrac{(2n - 2)!}{[(n - 1)!]^2} = \dfrac{2(2n - 1)}{n}\left(\dfrac{2[n - 1]}{n - 1}\right)$.

7. $v_n = v_0 + \dfrac{1}{2} + \dfrac{1}{4} + \cdots + \dfrac{1}{2^n} = 7 + \left(1 - \dfrac{1}{2^n}\right) = 8 - \dfrac{1}{2^n}$.

9. $v_n = v_0 + L_{n+2} + L_{n+1} - L_1 - L_2 = L_{n+3} - 4$.

11. $v_n = \dbinom{3}{3} + \dbinom{4}{3} + \cdots + \dbinom{n + 2}{3} = \dbinom{n + 3}{4} = \dfrac{(n + 3)(n + 2)(n + 1)n}{24}$. **13.** $v_n = [n - \frac{1}{2}]3^n + \frac{1}{2}$.

15. $y_n = \sqrt{(\frac{17}{4})3^n - (\frac{13}{4})(-1)^n}$. **17.** $y_n = (2^{n+3} - 7)n!$. **19.** $y_n = [3^n - 2^n + (-2)^n]n!$.

21. (i) $v_n = 3n$. (ii) $w_n = 3n \cdot 2^n$.

23. $S_0, S_1, \ldots$ satisfies the recursion $S_n - S_{n-1} = P(n)$. Then Theorem 2 of Section 9.5 with $p = d$, $r = 1$, and $m = 1$ tells us that S_n is a polynomial $P(0) + c_0 n + c_1 n^2 + \cdots + c_d n^{d+1}$.

25. $n + \dfrac{15}{2} n(n - 1) + \dfrac{25}{3} n(n - 1)(n - 2) + \dfrac{5}{2} n(n - 1)(n - 2)(n - 3) + \dfrac{1}{5} n(n - 1)(n - 2)(n - 3)(n - 4)$

$= \dfrac{1}{5} n^5 + \dfrac{1}{2} n^4 + \dfrac{1}{3} n^3 - \dfrac{1}{30} n$.

REVIEW PROBLEMS FOR CHAPTER 9

1. (a) $(3 + x)/(1 - x)^2$. (b) $4/(1 - 3x)$. **2.** $(5 - 11x)/(1 - 3x - x^2)$.

3. $(-2 + 11x)/(1 - 7x + 12x^2)$. **4.** (a) $2 \cdot 6^n - 4(-3)^n$. (b) $(\frac{22}{3})6^n - (\frac{1}{3})(-3)^n$. (c) $7(1 + n)5^n$.

5. $a_0, a_1 - 2a_0, a_2 - 2a_1 + a_0, \ldots, a_n - 2a_{n-1} + a_{n-2}, \ldots$. **6.** $1/(1 - x^2)^4$.

7. $u_n = 1.1^n u_0$. **8.** $3000(1.1^n)$.

9. (i) $x^2 - x - 42$. (ii) -6 and 7. (iii) $(-6)^n a + 7^n b$. (iv) $(\frac{90}{13})(-6)^n + (\frac{79}{13})7^n$. **10.** $(8 - 5n)4^n$.

11. (a) $u_n + 6u_{n-1} + 9u_{n-2} = 0$. (b) $u_n - 3u_{n-1} - 10u_{n-2} = 0$. **12.** $4^n a + (-4)^n b$.

13. (a) (i) $v_n = -2$, (ii) $v_n = -2 + 3^n a$, (iii) $v_n = -2 + 4 \cdot 3^n$.

(b) (i) $v_n = -10 \cdot 5^n$, (ii) $v_n = -10 \cdot 5^n + 6^n a$, (iii) $v_n = -10 \cdot 5^n + 12 \cdot 6^n$.

(c) (i) $v_n = 5n \cdot 6^n$, (ii) $v_n = (a + 5n)6^n$, (iii) $v_n = (4 + 5n)6^n$.

(d) (i) $v_n = -10 \cdot 5^n + 5n \cdot 6^n$, (ii) $v_n = -10 \cdot 5^n + (a + 5n)6^n$, (iii) $v_n = -10 \cdot 5^n + (16 + 5n)6^n$.

14. $1/(1 + 3x)^6$.

15. (i) 2, -2, -3; each with multiplicity 1; (ii) $u_n = 2^n a + (-2)^n b + (-3)^n c$;

(iii) $u_n = (\frac{2}{5})2^n + (-2)^n - (\frac{2}{5})(-3)^n$.

16. (a) $u_n = (a + bn + cn^2)(-2)^n$. (b) $u_n = (a + bn + cn^2)3^n$.

17. (a) $4(1 + n)(-3)^n$.   (b) $(5 + 3n)(-3)^n$.   (c) $4\binom{n + 3}{3}5^n - 7\binom{n + 5}{5}(-2)^n$.

18. (i) $v_n = -\frac{3}{2}$.   (ii) $v_n = -\frac{3}{2} + (a + bn)2^n + c \cdot 3^n$.   (iii) $v_n = -\frac{3}{2} + (1 + n)2^n + (\frac{1}{2})3^n$.

19. (a) $v_n = (\frac{125}{18})5^n + 2^n(a + bn) + 3^n c$.   (b) $v_n = 3^n(c + 9n) + 2^n(a + bn)$.   (c) $v_n = 2^n(a + bn - n^2) + 3^n c$.
(d) $v_n = -3 + 3^n(c + 36n) + 2^n(a + bn + 5n^2)$.

20. $v_n = \sqrt[5]{n} + 32$.   **21.** $u_n = (2^n + 3^n)^2$.

SECTION 10.1

1. **Basis** $\max(a_1) = a_1$.   **Inductive Part** Let $n \geq 2$ and $M = \max(a_1, \ldots, a_{n-1})$. Then
$$\max(a_1, \ldots, a_n) = \begin{cases} a_n & \text{if } M \leq a_n, \\ M & \text{if } M > a_n. \end{cases}$$

3.

n	1	2	3	4	5	6	7	8	9	10	11	12
$B(n)$	0	1	3	6	10	15	21	28	36	45	55	66
$D(n)$	0	1	3	5	8	11	14	17	21	25	29	33

5. $B(1024) = 523776$; $D(1024) = 9217$ is less than 2% of $B(1024)$.

7. (i) $(a_1) = (n + 1)$ and $(b_1, \ldots, b_n) = (1, 2, \ldots, n)$.   (ii) $(a_1) = (1)$ and $(b_1, \ldots, b_n) = (2, 3, \ldots, n + 1)$.

9. $(a_1, a_2) = (1, n + 2)$ and $(b_1, \ldots, b_n) = (2, 3, \ldots, n + 1)$.   **11.** (i) 2;   (ii) 3;   (iii) 7.

13. (i) 5;   (ii) 4.   **15.** (i) 17;   (ii) 12.

17. Using Algorithm 3, the merged vector $(s_1, \ldots, s_{n+1})$ will have $s_1 = b_1$, $s_2 = b_2, \ldots, s_{n-1} = b_{n-1}$, and $s_n = \min(a_1, b_n)$, with each of these s_i found using one comparison. The final s_{n+1} will not require any comparisons.

19. Algorithm 3 will use $m + k$ comparisons to determine that the merged vector $(s_1, \ldots, s_{m+n})$ has $s_1, \ldots, s_{m+k-1}$ as $a_1, \ldots, a_{m-1}, b_1, \ldots, b_k$ in some order and $s_{m+k} = a_m$. Then it will follow without any more comparisons that $s_{m+k+1} = b_{k+1}, s_{m+k+2} = b_{k+2}, \ldots, s_{m+n} = b_n$.

21.

n	0	1	2	3	4	5	6	7	8	9	10	11	12	13	14	15	16
$T(n)$	0	0	1	3	5	8	11	14	18	22	25	29	33	37	42	47	51

n	17	18	19	20	21	22	23	24	25	26	27
$T(n)$	56	61	65	70	75	80	86	92	97	103	109

23. (i) 3;   (ii) 22;   (iii) 109;   (iv) 460;   (v) 1783.

SECTION 10.2

1. $\det M = 1$, $\det M_1 = -53$, $\det M_2 = 87$, $x_1 = (\det M_1)/(\det M) = -53$, $x_2 = (\det M_2)/(\det M) = 87$.

3. $\det M = 2(60 + 63) - 5(-30 + 36) + 8(21 + 24) = 576$.   **5.** $(x_1, x_2, x_3) = (4, -3, -1)$.

7. More than $4.7 \times 10^8 = 470000000$ years.

9. This follows by repeated use of the formula in Display (15).

11. $a_{11}(a_{22}a_{33} - a_{32}a_{23}) - a_{21}(a_{12}a_{33} - a_{32}a_{13}) + a_{31}(a_{12}a_{23} - a_{22}a_{13})$.

15.

n	5	6	7
f_n	1235	8658	69279

17. $s = \frac{3}{2}$.　　**19.** $s = -\frac{3}{2}$.　　**21.** $\det M' = -(\det M)$.　　**23.** $\det K = k(\det M)$.
25. The largest n is 22103.

SECTION 10.3

1.

n	1	2	3	4	5	6	7	8	9	10
2^n	2	4	8	16	32	64	128	256	512	1024
$n!$	1	2	6	24	120	720	5040	40320	362880	3628800

3. (a) $r = 4$.　　(b) $s = 6$.　　(c) $t = 8$.
5. (i) $n = 41$, since the computer can do 3.6×10^{12} multiplications in an hour, $2^{41} < 2.2 \times 10^{12}$, and $2^{42} > 4 \times 10^{12}$.
　　(ii) $n = 15$.
7. Since $g(n)$ is $O[f(n)]$, there exist positive c and n_0 such that $g(n) \leq cf(n)$ for $n \geq n_0$. Let $k = c/r$. Then $g(n) \leq k[rf(n)]$ for $n \geq n_0$, and hence $g(n)$ is $O[rf(n)]$.
9. Theorem 2(d) tells us that 1000^n is $o[n!]$. Then it follows from Problem 8 with $r = .01$ that 1000^n is $o[.01(n!)]$.
11. $g_1(n) = n^{98} \log n$, $g_2(n) = .1(n^{99})$, $g_3(n) = .01(2^n)$, $g_4(n) = .001(100^n)$, $g_5(n) = .0001(n!)$, $g_6(n) = .00001(n^n)$.
13. Let $f(n) = 2n!$ and $g(n) = n!$. Then $f(n) \leq 2g(n)$ and $g(n) \leq f(n)$ for $n \geq 1$. Hence $f(n)$ is $O[g(n)]$ and $g(n)$ is $O[f(n)]$. These imply that $f \sim g$.

REVIEW PROBLEMS FOR CHAPTER 10

1. (i) $2A(m) + 1 = 2(m - 1) + 1 = 2m - 1$.　　(ii) They are equal.
2. 4.　　**3.** 7.　　**4.** (1, 2, 3) and (4, 5, 6, 7).　　**5.** (1, 2, 6) and (3, 4, 5, 7).
6. (i) $D(23) = 29 + 33 + 22 = 84$.　　(ii) $B(23) = \binom{23}{2} = 23 \cdot 22/2 = 253$.　　**7.** (i) 89.　　(ii) 276.
8. $(-2 - 3) - 2(4 + 1) + 3(6 - 1) = -5 - 10 + 15 = 0$.　　**9.** $x = \frac{61}{20}$, $y = -\frac{7}{20}$, $z = \frac{1}{4}$.
10. $s = -\frac{3}{2}$.　　**11.** $t = \frac{14}{3}$.　　**13.** 1235.　　**14.** 3594047771441.
15. Yes; n^{100} is $o[1.001^n]$ by Theorem 2(c) of Section 10.3, and then n^{100} is $o[.000001(1.001^n)]$ by Problem 8 of Section 10.3.
16. The inequality is easily seen to be true for all small values of n. There is a largest m_0 because m_0 is smaller than the n_0 of Problem 15.
17. $r = 7$, $s = 9$, $t = 11$.　　**18.** $g_1(n) = 8n^3 \log n$, $g_2(n) = n^4 - n^3 + 5$, $g_3(n) = 10(1.1^n)$, $g_4(n) = (2n)!$.
19. $d = 2$.　　**20.** $e = d + 1$.　　**21.** $b = 4$.

SECTION 11.1

1. (a) 3;   (b) 3;   (c) 4;   (d) 011101;   (e) 4.   **3.** 1; $d(011100, 011110) = 1$.
5. Let $\alpha = a_1 a_2 \ldots a_n$, $\beta = b_1 b_2 \ldots b_n$, and $\gamma = c_1 c_2 \ldots c_n$. For each i such that $a_i \neq c_i$, one must have either $a_i \neq b_i$ or $b_i \neq c_i$, because otherwise $a_i = b_i = c_i$ implies that $a_i = c_i$. Since $d(\alpha, \gamma)$ is the number of values of i in $\{1, 2, \ldots, n\}$ for which $a_i \neq c_i$, one has $d(\alpha, \gamma) \leq d(\alpha, \beta) + d(\beta, \gamma)$.
7. (a) 101010;   (b) 10;   (c) 10.   **9.** (a) and (d).

SECTION 11.2

1. (a) 01110;   (b) 11001;   (c) 11100;   (d) 11001.   **3.** 001000.   **5.** (a) 01000;   (b) 00100.
7. (a) 00001 00100 01010 01111 10011 10110 11000 11101.   (b) 01110.   (c) No.
9. This can be done by showing closure under $\oplus$ using an operation table.
11. 001001 000111 011010 010100 101100 100010 111111 110001.
13. The other strings of weight 2 in this coset are 010100 and 100010. Either of these could be the coset leader. The row using 010100 is 010100 011010 000111 001001 110001 111111 100010 101100. The row using 100010 is 100010 101100 110001 111111 000111 001001 010100 011010.
15. (a) 011101;   (b) 010011.
17. This follows from Definition 1 in Section 11.2 and Theorem 1 in Section 11.1.

REVIEW PROBLEMS FOR CHAPTER 11

1. (a) 001001001;   (b) 101101101;   (c) 100;   (d) 010.
3. It helps to detect errors but not to correct them.   **5.** 6.   **7.** 1, 2, and 3.
9. Yes; for example, $\{111, 100, 010\}$.

SECTION 12.1

1. Yes; A is a subset of A^*.
3. (b) and (c) are alphabets. (a) is not an alphabet because 12 is a word in $A - \{12\}$.

5.

·	ba	cb	ac
a	aba	acb	aac
b	bba	bcb	bac
c	cba	ccb	cac

7. $LL' = \{$aba, acb, aac, bba, bcb, bac, cba, ccb, cac$\}$.

9. (i) Yes.   (ii) Yes.   (iii) Yes.
11. (a) No; the production t → s does not satisfy condition (d) of Definition 4, "Phrase-Structure Grammar." (b) Yes.
13. (a) No; s → 0s.   (b) No; a → b.   (c) Yes.
15. s → 1b, b → 0a, a → 1b, b → 0a, a → 0a, a → 1.   **17.** No; 110001 is friendly (that is, not unfriendly).

19. 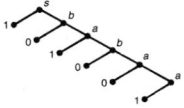 **21.** aaa, aab.

25. (A, S, T, P) with $A = \{s, a, 0, 1, 8, 9\}$, $S = \{s\}$, $T = \{0, 1, 8, 9\}$, and $P = \{s \to 1a89,\ a \to 1a8,\ a \to 0\}$.

SECTION 12.2

1.

State	Input	Output
0	10	1
0	00	0
0	01	1
0	11	0
1	00	1

$\gamma = 10101.$

3. (a)

State	Input	Output
0	1	1
1	0	1
1	1	0
0	1	1

(b)

State	Input	Output
0	0	0
0	1	1
1	1	0
0	0	0

5.

x \ i	0	1
0	0	1
1	1	0

7.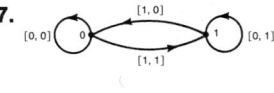

9. (X, I, F, G, U) with $X = \{s, a, b, r\}$, $I = U = \{0, 1\}$, and F and G given by the two tables below.

Next State Function F

x \ i	0	1
s	b	a
a	b	a
b	r	a
r	r	r

Output Function G

x \ i	0	1
s	0	0
a	0	0
b	1	0
r	1	1

11.

x \ i	0	1
s	b	c
b	d	e
c	f	g
d	d	e
e	f	g
f	d	r
g	f	g
r	r	r

REVIEW PROBLEMS FOR CHAPTER 12

1.

	012	120	201
01	01012	01120	01201
12	12012	12120	12201
20	20012	20120	20201

2. No; 12001 is in $L'L$ but is not in LL'.   **3.** Parts (b) and (c) are phrase-structure grammars.

4. In Part (a), $12 \rightarrow 0$ is the culprit because 12 is a word in T^*.   **5.** Part (b) gives a regular grammar.

6. In Part (c), the culprit is $s \rightarrow 0s$. The start symbol s is not allowed on the right-hand side of a production $\alpha \rightarrow \beta$ for a regular grammar.

7. Of these words, only ε, 00, and 010 are in L.   **8.** $s \rightarrow 0b$, $b \rightarrow 1b$, $b \rightarrow 1b$, $b \rightarrow 1b$, $b \rightarrow 0$.

9. (a) 2,   (b) 0,   (c) 1.   **10.** Yes, by having 0 as the final output symbol.

11.

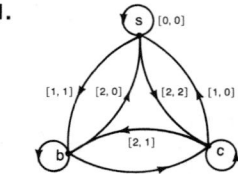

12. (A, S, T, P) with $A = \{s, a, b, c, 0, 1, 2\}$, $S = \{s\}$, $T = \{0, 1, 2\}$, and $P = \{s \rightarrow \varepsilon, s \rightarrow 0, s \rightarrow 0a, s \rightarrow 1b,$ $s \rightarrow 2c, a \rightarrow 0, a \rightarrow 0a, a \rightarrow 1b, a \rightarrow 2c, b \rightarrow 2, b \rightarrow 2a, b \rightarrow 0b, b \rightarrow 1c, c \rightarrow 1, c \rightarrow 1a, c \rightarrow 2b, c \rightarrow 0c\}$.

13. (A, S, T, P) with $A = \{s, 0, 1\}$, $S = \{s\}$, $T = \{0, 1\}$, and $P = \{s \rightarrow \varepsilon, s \rightarrow 0s0, s \rightarrow 1s1, s \rightarrow 0, s \rightarrow 1\}$.

14. (A, S, T, P) with $A = \{s, 0, 1\}$, $S = \{s\}$, $T = \{0, 1\}$, and $P = \{s \rightarrow \varepsilon, s \rightarrow 0s0, s \rightarrow 1s1\}$.

INDEX